Swaiman's
Pediatric
Neurology

Dedication

With pleasure and appreciation we dedicate this book to our spouses, Phyllis Sher, Eileen Ashwal, Thomas Rando, and Robert Schor, who made it possible for us to spend the enormous amount of time planning, reading, and editing that was necessary to bring this text to fruition. It is impossible to describe the value of their encouragement and support adequately.

Furthermore, no dedication of a book embracing this field would be meaningful without a tribute to the courage and perseverance of neurologically impaired children and their caretakers.

Commissioning Editor: Lotta Kryhl
Development Editor: Janice Gaillard
Editorial Assistant: Emma Cole
Project Manager: Frances Affleck
Design: Kirsteen Wright
Illustration Manager: Karen Giacomucci
Illustrator: Dartmouth Publishing and Joe Chovan
Marketing Manager (UK/USA): Gaynor Jones/Helena Mutak

Swaiman's
Pediatric
Neurology

FIFTH EDITION

Principles and Practice

Volume 1

Kenneth F. Swaiman MD
Director Emeritus, Division of Pediatric Neurology
Professor Emeritus of Neurology and Pediatrics
University of Minnesota Medical School
Minneapolis, MN, USA

Stephen Ashwal MD
Distinguished Professor of Pediatrics
Chief of the Division of Child Neurology and
Pediatrics
Loma Linda University School of Medicine
Loma Linda, CA, USA

Donna M. Ferriero MD MS
W.H. and Marie Wattis Distinguished Professor
and Chair Department of Pediatrics
Physician-in-Chief
UCSF Benioff Children's Hospital
University of California San Francisco
San Francisco, CA, USA

Nina F. Schor MD PhD
William H. Eilinger Chair of Pediatrics
Professor, Departments of Pediatrics, Neurology,
and Neurobiology and Anatomy
University of Rochester School of Medicine
and Dentistry
Rochester, NY, USA

ELSEVIER
SAUNDERS

SAUNDERS is an imprint of Elsevier Inc.

First edition 1989
Second edition 1994
Third edition 1999
Fourth edition 2006
Fifth edition 2012

Saunders

British Library Cataloguing in Publication Data

Swaiman's pediatric neurology. – 5th ed.
  1. Pediatric neurology.
  I. Ashwal, Stephen, 1945- II. Swaiman, Kenneth F., 1931-
  III. Pediatric neurology.
  618.9'28-dc22

ISBN-13: 9781437704358

Printed in China
Last digit is the print number: 9 8 7 6 5 4 3 2 1

Contents

 Available on-line at ExpertConsult.com. See inside cover for details

Video Table of Contents

Available on-line at ExpertConsult.com. See inside cover for details

Preface to the First Edition

It is concurrently tiring, humiliating, and intellectually revitalizing to compile a book containing the essence of the information that embraces one's life work and professional preoccupation. For me, there is a certain moth-to-the-flame phenomenon that cannot be resisted; therefore this new book has been produced.

Pediatric neurology has come of age since my initial interest and subsequent immersion in the field. Concentrated attention to the details of brain development and function has brought much progress and understanding. Studies of disease processes by dedicated and intelligent individuals accompanied by a cascade of new technology (e.g., neuroimaging techniques, positron emission tomography, DNA probes, synthesis of gene products, sophisticated lipid chemistry) have propelled the field forward. The simultaneous increase of knowledge and capability of pediatric neurologists and others who diagnose and treat children with nervous system dysfunction has been extremely gratifying.

Although once within the realm of honest delusion of a seemingly sane (but unrealistic) devotee of the field, it is no longer possible to believe that a single individual can fathom, much less explore, the innumerable rivulets that coalesce to form the river of knowledge that currently is pediatric neurology. Streams of information in certain areas sometimes peacefully meander for years; suddenly, when knowledge of previously obscure areas is advanced and the newly gained information becomes central to understanding basic pathophysiologic entities, a once small stream gains momentum and abruptly flows with torrential force.

This text is an attempt to gather the most important aspects of current pediatric neurology and display them in a comprehensible manner. The task, although consuming great energies and concentration, cannot be accomplished completely because new conditions are described daily.

The advancement of the field necessitated that preparation of this text keep pace with current knowledge and present new and valuable techniques. My colleagues and I have made every effort to discharge this responsibility. Because of continuous scientific progress, controversies are extant in some areas for varying periods; wherever possible, these areas of conflict are indicated.

This book is divided into four unequal parts. Part I contains a discussion of the historic and clinical examination. Part II contains information concerning laboratory examination. Chapters relating to the symptom complexes that often reflect the chief complaints of neurologically impaired children compose Part III. Part IV provides detailed discussion of various neurologic diseases that afflict children.

Although every precaution has been taken to avoid error, bias, and prejudice, inevitably some of these demons have become embedded in the text. The editor assumes full responsibility for these indiscretions.

It is my fervent hope that the reader will find this book informative and stimulating and that the contents will provide an introduction to the understanding of many of the conditions that remain mysterious and poorly explained.

Kenneth F. Swaiman, MD
Autumn 1988

Preface to the Fifth Edition

Since publication in 2006 of the fourth edition of *Pediatric Neurology: Principles & Practice*, the discipline of child neurology has progressed and reached new levels of complexity. Advances in molecular biology and neuroimaging have fueled an explosion of knowledge that has translated into a richer understanding of nervous system development and function. Researchers and clinicians alike believe that, during the next decade, novel and targeted treatments will be the product of such fundamental advances in knowledge. Successful treatment of children with both common and rare neurologic disorders is becoming a reality.

This fifth edition reflects the enormous growth and intricacy of the basic and clinical neurosciences. The entire text has been revised and reorganized. Many chapters have undergone extensive updating, as they reflect clinical areas of child neurology that are becoming even more relevant (e.g., neurogenetics, neuropsychopharmacology, neurorehabilitation), and new chapters are included on diseases that previously were given little attention in child neurology (e.g., channelopathies). Many chapters have new authors who bring to these discussions new insights into disease mechanisms. Also, the editors of the 2006 edition are extremely fortunate to have Nina Schor join us to provide her expertise to enhance the quality of this publication.

Several major and important changes are present in this edition. The first is that purchasers of the book will be able to access all chapters online through a website established by Elsevier. This innovation will allow readers to access contents from any location and it will also provide an online ability to search the text for specific topics – finding particular information about a disease or syndrome will be much easier. Second, because of the continued explosion in knowledge, we have decided to publish a group of chapters exclusively in the online version of the book (see below). This change will allow the hard-copy version to remain a two-volume work. The chapter on congenital malformations has been converted to a "book within a book" – contained as nine chapters in Part V of the text. Finally, we also have included three chapters on cutting edge neuroscience devoted to concepts of plasticity, cell-death mechanisms, and neuroinflammation, written by several of the leading authorities in their respective fields.

The two volumes are divided into 17 parts, encompassing 108 chapters as outlined in the table of contents. Parts I and II will be published on the book's website and contain information regarding selected aspects of the pediatric neurologic examination, as well as the different motor and sensory systems, and these discussions are followed by a comprehensive review of the pertinent neurodiagnostic testing procedures and their clinical application. Part III is a new section devoted to important concepts in the developmental neurosciences related to plasticity, cell-death mechanisms, and neuroinflammation – topics that are complex but very important for clinicians to understand as they try to apply this information to diseases that their patients endure. Part IV covers important aspects of neonatal neurology and the long-term sequelae of acquired and developmental abnormalities that can result in chronic disorders, such as cerebral palsy, developmental delay, and epilepsy. Part V is a new expanded section devoted to brain malformations. It includes an overview and classification of brain development, five chapters on specific groups of developmental malformations, and chapters on hydrocephalus, congenital skull anomalies, and prenatal diagnosis. Part VI documents the vast array of genetic and neurometabolic disorders that occur in infants and children; this section also provides many of the fundamental concepts of molecular biology and neurochemistry that constitute the scientific basis of these diseases. Part VII describes the major neurobehavioral disorders of childhood and includes chapters on autism and the neuropsychiatric problems that accompany Tourette's syndrome, and a newly revised chapter on neuropsychopharmacology. Part VIII focuses on pediatric epilepsy and contains revised chapters on the neurophysiology and neurogenetics of pediatric epilepsy. Also included are chapters on the various types of pediatric epilepsy, epileptiform disorders with cognitive symptomatology, the ketogenic diet, surgical treatment, and the learning and behavioral problems associated with epilepsy.

The second volume encompasses many of the serious and complex central and peripheral nervous system diseases that present to child neurologists and allied health professionals. Part IX reviews the nonepileptiform paroxysmal disorders, including headache, syncope, and sleep disorders. Parts X and XI deal with conditions that are degenerative in nature and cause severe loss of motor and mental function. These conditions include disorders of balance and movement in Part X (e.g., cerebellar disorders and hereditary ataxia, movement disorders, cerebral palsy, and Tourette's syndrome) and metabolic-genetic disorders, as well as acquired disorders of the white matter in Part XI. Part XII contains chapters on traumatic and nontraumatic brain injury in infants and older children. As neurologists frequently are asked to provide consultation for many of these conditions, chapters on disorders of consciousness, nonaccidental trauma, anoxic brain injury, and traumatic brain and spinal cord injury are included, as well as a current review of the issues related to brain death determination. Parts XIII (infection) and XIV (tumors and cerebrovascular and vasculitic disorders) extensively cover the major diseases that, directly or indirectly, cause serious neurologic symptoms and are discussed from a clinical perspective. In addition, a new chapter on paraneoplastic syndromes is included. The neuromuscular diseases are reviewed in Part XV, which contains chapters on the classic neuromuscular disorders, including the anterior horn cell diseases, disorders of the peripheral nervous system and neuromuscular junction, inflammatory neuropathies, metabolic myopathies, and channelopathies. Part XVI covers systemic and autonomic nervous systemic disorders. These include important chapters that review many pediatric systemic conditions (e.g., endocrine, renal, cardiac, gastrointestinal) that are known to cause neurologic symptoms, as well as chapters on poisonings, complications of immunizations, and autonomic nervous system disorders. This volume concludes with Part XVII, which is Web-based, and reviews the care of the child with neurologic diseases, revised extensively, and including updated chapters on pediatric neurorehabilitation, pain and palliative care management, ethical issues in child neurology, and the Internet as it relates to child neurology.

We hope that the reader will find this book a useful resource and that the information will benefit the many children who suffer from these conditions. It is our wish that the greater world community will increase support for the care of neurologically impaired children and the research necessary to provide further understanding of, and improved treatment and preventive measures for, neurologic diseases. This support will improve the survival and quality of life of these brave children and their families.

Kenneth F. Swaiman
Stephen Ashwal
Donna M. Ferriero
Nina F. Schor

Contributors

Amal Abou-Hamden MB BS BMedSc (Hons) FRACS
Paediatric Neurosurgery Fellow
Neurosurgery
Hospital for Sick Children
Toronto, Ontario, Canada

Anthony A. Amato MD
Vice-Chairman
Neurology
Brigham and Women's Hospital
Harvard Medical School
Boston, MA, USA

Stephen Ashwal MD
Distinguished Professor of Pediatrics
Chief of the Division of Child Neurology and
Pediatrics
Loma Linda University School of Medicine
Loma Linda, CA, USA

Felicia B. Axelrod MD
Carl Seaman Family Professor of Dysautonomia
Treatment and Research
Pediatrics and Neurology
New York University School of Medicine
New York, NY, USA

James F. Bale, Jr. MD
Professor and Associate Chair
Department of Pediatrics
University of Utah School of Medicine
Salt Lake City, UT, USA

Brenda Banwell MD FRCPC
Associate Professor of Pediatrics (Neurology)
Director
Pediatric Multiple Sclerosis Clinic
Senior Associate Scientist
Research Institute
Hospital for Sick Children
University of Toronto
Toronto, Ontario, Canada

Kristin W. Baranano MD PhD
Instructor
Department of Pediatric Neurology
Johns Hopkins University School of Medicine
Baltimore, MD, USA

A. James Barkovich MD
Professor of Radiology, Neurology, Pediatrics
and Neurosurgery
University of California San Francisco
San Francisco, CA, USA

Richard J. Barohn MD
Chairman
Gertrude and Dewey Ziegler Professor of
Neurology
University of Kansas Medical Center
Kansas City, KS, USA

Mark L. Batshaw MD
Chief Academic Officer
Children's National Medical Center
Professor and Chair, Department of Pediatrics
Associate Dean for Academic Affairs
George Washington University School of Medicine
and Health Sciences
Washington, DC, USA

Liat Ben-Sira MD
Doctor
Pediatric Radiology Unit,
Tel-Aviv Medical Center
Sackler School of Medicine
Tel-Aviv University
Tel-Aviv, Israel

Angela K. Birnbaum PhD
Associate Professor
Department of Experimental and Clinical
Pharmacology
College of Pharmacy
University of Minnesota
Minneapolis, MN, USA

Rose-Mary N. Boustany MD
Professor of Pediatrics and Biochemistry
American University of Beirut
Adjunct Professor of Pediatrics
Professor of Neurobiology and Associate in
Medicine
Duke University Medical Center
Beirut, Lebanon

Amy Brooks-Kayal MD
Chief and Ponzio Family Chair in Pediatric
Neurology
Children's Hospital of Colorado
Professor of Pediatrics
Neurology and Pharmaceutical Sciences
University of Colorado Schools of Medicine and
Pharmacy
Aurora, CO, USA

Lawrence W. Brown MD
Associate Professor of Neurology and Pediatrics
Children's Hospital of Philadelphia
Philadelphia, PA, USA

Carol S. Camfield MD
Professor Emeritus
Department of Pediatrics
Dalhousie University and the IWK Health Centre
Halifax, Nova Scotia, Canada

Peter R. Camfield MD FRCP(c)
Professor
Pediatrics
Dalhousie University and IWK Health Centre
Halifax, Nova Scotia, Canada

Margaretha L. Casselbrant MD PhD
Eberly Professor of Pediatric Otolaryngology
University of Pittsburgh School of Medicine
Director
Division of Pediatric Otolaryngology
Children's Hospital of Pittsburgh of UPMC
Pittsburgh, PA, USA

Claudia A. Chiriboga MD MPH
Associate Professor, Clinical Neurology and
Pediatrics
Interim Program Director of Pediatric Neurology
Columbia University Medical Center
New York, NY, USA

Susan L. Christian PhD
Laboratory Director
Center for Integrative Brain Research
Seattle Childrens Research Institute
Seattle, WA, USA

Maria Roberta Cilio MD PhD
Faculty
Bambino Gesù Children's Hospital
Rome, Italy
Associate Professor in Neurology
University of California San Francisco
San Francisco, CA, USA

Anne M. Connolly MD
Professor of Neurology and Pediatrics
Washington University School of Medicine
St. Louis, MO, USA

Jeannine M. Conway PharmD
Assistant Professor
Department of Experimental and Clinical
Pharmacology
College of Pharmacy
University of Minnesota
Minneapolis, MN, USA

Susannah Cornes MD
Assistant Professor of Clinical Neurology
Department of Neurology
University of California San Francisco
San Francisco, CA, USA

David L. Coulter MD
Associate Professor
Neurology
Harvard Medical School
Boston, MA, USA

Tina M. Cowan PhD
Associate Professor
Pathology
Stanford University
Stanford, CA, USA

Soma Das PhD
Professor of Human Genetics
University of Chicago
Chicago, IL, USA

Darryl C. De Vivo MD
Sidney Carter Professor of Neurology
Professor of Pediatrics
Columbia University College of Physicians and
Surgeons
New York, NY, USA

Linda S. de Vries MD
Professor in Neonatal Neurology
Department of Neonatology
Wilhelmina Children's Hospital
UMCU
Utrecht, The Netherlands

Jay Desai MD
Fellow
Division of Neurology
Children's Hospital Los Angeles
Los Angeles, CA, USA

Maria Descartes MD
Associate Professor Genetics and Pediatrics
Department of Genetics
University of Alabama at Birmingham
Birmingham, AL, USA

Gabrielle deVeber MD MHSc
Director
Children's Stroke Program
Neurology
Hospital for Sick Children
Toronto, Ontario, Canada

Salvatore DiMauro MD
Lucy G. Moses Professor of Neurology
Department of Neurology
Columbia University Medical Center
New York, NY, USA

William B. Dobyns MD
Professor
Departments of Pediatrics and Neurology
University of Washington and

Center for Integrative Brain Research
Seattle Children's Research Institute
Seattle, WA, USA

Qing Dong MD PhD
CEO and President
Sound Pediatrics
Daly City, CA, USA

**James M. Drake BSE MBBCh MSc
FRCSC FACS**
Professor and Divisions Head
Pediatric Neurosurgery
Harold Hoffman/Shopper's Drug Mart Chair
Hospital for Sick Children
University of Toronto
Toronto, Ontario, Canada

Ann-Christine Duhaime MD
Professor of Neurosurgery
Harvard Medical School
Attending Neurosurgeon
Massachusetts General Hospital
Boston, MA, USA

Adre J. du Plessis MBChB
Chief of Fetal and Transitional Medicine
Children's National Medical Center
Professor of Pediatrics and Neurology
George Washington University Medical School
Washington, DC, USA

Mohamad K. El-Bitar
c/o Rose-Mary N. Boustany

Gregory M. Enns MD
Associate Professor
Stanford School of Medicine
Palo Alto, CA, USA

Diana M. Escolar MD
Associate Professor of Neurology
Johns Hopkins School of Medicine
Neurology Department
Kennedy Krieger Institute
Baltimore, MD USA

Owen B. Evans Jr, MD
Professor of Pediatrics and Neurology
Department of Pediatrics
University of Mississippi School of Medicine
Jackson, MS, USA

S. Ali Fatemi MD
Assistant Professor of Neurology and Pediatrics
Johns Hopkins University School of Medicine
Pediatric Neurologist
Division of Neurology and Developmental
Medicine
Kennedy Krieger Institute
Baltimore, MD, USA

Donna M. Ferriero MD MS
W.H. and Marie Wattis Distinguished Professor
and Chair Department of Pediatrics
Physician-in-Chief
UCSF Benioff Children's Hospital
University of California San Francisco
San Francisco, CA, USA

Pauline A. Filipek MD
Director, Autism Center at the Children's Learning
Institute
Professor of Pediatrics
Children's Learning Institute and
Division of Child and Adolescent Neurology
UT Health Sciences Center at Houston
Houston, TX, USA

Yitzchak Frank MD
Professor
Pediatrics and Neurology
Mount Sinai Medical School
New York, NY, USA

Douglas R. Fredrick MD
Clinical Professor of Ophthalmology and
Pediatrics
Department of Ophthalmology
Stanford University
Stanford, CA, USA

Hudson H. Freeze PhD
Professor and Director
Genetic Disease Program
Sanford Children's Health Research Center
Burnham Institute for Medical Research
La Jolla, CA, USA

Neil R. Friedman MBChB
Staff Center for Pediatric Neurology
Neurological Institute
Cleveland Clinic
Cleveland, OH, USA

Joseph M. Furman MD PhD
Professor
Departments of Otolaryngology and Neurology
University Of Pittsburgh
Pittsburgh, PA, USA

Bhuwan P. Garg MB MS
Professor Emeritus
Department of Neurology
Indiana University School of Medicine
Indianapolis, IN, USA

Debabrata Ghosh MD DM
Staff, Center for Pediatric Neurology
Neurological Institute
Cleveland Clinic
Cleveland, OH, USA

Elizabeth E. Gilles MD
Assistant Professor of Pediatrics
University of Minnesota
Medical Director
Pediatric Neurology
Children's Hospitals and Clinics
St. Paul, MN, USA

Christopher C. Giza MD
Associate Professor in Residence
Division of Pediatric Neurology and Department
of Neurosurgery
UCLA Brain Injury Research Center
David Geffen School of Medicine at UCLA
Mattel Children's Hospital – UCLA
Los Angeles, CA, USA

Carol A. Glaser DVM MPVM MD
Chief of Encephalitis and Special Investigations
Section
Communicable Disease and Emergency Response
Branch
Division of Communicable Disease Control
California Department of Public Health
Richmond, CA, USA

Joseph G. Gleeson MD
Professor
Neurosciences and Pediatrics
University of California San Diego
La Jolla, CA, USA

John M. Graham, Jr. MD ScD
Director of Clinical Genetics and Dysmorphology
Professor of Pediatrics and Biomedical Sciences
Cedars Sinai Medical Center
Professor of Pediatrics
David Geffen School of Medicine at UCLA
Los Angeles, CA, USA

Pierre Gressens MD PhD
Laboratory Chief,
Paris 7 University,
Hôpital Robert Debré, Paris, France
Professor of Perinatal Neurology
Hammersmith Hospital
Imperial College of London
London, UK

Renzo Guerrini MD
Pediatric Neurology Unit and Laboratories
Children's Hospital
A. Meyer-University of Florence
Florence, Italy

Nalin Gupta MD PhD
Associate Professor
Neurological Surgery and Pediatrics
Chief, Pediatric Neurosurgery
UCSF Benioff Children's Hospital
University of California San Francisco
San Francisco, CA, USA

Jin S. Hahn MD
Professor of Neurology and Pediatrics
Department of Neurology and Neurological
Sciences
Stanford University School of Medicine
Stanford, CA, USA

Chellamani Harini MBBS MD
Clinical Instructor
Department of Neurology
Children's Hospital
Boston, MA, USA

Chad Heatwole MD
Assistant Professor of Neurology
Neurology
University of Rochester
Rochester, NY, USA

Deborah G. Hirtz MD
Program Director
Office of Clinical Research
National Institute of Neurological Disorders and
Stroke
National Institutes of Health
Bethesda, MD, USA

Gregory L. Holmes MD
Chair, Department of Neurology
Professor of Neurology and Pediatrics
Dartmouth Medical School
Dartmouth-Hitchcock Medical Center
Lebanon, NH, USA

Barbara A. Holshouser PhD
Professor of Radiology
Radiology
Loma Linda University Medical Center
Loma Linda, CA, USA

Rebecca N. Ichord MD
Associate Professor
Neurology and Pediatrics
Children's Hospital of Philadelphia
Philadelphia, PA, USA

Paymaan Jafar-Nejad MD
Post-doc fellow
Dr. Huda Zoghbi's laboratories
Jan and Dan Duncan Neurological Research
Institute
Baylor College of Medicine
Houston, TX, USA

Frances E. Jensen MD
Professor of Neurology
Neurology
Children's Hospital and Harvard Medical School
Boston, MA, USA

Michael V. Johnston MD
Chief Medical Officer
Kennedy Krieger Institute Children's Hospital
Professor of Neurology
Pediatrics and Physical Medicine and
Rehabilitation
Johns Hopkins University School of Medicine
Baltimore, MD, USA

Lori Jordan MD
Assistant Professor of Neurology and Pediatrics
Department of Neurology
Johns Hopkins University School of Medicine
Baltimore, MD, USA

Yasmin Khakoo MD
Pediatric Neurologist/Neuro-Oncologist
Departments of Pediatrics and Neurology
Memorial Sloan-Kettering Cancer Center
New York, NY, USA

Mustafa Khasraw MD MRCP FRACP
Clinical Fellow
Department of Neurology
Memorial Sloan-Kettering Cancer Center
New York, NY, USA

Adam Kirton MD MSc FRCPC
Assistant Professor
Pediatrics and Clinical Neurosciences
University of Calgary
Calgary, Alberta, Canada

John T. Kissel MD
Professor of Neurology and Pediatrics
Ohio State University and Nationwide Children's
Hospital
Columbus, OH, USA

Ophir Klein MD PhD
Assistant Professor
Departments of Orofacial Sciences and
Pediatrics
University of California San Francisco
San Francisco, CA, USA

Kelly Knupp MD
Neurology and Neurodiagnostics
Assistant Professor of Pediatrics
Children's Hospital
University of Colorado at Denver and Health
Sciences Center
Aurora, CO, USA

Bruce R. Korf MD PhD
Wayne H. and Sara Crews Finley Chair in Medical
Genetics
Professor and Chair
Department of Genetics
Director, Heflin Center for Genome
Sciences
University of Alabama
Birmingham, AL, USA

Suresh Kotagal MD
Professor
Division of Child Neurology
Consultant
Departments of Neurology and Pediatrics
Mayo Clinic
Rochester, MN, USA

Steven Leber MD PhD
Professor
Pediatrics and Neurology
University of Michigan
Ann Arbor, MI, USA

Ilo E. Leppik MD
Professor of Pharmacy
Adjunct Professor of Neurology
Director, Epilepsy Research and Education
Program
University of Minnesota
Minneapolis, MN, USA

Tally Lerman-Sagie MD
Associate Professor
Head, Pediatric Neurology Unit
Wolfson Medical Center
Holon, Israel

Jason T. Lerner MD
Assistant Professor
Director of Training
Division of Pediatric Neurology
Mattel Children's Hospital at UCLA
Los Angeles, CA, USA

Robert T. Leshner MD
Health Sciences Clinical Professor
Department of Neurosciences
University of California San Diego
San Diego, CA, USA

**Richard J. Leventer MBBS BMedSci
FRACP PhD**
Consultant Pediatric Neurologist
Children's Neuroscience Centre and Murdoch
Children's Research Institute
Royal Children's Hospital and Department of
Pediatrics
University of Melbourne
Melbourne, Victoria, Australia

Donald W. Lewis MD
Professor and Chairman
Department of Pediatrics
Children's Hospital of the King's Daughters
Eastern Virginia Medical School
Norfolk, VA, USA

Paul F. Lewis MD
Associate Professor
Pediatrics
Oregon Health and Sciences University
Portland, OR, USA

Uta Lichter-Konecki MD PhD
Director of the Metabolism Program
Children's National Medical Center
Associate Professor of Pediatrics
Department of Pediatrics
George Washington University
Washington, DC, USA

Catherine Limperopoulos PhD
Director, MRI Research of the Developing Brain
Associate Professor of Pediatrics
Diagnostic Imaging and Radiology
George Washington University Health Center
Children's National Medical Center
Washington, DC, USA

Janice K. Louie MD MPH
Chief, Surveillance and Epidemiology Section
Division of Communicable Disease Control
California Department of Public Health
Richmond, CA, USA

Quyen N. Luc MD
Clinical Fellow in Pediatric Movement Disorders
Division of Neurology
Children's Hospital Los Angeles
Los Angeles, CA, USA

Tobey J. MacDonald MD
Director, Pediatric Neuro-Oncology Program
Associate Professor of Pediatrics
Emory University School of Medicine
Atlanta, GA, USA

Naila Makhani MD FRCPC
Clinical Research Fellow
Pediatric Demyelinating Disease Program
Hospital for Sick Children
Toronto, Ontario, Canada

Gustavo Malinger MD
Professor
Fetal Neurology Clinic
Department of Obstetrics and Gynecology
Wolfson Medical Center
Holon, Israel
Sackler School of Medicine,
Tel-Aviv University,
Tel-Aviv, Israel

David E. Mandelbaum MD PhD
Professor
Neurology and Pediatrics
Alpert Medical School of Brown University
Providence, RI, USA

Charles J. Marcuccilli MD PhD
Assistant Professor of Neurology
Division of Pediatric Neurology
Medical College of Wisconsin
Milwaukee, WI, USA

Stephen M. Maricich MD PhD
Assistant Professor
Departments of Pediatrics, Neurosciences and
Otolaryngology
Case Western Reserve University School of
Medicine
Cleveland, OH, USA

Lee J. Martin PhD
Professor of Pathology and Neuroscience
Departments of Pathology and Neuroscience
Division of Neuropathology
Johns Hopkins University School of Medicine
Baltimore, MD, USA

Julie A. Mennella PhD
Member
Monell Chemical Senses Center
Philadelphia, PA, USA

Laura R. Ment MD
Professor
Pediatrics and Neurology
Associate Dean
Yale University School of Medicine
New Haven, CT, USA

David J. Michelson MD
Assistant Professor
Pediatrics, Division of Child Neurology
Loma Linda University School of Medicine
Loma Linda, CA, USA

Fady M. Mikhail MD PhD
Assistant Director
Cytogenetics Laboratory
Assistant Professor
Department of Genetics
University of Alabama at Birmingham
Birmingham, AL, USA

Kathleen J. Millen PhD
Associate Professor
Department of Pediatrics
Seattle Children's Hospital Research Institute
Center for Integrative Brain Research
University of Washington
Seattle, WA, USA

Steven P. Miller MDCM MAS FRCPC
Canada Research Chair in Neonatal Neuroscience
Senior Clinician Scientist
Child and Family Research Institute
Associate Professor of Pediatrics (Neurology)
University of British Columbia
Vancouver, British Columbia, Canada

Jonathan W. Mink MD PhD
Professor of Neurology
Chief, Child Neurology
Interim Chief, Movement Disorders
University of Rochester
Rochester, NY, USA

Ghayda Mirzaa MD FAAP
Fellow
Clinical Genetics
Department of Human Genetics
University of Chicago
Chicago, IL, USA

Wendy G. Mitchell MD
Professor
Neurology and Pediatrics
Keck School of Medicine
University of Southern California
Acting Division Head
Pediatric Neurology
Children's Hospital Los Angeles
Los Angeles, CA, USA

Manikum Moodley MD FRCP
Staff, Center for Pediatric Neurology
Neurological Institute
Cleveland Clinic
Cleveland, OH, USA

Lawrence D. Morton MD
Professor
Neurology and Pediatrics
Director, Clinical Neurophysiology
Virginia Commonwealth University Health
Systems
Richmond, VA, USA

Richard T. Moxley III MD
Professor of Neurology and Pediatrics
Director, Neuromuscular Disease Center
Associate Chair for Academic Affairs
Helen Aresty Fine and Irving Fine

Professor of Neurology
University of Rochester
Rochester, NY, USA

Srikanth Muppidi MD
Assistant Professor
Department of Neurology
UT Southwestern Medical Center
Dallas, TX, USA

Kendall Nash MD
Pediatric Neurophysiology/Epilepsy Fellow
Department of Neurology
University of California San Francisco
San Francisco, CA, USA

Ruth Nass MD
Professor of Child Neurology
Child and Adolescent Psychiatry and Pediatrics
NYU Langone Medical Center
New York, NY, USA

Michael J. Noetzel MD
Professor of Neurology and Pediatrics
Neurology and Pediatrics
Washington University School of Medicine
St. Louis, MO, USA

Douglas R. Nordli, Jr. MD
Lorna S. and James P. Langdon Chair of Pediatric Epilepsy
Professor
Department of Pediatrics
Northwestern University-Feinberg School of Medicine
Director, Epilepsy Center
Children's Memorial Hospital
Chicago, IL, USA

Frances J. Northington MD
Associate Professor of Pediatrics
Department of Pediatrics
Eudowood Neonatal Pulmonary Division and Neonatal Research Laboratory
Johns Hopkins University School of Medicine
Baltimore, MD, USA

Robert Ouvrier MD BS BSc (Med)
Petre Foundation Professor of Pediatric Neurology
Discipline of Pediatrics
University of Sydney
Children's Hospital at Westmead
New South Wales, Australia

Roger J. Packer MD
Senior Vice President
Neuroscience and Behavioral Medicine
Director, Brain Tumor Institute
Director, Gilbert Family Neurofibromatosis Institute
Children's National Medical Center
Washington, DC, USA

Seymour Packman MD PhD
Professor of Pediatrics
Department of Pediatrics
Division of Medical Genetics
University of California San Francisco
San Francisco, CA, USA

Julie A. Parsons MD
Assistant Professor of Pediatrics and Neurology
University of Colorado School of Medicine
Aurora, CO, USA

John C. Partridge MD MPH
Professor of Clinical Pediatrics
University of California San Francisco
San Francisco, CA, USA

Gregory M. Pastores MD
Associate Professor
Neurology and Pediatrics
NYU School of Medicine
New York, NY, USA

Marc C. Patterson MD FRACP
Professor of Neurology, Pediatrics, and Medical Genetics
Mayo Clinic College of Medicine
Chair, Division of Child and Adolescent Neurology
Departments of Neurology, Pediatrics, and Medical Genetics
Mayo Clinic
Rochester, MN, USA

John M. Pellock MD
Professor and Chairman
Division of Child Neurology
Virginia Commonwealth University/Medical College of Virginia Health System
Richmond, VA, USA

Ronald M. Perkin MD MA
Professor and Chairman
Department of Pediatrics
Brody School of Medicine at East Carolina University
Greenville, NC, USA

Isabelle Rapin MD
Professor
Saul R. Korey Department of Neurology and Department of Pediatrics
Albert Einstein College of Medicine
Bronx, NY, USA

Gerald V. Raymond MD
Professor of Neurology
Johns Hopkins University School of Medicine
Neurologist
Neurogenetics Research Center
Kennedy Krieger Institute
Baltimore, MD, USA

Rebecca Rendleman MD CM
New York Presbyterian Hospital/Weill Cornell Medical Center
New York, NY, USA

Jong M. Rho MD
Senior Staff Scientist
Neurology Research
Barrow Neurological Institute
Associate Director
Child Neurology
Barrow Neurological Institute
St. Joseph's Hospital and Medical Center
Phoenix, AZ, USA

Sarah M. Roddy MD
Associate Professor
Department of Pediatrics and Neurology
Loma Linda University School of Medicine
Loma Linda, CA, USA

Stephen M. Rosenthal MD
Professor of Pediatrics
Associate Program Director
Pediatric Endocrinology
Director
Pediatric Endocrine Outpatient Services
University of California San Francisco
San Francisco, CA, USA

N. Paul Rosman BSc MD CM
Professor
Departments of Pediatrics and Neurology
Boston University School of Medicine
Boston Medical Center
Boston, MA, USA

M. Elizabeth Ross MD PhD
Professor
Neurology and Neuroscience
Weill Cornell Medical College
New York, NY, USA

Robert S. Rust MA MD
Thomas E. Worrell Professor of Epileptology and Neurology
Professor of Pediatrics
Departments of Neurology and Pediatrics
University of Virginia
Charlottesville, VA, USA

Pedro A. Sanchez-Lara MD
Assistant Professor
Department of Pediatrics
University of Southern California
Keck School of Medicine
Director of Craniofacial Genetics
Medical Genetics
Children's Hospital Los Angeles
Los Angeles, CA, USA

Terence D. Sanger MD PhD
Associate Professor
Department of Biomedical Engineering
Child Neurology and Biokinesiology
University of Southern California
Los Angeles, CA, USA

Oranee Sanmaneechai MD
Pediatric Neurology Fellow
Neurology
Albert Einstein College of Medicine
Bronx, NY, USA
Assistant Professor in Pediatrics
Department of Pediatrics
Siriraj Hospital
Mahidol University
Bangkok, Thailand

Urs B. Schaad MD
Professor Emeritus
Pediatrics
Pediatric Infectious Diseases
University of Basel
Basel, Switzerland

Mark S. Scher MD
Professor of Pediatrics and Neurology
Department of Pediatrics
Division Chief, Pediatric Neurology
Director, Rainbow Neurological Center
Neurological Institute of University Hospitals
Director, Pediatric Neurointensive Care Program/
Fetal Neurology Program
Rainbow Babies and Children's Hospital
University Hospitals Case Medical Center
CWRU School of Medicine
University Hospitals of Cleveland
Cleveland, OH, USA

Nina F. Schor MD PhD
William H. Eilinger Chair of Pediatrics
Professor, Departments of Pediatrics, Neurology,
and Neurobiology and Anatomy
University of Rochester School of Medicine
and Dentistry
Rochester, NY, USA

Michael M. Segal MD PhD
Founder and Chief Scientist
SimulConsult, Inc.
Chestnut Hill, MA, USA

Bennett A. Shaywitz MD
Charles and Helen Schwab Professor in Dyslexia
and Learning Development
Chief, Pediatric Neurology
Yale University School of Medicine
New Haven, CT, USA

Sally E. Shaywitz MD
Audrey G. Ratner Professor in Learning
Development,
Co-Director, Yale Center for Dyslexia and
Creativity

Department of Pediatrics
Yale University School of Medicine
New Haven, CT, USA

Elliott H. Sherr MD PhD
Associate Professor
Neurology
University of California San Francisco
San Francisco, CA, USA

Michael I. Shevell MD CM FRCP FAAN
Professor, Departments of Neurology/
Neurosurgery and Pediatrics
McGill University
Director, Division of Pediatric Neurology
Montreal Children's Hospital
McGill University Health Centre
Montreal, Quebec, Canada

Shlomo Shinnar MD PhD
Professor of Neurology, Pediatrics, and
Epidemiology and Population Health
Hyman Climenko Professor of Neuroscience
Research
Director, Comprehensive Epilepsy Management
Center
Montefiore Medical Center
Albert Einstein College of Medicine
Bronx, NY, USA

Stanford K. Shu MD
Assistant Professor of Pediatrics and Neurology
Pediatrics
Loma Linda University School of Medicine
Loma Linda, CA, USA

Faye S. Silverstein MD
Professor
Pediatrics and Neurology
University of Michigan
Ann Arbor, MI, USA

Harvey S. Singer MD
Haller Professor of Pediatric Neurology
Johns Hopkins University School of Medicine
Director
Child Neurology
Johns Hopkins Hospital
Baltimore, MD, USA

John T. Sladky MD
Professor of Pediatrics and Neurology
Pediatrics
Emory University School of Medicine
Atlanta, GA, USA

Stephen A. Smith MD
Neurology
Gillette Children's Specialty Healthcare
Pathology
Hennepin County Medical Center
Minneapolis, MN, USA

Janet S. Soul MD CM FRCPC
Director, Clinical Neonatal Neurology
Director, Neonatal Neurology Clinic
Children's Hospital Boston
Assistant Professor of Neurology
Neurology
Harvard Medical School
Boston, MA, USA

Carl E. Stafstrom MD PhD
Chief, Pediatric Neurology
Professor
Neurology and Pediatrics
University of Wisconsin
Madison, WI, USA

Jonathan B. Strober MD
Director, Pediatric MDA Clinic
Associate Clinical Professor
Neurology and Pediatrics
Division of Child Neurology
University of California San Francisco
San Francisco, CA, USA

Joseph Sullivan MD
Director
UCSF Pediatric Epilepsy Center
Assistant Professor of Clinical Neurology and
Pediatrics
University of California San Francisco
San Francisco, CA, USA

Kenneth F. Swaiman MD
Director Emeritus, Division of Pediatric
Neurology
Professor Emeritus of Neurology and Pediatrics
University of Minnesota Medical School
Minneapolis, MN, USA

Matthew T. Sweney MD MS
Child Neurology Fellow
Division of Pediatric Neurology
University of Utah
Salt Lake City, UT, USA

Kathryn J. Swoboda MD FACMG
Associate Professor
Departments of Neurology and Pediatrics
Director
Pediatric Motor Disorders Research Program
University of Utah
Salt Lake City, UT, USA

Martin G. Täuber Dr. Med
Director and Chief
Institute for Infectious Diseases
University of Bern
and Inselspital University Hospital
Bern, Switzerland

Donald A. Taylor MD
Director of Pediatric Clinical
Neurophysiology
St. Mary's Hospital
Richmond, VA, USA

Ingrid Tein MD FRCP(C)
Associate Professor of Pediatrics, Laboratory
Medicine and Pathobiology
Director, Neurometabolic Clinic and Research
Laboratory
Staff Neurologist, Division of Neurology
Department of Pediatrics
Senior Scientist, Genetics and Genome Biology
Program
Research Institute
Hospital for Sick Children
University of Toronto
Toronto, Ontario, Canada

Elizabeth A. Thiele MD PhD
Director, Pediatric Epilepsy Program
Director, Herscot Center for Tuberous Sclerosis
Complex
Department of Neurology, Massachusetts General
Hospital
Harvard Medical School
Boston, MA, USA

Doris A. Trauner MD
Professor
Neurosciences and Pediatrics
University of California San Diego
La Jolla, CA, USA

Roberto Tuchman MD
Director
Autism Program
Neurology
Miami Children's Hospital Dan Marino Center
Weston, FL, USA

Adeline Vanderver MD
Assistant Professor of Neurology, Pediatrics and
Integrative Systems Biology
Department of Neurology
Children's National Medical Center
George Washington University School of Medicine
Washington, DC, USA

Michéle Van Hirtum-Das MD
Attending Physician
Neurology
Children's Hospital Los Angeles
Los Angeles, CA, USA

**V. Venkataraman Vedanarayanan MD
FRCPC**
Professor of Neurology, Pediatrics, and Pathology
University of Mississippi Medical Center
Jackson, MS, USA

Zinaida S. Vexler PhD
Professor of Neurology
University of California San Francisco
San Francisco, CA, USA

Gilbert Vezina MD
Director of Neuroradiology
Division of Radiology
Children's National Medical Center
Washington DC, USA

Emily von Scheven MD MAS
Professor of Clinical Pediatrics
Pediatric Rheumatology
University of California San Francisco
San Francisco, CA, USA

Ann Wagner PhD
Chief, Neurobehavioral Mechanisms Branch
Division of Developmental Translational Research
National Institute of Mental Health
Bethesda, MD, USA

Mark S. Wainwright MD PhD
Director, Pediatric Neurocritical Care Program
Children's Memorial Hospital
Associate Professor
Department of Pediatrics
Divisions of Neurology and Critical Care
Northwestern University Feinberg School of
Medicine
Chicago, IL, USA

John T. Walkup MD
Professor of Psychiatry
Vice Chair of Psychiatry and Director
Division of Child and Adolescent Psychiatry
Weill Cornell Medical College and New York
Presbyterian Hospital
New York, NY, USA

Laurence E. Walsh MD
Associate Professor of Clinical Neurology
Medical and Molecular Genetics
and Clinical Pediatrics
Child Neurology Section
Department of Neurology
Indiana University School of Medicine
Indianapolis, IN, USA

Ching H. Wang MD PhD
Associate Professor
Neurology and Pediatrics
Stanford University Medical Center
Stanford, CA, USA

James W. Wheless MD
Professor and Chief of Pediatric Neurology
LeBonheur Chair in Pediatric Neurology
University of Tennessee Health Science Center
Director, LeBonheur Comprehensive Epilepsy
Program & Neuroscience Institute
LeBonheur Children's Hospital
Clinical Chief & Director of Pediatric Neurology
St Jude Children's Research Hospital
Memphis, TN, USA

Nicole I. Wolf MD PhD
Assistant Professor
Child Neurology
VU University Medical Center
Amsterdam, The Netherlands

Gil I. Wolfe MD
Dr. Bob and Jean Smith Foundation Distinguished
Chair in Neuromuscular Disease Research
Professor of Neurology
University of Texas Southwestern Medical Center
Dallas, TX, USA

Yvonne W. Wu MD MPH
Professor
Neurology and Pediatrics
University of California San Francisco
San Francisco, CA, USA

Nathaniel D. Wycliffe MD
Associate Professor of Radiology
Division of Neuroradiology
Loma Linda University Medical Center
Loma Linda, CA, USA

Jerome Y. Yager MD FRCP(C)
Director of Research
Department of Pediatrics
Section of Pediatric Neurosciences
Stollery Children's Hospital
University of Alberta
Edmonton, Alberta, Canada

Jennifer A. Zimmer MD
Assistant Professor
Department of Child Neurology
Indiana University School of Medicine
Indianapolis, IN, USA

Huda Y. Zoghbi MD
Investigator, Howard Hughes Medical Institute
Professor
Baylor College of Medicine
Department of Pediatrics
Molecular and Human Genetics
Neurology and Neuroscience
Jan and Dan Duncan Neurological Research
Institute
Houston, TX, USA

Mary L. Zupanc MD
Professor
Department of Pediatrics and Neurology
University of California Irvine Children's Hospital
of Orange County
Chief
Division of Pediatric Neurology Director
Pediatric Comprehensive Epilepsy Program
Children's Hospital of Wisconsin
Milwaukee, WI, USA

Acknowledgments

We wish to thank the editorial and publishing staff at Elsevier, especially Janice Gaillard, Charlotta Kryhl, Frances Affleck, and Wendy Lee. Without their diligence and persistence, we would have never been able to complete this project.

Part I
Clinical Evaluation

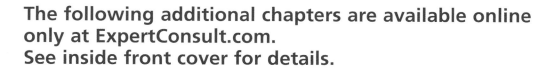

The following additional chapters are available online only at ExpertConsult.com.
See inside front cover for details.

Expert | CONSULT

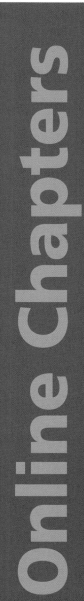

Online Chapters

Part II
Neurodiagnostic Testing

The following additional chapters are available online only at ExpertConsult.com.
See inside front cover for details.

Expert|CONSULT

Online Chapters

Brain Plasticity and its Disorders

Michael V. Johnston

Introduction

Brain plasticity is an important concept that plays a major role in the expression of many pediatric neurological disorders and strongly influences recovery from brain injuries in neonates, infants, and children. Plasticity refers to the brain's ability to change in response to experience, whether it is a positive experience such as education or practicing a skill, or an adverse event such as a stroke or other type of brain injury [Johnston, 2004]. The child's brain exhibits greater plasticity than the adult brain, and common examples of enhanced brain plasticity in children include their ability to learn new motor tasks quickly, such as playing a musical instrument, participating in a sport, or their ability to become fluent in a new language [Meltzoff et al., 2009]. Children and adolescents are also able to form memories more easily than adults and they recover more quickly from brain injuries. The mechanisms responsible for various kinds of brain plasticity are being uncovered at a rapid pace as are the defects in these steps that cause intellectual disability and other pediatric disorders [Johnston, 2009]. This chapter gives a brief overview of normal brain plasticity and its disorders that are relevant to pediatric neurology, and provides insight into the pathogenesis of a variety of disorders described in other sections.

It is useful to consider four aspects or types of plasticity in the developing brain in order to understand how this concept is integrated into many disorders of the child's nervous system (Box 13-1). The first type is generally referred to as adaptive plasticity, in which the nervous system changes in the process of learning new skills that have an adaptive advantage, such as learning to read or pass a test, learning to play a musical instrument, or learning to play a sport. Adaptive plasticity is also engaged when children recover from a brain injury, such as a stroke or extensive removal of brain tissue to cure epilepsy, and therapists try to harness this form of plasticity when providing speech, occupational, or physical therapy for a variety of disorders. In these cases, it is expected that normal childhood activities, such as attending school, music lessons, athletic practice, or therapies for cerebral palsy or other brain injuries, will activate normal plasticity programs to provide a good outcome that is beneficial for the child [Meltzoff et al., 2009]. Adaptive plasticity is generally enhanced in younger children compared with adults, and the genetically determined programs responsible for this kind of plasticity are heavily influenced by sensory input. Since learning and memory, as well as acquisition of physical skills, are very important for normal childhood development, genetic or acquired defects in the signaling pathways responsible for plasticity are reflected in a variety of developmental disability phenotypes [Johnston, 2004]. These disorders are best understood as examples of impaired plasticity.

Many types of intellectual disability are caused by genetic lesions in the signaling cascades that are normally responsible for activity-dependent synaptic plasticity (Table 13-1). For example, in fragile X syndrome (FraX), the most common form of inherited intellectual disability, a trinucleotide repeat in the gene for the fragile X mental retardation protein (FMRP) leads to its absence or reduction in the brain [Penagarikano et al., 2007]. FMRP is responsible for transport of certain messenger RNAs and translation of proteins within dendrites in response to synaptic activity, and its absence causes a reduction in long-term potentiation (LTP), a physiological form of synaptic plasticity involved in learning and memory [Huber et al., 2002]. Accordingly, the intellectual disability and other behavioral features of FraX can be considered to reflect a genetically determined form of impaired plasticity in synapses. Therapies aimed at restoring normal plasticity mechanisms to synapses in FraX show some promise in preclinical and small clinical trials [Wang et al., 2010].

Just as impaired plasticity is responsible for numerous brain disorders in children, maladaptive or excessive plasticity also can cause problems. When this phenomenon occurs, plasticity is misdirected or enhanced in a way that is harmful, or at least not beneficial. For example, children who have had strokes, traumatic brain injuries, or hypoxic-ischemic brain injuries sometimes develop delayed seizures that may result from formation of abnormal neuronal networks in damaged brain tissue [Kadam and Dudek, 2007]. In some cases, neurons in these networks have been shown to have functional changes in voltage-sensitive sodium channels that are similar to those found in certain forms of genetic epilepsy [Graef and Godwin, 2010]. Excessive plasticity may also be responsible for seizures and cognitive impairment in genetic disorders in which intracellular signaling pathways are enhanced, such as tuberous sclerosis and Costello's syndrome [Crino, 2010; Dileone et al., 2010]. Another example of enhanced, but maladaptive, plasticity that causes neurologic impairment is dystonia in the hand and fingers resulting from over-practice of the piano or another musical instrument requiring intense finger movement [Quartarone et al., 2006]. In patients with this disorder, functional imaging of the contralateral cortex has shown that the somatosensory map of the fingers is blurred in the musicians with dystonia compared to controls [Elbert et al., 1998]. This suggests that the somatosensory cortex is less able to distinguish precisely between individual finger movements, and an attempt to use the fingers leads to dystonic movements instead. Interestingly, selective injection of botulinum toxin into some of the fingers can compensate for the disrupted somatotopic map of the fingers and restore normal movement [Cole et al., 1995]. The immature brain may be especially

Box 13-1 Major Types of Plasticity in the Developing Brain

Adaptive Plasticity

- Plasticity that serves a useful purpose for learning or recovering from an injury or disability

Impaired Plasticity

- Disability due to a genetic or acquired disorder of brain plasticity

Excessive or Maladaptive Plasticity

- Disability that is due to a plastic response that leads to a new disorder, e.g., dystonia from over-practice

Plasticity as the Brain's Achilles' Heel

- A plasticity mechanism that creates a risk for injury, e.g., selective injury to a specific group of neuron circuits

Table 13-1 Pediatric Disorders Caused by Genetic Mutations of Signaling Pathways Involved in Neuronal Plasticity

Disorder	Mechanism of Disease
Neurofibromatosis 1	Ras too active, enhanced GABA activity
Tuberous sclerosis	Upregulated mTOR signaling pathway
Rett's syndrome	Mutations in MeCP2 transcription factor
Fragile X syndrome	Upregulated mGluR5 causes LTD
Coffin–Lowry syndrome	Mutations in RSK2 in Ras-MAPK pathway
Rubinstein–Taybi syndrome	Mutation in CREB binding protein (CBP)
X-linked intellectual disabilities	Mutation in PAK3 kinase: links RhoGTPases to dendritic cytoskeleton Mutation in oligophrenin, RhoGTPase Mutation in GluR3 AMPA receptor subunit
Costello's syndrome	Upregulated H-Ras signaling to MAPK (intellectual disability, heart, skeletal disorder)
Lead poisoning	Enhanced PKC activity, inhibited NMDA receptors; impairs maturation of dendritic spines

AMPA, α-amino-3-hydroxy-5-methyl-4-isoxazolepropionic acid; CREB, cyclic adenosine monophosphate response element binding protein; GABA, gamma-aminobutyric acid; MAPK, Ras-mitogen activated protein kinase; mTOR, mammalian target of rapamycin; NMDA, N-methyl-D-aspartate; PKC, protein kinase C.

susceptible to organizational changes in neuronal circuits that lead to acquired disorders associated with maladaptive or excessive plasticity.

A fourth aspect of plasticity that it is important to consider is its potential to create cell-specific selective vulnerabilities, leading to the understanding of plasticity as the brain's Achilles' heel. This concept is especially important in the developing brain, where different cells are undergoing dramatic shifts in their composition during growth and development. One example is the subplate neurons that are among the first to reach the cerebral cortex in the second trimester of pregnancy, providing targets for axons projected from neurons in the thalamus [McQuillen et al., 2003]. These neurons are selectively vulnerable to hypoxia-ischemia due to their enhanced expression of excitatory α-amino-3-hydroxy-5-methyl-4-isoxazolepropionic acid (AMPA)-type glutamate receptors during that time period [Nguyen and McQuillen, 2010]. Immature oligodendroglia are similarly more vulnerable to injury during the second trimester due to the subunit composition of their AMPA receptors that favors permeability to calcium [Volpe, 2009]. N-methyl-D-aspartate (NMDA) receptors also contribute to developmental vulnerability of immature oligodendroglia [Salter and Fern, 2005]. These age-dependent changes in excitatory amino acid receptors on neurons and oligodendroglia that favor excitation have a beneficial role in normal development, but they can also make cells vulnerable to death if they are accidentally exposed to hypoxia or ischemia [McDonald and Johnston, 1990]. In a similar way, developing neurons in the brain closer to term become more vulnerable to excitotoxicity mediated by NMDA receptors due to the fact that the receptors are genetically programmed at that time to be more excitable [Monyer et al., 1993]. NMDA receptors are easier to activate in the developing brain due to their subunit composition, which makes it easier to open their channels. However, this characteristic also creates a vulnerability to injury if the brain is exposed to hypoxia-ischemia, which can result in neuronal depolarization and calcium flooding through opening of the NMDA channels.

In addition, gamma-aminobutyric acid (GABA), which normally has an inhibitory effect on neuronal circuits in older children and adults, mediates excitation in the newborn period because of developmental changes in chloride pumps in GABAergic synapses [Ben-Ari, 2006]. Enhanced activity of the NKCC1 chloride transporter in the neonatal period leads to higher intraneuronal concentrations of chloride than are present later on, so that, when GABA opens chloride channels, the cation leaves the neuron rather than entering [Dzhala et al., 2005]. Therefore, GABA leads to depolarization rather than hyperpolarization, as it does at older ages. Later in development, activity of the NKCC1 pump declines, and expression of the NKCC2 pump, which pushes chloride out of neurons, increases, leading to lower baseline concentrations of chloride inside the neuron compared to outside, and to inhibition. Combined with the expression of NMDA receptors, which are more active and flux more calcium and sodium in the fetal and neonatal brain, developmental changes in the actions of GABA lead to the brain being more excitable. This enhanced excitability during development appears to play an important role in the establishment of normal neuronal circuitry, which is dependent on electrical activity [Penn and Shatz, 1999]. For example, production of growth factors, such as brain-derived neurotropic factor (BDNF), occurs in neurons and is dependent on neuronal activity [Lessmann and Brigadski, 2009]. Prolonged blockade of NMDA receptors, just like too much activity, can cause neuronal death because a minimum baseline amount of channel opening, with entry of calcium and sodium into neurons, is essential for neuronal survival [Hansen et al., 2004]. On the other hand, this bias towards excitement in the developing brain is probably responsible for the higher propensity for seizures in infants and children compared to adults, and the expression of some seizure types such as infantile spasms [Hablitz and Lee, 1992]. Therefore it is quite important for the molecular machinery responsible for balancing excitement and inhibition in the developing brain to operate properly in order to prevent it from becoming an Achilles' heel during periods of stress, such as hypoxia-ischemia or status epilepticus [McDonald and Johnston, 1990].

Basic Mechanisms for Plasticity in the Developing Brain

In addition to these four broad types of plasticity in the developing brain, there are at least six basic cellular mechanisms for plasticity (Box 13-2). The earliest mechanism is the overproduction of neurons and glia from stem cells, and then reduction of this population by apoptosis in the fetus [Haydar et al., 1999]. Most neurogenesis ceases after birth, but it continues in selected niches of stem-cell production in the subventricular zone of the lateral ventricles and the subgranular zone of the dentate gyrus of the hippocampus [Kernie and Parent, 2010]. These restricted zones of neurogenesis may contribute to recovery from brain injuries throughout life. Additional mechanisms for plasticity are:
1. activity-dependent plasticity that can vary the strength of information transfer across the synapse based on recent activity
2. activity-dependent production of growth factors, such as BDNF, that shape and stabilize neuronal circuits
3. overproduction of synapses and axodendritic connections in infancy, followed by pruning and selection of remaining synapses by adolescence
4. continued activity-dependent stabilization of synapses and dendrites, and turnover of new dendrites based on learning
5. epigenetic modification of DNA expression through modifications in histones that include methylation (generally inhibition) or acetylation (facilitation), as well as histone remodeling or variation.

Box 13-2 Basic Mechanisms for Plasticity in the Developing Brain

- Overproduction of neurons and glia from stem cells and reduction in programmed cell death
- Continued production of new cells from stem cells in the dentate gyrus of the hippocampus and the subventricular zone of the lateral ventricle
- Activity-dependent synaptic plasticity through receptor trafficking and related changes in synaptic chemistry and electrophysiology
- Activity-dependent production of growth factors, such as brain-derived neurotropic factor (BDNF)
- Overproduction of synapses and axonodendritic connections, followed by pruning and selection of remaining synapses
- Continued activity-dependent stabilization of synapses and dendrites, and turnover of new dendritic spines based on learning
- Epigenetic regulation of DNA expression through modification of histones, which includes modification by acetylation, methylation, or histone remodeling

Mechanisms of Synaptic Plasticity

Synaptic plasticity is the most important mechanism for everyday activities such as learning and memory, and acquiring new skills (Figure 13-1). The strength of the signals between axons and dendrites across synapses can be increased or decreased through processes called long-term potentiation (LTP) or long-term depression (LTD), and these processes are strongly influenced by previous synaptic activity [Malenka and Nicoll, 1993]. The most prominent examples of LTP and LTD occur in excitatory glutamate synapses, which account for about 75 percent of all synapses in the brain. However, LTP and LTD are also present in many different types of neurons, including inhibitory GABAergic neurons and dopaminergic neurons [Nugent and Kauer, 2008]. One of the best examples of LTP is mediated by the NMDA-type glutamate receptors, which are voltage-dependent, meaning that NMDA channel opening is dependent in part on membrane depolarization [Gilland et al., 1998]. Channel opening is also dependent on occupancy of receptors for glutamate and glycine by these amino acids. When multiple excitatory axons depolarize the neuronal membrane, and glycine and glutamate occupy their receptors, the NMDA-activated calcium channel opens, allowing a pulse of calcium to enter the neurons and, in turn, activating a cascade of biochemical events that encode a memory of the event [Johnston, 2004]. The NMDA receptor has been referred to as a coincidence detector because it requires both membrane depolarization, stimulated by multiple presynaptic inputs, and activation of glutamate and glycine receptors to open its channel [Brown and Milner, 2003]. NMDA receptor-mediated LTP results in a "step up" in the signal mediated by the synapse during subsequent synapse activations, and it becomes easier to activate. Neuronal stimulation can also activate another type of a glutamate receptor, called a metabotropic

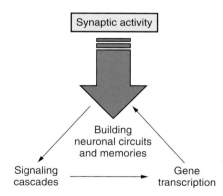

Fig. 13-1 Schematic of activity-dependent synaptic plasticity as it relates to genetic and acquired disorders of learning, memory, and behavior. Synaptic activity can change, based on previous experience, either to facilitate future transfer of information across the synapse (long-term potentiation, LTP), or to depress future neurotransmission (long-term depression, LTD). The synapse typically undergoes short-term changes in neurotransmission that do not require gene transcription, as well as longer-term changes that do require transcription. These longer-term changes activate signaling cascades from the synapse to the nucleus, where transcription and translation take place, to produce synaptic proteins that, in turn, contribute to expansion and remodeling of the structure of synapses. This relation between synaptic activity, gene transcription, and synaptic structure explains how many disorders of signaling pathways also disrupt the structure of synapses, dendrites, neuronal circuits, and white-matter pathways.

gluR5 (mGluR5) receptor because it activates the second messenger phosphoinositol turnover, rather than opening an ion channel, as NMDA receptors do [Antion et al., 2008].

Within synapses, a variety of mechanisms contribute to LTP and LTD, including an increase or decrease in neurotransmitter release from presynaptic nerve terminals, a change in reuptake of neurotransmitter by astroglia that surround each synapse, a change in the number of neurotransmitter receptors in the postsynaptic membrane, changes in the flux of calcium and other ions through membrane channels, and an activation of intracellular signaling cascades [Citri and Malenka, 2008]. One of the common mechanisms that synapses use to increase or decrease synaptic strength is to alter the number of receptors in the postsynaptic membrane through a process called "receptor trafficking" (Figure 13-2) [Keifer and Zheng, 2010; Conboy and Sandi, 2010]. In this process, receptors shuttle back and forth between the cytoplasm, where they do not have access to neurotransmitter in the synaptic cleft, postsynaptic density, and postsynaptic membrane, where they are positioned to interact with neurotransmitter. One excitatory receptor that is heavily regulated by receptor trafficking in synapses is the AMPA receptor, which is the ionotropic glutamate receptor that carries most of the fast excitatory current in the brain. AMPA receptors shuttle between the dendritic cytoplasm, where they are inaccessible to glutamate, to the postsynaptic membrane, where they can be stimulated by glutamate [Keifer and Zheng, 2010]. The number of receptors within the synaptic membrane determines the strength of the synapse when it is activated. Accordingly, LTP is associated with an increase in AMPA receptors inserted into the postsynaptic membrane, while a decrease in AMPA receptors in the postsynaptic membrane is associated with LTD. LTP can be induced by rapid stimulation of the postsynaptic membrane, leading to voltage-dependent opening of NMDA receptors and trafficking of AMPA receptors from the cytoplasm into the postsynaptic membrane. This makes the synapse better able to conduct a signal, in effect creating a fragment of a memory about that synapse's past experience. The mGluR5 metabotropic glutamate receptor also controls AMPA receptor trafficking, and an increase in mGluR5 activity leads to internalization of AMPA receptors, LTD, and weaker synaptic strength. In experimental models of fragile X syndrome, the activity of mGluR5 receptors has been reported to be increased, along with enhanced synaptic LTD, and antagonists of the mGluR5 receptor are able to restore LTP and improve abnormal behaviors and cognition (see Figure 13-2) [Muddashetty et al., 2007]. Fragile X syndrome is one example of a developmental brain disorder that can be understood at the level of the synapse. Synapses are thought to be the primary site of memory storage across large networks in which the strength of individual synapses is increased or decreased by the processes of LTP or LDP.

Production of nerve growth factors like BDNF is another mechanism by which previous synaptic activity can lead to plasticity in neuronal connections. BDNF is produced in neurons in response to neuronal activity, and it has been shown to increase and stabilize synaptic connections, as well as contribute to their maturation and integration into complex neuronal circuits [Yoshii and Constantine-Paton, 2010]. Learning has also been shown to increase neurotrophin signaling through the TrκB receptor, which mediates the actions of BDNF in the hippocampus in mice. BDNF has also been associated with cortical plasticity in humans. Kleim et al. reported that individuals with a val66met polymorphism (i.e., methionine codon substitution for valine codon at position 66 in the *BDNF* gene) showed reduced ability to reorganize their cortical motor map in response to a training exercise involving the fingers of one hand [Kleim et al., 2006]. In vitro studies showed that this mutation impairs the secretion of BDNF from neurons, but

IMPAIRED SYNAPTIC LTP IN FRAGILE X SYNDROME

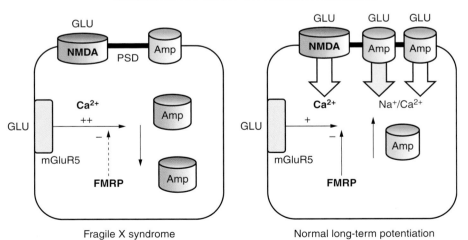

Fig. 13-2 Glutamate receptor trafficking at excitatory synapses. The diagram on the right shows movement of AMPA receptors (Amp) from the cytoplasm into the postsynaptic membrane in response to activation of NMDA receptors associated with long-term potentiation (LTP). This movement of receptors in and out of the postsynaptic membrane is called receptor trafficking. The potentiated electrophysiologic response across the synapse is mediated by extra sodium/calcium fluxed through additional AMPA channels that move into the postsynaptic membrane. Normally, the trafficking of AMPA receptors is regulated by metabotropic mGluR5 receptors, which stimulate receptor movement away from the postsynaptic membrane, and fragile X mental retardation protein (FMRP), which antagonizes the effect of mGluR5 and stimulates receptor movement into the postsynaptic membrane. In fragile X syndrome (left panel), the activity of FMRP is lost due to the presence of a trinucleotide repeat in its gene. This leaves the action of mGluR5 unopposed, resulting in AMPA receptor movement into the cytoplasm and impaired LTP. Trials of drugs that antagonize the mGluR5 receptor are in progress in persons with fragile X syndrome, after showing activity in fruit flies and mice with FraX. AMPA, α-amino-3-hydroxy-5-methyl-4-isoxazolepropionic acid; NMDA, N-methyl-D-aspartate; PSD, postsynaptic density.

its expression is normal. McHughen et al. used functional magnetic resonance imaging (fMRI) to show that subjects with this BDNF mutation made more errors and had poorer retention on a driver-based learning task, and had altered short-term plasticity [McHughen et al., 2010]. BDNF genotype has also been shown to be associated with anxiety and memory problems, as well as with impaired functional connectivity from the hippocampus to the amygdala, insula, and striatal regions in children studied with functional connectivity (FC) analysis on data obtained through whole-brain fMRI [Thomason et al., 2009].

Plasticity of Dendrites and Dendritic Spines

Activity-dependent plasticity in excitatory synapses is associated with physical changes in dendritic spines that are thought to reflect information storage (Figure 13-3) [Hotulainen and Hoogenraad, 2010]. Immature dendritic spines are long with a small head, but repeated activity during development, including LTP, leads to shortening of spine shafts and enlargement of spine heads. New learning in animals also has been shown to be associated with localized enlargement of some dendritic spines and loss of others. Remodeling of dendrite morphology occurs continuously in association with synaptic plasticity, and is mediated by the actin-rich cytoskeleton that fills dendrites [Hotulainen and Hoogenraad, 2010]. The actin cytoskeleton within spines containing excitatory synapses provides support for the postsynaptic density (PSD), which anchors glutamate receptors and cell adhesion molecules that span the synaptic cleft (see Figure 13-3). NMDA receptors within the PSD regulate actin signaling pathways within an endocytic zone just below the PSD. The purpose of this zone is to recycle the synaptic pool of AMPA-type glutamate receptors involved in trafficking between the cytoplasm and the PSD. Therefore, the actin cytoskeleton plays an important role in LTP, and it is not surprising that mutations in proteins involved in regulation of this cytoskeleton, such as small Rho and Ras GTPases, alter spine morphology and cause cognitive disorders and autistic spectrum disorders [Pinto et al., 2010]. Similarly, key proteins that make up the PSD and the scaffolding proteins beneath the PSD, such as SHANK and the cell adhesion proteins – neurexins, neuroligins, and cadherins – are associated with clinical disorders that impair learning (Table 13-2) [Durand et al., 2007; Johnston et al., 2001].

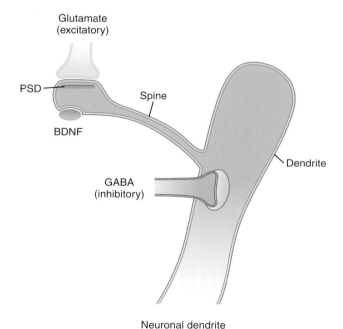

Fig. 13-3 Schematic drawing of the organization of excitatory and inhibitory synapses on dendrites and dendritic spines. Excitatory axons that contain glutamate synapse on the tips of dendritic spines, while inhibitory axons that contain gamma-aminobutyric acid (GABA) synapse on the shafts of dendrites. Excitatory synapses are asymmetric and contain a postsynaptic density (PSD), which anchors neurotransmitter receptors and a variety of other proteins that provide scaffolding for receptors (see Table 13-2). Typically, each dendritic spine contains only one excitatory synapse, while the shaft of the dendrite contains multiple inhibitory GABAergic synapses. This arrangement allows a single dendrite to receive and process information from many excitatory synapses on its dendritic spines. However, the summed output for each dendrite is controlled by inhibitory receptors on the shaft. The morphology of dendritic spines is controlled in part by age and activity, so that young spines are long and thin with narrow spine heads, while older spines that have experienced considerable activity become shorter with a broader spine head. These shape changes are mediated by an actin cytoskeleton that fills the spines, allowing them to change shape in response to synaptic activity. Abnormal morphology of dendrites, spines, and PSD proteins is commonly associated with syndromes that include intellectual disability, autism, and behavior disorders. BDNF, brain-derived neurotropic factor.

Table 13-2 Proteins Associated with the Postsynaptic Density of Excitatory Synapses and Possible Role in Neurologic Disease

Protein	Function	Connection with Neurological Disease
α-Actinin	Spine morphogenesis	Associated with faster-sprinting athletes
CaMKIIα/β	Activates gene expression	Major pathway to gene expression
Synapsins	Regulate neurotransmitter release	Seizures, cognitive disorders
N-cadherin	Adhesion molecule	Deafness, Usher's syndrome, epilepsy
Protocadherin	Adhesion molecule	Seizures, intellectual disability in females
GluR1,2,3	AMPA receptors	Cognitive impairment
Homer	Bind to mGluR5 receptors	Interacts with mGluR5 in fragile X syndrome
Neuroligin	Binds to presynaptic neurexin	Associated with autism
NR1-2A,B	NMDA glutamate subunits	Involved in learning and memory, autoimmune encephalopathy
PSD-95	Regulates synaptic plasticity	Major regulator of synapse development
Shank1/2/3	Scaffolding protein, promotes maturation of synapse	Associated with autism
SynGAP Ras GTPase activating protein	Controls signaling between synapse and nucleus to activate transcription	Regulates MAP kinases

In addition to the microscopic changes in synapses that occur during development, Huttenlocher has shown that there are large expansions of the number of synapses that occur during childhood, so that, by 2 years of age, there are approximately twice the number of synapses that will be present by age 16, when the number approximates adult levels [Huttenlocher, 1997]. This wave of expansion, overshoot, and then pruning begins earlier in the occipital lobe than in the frontal lobe, and pruning of synapses continues longest in the frontal lobes. Chugani and colleagues have shown, using positron emission tomography (PET), that glucose consumption of the cortex during childhood follows a curve that is similar to synapse number, consistent with the fact that synapses are the major site of energy consumption in the brain [Chugani et al., 1987]. These dynamic changes in synapse number probably support brain plasticity and growth of cognitive power in children because they allow synapses to be chosen from a surplus fairly late in childhood, based on synaptic activity provided by experience, and provide for redundancy of synapses if some injury does occur. Shaw et al. provided some evidence that these dynamic changes in synapse number may be functionally relevant in a study that used sequential MRI to measure cortical thickness in children of different intelligence levels [Shaw et al., 2006]. They found that children with superior intelligence had, on average, a higher peak and greater duration of peak cortical thickness than children of lower intelligence. The major differences in cortical thickness between groups of children with different levels of intelligence were found in the frontal cortex, which is the area that normally matures last. These results, as well as the earlier studies of glucose consumption and postmortem synaptic counting, suggest that cortical maturation in children moves like a wave of synapse proliferation and then pruning from back to front, and a higher, more prolonged wave is correlated with higher intelligence [Johnston, 2004]. These studies suggest that neuronal plasticity at multiple levels contributes to learning, memory, and higher intellectual function.

Intracellular Signaling Cascades and Gene Transcription

The changes in synapses, dendrites, and dendritic spines that accompany information storage in the developing brain require gene transcription and translation of proteins (Figure 13-4) [Johnston, 2004]. Several signaling cascades from the synaptic membrane to the nucleus are especially important in learning and memory; these include the calcium/calmodulin kinase II (CaMKII) pathway, the Ras-mitogen activated protein kinase II (MAP kinase II) pathway, and the protein kinase A (PKA) pathway. These pathways can all stimulate phosphorylation of the master transcription factor, cyclic adenosine monophosphate response element binding protein (CREB), which activates transcription of many genes that are important for learning, memory, and synaptic plasticity [Shalin et al., 2006]. CREB works closely with CREB binding protein (CBP), which has intrinsic histone acetylase activity that is required for DNA to unwind from histones in order to allow gene transcription [Roth et al., 2010]. The action of CREB is antagonized by transcriptional repressor proteins, including thyroid hormone receptor without thyroid hormone and MeCP2, the transcriptional factor that is mutated in Rett's syndrome. MeCP2 recruits transcriptional repressor Sin3 to block

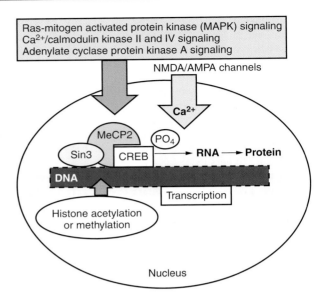

Fig. 13-4 Schematic of some important signaling pathways from the postsynaptic membrane and cell surface to the nucleus, where new genes are transcribed and proteins are produced in response to neuronal activity. This cellular machinery allows information to be stored for the long term within a distributed network of synapses, and it is essential for long-term memory. The pink box shows several important signaling cascades that activate transcription by phosphorylation of the master memory transcription factor, cyclic adenosine monophosphate response element binding protein (CREB). CREB enables the transcription of multiple genes and is assisted by CREB binding protein (CBP, not shown), which has histone acetylase activity that opens up DNA to allow transcription. Another important transcription factor is MeCP2, a transcriptional repressor that recruits other repressors such as Sin3, and controls activity-dependent transcription of brain-derived neurotropic factor (BDNF). Mutations in MeCP2 are the main cause of Rett's syndrome. Mutations in proteins involved in activity-dependent signaling within neurons are important causes of intellectual disability, autism, behavior disorders, and epilepsy (see Figure 13-2). AMPA, α-amino-3-hydroxy-5-methyl-4-isoxazolepropionic acid; NMDA, N-methyl-D-aspartate.

transcription of BDNF, although it has been shown also to activate many genes in the hypothalamus (see Figure 13-4) [Kaufmann et al., 2005]. Many other signaling cascades probably participate in activity-dependent transcription of genes that are involved in learning and memory and other aspects of brain plasticity.

Adaptive Plasticity

Adaptive plasticity includes the brain's ability to learn and remember information, and its capacity to change in response to practicing physical skills, such as playing the piano or a sport, as well as the ability to recover from a brain injury. The developing human brain has a greater capacity for adaptive plasticity than the adult brain, and several interesting examples have been reported. One of the earliest studies of morphologic changes in the developing brain in response to environment involved the ocular dominance columns in the visual cortex of monkeys in which one eye was occluded. These studies showed that reducing the visual input from one eye led to a reduction in thalamocortical axons from that eye, while the territory assigned to axons from the opposite eye expanded

[Tropea et al., 2008]. This process corresponds to the clinical scenario in which young children with strabismus develop amblyopia in one eye. Amblyopia can be corrected before about 10 years of age if the opposite eye is patched to restore balance in the visual inputs from the two eyes. Studies of plasticity in the occipital cortex of persons who were blind from birth have also provided insights into adaptive plasticity in the developing brain. Functional imaging using PET demonstrated that adults who were blind from birth activated the visual cortex in the occipital lobe, as well as somatosensory cortex representing their Braille-reading fingers [Sadato et al., 1996]. Other studies have shown that the occipital cortex of congenitally blind subjects is activated by nonvisual tasks, such as auditory processing, semantic processing, and verbal memory. Occipital lobe activity in these subjects seems to be functionally important for these nonvisual tasks because occipital strokes and temporary inactivation with repetitive transcranial magnetic stimulation (rTMS) have been shown to impair nonvisual skills such as Braille reading [Kupers et al., 2007]. It has also been shown that auditory association cortex is appropriated for visual processing in deaf children whose disability began at an age of less than 14 years [Weeks et al., 2000]. These examples demonstrate plasticity within one modality (vision) in response to differences between the eyes, and transmodal plasticity in which cortex assigned to another modality can be re-assigned if its intended sensory input is lost at an early age.

Although visual plasticity was one of the first types to be examined in humans, plasticity of the somatosensory cortex in response to the use of hands in musicians has also been explored. Taub and colleagues compared the differences in the contralateral somatosensory cortical maps for the fingers and thumb of the left hand between musicians who had played stringed instruments for many years versus nonplayers [Elbert et al., 1995]. Using a technique called magnetic source imaging to monitor effects of finger stimulation, they found that the expanse of cortex assigned to the fingers and thumb of the left hand used to finger the strings, as well as the strength of the signal, was greater than for nonplayers in direct proportion to the number of years they had been practicing. These data suggest that longer practice shapes and expands the cortical map in proportion to the amount of activity in the left hand. In another study of musicians, Schlaug et al. also reported that intense musical training for 29 months in children of 5–7 years of age, who played either piano or stringed instruments, was associated with an increase in volume of the anterior mid-body of the corpus callosum [Schlaug et al., 2009], compared to the same area of the corpus callosum in non-musician controls or musicians who practiced infrequently. The mid-body connects premotor and supplementary motor areas. Like the study of changes in the somatotopic map for string players, these results support the hypothesis that engagement of both hemispheres is important for musicians to process and play music, and that practice has a structural impact on the brain. Bengtsson et al. also found that extended piano practicing from childhood onward was strongly correlated with improved white-matter organization in the pyramidal and other white-matter tracts, as measured by increased fractional anisotropy on diffusion tensor imaging (DTI) [Bengtsson et al., 2005]. These results are consistent with classic experiments by Buonomano and Merzenich in primates, showing that the somatosensory map can be expanded by increased somatosensory stimulation of the fingers [Buonomano and

Merzenich, 1998]. Nudo et al. showed that sensory stimulation and retraining of the weak hand in a primate model of focal stroke prevented the shrinkage of the somatosensory area assigned to that hand that normally occurred [Nudo and Milliken, 1996]. As mentioned above, experiments in which subjects with a val66met polymorphism in the BDNF gene showed reduced ability to reorganize their cortical motor map in response to a training exercise involving the fingers of one hand show that adaptive plasticity is partially under genetic control [Kleim et al., 2006].

These results also agree with studies of the "barrel" field cortex in mice and rats, which represents a map of the animal's whiskers across the tangential expanse of somatosensory cortex [Nishimura et al., 2002]. Rodents depend on whiskers to navigate in the dark places where they live, as their visual system is less developed. Many experiments have shown that clipping a row of whiskers or enhancing whisker activity in neonatal rodents results in reassignment of the cortical map assigned to these whiskers. Specific neurotransmitters, such as glutamate, the inhibitory neurotransmitter GABA, and acetylcholine within the nucleus basalis projection from the basal forebrain to the cerebral cortex, have been shown to be important in this form of activity-dependent cortical plasticity [Inan and Crair, 2007]. Similar experiments, focused on the area of cortex that receives auditory inputs in developing rodents, have shown that a tonotopic map corresponding to sounds of different pitches is distributed across the surface of cortex, and can be altered markedly by exposing the animals to repeated monotonal sounds, together with a behavioral program and stimulation of the nucleus basalis [Barak et al., 2003]. These data are in agreement with those from children described above. The experiments in immature rodents show that structural brain plasticity is highly conserved across species and probably contributes to the enhanced functional plasticity seen in children.

Plasticity and Epilepsy in Children

A number of studies suggest that chronic epilepsy in children can disrupt learning and memory, as well as motor function [Holmes et al., 2002]. On the other hand, the child's brain can reorganize in response to epilepsy or extensive surgery for epilepsy to a greater extent than that of adults. Several studies indicate that motor and sensory functions in areas affected by focal epilepsy can be transferred from one hemisphere to the other. Boatman et al. reported a series of children who gained abilities in receptive language when a left hemispherectomy was performed for Rasmussen's syndrome in children aged 7–14 years [Boatman et al., 1999]. Hertz-Pannier et al. also reported a case of 9-year-old boy who had considerable improvement in speech after receiving a cortical resection in the left hemisphere for Rasmussen's encephalopathy [Hertz-Pannier et al., 2002]. In that case, speech improvement was associated with increased activity on fMRI scanning in the right hemisphere and both frontal lobes, suggesting that the epileptic activity in the left hemisphere led to migration of speech programs to the opposite side but was also impairing their expression. In this case, we can hypothesize that chaotic electrical activity impairs the expression of plasticity associated with movement of speech to the right hemisphere, and removal of the seizure focus is required to regain speech. Lippe et al. also recently reported that young children who underwent parieto-occipital lobe resection for intractable epilepsy due to cortical dysplasia had improved verbal and neuropsychological outcome when evaluated 3–7 years later [Lippe et al., 2010]. Roulet-Perez et al. also reported on cognitive functioning in a group of young children who had early surgery for severe intractable epilepsy, and found that cessation of epileptic activity can be associated with substantial cognitive gains, although not in all children [Roulet-Perez et al., 2010].

Plasticity in Older Children and Adults

Although children appear to have a greater degree of brain plasticity than adults, there is also evidence that the adult brain undergoes structural changes in response to experience and motor practice. For example, an MRI study of licensed taxi drivers in London found that their posterior hippocampi were larger than those in control subjects who did not drive taxis, and enlargement in the right, but not the left, hippocampus was directly related to their time as a taxi driver [Maguire et al., 2000]. The posterior hippocampus is an area that is associated with spatial representation of the environment, and this study suggests that a "mental map" of the city is stored there. Another study of young adults used voxel-based morphometry to examine their brains before and after they received instruction in learning to juggle for the first time [Draganski et al., 2004]. This study found an increase in parietal-occipital cortical gray matter assigned to visual motor processing after 3 months of practice compared with before practice. These changes persisted for several weeks after practice ended. Similar studies have revealed increases in gray matter in the auditory and visual-spatial cortex in professional musicians compared to non-musicians, increases in parietal lobe cortex in professional mathematicians, and thickening in the cortex of medical students studying for examinations [Draganski et al., 2006; Aydin et al., 2007].

Facilitating Adaptive Plasticity with Therapy Programs

Anecdotal and scientific evidence for plasticity in the nervous system has led to attempts to harness it to improve recovery from a variety of brain and spinal cord injuries and other disorders. One approach is generally referred to as constraint-based therapy or constraint-induced movement therapy (CIMT), used for patients with hemiparesis [Gauthier et al., 2008]. Another approach used for patients with spinal cord injury uses programmed, multi-electrode, direct stimulation of muscles above and below the level of injury in paralyzed individuals with spinal cord injury [Sadowsky and McDonald, 2009]. This type of stimulation simulates walking in order to improve muscle tone and cardiovascular function, as well as to enhance remyelination and neural stem-cell production at the site of partial spinal cord injury.

CIMT was developed for patients with hemiparesis for unilateral lesions such as stroke, and is based on the theory that using the good arm impairs movement of the hemiparetic side. Accordingly, the theory suggests that the good side should be constrained while movement of the hemiparetic arm is encouraged. In CIMT sessions, the less impaired hand is restrained using a mitt over the hand or a cast covering the arm and hand,

and a therapist directs repetitive movement of the hemiparetic side, along with behavioral shaping to encourage real-world use. EXCITE (Effect of Constraint-Induced Movement Therapy on Upper Extremity Function) was one of the first randomized controlled trials of this type of therapy, and it evaluated adults who had strokes more than 6–9 months prior to intervention [Park et al., 2008]. This trial demonstrated clinically relevant improvement in arm movement that lasted for more than a year. Subsequent trials in adults with stroke have shown that a behavioral program to promote use of the arm in real-world activities is important for a beneficial effect. Similar studies in rodents suggested that a behavioral program was important for changing the tonotopic map for sound, and this could be substituted by stimulation of the nucleus basalis that projects to the cortex [Buonomano and Merzenich, 1998].

MRI studies using voxel-based morphometry have shown that CIMT with a behavioral intervention produced bilateral gray matter increases in sensory and motor areas, as well as in the hippocampus [Gauthier et al., 2008]. In contrast to this study of CIMT, rehabilitation trials using bilateral arm movement while walking on a treadmill with auditory cueing did not improve arm use in adults with stroke, although it benefited their walking and cardiovascular fitness [Luft et al., 2004, 2008]. CIMT is also being applied to children with cerebral palsy with hemiparesis and has had some success [Cope et al., 2010; Eliasson et al., 2005]. One of the determinants of efficacy of CIMT in children with hemiplegia appears to be whether or not there is persistence of an ipsilateral corticospinal tract. Ipsilateral corticospinal tracts are normally present in the fetus and newborn, along with crossed corticospinal tracts, but then regress in infancy. Eyre et al. used TMS to study the development of the corticospinal tracts in infants who had unilateral or bilateral cerebral injuries in the neonatal period, and found that those with strong persistence of an ipsilateral CST had worse motor outcomes than those in which the ipsilateral tract regressed and the contralateral tract persisted [Eyre et al., 2007; Eyre, 2007]. Kuhnke et al. studied children with congenital hemiparesis and found that those with a single functional contralateral corticospinal tract responded better to CIMT than those with a persistent ipsilateral tract. Walther et al. recently reported a group of children with hemiparesis due to perinatal stroke, whose hand movements improved after CIMT [Walther et al., 2009]. TMS stimulation of the hemisphere contralateral to the hemiparetic limb in this group produced a stronger motor-evoked amplitude in the hemiparetic hand after CIMT treatment, suggesting increased synaptic excitability in the corticospinal tract pathway [Kuhnke et al., 2008]. These data suggest that CIMT is able to enhance plasticity and functional improvement in children with hemiparetic cerebral palsy, especially those who have an intact contralateral CST without input from a persistent ipsilateral CST.

Brain Stimulation and Adaptive Plasticity

As already discussed, brain plasticity is an activity-dependent process in which neurons that receive greater stimulation from the primary senses or other parts of the brain build larger, stronger network connections, but neurons deprived of activity lose their connections [Fregni and Pascual-Leone, 2007]. A relatively new form of therapy based on neural plasticity theory is referred to as electrical brain stimulation, and uses the techniques of TMS and transcranial direct current stimulation (tDCS) to control neuronal excitability in the brain [Fregni and Pascual-Leone, 2007]. TMS refers to the pulsatile magnetic stimulation delivered through the scalp and skull by an electromagnetic coil specially constructed for this purpose. The TMS coil is held over the scalp and generates an electrical current within the cortex that flows in the opposite direction to the current in the coil. The TMS pulse frequency can be controlled and pulse sequences have been discovered empirically that can be either inhibitory or excitatory for the cortex. This technique has been found generally to be safe in children and adults. One theory for the mechanism of impairment in patients with a hemiparesis after a stroke is that reduced function of the damaged hemisphere results in part from excessive neuronal inhibition from the opposite undamaged hemisphere. This is supported by reports that delivering inhibitory TMS sequences to the good hemisphere can improve function controlled by the opposite injured hemisphere. Excitatory TMS sequences delivered to the injured hemisphere, combined with paired retrograde stimulation of the same hemisphere via the contralateral median nerve, have also been found to produce functional improvement in patients with hemiparesis [Celnik et al., 2007]. The technique of tDCS uses a device that provides a constant level of direct current through the skull and brain, and has been shown to enhance neuronal plasticity in a variety of paradigms, including motor, language, and memory performance, as well as in the ability to form and retain motor memories [Galea and Celnik, 2009; Fregni and Pascual-Leone, 2007]. Experiments in mice show that tDCS depends on activity-dependent secretion of BDNF and augmentation of synaptic plasticity associated with TrκB receptor activation [Fritsch et al., 2010]. These electrical techniques appear to hold promise for improving outcome in children and adults with brain injury by enhancing brain plasticity.

Impaired Plasticity due to Genetic or Acquired Disorders

Many genetic and acquired disorders disrupt plasticity processes in the brain, leading to impaired learning, memory, behavior, and motor function, as well as brain and somatic growth abnormalities. Table 13-1 lists some prominent examples of disorders in which plasticity mechanisms are targeted. Neurofibromatosis 1 (NF-1) is a dominantly inherited disorder that is one of the most common single-gene abnormalities and is known for its café au lait skin lesions, plexiform neuromas, optic gliomas, skeletal manifestations, and learning problems. It is caused by mutations in neurofibromin, an oncogene and GTPase activating protein (GAP) that regulates the activity of Ras, a G-protein that mediates membrane receptor-mediated activation of MAPK signaling (see Figure 13-4). The Ras-MAPK signaling cascade normally leads to learning and memory formation and cellular growth, but excessive upregulation can lead to tumor formation and impaired cognition. At the synaptic level, mice with neurofibromin mutations show memory loss on water maze testing, and impaired LTP that is related to hyperactivity of inhibitory GABAergic interneurons [Staley and Anderson, 2009]. Cui et al. showed that GABAergic neurons in these animals released excessive GABA from inhibitory synapses due to

phosphorylation of synapsin 1, a protein that regulates neurotransmitter release [Cui et al., 2008]. Administration of low concentrations of a GABA antagonist has been shown to improve their memory problems and impaired LTP [Costa et al., 2002]. Lovastatin, an approved drug used to treat high cholesterol in adults, has also been shown to improve cognitive function by reducing elevated Ras-MAPK activity, and it is being studied as a treatment for cognitive and other manifestations of NF1 [Li et al., 2005].

Tuberous sclerosis (TSC) shares some features of NF-1, in that it is also an autosomal-dominant neurocutaneous disorder that results from overactivity in a signaling pathway that links extracellular signals, such as glucose, glutamate, other amino acids, and insulin, with pathways that regulate intracellular protein synthesis, cell growth, proliferation, and survival [Crino, 2010; Costa et al., 2002]. Two-thirds of individuals with TSC harbor sporadic mutations in one of two tumor suppressor genes, hamartin (TSC1) or tuberin (TSC2). These mutations result in upregulation of the small GTPase Rheb and its downstream binding partner, mammalian target of rapamycin (mTOR), an enzyme that regulates cell growth and transcription. Upstream signals that act on TSC proteins come from the Ras-MAPK and the phosphoinositide-3-kinase pathways. TSC is associated with skin and eye manifestations, as well as epilepsy, intellectual disability, and autism in a high percentage of cases. Subependymal nodules and tubers are typically present in the brain, and tumors or hamartomas are often found in the lung, kidney, and heart. mTOR has been implicated in synaptic plasticity through experiments showing that its inhibitor rapamycin can inhibit LTP and LTD in snails, crayfish, and mice [Ehninger et al., 2009]. Mice with mutations in *Tsc1* and *Tsc2* have abnormalities in synaptic plasticity, as well as in dendritic aborization, axonal outgrowth, neuronal migration, and behavior [Ehninger et al., 2009; Shilyansky et al., 2010]. It is interesting that a model of TSC has also been produced with homozygous mutations in the *Tsc1* gene in glia only, and these mice have low expression of the glutamate-1 transporter [Zeng et al., 2007]. The hypothesis that mTOR controls synaptic plasticity in brain is also supported by recent data showing that upregulation of mTOR by the anesthetic ketamine increases spine density and synaptic activity associated with an antidepressant effect in rats [Li et al., 2010]. Rapamycin is a clinically approved drug for immunosuppression for organ transplantation, and has been used in clinical trials to reduce tumor size in patients with TSC [Wong, 2010].

Impaired Plasticity in Fragile X and Rett's Syndromes

Fragile X syndrome and Rett's syndrome are X-linked disorders that cause intellectual disability, autistic-like behaviors, and other neuropsychiatric abnormalities, as well as abnormalities in synapse structure and plasticity in the brain. As described earlier, FraX is caused by a reduction in the FMRP protein, which binds to RNAs in the synapse, leading to abnormalities in translation of proteins regulated by synaptic activity (see Figure 13-2) [Penagarikano et al., 2007]. In contrast, Rett's syndrome is due to mutations in the MeCP2 transcription factor, which regulates gene transcription in the nucleus [Amir et al., 1999]. The primary role of MeCP2 is to silence expression of certain genes, including the growth factor *BDNF*; *UBE3A*, the gene involved in Angelman's syndrome; and the homeobox gene *DLX5*, which stimulates development of GABAergic neurons in the brain (see Figure 13-4) [Zhou et al., 2006]. Upregulation of glucocorticoid-regulated genes has also been reported in a mouse model of Rett's syndrome. In resting neurons, MeCP2 acts like a brake for BDNF transcription, but when neurons are activated, calcium-mediated phosphorylation of MeCP2 leads to de-repression of BDNF transcription and increased protein [Nuber et al., 2005; Stornetta and Zhu, 2010]. Both FraX and Rett's syndrome are associated with abnormalities in dendritic spines and synapses and with synaptic plasticity [Cruz-Martin et al., 2010; Fukuda et al., 2005]. In FraX, there is an excess of dendritic spines that are abnormally long and slender, probably reflecting their relative immaturity secondary to diminished excitatory neurotransmission (see Figure 13-2) [Pfeiffer et al., 2010]. Huber et al. also reported that LTD is selectively enhanced in the FraX mouse [Huber et al., 2002]. Several experimental drugs that inhibit mGluR5 receptors, such as fenobam, or their downstream signaling pathways, such as lithium or minocycline, have been reported to promote spine maturation and improve behavior in animal models [Berry-Kravis et al., 2008, 2009; Bilousova et al., 2009]. Some functional benefits have also been reported for these drugs in early clinical studies in adults with FraX [Wang et al., 2010]. In Rett's syndrome, the immature brain contains an excess of glutamate receptors that decrease later in life, and synaptic contacts in mice with Rett's syndrome have been reported to be immature, with reduced cross-sectional length of PSDs [Fukuda et al., 2005; Johnston et al., 2005; Blue et al., 1999]. Levels of glutamate have also been reported to be elevated in girls with Rett's syndrome, consistent with the seizures and hyperkinetic behavior they show [Horska et al., 2009]. Studies in Rett mice also indicate that neurons develop to the point of beginning to make synaptic connections but then cannot stabilize them [Belichenko et al., 2008; Smrt et al., 2007; Palmer et al., 2008]. Learning and memory, as well as synaptic plasticity as measured by LTP and LTD, are diminished in the hippocampus in a mouse model of Rett's syndrome [Moretti et al., 2006; Asaka et al., 2006]. Both insulin like growth factor (IGF-1) and BDNF have been reported partially to rescue the phenotype of Rett's syndrome [Kline et al., 2010; Tropea et al., 2009] Therefore, these two disorders represent variations on the theme of X-linked plasticity disorders.

Similar disorders that involve cell signaling pathways involved in neuronal plasticity are listed in Table 13-1, and others are likely to be described in the future. In addition to lesions in intracellular signaling cascades or defects in transcription or translation, recent genome microarray studies of children with intellectual disability or autistic spectrum disorders have found deletions and other copy number variations that include genes for glutamate receptors and other synaptic proteins [Miller et al., 2010]. These include presynaptic proteins or those localized to the PSD and associated scaffolding proteins, including SHANK2, SHANK3, SHANK4, SYNGAP1, NLGN3, NLGN4X, NRXN1, or DLGAP2. The Autism Genome Project Consortium (AGP) found rare gene deletions in individuals with autism that are enriched in functional networks, including those for GTPase/Ras signaling, cell proliferation and motility, central nervous system development, and cytoskeleton organization [Pinto et al., 2010] These genes can often be linked to both autism and intellectual disability.

Summary and Conclusion

Central nervous system plasticity is an important concept in child neurology because it is responsible for many features that distinguish the child's brain from that of the adult, such as the ability to learn languages, play music, and learn new information. Plasticity also influences the presentation of nervous system diseases in children, and the outcome from serious injuries and illnesses. Four major types of plasticity can be distinguished, including adaptive plasticity, impaired plasticity, excessive or maladaptive plasticity, and plasticity as the "Achilles' heel." Several major mechanisms for plasticity have been identified, including overproduction and apoptosis of neurons, activity-dependent plasticity in synapses, production of growth factors, overproduction and pruning of synapses followed by activity-dependent stabilization of remaining synapses, and epigenetic regulation of DNA expression. Adaptive plasticity is strongly influenced by repetitive activity and practice, and these activities are accompanied by plastic changes in neuronal networks, as well as in white-matter tracts. Some of these changes, such as expansion of the cortical area assigned to the fingers of one hand after a long period of practicing a stringed instrument, can be monitored noninvasively in humans. Rehabilitation techniques, such as CIMT, have been shown to improve the use of the hemiparetic hand in children with hemiplegic cerebral palsy. Other techniques, such as TMS, are also being used experimentally to enhance activity-dependent plasticity. Genetic disorders, such as fragile X syndrome, Rett's syndrome, neurofibromatosis 1, and tuberous sclerosis, as well as environmental insults, such as lead, impair cognition and behavior by disrupting signaling pathways that are responsible for plasticity. Rare genetic copy number variations associated with chromosomal deletions in genes connected with these signaling pathways have also been found in children with autistic spectrum disorders. Disorders of plasticity and mechanisms for enhancing plasticity are becoming increasingly important in pediatric neurology.

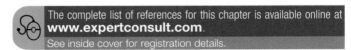
The complete list of references for this chapter is available online at **www.expertconsult.com**. See inside cover for registration details.

Neurodegeneration in the Neonatal Brain

Frances J. Northington and Lee J. Martin

Introduction

Underlying mechanisms of neuronal cell death are common to both immature and mature brains; however, important developmental differences in propinquity to cell cycle, metabolic requirements, connectivity, basal and stimulated expression of cell death proteins, excitatory receptor expression and subunit composition, antioxidant mechanisms, synaptic density, and neurotrophin requirement account for significant differences in injury response between the immature and mature central nervous system (CNS) [Corbett et al., 1993; Martin, 2001, 2002; Ferriero, 2004; Johnston, 2005, 2009; Northington et al., 2005; Zhu et al., 2005; Kostovic and Jovanov-Milosevic, 2006]. In this chapter, we will review information obtained on basic cell death processes from both mature and immature model systems, but highlight findings from studies on the response of the immature brain to injury. While clearly important to this topic, a discussion of the contribution of inflammation to injury, recovery, and developmental neuroplasticity following neonatal brain injury is outside the scope of this chapter. A recent review of this topic is available elsewhere [Vexler and Yenari, 2009] and in Chapter 15.

Types of Cell Death

Cells can die by different processes. These processes have been classified generally into two distinct categories, called necrosis and apoptosis. These forms of cellular degeneration were classified originally as different because they appeared different morphologically under a microscope (Figure 14-1). Necrosis is a lytic destruction of individual cells or groups of cells, while apoptosis (derived from a Greek word for "dropping of leaves from trees") is an orderly and compartmental dismantling of single cells or groups of cells into consumable components for nearby cells. Apoptosis is an example of programmed cell death (PCD) that is an adenosine triphosphate (ATP)-driven (sometimes gene transcription-requiring) form of cell suicide often committed by demolition enzymes called caspases, but other apoptotic and nonapoptotic, caspase-independent forms of PCD exist [Lockshin and Zakeri, 2002]. Apoptotic PCD is instrumental in developmental organogenesis and histogenesis and adult tissue homeostasis, functioning to eliminate excess cells. Each day in normal humans, estimates reveal that between 50 to 70 billion cells in adults and 20 to 30 billion cells in a child between the ages of 8 and 14 die due to apoptosis [Gilbert, 2006]. Another form of cell degeneration seen first with yeast and then in metazoans has been called autophagy [Klionsky and Emr, 2000]. Autophagy is an intracellular catabolic process that occurs by lysosomal degradation of damaged or expendable organelles. Necrosis and apoptosis both differ morphologically (see Figure 14-1) and mechanistically from autophagy [Klionsky and Emr, 2000; Lockshin and Zakeri, 2002].

More recently, the morphological and molecular regulatory distinctions between the different forms of cell death have become blurred and uncertain due to observations made on degenerating neurons in vivo and to a new concept that attempts to accommodate these observations. This concept, in its original form, posits that cell death exists as a continuum with necrosis and apoptosis at opposite ends of a spectrum, with hybrid forms of degeneration manifesting in between (see Figure 14-1) [Portera-Cailliau, et al., 1997a, b; Martin et al., 1998; Martin, 1999]. For example, the degeneration of neurons in diseased or damaged human and animal nervous systems is not always strictly necrosis or apoptosis, according to the traditional binary classification of cell death, but also occurs as intermediate or hybrid forms with coexisting morphological and biochemical characteristics that lie in a structural continuum, with necrosis and apoptosis at the two extremes [Portera-Cailliau et al., 1997a, b]. Thus, neuronal cell death can be syncretic. The different processes leading to the putative different forms of cell death can be activated concurrently with graded contributions of the different cell death modes to the degenerative process.

The in vivo reality of a neuronal cell death continuum was revealed first in neonatal and adult rat models of glutamate receptor excitotoxicity [Portera-Cailliau et al., 1997a, b] and then very nicely in rodent models of neonatal hypoxic-ischemic encephalopathy (HIE) [Nakajima et al., 2000; Northington et al., 2001b, 2007]. The hybrid cells can be distinguished cytopathologically by the progressive compaction of the nuclear chromatin into few, discrete, large, irregularly shaped clumps (see Figure 14-1). This morphology contrasts with the formation of few, uniformly shaped, dense, round masses in classic apoptosis and the formation of numerous, smaller, irregularly shaped chromatin clumps in classic necrosis. The cytoplasmic organelle pathology in hybrid cells has a basic pattern that appears more similar to necrosis than apoptosis, but is lower

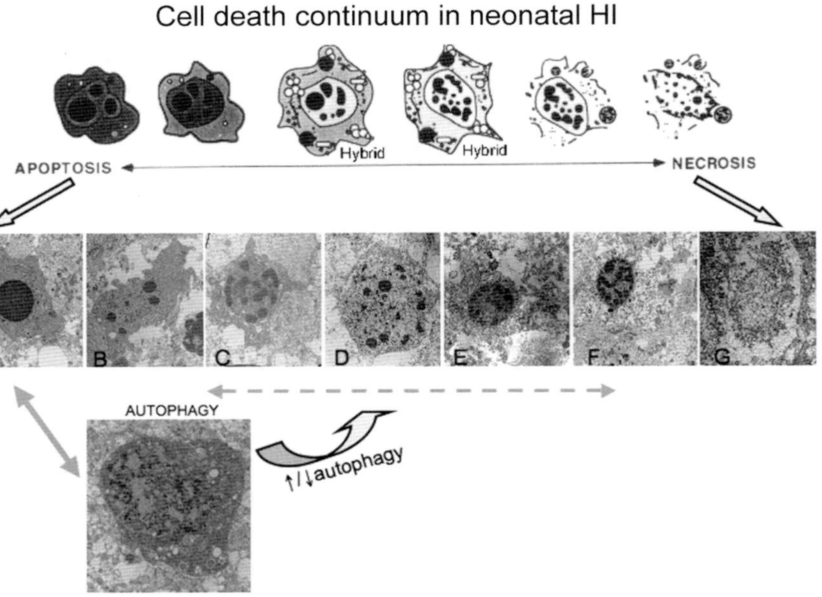

Cell death continuum in neonatal HI

Fig. 14-1 Cell death continuum. After its initial description by Portera-Cailliau et al., the continuum concept, in its original form, organized cell death as a linear spectrum with apoptosis and necrosis at the extremes and different syncretic hybrid forms in between (top) [Martin et al., 1998]. Subsequently we have found that this concept is fully realized in the neonatal rat brain following hypoxia-ischemia (HI), with clearly apoptotic **(A)** and necrotic **(G)** cells found intermixed with the hybrid forms **(B–F)**. Cells at the extremes have the well-described structures of necrosis (**G** – swelling and vacuolation of organelles, loss of cell membrane integrity, maintenance of nuclear membrane integrity, random digestion of chromatin) and apoptosis (**A** – condensation and darkening of cytoplasm within intact cell membrane, intact organelles until late phases of apoptosis, compaction of chromatin into few uniformly dense and rounded aggregates and loss of nuclear membrane). Cells with irregular chromatin condensation, organized in a "clockface" pattern around an intact nuclear membrane **(E, F),** may or may not have preservation of the cytoplasmic membrane, and their cytoplasmic organelles are disrupted. This structure has commonly been reported in models of excitotoxicity. Increasing organization of chromatin into regular crescenteric or rounded aggregates, dissolution of the nuclear membrane, and preservation of the cytoplasmic membrane, with or without swelling of cytoplasmic organelles **(B–D),** is the rule as cell death forms more closely mimic apoptosis. Autophagocytic neurons with large numbers of cytoplasmic vacuoles, partially condensed nuclear chromatin, and preservation of cellular integrity are found after neonatal HI (H). Autophagocytic cell death and apoptosis exist on a continuum. Drugs known to inhibit or promote autophagy can also modulate cell death along the apoptosis–necrosis continuum.

in amplitude than in necrosis (e.g., mitochondrial swelling). Toxicological studies of cultured cells have shown that stimulus intensity influences the mode of cell death [Lennon et al., 1991; Fernandes and Cotter, 1994; Bonfoco et al., 1995], such that apoptosis can be induced by injurious stimuli of lesser amplitude than insults causing necrosis [Raffray and Cohen, 1997], but the cell death modes were still considered distinct [Bonfoco et al., 1995].

Basic research is uncloaking the molecular mechanisms of cell death [Orrenius et al., 2003; Yuan et al., 2003], and, with this, the distinctiveness of different cell death processes, as well as the potential overlap among different cell death mechanisms. Experimental studies on cell death mechanisms, and particularly the cell death continuum, are important because they could lead to the rational development of molecular mechanism-based therapies for treating neonatal hypoxic-ischemic encephalopathy (HIE). The different categories of cell death are discussed below.

Necrosis

Cell death caused by cytoplasmic swelling, nuclear dissolution (karyolysis), and lysis has been classified traditionally as necrosis [Trump and Berezesky, 1996]. Cell necrosis (sometimes termed oncosis) [Majno and Joris, 1995], results from rapid

and severe failure to sustain cellular homeostasis, notably cell volume control [Trump et al., 1965]. The process of necrosis involves damage to the structural and functional integrity of the cell plasma membrane and associated enzymes, e.g., Na^+, K^+ ATPase, abrupt influx and overload of ions (e.g., Na^+ and Ca^{2+}) and H_2O, and rapid mitochondrial damage and energetic collapse [Bonfoco et al., 1995; Leist et al., 1997; Martin et al., 2000; Golden et al., 2001]. Metabolic inhibition and oxidative stress from reactive oxygen species (ROS) are major culprits in triggering necrosis. Inhibitory crosstalk between ion pumps causes pronecrotic effects when Na^+, K^+ ATPase "steals" ATP from the plasma membrane Ca^{2+} ATPase, resulting in Ca^{2+} overload [Castro et al., 2006].

The morphology and some biochemical features of classic necrosis in neurons are distinct (see Figure 14-1). The main features are swelling and vacuolation/vesiculation of organelles, destruction of membrane integrity, random digestion of chromatin due to activation of proteases and deoxyribonucleases (DNases), and dissolution of the cell. The overall profile of the moribund cell is maintained generally as it dissolves into the surrounding tissue parenchyma and induces an inflammatory reaction in vivo. In necrosis, dying cells do not bud to form discrete, membrane-bound fragments. The nuclear pyknosis and karyolysis appear as condensation of chromatin into many irregularly shaped, small clumps, sharply contrasting with the formation of few, uniformly dense and regularly shaped chromatin aggregates that occurs in apoptosis. In cells undergoing necrosis, genomic DNA is digested globally because protease that digest histone proteins that protect DNA, and DNases are coactivated to generate many randomly sized fragments seen as a DNA "smear." These differences in the cytoplasmic changes and condensation and digestion of nuclear chromatin in pure apoptosis and pure necrosis are very diagnostic.

Recent work has shown that cell necrosis might not be as chaotic or random as envisioned originally, but can involve the activation of specific signaling pathways to eventuate in cell death [Proskuryakov et al., 2003]. For example, DNA damage can lead to poly(ADP-ribose) polymerase activation and ATP depletion, energetic failure, and necrosis [Ha and Snyder, 2000]. Other pathways for "programmed" necrosis involve death receptor signaling through receptor interacting protein 1 (RIP1) kinase and mitochondrial permeability transition (Figure 14-2) [Crompton, 1999; Festjens et al., 2006; Hitomi et al., 2008].

Mitochondrial Ca^{2+} overload, excessive oxidative stress, and decreases in the electrochemical gradient, ADP and ATP, can favor mitochondrial permeability transition, which is defined by disruption of the proton-motive force [Crompton et al., 1998; Crompton, 1999; van Gurp et al., 2003]. This disruption involves the so-called mitochondrial permeability transition pore (mPTP), which functions as a voltage, thiol, and Ca^{2+} sensor. The mPTP is a large polyprotein transmembrane channel formed at contact sites between the inner mitochondrial membrane and the outer mitochondrial membrane

(Figure 14-3). The complete components of the mPTP are still controversial. The primary components of the mPTP are the voltage-dependent anion channel (VDAC; also called porin) in the outer mitochondrial membrane and the adenine nucleotide translocator (ANT) in the inner mitochondrial membrane [Crompton et al., 1998]. The VDAC makes the inner mitochondrial membrane permeable to most small hydrophilic molecules <5 kDa for free exchange of respiratory chain substrates. The ANT mediates the exchange of ADP for ATP. During normal mitochondrial function the intermembrane space separates the outer and inner mitochondrial membranes and the VDAC and the ANT do not interact, or interact only transiently in a state described as "flicker" [Crompton et al., 1998]. When the mPTP is in the open state, it permits influx of solutes of ≤1500 Da and H_2O into the matrix, resulting in depolarization of mitochondria and dissipated proton electrochemical gradient. Consequently, the inner mitochondrial membrane loses its integrity and oxidative phosphorylation is uncoupled. When this occurs, oxidation of metabolites by O_2 proceeds with electron flux not coupled to proton pumping, resulting in further dissipation of transmembrane proton gradient and ATP production, production of ROS, and large-amplitude mitochondrial swelling triggering necrosis or apoptosis [van Gurp et al., 2003]. Several proteins regulate the mPTP. Cyclophilin D is one of these proteins found in the mitochondrial matrix and it interacts reversibly with the ANT. Inactivation of cyclophilin D can block mitochondrial swelling and cellular necrosis induced by Ca^{2+} overload and ROS in the adult [Baines et al.,

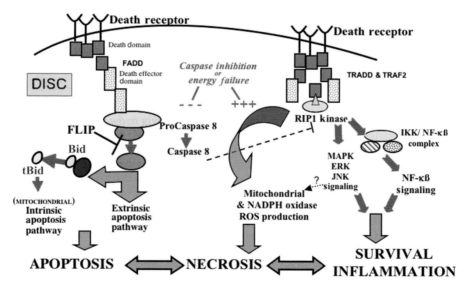

Fig. 14-2 Death receptor signaling. This diagram summarizes the pleiotropic outcomes possible following death receptor activation and the signaling pathways leading to these outcomes. Ligand binding to and trimerization of death domain containing members of the tumor necrosis factor receptor superfamily recruits Fas-associated death domain (FADD), a death effector domain containing adaptor protein and caspase 8, thus forming the "death-induced signaling complex" (DISC). Signaling for apoptosis then proceeds via the extrinsic or intrinsic pathway. In the extrinsic pathway, active caspase 8 directly cleaves caspase 3. Activation of the mitochondrial or intrinsic pathway proceeds via caspase 8-mediated cleavage of cytosolic Bid. The truncated form of BID then translocates to mitochondria, thereby functioning as a BH3-only transducer of the death receptor signal at the cell plasma membrane to mitochondria. Simultaneously, cleaved caspase 8 may inactivate death receptor signaling via receptor interacting protein 1 (RIP1) kinase, by cleaving and inactivating it. In the setting of caspase inhibition or energy failure, death receptor signaling may preferentially proceed via RIP1 kinase, a death domain containing protein, which binds the death receptor signaling complex containing the adaptor proteins TRADD and TRAF2. Signaling via RIP1 kinase, death receptor-mediated cell death occurs with reactive oxygen species (ROS) production and a cell death morphology resembling necrosis. Both mitochondrial and nicotinamide adenine dinucleotide phosphate (NADPH) oxidase may be the source of enhanced free radical production in this signaling paradigm. Through its kinase domain, RIP1 kinase can activate downstream kinase pathways, which may also contribute to ROS production and cleave the IKK subunit from the NF-κβ complex and initiate NF-κβ proinflammatory/prosurvival signaling.

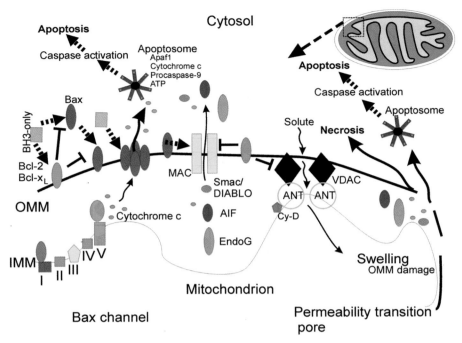

Fig. 14-3 Mitochondrial dysfunction and regulation of neuronal cell death after neonatal HI. Mitochondria (upper right) are multifunctional organelles, as illustrated. Oxygen is necessary to drive ATP production by the electron transport chain (lower left). Bcl-2 family members regulate apoptosis by modulating the release of cytochrome c from mitochondria into the cytosol. In the Bax channel model (left), Bax is a pro-apoptotic protein found in the cytosol that translocates to the outer mitochondrial membrane (OMM). Bax monomers physically interact and form tetrameric channels that are permeable to cytochrome c. The formation of these channels is blocked by Bcl-2 and Bcl-x_L at multiple sites. BH3-only members (Bad, Bid, Noxa, Puma) are pro-apoptotic and can modulate the conformation of Bax to sensitize this channel, possibly by exposing its membrane insertion domain, or by inactivating Bcl-2 and Bcl-x_L. The mitochondria apoptosis-induced channel (MAC) may be a channel similar to the Bax channel but possibly having additional components. Released cytochrome c participates in the formation of the apoptosome in the cytosol that drives the activation of caspase-3, leading to apoptosis. Second mitochondrial activator of caspases (Smac)/direct IAP-binding protein with low pI (DIABLO) are released to inactivate the anti-apoptotic actions of inhibitor of apoptosis proteins that inhibit caspases. Apoptosis inducing factor (AIF) and EndoG are released and translocate to the nucleus to stimulate DNA fragmentation. Another model for cell death involves the permeability transition pore (PTP). The PTP is a transmembrane channel formed by the interaction of the adenine nucleotide translocator (ANT) and the voltage-dependent anion channel (VDAC) at contact sites between the inner mitochondrial membrane (IMM) and the OMM, and is modulated by cyclophilin D (cy-D). Opening of the PTP induces matrix swelling and OMM rupture, leading to release of apoptogenic proteins (cytochrome c, AIF, EndoG) or to cellular necrosis. *(Adapted from Martin LJ. The mitochondrial permeability transition pore: a molecular target for amyotrophic lateral sclerosis therapy. Biochim Biophys Acta 2009.)*

2005; Nakagawa et al., 2005] but cyclophilin D appears to have prosurvival functions in the hypoxia-ischemia (HI)-injured immature brain [Wang et al., 2009]. Another protein that causes mPTP opening is BNIP3, which can integrate into the outer mitochondrial membrane and can trigger necrosis [Vande Velde et al., 2000].

Further comments on programmed necrosis, its regulation through death receptors and RIP1 kinase, and its possible contribution to experimental neonatal HI brain injury follow later in this chapter.

Apoptosis

Apoptosis is a form of PCD because it is carried out by active, intrinsic transcription-dependent [Tata, 1966] or transcription-independent mechanisms involving specific molecules. Apoptosis should not be used as a synonym for PCD because nonapoptotic forms of PCD exist [Schwartz et al., 1993; Amin et al., 2000]. Apoptosis is only one example of PCD. It is critical for the normal growth and differentiation of organ systems in vertebrates and invertebrates [see Jacobson, 1991, regarding Ernst's discovery of developmental PCD; Glucksmann, 1951; Lockshin and Williams, 1964; Saunders, 1966]. The structure of apoptosis

is similar to the type I form of PCD described by Clarke [Clarke, 1990]. In physiological settings in adult tissues, apoptosis is a normal process, occurring continuously in populations of cells that undergo slow proliferation (e.g., liver and adrenal gland) or rapid proliferation (e.g., epithelium of intestinal crypts) [Wyllie et al., 1980; Bursch et al., 1990]. Apoptosis is a normal event in the immune system when lymphocyte clones are deleted after an immune response [Nagata, 1999]. Kerr and colleagues were the first to describe apoptosis in pathological settings [Kerr et al., 1972], but many descriptions were made prior to this time in studies of developing animal systems [Lockshin and Zakeri, 2001].

Classical apoptosis has a distinctive structural appearance (see Figure 14-1). The cell condenses and is dismantled in an organized way into small packages that can be consumed by nearby cells. Nuclear breakdown is orderly. The DNA is digested in a specific pattern of internucleosomal fragments (see Figure 14-1), and the chromatin is packaged into sharply delineated, uniformly dense masses that appear as crescents abutting the nuclear envelope or as smooth, round masses within the nucleus (see Figure 14-1). The execution of apoptosis is linked to Ca^{2+}-activated DNases [Wyllie, 1980], one being DNA fragmentation factor 45 (DFF45) [Liu et al., 1997], which digests genomic DNA at internucleosomal sites only (because proteases that digest histone proteins remain inactivated and the DNA at these sites is protected from DNases) to generate a DNA "ladder" (see Figure 14-1). However, the emergence of the apoptotic nuclear morphology can be independent of the degradation of chromosomal DNA [Sakahira et al., 1999]. Cytoplasmic breakdown is also orderly. The cytoplasm condenses, (as reflected by a darkening of the cell in electron micrographs, see Figure 14-1), and subsequently the cell shrinks in size, while the plasma membrane remains intact. During the course of these events, it is believed that the mitochondria are required for ATP-dependent processes. Subsequently, the nuclear and plasma membranes become convoluted, and then the cell undergoes a process called budding. In this process, the nucleus, containing smooth, uniform masses of condensed chromatin, undergoes fragmentation in association with the condensed cytoplasm, forming cellular debris (called apoptotic bodies) composed of pieces of nucleus surrounded by cytoplasm with closely packed and apparently intact organelles. Apoptotic cells display surface markers (e.g., phosphatidylserine or sugars) for recognition by phagocytic cells. Phagocytosis of cellular debris by adjacent cells is the final phase of apoptosis in vivo.

Variants of classical or nonclassical apoptosis can occur during nervous system development [Pilar and Landmesser, 1976; Clarke, 1990] and also frequently in pathophysiological settings of nervous system injury and disease [Portera-Cailliau et al., 1997a, b; Martin et al., 1998]. Axonal damage (axotomy) and target deprivation in the mature nervous system can induce apoptosis in neurons that is similar structurally, but not identical, to developmental PCD [Martin et al., 1998]. Excitotoxins can induce readily and robustly nonclassical forms of apoptosis in neurons [Portera-Cailliau et al., 1997a, b]. Types of cell death similar to those seen with excitotoxicity occur frequently in pathological cell death resulting from neonatal HI [Martin et al., 2000; Nakajima et al., 2000; Northington et al., 2001b, 2007].

Cells can die by PCD through mechanisms that are distinct from apoptosis [Jacobson, 1991; Schwartz et al., 1993]. The structure of nonapoptotic PCD is similar to the type II or type III forms of cell death described by Clarke [Clarke, 1990]. Interestingly, there is no internucleosomal fragmentation of genomic DNA in some forms of nonapoptotic PCD [Schwartz et al., 1993; Amin et al., 2000].

Autophagy

Autophagy is a mechanism whereby eukaryotic cells degrade their own cytoplasm and organelles [Klionsky and Emr, 2000]. The degradation of organelles and long-lived proteins is carried out by the lysosomal system. Although autophagy functions as a cell death mechanism, it is primarily a homeostatic nonlethal stress response mechanism for recycling proteins to protect cells from low supplies of nutrients. Autophagy is classified as type II PCD [Clarke, 1990]. A hallmark of autophagic cell death is accumulation of autophagic vacuoles of lysosomal origin. Autophagy has been seen in developmental and pathological conditions. For example, insect metamorphosis involves autophagy [Lockshin and Zakeri, 1994], and developing neurons can use autophagy as a PCD mechanism [Schweichel and Merker, 1973; Xue et al., 1999]. Degeneration of Purkinje neurons in the mouse mutant *Lucher* appears to be a form of autophagy, thus possibly linking excitotoxic and autophagic cell

deaths to constitutive activation of the GluRδ2 glutamate receptor [Yue et al., 2002].

The molecular controls of autophagy appear common in eukaryotic cells from yeast to human, and it is believed that autophagy evolved before apoptosis [Yuan et al., 2003]. However, most of the work has been done on yeast, with detailed work on mammalian cells only beginning [Mizushima et al., 2002]. Double-membrane autophagosomes for sequestration of cytoplasmic components are derived from the endoplasmic reticulum (ER) or the plasma membrane. Tor kinase, phosphatidylinositol 3 (PI3) kinase, a family of cysteine proteases called autophagins, and death-associated proteins function in autophagy [Bursch, 2001; Inbal et al., 2002]. Autophagic and apoptotic cell death pathways crosstalk. The product of the tumor suppressor gene *Beclin1* (the human homolog of the yeast autophagy gene *APG6*) interacts with the anti-apoptosis regulator Bcl-2 [Liang et al., 1998]. Autophagy can block apoptosis by sequestration of mitochondria. If the capacity for autophagy is reduced, stressed cells die by apoptosis, whereas inhibition or blockade of molecules that function in apoptosis can convert the cell death process into autophagy [Ogier-Denis and Codogno, 2003]. Thus, a mechanistic continuum between autophagy and apoptosis exists (see Figure 14-1).

Autophagy appears to have a significant role in neurodegeneration after neonatal HI that may be insult severity-, time-, and region-specific [Lockshin and Zakeri, 1994; Koike et al., 2008; Ginet, et al., 2009]. Genetic deletion of the *atg7* gene results in near-complete protection from HI in adult mice [Koike et al., 2008], and pharmacologic inhibition of autophagy with 3-methyladenine up to 4 hours after focal ischemia is neuroprotective in p12 rats [Puyal et al., 2009]. Conversely, induction of autophagy immediately following neonatal global HI in mice appeared to be an endogenous neuroprotective mechanism in other studies [Carloni et al., 2008]. Pre-insult blockade of autophagy with methyladenine inhibited expression of autophagocytic proteins and switched cell death from apoptotic to necrotic; conversely, enhancing early autophagy with pre-insult administration of rapamycin provided neuroprotection in this model [Carloni et al., 2008]. Interestingly, known neuroprotective preconditioning strategies also increased markers of autophagy [Carloni et al., 2008] while providing the expected neuroprotection. Regional differences in induction of autophagocytic proteins, severity of insult, and timing of drug administration might account for these discrepant results.

Molecular and Cellular Regulation of Apoptosis

Apoptosis is a structurally and biochemically organized form of cell death. The basic machinery of apoptosis is conserved in yeast, hydra, nematode, fruitfly, zebrafish, mouse, and human [Ameisen, 2002]. Our current understanding of the molecular mechanisms of apoptosis in mammalian cells is built on studies by Robert Horvitz and colleagues on PCD in the nematode *Caenorhabditis elegans* [Metzstein et al., 1998]. They pioneered the understanding of the genetic control of developmental cell death by showing that this death is regulated predominantly by three genes (*ced-3*, *ced-4*, and *ced-9*) [Metzstein et al., 1998]. Several families of apoptosis-regulation genes have been identified in mammals, including the Bcl-2 family [Metzstein et al., 1998; Cory and Adams, 2002], the caspase family of cysteine-containing, aspartate-specific proteases [Wolf and Green, 1999], the p53 gene family [Levrero et al., 2000], cell surface death receptors [Nagata, 1999], and other apoptogenic factors, including cytochrome c, apoptosis inducing factor (AIF), and second mitochondrial activator of caspases (Smac) [Liu et al., 1996; Li et al., 1997; Hegde et al., 2002; Klein et al., 2002; Lockshin and Zakeri, 2002]. Moreover, a family of inhibitors of apoptosis proteins (IAPs) actively blocks cell death, and IAPs are inhibited mitochondrial proteases [Hegde et al., 2002]. Specific organelles have been identified as critical for the apoptotic process, including mitochondria and the ER (see Figure 14-3). In seminal work by Li, Wang, and colleagues, it was discovered that the mitochondrion integrates death signals mediated by proteins in the Bcl-2 family and releases molecules residing in the mitochondrial intermembrane space, such as cytochrome c, which complexes with cytoplasmic proteins (e.g., apoptotic protease activating factor-1 [Apaf-1]) to activate caspase proteases, leading to internucleosomal cleavage of DNA [Liu et al., 1996; Li et al., 1997]. The finding that cytochrome c has a function in apoptosis, in addition to its better-known role in oxidative phosphorylation, was astounding, although foreshadowing clues were available. The release of cytochrome c from mitochondria to the cytosol with concomitant reduced oxidative phosphorylation was described as the "cytochrome c effect" in irradiated cancer cells [van Bekkum, 1957]. The ER, which regulates intracellular Ca^{2+} levels, participates in a loop with mitochondria to modulate mitochondrial permeability transition and cytochrome c release through the actions of Bcl-2 protein family members [Scorrano et al., 2003].

Bcl-2 Family of Survival and Death Proteins

The *bcl-2* proto-oncogene family is a large group of apoptosis regulatory genes encoding about 25 different proteins, defined by at least one conserved B-cell lymphoma (Bcl) homology domain (BH1–BH4 can be present) in their amino acid sequence that functions in protein–protein interactions [Metzstein et al., 1998; Cory and Adams, 2002]. Some of the protein products of these genes (e.g., Bcl-2, Bcl-x_L, and Mcl-1) have all four BH1–BH4 domains and are anti-apoptotic. Other gene products, which are pro-apoptotic, are multidomain proteins possessing BH1–BH3 sequences (e.g., Bax and Bak), or proteins with only the BH3 domain (e.g., Bad, Bid, Bim, Bik, Noxa, and Puma) that contains the critical death domain. Bcl-x_L and Bax have α-helices resembling the pore-forming subunit of diphtheria toxin [Muchmore et al., 1996]; thus, Bcl-2 family members appear to function by conformation-induced insertion into the outer mitochondrial membrane to form channels or pores that can regulate the release of apoptogenic factors (see Figure 14-3).

The expression of many of these proteins is regulated developmentally, and the proteins have differential tissue distributions and subcellular localizations. Most of these proteins are found in the CNS, but the relative quantities of pro- and anti-apoptotic family members change over time [Li et al., 1997; Shimohama et al., 1998]. It appears that in mouse brain, the relative abundance of the pro-apoptosis Bcl-2 family members declines markedly after the perinatal period, while the anti-apoptotic Bcl-2 family members exhibit stable expression over time in the brain [Shimohama et al., 1998]. The subcellular distributions of Bax, Bak, and Bad in healthy adult rodent CNS tissue [Martin et al., 2003] are consistent

with in vitro studies of non-neuronal cells [Wolter et al., 1997; Nechushtan et al., 2001]. Bax, Bad, and Bcl-2 reside primarily in the cytosol, whereas Bak resides primarily in mitochondria (see Figure 14-3). Bcl-2 family members can form homodimers or heterodimers and higher-order multimers with other family members. Bax forms homodimers or heterodimers with Bak, Bcl-2, or Bcl-x_L. When Bax and Bak are present in excess, the anti-apoptotic activity of Bcl-2 and Bcl-x_L is antagonized. The formation of Bax homo-oligomers promotes apoptosis, whereas Bax heterodimerization with either Bcl-2 or Bcl-x_L neutralizes its pro-apoptotic activity. Neonatal HI enhances the relative pro-apoptosis balance of Bcl-2 family proteins. Marked increases in mitochondrial Bax occur within 24 hours of HI in neonatal rats, during which time there is no change in the relative amount of Bcl-x_L [Northington et al., 2001a] and changes in the subcellular distribution of Bax occur rapidly, prior to the activation of downstream apoptosis-effector mechanisms [Lok and Martin, 2002].

Release of cytochrome c from mitochondria may occur through mechanisms that involve the formation of membrane channels comprised of Bax or Bak [Antonsson et al., 1997] and Bax and the VDAC [Shimizu et al., 2000] (see Figure 14-3). Cytochrome c triggers the assembly of the cytoplasmic apoptosome (a protein complex of Apaf1, cytochrome c, and procaspase-9), which is the engine driving caspase-3 activation in mammalian cells [Li et al., 1997]. Bcl-2 and Bcl-x_L block the release of cytochrome c [Kluck et al., 1997; Yang et al., 1997] from mitochondria, and thus the activation of caspase-3 [Liu et al., 1996; Li et al., 1997]. The blockade of cytochrome c release from mitochondria by Bcl-2 and Bcl-x_L [Liu et al., 1996; Vander Heiden et al., 1997] is caused by inhibition of Bax channel-forming activity in the outer mitochondrial membrane [Antonsson et al., 1997] or by modulation of mitochondrial membrane potential and volume homeostasis [Vander Heiden et al., 1997]. Bcl-x_L also has anti-apoptotic activity by interacting with Apaf-1 and caspase-9, and inhibiting the Apaf-1-mediated autocatalytic maturation of caspase-9 [Hu et al., 1998]. Boo can inhibit Bak- and Bik-induced apoptosis (but not Bax-induced cell death), possibly through heterodimerization and by interactions with Apaf-1 and caspase-9 [Song et al., 1999]. Bax and Bak double-knockout cells are completely resistant to mitochondrial cytochrome c release during apoptosis [Wei et al., 2001]. BH3-only proteins, such as Bim, Bid, Puma, and Noxa, appear to induce a conformational change in Bax or they serve as decoys for Bcl-x_L, allowing Bax to form pores in the outer mitochondrial membrane [Letai et al., 2002]. The role of the BH3-only proteins in neonatal HI brain injury is unclear. There are no reports of Bid activation in neonatal HI, and in a single study using Bid-deficient mice no protection from neonatal HI brain injury was found [Ness et al., 2006].

Although many studies have focused on how Bcl-2 family members regulate mitochondrial apoptosis, it is now evident that Bcl-2 proteins localize to the ER and also translocate to the nucleus [Lithgow et al., 1994; Zhu et al., 2009]. This finding is relevant to neonatal HIE and excitotoxicity, where ER abnormalities may be particularly important to pathogenesis [Portera-Cailliau et al., 1997a, b; Martin et al., 2000; Puka-Sundvall et al., 2000]. The ER functions to fold proteins, and when this capacity is compromised, an unfolded protein response (UPR) is engaged. The UPR can lead to a return to homeostasis or to cell death. Bak and Bax also operate in the ER and function in the activation of ER-specific caspase-12 [Zong et al., 2003]. Cells lacking Bax and Bak are resistant to ER stress-induced apoptosis [Wei et al., 2001]. Translocation and accumulation of Bcl-2 in the nucleus occurs during a period when the total amounts of Bcl-2 decrease via calpain-dependent mechanisms following neonatal HI in mice [Hu et al., 1998; Zhu et al., 2009]. Overexpression of Bcl-2 and Bcl-x_L can block ER stress-induced apoptosis [Murakami et al., 2007], but the function of nuclear Bcl-2 is not known.

Protein phosphorylation regulates the functions of some Bcl-2 family members. Bcl-2 loses its anti-apoptotic activity following serine phosphorylation, possibly because its antioxidant function is inactivated [Haldar et al., 1995]. Bcl-2 phosphorylation at serine 24 in the BH4 domain precedes caspase-3 cleavage following cerebral HI in neonatal rat [Hallin et al., 2006]. In addition to interacting with homologous proteins, Bcl-2 can associate with nonhomologous proteins, including the protein kinase Raf-1 [Wang et al., 1996]. Bcl-2 is thought to target Raf-1 to mitochondrial membranes, allowing this kinase to phosphorylate Bad at serine residues. The phosphatidylinositol 3-kinase (PI3-K)–Akt pathway also regulates the function of Bad [Datta et al., 1997; del Peso et al., 1997] and caspase-9 [Cardone et al., 1998] through phosphorylation. In the presence of trophic factors, Bad is phosphorylated. Phosphorylated Bad is sequestered in the cytosol by interacting with soluble protein 14-3-3 and, when bound to protein 14-3-3, Bad is unable to interact with Bcl-2 and Bcl-x_L, thereby promoting survival [Zha et al., 1996]. Conversely, when Bad is dephosphorylated by calcineurin [Wang et al., 1999], it dissociates from protein 14-3-3 in the cytosol and translocates to the mitochondria, where it exerts pro-apoptotic activity. Nonphosphorylated Bad heterodimerizes with membrane-associated Bcl-2 and Bcl-x_L, thereby displacing Bax from Bax-Bcl-2 and Bax-Bcl-x_L dimers and promoting cell death [Yang et al., 1995]. The phosphorylation status of Bad helps regulate glucokinase activity, thereby linking glucose metabolism to apoptosis [Danial et al., 2003].

Caspases: Cell Demolition Proteases

Caspases (*c*ysteinyl *asp*artate-specific protein*ases*) are cysteine proteases that have a near-absolute substrate requirement for aspartate in the P_1 position of the peptide bond. Fourteen members have been identified [Wolf and Green, 1999]. Caspases exist as constitutively expressed inactive proenzymes (30–50 kDa) in healthy cells. The protein contains three domains: an amino-terminal prodomain, a large subunit (approximately 20 kDa), and a small subunit (approximately 10 kDa). The inactive proenzymes are present at detectable levels under basal conditions, but at least one study suggests that transcription and increased expression of the proenzyme occur following neonatal hypoxia [Deliveria-Papadopoulos et al., 2008]. By far the greatest control of caspase activity occurs through regulated proteolysis of the proenzyme with "initiator" caspases activating "executioner" caspases, although some caspase proenzymes (e.g., caspase-9) have low activity without processing [Stennicke et al., 1999]. Other caspase family members function in inflammation by processing cytokines [Wolf and Green, 1999]. The prodomain of initiator caspases contains amino acid sequences that are caspase recruitment domains (CARD) or death effector domains (DED), which enable the caspases to interact with other molecules that regulate their activation. Activation of caspases involves proteolytic

processing between domains, and then association of large and small subunits to form a heterodimer with both subunits contributing to the catalytic site. Two heterodimers associate to form a tetramer that has two catalytic sites that function independently. Active caspases have many target proteins [Schwartz and Milligan, 1996] that are cleaved during regulated and organized cell death. Caspases cleave nuclear proteins (e.g., DNases, poly(ADP) ribose polymerase, DNA-dependent protein kinase, heteronuclear ribonucleoproteins, transcription factors or lamins), cytoskeletal proteins (e.g., actin and fodrin), and cytosolic proteins (e.g., other caspases, protein kinases, Bid).

In cell models of apoptosis using human non-neuronal cell lines, activation of caspase-3 occurs when caspase-9 proenzyme (also known as Apaf-3) is bound by Apaf-1, which then oligomerizes in a process initiated by cytochrome c (identified as Apaf-2) and either ATP or dATP [Li et al., 1997] (see Figure 14-3). Cytosolic ATP or dATP is a required co-factor for cytochrome c-induced caspase activation. Apaf-1, a 130 kDa cytoplasmic protein, serves as a docking protein for procaspase-9 (Apaf-3) and cytochrome c [Li et al., 1997]. Apaf-1 becomes activated when ATP is bound and hydrolyzed, with the hydrolysis of ATP and the binding of cytochrome c promoting Apaf-1 oligomerization [Zou et al., 1999]. This oligomeric complex recruits and mediates the autocatalytic activation of procaspase-9 (forming the apoptosome), which disassociates from the complex and becomes available to activate caspase-3. In the newborn brain, HI in rat pups and hypoxia in piglets induced caspase 9-mediated caspase 3 activation, which is modulated by neuronal and inducible nitric oxide synthase (nNOS and iNOS) derived-NO and by neuronal nuclear Ca^{2+} influx [Zhu et al., 2004a; Deliveria-Papadopoulos et al., 2008]. These effects appear to occur at both transcriptional and post-translational levels. Once activated, caspase-3 cleaves multiple proteins, including a protein with DNase activity (i.e., DFF-45). DFF-45 cleavage activates a process leading to the internucleosomal fragmentation of genomic DNA [Liu et al., 1997].

So far, three caspase-related signaling pathways have been identified that can lead to apoptosis [Liu et al., 1996, 1997; Liu et al., 1997, 1998], but crosstalk among these pathways is possible. The intrinsic mitochondria-mediated pathway is controlled by Bcl-2 family proteins. It is regulated by cytochrome c release from mitochondria, promoting the activation of caspase-9 through Apaf-1 and then caspase-3 activation. The extrinsic death receptor pathway involves the activation of cell-surface death receptors, including Fas and tumor necrosis factor (TNF) receptor, leading to the formation of the death-inducible signaling complex (DISC) and caspase-8 activation, which in turn cleaves and activates downstream caspases such as caspase-3, 6, and 7. Caspase-8 can also cleave Bid, leading to the translocation, oligomerization, and insertion of Bax or Bak into the mitochondrial membrane. Another pathway involves the activation of caspase-2 by DNA damage or ER stress as a premitochondrial signal [Robertson et al., 2002].

Caspases are also critical regulators of nondeath functions in cells, notably some maturational processes. These nonapoptotic functions include modulation of synaptic plasticity via involvement in long-term potentiation [Gulyaeva, 2003] and cleavage of AMPA receptor subunits [Lu et al., 2002], and normal differentiation and migration of neurons to the olfactory bulb [Yan et al., 2001]. Transient caspase inactivation for the purpose of neuroprotection following neonatal HI may interfere with ongoing, normal nondeath-related functions of caspases. It is unknown whether inhibition of caspase activity in the acute setting of injury impairs similar functions or interferes with axonal sprouting, and whether there are long-term changes in brain structure or function as a result of acute caspase inhibition. Because of the potential importance of the nonapoptotic functions of caspase-3, it might be more appropriate to block the formation of "stress-induced", cleaved caspase-3 following injury with selective caspase-8 and 9 inhibitors that would not interfere with basal levels of caspase-3 activity. However, the nonapoptotic functions of caspase-8 and 9 are unknown, and the effects of acute caspase-8 and 9 inhibition on the developing brain, other than neuroprotection, are similarly unknown.

Caspases seem to be involved in the evolution of neonatal brain injury caused by HI, although this may vary between models. Caspase-3 cleavage and activation occur in brain after HI and trauma in neonatal rodents [Hu et al., 2000; Blomgren et al., 2001; Northington et al., 2001a; Felderhoff-Mueser et al., 2002], and after hypoxia in neonatal piglets [Delivoria-Papadopoulos et al., 2008]. The extent of caspase-3 cleavage and activation following brain injury is clearly greater in developing rodents compared to adults [Hu et al., 2000; Zhu et al., 2005]. This principle is replicated in immature and mature neuronal culture systems [Lesuisse and Martin, 2002]. Cerebroventricular injection of a pan-caspase inhibitor or intraperitoneal injection of a serine protease inhibitor 3 hours after neonatal HI in rat has neuroprotective effects [Cheng et al., 1998; Feng and LeBlanc, 2003]. Subsequent studies have shown 30–50 percent decreases in HI-induced tissue loss in neonatal rat brain at 15 days after the insult with non-selective inhibitors of caspase-8 and caspase-9 [Feng et al., 2003a, b]. However, the lack of enzyme specificity of caspase inhibitor drugs prevents unambiguous identification of caspases in mediating brain injury in most studies. The class of irreversible tetrapeptide caspase inhibitors covalently coupled to chloromethylketone, fluoromethylketone, or aldehydes efficiently inhibits other classes of cysteine proteases like calpains [Rozman-Pungercar et al., 2003]. Calpains, Ca^{2+}-activated, neutral, cytosolic cysteine proteases, are highly activated following neonatal HI in rats [Ostwald et al., 1993; Blomgren et al., 2001]. MDL28170, a drug that inhibits calpains and caspase-3, exerts neuroprotective actions in the neonatal rat brain by decreasing necrosis and apoptosis [Kawamura et al., 2005] and thus may be a particularly valuable tool for the treatment of neonatal HI. Cathepsins, cysteine proteases concentrated in the lysosomal compartment, are also likely to be activated based on electron microscopy evidence of lysosomal and vacuolar changes found following neonatal HI [Martin et al., 2000]. More potent, selective, and reversible nonpeptide caspase-3 inhibitors have been developed [Han et al., 2005] and used to protect against brain injury following neonatal HI in rats [Han et al., 2002], but the protective effects were more modest compared to initial reports with nonselective pan-caspase inhibition [Cheng et al., 1998].

Not all forms of apoptotic cell death are caspase-dependent [Beresford et al., 2001; Fan et al., 2003]. The serine protease granzyme A (GrA) mediates a caspase-independent apoptotic pathway [Beresford et al., 2001]. GrA is delivered to target cells through Ca^{2+}-dependent, perforin-generated pores, and activates a DNase (GrA-DNase, non-metastasis factor 23, NM23) that is sequestered in the cytoplasm. NM23 activity is inhibited by the SET complex, which is located in the ER and comprised of the nucleosome assembly protein SET, an inhibitor of protein phosphatase 2A, apurinic endonuclease-1, and a high-mobility group protein (a nonhistone DNA-binding protein that induces alterations in DNA architecture). GrA cleaves components of the SET complex to release activated NM23, which translocates to the nucleus to induce single-strand DNA nicks and cell death that can be apoptotic or nonapoptotic [Fan et al., 2003]. To date, there are no studies of this pathway in neonatal HI.

Inhibitor of Apoptosis Protein Family

The activity of pro-apoptotic proteins must be placed in check to prevent unwanted apoptosis in normal cells. Apoptosis is blocked by the IAP family in mammalian cells [Deveraux et al., 1998; LaCasse et al., 1998; Holcik, 2002]. This family includes X chromosome-linked IAP (XIAP), IAP1, IAP2, neuronal apoptosis inhibitory protein (NAIP), Survivin, Livin, and Apollon. These proteins are characterized by 1–3 baculoviral IAP repeat domains consisting of a zinc finger domain of approximately 70–80 amino acids [Holcik, 2002]. Apollon is a huge (530 kDa) protein that also has a ubiquitin-conjugating enzyme domain. The main identified anti-apoptotic function of IAPs is the suppression of caspase activity [Deveraux et al., 1998]. Procaspase-9 and procaspase-3 are major targets of several IAPs. IAPs reversibly interact directly with caspases to block substrate cleavage. Apollon also ubiquitylates and facilitates proteosomal degradation of active caspase-9 and Smac [Hao et al., 2004]. However, IAPs do not prevent caspase-8-induced proteolytic activation of procaspase-3. IAPs can also block apoptosis by reciprocal interactions with the nuclear transcription factor NF-κβ [LaCasse et al., 1998].

Scant information is available on IAPs in the nervous system and in neonatal brain injury. Survivin is essential for nervous system development in mouse because conditional deletion of *survivin* gene in neuronal precursor cells causes death shortly after birth, and reduced brain size and severe multifocal degeneration [Jiang et al., 2005]. NAIP is expressed throughout the CNS in neurons [Xu et al., 1997]. XIAP is highly enriched in mouse spinal motor neurons [Martin et al., 2007]. The importance of the IAP gene family in human pediatric neurodegeneration is underscored by the finding that NAIP is partially deleted in a significant proportion of children with spinal muscular atrophy [Roy et al., 1995]. Studies in transgenic XIAP mice indicate that XIAP plays an important role in regulating caspase activity after neonatal HI. Overexpression of XIAP virtually abolished activation of both caspase-9 and 3, and provided a 40 percent reduction in tissue loss in forebrain following neonatal HI in mouse [Wang et al., 2004].

Proteins exist that inhibit mammalian IAPs. A murine mitochondrial protein called Smac and its human ortholog, DIABLO (for direct IAP-binding protein with low pI), inactivate the anti-apoptotic actions of IAPs and thus exert pro-apoptotic actions [Du et al., 2000; Verhagen et al., 2000]. These IAP inhibitors are 23 kDa mitochondrial proteins (derived from 29 kDa precursor proteins processed in the mitochondria) that are released from the intermembrane space and sequester IAPs. High temperature requirement protein A2 (HtrA2), also called Omi, is another mitochondrial serine protease that exerts pro-apoptotic activity by inhibiting IAPs [Suzuki et al., 2004]. HtrA2/Omi functions as a homotrimeric protein that cleaves IAPs irreversibly, thus facilitating caspase activity. The intrinsic mitochondrial-mediated cell death pathway is regulated by Smac and HtrA2/Omi, and both of these proteins co-localize with XIAP in injured brain neurons after neonatal HI in mouse [Wang et al., 2004].

Apoptosis Inducing Factor

AIF is a mammalian cell mitochondrial protein identified as a flavoprotein oxidoreductase [Susin et al., 1999]. AIF has an N-terminal mitochondrial localization signal, and after import into the intermitochondrial membrane space the mitochondrial localization signal is cleaved off to generate a mature protein of 57 kDa. Under normal physiological conditions AIF might function as a ROS scavenger, targeting H_2O_2 [Klein et al., 2002], or in redox cycling with NAD(P)H [Mate et al., 2002]. With apoptotic stimuli (see Figure 14-3), AIF translocates to the nucleus [Susin et al., 1999]. Overexpression of AIF induces cardinal features of apoptosis, including chromatin condensation, high molecular weight DNA fragmentation, and loss of mitochondrial transmembrane potential [Susin et al., 1999]. Nuclear translocation of AIF plays a central role in neuronal loss induced by neonatal HI in mouse, particularly in males [Zhu et al., 2003, 2006, 2007]. These studies further showed that a substantial portion of the neurodegeneration following neonatal HI in mouse is caspase-independent [Zhu et al., 2003].

Cell Surface Death Receptors

Cell death by apoptosis can also be initiated at the cell membrane by surface death receptors of the tumor necrosis factor (TNF) receptor family. Fas (CD95/Apo-1) and the 75-kDa neurotrophin receptor (p75^{NTR}) are members of the large TNF receptor family [Nagata, 1999]. The signal for apoptosis is initiated at the cell surface by aggregation (trimerization) of the death domain containing members of this receptor family by their specific ligand. Fas death receptor-mediated apoptosis is the best described of these death receptor signaling pathways. Activation of Fas is induced by binding of the multivalent Fas ligand (FasL), a member of the TNF-cytokine family. FasL is expressed on activated T cells and natural killer cells. Clustering of Fas on the target cell by FasL recruits Fas-associated death domain (FADD), a cytoplasmic adapter molecule that functions in the activation of the caspase-8–Bid pathway, thus forming the "death-induced signaling complex" (DISC) [Li et al., 1998] (see Figure 14-2). Signaling for apoptosis then proceeds via the extrinsic or intrinsic pathway. In the extrinsic pathway, active caspase-8 then directly cleaves caspase-3 [Nagata, 1999]. Activation of the mitochondrial or intrinsic pathway proceeds via caspase-8-mediated cleavage of cytosolic Bid (a pro-apoptotic Bcl$_2$ family member) [Li et al., 1998] (see Figure 14-2). The truncated form of Bid then translocates to mitochondria, thereby functioning as a BH3-only transducer of Fas activation signal at the cell plasma membrane to mitochondria [Li et al., 1998]. Bid translocation from the cytosol to mitochondrial membranes is associated with a conformational change in Bax (that is prevented by Bcl-2 and Bcl-x$_L$), and is accompanied by release of cytochrome c from mitochondria [Desagher et al., 1999]. Apoptosis through Fas is independent of new RNA or protein synthesis. Evidence for the importance of these signaling pathways in experimental neonatal brain injury is growing. Activation of multiple components of the Fas death receptor signaling pathway have been found in neonatal rat and mouse models of HI and hyperoxic brain injury [Northington et al., 2001a; Graham et al., 2004; Dzietko et al., 2008], and blocking Fas death receptor signaling by either pharmacologic or genetic means affords protection in these models [Feng et al., 2003a; Graham et al., 2004; Dzietko et al., 2008]. Concurrent with activation of Fas death receptors, levels of Bax in mitochondrial-enriched cell fractions increase, and cytochrome c accumulates in the soluble protein compartment. Increased levels of Fas death receptor and Bax, cytochrome c accumulation, and activation of caspase-8 precede the marked activation of caspase-3 and the occurrence of neuronal apoptosis in the thalamus in neonatal rat HI [Northington et al., 2001a]. This thalamic neuronal apoptosis in the neonatal rat brain after HI is identical structurally to the apoptosis of thalamic neurons after cortical trauma [Natale et al., 2002]. HI in the neonatal rat causes severe infarction of cerebral cortex [Northington et al., 2001b], and it is assumed that this thalamic neuron apoptosis is caused by target deprivation via a Fas-dependent pathway.

Apoptosis can also be mediated by p75^{NTR} [Troy et al., 2002]. Activation of p75^{NTR} occurs through binding of nerve growth factor. When p75^{NTR} is activated without Trk receptors, neurotrophin binding induces homodimer formation and activates an apoptotic cascade. Activation of p75^{NTR} leads to the generation of ceramide through sphingomyelin hydrolysis. Ceramide production is associated with the activation of Jun N-terminal kinase (JNK), which phosphorylates and activates c-Jun and other transcription factors. p75 mediates hippocampal neuron death in response to neurotrophin withdrawal, involving cytochrome c, Apaf1, and caspases-9, 6, and 3 (but not caspase-8), and thus is different from Fas-mediated cell death [Troy et al., 2002].

Information on the role of death receptor activation in human and experimental neonatal brain injury, although relatively sparse, has been recently reviewed [Northington et al., 2007]. Inflammatory cytokines, especially TNFα, clearly play a role in the pathogenesis of ischemic brain injury in the human newborn [Nelson et al., 1998; Savman et al., 1998; Shalak et al., 2002; Bartha et al., 2004], suggesting that understanding death receptor signaling pathways is critical. Furthermore, activation of Fas death receptor pathways has been found in hydrocephalus, hemorrhagic and focal ischemic brain injury, and following neonatal asphyxia in human newborns [Felderhoff-Mueser et al., 2001, 2003; Mehmet, 2001; Van Landeghem et al., 2002]. The importance of these pathways in human neonatal brain injury may become even more prominent as the contributions of programmed necrosis and on-going/delayed inflammation to initiation and propagation of injury in the developing brain are understood.

p53 Family of Tumor Suppressors

Cell death by apoptosis can be triggered by DNA damage. p53 and related DNA binding proteins identified as p73 and p63 are involved in this process [Levreroi et al., 2000]. p53, p73, and p63 function in apoptosis or growth arrest and repair. They can commit to death cells that have sustained DNA damage from ROS, irradiation, and other genotoxic stresses [Levrero et al., 2000]. p53 and p73 have similar oligomerization and DNA sequence transactivation properties. p73 exists as a group of full-length isoforms (including p73α and p73β), and as truncated isoforms that lack the transactivation domain ($\triangle$N-p73). p53 is the best-studied of this family of proteins.

p53 is a short-lived protein with a half-life of approximately 5–20 min in most types of cells studied. p53 rapidly accumulates several-fold in response to DNA damage. This rapid regulation is mediated by post-translational modification such as phosphorylation and acetylation, as well as intracellular redox state [Giaccia and Kastan, 1998]. The elevation in p53 protein levels occurs through stabilization and prevention of degradation that is under partial control of hypoxia-inducible factor-1α [Calvert et al., 2006; Fan et al., 2009]. p53 is degraded rapidly in a ubiquitination-dependent proteosomal pathway [Maki et al., 1996; Chang et al., 1998]. Murine double minute 2 (Mdm2; the human homolog is Hdm2) has a crucial role in this degradation pathway [Shieh et al., 1997]. Mdm2 functions in a feedback loop to limit the duration or magnitude of the p53 response to DNA damage. Expression of the *Mdm2* gene is controlled by p53 [Shieh et al., 1997]. Mdm2 binds to the N-terminal transcriptional activation domain of p53 and regulates its DNA binding activity and stability by direct association. Mdm2 has ubiquitin ligase activity for p53 through the ubiquitin-conjugating enzyme E2. Stabilization of p53 is achieved through phosphorylation of serine^{15}, resulting in inhibition of formation of Mdm2–p53 complexes. Activated p53 binds the promoters of several genes encoding proteins associated with growth control and cell cycle checkpoints (e.g., p21, Gadd45, Mdm2) and apoptosis (e.g., Bax, Bcl-2, Bcl-x$_L$, and Fas). The BH3-only proteins Puma and Noxa are critical mediators of p53-mediated apoptosis [Villunger et al., 2003].

p53 and p73 regulate neuronal cell survival. p53 has a critical apoptotic role in cultured sympathetic ganglion neurons in response to neurotrophin withdrawal [Aloyz et al., 1998]. p53 deficiency protects against neuronal apoptosis induced by axotomy and target deprivation in vivo [Martin et al., 2001; Martin and Liu, 2002]. p53-mediated neuronal apoptosis can be blocked by the $\triangle$N-p73 isoform by direct binding and inactivation of p53 [Pozniak et al., 2000]. Little is known about the roles of p53 in neurodegeneration following neonatal HI, except that p53 levels increase [Calvert et al., 2006], and acute inhibition of NF-$\kappa\beta$ following neonatal HI prevents both nuclear and mitochondrial accumulation of p53 and provides significant sustained neuroprotection [Nijboer et al., 2008].

Excitotoxic Cell Death

Neuronal death can be induced by excitotoxicity. This observation was made originally in 1957 [Lucas and Newhouse, 1957], formulated into a concept by John Olney after showing that glutamate can kill neurons in brain [Olney, 1971], and then examined mechanistically by Dennis Choi [Choi, 1992]. This concept has fundamental importance to a variety of acute neurological insults, such as cerebral HI, epilepsy, trauma, and hypoxia [Delivoria-Papadopoulos and Mishra, 1998; Martin et al., 1998, 2000; Martin, 2003; Johnston, 2005]. This pathologic neurodegeneration is mediated by excessive activation of glutamate-gated ion channel receptors and voltage-dependent ion channels. Increased cytosolic free Ca^{2+} causes activation of Ca^{2+}-sensitive proteases, protein kinases/phosphatases, phospholipases, and NOS when glutamate receptors are stimulated. The excessive interaction of ligand with subtypes of glutamate receptors causes pathophysiological changes in intracellular

ion concentrations, pH, protein phosphorylation, and energy metabolism [Choi, 1992; Lipton and Rosenberg, 1994]. The precise mechanisms of excitotoxic cell death are still being examined intensively, driven by the hope of identifying therapeutic targets for neurological disorders with putative excitotoxic components. Yet, in vitro and in vivo experimental data are discordant with regard to whether excitotoxic neuronal death is apoptotic or necrotic, or perhaps even a peculiar form of cell death that is unique to excitotoxicity.

The contribution of apoptotic mechanisms to excitotoxic death of neurons has been examined in cultured neurons. However, these studies provide conflicting results. Excitotoxicity can cause activation of endonucleases and specific internucleosomal DNA fragmentation in cultures of cortical neurons [Kure et al., 1991; Gwag et al., 1997] and cerebellar granule cells [Ankarcrona et al., 1995; Simonian et al., 1996]. Internucleosomal fragmentation of DNA was not seen in other studies of cerebellar granule cell cultures [Dessi et al., 1993]. Excitotoxic cell death in neuronal cultures is prevented [Kure et al., 1991] or unaffected [Dessi et al., 1993; Simonian et al., 1996; Gwag et al., 1997] by inhibitors of RNA or protein synthesis, and sensitive [Kure et al., 1991; Simonian et al., 1996] or insensitive [Dessi et al., 1993] to the endonuclease inhibitor aurintricarboxylic acid. In primary cultures of mouse cortical cells, the non-N-methyl-D-aspartic acid (NMDA) glutamate receptor agonist kainic acid (KA) induces increases in Bax protein, and *bax* gene deficiency significantly protects cells against KA receptor toxicity [Xiang et al., 1998]. However, NMDA receptor toxicity in mouse cerebellar granule cells [Miller et al., 1997] and mouse cortical cells [Dargusch et al., 2001] was not Bax-related. These results support our expectation that non-NMDA glutamate receptor excitotoxicity is more likely than NMDA receptor-mediated excitotoxicity to induce apoptosis or continuum cell death [Portera-Cailliau et al., 1997a, b]. Glutamate (100 μM) stimulation of mouse cortical cells did not cause an increase in caspase activity [Johnson et al., 1999], but NMDA-treated rat cortical cells showed increased caspase activity [Tenneti and Lipton, 2000]. In cerebellar granule neurons, glutamate (100 μM to 1 mM) did not activate caspase activity, and adenoviral-mediated expression of IAPs did not influence excitotoxic cell death [Simons et al., 1999]. These conflicting results can also be related to the finding that activation of different subtypes of glutamate receptors appears to activate different modes of cell death [Portera-Cailliau et al., 1997a, b].

The morphological characteristics of excitotoxicity in many neurons in vivo include somatodendritic swelling, mitochondrial damage, and chromatin condensation into irregular clumps [Olney, 1971; van Lookeren Campagne et al., 1995; Portera-Cailliau et al., 1997a, b], features that are thought to be typical of cellular necrosis; however, in other neurons, excitotoxicity causes cytological features more like apoptosis [van Lookeren Campagne et al., 1995; Portera-Cailliau et al., 1997a, b]. Excitotoxic degeneration of CA3 neurons in response to KA is increased in NAIP-deleted mice, further supporting a contribution of apoptosis [Holcik et al., 2000]. Excitotoxic neurodegeneration in vivo has been shown to be either sensitive [Schreiber et al., 1993] or insensitive [Leppin et al., 1992] to protein synthesis inhibition; therefore, a role for de novo protein synthesis in the expression of a PCD cascade in excitotoxicity is uncertain.

The precise mechanisms of excitotoxic neuronal apoptosis in vivo have not been identified specifically. Neurons in the immature rodent CNS undergo massive apoptosis in response to glutamate receptor excitotoxicity [Portera-Cailliau et al., 1997a, b]. Apoptosis is much more prominent after excitotoxic injury in the immature brain compared to the mature brain [Portera-Cailliau et al., 1997a, b]. Intrastriatal administration of KA in newborn rodents causes copious apoptosis of striatal neurons [Ginsberg and Busto, 1989; Portera-Cailliau et al., 1997a, b], serving as an unequivocal model of apoptosis in neurons that are selectively vulnerable in HIE. This apoptosis has been verified structurally with light microscopy and electron microscopy, and by immunolocalization of cleaved caspase-3 [Lok and Martin, 2002]. Ubiquitous apoptosis is observed at 24 hours after the insult. DNA degradation by internucleosomal fragmentation further confirms the presence of apoptosis. Excitotoxic neuronal apoptosis is associated with rapid (within 2 hours after neurotoxin exposure) translocation of Bax and cleaved caspase-3 to mitochondria [Lok and Martin, 2002]. Moreover, this study revealed that the ratio of mitochondrial membrane-associated Bax to soluble Bax in normal developing striatum changes prominently with brain maturation. Newborn rat striatum has a much greater proportion of Bax in the mitochondrial fraction, with lower levels of soluble Bax. Mature rat striatum has a much larger proportion of Bax in the soluble fraction and low amounts of Bax in the mitochondrial fraction. With brain maturation there is a linear decrease in the ratio of mitochondrial Bax to soluble Bax. This developmental subcellular redistribution of Bax might be a reason why immature rodent neurons exhibit a more robust classical apoptosis response compared to adult neurons after brain damage [Martin, 2001].

The therapeutic potential of NMDA receptor blockade for neonatal HI and excitotoxic insults, in rat, was initially reported by McDonald et al. [McDonald et al., 1987]. MK-801 (dizocilpine, (5R,10S)-(+)-5-Methyl-10,11-dihydro-5H-dibenzo[a,d]cyclohepten-5,10-imine hydrogen maleate), a noncompetitive antagonist of NMDA receptors, provided near-complete neuroprotection but only when given as an immediate pretreatment and during the insult [McDonald et al., 1987]. Pretreatment with MK-801 also protected against hippocampal neurodegeneration and improved performance in memory tasks following neonatal HI [Ford et al., 1989]. These studies were followed by evidence that MK-801, given immediately prior to excitotoxin injection, completely blocks NMDA and partially blocks quisqualic acid excitotoxicity in neonatal rats [McDonald et al., 1990b], and blocks both NMDA-mediated lesions and associated hyperemia in the newborn lamb [Taylor et al., 1995]. Although, at low doses, MK-801 is highly effective as a neuroprotectant in neonatal HI [Hagberg et al., 1994], it is not a therapeutically useful agent because it exacerbates injury when given 24 hours prior to HI [McDonald et al., 1990a], and even brief exposure causes massive apoptosis in the developing brain when given at p7 to the rat in the absence of an acute injury [Ikonomidou et al., 1999]. This neuroprotection/neurodevelopmental apoptosis paradox also extends to other NMDA receptor antagonists, including magnesium, which provides neuroprotection to the p7 rat receiving intrastriatal NMDA but results in widespread neuronal apoptosis when given at p3 and p7 to naïve uninjured mice [McDonald et al., 1990; Dribben et al., 2009].

Other attempts to interrupt NMDA excitotoxicity circumvent direct NMDA receptor blockade or use novel pharmacologic agents unrelated to MK-801. Xenon, an NMDA receptor antagonist, provides both in vivo and in vitro neuroprotection against neonatal HI in the rat and oxygen-glucose deprivation in neuronal-glial co-culture experiments, and these effects are accentuated by dexmedetomidine [Rajakumaraswamy et al., 2006]. Memantine, a low-affinity voltage-dependent channel NMDA receptor antagonist, shows promise in the neonatal rat HI model, in vitro in organotypic slices and neuronal culture models [Volbracht et al., 2006], and most recently in the neonatal rat HI model modified to produce a more selective white matter injury [Manning et al., 2008]. Unlike MK-801, memantine appears to permit neuronal signaling, which may be crucial to prevent the neurodevelopmental apoptosis caused by MK-801 [Volbracht et al., 2006]. Other potentially useful targets for neuroprotection after neonatal HI include non-NMDA glutamate receptors and sodium channels.

The Cell Death Continuum

Using animal models of neurodegeneration, we discovered that cell death exists as a continuum of necrosis and apoptosis at opposite ends of a degenerative spectrum; numerous hybrid forms of degeneration manifest between necrosis and apoptosis (see Figure 14-1) [Portera-Cailliau et al., 1997a, b; Martin et al., 1998]. The age or maturity of brain, and the subtype of excitatory glutamate receptor that is activated influence the mode and speed of neuronal cell death [Portera-Cailliau et al., 1997a, b; Martin, 2001; Natale et al., 2002] (Figure 14-4). This structural and temporal diversity of neuronal cell death is seen with a variety of brain injuries, including excitotoxicity, HI, target deprivation, and axonal trauma. Biochemical evidence for the existence of an intermediate "continuum" form of cell death is verified by the coexpression of markers for both apoptosis and necrosis in neurons in the injured forebrain at 3 hours following HI in neonatal rat [Ostwald et al., 1993; Blomgren et al., 2001], and evidence for crosstalk between calpain and caspase pathways as a fundamental mechanism contributing to "continuum" cell death is found [Blomgren et al., 2001]. The significance of this finding is evident from the demonstration that caspase-3 inhibition provides complete blockade of caspase activation but only partial neuroprotection. Caspase-3 inhibitors fail to prevent the necrotic mode of cell death induced by HI, as revealed by the presence of necrosis markers, and, thus, the forebrain still sustains significant injury [Han et al., 2002].

This diversity of cell death is one of the fundamental differences in injury-associated neuronal death in immature and mature CNS, manifesting much more often in the injured immature brain [Northington et al., 2007]. Additionally, cell death is clearly pleiomorphic in neurons within the same brain [Sheldon et al., 2001; Blomgren et al., 2007; Northington et al., 2007]. To help explain these data we formulated the concept of the cell death continuum (see Figure 14-1). A fundamental cornerstone of the continuum is thought to be gradations in the responses of cells to stress. Some specific mechanisms thought to be driving the continuum are the developmental expression of different subtypes of glutamate receptors, mitochondrial energetics (see Figure 14-3), the propinquity of developing neurons to the cell cycle, neurotrophin requirements, DNA damage

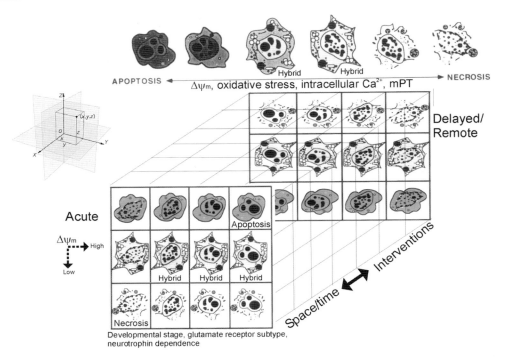

Fig. 14-4 Cell death matrix. This diagram summarizes, in linear (top) and three-dimensional matrix (bottom) formats, the concept of the apoptosis–necrosis continuum of cell death. The concept, as proposed in its original form, organized cell death as a linear spectrum, with apoptosis and necrosis at the extremes and different syncretic hybrid forms in between (top). A hypothetical dying neuron in the brain is illustrated at coordinates (x,y,z) in the Euclidian coordinate system (at left). The front matrix of the cube shows some of the numerous possible structures of neuronal cell death near or at the terminal stages of degeneration. Combining different nuclear morphologies and cytoplasmic morphologies generates a nonlinear matrix of possible cell death structures. In the cell at the extreme upper right corner, nuclear and cytoplasmic morphologies combine to form an apoptotic neuron that is typical of naturally occurring PCD during nervous system development. This death is classical apoptosis. In contrast, in the cell at the extreme lower left corner, the merging of necrotic nuclear and necrotic cytoplasmic morphologies forms a typical necrotic neuron resulting from NMDA receptor excitotoxicity and cerebral HI. Between these two extremes hybrids of cell death can be produced with varying contributions of apoptosis and necrosis. The typical apoptosis–necrosis hybrid cell death structure is best exemplified by neurons in the CNS dying from HI or non-NMDA glutamate receptor-mediated excitotoxicity. The death forms shown in the front matrix of the cube represent only a small number of the possible forms of cell death that we can envision to fill the empty cells of the matrix. Neuronal maturity and the subtypes of glutamate receptors that are overactivated are known to influence where an injured/degenerating neuron falls within the matrix. The types and levels of DNA damage that are sustained by a cell might also influence the position of a degenerating cell within the death matrix and in the brain Euclidian coordinate system. The back panel represents the possible cell death forms occurring in space/time over a delayed period or after administration of therapeutic interventions. The matrix predicts that the cell death patterns could change over time from apoptosis to apoptosis–necrosis variants or necrosis, and from necrosis to apoptosis–necrosis variants or apoptosis. This concept may also be relevant to cell death in general, and thus may be widely applicable to cell biology outside the nervous system. *(Adapted from Martin, LJ. Excitotoxicity. Encyclopedia of Neuroscience, CD-ROM. G Adelman and BH Smith (eds). Elsevier, Philadelphia, PA 2004.)*

vulnerability, and the degree of axonal collateralization [Martin, 2001, 2002]. Although the molecular mechanisms that drive this cell death continuum in the brain are currently uncertain, cell culture data hint that ATP levels [Leist et al., 1997], intracellular Ca^{2+} levels [Trump and Berezesky, 1996], level of caspase activity [Lin et al., 1999], and mitochondrial permeability transition [Crompton, 1999] could be involved (see Figure 14-4). In vivo experiments so far suggest that the relative level of Bax in the outer mitochondrial membrane could regulate the cell death continuum in neurons [Lok and Martin, 2002] (see Figure 14-3). In the newborn brain with its proclivity to apoptotic cell death, the concept that energy failure interrupts and prevents successful completion of apoptosis with a resultant increase in necrotic cell death forms is an appealing explanation for the abundant expression of biochemical markers of apoptosis and the paucity of evidence for complete execution of apoptosis [Northington et al., 2007]. This

suggests that the concept of the cell death continuum is particularly pertinent to neuron degeneration in the immature brain (see Figure 14-1), although it might be applicable to cytopathology in general.

Recent data now suggest that, under certain conditions and perhaps in specific brain regions, autophagy is also part of the complex continuum of neurodegeneration following neonatal HI in mice [Ginet et al., 2009]. Pharmacologic inhibition of autophagy prior to neonatal HI worsens injury and shifts the cell death continuum from apoptosis to necrosis in p7 rats [Carloni et al., 2008]. One possible explanation for these results is that autophagy may play an important role in maintaining cellular energy stores at adequate levels soon after a severe HI insult, and thus allows for successful completion of apoptosis. Clearly, autophagocytic and apoptotic markers are often coexpressed following neonatal HI [Ginet et al., 2009]. Early on, without the energy savings provided for by induction of autophagocytic mechanisms, ATP levels may fall below the critical threshold required for completion of apoptosis, and forms of necrosis ensue. Conversely, inhibition of autophagy appears to be neuroprotective at later time points and in less severe insults [Puyal et al., 2009]. In these settings, maintenance of cellular energy may not be as critical and autophagocytic mechanisms may be activated in stressed but possibly still viable neurons. Crosstalk between autophagic and apoptotic pathways may then result in the cells ultimately being eliminated by apoptotic mechanisms [Maiuri et al., 2007]. Under these conditions, inhibition of autophagy would provide much earlier and perhaps more effective interruption of cell death pathways. It remains to be seen whether inhibiting delayed autophagy provides functional benefits. Moreover, it is clearly evident that timing and energy state are critical variables in any attempt to modulate autophagy following neonatal HI.

Despite the mounting evidence for the cell death continuum, the concept has been challenged and deemed confusing by some investigators [Ishimaru et al., 1999; Fujikawa, 2000; Sloviter, 2002]. Opponents of the cell death continuum assume that morphology and underlying biochemical processes remain binary and discrete [Fujikawa, 2000]. While this is the case at the extremes of the cell death continuum, absolute discreteness ignores the observable features of cell degeneration seen in the injured and diseased CNS, particularly in the immature brain (see Figure 14-1). Experiments done by us [Martin, 2001; Northington et al., 2005] and others [Sheldon et al., 2001; Wei et al., 2004; Baille et al., 2005; Zhu et al., 2005] have shown that neuronal degeneration triggered by excitotoxicity and HI can be apoptotic, apoptosis-necrosis hybrids, necrotic, and possibly autophagocytic-apoptosis hybrids. Rigid conceptualization regarding cellular pathology is not realistic and is misleading, and can hinder our goal of the identification of relevant molecular mechanisms in complex biological systems, especially in the injured perinatal brain, and ultimately limit the realization of therapeutic opportunities. This view is now supported by recommendations of the Nomenclature Committee on Cell Death 2009 [Kroemer et al., 2009]. In comments reminiscent of the above reasoning for discarding the rigid/non-overlapping conceptual framework of neuronal cell death, the primary conclusion, of the panel addressing cell death in general, is that, if there is no clear equivalence between morphology and biochemistry, then rigid morphologic classifications are not useful. Conversely, cell death nomenclature is most useful when it predicts the possibilities of pharmacologic or genetic modulation of cell death or when it predicts the consequences of cell death in vivo [Kroemer et al., 2009].

Programmed Cell Necrosis

Forms of neurodegeneration in the developing brain similar to "continuum" cell death have been previously described and termed "pathological apoptosis" [Blomgren et al., 2007] and excitotoxic neurodegeneration [Ishimaru et al., 1999]. In vitro, similar hybrid forms of neurodegeneration are termed necroptosis, programmed necrosis, paraptosis, oncosis, and aponecrosis [Degterev et al., 2008]. The important contribution of these regulated but morphologically hybrid forms of cell death to neurodegeneration and stroke has recently been extensively reviewed [Yuan et al., 2003; Festjens et al., 2006; Bredesen, 2008; Henriquez et al., 2008], but their importance in neonatal brain injury is just now emerging [Blomgren et al., 2007]. In 2007, we identified the morphologic hallmark of delayed-ongoing neurodegeneration in the neonatal brain as the "apoptotic–necrotic continuum cell" [Northington et al., 2007]. After its initial description by Portera-Cailliau et al. [Portera-Cailliau et al., 1997a, b], continuum cell and similar hybrid forms of neurodegeneration have been identified in neonatal animal models of excitotoxicity and HI [Northington et al., 2001b; Sheldon et al., 2001; Blomgren et al., 2007] and in cell culture models [Formigli et al., 2000]. "Continuum" cell neurodegeneration may fundamentally result from failure to complete caspase-dependent apoptotic cell death following neonatal HI [Northington et al., 2007] (see Figure 14-2). The abundance of biochemical evidence for activation of caspase-dependent pathways following neonatal HI [Nakajima et al., 2000; Blomgren et al., 2001; Northington et al., 2001a; Han et al., 2002; Feng et al., 2003a; Feng et al., 2003b; Zhu et al., 2006], and the paucity of evidence that apoptosis is fully executed following neonatal HI [Ishimaru et al., 1999; Martin et al., 2000; Blomgren et al., 2007; Northington et al., 2007], lend credence to this argument.

A recently described small-molecule inhibitor of programmed cell necrosis will likely shed light on mechanisms relevant to these regulated hybrid forms of cell death. Necrostatin was first described as a specific antagonist of programmed cell necrosis or necroptosis in cell culture models. This regulated form of "necrotic" cell death is a good example of molecular switching between modes of cell death and a "backup" mechanism generally avoided but activated when other less injurious cell death mechanisms fail [Henriquez et al., 2008]. Necroptosis is defined as "nonapoptotic" death with necrotic features, and occurs optimally when death receptors are activated in the presence of caspase inhibition [Yuan et al., 2003; Degterev et al., 2005]. The death domain containing kinase, RIP1, appears to be a key signaling intermediate in this programmed necrosis and is inhibited by necrostatin [Festjens et al., 2007; Degterev et al., 2008] (see Figure 14-2). Necrostatin has shown promise as a neuroprotectant in adult animal models of myocardial ischemia and traumatic and ischemic brain injury [Degterev et al., 2005; Lim et al., 2007; You et al., 2008], and we have shown that it provides robust sustained neuroprotection following neonatal HI in mice [Graham et al., 2009].

Necrostatin's primary mechanism of action is allosteric inhibition of RIP1 kinase [Degterev et al., 2008] with possible downstream anti-inflammatory effects [You et al., 2008] and perhaps other mechanisms. Depending on the experimental conditions, RIP1 functions as the crucial adaptor kinase at the crossroads of a death receptor-stimulated cell's decision to live or die, and also at a critical juncture determining whether programmed cell apoptosis or necrosis is predominant after death receptor activation [Lin et al., 1999; Festjens et al., 2007]. RIP1 is one of seven known members of a family of serine/threonine kinases, and is constitutively expressed in many tissues, including the brain [Festjens et al., 2007]. Importantly, RIP1 contains a caspase recruitment domain and a death domain within its C-terminal region. It is the death domain that allows RIP1 to be recruited to death receptor-initiated protein complexes, which then propagate either prosurvival, proinflammatory, pro-apoptotic, or pronecrotic signals [Festjens et al., 2007] (see Figure 14-2). RIP1-mediated activation of the regulated necrosis-signaling pathway preferentially occurs in the presence of caspase inhibition [Shen and Pervaiz, 2006; Festjens et al., 2007]. Inhibition of endogenous caspase-8-mediated cleavage of RIP1 is essential for maximal execution of death receptor-mediated programmed necrosis. Caspase inhibition can also occur in the setting of significant energy failure [Eguchi et al., 1997; Leist et al., 1997, 1999; Leist and Jaattela, 2001], such as that which occurs following neonatal HI (see Figure 14-2). It has been hypothesized that this energy failure interrupts the neonatal brain's proclivity to apoptosis [Leist et al., 1999; Leist and Jaattela, 2001; Blomgren et al., 2007; Northington et al., 2007] and results in the hybrid, continuum cell death morphology.

Although necrostatin has no known direct antioxidant effect, and does not prevent cell death in vitro caused by hydrogen peroxide, it clearly modulates redox mechanisms in experimental systems [Xu et al., 2007]. Necrostatin inhibition of glutamate excitotoxicity occurs with an increase in glutathione levels and a decrease in ROS production [Xu et al., 2007]. It remains controversial, but necrostatin may also delay opening of mitochondrial permeability transition pores (see Figure 14-3) [Lim et al., 2007; Smith et al., 2007], or block the reduction in mitochondrial membrane potentials caused by excitotoxic stimuli [Hsu et al., 2009]. Furthermore, RIP1 is an essential component of the complex formed by TRADD, RIP1, and Rac1 upon death receptor activation [Shen et al., 2004] (see Figure 14-2). This complex then activates membrane-bound NOX1 NADPH oxidase to produce O_2^- [Kim et al., 2007]. Superoxide radical formation is critical to TNF and Fas-induced necrotic cell death in L929 (fibrosarcoma cells), and is potentiated in the presence of pan-caspase inhibition, the exact setting in which necrostatin has maximal effect to block cell death [Vercammen et al., 1998; Shen and Pervaiz, 2006].

Necrostatin appears to be a useful tool to direct therapy at "continuum" and other hybrid forms of neurodegeneration, and may allow improved understanding of some of the complex interactions and ordering of key components of death receptor-mediated injury mechanisms that result from HI injury to the immature brain. Importantly, it may additionally clarify the contribution of hybrid or continuum forms of neurodegeneration to HI neonatal brain injury. This task is likely to be simplified by the recent identification of the genes most important to the cellular signaling network that regulates necroptosis and the molecular bifurcation that controls the choice of apoptotic vs hybrid forms of cell death [Hitomi et al., 2008].

The Cell Death Matrix

Studies show that the morphologic appearance of the dying cell is a valuable tool for providing hints about the biochemical and molecular events responsible for cell death [Portera-Cailliau et al., 1997]. When studying mechanisms of cell death in human disease and in animal/cell models of disease, we believe that it is helpful to embrace the idea that apoptosis, necrosis, autophagy, and nonapoptotic PCD are not strictly "black and white." For the nervous system, this complexity is overlaid with cell death mechanisms that are influenced by brain

maturity, capacities for protein/RNA synthesis and DNA repair, antioxidant status, neurotrophin requirements, location in brain, and location relative to the primary sites of injury, as well as intensity of the insult. These factors that influence nervous system damage, at least in animal models, can make the pathobiology of perinatal HIE seem to abandon strict certainty and causality, thus yielding a neuropathology that is probabilistic and uncertain.

To help organize neurodegeneration and discover laws that determine causes and effects in neurodegenerative settings, the concept of the cell death continuum was extended to a hypothetical cell death matrix to embrace the "fuzziness" and spatiotemporal dynamics of cell death in the injured CNS (see Figure 14-4). A matrix might be a useful tool for pathology in general, and specifically for delineating and mathematically modeling the contributions and temporal/spatial emergence of the different forms of cell death, and the possible identification and prediction of previously unrecognized forms of cell death in human neurological disorders and in their animal/cell models. Our cell death matrix draws on the framework of biological space/time. It integrates space (location in brain, location of primary insult) and time into a continuum; thus, cell death manifests in a brain regional three-dimensional context, with time playing the role of a fourth dimension that is of a different context than the spatial dimension. By combining space and time into a single matrix we can potentially organize a large number of cell death phenotypes and mechanisms into a manageable frame of reference to reveal the potential early and delayed responses of the brain to injury.

A cell death matrix could also be useful for modeling how drugs and other treatments can influence outcomes. We need to identify better the relationships between mechanisms of cell death and the structure of dying cells in human pathology, in developing and adult CNS, as well as in animal and cell models of neurotoxicity in undifferentiated immature and terminally differentiated cells. It must be emphasized strongly that much more work needs to be done on the pathobiology of human HIE to define its cell death types better. To help with this necessity, perinatal intensivists and pediatric neurologists must encourage autopsy. The concept of a cell death matrix could be important for understanding neuronal degeneration in a variety of pathophysiological settings, and thus may be important for mechanism-based neuroprotective treatments in neurological disorders in infants, children, and adults. If brain maturity and brain location dictate how and when neurons die relative to the insult [Martin et al., 1998; Martin, 2001], then the molecular mechanisms responsible for neuronal degeneration in different brain regions (and at different times after the injury) in infants and children might be different from the mechanisms of neuronal degeneration in adults; hence, therapeutic targets will differ, and, thus, therapies will need to be customized for different brain regions, postinsult time, and age groups.

Effects of Hypothermia on Neuronal Cell Death Following HIE

Hypothermia is the only effective method of neuroprotection currently available for the clinical treatment of neonatal HIE [Gunn et al., 1998; Gluckman et al., 2005; Shankaran et al., 2005; Thoresen and Whitelaw, 2005; Jacobs et al., 2007; Azzopardi et al., 2009]. The neuroprotective clinical effects appear to derive from the ability of hypothermia to interrupt cell death cascades at multiple levels in non-neuronal and neuronal cells [Thoresen and Whitelaw, 2005; Zhao et al., 2007]. Specifically, hypothermia results in a reduction in cerebral metabolism that slows cell depolarization, prevents ATP depletion, reduces accumulation of excitotoxic neurotransmitters, preserves blood–brain barrier integrity, suppresses oxygen and nitrogen free radical release and lipid peroxidation of cell membranes, blocks postischemic inflammation by suppressing microglial activation and cytokine release, and may effect gene and protein expression in a positive manner [Mitani and Kataoka, 1991; Thoresen et al., 1997; Gunn and Bennet, 2002; Colbourne et al., 2003; Erecinska et al., 2003; Zhao et al., 2007; Gonzalez and Ferriero, 2008; Polderman, 2009]. The effect of cooling on non-neuronal cells in the brain is also likely important to its overall efficacy. Endothelial cells are a front-line target for reperfusion injury, and in vitro hypothermia blocks activation of both extrinsic and intrinsic apoptosis cascades, suppresses Fas-mediated caspase-8 activation, returns levels of Bax and Bcl-2 to control levels, blocks expression of cleaved caspase-3, and inhibits activation of JNK1/2 in endothelial cells [Yang et al., 2009]. A full review of the effects of hypothermia on non-neuronal cells is beyond the scope of this chapter; however, these new data suggest that many additional studies of the effect of hypothermia on non-neuronal cell death in the neonatal brain are needed.

Despite the effects of hypothermia on excitotoxic and oxygen free radical release, initial animal studies suggested that hypothermia specifically blocked apoptotic cell death but not necrotic cell death following transient HI in the neonatal piglet [Edwards et al., 1995]. Many subsequent mechanistic studies have followed this observation by focusing primarily on effects of hypothermia to block caspase-3 activation. Both intra-ischemic and postischemic hypothermia block cytochrome c release from mitochondria, caspase-3 activation and apoptotic cell death as determined with TUNEL (terminal deoxynucleotidyl transferance duTP nick end labelling) labeling [Zhu et al., 2004b, 2006], which is not specific for apoptosis [Martin et al., 1998]. Intra-ischemia hypothermia additionally blocks translocation of AIF to nuclei and supports cell survival by inhibiting dephosphorylation of Akt [Zhu et al., 2006]. Postischemic hypothermia may not have the same effect on Akt phosphorylation [Tomimatsu et al., 2001]. A combination of intra-ischemic hypothermia and pan-caspase inhibition pretreatment provides robust and additive neuroprotection in the Vannucci model [Adachi et al., 2001] suggesting that hypothermia is also blocking non-caspase-mediated cell death pathways. Recent studies now confirm that hypothermia blocks necrosis as well as apoptosis following neonatal HI in rat [Ohmura et al., 2005]. This is consistent with our findings that 24 hours of mild, whole-body hypothermia with sedation and paralysis has profound, perhaps sustained, neuroprotective effects on the HI piglet striatum where we find necrosis to be the major form of neurodegeneration and minimal evidence for apoptosis [Agnew et al., 2003]. Hypothermia-mediated striatal neuroprotection may result from blocking NMDA receptor activation and

oxidative damage to proteins [Mueller-Burke et al., 2008], as well as preventing ischemia-induced downregulation of the GluR2 AMPA receptor subunit that limits Ca^{2+} influx [Colbourne et al., 2003].

In an important study, it was shown that experimental asphyxia causes long-lasting morphologic modification of postsynaptic densities. These damaged postsynaptic densities stained intensely for ubiquitin, and hypothermia effectively blocked both the morphological and molecular changes [Capani et al., 2009]. Whether neurons with damaged synapses are ultimately targeted for premature cell death is unknown. It is also important to note that it is not known if neurons salvaged by treatment with hypothermia are normal. We have found that neurons can exist in damaged atrophic states with few synaptic contacts for months after injury [Ginsberg and Martin, 1998]. Determining the functionality of rescued neurons will have important implications for neurologic function following neonatal HI. The panoply of neuroprotective effects of hypothermia suggests that it may work to prevent neuronal cell death along the cell death continuum and throughout our hypothetical cell death matrix.

Conclusion

It will be extremely important to combine data from biochemical studies with information on cell death structure following different degrees and types of perinatal brain injury to understand better which insults are most likely to respond to antinecrosis, anti-apoptosis, anti-autophagy, or combination therapies, and whether these therapies actually ameliorate injury or simply delay or change the mode of cell damage. Animal studies predict that apoptosis inhibitors alone will be inadequate to ameliorate most of the early brain damage following neonatal HI [Martin et al., 2000; Northington et al., 2001b], and the cell death continuum predicts that apoptosis inhibitor drugs administered at acute and perhaps delayed time points may push cell degeneration from apoptosis to apoptosis-variant or necrotic cell death, as seen in vitro with caspase inhibitors applied following chemical hypoxia [Formigli et al., 2000]. When given as a pretreatment, inhibitors of autophagy may also push neurodegeneration along the cell death continuum in a deleterious manner [Carloni et al., 2008]. No studies to date have shown this; however, inhibitors of programmed necrosis may actually afford the opportunity to push neurodegeneration from necrosis to apoptosis. In settings where postinjury inflammation contributes to delayed neurodegeneration, this may actually be beneficial. Using concepts from the cell death matrix, we predict that it will be difficult to pinpoint appropriate times for effective mechanism-based, spatially directed drug therapy, particularly for neonatal HIE. It is especially important to prepare for the possibility that pharmacological interventions directed against a single mechanism of injury might only delay, convert, or worsen the evolving brain damage associated with HIE in newborns. For this reason, hypothermia might be an ideal strategy because it appears to protect against necrosis and apoptosis [Ohmura et al., 2005], and may be working along both the cell death continuum and possibly the space/time gradient that defines the matrix of cell death. Clearly, much more experimental and clinical work needs to be done. In light of these difficulties, it is clear that combination therapies with broad neuroprotective properties, acting at early and late time points, and alternative therapeutic approaches using stem and progenitor cells should be investigated for the treatment of perinatal HIE.

Dedication

This chapter is dedicated to the memory of Dr. Michael LeBlanc, Neonatology, University of Mississippi.

Acknowledgments

The authors are supported by the March of Dimes Foundation (6-08-275) and NS 059529- (FJN), AG 016282 (LJM), NS 060703 (LJM), NS 052098 (LJM), and by a grant from the Broccoli Foundation (FJN).

 The complete list of references for this chapter is available online at **www.expertconsult.com**. See inside cover for registration details.

Neuroinflammation

Pierre Gressens and Zinaida S. Vexler

Introduction

Inflammation and the developing brain

Until recently, the central nervous system (CNS) has been thought to be an immune privileged organ. However, neuronal injury or a potent immune stimulation can induce a cascade of immune responses within the CNS. It is now clear that neuroinflammation is linked with the development of several diseases affecting the adult and developing CNS, including infectious, autoimmune, degenerative, ischemic, and traumatic disorders. The impact and mechanisms of action of neuroinflammation might be different in the developing brain, as compared to the adult CNS. In addition, there is growing evidence that, in the context of inflammation, there is important crosstalk between the CNS and the periphery, and that systemic inflammation can have deleterious effects on the developing brain, further extending the concept of neuroinflammation. In the developing brain, these different aspects of neuroinflammation have been particularly well characterized in the context of perinatal brain damage; they will be further described in the present chapter in models of developmental neuroinflammation.

Perinatal Brain Damage

The consequences of perinatal injury include a spectrum of disorders, such as mental retardation, cerebral palsy, epilepsy, vision and hearing loss, learning difficulties, and school failure. Periventricular white matter damage, including periventricular leukomalacia, is most frequently observed in human preterm neonates [Volpe, 2009]. Full-term neonates with perinatal encephalopathy generally develop gray matter damage that most frequently affects the neocortex, basal ganglia, and hippocampus [Volpe, 2001]. Cerebrovascular occlusion leading to perinatal stroke may be arterial or venous, but excludes global injuries due to hypoxic-ischemic injury. Neurodevelopmental disability, including cerebral palsy, epilepsy, and behavior disorders, as well as impaired vision and language, is common after perinatal stroke [Kirton and deVeber, 2009].

The pathophysiology of perinatal brain damage (see Chapters 17 and 18) has proven to be multifactorial, with sensitizing factors occurring in utero that make the brain more vulnerable to secondary insults occurring around birth, such as hypoxia-ischemia (HI), and excess release of glutamate leading to excitotoxicity [Dammann et al., 2002; Mesples et al., 2005b; Nelson and Chang, 2008; Degos et al., 2008]. Systemic inflammation linked to chorioamnionitis has been recognized as a key sensitizing factor, while CNS inflammatory responses have been shown to play a key modulatory role in the amplitude of brain damage and subsequent adverse neurological outcome.

Systemic Inflammation and Perinatal Brain Damage

Epidemiological studies have shown a strong association between fetal infection/inflammation (chorioamnionitis) and brain damage in the newborn and/or neurological handicap in survivors [Dammann and Leviton, 2007]. Experimental studies have confirmed a sensitizing effect of systemic inflammation on perinatal brain lesions induced by hypoxic-ischemic or excitotoxic insults [Dommergues et al., 2000; Eklind et al., 2005]. In addition, some experimental data also suggest that perinatal exposure to infectious/inflammatory factors can alter, in a more or less subtle manner, the programs of brain development that will result in lasting neurological deficits. The relationship between this latter observation and human diseases remains to be fully demonstrated, although clinical evidence is supportive of this hypothesis [Volpe, 2009].

Sensitizing Effect

As mentioned above, perinatal brain damage may be caused by a combination of several insults. In this so-called multiple hit hypothesis, systemic infection/inflammation linked to chorioamnionitis can act as predisposing factors, making the brain more susceptible to a second stress (sensitization process). Indeed, systemic injection of low doses of lipopolysaccharide (LPS) to developing rats makes the newborn brain significantly more susceptible to hypoxic-ischemic insult [Eklind et al., 2005]. Similarly, systemic injection of interleukin-1-beta (IL-1β) or LPS to newborn mice or rats makes the brain much more sensitive to an excitotoxic insult [Dommergues et al., 2000]. The mechanisms by which sensitization is working are not yet fully understood, but could include changes in gene transcription and modifications of glutamate receptor activity.

Disruption of Brain Programming

Systemic infection/inflammatory factors can also alter brain development by themselves, even if they do not induce major clastic lesions. Accordingly, injection of *Escherichia coli* to pregnant rabbits induces diffuse white matter cell death [Debillon et al., 2000], and injection of *Ureaplasma parvum*, a pathogen frequently observed in chorioamnionitis, to pregnant mice induces myelin defects and loss of interneurons in the offspring [Normann et al., 2009]. Similarly, injection of LPS to pregnant rats induces transient central inflammation and myelination defects in the offspring [Rousset et al., 2006]. Of major concern, exposure of newborn mice to low doses of systemic IL-1β induces a moderate and transient inflammatory response during the neonatal period, that may be sufficient to disrupt oligodendrocyte maturation, myelin formation, and axonal development [Favrais and Gressens, personal communication]. These white matter abnormalities are moderate during the developmental period but persist until adulthood. They lead to permanent deficiencies in cognitive testing without detectable effects on motor function. The relevance of these abnormal behaviors to human pathology remains to be confirmed. The underlying molecular mechanisms include alterations of the transcription of genes implicated in oligodendrogenesis, myelin formation and axonal maturation.

Blood–Brain Barrier

At birth, the blood–brain barrier (BBB) in the neonate is substantially more mature than is commonly thought. The tight junctions are present early in embryonic development [Kniesel et al., 1996], restricting entrance of proteins into the brain in a controllable fashion, and by birth the BBB is functional with no fenestrations [Engelhardt, 2003]. The presence of the barrier substantially affects leukocyte passage but does not guarantee minimal leukocyte transmigration. The use of direct inflammatory challenge, such as intrastriatal injections of IL-1β or tumor necrosis factor alpha (TNFα) in rats of different ages, does not show a linear decline of leukocyte transmigration with age [Anthony et al., 1997], but rather that the newborn CNS is more resistant to inflammatory stress than the juvenile brain. The reported magnitude of BBB disturbance following HI or focal stroke in neonatal rodents varies and depends on the aspect of barrier studied [Svedin et al., 2007; Faustino et al., 2009]. Degradation of the extracellular matrix plays a role in neonatal ischemic injury. Excessive activation of matrix metalloproteinase-9 (MMP-9) early after HI is deleterious to the immature brain, as demonstrated by smaller injury size in MMP-9 knockout mice [Svedin et al., 2007] and following pharmacological inhibition of this protease [Leonardo et al., 2008].

Crosstalk between the Periphery and the CNS

The precise molecular mechanisms by which circulating mediators of inflammation have a deleterious effect on perinatal brain lesions remain a matter for debate [Hagberg and Mallard, 2005]. Circulating cytokines do not seem to cross the intact BBB easily, although this issue is contested. Different alternative pathways have been proposed to link serum cytokines with brain damage [Malaeb and Dammann, 2009]. Several major crosstalk mechanisms are outlined in Figure 15-1. Circulating cytokines could initially alter the permeability of the BBB to inflammatory mediators and cells. They could also act directly on parts of the brain lacking the BBB, such as the circumventricular organs, meninges, and choroid plexus, or, as demonstrated in the adult brain, indirectly through activation of the vagal nerve. Cytokine effects also could be mediated by cyclo-oxygenases (Cox) located in the BBB. In particular, cytokines could activate the inducible isoform Cox-2 to enhance the local production of prostaglandin E_2 (PGE$_2$), which could have deleterious effects on the developing brain. This latter mechanism has been demonstrated in a mouse model of perinatal excitotoxic brain damage [Favrais et al., 2007]. Some of these deleterious effects could involve an autocrine/paracrine loop, leading to excess production of inflammatory cytokines by brain cells.

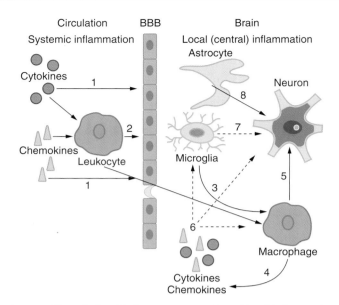

Fig. 15-1 The relationship between systemic and local inflammation after neonatal brain injury, and the key inflammatory mechanisms that contribute to neonatal brain injury and modulate the role of sensitization. 1, Direct effect of the systemic inflammatory mediators on brain endothelium. 2, The effect of the systemic inflammatory mediators on leukocyte-mediated activation of local inflammation. 3, Microglia activation. 4, Propagation of neuroinflammation by release of toxic species, including cytokines and chemokines from macrophages, both endogenous and invading. 5, Direct injurious effects of microglial cells. 6, Effects of locally produced inflammatory mediators to propagate injury and directly affect neurons. 7, Protection by microglia-produced growth factors and cytokines. 8, Astrocyte-mediated effects. BBB, blood–brain barrier.

Glial Cells

Macrophages are seen in abundance following neonatal HI [McRae et al., 1995; Ivacko et al., 1996] and focal stroke [Dingman et al., 2006; Denker et al., 2007], producing inflammatory cytokines, high levels of nitric oxide, MMPs, and complement molecules. The early postinjury macrophage population is predominantly comprised of resident microglia rather than invading monocytes [Denker et al., 2007]. The notion that microglia contribute to, rather than limit, acute ischemic injury in the immature brain comes from findings that reduction in injury is associated with diminished microglial activation/monocyte infiltration [Arvin et al., 2002; Dommergues et al., 2003]. At the same time, several studies have shown that anti-inflammatory drugs thought to protect adult brain by reducing macrophage accumulation after stroke protect neonatal brain without directly affecting inflammatory mechanisms associated with microglial activation [Tikka et al., 2001; Fox et al., 2005; van den Tweel et al., 2005; Dingman, et al. 2006]. Distinct steps of microglial maturation and differentiation (such as expression of class II histocompatibility complex [MHC], cathepsin, and other molecules), and the propensity of neurons to undergo apoptosis in the developing brain, may account for this age-dependence of the microglial response. Complement activation – C3 and C1q deposition in particular – is deleterious after HI, whereas sensitizing of neonatal rodents with cobra venom factor or deletion of the C1q gene confers protection [Cowell et al., 2003; Ten et al., 2005]. The mechanisms of protection are not completely understood but may include decreased C3 deposition and reduction in neutrophil activation [Ten et al., 2005].

The relative contribution of proinflammatory mechanisms in astrocytes, as opposed to other roles of these cells in ischemic injury, is not well understood but astrocytes express MHC and can upregulate inducible nitric oxide synthase (iNOS) and increase cytokine production. Mast cells have been shown to play an injurious role in neonatal HI [Jin et al., 2007] and focal stroke [Biran et al., 2008]. The injurious effects of these cells are thought to depend on TGF-β and IL-9 [Mesples et al., 2005a]. Less is known about the contribution of the T and B cell infiltration that is seen at later time points after injury.

Individual Inflammatory and Cell Signaling Molecules

Cytokines and Chemokines

Clinical data on the pathophysiological role of inflammatory cytokines in perinatal brain damage, including in term babies, continue to emerge [Grether and Nelson, 1997; Foster-Barber and Ferriero, 2002; Bartha et al., 2004].

Overall, it appears that IL-1 potentiates ischemic brain injury. Following HI or transient middle cerebral artery occlusion (MCAO) in neonatal rats, brain IL-1β expression is increased rapidly [Hagberg et al., 1996; Denker et al., 2007] following a major rapid systemic increase of IL-1β protein [Denker et al., 2007]. Brain IL-1β levels can be further amplified by concomitant infection or manipulations within the oxidant pathways [Doverhag et al., 2008; Girard et al., 2008]. The pro-inflammatory shift in balance between IL-1β and IL-1ra following HI when combined with infection (modeled by endotoxin or LPS exposure) can play a role in the initiation of perinatal brain damage [Girard et al., 2008]. IL-1β-induced local inflammatory reaction and chemokine expression, with the consequent leukocyte attraction and BBB disruption, is age-dependent [Anthony et al., 1997]. Studies that use genetic deletion of IL-1β or IL-1α alone, or in combination (IL-1αβ knockout), however, show no protection after HI injury [Hedtjarn et al., 2005], indicating the presence of multiple or desynchronized pro- and anti-injurious effects of IL-1, which are all abrogated in knockout mice. IL-18, a pro-inflammatory cytokine from the IL-1 family, also contributes to HI injury [Hedtjarn et al., 2002].

TNFα can exhibit pleiotropic functions in the ischemic adult brain. It may lead to apoptosis by reacting with Fas-associated death domain (FADD) and caspase-8, whereas signaling through TNFR2 can lead to anti-inflammatory and anti-apoptotic functions, depending on the cell origin of TNFα production and the type of receptor involved. In adult, TNFα-induced sensitization prior to cerebral ischemia is shown to be associated with a preconditioning response, whereas TNFα sensitization post stroke is detrimental [Hallenbeck, 2002]. In neonatal brain injury the pathophysiological role of TNFα may also be complex. A key role of TNFα in injury in an excitotoxic model combined with prior inflammatory challenge (IL-1β) has been recently demonstrated [Aden et al., 2009]. A TNFα blocker, etanercept, did not affect brain damage when given before injury, but substantially ameliorated injury when given after the combined inflammatory and excitotoxic insult, suggesting that TNFα may act by producing

an imbalance between pro- and anti-inflammatory cytokines in injured brain [Aden et al., 2009].

Type 2 T helper (Th2) cytokines play multiple roles in neonatal brain injury. The IL-9/IL-9 receptor pathway, which is most active in the newborn brain, has a direct anti-apoptotic action in the newborn neocortex [Fontaine et al., 2008], and contributes to HI and excitotoxic injury in the developing brain, presumably by activating mast cells [Dommergues et al., 2000; Patkai et al., 2001]. IL-10, a Th2 cytokine that is synthesized in the CNS and can act on hematopoietic and nonhematopoietic cells, can reverse injury caused by IL-1β, TNFα, and IL-6. In a white matter lesion model in P5 rats, protection is seen when IL-10 is administered post insult, whereas treatment prior to or at the time of insult is ineffective [Mesples et al., 2003].

Chemokines play a key role in crosstalk between peripheral and local responses. The pathophysiological role of the CC-class chemokine, monocyte chemoattractant protein 1 (MCP-1), in neonatal brain injury is evident from protection by functional inactivation of MCP-1 post insult [Galasso et al., 2000] or in mice with depleted IL-1 converting enzyme [Xu et al., 2001]. The role of the CXC-(Cys-X-Cys chemokine) family chemokines after neonatal brain injury is less understood but may be crucial for BBB modulation after inflammatory challenge of injured immature brain [Anthony et al., 1998]. Information on SDF-1 (CXCL12), which has been suggested to play a role in homing stem cells to regions of ischemic injury and repair in the adult, is rather scarce in the neonate but the timing for SDF-1-mediated chemotaxis and recruitment of reparative cells in the neonate may be narrow [Miller and Tran, 2005].

Intracellular Reactive Oxidant Metabolism

Oxidative stress and inflammation are tightly linked. Once activated, the inflammatory cells generate reactive oxygen species (ROS), which, in turn, trigger an inflammatory response. Superoxide anion, which is generated via Cox, xanthine oxidase, and NADPH (nicotinamide adenine dinucleotide phosphate) oxidase and is utilized via superoxide dismutase (SOD) in the cytosol and mitochondria, plays an important role in ischemic injury. Copper Zinc (CuZn) SOD overexpression exacerbates brain injury after HI by increased superoxide utilization and hydrogen peroxide (H_2O_2) accumulation in injured developing brain [Fullerton et al., 1998; Sheldon et al., 2004]. Enhanced activity of anti-oxidative metabolism is protective [Sheldon et al., 2008], supporting the notion of the pro-injurious role of oxidative stress in neonatal ischemic brain injury.

The role of NADPH oxidase in neonatal brain injury is now better understood. Genetic deletion of gp91-phox (the catalytic subunit of nicotinamide adenine dinucleotide phosphate) increases the extent of brain injury in two neonatal models, the HI model in P9 mice and an excitotoxic model in P5 mice [Doverhag et al., 2008], rather than decreasing injury, as seen in adult stroke. More severe HI injury parallels reduced NADPH oxidase activity and enhanced local neuroinflammation.

NO generation can have opposing roles in the process of ischemic injury, depending on the NOS isoform and cell type. iNOS inhibition is neuroprotective in neonatal HI models [Peeters-Scholte et al., 2002; Dingman et al., 2006], but inhibition is not necessarily associated with reduced proliferation of microglial cells.

Intracellular Inflammatory Signaling Pathways

The transcription factor nuclear factor-κβ (NF-κβ) is involved in the regulation of inflammation and neuronal death after stroke. It is normally located in the cytoplasm as a heterodimer composed of p65 and p50 subunits, bound to the endogenous inhibitor protein Iκβ (Nfκβ subunit). Dissociation of this complex by phosphorylation of Iκβ allows it to translocate to the nucleus, bind to functional κβ sites, and induce an array of genes involved in inflammation. NF-κβ plays a dual role in HI [Nijboer et al., 2008a, b]. NF-κβ inhibition during the early peak of activation prevents upregulation and accumulation of p53 in the nucleus and caspase-3 activation, and results in major neuroprotection weeks after injury [Nijboer et al., 2008a], whereas prolongation of inhibition abolishes the effect on neuronal apoptosis and even exacerbates injury [Nijboer et al., 2008a]. Taken together, these results demonstrate the crucial role of timing in the effects of potentially neuroprotective strategies.

Data on the contribution of mitogen-activated protein kinases (MAPK) to neonatal ischemic injury continue to accumulate. The extracellular signal-regulated kinase (ERK1/2) activation is generally neuroprotective in brain injury, whereas MAPK p38 activation is deleterious after HI [Hee Han et al., 2002]. The contribution of p38 to injury may depend on the model used, however [Fox et al., 2005]. Targeted deletion of the brain-specific c-Jun N-terminal kinase (JNK) isoform has been shown to reduce the overall JNK activity and protect mice against HI [Pirianov et al., 2007].

Anti-Inflammatory Strategies and Neuroprotection

The progressive elucidation of the pathophysiological mechanisms by which inflammation can harm the developing brain allows the design of new neuroprotective strategies specifically targeting mediators of neuroinflammation. Different strategies have been tested in relevant animal models; some of them, especially those for which clinically relevant drugs are available [Wolfberg et al., 2007], are summarized in Table 15-1.

Although some of these strategies offer the potential to limit brain damage in the newborn and other neuroinflammatory diseases affecting the developing brain, several points need to be considered before moving towards clinical trials. The developing brain is very different from the adult brain and therefore data from the adult literature cannot be extrapolated without confirmatory developmental studies. Some inflammatory mediators, such as microglia, have deleterious or beneficial roles, depending on the timing after the insult and/or the cellular/molecular context in which they are administered. Therefore, the timing of intervention might be critical for outcome. Use of some of these agents also has to be evaluated in the context of their systemic and nervous system side effects during maturation, and balanced with their potential benefits.

Table 15-1 Potential Targets and Drugs for Protection Against Neuroinflammation

Target	Examples of Drugs with Potential Clinical Use
Inflammation	Glucocorticoids, hypothermia
BBB integrity	?
MMP-9	?
Cox	Nonsteroidal anti-inflammatory drugs (Cox-2 inhibitors)
Microglia	Minocycline, melatonin, cannabinoids, hypothermia
Mast cells	Cromolyn, histamine receptor blockers
Cytokines	Etanercept (soluble TNFα receptor), IL-1 receptor antagonist, IL-10, tianeptine
Chemokines	Broad-spectrum chemokine inhibitors
ROS	N-acetyl-cysteine, melatonin, hypothermia
iNOS	Aminoguanidine, tilarginine acetate
NF-κβ	?
JNK	JIP peptide
Mitochondria	Caspase antagonists, minocycline
Multiple known targets	Hypothermia, erythropoietin, topiramate

BBB, blood–brain barrier; IL, interleukin; iNOS, inducible nitric oxide synthase; JIP, jnk interacting protein; JNK, Jun N-terminal kinase; MMP, matrix metalloproteinase; NF, nuclear factor; ROS, reactive oxygen species; TNF, tumor necrosis factor.

Conclusions and Areas of Future Development

Neuroinflammation has emerged as a key pathophysiological mechanism in a myriad of neurological disorders affecting the adult and the developing brain. Cellular and molecular players are being indentified, allowing the design of new potential targets for neuroprotection. In parallel, the concept of inflammation as a sensitizing process for the developing brain has emerged in the last decade, opening the possibilities for linking pre- or perinatal events with somewhat remote brain diseases. Despite these major advances, several areas remain rather poorly explored, such as the impact of sensitization processes on postlesional plasticity or the impact of systemic inflammation on epigenetic mechanisms.

 The complete list of references for this chapter is available online at **www.expertconsult.com**.
See inside cover for registration details.

Neonatal Seizures

Frances E. Jensen and Faye S. Silverstein

Neonatal seizures are common, subtle, difficult to diagnose and treat, and associated with a greater long-term risk of neurodevelopmental disabilities. This chapter provides a comprehensive overview of the epidemiology, diagnosis, pathophysiology, electrophysiology, etiologies, treatment, and prognosis of neonatal seizures. We also discuss current controversies regarding the optimal diagnosis and treatment of neonatal seizures and highlight recent advances in understanding the basic mechanisms that underlie the distinctive features of neonatal seizures. Since neonatal seizures are inextricably linked with their etiologies, several other chapters also include discussion of their diagnostic evaluation, treatment, and prognosis.

Epidemiology

Estimates of the incidence of neonatal seizures range from 1 to 3.5/1000 term births in the United States and similar rates have been reported from other developed countries. The incidence of neonatal seizures is substantially higher in premature infants, approaching rates as high as 5.8 percent in preterm neonates with birth weights less than 1500 g [Lanska et al., 1995].

Diverse case detection methods have been utilized in epidemiologic studies to determine the incidence of and associated risk factors for neonatal seizures. Lanska et al. [1995] attempted to identify all potential cases in one Kentucky county over 4 years [Lanska et al., 1995; Lanska and Lanska, 1996]. Their strategy was to search hospital-based medical record systems, regional birth certificate data files, and National Center for Health Statistics multiple-cause-of-death mortality data files, and couple these data with independent review of abstracted medical records for potential cases by three neurologists using prospectively determined case-selection criteria; they found 3.5 cases/1000 live births. Saliba et al. [1999] estimated the incidence of clinical neonatal seizures among newborns born between 1992 and 1994 in Harris County, Texas, by incorporating cases from four sources: hospital discharge diagnoses, birth certificates, death certificates, and a clinical study conducted concurrently at a tertiary care center in Houston, Texas; they reported 1.8 cases/1000 live births [Saliba et al., 1999]. In contrast, Ronen et al. performed a prospective study that included all obstetrical and neonatal units in Newfoundland, Canada [Ronen et al., 1999]. All units were given educational sessions on neonatal seizure symptoms, and detailed questionnaires were prospectively collected for all infants with probable neonatal seizures over a 5-year period; their reported rate was 2.6/1000 births. Glass et al. [2009] used a California Office of Statewide Planning and Development-linked Vital Statistics/Patient Discharge Data file created specifically to study perinatal outcomes, based on a cohort of 2.3 million California children born at >36 weeks' gestation between 1998 and 2002 [Glass et al., 2009]. The matched file linked 97 percent of California birth certificates to the corresponding newborn and maternal hospital discharge record. The resulting data set included demographic data and up to 25 International Classification of Diseases, Ninth Revision, Clinical Modifications (ICD-9-CM) maternal and infant discharge diagnoses [Martin et al., 2008]. These approaches have all yielded rates in a relatively similar range. An important caveat that must be recognized in interpretation of all these reports is that they are invariably based on the clinical diagnoses of seizures. Later in this chapter, we will discuss the limitations inherent in reliance on clinical (rather than electroencephalographic) criteria for the diagnosis of neonatal seizures. None the less, there is substantial concordance among many studies regarding the relatively high incidence of neonatal seizures and the increased risk in premature infants. Among the studies cited above, the most recent one, that in which California births from 1998 to 2002 were analyzed, reported that the incidence of seizures during the birth admission was 0.95/1000 live births, i.e., at the low end of prior estimates [Glass et al., 2009]. Whether this rate reflects a significant decline in neonatal seizure frequency remains to be determined.

A consistently identified trend is the greater risk for seizures in premature than in term infants. Some studies have reported an inverse relationship between birth weight category (or degree of prematurity) and seizure risk. Neonatal seizure rates of 57.5/1000 live births have been reported among very low birth weight infants (less than 1500 g), compared with 4.4/1000 for infants with moderately low birth weight (1500–2499 g), 2.8/1000 for those with normal birth weight (2500–3999 g), and 2.0/1000 for those with high birth weight (4000 or more grams) [Lanska et al., 1995; Lanska and Lanska, 1996]. This was corroborated by another study that found that seizure incidence was highest among infants weighing less than 1500 g (19/1000) and decreased as birth weight increased [Saliba et al., 1999]. In the prospective study from Newfoundland, the rates reported were 11.1/1000 for preterm neonates, and 13.5/1000 for infants weighing less than 2500 g at birth (presumably including both preterm and small-for-gestational-age neonates) [Ronen et al., 1999]. Analysis of a recent population-based cohort of very low birth weight infants in Israel reported that the incidence of neonatal seizures was 5.6 percent (i.e. the same as in the study from Kentucky cited above, in the preceding decade). In the study from Israel, male sex, and major systemic and neurological comorbidities (e.g., intraventricular hemorrhage or periventricular leukomalacia) were independent predictors of neonatal seizures. Male gender was also identified as a risk factor in preterm infants with seizures in the Harris County, Texas, cohort (relative risk = 1.8, 95 percent confidence interval: 1.0, 3.4) [Saliba et al., 2001]. Gender differences in seizure incidence have also been identified in term infants; in the northern California cohort cited earlier, the proportion of males was higher in the seizure group than in the overall cohort (57.3 percent vs. 50.9 percent) [Glass et al., 2009]. Ethnicity-related risk factors for neonatal seizures have not been reported.

In the Texas cohort [Saliba et al., 2001], multivariate analysis identified several additional risk factors for term infants, including birth by cesarean section, low birth weight for gestational age, birth in a private/university hospital, and maternal age of 18–24, compared with 25–29 years. In the California cohort study, using multivariable logistic regression analysis, neonates of women aged 40 years and older who were nulliparous, or had diabetes mellitus, intrapartum fever, or infection, or delivered at > 42 weeks were at increased risk for seizures [Glass et al., 2009].

Pathophysiology

Since neonatal seizures are refractory to conventional antiepileptic drugs (AEDs) and can have severe consequences for long-term neurologic status, there is a growing body of research directed at defining age-specific mechanisms of this disorder to identify new therapeutic targets and biomarkers. There have been substantial advances with regard to understanding pathophysiology, particularly with respect to identification of the developmental stage-specific factors that influence mechanisms of seizure generation, responsiveness to anticonvulsants, and the impact of seizures on central nervous system (CNS) development (for detailed review, see Rakhade and Jensen [2009]). In addition, experimental data have raised concerns about the potential adverse effects of current treatments with barbiturates and benzodiazepines on brain development. Improved understanding of the unique age-specific mechanisms should yield new therapeutic targets with clinical potential. However, to date, no novel compounds have been specifically developed or achieved Food and Drug Administration (FDA) approval for treatment of neonatal seizures [Sankar and Painter, 2005].

Developmental age-specific mechanisms influence the generation and phenotype of seizures, the impact of seizures on brain structure and function, and the efficacy of anticonvulsant therapy. Factors governing neuronal excitability combine to create a relatively hyperexcitable state in the neonatal period, as evidenced by the extremely low threshold for seizures and reflected by the fact that, across the life span, this is the period when seizures occur most commonly [Hauser et al., 1993; Aicardi and Chevrie, 1970]. Similarly, in the rodent, seizure susceptibility peaks in the second postnatal week in many models, a time period compatible with the neonatal period in humans [Sanchez and Jensen, 2001; Sanchez et al., 2005b; Rakhade and Jensen, 2009]. In addition, the incomplete development of neurotransmitter systems results in a lack of "target" receptors for conventional AEDs. Finally, the relatively limited degree of cortical and subcortical myelination results in the multifocal nature or unusual behavioral correlates of seizures at this age [Haynes et al., 2005; Talos et al., 2006a].

The neonatal period is a period of intense physiological synaptic excitability, as synaptogenesis is wholly dependent upon activity. In the human, synapse and dendritic spine density are peaking around birth and into the first months of life [Takashima et al., 1980; Huttenlocher et al., 1982]. In addition, the balance between excitatory versus inhibitory synaptic activity is tipped in favor of excitation to permit robust activity-dependent synaptic formation, plasticity, and remodeling [Rakhade and Jensen, 2009]. Glutamate is the major excitatory neurotransmitter in the CNS, while gamma-aminobutyric acid (GABA) is the major inhibitory neurotransmitter. There is considerable and growing evidence from animal models and human tissue studies that neurotransmitter receptors are highly developmentally regulated [Sanchez and Jensen, 2001; Rakhade and Jensen, 2009; Johnston, 1995] (Figure 16-1). Studies of cell morphology, myelination, metabolism and, more recently, neurotransmitter receptor expression suggest that the first 1–2 weeks of life in the rodent constitute an analogous stage to the human neonatal brain, and Figure 16-1 shows that both species reveal similar patterns of changes in neurotransmitters during this stage.

Enhanced Excitability of the Neonatal Brain

Glutamate receptors are critical for plasticity and are transiently overexpressed during development in animal models and human tissue studies. A relative overexpression of certain glutamate receptor subtypes in rodent and human developing cortex coincides with the ages of increased seizure susceptibility

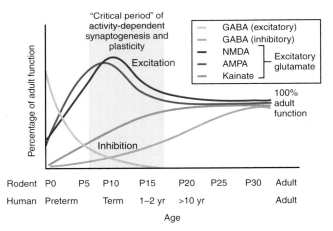

Fig. 16-1 Schematic depiction of the developmental profile of glutamate and GABA receptor expression and function. Equivalent developmental periods are displayed for rats and humans on the top and bottom x-axes, respectively. Activation of GABA receptors is depolarizing in rats early in the first postnatal week, and in humans up to and including the neonatal period. Functional inhibition, however, is gradually reached over development in rats and humans. Prior to full maturation of GABA-mediated inhibition, the NMDA and AMPA subtypes of glutamate receptors peak between the first and second postnatal weeks in rats, and in the neonatal period in humans. Kainate receptor binding is initially low and gradually rises to adult levels by the fourth postnatal week. Neonatal seizures emerge within the "critical period" of synaptogenesis and cerebral development. AMPA, alpha-amino-3-hydroxy-5-methyl-4-isoxazole propionate; GABA, gamma-aminobutyric acid; NMDA, N-methyl-D-aspartate; P, postnatal day. *(Reprinted from Rakhade and Jensen, 2009. Permission obtained from Nature Reviews Neurology.)*

(see Figure 16-1) [Sanchez and Jensen, 2001; Talos et al., 2006b; Sanchez et al., 2001]. Glutamate receptors include ligand-gated ion channels, permeable to sodium, potassium, and in some cases calcium, and metabotropic subtypes [Hollmann and Heinemann, 1994]. They are localized to synapses and extrasynaptic sites on neurons, and are also expressed on glia. The ionotropic receptor subtypes are classified based on selective activation by specific ligands:

- N-methyl-D-aspartate (NMDA)
- α-amino-3-hydroxy-5-methyl-4-isoxazolepropionic acid (AMPA)
- kainate.

NMDA receptors are heteromeric, including an obligate NR1 subunit, and their structure is developmentally regulated. In the immature brain, the NR2 subunits are predominantly those of the NR2B subunit type, with the functional correlate of longer current decay time compared to the NR2A subunit, which is the form expressed in later life on mature neurons [Jiang et al., 2007]. Other developmentally regulated subunits with functional relevance include the NR2C, NR2D, and NR3A subunits. Rodent studies show that these are all increased in the first 2 postnatal weeks, and this is associated with lower sensitivity to magnesium, the endogenous receptor channel blocker that in turn results in increased excitability (Figure 16-1 and Figure 16-2) [Hollmann and Heinemann, 1994; Wong et al., 2002]. NMDA receptor antagonists administered to immature rat pups are highly effective against a variety of hypoxic/ischemic insults and seizures in the immature brain [Stafstrom et al.,

1997; Chen et al., 1998; Mares and Mikulecka, 2009]. However, the clinical potential of NMDA antagonists may be limited due to their severe sedative effects and a propensity possibly to induce apoptotic death in the immature brain [Ikonomidou et al., 1999; Bittigau et al., 2003]. Importantly, memantine, an agent currently in clinical use as a neuroprotectant in Alzheimer's disease, may be an exception with fewer side effects, owing to its use-dependent mechanism of action [Chen et al., 1998; Manning et al., 2008; Mares and Mikulecka, 2009].

While the NMDA receptor is selectively activated in processes related to plasticity and learning, the AMPA subtype of glutamate receptor subserves most fast excitatory synaptic transmission. In addition, unlike the NMDA receptor, most AMPA receptors are not calcium-permeable in the adult. AMPA receptors are heteromeric and consist of four subunits, including combinations of the GluR1, GluR2, GluR3, or GluR4 subunits [Hollmann and Heinemann, 1994]. However, in the immature rodent and human brain, AMPA receptors are calcium-permeable because they lack the GluR2 subunit (see Figure 16-2) [Sanchez et al., 2001; Kumar et al., 2002]. AMPA receptor subunits are developmentally regulated, with GluR2 expressed only at low levels until the third postnatal week in rodents and later in the first year of life in human cortex [Talos et al., 2003, 2006b]. Hence AMPA receptors in the immature brain, owing to their enhanced calcium permeability, may play an important role in contributing not only to excitability but also to activity-dependent signaling downstream of the receptor. Both NMDA and AMPA receptors are expressed at

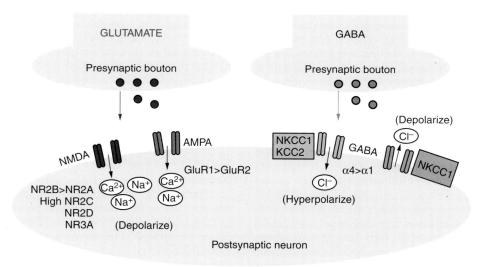

Fig. 16-2 Dynamics of synaptic transmission at cortical synapses in the neonatal period. Depicted are an excitatory glutamatergic synapse (left panel) and a GABAergic inhibitory synapse (right panel). Presynaptic release of glutamate results in depolarization (excitation) of the postsynaptic neuron (left panel) by activation of NMDA and AMPA receptors. In contrast, release of GABA (right panel) results in hyperpolarization (inhibition) when the postsynaptic neuron expresses sufficient quantities of the Cl⁻ transporter KCC2, but depolarization (excitation) when intracellular Cl⁻ accumulates as a result of unopposed action of the Cl⁻ importer NKCC1. The immature glutamatergic receptors (left panel) are comprised of higher levels of NR2B, NR2C, NR2D, and NR3A subunits of the NMDA receptor, enhancing influx of Ca^{2+} and Na^+ compared with mature synapses. In addition, AMPA receptors are relatively deficient in GluR2 subunits, resulting in increased Ca^21 permeability compared with mature synapses. Hence, specific NMDA receptor antagonists and AMPA receptor antagonists may prove to be age-specific therapeutic targets for treatment development. In addition, although GABA_A receptor activation normally results in hyperpolarization and inhibition at mature synapses, because of the coexpression of NKCC1 and KCC2, the expression of KCC2 is low in the neonatal period compared with later in life and thus Cl⁻ levels accumulate intracellularly; opening of GABA_A receptors allows the passive efflux of Cl⁻ out of the cell, resulting in paradoxic depolarization. GABA_A receptor subunit expression in the immature brain is typified by higher levels of the α4 subunit, which is functionally associated with diminished benzodiazepine sensitivity. Both these attributes of the GABA_A receptor make classic GABA agonists such as barbiturates and benzodiazepines less effective in the neonatal brain. The NKCC1 channel blocker bumetanide has anticonvulsant efficacy when administered with phenobarbital, suggesting a synergistic effect.

levels and with subunit composition that enhance excitability of neuronal networks around term in the human and in the first 2 postnatal weeks in the rodent (see Figure 16-2).

Rodent studies show that AMPA receptor antagonists are potently effective against neonatal seizures, even superior to NMDA receptor antagonists or conventional AEDs and GABA agonists. Topiramate, which is FDA-approved for the treatment of seizures in children and adults, is an AMPA receptor antagonist, in addition to several other potential anticonvulsant mechanisms [Shank et al., 2000]. Topiramate is effective in suppressing seizures and long-term neurobehavioral deficits in a rodent neonatal seizure model, even when administered following seizures [Koh and Jensen, 2001; Koh et al., 2004]. In addition, topiramate in combination with hypothermia was neuroprotective in a rodent neonatal hypoxia-ischemia model [Liu et al., 2004]. Finally, the specific AMPA receptor antagonist talampanel, currently in phase II trials for epilepsy in children and adults, as well as for amyotrophic lateral sclerosis, was recently shown to protect against neonatal seizures in a rodent model [Aujla et al., 2009].

Decreased Efficacy of Inhibitory Neurotransmission in the Immature Brain

Expression and function of the inhibitory GABA$_A$ receptors are also developmentally regulated. Rodent studies show that GABA receptor binding, synthetic enzymes, and overall receptor expression are reduced early in life compared to later [Sanchez and Jensen, 2001; Swann et al., 1989]. GABA receptor function is regulated by subunit composition, and the $\alpha 4$ and $\alpha 2$ subunits are relatively overexpressed in the immature brain compared to the $\alpha 1$ subunit (see Figure 16-2) [Brooks-Kayal et al., 1998]. Notably, when the $\alpha 4$ subunit is expressed, the receptor is less sensitive to benzodiazepines compared to receptors containing $\alpha 1$ [Kapur and Macdonald, 1999], and as is often the case clinically, seizures in the immature rat respond poorly to benzodiazepines [Jensen et al., 1995; Swann et al., 1997].

Receptor expression and subunit composition can partially explain the resistance of seizures in the immature brain to conventional AEDs that act as GABA agonists. However, inhibition of neuronal excitability via GABA agonists relies on the ability of GABA$_A$ receptors to cause a net influx of chloride (Cl$^-$) from the neuron, resulting in hyperpolarization [Dzhala and Staley, 2003]. In the immature rodent forebrain, GABA receptor activation can cause depolarization rather than hyperpolarization [Khazipov et al., 2004; Loturco et al., 1995; Owens et al., 1996]. GABA$_A$-mediated depolarization occurs because the chloride (Cl$^-$) gradient is reversed in the immature brain: chloride (Cl$^-$) levels are high in the immature brain due to a relative underexpression of the Cl$^-$ exporter KCC2 compared to the mature brain (see Figure 16-1 and Figure 16-2) [Dzhala et al., 2005]. Recent studies in human brain have shown that KCC2 is virtually absent in cortical neurons until late in the first year of life, and gradually increases, while the Cl$^-$ importer NKCC1 is overexpressed in the neonatal human brain and during early life in the rat when seizures are resistant to GABA agonists [Dzhala et al., 2005]. The NKCC1 inhibitor, bumetanide, shows efficacy against kainate-induced seizures in the immature brain [Dzhala et al., 2008]. This agent, already FDA-approved as a diuretic in neonates, is currently under investigation in a phase I/II clinical trial as an add-on agent

for the treatment of neonatal seizures (www.clinicaltrials.gov; trial ID: NCT00830531).

Ion Channel Configuration Favors Depolarization in Early Life

Ion channels also regulate neuronal excitability and, like neurotransmitter receptors, are developmentally regulated. Mutations in the K$^+$ channels KCNQ2 and KCNQ3 are associated with benign familial neonatal convulsions [Cooper and Jan, 2003]. These mutations interfere with the normal hyperpolarizing K$^+$ current that prevents repetitive action potential firing [Yue and Yaari, 2004]. Hence, at the time when there is an overexpression of GluRs and incomplete network inhibition, a compensatory mechanism is not available in these mutations. Another K$^+$-channel superfamily member, the HCN (or h) channels, is also developmentally regulated. The h currents are important for maintenance of resting membrane potential and dendritic excitability [Pape, 1996], and their function is regulated by isoform expression. The immature brain has a relatively low expression of the HCN1 isoform, which serves to reduce dendritic excitability in the adult brain [Bender et al., 2001]. Ion channel maturation can thus also contribute to the hyperexcitability of the immature brain and can also have a cumulative effect when occurring in combination with the aforementioned differences in ligand-gated channels. Recently, selective blockers of HCN channels have been shown to disrupt synchronous epileptiform activity in the neonatal rat hippocampus [Bender et al., 2005], suggesting that these developmentally regulated channels may also represent a target for therapy in neonatal seizures. Both N- and P/Q-type voltage-sensitive calcium channels regulate neurotransmitter release [Iwasaki et al., 2000]. With maturation, this function is exclusively subsumed by the P/Q-type channels, formed by Cav2.1 subunits, a member of the Ca^{2+} channel superfamily [Noebels, 2003]. Mutations in Cav2.1 may be involved in absence epilepsy, suggesting a failure in the normal maturational profile [Chen et al., 2003].

A Role for Neuropeptides in the Hyperexcitability of the Immature Brain

Neuropeptide systems are also dynamically fluctuating in the perinatal period. An important example is corticotropin releasing hormone (CRH), which elicits potent neuronal excitation [Baram and Hatalski, 1998; Ju et al., 2003]. CRH and its receptors are expressed at higher levels in the perinatal period, specifically in the first 2 postnatal weeks in the rat, than later in life [Brunson et al., 2001b]. CRH levels increase during stress, and seizure activity in the immature brain may exacerbate subsequent seizure activity. Notably, adrenocorticotropic hormone, which has demonstrated efficacy in infantile spasms, also downregulates CRH gene expression [Brunson et al., 2001a]. Neuropeptide modulation may be an area of future clinical import in developing novel treatments for neonatal seizure.

Enhanced Potential for Inflammatory Response to Seizures in the Immature Brain

Neonatal seizures can occur in the setting of inflammation, either due to an intercurrent infection or secondary to hypoxic-ischemic injury. Experimental and clinical evidence exists for early microglial activation and inflammatory cytokine production in the developing brain when hypoxia-ischemia [Ivacko et al., 1996; Dommergues et al., 2003] or inflammation [Saliba and Henrot, 2001; Debillon et al., 2003] occurs. Importantly, microglia are highly expressed in immature white matter in rodents and humans during cortical development [Billiards et al., 2006]. Anti-inflammatory compounds or agents that inhibit microglial activation, such as minocycline, attenuate neuronal injury in some models of excitotoxicity and hypoxia-ischemia [Tikka et al., 2001]. During the term period, microglia density in deep gray matter is higher than at later ages; that is likely due to migration of the population of cells en route to more distal cortical locations. Experimental models demonstrate microglia activation, as seen by morphologic changes and rapid production of proinflammatory cytokines, occurring after acute seizures in different epilepsy animal models [Shapiro et al., 2008; Vezzani et al., 2008]. During development, microglia show maximal density simultaneous with the period of peak synaptogenesis [Dalmau et al., 2003]. During normal development, as well as in response to injury, microglia participate in "synaptic stripping" by detaching presynaptic terminals from neurons [Pfrieger and Barres, 1997; Stevens et al., 2007]. Importantly, the microglial inactivators, minocycline and doxycycline, are protective against seizure-induced neuronal death [Heo et al., 2006] and also protective in some neonatal stroke models [Jantzie et al., 2005; Lechpammer et al., 2008].

Selective Neuronal Injury in the Developing Brain

While many studies suggest that seizures, or status epilepticus, induce less death in the immature than in the adult brain, there is evidence that some neuronal populations are vulnerable. Similar to the sensitivity of subplate neurons, hippocampal neurons in the perinatal rodent undergo selective cell death, as well as oxidative stress, following chemoconvulsant-induced cell death [Wasterlain et al., 2002]. Stroke studies in neonatal rodents also suggest that there can be selective vulnerability of specific cell populations in early development [Stone et al., 2008]. Subplate neurons are present in significant numbers in the deep cortical regions during the preterm and neonatal period [Kinney et al., 2004]. These neurons are critical for the normal maturation of cortical networks [Lein et al., 1999; Kanold et al., 2003]. Importantly, in both humans and rodents, these cells possess high levels of both AMPA receptors and NMDA receptors [Talos et al., 2006a, b]. These cells may also lack oxidative stress defenses present in mature neurons. Animal models have revealed that these neurons are selectively vulnerable compared to overlying cortex following an hypoxic-ischemic insult [McQuillen et al., 2003]. Indeed, chemoconvulsant-induced seizures in rats, provoked by the convulsant kainate in early postnatal life, produced a similar loss of subplate neurons with consequent abnormal development of inhibitory networks [Lein et al., 1999].

A number of studies have shown that the application of clinically available antioxidants, such as erythropoietin, is protective against neuronal injury in neonatal stroke [Chang et al., 2005; Gonzalez et al., 2007]. Recently, erythropoietin was shown to reduce later increases in seizure susceptibility of hippocampal neurons following hypoxia-induced neonatal seizures in rats [Mikati et al., 2007].

Seizure-Induced Neuronal Network Dysfunction: Potential Interaction Between Epileptogenesis and Development of Neurocognitive Disability

Given that there is minimal neuronal death in most models of neonatal seizures, the long-term outcome of neonatal seizures is thought to be due to seizure-induced alterations in surviving networks of neurons. Evidence for this theory comes from several studies that reveal disordered synaptic plasticity and impaired long-term potentiation, as well as learning later in life, in rodents following brief neonatal seizures [Sayin et al., 2004; Ben Ari and Holmes, 2006]. The neonatal period represents a stage of naturally enhanced synaptic plasticity when learning occurs at a rapid pace [Silverstein and Jensen, 2007; Maffei and Turrigiano, 2008]. A major factor in this enhanced synaptic plasticity is the predominance of excitation over inhibition, which also increases susceptibility to seizures, as mentioned above. However, seizures that occur during this highly responsive developmental window appear to access signaling events that are central to normal synaptic plasticity. There are rapid increases in synaptic potency that appear to mimic long-term potentiation, and this pathologic activation may contribute to enhanced epileptogenesis [Rakhade et al., 2008]. In addition, GluR-mediated molecular cascades associated with physiological synaptic plasticity may be overactivated by seizures, especially in the developing brain [Cornejo et al., 2007; Rakhade et al., 2008]. Rodent studies demonstrate a reduction in synaptic plasticity in neuronal networks such as hippocampus following seizures early in life, suggesting that the pathologic plasticity may have occluded normal plasticity, and this mechanism could contribute to the impaired learning [Rakhade et al., 2008]. Many models reveal that neonatal seizures alter synaptic plasticity [Stafstrom et al., 2006], and recent studies are delineating the molecular signaling cascades that are altered following early-life seizures [Sanchez et al., 2005a; Raol et al., 2006]. In addition to glutamate receptors, inhibitory $GABA_A$ receptors can also be affected by seizures in early life, resulting in long-term functional impairments. Early and immediate functional decreases in inhibitory GABAergic synapses mediated by post-translational changes in $GABA_A$ subunits are seen following hypoxia-induced seizures in rat pups [Sanchez et al., 2005a]. Flurothyl-induced seizures result in a selective impairment of GABAergic inhibition within a week [Isaeva et al., 2006]. Importantly, there is evidence that some of these changes may be downstream of Ca^{2+} permeable glutamate receptors and Ca^{2+} signaling cascades, and that early postseizure treatment with GluR antagonists or phosphatase inhibitors may interrupt these pathologic changes that underlie the long-term disabilities and epilepsy [Sanchez et al., 2005a; Rakhade et al., 2008].

Diagnosis

Neonatal seizures can be difficult to diagnose, as there are often no clinical correlates of the electrographic seizures, a phenomenon called electroclinical dissociation. Regional interconnectivity, including interhemispheric as well as corticospinal, is not fully mature due to incomplete myelination of white matter tracts, leading to only modest behavioral manifestations of these seizures. Infants can show no signs or very subtle tonic or clonic movements, often limited to only one limb, making

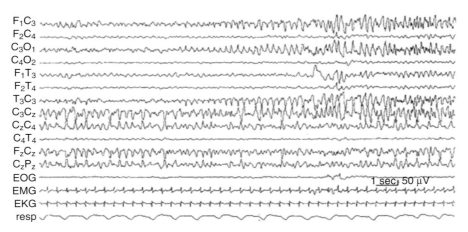

Fig. 16-3 Electroencephalographic appearance of neonatal seizures. Electrical seizure activity begins in the midline central region (CZ) and then shifts to the left central region (C3). Toward the end of the seizures, as the electrical activity persists in the left central region, the midline central region becomes uninvolved. This electrical seizure activity occurred in the absence of any clinical seizure activity in this 40-week gestational age female infant with hypoxic-ischemic encephalopathy. She was initially comatose and hypotonic, and, at the time of EEG recording, had been treated with phenobarbital. *(Reprinted with permission from Mizrahi EM, Kellaway P. Characterization and classification of neonatal seizures. Neurology 1987;37:1837–1844.)*

the diagnosis difficult to discern from myoclonus or other automatisms [Mizrahi and Kellaway, 1998]. A recent study revealed that approximately 80 percent of EEG-documented seizures were not accompanied by observable clinical seizures [Clancy, 2006a]. Hence, EEG is essential for diagnosis and for assessing treatment efficacy in this group (see Chapter 12). Full 20-lead EEGs are most sensitive in detecting these, often multifocal, seizures (Figure 16-3). As full-lead EEGs can be difficult to obtain on an emergent basis in many neonatal intensive care units, amplitude-integrated EEG (aEEG) devices are becoming increasingly utilized. aEEG is usually obtained from a pair or limited number of leads and is displayed as a fast Fourier spectral transform. With aEEG, seizures are detected by acute alterations in spectral width, and a raw EEG from the single channel can be accessed by the viewer for confirmation [Lawrence et al., 2009]. Several reports now indicate that aEEG has relatively high specificity but compromised sensitivity, detecting approximately 75 percent of that of conventional full-lead montage EEG [Tekgul et al., 2005a, b; Clancy, 2006b; Navakatikyan et al., 2006; Shellhaas and Clancy, 2007; Shellhaas et al., 2007; de Vries and Toet, 2006]. Chapter 12 discusses in detail the ontogeny of EEG development, the types of EEG patterns that can occur, and characteristic EEG abnormalities reported in various neonatal disorders.

Once neonatal seizures are confirmed, treatable metabolic, genetic, or symptomatic causes need to be identified. Serologic studies include blood and serologic studies to assess for systemic infection, and metabolic derangements such as electrolyte disturbances, acidosis and hypoglycemia. The timing of seizures can be a helpful indicator, such as in the case of "fifth day fits" or seizures due to hypocalcemia. Pyridoxine-dependent seizures present as refractory early neonatal seizures that uniquely respond to pyridoxine administration [Baxter, 2001; Grillo et al., 2001]. Seizures that continue to be refractory in the setting of a history consistent with hypoxic-ischemic encephalopathy (HIE) manifest within the first 24–48 hours of life, and persist over several days, then may gradually remit. Chapter 20 reviews metabolic disorders that can cause neonatal seizures.

Brain imaging is often the next step in the diagnostic evaluation. The type of brain imaging acquired depends on the clinical setting, institutional resources, and the infant's medical status. In premature infants, who are at greatest risk for intraventricular hemorrhage, cranial ultrasound is often the most appropriate initial neuroimaging modality. Computed tomography (CT) can provide useful complementary radiological information, but magnetic resonance imaging (MRI) may yield the most information concerning the etiology of neonatal seizures (see Chapter 11). Figure 16-4 illustrates how MRI, in some cases complemented by MR spectroscopy, can be informative with regard to the etiology of seizures.

MRI provides an important assessment of risk in infants with neonatal seizures. Imaging can identify cerebral dysgenesis and gross structural malformations that can be associated with neonatal seizures, such as that seen in association with tuberous sclerosis, hemimegalencephaly, or cortical dysplasias. For symptomatic seizures due to hypoxia-ischemia, abnormal T2, fluid-attenuated inversion-recovery (FLAIR) and diffusion-weighted imaging can localize regional injury and determine its severity [Grant and Yu, 2006]. MR spectroscopy can provide data estimating the severity of neuronal injury and may be an important prognostic indicator. A previous study has shown that in neonates with hypoxic-ischemic injury and seizures, an increased lactate to choline ratio, as well as reduced *N*-acetyl-aspartate ratios, was more abnormal in patients with a greater seizure burden [Miller et al., 2005]. Another study of term infants with asphyxia and/or seizures [Glass et al., 2009] demonstrated that, after adjusting for the degree of MRI abnormality, seizure severity was associated with a higher risk of neuromotor abnormalities at 4 years of age than in those without seizures. These results suggest that neonatal seizures may independently be associated with a poorer outcome, even when MRI lesions are present.

Etiology

Box 16-1 summarizes the general categories of disorders that can cause neonatal seizures. A step-wise diagnostic approach to determine the etiology of neonatal seizures will prioritize identification of treatable causes; however, clinical judgment and resource availability, among many factors, will influence

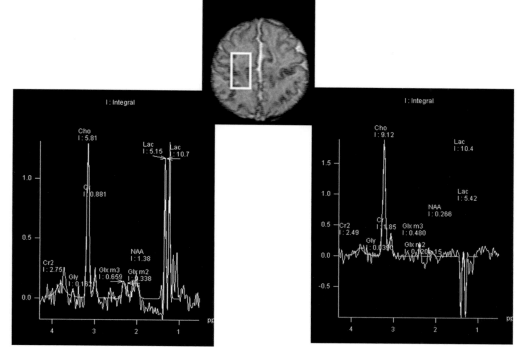

Fig. 16-4　An MRI performed on day 10. Diffuse signal abnormalities consistent with hypoxia-ischemia were shown, but the most distinctive finding was markedly elevated lactate peaks on MR spectroscopy (TE = 288 ms on left [lactate up] and TE = 144 ms on right [lactate down]). This infant died in the neonatal period. *(Images were generously provided by Drs. K. Poskitt and S. Miller, University of British Columbia.)*

Box 16-1　Etiologies of Neonatal Seizures

Acute Metabolic

- Hypoglycemia
- Hypocalcemia
- Hypomagnesemia
- Hypo- or hypernatremia
- Withdrawal syndromes associated with maternal drug use
- Iatrogenic associated with inadvertent fetal administration of local anesthetic
- Rare inborn errors of metabolism (including pyridoxine-responsive)

Cerebrovascular

- Hypoxic ischemic encephalopathy
- Arterial and venous ischemic stroke
- Intracerebral hemorrhage
- Intraventricular hemorrhage
- Subdural hemorrhage
- Subarachnoid hemorrhage

CNS infection

- Bacterial meningitis
- Viral meningoencephalitis
- Fetal infections

Developmental

- Multiple forms of cerebral dysgenesis

Other

- Rare genetic disorders (inborn errors of metabolism; vitamin dependency)
- Benign neonatal familial convulsions (sodium and potassium channel mutations)
- Early myoclonic encephalopathy

the sequence, extent, and rapidity of testing decisions. Assessment of the cause(s) and initiation of treatment(s) should occur concurrently. The cause of neonatal seizures is sometimes easily determined and in these cases little additional laboratory testing may be needed. Neurodiagnostic testing should proceed in a step-wise fashion, geared initially to confirm the diagnosis of seizures (discussed in the preceding section) and to identify disorders with specific effective treatments. The highest priorities are the identification of reversible, acute metabolic derangements and treatable infections. In neonates with unexplained seizures and depressed mental status, a lumbar puncture is an essential component of the initial diagnostic evaluation. Interpretation of cerebrospinal fluid abnormalities and the range of bacterial, viral, and other pathogens that cause neonatal CNS infections and their treatments are discussed in Chapters 10 and 80–82.

It is important to be cognizant of rare, potentially treatable conditions that can present with neonatal seizures (e.g. pyridoxine-dependent seizures), particularly if the seizures do not respond to conventional AED treatment and the underlying cause is not readily identified. In some cases (if seizures persist and are associated with unexplained encephalopathy), continuing the neurodiagnostic evaluation is warranted, including consideration of very rare disorders – identification of which may help illuminate prognosis and/or genetic recurrence risk. The general principles discussed in Chapter 20 on perinatal metabolic encephalopathies are applicable to this diagnostic approach.

Acute Metabolic Abnormalities

In neonates, poor feeding, as well as a broad range of systemic disorders, can result in hypoglycemia and seizures; the types of seizures vary and no features are pathognomonic. In a neonate with new-onset seizures, checking serum glucose concentrations and providing supplemental glucose, if warranted, should precede administration of AEDs. Although it is impossible to provide precise serum glucose values below which it is likely that seizures are attributable to hypoglycemia, commonly applied values are as follows: less than 45 mg% in term infants, and less than 30 mg% in premature infants. Unexplained or persistent hypoglycemia should prompt evaluation for an underlying endocrinopathy.

In neonates, total serum calcium values may be difficult to interpret, and free ionized calcium measurement provides a more accurate assessment to detect clinically significant hypocalcemia. Early (first 3 days of life) hypocalcemia can occur transiently in asphyxiated infants and in infants of mothers with diabetes or other endocrinopathies. In somewhat older infants, hypocalcemia can result from feeding with high phosphorus-containing formulas, and may be associated with low magnesium levels; this syndrome is currently very unusual in North America. Persistent neonatal hypocalcemia raises concerns about hypoparathyroidism (most commonly in association with other features of DiGeorge syndrome). Hyponatremia or hypernatremia can also result in seizures; both iatrogenic and endocrine etiologies should be considered.

Other acute metabolic derangements that can result in neonatal seizures are withdrawal syndromes associated with maternal therapeutic or illicit drug use. Rarely, neonatal seizures can result from abrupt withdrawal from a drug that was administered therapeutically to the mother; for example, otherwise unexplained seizures were described in a neonate whose mother was being treated for spasticity with baclofen [Ratnayaka et al., 2001]. Convulsions are an uncommon but well-recognized complication of the neonatal abstinence syndrome that is attributable to withdrawal from maternally administered opiates [Kaltenbach and Finnegan, 1986]; other neurological findings include frequent myoclonic jerks, tremor, irritability, poor sleep, a high-pitched cry, and autonomic instability. The combination of a relevant maternal history and associated clinical findings raises the index of suspicion for this etiology.

Exposure to anesthetics such as lidocaine and mepivacaine, accidentally injected into the fetal scalp with administration of local anesthesia during labor, has been described as a cause of neonatal seizures [Hillman et al., 1979; Kim et al., 1979].

Rare Inborn Errors of Metabolism and Genetic Disorders

There is an ever-expanding list of very rare metabolic and other genetic disorders that can present with neonatal seizures. Of particular clinical importance are those disorders for which specific biochemically targeted treatments are available (reviewed in Pearl [2009]). The prototypical disorder in this category is pyridoxine-dependent epilepsy (PDE) due to antiquitin deficiency (see Chapter 52). The clinical syndrome of refractory neonatal seizures that rapidly abated with intravenous administration of pyridoxine was well described for many years. The underlying genetic abnormality, alpha-aminoadipic semialdehyde dehydrogenase (antiquitin) deficiency, was recently delineated, and it was subsequently reported that folinic acid-dependent seizures were allelic with pyridoxine dependency. These disorders can be diagnosed by measurement of alpha-aminoadipic semialdehyde in urine; alternatively, seizure cessation in response to an empiric trial of intravenous pyridoxine with EEG (and EKG) monitoring can provide the initial

diagnosis. A related condition, pyridox(am)ine-5′-phosphate oxidase (PNPO) deficiency, also presents in neonates with a severe epileptic encephalopathy and is responsive to pyridoxal phosphate but not to pyridoxine. Consideration must be given in those neonates who have medically refractory epilepsy and who do not respond to pyridoxine, to using pyridoxal phosphate, which is not readily available for clinical use. Serine-dependent seizures (see Chapters 20 and 32) and glucose transporter deficiency (see Chapters 20 and 34) are similarly very rare causes of neonatal seizures that have specific treatments.

Inherited disorders of amino acid and organic acid metabolism can present with refractory neonatal seizures. Typically, encephalopathy (depressed mental status, hypotonia, and sometimes evidence of cerebral edema and increased intracranial pressure) is the most prominent clinical feature. Some of these infants are initially indistinguishable from those with HIE, and the persistence of refractory seizures beyond the first few days of life, coupled with lack of a history of a perinatal sentinel event, are often sufficient factors to warrant further diagnostic testing. Alternatively, affected infants may have a history of initial normal behavior and progression of symptoms after several feedings.

One of the best-characterized inborn errors of metabolism that can present with refractory neonatal seizures is glycine encephalopathy (nonketotic hyperglycinemia) [Hoover-Fong et al., 2004]. This disorder is caused by a defect in the glycine cleavage system; typical features in affected neonates include apnea, hypotonia, and persistent seizures. The diagnosis is established by detection of marked elevation in cerebrospinal fluid glycine concentrations, and more specifically, elevated ratio of cerebrospinal fluid:plasma glycine concentration (>0.08). Seizures may be attributable to overactivation of N-methyl-D-aspartate-type excitatory amino acid receptors (at a glycine regulatory site), and in some cases treatment with dextromethorphan, a clinically available weak NMDA antagonist, along with sodium benzoate, can help control refractory seizures in affected infants.

Peroxisomal biogenesis disorders (Zellweger's syndrome, neonatal adrenoleukodsytrophy, infantile Refsum's syndrome) can also present with persistent neonatal seizures and severe encephalopathy; there are typically associated subtle dysmorphic features (see Chapter 38) that prompt consideration of these disorders. The initial diagnostic testing includes measurement of serum very long chain fatty acids.

There are also other neurometabolic disorders that elude even the most advanced newborn screening assays and that can result in persistent neonatal seizures. Molybdenum cofactor deficiency, a very rare inherited metabolic disorder in which there is combined deficiency of aldehyde oxidase, xanthine dehydrogenase, and sulfite oxidase, typically presents soon after birth with intractable seizures; isolated sulfite oxidase deficiency is similarly very rare, and can also present with intractable neonatal seizures. An interesting feature of these two disorders is that their clinical manifestations, as well as neuroimaging features, can mimic hypoxic-ischemic injury, and this may lead to misdiagnosis and delayed awareness of genetic recurrence risks [Eichler et al., 2006]. However, neuroimaging with proton MR spectroscopy can provide important diagnostic clues [Basheer et al., 2007]. Proton MR spectroscopy demonstrates profound metabolic abnormalities with very high lactate peaks (see Figure 16-4), and MRI may demonstrate evolution of cystic white matter damage.

Benign Familial Neonatal Convulsions

These genetic disorders, typically inherited in an autosomal-dominant fashion, present with early neonatal seizures that typically remit within a few months of life, and are commonly associated with good neurological outcomes (see Chapter 52). Several mutations of potassium channel genes *KCNQ2* and *KCNQ3* have been identified in affected individuals [Coppola et al., 2003, 2006; Singh et al., 2003]. Another benign syndrome possibly associated with a mutation in *KCNQ2* is that of "fifth day fits," which transiently occur for a day or so around the fifth or sixth postnatal day [Claes et al., 2004]. Berkovic et al. have also identified mutations in the sodium channel gene *SCN2A* in families with autosomal-dominant "benign familial neonatal-infantile seizures." In these families, seizures began as early as day 2, but also as late as 7 months of age; in all reported cases, the seizures stopped by age 12 months [Berkovic et al., 2004].

Infection

Both neonatal sepsis and meningoencephalitis are often complicated by seizures. The most likely pathogens vary, depending on clinical setting (gestational age, postnatal age, geographic location). Empiric broad-spectrum antibiotic and antiviral therapy is usually initiated rapidly when infection is suspected, and if no pathogen is identified, the appropriate duration of therapy is a resulting clinical dilemma. Neonatal CNS infections are discussed in detail in Chapter 16.

Infections of the CNS, acquired prenatally, can also present in the neonatal period with seizures. These diverse infections, collectively classified as "TORCH" infections, are suspected in neonates with intracranial calcifications, unexplained hydrocephalus, and specific disease-associated systemic abnormalities. These are discussed in Chapters 80–82.

Hypoxic-Ischemic Encephalopathy

Term infants with neonatal encephalopathy as a result of hypoxia-ischemia are at particularly high risk for seizures (see Chapter 17). In two recent clinical trials of hypothermia for treatment of neonatal HIE, seizures were frequent at the time of randomization (40–60 percent) [Gluckman et al., 2005; Shankaran et al., 2005]. Clinically apparent seizures typically begin 6–12 hours after the asphyxial event; the pathophysiological mechanisms underlying this lag period are uncertain. Seizures are often difficult to control with medication for 2–3 days, and then often wane.

A subject of considerable controversy is whether seizures contribute to the progression of hypoxic-ischemic brain injury, and whether more rapid and effective control of seizures could improve neurodevelopmental outcome. Several studies provide evidence that seizures do, in fact, contribute to poor outcomes in affected neonates; however, to date, there is no evidence that seizure treatment is of long-term benefit [Booth and Evans, 2004].

Cerebrovascular Disorders

There is increasing recognition of the broad range of cerebrovascular pathology in neonates, and seizures are often the initial symptom of ischemic or hemorrhagic brain injury. Neonatal cerebrovascular disorders include arterial and venous infarction, and intracranial hemorrhage (intraparenchymal, intraventricular, subarachnoid, and/or subdural). These disorders are discussed in Chapter 18 and 19.

In term infants, perinatal arterial strokes most commonly occur in the left middle cerebral artery distribution and present with seizures in the first 2 days of life; seizures are often easily controlled, although there is a significant risk for later onset of epilepsy. Cerebral sinovenous thrombosis can occur in neonates with severe systemic illness or thrombophilic disorders, and can be complicated by the development of venous infarctions (cortical or deep) that result in seizures, which may be difficult to control.

The classic clinical presentation of subarachnoid hemorrhage in term infants is with seizures on the second day of life in an otherwise well-appearing infant. When a lumbar puncture is performed, the bloody fluid obtained is sometimes inappropriately attributed to procedure-related bleeding ("traumatic tap"); CT can confirm the diagnosis. Typically, no treatment beyond AEDs is required. Seizures are usually easily controlled, although there is no information available about the optimal duration of drug therapy when seizures occur as a result of subarachnoid hemorrhage.

Intraparenchymal hemorrhages, as a result of trauma, coagulopathy, vascular malformation, or unknown causes, may also present with seizures. There is an unusual reported association between temporal lobe hemorrhages and apneic seizures in full-term neonates [Sirsi et al., 2007]. Progression of intraventricular hemorrhage may provoke seizures in premature infants, sometimes in association with periventricular hemorrhagic infarction.

Congenital Heart Disease

Neonates with complex congenital heart disease are at high risk for seizures. Risk factors include coexistent CNS developmental anomalies, pre- and postnatal cerebrovascular compromise, hypoparathyroidism with DiGeorge syndrome complex, complications of cardiac catheterization including therapeutic interventions such as atrial septostomy, cardiopulmonary bypass intraoperatively, and diverse postoperative complications. These are reviewed in Chapter 101.

In the acute postoperative period, accurate seizure detection requires electrophysiological monitoring. In a study of 183 consecutive infants undergoing heart surgery who were monitored by video-EEG for 48 hours postoperatively, electrographic neonatal seizures occurred in 21 (11.5 percent); none had clinically visible seizure, while some of the affected infants had numerous seizures [Clancy et al., 2005]. Whether more rapid and effective treatment of seizures would improve neurodevelopmental outcome in these infants is an important unanswered question.

Developmental Disorders

Many types of cerebral dysgenesis present with neonatal seizures. Infants with CNS developmental anomalies may tolerate labor and delivery poorly, and initially, their seizures and encephalopathy may be attributable to perinatal asphyxia. Often, it is persistence of seizures or atypical manifestations (e.g., sustained unilateral focal motor seizures) that raise suspicion of underlying neurodevelopmental anomalies, and these are best delineated with MRI (as illustrated in Figure 16-5). These disorders are discussed in Part IV.

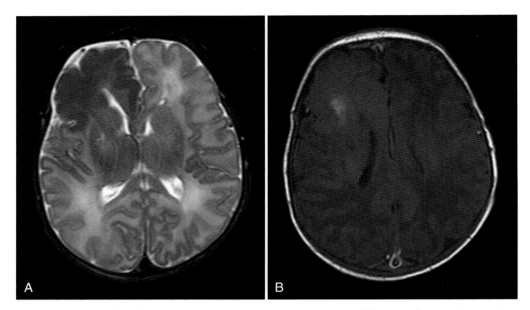

Fig. 16-5 Neonatal seizures resulting from focal cortical dysplasia. Brain MRI on day 2 of life in a full-term infant who began to have seizures, characterized by bilateral clonic movements of both arms (right greater than left, and deviation of the eyes to the right) within several hours of an uneventful birth (Apgars 9 and 9, at 1 and 5 min). A standard protocol brain MRI with and without IV contrast was performed on a 1.5 Tesla scanner. **A,** Abnormal cortical thickening of the right frontal lobe is demonstrated, with decreased white matter and dysmorphic frontal horn of right lateral ventricle. **B,** Abnormal increased T1 signal is demonstrated in this region, along with absence of mass effect or pathological enhancement after contrast administration. Seizures were refractory to multiple antiepileptic drugs, and this dysplastic lesion was surgically resected when the infant was 2 months old.

Treatment

Although the preceding sections highlighted the importance of electrophysiology in confirmation of the diagnosis of neonatal seizures, in practice, treatment is commonly based on clinical diagnosis (or high index of suspicion for seizures). In neonatal intensive care units, treatable common metabolic causes such as hypoglycemia, hypocalcemia, and hypomagnesia have become infrequent but, none the less, must not be overlooked. In fact, initial diagnostic evaluation (described in the preceding section) and treatment should occur concurrently. The treatment of neonatal seizures is related, at least in part, to an understanding of the underlying cause in each infant, and correction of identified metabolic derangements, along with ensuring adequate ventilation and support of circulation, should precede consideration of AED therapy.

In neonates, single seizures are unusual, and recurrence is expected. Single seizures are treated in a similar fashion to status epilepticus in older age groups, i.e., with rapid intravenous administration of a full loading dose of an AED, most commonly phenobarbital (20–30 mg/kg) [Bartha et al., 2007; Blume et al., 2009]. There is no consensus regarding the optimal second-line therapy, if seizures persist. Options include additional phenobarbital, phenytoin or fosphenytoin, lorazepam or midazolam, and lidocaine (Table 16-1).

Systematic assessment of AED efficacy for treatment of neonatal seizures is extremely challenging and very limited data are available. There is consensus that such studies need to incorporate continuous EEG monitoring, both for confirmation of the diagnosis and also for assessment of the efficacy of treatment [Silverstein et al., 2008]. Studies that include evaluation of long-term outcomes also require selection of uniform or well-matched populations with respect to gestation, gender, and neurological and systemic disease. The classic study of Painter and colleagues compared the efficacy of loading doses of phenobarbital and phenytoin for treatment of EEG-confirmed seizures in term infants [Painter et al., 1999]. Their major findings were that these drugs were equally but incompletely effective, that either drug alone controlled seizures in fewer than half of the patients, and that adding the second drug conferred some additional benefit (overall rate of seizure control was about 60 percent). Although the two agents are equipotent, phenobarbital is used much more widely in neonatal intensive care units. In many centers, fosphenytoin has replaced phenytoin as the second-line intravenous drug, since it is considered much less likely to cause local injury if there is tissue extravasation.

Benzodiazepines are often used for treatment of refractory seizures. Hypotension and respiratory depression may complicate treatment, and midazolam has gained more widespread usage in intensive care unit settings because of its short half-life. Variable efficacy (ranging from minimal to 100 percent) has been reported for midazolam as a second-line or third-line medication. A recent study reported that in 10 of 13 neonates with EEG-confirmed status epilepticus that had been refractory to conventional therapy (40 mg/kg phenobarbital ± phenytoin 20 mg/kg), treatment with midazolam infusion was effective within an hour [Castro Conde et al., 2005]. A favorable response to treatment was defined as no more than two electrical seizures per hour lasting less than 30 seconds. Their midazolam dose was an initial intravenous bolus of 0.15 mg/kg, followed by continuous infusion (1 μg/kg/min), increasing by 0.5–1 μg/kg/min every 2 minutes until a favorable response or a maximum of 18 μg/kg/min was attained; if status epilepticus persisted after the initial bolus, another bolus of 0.10–0.15 mg/kg was administered 15–30 minutes later.

Table 16-1 Current Drug Therapy for Neonatal Seizures

Drug	Route of Administration	Initial Dose	Comments
Phenobarbital	Intravenous or oral	20–40 mg/kg	Most widely used initially; substantial dosing variation
Fosphenytoin or phenytoin	Intravenous	20 mg/kg phenytoin equivalents	Must be given slowly to avoid cardiac arrhythmias
Midazolam	Intravenous	0.15 mg/kg bolus, followed by infusion of 1 µg/kg/min up to 18 µg /kg/min*	Careful monitoring of cardiorespiratory status required
Lorazepam	Intravenous	0.05–0.1 mg/kg	Careful monitoring of cardiorespiratory status required
Lidocaine	Intravenous	2 mg/kg over 10 min, followed by 6 mg/kg/h for 6 h, with subsequent wean†	Contraindicated with congenital heart disease or prior phenytoin
Levetiracetam	Intravenous or oral	Uncertain	More neonatal data needed
Topiramate	Oral	Uncertain	More neonatal data needed

* See text and Castro Conde et al. [2005] for additional details.
† See text and Malingre et al. [2006] for additional details.

Lidocaine infusion can also be effective for treatment of refractory neonatal seizures, but concerns about cardiac toxicity have limited widespread adoption of this agent. A recent European study provided a detailed protocol [Malingre et al., 2006] that recommended a loading dose of 2 mg/kg in 10 minutes, followed by the continuous infusion of 6 mg/kg per hour for 6 hours, 4 mg/kg per hour for 12 hours, and finally 2 mg/kg per hour for 12 hours. The authors provided specific guidelines for its usage, including that it only be used in a neonatal intensive care unit with continuous cardiac monitoring, that the infusion be stopped if any cardiac arrhythmia develops, that it be used only for seizures that have not responded to phenobarbital and midazolam, and that it not be used in infants with congenital heart disease or prior treatment with phenytoin.

In older age groups, the intravenous formulation of levetiracetam is gaining acceptance for rapid treatment of seizures and status epilepticus; there is insufficient information about pharmacokinetics and safety in neonates to recommend its utilization currently.

Metabolic Therapies

Administration of pyridoxine is often considered in neonates with unexplained refractory seizures. There are no widely accepted clinical criteria that mandate this treatment trial and practice varies. Intravenous administration of 100 mg pyridoxine with continuous EEG and cardiac monitoring should result in a marked attenuation of epileptiform activity within 15 minutes in responders; doses as high as 500 mg have been suggested. Rarely, treatment is associated with adverse effects, including onset of respiratory depression up to a day later [Pearl, 2009]. Of interest, a recent report described the novel strategy of antenatal pyridoxine supplementation in a pregnant woman with a family history of pyridoxine-dependent neonatal seizures [Bok et al., 2010].

Although recent work indicates genetic overlap between pyridoxine-responsive and folinic acid-responsive neonatal seizures, infants who respond preferentially to folinic acid (2.5–5 mg/day) have been described. There are recently described cases of mutations in the pyridox(am)ine-5′-phosphate oxidase gene, in which affected individuals presented with neonatal seizures unresponsive to pyridoxine and anticonvulsant treatment but responsive to pyridoxal phosphate. Pyridox(am)ine-5′-phosphate oxidase converts pyridoxine phosphate and pyridoxamine phosphate to pyridoxal phosphate, which is the biologically active form [Bagci et al., 2008].

Chronic Therapy

An important unresolved issue is whether chronic AED therapy is warranted in neonates. In many term neonates whose seizures are attributable to acute brain injury, seizures stop by the end of the first week of life. There is less information available about the natural history of seizures in premature infants. Although there is a significant risk for development of epilepsy after neonatal seizures, there is no evidence that AED therapy modifies this risk. None the less, continuation of AED therapy after hospital discharge is common [Bartha et al., 2007].

Hellstrom-Westas et al. evaluated the risk of seizure recurrence within the first year of life in 31 neonates for whom antiepileptic treatment was discontinued after 1–65 days (median 4.5 days) [Hellstrom-Westas et al., 1995]. Seizures recurred in only three – one infant receiving prophylaxis, one treated for 65 days, and one infant treated for six days – and in this small group, no clinical features were predictive of recurrence. A retrospective study that attempted to evaluate whether chronic phenobarbital treatment influenced seizure recurrence or neurological development found no benefit [Guillet and Kwon, 2007]. These investigators are now undertaking a prospective study to address this issue (www.clinicaltrials.gov; trial ID: NCT01089504).

The Interaction Between Anticonvulsants and the Developing Brain

Emerging identification of age-specific mechanisms for neonatal seizures is pointing to the use of novel therapeutic targets. Caution must be exercised when devising new therapies, as the target may indeed be essential for normal brain development, albeit a contributor to neuronal hyperexcitability. Over two decades ago, experimental data emerged demonstrating that phenobarbital exposure had adverse effects on survival and morphology of cultured neurons, derived from fetal mouse tissue, and these observations raised concerns about risks of this drug for treatment of neonatal seizures [Bergey et al., 1981; Serrano et al., 1988]. Subsequent studies in neonatal rats demonstrated that daily treatment with phenobarbital or diazepam in the first postnatal month resulted in measurable changes in regional cerebral metabolism and behavior [Pereira et al., 1990; Schroeder et al., 1995].

More recently, evidence emerged that brief systemic treatment with conventional AEDs, such as phenobarbital, diazepam, phenytoin, and valproate, increases apoptotic neuronal death in normal immature rodents [Bittigau et al., 2002]. Similarly, NMDA receptor antagonists also induce an increase in constitutive apoptosis in the developing rodent brain [Ikonomidou et al., 1999]. Yet, the AMPA receptor antagonists NBQX and topiramate do not cause such adverse effects [Ikonomidou et al., 1999; Glier et al., 2004], although the mechanism for this relative safety over the other agents is not understood. The novel AED levetiracetam also has no effect on apoptosis in the developing brain [Manthey et al., 2005].

Despite these data on adverse effects or lack thereof in rodents, minimal evidence of similar phenomena exists for other species, and it remains unknown if these toxicity mechanisms are relevant for human neonates. Moreover, interpretation of AED toxicity studies must be tempered by the consideration that these experiments are typically performed in normal animals, and that the impact of AED administration may well differ in normal animals and in those with seizures.

Prognosis

Neonatal seizures are associated with high neonatal mortality. In survivors, there is a significant risk for the development of epilepsy and subsequent motor and cognitive deficits. Although population risks for adverse outcomes can be ascertained, it is very challenging to predict neurodevelopmental outcome in individual neonates with seizures. Clinicians need to consider seizure manifestations, etiology, response to treatment, gestational age, and the results of clinical examination, electrophysiology, and brain imaging studies in formulating their predictions. This approach stems from clinical experience and trends that have emerged from studies reported over the past 25–30 years. Prematurity, neonatal encephalopathy ("hypoxia-ischemia"), cerebral dysgenesis, and frequent, prolonged, or medically refractory seizures are associated with worse neurodevelopmental prognosis.

Holden et al. (1982) reviewed the prognosis of 277 newborns with seizures who were enrolled in the National Collaborative Perinatal Project (data collected about 50 years ago) [Holden et al., 1982]; gestational age was less than 36 weeks in about 30 percent. There was 35 percent mortality, and 30 percent of survivors had adverse neurological outcomes at age 7 years; these included cerebral palsy (13 percent), intelligence quotient less than 70 (19 percent), and epilepsy (20 percent), alone or in combination. Bergman et al. [1983] evaluated outcomes in 131 children, aged 1–5 years old, who had neonatal seizures, and were treated in a single intensive care unit from 1976 to 1979. Half were born at less than 37 weeks' gestation (28 percent at or below 31 weeks). Fifty-one of 131 were normal, 42 had minor to moderate disabilities, 30 had severe disabilities, and 6 had died (2 were lost to follow-up); 26 had epilepsy.

Of 77 with neonatal asphyxia and seizures, 41 developed moderate or severe disabilities. Significant neonatal predictors of poor outcome included later onset of seizures, tonic seizures, and seizures lasting for many days. Although seizure frequency and neonatal mortality were greatest in very premature infants, the outcome in survivors did not differ from that in term infants.

In a study of 90 infants with prospectively diagnosed clinical neonatal seizures, born in Newfoundland between 1990 and 1995, trends were similar [Ronen et al., 2007]. Among term infants, 28 of 62 (45 percent) were normal, whereas only 3 of 15 (20 percent) surviving preterm infants were normal. Of survivors, 17 (27 percent) developed epilepsy, 16 (25 percent) had cerebral palsy, 13 (20 percent) had mental retardation, and 17 (27 percent) had learning disorders. Variables associated with poor prognosis were severe encephalopathy, cerebral dysgenesis, complicated intraventricular hemorrhage, infections in preterm infants, abnormal neonatal EEGs, and the need for multiple drugs to treat the neonatal seizures. Pure clonic seizures without facial involvement in term infants suggested favorable outcome, whereas generalized myoclonic seizures in preterm infants were associated with mortality.

Brunquell et al. [2002] performed a retrospective review of 77 cases of neonatal seizures (2.2 percent of their neonatal intensive care unit admissions over 7 years), and also found that clinical seizure semiology (determined from review of medical records) was predictive of outcomes. Neonatal mortality was high (30 percent). Of 53 survivors with mean 3.5-year follow-up, 59 percent had abnormal neurological examinations, 40 percent were mentally retarded, 43 percent had cerebral palsy, and 21 percent had epilepsy. Compared with patients with other seizure types, those with subtle and generalized tonic seizures or two or more seizure types had a higher prevalence of adverse outcomes.

In a recent study of 89 term infants with clinical seizures evaluated at the Children's Hospital in Boston, neonatal mortality was 7 percent, and long-term neurological outcome was poor in 28 percent. Cerebral dysgenesis and global hypoxia-ischemia were associated with poor outcome. Normal neonatal/early infancy neurological examination and normal/mildly abnormal neonatal EEG were associated with a favorable outcome, particularly if neonatal neuroimaging was normal [Tekgul et al., 2005b, 2006].

A recent study from Italy is noteworthy because enrollment was restricted to infants with video-EEG-confirmed seizures; 106 neonates, admitted to a single neonatal intensive care unit from 1999 to 2004, were enrolled (51 preterm, 55 full-term) [Pisani et al., 2007]. They also evaluated the prognostic significance of neonatal status epilepticus, defined as continuous seizure activity for 30 minutes or recurrent seizures lasting more than 30 minutes without definite return to baseline neurological condition between seizures. At age 24 months, 34 percent were normal, 19 percent had died, and 47 percent had an adverse outcome. Of those with neonatal status epilepticus, 25 of 26 had adverse outcomes. Birth weight, severely abnormal cerebral ultrasound scans, and status epilepticus were independent predictors of abnormal outcome.

A critical unanswered question is whether effective treatment of seizures could improve outcomes. A recent Cochrane analysis concluded that there was no evidence that treatment of neonatal seizures improved outcome; however, this analysis was based on evaluation of conventional AEDs with limited efficacy in neonates [Booth and Evans, 2004]. Moreover, it is evident that the underlying cause is a major determinant both of medical "refractoriness" and of neurodevelopmental outcome. The converse, however, is also true, and the deleterious effects of seizures may be most pronounced in the setting of underlying hypoxic-ischemic brain injury.

Miller et al. used MR spectroscopy to evaluate brain metabolism and integrity in neonates with asphyxia and (clinically detected) seizures [Miller et al., 2002]. This analysis demonstrated that seizures contributed to abnormal metabolism (as measured by the lactate/choline ratio) and tissue injury (as measured by the N-acetyl-aspartate/choline ratio). In neonates with neonatal hypoxic-ischemic brain injury (based on neonatal MRI measures), neonatal seizures (again, clinically detected) were an independent risk factor for adverse neurodevelopmental outcome at age 4 years [Glass et al., 2009]. Similarly, in the CoolCap neonatal asphyxia and hypothermia treatment trial, the absence of seizures was a predictor of better outcome [Wyatt et al., 2007]. Mechanisms that could account for seizure-induced amplification of ischemic injury include increases in brain temperature and metabolic demands, generation of mediators (such as reactive oxygen species) that contribute to tissue damage, and disruption of endogenous protection and repair mechanisms [Silverstein, 2009].

Underlying CNS pathology influences the prognosis of neonatal seizures, but it is also possible that neonatal seizures have complex effects on the impact of and recovery from neonatal brain injury (distinct from amplification of hypoxic-ischemic injury). In a recent study of cognitive outcome after unilateral perinatal ischemic stroke that included longitudinal testing of intellectual and cognitive abilities at two time points in 29 children, one of the most remarkable and unexpected findings was that the presence of seizures had an adverse effect on cognitive outcome. The mechanisms underlying this limitation of plasticity and reorganization after neonatal brain injury remain uncertain, and the effects of seizures and their treatment with AEDs could not be distinguished [Ballantyne et al., 2008].

Future Directions

Effective prevention and more effective early treatment of HIE could reduce the incidence of newborn seizures and their adverse impact. Similarly, since preterm infants have a higher risk for seizures, interventions that reduce rates of premature birth would also contribute to reduced frequency of neonatal seizures. Pediatric neurologists can work collaboratively to help achieve these goals. Concurrently, there will be opportunities to improve the diagnosis and treatment of neonatal seizures, and to develop and refine experimental models that can yield new insights about mechanisms of seizure-related brain injury and neuroprotection.

There are many practical challenges that must be addressed to implement clinical trials of new AEDs in neonates. Incorporation of continuous EEG monitoring into clinical studies of neonatal seizure therapy is a daunting task. Delineation of reasonably homogeneous clinical populations for study and practical stratification strategies that take into account the critical factors that contribute to outcome, including gestational age, seizure cause, and systemic disorders, and their treatments are prerequisites for trials of anticonvulsant efficacy, as well as neurological outcomes. It also will be essential to assess AED interactions with other therapies (e.g., induced hypothermia) in critically ill neonates. There will be opportunities to perform therapeutic trials of new agents with well-defined clinical outcome measures. Systematic evaluation of safety and pharmacokinetics in the appropriate study populations must precede analysis of efficacy, and this is particularly challenging in neonates. Multicenter and interdisciplinary collaborations are essential for the success of such studies.

Clinical therapeutic trials in neonates would be greatly improved if there were accurate biomarkers of acute and chronic therapeutic efficacy, yet none exists other than the EEG. There is no widely approved consensus regarding optimal "standard" lead montage for EEG monitoring in neonates, although fewer leads may be more appropriate clinically. There is considerable enthusiasm for introduction of aEEG devices into neonatal intensive care units, although their sensitivity and specificity for seizure detection are imperfect.

Measures of brain metabolic integrity such as MR spectroscopy or near-infrared spectroscopy, when combined with EEG data, may provide surrogate measures of treatment efficacy.

Although the experimental data regarding the potential efficacy of agents such as bumetanide, topiramate, and levetiracetam are encouraging, the duration of use of these agents may be limited by safety concerns related to their effects on long-term brain development. Animal model trials and human studies must be aligned in order to understand how data obtained from rodent and nonhuman primates predict human responses. Whether early-life seizure models in which there are long-term deleterious effects on learning can be used to determine the effects of AED treatment on cognitive development in humans is uncertain. Indeed, there is now an FDA-approved investigational new drug (IND) for a clinical trial assessing the pharmacokinetics and safety of bumetanide in combination with standard phenobarbital treatment of early neonatal seizures (http://www.clinicaltrials.gov). In this study, neonates who have had a breakthrough seizure after a first loading dose of phenobarbital are enrolled for full-lead EEG monitoring, and receive randomized treatment with a second dose of phenobarbital in combination with bumetanide or vehicle.

New Therapeutic Targets

Refractory neonatal seizures remain a significant clinical problem, and no new treatments for this condition have been introduced for decades. Many new mechanisms and components of neonatal seizures have been uncovered and present important possibilities for novel therapeutic strategies in the population of neonates at risk for acute and long-term neurologic damage from neonatal seizures. Several major classes of agents with possible age-specific effects have emerged and are summarized in Table 16-2. These include modulators of neurotransmitter receptors and ion channels and transporters, anti-inflammatory compounds, neuroprotectants, and antioxidants. Interdisciplinary collaboration between neonatologists and neonatal neurologists is essential for the success of such studies. As basic research reveals

Table 16-2 **Candidate Potential Targets and Therapies from Emerging Experimental and Clinical Literature**

Temporal Profile	Mechanism Targeted	Potential Therapeutic Options
Acute changes	Immediate early genes	Chromatin acetylation modifiers/histone deacetylation inhibitors (valproate)
	NMDA receptors	NMDA receptor inhibitors (memantine, felbamate) NR2B-specific inhibitors (ifenprodil)
	AMPA receptors	AMPA receptor antagonists (topiramate, talampanel, GYKI compounds)
	NKCC1 chloride transporters	NKCC1 inhibitor (bumetanide – in combination with GABA agonists phenobarbital, benzodiazepines)
	GABA receptors	GABA receptor agonists (phenobarbital, benzodiazepines)
	Phosphatases (e.g., calcineurin)	Phosphatase inhibitors (FK-506)
	Kinases (activation of PKA, PKC, CaMKII, Src kinases, etc.)	Kinase inhibitors (CaMKII inhibitor KN-62, PKA inhibitor KT5720, PKC inhibitor chelerythrine)
Subacute changes	Inflammation	Anti-inflammatory compounds (ACTH), microglial inactivators (minocycline, doxycycline)
	Neuronal injury	Erythropoietin, antioxidants, NO inhibitors, NMDA receptor antagonists (memantine)
	HCN channels	I(h)-blocker ZD7288
	CB1 receptor	CB1 receptor antagonists (SR 14176A, rimonabant)
Chronic changes	Sprouting	Protein synthesis inhibitors (rapamycin, cycloheximide)
	Gliosis	Anti-inflammatory agents, (Cox-2 inhibitors, minocycline, doxycycline)

(Reprinted with permission from Rakhade SN, Jensen FE. Epileptogenesis in the immature brain: emerging mechanisms. Nat Rev Neurol 2009;5:380–391.)

new age-specific therapeutic targets, these targets can be validated with analysis of cell-specific gene and protein expression in human autopsy samples. Experimental data regarding the potential efficacy of agents such as bumetanide, topiramate, and levetiracetam are encouraging, but the duration of use of these agents may be limited by safety concerns related to their effects on long-term brain development. Incorporation of continuous EEG monitoring into clinical studies of neonatal seizure therapy will be essential. Seizure cessation is an important therapeutic goal; yet, improved neurodevelopmental outcome is clearly of critical importance.

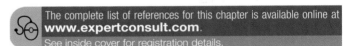

The complete list of references for this chapter is available online at **www.expertconsult.com**.
See inside cover for registration details.

Hypoxic-Ischemic Brain Injury in the Term Newborn

Steven P. Miller and Donna M. Ferriero

Scope of the Problem

The syndrome of neonatal encephalopathy in the term newborn occurs in up to 6 per 1000 live term births and is a major cause of neurodevelopmental disability, with one-quarter of survivors sustaining permanent neurological deficits [Volpe, 2008]. While the syndrome of neonatal encephalopathy may result from a number of causes, this chapter will focus on the etiology, pathophysiology, and management of hypoxic-ischemic brain injury in the term newborn. Hypoxic-ischemic brain injury is recognized clinically by a characteristic encephalopathy with either a lack of alertness or hyperalertness, abnormal tone, abnormal reflex function, poor feeding, compromised respiratory status, and seizures [Miller et al., 2004]. Brain imaging has revealed patterns of brain injury following a hypoxic-ischemic insult that are unique to the immature brain; they depend on the age at which it occurs and on the severity and duration of the insult (Figure 17-1) [Miller et al., 2005; Cowan et al., 2003]. The capacity to repeat brain imaging safely in the newborn following hypoxia-ischemia has enabled studies confirming the clinical and experimental observations that neonatal brain injury evolves over days, if not weeks [Ferriero, 2004]. These clinical investigations are consistent with the prolonged temporal evolution of brain injury in neonatal animal models [Ferriero, 2004]. This time-course "opens the door" for therapeutic interventions instituted not only hours, but also days, after the hypoxic-ischemic insult, with different interventions needed as the injury evolves [Ferriero, 2004].

Etiology of Brain Injury in the Term Newborn

There is increasing recognition that neonatal brain injury is related to antenatal, perinatal, and postnatal factors, and is not always the result of "birth asphyxia" [Badawi et al., 1998]. While hypoxia-ischemia accounts for a substantial fraction of neonatal brain injury, a documented hypoxic-ischemic insult is lacking in many term newborns with encephalopathy [Volpe, 2008; Ferriero, 2004]. Many risk factors for neonatal encephalopathy are clearly prenatal [Badawi et al., 1998], such as maternal hypotension, infertility treatment, and thyroid disease. A minority of cases have only intrapartum risk factors, such as breech extraction, cord prolapse, or abruptio placentae [Badawi et al., 1998]. However, recent cohorts evaluated with magnetic resonance imaging (MRI) studies demonstrate that

brain injury actually happens at or near the time of birth [Cowan et al., 2003; Miller et al., 2005]. It is also important to recognize that postnatal causes may account for up to 10 percent of neonatal encephalopathy in the *term* infant. Therefore, metabolic abnormalities such as acute bilirubin encephalopathy and inborn errors of metabolism, infection, severe respiratory distress, and trauma should be considered in the clinical evaluation.

Clinical Syndromes and Natural History

Clinical Syndromes

Neonatal encephalopathy and seizures are the most overt manifestation of the severity of brain injury. Clinical signs and symptoms depend on the severity, timing, and duration of the insult, as well as the newborn's maturity, even within ages considered "full term." It is equally important to note that not all newborns with significant acquired brain injuries present with an easily recognizable encephalopathy or seizures. Some conditions, such as stroke and perinatal white matter injury, discussed in Chapters 18 and 19, may only have subtle manifestations that may not be recognized on clinical examination. This chapter will focus on the clinical syndrome of neonatal encephalopathy secondary to hypoxia-ischemia. The diagnosis and management of neonatal seizures is discussed in Chapter 16.

Neonatal Encephalopathy

The major components of the syndrome of "neonatal encephalopathy" include: alertness, tone, respiratory status, reflexes, feeding, and seizures (Table 17-1). The severity of brain injury, reflecting the duration and magnitude of the hypoxic-ischemic insult, determines the severity of evolution of this clinical encephalopathy. In newborns with moderate to severe encephalopathy, symptoms usually evolve over days, making *serial* detailed examinations important. As with any neurologically ill newborn, the baby's gestational age must be considered in the interpretation of physical findings. As described by Volpe, there is a characteristic progression of signs in newborns with a severe hypoxic-ischemic insult [Volpe, 2008]. The affected neonate exhibits a depressed level of consciousness from the very first hours of life. Periodic breathing with apnea and bradycardia often heralds this initial presentation. Hypotonia with

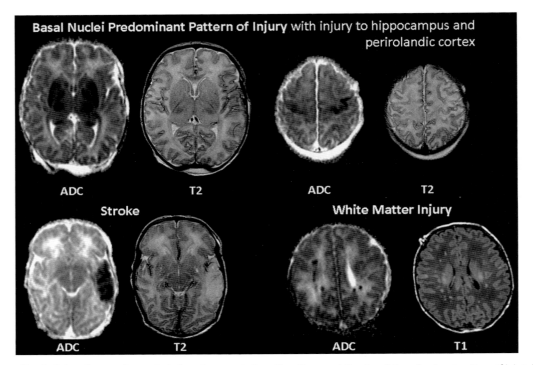

Fig. 17-1 Patterns of brain injury in term hypoxic-ischemic encephalopathy. *Top panel*: Basal nuclei-predominant pattern of injury in a newborn with perinatal asphyxia imaged on the third day of life. Brain injury is demonstrated on apparent diffusion coefficient (ADC) maps as areas of restricted diffusion (hypointense, dark areas) and on T2-weighted images as areas of hyperintensity (bright areas). Note involvement of the basal ganglia, thalamus, hippocampus, and perirolandic cortex. *Bottom panel*: Stroke: focal infarct in the left middle cerebral artery territory in a a newborn with perinatal asphyxia demonstrated on the ADC as areas of restricted diffusion (hypointense, dark areas) with a corresponding area of hyperintensity on the T2-weighted image. White matter injury: multifocal white matter injury in the periventricular and subcortical white matter in a newborn with perinatal asphyxia demonstrated on the ADC as areas of restricted diffusion (hypointense, dark areas) with corresponding areas of hyperintensity on the T1-weighted image.

Table 17-1 The Encephalopathy Score

Sign	Score = 0	Score = 1
Feeding	Normal	Gavage feeds, gastrostomy tube, or not tolerating oral feeds
Alertness	Alert	Irritable, poorly responsive, or comatose
Tone	Normal	Hypotonia or hypertonia
Respiratory status	Normal	Respiratory distress (need for continuous positive airway pressure or mechanical ventilation)
Reflexes	Normal	Hyperreflexia, hyporeflexia, or absent reflexes
Seizure	None	Suspected or confirmed clinical seizure

(From Miller et al. Clinical signs predict 30-month neurodevelopmental outcome after neonatal encephalopathy. Am J Obstet Gynecol 2004;190(1):93–99.)

decreased movement is almost universally found. In the first day of life, the pupillary response is often preserved and abnormalities of eye movements are not detected. In severely injured newborns, seizures may be seen within 6–12 hours after birth. Seizures at this stage are often subtle, manifesting as ocular movements, lip smacking, apnea, or bicycling movements of the extremities. The nursing staff should be alerted to identify and document paroxysmal behaviors. Multifocal or focal clonic seizures may also occur, and often indicate focal cerebral infarction. In the latter hours of the first day of life, there may be a transient increase in the level of alertness that is not accompanied by other signs of neurological improvement. This should not be falsely reassuring, as this apparent increase in alertness is frequently accompanied by more seizures and apnea, a shrill cry, and jitteriness. With careful bedside examination, weakness in the proximal limbs and increased muscle stretch reflexes may be observed, but in the very severely injured newborn, diffuse weakness with absent movements and reflexes is common.

By the third day of life in newborns with severe brain injury, the level of consciousness deteriorates with symptoms of respiratory failure and other signs of brainstem dysfunction. During this period, cerebral edema resulting from hypoxia-ischemia is maximal and can further impair cerebral blood flow secondary to increased intracranial pressure. Most clinicians avoid treatment of cerebral edema in this setting, as many interventions such as corticosteroids, hyperventilation ($PaCO_2$ 20–25 mmHg), furosemide, or mannitol, may be harmful and no studies have shown proven benefit. Those newborns surviving beyond the third day of life begin to show improved alertness. Yet hypotonia and weakness in proximal limbs, face, and bulbar musculature persist. While less intensive care may be required with this improved level of consciousness, the clinician must be vigilant for feeding difficulties and the risk of aspiration as the newborn's suck and swallow responses often remain impaired.

Documenting this clinical evolution is a critical component of the evaluation, and use of a simple encephalopathy score as a bedside tool can help the clinician standardize assessment of encephalopathic newborns, monitor the evolution of the clinical syndromes, and help in systematically identifying neonates who require therapeutic intervention (see Table 17-1) [Miller et al., 2004].

Subtle Neonatal Syndromes

Stroke and white matter injury in the term newborn may present with clinical signs that are so subtle that they remain undetected for months or years. Advances in brain monitoring (amplitude integrated EEG, prolonged video-EEG monitoring) and brain imaging (MRI) in the neonatal intensive care unit have increased recognition of these injuries. However, both stroke and white matter injury may present in the neonatal period with an overt encephalopathy [Li et al., 2009; Ramaswamy et al., 2004]. These conditions share many of the risk factors of "global" hypoxic-ischemic brain injury considered in this chapter.

Management of Neonatal Encephalopathy

Clinical Management

As many etiologies of neonatal encephalopathy have specific therapies, the clinician's initial task is to determine the underlying etiology through careful history taking, neurological examination, and laboratory and brain imaging studies. The history should elicit indicators of intrauterine distress that may have contributed to decreased placental or fetal blood flow: fetal heart tracing abnormalities, passage of meconium, or a history of a difficulty in labor or delivery. The Apgar score will indicate who is at risk for mortality. The details of the delivery-room resuscitation, medications, and ventilatory support should be noted. Because the clinical signs of encephalopathy and seizures are often not specific for an etiology, laboratory tests are critical to exclude reversible causes of neonatal encephalopathy. The management of moderate or severe encephalopathy should occur in a neonatal intensive care unit in close collaboration with a neonatologist. Immediate management requires securing an appropriate airway and maintaining adequate circulation. Ventilatory support with mechanical ventilation or continuous positive airway pressure (CPAP) is often required. Metabolic complications, such as hypoglycemia, hypocalcemia, hyponatremia, and acidosis, frequently accompany hypoxic-ischemic encephalopathy (HIE), and should be identified and treated. Liver enzymes and serum creatinine levels should be performed to detect injury to other organs, while serum ammonia and lactate levels can screen for possible inborn errors of metabolism. Lumbar puncture to evaluate for intracranial infections should be performed if the history is not typical for HIE, or if a clinical suspicion of infection exists. If infection is suspected, ampicillin and gentamicin are started in addition to acyclovir if herpes simplex virus infection is a consideration. If the history, examination, or initial laboratory investigation points to an inborn error of metabolism, early treatment is crucial and a biochemical geneticist should be consulted. Additional diagnostic tests, such as serum amino acids and urine organic acids, as well as specific management strategies, are required (detailed in Chapter 20). The diagnosis of a severe intracranial hemorrhage should prompt consultation with a neurosurgeon to manage raised intracranial pressure from mass effect or hydrocephalus; platelet levels and coagulation function should be measured. Since the clinical syndrome evolves considerably over the first 72 hours of life, management of specific complications, such as respiratory compromise or seizures, can often be anticipated.

Investigation of term newborns with encephalopathy addresses three primary questions:
1. identifying the underlying etiology
2. determining the timing and severity of the brain injury
3. predicting the neurodevelopmental outcome of the affected newborn.

Addressing these questions is critical for the application of "neuroprotection" strategies, such as hypothermia [Eicher et al., 2005; Gluckman et al., 2005; Shankaran et al., 2005; Azzopardi et al., 2009]. To assess the encephalopathic term newborn, diagnostic tools available to the clinician include clinical features and biochemical and electrophysiological tests. However, the severity of brain injury in term asphyxiated newborns is not reliably predicted by clinical indicators commonly used during the first days of life, such as umbilical cord pH and Apgar scores [Shevell et al., 1999]. On the other hand, the severity of clinical encephalopathy is a strong predictor of neurodevelopmental outcome [Miller, 2004]. However, while the risk of motor and cognitive deficits appears to be minimal in mild encephalopathy, and pronounced at the severe end of the spectrum, it is inconsistent in neonates with moderate encephalopathy [Sarnat and Sarnat, 1976; Robertson et al., 1989; Dixon et al., 2002; Marlow et al., 2005]. Newborns with moderate encephalopathy are thus the most likely to benefit from the improved prognostic capabilities of brain imaging.

Brain Imaging of Newborns with Encephalopathy

Current guidelines for neuroimaging term newborns with encephalopathy suggest a noncontrast computed tomography (CT) scan to detect hemorrhage in infants with a history of significant birth trauma, and evidence of low hematocrit or coagulopathy [Ment et al., 2002]. If CT findings cannot explain the newborn's clinical status, then MRI is recommended. For other encephalopathic term newborns, MRI is recommended between days 2 and 8 to assess the location and extent of injury [Ment et al., 2002]. In a recent study, the neuroimaging findings from a group of 48 term newborns with encephalopathy uniformly scanned with CT and MRI (T1 and T2-weighted images) with diffusion-weighted imaging (DWI) on the third day of life were compared [Chau et al., 2009]. On the third day of life, both CT and MRI with DWI reliably identify injury to the basal nuclei. However, DWI more readily detects cortical injury and focal and multifocal lesions, such as strokes and white matter injury, than either CT or conventional MRI. The choice of the best neuroimaging technique must balance the risk of transport and sedation involved in MRI against the risk of ionizing radiation with CT [Brenner et al., 2003; Berrington de Gonzalez and Darby, 2004; Hall et al., 2004]. With the development of MR-compatible incubators and monitoring equipment [Dumoulin et al., 2002; Bluml et al., 2004], as well as improved capacity to scan newborns without pharmacological sedation, MRI should now be the modality of choice when possible. MRI with DWI appears to be the most sensitive imaging study to detect abnormalities associated with other causes of neonatal encephalopathy, such as cerebral dysgenesis, infections, stroke, and metabolic disorders [Volpe, 2008; Cowan et al., 2003]. In order to confirm the diagnosis of hypoxic-ischemic brain injury and determine the extent of injury, MRI and DWI are optimally obtained between 3 and 5 days of life in term newborns with encephalopathy [Chau et al., 2009; Barkovich, 1997; Rutherford et al., 2004; Barkovich et al., 2006]. In newborns treated with hypothermia, further studies are needed to determine the optimal timing of MRI. The importance of rigorous imaging protocols with appropriate quality controls, and high quality neuroradiological review, must be emphasised.

Advanced MR Techniques

Advanced MR techniques, such as diffusion and spectroscopic imaging, allow us to observe the progression of neonatal brain injury. Diffusion MRI and MR spectroscopy (MRS) can be used to measure brain maturation and also provide important measures of brain microstructure and metabolism following injury. Given the widespread availability of these techniques on current MR scanners, their application will be discussed below. In addition to diffusion MRI and MRS, other advanced MR techniques are emerging. Computer-assisted morphometric techniques, including voxel-based and deformation-based morphometry, are used to correlate regional brain volumes in newborns, children, and adolescents with a history of neonatal encephalopathy with their neurodevelopmental outcomes [Maneru et al., 2003; Nishida et al., 2006; Srinivasan et al., 2007]. Moreover, diffusion tensor tractography, an extension of diffusion MRI, is providing new insights into recovery and resilience by measuring microstructural development of specific functional pathways [Glenn et al., 2007]. Together, these quantitative techniques are helping to identify injuries and abnormalities of subsequent brain development that may not be apparent on conventional MRI.

MAGNETIC RESONANCE SPECTROSCOPY IMAGING

MRS can be used to measure changes in certain brain metabolites from a given brain region. Of the compounds measured by MRS at long echo times, N-acetylaspartate (NAA) and lactate are the most useful in assessing brain injury. NAA is an acetylated amino acid found in high concentrations in neurons of the central nervous system (CNS). NAA levels increase with advancing cerebral maturity [Barkovich, 2000; Novotny et al., 1998], and decrease with cerebral injury or impaired cerebral metabolism [Barkovich, 2000; Novotny et al., 1998]. Lactate is normally produced in the brain by astrocytes and used as fuel by neurons to replenish energy stores via oxidative phosphorylation [Pellerin and Magistretti, 2004]. Lactate levels are elevated with disturbed brain energy substrate delivery and oxidative metabolism, as seen with hypoxia-ischemia. Elevated lactate and reduced NAA levels are highly predictive of neurodevelopmental outcome following neonatal brain injury [Barkovich, 2000; Novotny et al., 1998]. Given this, lactate/NAA ratios are especially discriminatory of newborns with adverse outcomes [Shanmugalingam et al., 2006; Thayyil et al., 2010]. Myo-inositol, one of the major brain osmolytes, is best measured with MRS at short echo times, and is elevated with neonatal hypoxic-ischemic brain injury [Robertson et al., 2001].

DIFFUSION IMAGING

Diffusion-weighted MR imaging (DWI) detects alterations in free water diffusion. Diffusion tensor imaging (DTI) measures the amount (apparent diffusion coefficient [ADC] or average diffusivity) and directionality of water motion (fractional anisotropy [FA]). With brain maturation, ADC decreases in gray and white matter, presumably due to a reduction in water content and the development of cell membranes that restrict water diffusion [Mukherjee et al., 2002; Beaulieu, 2002, Coats et al., 2009]. Over this period, FA increases in white matter, even before myelin is evident on T1 and T2-weighted images [Miller et al., 2002b; Drobyshevsky et al., 2005; Prayer et al., 2001]. DWI and DTI also provide sensitive measures of brain injury [Barkovich et al., 2001; McKinstry et al., 2002]. With acute injury, intracellular water increases and water movement are "restricted" by the cell membrane when a diffusion gradient is applied. The DWI image will show an area of restricted diffusion as increased signal intensity that is a complicated product of T2* properties and restricted diffusion. The ADC or average diffusivity map (D_{av}) is a quantitative water diffusion map that shows restricted diffusion as areas of diminished signal intensity. Reduced ADC values in the posterior limb of the internal capsule are associated with a greater risk of adverse neurodevelopmental outcome in term newborns with encephalopathy [Hunt et al., 2004]. FA values in the white matter and basal nuclei are decreased with significant injury during the first week of life in term newborns with encephalopathy [Ward et al., 2006]. In newborns with brain injury, DTI also detects abnormalities of microstructural brain development remote from the primary injuries, in areas of the brain that are normal on T1 and T2-weighted images [Miller et al., 2002b].

Patterns of Brain Injury

In a primate model of brain injury in the "term newborn," the distribution of injury was associated with the duration and severity of ischemia. While acute-profound asphyxia produced injury in the basal ganglia and thalamus, partial asphyxia caused white matter injury [Myers, 1972, 1975]. Similar patterns of injury are found in term newborns following hypoxia-ischemia (see Figure 17-1). *The* basal ganglia-predominant pattern involves both the basal ganglia and thalamus, and perirolandic cortex [Miller et al., 2005; Sie et al., 2000; Chau et al., 2009]. The watershed pattern predominantly involves the vascular watershed, from the white matter and extending to the cerebral cortex [Miller et al., 2005; Sie et al., 2000]. Maximal injury in both the watershed region and basal nuclei results in the total pattern of brain injury [Miller et al., 2005; Sie et al., 2000]. Identifying the predominant pattern of brain injury is helpful to the clinician caring for a term newborn with encephalopathy, as the predominant pattern is more strongly associated with neurodevelopmental outcome than the severity of injury in any given region [Miller et al., 2005].

The final pattern of injury, increasingly recognized by MRI, is the "focal- or multifocal" pattern of injury: stroke or white matter injury (WMI). Recent data suggest that strokes (arterial or venous) are also associated with neonatal encephalopathy in the term newborn [Cowan et al., 2003]. Many newborns with stroke have *multiple* risk factors for brain injury, including intrapartum complications.

While WMI is the characteristic pattern of brain injury in premature newborns, it is increasingly recognized in term newborns with encephalopathy, identified in 23 percent in one series (see Figure 17-1) [Li et al., 2009]. In this series, WMI demonstrated restricted diffusion on ADC maps in almost all newborns, suggesting that these lesions were acquired near birth. As newborns with WMI had milder encephalopathy relative to other newborns in the cohort, these lesions may have been underdetected in the past. Lower gestational age at birth, within the range of term birth, was associated with an increasing severity of WMI, suggesting a role for brain maturation in the etiology of this injury pattern [Li et al., 2009]. In sequential studies of term newborns with encephalopathy, delayed white matter degeneration, extending past the first week of life, is also seen [Barkovich et al., 2006; Neil and Inder, 2006]. This delayed WMI might follow injury to the basal nuclei, just as Wallerian degeneration of the corticospinal tract is found following some middle cerebral artery strokes in the term newborn [De Vries et al., 2005; Kirton et al., 2007]. It should be noted that full-term infants with congenital heart disease also have a strikingly high incidence of WMI on MRI and at autopsy [McQuillen et al., 2007; Mahle et al., 2002; Galli et al., 2004; Gilles et al., 1973; Kinney et al., 2005]. Similar to premature newborns and term newborns with encephalopathy, those with congenital heart disease are at risk of impaired delivery of energy substrates due to ischemia, inflammation, and oxidative stress, particularly with cardiopulmonary bypass. Recent data from autopsy and brain imaging studies suggests that in utero brain development is delayed in newborns with some forms of serious congenital heart disease [Miller et al., 2007; Rosenthal, 1996; Licht et al., 2009]. These abnormalities in early brain development might explain the predominance of WMI in term newborns with congenital heart disease, as opposed to the more expected "term" predominance of injury to the basal nuclei or watershed regions predominantly.

Progression of Neonatal Brain Injury

Timing the onset and determining the progression of brain injury have been greatly facilitated with the use of diffusion MR techniques and MRS. Recent studies have shown that the reduction in ADC on diffusion imaging due to brain injury in term newborns evolves over the initial days of life, reaching their nadir by 2–4 days after injury [Barkovich et al., 2006; McKinstry et al., 2002]. Thus, MR diffusion images obtained prior to the nadir, as in the first day following an injury, may not show the full extent of injury. Importantly, diffusion abnormalities persist for 7–8 days in the newborn before returning towards normal values (pseudonormalization) and ultimately reflect increased diffusion [Barkovich et al., 2001; McKinstry et al., 2002; Coats et al., 2009]. In a proportion of patients, brain injury will progressively worsen over the first 2 weeks of life to involve new brain areas, particularly the white matter tracts [Barkovich et al., 2006]. It is critical to interpret diffusion imaging in the context of the time between injury and the acquisition of the scan [Barkovich et al., 2001; McKinstry et al., 2002]. MRS data in newborns mirror this time course of injury progression. In the first 24 hours following brain injury in the term newborn, lactate increases, followed by a decrease in NAA in the 3 days after injury [Barkovich, 2000; Barkovich et al., 2001; Novotny et al., 1998]. The prolonged progression of neonatal brain injury is consistent with the mechanisms of cell injury, discussed below, that persist for days following hypoxic-ischemic brain injury in the newborn. These observations also suggest that the opportunity to intervene to prevent or ameliorate brain injury may extend over *days* in the term newborn, if not weeks. These quantitative MR techniques

now offer a dynamic measure of brain injury in the newborn that can be safely used to determine the short-term effects of novel intervention strategies.

Outcomes

Neurodevelopmental outcomes following neonatal encephalopathy depend on the pattern and severity of the brain injury. Neurodevelopmental deficits may involve motor, visual, and cognitive functions. Both genetic and postnatal variables such as socioeconomic factors (e.g., environmental exposures and parental education) likely modify an individual's neurodevelopmental outcome following neonatal brain injury [Miller et al., 2002a; Robertson and Finer, 1993]. Given the broad spectrum of neurodevelopmental impairments following neonatal encephalopathy, follow-up of these newborns should include assessment of motor function, vision and hearing, cognition, behavior, and quality of life, through infancy and childhood. Epilepsy is identified in up to one-half of survivors from moderate to severe neonatal encephalopathy [Brunquell et al., 2002; Clancy and Legido, 1991], and is particularly common in those infants with cerebral palsy and developmental delay [Toet et al., 2005].

The American College of Obstetricians and Gynecologists (ACOG) Task Force on Neonatal Encephalopathy concluded that an acute intrapartum event could result in cerebral palsy of the spastic quadriplegic or dyskinetic type, but could not account for isolated cognitive deficits [ACOG, 2004]. Recently reviewed data [Gonzalez and Miller, 2006] indicate that cognitive deficits may feature prominently following term neonatal encephalopathy of presumed hypoxic-ischemic brain injury, even in the absence of cerebral palsy. This pattern of neurodevelopmental deficits follows an overt neonatal encephalopathy, often in the context of a critical illness, and is most commonly associated with the watershed pattern of injury and white matter damage, rather than the basal nuclei-predominant pattern of injury. A complete assessment of neurodevelopmental outcome must include aspects of cognition most readily assessed at school age: learning, executive function, behavior, and social competence. In addition, developmental coordination disorder, autism spectrum disorder, or specific language impairments should be considered as possibilities in follow-up of newborns with a history of encephalopathy [van Handel et al., 2007]. Finally, "quality of life," an individual's subjective perception of physical and psychological health, should be evaluated by the clinician assessing outcomes to tailor rehabilitation and monitoring services best.

Motor Function

In term survivors of hypoxic-ischemic brain injury, the risk of cerebral palsy or severe disability may involve more than one-third of affected newborns, and is most common in those with a severe encephalopathy [Volpe, 2008; Dixon et al., 2002; Barnett et al., 2002]. Spastic quadriparesis is the most common type of cerebral palsy, although athetoid or spastic hemiparesis also occurs. The diagnosis and management of cerebral palsy are addressed in Chapter 69. A complete assessment of neurosensory and cognitive functions is critical in children with cerebral palsy [Marlow et al., 2005]. Minor motor impairments that do not meet diagnostic criteria for cerebral palsy [Shevell et al., 1999] are diagnosed in more than one-third of children with moderate encephalopathy, and in more than one-quarter of children with mild encephalopathy [Van Kooij et al., 2008].

Vision and Hearing

Severe visual impairment occurs in up to one-quarter of children after moderate or severe encephalopathy [Robertson and Finer, 1985; Shankaran et al., 1991]. This may be due to injury to the posterior visual pathway, including the primary visual cortex, resulting in "cortical visual impairment" [Van Hof-van Duin and Mohn, 1984]. Injuries to the basal nuclei may also affect acuity, visual fields, or stereopsis (depth perception) [Mercuri et al., 1997]. Sensorineural hearing loss, likely secondary to brainstem injury, is also seen following neonatal encephalopathy [Robertson and Finer, 1985; Robertson et al., 1989], affecting 18 percent of survivors of moderate encephalopathy without cerebral palsy [Lindstrom et al., 2006].

Cognition

Overall, cognitive deficits are seen in 30–50 percent of childhood survivors of moderate neonatal encephalopathy [Dilenge et al., 2001]. Intellectual performance in children with severe encephalopathy *without* cerebral palsy is also affected [Marlow et al., 2005]. School-age survivors of moderate neonatal encephalopathy are more likely to have difficulties with reading, spelling, and arithmetic, or require additional school resources [Moster et al., 2002; Robertson et al., 1989]. Cognitive deficits, such as those in language and memory, may be seen, even when IQ scores are "normal." [Marlow et al., 2005]. Behavioral difficulties, such as hyperactivity and emotional problems, should also be considered, even in individuals without motor disability [Marlow et al., 2005].

Brain Imaging and Outcome

The pattern of brain injury on neuroimaging conveys important prognostic information regarding the "pattern" of neurodevelopmental abnormalities. The basal nuclei pattern of injury and abnormal signal intensity in the posterior limb of

the internal capsule are both predictive of severely impaired motor and cognitive outcomes [Rutherford et al., 1998; Miller et al., 2005]. The cognitive deficits associated with this pattern are not surprising, given the common involvement of the cerebral cortex [Miller et al., 2005] and cerebellum [Le Strange et al., 2004; Sargent et al., 2004]. In contrast, the watershed pattern is associated with cognitive impairments that are not necessarily accompanied by major motor deficits [Miller et al., 2005]. Importantly, the cognitive deficits following the watershed pattern may only be evident after 2 years of age [Miller et al., 2005]. In survivors of neonatal encephalopathy without functional motor deficits assessed at 4 years of age, the severity of watershed-distribution injury was most strongly associated with impaired language skills [Steinman et al., 2009]. While neurodevelopmental outcomes may be significantly better than anticipated, neurological deficits may also be found in some newborns whose brain imaging studies are normal [Bax et al., 2006]. More subtle brain injuries associated with later neurodevelopmental deficits, such as white matter injuries or hippocampal volume loss, may only be detectable with quantitative brain imaging techniques [Miller et al., 2002a; Nagy et al., 2005; Gadian et al., 2000].

Pathophysiology of Neonatal Hypoxic-Ischemic Brain Injury

In term infants with neonatal encephalopathy, perinatal hypoxia-ischemia predominates as the major cause of future neurologic disability. The adverse consequences of cerebral ischemia include deprivation of energy substrates and oxygen, and an inability to clear accumulated, potentially toxic metabolites. Although linear flow charts cannot accurately convey the complex cascade of interrelated molecular pathways that lead to hypoxic-ischemic neurodegeneration, Figure 17-2 highlights some of the critical mechanisms.

Over the past 20 years, considerable information has emerged about the cellular and molecular consequences of cerebral hypoxia-ischemia and the molecular events that lead to neuronal cell death. The underlying rationale for this scientific

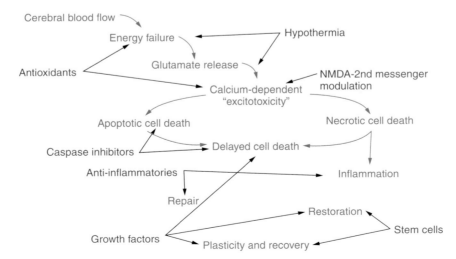

MOVING BEYOND A SINGLE TREATMENT FOR NEONATAL NEUROPROTECTION

Fig. 17-2 Some of the key molecular mechanisms that contribute to hypoxic-ischemic neurodegeneration and opportunities for neuroprotection.

focus is the hope that a better understanding of the basic molecular mechanisms of neurodegeneration may provide ways to modulate these events pharmacologically to limit their adverse consequences and to protect the brain from irreversible damage. A complementary focus that has emerged – and will likely become particularly important in the setting of neonatal brain injury – is the delineation of the intrinsic neuronal mechanisms of adaptation and repair after hypoxic-ischemic brain injury. Despite the traditional view of greater resistance to CNS injury in the neonate because of lower metabolic demands and the greater plasticity of the developing CNS, at specific stages of brain maturation, susceptibility to hypoxia-ischemia may be amplified. Clinical and experimental data have demonstrated that specific brain structures and neural cells in the developing brain may be selectively vulnerable to hypoxic-ischemic injury [McQuillen and Ferriero, 2004]. One of the best-characterized examples is the increased vulnerability of immature oligodendroglia to hypoxic-ischemic injury, which is evident clinically in premature infants and which has been successfully demonstrated in fetal and neonatal animal models [Back et al., 2002; Segovia et al., 2008].

Risk of injury to the immature brain may be heightened by certain therapeutic interventions; this risk stems from the complex roles that pivotal molecular mediators of hypoxic-ischemic injury (e.g., glutamate, calcium) play in brain development. For example, some studies have provided compelling experimental evidence of maturational stage-dependent deleterious effects of several commonly used antiepileptic drugs [Ikonomidou and Turski, 2009].

This section reviews information about the pathophysiology of hypoxic-ischemic brain injury, integrates data obtained from experimental and clinical studies, and highlights mechanisms that are particularly relevant to understanding perinatal brain injury and repair. Several reviews can provide complementary perspectives [Gonzalez and Ferriero, 2008; Vexler and Yenari, 2009; Northington et al., 2005; Pediatric Neurology, 2009]. Please also see Part III of this book on emerging neuroscience concepts (Chapters 13, 14, and 15).

Cerebral Blood Flow and Energy Metabolism

Disruption of cerebrovascular autoregulation has been implicated as an important factor in the pathophysiology of neonatal hypoxic-ischemic brain injury. It is widely accepted that preterm infants have a "pressure-passive" cerebral circulation; however, term infants may remain at risk for impairment of cerebrovascular autoregulation [Boylan et al., 2000] and susceptibility to cerebral ischemia with fluctuations in systemic blood pressure. Several basic physiologic mechanisms may contribute to impaired autoregulation in the neonate. Increased expression of inducible and neuronal isoforms of nitric oxide synthase (iNOS and nNOS), as well as endothelial NOS, may narrow the autoregulatory window, and downregulation of prostaglandin receptors in response to high circulating prostaglandin levels may blunt the prostaglandin-mediated vasoconstrictive response to hypertension and thereby contribute to inappropriately increased cerebral blood flow [Chemtob et al., 1996]. After an ischemic insult, the neonate remains at high risk for further damage in the acute recovery phase because neonatal encephalopathy is often associated with blood pressure fluctuations.

An inadequate supply of glucose or alternate substrates plays a pivotal role in hypoxic-ischemic neuronal cell death.

Although overall metabolic demands are lower in the neonatal than in the adult brain, during periods of rapid brain growth, particularly the perinatal period, metabolic needs rise. The pattern of injury after hypoxia-ischemia can be explained in part on the basis of this metabolic demand; brain regions most susceptible to hypoxic-ischemic injury in the term infant (e.g., subcortical gray matter structures such as the basal ganglia and thalamus) are the same regions that are most vulnerable to mitochondrial toxins. Brain development is associated with a transition from the ability to use glucose and ketones as energy substrates in the neonate to an absolute requirement for glucose in the adult. The immature brain can use lactate as an alternate fuel source to some degree, and the deleterious effects of lactate accumulation after hypoxia-ischemia therefore may be attenuated in the neonate compared with the adult. However, normal maturation is characterized by limitations in glucose transport capacity and increased use of these alternative fuels such as lactate. The inability to transport glucose across the blood–brain barrier threatens cerebral glucose utilization. These factors illustrate the importance of understanding the use of glucose, lactate, and ketones in the newborn brain under normal and pathologic conditions [Vannucci and Vannucci, 2000; Vannucci and Hagberg, 2004].

Excitotoxicity

Glutamate can activate a variety of excitatory amino acid receptors that are broadly classified based on their selective responses to specific agonists (e.g., NMDA, α-amino-3-hydroxy-5-methyl-4-isoxazole propionic acid [AMPA], kainate) or their signaling mechanisms (i.e., ionotropic [ligand-gated ion channel] or metabotropic [G-protein-coupled]). Excitatory amino acid neurotransmission plays a pivotal role in brain development and in learning and memory. A substantial body of data has emerged over the past 30 years documenting the fact that overactivation of excitatory amino acid receptors (i.e., excitotoxicity) contributes to neurodegeneration in a broad range of acute and chronic neurologic disorders [Johnston, 2005].

Most information about mechanisms of excitotoxicity comes from experimental studies, but studies in the human neonate have provided some evidence to support the hypothesis that hypoxic-ischemic brain injury disrupts brain glutamate metabolism. Elevated levels of cerebrospinal fluid glutamate have been documented (by direct cerebrospinal fluid measurements and by proton MRS) in infants with severe hypoxic-ischemic injury [Pu et al., 2000]; cerebrospinal fluid levels of excitatory amino acids are directly proportional to the severity of clinical encephalopathy [Hagberg et al., 1997; Riikonen et al., 1992].

Two closely linked mechanisms contribute to ischemia-induced increases in synaptic glutamate: increased efflux from presynaptic nerve terminals and impaired reuptake by glia and neurons. The initial increase in efflux is mediated by a calcium-dependent process through activation of voltage- dependent calcium channels; later, calcium-independent efflux is thought to be mediated primarily by functional reversal of glutamate transporters. Removal of glutamate from the synaptic cleft depends primarily on energy-dependent glutamate transporters, which are predominantly glial. Any pathophysiologic process that depletes energy supply (e.g., hypoxia-ischemia, hypoglycemia, prolonged seizures) will disrupt these mechanisms and result in increased synaptic glutamate accumulation [Johnston, 2005].

The structure and function of the NMDA receptor channel complex are developmentally regulated. The receptor possesses multiple functional sites that recognize glutamate, co-agonists, modulatory molecules such as glycine, dissociative anesthetics, redox agents, steroids, zinc, magnesium (which blocks permeability to calcium), and a cation-selective ion channel that admits Na^+, K^+, and Ca^{2+}. When the neurotransmitter recognition site is activated by glutamate, the ion channel allows influx of calcium and sodium. The resulting increase in intracellular calcium is the stimulus for a multitude of downstream events, including transcription factor modulation, cell cycle regulation, and DNA replication. The NMDA receptor is relatively overexpressed in the developing brain compared with the adult brain; in postnatal day 6–14 rats (which approximates to the term human neonate), the NMDA receptor is expressed at 150–200 percent of adult levels. In humans, receptor expression is significantly higher at term than in the adult [Johnston, 2005]. The particular combination of subunits determines the NMDA receptor's functional state, and the predominating combination in the perinatal period seems to favor a more prolonged and pronounced calcium influx. In the setting of hypoxia-ischemia, NMDA receptor overactivation leads to massive Na^+ and water influx, cell swelling, elevated intracellular calcium and its associated mitochondrial dysfunction, increased nitric oxide production, increased phospholipid turnover and accumulation of potentially toxic free fatty acids, and cell death by apoptotic or necrotic mechanisms. However, ischemia and energy failure also result in cation influx by non-NMDA-mediated mechanisms.

In experimental rodent models, there is compelling evidence that susceptibility to NMDA- and AMPA-mediated excitotoxicity peaks in the immature and that treatment with NMDA and AMPA receptor antagonists confers robust protection against neonatal hypoxic-ischemic brain injury [Johnston et al., 2001]. However, concerns have been raised that NMDA receptor antagonists might have specific risks in the immature brain; blockade of NMDA synaptic activity could disrupt critical neurodevelopmental processes. Whether AMPA antagonists, which can block neuronal and white matter hypoxic-ischemic damage in neonatal rodent models, have fewer potential risks in the immature brain than do NMDA antagonists is an important question for study [Silverstein and Jensen, 2007].

There has been considerable interest in evaluating the neuroprotective efficacy of magnesium sulfate in experimental and clinical models of neonatal brain injury. This interest stems from the intrinsic potentially neuroprotective properties of Mg^{2+} (including blockade of NMDA receptor activation), and the many years of clinical experience in safe use of magnesium sulfate in obstetric practice. Experimental studies provide evidence that pretreatment with magnesium sulfate can limit subsequent neonatal hypoxic-ischemic injury, but treatment after hypoxia-ischemia is of limited benefit [Greenwood et al., 2000; Turkyilmaz et al., 2002]. Magnesium sulfate has many effects, including blockade of NMDA receptors. It has been found give protection in some animal models of white matter damage [Turkyilmaz et al., 2002; Marret et al., 1995; Spandou et al., 2007], but did not affect cerebrospinal fluid levels of excitatory neurotransmitters in asphyxiated human neonates [Khashaba et al., 2006]. In addition, in a multicenter clinical trial of mothers treated with magnesium who were at risk for preterm delivery, no perinatal side effects were seen and there was some benefit in the neurodevelopment of survivors [Crowther et al., 2003]. A recent study, the BEAM trial, showed that exposure to magnesium sulfate before anticipated early preterm delivery did not reduce the combined risk of moderate or severe cerebral palsy or death, although the rate of cerebral palsy was reduced among survivors [Rouse et al., 2008].

Oxidative Stress

Oxidative stress describes the alterations in cellular milieu that result from an increase in free radical production as a result of oxidative metabolism under pathologic conditions. In the brain injured by hypoxia-ischemia, excitotoxicity and oxidative stress are inextricably linked. In cells with normally functioning mitochondria, more than 80 percent of available oxygen is reduced to energy equivalents (ATP) by cytochrome oxidase. The rest is converted to superoxide anions, which, under physiologic conditions, are reduced to water by enzymatic and nonenzymatic antioxidant mechanisms. An inevitable consequence of mitochondrial dysfunction is an accumulation of superoxide, and any process that depletes antioxidant defenses will result in the default conversion of superoxide to even more reactive species, such as the hydroxyl radical [Ferriero, 2001]. The concept of ischemia-reperfusion injury (i.e., progression of tissue injury with reoxygenation after ischemia) [Inder and Volpe, 2000] is fundamental to the understanding of oxidative stress. This mechanism is not limited to the brain, but excitotoxic mechanisms in the brain can amplify these processes. Excitotoxicity causes energy depletion, mitochondrial dysfunction, and cytosolic calcium accumulation, leading to the generation of free radicals, such as superoxide, nitric oxide derivatives, and the highly reactive hydroxyl radical.

With reoxygenation, mitochondrial oxidative phosphorylation is overwhelmed and reactive oxygen species accumulate. Intrinsic antioxidant defenses are depleted, and free radicals directly damage multiple cellular constituents (lipids, DNA, protein) and can activate pro-apoptotic pathways. The brain is particularly susceptible to free radical attack and lipid peroxidation, and vulnerability is magnified in the immature brain. Contributing factors include a high polyunsaturated fatty acid content, high level of lipid peroxidation (particularly in response to hypoxic stress), immaturity of antioxidant defense enzymes, and high free iron concentrations, compared with the adult brain [Ferriero, 2001]. The level of free iron, which catalyzes the production of various reactive oxygen species, is increased in the plasma and cerebrospinal fluid of asphyxiated newborns [Ogihara et al., 2003]. The deleterious effects of abundant iron and immaturity of the enzymatic oxidant defenses of the immature brain are tightly interrelated. Free radical scavengers (e.g., alpha-phenyl-*n*-tert-butyl-nitrone [PBN], a spin-trap agent that converts free radicals to stable adducts) and metal chelators (e.g., deferoxamine) can protect neurons from injury mediated by hydrogen peroxide in vitro and in vivo. These agents also protect neurons from NMDA-induced toxicity, providing complementary evidence of the pathophysiologic link between excitotoxicity and oxidative stress [Peeters-Scholte et al., 2003].

Nitric oxide metabolism provides another critical link between excitotoxicity and oxidative injury in the hypoxic-ischemic injured brain. Nitric oxide is produced constitutively in endothelium, astrocytes, and neurons in response to an increase in intracellular calcium. Hypoxic-ischemic increases in nitric oxide production have multiple potential beneficial and detrimental effects. Nitric oxide regulates vascular tone, influences inflammatory responses to injury, and directly modulates NMDA receptor function [Sorrentino et al., 2004]. In neonatal rodent brain, striatal neurons that express nNOS are selectively resistant to hypoxia-ischemia injury, providing a source for NMDA receptor-mediated regulation of nitric oxide production. Disruption of the nNOS gene and pharmacologic inhibition of nNOS (reviewed in Gonzalez and Ferriero) ameliorate neonatal hypoxia-ischemia injury [Gonzalez and Ferriero, 2008]. Other nitric oxide synthase isoforms contribute to injury via inflammation (iNOS) and may potentially provide another crosstalk for protection therapies. Early endothelial NO is protective by maintaining blood flow, but early neuronal NO and late inducible NO are neurotoxic by promoting cell death [Iadecola et al., 1997]. Brain iNOS is induced in multiple cell types during upregulation of the pro-inflammatory pathway after brain injury [Higuchi et al., 1998], enhancing excitotoxicity by modifying binding to NMDA receptors [Ishida et al., 2001].

Neuroprotection by selective inhibition of nNOS or iNOS has been demonstrated [van den Tweel et al., 2005]. Regions expressing nNOS correspond to those that express NMDA receptors and correlate with regions of neurotoxicity both in vivo and in vitro [Black et al., 1995; Ferriero et al., 1996; Dawson et al., 1993]. Destruction of neurons containing nNOS with local injections of quisqualate prior to hypoxia-ischemia results in lower injury scores and less infarction [Ferriero et al., 1995]. Likewise, neonatal mice with targeted disruption of the nNOS gene, when subjected to a similar hypoxic-ischemic insult, are markedly protected from injury [Ferriero et al., 1996], but nonspecific blockade of both nNOS and eNOS (endothelial NOS) in sheep with NG-nitro-L-arginine (L-NNA) was not protective [Marks et al., 1996]. Few studies have been performed in asphyxiated human newborns in relation to cerebral NO production. Cerebrospinal fluid NO levels increase with severity of HIE at 24–72 hours after asphyxia [Ergenekon et al., 1999], with increased NO and nitrotyrosine levels in spinal cord as well [Groenendaal et al., 2008]. Initial results in premature infants treated with inhaled NO for prevention of bronchopulmonary dysplasia showed reductions in ultrasound-diagnosed brain injury and improvements in neurodevelopmental outcomes at 2 years of age, but long-term results are pending [Schreiber et al., 2003; Ballard et al., 2006].

Several other antioxidant strategies that either block free radical production or increase antioxidant defenses have been studied. Melatonin is an indoleamine that is formed in higher quantities in adults and is a direct scavenger of reactive oxygen species and NO. It has been found to provide long-lasting neuroprotection in experimental hypoxia-ischemia and focal cerebral ischemic injury [Carloni et al., 2008; Koh, 2008]. Human neonates treated with melatonin were also found to have decreased proinflammatory cytokines [Gitto et al., 2004, 2005]. Allopurinol has mixed effects which have shown promise in animal and human studies. Xanthine oxidase-derived superoxide and H_2O_2 react with NO to form damaging RNS (reactive nitrogen species). Allopurinol functions by reducing free radical production via xanthine oxidase inhibition, while also scavenging hydroxyl radicals. Short-term benefits have also been seen in neonates undergoing cardiac surgery for hypoplastic left heart syndrome [Clancy et al., 2001]. Early allopurinol in asphyxiated infants improved short-term neurodevelopmental outcomes and decreased serum NO levels after administration; however, no improvement in long-term outcomes was seen for later treatment

after birth asphyxia, perhaps because only a very brief window for benefit exists [Benders et al., 2006].

Inflammation

Nelson and colleagues first reported a link between elevated neonatal blood levels of a broad range of serum proinflammatory cytokines and subsequent diagnosis of spastic diplegia [Nelson et al., 1998]. Cytokines are polypeptides that act systemically and locally to mediate and regulate multiple components of inflammation. Cytokines that have been strongly implicated as mediators of brain inflammation in neonates include interleukin (IL)-1β, tumor necrosis factor (TNF)α, IL-6, and membrane co-factor protein-1 [Foster-Barber and Ferriero, 2002]. After an asphyxial episode, there are many potential sources of plasma cytokines, including injured endothelium and acutely injured organs, such as the brain by means of a disrupted blood–brain barrier. Measurements of cerebrospinal fluid and plasma levels of several cytokines in asphyxiated term infants suggest that the injured brain can be the source of acutely elevated cytokine levels [Silveira and Procianoy, 2003]. A more recent study links IL-6 with cerebral palsy, giving credence to the fact that there is an underlying genetic susceptibility in at-risk newborns [Wu et al., 2009].

The observed relation between maternal infection and neonatal brain injury could be explained by a number of mechanisms. Experimental studies provide support for the hypothesis that a proinflammatory milieu increases the susceptibility of the neonate to hypoxic-ischemic brain injury. In fetal or neonatal models, maternal infection is commonly simulated by injecting the potent proinflammatory agent, lipopolysaccharide (i.e., endotoxin derived from *Escherichia coli*). Systemically administered endotoxin amplifies neonatal hypoxic-ischemic brain injury in rodent and sheep models; some of these deleterious effects are mediated, at least in part, by systemic mechanisms (e.g., hypotension, hypoglycemia) [Lehnardt et al., 2003].

Drugs that block microglial activation and cytokine release protect the brain from excitotoxic damage [Dommergues et al., 2003]. Minocycline is a tetracycline derivative that crosses the blood–brain barrier and has been postulated to confer anti-inflammatory effects on microglia, as well as modulate immune cell activation, and cytokine and NO release, while also decreasing apoptosis. In the neonatal brain, minocycline appears to block hypoxia-ischemia-induced tissue damage and caspase-3 activation in rodents when given immediately before or after injury, but results are inconsistent [Arvin et al., 2002; Fox et al., 2005; Cai et al., 2006]. Minocycline attenuates lipopolysaccharide-induced brain injury and improves neurobehavioral outcomes in P5 rats via inhibition of microglial activation with resultant decreases in IL-1β and TNFα [Fan et al., 2005]. Low- and high-dose regimens were effective in reducing short-term hypoxia-ischemia-induced inflammation, protecting developing oligodendrocytes [Cai et al., 2006] and myelin content in neonatal rats [Carty et al., 2008], but this effect was only transient in another study of neonatal rodent stroke [Fox et al., 2005]. Following stroke, it decreases postischemic brain inflammation via inhibition of 5-LOX and enzymatic activation. Delayed therapy was found to decrease TNFα and matrix metalloproteinase (MMP)-12, but efficacy was lost when treatment was extended for a week after stroke [Wasserman et al., 2007]. These effects also appear to be species-dependent, with an increase in injury in developing C57B1/6 mice [Tsuji et al., 2004].

Apoptosis

Apoptosis is critical for normal brain development, but it is also an important component of injury following neonatal hypoxia-ischemia and stroke [Northington et al., 2005]. Activation of intrinsic or extrinsic apoptotic pathways leads to cleavage and activation of caspase 3, which is maximally produced in the neonatal period [Hu et al., 2000]. Pro-apoptotic Bax is present in high concentrations during the first 2 postnatal weeks [Lok and Martin, 2002]. While necrosis plays a major role in early neuronal death in both the immature and mature brain [Northington et al., 2001], there appears to be some aspect of apoptosis within the first 24 hours following neonatal hypoxia-ischemia [Portera-Cailliau et al., 1997], with a spectrum of cell death present that may result in heterogenous responses to anti-apoptotic therapies [Northington et al., 2005]. It is likely that apoptosis is not the cause of most acute cell death, but rather of delayed phases of injury and neurodegeneration. This delayed apoptotic cell death likely relates to target deprivation and loss of neurotrophic support [Northington et al., 2005]. Specific and nonspecific inhibition of caspases or cysteine proteases, which are highly activated after hypoxia-ischemia, has also been attempted with some success [Feng et al., 2003; Han et al., 2002; Blomgren et al., 2001; Ostwald et al., 1993]. See Chapter 14 for more details.

Brain Protection

Neuroprotection

In addition to manipulating some of the mechanisms described above, there has been a recent focus on using hypothermia, which may reduce injury at multiple steps. Although neuroprotective interventions consisting of pharmacologic antagonism of glutamate, free radicals, inflammatory mediators, and apoptosis have been successful to some degree in experimental neonatal and adult animal models of hypoxic-ischemic brain injury, none of these other strategies has been successfully translated into clinical practice. Perhaps it is time to consider syngeristic and combinatorial therapies with hypothermia.

A recent therapy that is becoming standard of care for selected newborns is the use of therapeutic hypothermia for brain injury. It is postulated to work by modifying apoptosis and interrupting early necrosis [Edwards et al., 1995], reducing cerebral metabolic rate and the release of excitotoxins, NO, and free radicals [Globus et al., 1995]. Multiple animal models of perinatal brain injury demonstrate histological and functional benefit of early initiation of hypothermia [Laptook et al., 1994, 1997; Thoresen et al., 1995; Gunn et al., 1997; Gunn et al., 1998b]. Brief hypothermia initiated early after injury provided partial neuroprotection [Laptook and Corbett, 2002; Towfighi et al., 1994], but prolonged moderate hypothermia to 32–34°C for 24–72 hours results in sustained improvement in behavioral performance in newborn and adult animals [Gunn et al., 1997, 1998b]. The only complications were transient reductions of heart rate and blood pressure [Thoresen and Whitelaw, 2000].

Review of human neonatal studies shows reduction in mortality and long-term neurodevelopmental disability at 12–24 months of age, with more pronounced effects in moderately encephalopathic infants [Gunn et al., 1998a; Eicher et al., 2005; Gluckman et al., 2005; Shankaran et al., 2005; Azzopardi et al., 2009]. Sustained protection does depend on the degree of hypothermia, with maximum benefit obtained with cooling to 33–34°C, as well as in minimizing delay time to treatment [Bona et al., 1998; Gunn et al., 1997]. Mild hypothermia to this level appears to be well tolerated without serious adverse effects if initiated within the first 6 hours of life [Gunn et al., 1998a; Azzopardi et al., 2000; Thoresen, 2000; Shankaran et al., 2002]. In selective head cooling, treatment benefited infants with moderate but not severe amplitude integrated EEG changes, improving survival without severe neurodevelopmental deficits or an increase in complications [Gluckman et al., 2005]. In addition to severity of encephalopathy, larger infants were more responsive to hypothermia and at higher risk for injury if hyperthermic at any point [Wyatt et al., 2007]. In a second multicenter trial, whole-body cooling to 33.5°C, initiated within 6 hours and continued for 72 hours, resulted in less death and severe disability at 18 months. In a piglet model, the degree of hypothermia altered the amount of protection in the cortical gray matter relative to the deep gray matter [Iwata et al., 2005]. Whole-body cooling may be more effective in reducing temperature in the deep brain structures [Van Leeuwen et al., 2000]. Most recently, another whole-body cooling trial was completed (TOBY) and the results were consistent with the other two major trials, with a significant number of treated babies showing survival without neurodevelopmental sequelae (Figure 17-3) [Azzopardi et al., 2009].

Three Published Trials of Hypothermia for Neuroprotection in the Newborn			
Outcome	Coolcap	TOBY	NICHD
Death or severe disability	66% v. 55% p = 0.1 P = 0.04 ADJUSTED	53% v. 45% p = 0.17	62% vs. 44% p <0.01
Disabling CP	31% v. 19% p = 0.12	41% v. 28% p = 0.03	30% vs. 19% p = 0.20
Survival without neurological abnl		28% v. 44% p = 0.003	

Gluckman et al Lancet 2005
Shankaran et al NEJM 2005
Azzopardi et al NEJM 2009

Fig. 17-3 Summary of published trials of hypothermia for neuroprotection in the newborn. CP, cerebral palsy.

Combinatorial therapy may provide more long-lasting neuroprotection, salvaging the brain from severe injury while also enhancing repair and regeneration, and hopefully providing additive, if not synergistic, protection.

Xenon is approved for use as a general anesthetic in Europe, and has shown promise as a protective agent. It is an NMDA antagonist, preventing progression of excitotoxic damage. It appears to be superior to other NMDA antagonists, possibly through inhibition of AMPA and kainite receptors, reduction of neurotransmitter release, or effects on other ion channels [Ma and Zhang, 2003; Dinse et al., 2005; Gruss et al., 2004]. The combination of xenon and hypothermia initiated 4 hours after neonatal hypoxia-ischemia provided synergistic histological and functional protection when evaluated at 30 days after injury in rodents [Ma et al., 2005]. More recently, an additive effect was shown after hypoxia-ischemia in P7 rats that were cooled to 32°C and received 50 percent xenon, with improvement in long-term histology and functional performance that exceeded the individual benefit of either [Hobbs et al., 2008]. Studies on xenon use in human neonates are under way.

N-acetylcysteine (NAC) is a medication, approved for neonates, that is a scavenger of oxygen radicals and restores intracellular glutathione levels, attenuating reperfusion injury and decreasing inflammation and NO production. Adding NAC therapy to systemic hypothermia reduced brain volume loss at both 2 and 4 weeks after neonatal rodent hypoxia-ischemia, with increased myelin expression and improved reflexes [Jatana et al., 2006]. Inhibition of inflammation with MK-801 has also been effective when combined with hypothermia in neonatal rats post hypoxic-ischemic injury [Alkan et al., 2001]. In P7 rats who underwent hypoxia-ischemia, followed by early topiramate and delayed hypothermia, improved short-term histology and function was seen [Liu et al., 2004]. This may provide a window for protection if hypothermia is delayed, which is possible, given the difficulty in initiation of cooling if infants are born outside hospital or transport is delayed.

Neurotrophic Factors

EPO is a 34-kDa glycoprotein that was originally identified for its role in erythropoiesis, but has since been found to have a variety of other roles. The pleiotropic functions of this cytokine include modulation of the inflammatory and immune responses [Villa et al., 2003], and vasogenic and pro-angiogenic effects through its interaction with vascular endothelial growth factor (VEGF) [Wang et al., 2004; Chong et al., 2002], as well as effects on CNS development and repair. EPO and EPO receptors are expressed by a variety of different cell types in the CNS, with changing patterns during development [Juul et al., 1999]. EPO plays a vital role in neural differentiation and neurogenesis early in development, promoting neurogenesis in vitro and in vivo [Shingo et al., 2001].

Recent evidence suggests that exogenously administered EPO has a protective effect in a variety of different models of immature brain injury [Sola et al., 2005b]. In newborn rodents, pretreatment with EPO before injury has a protective effect [Sola et al., 2005b]. In addition, postinjury treatment protocols have demonstrated both short- and long-term histological and behavioral improvement. A single dose of exogenous EPO administered immediately after neonatal hypoxic-ischemic injury in rats significantly reduced infarct volume and improved long-term spatial memory after injury [Kumral et al., 2004].

Single- and multiple-dose treatment regimens of EPO following neonatal focal ischemic stroke in rats also reduced infarct volume [Sola et al., 2005a] and improved short-term sensorimotor outcomes [Chang et al., 2005], but there may be more long-term behavioral benefit in female rats [Wen et al., 2006]. EPO treatment that was delayed 24 hours after neonatal hypoxia-ischemia also attenuated brain injury [Sun et al., 2005]. In addition, EPO enhances neurogenesis and directs multipotential neural stem cells toward a neuronal cell fate [Shingo et al., 2001; Wang et al., 2004; Gonzalez et al., 2007]. Following transient ischemic stroke, there is temporary precursor cell proliferation in the rodent subventricular zone (SVZ), with this precursor cell proliferation and differentiation favoring gliogenesis [Plane et al., 2004]. EPO has been shown to enhance neurogenesis in vivo in the SVZ following stroke in the adult rat [Wang et al., 2004]. Neurogenesis has also been demonstrated following EPO treatment with an increase in newly generated cells from precursors [Wang et al., 2004; Lu et al., 2005; Shingo et al., 2001], and possibly also an effect on cell fate commitment [Wang et al., 2004; Shingo et al., 2001] in vitro.

In humans, EPO is safely used for treatment of anemia in premature infants [Aher and Ohlsson, 2006]. EPO for neuroprotection is given in much higher doses (1000–5000 U/kg/dose) than that given for anemia [Chang et al., 2005; Demers et al., 2005; McPherson and Juul, 2007] to enable crossing of the blood–brain barrier, with unknown pharmacokinetics in humans. Recently, extremely low birth weight infants tolerated doses between 500 and 2500 U/kg/dose [Juul et al., 2008]. A recent trial of EPO for neonatal asphyxia showed that repeated low-dose therapy (300–500 U/kg every other day for 2 weeks) reduced the risk of disability for infants with moderate HIE and no negative hematopoietic side effects were observed [Zhu et al., 2009].

VEGF is a regulator of angiogenesis that also promotes neuronal cell proliferation and migration [Zachary, 2005]. The endothelial microenvironment establishes a vascular niche to promote survival and proliferation of progenitor cells, which is tightly coordinated with angiogenesis [Palmer et al., 2000]. VEGF-A is the most important member of a family of growth factors that also includes placental growth factor (PLGF) and VEGFs B, C, and D. VEGF-A expression occurs in cortical neurons during early development, switching to mature glial cells near vessels during later development. Following exposure to hypoxia, there is increased neuronal and glial expression [Krum and Rosenstein, 1998], directing vascularization and stimulating proliferation of astrocytes, microglia, and neuronal cell types [Forstreuter et al., 2002; Mu et al., 2003; Jin et al., 2002]. VEGF also has chemotactic effects on neurogenic zones in the brain [Yang and Cepko, 1996], increasing migration of stem cells during anoxia [Bagnard et al., 2001; Maurer et al., 2003]. VEGF knockout mice have severe impairments in vascularization, neuronal migration, and survival [Raab et al., 2004].

VEGF appears to play an essential role in the beneficial and protective effects of hypoxic preconditioning in neonatal mice [Laudenbach et al., 2007]. VEGF-R2 inhibition increases tissue injury and cell death in a neonatal stroke model, as well as reducing endothelial cell proliferation in the injured core [Shimotake, 2010].

Other trophic factors have also shown promise in reducing brain injury but, given their role in normal neurodevelopment, the effects of treatment are not known. Insulin-like growth factor-1 (IGF-1) has prosurvival properties that can prevent perinatal hypoxic or excitotoxic injury [Johnston et al., 1996; Pang et al., 2007]. Brain-derived neurotrophic factor (BDNF) is a neurotrophin that also provides neuroprotection in neonatal hypoxia-ischemia [Cheng et al., 1997, 1998; Holtzman et al., 1996; Husson et al., 2005]. It prevents spatial memory learning impairments after insult, but its effectiveness is limited by the stage of development [Husson et al., 2005; Cheng et al., 1998]. While protective in mice at P5, it exacerbates excitotoxicity at P0 and has no effect at later time points [Husson et al., 2005].

Stem Cells

Neural stem cells (NSCs) are multipotent precursors that self-renew and retain the ability to differentiate into a variety of neuronal and non-neuronal cell types in the CNS. They reside in neurogenic zones throughout life, such as the SVZ and sub-granular zone of the dentate gyrus in rodent models, and help maintain cell turnover at baseline and replace injured cells by migrating to penumbral tissue after injury. NSC transplantation has shown potential as a therapeutic strategy in adult animal models of stroke and hypoxia-ischemia. Implanted cells integrate into injured tissue [Park et al., 2002], decreasing volume loss [Hoehn et al., 2002; Park et al., 2006a, b] and improving behavioral outcomes [Capone et al., 2007; Hicks et al., 2007]. In neonatal models, intraventricular implantation of NSCs after hypoxia-ischemia results in their migration to areas of injury [Park et al., 2006a, b]. These stem cells differentiate into neurons, astrocytes, and oligodendrocytes, as well as undifferentiated progenitors. These cells not only promote regeneration, but non-neuronal phenotypes inhibit inflammation and scar formation, while promoting angiogenesis and neuronal cell survival in both rodent and primate models [Imitola et al., 2004; Mueller et al., 2006]. While no adverse effects have been noted, efficacy is dependent on time of implantation, and the therapeutic window is not known. More recent technology enables labeling of stem cells, which can then be tracked from their site of implantation through their migratory path into the ischemic tissue [Modo et al., 2004; Guzman et al., 2007; Rice et al., 2007; Obenaus et al., 2007], which will make tracking of these cells in humans possible [Ashwal et al., 2009].

Future Directions

In clinical practice, there is unexplained variation in the severity of acute encephalopathy and in the ultimate neurologic outcome among infants who have incurred apparently equivalent hypoxic-ischemic insults. It is attractive to speculate that genetic variation with respect to any of the mechanisms discussed in this chapter may account for these divergent outcomes. Experimental data provide compelling evidence that genetic factors influence susceptibility to hypoxic-ischemic brain injury; for example, in neonatal mice, there is wide interstrain variability in the severity of injury after the same hypoxia-ischemia insult. Sources of genetic variation that contribute to differential sus-

ceptibility, including sex, to a broad range of illnesses are a subject of intense investigation, and many specific examples are likely to emerge. Similarly, genetic variations in the metabolism and efficacy of neuroactive drugs will be important to delineate.

A major challenge for future studies will be to establish meaningful links between experimental and clinical data, and to identify clinically important developmental stage-specific risks and benefits of specific treatment modalities that emerge. The use of advanced brain imaging may improve the application of newborn protective strategies by the early identification and stratification of injury severity, as well as providing a non-invasive method to monitor early responses to new treatments. Brain imaging may also provide important insight into how therapeutic hypothermia is acting so that its use can be optimized and synergistic therapies added. For example, in two recent studies of cooled newborns, one showed that systemic cooling reduced cortical injury [Inder et al., 2004], while a more recent one demonstrated a decrease of injury in the basal nuclei and white mater. Importantly, therapeutic hypothermia did not limit the predictive value of MRI for subsequent neurological impairment [Rutherford et al., 2010.] Studies are needed to determine whether applying a specific method of cooling to a defined pattern of injury will enable individualized treatment. Complementary investigations in neonatal animal models and in the neonatal intensive care unit should continue to provide insights about basic mechanisms of neurodegeneration and repair that are particularly important in the developing nervous system.

Conclusions

The last decade has seen tremendous advances in our understanding of neonatal hypoxic-ischemic brain injury, including the application of therapeutic hypothermia as a clinical brain protection strategy. There remains a critical need to establish the causal link between antenatal and perinatal risk factors to the genesis of brain injury in the newborn so that preventive strategies can be implemented. Achieving this goal may be facilitated with the application of more accurate in utero measures of brain injury, such as fetal MRI. A better understanding of the mechanisms that underlie injury to the developing brain may provide opportunities to intervene with novel synergistic therapies that optimize existing therapies. Early recognition of newborns with hypoxic-ischemic brain injury, via detailed clinical assessment and high-quality MRI protocols, may improve our ability to implement neonatal intervention and optimize long-term rehabilitation therapies. Ultimately, the improved care of affected newborns should result in the reduction of life-long disabilities such as cerebral palsy, epilepsy, and behavioral and learning disorders.

Neonatal Brain Injury

Adam Kirton, Linda S. de Vries, Lori Jordan, and Jerome Y. Yager

Neonatal brain injury encompasses a wide variety of conditions that result in damage to the nervous system. This chapter focuses on only the conditions thought to be acquired at or near the time of birth – neonatal stroke and trauma – rather than diseases that manifest at birth with similar clinical presentations (e.g., neonatal encephalopathy) but are caused by metabolic diseases, genetic malformations, or early intrauterine ischemic events.

Although neonatal stroke and trauma are not uncommon, data about risk factors, causes, and outcomes are still scarce because of a paucity of population-based studies. However, emerging data are changing previous concepts regarding pathophysiology, especially for neonatal stroke. In the past, outcomes for these conditions have been primarily focused on the major neurologic residua of cerebral palsy (see Chapter 69). However, data from the Canadian Pediatric Stroke Registry and the German Childhood Stroke Study Group [deVeber et al., 2000; Kurnik et al., 2003] and from recent longitudinal studies [Westmacott et al., 2009a, b; Ballantyne et al., 2008; Ricci et al., 2008] suggest that cognitive deficits only become apparent during early childhood. This chapter reviews what is known regarding the incidence, causes, risk factors, and outcome of stroke and traumatic brain injury, with attention to the clinical presentations and methods of diagnosis and management after these conditions occur. Pathophysiology is discussed in more detail in Chapter 17 because hypoxic-ischemic injury and focal ischemia-reperfusion injury in the setting of stroke are thought to have common pathogenetic mechanisms. However, pathophysiology of trauma in the newborn period is relatively unstudied, and only broad assumptions can be made for these conditions.

Perinatal Arterial Ischemic Stroke

Definitions and Epidemiology

A recent National Institute of Neurological Disorders and Stroke workshop on perinatal stroke provided consensus recommendations on the definition and classification of ischemic perinatal stroke (Raju et al., 2007). Agreement about the following working definition was obtained during the workshop: "a group of heterogeneous conditions in which there is a focal disruption of cerebral blood flow secondary to arterial or cerebral venous thrombosis or embolization, occurring between 20 weeks of fetal life through the 28th postnatal day and confirmed by neuroimaging or neuropathology studies." The two major subtypes, ischemic (including cerebral venous thrombosis) and hemorrhagic perinatal stroke, will be discussed separately. Time of onset can be considered as "late fetal" (28 weeks to birth), "perinatal" (28 weeks to 7 days after birth), "neonatal" (0–28 days after birth), and "presumed perinatal" (symptoms presenting beyond day 28 of life). This part of the chapter will focus on perinatal arterial ischemic stroke (PAIS).

Brain infarction due to occlusion of a major artery or one of its territorial branches is now recognized in an increasing number of full-term infants, with an incidence of approximately 1 per 2300–4000 live births, not dissimilar to that of stroke in the elderly [Estan and Hope, 1997; Nelson and Lynch, 2004; Schulzke et al., 2005; Schneider et al., 2004; Kirton and deVeber, 2009]. Data in preterm infants are scarce, but have recently been reported with an estimated incidence of 0.7 percent in a hospital-based case-control study [Benders et al., 2007].

Stroke in newborns is reported to have a male predominance [Chabrier et al., 2009], but this was not seen in a recent study from the International Pediatric Stroke Study (IPSS) registry data, of 249 infants aged less than 29 days with arterial ischemic stroke. Just over half of the patients (57 percent) were male, with a 1.3:1 male:female ratio, which is not significant [Golomb et al., 2009]. There is a tendency toward involvement of left-sided lesions within territories of the middle cerebral artery [Golomb et al., 2009; Trauner et al., 1993]. This is thought to be due to hemodynamic differences in cerebral blood flow between the right and left carotid arteries due to the hemodynamic effects of a patent ductus arteriosus or possibly due to preferential flow of placental emboli into the left-sided cerebral vessels.

Despite relatively low mortality (3–10 percent in the Canadian Stroke Register) [deVeber et al., 2000] and low recurrence rates (1.1–5 percent) [deVeber et al., 2000; Fullerton et al., 2007; Kurnik et al., 2003], there is a significant risk of developing adverse neurologic sequelae. Unilateral spastic cerebral palsy develops in about one-third of infants, and impairments in vision, cognition, language, and behavior are common [Lee et al., 2005; Westmacott et al., 2009].

The infant mortality rate in the United States for 1995–1998 due to stroke (ICD-9 CM 430–437) is reported to be 5.33 deaths per 100,000 per year, the perinatal mortality rate is 2.21 per 100,000, and the neonatal mortality rate is 3.49 per 100,000 live births per year [Lynch and Nelson, 2001]. The National Hospital Discharge Survey (1980–1998) determined that, for infants younger than 30 days of age, the hospital mortality rate for neonatal stroke is 10.1 percent, or 2.67 deaths per 100,000 live births [Lynch and Nelson, 2001; Lynch et al., 2002], which is similar to a more recent review, in which the infant death rate due to cerebrovascular disorders was 3 per 100,000 in the United States in 2005 [Kung et al., 2008].

Pathophysiology and Risk Factors

Many maternal, fetal, and neonatal risk factors are associated with neonatal arterial ischemic strokes, but evidence for true causation is lacking in most cases. Often, more than one potential risk factor can be identified (Figure 18-1).

Maternal Risk Factors

A history of infertility was identified as a risk factor in two recent studies (7–11 percent) [Lee et al., 2005; Curry et al., 2007]. An assumption is made that ovarian stimulation drugs would result in a hypercoagulable state, leading to placental thrombosis, but this still has to be confirmed with placental examination. Other maternal conditions, such as thyroid disease, diabetes mellitus, and gestational diabetes, were noted, but have not been identified as independent risk factors.

Antepartum Risk Factors

Pre-eclampsia was identified as a consistent independent risk factor in several studies (15–25 percent) [Lee et al., 2005; Curry et al., 2007]. This condition is known to affect uteroplacental blood flow. Oligohydramnios and decreased fetal movements have also been identified as risk factors, but both have no longer found to be significant in multiple regression analyses [Lee et al., 2005; Curry et al., 2007].

Intrapartum Risk Factors

While Ramaswamy et al. [2004] found only six cases with neonatal arterial ischemic stroke among 124 infants admitted with neonatal encephalopathy, the birth process tends to be reported as being 'complicated' and an intervention to deliver the infant is often required. Infants were not often severely depressed at birth, however, and were often well enough to stay with their mothers rather than in a neonatal intensive care unit. Factors

that emerged after multivariate analysis were a prolonged second stage of labor (OR = 8.8; P = 0.001) and prolonged rupture of membranes (OR = 3.4; P = 0.05) [Lee et al., 2005]. More general signs of fetal distress (fetal heart-rate abnormalities, meconium-stained amniotic fluid, an Apgar score <7 at 5 minutes), cord abnormalities (tight nuchal cord), and need for intervention during delivery (instrumental delivery or need for emergent cesarean section) were more common in cases compared to controls, but were not identified as independent risk factors. A combination of three or more risk factors led to an odds ratio of 25.3. This implied a risk of 1 in 200 when three or more of the following risk factors were present: primiparity, infertility, oligohydramnios, pre-eclampsia, chorioamnionitis, prolonged rupture of membranes, decreased fetal movements, prolonged second stage of labour, and fetal heart-rate abnormalities [Lee et al., 2005].

Although the placenta is the most likely source of emboli to the fetal brain, data about the placenta are scarce, mainly because the placenta is often unavailable by the time the infant develops symptoms. Several placental abnormalities have been reported in infants with perinatal stroke, such as placental thrombosis, infarction, chorioamnionitis, funisitis, and placental chorioangiomas [Benders et al., 2007; Burke et al., 1997; Kraus et al., 1999; Elbers et al., 2011].

Postnatal Risk Factors

PROTHROMBOTIC RISK FACTORS

The peripartum period is a prothrombotic state in both the mother and fetus. Prothrombotic factors have been reported to play a possible role in the child, and more recently, it also has been shown that a prothrombotic factor is more often present in both mother and child [Simchen et al., 2009]. Gunther et al. [2000] performed a case-control study in 91 cases

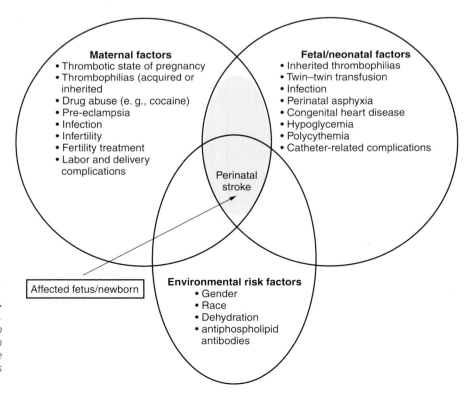

Fig. 18-1 Risk factors for perinatal arterial stroke. *(Adjusted from Raju TN, Nelson KB, Ferriero D et al. Ischemic perinatal stroke: summary of a workshop sponsored by the National Institute of Child Health and Human Development and the National Institute of Neurological Disorders and Stroke. Pediatrics 2007;120:609.)*

and showed that the percentage of prothrombotic risk factors was significantly higher in affected infants (68 percent compared to 24 percent; OR = 6,7, CI = 3,8–11,7). The most commonly found prothrombotic factors were elevated lipoprotein(a) and factor V Leiden, but hyperhomocysteinemia and mutations in the methyltetrahydrofolate reductase (*MTHFR*) gene also have been identified as associated factors. In two recent studies, high percentages of prothrombotic factors were found in both the neonate and the mother, as well as in mother–infant pairs, demonstrating the importance of also performing a thrombophilia screen in the mother [Curry et al., 2007; Simchen et al., 2009]. Simchen et al. [2009] noted a 8.5-fold increased risk for arterial ischemic stroke in a mother carrying factor V *G1691A* mutation (FVL), and a 2.1- and 3.8-fold increased risk in mothers with factor II *G20210A* mutation, or acquired antiphospholipid antibodies (APA) as compared to controls. In the study by Curry et al. [2007], a heterozygous or homozygous *MTHFR* C677T mutation was most common, seen in 41 of 60 neonates (68 percent). However, no significant differences between frequencies of prothrombotic coagulation defects were found in another recent cohort study [Miller et al., 2006].

OTHER NEONATAL RISK FACTORS

Arterial ischemic stroke is found in almost 40 percent of a series of infants preceding repair of congenital heart disease, and this is especially common in those infants who require atrial septostomy [McQuilllen et al., 2006]. In a more recent study, 10 percent of 122 patients with congenital heart disease were diagnosed with stroke, and in 6 patients the stroke occurred preoperatively. Stroke was clinically silent in 11 of the 12 infants [Chen et al., 2009]. Newborn infants undergoing extracorporeal membrane oxygenation are also at increased risk for developing arterial ischemic stroke (Wu et al., 2005).

Early-onset infection and bacterial meningitis have been associated with arterial and venous stroke. Maternal use of drugs, toxins, and alternative medication have all been reported in neonates with arterial ischemic stroke.

PAIS IN THE PRETERM INFANT

Independent risk factors identified in a case-control study of 31 preterm infants with stroke, using multivariate risk factor analysis, were different from risk factors identified in full-term infants. Twin-to-twin transfusion syndrome (TTTS) (OR = 31,2; 95 percent CI = 2.9–340.00), abnormal heart rate pattern (5,2; 1,5–17,6), and hypoglycaemia (<2 mmol/L) (3.9, 1,2–12,6) were independently associated with PAIS [Benders et al., 2007].

Perinatal Hemorrhagic Stroke

In a population-based cohort over a period of 10 years, a prevalence of 6.2 in 100,000 live births was observed for perinatal hemorrhagic stroke (PHS) [Armstrong-Wells et al., 2009]. A case-control study was performed with three controls per case. In contrast to what is known in infants with PAIS, all newborn infants with PHS presented with encephalopathy and more than half with seizures (65 percent). PHS was typically unifocal (74 percent) and unilateral (83 percent). Etiologies included thrombocytopenia (n = 4) and cavernous malformation (n = 1); 15 (75 percent) were idiopathic. Fetal distress and postmaturity were identified as independent predictors in a multivariate analysis.

Clinical Presentation and Diagnosis

PAIS in the newborn often manifests with seizures. The infants are initially well and have stayed with their mother on the ward, or can even be admitted from home. Whereas seizures associated with other forms of neonatal encephalopathy tend to be multifocal or myoclonic, seizures associated with arterial ischemic stroke tend to be persistently focal motor, usually involving only one upper extremity. Seizures tend to occur later than in neonates with hypoxic-ischemic encephalopathy (HIE) [Rafay et al., 2009]. Using multivariate analysis in 27 with PAIS and 35 with HIE, delayed seizure onset (≥12 hrs after birth) (p <0.0001; OR = 39.7; CI = 7.3, 217) and focal motor seizures (p = 0.007; OR = 13.4; 95 percent CI = 2.1,87.9) predicted stroke. Other more subtle symptoms observed in a large cohort of 215 newborn infants included poor feeding, hypotonia, and apnea [Kurnik et al., 2003; Redline et al., 2008].

In a population-based study of PAIS in children with motor impairment, most of the children presented after 3 months of life with hemiparesis (first recognized as early hand preference) or seizures [Wu et al., 2004]. These children are considered to have so-called "presumed perinatal ischemic stroke" (PPIS) [Kirton et al., 2008], which is diagnosed as a term (>36 weeks) infant older than 28 days with a normal neonatal neurologic history presenting with a neurological deficit or seizure referable to focal, chronic infarction on neuroimaging. Focal infarction specifies stroke (without limiting lesions to arterial territories) and includes unilateral/multiple/bilateral infarcts while excluding global injuries (HIE, watershed infarction, and periventricular leukomalacia [PVL]). Lesion chronicity is implied by imaging (restricted diffusion absent, encephalomalacia, gliosis, and atrophy of connected structures or Wallerian degeneration).

Infants with PPIS are less likely to have cortical involvement and more often show involvement of one or more of the lenticulostriate arteries. In a recent study, only 40 percent of late-diagnosed cases showed cortical involvement [Laugesaar et al., 2007]. In a large series of 59 cases with PPIS, venous periventricular venous infarction (PVI) was included in the spectrum of presumed perinatal stroke. Arterial proximal middle cerebral artery M1 segment infarction was most common (n = 19; 35 percent), and venous PVI was second (n = 12; 22 percent) and accounted for 75 percent of subcortical injuries [Kirton et al., 2008]. When risk factors are studied and outcome is reported, it is better to report children who are diagnosed in the neonatal period separately from those diagnosed later, referred to as PPIS.

Imaging

Cranial ultrasound studies (Box 18-1) may be normal if the stroke is superficial and ischemic, or they may reveal a wedge-shaped area of increased echogenicity with a linear demarcation line, usually within the territory of the middle cerebral artery. The echogenicity tends to become visible during the second half of the first week. Magnetic resonance imaging (MRI), including diffusion-weighted imaging (DWI), and MR angiography, is superior to head ultrasound, and should be performed in any newborn presenting with focal neonatal seizures.

The role of DWI in the prediction of motor outcome was first shown by Mazumdar et al. [2003] and subsequently by others [de Vries et al., 2005; Kirton et al., 2007], showing restricted diffusion within the descending corticospinal tracts. Restricted diffusion at the level of the internal capsule and especially the

---

Box 18-1 Evaluation of Neonates with Arterial Ischemic Stroke or Cerebral Sinovenous Thrombosis*

Prothrombotic Risk Factors

Probably Useful

- Complete blood count with differential (to screen for polycythemia and anemia)
- Prothrombin time (PT) with international normalized ratio (INR)
- Partial thromboplastin time (PTT)
- Serum electrolytes (to screen for dehydration)
- Protein C activity, protein S activity, antithrombin III activity†
- Activated protein C resistance (APCR) screen
- Lipoprotein(a)
- Homocysteine
- Factor V Leiden mutation
- Prothrombin 20210 gene defect
- Methylene tetrahydrofolate reductase (MTHFR) C677T gene defect
- Antiphospholipid antibody testing including:
  - Dilute Russell's viper venom time
  - Beta$_2$ glycoprotein immunoglobulin (Ig) G and IgM
  - Anticardiolipin antibodies IgG and IgM

Possibly Useful

- Factor VIIIc
- MTHFR A1298C gene defect
- Plasminogen activator inhibitor-1 gene 4G/5G polymorphism

Cranial Imaging

- Head CT; CT angiography or venography, as appropriate and available
- MRI; diffusion-weighted imaging (DWI), MR angiography or venography, as appropriate and available

Echocardiography

- Transthoracic echocardiography

Possibly Useful

- Follow-up transthoracic echocardiography with injection of agitated saline after 1 year of age; transesophageal echocardiography in rare cases to screen for patent foramen ovale (PFO) because all neonates will have a PFO detected if echocardiography is done too early

---

* There are few studies in this area, and there are no universally accepted guidelines.
† Normal levels (determined by antigen measurement and activity) for neonates are lower than for older children and adults. Levels may be temporarily low in the setting of acute illness; the significance of this is unclear.
(Data from Debus OM et al. The factor V G1691A mutation is a risk for porencephaly: A case-control study. Ann Neurol 2004;56:287; Manco-Johnson MJ, Grabowski EF, Hellgreen M et al. Laboratory testing for thrombophilia in pediatric patients. On behalf of the Subcommittee for Perinatal and Pediatric Thrombosis of the Scientific and Standardization Committee of the International Society of Thrombosis and Haemostasis [ISTH]. Thromb Haemost 2002;88:155–156.)

---

middle part of the cerebral peduncle is now referred to as "pre-Wallerian degeneration," as it is followed by Wallerian degeneration at 6–12 weeks and beyond (Figure 18.2).

A simple classification has been used, based on the primary artery involved [de Vries et al., 1997; Mercuri et al., 2004]. Infarcts in the territory of the middle cerebral artery were further subdivided into main branch, cortical branch, and lenticulostriate branch infarctions. Others have used a different classification, making a distinction between proximal M1 (PM1) of the middle cerebral artery that includes the lateral lenticulostriate (LLS) arteries, associated with infarction of the basal ganglia or distal M1 (DM1), in which compromised flow occurs distal to LLS and spares the basal ganglia while infarcting distal (cortical) middle cerebral artery territory. A third type of occlusion involves the anterior trunk of the middle cerebral artery, which is a superior middle cerebral artery division infarction that includes the frontal lobe (anterior-to-central sulcus) and the anterior temporal lobe (distal anterior trunk branch occlusions included). A fourth type involves the posterior trunk of the middle cerebral artery and is an inferior middle cerebral artery division infarction that includes parietal (posterior-to-central sulcus) and posterior temporal lobes (distal posterior trunk branch occlusions included). Finally, a fifth type, LLS infarcts, affects the basal ganglia (putamen and caudate body) and posterior limb of internal capsule (PLIC), with sparing of the subcortical white matter and cortex [Kirton et al., 2008]. Comparison of full-term and preterm infants showed that main branch involvement is rare in preterm infants, who tend to have LLS infarcts and less often show cortical involvement [Benders et al., 2009].

Newly developed techniques, such as diffusion tensor imaging (DTI), which allows quantification and visualization of white matter pathways in vivo, are more frequently being used in the evaluation of neonatal stroke [Lequin et al., 2009]. DTI characterizes the three-dimensional spatial distribution of water diffusion in each MRI voxel (see Chapter 11). Water diffuses preferentially along the direction of the axons and is restricted perpendicular to axons by myelin. This directional dependency is referred to as anisotropy. Directionality-encoded color maps (red–green–blue, RGB) or fiber tracking are commonly used. A fractional anisotropy (FA) map can show asymmetry of the PLIC as early as the neonatal period. In a study of 15 patients with congenital hemiparesis of different etiologies, studied at a median age of 2 years and compared with 17 age-matched controls, the clinical severity of hemiparesis was noted to correlate with asymmetry in FA (p <0.0001), transverse diffusivity (p <0.0001), and mean diffusivity (p <0.03) [Glenn et al., 2007]. Another promising technique is volumetric determination of stroke volumes, which was noted to predict motor outcome in animal studies [Ashwal et al., 2009]. Functional MRI (fMRI) tends to be used in childhood or adolescence to study reorganization of the sensorimotor cortex [Staudt et al., 2002; Seghier et al., 2005], but it was recently shown that passive unilateral sensorimotor stimulation is feasible, even in the preterm infant, resulting in bilateral activation of the sensorimotor cortex [Arichi et al., 2009; Heep et al., 2009].

Management/Treatment

Acute Period

For all types of perinatal stroke, supportive care with particular attention to monitoring of intracranial pressure is essential [Roach et al., 2008]. The use of continuous EEG monitoring

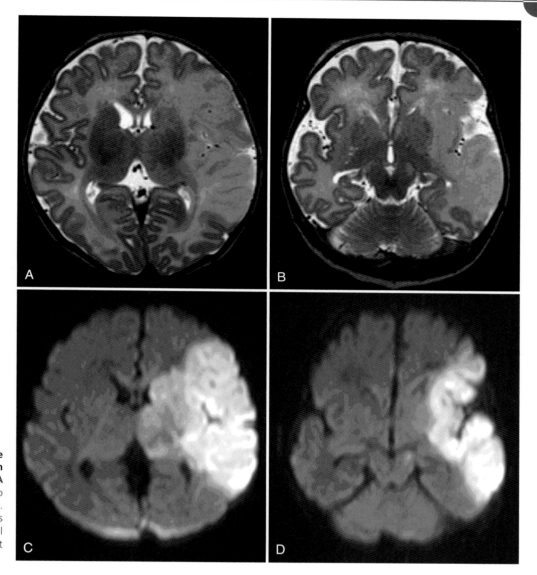

Fig. 18-2 Main branch middle cerebral artery infarct in a term infant with hemiconvulsions. A and **B,** T2 weighted spin eccho sequence (T2SE) (TR/TE = 7650/150). **C** and **D,** Diffusion-weighted images (b = 800). Involvement of basal ganglia and cerebral peduncle is best appreciated with DWI.

or amplitude integrated EEG (aEEG) may be helpful for recognizing and treating neonatal seizures. Unilateral ictal discharges can be identified using two-channel aEEG, often suggesting a unilateral parenchymal lesion, usually PAIS or PHS before an MRI can be acquired [van Rooij et al., 2009]. Guidelines on the management and treatment of PAIS were published in 2008 [Roach et al., 2008; Monagle et al., 2008]. The American College of Chest Physicians (ACCP) only recommends administration of unfractionated heparin (UFH) or low molecular weight heparin (LMWH) in neonates with their first PAIS and an on-going documented cardioembolic source. Thrombolytic agents are not recommended.

Outcomes

Perinatal stroke in the term and near-term neonate may result in significant long-term morbidities, including cerebral palsy, cognitive delay, epilepsy, and sensory deficits. Many variables, including the extent of injury and the presence of coexistent conditions, may help predict the eventual outcome. Impairments may only become apparent after several years.

Motor Effects

Arterial ischemic stroke may lead to permanent motor impairment or cerebral palsy. Estimates of motor impairment after neonatal arterial ischemic stroke range from 9 percent to 91 percent [Clancy et al., 1985; deVeber et al., 2000; de Vries et al., 1997; Golomb et al., 2008, Koelfen et al., 1995; Lee et al., 2005; Mercuri et al., 2004; Sran and Baumann, 1988; Trauner et al., 1993]. In a study by Lee et al. [2005], 58 percent of 40 children developed cerebral palsy and a delayed presentation was associated with increased risk for cerebral palsy (relative risk [RR], 2.2; 95 percent CI = 1.2–4.2). Cerebral palsy occurred in 68 percent of the largest cohort studied so far, and 87 percent of these children developed hemiplegia. This large cohort also consisted of infants with PAIS, with 47 percent developing cerebral palsy, as well as infants with PPIS, with 91 percent developing cerebral palsy. Most children with ischemic stroke diagnosed in the neonatal period attain independent walking, with the median time to taking first steps for the whole cohort, including infants with cerebral sinovenous thrombosis, being 13 months [Golomb et al., 2003]. In a study looking specifically at children with PPIS, motor outcomes (mean follow-up, 5.3 years) that were predicted by basal ganglia involvement included leg hemiparesis, spasticity, and need for assistive devices (p <0.01) [Kirton et al., 2008].

Sensory Deficits

Children with hemiplegic cerebral palsy are known to have sensory impairments but there are few detailed studies, in part because it is difficult to assess sensory function in young children [Cooper et al., 1995]. Thalamic atrophy has been seen in children with neonatal middle cerebral artery infarction, but whether this atrophy has long-term implications for sensory perception or memory is unclear [Giroud et al., 1995]. When children are carefully studied for visual field defects, hemianopia or quadrantanopia is not uncommon. Six (28 percent) of 16 school-age children with perinatal stroke had impaired visual function [Mercuri et al., 2003]. Children with unilateral pre- or perinatal stroke have more difficulty with facial recognition [Ballantyne and Trauner, 1999] and other visuospatial tasks [Schatz et al., 2000; Stiles et al., 1996, 1997].

Cognitive Effects

In some studies, most children with PAIS were noted to have intelligence within the normal range [Ricci et al., 2008; Trauner et al., 1993]. Cognitive impairment tends to be more common in the presence of hemiplegia and/or epilepsy. In a larger study of 46 infants, studied at a mean age of 42 months, cognitive impairment was present in 41 percent [Sreenan et al., 2000]. Cognitive outcome has only more recently been studied into childhood, showing more problems than intitially reported in small groups of infants studied early in life. Westmacott et al. [2009] studied 26 children with a history of acutely diagnosed unilateral PAIS as preschoolers (3 years 6 months to 5 years 11 months) and again as grade-school students (6 years 1 month to 12 years 5 months). While patients' performance did not differ from the normative sample for full-scale IQ, verbal IQ, or performance IQ, and there were no significant differences associated with infarct laterality as preschoolers, performance was significantly lower than the normative sample for full-scale IQ working memory and processing speed, but not for verbal IQ or performance IQ at school age. Contrasts between preschool evaluation and grade-school evaluation revealed a significant decline in full-scale IQ, which reflected emerging deficits in nonverbal reasoning, working memory, and processing speed. Individual subject analyses revealed that 69 percent of the children showed significant declines in one or more IQ index measures. There were no significant differences in cognitive performance associated with lesion laterality, although males performed more poorly than females on several cognitive measures at grade school. These data are not in agreement with a study by Ballantyne et al. [2008], who found no evidence of a decline in cognitive function over time in children with perinatal unilateral brain damage, suggesting that there was sufficient on-going plasticity in the developing brain following early focal damage to result in the stability of cognitive functions over time. The time span between the two tests was shorter than in the study by Westmacott et al. [2009], and the time at first test was later, which could explain some of the differences. In another study by the same group, comparing effects of age at stroke and lesion location, it was found that the perinatal group performed more poorly than the childhood group, regardless of lesion location [Westmacott et al., 2009].

Language delay is not uncommon after perinatal stroke and was found in 25 percent of 36 survivors of the Kaiser Permanente study [Lee et al., 2005]; lesion laterality does not appear to predict degree of language impairment, but development of postneonatal epilepsy was a major contributor to language outcome [Ballantyne et al., 2008]. Above-average academic performance is, however, also possible in the setting of large middle cerebral artery strokes and hypsarrhythmia [Golomb et al., 2005]. In children with presumed perinatal stroke, nonmotor outcomes were associated with cortical involvement, including cognitive/behavioral outcomes, visual deficits, and epilepsy (p <0.01) [Kirton et al., 2008].

Epilepsy

Data about rates of childhood epilepsy after PAIS are still scarce. The longer the follow-up period, the greater the risk that there has been a recurrence of epilepsy following seizures seen in the neonatal period. During the first year there is a subset of children who will develop hypsarrhythmia, usually associated with cerebral palsy and cognitive impairment [Golomb et al., 2006]. Infants with hypsarrhythmia following "presumed perinatal stroke" appeared to have a better cognitive outcome. The highest rate of epilepsy after the neonatal period for neonates with arterial ischemic stroke reported is 67 percent, established in a group of 64 children, with resolution of their epilepsy in 32 percent [Golomb et al., 2007]. In a series of 46 children with a mean follow-up duration of 42.1 months (range 18–164 months), 46 percent developed epilepsy [Sreenan et al., 2000]. In a series of 67 preterm and full-term infants with PAIS, epilepsy occurred in 16 percent and was seen most often in children following main branch middle cerebral artery infarction (7/15, 47 percent) [Benders et al., 2009].

Recurrence

The recurrence rate after PAIS is low. The largest prospective study, which followed 215 neonates with arterial ischemic stroke for a median of 3.5 years, found that only 1.8 percent of children developed a recurrent stroke and 3.3 percent a recurrent symptomatic thromboembolism. Prothrombotic risk factors and the presence of additional morbidities, such as complex congenital heart disease or dehydration, were associated with an increased recurrence risk [Kurnik et al., 2003]. More recently a similar 5-year cumulative recurrence rate of 1.2 percent was reported (1 of 84 infants with PAIS) [Fullerton et al., 2007]. Also observed was the fact that children whose stroke occurred later in childhood had a 16-fold increased recurrence risk compared with the neonates (HR = 16; 95 percent CI = 2.1–120; p = 0.008).

Predictors of Outcomes

VASCULAR TERRITORY

The vascular territory that is infarcted aids in predicting outcome but is not highly accurate. One study of 24 children with perinatal stroke reported that concomitant involvement of cortex, basal ganglia, and internal capsule on MRI predicted hemiplegia more strongly than involvement of just one of these territories [Mercuri et al., 1999]. Two studies of initially 23 and subsequently 54 preterm and term neonates with middle cerebral artery ischemic stroke found that involvement of the main branch territory was predictive of hemiplegia [de Vries et al., 1997; Benders et al., 2009]. In a study of 62 children with neonatal arterial ischemic stroke, the presence of bilateral infarctions predicted a lower probability of walking [Golomb et al., 2003]. Another study found that large stroke size (RR = 2.0; 95 percent CI = 1.2–3.2) and injury to Broca's area (RR = 2.5; 95 percent CI = 1.3–5.0), internal capsule (RR = 2.2; 95 percent CI = 1.1–4.4), Wernicke's area (RR = 2.0; 95 percent CI = 1.1–3.8), or basal ganglia (RR = 1.9; 95 percent CI = 1.1–3.3) were predictors of hemiplegia [Lee et al., 2005]. Using DWI, "pre-Wallerian degeneration" can be recognized as restricted diffusion involving the descending corticospinal tracts. Restricted diffusion of the internal capsule and especially the cerebral peduncles is now considered to be the best and earliest predictor of hemiplegia [de Vries et al., 2005; Kirton et al., 2007]. In the small series of 14 infants studied by Kirton et al. [2007], percentage of peduncle being affected (p = 0.002), length of descending corticospinal tracts (p <0.001), and volume of descending corticospinal tracts (p = 0.002) were significantly associated with subsequent development of hemiplegia.

NEONATAL SEIZURES AND EARLY ELECTROENCEPHALOGRAM

In one study of 46 neonates with arterial ischemic stroke, the presence of seizures in the neonatal period was predictive of one or more disabilities in the first years of life [Sreenan et al., 2000]. The presence of an abnormal background EEG pattern was a predictor of hemiplegia in another study [Mercuri et al., 1999].

PROTHROMBOTIC COAGULATION FACTORS

Two studies showed an association between the presence of prothrombotic coagulation factors and neurological outcome. Among the 24 children studied by Mercuri et al. [2001], 9 developed hemiplegia and 8 had at least one prothrombotic coagulation factor (FVL or increased factor VIIIc), compared to only 2 (factor VIIIc) of the 13 with a normal outcome. In the study by Suppiej et al. [2008], inherited thrombophilia was significantly more common in patients with a poor neurologic outcome (Fisher's exact test, p = 0.002), but this only applied to the children with PPIS.

REHABILITATION

As PAIS usually involves the middle cerebral artery, the upper extremity tends to be more severely affected than the lower extremity. Most children will be able to walk and first steps were taken at a mean age of 13 months, but this cohort consisted of children with PAIS (n = 62) or cerebral sinovenous thrombosis (n = 25) [Golomb et al., 2003]. Performing the assisting hand assessment (AHA) at 18 months can, to a certain degree, predict function of the assisting hand [Holmefur et al., 2009]. Until recently, treatment has been aimed at reducing spasticity and improving range of motion and function, using serial casting or botulinum toxin injections to reduce increased tone [Russo et al., 2007]. More recently, novel strategies have been used, such as constraint-induced movement therapy (CIMT), which involves restraining the unaffected arm to force use of the plegic arm, and this treatment strategy has been shown to be promising for improving function in hemiplegic

cerebral palsy [Taub et al., 2004; Deluca et al., 2006]. In 4 out of 10 patients (age range 10–30 years) with hemiplegia following PAIS and preserved corticospinal projections from the affected hemisphere, increases in fMRI activation at the level of the primary sensorimotor cortex, as well as in the supplementary motor areas, were seen [Juenger et al., 2007]. In subsequent studies by the same group it was noted that improvement only occurred in patients with preserved crossed projections, with increased amplitude shown with transcranial magnetic stimulation (TMS) when stimulating the ipsilesional hemisphere [Kuhnke et al., 2008; Walther et al., 2009]. These studies, involving only small groups of children, do suggest that CIMT in PAIS with preserved crossed corticospinal projections induces neuroplastic changes in the primary motor cortex of the lesioned hemisphere, detected as increased cortical excitability (TMS) and increased task-related cortical activation (fMRI).

Neonatal Cerebral Sinovenous Thrombosis

Epidemiology

Population-based studies of neonatal cerebral sinovenous thrombosis (CSVT) are rare. Based on data from the Canadian Pediatric Stroke Registry, the incidence of CSVT in children is 0.67 per 100,000, and in neonates is 0.41 per 100,000 [deVeber et al., 2001]. This study included 69 neonates and is one of the larger studies in this population. A study from the Netherlands included 52 infants, admitted to five neonatal intensive care units [Berfelo et al., 2010]. The largest study to date, which was not population-based, included 84 neonates with symptomatic CSVT [Jordan et al., 2010]; 61 percent presented during the first week of life.

Pathophysiology and Risk Factors

The cerebral veins drain into the dural venous sinuses and this slowly flowing blood is presumably more susceptible to thrombosis. The dural venous sinuses are near suture lines and this location may result in trauma at the time of birth [Shroff et al., 2003]. Occlusion of venous sinuses results in cerebral venous congestion and persumably is the cause of brain injury [Adams, 2007]. Increased venous pressure may cause cerebral edema, venous infarction with or without hemorrhagic conversion, and intraventricular hemorrhage [Wu et al., 2002]. Wu et al. first pointed out that CSVT should always be considered in the presence of an intraventricular hemorrhage (IVH) occurring at term, especially when this is associated with a unilateral thalamic hemorrhage. Thirty-one percent of 29 infants born > 36 weeks' gestation, who were diagnosed with CSVT, presented with an IVH. Thalamic hemorrhage was diagnosed in 16 percent of infants with CSVT [Wu et al., 2002]. Intracranial hypertension is often present due to venous congestion and to impaired cerebrospinal fluid reabsorption through the arachnoid granulations that are within the venous sinuses [Adams, 2007].

Risk factors for CSVT during the first 28 days of life include dehydration, infection, maternal fever/chorioamnionitis, hypoxic-ischemic injury, and thrombophilia [Fitzgerald et al., 2006; Kenet et al., 2007]. Often, neonates have more than one risk factor [Wu et al., 2002].

Clinical Presentation and Diagnosis

Seizures are the most common presentation in a neonate, followed by nonspecific signs such as lethargy, hypotonia, feeding difficulties, respiratory distress, and apnea [deVeber et al., 2001; Fitzgerald et al., 2006; Wasay et al., 2008]. Focal deficits are present in very few neonates: 6 percent in two different studies [deVeber et al., 2001; Jordan et al., 2010]. With an extensive CSVT, neonates will present with tense or bulging fontanels, splaying of the cranial sutures, and prominent scalp veins. These are signs of poor cerebral venous drainage and increased intracranial pressure.

Cranial ultrasound may detect CSVT, particularly in the presence of a midline thrombus in the superior sagittal sinus, or a unilateral thalamic hemorrhage. Power Doppler may be superior to color Doppler when available [Govaert et al., 1992a; Tsao et al., 1999]. Additional imaging is required to exclude CSVT in more peripheral locations and to confirm the extent of the thrombus. Unenhanced CT may detect a thrombus, and contrast-enhanced CT may show the "empty delta" sign which is a filling defect in the posterior portion of the superior sagittal sinus due to thrombus. Radiologically based false-positive or missed diagnoses have been reported in up to 40 percent of children with CSVT [Davies and Slavotinek, 1994]. MRI of the brain and MR or computed tomography (CT) venography are needed to confirm the diagnosis [Eichler et al., 2007] (Figure 18-3 and Figure 18-4). Susceptibility-weighted imaging (SWI) has recently been reported as another useful sequence in confirming the presence of CSVT and for following to establish progression or resolution [Takekawa et al., 2008; Kawabori et al., 2009].

Management/Treatment

Published consensus-based guidelines for antithrombotic treatment of neonatal CSVT are not in agreement. The American College of Chest Physicians guidelines, published in 2004 [Monagle et al., 2004] and updated in 2008 [Monagle et al., 2008], suggest anticoagulation for neonates without significant intracranial hemorrhage, while the American Heart Association (AHA) guidelines, published in 2008 [Roach et al., 2008], recommend anticoagulation only

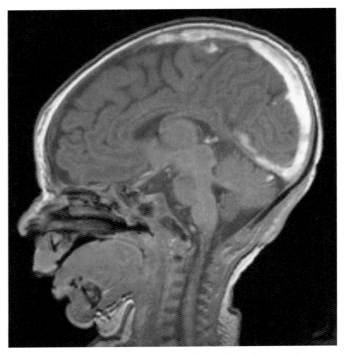

Fig. 18-3 Sagittal T1 MRI shows extensive T1 hyperintense thrombus within the superior sagittal sinus, straight sinus, and the vein of Galen in a 2-week-old neonate who presented with seizure.

when there is evidence of thrombus propagation, multiple cerebral or systemic emboli, or a severe prothrombotic state. From the Canadian Pediatric Ischemic Stroke Registry, only 25 of 69 neonates (36 percent) with CSVT, diagnosed between 1992 and 1998, were anticoagulated [deVeber et al., 2001]. Most treated neonates received low molecular weight heparin (LMWH; 20 of 25). None had hemorrhagic complications associated with death or neurologic deterioration. Hemorrhagic infarction was reported in 24 of 69 neonates (35 percent), while ischemic infarction was reported in 5 of 69 (7 percent). Similar data were obtained in the Netherlands, where 23 of 52 infants received anticoagulation without any hemorrhagic complications [Berfelo et al., 2010]. In a European collaborative study

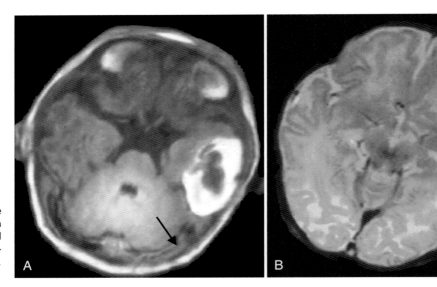

Fig. 18-4 In a 6-day-old neonate with focal seizures, MRI reveals a venous infarct in the temporal lobe with a thrombosed left transverse sinus (arrow). A, SE = 500/15. **B**, SE = 3000/120.

of childhood CSVT, 75 neonates were included [Kenet et al., 2007]. Specific data for neonates were not reported in detail, but there was no significant difference in treatment for children younger versus those older than age 2 years. If anticoagulation is deferred in a neonate with a CSVT, then follow-up neuroimaging should be performed after 5–7 days of supportive care to assess for thrombus propagation. If anticoagulation is used, the duration of therapy is typically 6 weeks to 3 months [Shroff et al., 2003; Moharir et al., 2010].

A recent small series (n = 10) of neonates with CSVT and intracerebral hemorrhage (unilateral thalamic hemorrhage) showed that 7 out of 10 neonates who were treated with anticoagulation did not show an increase of the thalamic hemorrhage [Kersbergen et al., 2009]. There are insufficient data to recommend thrombolysis; however, there are case reports of thrombolysis in the setting of progressive CSVT despite anticoagulation [Wasay et al., 2006; Wong et al., 1987].

Outcomes

There is significant risk of adverse outcome. There are few studies with detailed long-term outcomes, but even in younger children, motor and cognitive impairments, as well as epilepsy, are frequent. In series of 42 neonates with CSVT, only 6 of 29 (21 percent) children available for follow-up were neurologically normal at a median age of 2 years. The others had some impairment, such as persistent seizures or motor or cognitive problems [Fitzgerald et al., 2006]. Other studies have reported developmental delays or neurologic deficits in 35–50 percent of individuals [Carvalaho et al., 2001; Jordan et al., 2010]. Not surprisingly, the presence of cerebral venous infarction is one predictor of poor outcome, particularly when infarction is bilateral [deVeber et al., 2001; Golomb et al., 2003].

Data on recurrence risk after neonatal CSVT are limited. In the Canadian Pediatric Stroke Registry, 5 of 69 (7 percent) neonates had a recurrent systemic or cerebral thrombosis at a mean follow-up time of 1.6 years [deVeber et al., 2001].

Motor Effects

Hemiparesis, cerebral palsy, and nonspecific motor effects have all been reported after neonatal CSVT, with estimates ranging from 6 to 67 percent [deVeber et al., 2000, 2001; Fitzgerald et al., 2006]. The median length of follow-up in these studies ranged from 1.6 to 2 years. Most children with a history of perinatal ischemic stroke (including CSVT) eventually walk. In a Canadian cohort of 88 term or near-term neonates with CSVT or arterial ischemic stroke, 100 percent of those with CSVT without parenchymal infarction walked [Golomb et al., 2003]. Of those with infarction (due to arterial ischemic stroke or CSVT), 95 percent with unilateral infarcts and 67 percent with bilateral infarcts walked. The median age of first steps for the cohort was 13 months.

Cognitive Effects

Many studies combined PAIS and CSVT when looking at outcomes. In one study that focused specifically on CSVT, 1 of 19 neonates had a learning disability, and generalized developmental delays were reported in up to 58 percent; the median length of follow-up was 5 years [Carvalho et al., 2001].

Epilepsy

The risk of epilepsy after neonatal CSVT has been estimated at 6–18 percent [deVeber et al., 2001; Shevell et al., 1989]. When no parenchymal infarct is present after neonatal CSVT, epilepsy is less likely [Fitzgerald et al., 2006].

Rehabilitation

Rehabilitation strategies for neonatal CSVT are the same as those for PAIS. No studies specifically targeted the neonatal CSVT population.

Perinatal Birth Trauma

Perinatal traumatic injuries were first reported almost 2 centuries ago. In 1819, the occurrence of subgaleal hematoma was described by Naegele [Amar et al., 2003]. Salmonsen described cranial birth injuries after normal spontaneous vaginal deliveries in 1928 [Pollina et al., 2001]. Perinatal spinal cord injury was reported as early as 1869, when Parrot described an infant with difficult delivery requiring significant traction to the head, which resulted in rupture of the spinal cord at C6–7. In the 1920s, several classic articles on spinal cord injury were published [Blount et al., 2004; Filippigh et al., 1994; Rossitch and Oakes, 1992]. With recognition of the risk of significant perinatal central nervous system (CNS) injuries and improvements in obstetrical techniques, the incidence of such injuries has decreased but remains a significant cause of neonatal morbidity and mortality.

Definition and Epidemiology

Although cranial birth injuries in newborn infants are rare, they are potentially life-threatening. Major birth trauma, defined as "any condition that affects the fetus adversely during delivery" [Hughes et al., 1999], occurs in approximately 3.2 percent of births. Mechanical forces and hypoxia can contribute to birth injury. Mechanical trauma can result in damage to the extracranial, cranial, or intracranial structures; spinal cord; or peripheral nerves. Most birth injuries are clavicular fractures, accounting for more than 94 percent of injuries [Medlock and Hanigan, 1997]. However, 2 percent of all neonatal deaths and 10 percent of all neonatal deaths of term infants are the result of birth injury [Hughes et al., 1999; Pollina et al., 2001]. Injury-related neonatal death can result from intracranial hemorrhage, massive blood loss as a result of subgaleal hemorrhage, or cervical spinal cord injury.

Risk Factors

A variety of factors predisposing infants to birth trauma have been reported. These include fetal macrosomia, breech or footling presentation, shoulder dystocia, prolonged labor, primiparity, and forceps- or vacuum-assisted delivery [Hughes et al., 1999; Medlock and Hanigan, 1997; Perrin et al., 1997; Pollina et al., 2001]. There also have been reports of significant perinatal injury, even in the setting of seemingly uncomplicated delivery [Chamnanvanakij et al., 2002; Medlock and Hanigan, 1997; Pollina et al., 2001]. During the normal birth process, the fetal head is subjected to significant intrauterine pressure, ranging from 38 to 390 mmHg, with an average of 158 mmHg [Medlock and Hanigan, 1997]. These pressures can result in overriding sutures, which may cause direct cerebellar trauma, and rupture or tearing of large venous channels, bridging veins, or tentorial leaflets [Chamnanvanakij et al., 2002; Hayashi et al., 1987; Perrin et al., 1997]. Traction and torsion injuries may result in cervical spinal cord and brachial plexus injury [Filippigh et al., 1994; Menticoglou et al., 1995; Rehan and Seshia, 1993; van Ouwerkerk et al., 2000].

There is controversy about the effect of mode of delivery on the incidence of significant neonatal injury. In a large study of 583,340 live-born singleton infants born to nulliparous women and weighing between 2500 and 4000 g, Towner et al. [1999] found that the incidence of neonatal intracranial injury (including subdural, intracerebral, intraventricular, and subarachnoid hemorrhage) was significantly higher with vacuum extraction, forceps delivery, and cesarean delivery during labor (odds ratios of 1.9–3.4), compared with spontaneous vaginal delivery or cesarean section with no labor. The investigators concluded that the increased risk of injury resulted from abnormal labor requiring intervention, rather than vacuum extraction or forceps delivery [Towner et al., 1999]. In another study, Pollina et al. [2001] conducted a retrospective chart review of 41 children with cranial birth injuries (i.e., skull fracture, epidural or subdural subarachnoid intracerebral intraventricular hemorrhage, or intraparenchymal brain injury) over a 9-year period. They found that birth weight, Apgar scores, and mode of delivery were independently associated with cranial injury. However, in contrast with the previous study, these investigators found that the incidence of cranial trauma was only slightly higher with delivery by cesarean section compared with spontaneous vaginal delivery, whereas it was markedly higher for infants delivered by means of forceps- or vacuum-assisted delivery [Pollina et al., 2001].

Clinical Presentation and Management by Diagnosis

The clinical presentation of neonatal traumatic CNS injury varies according to the type of injury. Most commonly, cranial birth injuries manifest with apnea and seizures [Pollina et al., 2001]. Clinical presentations of the different types of injuries are discussed in more detail in later sections. A neonate presenting with signs and symptoms of cranial birth injury should be evaluated for anemia, thrombocytopenia, and coagulopathy. Laboratory tests should include complete blood count, prothrombin time, partial thromboplastin time, fibrinogen, and blood typing in anticipation of possible transfusion in more severe cases. Because of the difficulty in distinguishing between neonatal sepsis and cranial trauma on presentation, blood and urine cultures and a lumbar puncture are often performed during the initial evaluation [Chamnanvanakij et al., 2002]. Results of these initial evaluations usually reveal predisposing factors, such as vitamin K deficiency, hemophilia, thrombocytopenia, sepsis, or disseminated intravascular coagulopathy [Haase et al., 2003].

Radiographic studies that should be considered depend on the presentation and suspected site of injury. CT scanning is useful in the acute phase when neurosurgical intervention is considered. Depressed skull fractures, large subgaleal hematomas, and intracranial hemorrhage will be recognized. MRI can further elucidate parenchymal injury and underlying bony fractures revealed by CT.

Extracranial Injury

Scalp electrode injury is a possible effect of monitoring. Use of scalp electrodes for fetal monitoring has increased along with fetal blood sampling for blood gas measurement. The site of insertion can become a site of infection or bleeding. Although generally benign, scalp electrodes are associated with infection in 1 percent of cases, and in rare cases (usually in preterm infants), they can cause severe bleeding leading to hypotension.

Caput succedaneum refers to the soft tissue swelling that is often associated with bruising over the molded region. Although the condition is generally benign and resolves over time, abrasions over the area can become infected, and absorption of blood from bruising can result in hyperbilirubinemia.

Cephalohematoma is the term for hemorrhage into the subperiosteum as a result of separation of the pericranium from the skull during birth. It does not cross suture lines and does not transilluminate (in contrast to caput succedaneum). The incidence ranges from 0.4 to 2.49 percent of live births [Hughes et al., 1999]. Ultrasound may distinguish between cephalohematomas and subgaleal hematomas, and detect coexisting intracranial hemorrhage. Spontaneous resolution usually occurs, with calcification appearing as a rim of curvilinear new bone that resorbs within 2–8 weeks (Figure 18-5). Rarely, a cephalohematoma may become infected [King and Boothroyd, 1998].

Skull fracture is associated with cephalohematoma in up to 25 percent of neonates [Hughes et al., 1999], and skull radiography or CT is indicated when a fracture is suspected. Significant cephalohematoma may result in symptomatic anemia or hyperbilirubinemia, or both. Aspiration of a cephalohematoma is indicated only in the presence of increasing size, increasing erythema, or suspected infection [Medlock and Hanigan, 1997].

Neonates with subgaleal hematomas present initially with fluctuant scalp swelling that may progress to skin discoloration

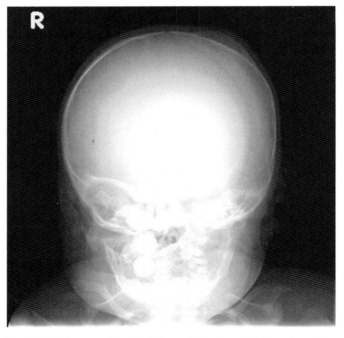

Fig. 18-5 Plain x-ray film depicts a calcified cephalohematoma in a 6-week-old infant.

of the frontal and suboccipital areas, and obscuration of the fontanel. In contrast to cephalohematoma, subgaleal hematomas may cross suture lines and extend to the nape of the neck. Most subgaleal hematomas are benign and do not require treatment [Medlock and Hanigan, 1997]. If the hematoma is large enough to cause cerebral injury, irritability, lethargy, poor feeding, and other signs of CNS depression may ensue [Amar et al., 2003]. A rough estimate of blood loss can be made by equating a 1-cm increase in head circumference to a 40-mL blood loss. In severe cases, it is a potentially fatal condition. Diffuse swelling of the head occurs and there is evidence of hypovolemic shock; mortality rate is estimated at 20–25 percent. Subgaleal hemorrhages are caused by rupture of the emissary veins, which are connections between the dural sinuses and the scalp veins. Blood accumulates between the epicranial aponeurosis of the scalp and the periosteum. Most cases of subgaleal hemorrhage reported have been associated with use of a vacuum extractor. The incidence of subgaleal hemorrhage is estimated to occur in 4–6 of 10,000 spontaneous vaginal deliveries and in 46–59 of 10,000 vacuum-assisted deliveries [Chadwick et al., 1996; Uchil et al., 2003]. In a study by Kilani et al. [2006], associated intracranial hemorrhage was present in half of the 34 infants studied, and four (11.8 percent) of infants died. In yet another study, 31 percent had a poor outcome (five died, four had epilepsy, three with severe auditory dysfunction, two with cerebral palsy, and one with renal vein thrombosis) [Chang et al., 2007]. The group with the poor outcome had significantly more patients who had been transferred from other hospitals (p <0.001). Those with a poor outcome had significantly more hypotension (p <0.001) and seizures (p <0.05). Other reported risk factors are vacuum extraction, prematurity, male gender, African lineage, primiparity, macrosomia, positional dystocia, and hypoxia [Amar et al., 2003]. Prompt and aggressive administration of blood products and treatment of associated coagulopathy are recommended to improve outcome.

Cranial Injuries

Skull fractures should be suspected in any neonate with a cephalohematoma or subarachnoid hemorrhage. Skull fractures may be linear, most commonly involving the parietal bone, or depressed, resulting in the so-called "ping-pong" fracture. Although fractures due to fetal compression against the bones surrounding the birth canal may occur during normal delivery, they are often associated with application of forceps or other assisted deliveries [Hughes et al., 1999; Medlock and Hanigan, 1997; Papaefthymiou et al., 1996]. Isolated depressed skull fractures can be diagnosed on physical examination as a shallow depression, usually in the parietal region [Tavarez et al., 1989]. The presence of a concomitant caput, cephalohematoma, or subgaleal hematoma may mask the fracture, which can be diagnosed by radiographic imaging.

Depressed skull fractures should prompt neurosurgical evaluation, although not all fractures require elevation [Medlock and Hanigan, 1997; Tavarez et al., 1989]. Surgical intervention is indicated in the setting of associated complications, such as increased intracranial pressure, cortical compression, or underlying hematoma [Tavarez et al., 1989]. Other complications of depressed skull fractures include sagittal sinus thrombosis associated with an occipital depressed skull fracture [Medlock and Hanigan, 1997], osteodiastasis (i.e., separation between the temporal squama and occipital bone at the lambdoid

suture) associated with breech presentation and significant neck hyperextension [Pollina et al., 2001], and "growing skull fracture," or leptomeningeal cyst. This latter entity occurs as a result of a dural tear allowing free communication of the subarachnoid space and herniation of the meninges through the bony defect accompanied by rapid growth of the brain. Neurologic symptoms, such as seizures, behavioral disturbances, and motor weakness, may appear months to years after the injury. Some investigators advocate close follow-up of conservatively managed fractures with serial radiographs and CT [Papaefthymiou et al., 1996]. Ultrasound and MRI are also useful for evaluation of a leptomeningeal cyst [King and Boothroyd, 1998].

Intracranial Injuries

PATHOGENESIS

A paucity of studies have examined the underlying mechanisms of brain injury in the newborn and premature infant following traumatic delivery. Most information regarding the cellular mechanisms responsible for cell death are based on investigation of traumatic brain injury in older infants, toddlers, and children following accidental or nonaccidental injury. None the less, important information and lessons can be learned from these studies and are transferable to the newborn in terms of our general understanding of the evolution of injury and of how this can relate to treatment.

Traumatic injury to the brain involves three main mechanisms acting in concert to influence outcome. These include:
1. focal hemorrhagic or nonhemorrhagic lesions, which mainly occupy space intrinsic or extrinsic to the cortical gray matter
2. diffuse axonal injury, primarily to white matter
3. secondary injury associated with edema formation and subsequent reduction in surrounding tissue perfusion.

The mechanisms by which cell death occurs following traumatic brain injury, at the cellular level, are in some ways similar to those processes occurring after an hypoxic-ischemic event in the immature brain and are referred to in greater detail in Chapter 17. Direct impact to the developing brain as a result of trauma, the release of blood, and contusive disruption of cell membranes leads to the release of excitatory amino acids and calcium, and inflammatory responses that characterize those processes, leading to cell death along the necrotic/apoptotic continuum [Lea and Faden, 2001].

Each of these responses to injury is influenced significantly by the effects of age and maturational capacity of the developing nervous system. In this regard, it is known that the nervous system of the newborn infant has a reduced capacity for glutamate clearance from the synaptic cleft due to the decreased expression of glutamate transporters, near-adult levels of NMDA receptors, and increased permeability to calcium influx [Statler, 2006].

In addition, the immature brain is less able to quench free radicals. Traumatic brain injury, resulting in tissue disruption, results in the release of transition metals, such as iron and heme, originating from the degradation of intracellular and extracellular heme proteins. Iron is in very high concentrations in human developing oligodendroglia and is a huge source for the production of free radicals [Hussain and Juurlink, 1995; Thorburne and Juurlink, 1996]. Metallothioneins are among a number of proteins that reduce redox activity of transition metals; however, they are inadequately expressed in the developing brain, compared to adults. Similarly, the breakdown of heme is catalyzed by heme oxygenases (HO) found in neurons and glia, but in lower concentrations in the newborn than in the adult. Indeed, essentially all of the endogenous free radical scavenging proteins, including superoxide dismutase and glutathione reductase, are in reduced concentrations in the newborn compared to the adult brain [Bavir et al., 2006; Robertson et al., 2006].

Enhanced exposure to the putative amino acids, increased permeability to calcium influx, and the reduced capacity to scavenge free radicals, likely make the newborn brain more sensitive to the damaging effects of trauma than the adult brain, although this remains controversial. Additional potential contributing factors include the rapid and extensive brain swelling and edema that is seen in the younger infant, compared to the adult [Duhaime and Durham, 2007; Vannucci et al., 1993]. Although the cause for these age-related changes remains unknown, several theories have been proposed. Studies point to the relatively compliant skull and membranous suture properties of the newborn skull that are associated with an increased likelihood of brain distortion. Other studies have suggested that the blood–brain barrier is more permeable in the immature compared to the adult brain after injury [Grundl et al., 1994], and that inflammatory responses and diffusion of excitotoxic neurotransmitter release are greater in the developing brain [van Lookeren Campagne et al., 1994]. Increased brain swelling in newborns can cause secondary injury due to patchy cerebral hypoperfusion and surrounding ischemia, presumably augmenting the region of vulnerability. Duhaime et al. [2007] describe the MRI appearance of the "big black brain" in infants following nonaccidental traumatic injury as being due to excessive edema formation seen with subdural hemorrhages in contrast to the adult. This was thought to be secondary to a combination of clinical events, including apnea, seizures, and patchy areas of ischemia. Several pathologic studies have pointed to an increased number of "ischemic" changes in these postmortem brains that may contribute to the production of cell swelling [Geddes et al., 2001a; Geddes et al., 2001b].

The question as to whether the immature brain is more sensitive or resistant to injury compared to the adult continues to be debated [Kochanek, 2006]. The developing brain may well be more sensitive to injury, simply based on the immature nature of its endogenous protective mechanisms. Pragmatically, several laboratories have shown that the immature brain is more sensitive to injury. Following a focal contusion in newborn rats between 3 (preterm human equivalent) and 30 (juvenile human equivalent) postnatal days, investigators found widespread cell death which first appeared at 6 hours post injury, peaked at 24 hours, and subsided by 5 days after the injury. The extent of injury, which was uniformly apoptotic in nature, peaked at 3–7 postnatal days (term newborn human equivalent), and subsequently diminished [Bittigau et al., 1999; Pohl et al., 1999]. The authors concluded that the prognosis for traumatic brain injury is age-dependent, with the newborn being most sensitive. Similar findings were shown in an excitotoxic model of cell death. McDonald et al. [1988, 1992] injected NMDA into the brains of rat pups aged 7–42 postnatal days, and found that the volume of injury in the younger, immature rat was 21 times greater than that seen in their adult counterparts. Kolb et al. (1987, 2003) found that, after

surgically removing sections of the frontal lobe in rats of varying ages, both neurogenesis and functional recovery were age-dependent. Therefore, 1-day-old rats (very preterm human equivalent) had more extensive behavioral impairments than any of the other older groups of animals. Ten-day-old rats (term human equivalent) showed the greatest degree of behavioral sparing' and adult animals were less affected. Yager et al. (1996, 1997) showed that the newborn rat brain was more sensitive to injury following hypoxia-ischemia than older rats given the same insult. However, during recovery, younger rats showed a greater degree of behavioral functional recovery than did the adult animals, suggesting a greater degree of plasticity in the younger rats [Yager et al., 2005, 2006; Saucier et al., 2007].

Pathophysiologically, there is substantive evidence to suggest that the newborn brain, following traumatic injury, suffers the consequences of profound edema, leading to secondary ischemic injury and early extensive apoptotic cell death. The immature brain also appears to have a greater capacity for plasticity and potential recovery than the adult's. However, these relationships are clearly not fully elucidated; nor do they behave in a linear fashion [Giza and Prins, 2006]. Much research needs to be done before we fully understand the effect of traumatic brain injury in the newborn and how age influences outcomes and approaches to therapy.

Recent literature has further elucidated biomarkers of injury that may be used as surrogates for outcome determination and indicators for therapy. Berger et al. (2007) have determined serum levels of neuron-specific enolase (NSE), S100B, and myelin basic protein in groups of children following hypoxic-ischemic injury, inflicted traumatic brain injury (iTBI), and noninflicted traumatic brain injury (nTBI). This group found significant correlation between the three markers and outcome at 6 months of age [Beers et al., 2007], and between iTBI and hypoxic-ischemic insults [Berger et al., 2007]. Similarly, new neuroimaging techniques involving SWI, MR spectroscopy (MRS), and DTI are being used to determine the extent and diversity of early injury as markers of blood deposition (SWI) with greater sensitivity, metabolic perturbations (MRS), and long-term plasticity (DTI). These techniques, although being used in older children at present, have great capacity for use in the newborn [Ashwal et al., 2004a, b, 2006a, b].

EPIDURAL HEMATOMAS

Epidural hematomas in the neonate occur only rarely, even in the setting of intracranial hemorrhage [Park et al., 2006]. In one postmortem examination series, only 2 percent of neonatal intracranial hemorrhages were epidural in location. In a series of 41 patients with cranial injuries monitored over an 8-year period, no epidural hematomas were reported. The investigators postulated that this was because most epidural hematomas are asymptomatic and therefore unrecognized [Pollina et al., 2001]. Moreover, the bleeding is venous, resulting in the slow development of a hematoma and less dramatic presentation. Others have postulated that, because the dura mater does not separate from the skull as easily in neonates and the middle meningeal artery has not yet developed, neonates are at lower risk for epidural hematomas. Unlike epidural hematomas in older children, associated skull fractures are often absent [Park et al., 2006].

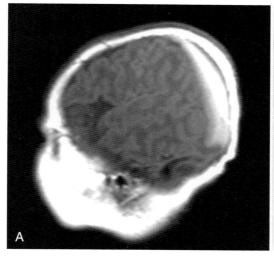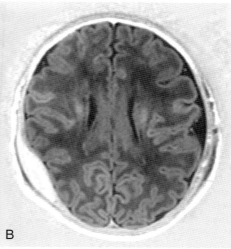

Fig. 18-6 MRI of a term infant who made a fall from her parent's shoulder, showing an epidural hematoma. A, Sagittal T1 (TR/TE = 512/15). **B,** Axial inversion recovery sequence (TR/TE = 4140/30).

Clinical presentation can include increasing head circumference, altered level of consciousness, or focal neurologic signs. Evaluation consists of obtaining a complete blood count, coagulation studies, and head CT or MRI (Figure 18-6). Neurosurgical evacuation of symptomatic epidural hematoma is required by craniotomy or by ultrasound-guided needle aspiration [Vachharajani and Mathur, 2002]. Neonates with isolated epidural hematomas have a good prognosis. In a review of several case series, Akiyama et al. [2001] found that, of 18 children with neonatal epidural hematomas, 5 (28 percent) died, and 3 of those who died had associated injuries, including subdural hematoma, intraventricular hemorrhage, or subarachnoid hemorrhage. The survivors all had good outcomes, with the exception of one child who had psychomotor delay. However, in this report, the length of follow-up and method of developmental assessment were not enumerated.

SUBDURAL HEMATOMAS

Subdural hematomas are the most common intracranial birth injury, accounting for 73 percent of neonatal intracranial hemorrhage [Pollina et al., 2001]. In a study of 583,340 live births of singleton newborns weighing between 2500 and 4000 g and excluding breech presentation, the incidence of subdural or cerebral hemorrhage was 2.9 per 10,000 for spontaneous vaginal delivery, 4.1 per 10,000 for cesarean section without labor, 21.3 per 10,000 with combined vacuum- and forceps-assisted delivery, and 25.7 per 10,000 for cesarean section after failed vaginal delivery [Towner et al., 1999]. Antenatal subdural hematomas and subdural hematomas after normal spontaneous vaginal delivery have been described [Chamnanvanakij et al., 2002]. While a significant subdural hemorrhage is most often related to birth trauma, a small subdural was noted to be common when MRI was performed routinely in 111 consecutive, asymptomatic full-term infants [Whitby et al., 2004]. Nine infants had a subdural hemorrhage: three following a normal vaginal delivery (6.1 percent) and five following a forceps after an attempted ventouse delivery (27.8 percent), and only one after a traumatic ventouse (i.e., vacuum device) delivery (7.7 percent). A similar incidence of a 26 percent prevalence rate for intracranial hemorrhage was determined in 88 newborns following vaginal births. However, in this group, no

association was seen with traumatic or assisted birth compared to an uncomplicated vaginal birth. All newborns were asymptomatic [Looney et al., 2007]. Risk factors include primiparity, vacuum- or forceps-assisted delivery, traumatic or breech delivery, asphyxia, shock, and coagulopathy [Chamnanvanakij et al., 2002; Haase et al., 2003; Hayashi et al., 1987]. Occipital diastasis can occur during a vaginal breech delivery with excessive extension of the newborn's neck. Vaginal breech deliveries are not commonly performed as a consequence of results of multicenter, randomized studies [Hofmeyr et al., 2003].

Neonatal subdural hematomas are thought to result from tearing of the falx and tentorium or bridging cortical veins due to stretching associated with labor. Hemorrhage is therefore most commonly seen in tentorial or interhemispheric areas [Haase et al., 2003; Perrin et al., 1997; Pollina et al., 2001]. Intraventricular, subarachnoid, or intraparenchymal hemorrhage may occur [Chamnanvanakij et al., 2002; Medlock and Hanigan, 1997]. Secondary cerebral infarction has also been reported and has been related to prolonged arterial compression [Govaert et al., 1992b]. The majority of the subdural hemorrhages are infratentorial (Figure 18-7), but a supratentorial location can also be noted and is sometimes associated with a lobar hemorrhage, which can be large and associated with a midline shift, requiring neurosurgical intervention.

Clinical presentation may vary from asymptomatic to severe mass effect with neurologic symptoms. When symptomatic, patients may present with irritability, poor feeding, apnea, seizures, or bradycardia [Perrin et al., 1997]. In one series of 26 infants with subdural hematoma, 60 percent had respiratory symptoms (e.g., cyanotic episodes, apnea), and the remainder had neurologic symptoms, including seizures, hypotonia, or both [Chamnanvanakij et al., 2002]. An overlying cephalohematoma, subgaleal hematoma, or skull fracture may be present. Other birth injuries, such as a brachial plexopathy (e.g., Erb's palsy) or clavicular fracture, may be present and are indicative of a difficult labor and delivery [Perrin et al., 1997]. Rarely, an infant with a subdural hematoma may present with signs of impending herniation or cerebral infarction [Govaert et al., 1992b; Haase et al., 2003; Perrin et al., 1997].

Appropriate laboratory evaluation includes a complete blood count and coagulation profile. Subdural hematomas may be diagnosed by head ultrasound, but definitive diagnosis, including the presence of intracerebral hemorrhage, cerebral

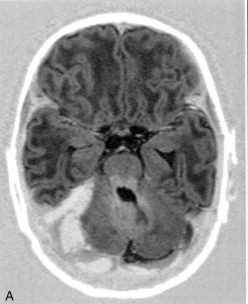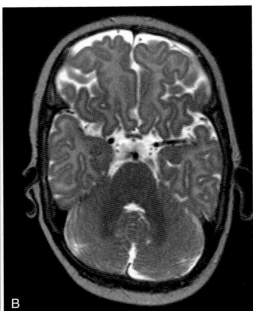

Fig. 18-7 MRI, axial inversion recovery sequence (TR/TE = 4140/ 30) and axial T2SE (TR/TE = 7650/ 150) of a term infant who had a planned home delivery and was jittery after birth, subsequently developing seizures. A, A large right-sided subdural hemorrhage is seen in the posterior fossa, causing a shift of the cerebellum. **B,** MRI at 3 months does not show clear injury of the cerebellum and the child is developing well at 2 years.

edema, hydrocephalus, or cerebral infarction, requires CT or MRI [Chamnanvanakij et al., 2002; Hayashi et al., 1987; Perrin et al., 1997]. MRI angiography or cerebral angiography may be considered as secondary imaging studies [Perrin et al., 1997]. MRI provides superior imaging of tentorium tears, as well as better delineation of posterior fossa injury [King and Boothroyd, 1998].

Management is generally supportive, with maintenance of circulating blood volume, correction of significant anemia and coagulopathy, and treatment of seizures. Most often, neurosurgical intervention is unnecessary. If there are signs of transtentorial herniation, percutaneous needle aspiration of the subdural hematoma may be attempted, which was successful in 5 out of 7 neonates and was recommended as the treatment of choice [Vinchon et al., 2005]. In one series of 26 neonates with subdural hematomas, only 1 required surgery for elevation of a depressed skull fracture [Chamnanvanakij et al., 2002]. Perrin et al. [1997] studied a series of 15 neonates with posterior fossa subdural hematomas for whom neurosurgical consultation was obtained. In this series, 8 of 15 patients underwent surgical evacuation. Indication for surgery included development of signs of progressive brainstem compression [Perrin et al., 1997]. In another case series of 48 neonates with subdural hematomas, 13 underwent neurosurgical intervention, consisting of burr holes, craniotomy, or placement of a ventriculoperitoneal shunt. The investigators recommend surgical intervention for increased intracranial pressure, obstructive hydrocephalus, or accompanying intracerebral hemorrhage [Hayashi et al., 1987].

Short-term outcome in children with an isolated infratentorial subdural hemorrhage, and also in those with a lobar hemorrhage, has often been reported to be more favourable than expected [Govaert et al., 1992b; Hanigan et al., 1995].

Neurologic sequelae after perinatal subdural hematoma depend on the location of the hematoma, associated cerebral injury, and accurate diagnosis and management. In one study of 26 infants with subdural hematoma, 9 (34.6 percent) had an abnormal neurologic examination at discharge, with 7 infants

exhibiting mild hypotonia and 2 infants with Erb's palsy. There were no deaths in this series [Chamnanvanakij et al., 2002]. In another series, Perrin et al. [1997] retrospectively reviewed charts of 15 children with perinatal subdural hematoma. Follow-up ranged from 2 to 10 years, with a mean of 4.5 years. There were no deaths in this series, but 3 children were profoundly delayed, 2 were moderately delayed, 3 were mildly delayed, and 7 were neurodevelopmentally normal. Hayashi et al. [1987] found that 8 (17 percent) of 46 neonates with subdural hematomas had some developmental abnormalities 6 months to 3 years after injury.

Intracerebral hemorrhage may occur in isolation or in association with other cranial birth injuries, including subdural hematomas or cerebral vascular injuries. Possible mechanisms of injury include direct compression of the brain as a result of molding, forcing the frontal bone under the parietal bone during passage through the birth canal, occipital osteodiastasis resulting in intracerebellar hemorrhage, asphyxia inducing hemorrhagic arterial infarct, or venous infarct due to sagittal sinus thrombosis [Govaert et al., 1992a; Hayashi et al., 1987].

Intracerebral hemorrhage occurs in 7–20 percent of full-term infants with intracranial hemorrhage [Hanigan et al., 1995; Pollina et al., 2001; Sandberg et al., 2001]. In one report, 31 percent of infants had risk factors for intracerebral hemorrhage, including perinatal asphyxia, coagulopathy, complicated delivery, or hyperviscosity. However, up to 50 percent of neonates with intracerebral hemorrhage in this series did not have any identifiable risk factors [Hanigan et al., 1995]. The most common presentation for intracerebral hemorrhage is seizures within 48 hours of birth [Govaert et al., 1992b; Hanigan et al., 1995; Medlock and Hanigan, 1997]. In a recent study by Armstrong-Wells et al. [2009], this lesion was referred to as perinatal hemorrhagic stroke (PHS). They identified 20 cases among 323,532 live births (19 intracerebral hemorrhage and 1 subarachnoid hemorrhage), which gave a prevalence of 6.2 in 100 000 live births. Infants presented with encephalopathy (100 percent) and seizures (65 percent). PHS was typically unifocal (74 percent) and unilateral (83 percent). Etiologies

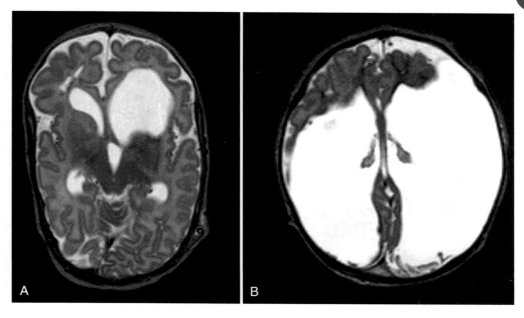

Fig. 18-8 MRI, axial T2SE (TR/TE = 7650/150), of two newborn infants, both with *COL4A1* mutation, illustrating the wide spectrum of severity of the lesions. A, Born at 33 weeks gestational age. **B,** Born at 40 weeks.

included thrombocytopenia (n = 4) and cavernous malformation (n = 1), but most 15 (75 percent) were idiopathic. Fetal distress and postmaturity were identified as independent risk factors. Antenatal onset of parenchymal hemorrhage can be associated with a mutation in the *COL4A1* gene [de Vries et al., 2009; Meuwissen et al., 2011]. The lesions can be severe, with almost complete destruction of both hemispheres, and the cerebellum can be involved as well (Figure 18-8). In the study by Sandberg et al. [2001], only 11 infants were identified from January 1960 to February 2000, and most presented within the first 2 days of life (6 of 11 patients); the most common presenting sign was seizure (7 of 11 patients). No cause was identified in 6 of 11 patients; the remainder were attributed to coagulopathy (n = 3), ruptured intracranial aneurysm (n = 1), or hemorrhagic infarction (n= 1). Eight patients underwent surgical hematoma evacuation on the basis of radiographic evidence of significant mass effect, evidence of signs of elevated intracranial pressure, or both. Four patients had normal neurologic outcomes, 4 had motor deficits (one of whom additionally demonstrated cognitive delay), and 3 had delayed speech. Outcome is often reported to be better, even in the context of large intracerebral lesions [Brouwer et al., 2010; Huang et al., 2004; Sandberg et al., 2001]. In a subgroup of infants with intracerebral lesions, the temporal lobe is affected; these infants tend to present with apnea as the initial manifestation [Sirsi et al., 2007; Slaugther et al., 2009; Hoogstraate et al., 2009]. Slaughther et al. [2009] suggested that neonatal temporal lobe hemorrhagic infarct could be secondary to suspected superficial temporal venous thrombosis but this was not confirmed in all patients with MR venography. In spite of often dramatic imaging abnormalities, a good clinical outcome was noted. The frontal lobe has been recognized as another predilection site, often following an uncomplicated vaginal delivery.

In a recent series of 53 infants with a subdural hemorrhage associated with an infra- or supratentorial intracerebral hemorrhage, mortality was high (24.5 percent), with the lowest mortality in infants with a supratentorial intracerebral hemorrhage (10 percent). Three infants with a midline shift required a craniotomy; 6 infants needed a subcutaneous reservoir due to

outflow obstruction and 3 subsequently required a ventriculoperitoneal shunt. The group with a poor outcome (death or developmental quotient <85) had a significantly lower 5-minute Apgar score (p = 0.005). Follow-up was available in 36 of 40 survivors, at an age of at least 15 months. Patients were assessed with the Griffiths' Mental Developmental Scale, and the mean DQ of all survivors was 97. Six infants (17 percent) had a DQ below 85 (2 of them had cerebral palsy). Three infants developed cerebral palsy (8.6 percent); 1 had cerebellar ataxia and 2 a hemiplegia (Brouwer et al., 2010).

SUBARACHNOID HEMORRHAGE

Subarachnoid hemorrhage is a relatively common neonatal intracranial injury and occurs as a result of tearing of veins traversing the subarachnoid space [Hughes et al., 1999; King and Boothroyd, 1998]. With the increased use of CT and MRI, clinically insignificant subarachnoid hemorrhage has been diagnosed with increasing frequency [Whitby et al., 2004]. In their study of 583,340 singleton live births, Towner et al. [1999] found the incidence of subarachnoid hemorrhage varied from 0.9 per 10,000 infants born by cesarean section to as high as 10.7 per 10,000 infants born by vacuum- and forceps-assisted delivery. In Pollina's series of 41 infants with cranial birth injury, 20 percent had subarachnoid hemorrhage [Pollina et al., 2001].

Presenting symptoms include decreased level of consciousness, hypotonia, and seizures [Hughes et al., 1999]. Hydrocephalus may develop because of obstruction of the fourth ventricle by clot formation or by subarachnoid adhesions over the convexities [Hayashi et al., 1987; King and Boothroyd, 1998]. Subarachnoid hemorrhage may cause cerebral vasospasm, leading to infarction [Medlock and Hanigan, 1997] (Figure 18-9).

Diagnosis is difficult using cranial ultrasound and is best made by CT, but subarachnoid hemorrhage should be suspected when frank blood or blood-tinged fluid and an elevated cerebrospinal fluid protein level are found on lumbar puncture. Unless there is evidence of hydrocephalus, no treatment is

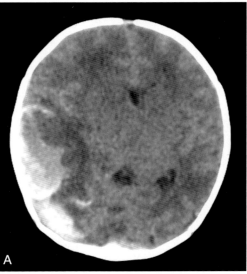
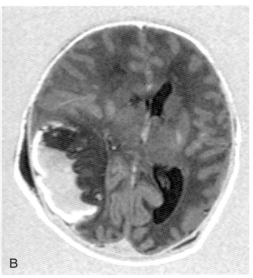

Fig. 18-9 An infant born at 38 weeks with a birth weight of 2230 g (<2.3 centile), who developed a petechial rash and had a platelet count below 5×10^9/L); she was diagnosed as having Neonatal Alloimmune Thrombocytopenia. **A,** CT. **B,** MRI, inversion recovery (TR/TE = 4140/30). The infant developed seizures, and a large subarachnoid hemorrhage with adjacent edema of the parenchyma was revealed with both imaging modalities. Also note the shift of the midline.

needed because the condition generally resolves spontaneously. Outcome is related to associated conditions, such as subdural hematoma or stroke.

Cranial Nerve Injuries

Acquired facial nerve palsy occurs in 1.8–7.5 per 1000 deliveries and is more common in males than females (2:1 in one study). Most cases are associated with forceps deliveries, but 33 percent occur after spontaneous delivery. The mechanism of injury in either case is similar, with compression of the facial nerve at the stylomastoid foramen either by the posterior forceps blade or by compression against the maternal sacral promontory [Hughes et al., 1999; Medlock and Hanigan, 1997].

Signs and symptoms include difficulty in closing the eyelid on the affected side, loss of the nasolabial fold, and an asymmetric crying facies. Electromyography and auditory brainstem response testing are recommended for neonates in whom there is no improvement over 3–4 days. Surgical intervention usually is deferred until 1–2 years of age [Hughes et al., 1999].

Other cranial nerve injuries include abducens nerve palsies, hypoglossal nerve palsies, and recurrent laryngeal nerve palsies [Medlock and Hanigan, 1997].

Spinal Cord Injuries

Cervical spinal cord injury is an important, although rare, cause of neonatal morbidity and mortality, for which the diagnosis is often delayed or overlooked during the initial evaluation. The incidence is difficult to ascertain because examination of the spinal cord is not routinely done at postmortem examination. In one series, 45 percent of neonates undergoing postmortem examination had evidence of distortional trauma to the spinal cord [Yates, 1959]; in a second series, the incidence of significant spinal or brainstem injury was greater than 10 percent [Towbin, 1969]. In a Canadian study from 1993, the investigators cite an incidence of 1 case in 29,000 live births [Rehan and Seshia, 1993], whereas another study reported an incidence of upper cervical spinal cord injury of 1 in 80,000 [Menticoglou et al., 1995].

Spinal cord injury may occur as a result of longitudinal traction, hyperextension or hyperflexion of the neck, excessive rotational force, or ischemic damage to the spinal cord [Filippigh et al., 1994; Morota et al., 1992; Rossitch and Oakes, 1992]. Because the interspinous ligaments, posterior joint capsule, and cartilaginous end plates of the neonate are elastic and redundant, the spine is more deformable in the child than in the adult. The facet joints are more horizontally oriented and therefore less stable. These factors make the pediatric spine more susceptible to hyperextension injury. This type of injury may occur in utero and usually results in a high spinal cord lesion [Rossitch and Oakes, 1992]. The neonatal spinal column is quite elastic, but the spinal cord can be stretched only 0.25 inch before rupturing. This difference in elasticity can result in spinal cord injury without radiographic abnormality (SCIWORA) because the bony and ligamentous elements may remain intact, even when the spinal cord has been ruptured. Forceful longitudinal traction during difficult breech delivery may cause this type of injury, and results in lower cervical to high thoracic spinal cord injury [Morgan and Newell, 2001; Rossitch and Oakes, 1992, Vialle et al., 2008]. Torsional forces during instrumentation with forceps, with head rotation of 90° or more, may cause rotational injury during delivery with cephalic presentation [Medlock and Hanigan, 1997]. This type of injury typically results in high cervical cord lesions [Rossitch and Oakes, 1992].

Diagnosis of spinal cord injury is often delayed because of the variable presentation and frequent presence of confounding factors. There is often concomitant perinatal asphyxia, respiratory distress, and brachial plexus injury [Mills et al., 2001; Onal et al., 2002; Rossitch and Oakes, 1992]. Neonates with spinal cord injury are flaccid, with absent spontaneous movements and absent deep tendon reflexes. Complex spinal reflexes may be present and misleading. Apnea may occur in high cervical cord injury, requiring intubation and mechanical ventilation. A sensory level can be detected by lack of facial response to painful stimuli below the level of injury [Filippigh et al., 1994; MacKinnon et al., 1993; Rossitch and Oakes, 1992]. The differential diagnosis includes HIE, spinal muscular atrophy, congenital myopathies, brachial plexus injury, congenital intraspinal tumors, myelodysplasia, and sepsis. Unaffected facial muscles and presence of a sensory level can distinguish spinal cord injury from spinal muscular atrophy and cerebral diplegia [Filippigh et al., 1994]. Radiographic evaluation can elucidate the cause in most neonates.

A variety of radiographic tests can be useful in the setting of suspected spinal cord injury. Plain films of the spine are often normal because of the deformability of the neonatal spine [Rehan and Seshia, 1993; Rossitch and Oakes, 1992]. Ultrasonography is useful in initial evaluation as a noninvasive test that may be done at the bedside. Due to incomplete ossification of the vertebral arch in neonates, the spinal cord may be visualized, and edema, hematomyelia, extraspinal hematoma, and avulsion of a nerve root may be revealed [Filippigh et al., 1994; Rehan and Seshia, 1993; Simon et al., 1999]. CT delineates the spinal column better than the cord itself, but bony abnormalities are relatively uncommon. CT myelography is invasive and may lead to false-negative or false-positive results [MacKinnon et al., 1993]. If the infant is stable enough for transport, MRI is the imaging modality of choice. It provides excellent soft-tissue delineation and can distinguish edema from hemorrhage, infarction, vascular anomalies, or congenital anomalies [Blount et al., 2004; Mills et al., 2001; Onal et al., 2002; Rehan and Seshia, 1993]. Somatosensory-evoked potentials may provide additional useful information [Rehan and Seshia, 1993].

The long-term outcome of neonatal spinal cord injury depends on the location of the injury. Infants with a lesion above C4 who display recovery of breathing movements in the first day with continued rapid recovery generally have a good outcome [MacKinnon et al., 1993]. Perinatal spinal cord injury usually results in some degree of permanent neurologic deficit (Figure 18-10). In one retrospective series of 22 patients, all had at least mild disability. Seven patients with upper cervical cord lesions died, and four with cervicothoracic or thoracolumbar injuries died [MacKinnon et al., 1993]. Postmortem examination of the spinal cord in three neonates with intramedullary cord hemorrhage revealed irreversible spinal cord trauma,

whereas a fourth neonate in the same case series, who had presented identically with quadriparesis, had only cord edema without hemorrhage and made a complete recovery. Similar to adult spinal cord injury, edema of the spinal cord without intramedullary hemorrhage on MRI is associated with a good outcome [Mills et al., 2001].

Brachial Plexus Injury

Brachial plexus injury is a relatively common birth injury. The reports of the largest populations found incidences occurring in 0.42 and 1.5 per 1000 live births (Gilbert et al., 1999; Donnelly et al., 2002; Evans-Jones et al., 2003; Andersen et al., 2006; McNeely and Drake, 2003; Medlock and Hanigan, 1997; van Ouwerkerk et al., 2000).

Despite improved perinatal care, the incidence of brachial plexus injury has not declined, possibly because of increasing birth weights. Predisposing factors include macrosomia, breech presentation, shoulder dystocia, and assisted delivery with forceps or vacuum extraction [McNeely and Drake, 2003; van Ouwerkerk et al., 2000]. In the study by Evans-Jones et al. [2003], significant associated risk factors were compared with the normal population: shoulder dystocia (60 percent vs. 0.3 percent); high birth weight, with 53 percent infants weighing more than the 90th percentile; and assisted delivery (relative risk [RR] 3.4, 95 percent confidence interval [CI] 2.9–3.9, p = 0.0001). There was a considerably lower risk of brachial plexus palsy in infants delivered by cesarean section (RR = 7, 95 percent CI 2–56, p = 0.002).

The mechanism of injury is thought to be excessive traction on the brachial plexus caused by lateral flexion and traction on the head during a difficult delivery with shoulder dystocia. In cases of breech presentation, bilateral injury may exist [van Ouwerkerk et al., 2000]. Four types of injury have been

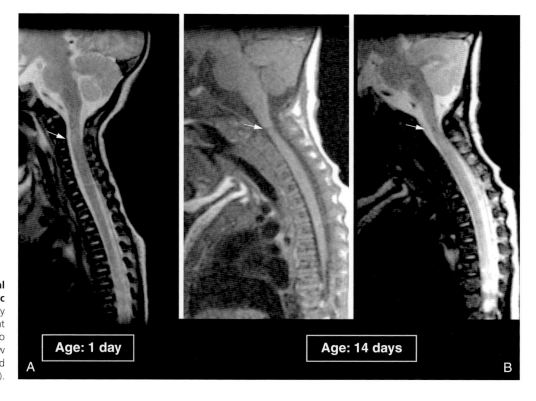

Fig. 18-10 Term infant with spinal cord injury caused by a traumatic delivery. A, Image obtained at day 1 demonstrates slight hyperintensity at the craniocervical junction. **B,** Two images obtained at 14 days show volume loss and a little blood (hypointensity on T2-weighted images).

Age: 1 day

Age: 14 days

A

B

described: neuropraxia, or temporary conduction block; axonotmesis, in which the axon is severed but surrounding neural elements are intact; neurotmesis, or complete postganglionic disruption of a nerve; and avulsion, or preganglionic disconnection from the spinal cord [van Ouwerkerk et al., 2000]. Brachial plexus injury may also be classified as complete, upper, or lower palsies [Medlock and Hanigan, 1997].

Diagnosis is generally made by noticing an asymmetric Moro reflex. Erb's palsy is characterized by injury to C5 and C6, resulting in paralysis of the deltoid, biceps, brachioradialis, and supinator muscles. Grasp is preserved, and the arm is held in the "waiter's tip" position. This accounts for 90 percent of brachial plexus injuries. Klumpke's paralysis involves C7 and results in loss of the grasp reflex in addition to the previously described symptoms. With involvement of the sympathetic fibers from the first thoracic root, Horner's syndrome may be identified [Hughes et al., 1999]. Complete plexus injury results in atonic "flail limb" and a Horner's sign. Differential diagnosis includes arthrogryposis, sepsis or osteomyelitis of the shoulder joint, fractures of the humerus or clavicle, upper motor neuron injury, and spinal cord injury [van Ouwerkerk et al., 2000]. Electromyography and nerve conduction studies may be considered to assess the degree of injury and to guide therapy for future management [Hughes et al., 1999; Medlock and Hanigan, 1997]. MRI can delineate the extent of injury and distinguish between brachial plexus and spinal cord injury or congenital anomalies [Medlock and Hanigan, 1997]. MR neurography enables localization of injured nerves and characterization of associated pathology, and is a useful adjunct in treatment planning [Smith et al., 2008].

Management is controversial. Most injuries resolve spontaneously and require only supportive care with physical therapy and application of dynamic splints [Hughes et al., 1999]. In a systematic review of brachial plexus surgery, McNeely and Drake [2003] conclude that there is no definitive advantage to surgery over conservative management. Results of surgical intervention were variable, and patients frequently did not regain normal function. They recommend waiting at least 3–6 months before proceeding with surgical intervention. Andersen et al. [2006] reviewed data from nonrandomized studies and these indicated that children with severe injuries do better with surgical repair. Malessy and Pondaag [2009] recommend restricting surgery to severe cases in which spontaneous restoration of function is unlikely to occur (i.e., in neurotmesis or root avulsions).

Brachial plexus injuries often resolve spontaneously, but in 5–25 percent of children, there is residual extremity weakness [Andersen et al., 2006; Hughes et al., 1999; McNeely and Drake, 2003; van Ouwerkerk et al., 2000]. In a prospective observational study of the natural history of brachial plexus injuries, Noetzel et al. [2001] found that, for infants who had not recovered antigravity movement at the shoulder at 2 weeks of age, the degree of residual weakness at 6 months was highly predictive of eventual recovery. Permanent weakness or disability was highly likely in those children who had less than antigravity strength in the biceps, triceps, and deltoid muscles, or absence of active wrist extension. From the review by Andersen et al. [2006], it was noted that 75 percent of affected infants recover completely within the first month of life. Permanent impairment and disability are experienced by 25 percent of affected infants. Andersen et al. recommended referral to a multidisciplinary brachial plexus team if a physical examination demonstrated an incomplete recovery by the end of the first month.

 The complete list of references for this chapter is available online at **www.expertconsult.com**.
See inside cover for registration details.

Injury to the Developing Preterm Brain: Intraventricular Hemorrhage and White Matter Injury

Laura R. Ment and Janet S. Soul

Introduction

As newborn intensive care approaches its sixth decade, preterm birth has emerged as a major pediatric public health problem [Behrman and Stith Butler, 2007]. There were almost 129 million births worldwide in 2005, and 9.6 percent of them were premature [Beck et al., 2010]. Survival is increasing for neonates of all gestational ages, and the prevalence of children with cognitive impairments at school age continues to rise [Allen, 2008; Behrman and Stith Butler, 2007; Hack et al., 2009; Robertson et al., 2009]. At age 8 years, more than 50 percent of infants with birth weights < 1000 g require special classroom assistance in the classroom, 20 percent are in special education, and 15 percent have repeated at least one school grade [Allen, 2008; Aylward, 2005; Bhutta et al., 2002; Larroque et al., 2008; Neubauer et al., 2008; Saigal and Doyle, 2008; Voss et al., 2007]. In addition, 10–20 percent have cerebral palsy [Larroque et al., 2008].

Brain injury is common in preterm neonates and may perturb the genetically prescribed program of cerebral development in the prematurely born [Volpe, 2009a]. Magnetic resonance imaging (MRI) has permitted noninvasive high-resolution evaluation of the developing brain, and numerous investigators have reported that very low birth weight (VLBW) preterm infants experience both macrostructural alterations in postnatal brain development, as well as in microstructural connectivity when compared to term neonates [De Vries et al., 1999; Hagmann et al., 2009; Huppi et al., 1996; Maalouf et al., 1999; Mercuri et al., 1996; Woodward et al., 2006]. To date, however, both the pathophysiology of these changes and the relationship of MRI studies to neurodevelopmental outcome data remain poorly understood [Allin et al., 2004; Boardman et al., 2007; Huppi et al., 1998; Inder et al., 1999, 2005; Mewes et al., 2006; Peterson et al., 2000]. These data suggest that strategies for identifying and preventing causes of disability in this patient population are critically important to both physicians and parents.

The neuropathologic processes that most commonly affect the prematurely born neonate include intraventricular hemorrhage (IVH) and white matter injury, or the periventricular leukomalacia complex [Volpe, 2009a]. IVH, or hemorrhage into the germinal matrix tissues of the developing brain, is detected in approximately 10–25 percent of VLBW neonates [Fanaroff et al., 2007; O'Shea et al., 2008], while white matter injury (WMI) and the global neuronal and axonal deficits that may accompany it are found in 50 percent or more of this vulnerable population [Dyet et al., 2006; Maalouf et al., 1998; Woodward et al., 2006]. Because both IVH and WMI are unique to the preterm population and represent a significant burden of disease, the pathophysiology, outcome, and prevention of these two injuries will be reviewed separately.

Intraventricular Hemorrhage

Although IVH occurs in 10–25 percent of all VLBW neonates, it is most significantly a problem for those infants at the lowest limits of viability [Fanaroff et al., 2007]. Both the incidence and the severity of IVH are inversely related to birth weight and gestational age, and almost 25 percent of neonates of 501–750 g birth weight experience the highest grades of hemorrhage [Fanaroff et al., 2003, 2007]. High-grade IVH is more common in male infants than females [Hintz et al., 2006; Synnes et al., 2001; Tioseco et al., 2006], and although the risk period for IVH is in the first 4–5 postnatal days, data from several centers indicate that approximately half of all hemorrhages occur within the first 6–8 postnatal hours [Dolfin et al., 1983; Ment et al., 1993; Perlman and Volpe, 1986; Perlman and Rollins, 2000; Shaver et al., 1992] – a time of intense medical instability for those neonates with the lowest gestational ages.

Many neonatal intensive care units perform routine head ultrasound screening of preterm neonates using the system developed by Papile for grading IVH, as shown in Table 19-1 [O'Shea et al.,

Table 19-1 **Grading Systems for Germinal Matrix Intraventricular Hemorrhages**

Papile*		Volpe†	
Grade	**Description**	**Grade**	**Description**
Grade 1	Germinal matrix hemorrhage	Grade I	Germinal matrix hemorrhage with no or minimal hemorrhage
Grade 2	Blood within but not distending ventricular system	Grade II	IVH (10–50% of ventricular area)
Grade 3	Blood filling and distending ventricular system	Grade III	IVH (>50% of ventricular area; usually distends ventricle)
Grade 4	Parenchymal involvement of hemorrhage	Severe + periventricular hemorrhagic infarction	Grade III IVH with periventricular hemorrhagic infarction

* (Data from Papile LS, Burstein J, Burstein R. Incidence and evolution of the subependymal intraventricular hemorrhage: A study of infants with weights less than 1500 grams. J Pediatr 1978;92:529.)
† (Data from Volpe JJ. Neurology of the newborn, 3rd edn. Philadelphia: WB Saunders, 1995:424–428.)

2008; Papile et al., 1978]. Employing this nomenclature, grade 1, or germinal matrix hemorrhage (GMH), describes blood in the germinal matrix only. Grade 2 is blood filling the lateral ventricles without distension, grade 3 is blood filling and acutely distending the ventricular system, and grade 4 describes hemorrhages with parenchymal involvement of hemorrhage. When associated with grades 1–3 IVH, unilateral grade 4 hemorrhages are considered in most cases to represent venous infarction of the periventricular white matter [de Vries et al., 2001], and the nomenclature of Volpe [Volpe, 2001], also shown in Table 19-1, provides a more pathophysiologic approach to parenchymal events.

In the newborn period, 5–10 percent of preterm infants with IVH suffer seizures and as many as 50 percent of infants with grade 4 IVH experience posthemorrhagic hydrocephalus [Volpe, 2009a]; mortality is also higher in those infants with IVH. Finally, although the long-term neurodevelopmental outcome for infants with lower grades of hemorrhage remains uncertain at this time, most observers agree that infants with parenchymal hemorrhage are at high risk for neurodevelopmental handicap (Figure 19-1) [Luu et al., 2009a; Saigal et al., 2003; Sherlock et al., 2005, 2008].

Pathophysiology

Intraventricular Hemorrhage is a Complex Disorder

IVH has been attributed to alterations in cerebral blood flow to the immature germinal matrix microvascular network [Shalak and Perlman, 2002; Whitelaw, 2001], as shown in Figure 19-2, and studies addressing the etiology of IVH have identified numerous environmental and medical risk factors (Box 19-1). These include low gestational age, absence of antenatal steroid exposure, maternal antenatal hemorrhage, chorioamnionitis/infection/inflammation and/or fertility treatment, neonatal transport to a tertiary care center following birth, maternal sepsis, seizures, hypotension requiring medical therapy, hypoxemia, hypercapnia, and acidosis [du Plessis, 2008; Fabres et al., 2007; Limperopoulos et al., 2008; McCrea and Ment, 2008; O'Leary et al., 2009]. As this lesion is unique to preterm infants,

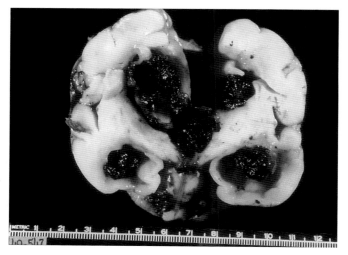

Fig. 19-1 Coronal cross-section of a 28-week preterm infant brain with intraventricular hemorrhage and marked ventricular enlargement. *(From Ment LR, Schneider K. Intraventricular hemorrhage of the preterm infant. Semin Neurol 1993b;13:42.)*

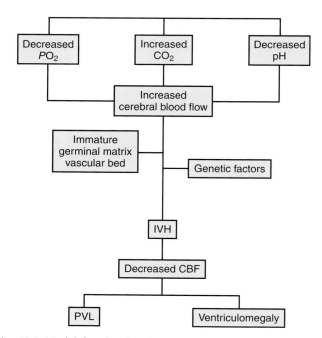

Fig. 19-2 Model for the development of intraventricular hemorrhage in the preterm infant. CBF, cerebral blood flow; IVH, intraventricular hemorrhage; PVL, periventricular leukomalacia.

Box 19-1 Clinical Risk Factors for Intraventricular Hemorrhage

Early Onset

- Low birth weight, low gestational age
- Maternal fertility treatment
- No antenatal steroid exposure
- Maternal antenatal hemorrhage
- No maternal pre-eclampsia
- Maternal chorioamnionitis and/or infection
- No tertiary care delivery
- Vigorous resuscitation
- Neonatal transport following delivery

Onset after 6–8 Postnatal Hours

- Hypotension requiring medical therapy
- Respiratory distress syndrome
- Acidosis
- Hypoxemia
- Extremes of PCO_2 levels (both high and low)
- Sodium bicarbonate exposure
- Pneumothoraces
- Seizures

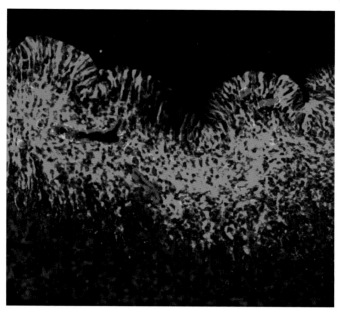

Fig. 19-3 Morphology of the germinal matrix. Immunofluorescence of cryosection from the germinal matrix of a 24 week preterm infant labeled with DAPI (blue), GFAP (green), and CD34 (red). The germinal matrix is highly vascular and contains many glial cells. *(Courtesy of Praveen Ballabh, M.D., Department of Pediatrics, Anatomy, and Cell Biology, New York Medical College-Westchester Medical Center, Valhalla, NY.)*

examination of those developmental, environmental, and genetic events that result in IVH is critical. These include anatomic, physiologic, and genetic factors.

Anatomic Factors are Permissive for Hemorrhage

During the late second and third trimesters, the developing brain almost triples in volume, and there are multiple developmental events that occur during this time interval. The germinal matrix and the adjacent subventricular zone (SVZ) are the sites of proliferation of both glial and neuronal precursors. The SVZ generates predominately GABAergic cortical interneurons, although recent data suggest that the germinal matrix also produces GABAergic neurons that migrate to the dorsal thalamus during the risk period for IVH. (For review, please see Volpe [2009a].)

By 24 weeks of gestation, almost but not all of the cortical neurons have migrated from the germinal zones and axonal ingrowth begins [Kostovic, 1990; Kostovic and Rakic, 1990; Kostovic et al., 2002, 1989]. The elaboration of dendritic arbors is at an active stage and synaptic contacts are beginning to form [Huttenlocher and de Courten, 1987; Huttenlocher and Dabholkar, 1997; Huttenlocher et al., 1982]. The germinal matrix remains relatively robust through 32–34 weeks of gestation but almost completely involutes by term [Donat et al., 1978; Rorke, 1982; Whitelaw, 2001].

During this period of rapid cell genesis, the metabolically active germinal matrix requires a rich blood supply, as shown in Figure 19-3, yet its vessels are neuropathologically immature and present numerous risk factors for hemorrhage (Table 19-2). The developing blood–brain barrier is characterized by basement membrane proteins, endothelial tight junctions, capillary pericytes, and astrocytic endfeet [Ballabh et al., 2004]. Immunohistologic and electron microscopic examinations comparing germinal matrix microvessels with those in the periventricular

Table 19-2 Germinal Matrix Risk Factors for Intraventricular Hemorrhage

Factor	Developmental Regulation in GM	Changes in GM
Vascular density and area	Increase with GA	GM > cortex, WM
BLOOD–BRAIN BARRIER		
Tight junction proteins	No change	No differential expression
Claudin-5	No change	No differential expression
Occludin	No change	No differential expression
Junction adhesion molecule 1		No differential expression
Basement membrane proteins	No change	GM > cortex, WM
Laminin	Increase with GA	No change
Collagen IV	No change	GM < cortex, WM
Fibronectin		
Glial endfeet		
Glial fibrillary acidic protein	Increase with GA	GM < cortex, WM
Pericytes		
Vascular coverage	Increase with GA	GM < cortex, WM
Angiogenic factors	N/a	GM > cortex, WM
VEGF	N/a	GM > cortex, WM
Angiopoietin-2		

GA, gestational age; GM, germinal matrix; N/a, not available; VEGF, vascular endothelial growth factor; WM, white matter.

white matter and cortical mantle demonstrate a paucity of fibronectin, fewer pericytes, and decreased perivascular coverage by glial fibrillary acidic protein (GFAP)-positive astrocytic endfeet [Ballabh et al., 2005; Braun et al., 2007; El-Khoury et al., 2006; Wei et al., 2000; Xu et al., 2008]. Since GFAP provides both shape and mechanical strength to the endfeet of astrocytes, its decrease, in combination with alterations in basement membrane proteins and pericyte investiture, suggests a structural weakening of the germinal matrix blood–brain barrier. In contrast, studies of fetuses and preterm neonates during the second and third trimesters of gestation have demonstrated no difference in the primary endothelial tight junction molecules, claudin-5, occludin, and JAM-1, in the germinal matrix compared to cortical gray and white matter regions [Ballabh et al., 2005; Xu et al., 2008].

The germinal matrix has a greater vascular density than other developing brain regions, and recent reports suggest rapid angiogenesis in the germinal matrix, perhaps to support its greater metabolic rate and oxygen requirement [Ballabh et al., 2004]. This angiogenesis is induced by the high levels of vascular endothelial growth factor (VEGF) and angiopoietin (ANGPT)-2 found selectively in the germinal matrix compared to both the cortex and periventricular white matter [Carmeliet, 2003; Ferrara et al., 2003]. Since preclinical studies demonstrate that an increase in the expression of ANGPT-2 in the presence of VEGF promotes the sprouting of immature vessels lacking both basement membrane proteins and pericyte investiture [Carmeliet, 2003; Yancopoulos et al., 2000], the increased presence of these factors in the highly vascular germinal matrix provides further evidence for microvessels lacking a competent blood–brain barrier [Ballabh et al., 2007].

Finally, the venous circulation of the preterm brain may also contribute to the susceptibility to intraparenchymal hemorrhage. Venous blood from the periventricular white matter flows through a fan-shaped array of both short and long medullary veins into the veins of the germinal matrix, and subsequently into the terminal veins found inferior to this highly proliferative zone. The somewhat tortuous anatomy of these veins permits venous stasis, with subsequent hemorrhagic venous infarction of the periventricular white matter [Gould et al., 1987; Takashima et al., 1986; Taylor, 1995].

Alterations in Cerebral Blood Flow Contribute to IVH

Both experimental animal models (i.e., "preclinical data") and clinical data suggest that alterations in cerebral blood flow may play an important role in the pathophysiology of IVH. (For review see du Plessis [2008].) Cerebral blood flow was reported to be pressure-passive in the asphyxiated preterm infant over four decades ago [Lou et al., 1979], yet the factors that contribute to cerebral autoregulatory systems in the prematurely born are just beginning to be explained. Further, the definition of the cerebral pressure-flow autoregulatory plateau, or that range of cerebral perfusion pressures (mean arterial pressure − cerebral venous pressure) over which cerebral blood flow is normally maintained, is poorly defined for the critically ill, extremely low birth weight preterm neonate. None the less, experimental animal data suggest that at perfusion pressures above this reportedly relatively narrow plateau, cerebral blood flow becomes pressure-passive.

Changes in perfusion pressure, alterations in circulating oxygen and carbon dioxide levels, and the magnitude of these respiratory fluctuations are perhaps the most important regulators of cerebral blood flow in the preterm neonate. In response to these physiologic alterations, cerebral blood flow rises, hemorrhage begins within the germinal matrix, and blood may rupture into the ventricular system. After ventricular distension by an acute hemorrhage event, cerebral blood flow falls. Venous stasis within the periventricular white matter ensues, and parenchymal venous infarction may soon develop [McCrea and Ment, 2008; Volpe, 2001].

Prostaglandins, and particularly the cyclo-oxygenase 2 (COX-2) system, are important modulators of cerebral blood flow in the developing brain [Leffler et al., 1985, 1986]. Hypoxia, hypotension, growth factors, including transforming growth factor-β and epidermal growth factor, and inflammatory modulators, such as interleukin (IL)-6, IL-1β, tumor necrosis factor α (TNFα), and nuclear factor κβ, may all induce COX-2 [Baier, 2006; Dammann and Leviton, 2004; Heep et al., 2003, 2005; Ribeiro et al., 2004]. The resultant increase in prostanoids results in the release of VEGF, the potent angiogenic factor associated in preclinical and clinical studies with IVH.

Following hemorrhage, these same triggers set into motion a cascade of events leading to disruption of tight junction proteins, increased blood–brain barrier permeability, and microglial activation within the developing white matter. The damaged endothelium releases IL-1β and TNFα, and these cytokines promote transmigration of leukocytes across the emerging blood–brain barrier. The activated microglia release reactive oxygen species (ROS), which in turn promote endothelial damage, alter hemostasis, and increase metabolism. (For review, please see du Plessis [2008] and Chua et al. [2009].) The preterm brain is very sensitive to ROS because of the immaturity of those enzyme systems designed to detoxify them, and experimental animal studies suggest that ROS play a significant role in the generation of periventricular parenchymal infarction [Zia et al., 2009].

Clinical events believed to be associated with increases in cerebral blood flow in the preterm infant and the presumed postnatal onset of IVH include endogenous and exogenous events. Vigorous resuscitation, rapid volume re-expansion, endotracheal tube repositioning, recurrent suctioning, complex nursing care procedures, and the administration of sodium bicarbonate, as well as respiratory distress syndrome, hypoxemia, extremes of PCO_2 levels (i.e., both hypo- and hypercapnia), and acidosis have all been associated with IVH [Ancel et al., 2005; Hall et al., 2005; Kaiser et al., 2006; Kluckow, 2005; Kuint et al., 2009; Linder et al., 2003; O'Leary et al., 2009; Osborn and Evans, 2004; Synnes et al., 2001; Whitelaw, 2001] (Box 19-2). Routine screening by bedside cranial ultrasonography has demonstrated IVH after seizures and pneumothoraces in infants who were previously known to have no evidence of hemorrhage [Cooke, 1981; Hill and Volpe, 1981; Hill et al., 1982]. Finally, cerebrovasoactive cytokines are released in association with sepsis and may contribute to IVH.

Cerebral blood flow is markedly diminished after hemorrhage [Del Toro et al., 1991; Volpe, 1997]. Both xenon-133 inhalation and positron emission tomography (PET) have demonstrated significant hypoperfusion for longer than the first postnatal week in preterm infants with IVH [Ment et al., 1984; Volpe et al., 1983]. The cerebral hypoxemia and ischemia that accompany this depression in flow may result in damage

Box 19-2 Events Associated with Increased Cerebral Blood Flow

- Vigorous resuscitation
- Endotracheal tube repositioning
- Recurrent suctioning
- Complex medical and nursing procedures
- Acute hypoxemia
- Acute hypercarbia
- Apnea
- Pneumothorax
- Rapid volume re-expansion

not only to the periventricular white matter but also to those neural and glial precursors still residing in the germinal matrix and SVZ. Oligodendroglia and their precursors are among the cells in the developing cortex most sensitive to hypoxia, and their loss is postulated to result in secondary, gestational age-dependent alterations in connectivity in the developing brain [Gimenez et al., 2006; Miller et al., 2002; Nosarti et al., 2009]. Consistent with this hypothesis are reports of significantly decreased cortical gray matter volumes at term equivalent in VLBW preterm infants with grades 1–3 IVH compared to those with no IVH [Vasileiadis et al., 2004], and of decreases in cortical gray and white matter volumes, as well as callosal areas, in preterm subjects at 8–15 years of age [Kesler et al., 2004; Nosarti et al., 2008].

Candidate Genes for IVH

Although the environmental risk factors for IVH have been well studied, not all infants of a given birth weight range or those who suffer a known hypoxemic event experience IVH. Further, the incidence of high-grade IVH has not changed during the past 10 years despite improvements in care (Table 19-3) [Fanaroff et al., 2003, 2007]. Finally, twin analyses show that intraventricular hemorrhage is familial in origin, and over 40 percent of the variance in liability for IVH can be accounted for by shared

Table 19-3 Selected Perinatal Information for Infants Born with Birth Weights 500–1000 g in the National Institute of Child Health and Human Development (NICHD) Neonatal Research Network in Three Epochs

Birth Years	1987–1988*	1997–2002*	2005–2009†
Number	731	8312	1316
Antenatal steroids (%)	14	77	96
Delivery: cesarean section (%)	43	55	N/a
Grades 3–4 IVH (%)	26	19	12

* Birth weight 500–1000 g.
† Gestational age 24 weeks 0 days to 27 weeks 6 days.
(Adapted from Fanaroff AA et al., The NICHD neonatal research network: changes in practice and outcomes during the first 15 years. Sem Perinatol 2003;27:281; Fanaroff AA et al., Trends in neonatal morbidity and mortality for very low birthweight infants. Am J Obstet Gynecol 2007;196:147.e1.

Table 19-4 Susceptibility Genes for IVH

Gene	Allele	Effect
THROMBOPHILIA AND COAGULATION GENES		
Factor V Leiden	Gln506-FV	Decreased inactivation of factor V Increased thrombin generation Candidate gene for perinatal stroke and IVH
Prothrombin	G20210A	Increased thrombin Candidate gene for perinatal stroke and IVH
Factor XIII	34 Leu allele	High fibrinolytic activity in germinal matrix Associated with hemorrhagic events in adults Candidate gene for IVH
MTHFRC mutations		Result in increased plasma homocysteine Increased thrombosis Candidate gene for IVH
VASCULAR STABILITY GENES		
COL4A1		Decreased vascular stability Candidate gene for fetal stroke and IVH
PROINFLAMMATORY CYTOKINES		
TNF-α	Biallelic G to A at -308	A allele confers high gene transcription A allele is candidate gene for IVH
IL-1β	-511 CT	Increased production T allele is a candidate gene for IVH
IL-6	174 G or C	CC genotype increases production CC genotype is candidate gene for IVH

genetic and environmental factors [Bhandari et al., 2006]. For these reasons, several investigators have tested the hypothesis that the etiology of IVH is multifactorial, involving both environmental and genetic events.

The description of the thrombophilias associated with the factor V Leiden and prothrombin *G2021A* mutations, and the implication of both abnormalities in fetal and neonatal stroke, suggested to several investigators that these might also be candidate genes for IVH [Debus et al., 1998; Gopel et al., 2001, 2002; Petaja et al., 2001]. Examination of other target genes in the presumptive pathway to IVH shortly followed. As shown in Table 19-4, these include genes contributing to hemostasis, vascular stability, and inflammation [Baier, 2006].

THROMBOPHILIA AND COAGULATION GENES

Numerous investigators have examined the role of factor V Leiden (FVL) mutation, polymorphisms in those genes responsible for prothrombin, factor XIII, *MTHFRC*, and total homocysteine in the genesis of IVH [Debus et al., 1998; Gopel et al., 2001, 2002; Komlosi et al., 2005; Petaja et al., 2001].

A point mutation in the factor V gene resulting in the arginine 506 to glutamine substitution in factor V (Gln506-FV) is known as the FVL mutation. FVL is common in the Caucasian population and causes decreased inactivation of factor V, leading to markedly increased thrombin generation [Bertina et al.,

1994]. Importantly, FVL has been associated with thrombotic conditions in both adult and pediatric populations.

The G20210A polymorphism in the prothrombin gene results in a G to A substitution at nucleotide 20210; this mutation increases thrombin and thus also increases the risk for thrombosis. FVL and prothrombin G20210A have been reported in children and infants with ischemic stroke, porencephaly, and other thromboembolic events. Gopel hypothesized that relative hypercoagulability would protect preterm neonates from the extension of grade 1 IVH to higher grades of hemorrhage [Gopel et al., 2001]. In this study of 305 infants with birth weights <1500 g, the FVL mutation was protective for grades 2–4 IVH. In contrast, Petaja hypothesized that the hypercoagulable state associated with FVL would promote periventricular venous infarction and render the infant susceptible to parenchymal involvement of IVH; this study of 51 infants of <32 weeks gestational age suggested that FVL was associated with grade 4 IVH (odds ratio 5.9) [Petaja et al., 2001]. Aronis evaluated 55 preterm infants of <32 weeks gestational age for FVL and prothrombin mutations, and noted a "trend" for thrombophilias among infants with the latter mutation [Aronis et al., 2002].

Factor XIII levels are low in the preterm neonate, and this finding may result in high fibrinolytic activity in the germinal matrix. The factor XIII 34 Leu allele has been reported to cause hemorrhage events in adults and increased IVH in preterm neonates [Gopel et al., 2002].

Finally, mutations in the 5,10 methylenetetrahydrofolate reductase gene (*MTHFRC*) lead to increased plasma homocysteine levels, a well-recognized risk factor for increased thrombosis. None the less, several authors have reported no association with either these mutations or total homocysteine levels at birth in preterm neonates with IVH [Aronis et al., 2002; Gopel et al., 2001].

MUTATIONS IN VASCULAR STABILITY GENES

Numerous vascular, astrocytic, and pericytic proteins contribute to the maturation of the developing blood–brain barrier, and allelic alterations in these genes and their impact on IVH are just beginning to be described. Recent data suggest that mutations in collagen IVA1 result in IVH in neonatal mice, and fetal stroke and porencephalies in human infants [de Vries et al., 2009; Gould et al., 2005, 2006]. More recently, a mutation in this important vascular structural protein has been reported in preterm twins with grade 4 IVH [Bilguvar et al., 2009].

MUTATIONS IN PROINFLAMMATORY CYTOKINES

Proinflammatory cytokines are believed to represent important mediators of perinatal brain injury, and TNFα is known to be a central mediator in the inflammatory cascade. The degree of TNFα production may in part be genetically driven. A biallelic G to A polymorphism at position −308 in the TNFα promoter region confers either high (A) or low (G) gene transcription [Kroeger et al., 1997]. Hypoxia and ischemia, both of which are known to contribute to the pathogenesis of IVH, are associated with the upregulation of TNFα. Baier examined the role of this mutation in ventilated VLBW preterm neonates and found that the TNFα-308A allele was associated with an increased risk of IVH (40 percent for infants with an A allele compared to 24 percent with the GG genotype) [Adcock et al., 2003].

Polymorphisms in interleukins may also be possible genetic modifiers for IVH, although the results require further validation. These include mutations in IL-1β, IL-6, and IL-4. The IL-1β-511 CT mutation results in increased production of this proinflammatory cytokine and has been reported to increase the risk of IVH in ventilated preterm neonates with the T allele (33 percent vs. 14 percent for neonates with the C allele) [Baier, 2006]. Similarly, IL-6 mutations are believed to be strong candidate genes for IVH. Position 174 can be either a G or a C, and IL-6 production is greater in neonates with the CC genotype, but studies investigating IVH rates and/or and neurodevelopmental outcome in this subject population are contradictory [Gopel et al., 2006; Harding et al., 2004]. Similarly, a polymorphism at position 472 of the IL-6 gene has been shown in a small study to be associated with alterations in neurodevelopmental outcome in preterm infants at 2 years of age, although the study infants did not appear to have an increased incidence of IVH [Harding et al., 2005]. Finally, in a single study, mutations in IL-4 have been associated with a decreased incidence of IVH in African-American neonates [Baier, 2006].

Neuropathology

Over 90 percent of all IVH in preterm infants originates in the germinal matrix tissues located between the caudate nucleus and the thalamus at the level of, or slightly posterior to, the foramen of Monro in the developing brain [Donat et al., 1978; Volpe, 1997]. A small percentage of hemorrhages in preterm neonates may also originate from the choroid plexus, which is the most common site of IVH in term infants [Rorke, 1982].

Although it is often difficult to differentiate the neuropathologic findings that are directly attributable to IVH from those that frequently accompany it, most authors would agree that germinal matrix destruction, periventricular hemorrhagic infarction, porencephaly, and posthemorrhagic hydrocephalus (PHH) are the direct neuropathologic consequences of IVH [Shalak and Perlman, 2002; Whitelaw, 2001]. In contrast, periventricular leukomalacia and ventriculomegaly, to be described later in this chapter, are frequently detected in infants with IVH but are multifactorial in etiology.

Germinal matrix hemorrhage (GMH), solely confined to the germinal layer, occurs equally in both hemispheres and is found to be bilateral in approximately half of cases [Leech and Kohnen, 1974]. Not infrequently, there are multiple hemorrhages over one caudate nucleus, and injection techniques have demonstrated that all of the major vessels supplying the germinal matrix, including the artery of Heubner, the anterior choroidal artery, the lateral striate arteries, and the terminal vein, remain intact after an initial GMH [Pape and Wigglesworth, 1979]. Such a hemorrhage is associated with destruction of the capillary bed, and secondary germinal matrix cyst formation is common [Hambleton and Wigglesworth, 1976].

After rupture of a GMH, the spread of blood throughout the ventricular system is variable. Sonograms may demonstrate clots attached not only to the site of rupture but also to the choroid plexus, and variable spread of blood throughout the entire ventricular system. A characteristic pathologic finding is a mass of clot within the subarachnoid spaces at the base of the brain (Figure 19-4), and extension of blood through the subarachnoid pathways into the sylvian fissure and over the convexities of the developing hemispheres.

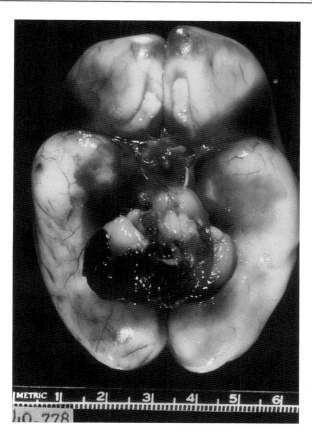

Fig. 19-4 A 28-week preterm brain with intraventricular hemorrhage and mass of a clot within the subarachnoid spaces at the base of the brain.

Serial cranial sonograms suggest that as many as 10–20 percent of preterm infants with GMH develop intraparenchymal abnormalities [Fanaroff et al., 2003]. The neuropathologic correlates of these abnormalities are most easily understood as arising not only from the acute increase in intracranial pressure attributable to the GMH itself, but also from the profound decreases in regional blood flow that may follow it. In 10–20 percent of infants with extensive GMH, the branches of the terminal vein that typically drain through the area of hemorrhage become grossly congested, and venous hemorrhagic infarction of the periventricular white matter and even cortical tissues may occur during the first several days after IVH [Pape and Wigglesworth, 1979]. These periventricular white matter infarctions are frequently termed intraparenchymal echodensities (IPE) when examined by cranial ultrasonography or MRI. In addition, some investigators believe that the parenchymal involvement of IVH readily visible by cranial ultrasonography represents a direct pressure-mediated extension of hemorrhage from either a massive GMH or blood within the ventricular system, but the close clinical association of ischemia and hemorrhage and the timing of the development of intraparenchymal echodense lesions on ultrasonography suggest that these lesions represent venous infarction of the periventricular white matter. These lesions are difficult to distinguish at the time of postmortem examination and have been variously named hemorrhagic intracerebral involvement, parenchymal involvement of hemorrhage, or grade 4 IVH. As proposed by Volpe, while GMH may result in the destruction of the germinal

matrix and loss of neuronal and glial cells residing there, extension of hemorrhage into the SVZ and periventricular white matter is associated with not only the loss of additional precursor cells but also axonal and glial necrosis [Volpe, 2009a].

Following grade 4 IVH or intraparenchymal hemorrhagic infarction, a cavitary lesion, or porencephaly, may result. Porencephalies generally have hemosiderin in the walls lining them and they are frequently freely communicating with the ventricular system, although a rare porencephaly may appear to be a fluid-filled parenchymal cyst on imaging and obstruct the ventricular system.

PHH represents a not uncommon sequela of IVH [Whitelaw, 2001; Whitelaw et al., 2004]. The meninges are thickened and show an infiltration by hemosiderin-laden macrophages [Deonna et al., 1975; Larroche, 1972]. These findings result in occlusion of the arachnoid villi, obstruction to flow of cerebrospinal fluid (CSF) through the foramina of Luschka and Magendie, and impairment of flow through the tentorial notch (see Figure 19-4). Occasionally, aqueductal obstruction is caused by an acute blood clot, ependymal disruption, or reactive gliosis [Cherian et al., 2004; Whitelaw, 2001].

Neuroimaging

Intraventricular Hemorrhage

Routine cranial ultrasonography via the anterior fontanel is performed in neonatal intensive and special care units around the world, and this modality represents the method of choice for the diagnosis and monitoring of IVH and its complications in preterm infants. Most nurseries use the standard grading system found in Table 19-1, which was originally developed for computed tomography (CT) scanning but fairly quickly applied to ultrasonography (Figure 19-5) [Papile et al., 1978]. Although grade 4 hemorrhages (shown in Figure 19-6) have been noted within the first 6 postnatal hours, most infants initially experience low-grade hemorrhage, which can be seen to progress over the course of time by ultrasonography. The most common sites for parenchymal hemorrhage are the frontal and parietal regions; approximately 50 percent of such hemorrhages occur bilaterally [Shalak and Perlman, 2002].

Intraparenchymal Echodensities

Cranial ultrasonography and MRI are also used for the diagnoses of IPE and porencephaly. IPE has been described as an asymmetric white matter lesion that may accompany the onset of IVH or follow it. Rarely found without GMH or IVH, IPE is believed to represent hemorrhagic venous infarction of the periventricular white matter and generally occurs in infants of the youngest gestational ages during the first postnatal week [de Vries et al., 2001]. The ultrasound appearance, found in Figure 19-7, is an echogenic juxtaventricular white matter lesion superior and lateral to the lateral ventricle and extending toward the cortex in a flare pattern without evidence for mass effect on the surrounding brain. Most often, IPE eventually cavitates or atrophies to form either a porencephaly or adjacent ex vacuo ventriculomegaly [De Vries et al., 2004].

Improvements in MRI technology and the use of special MRI-compatible incubators and ventilators have permitted MR imaging of hemorrhage in the developing brain. In the newborn period, MR studies demonstrate a single hemorrhagic

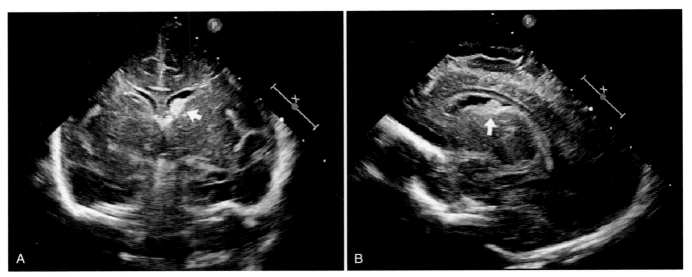

Fig. 19-5 Germinal matrix hemorrhage (GMH). A, Coronal view demonstrates a focus of increased echogenicity (arrow) between the head of the caudate and the thalamus in the caudothalamic groove. **B,** Parasagittal view shows the GMH (arrow) at its usual location along the posterior aspect of the caudothalamic groove. *(Courtesy of Walter C Allan, M.D., Maine Medical Center, Portland, ME.)*

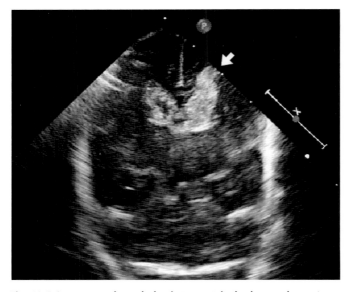

Fig. 19-6 Intraparenchymal plus intraventricular hemorrhage. Large hemorrhage emanating from the left and right germinal matrix destroys the ventricular anatomy bilaterally and merges with parenchymal hemorrhage in the left frontoparietal region (arrow). *(Courtesy of Walter C Allan, M.D., Maine Medical Center, Portland, ME.)*

lesion adjacent to or communicating with the lateral ventricle in addition to IVH [Dyet et al., 2006] (Figure 19-8).

Porencephaly

Porencephalies (Greek for "holes in the brain") are hemispheric cavitary lesions. In neonates, porencephalies follow grade 4 hemorrhages, IPEs, or periventricular venous infarctions. Although most porencephalies are freely communicating with the ventricular system, a porencephaly may present as a fluid-filled cyst that causes increased intracranial pressure in the preterm infant. A typical porencephaly is shown by ultrasound and MRI in Figure 19-9.

Clinical Findings

Incidence

While the incidence of IVH depends on a number of factors previously discussed, most centers report that 20–25 percent of VLBW neonates experience IVH, and 6 to more than 20 percent experience grades 3–4 IVH [Fanaroff et al., 2007; Zeitlin et al., 2009]. The incidence of IVH is inversely related to birth weight and gestational age [Sarkar et al., 2009], and data for 18,153 neonates of 501–1500 g birth weight from the National Institute of Child Health and Human Development (NICHD) Neonatal Network between 1 January 1997 and 12 December 2002 suggest that 24 percent of infants of 501–750 g birth weight, 14 percent of infants of 751–1000 g birth weight, 9 percent of those with 1001–1250 g birth weight, and 5 percent of infants with birth weights between 1251 and 1500 g experienced grades 3–4 IVH [Fanaroff et al., 2003, 2007]. Grades 3–4 IVH are more common in male neonates [Leijser et al., 2009]; when Synnes evaluated 3772 neonates of <33 weeks gestational age, 317 (8.3 percent) were found to have grade 3–4 IVH. In this cohort, male gender was an independent and important predictor of IVH (OR = 1.5, 95 percent CI = 1.1–1.9) [Synnes et al., 2006].

Timing of IVH

The risk period for IVH for preterm infants is the first 4–5 postnatal days [Ment et al., 2002; Perlman and Rollins, 2000]. Over 50 percent of all hemorrhages are detectable within the first 6 postnatal hours, and the work of Shaver suggests that almost all of these early hemorrhages are in fact detectable within the first postnatal hour [Shaver et al., 1992]. Less than 5 percent of hemorrhages occur after the fourth or fifth postnatal day (see Figure 19-9). The risk period for IVH is independent of gestational age, and between 10 and 65 percent of infants experience progression, or extension, of their hemorrhages over the first several postnatal days [Whitelaw, 2001]. Extension of IVH and the development of high-grade IVH are twice as common in those infants with the earliest onset of IVH. This progression

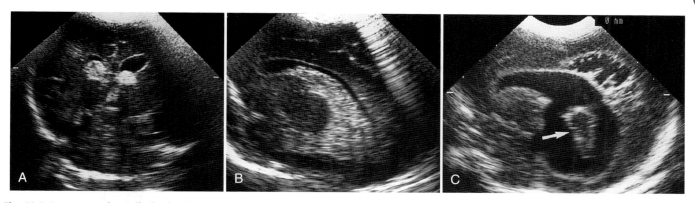

Fig. 19-7 Intraparenchymal echodensity. A sizable amount of blood has ruptured from both germinal matrices into the lateral ventricles and the third ventricle, creating acute hemorrhagic distension. **A,** Coronal view. **B,** Parasagittal view. **C,** Follow-up study demonstrates that, in the deep peritrigonal white matter on the left side, a cavity with an echogenic rim has developed in the deep white matter as a result of secondary infarction. Residual clot in the trigone (arrow) has evolved in the typical way, demonstrated by a hypoechoic center surrounded by an echogenic rim.

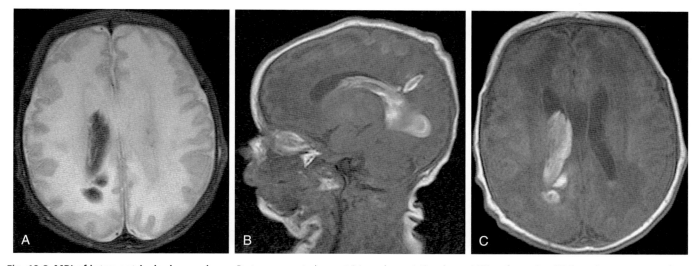

Fig. 19-8 MRI of intraventricular hemorrhage. Preterm neonate born at 34 weeks gestational age: MRI performed at 35.5 weeks postmenstrual age. **(A)** T1-weighted images demonstrate significant IVH with ventriculomegaly and intraparenchymal hemorrhage, consistent with grade IV IVH. **(B, C)** T2-weighted images confirm the IVH, now seen as hypointense, as well as several periventricular foci of intraparenchymal hemorrhage. *(Courtesy of Gordon Sze, MD, Department of Diagnostic Imaging, Yale University School of Medicine, New Haven, CT.)*

Fig. 19-9 Neuroradiologic demonstration of the development of a porencephaly. A, Coronal cranial ultrasound of a 26-week-gestation male triplet at 2 weeks of age demonstrates a large left-sided parenchymal hemorrhage. **B,** Axial MR image at term equivalent shows a left-sided porencephaly with mild ventriculomegaly. At the corrected age of 18 months, this child has hemiplegia but normal cognitive function. *(Courtesy of Linda S. De Vries, MD, Wilhelmina Children's Hospital, UMC, Utrecht, The Netherlands.)*

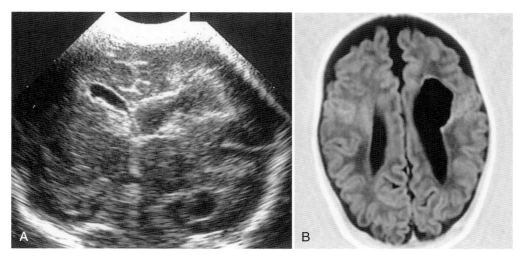

Table 19-5 **Clinical Symptoms of High-Grade Intraventricular Hemorrhage**

Symptom	Incidence
Decrease in hematocrit	75%
Seizures	10–15%
Changes in tone	75–90%
Abnormal eye signs	33–95%
Apnea/bradycardia	50–75%
Hyperglycemia	>50%
Hyponatremia	>50%
Metabolic acidosis	>75%

Ment unpublished data, NS27116 Randomized Indomethacin IVH Prevention Trial, 1997.

of hemorrhage has been linked to known clinical events, such as pneumothoraces and seizures, which have been demonstrated to increase cerebral blood flow [du Plessis, 2008].

Clinical Manifestations

The clinical manifestations of IVH are variable, and in one large series of postmortem examinations, over 75 percent of hemorrhages were clinically unrecognized [Allan and Sobel, 2004; Perlman and Rollins, 2000; Volpe, 1997]. None the less, as shown in Table 19-5, infants with large hemorrhages generally are noted to suffer a profound decrease in peripheral hematocrit and may experience coma, seizures, abnormal eye findings, including dilated and nonreactive pupils and loss of eye movements, and changes in tone and reflexes [Dubowitz et al., 1998]. Apneic and bradycardic spells may be attributable to either increased intracranial pressure or changes in cerebral blood flow to brainstem respiratory control centers. Of note, infants with even low-grade IVH may have significantly elevated serum glucose values and evidence for inappropriate secretion of antidiuretic hormone [Moylan et al., 1978; Shalak and Perlman, 2002]. Finally, persistent, unremitting metabolic acidosis unresponsive to alkali therapy or pressor agents is the hallmark of high-grade hemorrhage.

Cerebrospinal Fluid Studies

Several authors have demonstrated that examination of the CSF in preterm infants undergoing unremarkable sepsis evaluations routinely reveals 0–20 white blood cells (predominantly lymphocytes and monocytes per high-power filed), the absence of red blood cells, and protein values of 100–200 mg%. In patients with new-onset IVH, CSF findings include large numbers of red blood cells, white cells in direct proportion to the peripheral red blood cell/white blood cell ratio, elevations of protein, and low glucose values. In addition, CSF protein levels and red blood cell counts have been reported to correlate with the grade of IVH. Subjects with grades 3–4 IVH generally are found to have CSF protein levels of 500–1000 mg% and red blood cell values in excess of $1,000,000/mm^3$. In contrast, patients with grade 2 IVH generally demonstrate CSF protein values of less than 500 mg% and red blood cell values of $10,000–250,000/mm^3$. Patients with GMH, or grade 1 IVH, generally have no evidence for red blood

cells within the CSF unless they have also experienced a subarachnoid bleed; similarly, infants with grade 1 IVH are usually found to have normal values for CSF protein. Profound hypoglycorrhachia, with CSF glucose values below 10 mg%, may be found in infants with all grades of hemorrhage, although this is also more common in patients with high-grade hemorrhage.

Days to weeks after the primary hemorrhage, examination of the CSF demonstrates decreasing red blood cell numbers but elevated white blood cell counts in excess of $500–1000/mm^3$ and persistent hypoglycorrhachia. The latter two findings may lead the clinician to suspect bacterial meningitis, a diagnosis that can only be determined by cerebrospinal culture studies.

Neonatal Outcome

In the neonatal period, infants with IVH are at risk for the development of seizures and PHH [Allan and Sobel, 2004; Whitelaw et al., 2004]. Depending on the birth weights and gestational ages of the cohorts studied and the investigator's method for determining seizures, the incidence of seizures in preterm infants with IVH has been reported to range from 5 to 45 percent. Of note, a recent continuous amplitude-integrated EEG (aEEG) study of preterm neonates suggests that the mean age of seizure detection is 28 hours in infants with IVH, and only 2 of 8 neonates with IVH and seizures detected by aEEG had clinically recognizable events [Shah et al., 2010].

Similarly, the incidence of PHH depends not only on the gestational age of the population reported and the author's diagnoses, but also on grade of IVH; as many as 25–50 percent of infants with grades 3 and 4 IVH may experience PHH. Mortality is also higher in those infants with IVH when compared with their gestational age-matched peers without hemorrhage. Finally, IVH is believed to disrupt the genetically proscribed pattern of cerebral development in the preterm brain, and infants with hemorrhage are more likely to exhibit both macro- and microstructural changes on MRI than their nonhemorrhage peers.

Posthemorrhagic hydrocephalus

Posthemorrhagic hydrocephalus, shown by ultrasound in Figure 19-10, is diagnosed in the infant who meets all of the following criteria: presence of intraventricular blood, increasing ventriculomegaly (most commonly diagnosed by cranial ultrasonography), and evidence of increased intracranial pressure (defined as an opening pressure of greater than 140 mm H_2O by either lumbar puncture or, if indicated, cerebral ventricular tap) [McCrea and Ment, 2008; Whitelaw, 2001; Whitelaw et al., 2004]. In addition, in infants with PHH, the ventricular width at the intraventricular foramen by sonographic measurement exceeds 4 mm over the 97th percentile for gestational age [Levene, 1981]. PHH is most common in those infants with high grades of hemorrhage and less frequent in infants with the lowest gestational ages [Kazan et al., 2005]. Because of the compliance of the neonatal brain, the signs and symptoms of hydrocephalus may not be evident for several weeks following hemorrhage, and routine ultrasonographic monitoring is recommended in those infants at risk for PHH.

In most instances, the sequence of events resulting in PHH begins with multiple small clots throughout the ventricles. Although PHH is traditionally thought to represent a communicating hydrocephalus with obstruction to the passage of CSF at the level of the arachnoid villi, it is also probable that the CSF is reabsorbed across the ependyma into small penetrating vessels within the developing white matter. Obstruction to flow may

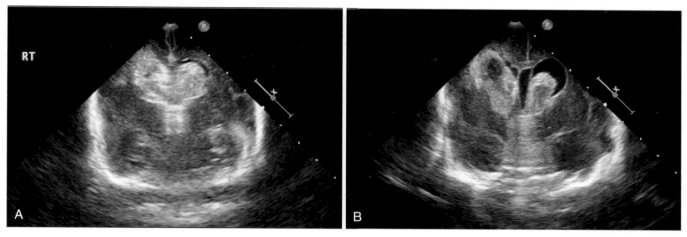

Fig. 19-10 Intraventricular hemorrhage leading to posthemorrhagic hydrocephalus. A, Coronal view of a 3-day-old, 29-week preterm neonate with intraventricular blood and right-sided parenchymal hemorrhage. **B,** Ultrasound performed at age 10 days to follow grade 4 IVH demonstrates significant ventriculomegaly; the patient developed clinical signs of increased intracranial pressure at postnatal day 14–16. *(Courtesy of Walter C Allan, MD, Maine Medical Center, Portland, ME.)*

thus also occur at the level of these vessels, or less commonly, at the foramina of Luschka and Magendie in the posterior fossa [Cherian et al., 2004]. In the presence of an obstruction in the normal CSF flow pathways, ventriculomegaly develops and periventricular white matter damage may ensue. Suggested mechanisms for periventricular white matter injury following PHH include raised pressure and edema, damaging effects of the free iron released into the CSF during clot lysis, and/or proinflammatory cytokines [Savman et al., 2001]. In addition, a small percentage of infants with IVH may develop acute obstruction at either the foramen of Monro, as shown in Figure 19-11, or the aqueduct

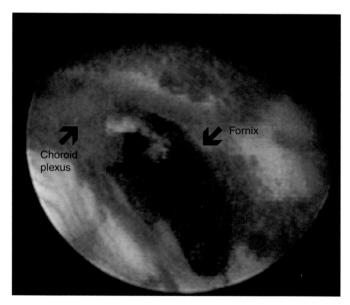

Fig. 19-11 Endoscopic view of the foramen of Monro. Endoscopic view of the foramen of Monro in a preterm neonate with IVH. The third ventricle is central in the image and is filled with clot. To the right of the third ventricle, the ependyma underlying the fornix contains residual clot and hemosiderin, while the thalamus can be seen in the lower left corner and the choroid plexus is visualized in the superior left quadrant. *(Courtesy of Charles C Duncan, MD, Department of Neurosurgery, Yale University School of Medicine, New Haven, CT.)*

secondary to the presence of clots obstructing CSF flow; these infants present with signs of acutely increased intracranial pressure (i.e., apnea, bulging fontanel, split sutures, and lethargy or coma). These infants require immediate neurosurgical attention, as shown in Video 19-1.

Randomized controlled trials have evaluated several treatment strategies either to prevent or to reduce the extent of PHH. These include intraventricular streptokinase, repeated lumbar or ventricular punctures, and DRIFT (drainage, irrigation and fibrinolytic therapy), but none of these has yet proved effective [Shooman et al., 2009; Whitelaw, 2000a, 2000b; Whitelaw and Odd, 2007; Whitelaw et al., 2001, 2007].

When treating infants with PHH, the physician must both protect the neonate from damage secondary to increased intracranial pressure and avoid the need for permanent CSF drainage procedures. (For review see Shooman et al. [2009].) Infants with intraventricular and/or intraparenchymal hemorrhage should undergo frequent determinations of occipitofrontal circumference and ultrasonographic determinations of ventricular size. Because prolonged increased intracranial pressure may result in poor feeding, lethargy, apnea, and, ultimately, optic atrophy, if ventricular size increases, neurosurgical consultation is recommended. Further, although some investigators have recommended ventricular puncture with the acute removal of 10–20 mL/kg of CSF for symptomatic infants with PHH, others have explored temporizing measures, such as subgaleal shunt placement, ventricular reservoir placement for intermittent tapping, or third ventriculostomy (Video 19-2). These strategies aim to avoid permanent ventriculoperitoneal shunt placement, and a small retrospective review of these interventions in neonates with IVH reported that 91 percent of those infants with subgaleal shunt placement and 62 percent of those with reservoir taps required permanent shunt placement. Of importance, infection rates were similar in the two populations, but future randomized trials are required to explore these treatment options.

Finally, those infants with acute signs of increased intracranial pressure and ventriculomegaly with blockage at the aqueduct will require immediate neurosurgical intervention.

Long-Term Outcome

Although recent advances in neonatal intensive care have resulted in increased survival rates for many critically ill and very preterm neonates, the neurodevelopmental fate of VLBW infants remains uncertain. Depending on the birth weight of the patient cohort and the years in which they were born, the incidence of minor developmental impairment is diagnosed in 30–40 percent and major disabilities are found in almost 20 percent of preterm children [Allen, 2008; Larroque et al., 2008; Neubauer et al., 2008; Saigal and Doyle, 2008; Voss et al., 2007]. Over half require special assistance in the classroom, 20 percent are in special education, and 15 percent have repeated at least one grade in school [Aylward, 2005; Bhutta et al., 2002]. Cerebral palsy has long been recognized as a frequent sequela of preterm birth, but significant cognitive and behavioral abnormalities are also being recognized at school age and beyond [Allen, 2008; Hack et al., 2009; Marlow et al., 2005; Robertson et al., 2009; Taylor et al., 2004].

Cerebral Palsy

Cerebral palsy (CP) is an important and well-established outcome of preterm infants that, in some centers, has been monitored for more than 45 years [Saigal and Doyle, 2008]. Recent data suggesting that the prevalence of neurodevelopmental handicap is increasing in the United States have attributed this finding to the increasing survival rates of many preterm and VLBW infants [Allen, 2008; Behrman and Stith Butler, 2007; Larroque et al., 2008].

Several recent studies have assessed the incidence of CP in children solely with IVH. In all, the incidence of CP is reported to increase with the grade of IVH. In pre-surfactant era studies, Pinto Martin reported that grade 4 IVH was strongly associated with CP (odds ratio = 15.4; 95 percent CI = 7.6–31.1), and in the study of Hansen and colleagues, the odds ratio for CP with grades 3 or 4 IVH was 19.9 (CI = 6.1–64.8) [Hansen et al., 2004; Pinto-Martin et al., 1999]. Further, in Pinto-Martin's study, any grade IVH alone was associated with CP (odds ratio = 3.14; 95 percent CI = 1.5–6.5).

More recently, Sherlock evaluated 270 neonates of <1000 g birth weight or <28 weeks gestational age at 8 years of age and found CP in 100 percent of those children with grade 4 IVH [Sherlock et al., 2005, 2008]. In contrast, approximately one-fifth of neonates with grades 2 or 3 IVH developed CP, and those with grade 1 hemorrhage experienced no increase in incidence of motor handicap when compared to children with no IVH. Similarly, Patra examined 362 children with birth weights <1000 g at 20 months of age; 104 had experienced grade 1–2 IVH [Patra et al., 2006]. Abnormal neurological examinations, including CP, were significantly more common in the IVH group (odds ratio = 2.60, 95 percent CI = 1.06–6.36).

Although most investigators include the results of all scans performed during the infant's hospitalization, Allan has reported that CP can be predicted from postnatal day 3 onward in preterm infants in whom serial ultrasonography is performed [Allan et al., 1997]. Further, although preterm infants with CP have traditionally been found to suffer spastic diplegia, concomitant with the rising rate of disabling spastic motor handicap, several investigators have also noted that CP among preterm infants is almost equally divided among the three classical forms: spastic diplegia, hemiplegia, and quadriplegia [Allan et al., 1997; Saigal and Doyle, 2008]. It is believed that this change in distribution reflects more focal and diffuse CNS injuries producing proportional increases in hemiplegias and quadriplegia.

Cognitive Outcome in Neonates with Intraventricular Hemorrhage

IVH is a significant cause of disability in the prematurely born. As shown in Figure 19-12, preterm subjects with grade 4 IVH have significantly worse cognitive abilities and educational performance when compared to those without IVH, as well as to those with lesser grades of hemorrhage [Luu et al., 2009a; Neubauer et al., 2008]. In Sherlock's study of 298 infants with birth weight <1000 g or gestational age <28 weeks, 100 percent of children with grade 4 IVH had full-scale IQ scores more than 1 SD below the population mean, compared to 60 percent of subjects with grade 3 IVH and approximately 40 percent of all other study participants (no IVH, grade 1 IVH, and grade 2 hemorrhage) [Sherlock et al., 2005, 2008]. Similarly, in Patra's study of 362 preterm neonates of the same birth weight, 45 percent of children with grades 1–2 IVH had mental scores >2 SD below the population mean, compared to 25 percent for those with no evidence of hemorrhage in the newborn period (odds ratio = 2.0, 95 percent CI = 1.20–3.60) [Patra et al., 2006].

Alterations in Brain Development

The advent of MRI has permitted assessment of the long-term influence of a neonatal injury such as IVH on the developing brain [Mewes et al., 2006; Nosarti et al., 2002; Reiss et al., 2004; Woodward et al., 2006]. Preterm children have smaller brain volumes at adolescence and beyond, and lower cortical gray, cortical white, deep gray, and cerebellar volumes when compared to term controls. In addition, IVH has been associated with significant additional reductions in cerebral gray volumes in preterm subjects during childhood and adolescence

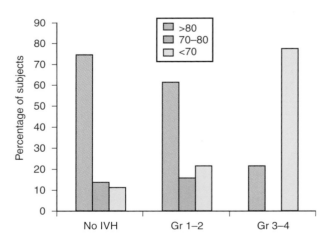

Fig. 19-12 Cognitive outcome of intraventricular hemorrhage at adolescence. Cognitive outcomes at 16 years of 315 subjects with birth weights between 600 and 1250 g, who participated in the Multicenter Randomized Indomethacin IVH Prevention Trial (NS 27116). The graph demonstrates the percentage of subjects with normal full-scale IQ scores (>80), borderline scores (70–80), and scores in the mentally retarded range (<70); p = 0.005 for differences among the groups. Gr, grade; IVH, intraventricular hemorrhage.

[Kesler et al., 2008; Nosarti et al., 2008; Reiss et al., 2004; Vasileiadis et al., 2004]. Studying the largest cohort of subjects born preterm at age 14 years and comparing them with age-matched and socioeconomically matched term adolescents, Nosarti also noted widespread alterations in white matter volumes throughout the developing hemispheres [Nosarti et al., 2008]. All areas of differential volumes between the preterm and term subjects were functionally related, and subjects with IVH and ventriculomegaly had the greatest white matter changes.

Prevention of Intraventricular Hemorrhage

The increasing rates of preterm birth and handicap for preterm neonates, and particularly those at the lower limits of viability, enforce the importance of preventing injury in the developing brain. Although the most efficacious means for preventing IVH would be the prevention of preterm birth [Behrman and Stith Butler, 2007], environmental, genetic, and pharmacologic interventions must be considered (Table 19-6).

Environmental Prevention Strategies

The risk factors for IVH have been well described [du Plessis, 2008; Leijser et al., 2009; Shalak and Perlman, 2002; Soraisham et al., 2009; Synnes et al., 2001, 2006]. When preterm birth is certain, transport of the mother and fetus to a tertiary perinatal center specializing in high-risk obstetric care is mandatory; for over three decades, neonatologists have recognized that those infants who were "outborn" and required transport to the neonatal intensive care unit have consistently higher rates of IVH than "inborn" patients [Hohlagschwandtner et al., 2001].

Abrupt increases in blood pressure, either by volume re-expansion or pharmacologic means, result in the loss of cerebral autoregulation and thus increased cerebral blood flow and are to be avoided. Blood pressure and transcutaneous oxygen pressure should be continuously monitored to prevent hypoxemia, hypotension, and secondary acidosis. Similarly, hypocarbia with $PaCO_2$ levels below 30 mmHg have also been significantly associated with severe IVH. (For review please see du Plessis [2008].) Depending on the gestational age and the postnatal day, preterm infants are known to have a high

Table 19-6 Prevention of IVH

Etiology	Strategies
Environmental	Maternal transport Bag and mask ventilation, early CPAP Monitoring of blood gases to prevent hypoxemia, hypocarbia, hypercarbia, and/or acidosis Continuous blood pressure monitoring – prevention of arterial hypotension No routine tracheal suctioning or chest physical therapy
Pharmacologic	Complete course of antenatal steroid exposure Administration of surfactant within the first 15 min Postnatal indomethacin Avoid sodium bicarbonate exposure

CPAP, continuous positive airways pressure.

incidence of patent ductus arteriosus, and previous studies have suggested that the pharmacologic closure of this lesion is less likely to be associated with abrupt changes in cerebral blood flow than the surgical approach might produce [Weiss et al., 1995].

Pharmacologic Prevention

The well-known sequelae of IVH have prompted the development of pharmacologic prevention strategies. The hallmark of antenatal prevention is corticosteroid therapy, while current potential postnatal strategies include indomethacin, activated factor VIIa, and erythropoietin.

ANTENATAL CORTICOSTEROID EXPOSURE

Corticosteroids administered prior to preterm birth have been shown both to lower the incidence of respiratory distress syndrome and to decrease neonatal mortality [Crowley, 2000, 2003]. The incidence of IVH is also reported to be lower in infants with antenatal corticosteroid exposure. In the Cochrane Review of 13 trials including 2827 neonates, corticosteroid therapy consisted of 24 mg of betamethasone, 24 mg of dexamethasone, or 2 g of hydrocortisone. In this large meta-analysis, the fetal exposure to antenatal steroids was associated with a relative risk of any IVH of 0.54 (CI = 0.43–0.69), and the relative risk for severe IVH was 0.28 (95 percent CI = 0.16–0.05). These benefits extend to a broad range of gestational ages and are not limited by gender or race. Further, no adverse consequences of a single course of prophylactic corticosteroid for preterm birth have been reported, although the action and long-term consequences of multiple courses of antenatal steroid exposure have been reported to result in decreases in weight length and head circumference at birth. For these reasons, the National Institutes of Health Consensus Development Conference recommended the widespread use of antenatal steroids for all preterm infants and stated that the significant benefits of this therapy outweigh possible adverse outcomes [Crowley, 1994, 1995].

INDOMETHACIN

Indomethacin, a potent inhibitor of the cyclo-oxygenase pathway of prostaglandin synthesis, decreases both the incidence and severity of IVH in VLBW preterm infants [Ment et al., 1994; Schmidt et al., 2001; Yanowitz et al., 2003]. In Fowlie's meta-analysis of 19 clinical trials looking at the postnatal use of indomethacin in 2872 infants, postnatal indomethacin treatment reduced the overall risk for IVH by almost 50 percent and was found to be most efficacious for prevention of grades 3–4 IVH [pooled RR = 0.66 (90.53, 0.82)] [Fowlie and Davis, 2002; 2003]. In addition, the ability of indomethacin to decrease both the incidence and severity of IVH was not found to be gestational age-dependent.

A synthetic indole derivative with a half-life of 11–30 hours in preterm infants, indomethacin decreases cerebral blood flow and blood-flow velocity in both animal and human studies [Hammerman et al., 1995; McCormick et al., 1993]. Experimental animal studies have demonstrated a reduction in the normal pattern of cerebral blood flow reactivity to episodes of asphyxia or hypertension, including reducing the normal hyperemia induced by asphyxia [Leffler et al., 1985, 1986; van Bel et al., 1993]. None the less, Fowlie's meta-analysis demonstrated no evidence of difference in rates of necrotizing enterocolitis, excessive bleeding, or sepsis in treated infants compared to controls [Fowlie and Davis, 2002, 2003]. An increased incidence of oliguria was seen with prophylactic indomethacin [RR = 1.90 (1.45, 2.47)], but there was no evidence for major renal impairment.

Despite the obvious effect in preventing IVH and the low incidence of sequelae, the long-term cognitive benefit of indomethacin therapy has become more controversial. Although Luu found improved cognitive testing scores for preterm males randomized to indomethacin [Luu et al., 2009b], Schmidt reported that indomethacin did not prevent a combined outcome of neonatal death or developmental delay in preterm neonates at 18 months corrected age [Schmidt et al., 2001]. Similarly, Harding noted that prematurely born subjects with a COX-2 C765 allele, associated with reduced COX-2 activity, had decreased cognitive performance at school age and may be vulnerable to the cerebral blood flow effects of indomethacin [Harding et al., 2007].

None the less, current recommendations in many neonatal intensive care units around the world suggest that all infants of 1250 g birth weight or less who are clinically stable and lack contraindications for indomethacin treatment be treated with prophylactic indomethacin 0.1 mg/kg/dose beginning at 6–12 postnatal hours, and with two additional doses 24 and 48 hours after the first administration. Indomethacin might be best administered after the administration of surfactant when there is evidence for acceptable oxygenation and ventilation; indomethacin should be infused slowly, preferably over 30 minutes or more [Bada, 1996; Clyman, 1996].

ACTIVATED FACTOR VII

Recombinant activated factor VII (rFVIIa) was originally developed as a hemostatic agent for patients with hemophilia and acts in the clotting cascade, through a variety of tissue factor-dependent and independent mechanisms, to accelerate the formation of thrombin clot in damaged tissues [Labattaglia and Ihle, 2007; Macik et al., 1993]. Because factor VII has been shown to be an effective agent for the prevention of bleeding in a diverse array of situations [Ghorashian and Hunt, 2004], it has also been proposed as a potential treatment for neonates with low-grade IVH, but large-scale safety and efficacy trials have yet to be reported [Greisen and Andreasen, 2003; Mitsiakos et al., 2007; Robertson, 2006].

ERYTHROPOIETIN

In preclinical studies, in vitro experiments, and adult human trials, erythropoietin (EPO) has been shown to be protective against both hypoxic-ischemic and inflammatory-mediated cerebral injury. Numerous safety trials of EPO suggest no adverse effects in the preterm population, and multicenter trials have been proposed to test the ability of EPO to prevent IVH and adverse neurodevelopmental outcome in the prematurely born [Fauchere et al., 2008; Strunk et al., 2004].

OTHER PHARMACOLOGIC PREVENTION STRATEGIES

Additional agents evaluated have included antenatal and postnatal phenobarbital, ibuprofen, ethamsylate, vitamin E, and pavulon. After over 15 years of study, the first two agents have been found not to influence the incidence of IVH in preterm infants [Donn et al., 1981; Shankaran et al., 1996].

Ibuprofen has been shown in preclinical studies to prevent cerebral blood flow autoregulation and close the patent ductus arteriosus. However, one study has found that ibuprofen was not effective with respect to IVH prevention in preterm neonates [Aranda and Thomas, 2006].

Ethamsylate is a water-soluble, nonsteroidal drug that has been used in Europe for several decades to reduce capillary bleeding during surgery. There is some evidence that it may increase platelet adhesiveness and capillary resistance by causing polymerization of hyaluronic acid in the capillary basement membrane and may also modify prostaglandin biosynthesis [Vinazzer, 1980]. Several clinical studies have been performed in Europe to evaluate the efficacy of postnatally administered ethamsylate in preventing IVH [Benson et al., 1986; Morgan et al., 1981; EC Ethamsylate Trial Group, 1994]. In these trials, ethamsylate reduced the risk of overall IVH without significant reduction in severe IVH, death, or neurological abnormality. Similarly, vitamin E, a well-recognized antioxidant, has also been shown to decrease the rate of IVH, although the effect on high-grade IVH has not been specifically examined [Chiswick et al., 1991]. Finally, pavulon (pancuronium) also has been evaluated for the prevention of IVH in mechanically ventilated newborns. By inducing muscular paralysis, pavulon is believed to prevent asynchronous breathing and the hypoxemia and secondary increases in cerebral blood flow associated with this phenomenon in the prematurely born [Cools and Offringa, 2005].

Combined Environmental and Pharmacologic Strategies

Repeated reports from numerous investigators have documented the variations in IVH rate and grade from institution to institution across Europe and the United States [Express Group et al., 2009; Fanaroff et al., 2007; Zeitlin et al., 2009]. Variances in patient populations, availability of prenatal care, and perinatal strategies may all contribute to these findings. Most recently, Obladen reported the results of a prospective monitoring trial for neonates of <1000 g birth weight [Obladen et al., 2008]. Monthly care conferences including all obstetric and neonatology personnel were held, and the hypothesis was that a rigidly adhered-to standard of care would lower the incidence of IVH in this vulnerable patient population. Mandatory care strategies included the following:

1. completion of a full course of antenatal steroid exposure for as many infants as possible
2. resuscitation by an attending neonatologist, to include bag and mask ventilation with air only, early continuous positive airways pressure (CPAP), and the delivery of surfactant within the first 15 postnatal minutes
3. careful monitoring of arterial blood gases to maintain acid–base balance without the use of sodium bicarbonate
4. no routine tracheal suctioning or vigorous chest physical therapy
5. prevention of arterial hypotension (i.e., mean arterial blood pressure <25 mmHg)
6. early indomethacin or ibuprofen at 12–36 hours for clinically significant patent ductus arteriosus.

Employing this strategy, Obladen noted a decrease in IVH rate from 34 to 13 percent.

Cerebellar Hemorrhage

Hemorrhage into the developing cerebellum is a recently described complication of prematurity. Cerebellar hemorrhage (CBH), shown in Figure 19-13, has been reported in 20 percent or more of VLBW preterm neonates, and as many as three-quarters of neonates with cerebellar hemorrhages also experience IVH [Limperopoulos et al., 2005; Sehgal et al., 2009; Steggerda et al., 2009]. The timing of these hemorrhages may differ, however, suggesting differences in pathophysiology of these injuries in the developing brain; Limperopoulos has reported that the mean age for diagnosis of CBH is 5.2 days, compared to 1.7 days for IVH [Limperopoulos et al., 2005]. The risk factors for CBH include lack of antenatal steroid exposure, emergent cesarian section, hypotension requiring medical therapy, sepsis, patent ductus arteriosus, and lower 5-day minimum pH values for the neonates with CBH.

Infants who experience CBH are at high risk for neurodevelopmental handicap [O'Shea et al., 2008]. Limperopoulos reported that children with CBH had significantly more severe motor disabilities, language delays, and cognitive deficits at 2–3 years of age than preterm control subjects of similar gestational age, although preterm infants with CBH and grade 4 IVH were not at overall greater risk for neurodevelopmental disabilities [Limperopoulos et al., 2007].

White Matter Injury of the Premature Newborn

White matter injury (WMI) is the predominant lesion of the premature newborn brain, resulting in much of the cognitive and behavioral impairments seen in children born prematurely, and to a lesser extent, the motor impairments. Notably, the true incidence of this injury is not known, largely because detection of the mild form of this lesion is difficult using conventional neuroimaging and because the threshold for determining signal abnormality in the cerebral white matter has not been rigorously defined. Studies have shown a decline in the incidence of cystic WMI, which is easily detected by ultrasound, but the incidence of clinically important noncystic WMI is unknown [Groenendaal et al., 2010; Hamrick et al., 2004]. White matter injury is used increasingly in place of the traditional term periventricular leukomalacia (PVL) or periventricular leukoencephalopathy, although the term PVL is still commonly used. WMI is a somewhat broader term than PVL in that it denotes the diffuse lesion of the cerebral white matter that extends beyond the periventricular regions defined in initial neuropathologic and ultrasonographic studies, and is often a noncystic lesion. An even more encompassing term, "encephalopathy of prematurity," was proposed by Volpe to include the findings of neuronal abnormalities in gray matter structures demonstrated by neuropathology and neuroimaging studies in addition to the white matter injury [Volpe, 2005, 2009a]. This term is not yet in widespread use in the literature, but it reflects increasing evidence that premature newborns suffer a brain injury that affects many gray matter structures in addition to the cerebral white matter. Although WMI with a similar imaging pattern to WMI in the preterm infant has been reported in infants born at term [Kwong et al., 2004] and in term newborns with congenital heart disease [Galli et al., 2004], this section of the chapter will focus exclusively on the pathology, pathogenesis, and clinical features of WMI of the premature newborn.

Neuropathology

The neuropathology of WMI was first described by Banker and Larroche in their classic 1962 report detailing the histological findings in 51 autopsy specimens [Banker and Larroche, 1962]. They described PVL as including bilateral areas of focal necrosis, gliosis, and disruption of axons, with the so-called "retraction clubs and balls." They noted the topographical distribution of the lesions to be in the periventricular white matter dorsolateral to the lateral ventricles, primarily anterior to the frontal horns and dorsolateral to the occipital horns. They noted that a severe anoxic episode occurred in 50 of 51 infants and that the lesions were consistently observed in the location

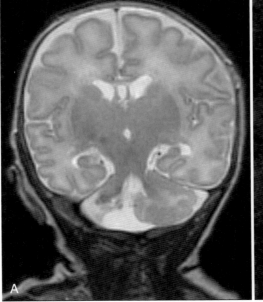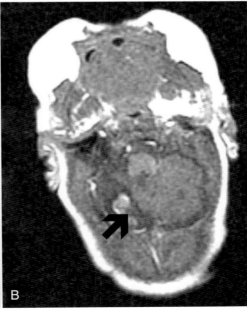

Fig. 19-13 Cerebellar hemorrhage. **A,** T2 MR image of a 25-week preterm neonate with right-sided cerebellar hemorrhage demonstrates diffuse loss of cerebellar tissue. **B,** T1 image shows persistent blood within the cerebellar space (arrow).

of the border zone of the vascular supply, which they suggested indicated that hypoxia-ischemia affecting the watershed regions of the white matter was a major pathogenetic factor. Second, their observation that 75 percent of the infants were born prematurely suggested a particular vulnerability of the periventricular white matter of the immature brain.

Further neuropathological studies extended these initial observations, demonstrating that, in many cases, WMI consists of areas of both focal necrosis (which become cystic) in the deep periventricular white matter, and a diffuse gliosis of the cerebral white matter, often extending well beyond the periventricular region [Deguchi et al., 1997; Gilles and Murphy, 1969; Takashima et al., 2009]. The acute lesions of WMI are characterized by axonal swellings, microglial activation, and reactive astrocytosis [Takashima et al., 2009]. Older lesions of remote WMI consist of astrogliosis, microgliosis, and loss of myelination, and may contain cystic foci. The cysts may be quite small, measuring <1 mm in some cases [Pierson et al., 2007], which may not be detectable by conventional imaging studies. In addition, there may be neovascularization around necrotic foci [Takashima et al., 2009]. The diffuse gliotic lesion of WMI consists of proliferation of hypertrophic, reactive astrocytes and activated microglia, loss of oligodendrocytes, and axonal damage. Both the cystic and gliotic white matter lesions are followed by an overall decrease in the volume of myelin (hypomyelination), and often a decrease in cerebral white matter volume with accompanying increase in ventricular volume (atrophic ventriculomegaly). Immunomarkers of axonal pathology, such as β-amyloid precursor protein and fractin, show that this reduction in white matter volume is related to a diffuse injury to axons beyond necrotic regions, and not only to loss of oligodendrocytes and subsequent hypomyelination [Arai et al., 1995; Haynes et al., 2008].

The recognition of a significant component of neuronal loss and injury occurred relatively recently, as early neuropathological studies were focused on the obvious white matter pathology and reported little in the way of overt neuronal injury in premature newborns [Banker and Larroche, 1962; Gilles and Murphy, 1969]. Findings from neuroimaging research studies were a factor that prompted re-examination of neuronal injury in preterm newborns with WMI, since quantitative MRI studies showed that WMI injury was accompanied by marked reductions in the volume of cortical and subcortical gray matter, with relatively smaller reductions in white matter volume [Boardman et al., 2006; Inder et al., 1999, 2005; Kapellou et al., 2006]. Recent neuropathologic studies have now demonstrated that there is significant neuronal loss and gliosis in the thalamus, basal ganglia, and cerebral cortex associated with WMI in human infants born prematurely [Andiman et al., 2010; Ligam et al., 2008; Pierson et al., 2007]. In addition, gliosis and neuronal loss were found in the cerebellar white matter, cortex, and nuclei, and selected brainstem nuclei of some infants with WMI [Pierson et al., 2007].

It is still not entirely clear whether the neuronal loss and gliosis are predominantly a consequence of a primary injury to axons of the cerebral white matter, or whether there is a separate direct injury to neurons of the cortical, subcortical, and cerebellar gray matter, or both. Volpe's elegant review synthesizes the neuropathologic findings of WMI in the preterm brain, together with the current understanding of brain development at this age to present a comprehensive thesis of how the interaction of these destructive and developmental processes produces the "encephalopathy of prematurity" [Volpe, 2009a]. He proposes that WMI in the preterm brain involves primary destructive effects, as well as widespread disturbances of brain maturation and development, producing a diffuse brain "lesion." Volpe introduced the term "encephalopathy of prematurity" to reflect the widespread nature of this combined gray and white matter pathology of the immature brain. In particular, he explained how the numerous critical developmental processes occurring during the vulnerable period of 24–36 weeks' gestation may be disturbed by WMI, affecting specific cortical, subcortical, and cerebellar neurons by direct and indirect mechanisms. He proposed that primary axonal injury and loss in the cerebral white matter are likely responsible for some degree of secondary neuronal injury and loss in the cortex, thalamus, and cerebellum. An autopsy study demonstrated that there is a marked reduction of pyramidal neurons in layer V of the cortex of preterm newborns, which was hypothesized to occur secondary to axonal injury and loss [Andiman et al., 2010]. However, there may also be direct injury to and loss of developing neurons, such as subplate neurons located in the subcortical white matter [Volpe, 2005], which peak at gestational age 26–29 weeks and have been shown to be particularly vulnerable to hypoxia-ischemia in the rodent [McQuillen et al., 2003]. Similarly, a small autopsy series of preterm newborns showed a loss of cortical GABAergic neurons that normally migrate through the cerebral white matter in the third trimester [Robinson et al., 2006]. Further work is needed to delineate the precise nature and etiology of the neuronal abnormalities in preterm WMI, but it is now clear that the "injury" to the developing brain of the preterm newborn extends beyond the well-recognized white matter pathology.

Pathogenesis

The distinctive lesion of WMI found in the immature white matter of preterm newborns likely results from the interaction of multiple pathogenetic factors. Numerous risk factors for the development of WMI have been identified, but in most cases three major factors contribute to the pathogenesis of WMI in premature newborns (Box 19-3):

1. hypoxia-ischemia
2. inflammation/infection
3. vulnerability of immature white matter, particularly immature oligodendrocytes.

These three categories, as well as additional individual risk factors for WMI that have been identified, are discussed in detail below.

Hypoxia-Ischemia

Banker and Larroche originally suggested that WMI occurred in the regions of vascular border zones in the cerebral white matter, and that ischemia would thus be expected to affect these zones preferentially [Banker and Larroche, 1962]. Subsequent neuropathological studies employed postmortem injections of the vessels to demonstrate vascular border and end zones in the periventricular white matter where WMI is typically found [De Reuck, 1984; Takashima and Tanaka, 1978]. These watershed zones are thought to render the periventricular white matter vulnerable to ischemic injury during periods of low cerebral perfusion. This tenuous vascular structure is notable, given that

Box 19-3 Factors in the Pathogenesis of White Matter Injury

Hypoxia-ischemia

- Arterial watershed zone in periventricular white matter
- Low cerebral blood flow in cerebral white matter
- Impaired autoregulation – pressure-passive cerebral circulation
- Patient ductus arteriosus
- Acute/chronic lung disease, including hypoxia, hypocarbia
- Sepsis/infection causing hypotension, impaired autoregulation

Inflammation/Infection

- Chorioamnionitis
- Maternal/intrauterine infections (other than chorioamnionitis)
- Neonatal infections, (e.g., necrotizing enterocolitis)
- Abundance of activated microglia in immature white matter

Intrinsic Vulnerability of Immature White Matter and Oligodendrocytes

- Impaired antioxidant defense in immature oligodendrocytes
- Exuberant production of reactive oxygen and nitrogen species by reactive astrocytes, oligodendroglia, and microglia
- Susceptibility to excitotoxicity through high expression of glutamate transporter and receptors

cerebral blood flow is quite low in the white matter of preterm newborns [Borch and Greisen, 1998]. Moreover, there is evidence to suggest that critically ill premature newborns may have at least an intermittently pressure-passive circulation, which puts them at risk for episodes of cerebral ischemia [Lou et al., 1979; Soul et al., 2007]. Indeed, a higher incidence of WMI (as well as IVH) was found in one study of newborns who demonstrated evidence of a pressure-passive circulation [Tsuji et al., 2000]. In a larger prospective study, episodes of pressure-passivity were found in the first 5 days after birth in 97 percent of critically ill newborns with birth weights of <1500 g, with some of the sickest newborns of gestational age <29 weeks showing frequent episodes of pressure-passivity (>50 percent) and hypotension (>40 percent) [Soul et al., 2007]. Notably, these fluctuations in pressure-passivity did not necessarily correlate with periods of hypotension, which occurred less often than episodes of pressure-passivity. These data suggest that a normal blood pressure does not necessarily guarantee adequate cerebral perfusion, particularly given the uncertainty regarding normal or ideal blood pressure ranges for preterm newborns [Laughon et al., 2007].

In addition to the intrinsic properties of the cerebral circulation in preterm newborns, the occurrence of other medical illnesses may contribute to episodes of cerebral ischemia. Newborns are often hypotensive in the first hours and days after birth for a variety of reasons, and a patent ductus arteriosus in particular may contribute to systemic and cerebral hypoperfusion. Serious postnatal infections, such as necrotizing enterocolitis, sepsis, and/or meningitis often affect both systemic and cerebral hemodynamics. Hypoxia and hypercarbia from acute and chronic lung disease, and the impact of various ventilation strategies, suctioning, medications, infusions, transfusions, and other interventions may all exert a deleterious effect on cerebral hemodynamics and contribute

to the pathogenesis of WMI [Greisen et al., 1987a; Hoecker et al., 2002; Murase and Ishida, 2005; Patel et al., 2000; Perlman and Volpe, 1983; Perlman et al., 1983; van Alfen-van der Velden et al., 2006].

Inflammation/Infection

Both epidemiological and experimental studies suggest a role for inflammation and/or infection in the pathogenesis of WMI [Dammann and Leviton, 1997; Leviton et al., 1999b, 2010; Van Marter et al., 2002; Wu and Colford, 2000; Yoon et al., 1996]. Studies have shown an association between maternal infection, prolonged rupture of membranes, cord blood IL-6 levels, placental inflammation/infection, and WMI, suggesting that maternal infection is an important etiologic factor in the pathogenesis of WMI [Dammann and Leviton, 1997; Yoon et al., 1996]. Similarly, postnatal infection has been found to be associated with WMI [Shah et al., 2008; Van Marter et al., 2002]. Neuropathologic data showing that there is an abundance of activated microglia in the white matter of the preterm brain suggest a potential mechanism by which WMI may be mediated [Billiards et al., 2006]. Indeed, rodent studies show that activated microglia are necessary to mediate impaired development and death of immature oligodendrocytes by lipopolysaccharide [Lehnardt et al., 2002; Pang et al., 2010]. Peroxynitrite produced by inducible nitric oxide synthase and nicotinamide adenine dinucleotide phosphate (NADPH) oxidase in activated microglia likely plays a role in lipopolysaccharide-induced death of oligodendroglia [Li et al., 2005], and excitotoxicity mediated by N-methyl-D-aspartate (NMDA) receptors on microglia appears to mediate astrocyte death [Tahraoui et al., 2001]. Experimental studies suggest a role for cytokines, such as interferon-γ, in the pathogenesis of WMI. For example, apoptotic death of immature oligodendrocytes has been demonstrated in the presence of interferon-γ, a cytokine generated by macrophages and reactive astrocytes that likely acts on the premyelinating oligodendrocytes through receptor-mediated mechanisms [Baerwald and Popko, 1998; Folkerth et al., 2004a]. These experimental data demonstrate mechanisms by which inflammation/infection may result in WMI, given the observed association between infection and WMI in human epidemiological studies. It should be noted that hypoxia-ischemia can result in activation of microglia, providing another mechanism for oligodendrocyte injury and death, and that significant infection may result in hypoxia-ischemia; thus there is likely an interaction or even synergism between these two mechanisms of injury. There are likely to be genetic factors that modify the degree to which inflammation/infection contributes to WMI, as demonstrated by a study where specific IL-6 genotypes were associated with mental retardation in children with WMI [Resch et al., 2009]. Thus there is increasing evidence of the important role of antenatal and postnatal inflammation/infection in the pathogenesis of WMI; further work is needed to elucidate the specific mechanisms involved and potential preventive therapies.

Vulnerability of Immature White Matter, Particularly Immature Oligodendrocytes

The hypothesis that the periventricular white matter of the premature newborn may be more vulnerable to anoxia than the mature brain was also proposed by Banker and Larroche in their seminal paper [Banker and Larroche, 1962]. A maturational vulnerability of the periventricular white matter is suggested by the finding that WMI occurs much more commonly in the preterm newborn than in the term newborn. Specifically, the observation that the diffuse gliotic lesion of WMI affects the immature oligodendrocyte predominantly, with relative preservation of other cellular elements, suggests that the immature (premyelinating) oligodendrocyte is the cell most vulnerable to injury at this age. Immature oligodendrocytes are susceptible to injury and apoptotic cell death by free radical attack [Back et al., 1998; Oka et al., 1993]. Indeed, apoptosis was demonstrated to be the mechanism of free radical-mediated cell death by cystine deprivation [Back et al., 1998], which was an important finding because apoptosis is postulated to be the mechanism of cell death by moderate ischemia, rather than necrosis, which typically results from severe ischemic insults [Ankarcrona et al., 1995]. A relative lack of antioxidant defenses in the immature oligodendrocyte is one reason why this cell population is particularly vulnerable to free radical attack [Folkerth et al., 2004b]. In addition to free radical attack, premyelinating oligodendrocytes are also susceptible to injury or death by excitotoxicity [Deng et al., 2006; Follett et al., 2004; Husson et al., 2005]. This vulnerability to excitotoxicity likely results from high levels of extracellular glutamate due to high expression of glutamate transporter and because of high expression of glutamate receptors (AMPA and NMDA) by immature oligodendrocytes [Deng et al., 2006; Desilva et al., 2007; Follett et al., 2004; Husson et al., 2005; Karadottir and Attwell, 2007; Rosenberg et al., 2003]. Thus there is cellular and biochemical evidence to support the original postulate that the preterm newborn's white matter displays a maturational vulnerability that contributes to the high incidence of WMI.

Additional Risk Factors

There are numerous risk factors for WMI that have been identified in epidemiologic and prospective studies of preterm newborns, but the precise mechanism by which each risk factor exerts its effect is not always clear. Lower gestational age at birth and birth weight are associated with a higher risk of WMI and associated neuronal abnormalities, but these two factors are likely related to the three major pathogenetic factors listed above, as well as to other genetic and acquired risk factors [Inder et al., 2003b, 2005]. Chronic ventilation for chronic lung disease in preterm newborns has been identified as a risk factor for later neurodevelopmental deficits [Short et al., 2003], which may be mediated by the respiratory, hemodynamic, and inflammatory disturbances known to be associated with chronic lung disease and ventilator support.

INTRAVENTRICULAR HEMORRHAGE

As described in the previous section on IVH, it is difficult to separate IVH and WMI in many neuropathology, imaging, and clinical studies of preterm newborns because they are often both present [Armstrong et al., 1987; Takashima et al., 1989]. In fact, it is likely that IVH increases the risk of WMI, not only because these two entities share some of the same pathogenetic risk factors, but also because IVH may exacerbate WMI [Takashima et al., 1989]. For example, one study showed that ventricular dilatation in the presence of IVH by neonatal ultrasonography was associated with worse cognitive and motor outcome when compared with isolated ventricular dilatation,

suggesting that IVH may increase the severity of WMI [Vollmer et al., 2006]. One hypothesis to explain this observation is that non-protein-bound iron from IVH contributes to the generation of free radicals, which causes or exacerbates WMI via free radical attack [O'Donovan and Fernandes, 2004; Savman et al., 2001].

POSTNATAL CORTICOSTEROID USE

Clinical studies of postnatal corticosteroids given to treat lung disease have shown an association with worse neurodevelopmental outcome in preterm treated compared to untreated newborns [Barrington, 2001; Wood et al., 2005]. Postnatal hydrocortisone may have a less deleterious effect on the developing brain than dexamethasone [Lodygensky et al., 2005; Watterberg et al., 2007]. It is currently unclear how postnatal steroids exert their effect on the brain: for example, whether steroids contribute to WMI or whether steroids have an independent deleterious effect on the developing brain. Dexamethasone may exacerbate WMI through mechanisms such as exacerbation of ischemic injury, but may also directly impair neurogenesis and neuronal maturation [Baud, 2004]. As a result of published data showing the adverse effect of postnatal steroids on neurodevelopmental outcome, there has been a significant decline in the routine use of steroids to treat lung disease in most centers, except in cases of very severe lung disease. In contrast, antenatal steroid use decreases neonatal death and does not worsen neurodevelopmental outcome [Foix-L'Helias et al., 2008], and thus is administered routinely to women in preterm labor.

NUTRITION

Relatively little attention has been paid to the effects of nutrition on brain injury and development in preterm newborns, but it is likely that nutritional factors, such as total caloric intake, as well as specific vitamins and nutrients, are key to optimal brain development and neurologic outcome. A trial comparing two nutritional approaches demonstrated that energy deficit at 28 days of age correlated with total brain volume and developmental outcome, even though there was no difference in measures of brain volumes or outcome between the two groups [Tan et al., 2008]. Further work is needed in this critically important field of early life nutrition and its impact on brain development.

Clinical and EEG Findings

WMI is a typically a clinically silent lesion, evolving over days to weeks with few or no outward neurologic signs until weeks to months later when spasticity is first detected, or at an even later age when children present with cognitive difficulties at preschool or school age. With moderate to severe WMI, some degree of spasticity in the lower extremities may be detected by careful examination by term age or earlier, and there may be axial flexor weakness or proximal appendicular weakness when WMI is severe. Most commonly, however, WMI is diagnosed in the neonatal period by routine cranial ultrasonography or by MRI [Maalouf et al., 2001]. Since detection of WMI is not possible by routine clinical examination during the newborn period in the majority of cases, imaging studies are needed to detect WMI (as well as IVH), as recommended in standard published guidelines [Ment et al., 2002]. The importance of detecting WMI in the newborn period relates to the institution of early monitoring and intervention services, which may improve the care and long-term outcome of children born prematurely.

There have been numerous reports regarding the utility of EEG in the identification of brain injury by background or focal abnormalities, such as the transient appearance of sharp waves. Although there has been increasing use of one- or two-channel EEG monitoring (aEEG), this reduced montage EEG is most useful for identifying significant abnormalities of background patterns or trends over time, rather than focal abnormalities such as positive rolandic sharp waves [Greisen et al., 1987b]. Early conventional EEG studies reported that positive rolandic sharp waves appeared to be a highly specific but not highly sensitive marker of WMI in premature newborns [Aso et al., 1989; Clancy and Tharp, 1984; Marret et al., 1992; Novotny et al., 1987]. Positive rolandic sharp waves have also been observed in some newborns with large IVH, although this finding is likely related to coexisting WMI rather than IVH alone [Clancy and Tharp, 1984; Novotny et al., 1987]. Significant abnormalities of the EEG background pattern, particularly in the first days after birth, also have been shown to correlate with WMI and later neurodevelopmental impairments. In particular, the severity of EEG abnormalities has been shown to correlate with the severity of WMI [Aso et al., 1989; Kidokoro et al., 2009]. Serial EEG studies are more useful than a single EEG for the identification of either the rolandic sharp waves or background abnormalities that correlate with WMI and long-term neurologic deficits [Hellstrom-Westas

and Rosen, 2005; Kidokoro et al., 2009]. In particular, the combination of an early EEG in the first days after birth to identify acute abnormalities, followed by EEG in the second week and 1–2 months later, is best for identifying the evolution of EEG abnormalities associated with WMI [Kidokoro et al., 2009]. Interestingly, the observation that WMI is associated with early acute EEG changes, followed by later chronic abnormalities (coinciding with cyst formation, when that occurs), supports the idea that the insult resulting in WMI occurs around or very soon after birth [Volpe, 2009b].

Neuroimaging

Ultrasound

The evolution of echogenic (or hyperechoic) lesions in the periventricular white matter over the first few weeks after birth, with or without cyst formation (which are echolucent, or hypoechoic), is the classic description of WMI detected by serial cranial ultrasound studies (Figure 19-14). None the less, the detection of WMI by cranial ultrasound remains problematic, in that interobserver variability is high even in rigorous studies of WMI by cranial ultrasound, particularly with regard to the detection of hyperechoic lesions, with less than 50 percent agreement among observers in one study [Kuban et al., 2007]. Furthermore, there is no general agreement regarding the number, size, location, and persistence of hyperechoic lesions defining WMI diagnosed by serial cranial ultrasound [Kuban et al., 2001]. In contrast, hypoechoic or echolucent

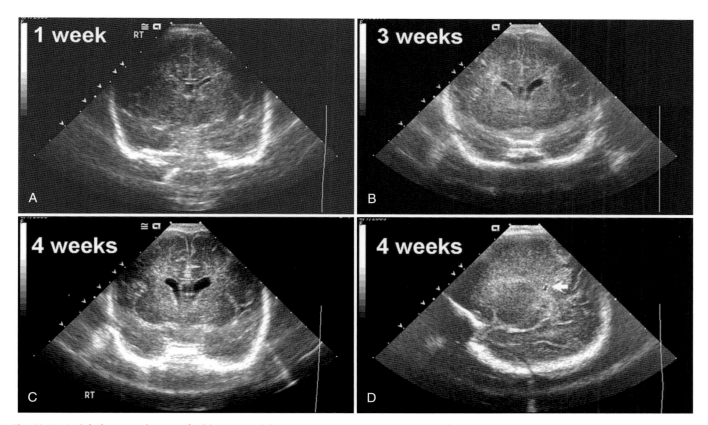

Fig. 19-14 Serial ultrasound scans of white matter injury. A–D, Cranial ultrasound scans performed at 1, 3, and 4 weeks of age show the progressive evolution of WMI, with a progressive increase in echogenicity in the periventricular white matter, an increase in ventricular size (atrophic ventriculomegaly) and extra-axial cerebrospinal fluid volume, and the appearance of a small cyst (arrow) at 4 weeks of age.

lesions denoting cysts and the presence of ventriculomegaly are easily and reliably detected by readers of cranial ultrasound [Kuban et al., 2007]. Notably, cystic lesions and significant ventriculomegaly are significantly associated with later cerebral palsy [Kuban et al., 2009]. Ventriculomegaly resulting from atrophy of the periventricular white matter (i.e., volume loss) is usually present within weeks after birth (see Figure 19-14), although it may not be observed by cranial ultrasound until late in the newborn period, suggesting that a cranial ultrasound performed prior to discharge from the neonatal intensive care unit provides additional diagnostic benefit, particularly when previous studies have been normal. Notably, isolated ventriculomegaly is associated with an increased risk of CP [Allan et al., 1997], suggesting that ventriculomegaly without radiologically evident white matter abnormalities likely indicates WMI, particularly in the absence of IVH. Studies correlating ultrasound and autopsy data have demonstrated that the incidence of WMI is underestimated by cranial ultrasound [Carson et al., 1990; Hope et al., 1988], and in the living newborn, MRI has been shown to be superior for the detection of WMI and other brain lesions in the preterm newborn.

Magnetic Resonance Imaging

MRI has been increasingly used to detect WMI in newborns and children born prematurely, although cranial ultrasound remains the preferred imaging modality for most centers because of its portability, safety, and lower cost. Conventional T1- or T2-weighted MRI sequences easily demonstrate cystic lesions that are the hallmark of the focal necrotic lesions of WMI. Noncystic WMI is also detected by MRI, evident as high signal intensity in the cerebral white matter by T2-weighted MRI, and low signal intensity by T1-weighted sequences in the newborn period. Diffusion weighted imaging (DWI) shows restricted diffusion if the MRI is obtained very early in the newborn period [Bozzao et al., 2003], but scans at later ages show increased diffusion in areas of WMI [Counsell et al., 2003]. Punctate lesions have also been detected by MRI in the white matter, often in the corona radiata and posterior periventricular white matter (and occasionally the gray matter) [Dyet et al., 2006; Ramenghi et al., 2007]. The etiology and neuropathology of these punctate lesions are currently unknown, although they have been hypothesized to represent tiny infarctions (possibly venous infarcts), small hemorrhages, or areas of activated microglia or increased cellularity [Rutherford et al., 2010]. Similarly, the clinical significance of these punctate lesions is unknown and follow-up studies are needed to determine if these lesions are associated with neurodevelopmental impairments. MRI performed in infancy or childhood can be useful for the detection of WMI, particularly for children who present with neurodevelopmental impairments but whose neonatal cranial ultrasound studies were normal or only mildly abnormal. MRI studies beyond the newborn period rarely show cysts but typically show increased signal intensity on T2-weighted and fluid-attenuated inversion-recovery (FLAIR) images in areas of gliotic white matter with delayed or decreased myelination (Figure 19-15). Thinning of the corpus callosum usually indicates a decrease in cerebral white matter volume (atrophy) associated with WMI.

MRI has been demonstrated to be more sensitive than cranial ultrasound for the detection of WMI in preterm newborns, especially for the noncystic form of WMI [Inder et al., 2003a;

Maalouf et al., 2001; Roelants-van Rijn et al., 2001]. As for cranial ultrasound studies, there is no universally accepted measure of the severity or extent of signal abnormality by MRI that defines WMI. While it is clear that greater severity of WMI is correlated with a higher incidence of later neurodevelopmental deficits, there is a broad range of outcomes for mild, moderate, and severe WMI [Woodward et al., 2006], and the threshold for defining clinically significant WMI has not been determined. For example, one study reported diffuse excessive high signal intensity (DEHSI) by T2-weighted MRI within the cerebral white matter at term age in 80 percent of infants born at 23–30 weeks gestational age [Dyet et al., 2006]. It has not yet been demonstrated that this high signal intensity on T2-weighted MRI is correlated with either neuropathological correlates of WMI (such as gliosis) or clinically significant WMI, although the authors reported a correlation between DEHSI and mild developmental delay at 18 months of age [Dyet et al., 2006]. Thus caution is needed when prognosticating outcome based on neuroimaging findings in preterm newborns.

Numerous MRI research studies have been helpful in elucidating the timing, distribution, and effects of WMI in children born prematurely. MRI scans performed soon after birth may be useful for demonstrating acute evidence of WMI, although later MRI studies (e.g., at term age) are superior for demonstrating the full extent of any WMI, gray matter abnormalities, or other congenital or acquired structural brain abnormalities. Diffusion tensor imaging (DTI) has been useful to demonstrate normal white matter development, as well as acute and chronic white matter abnormalities, showing the disruption of normal white matter architecture with WMI [Counsell et al., 2003; Huppi et al., 2001; Yoo et al., 2005]. These DTI abnormalities also have been shown to correlate with developmental outcome [Krishnan et al., 2007]. Similarly, volumetric analysis of brain MRI data has been used to demonstrate normal brain development and the specific gray and white matter volume changes related to WMI. Volumetric MRI data analysis was key to the discovery of the marked reduction in cortical and subcortical gray matter volumes accompanying WMI that had been underappreciated prior to the availability of these quantitative measurement techniques [Abernethy et al., 2004; Inder et al., 2005; Peterson et al., 2000]. Volumetric MRI studies of older children born preterm have been particularly useful in determining the clinical correlates of these volumetric changes, since the larger, mostly myelinated brain of the older child or adolescent can be analyzed in greater detail and more precisely than that of the newborn, and cognitive, social, and behavioral outcome measures are also more definitive and specific than at the young ages often used in neonatal outcome studies [Abernethy et al., 2002; Nosarti et al., 2008; Peterson et al., 2000]. Such studies have demonstrated that, compared with term-born matched controls, children born preterm showed reduced volumes of the white matter, hippocampus, parieto-occipital and sensorimotor cortex, cerebellum, and basal ganglia, and larger ventricular volumes [Nosarti et al., 2008; Peterson et al., 2000]. There was some variability in the findings among studies, which may be related to differences in study populations and measurement techniques, but volumes of the hippocampus, caudate, and sensorimotor cortex correlated with measures of cognitive outcome such as IQ [Nosarti et al., 2008; Peterson et al., 2000]. There is much more to be learned about the pathogenesis and outcome of WMI by detailed quantitative analysis of volumetric, DTI, and functional MRI data obtained at both newborn and later ages, particularly when correlated with perinatal/neonatal risk factors for WMI and with functional outcome measures.

Recommendations for Imaging the Preterm Neonate and Child Born Preterm

Current recommendations for imaging the preterm neonate suggest that screening cranial ultrasound should be performed on all infants with gestational ages <30 weeks at 7–14 days of age, and should be repeated at 36–40 weeks postmenstrual age [Ment et al., 2002]. This recommendation by the Quality Standards Subcommittee of the American Academy of Neurology and the Practice Committee of the Child Neurology Society is designed to detect both clinically unsuspected IVH, which may require additional clinical and/or radiologic monitoring and changes in management plans, and evidence for PVL

and/or ventriculomegaly, which are useful for prognosis and best seen when the infants are examined at term. Although older published guidelines do not recommend routine MRI scans for all premature newborns [Ment et al., 2002], emerging data suggest that cerebral MRI with DTI at term equivalent age may provide important prognostic information about developmental and motor handicap in the prematurely born. A brain MRI may also be performed in an older infant or child born prematurely to confirm clinically suspected WMI when there are cognitive, motor, and/or sensory impairments of unclear etiology (see Figure 19-15).

Outcome

WMI is the principal cause of the cognitive, behavioral, motor, and sensory impairments found in children born at <32 weeks gestational age [Volpe, 2003] (Box 19-4). Most outcome studies of children born prematurely are not restricted just to children

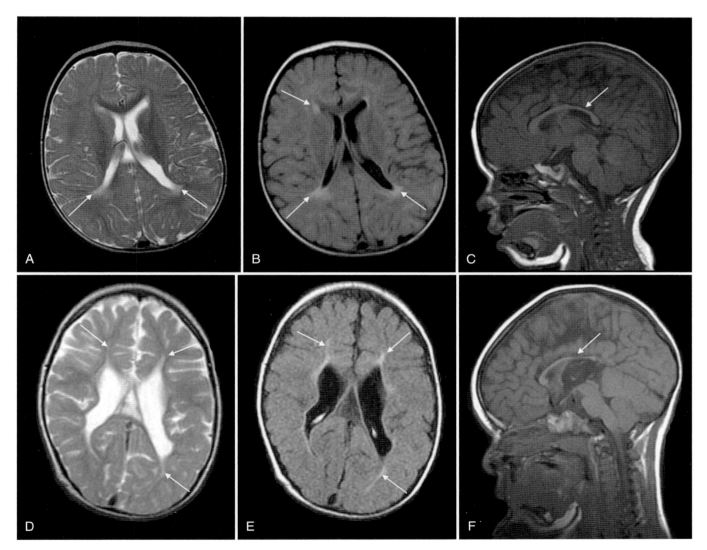

Fig. 19-15 MRI of mild and severe white matter injury in young children. A–C, Axial T2-weighted **(A)** T2 fluid-attenuated inversion-recovery (FLAIR) **(B)** and sagittal T1-weighted **(C)** images demonstrating mild WMI in an 12-month-old born at 30 weeks gestational age; at age 3 years this patient had mild spastic diparesis with accompanying gross and fine motor impairments/delays. **D–F,** Axial T2-weighted **(D),** T2 FLAIR **(E)** and sagittal T1-weighted **(F)** images demonstrating severe WMI in a 2-year-old boy born at 29 weeks gestational age; this patient had severe diplegia (quadriplegia), infantile spasms, severe cognitive impairment with IQ <70, and cerebral visual impairment. Arrows demonstrate areas of signal abnormality in the white matter on axial sequences and thinning of the corpus callosum on the sagittal sequence.

Box 19-4 Neurologic Problems Likely Related to White Matter Injury

Cognitive

- Low full-scale and performance IQ
- Difficulties with reading comprehension
- Difficulties with math
- Impaired executive function

Social/Behavioral

- Impaired attention, impulse control disorders
- Anxiety, emotional disorders
- Autism, autism spectrum disorders
- Conduct or oppositional disorders (uncommon)

Visual

- Ocular motility disorders
- Decreased visual acuity
- Lower visual field deficits
- Visual perceptual impairments

Motor

- Spastic diplegia, or quadriplegia when severe
- Motor coordination problems
- Dysphagia, articulation difficulties
- Hypotonia, ataxia (uncommon)

Epilepsy

- Generalized or focal epilepsy (uncommon)

with WMI, so it is difficult to quantify precisely the specific outcome attributable to WMI alone. That being said, it is likely that the great majority of cognitive, behavioral, motor, and sensory impairments and disabilities are related to WMI, with hemorrhagic venous infarction (grade 4 IVH) being the other major lesion that contributes significantly to neurologic disabilities in children born prematurely. In general, children with a severe neurologic disability in one domain often have multiple disabilities; for example, children with severe CP are more likely to have cognitive and sensory impairments than children without CP. The incidence of neurologic impairments increases with lower gestational age and birth weight, but there are many other antenatal and neonatal risk factors related to later neurodevelopmental impairments, including postneonatal factors, such as chronic medical illness, and environmental factors, such as socioeconomic status and maternal education [Vohr et al., 2003].

Cognitive

Lower overall IQ and many specific types of cognitive impairments have been found in children born prematurely when compared with term-born children. Lower gestational age and birth weight are major risk factors for cognitive impairments, as demonstrated in a study of extremely low birth weight infants (<1000 g) showing that only 30 percent of such children were performing at grade level without extra support at 8 years of age [Bowen et al., 2002]. Chronic lung disease, in particular, has been associated with worse cognitive function and greater need for special education and therapies when comparing children born prematurely with and without lung

disease [Short et al., 2003]. Deficits of attention and organization, math skills, and reading comprehension are much more common in children born prematurely than in term-born age-matched controls [Johnson et al., 2009]. Most large prospective studies of the cognitive outcome of older children born prematurely do not associate cognitive measures with specific brain lesions (such as WMI) by neonatal cranial ultrasound studies, but quantitative imaging studies to date suggest that it is indeed WMI and its gray matter correlates that underlie much of these cognitive impairments (see Neuroimaging section above) [Abernethy et al., 2002; Nosarti et al., 2008; Peterson et al., 2000]. Knowledge of neuroanatomy and the distribution of abnormalities with WMI allows for hypotheses regarding the potential neural substrate of various types of cognitive impairments. For example, deficits of attention and working memory may relate, at least in part, to involvement of the mediodorsal and reticular nuclei of the thalamus noted in one neuropathologic study of WMI [Ligam et al., 2008].

Social/Behavioral

There has been increasing recognition that children born prematurely have higher rates of social and behavioral difficulties than do term-born children [Delobel-Ayoub et al., 2006]. These include attention deficit/hyperactivity, emotional, anxiety, autism spectrum, and perhaps conduct disorders, particularly in children born extremely prematurely [Delobel-Ayoub et al., 2006; Johnson et al., 2010]. Of these, attentional problems are the most commonly recognized, with anxiety and other similar emotional disorders being increasingly identified and diagnosed. Various rates of these disorders have been reported, likely related in part to the age at evaluation and the method used to define or test for these disorders.

Motor

Lower gestational age at birth is also a risk factor for motor disability. The incidence of CP is much higher in children born extremely prematurely, occurring in approximately 20 percent of children born at ≤26 weeks gestational age, but in only 4 percent of children born at 32 weeks gestational age [Ancel et al., 2006; Wood et al., 2000]. Notably, one study showed that 25 percent of newborns diagnosed with WMI by neonatal cranial ultrasound had later CP, whereas only 4 percent with normal neonatal cranial ultrasound had CP, supporting the notion that significant motor impairments are typically related to WMI [Ancel et al., 2006]. Spastic diparesis is the most common form of CP in children born prematurely, which may present as quadriparesis when severe [Ancel et al., 2006; Kuban et al., 2008]. Hemiparesis is found less frequently than spastic diparesis, and is more likely to result from periventricular hemorrhagic infarction, but may result from asymmetric WMI [Ancel et al., 2006]. The topography of the cerebral white matter is such that the axons subserving the lower extremities are located closest to the ventricle, the axons of the upper extremities are situated lateral to them, and the axons of the facial musculature are located furthest from the ventricle. Since WMI is typically more severe proximal to the ventricle, WMI results in greater abnormalities of tone and power in the lower extremities than the upper extremities and face, i.e., a spastic diparesis. Dystonia is a frequent component of spastic diparesis caused by PVL, and occasionally hypotonia, ataxia, or some other motor abnormality is observed. In the absence of overt CP, coordination difficulties and other abnormalities of motor function or development may be found in children born prematurely.

Visual

While some children born prematurely have retinopathy of prematurity affecting their vision, WMI and other cerebral lesions alone can result in strabismus, nystagmus and other disorders of ocular motility, decreased acuity, visual field deficits, and perceptual difficulties, some of which may not be recognized until school age or later [Jacobson et al., 2002; Jacobson and Dutton, 2000; Pike et al., 1994]. Inferior visual field deficits may be found as a result of WMI, particularly since the optic radiations subserving the lower visual field and the white matter of the association areas of visual cortical regions are frequently affected by WMI [Jacobson et al., 1998]. Thalamic injury has also been shown to be associated with cerebral visual impairment in infants with WMI, separate from the effect of WMI alone on visual function [Ricci et al., 2006]. Children with WMI may have later visual perceptual defects or other higher-order visual impairments that contribute to their cognitive impairments, or in other words, worsen their cognitive and school function, so these are particularly important to detect [Jacobson et al., 1996].

Epilepsy

Children with severe WMI occasionally develop epilepsy, although epilepsy is more commonly related to gray matter lesions, such as periventricular venous infarction. In one study of 5-year-old children born at <26 weeks gestational age, 6 percent developed recurrent nonfebrile seizures [Wood et al., 2000]. Those premature newborns who develop later epilepsy likely have significant neuronal injury, such as the child whose MRI is shown in Figure 19-14, who developed infantile spasms.

Prevention

At the time of writing, there are no specific neuroprotective therapies or medications available during the newborn period to prevent or minimize WMI. Experimental data from animal models of WMI suggest promising neuroprotective agents to prevent or minimize WMI [Deng et al., 2006; Follett et al., 2004; Husson et al., 2005; Oka et al., 1993], but human trials of such agents are probably still years away. Current efforts are directed at prevention of WMI by addressing the known modifiable risk factors and pathogenetic mechanisms described above.

Preventive efforts ideally should begin antenatally, with prevention of maternal infection and other antenatal risk factors for the development of WMI. While known bacterial infections (such as group B streptococcus) are routinely treated by most obstetricians, there are no randomized trials to show that routine administration of antibiotics to women in preterm labor can prevent or minimize WMI in their newborns. Antenatal steroid administration appears to have a protective effect on the development of WMI, but this therapy is already administered to the vast majority of mothers in preterm labor as standard care [Foix-L'Helias et al., 2008; Leviton et al.,

1999a]. After birth, maintenance of normal cerebral perfusion should be attempted by careful management of systemic hemodynamics, including blood pressure, intravascular volume, oxygenation, and ventilation, and avoidance of treatments or procedures that result in sudden changes in systemic and cerebral hemodynamics. There is significant controversy about management of blood pressure in the premature infant and even about what constitutes a normal or "ideal" blood pressure for a given gestational and postnatal age [Laughon et al., 2007]. Furthermore, a normal blood pressure does not necessarily imply normal cerebral perfusion, given the known impairments of cerebral pressure autoregulation in some premature newborns [Soul et al., 2007]. In addition, medications that improve blood pressure and systemic perfusion may have little or no effect on cerebral perfusion [Lundstrom et al., 2000]. The management of systemic and cerebral hemodynamics remains an area of active research, as studies have yet to provide guidelines to improve neurologic outcome. Avoidance and prompt treatment of infection may also minimize WMI, although no studies have demonstrated the effect of such interventions on WMI.

Management of infants with WMI after discharge from the neonatal intensive care unit is directed at careful monitoring for and identification of any cognitive, behavioral, sensory, or motor impairments with implementation of appropriate therapies for any such impairments. Monitoring head circumference/growth during and after the newborn period can be useful to detect a deceleration in head growth signifying loss of brain volume related to WMI. Follow-up by pediatric neurologists or other pediatric physicians trained in infant and child development should be provided for children born prematurely, particularly those born at <32 weeks gestational age. Early intervention services in developmental monitoring and therapy, and additional specific services such as physical, occupational, speech and language, behavioral/social, and visual therapies, should be provided as needed to address specific developmental delays or impairments. Auditory and visual evaluations should be performed at older ages; most children born at <32 weeks will have had routine ophthalmologic examinations in the neonatal intensive care unit, with follow-up examinations in infancy. However, it is important to assess for visual impairments in preterm infants up to and including school age, which may require specialized testing of visual function and perception beyond routine ophthalmological evaluations. Similarly, assessment of cognitive and social function of school-age children may be needed, given the known risks of cognitive and behavioral difficulties in these children, even in the absence of early developmental delay or other neurodevelopmental impairments.

Acknowledgments

This work was supported by NS 27116 (LRM), NS 53865 (LRM), NINDS 1P01-NS38475, the Charles H Dana Foundation (JSS) and the March of Dimes (JSS). The authors thank Walter C Allan, M.D., Praveen Ballabh, M.D., Charles C Duncan, M.D., Gordon Sze, M.D., and Joseph J Volpe, M.D., for scientific advice.

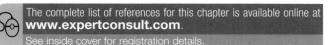

The complete list of references for this chapter is available online at **www.expertconsult.com**.
See inside cover for registration details.

Perinatal Metabolic Encephalopathies

Rebecca N. Ichord

Introduction

Neurologic disease in the newborn poses great peril and great opportunity. Knowledge of the pathophysiologic basis for neurologic disease of metabolic origin in newborns has grown rapidly as a result of applying advanced molecular biological approaches to these conditions. Improved availability of specific metabolic testing provides the means to institute specific treatments that can be life-saving and protective of the developing brain. In the many diseases where specific curative treatments are not available, knowledge of underlying molecular and cellular defects provides a starting point for further evaluation of the links between molecular defect and clinical syndrome.

This chapter provides a general summary of metabolic encephalopathies in the newborn, divided into two broad categories:

1. correctable disturbances in glucose metabolism and ion balance that accompany other illnesses
2. genetically determined inborn errors of metabolism.

Genetically determined metabolic diseases are grouped according to predominant type and tempo of clinical symptomatology into one of four groups:

1. acute fulminant illnesses with metabolic crisis
2. epileptic encephalopathies
3. chronic encephalopathies with multi-organ involvement
4. chronic encephalopathies without multi-organ involvement (Box 20-1).

A brief synopsis of each condition is provided, with emphasis on distinctive clinical features, diagnostic approach, and management. Comprehensive discussion of the molecular biology, pathophysiology, and genetics of these disorders may be found in several excellent reviews [Scriver et al., 2001; Hoffmann et al., 2010].

General Approach

Metabolic disease should be considered in the differential diagnosis of any newborn demonstrating symptoms or signs of encephalopathy, which are summarized in Table 20-1. While none of these abnormalities is specific to metabolic disease, the temporal pattern and specific constellation of symptoms taken together often suggest a metabolic disease. Encephalopathies caused by acute correctable metabolic perturbations, such as in hypoglycemic encephalopathy, typically follow a monophasic course that resolves in proportion to the timeliness of correction of the metabolic perturbation. The tempo of genetically determined metabolic diseases is more variable than acquired acute injury such as hypoxia or trauma. It often has a delayed or subacute presentation with unexplained disturbances in state of arousal or neonatal behaviors, such as feeding or visual attentiveness, or with the emergence of myoclonic seizures or movement disorder. Chronic encephalopathies that initially manifest in the newborn period are increasingly being linked to determine metabolic disease genetically. These disorders may have few or no features that distinguish them as metabolic, presenting with nonspecific signs such as hypotonia, depressed neonatal behaviors, or poor feeding. Nervous system manifestations of metabolic disease are generalized in nature, with depression of consciousness or irritability. Motor abnormalities and brainstem dysfunction parallel the severity of disturbed consciousness in a nonlocalizing manner. Suspicion of an inborn error of metabolism should be elevated by any of the following patterns:

1. involvement of multiple components of the nervous system (brain, special senses, peripheral nerves, skeletal muscle, autonomic nervous system)
2. involvement of multiple organ systems
3. systemic symptoms such as prominent unexplained vomiting, hyperpnea in the absence of lung disease, or unusual body or urine odors.

Once a metabolic encephalopathy is suspected, further evaluation should proceed urgently. The most common causes of acute encephalopathy not due to metabolic disease can usually be identified based on history, known risk factors, and the results of first-stage laboratory and imaging studies. These include hypoxic-ischemic injury, intracranial hemorrhage, trauma, stroke, venous thrombosis, effects of congenital heart disease on brain function (e.g., hypoxia, ischemia), central nervous system (CNS) infection, and intoxication. It should be emphasized that many neonates with encephalopathy are assumed incorrectly to have suffered "asphyxia" when, in fact, they have a static disease of prenatal origin, or a metabolic disease that decompensated in the face of the metabolic stress of birth. A diagnosis of perinatal hypoxic-ischemic encephalopathy should be made with certainty only when there is unequivocal evidence of severe compromise of circulation and gas exchange in the peripartum period, such as in the case of uterine rupture, placental separation, or fetal or neonatal circulatory arrest. In the absence of such certainty, the differential diagnosis should remain broad until a comprehensive evaluation is complete.

Box 20-1 Predominant Presenting Clinical Features in Neonatal Genetic Metabolic Disorders

Acute fulminant metabolic crisis

- Urea cycle defects
- Maple syrup urine disease (MSUD)
- Organic acidopathies: isovaleric, propionic, methylmalonic
- Oxidative phosphorylation disorders (OxPhos defects): pyruvate dehydrogenase (PDH) deficiency, pyruvate carboxylase (PC) deficiency, electron transport defects
- Fructose-1,6-biphosphatase deficiency
- Glutamine synthetase deficiency
- Fatty acid oxidation defects: carnitine palmitoyltransferase deficiency type II (CPT II), mitochondrial trifunctional protein deficiency (MTP defects), malonyl CoA decarboxylase (MCD)

Subacute progressive epileptic encephalopathy

- Glycine cleavage defects
- Pyridoxine and pyridoxal 5′-phosphate (PLP) dependency
- Sulfite oxidase and molybdenum co-factor deficiency (Sulf Ox, Moco)
- Menkes' disease
- Cytochrome oxidase (COX) deficiency
- L-amino acid decarboxylase (L-AAD) deficiency

- Methyl-CpG-binding protein-2 (MECP2)
- Glucose transporter type 1 deficiency syndrome (GLUT1 DS)
- 5-amino-4-imidazolecarboxamide ribosiduria/succinyl-5-amino-4-imidazolecarboxamide ribosiduria (AICAR/SAICAR)
- Serine biosynthesis defects

Chronic encephalopathy with multiple organ involvement

- Mitochondrial disorders
- Congenital defects of glycosylation (CDG)
- Peroxisomal disorders
- Cholesterol biosynthesis defects

Chronic encephalopathy without multiple organ involvement

- L-amino acid decarboxylase (L-AAD) deficiency
- Glutaric aciduria
- GTP cyclohydrolase deficiency
- Phenylketonuria (PKU)
- Succinic semialdehyde dehydrogenase (SSADH) deficiency

Table 20-1 Neurologic Signs and Symptoms of Neonatal Metabolic Disease

Neurologic Examination Category	Finding in Affected Infant with Metabolic Disease

Alterations in consciousness
  Mild to moderate
  Severe
	Excessively irritable, or somnolent but awakens with light stimulation
	Unarousable, but withdraws purposefully
	Comatose, responds to pain only by posturing, or not at all

Brainstem dysfunction	Pupillary abnormalities Oculomotor deficits Depressed or disordered suck and swallow function Disordered control of breathing (hyperpnea, apnea) High-pitched ("cerebral") cry
Cortical special senses	Absent arousal to sound, poor or absent visual fixation
Tone and movement abnormalities	Generalized hypotonia or hypertonia Nonepileptic myoclonus Dystonia, rigidity, opisthotonus, oculogyric crises
Reflex abnormalities	Exaggerated deep tendon reflexes Disturbed neonatal reflex behaviors (e.g., Moro, grasp)
Seizures	Myoclonic, clonic, tonic, subtle, apnea
Neuromuscular abnormalities	Diffusely absent tendon reflexes, bilateral symmetric facial or limb weakness, respiratory insufficiency
Autonomic dysfunction	Temperature instability, gastrointestinal dysmotility

Diagnosis is further delineated by appropriate staged laboratory studies, as shown in Table 20-2. The aim of the initial evaluation is to narrow down the differential diagnosis and simultaneously treat potentially life-threatening or handicapping conditions as quickly as possible. The results of "first-stage" studies will reveal abnormalities requiring immediate correction, such as hypoglycemia, hyponatremia, hypocalcemia, or hypoxia. They will further define other organ involvement, such as renal, cardiac, or hepatocellular dysfunction. A constellation of abnormalities on the initial screening testing may suggest a particular inborn error of metabolism (Figure 20-1). If the results of first-stage assessment, combined with clinical history, examination,

and neuroimaging, do not provide a specific diagnosis, they should provide the rationale for choosing appropriate "second-stage" studies. These are aimed at identifying the category of metabolic defect, and in some cases provide a probable specific diagnosis that can be verified in "third-stage" studies, in which DNA or tissue sampling provides material for enzyme quantification or genetic analysis. A careful family history should be obtained to ascertain consanguinity, known inherited metabolic disease, excess fetal loss, or infant demise in a sibling under similar circumstances.

Neuroimaging should be obtained early in the course of diagnostic evaluation. While head cranial ultrasound or

Table 20-2 Laboratory Evaluation of the Infant with Suspected Metabolic Encephalopathy

First Stage Survey and Screening	Second Stage Identify Category of Metabolic Defect	Third Stage Verify Enzyme or Gene Defect

Blood
  Glucose
  Electrolytes
  Mg^{++}, Ca^{++}, PO_4
  BUN, creatinine
  Liver enzymes
  CBC, platelets, PT, PTT
  Arterial blood gas
  Ammonia
  Lactate, pyruvate
	Blood
	  Quantitative plasma amino acids
	  Very long chain fatty acids
	  Acyl carnitine profile
	  Isoelectric transferrin point
	  Copper, ceruloplasmin levels
	  Cholesterol
	  Uric acid
		Tissue biopsy (muscle, liver) for enzyme assay
		Skin fibroblast culture for enzyme assay
		DNA studies and specific gene mutation probes
		Family studies

Urine
  Ketone bodies, reducing substances
  Protein, blood
  Cells
	Urine
	  Quantitative amino acids
	  Organic acids
	  Galactose
	  Sulfites
	  Xanthine, hypoxanthine
	  Uric acid
	  Ribosides	

CSF
  Glucose, protein
  Cell count
  Microbiology
	CSF
	  Quantitative amino acids
	  Neurotransmitters - Biopterin metabolites
	  Lactate, pyruvate	

BUN, blood urea nitrogen; CBC, complete blood count; CSF, cerebrospinal fluid; PT, prothrombin time; PTT, partial thromboplastin time.

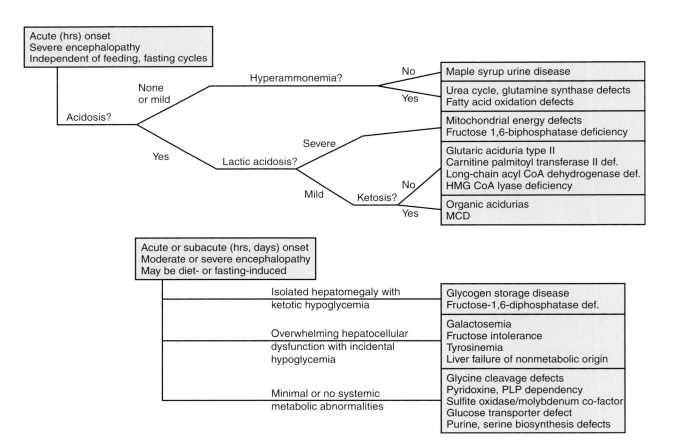

Fig. 20-1 Algorithm for evaluation of suspected metabolic encephalopathy in neonates. MCD, malonyl CoA decarboxylase deficiency; PLP, pyridoxine and pyridoxal 5′-phosphate dependency.

computed tomography (CT) can provide diagnostic clues and are sensitive to hemorrhage and major malformations, magnetic resonance imaging (MRI) is the preferred modality. Diffusion-weighted sequences add sensitivity, and when combined with standard anatomical imaging sequences and vascular studies such as MR angiography or venography, may provide a definitive diagnosis in many cases with nonspecific clinical findings. MR spectroscopy should be considered as part of the comprehensive imaging evaluation for children with encephalopathy of uncertain cause, as it can provide supportive evidence of primary metabolic disease.

Correctable Disturbances of Glucose and Salt Balance

Hypoglycemia

Hypoglycemia is common among critically ill newborns and is a frequent manifestation of inborn errors of metabolism. The definition of hypoglycemia is controversial. Blood glucose values reflect a dynamic balance between substrate availability and utilization, and in healthy newborns vary across a broad range, typically >2.2 μM (36 mg/dL), but reported as low as 1.3 μM (23 mg/dL) in healthy breastfed infants in the first few days of life. The risk of neurologic injury from hypoglycemia depends on multiple factors, including gestational age, availability of alternate substrates, metabolic rate, maturity and efficiency of glucose transport systems, status of oxidative metabolism, and differences in regional brain metabolic activity. As such, clinical factors such as coexistent hypoxic-ischemic injury, seizures, and the presence of hyperinsulinism strongly influence the occurrence and nature of hypoglycemia-related neuronal injury. These observations have led a number of investigators to propose an "operational" definition, whereby threshold blood glucose value, for example, 2.5 mmol/L (46 mg/dL), prompts treatment and further evaluation. This threshold may be modified up or down in individual cases, depending on clinical symptoms and factors likely to affect brain substrate demand, such as seizures or hypoxia, and alternative substrate availability, such as lactate or ketones or the effects of hyperinsulinism. Presently, there is insufficient evidence to define specific threshold values as predictive of neurologic injury in all clinical settings, and further research is needed on this point [Hay et al., 2009].

Disorders leading to neonatal hypoglycemia may be grouped into four broad categories: maladaptation to extrauterine life, hyperinsulinism, increased glucose consumption due to prior or intercurrent illness, and inborn errors of metabolism (Table 20-3). Maladaptation to extrauterine life affects premature infants and small-for-gestational-age infants due to low stores of fat, protein, and glycogen; inefficient ketogenesis and gluconeogenesis; or diminished tolerance of feedings. Hyperinsulinism is associated with maternal diabetes and gene defects affecting regulation of insulin production [Kapoor et al., 2009], and should be suspected when severe hypoglycemia (<2.6 mmol/L) without ketonuria in a well-nourished infant persists beyond the first 2 postnatal hours despite initiation of enteral feeds. Hypoglycemia from increased substrate utilization occurs during hypoxia or ischemia due to a shift from aerobic to anaerobic metabolism, sometimes compounded by decreased hepatic gluconeogenesis

Table 20-3 Causes of Neonatal Hypoglycemia

Category	Specific Disorders
Disorders of adaptation to extrauterine life	Prematurity Intrauterine growth retardation

Hyperinsulinism	Infants of diabetic mothers
	Maternal isoimmune disease
	Genetic defects of insulin secretion
	  ABCC8, ATP binding cassette C
	  KCNJ11, potassium channel J11
	  GLUD1, glutamate dehydrogenase
	  GCK, glucokinase
	  HADH, OH-acyl-CoA dehydrogenase
	  SLC16A1, solute carrier 16-1
	  HNF4A, hepatocyte nuclear factor 4 alpha
	Beckwith–Wiedemann syndrome
	Maternal isoimmune disease
	Congenital disorders of glycosylation

Elevated glucose consumption	Hypoxia Global ischemia Seizures
Acquired or transient hepatic dysfunction	Post hypoxic-ischemic hepatocellular injury Infectious hepatitis Any cause of liver failure
Primary endocrine disorders	Hypopituitarism due to brain malformation Congenital adrenal insufficiency Adrenal hemorrhage Hypothyroidism
Inborn errors of metabolism	See Table 20-4

and ketogenesis. Brain glucose consumption is dramatically increased by seizures from any cause, and may exceed the capacity of cerebral energy metabolism in brain regions compromised by a recent ischemic insult. Inborn errors of metabolism may cause hypoglycemia due to enzyme deficiencies in glycogenolysis or gluconeogenesis, or as a result of hepatocellular dysfunction. The neurologic manifestations in these cases represent combined effects of the hypoglycemia and the metabolic disorder. Table 20-4 lists inborn errors of metabolism commonly associated with neonatal hypoglycemia. Neonatal hypoglycemia may be associated with congenital endocrinopathies affecting the hypothalamic-pituitary-adrenal axis as a result of major brain malformations of the hypothalamic-pituitary region, congenital adrenal hypoplasia, or hypothyroidism.

The clinical signs and symptoms of hypoglycemia in the neonate are variable and nonspecific, exemplified by infants with hyperinsulinism. Signs and symptoms in the early stages may be dominated by signs of elevated circulating catecholamines: tachycardia, pallor, diaphoresis, irritability, jitteriness or tremor, and exaggerated tendon reflexes and neonatal reflexes (e.g., Moro reflex). Progressive depression of consciousness occurs as cerebral glucose stores are exhausted, associated with hypotonia, depressed reflexes, hypothermia, and often seizures. At its worst, uncorrected hypoglycemia at levels <1.0 μM in the absence of circulating ketone bodies will progress to coma, characterized by isoelectric electroencephalogram (EEG), cerebral edema, flaccid unresponsiveness, apnea, loss of brainstem reflexes, and circulatory collapse. Mild and moderate degrees of symptoms are rapidly reversed with

Table 20-4 Inborn Errors of Metabolism in which Neonatal Hypoglycemia is a Common Symptom

Category	Specific Disorders
Disorders of carbohydrate metabolism	Hereditary fructose intolerance Fructose 1,6-biphosphatase deficiency Glycogen storage diseases, esp. I and III
Fatty acid oxidation defects	Medium-chain and long-chain acyl-CoA dehydrogenase deficiencies Carnitine palmitoyl transferase II deficiency Mitochondrial trifunctional protein deficiency Malonyl-CoA decarboxylase deficiency (MCD)
Defects in ketone body synthesis	HMG CoA lyase deficiency
Gluconeogenesis defects	Holocarboxylase synthetase deficiency (multiple carboxylase deficiency) Pyruvate carboxylase deficiency
Disorders of branched chain amino acid catabolism and related organic acidurias	Maple syrup urine disease Propionic acidemia Methylmalonic acidemia Isovaleric acidemia Ethylmalonic aciduria 3-methyl-glutaconic aciduria 2-methyl-3-OHbutyryl-CoA dehydrogenase deficiency (MHBD)

glucose administration, whereas severe encephalopathy reflecting irreversible neuronal injury is not. Hypoglycemic coma is associated with irreversible neuronal necrosis and lasting neurologic deficits, with a predilection for parietal-occipital cortex and periventricular white matter [Burns et al., 2008]. Long-term sequelae may include microcephaly, cortical visual impairment, combined motor and cognitive handicap, and, in some cases, epilepsy [Tam et al., 2008].

The management of neonatal hypoglycemia remains a controversial subject [Hay et al., 2009]. High-risk infants should be screened for hypoglycemia, and provided exogenous feeds, intravenous or enteral, at rates and concentrations sufficient to maintain adequate blood glucose concentrations. Bedside screening for low blood glucose should be performed in any infant who develops signs and symptoms of acute encephalopathy. Symptomatic infants should be treated while the first-stage evaluation proceeds, as outlined in Table 20-2. If ketones are absent and the exogenous glucose requirement is high (>10 mg/kg/min), then hyperinsulinism should be suspected and further evaluated by measuring insulin levels. A paradigm for assessment of hypoglycemia in neonates is shown in Figure 20-2. According to the "operational" approach to the definition of hypoglycemia, treatment of acute symptomatic hypoglycemia should proceed immediately for any infant with a blood glucose <2.5 mmol/L (46 mg/dL), with a minibolus of 200 mg/kg using 10 percent dextrose infused over 2 minutes, followed by continuous infusion of 10 percent dextrose starting at 8 mg/kg/min and increasing as necessary to maintain stable blood glucose levels >2.6 mmol/L. Monitoring the effect of glucose administration on clinical symptoms, particularly the level of consciousness, can help clarify the neurologic significance of the hypoglycemia, and the need for evaluation for other causes of encephalopathy.

Disturbances of Sodium Balance

The function of excitable membranes depends on the regulation of concentrations and fluxes of sodium, potassium, and calcium within narrow limits. Sodium plays a critical role in synaptic transmission as a co-transported ion in neurotransmitter reuptake systems for glutamate, gamma-aminobutyric acid (GABA), glycine, and serotonin. Sodium accounts for the vast majority (>90 percent) of body fluid osmoles, and as such plays a critical role in regulating cell volume and water metabolism. Cell volume is largely determined by passive diffusion of water, which is determined by extracellular sodium and intracellular potassium concentrations, as well as by the effects of aquaporins. In the acute phase, hypotonic serum

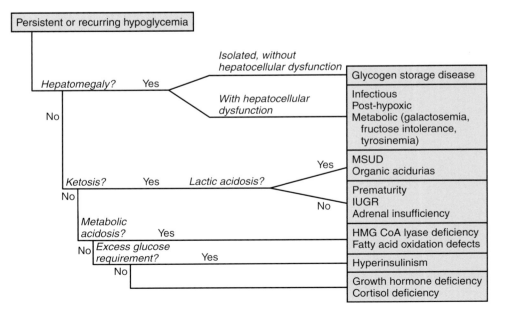

Fig. 20-2 Algorithm for evaluation of hypoglycemia in neonates. IUGR, intra-uterine growth retardation; MSUD, maple syrup urine disease.

sodium concentrations cause cell swelling, while hypertonic serum sodium concentrations cause cell shrinkage. Cell swelling may worsen neurologic dysfunction by causing an increase in intracranial pressure, which may lead to secondary ischemia. Cell swelling from hypotonic serum sodium concentrations provokes cellular counter-regulatory mechanisms to extrude potassium and amino acids, returning the osmoles and cell volume to normal levels.

Hyponatremia

The clinical effects of hyponatremia depend on the rapidity of the change, the absolute level of abnormality, and the effectiveness of cellular counter-regulatory responses. Acute decreases in sodium, occurring over hours or days, can cause mild symptoms at serum concentrations between 120 and 130 mEq/L, and severe symptoms at concentrations <120 mEq/L. Mild symptoms include irritability, apathy, excessive somnolence, and hypotonia. As the degree of hyponatremia worsens, seizures may occur, culminating in coma if uncorrected or if complicated by severe cerebral edema and intracranial hypertension. Osmotic demyelination, or central pontine myelinolysis, due to overly rapid correction of hyponatremia, has not been described in neonates. It would be difficult to isolate osmotic demyelination as a cause of white matter injury in neonates, most notably premature infants, who are vulnerable to white matter injury from other causes.

Hyponatremia occurs when sodium losses exceed sodium or water intake, or reabsorption exceeds water excretion, or both. Hyponatremia is common in sick neonates due to immature or damaged renal mechanisms of salt and water balance or to perturbations in the hypothalamic-pituitary mechanisms regulating volume and osmolar status. Hyponatremia during the first 1–2 weeks of life in sick neonates is most commonly due to excess arginine vasopressin (AVP) secretion in association with other diseases such as lung disease, intracranial hemorrhage, pain, and surgical procedures, and rarely is due to congenital adrenal insufficiency. Causes of hypo- or hypernatremia are summarized in Box 20-2.

The management of hyponatremic encephalopathy in neonates depends on the cause, the chronicity, and the severity of symptoms. Subacute or chronic (days to weeks) hyponatremia of mild degree (>120 mEq/L) should be treated by determining and correcting the underlying cause. Controversy surrounds the treatment of acute severe hyponatremic encephalopathy, which is usually associated with serum sodium concentrations <120 mEq/L. In such cases, seizures are usually resistant to standard anticonvulsants, and the encephalopathy frequently depresses respiratory drive and airway protective reflexes, all of which constitute a degree of urgency in favor of rapid correction. Rapid correction of hyponatremic seizures in infants and young children can be accomplished without neurologic complications by the use of 3 percent saline [Sarnaik et al., 1991]. The fact remains, however, that very little is known about neurologic complications from rapid correction of acute symptomatic hyponatremia in premature infants and critically ill term neonates who are already at high risk for neurologic injury from other causes. Until better data are available in this population, treatment should proceed with caution.

Hypernatremia

Neurologic manifestations of hypernatremia arise from hypertonic dehydration of neurons and glia, and may be compounded by secondary ischemic injury from hyperviscosity, cerebral venous thrombosis, or intracranial hemorrhage. Mild symptoms accompany mild elevations of serum sodium, generally <160 mEq/L, while severe encephalopathy usually occurs with

---

Box 20-2 Causes of Hyponatremia and Hypernatremia in Neonates

Causes of Hyponatremia

Disorders causing positive water balance
- Excessive AVP secretion
  - Systemic hypoxia, ischemia
  - Mechanical ventilation
  - Pneumothorax
  - Intracranial hemorrhage
  - Septic shock
  - Neonatal drug withdrawal
  - Hypothyroidism
- Water intoxication
  - Inappropriately dilute intravenous fluids
  - Inappropriately dilute formula feedings

Disorders causing negative sodium balance
- Abnormal renal salt handling
  - Chronic renal insufficiency
  - Adrenal insufficiency
  - Acute pyelonephritis
  - Acute obstructive uropathy
  - Urinary ascites

- Insufficient salt intake relative to losses
  - High insensible fluid/electrolyte losses
  - Vomiting, diarrhea
  - Low-salt-containing infant formulas

Causes of Hypernatremia

Disorders causing negative water balance
- Deficient AVP secretion (central diabetes insipidus)
  - Meningitis, encephalitis
  - Hypoxic-ischemic encephalopathy
  - Midline CNS malformations with pituitary insufficiency
- Renal unresponsiveness to AVP
  - Obstructive uropathy
  - Renal dysplasia
  - Drugs
- Excess water losses
  - Extensive skin disease
  - Osmotic diuresis

Disorders causing positive sodium balance
- Administration of hypertonic salt solutions
- Ingestion of hypertonic feedings

AVP, arginine vasopressin.

elevations >170 mEq/L. The causes of hypernatremia are the inverse of those causing hyponatremia: excess sodium intake relative to sodium losses, or excess water losses relative to water intake or reabsorption, or both (see Box 20-2). Excess sodium intake occurs with administration of hypertonic intravenous solutions or from hypertonic oral feedings. Negative water balance is the most common cause of hypernatremia, caused by excess losses of hypotonic body fluids, defective renal water absorption due to nephrogenic diabetes insipidus, deficient pituitary secretion of AVP, or cerebral salt wasting. Hypothalamic-pituitary insufficiency is caused by acquired brain insults, such as meningitis or hypoxic-ischemic encephalopathy, and by midline brain malformations. Management of hypernatremia begins with assessment and correction of intravascular volume deficits with normotonic solutions or plasma expanders in sufficient amounts to restore perfusion to normal levels and to maintain urinary output. The guiding principle in treatment is to prevent cerebral edema by correcting the hypernatremia over 48–72 hours, decreasing the serum sodium concentration at a rate not exceeding 10–15 mEq/L per 24 hours.

Inborn Errors of Metabolism

Neonatal encephalopathies due to genetically determined errors of metabolism comprise a rapidly growing class of diseases, as the powerful tools of molecular biology are applied to the evaluation of infants with previously ill-defined neurologic syndromes. The approach to diagnosis taken in this chapter is to classify diseases into one of four groups based on predominant clinical pattern and tempo of illness:

1. acute fulminant illnesses with metabolic crisis
2. subacute epileptic encephalopathies
3. chronic encephalopathies with multi-organ involvement
4. chronic encephalopathies without multi-organ involvement (see Box 20-1).

Patterns of clinical features may be helpful in recognizing characteristic patterns associated with specific disorders, as shown in Table 20-5 and Table 20-6. Specific diagnoses can be suspected based on the predominant clinical features and results of first-stage assessments, then verified by definitive second- or third-stage studies, as described in Table 20-2. Many of the subacute epileptic encephalopathies and chronic disorders are less common and less well characterized. The full range of phenotypic variation remains to be fully elucidated in more recently described disorders. The widespread availability of MRI has provided new insights concerning the nature and anatomic distribution of brain abnormalities in these disorders, as well as in more classic metabolic diseases. Some disorders are associated with distinctive MRI findings, such as the cavitary leukomalacia seen in sulfite oxidase deficiency (Table 20-7). A brief summary follows for genetically determined metabolic encephalopathies that are reported to present

Table 20-5 Clinical Neurologic Features of Neonatal Genetic Metabolic Encephalopathies

Disorder	Hypotonia	Seizures	Microcephaly	Movement Disorder	Retina, Optic Nerve	Myopathy	Neuropathy
AICAR/SAICAR	+	+			+		
CDG	+	+	+		+		+
Cholesterol biosynthesis	+		+				
COX	+	+			+	+	+
CPT II	+	+					
Glutamine synthetase	+	+	+				
GLUT1 DS	+	+		+			
Glutaric aciduria I	+	+		+			
Glycine cleavage	+	++					
GTPC	+	+		+			
L-AAD	+			+			
MECP2	+	+	+				
Menkes' disease	+	+					
Methylmalonic aciduria	+						
Mitochondrial disorders	+	+				+	
MTP defects	+				+	+	+
Pyruvate carboxylase	+			+			
Serine biosynthesis	+	+	+				
SSADH	+	+		+			+
Sulf Ox, Moco	+	++	+				
Urea cycle			+/−				

AICAR/SAICAR, 5-amino-4-imidazolecarboxamide ribosiduria and succinyl-5-amino-4-imidazolecarboxamide ribosiduria; CDG, congenital defects of glycosylation; COX, cytochrome oxidase deficiency; CPT II, carnitine palmitoyl transferase deficiency type II; GLUT1 DS, glucose transporter deficiency syndrome; GTPC, GTP cyclohydrolase defect; L-AAD, L-amino acid decarboxylase deficiency; MECP2, methyl-CpG-binding protein-2; MTP, mitochondrial trifunctional protein deficiency; SSADH, succinyl semialdehyde dehydrogenase defect; Sulf Ox, Moco, sulfite oxidase and molybdenum co-factor deficiency.

Table 20-6 Non-neurologic and Metabolic Abnormalities in Neonatal Genetic Metabolic Disorders

Disorder	Other Organ Involvement	Associated Metabolic Findings	Other Features
CPT II	Heart, kidneys, liver	Hypoglycemia (nonketotic), metabolic acidosis, ketonuria, hyperammonemia, low carnitine	Myopathy, neuropathy
CDG	Heart failure, thrombophilia	Abnormal transferrin isoelectric focus point (may be delayed finding)	Inverted nipples, subcutaneous fat pads, growth failure
COX deficiency	Heart	Lactic acidosis	Dysmorphic facies
Cholesterol biosynthesis	Heart, kidneys, lungs, gastrointestinal tract, genital, digital anomalies	Low serum cholesterol, high 7-dehydrocholesterol	Dysmorphic facies, cleft palate
Urea cycle defects		Elevated plasma ammonia	
Sulf Ox, Moco		Low serum uric acid, high urinary sulfites, high urinary xanthine and hypoxanthine	
GTPC		Hyperphenylalaninemia	
AICAR/SAICAR		Hypoglycemia, high uric acid and ribosides in urine	Dysmorphic facies, growth failure
GLUT1 DS		Low CSF glucose	Apnea
MECP2 mutation (in males)			Polymicrogyria (bilateral perisylvian), central hypoventilation, growth failure
L-AAD		Hypoglycemia, metabolic acidosis	Autonomic dysfunction
Glutaric aciduria I		High glutaric acid in urine	Macrocephaly
Glycine cleavage defects		Elevated CSF and plasma glycine, and high CSF/plasma ratio for glycine	Rapidly progressive to coma, burst suppression on EEG
Mitochondrial disorders	Heart, muscle	Lactic acidosis	Growth failure
Methylmalonic aciduria	Bone marrow, liver	Metabolic acidosis, hyperammonemia, hypoglycemia	Growth failure
MTP deficiency	Heart, liver	Lactic acidosis, hypoketotic hypoglycemia, dicarboxylic aciduria, transaminitis, elevated CK, hyperammonemia, hypocalcemia	IUGR, hydrops
Menkes' disease	Coarse brittle hair, lax skin		Hypothermia
Serine biosynthesis defect		Low serum and CSF serine and glycine, low CSF 5-MTHF	IUGR, hypogonadism, cataracts
SSADH defect		High GABA in CSF and urine, high 4-OH-butyric acid in urine	

AICAR/SAICAR, 5-amino-4-imidazolecarboxamide ribosiduria and succinyl-5-amino-4-imidazolecarboxamide ribosiduria; CDG, congenital defects of glycosylation disorder; CK, creatine kinase; COX, cytochrome oxidase deficiency; CPT II, carnitine palmitoyl transferase deficiency type II; CSF, cerebrospinal fluid; GABA, gamma-aminobutyric acid; GLUT1 DS, glucose transporter type I deficiency syndrome; GTPC, GTP cyclohydrolase defect; IUGR, intrauterine growth retardation; L-ADD, L-amino acid decarboxylase deficiency; MECP2, methyl-CpG-binding protein-2; 5-MTHF, 5-methyltetrahydrofolate; MTP, mitochondrial trifunctional protein deficiency; SSADH, succinyl semialdehyde dehydrogenase; Sulf Ox, Moco, sulfite oxidase and molybdenum co-factor deficiency.

predominantly, or in variant form, in the neonatal period. The reader is referred to excellent reviews for comprehensive discussions of inherited metabolic diseases [Saudubray et al., 2002].

Acute Fulminant Metabolic Diseases

Maple Syrup Urine Disease

Maple syrup urine disease (MSUD) is an autosomal-recessive disorder due to deficient activity of branched chain keto-acid dehydrogenase (BCKAD); it causes accumulation in plasma of leucine, isoleucine, and valine, and their corresponding keto-acids (Figure 20-3). Of the five clinical phenotypes, the severe neonatal form is the most common [Morton et al., 2002]. After a normal interval of 4–7 days after birth, affected infants develop progressive lethargy and hypotonia, evolving to coma and decerebrate posturing, sometimes with seizures. Cerebral edema, particularly involving white matter, appears in the early stages, giving rise to a distinctive pattern of abnormalities on MRI, with pronounced T2 hyperintensity and restricted diffusion in the brainstem, cerebellar dentate nuclei, deep gray nuclei, and periventricular white matter [Jan et al., 2003]. Biochemical abnormalities include ketoacidosis, ketonuria, and hypoglycemia, often complicated by hyponatremia. Neuropathology consists of spongiform degeneration or

Table 20-7 Summary of MRI Findings in Neonatal Genetic Metabolic Encephalopathies

Disorder	Malformative Abnormalities				Destructive Abnormalities				Other
	Cortical Dysplasia	Cerebral Atrophy*	Cerebellar Atrophy	Corpus Callosum	Cortex	Basal Ganglia	White Matter	Brainstem	
Sulf Ox, Moco					+	+	+		Mimics hypoxic-ischemic injury; severe diffuse cystic leukomalacia in chronic stage
Urea cycle					+	+	+		Diffuse cytotoxic edema, then atrophy/gliosis
MSUD						+	+	+	Edema subcortical and brainstem nuclei, periventricular white matter
Glycine cleavage defect		+ D					+	+	Vacuolated degeneration of myelinated tracts in pyramidal tracts, cerebellar peduncles, dentate nuclei
Glutaric aciduria I		+ FT				+	+		Communicating hydrocephalus, SDH, arachnoid cysts
COX deficiency			+			+	+		White matter lesions mimic PVL
PKU				+			+		Progressive dysmyelination
AICAR/ SAICAR		+ D							
Menkes' disease			+	+					Tortuous arteries
Cholesterol synthesis		+ F	+	+					Holoprosencephaly, microcephaly
MMA						+			
Serine defects		+ WM							Microcephaly, hypomyelination
GLUT1 DS									Microcephaly
CPT II		+ D		+					Cortical dysgenesis: pachygyria, gray matter heterotopia
CDG	+		+	+					Dandy–Walker anomaly
MECP2	+								Bilateral perisylvian polymicrogyria
SSADH defect			+			+			

AICAR/SAICAR, 5-amino-4-imidazolecarboxamide ribosiduria and succinyl-5-amino-4-imidazolecarboxamide ribosiduria; CDG, congenital defects of glycosylation; COX, cytochrome oxidase deficiency; CPT II, carnitine palmitoyl transferase deficiency type II; GLUT1 DS, glucose transporter type I deficiency syndrome; MECP2, methyl-CpG-binding protein-2; MMA, methyl malonic acidurias; MSUD, maple syrup urine disease; PKU, phenylketonuria; SDH, subdural hematoma; SSADH, succinic semialdehyde dehydrogenase deficiency; Sulf Ox, Moco, sulfite oxidase and molybdenum co-factor deficiency.
* Regions affected by atrophy: D, diffuse; F, frontal; FT, frontotemporal; WM, white matter.

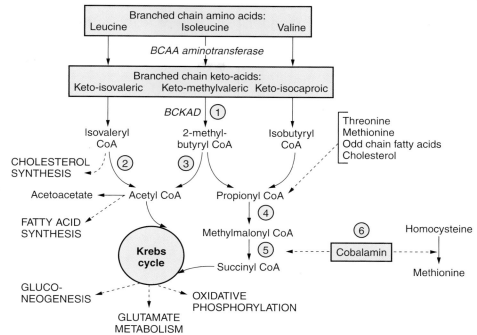

Fig. 20-3 Biochemical pathways affected by defects in branched chain amino acid (BCAA) and organic acid metabolism. Disorders and their corresponding enzyme defects: 1, Maple syrup urine disease, branched chain keto-acid dehydrogenase (BCKAD). 2, Isovaleric acidemia, isovaleryl CoA dehydrogenase. 3, Isoleucine defects, mitochondrial acetoacetyl CoA thiolase. 4, Propionic acidemia, proprionyl CoA carboxylase. 5, Methylmalonic acidemia, methylmalonyl. 6, CoA mutase or defective cobalamin metabolism.

delayed myelination of white matter with oligodendroglial cell loss, and cerebellar granular cell necrosis. The EEG during metabolic decompensation may show characteristic central sharp waves, or diffuse slowing to burst suppression as the symptoms progress. Diagnosis rests on the detection of marked elevations of plasma leucine (up to 1000–5000 μM during acute decompensation), isoleucine, and valine. Detection of L-alloisoleucine in plasma is pathognomonic for this disorder. An elevated ratio of leucine:alanine has been described as a sensitive and specific marker for MSUD, along with appreciation of the distinctive maple syrup odor in cerumen, allowing for earlier diagnosis of newborns in the presymptomatic stage. Urine organic acid profiles reveal elevated 3-hydroxyvaleric acid. BCKAD assay in cultured skin fibroblasts reveals activity at less than 2 percent of normal levels, and confirms the diagnosis. Treatment for acute severe decompensation requires metabolite removal via peritoneal dialysis or hemodialysis, along with supportive and nutritional measures to induce an anabolic state. Morton et al. reported that infants diagnosed in the first 72 hours of life, before becoming symptomatic, can be managed readily with enteral MSUD formula, thereby preventing acute metabolic decompensation and the associated neurologic injury [Morton et al., 2002]. Long-term management consists of dietary restriction of leucine, good nutritional support, and avoidance of catabolic stresses. Long-term outcome is related to the number and severity of metabolic decompensations.

The pathophysiology of the neurologic manifestations is incompletely understood, and is likely multifactorial and related to the roles of branched chain amino acids and their metabolites in cellular energetics, glutamate and GABA metabolism, fatty acid and cholesterol synthetic pathways, and the regulation of neuronal cytoskeleton development [Pessoa-Pureur and Wajner, 2007]. It has been suggested that acute symptoms reflect toxic effects of the keto-isocaproic acid (KIC) metabolite on glutamate, glutamine, and GABA signaling pathways and energy metabolism. Long-term effects of KIC may be related to altered phosphorylation of cytoskeletal proteins, which is

influenced by glutamatergic and GABAergic receptor activation in a developmentally regulated manner. A further potential mechanism for toxicity of branched chain keto-aciduria (BCKAs) is via inhibition of glutamate reuptake (see Figure 20-3). Deficiencies in transmitter pools of glutamate, aspartate, and GABA, along with deficient GABA receptors, have been demonstrated in an animal model [Dodd et al., 1992], while human neuropathologic analysis has revealed reduced myelin lipids in untreated patients.

Organic Acidopathies due to Defects in Branched Chain Amino Acid Metabolism

BCKAs are autosomal-recessive disorders due to defects in the catabolism of branched chain amino acids. MSUD is a prominent example of an organic aciduria, as described in the preceding section. Defects in the downstream degradation of branched chain ketoacids of leucine, valine, and isoleucine cause accumulation of one or more branched chain organic acid intermediates (see Figure 20-3). While isovaleric, propionic, and methylmalonic aciduria are the best known of these disorders, several others have been described (Table 20-8). Clinical symptoms first appear from the neonatal period to early infancy, characterized by acute onset of severe metabolic acidosis with ketoacidosis, hypoglycemia, and hyperammonemia, which may progress to seizures and coma. Associated features may include growth failure, vomiting, diarrhea, hepatic dysfunction, circulatory collapse, neutropenia, and thrombocytopenia. Pathogenesis of clinical symptoms has been attributed to a combination of direct toxic effects of accumulated metabolites and compensatory responses. Energy metabolism may be compromised as a result of deficient substrates for gluconeogenesis and limited availability of free CoA for mitochondrial fatty acid oxidation. Accumulation of acyl-CoA intermediates inhibits the urea cycle, resulting in hyperammonemia.

Diagnosis should be suspected when first-stage screening reveals prominent metabolic acidosis with variable combinations

Table 20-8 Biochemical Diagnosis of Organic Acidopathies

Disorder	Enzyme Deficiency	Urinary Organic Acid Profile	Associated Biochemical Abnormalities
Isovaleric acidemia	Isovaleryl CoA dehydrogenase	Isovaleryl glycine 3-OH-isovaleric acid 3-OH-butyrate	Metabolic acidosis (ketones, lactate) Hyperammonemia Low plasma glycine Pancytopenia
3-OH-3-methyl-glutaric aciduria	Hydroxymethylglutaric CoA Lyase	3-OH-3-methyl glutaric acid 3-methyl glutaconic acid 3-OH-isovaleric acid 3-methyl glutaric acid	Severe hypoglycemia No ketosis Lactic acidosis
Isoleucine defects	Mitochondrial acetoacetyl CoA thiolase	2-methyl-3-OH-butyric acid 2-methyl acetoacetic acid 2-butanone Acetoacetic acid 3-OH-butyric acid	Similar to isovaleric acid
Propionic acidemia	Propionyl CoA carboxylase	Propionic acid Methylcitrate β-OH-propionic acid Tiglic acid	Severe acidosis with ketosis Variable elevations of plasma branched chain amino acids Hyperglycinemia
Methylmalonic acidemia	Methylmalonyl CoA mutase, defective cobalamin metabolism	Methylmalonic acid	Severe acidosis with ketosis Hyperammonemia Thrombocytopenia Pancytopenia

of ketosis, lactic acidosis, hypoglycemia, and hyperammonemia. Specific diagnosis rests on specific urinary organic acid profiles, and can be confirmed by enzyme assay in cultured skin fibroblasts (see Table 20-8). Management consists of glucose administration, with insulin if necessary, to reverse catabolic states, and protein restriction, along with respiratory and circulatory support. Peritoneal dialysis may be necessary in the most severe cases with acute metabolic coma. L-carnitine and N-carbamylglutamate (NCG) supplementation respectively have been used to mitigate excessive ketogenesis and the inhibitory effects of high propionic acid levels on urea cycle function [Tuchman et al., 2008]. Carnitine and glycine supplementation may improve clearance of toxic metabolites in isovaleric acidemia. Co-factor supplementation can be helpful in subgroups characterized by primary defects in the co-factor metabolism using pharmacologic doses of cobalamin in some cases of methylmalonic acidemia, or biotin in some cases of propionic acidemia. Long-term management includes protein-restricted, high-carbohydrate diets and avoidance of catabolic stresses. Several case reports and case series have described improved long-term outcome following liver transplantation for some organic acidopathies [Morioka et al., 2007]. Long-term outcome can be normal if decompensations are minimized in frequency and treated aggressively when they occur.

Primary Lactic Acidosis due to Defects in Oxidative Phosphorylation

Primary lactic acidosis causes a severe metabolic encephalopathy in neonates with several types of defects in energy metabolism, including defects of pyruvate dehydrogenase complex, pyruvate carboxylase, and the respiratory chain. Figure 20-4 illustrates these pathways in relation to cellular energy and lactate metabolism. Secondary lactic acidosis is common in hypoxia or ischemia, and in other inborn errors of metabolism that secondarily affect energy metabolism, including organic

acidopathies, urea cycle disorders, and fatty acid oxidation defects. Changes in the flux of citric acid cycle intermediates produce a multitude of downstream effects on energy substrate availability, precursors of neurotransmitters, and protein synthesis pathways. In the developing brain, these metabolic shifts have profound effects on immediate cellular functional integrity, as well as transcriptional and translational processes central to cell proliferation and differentiation. Advances in the understanding of the role of cellular energetics in the regulation of the cell cycle and differentiation have shed new light on the mechanisms of neurologic effects of these disorders (Figure 20-5). Energy substrate deficiency shifts the ratio of adenosine monophosphate (AMP):adenosine triphosphate (ATP), which is a key regulator of the intracellular signaling system involving mammalian target of rapamycin (mTOR). The state of activation of mTOR broadly modulates protein synthesis and cell proliferation [Fingar and Blenis, 2004]. Under conditions of energy substrate deprivation, changes in mTOR signaling shift protein metabolism from an anabolic to a catabolic state, initiating a cascade of events with major implications for subsequent growth and development.

Improved understanding of the molecular and cellular pathophysiology of metabolic disease has led to the development of "anaplerotic" therapeutic strategies [Roe and Mochel, 2006]. These interventions aim to restore a more physiologic state of cellular energetics and protein synthesis, and go beyond replacement of deficient metabolites or removal of toxins by providing alternative substrates for the citric acid cycle and respiratory chain. This approach is exemplified by use of the triglyceride triheptanoin as an alternative source of citric acid cycle substrates in the treatment of pyruvate carboxylase deficiency, further discussed below. As such, these strategies are most relevant for defects of oxidative phosphorylation and the respiratory chain, but can theoretically play a role in any metabolic disorder that disrupts energy metabolism.

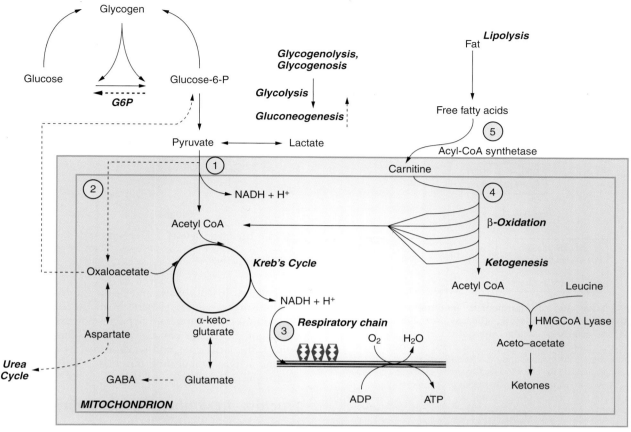

Fig. 20-4 Schematic of intermediate metabolism. Selected disorders and their corresponding enzyme deficiencies are indicated as follows. Defects in oxidative phosphorylation include: 1, pyruvate dehydrogenase; 2, pyruvate carboxylase; 3, respiratory chain. Fatty acid oxidation defects include: 4, carnitine palmitoyl transferase (CPT); 5, malonyl CoA decarboxylase (MCD). ADP/ATP, adenosine monophosphate/triphosphate; GABA, gamma-aminobutyric acid; NADH, nicotine adenine dinucleotide.

Pyruvate dehydrogenase (PDH) defects are the most common of the primary congenital lactic acidoses, and include multiple subtypes depending on which component of this large enzyme complex is affected. E_1 component defects are the most common, and are inherited as X-linked dominants. The most severe form presents in newborns with permanent lactic acidosis, often >7 μM, which is maximal in the fed state, and a fulminant severe encephalopathy progressing to death in the first months of life. Intrauterine growth retardation, subtle facial and limb anomalies, and minor signs of brain dysgenesis (absent corpus callosum) illustrate the fetal effects of this disorder. Postnatal evolution of the neurologic symptoms is associated with necrotic changes and cavitation in cortical white matter, basal ganglia, and brainstem nuclei. Treatment options are limited, although some success has been reported with institution of a ketogenic diet and thiamine and carnitine supplements.

Pyruvate carboxylase (PC) converts pyruvate to oxaloacetate. It plays a critical role in hepatic gluconeogenesis and in maintaining a stable supply of citric acid cycle intermediates influencing energy metabolism, the function of the urea cycle, and substrate availability for neurotransmitter pools of glutamate and GABA. PC deficiency has several subtypes with a broad spectrum of clinical manifestations. PC deficiency type B (the French subtype) is the severe neonatal form, and presents with a fulminant neonatal encephalopathy with permanent severe lactic acidosis, hypoglycemia, citrullinemia, and hyperammonemia, and is usually fatal in early infancy. The neurologic symptoms include variably depressed mental status, hypotonia, high-amplitude tremors and dystonic movements, and a variety of paroxysmal eye movement abnormalities (gaze defects, pendular nystagmus) [Garcia-Cazorla et al., 2006]. Imaging shows cystic periventricular leukomalacia. Autopsies in these patients show widespread neuronal death and arrest of myelination, leading to cortical and white matter atrophy or cystic encephalomalacia. Treatment strategies with high carbohydrate diets have been used in these patients to avoid dependence on the defective gluconeogenic pathways. Early administration of triheptanoin as a form of anaplerotic therapy may rapidly reverse the metabolic crisis and ameliorate neurologic symptoms in symptomatic newborns.

Respiratory chain defects comprise a large spectrum of disorders in oxidative phosphorylation, which have a highly variable and rapidly expanding phenotype. The phenotypic complexity arises in part from the fact that both nuclear and mitochondrial genes determine these structures. This group of disorders should be considered in infants with either severe intractable lactic acidosis, or a cardinal clinical feature with or without lactic acidosis. Cardinal clinical features include external ophthalmoplegia, myopathy, or cardiomyopathy, often with variable encephalopathy. Involvement of other organs is common, such as hepatic dysfunction, renal tubular

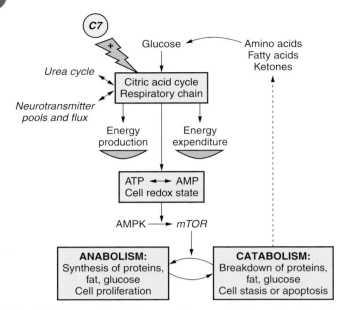

Fig. 20-5 Schematic of intermediate metabolism, showing the potential role of anaplerotic therapy for inborn errors of metabolism affecting cellular energetics. Energy status regulates anabolic vs. catabolic state of cellular systems via ratio of adenosine monophosphate (AMP):adenosine triphosphate (ATP), activation of AMP-mediated protein kinase (AMPK), and mammalian target of rapamycin (mTOR) activity. Anaplerotic therapeutic strategies may restore deficiencies in the supply of substrates for the Krebs cycle caused by some inborn errors, and indirectly affect downstream anabolic vs. catabolic state and cellular proliferation. C7 is heptanoin, a triglyceride, given as anaplerotic therapy; it is metabolized through the fatty acid oxidation pathway to produce acetyl-CoA and ketone bodies, restoring cellular metabolism toward an anabolic state.

abnormalities, or growth failure. When lactic acidosis is present, the lactate:pyruvate ratio is increased (>25) in disorders of oxidative phosphorylation, as compared to PDH complex disorders where the lactate:pyruvate ratio is usually normal. The clinical course may be benign in cases with only skeletal muscle involvement (benign infantile mitochondrial myopathy), or intractable and fatal in cases with intractable acidosis (lethal infantile mitochondrial disease). Diagnosis is difficult because of the extreme phenotypic and genotypic variability, and because histologic and histochemical diagnostic techniques are difficult and not widely available. Treatment options are limited, and have generally relied on supportive strategies to minimize catabolic stresses, and administration of carnitine and the respiratory chain co-factors nicotinamide and riboflavin.

Glutamine Synthetase Deficiency

Glutamine synthetase (GS) forms glutamine from glutamate and ammonia (Figure 20-6). Glutamine is the most abundant amino acid in plasma, and functions as an amino-group donor in the synthesis of several amino acids and nucleotides. GS plays a critical role in the brain to detoxify ammonia and regulate the concentration and compartmentalization of neurotransmitter pools of glutamate and GABA (see Figure 20-6). GS deficiency has been described as a rare autosomal-recessive condition manifest as profound neonatal encephalopathy with coma, quadriparesis, severe bulbar

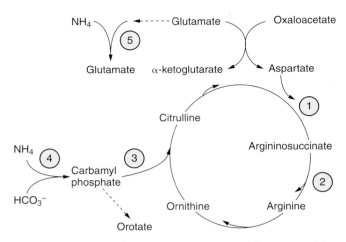

Fig. 20-6 Urea cycle defects. 1, Argininosuccinate synthetase. 2, Argininosuccinase. 3, Ornithine transcarbamylase. 4, Carbamyl phosphate synthetase. 5, Glutamine synthetase.

dysfunction, lissencephaly, and death shortly after birth due to multi-organ failure [Haberle et al., 2006]. Diagnosis rests on the finding of moderate hyperammonemia, and very low or absent glutamine concentration in blood, cerebrospinal fluid (CSF), and urine, and is confirmed by severely deficient enzyme activity in cultured fibroblasts. There is no effective treatment.

Fructose-1,6-Biphosphatase Deficiency

Fructose-1,6-biphosphatase (FDPase) deficiency is an autosomal-recessive disorder causing a profound defect in gluconeogenesis. It presents as a severe acute metabolic encephalopathy in the first month of life, with fasting-induced marked lactic acidosis and ketoacidosis and hypoglycemia, usually without other organ involvement, except for hepatomegaly. The characteristic clinical and biochemical features should suggest the diagnosis, but confirmation rests on enzyme assay on a liver biopsy specimen. Treatment is similar to that for type I glycogenosis, in addition to restriction of fructose and sucrose intake.

Fatty Acid Oxidation Defects

Fatty acid oxidation defects comprise a broad spectrum of disorders, most of which present beyond the neonatal period as acute encephalopathies with nonketotic hypoglycemia provoked by fasting or catabolic stress. In these disorders, one of several enzymes is deficient in the pathway for degradation of lipids to fatty acids to acetyl CoA or ketone body production (see Figure 20-4). Several of these disorders have been reported with prominent and distinctive presentations in neonates. These include carnitine palmitoyl transferase II (CPT II) deficiency, mitochondrial trifunctional protein deficiency (MTP) and malonyl CoA decarboxylase deficiency (MCD). Acyl CoA dehydrogenase deficiencies (long-chain or LCAD, medium-chain or MCAD, short-chain or SCAD) more typically present outside the neonatal period. These disorders share a constellation of clinical features, which include the rapid onset of a fulminant metabolic encephalopathy with hypoglycemia, moderate hyperammonemia, low or moderate ketonuria (disproportionately low for the degree of hypoglycemia), and metabolic acidosis. Associated clinical features may include hepatomegaly, cardiomyopathy, and myopathy.

Patients with MCD deficiency have been reported to have cortical dysgenesis, manifest as pachygyria, white matter atrophy, and gray matter heterotopias. The pathogenesis of neurologic symptoms has been attributed to the combined effects of direct toxicity from accumulated free fatty acids, as well as insufficient glucose and ketones to fuel the Krebs cycle, and inhibition of mitochondrial energy production by the disturbed ratio of acyl CoA:free CoA. The characteristic clinical features should suggest the diagnosis, which can be further supported by finding decreased total plasma carnitine levels and specific patterns of elevated plasma acylcarnitine intermediates as follows: C16 and C18 species in CPT II deficiency; C14 species in LCAD; C6–C8 species in MCAD; C4 species in SCAD. MCD deficiency is identified by the finding of elevated urinary malonic acid. Definitive diagnosis rests on assay of enzyme activity from cultured skin fibroblasts, and identification of specific mutations by genomic sequence analysis. Treatment involves supportive measures, glucose administration, and carnitine supplementation, and modification of feeding schedules to minimize fasting states. Creatine supplements have been suggested for patients with MTP deficiency. Recurrent decompensations can be minimized by early initiation of intravenous glucose during intercurrent illnesses and avoidance of fasting. Long-term outcome depends on the frequency and severity of decompensations.

MTP is distinguished among these disorders by the high proportion of cases (about 50 percent) presenting in the neonatal period [den Boer et al., 2003]. It has two types of presentations:

1. a neonatal presentation consisting of fulminant acute illness with rapid onset of depressed consciousness, heart failure, diffuse hypotonia and weakness with absent tendon reflexes, severe lactic acidosis, and death in a majority of patients due to heart failure
2. a subacute infantile presentation with gradually progressive hypotonia, diffuse weakness, and cardiomyopathy.

Multisystem involvement has been reported, including retinopathy, peripheral neuropathy, myopathy, cardiomyopathy, and liver disease.

CPT II deficiency has several phenotypes, with onset in adulthood, infancy, or the neonatal period. The latter is the least common and most severe form [Sigauke et al., 2003], and is reported to be universally fatal. Affected infants often have prenatally detected cerebral lesions and malformations, including ventriculomegaly, agenesis of the corpus callosum, polymicrogyria, periventricular cystic leukomalacia, and subependymal hemorrhages. Neurologic symptoms appear at birth or within the first few days of life, including seizures, depressed consciousness, and hypotonia with myopathic features. Cardiomyopathy leading to circulatory failure is common. The metabolic findings are typical of fatty acid oxidation defects, as described above. Management is supportive and symptomatic, but ineffective in most cases. Definitive biochemical diagnosis is a prelude to genetic testing, which can provide a basis for family counseling and management of future pregnancies. A number of US states have incorporated CPT II in neonatal metabolic screening programs in hopes of promoting early diagnosis.

Urea Cycle Disorders

Urea cycle defects presenting in the neonate are characterized by the onset, between 1 and 4 days of age, of severe hyperammonemia with rapidly progressive lethargy and vomiting, progressing to coma with signs of cerebral edema [Summar et al., 2008]. Associated features may include respiratory alkalosis and hypothermia. First-stage laboratory assessments reveal no other major abnormalities. A presumptive diagnosis can be made from results of plasma amino acid, urine organic acid, and urinary orotate excretion profiles (see Figure 20-6). Elevated plasma glutamine levels are common to all the urea cycle disorders. Organic acidopathies and congenital lactic acid disorders that may cause hyperammonemia can be distinguished from urea cycle disorders by the presence in the former of acidosis, ketosis, or lactic acidosis, as well as by specific metabolites in urinary organic acid profiles, as described in previous sections. Transient hyperammonemia of the newborn is a poorly understood disorder, characterized by severe transient hyperammonemia associated with respiratory distress syndromes or herpes simplex infection. It is distinguished from the genetically determined enzyme defects by its earlier onset (first 24 hours of life) and its association with prematurity and pulmonary disease. The pathophysiology of hyperammonemic encephalopathy is complex, involving astrocyte swelling and dysfunction due to excessive glutamine accumulation [Takahashi et al., 1991] and disturbed regulation of nitric oxide synthesis [Nagasaka et al., 2009]. Treatment of acutely symptomatic infants includes administration of sodium benzoate, phenylacetate, and arginine. Infants unresponsive to these measures or those presenting with acute severe hyperammonemic coma are treated with hemodialysis to reduce plasma ammonia levels rapidly [Enns et al., 2007]. Use of pressors and volume to maintain adequate cerebral perfusion pressure is preferable to the use of hyperventilation or osmotic diuresis in managing intracranial hypertension. Careful protein restriction, providing adequate calories to prevent catabolic state, and administration of drugs to enhance excretion of excessive metabolites are tailored according to the specific enzyme defect. Orthotopic liver and liver cell transplantation have been reported with some success in stabilizing the disease process and improving outcome in some cases [Meyburg et al., 2009]. Long-term outcome is variable, with motor and cognitive deficits dependent on the severity and frequency of hyperammonemic decompensations.

Subacute Epileptic Encephalopathies

Glycine Cleavage Defects

Glycine cleavage defects are a group of autosomal-recessive disorders that lead to accumulation of glycine (Figure 20-7). The most common form is a neonatal-onset progressive encephalopathy with depressed consciousness, apnea, and seizures, usually myoclonic, associated with a pattern of burst suppression on EEG. A transient form of nonketotic hyperglycinemia has been reported, in which symptoms similar to the classic form appear in the neonatal period, but which may resolve at 1–3 months of age when the glycine levels spontaneously normalize. In such children, enzyme activity measured from liver biopsy is normal, and long-term outcome is normal in the majority of individuals [Lang et al., 2008]. Glycine toxicity appears to be maximal in the neonatal period, and may spontaneously diminish after 1 month of age. Lifelong severe cognitive and motor handicap and intractable epilepsy are the rule among survivors, although there is considerable variability. Factors that predict a poorer outcome include

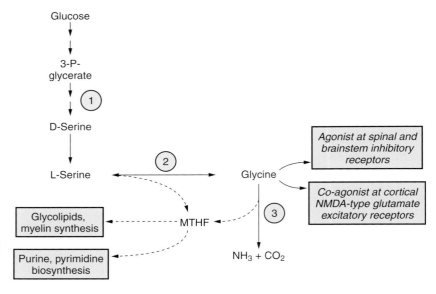

Fig. 20-7 Disorders of serine and glycine metabolism. 1, 3-phosphoglycerate dehydrogenase. 2, Serine hydroxymethyl transferase. 3, Glycine cleavage system. MTHF, methylenetetrahydrofolate; NMDA, *N*-methyl-D-aspartate.

earlier age of symptom onset, presence of cerebral dysgenesis, and degree of glycine elevation. Neurologic manifestations occur as a result of excessive stimulation of CNS glycine receptors, which are inhibitory in spinal cord and brainstem and excitatory in brain via a co-agonist effect at the *N*-methyl-D-aspartate (NMDA) subtype of glutamate receptors. Neuroimaging findings are varied, and may include cerebral dysgenesis of prenatal origin related to disturbed neuronal proliferation and differentiation, evolving to a progressive vacuolating myelinopathy in the postnatal period [Mourmans et al., 2006]. Biochemical abnormalities are limited to the finding of elevated glycine levels in plasma (1–8-fold above normal) and CSF (15–30-fold above normal). In cases with equivocal plasma elevations of glycine, the diagnosis can be made by finding a CSF:plasma ratio >0.06. Definitive diagnosis can be made by demonstrating absent or very low activity of the glycine cleavage system enzyme in liver biopsy or autopsy. Glycine cleavage defects can be distinguished from the hyperglycinemia that accompanies organic acidopathies by the presence of ketosis in the latter, and by characteristic organic acid excretion profiles. There are no proven therapies. Seizures have generally been resistant to standard anticonvulsants. Treatment with dextromethorphan, an NMDA-receptor antagonist, or with ketamine and benzoate has been reported in a small number of cases with limited success [Korman et al., 2006].

Pyridoxine and Pyridoxal Phosphate Dependency Epileptic Encephalopathies

Pyridoxine is the precursor for pyridoxal-5-phosphate (PLP), an essential co-factor for multiple enzymes in brain metabolism. There are two known enzyme defects with distinct gene mutations that result in depletion or deficient production of PLP. These are pyridoxine-dependent epilepsy (PDE) and pyridoxal phosphate-dependency disorder, known as PNPO deficiency. The biochemical and genetic basis for PDE has been defined, and involves depletion of PLP as a result of binding with 1-piperideine 6-carboxylate, a byproduct of defective lysine metabolism (Figure 20-8). The defect in the lysine pathway enzyme, alpha-aminoadipic semialdehyde dehydrogenase (AASAD), arises from mutation of the gene *antiquitin*

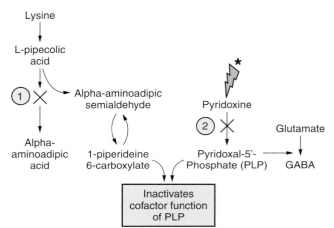

Fig. 20-8 Pyridoxine dependency/deficiency. 1, This is due to depletion of the active form of pyridoxine–pyridoxal-5′-phosphate (PLP), as a result of binding with 1-piperideine 6-carboxylate, a byproduct of lysine metabolism that builds up from deficiency of α-aminoadipic semialdehyde dehydrogenase (α-AASAD). *Effects of AASAD deficiency may be partially or wholly overcome by pyridoxine administration. 2, Pyridoxal phosphate-dependency disorder is due to deficient activity of pyridox(am)ine-5′-phosphate oxidase (PNPO), which converts pyridoxine to PLP.

(ALDH7A1) [Mills et al., 2010]. Pyridoxal phosphate-dependency disorder involves mutations in the gene for pyridox(am)ine-5′-phosphate oxidase (PNPO), which converts pyridoxine to PLP [Bagci et al., 2008]. The pathophysiology of the encephalopathy is not fully defined, but likely involves multiple pyridoxine-dependent pathways in brain metabolism. Prominent among these is glutamic acid decarboxylase (GAD), which converts glutamate to GABA, the major inhibitory neurotransmitter in mammalian brain (Figure 20-9). A disruption of this pathway alters GABA-related neurotransmission, and may contribute to the clinical manifestations of intractable seizures and severe cortical dysfunction.

Affected infants with either disorder have a similar clinical presentation, dominated by neonatal-onset seizures, or in some cases in utero-onset seizures, and chronic encephalopathy, with no other metabolic abnormalities. Seizures are usually

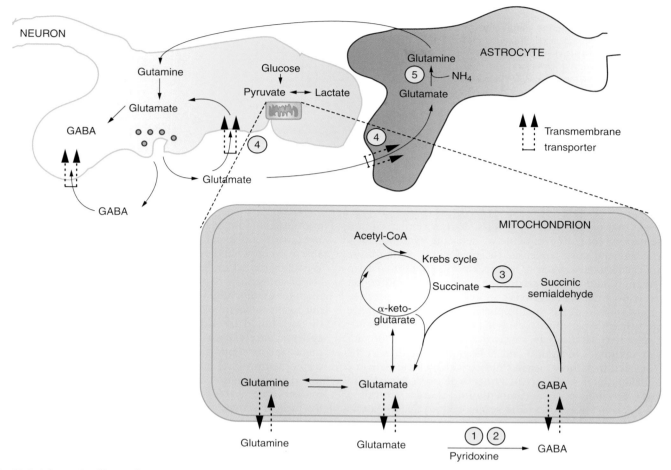

Fig. 20-9 Schematic of interrelationships between intermediate metabolism and the major neuronal neurotransmitters glutamate and GABA. Selected defects affecting neurotransmitter metabolism include: 1, pyridoxine dependency/deficiency, due to α-aminoadipic semialdehyde dehydrogenase (α-AASAD) deficiency; 2, pyridox(am)ine-5'-phosphate oxidase (PNPO) deficiency; 3, succinic semialdehyde dehydrogenase deficiency; 4, glutamate transporter defects; 5, glutamine synthetase defects. Alpha-AASAD may be partially or wholly responsive to pyridoxine or folinic acid administration.

unresponsive to standard anticonvulsants. EEG is typically severely abnormal, with any of several types of epileptiform patterns including hypsarrhythmia, burst suppression, or generalized spike-wave activity. The diagnosis of either disorder starts with clinical suspicion in the setting of refractory neonatal-onset seizures. Diagnosis of PDE can be confirmed by finding elevated levels of α-aminoadipic semialdehyde and pipecolic acid in urine, blood, and CSF. It can be further defined by mutation analysis of the *antiquitin* gene in affected children and their parents [Mills et al., 2006, 2010]. Diagnosis of pyridoxal phosphate-dependency disorder should be considered in infants with the clinical features of pyridoxine dependency, but who are unresponsive to pyridoxine, lack the confirmatory biochemical markers (elevated urinary AASA), and who respond to PLP.

Folinic acid-responsive neonatal epileptic encephalopathy resembles PDE clinically and electrographically. Gallagher et al. demonstrated that folinic acid-responsive epileptic encephalopathy is identical biochemically and genetically to PDE [Gallagher et al., 2009]. The biochemical basis for the favorable response to folinic acid is unknown.

Treatment recommendations for infants with clinically suspected or proven pyridoxine-dependency disorders include supplementation with both pyridoxine and folinic acid, as

there is variable response to either agent. Institution of a lysine-restricted diet has also been suggested. For infants with clinical features resembling pyridoxine-dependency disorder, but who are not responsive to pyridoxine and folinic acid, a trial of pyridoxal supplementation may be considered while awaiting results of genetic testing for PNPO deficiency.

Sulfite Oxidase and Molybdenum Co-factor Deficiency

Molybdenum co-factor deficiency and isolated sulfite oxidase deficiency are closely related autosomal-recessive diseases involving defects in xanthine metabolism and sulfite degradation pathways [Schwarz et al., 2009]. Molybdenum co-factor (Moco) is essential for the function of xanthine dehydrogenase and sulfite oxidase. Synthesis of Moco involves conversion of guanosine triphosphate (GTP) to a pterin-containing intermediate (cPMP) (Figure 20-10). The mechanism of the brain injury is multifactorial, involving direct toxic effects of xanthines and sulfite metabolites on cellular architecture, damage to mitochondria, thiamine degradation, and impaired mucopolysaccharide synthesis. Moco deficiency leads to accumulation of *S*-sulfocysteine, which activates the glutamate receptor, and may contribute to the prominent epileptic features of affected patients.

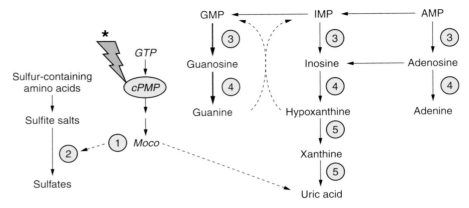

Fig. 20-10 Defects in purine metabolism and sulfur-containing amino acids. These are caused by deficiencies in: 1, molybdenum co-factor (Moco); 2, isolated sulfite oxidase deficiency. Enzymes in purine metabolism are shown as: 3, 5'-nucleotidase; 4, purine nucleoside phosphorylase; 5, xanthine dehydrogenase, which requires molybdenum as a co-factor. Synthesis of Moco involves conversion of guanosine triphosphate (GTP) to a pterin-containing intermediate (cPMP). *Administration of cPMP in animal models of Moco deficiency has been effective in normalizing the phenotype. AMP, adenosine monophosphate; GMP, guanosine monophospate; IMP, inosine monophosphate.

These two distinct genetic defects share a similar clinical presentation, consisting of acute or subacute evolution of a severe neonatal-onset epileptic encephalopathy with diffuse severe cavitary leukomalacia. Infants are usually born at term uneventfully, and develop seizures in the first week of life that progress over the ensuing weeks in association with arrested development, acquired microcephaly, and early appearance of generalized hypertonicity, evolving to a severe mixed motor and cognitive handicap in survivors. Most children do not survive infancy. The clinical and radiographic features in the early stages mimic those seen in children with hypoxic-ischemic encephalopathy. The absence of a history of severe peripartum hypoxia or circulatory decompensation should prompt a search for other diagnoses. The severe cavitary leukomalacia seen in these patients is very distinctive and not typically seen after perinatal hypoxia-ischemia. It is more severe in isolated sulfite oxidase deficiency than in Moco deficiency. There are no associated malformative anomalies, systemic metabolic perturbations, or abnormalities affecting other organ systems.

Diagnostic biochemical characteristics include increased urinary excretion of sulfites, thiosulfate, S-sulfocysteine, and taurine. Patients with Moco deficiency have low serum and urinary uric acid levels, and increased urinary xanthine and hypoxanthine levels. These findings may vary according to protein intake and nutritional status. Patients with isolated sulfite oxidase deficiency have normal uric acid metabolite levels. The diagnosis may be confirmed by enzyme assay of biopsied liver or cultured skin fibroblasts. Treatment is supportive with an emphasis on optimizing anticonvulsant therapy. Dietary intervention with cysteine and thiamine supplementation and methionine restriction has been reported to be beneficial in isolated cases [Boles et al., 1993]. Administration of cPMP in animal models of Moco deficiency has been effective in normalizing the phenotype, but has not been evaluated in humans [Schwarz et al., 2004].

Menkes' disease

Menkes' disease is an X-linked recessive disorder of the *ATP7A* gene, which results in defective function of the intestinal copper transport protein [Tumer and Moller, 2010]. This causes low tissue levels of copper and secondarily deficient function of numerous enzymes for which copper is a co-factor, including dopamine-β-hydroxylase, cytochrome c oxidase, and lysyl oxidase. The clinical phenotype invariably consists of severe neonatal-onset chronic encephalopathy with refractory epilepsy. Infants typically have central hypotonia and developmental arrest with microcephaly. Distinguishing findings on

examination, outside of neurologic abnormalities, include redundant and hyperelastic skin, coarse brittle hair, thin or absent eyebrows and eyelashes, and poor temperature stability. When examined under a microscope, hair fibers display the classic appearance of pili torti. Non-neurologic manifestations include vasculopathy with excess tortuosity and fragility, leading to thromboembolic stroke or subdural hemorrhage. This disease should be suspected in the setting of early infantile epileptic encephalopathy with the characteristic physical stigmata, and is supported by the biochemical findings of low ceruloplasmin level and low serum copper. Confirmation of the diagnosis based on serum ceruloplasmin and copper markers is unreliable in the newborn period. Distinctive abnormalities in serum profiles of catecholamines, on the other hand, provide a sensitive and specific diagnostic approach in the presymptomatic neonates [Kaler et al., 2008]. Correction of serum copper levels with dietary supplements may be helpful if started in presymptomatic infants. Otherwise, treatment is supportive with an emphasis on anticonvulsant management.

Glucose Transporter Defects

DeVivo et al. characterized a disorder arising from mutations in the neuronal glucose transporter, known as GLUT1 deficiency syndrome (GLUT1 DS) [De Vivo et al., 2002]. The disease manifests as early infantile-onset epileptic encephalopathy associated with a low CSF glucose concentration (mean 30 mg/dL). Seizures have their onset from age 4 weeks to 18 months, with a mean of 5 months, include all clinical seizure types (focal, generalized, myoclonic), and are resistant to anticonvulsant drugs. Affected infants have neurodevelopmental impairment of variable severity, and acquired microcephaly. The cardinal biochemical feature is a decreased ratio of CSF glucose relative to plasma glucose, typically <33 percent, which contrasts with the relatively high ratio of CSF/blood glucose seen in term and premature newborns of 70–80 percent, accompanied by low levels of the GLUT1 glucose transporter assayed in red blood cells. Conventional anatomical neuroimaging with CT or MRI is typically normal, while metabolic imaging with ^{18}F-fluorodeoxyglucose positron emission tomography (FDG-PET) reveals a distinctive pattern of hypometabolism in the thalami and mesial temporal regions [Pascual et al., 2002]. The ketogenic diet is the mainstay of treatment, resulting in good control of seizures in most patients but limited benefit for the neurodevelopmental disability. Long-term outcome is variable, with most children affected by some degree of cognitive impairment.

Serine Biosynthesis Defects

Defects in serine biosynthesis have been described that present as neonatal-onset chronic encephalopathies with prominent refractory epilepsy [de Koning and Klomp, 2004]. Affected infants are neurologically abnormal at birth with intrauterine growth retardation (IUGR), congenital microcephaly, cataracts, seizures, and neurodevelopmental impairment. A distinctive pattern of leukoencephalopathy is seen on MRI, characterized by hypomyelination, vacuolar changes, and gliosis, which may improve after treatment with serine and glycine supplementation. The disease involves defective serine biosynthesis due to 3-phosphoglycerate dehydrogenase deficiency (see Figure 20-7). Clinical manifestations have been attributed to multiple mechanisms, including loss of neurotrophic effects of serine, impaired synthesis of glycine, which acts as a glutamate receptor co-agonist, and impaired synthesis of 5-methyltetrahydrofolate (5-MTHF), which is a co-factor for numerous brain enzyme pathways. Diagnosis can be made by finding low CSF concentrations of serine, glycine, and 5-MTHF. In contrast to many inborn errors of metabolism, this disorder is potentially treatable by high-dose dietary supplementation of serine (200–600 mg/kg/day) and glycine (200 mg/kg/day).

Purine Biosynthesis Defects

Defects of purine biosynthesis have recently been described, with clinical presentation in the neonatal period involving adenylosuccinate lyase, or riboside transformylase enzyme deficiencies [Jurecka, 2009] (Figure 20-11). These infants are typically born uneventfully at term, and manifest a severe neonatal encephalopathy with hypotonia, seizures, and mildly dysmorphic facies. Neuroimaging initially may be normal, and over time discloses diffuse atrophy. The long-term course is characterized by persistent severe static encephalopathy with profound mental retardation, blindness due to optic atrophy, refractory epilepsy, and growth failure. The cardinal biochemical features include massive urinary excretion of the riboside metabolites 5-amino-4-imidazolecarboxamide ribosiduria (AICA) and succinyl-5-amino-4-imidazolecarboxamide ribosiduria (SAICA) in urine and CSF. These metabolites give a positive result on the Bratton–Marshall test, which screens for high concentrations of succinyl purines. Diagnosis is confirmed by high-resolution thin-layer chromatography analysis of urine for succinyl purines. In addition, affected infants may have disturbed glucose and lipid metabolism as a result of impaired hepatic gluconeogenesis, fatty acid, and cholesterol synthesis. Management is symptomatic and supportive, as there is no definitive or curative treatment.

L-Amino Acid Decarboxylase Deficiency

L-ADD is a defect of biogenic amine neurotransmitter metabolism, causing a combined deficiency of brain dopamine, serotonin, norepinephrine, and epinephrine [Swoboda et al., 2003] (Figure 20-12). Patients commonly present in the first weeks of life with a progressive disorder affecting multiple levels of the nervous system. Symptoms and signs include lethargy, hypotonia, suck/swallow dysfunction, and seizures, sometimes associated with hypoglycemia and acidosis. Autonomic dysfunction leads to ptosis, hypotension, gastric and intestinal dysmotility, and poor temperature regulation. With advancing age, a distinctive movement disorder appears, consisting of dystonia, athetosis, oculogyric crises, and nonepileptic myoclonus. Diagnosis rests on evaluation of CSF neurotransmitter profiles, which show increased levels of biogenic amine precursors L-DOPA and 5-hydroxytryptamine, and decreased levels of the neurotransmitter metabolites homovanillic acid (HVA) and 5-hydroxy-indole-acetic acid (5-HIAA). Similar profiles of neurotransmitter amino acids are measured in plasma and urine. A clue to this disorder would be the finding on a urine organic acid profile of elevated vanillactic acid (VLA), a breakdown product from an alternate degradative

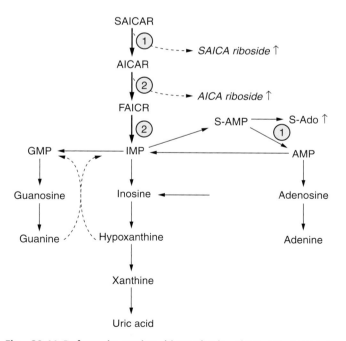

Fig. 20-11 Defects in purine biosynthesis. These are caused by deficiencies in: 1, adenylosuccinate lyase; 2, 5-amino-4-imidazolecarboxamide riboside transformylase. AICAR, 5-amino-4-imidazolecarboxamide riboside; AMP, adenosine monophosphate; FAICR, formyl-5-amino-4-imidazolecarboxamide riboside; GMP, guanosine monophosphate; IMP, inosine monophosphate; S-Ado, succinyl-adenosine; SAICAR, succinyl-5-amino-4-imidazolecarboxamide riboside.

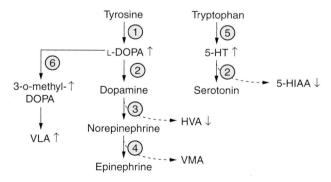

Fig. 20-12 Defects in biogenic amine neurotransmitter metabolism. 1, Tyrosine hydroxylase + BH_4. 2, Aromatic L-amino acid decarboxylase + B_6. 3, Dopamine β-hydroxylase. 4, Phenylethanolamine-N-methyl-transferase. 5, Tryptophan hydroxylase + BH_4. 6, Catechol-ortho-methyl transferase (COMT). Affected metabolites and co-factors include homovanillic acid (HVA), vanillylmandelic acid (VMA), vanillactic acid (VLA), 5-hydroxytryptamine (5-HT), 5-hydroxy-indole-acetic acid (5-HIAA), and tetrahydrobiopterin (BH_4).

pathway for L-DOPA. Management is symptomatic and supportive. Attempts to treat by replacing deficient neuroactive amines have been hindered by the lack of an effective targeted delivery system. Outcome is poor in most patients, who develop mixed severe motor and cognitive disability and chronic movement disorders that are refractory to symptomatic treatment.

Chronic Encephalopathies without Multi-Organ Involvement

Hyperphenylalaninemia

Hyperphenylalaninemia causes a chronic encephalopathy with neonatal onset due to one of several defects in the metabolism of phenylalanine. These include phenylalanine hydroxylase (PAH) deficiency, tetrahydrobiopterin (BH$_4$) synthesis deficiency, and GTP cyclohydrolase deficiency (Figure 20-13). In classical phenylketonuria (PKU) caused by PAH deficiency, plasma phenylalanine levels exceed 1000 μM, and PAH activity in liver biopsy is severely deficient (<1 percent of normal). In a milder form of the disease, designated non-PKU hyperphenylalaninemia, plasma phenylalanine levels are <1000μM and PAH activity is less severely deficient (5–30 percent of normal). Clinical symptoms in untreated classical PKU evolve with age to include irritability, hyperkinesis, acquired microcephaly, and severe cognitive deficiency. Infants with GTP cyclohydrolase deficiency have a neonatal-onset chronic encephalopathy with severe hypotonia, bulbar dysfunction, and seizures. Symptoms may evolve over time to a pattern of rigidity, hyperkinesia, and oculomotor abnormalities. Treatment with L-DOPA has been beneficial in some patients [Nardocci et al., 2003]. Diagnosis is made by newborn metabolic screening in most countries. After identification of newborns with hyperphenylalaninemia, further quantitation of plasma phenylalanine and tyrosine, and of urinary and CSF biopterin metabolites at baseline and after phenylalanine loading is necessary to distinguish classical PKU from BH$_4$ and GTP cyclohydrolase disorders. Treatment consists of the use of a semisynthetic diet low in phenylalanine that is carefully titrated according to plasma amino acid levels.

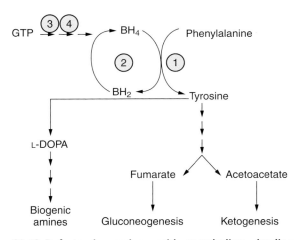

Fig. 20-13 Defects in amino acid metabolism leading to hyperphenylalaninemia. 1, Phenylalanine hydroxylase. 2, Dihydropterin reductase. 3, GTP cyclohydrolase. 4, 6-pyruvoyltetrabiopterin synthase. BH$_2$, dihydrobiopterin; BH$_4$, tetrahydrobiopterin.

Patients with BH$_4$ disorders require folate and BH$_4$ replacement. A subset of patients with milder forms of PKU, and some residual PAH enzyme activity, may respond to BH$_4$ supplementation. In these patients, BH$_4$ responsiveness is associated with missense mutations of PAH [Sarkissian et al., 2009]. A trial of L-DOPA and 5-hydroxytryptophan replacement to restore brain monoamine levels may prove helpful in some patients for symptoms of the dystonia and rigidity. Gene therapy and enzyme replacement therapy, while conceivable, are not yet clinically available, and are the focus of intensive experimental study.

Succinic Semialdehyde Dehydrogenase Deficiency

Succinic semialdehyde dehydrogenase deficiency is a defect of GABA degradation that results in elevated brain GABA levels (see Figure 20-9). The clinical presentation is variable. Some patients present in the neonatal period with a chronic encephalopathy and later symptoms of diffuse hypotonia, neurodevelopmental impairment, and epilepsy. An important clue to the diagnosis in this otherwise nonspecific clinical pattern is the finding on brain MRI of T2 hyperintensity in the globus pallidus. Diagnosis rests on the finding of elevated urinary 4-hydroxybutyric acid, and is associated with high levels of GABA in CSF and urine. Treatment with vigabatrin, a selective inhibitor of GABA transaminase, has been suggested, though results are mixed [Pearl et al., 2009].

Glutaric Aciduria

Glutaric aciduria (GA) is an autosomal-recessive defect in degradation of 2-keto-adipic acid, a metabolite in lysine and tryptophan degradation pathways. The neonatal and early infantile presentation occurs in type I GA, which is due to glutaryl-CoA dehydrogenase deficiency. Affected infants have a chronic progressive encephalopathy of neonatal or early infantile onset with macrocephaly, hypotonia evolving to rigidity and dystonia, developmental regression, and epilepsy. There may be episodic decompensations with vomiting, ketotic hypoglycemia, acidosis, hyperammonemia, hepatomegaly, and depressed consciousness triggered by intercurrent illness. MRI abnormalities are distinguished by the finding of selective frontotemporal atrophy, especially involving subcortical white matter, with prominent extra-axial CSF collections, and in some cases subdural hemorrhage. Metabolic crises are associated with acute bilaterally symmetric striatal necrosis in a large proportion of these patients, leading to permanent neuromotor disability. Diagnosis rests on the finding of elevated urinary glutaric acid and 3-OH-glutaric acid, and confirmed if needed in equivocal cases by enzyme assay in cultured fibroblasts. Treatment involves dietary protein restriction, in particular L-lysine and tryptophan, and supplementation with L-carnitine and riboflavin. Timely supportive care with intravenous fluids and dextrose during intercurrent illness can minimize the risk of metabolic decompensations and striatal necrosis. Type II GA involves multiple acyl-CoA dehydrogenase deficiencies, which lead to elevations of multiple organic acids (glutaric, lactic, ethylmalonic, butyric, isobutyric, 2-methyl-butyric, and isovaleric). The clinical picture in the neonatal-onset form of type II GA is typically severe, with nonketotic hypoglycemia, metabolic acidosis, vomiting, depressed consciousness, and multi-organ dysfunction.

Chronic Encephalopathies with Multi-Organ Involvement

Congenital Disorders of Glycosylation

Congenital disorders of glycosylation (CDG) comprise a group of genetically determined metabolic diseases characterized by abnormalities in protein glycosylation, which is a cotranslational modification step in the synthesis of most secretory and membrane-bound proteins (see Chapter 35). The nervous system is prominently affected, in association with abnormalities in multiple other organ systems, including liver, kidney, heart, and bone [Haeuptle and Hennet, 2009]. Two main subgroups have been described: type I, involving defects in assembly of the oligosaccharide precursors; and type II' involving processing of the oligosaccharide. CDG Ia is the most common and best described of these disorders, and has two types of presentations: a neurologic and a multisystem pattern. The neurologic presentation is one of chronic severe neurologic disability punctuated by episodic acute deterioration resembling stroke. There is usually prominent cerebellar dysfunction, with severe cerebellar atrophy detected on brain MRI. Usually normal at birth, some patients present with hypotonia and oculomotor abnormalities. Over time, patients display persisting ataxic hypotonic motor impairment and severe cognitive deficiency, retinopathy, epilepsy, acquired microcephaly, thromboembolic strokes, and weakness due to polyneuropathy. Associated non-neurologic findings include growth failure, protein-losing enteropathy, obstructive cardiomyopathy, nephrotic syndrome, deficient antithrombin III or protein C or S. Inverted nipples and subcutaneous fat pads are distinctive physical stigmata that may serve as clues to the disorder. Diagnosis is made by measuring transferrin isoelectric focusing using mass spectrometry, which may not become abnormal until the second or third week of life. Associated biochemical findings include elevated liver transaminases, low serum proteins, anemia, leukopenia, and low serum cholesterol. Treatment with high-dose mannose supplementation may ameliorate systemic symptoms, but the benefit for neurologic and neuromuscular manifestations is uncertain [Sparks and Krasnewich, 2009].

Peroxisomal Disorders

Peroxisomal disorders comprise a group of progressive neurologic diseases with variable age of onset and severity (see Chapter 38). Neonatal forms with prominent neurologic involvement include Zellweger's syndrome and neonatal adrenoleukodystrophy, both of which are inherited as autosomal-recessive disorders [Steinberg et al., 2006]. Infants with classic Zellweger's syndrome have multi-organ involvement with typical facial dysmorphic features, ocular anomalies (cataracts, glaucoma, pigmentary retinopathy), hepatic fibrosis, cystic kidney disease, subclinical adrenocortical insufficiency, and cardiac anomalies. Neurologic features include seizures, cranial nerve dysfunction, optic atrophy, and diffuse myopathic weakness. Survivors are multiply and profoundly handicapped. Neuroimaging and pathologic studies have revealed cortical and cerebellar migrational abnormalities and a central white matter demyelinating process. The pathogenesis relates to near-complete failure of peroxisomal function as a result of defective transport of proteins into the peroxisomal matrix. This results in defective oxidation and abnormal accumulation of very long chain fatty acids (VLCFAs), phytanic acid, pipecolic acids, and deficient synthesis of plasmalogens. The typical clinical features should suggest the diagnosis, which is supported by finding markedly elevated plasma VLCFA and decreased plasmalogen levels. Neonatal adrenoleukodystrophy resembles Zellweger's syndrome in many respects, but is less severe. There are no proven definitive treatments. Trials are under way to evaluate strategies aimed at modifying lipid and fatty acid composition of the diet.

Cholesterol Biosynthesis Defects (Smith–Lemli–Opitz Syndrome)

The molecular defect in Smith–Lemli–Opitz syndrome was recently characterized as a disorder of cholesterol biosynthesis. This condition presents in the neonatal period with a constellation of multiple congenital anomalies and a chronic static encephalopathy [Herman, 2003]. Infants present with microcephaly, abnormal facies with ptosis and micrognathia, genital anomalies, and growth retardation. Less frequent abnormalities include cataracts, congenital heart defects, digital anomalies, and cleft palate. Neurologic features include hypotonia, sensori-neural deafness, feeding and swallowing dysfunction, and severe cognitive deficiency. Cerebral malformations are common, including holoprosencephaly, agenesis of the corpus callosum, frontal hypoplasia, and cerebellar hypoplasia. Serum cholesterol is low in 90 percent of cases, but definitive diagnosis rests on finding elevated serum levels of 7- and 8-dehydrocholesterol measured by GC mass spectrometry. Treatment is supportive and symptomatic. Enteral supplements of cholesterol may mitigate some of the symptoms.

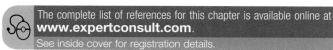

Overview of Disorders of Brain Development

William B. Dobyns, Renzo Guerrini, and A. James Barkovich

Introduction

This section of the book reviews a large and growing number of complex developmental disorders of the brain, often associated with malformations of the spinal cord and skull and recognizable on clinical examination or imaging studies, encompassing a field of knowledge that has expanded dramatically over the past several decades. But the field has not expanded in isolation. From our collective experience over several decades, we have observed that brain malformations:

- largely (but not exclusively) represent defects during the earliest stages of brain development, and thus reflect the underlying embryology and developmental genetics of the nervous system
- provide an important window into normal brain development and into the genetic regulation of brain development and function
- frequently co-occur with other diverse developmental brain disorders both with and without recognized structural defects
- are often associated with a wide spectrum of functional deficits, including intellectual disability, developmental language disorders, epilepsy, social and behavioral disabilities, numerous other specific learning disabilities, attention deficits, motor deficits connected with abnormal motor tone and posture or dyskinesias, and a host of problems associated with sleep, feeding, mood, and hormonal and autonomic dysregulation.

Thus, an understanding of brain malformations is important in assessing almost all types of neurological disorders in children. On a practical basis, we have separated brain malformations into disorders involving development of the neural tube (Chapter 22), forebrain (Chapter 23), and mid-hindbrain (Chapter 24); disorders of cortical development, separated into those of brain size (Chapter 25) and those of migration and later cortical development (Chapter 26); disorders predisposing to hydrocephalus (Chapter 27); and disorders of skull development (Chapter 28). We end with an overview of prenatal diagnosis for all brain malformations (Chapter 29). Here, we will address a few topics relevant to brain malformations generally, including epidemiology, classification, clinical recognition, relationship to other neurological disorders and selected environmental factors, and genetic counseling.

Epidemiology

The incidence of brain malformations has been estimated to be approximately 3.32 per 1000 and the prevalence approximately 2.21 per 1000 at age 14 years from studies of a 1-year birth cohort from northern Finland [Von Wendt and Rantakallio, 1986]. These are much higher rates than were recognized in the era before magnetic resonance imaging (MRI) and recent increases in surgical treatment of hydrocephalus and epilepsy [Kuzniecky et al., 1993; Massimi et al., 2009; Warkany et al., 1981]. Not surprisingly, the incidence is much higher (i.e., approximately 88 per 1000) in studies of children with cerebral palsy [Rankin et al., 2010]. This is an important point. To emphasize this, a boy was recently evaluated with apparent cerebral palsy attributed to prematurity at approximately 29 weeks' gestation. But his brain MRI revealed mild callosal- and cerebellar vermis hypoplasia, and chromosome microarray revealed a small deletion in 22q11.2, which implies either a genetic or a mixed pathogenesis.

Classification

While the chapters that follow review many different malformations, they are not complete, as the number of recognized malformations continues to grow steadily. Presenting these data is also complicated by the tendency for malformations to co-occur in some patients. For example, Figure 21-1 shows a striking example of a boy with malformations of the forebrain (agenesis of the corpus callosum), mid-hindbrain (severe cerebellar hypoplasia and mega-cisterna magna), brain size (megalencephaly), neuronal migration (periventricular nodular heterotopia), and cortical organization (polymicrogyria overlying the heterotopia).

From time to time, flexible classification schemes have been constructed for many of these malformations that primarily rely on traditional concepts such as embryology and anatomy, with a contribution from genetic discoveries. While recent discoveries are leading us to think more of genes and gene pathways than of embryology and anatomy, a more traditional classification scheme is presented in this and the following chapters. The most current outline for brainstem and cerebellar (mid-hindbrain) malformations is shown in Box 21-1, and an outline for cortical malformations in Box 21-2. Further details regarding most subgroups of

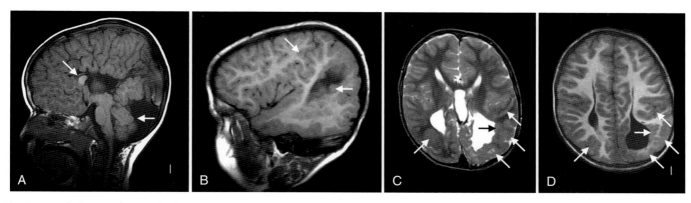

Fig. 21-1 Brain images from a single patient showing multiple malformations. A and **B,** T1-weighted sagittal images demonstrate severe callosal hypogenesis with a small anterior remnant (angled arrow in **A**), very small cerebellar vermis (horizontal arrow in **A**) in an enlarged posterior fossa, extended sylvian fissure with cortex connecting the perisylvian and superior parietal regions (angled arrow in **B**), and periventricular nodular heterotopia in the trigone (horizontal arrow in **B**). **C** and **D,** T2- and T1-weighted axial images show periventricular nodular heterotopia adjacent to the posterior portion of the lateral ventricles (horizontal arrows in **C** and **D**), and infolded gyri with mildly thick cortex overlying the heterotopia (angled arrows in **C** and **D**). *(Courtesy of WB Dobyns, research subject LR00-086.)*

Box 21-1 Classification Scheme for Mid-Hindbrain Malformations

I. Malformations Secondary to Early Anteroposterior and Dorsoventral Patterning Defects, or to Mis-Specification of Mid-Hindbrain Germinal Zones

A. Anteroposterior patterning defects
1. Gain, loss, or transformation of the diencephalon and midbrain
2. Gain, loss, or transformation of the midbrain and rhombomere 1
3. Gain, loss, or transformation of lower hindbrain structures

B. Dorsoventral patterning defects
1. Defects of alar and basal ventricular zones
2. Defects of alar ventricular zones only
3. Defects of basal ventricular zones only

II. Malformations Associated with Later Generalized Developmental Disorders that Significantly Affect the Brainstem and Cerebellum (and have Pathogenesis at Least Partly Understood)

A. Developmental encephalopathies associated with mid-hindbrain malformations

B. Mesenchymal-neuroepithelial signaling defects associated with mid-hindbrain malformations

C. Malformations of neuronal and glial proliferation that prominently affect the brainstem and cerebellum

D. Malformations of neuronal migration that prominently affect the brainstem and cerebellum
1. Lissencephaly with cerebellar hypoplasia
2. Neuronal heterotopia with prominent brainstem and cerebellar hypoplasia
3. Polymicrogyria with cerebellar hypoplasia

4. Malformations with basement membrane and neuronal migration deficits

E. Diffuse molar tooth-type dysplasias associated with defects in ciliary proteins
1. Syndromes affecting the brain with low-frequency involvement of the retina and kidney
2. Syndromes affecting the brain, eyes, kidneys, liver, and variable other systems

III. Localized Brain Malformations that Significantly Affect the Brainstem and Cerebellum (Pathogenesis Partly or Largely Understood; Includes Local Proliferation, Cell Specification, Migration, and Axonal Guidance)

A. Multiple levels of mid-hindbrain
B. Midbrain malformations
C. Malformations of rhombomere 1, including cerebellar malformations
D. Pons malformations
E. Medulla malformations

IV. Combined Hypoplasia and Atrophy in Putative Prenatal-Onset Degenerative Disorders

A. Pontocerebellar hypoplasia
B. Mid-hindbrain malformations with congenital disorders of glycosylation
C. Other metabolic disorders with cerebellar or brainstem hypoplasia or disruption
D. Cerebellar hemisphere hypoplasia (rare, more commonly acquired than genetic, often associated with clefts or cortical malformation)

---

malformations and the basis for the classification are given in the primary references [Barkovich et al., 2005, 2009]. These schemes were constructed relying on – in decreasing order of priority – the underlying genetic basis when known, the relevant embryology, brain imaging features, and miscellaneous other clinical features.

Brain Imaging Recognition

The improved quality of brain imaging studies, especially advances in MRI technology, has led directly to increased recognition and more accurate classification of brain malformations. Still, several recurrent types of classification errors continue to occur, based

Box 21-2 Classification Scheme for Malformations of Cortical Development

I. Malformations Due to Abnormal Neuronal and Glial Proliferation or Apoptosis

A. Decreased proliferation or increased apoptosis, or increased proliferation or decreased apoptosis
1. Microcephaly with normal to thin cortex
2. Microlissencephaly (extreme microcephaly with thick cortex)
3. Microcephaly with polymicrogyria
4. Megalencephaly

B. Abnormal proliferation (abnormal cell types)
1. Non-neoplastic
   a. Cortical hamartomas of tuberous sclerosis
   b. Cortical dysplasia with balloon cells
   c. Hemimegalencephaly
2. Neoplastic (with disordered cortex)
   a. Dysembryoplastic neuroepithelial tumor
   b. Ganglioglioma
   c. Gangliocytoma

II. Malformations Due to Abnormal Neuronal Migration

A. Lissencephaly and subcortical band heterotopia spectrum
B. Cobblestone malformation syndromes
C. Heterotopia

1. Subependymal (periventricular)
2. Subcortical (other than band heterotopia)
3. Marginal glioneuronal

III. Malformations Due to Abnormal Cortical Organization (Including Late Neuronal Migration)

A. Polymicrogyria and schizencephaly
1. Bilateral polymicrogyria syndromes
2. Schizencephaly (polymicrogyria with clefts)
3. Polymicrogyria as part of multiple congenital anomaly/mental retardation syndromes
B. Cortical dysplasia without balloon cells
C. Microdysgenesis

IV. Malformations of Cortical Development, Not Otherwise Classified

A. Malformations secondary to inborn errors of metabolism
1. Mitochondrial and pyruvate metabolic disorders
2. Peroxisomal disorders
B. Other unclassified malformations
1. Sublobar dysplasia
2. Others

---

on studies sent to the authors for review. First, pachygyria appears to be the best known of the severe cortical malformations, and accordingly all types of severe cortical malformations are often interpreted as "pachygyria." The prime examples of malformations mistaken for pachygyria include severe congenital microcephaly (but here the cortex is thin rather than thick), polymicrogyria, and cobblestone malformations (for these, the cortex is moderately thick but the surface and cortex–white matter interface are irregular rather than smooth). This unfortunately often leads to testing of the "lissencephaly" genes in patients with these other cortical malformations, with uniformly negative results. Second, a thin corpus callosum may result from reduced volume of white matter due to abnormal development of white matter, progressive white-matter dysgenesis, or white-matter injury. However, this appearance is sometimes interpreted as agenesis of the corpus callosum. Next, diverse causes of cerebellar hypoplasia are often interpreted as Dandy–Walker malformation (when associated with a large posterior fossa and an enlarged fourth ventricle) or the so-called "Dandy–Walker variant" (equated with isolated cerebellar vermis hypoplasia). The latter is so overused and misapplied that the authors have abandoned the term. Finally, enlarged fluid collections below and especially behind the cerebellum are interpreted as arachnoid cysts or as "mega-cisterna magna," considering the latter a nonpathogenic variant. In the authors' experience, mega-cisterna magna with fluid both below and behind the cerebellum sometimes represents a developmental disorder that belongs in the Dandy–Walker spectrum [Aldinger et al., 2009], and may be incorrectly interpreted as an arachnoid cyst.

Relationships to Other Neurologic Disorders

The close connection between brain malformations and other classes of developmental disorders is conceptually important. A few examples include agenesis of the corpus callosum

associated with nonketotic hyperglycinemia [Dobyns, 1989], cerebellar vermis hypoplasia or heterotopia with multiple acyl-CoA dehydrogenase deficiency, also known as glutaric aciduria type 2 [Bohm et al., 1982; Lehnert et al., 1982], cobblestone malformations and cerebellar hypoplasia with congenital disorders of glycosylation [Aronica et al., 2005; Morava et al., 2009; Van Maldergem et al., 2008], pachygyria variants with severe peroxisomal disorders such as Zellweger's syndrome [Barkovich and Peck, 1997; Van Der Knaap and Valk, 1991], and cerebellar hypoplasia or agenesis of the corpus callosum with either autism or infantile spasms [Chugani and Conti, 1996; Courchesne et al., 1988; Kato et al., 2004; Manes et al., 1999; Schiffmann et al., 1993]. Further, most malformations of cortical development are associated with epilepsy, which may be severe [Guerrini, 2005; Leventer et al., 2008]. Observations in these and many other disorders collectively lead us to hypothesize that brain malformations represent the most severe expression or "tip of the iceberg" of a host of developmental brain disorders. Of course, this is much more than a hypothesis, as it has already been proven for disorders reviewed in chapters throughout this text.

Relationship to Environmental Factors

The genetic basis for many brain malformations has been known for years, and new genes are constantly being discovered. The question arises: are all brain malformations genetic? While easy to overlook, substantial data exist to support environmental (extrinsic) causes for several brain malformations. Both microcephaly and hydrocephalus can result from numerous prenatal and early-life diseases, such as intraventricular hemorrhage in premature infants, other causes of intracranial bleeding, hypoxic-ischemic injury, central nervous system infections, and a host of other disorders reviewed throughout this text. Holoprosencephaly has been associated with pregestational diabetes and with structural analogs of cholesterol that interfere with cholesterol metabolism or uptake in humans and animals [Edison and Muenke, 2004; Haas and Muenke, 2010; Johnson and Rasmussen, 2010; Lipinski et al., 2010]. Periventricular nodular heterotopia has been seen in mice and rats following prenatal exposure to high-dose ionizing radiation, and possibly in humans as well [Barth, 1987; Dekaban, 1968; Ferrer et al., 1993]. Schizencephaly and polymicrogyria have been associated with second trimester (13–21 weeks' gestation) prenatal vascular disruption and with intrauterine cytomegalovirus infections [Barth and Van Der Harten, 1985; Curry et al., 2005; Marques Dias et al., 1984; Mcbride and Kemper, 1982; Pati and Helmbrecht, 1994; Sherer and Salafia, 1996; Suchet, 1994].

Genetic Counseling

While the genetic basis for more and more brain malformations and malformation syndromes is being uncovered, few studies examining the overall contribution of genetic disorders to brain malformations have been reported. Accordingly, only partial and selective information about the genetic recurrence risk for different brain malformations is available. While the authors have conducted only a few formal studies of recurrence risk, we collectively have several decades of experience with these disorders and can provide some general guidelines, which are listed in Table 21-1.

For example, the recurrence risk for holoprosencephaly reported in the literature is approximately 6 percent [Roach et al., 1975]. This report dates from more than 35 years ago, and we are now aware of frequent mild expression or "formes frustes" of this malformation, and accordingly we suggest using a higher recurrence risk of 13 percent for isolated holoprosencephaly without known chromosome imbalances [Mercier et al., 2010]. For several malformations such as agenesis of the corpus callosum and polymicrogyria, single-gene inheritance has been reported, but only rarely, and no formal studies are available. We therefore suggest a "generally low" risk, and counseling for some uncertainty, given that the experience is limited and exceptions occur. For some other malformations, such as rhombencephalosynapsis, hemimegalencephaly, and focal cortical dysplasia, no examples of familial recurrence have

Table 21-1 Probable Genetic Recurrence Risks for Major Classes of Brain Malformations

Malformation Groups	Pattern of Inheritance					Recurrence Risk/Comments
	Sp	**Ch**	**AD**	**AR**	**XL**	
FOREBRAIN MALFORMATIONS						
Holoprosencephaly	++	++	++	±	±	Risk is variable, may be high
Agenesis of corpus callosum	++	++	±	±	++	Risk is generally low
Septo-optic dysplasia	++	–	–	±	–	Risk is very low, has occurred
MID-HINDBRAIN MALFORMATIONS						
Pontocerebellar hypoplasia	–	–	–	++	–	Risk is 25%, all forms are AR
Cerebellar hypoplasia (diffuse)	++	++	±	++	+	Risk is variable, need diagnosis
Cerebellar hypoplasia (vermis)	++	++	±	+	+	Risk is variable, need diagnosis
Dandy–Walker malformation	++	+	±	±	±	Risk is very low, has occurred
Molar tooth malformation	–	–	–	++	–	Risk is 25%, all forms are AR
Rhombencephalosynapsis	++	–	–	–	–	No recurrences reported
CORTICAL MALFORMATIONS						
Microcephaly, congenital	–	–	–	++	–	Risk is 25%, most forms are AR
Microcephaly, postnatal	++	++	+	+	+	Risk is variable, includes XL
Megalencephaly	++	–	–	–	–	Risk is low (except for PTEN)
Lissencephaly and SBH	++	++	–	+	++	Risk is variable, includes XL
Cobblestone malformation	–	–	–	++	–	Risk is 25%, all forms are AR
Heterotopia, periventricular	++	++	+	±	++	Risk is variable, may be high
Heterotopia, subcortical	++	–	–	–	–	No recurrences reported
Polymicrogyria, perisylvian	++	++	±	±	+	Risk is low, XL may be important
Polymicrogyria, other forms						Risk is generally low
Schizencephaly	++	–	–	±	–	Risk is very low, has occurred
Focal cortical dysplasias	++	–	–	–	–	No recurrences reported
Hemimegalencephaly	++	–	–	–	–	No recurrences reported

AD, autosomal-dominant; AR, autosomal-recessive; Ch, chromosome imbalance; PTEN, phosphatase and tensin homolog, Risk, recurrence risk for siblings or other relatives; SBH, subcortical band heteropia, Sp, sporadic occurrence; XL, X-linked; +, occasionally observed; ++, commonly observed; ±, rarely observed and often poorly documented; –, never observed.

ever been reported, despite clinical recognition for decades. We therefore suggest that the recurrence risk is very low. The most difficult malformations are those with significantly different recurrence risks for different subtypes and syndromes, such as diffuse and vermis-predominant cerebellar hypoplasia. These estimates are largely anecdotal in origin, so treating physicians and genetic counselors are encouraged to review information on the specific disorder at hand when counseling families.

The complete list of references for this chapter is available online at **www.expertconsult.com**.
See inside cover for registration details.

Disorders of Neural Tube Development

Nalin Gupta and M. Elizabeth Ross

Introduction

Neural tube defects (NTDs) are among the most frequently encountered congenital anomalies involving the central nervous system (CNS). Indeed, NTDs are second only to congenital heart defects as the most common serious birth defect, affecting between 0.5 and 10 per 1000 live births, depending on the population studied [Gelineau-van Waes and Finnell, 2001]. Rostral NTDs, such as anencephaly, that lead to an absent cranial vault and exposed brain are uniformly fatal. In contrast, most children born with posterior NTDs confined to the spinal column will survive with varying degrees of functional disability and shortened life span. NTDs may be classified in a number of ways but the most useful strategy is to assign the observed defect according to the suspected developmental abnormality. This allows a better appreciation of the severity of the CNS anomaly, which often correlates with the clinical picture and expected outcome. In this chapter, the term NTD will be used to encompass all defects that involve neural tube formation and differentiation. NTDs are also referred to as spinal or cranial dysraphism, depending on the level of the defect. Spina bifida formally refers to all types of spinal dysraphism, though it is often used synonymously with myelomeningocele (MMC), which is a severe and common form of spinal dysraphism in which meninges, along with spinal cord or axons, protrude outside of the vertebral column.

NTDs have been the subject of intensive research for decades and are considered to result from complex interactions of genes and environmental conditions. Indeed, over 200 gene defects in the mouse have now been associated with failed neural tube closure, and a number of these genes are likely to be involved in human NTDs as well [Harris and Juriloff, 2007; Gray and Ross, 2009; Harris, 2009]. This class of neurodevelopmental defect is particularly important to understand because a significant proportion of NTDs may be preventable with measures like prenatal maternal folic acid (FA) supplementation [MRC, 1991], by avoiding prenatal exposure to known teratogens like retinoids, and because medications often used in the treatment of epilepsy and neuropsychiatric disorders can increase the risk to pregnancies conceived while taking the drug [Ross, 2010]. This chapter will discuss the pathogenesis, risk factors, complications, and management of NTDs in children.

Anatomy and Embryology

Formation of the Neural Tube

Among the earliest morphological specializations in the embryo is the formation of the neural placode, followed by neural plate and then neural tube [Sadler, 2005]. At the end of the second gestational week, the human embryo is a bilaminar disc of epiblast cells overlying hypoblast cells [Sadler, 2004]. At the beginning of the third week, the disc develops a midline groove, the primitive streak, in the caudal third (Figure 22-1A), which marks the initiation of gastrulation and the formation of three germ layers – ectoderm (giving rise to skin and the nervous system), mesoderm (providing inductive signals to ectoderm and contributing to morphogenesis), and endoderm (giving rise to viscera). The primitive node at the cranial end of the streak contains cells that act to organize the embryonic axes (see Figure 22-1). At the same stage, thickening of the rostral ectoderm by the apical–basal elongation of cells into a pseudostratified columnar shape produces the neural placode that marks the initiation of neurulation (see Figure 22-1B) [Schoenwolf and Powers, 1987; Schoenwolf, 1988; Colas and Schoenwolf, 2001]. Cells migrating through the primitive streak and node displace the hypoblast cells to form endoderm and subsequently middle layer mesoderm. Cells that migrate through the node in the midline form the prechordal plate and notochord (Figure 22-2), which are important for induction of the ventral CNS structures, starting with the neural plate. The remainder of ectoderm surrounding the neural plate becomes epidermis.

Neural plate formation is actually a default state of the ectoderm, and formation of epidermis involves the inhibition of bone morphogenetic protein (BMP) and the wingless (Wnt) signaling pathway [Harland, 2000]. As the plate begins to emerge, morphogenesis, or shape changes, involving groups of cells in the neuroepithelium and surround, is essential to formation of brain and spinal cord (Figure 22-3). By 20 days of gestation, the neural plate appears indented in the midline, forming a groove or medial hinge region flanked by ridges – the neural folds. These folds elevate from the plane of the neural plate through the combined influences of proliferation of neural cells and underlying mesenchymal cells [Greene and Copp, 2009]. Bending inward of the neural folds at the dorsolateral hinge points occurs through morphological shape

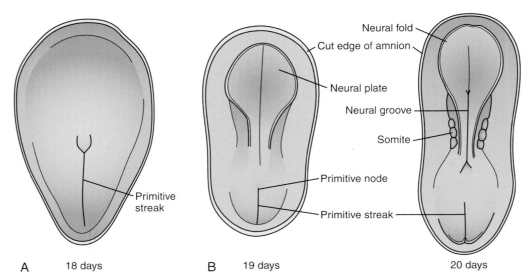

Fig. 22-1 Early stages of gastrulation and neurulation in human embryogenesis: views of the dorsal surface. A, The primitive streak emerges as a groove at the caudal pole of the embryo, with the primitive node at the cranial pole. Epiblast cells moving through the primitive streak and node form the three germ layers – ectoderm, mesoderm, and endoderm. **B,** A thickening of the ectoderm forms the neural plate, initiated at the cranial pole, while the primitive streak at the caudal end initiates gastrulation. By 20 days' gestation, the neural folds have elevated from the neural plate, and tips of the folds are closing. Somites, comprised of mesoderm cells, support the elevation of the neural folds and are the precursors of vertebrae. *(Adapted from Sadler TW. Embryology of neural tube development. Am J Med Genet C Semin Med Genet 2005;135C:2–8.)*

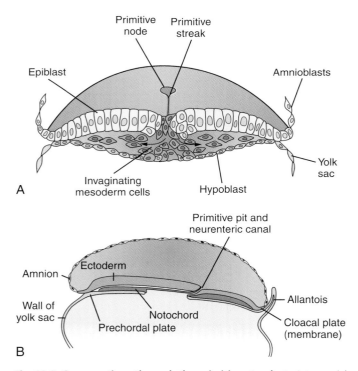

Fig. 22-2 Cross-sections through the primitive streak. A, A transaxial view shows movement of epiblast cells through the streak to form a mesodermal layer between the original epiblast (becoming the ectodermal layer) and hypoblast cells (becoming the endoderm). **B,** A midsagittal section shows the disc-shaped embryo suspended between yolk sac and amniotic cavities. The notochord and prechordal plate have formed by the displacement of cells through the primitive node. *(Adapted from Sadler TW. Embryology of neural tube development. Am J Med Genet C Semin Med Genet 2005;135C:2–8.)*

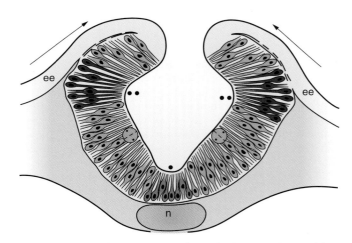

Fig. 22-3 A coronal cross-section through the cranial neural folds as they come together in the midline. The pseudostratified appearance of the neuroepithelium is due to the translocation of cell nuclei (interkinetic nuclear migration) during cell-cycle progression, in which M-phase nuclei are at the apical (central) surface and S-phase nuclei are at the basal (outer) surface. Bending of the folds takes place at a midline, median hinge point (black dot) and at two dorsolateral hinge points (double black dots). Bending of the dorsolateral hinge points is facilitated by cell-shape changes, in which the apical poles are narrowed by actin-myosin-dependent constriction and basal expansion of cells, more of which contain translocated, S-phase nuclei. Closure is also facilitated by the movement toward the midline of surface ectoderm (ee) cells. n, notochord. *(Adapted from Sadler TW. Embryology of neural tube development. Am J Med Genet C Semin Med Genet 2005;135C:2–8.)*

changes of the neural cells, which become radially elongated, while their apical (luminal) poles constrict, through a combination of cell-cycle regulation that moves nuclei to the basal end of cells in the hinge region, and actin-myosin contraction at the apical poles of cells in the hinge region, to bring the tips of the neural folds into apposition [Greene and Copp, 2009]. In the head region, proliferation and movement of epidermis and mesenchyme cells also help to push the neural folds into apposition, while at spinal levels, neighboring mesenchyme may be less critical to neural tube closure [Greene and Copp, 2009]. In addition to cell elongation and proliferation, the shape changes in the neural plate are affected by cell motility in the form of convergent extension, in which laterally placed cells move to the midline and migrate rostrocaudally in a process that is mediated by noncanonical Wnt signaling (Figure 22-4) [Wallingford and Harland, 2001; Wallingford et al., 2002]. Thus, once elevation and bending of the neural folds occur, the lateral margins or tips of the folds join and then fuse in the midline to become the neural tube.

In order to achieve this rising and bending inward of the neural folds, the cells of the neural plate must proliferate in an ordered manner, called interkinetic nuclear migration of progenitors, forming a pseudostratified epithelium in which S-phase occurs at the basal (outer) surface of the neural folds, mitosis (M-phase) occurs at the apical (central or luminal) surface, and G1 and G2 phase nuclei are positioned at intermediate locations. In addition, in the process of convergent extension, cells move medially and through the medial hinge region to migrate rostrocaudally and elongate the neuraxis, narrowing the ventral floorplate (see Figure 22-3). If the floorplate is too wide or the neural folds fail to elevate and bend, the folds will not appose and NTDs will ensue (see Figure 22-4). The broadening of the ventral floorplate and shortening of the rostrocaudal axis reflect impaired convergent extension; they are demonstrated in the looptail mouse mutant, which bears a mutation in the *Van Gogh-like 2* (*Vangl2*) gene that functions in the planar cell polarity

(PCP) pathway [Ybot-Gonzalez et al., 2007]. When apposition is successful, midline fusion of the neural folds, a process known as neurulation, occurs first at primary closure points, and extends by adding multiple closure points like the teeth of a zipper rostrally and caudally from each node to complete neural tube closure [Pyrgaki et al., 2010]. In the mouse, there are typically three closure points:

1. hindbrain level
2. midbrain
3. frontal neuropore.

In humans, there are two, points 1 and 3, which are located at the hindbrain–spine junction and the frontal neuropore, respectively. The anterior neuropore, the region that will eventually give rise to the brain, closes approximately by day 26 of human gestation. The posterior neuropore, the region that will give rise to the caudal spinal column, closes approximately at day 29 of human embryogenesis. After the neural tube closes, it separates from the overlying ectoderm in a process termed dysjunction. Cells of the somitic mesoderm invade the space between the ectoderm and neural tube to form somites that eventually give rise to the posterior elements of the vertebral bodies and the paraspinal muscles. Specific neural cells at the tips of the folds are excluded from the neural tube; these cells form the neural crest, which is the anlage of the peripheral and autonomic nervous systems, and which also contributes the meninges, and portions of the skull and face.

Molecular Patterning of the Neural Tube

Work on frog, mouse, and zebrafish species has identified a host of factors that are necessary for proper neurulation and neural tube closure. These data have direct implications for human disease because vertebrates display a conserved body plan. A key observation was that a small fragment of non-neural tissue (mesoderm), when transplanted, was capable of duplicating the neural tube, indicating that secreted

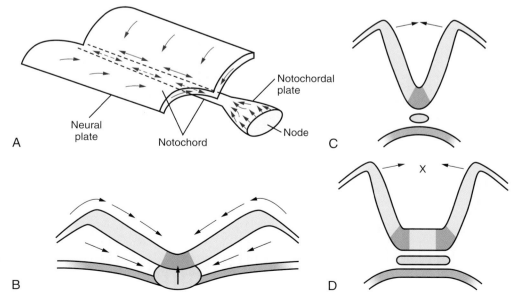

Fig. 22-4 Cell movements affecting planar cell polarity (PCP) signaling in the early developing nervous system. A and **B,** Schematics showing cell movement toward the midline into the neural groove and longitudinally to narrow and elongate the embryo. **C,** This movement serves to narrow the ventral floorplate (red), facilitating median hinge-point bending and apposition of the neural folds. **D,** When PCP signaling is impaired, as in the looptail mouse-bearing mutation in *Vangl2*, the floorplate is wider (intervening cells remain in the floorplate region), which prevents the folds from meeting in the midline. (**A,** *From Ybot-Gonzalez P et al. Convergent extension, planar-cell-polarity signalling and initiation of mouse neural tube closure. Development 2007;134:789–799.* **B–D,** *From Copp AJ et al. Trends Neurosci: Dishevelled: Linking convergent extension with neural tube closure, 2003;26:453–455.*)

Neural plate

Notochordal plate

Node

Notochord

X

factors from mesoderm are sufficient to induce neurulation. Thus, the factors necessary for neurulation are intrinsic to and secreted from this mesodermal region. These factors include chordin, noggin, sonic hedgehog (SHH), and several others, which are both necessary and sufficient for proper neurulation and control of the amount and fate of the neuroectoderm (reviewed in De Robertis and Kuroda [2004]). In mammals, two distinct groups of non-neural cells appear to provide these early patterning signals: axial mesodermal cells of the notochord, which underlie the midline of the neural plate, and the cells of the epidermal ectoderm, which flank its lateral edges. The notochord is the source of ventralizing inductive factor, and the epidermal ectoderm is the source of dorsalizing factors. Opposing actions of these two signals appear to be critical in establishing the identity and pattern of cell types generated along the dorsal–ventral axis of the neural tube.

The nervous system is patterned along the anteroposterior, dorsal–ventral, and right–left axes in response to the expression of intrinsic patterning genes and critical embryonic signaling pathways involving secreted factors and cell–cell interactions [Altmann and Brivanlou, 2001]. The homeotic, Hox, transcription factor genes provide a positional "address" or identity of spinal cord and hindbrain neurons [Carpenter, 2002]. Fate determination along the dorsal–ventral axis also requires the action of three opposing signaling pathways:

1. sonic hedgehog (SHH), produced ventrally by the notochord
2. Wnt, in which pathway different Wnts define dorsoventral regions of neural tube
3. bone morphogenetic protein (BMP), in which pathway different BMPs are secreted by dorsally placed cells from the boundary of the neural and non-neural ectoderm [Takahashi and Liu, 2006; Ulloa and Marti, 2010].

In this model, SHH released by the notochord diffuses toward the ventral neural tube and induces the differentiation of the floor plate. The floor plate then becomes capable of producing additional SHH, which diffuses and establishes a gradient along the dorsal–ventral axis of the neural tube. Differentiation of cells in the dorsal half of the neural tube depends on signals such as BMPs provided by the lateral epidermal ectoderm. BMP4 and BMP7, released by the epidermal ectoderm, diffuse toward the dorsal neural tube and induce the differentiation of the roof plate. The roof plate then becomes capable of producing additional BMPs, which diffuse and establish a gradient along the ventral–dorsal axis of the neural tube. Regions of the spinal cord that are exposed to the highest concentrations of SHH and lowest concentrations of BMPs give rise to cells of ventral fate, including motor neurons, whereas cells exposed to lowest SHH and highest BMP concentrations give rise to cells of dorsal fate, such as commissural projection neurons [Cowan et al., 1997]. Fibroblast growth factor (FGF), NOTCH, and retinoic acid (RA) signaling is also known to act in dorsal–ventral patterning and neural fate determination, though their roles are less well understood. Rostrocaudally, the neural tube is regionalized into four major divisions: forebrain, midbrain, hindbrain, and spinal cord. Actions of FGF, Wnt and RA pathways confer a caudal identity [Diez del Corral and Storey, 2004; Aboitiz and Montiel, 2007] and also impact telencephalic patterning [Takahashi and Liu, 2006]. Homeotic Hox and Engrailed

family transcription factors are particularly important for establishing segmental identities and morphogenetic features of hindbrain [Barrow et al., 2000; Cheng et al., 2010] (see also Chapter 24).

Epidemiology and Pathogenesis

Incidence

Among live births, females are more affected by NTDs than males by 2:1 [Elwood and Little, 1992; Little and Elwood, 1992; Shaw et al., 1994]. Additionally, the prevalence of NTDs varies across time, by region, and by ethnicity, and approximates 0.5 cases per 1000 in the United States but 10 per 1000 in parts of China and India [Northrup and Volcik, 2000; Gelineau-van Waes and Finnell, 2001]. These numbers do not reflect the decrease in incidence that has followed FA supplementation – with current estimates of 0.37 cases per 1000 reported in the US [Mills and Signore, 2004] – or the availability of prenatal diagnosis and the elective termination of some pregnancies with affected fetuses. The geographic and population variabilities in NTD rates are in keeping with the complexities of the etiology of neural tube closure failure, which involve both genetic and environmental factors [Janerich and Piper, 1978; Ross, 2010].

Over 30 years of clinical and basic science investigation are behind the insight that NTDs in humans are not caused by a single-gene defect but instead arise from the interplay of multiple genes, as well as gene–environment interactions [Holmes et al., 1976]. The twin concordance rate among same-sex twins (presumed monozygotic) is significantly increased (to 6.8 percent), supporting a genetic contribution [Janerich and Piper, 1978]. Furthermore, compared to an incidence in the general population of 1 per 1000, the risk of NTD recurrence in a family with one affected child increases to 1.8 per 100, but does not approach the 1 in 4 recurrence risk of an autosomal-recessive mutation with complete penetrance. Studies have documented the higher occurrence rate of NTDs in females compared to males, and the significantly higher incidence of consanguinity among parents of infants with NTDs [Elwood and Little, 1992; Shaw et al., 1994]. These and many other studies indicate prominent genetic, heritable contributions to failed neural tube closure that may well require the concerted action of multiple gene polymorphisms to manifest the disorder.

Complex Genetic Contributions

The complexity of the genetic underpinnings of neurulation is reflected in the NTD-prone mouse lines, for which over 200 mutations have been associated with failure of neural tube closure [Harris and Juriloff, 2007; Harris, 2009]. Despite this wealth of information, there is no single-gene polymorphism in the human homologs of these mouse genes that confers a robust, broadly reproducible enhanced risk of developing an NTD [Greene et al., 2009; Ross, 2010]. This has led to the supposition that either neurulation in the mouse is significantly different from that in humans, despite the similarities in morphogenesis and cell behaviors, or the genesis of NTDs requires the compounding of multiple gene polymorphisms. Supporting this latter premise, there are a number of examples in which modifier loci have been detected that increase the penetrance of NTD in mutant mouse models. A classic example is found the curly tail (ct) mouse, in which spina bifida is associated with a primary risk gene and at least three distinct modifier loci [Neumann et al., 1994]. The hypomorphic, partial loss-of-function mutation most responsible for NTDs in ct/ct mouse embryos occurs in a transcription factor called Grainy-head-like 3 (Grhl3). Another mutant with demonstrated multiple gene interactions is the SELHBc mouse, for which four loci have been mapped that conspire to result in exencephaly [Harris and Juriloff, 2007]. There are also examples of digenic mutations, or mutations in two genes, that must occur together to produce NTD in the mouse [Harris and Juriloff, 2007]. These digenic mutations in compound heterozygous mice affect processes from cell polarity (Cobl/Vangl2, Dvl1/Dvl2, Fzd3/Fzd6, Vangl2/Celsr1, Vangl2/Scrb, Vangl2/Ptk7), to actin cytoskeletal regulation (Enah/Vasp, Enah/Pfn1), to cell–cell adhesion (Gja1/Gja5, Itga1/Itga6), intracellular protein transport (Snx1/Snx2), intracellular signaling (Jnk1/Jnk2, Prkaca/Prkacb), or transcription regulation (Msx1/Msx2, Rara/Rarg). Genetic interactions that increase NTD risk certainly do occur in mice and can be expected to occur in humans as well [Ross, 2010].

The several hundred genes that have been associated with NTDs in mouse models are beginning to provide insights into molecular networks that are critically important for neurulation and may become clinically useful [Ross, in press]. For example, just as mutation in *Vangl2* renders the looptail mouse prone to NTD, polymorphisms in human *Vangl1* [Kibar et al., 2007] and *Vangl2* [Lei et al., 2010] have recently been implicated in NTD patients. However, evidence that these single nucleotide polymorphisms (SNPs) can occur in unaffected individuals as well suggests that the picture is too incomplete at present to permit using these SNPs for risk assessment. The context of the SNP or genetic background and environmental factors must be taken into consideration. Toward establishing this capability, pathway relationships associated with NTDs are emerging that include PCP signaling pathways encompassing Wnt and SHH pathways, chromatin remodeling and DNA methylation pathways, cell-cycle regulation, apoptosis, and cytoskeletal regulation, as well as transcription factors [Harris and Juriloff, 2007; Harris, 2009; Ross, 2010]. The complexity of the genetic underpinnings of NTD indicates that meeting the challenge for determining individual risk – and the optimal preventative therapy – will require evaluation of multiple genes (in signaling, metabolic, and transcriptional pathways) in a single person to detect compounding effects of gene polymorphisms that alone might not be significant [Greene et al., 2009; Ross, 2010]. Advanced technologies for high-throughput genomic DNA sequencing and analysis, and detection of the epigenome and perhaps the microbiome, as well as untargeted metabolomic screening, will all play a role in the clinical evaluation of individual patient assessments of NTD risk and prevention.

Gene–Environment Interactions Influencing Neural Tube Defects

Environmental influences contributing to NTDs have long been recognized [Janerich and Piper, 1978; Zhu et al., 2009]. The variables that have been implicated as risk factors for nonsyndromic forms of spina bifida are listed in Table 22-1. Risk factors include maternal diabetes, in which both hyperglycemia

Table 22-1 Risk Factors for Spina Bifida

Risk Factor	Relative Risk (-Fold Increase)
ESTABLISHED RISK FACTORS	
History of previous affected pregnancy with same partner	30
Inadequate maternal intake of folic acid	2–8
Pregestational maternal diabetes	2–10
Valproic acid and carbamazepine	10–20
SUSPECTED RISK FACTORS	
Maternal vitamin B$_{12}$ status	3
Maternal obesity	1.5–3.5
Maternal hyperthermia	2
Maternal diarrhea	3–4
Gestational diabetes	NE
Fumonisins	NE
Paternal exposure to Agent Orange	NE
Chlorination disinfection byproducts in drinking water	NE
Electromagnetic fields	NE
Hazardous waste sites	NE
Pesticides	NE

NE, not established.
(From Mitchell LE et al. Spina bifida. Lancet 2004;364:1885–1895.)

and associated hyperinsulinemia increase NTD risk [Eriksson et al., 2003]. Maternal obesity and pre-pregnancy weight gain are also associated with increased NTD risk [Werler et al., 1996; Hendricks et al., 2001]. Moreover, maternal periconceptional elevations in simple sugars that raise the glycemic index have been associated with increased NTD risk, even among nondiabetic women [Shaw et al., 2003]. In animal models, exposing rat embryos to a hyperglycemic environment induces dysmorphisms, accompanied by increases in biomarkers of oxidative stress and inositol depletion [Wentzel et al., 2001].

Gene–Diet Interactions in Neural Tube Defects: Role of Metabolism of Folic Acid and Other Nutrients

The important role of the folate pathway in the pathogenesis of NTDs has steadily gained acceptance since the landmark clinical investigations of Smithells and colleagues in the early 1980s prompted a large randomized trial of prenatal FA supplementation for women with previous NTD-affected pregnancies [Smithells et al., 1976; Smithells et al., 1983; MRC, 1991; Czeizel and Dudas, 1992]. Studies in the United Kingdom, later corroborated in Eastern Europe and elsewhere, indicated that the prevalence of NTDs could be reduced by 70 percent or more by prenatal supplementation with FA, even in the absence of maternal folate deficiency [MRC, 1991; Czeizel and Dudas, 1992]. However, some populations demonstrated only a small or no significant reduction in NTD rates with prenatal FA supplementation [Shaw et al., 1995], suggesting that differences in genetic background, diet, or other environmental exposures could impact the efficacy of folate supplementation. Inadequate intake of natural folate before and during early pregnancy is associated with a 2- to 8-fold increased risk of MMC and anencephaly, as indicated by several series of case-controlled, randomized clinical trials and community-based interventions [Wald, 1993]. Moreover, the risk of having a child affected by an NTD is indirectly related to both maternal folate intake and maternal folate intracellular level [Daly et al., 1995; Wald et al., 2001; Moore et al., 2003].

The mechanism underlying the association between NTDs and folate has not been established [Blom et al., 2006]. In view of the extraordinary variety of genes and molecular pathways contributing to NTD formation, perhaps the success of FA supplementation is due to the many biological functions to which folate metabolism contributes [Beaudin and Stover, 2009; Ross, 2010]. The exchange of single carbon units takes place in part in mitochondria, where serine cleavage generates glycine and formate, and glycine cleavage enzymes also generate formate that is transported to the cytoplasm. In the cytoplasm, formate enters the folate pathway for one-carbon metabolism (OCM) as formyl and then methenyl and methylene groups, added to or donated by dihydrofolates and tetrahydrofolates [Beaudin and Stover, 2007, 2009]. In the cytoplasm, the FA metabolic pathway is needed for physiological processes ranging from nucleotide biosynthesis, crucial for proliferation, to generation of pterin coactors impacting biochemical reactions, and generation of the body's principal methyl donor, S-adenosyl methionine (SAM or Ado-met), which participates in methylation of DNA and histones modulating gene expression, and methylation of proteins and lipids [Blom et al., 2006; Beaudin and Stover, 2007; Miller, 2008].

Recent studies have demonstrated that NTDs can occur in the offspring of pregnant women who had maternal auto-antibodies against folate receptors [Rothenberg et al., 2004]. These autoantibodies blocked the binding of [3H]FA to folate receptors on placental membranes, presumably resulting in reduced levels of CNS folate that contributed to development of the NTD. This result was not replicated in a population study of a large Irish cohort [Molloy et al., 2009]. However, that research was weakened by the fact that a number of serum samples were taken from women up to 10 years after pregnancy. Another study, which was confined to measuring folate receptor antibodies in samples drawn during midgestation, found a significant association between antibody levels, the folate transport-blocking capability of the antibody, and NTD occurrence [Cabrera et al., 2008]. This may lead in future to clinical testing during first pregnancies that will be used to adjust the recommended level of FA supplementation in subsequent pregnancies.

Teratogens

RA is a well-known teratogen when administered to nonhuman embryos, in which one of its many effects is to induce NTDs, including spina bifida, exencephaly, and anencephaly in several different species [Shenefelt, 1972; Tibbles and Wiley, 1988; Yasuda et al., 1989]. Exposure to excess RA has also been implicated in human embryopathy [Lammer et al., 1985; Rosa et al., 1986]. In contrast, inactivation of RA-synthesizing enzyme genes or receptor genes in mice leads to significantly increased rates of NTDs. High doses of RA (vitamin A) or retinoids in medications such as isotretinoin (Accutane) are to be avoided during pregnancy, although vitamin A deficiency can also increase NTD risk [Azais-Braesco and Pascal, 2000].

Most, if not all, antiepileptic drugs (AEDs) are known teratogens [Ornoy, 2006]. Different AEDs, however, are associated with different constellations of malformations. An increased risk of MMC is associated with in utero exposure to valproic acid or carbamazepine alone, or in combination with other AEDs [Lammer et al., 1987; Dansky and Finnell, 1991; Matalon et al., 2002]. In infants exposed to valproic acid or carbamazepine, the risk of MMC can be as high as 1–2 percent [Koren and Kennedy, 1999; Zhu et al., 2009]. Women who use these drugs for indications other than epilepsy (e.g., bipolar disease, migraine, chronic pain) also are at increased risk of having a child with MMC if they become pregnant while taking these drugs. The mechanisms by which valproic acid and carbamazepine increase the risk of NTD have not been established, but there is general consensus that genetic predisposition to its teratogenic effect is required for valproate to promote NTDs. Among the pathogenic mechanisms associated with valproic acid are increased homologous recombination that induces mutations in the genome, generation of reactive oxygen species, and epigenetic reprogramming through direct inhibition of histone deacetylases by valproate (reviewed in Ross, 2010). Folate administration does not appear to protect against the effects of valproic acid or carbamazepine on neural tube closure.

Classification of Neural Tube Defects

Nomenclature

The historical nomenclature of NTDs is imprecise. Many terms are based upon older descriptive terms that were derived with limited knowledge of the underlying embryologic defect. Broadly speaking, it is useful to separate those anomalies that arise from an early failure of neural tube formation, and those that arise from defects in subsequent developmental steps. MMC refers to the commonest form of spina bifida, in which the specific developmental defect is the presence of a flat neural placode, the unfolded derivative of the neural plate, elevated above a sac containing cerebrospinal fluid and continuous with the skin. Rather than representing a simple failure of fusion of the edges of the neural tube, the typical gross appearance of the neural placode of an MMC is most consistent with failure of folding of the neural plate at the median and dorsolateral hinge points.

Neural tube closure is usually required for subsequent developmental steps, such as the formation of mesodermal structures (e.g., dura, posterior spinal elements, and muscle). If the neural tube does not fold or close, the subsequent steps of mesodermal formation and ectodermal fusion at that segmental level do not occur. Milder NTDs will often result in near-normal formation of mesodermal structures and closure of the overlying skin. This basic difference, the presence or absence of skin, has led to the designation of spina bifida into open forms, spina bifida aperta, or closed forms, spina bifida occulta. Spina bifida occulta is a confusing term, since it can refer to either a broader group of anomalies that have normal skin overlying the spinal defect, or a specific anomaly that indicates a lack of fusion of the spinous processes in the lumbar area and has limited clinical significance (see below). Fortunately, both of these terms are not commonly used in the current era.

Embryologic Classification of Neural Tube Defects

One of the first visible steps in neurulation is the thickening of the ectoderm into the neural plate. In mammalian embryos, this is rapidly followed by a change in shape of the columnar epithelium in specific areas of the neural plate, resulting in formation of the neural tube. Once the edges of the neural groove fuse, the neural tube separates from the overlying ectoderm in a process known as dysjunction. This allows para-axial mesoderm to fill in the space between the neural tube and the ectoderm. This simplified series of events can be used to divide the commonly encountered NTDs on the basis of the embryologic defect:

- anomalies due to defects of neural folding and formation – myelomeningocele and anencephaly
- anomalies due to disordered postneurulation development – encephaloceles
- anomalies due to incomplete dysjunction – dermal sinus and associated dermoid and epidermoid tumors
- anomalies due to premature dysjunction – spinal cord lipomas
- anomalies due to disorders of gastrulation – split cord malformation, neurenteric cysts
- anomalies due to disordered secondary neurulation – thickened filum terminale, myelocystocele
- anomalies due to failure of caudal neuraxial development – sacral agenesis.

Myelomeningocele

Myelomeningocele (MMC), the most complex of congenital spinal deformities, involves all tissue layers dorsal to and including the neural tube (i.e., spinal cord, nerve roots, meninges, vertebral bodies, skin). The dysplastic neural tube is a flat, disorganized segment of tissue located at the middle and most superficial portion of a cerebrospinal fluid-containing sac (Figure 22-5A, B). The surrounding epithelium may, in some cases, grow over the placode or, in some cases, the neural placode may remain in the spinal canal without a sac present. This condition is referred to as myeloschisis (Figure 22-5C), but probably is not substantially different from a typical MMC in embryologic terms. The absence of a sac probably occurs if cerebrospinal fluid flow in the spinal canal is obstructed, or if cerebrospinal fluid leaks from the spinal subarachnoid space into the amniotic cavity.

Antenatal Diagnosis

Maternal serum α-fetoprotein (AFP) determination and ultrasound examination are used to identify fetuses that have or are likely to have spina bifida or anencephaly [Drugan et al., 2001]. Positive findings from either of these two screening tests can be monitored with amniocentesis and detailed sonography [Kooper et al., 2007]. AFP is a component of fetal cerebrospinal fluid, and it may leak into the amniotic fluid from the open

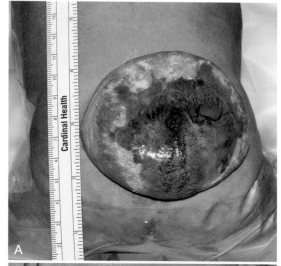
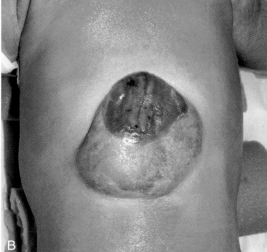
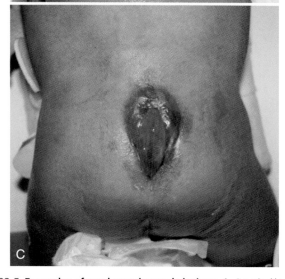

Fig. 22-5 Examples of myelomeningocele lesions. A, A typical lesion in the lumbar area with a large cerebrospinal fluid-containing sac. The structure in the center of the sac is the neural placode, which is continuous with the epithelium. The skin extends for a variable distance upwards along the wall of the sac. **B,** A thoracic lesion with an upwards-directed placode. **C,** A flat lesion, also known as myeloschisis.

neural tube. Elevated amniotic AFP concentrations correlate with open NTDs, while closed lesions usually do not lead to increased AFP concentration. Detection of NTDs correlates with the magnitude of increase in the amniotic fluid AFP level; NTDs are associated in a minority of pregnancies with mildly elevated AFP levels, in a majority of those with moderately elevated levels, and overwhelmingly in those with very elevated AFP levels [Canick et al., 2003]. An AFP level of two times the normal median or higher is found in approximately 2 percent of unaffected pregnancies, 80 percent of open spina bifida pregnancies, and 95 percent of anencephalic pregnancies.

Elevations in amniotic fluid acetylcholinesterase, produced by the fetal nervous system, correlate with maternal serum or amniotic fluid AFP, and can provide additional specificity and sensitivity in this screening approach. When acetylcholinesterase is elevated, more than 95 percent of patients with moderately or very elevated AFP levels had evidence of an NTD. Thus, it can differentiate between open ventral wall defects (i.e., gastroschisis and omphalocele), which will have normal acetylcholinesterase, and open NTDs, which will have elevated acetylcholinesterase.

Sonography also can be used to differentiate between ventral wall defects and NTDs [Lennon and Gray, 1999], and to identify additional structural malformations that are characteristic of fetuses with chromosomal abnormalities [Sepulveda et al., 2004]. When a diagnosis of spina bifida is confirmed, ultrasound examination is used to assess spontaneous leg and foot motion and to screen for leg and spine deformities, a Chiari II malformation, and other physical defects. Ultrasonography can detect or confirm the extent of the NTDs [Watson et al., 1991] and has had an enormous impact on the number of liveborn infants among populations in which termination of pregnancy is accepted [Zlotogora et al., 2002]. It is 60 percent accurate in low-risk pregnancies, which is equivalent to the accuracy of serum AFP screening (64 percent), 89 percent accurate in high-risk pregnancies, and 100 percent accurate for women referred for confirmation of a suspected spina bifida by another ultrasonographer [Chan et al., 1993, 1995]. The data indicate that neither sonography nor AFP screening alone provides sufficient sensitivity or specificity, but that, when these studies are used together, the predictive value is much higher [Chan et al., 1995].

Prenatal magnetic resonance imaging (MRI), with ultra-fast T2-weighted sequences, also can be used to characterize the Chiari II and other malformations (Figure 22-6). Such prenatal imaging studies might help to predict neurologic deficit [Cochrane et al., 1996] and ambulatory potential [Biggio et al., 2001]. Most fetuses with spina bifida that are not electively terminated receive no treatment until after birth. Several studies have investigated whether method of delivery influences the outcome for infants with the disorder. A study based on a review of this work concluded that, in general, conclusive evidence is lacking that, relative to vaginal delivery, cesarean section improves the outcome in children with spina bifida [Anteby and Yagel, 2003]. Cesarean section, however, might be justified for large lesions, to reduce the risk of trauma, and is done after in utero treatment of spina bifida because the forces of labor are likely to produce a wound dehiscence.

Additionally, the fetal karyotype can be examined to rule out chromosomal anomalies. Cytogenetic analysis is justified in the setting of prenatally detected spina bifida based on the prevalence of chromosome abnormalities in 17 percent of fetuses (trisomy 18, trisomy 13, triploidy, and translocation).

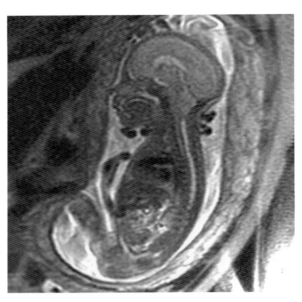

Fig. 22-6 A T2-weighted magnetic resonance image of a 22-week-old fetus with an open neural tube defect and cerebellar tonsils descended into the upper cervical canal. These features are consistent with a Chiari II malformation.

Prevention

NTDs occur during early pregnancy, often before a woman knows she is pregnant; 50–70 percent of these defects can be prevented if a woman consumes sufficient FA daily before conception and throughout the first trimester of her pregnancy. Two landmark studies in the early 1990s found that administration of FA had a profound effect on the risk of NTDs [MRC, 1991; Czeizel and Dudas, 1992]. In 1992, to reduce the number of cases of MMC, the U.S. Public Health Service recommended that all women capable of becoming pregnant consume 400 µg of FA daily. Because approximately 50 percent of pregnancies in the United States are unplanned and the neural tube develops before most women know they are pregnant, it was also recommended that women consume this amount of FA routinely. Three approaches to increase FA consumption were cited:
1. Improve dietary habits.
2. Fortify foods with FA.
3. Use dietary supplements containing FA.

Mandatory fortification of cereal grain products was legislated in the U.S. in 1996 and fully implemented as of January 1998. The estimated number of NTD-affected pregnancies in the U.S. declined from 4000 in the period 1995–1996 to 3000 in 1999–2000 [CDC, 2004; Mills and Signore, 2004]. This analysis controlled for declines in live births with NTDs as a result of recently implemented screening programs. Since the overall reduction of 25–30 percent in NTD rates in the U.S. since fortification was put into effect is below the expected 70 percent reduction, the debate continues regarding whether the fortification standard should be raised [Pitkin, 2007; Smith et al., 2008; Oakley, 2010].

Regardless of whether the optimal regimen for prenatal FA supplementation has been determined, there is still a significant proportion of pregnancies at risk for NTD for which FA will not effectively prevent NTD. Evidence in mouse models indicates that certain genetic backgrounds may include partial block in folate metabolism that can be circumvented by using alternative supplements. For example, the NTDs in the mouse mutant, Axial defects (Axd), are resistant to FA supplementation, but methionine – which will contribute to the methylation arm of the folate metabolic pathway – can reduce the occurrence of neurulation failure [Essien and Wannberg, 1993]. Another mouse mutant, curly tail (ct), which is prone to spina bifida that is not rescued by FA, can be protected against NTD by supplementation with myo-inositol [Greene and Copp, 1997]. Currently, clinical trials of prenatal inositol supplementation for the prevention of NTD are under way in the U.K. It appears likely that additional options for prevention of NTD will be available in the foreseeable future.

Clinical Features

The mortality rate for MMC is approximately 50 percent in the absence of therapy. Early surgery for closure of the lumbosacral defect is required to prevent meningitis. Later causes of death include hydrocephalus and renal failure. The renal complications are induced by chronic urinary tract infections, abnormal urodynamic function, and genitourinary tract abnormalities, such as progressive hydronephrosis. Patients at particular risk are the subgroup with high pressure within the bladder [Snodgrass and Adams, 2004].

MMCs may be situated at any longitudinal level of the neuroaxis. The location and extent of the defect determine the nature and degree of neurologic impairment; rating scales have been developed in an attempt to standardize the evaluation of affected children [Oi and Matsumoto, 1992]. Lumbosacral involvement is most common. Thoracic defects are the most complex and frequently are associated with serious complications. Cervical cord involvement is different from MMC of the lower spine and can be differentiated into two types:

1. myelocystocele herniating posteriorly into a meningocele
2. meningocele with or without an underlying split cord malformation [Steinbok, 1995; Steinbok and Cochrane, 1995].

Cervical lesions are clearly protuberant, covered at the base by full-thickness skin, and covered on the dome by a thick epithelium. Neural tissue is not superficially exposed but usually is tethered to adjacent dural or intrasaccular tissues. These differences likely are responsible for the more favorable outcome in cervical lesions [Meyer-Heim et al., 2003]. Varying degrees of paresis of the legs, usually profound, and sphincter dysfunction are the major clinical manifestations. Congenital dislocation of the hips or deformities of the feet, such as clubbing, may also occur. Severe sensory loss and accompanying trophic ulcers may complicate the condition. Occasionally, only sphincter disturbances are present. Radiographs reveal the primary defect of the vertebral arch.

Hydrocephalus is present in about 70–85 percent of patients with MMC, and occurs most frequently when the lesion is situated in the thoracolumbar area [Rintoul et al., 2002], which is the case in 90 percent of patients. Most persons with spina bifida have normal intelligence, but specific cognitive disabilities and language difficulties are common and can adversely affect educational and occupational achievements and the ability to live independently [Northrup and Volcik, 2000; Vachha and Adams, 2003].

Secondary Abnormalities

Central Nervous System Complications

Seizures have been reported in up to 17 percent of patients with MMC and almost always occur in those with shunted hydrocephalus [Talwar et al., 1995]. Electroencephalographic (EEG) abnormalities are nonspecific. Additional CNS abnormalities seen in these patients are believed to explain the cause of seizures, and include encephalomalacia, previous stroke, malformations, and intracranial calcifications. Seizures may be difficult to control, and frequently, exacerbation of seizures is associated with shunt malfunction or ventriculitis.

Bladder and Bowel Dysfunction

Bladder dysfunction and urinary incontinence pose major management problems and may be present at birth in the form of hydronephrosis [Stone, 1995; Silveri et al., 1997]. Interruption of sacral nerve roots and fiber connections between the brainstem and sacral cord causes the dysfunction. Loss of sphincter tone, overflow incontinence, sacral and rectal loss of sensation, and loss of detrusor activity on cystometry are seen. In other patients with higher lesions, dyssynergia of reflex pathways results in irregular contractions of the bladder in conjunction with outlet obstruction. Normal bladder control occurs in 10 percent of children with MMC. Prevention of bladder infection requires intermittent catheterization to maintain low residual urine volumes and prophylactic antibacterial drugs [Buyse et al., 1995]. Vesicoureteral reflux often develops during the second and third years of life, and assessment for this problem must be on-going. Re-implantation of the ureters into the bladder, or external drainage of the ureters either directly or through an ileal conduit, may be helpful. Transurethral resection of the external sphincter has been recommended when ureteral dilatation occurs. The use of prosthetic devices emulating sphincters has been useful in highly selected patients [Simeoni et al., 1996], as has selective sacral rhizotomy [Schneidau et al., 1995].

Constipation and fecal incontinence are common problems in children with spinal dysraphism and usually can be managed medically [Knab et al., 2001]. Dietary manipulation, oral and rectal laxatives, and manual evacuation are common treatments. Retrograde colonic enemas also may be successful.

Orthopedic Problems

It is important to consider that the paralysis below the cord lesion associated with spina bifida will be hypotonic, which predicts the types of orthopedic problems. Orthopedic defects associated with this paralysis, muscle imbalance, and accompanying regional spasticity may be severe and necessitate early intervention. Hip subluxation usually is treated with prosthetic splints or plaster casting [Heeg et al., 1998]. Sensory deficits of the casted skin areas frequently enhance the likelihood of skin ulcers. Severe foot deformities are seen in up to 80 percent of children and are treated with splinting or casting; neither age nor segmental level influences outcome of the foot deformity [Flynn et al., 2004]. Physical therapy may help to preserve and extend the range of motion of the joints [McDonald, 1995].

In infants and children, progressive leg or foot deformity, weakness, pain, or deterioration of gait or bladder function implies restricted growth or tethering of the spinal cord. Cord tethering may be found in many older children with spina bifida who are neurologically stable, however. Evidence of brainstem dysfunction may be recorded by means of respiratory pneumograms with a carbon dioxide challenge [Petersen et al., 1995] or by using brainstem auditory-evoked response testing [Docherty et al., 1987]. These signs and symptoms indicate the possibility of a Chiari II malformation or a tethered spinal cord.

Considerations in the differential diagnosis of delayed deterioration in a child with repaired MMC include a malfunctioning or infected shunt, seizures, scoliosis, hydrocephalus, hydromyelia, and an undetected second lesion of occult spinal dysraphism, such as a dermoid, epidermoid, or arachnoid cyst. Of course, intercurrent illness or drug toxicity should be considered. Surgical repair of a worsening tethered spinal cord and shunting or fenestration of syringomyelia can prevent decline of function [Iskandar et al., 1994].

Chiari II Malformation

CLASSIFICATION

Chiari was among the first to recognize multiple hindbrain malformations associated with congenital hydrocephalus [Arnett, 2003]. Four types of Chiari malformation have been characterized. Chiari I malformation is a downward displacement of the cerebellum and cerebellar tonsils. Chiari II malformation, also known as the Arnold–Chiari malformation, is a complex malformation that includes downward displacement of the cerebellar vermis and tonsils, and is encountered almost exclusively in patients with MMC. Chiari III is an encephalocervical meningocele, and Chiari IV refers to hypoplasia of the cerebellum. The differentiating features are indicated in Table 22-2.

The major features of the Chiari II malformation include:
1. inferior displacement of the medulla and the fourth ventricle into the upper cervical canal
2. elongation and thinning of the upper medulla and lower pons, persistence of the embryonic flexure of these structures, and the appearance of a "beaking" of the tectum
3. inferior displacement of the lower cerebellum through the foramen magnum into the upper cervical regions
4. a variety of bone defects of the foramen magnum, occiput, and upper cervical vertebrae (Figure 22-7).

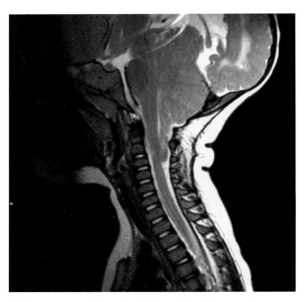

Fig. 22-7 A postnatal sagittal T2-weighted magnetic resonance image of a child with a Chiari II malformation. The cerebellar tonsils are descended to C3, the posterior fossa is small, and the brainstem is dysmorphic.

Hydromyelia and syringomyelia of the cervical spinal cord occur in 20–50 percent of patients.

PATHOPHYSIOLOGY

The precise mechanism causing Chiari II malformation is unknown. The most parsimonious theory is that the open neural tube fusion to the overlying skin produces downward traction on the neural axis, resulting in herniation of the brainstem and cerebellum through the foramen magnum. This herniation results in obstruction of hindbrain cerebrospinal fluid outflow, which leads to hydrocephalus. This theory is in keeping with the observation that the Chiari II malformation precedes the development of hydrocephalus. Hydrocephalus associated with the Chiari II malformation probably results primarily from one or both of two basic causes. The first is the hindbrain malformation that blocks either the fourth ventricular outflow or the cerebrospinal fluid flow through the posterior fossa. The

Table 22-2 Classification of Chiari Malformations

Type	Anatomic Abnormalities	Neurologic Findings
I	Downward displacement of the cerebellum and cerebellar tonsils, elongated brainstem fourth ventricle	Mild and delayed onset of headache and brainstem symptoms, usually beginning in adolescence; symptoms secondary to hydrocephalus or syringomyelia
II (Arnold–Chiari malformation)	Downward displacement of the cerebellar vermis and cerebellar tonsils; thinned and elongated medulla may actually be positioned side by side with upper segments of the atrophic cervical spinal cord	Associated with myelomeningocele in more than 95 percent of patients; symptoms resulting from progressive hydrocephalus and secondary brainstem dysfunction; feeding and respiratory complications are common, including apnea
III	Encephalocervical meningocele with spina bifida over the cervical area and protrusion of cerebellum through posterior encephalocele	Features as for Chiari II, without the same degree of association with myelomeningocele
IV	Hypoplasia of the cerebellum	Variable, ranging from asymptomatic to classic cerebellar dysfunction

(Data from Friede [1989]; Norman et al. [1995]; Sarnat [1992].)

second is aqueductal stenosis or atresia that may be associated with the malformation in approximately 50–85 percent of cases [Peach, 1965; Stein and Schut, 1979; Bell et al., 1987]. Further insights into the pathogenesis of the Chiari II malformation will come from study of animal models of NTDs. It has been possible to examine the developmental progression of this constellation of malformations in the Splotch animal model of spina bifida due to mutations in the *PAX3* gene [McLone and Dias, 2003].

CLINICAL FEATURES

The symptoms associated with Chiari II malformations include apnea, swallowing difficulties, and stridor in the newborn, and headache, quadriparesis, scoliosis, and balance and coordination difficulties in the older child; they are present in up to one-third of persons with the disorder. It is often difficult to differentiate between symptoms related to the hydrocephalus and those related to the Chiari II malformation, but several features are uniformly seen in this condition (Box 22-1). These symptoms are directly referable to cerebellar, brainstem, and cranial nerve dysfunction. More than one-third of affected infants display feeding disturbances associated with reflux and aspiration. Other features include vocal cord paralysis with stridor and abnormalities of ventilation, including both obstructive and central apnea.

The causes of the clinical abnormalities of brainstem function are threefold. First, they relate in part to the brainstem malformation, which involves cranial nerves and other nuclei, and which are present in the large majority of NTDs [Gilbert et al., 1986]. Second, compression and traction of the anomalous caudal brainstem by hydrocephalus and increased intracranial pressure also may play a role, especially in the vagal nerve disturbance that results in vocal cord paralysis and stridor. Third, ischemic and hemorrhagic necrosis of the brainstem often is present also, and may be secondary to the

---

Box 22-1 Clinical Manifestations of Chiari II Malformation

- Apnea
- Tongue fasciculations
- Stridor
- Facial palsy
- Gastroesophageal reflux
- Swallowing difficulties
- Poor feeding
- Ataxia
- Hypotonia
- Upper extremity weakness
- Hydrocephalus
- Syringomyelia
- Attention deficit
- Seizures
- Extraocular movement abnormalities
- Nystagmus
- Increased mortality

(From McLone DG, Dias MS. The Chiari II malformation: Cause and impact. Childs Nerv Syst 2003;19:540–550.)

---

disturbed arterial architecture of the caudally displaced vertebrobasilar circulation [Charney et al., 1987].

Management

Management of a child with a MMC requires the efforts of a multidisciplinary team involving many specialists. Treatment includes surgical reduction and other associated defects, such as syringomyelia, prevention of infection, covering of the MMC, control of hydrocephalus, management of urinary dysfunction, and treatment of the paralysis and abnormalities of the hips and feet.

Fetal Repair of Myelomeningocele

Animal studies, in which a model for spina bifida is created by laminectomy and exposure of the spinal cord to amniotic fluid, demonstrate that function can be retained if the lesion is closed before birth [Michejda and Bacher, 1985; Meuli et al., 1995]. Other evidence indicates that the Chiari II malformation, which occurs in almost all persons with spina bifida, is acquired and could potentially be prevented by in utero closure [Osaka et al., 1978; Paek et al., 2000].

Some evidence suggests that surgical treatment in utero results in improved outcomes. In 1998, in utero repair of MMC by hysterotomy was reported [Adzick et al., 1998; Tulipan and Bruner, 1998]. Early experience suggested that infants with MMC treated by hysterotomy had at least partial correction of hindbrain herniation [Tulipan et al., 1998], and possibly a diminished need for shunting relative to infants who received postnatal treatment [Bruner et al., 1999]. Compared with historical controls, infants given treatment in utero have a lower incidence of moderate to severe hindbrain herniation and hydrocephalus requiring shunting (Figure 22-8) [Tulipan and Bruner, 1999]. In a series of 50 MMC cases treated in utero, reversal of hindbrain herniation was reported in all patients, and the proportion requiring shunting was less than in historical control subjects (43 versus 85 percent) [Johnson et al., 2003]. A similar proportion requiring shunting (54 percent) also was noted in a second series of 116 spina bifida cases treated in utero at Vanderbilt University Medical Center [Bruner et al., 2004]. Comparisons between infants with spina bifida treated in utero and historical control subjects are, however, subject to substantial bias. The approach is being tested in a prospective randomized clinical trial.

Management in the Newborn Period

Without treatment, the mortality rate is extremely high (approximately 85 percent) during the first year of life and usually results from infection. Standard treatment includes closure of skin lesions overlying MMCs and treatment of hydrocephalus.

Neonates with spina bifida should undergo baseline imaging studies of the CNS with subsequent serial head measurements to assess the velocity of head growth and the need for shunting. Orthopedic deformities also should be treated shortly after birth, and ultrasonography and urodynamic studies should be carried out to assess the status of the urinary tract and provide a baseline for continuing assessment. At this age, bowel function is usually not a substantial difficulty, because affected infants have the gastrocolic reflex and pass stools with most feedings. Medical care and monitoring of patients with spina bifida are best provided by regular assessments by a

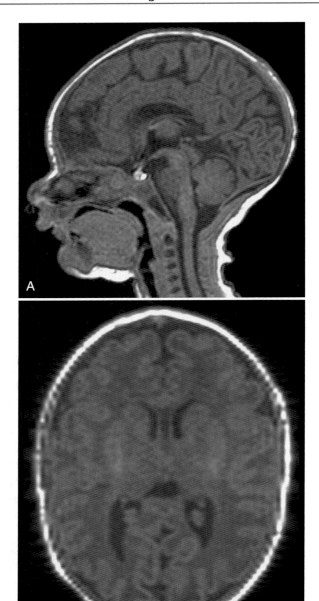

Fig. 22-8 Postnatal magnetic resonance images of a child who underwent fetal repair of a myelomeningocele. (The fetal MRI is shown in Figure 22-6). There is resolution of the Chiari II malformation and the ventricular size is normal.

multidisciplinary team. This team should be under the direction of a skilled physician with training in the care of children who have multiple disabilities, and should include a nurse specializing in the care of children with multiple handicaps, a pediatric neurosurgeon, a urologist, an orthopedic surgeon, a physical therapist, and a social worker.

The value of immediate correction of the defect within 48 hours of birth is widely accepted. Even when cerebrospinal fluid leakage occurs, however, a delay in closure for up to 48 hours does not increase the risk of infection or worsen the neurologic deficit [McComb, 1997]. In such cases, the patient is given antibiotics, and the exposed placode is kept clean and moist. When primary closure is impossible because of the large cutaneous area involved, epithelialization must be encouraged, and surgery performed later. The decision to give vigorous therapy for the most severely affected infants with MMC is beset by moral and medical considerations; restricted therapy often is associated with survival but poor outcome. Appropriate treatment of newborns with MMC increases the number of survivors and perhaps the quality of survival. Early surgical repair is appropriate for most newborns with myelodysplasia [McComb, 1997]. Each patient must be assessed individually in the context of advances in technology and medical care.

Treatment of Chiari II Malformation

Careful monitoring of infants with known Chiari II malformations is advocated [Cai and Oakes, 1997; Stevenson, 2004]. Evaluation with MRI is the procedure of choice. Before surgical decompression of the posterior fossa in symptomatic patients is considered, it is important to treat hydrocephalus if present. A properly functioning ventricular shunt often can obviate the need for decompression of hindbrain herniation. Many patients will have resolution of brainstem symptomatology once a shunt is placed [Caldarelli et al., 1995]. Significant improvement in the size of the accompanying spinal syrinx may occur after ventriculoperitoneal shunting or shunt revision [Milhorat et al., 1992].

Suboccipital craniectomy to decompress the suboccipital and cervical areas may be warranted to reduce the progressive compression of neural and vascular structures. Studies have suggested that early surgical intervention to alleviate brainstem compression is associated with improved long-term neurologic outcome and a decreased need for tracheostomy or gastrostomy [Pollack et al., 1992, 1996]. Alleviation of fourth ventricle outflow obstruction by foraminal fenestration or shunting may be required in rare cases. In one series of 50 symptomatic Chiari II patients, surgical treatment resulted in complete relief of symptoms in 20 percent, improvement in 66 percent, stabilization in 8 percent, and worsening in 6 percent [Dyste et al., 1989]. Despite these data, no standards for treatment have yet been established because the current neurosurgical literature is characterized by significant debate and variable results [Tubbs et al., 2004].

Outcome

Short-term and long-term survival of patients with spina bifida has increased with improvements in medical and surgical management. The most recent population-based data indicate that the 1-year survival rate is about 87 percent, and that roughly 78 percent of all persons with MMC survive to the age of 17 years [Wong and Paulozzi, 2001]. Unfortunately, these patients continue to be subject to excess morbidity and mortality throughout adulthood [Singhal and Mathew, 1999; McDonnell and McCann, 2000; Bowman et al., 2001]. Patients with MMC are at substantial risk for leg weakness and paralysis, sensory loss, bowel and bladder dysfunction, and orthopedic abnormalities (e.g., clubfoot, contractures, hip dislocation, scoliosis, kyphosis). In general, the functional level of the defect corresponds to the anatomic level of the bony spinal defect, as determined by radiologic studies. Patients with MMC also develop symptoms from associated malformations of the CNS, including hydrocephalus, syringomyelia, and Chiari II malformations. Almost all patients with thoracic level lesions require a ventricular shunt, whereas shunting is required in less than 70 percent of those with sacral level lesions [Rintoul et al., 2002]. Radiographic evidence of Chiari II malformations is present in more than 75 percent of affected persons [Just et al., 1990].

Virtually all infants and children born with NTDs are provided with surgical and medical treatment. Previous studies reported that the 5-year survival rate for children with sacral lesions was in the range of 80–90 percent, with increased mortality among children with lesions located more superiorly along the neuraxis [Honein et al., 2001]. Studies of the long-term outcome in children born with MMC have demonstrated an improved outcome that coincides with medical advances [Wong and Paulozzi, 2001]. Among 101 patients assessed at birth, the mortality rate was 18 percent; 53 percent were community ambulators, 58 percent attended normal school and were grade-appropriate, 75 percent were continent of urine, and 86 percent were continent of stool. Hydrocephalus was present in 93 children, and 85 required shunting. The shunt revision rate in the first year of life was 50 percent and, after 2 years, decreased to 10 percent per year [Steinbok et al., 1992]. Of note, an increased risk of shunt infections follows new abdominal surgery for renal complications [Aldana et al., 2002].

Counseling

Counseling is essential to ensure that parents understand the nature and severity of the deformities and the necessary surgical and long-term rehabilitative efforts [Liptak et al., 1988]. Parents also should be aware of the patient's potential for intellectual and physical development. In addition, parents should be educated about the higher incidence of late medical complications that can arise, such as latex allergy, and their warning signs in children with spina bifida [Konz et al., 1995]. It is important to communicate these potential problems to family members and others involved in their care.

Anencephaly

Anencephaly is a congenital malformation in which both cerebral hemispheres are absent [MTFA, 1990]. Most anencephalic infants are stillborn, and those infants born alive die shortly after birth [Walters et al., 1997]. Epidemiologic studies demonstrate a striking variation in prevalence rates. The highest incidence is in Great Britain and Ireland, and the lowest incidence is in Asia, Africa, and South America. Other countries have intermediate incidence rates. Anencephaly occurs six times more frequently in whites than in blacks. Female fetuses are more often affected than males.

Antenatal diagnosis is possible using assays of AFP or acetylcholinesterase, which are increased in maternal serum and amniotic fluid [Brock et al., 1985; Wald et al., 1989; Loft et al., 1993; Crandall and Chua, 1995]. Antenatal diagnosis also is feasible through the use of fetal ultrasonography [Birnbacher et al., 2002]. In the past two decades, prenatal screening with ultrasound examination during the first trimester, which is nearly 100 percent accurate, and maternal AFP determinations have resulted in earlier detection of anencephaly [Aubry et al., 2003]. Earlier detection has resulted in a dramatic decrease in the average gestational age at birth, from 35.6 weeks in the 1970s to 19.6 weeks in 1988 to 1990, with virtually no term liveborn anencephalic infants born after 1990 in those pregnancies

in which a prenatal diagnosis of anencephaly had been made [Drugan et al., 2001].

Pathogenesis

Anencephaly follows failure of closure of the anterior neural tube. The embryonic defect probably occurs before closure of the anterior neuropore on day 26. Two mechanisms leading to anterior NTDs have been proposed: Anencephaly could result from failure of neural folds to come together at a discrete site, or from a failure of apposed neural folds to remain closed and fuse in the midline. The causes of anencephaly remain unknown but, of importance, they mirror the causes of spina bifida and, similarly, folate has reduced the incidence of disease significantly. Indeed, both spina bifida and anencephaly can occur in the same family, reflecting the stochastic nature of where and when neural tube closure may fail. Risk factors discussed above apply to both spina bifida and anencephaly.

Differential Diagnosis

In anencephaly, the absence of the brain and calvaria can be total or partial. Acrania is defined as congenital partial or total absence of the skull. Craniorachischisis is characterized by anencephaly, accompanied by a contiguous bony defect of the spine and exposure of neural tissue. Craniorachischisis is typically, an extremely thin and flattened spinal cord, accompanied by foreshortening of the neuraxis and is thought to result from impaired convergent extension during embryogenesis. In iniencephaly, dysraphism in the occipital region is accompanied by severe retroflexion of the neck and trunk, with three cardinal features: deficiency of the occipital bone, cervicothoracic spinal retroflexion, and rachischisis. Iniencephaly differs from anencephaly in that the cranial cavity is present and skin covers the head and retroflexed region. Severe retroflexion of the neck present on fetal ultrasound examination may suggest the diagnosis. A majority of the patients also have visceral and other severe CNS malformations. Another related condition is meroanencephaly. Meroanencephaly is a rare form of anencephaly characterized by malformed cranial bones and a median cranial defect, through which protrudes the area cerebrovasculosa. In encephalocele, the brain and meninges herniate through a defect in the calvaria [Botto et al., 1999].

Pathology

The cranial vault is defective over the vertex, exposing a soft, angiomatous mass of neural tissue covered by a thin membrane continuous with the skin. The cranial abnormality may extend inferiorly to the cervical region, with formation of a complete spina bifida. The extremely thin and flattened spinal cord is readily observed. The optic globes usually are protuberant because of inadequate bony orbits.

Encephalocele

An encephalocele is a herniation of intracranial contents through a midline skull defect. Also known as cephaloceles, these lesions are classified by their contents and location [David, 1993]. Cranial meningoceles contain only leptomeninges and cerebrospinal fluid, whereas encephaloceles also contain brain parenchyma. The incidence of cephaloceles is approximately 0.8–5 per 10,000 live births, with encephaloceles being the most common form [Siffel et al., 2003].

Encephaloceles usually are located in the occipital (75 percent) or frontal areas (25 percent). Basal and trans-sphenoidal encephaloceles are rare; they may appear between the ethmoid and sphenoid bones and extend into the upper pharynx [Harley, 1991]. Encephaloceles that extend from the area of the orbit, nose, or forehead are termed sincipital encephaloceles; those in the occipital region are termed notencephaloceles. Exencephaly consists of a large outpouching of brain tissue with surrounding thick walls. This defect may involve the spinal cord, forming an encephalomyelocele. Cranial encephalocele may contain a combination of meninges, ventricles, and brain parenchyma [Wininger and Donnenfeld, 1994].

Etiology

The etiology of encephaloceles is not known but likely is multifactorial [Van Allen et al., 1993; Golden and Chernoff, 1995; Martinez-Lage et al., 1996; McComb, 1997]. Studies have indicated that consumption of FA during the periconceptional period can reduce the risk of anencephaly, as well as spina bifida [Botto et al., 1999; Honein et al., 2001]. A similar protective effect, however, has not been noted for encephalocele [Stevenson et al., 2000], suggesting that efforts to increase FA consumption among women of reproductive age are not likely to have any influence on the incidence of encephaloceles. Although some affected fetuses are stillborn, or some affected pregnancies are terminated as a consequence of increased prenatal diagnosis of NTDs, a substantial proportion of affected infants are live-born [Allen et al., 1996]. Although the etiology in most cases likely is multifactorial, some cases display likely monogenetic causes [Van Esch et al., 2004) that are associated with well-defined syndromes (Table 22-3).

Clinical Characteristics

A fluctuant, round, balloon-like mass that protrudes from the cranium, usually posteriorly, is the most typical manifestation of encephaloceles (Figure 22-9). The mass may pulsate and be

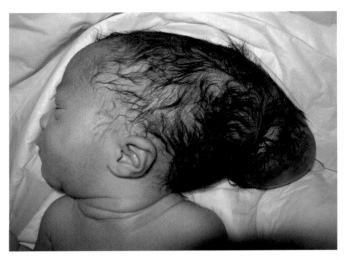

Fig. 22-9 A typical occipital encephalocele. There is a cerebrospinal fluid-containing sac that extends beyond the calvarium through a bony defect.

covered by an erythematous, translucent, or opaque membrane, or by normal skin. The covering may not be uniform throughout its surface. The amount of compromised and deformed neural tissue and the degree of resultant microcephaly determine the extent of cerebral dysfunction [Lorber and Schofield, 1979], but otherwise little has been published about prognosis. Brain tissue not extending into the encephalocele (i.e., retained within the intracranial cavity) may be deformed and functionally impaired.

Severe intellectual and motor delays typically occur in association with microcephaly; motor delay is accompanied by weakness and spasticity. Intellectual impairment is more prevalent in patients with posterior encephaloceles than in those with anterior encephaloceles [Hockley et al., 1990]. Some patients, however, may have fairly normal development. Occipital lobe destruction is associated with various degrees of visual impairment. When the deformity extends into the

Table 22-3 Selected Syndromes Associated with Encephaloceles

Syndrome	Clinical Features
Walker–Warburg syndrome	Hydrocephalus, severe neurologic impairment, vermian agenesis, type II lissencephaly, autosomal-recessive inheritance
Meckel–Gruber syndrome	Polycystic kidney, sloping forehead, polydactyly, hepatobiliary fibrosis, cleft lip and palate, autosomal-recessive inheritance
Dandy–Walker syndrome	Hydrocephalus, partial or complete absence of cerebellar vermis, posterior fossa cyst contiguous with fourth ventricle, cranial nerve palsies, nystagmus, truncal ataxia, sporadic occurrence
Joubert's syndrome	Cerebellar vermian aplasia, episodic hyperpnea, abnormal eye movements, rhythmic protrusion of tongue, ataxia, retardation, coloboma, retinal dystrophy, renal cysts, autosomal-recessive inheritance
Goldenhar–Gorlin syndrome	Orofacial abnormalities, pre-auricular tags, epibulbar dermoids, sporadic occurrence
Knobloch's syndrome	Vitreoretinal degeneration with retinal detachment, high myopia, and occipital encephalocele, normal intelligence, gene localized to 21q22.3
Robert's syndrome	Anterior encephalocele, autosomal-recessive inheritance
Median cleft face syndrome	Anterior encephalocele, autosomal-dominant inheritance

(Data from Online Mendelian Inheritance in Man [OMIM], http://www.ncbi.nim.nih.gov/omim, accessed 2005.)

ventricle, hydrocephalus is almost inevitable. Because of increased intracranial pressure, the encephalocele may become stretched until the rim of neuronal tissue is infarcted, with resultant infection and rupture if the problem is not surgically corrected.

Other malformations may accompany encephaloceles, including Dandy–Walker syndrome, Klippel–Feil syndrome, Arnold–Chiari malformation, porencephaly, agenesis of the corpus callosum, myelodysplasia, optic nerve dysplasia, cleft palate, and others [Mecke and Passarge, 1971; Lieblich et al., 1978; Pagon et al., 1978; Fisher and Smith, 1981; Cohen and Lemire, 1982; Koenig et al., 1982; Aleksic et al., 1983; Waterson et al., 1985; Sertie et al., 1996; Wang et al., 1999; Joy et al., 2001; Van Esch et al., 2004] (see Table 22-3). Although ultrasonography may be helpful, the clinical diagnosis is confirmed by computed tomography (CT) or MRI (Figure 22-10).

Neuroendocrine disturbances occur, particularly with basal encephaloceles that involve the sella turcica or sphenoid sinus [Lieblich et al., 1978]. These conditions may be undetectable by gross inspection. Intranasal mass or endocrine dysfunction is the cardinal feature. Encephaloceles are seen with a variety of chromosomal disorders (e.g., trisomy 13 or 18; 13q or 16q deletion) and syndromes (see Table 22-3). Occipital encephalocele, microcephaly, cleft palate or lip, polydactyly, holoprosencephaly, and polycystic kidneys constitute Meckel–Gruber syndrome [Chao et al., 2005]. Retinal degeneration with detachment and occipital encephalocele (Knobloch's syndrome) is another autosomal-recessive condition [Wilson et al., 1998].

Nasal glioma, a congenital tumor, appears as a frontonasal mass that mimics an encephalocele [Rahbar et al., 2003]. The tumor is derived from herniated brain tissue that has lost its connection to the brain; this relation can be demonstrated by neuroimaging techniques.

Management

Prenatal diagnosis of encephaloceles may be established with determination of increased amniotic AFP content and ultrasound studies [Graham et al., 1982]. Surgical correction of all but the smallest encephaloceles is necessary. Accompanying hydrocephalus may require ventriculoperitoneal shunting. Associated systemic abnormalities are present in approximately half of the patients, depending on the syndromic nature of the condition. A full battery of endocrinologic screens should be performed to evaluate basal encephaloceles.

Occult Forms of Spinal Dysraphism

The spectrum of occult spinal dysraphism includes anomalies where the overlying skin is mostly normal and covers the underlying NTD. These anomalies include distortion of the spinal cord or roots by fibrous bands and adhesions, intraspinal lipomas, dermoid or epidermoid cysts, fibrolipomas, spinal cord lipomas, lipomyelomeningocele, and split cord malformations [Anderson, 1975; Byrd et al., 1991; Kriss et al., 1995].

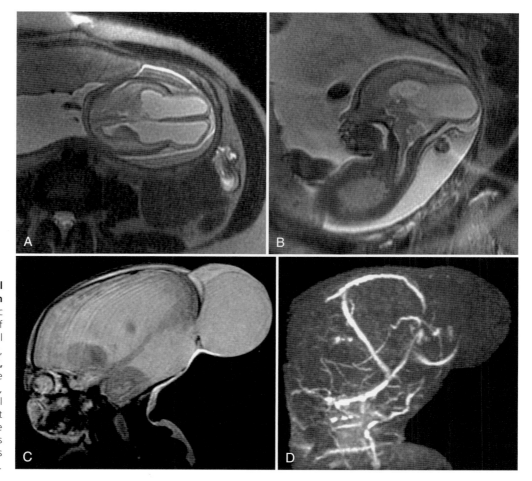

Fig. 22-10 Prenatal and postnatal images of the patient shown in Figure 22-9. A and **B,** Fetal magnetic resonance images show extension of the ventricles through the occipital defect. Note that the occipital cortex, although thinned, is still present. **C,** Postnatal MRI shows extension of the ventricle through the bony defect, which is now smaller. The occipital cortex is now so thin that it is not visible on the sagittal image. **D,** The magnetic resonance venogram shows displacement of the venous sinuses around the origin of the encephalocele.

Symptoms of occult spinal dysraphism may be absent, minimal, or severe, depending on the degree of neural involvement. The patient may exhibit static or slowly progressive weakness, spasticity, or sensory loss in the legs or feet, gait difficulty, and foot deformity. Bowel and bladder dysfunction, such as incontinence, repeated bladder infection, and enuresis, also may occur. Symptoms are caused by abnormally formed neural tissue or pressure on the spinal cord or nerve roots. Common findings include diminished Achilles tendon reflexes, contracted heel cords, high arches, equinovarus deformity of the feet, decreased rectal sphincter tone, unequal leg or foot length, scattered sensory loss, Babinski signs, and trophic ulcers. Because many of these patients have associated posterior fossa or cervical cord malformations, neurologic involvement of the upper extremities may occur in the form of partial paralysis or spasticity. Ophthalmologic complications, usually observed when hydrocephalus is present, also are common and require careful evaluation and follow-up. Ultrasonography and MRI have greatly facilitated the diagnosis and management of these occult lesions. A tethered spinal cord, lipoma, or fatty filum terminale can be detected without invasive myelography. Ultrasonography can demonstrate a poorly pulsatile, low-lying, or thickened conus medullaris in infants. The decision to proceed to surgery is based on progressive symptomatology.

Spinal Cord Lipoma

Spinal cord lipomas are a continuum of developmental anomalies that range from a small fatty mass attached to the distal spinal cord to very complex anomalies that involve all spinal structures. In some cases, the lipoma is entirely intraspinal and extends through a limited defect in the posterior elements of the spine into the subcutaneous tissues (Figure 22-11). In other cases, the spinal cord lipoma is continuous with the caudal spinal cord, and the spinal cord itself extends into the subcutaneous tissues, along with the meninges. If the spinal cord extends into the subcutaneous tissues along with a cerebrospinal fluid-containing space, this is usually referred to as a lipomyelomeningocele.

Spinal cord lipomas are considered more complex forms of spinal dysraphism. Despite this, they can present with either no symptoms, or symptoms over long periods of time. In general, if untethering of the spinal cord can be accomplished with low morbidity, then a surgical procedure should be considered early in life. For large and complex lesions, particularly in patients with normal function, serious consideration should be given to observation, since deficits can evolve that may have substantial functional effects.

Dermal Sinus Tract

Recurrent meningitis from external contamination of cerebrospinal fluid may result from occult congenital malformations along the spinal canal and neuroaxis. These external connections include midline dermal sinus; temporal bone fistula to the middle ear, eustachian tube, or nasopharynx; neurenteric fistula; and basal encephalocele or meningocele involving the cribriform plate, sphenoid bone, or clivus. From an embryological perspective, sinus tracts consist of epithelial-lined canals that probably represent persistence of an ectodermal-derived pathway from the skin to the CNS (Figure 22-12). In most cases, the spinal cord appears largely normal, implying that neural tube formation is complete but a persistent communication is still present. The spinal cord may be low or deformed by the presence of the sinus tract.

Dermal sinus tracts are seen in approximately 1 in 2500 live births. A rapid test for whether clear discharge from a dermal pit is cerebrospinal fluid is to analyze the fluid for glucose; results will be positive with cerebrospinal fluid but negative with most other body fluids. An MRI scan should be obtained, followed by surgical treatment to eliminate this connection and remove the risk of meningitis.

Spina Bifida Occulta

Spina bifida occulta, a confusing term, is defined as a defect in the posterior bony components of the vertebral column without involvement of the cord or meninges (Figure 22-13). It occurs in at least 5 percent of the population but most often is asymptomatic. This defect often is found incidentally on radiographic studies, or is diagnosed because of a subtle clinical finding such as a tuft of hair or a cutaneous angioma or lipoma in the midline of the back, marking the location of the defect. The presence of such a cutaneous lesion is associated with spina bifida occulta in only approximately 10 percent of cases, although the percentage increases to approximately 50 percent when two or more skin lesions are present [Guggisberg et al., 2004]. This defect is located most often in the lower lumbar area, involving the lamina of L5 and S1. The presence of a bifid spinous process is not associated with neurologic deficits or spinal instability. No treatment or intervention is required.

Meningocele

Meningocele, a protrusion of meninges without accompanying nervous tissue, is not associated with neurologic deficit. The mass usually is evident as a fluid-filled protrusion covered by skin or membrane in the midline. Membranous lesions are

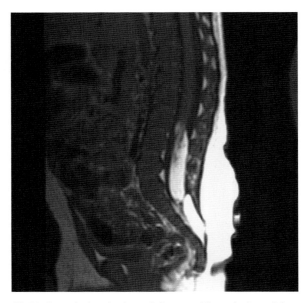

Fig. 22-11 A typical spinal cord lipoma. The spinal cord becomes continuous with a fatty structure, which then continues through a fascial defect into the subcutaneous tissues. There is no protrusion of the spinal cord or meninges through the defect.

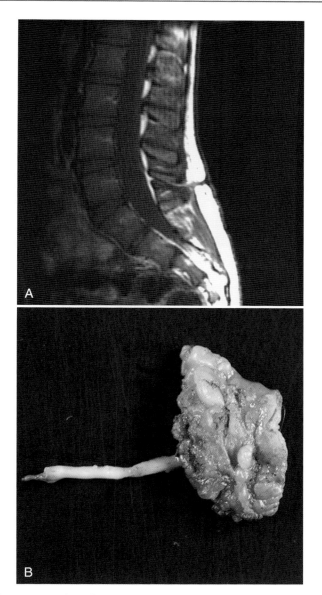

Fig. 22-12 A dermal sinus tract. A, The sagittal magnetic resonance image clearly shows a tract leading from the skin through a spinous process into the spinal canal and extending upwards to the spinal cord. **B,** The excised surgical specimen shows the ellipse of skin (to the right) surrounded by subcutaneous tissue, and the epithelial-lined tract that extends to the dorsal surface of the spinal cord.

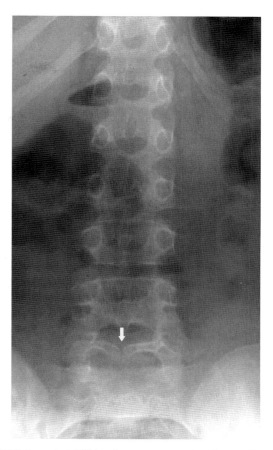

Fig. 22-13 A typical bifid spinous process that is usually termed spina bifida occulta. It has no clinical significance.

A meningocele in the cranial or high cervical area may coexist with aqueductal stenosis, hydromyelia, or a Chiari II malformation. Membrane-covered meningoceles are more likely to be accompanied by severe abnormalities; lesions covered with normal skin often are free of associated abnormalities. Elective surgical treatment is recommended, except for very small lesions [Feltes et al., 2004].

Split Cord Malformations

Embryology

In split cord malformations, previously known as diastematomyelia, a midline septum divides the spinal cord longitudinally into two, usually unequal portions extending up to ten thoracolumbar segments. The septum may span the entire width of the spinal canal and is anchored to the ventral dura mater on the posterior aspect of the vertebral bodies. It may be attached posteriorly to the vertebral arch or dura mater. The septum is derived from mesoderm and is composed of fibrous tissue, cartilage, or bone. The etiology of split cord malformations is currently unknown.

Split cord malformations can be divided into two different types. In type I, present in 50 percent of cases, a split spinal cord is surrounded by a normal undivided arachnoid-dural sleeve without a septum. In type II, present in the other 50 percent, each hemicord is invested by a separate dural sleeve, divided by a fibrous, cartilaginous, or bony septum [Pang et al.,

found rostrally, and skin-covered lesions are more evenly distributed along the neuraxis. MRI analysis is helpful in determining the contents of a mass along the spine and in differentiating meningocele from MMC (Figure 22-14). Very small subcutaneous lesions may remain undetected for prolonged periods and typically require no specific treatment, but must be differentiated from small encephaloceles.

When careful examination of patients with suspected meningocele reveals significant neurologic abnormality (e.g., equinovarus deformity, gait disturbance, abnormal bladder function), the diagnosis of MMC is appropriate. These patients likely have entrapped nerve roots within the defect that can be identified during surgery.

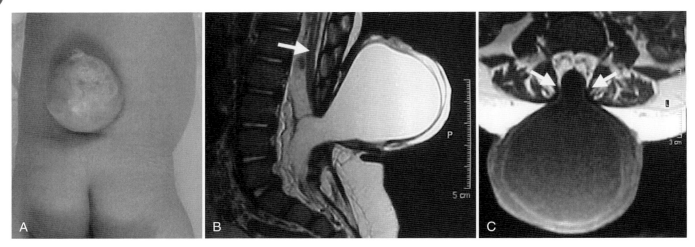

Fig. 22-14 Lumbar meningocele in a newborn. A, External appearance of the skin. **B,** Midline sagittal view from T2-weighted MRI study depicts a fluid-filled cystic lesion, measuring 5 cm by 5 cm. Note homogeneous water signal within the lesion, confirming the diagnosis of meningocele, rather than meningomyelocele. The spinal cord terminates appropriately at T1 (arrow). **C,** Axial view of the lesion from T1-weighted MRI study. Note the defect in the posterior spinal process (arrows), with extrusion of contents into the cyst. *(From http://www.neurocirugia.com/intervenciones/ meningocele/ Meningocele.htm, with permission.)*

1992]. The bony septum can be visualized on CT, which may be helpful if surgery is required (Figure 22-15). These conditions are differentiated from diplomyelia (see below) on the basis of the integrity of the spinal cord; in diastematomyelia, only a single central canal that is split at or near the midline is present.

Diplomyelia is a side-by-side or anteroposterior duplication of the spinal cord [Dias and Pang, 1995]. It is differentiated from diastematomyelia by the presence of two central canals, each surrounded by gray and white matter arranged in the normal pattern. The two cords often are completely reunited caudally but may remain separated to the tip of the conus medullaris. A bony septum may partly intervene between the duplicated cords. The two cords are often unequal and may be side by side (the most common position), or one may be dorsal to the other. These malformations are compatible with normal function; deterioration suggests the presence of diastematomyelia or tethering. The etiology of this condition also remains unknown.

Clinical Characteristics

Patients with split cord malformations present with a congenital scoliosis, hydrocephalus, or cutaneous lesion such as hairy patch, dimple, hemangioma, subcutaneous mass, or teratoma [Kothari and Bauer, 1997]. A progressive myelopathy, with deformities of the feet, scoliosis, kyphosis, or discrepancy in leg length, may develop. Resection of the spur frequently does not result in clinical improvement, but may prevent further deterioration. The intervening mesenchymal elements appear to contribute to progressive neurologic, urologic, and orthopedic deterioration from spinal cord tethering. Resection of the spur should be performed in patients who have progressive neurologic manifestations; those without worsening symptoms should be observed until progression occurs and then resection performed [Miller et al., 1993]. Split cord malformations can be detected prenatally by ultrasonography [Anderson et al., 1994; Sonigo-Cohen et al., 2003]. MRI is the preferred neuroimaging study for the evaluation of patients suspected of having this condition. Although most lesions occur in the

lumbosacral region, presentations involving the cervical cord are reported. Split cord malformations are more common in females (female to male ratio of greater than 3:1) [Mathieu et al., 1982]. Urodynamic and electrophysiologic studies are abnormal in approximately 80 percent of patients [Kothari and Bauer, 1997].

Disorders of Secondary Neurulation

Fibrofatty Filum Terminale

The filum terminale is the nonfunctional continuation of the end of the spinal cord. It usually consists of fibrous tissue without functional nervous tissue. Although its embryologic origin is unclear, it probably represents the termination of the neural tube and its most caudal link to the rest of the embryonic tissues. The filum can be enlarged either with fibrous tissue only or with fat (Figure 22-16). If the filum is thicker than 2 mm, it is usually defined by radiologists as being "associated with tethered spinal cord." A thickened or fatty filum terminale may be associated with a low conus and a spectrum of clinical findings, including bladder dysfunction, leg numbness and weakness, and scoliosis. In the presence of neurologic findings and a fatty filum, an untethering procedure may be considered.

Sacral Agenesis

Sacral agenesis is defined as congenital absence of the whole or part of the sacrum (Davidoff et al., 1991; Towfighi and Housman, 1991). It has a heterogeneous etiology. In its classic form, often described as the caudal regression syndrome, malformations of most or all structures derived from the caudal region of the embryo, including the urogenital system, the hindgut, caudal spine, spinal cord, and the lower limbs, may be seen. Approximately 15 percent to 25 percent of mothers of these children have insulin-dependent diabetes mellitus.

An autosomal-dominant form of sacral agenesis, sometimes described as a partial sacral dysgenesis, ASP (anal atresia, sacral anomalies, presacral mass) syndrome, or Currarino's

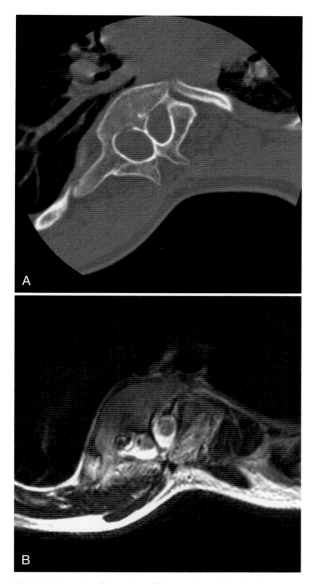

Fig. 22-15 A type II split cord malformation. A, A clear bony septum. **B,** Two spinal hemicords.

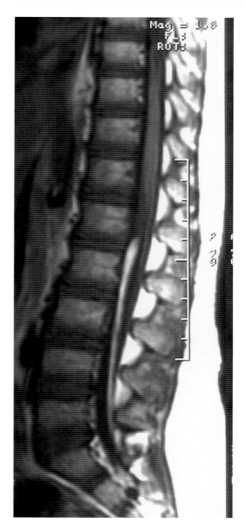

Fig. 22-16 A fibrofatty filum terminale extending from the end of the conus to the end of the thecal sac. Of note, the dorsal structures, such as the spinous processes and lamina, are usually intact in this condition.

syndrome, also exists. Typical features include hemisacrum with preservation of the first sacral vertebra [Lynch et al., 2000]. The defect usually takes the form of a sickle-shaped or crescent-shaped deformity of the sacrum; the hemisacrum or so-called scimitar sign is present in approximately 75 percent of patients (Figure 22-17). In its most severe presentation, the hemisacrum is associated with a presacral mass (anterior meningocele, enteric cyst, and/or presacral teratoma) and anorectal stenosis. Autosomal-dominant inheritance, localization to 7q36, and mutations in a homeobox gene, *HLXB9*, have been identified in several affected patients [Ross et al., 1998; Belloni et al., 2000]. Mutations in the coding sequence of *HLXB9* have been identified in nearly all cases of familial Currarino's syndrome and in approximately 30 percent of patients with sporadic Currarino's syndrome.

The neurologic findings are similar to those in MMC, ranging from a minimal deficit to equinovarus deformity of the feet, to more extensive sensory and motor deficits of the lower extremities. The level of bone anomaly corresponds well to the level of weakness but not to sensory loss, as sensation usually is preserved. The caudal spinal cord often is truncated, dysraphic, and tethered [Estin and Cohen, 1995]. Most patients have neurogenic urinary tract and bowel impairment, visceral abnormalities, flattened buttocks, and prominent iliac crests. Constipation and perianal sepsis are common complaints. Ascending infection resulting in bacterial meningitis also has been reported.

Some patients experience progressive neurologic deficits, demonstrating that sacral agenesis is not always a static disability [O'Neill et al., 1995]. Slow deterioration of neurologic function may masquerade as an orthopedic or urologic problem, unless the potential for progressive lesions is appreciated. Dural sac stenosis, tethered spinal cord, diastematomyelia, and cauda equina lipomas and dermoids also have been associated with sacral agenesis. Although plain radiographs demonstrate the degree of sacral agenesis, CT or MRI is necessary to delineate the underlying spinal cord anomalies (Figure 22-18). Surgical intervention is indicated in patients

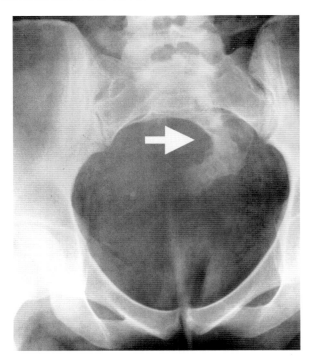

Fig. 22-17 Partial sacral dysgenesis, or Currarino's syndrome. Note the scimitar sacrum (arrow) with a right-sided defect. *(From Lynch SA et al. Autosomal dominant sacral agenesis: Currarino syndrome. J Med Genet 2000;37:561–566. Reproduced by permission from BMJ Publishing Group.)*

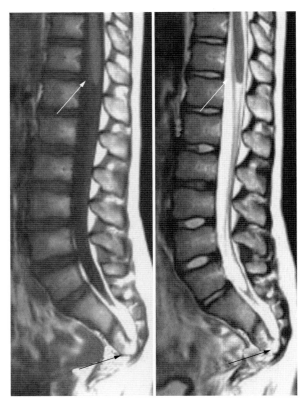

Fig. 22-18 Partial absence of distal sacrum (black arrows) and abrupt wedge-shaped truncation of the tip of the conus (white arrows). No tethered cord is noted. These findings are consistent with caudal regression syndrome (also known as sacral agenesis). *(From http://www.aiclancaster. com/nl/nl_0036.htm.)*

with progressive neurologic deficits associated with occult spinal cord lesions [Pang, 1993]. Treatment is similar to that for patients with myelodysplasia, particularly for the problems of urinary incontinence, constipation, progressive urinary tract and renal dysfunction, and orthopedic abnormalities.

Sirenomelia is a condition typically characterized by fusion of the lower limbs, single umbilical artery, and severe malformations of the urogenital and lower gastrointestinal tracts. Controversy exists in the literature regarding whether sirenomelia occurs as a separate entity or represents the extreme form of caudal regression syndrome. The presence of two umbilical arteries, nonlethal renal anomalies, nonfused lower limbs, abdominal wall defects, and abnormalities of tracheoesophageal tree, neural tube, and heart serves to differentiate caudal

regression syndrome from sirenomelia, however. In addition, caudal regression syndrome is strongly associated with maternal diabetes, whereas sirenomelia is typically due to bilateral renal agenesis and associated severe pulmonary hypoplasia [Das et al., 2002].

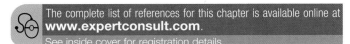

The complete list of references for this chapter is available online at **www.expertconsult.com**. See inside cover for registration details.

Disorders of Forebrain Development

Elliott H. Sherr and Jin S. Hahn

Introduction

The prosencephalon forms at the end of primary neurulation as one of three principal vesicles: the hindbrain, the midbrain, and the forebrain (prosencephalon). Detailed embryology of the normal prosencephalon is beyond the scope of this chapter, but is covered comprehensively in Rao and Jacobson [2005]. The primary disorders of prosencephalic formation, prosencephaly and atelencephaly, are extremely rare and not further discussed in this chapter. The major disorders of prosencephalic formation, holoprosencephaly, agenesis of the corpus callosum, and septo-optic dysplasia, are discussed below, after a brief introduction to prosencephalic development.

Prosencephalon Patterning

Prosencephalic development occurs by inductive interactions under the primary influence of the prechordal mesoderm. The peak time period of development is the second and third months of gestation, with the earliest prominent phases in the fifth and sixth weeks of gestation. The major inductive relationship of concern is between the notochord/prechordal mesoderm and the forebrain. This interaction occurs ventrally at the rostral end of the embryo, and thus the term ventral induction is sometimes used. The inductive interaction influences formation of much of the face and of the forebrain; accordingly, severe disorders of brain development at this time usually result in striking facial anomalies. Development of the prosencephalon is considered best in terms of three sequential events: prosencephalic formation, prosencephalic cleavage, and midline prosencephalic development (Figure 23-1). Prosencephalic formation begins at the rostral end of the neural tube at the end of the first month and the beginning of the second month of gestation. It consists of segmentation of the prosencephalon into three major domains, termed prosomeres (P1–P3). P1 gives rise to the pretectum, the region of brain immediately rostral to the midbrain-derived tectum. P2 is associated with development of the thalamus, and P3 gives rise to the prethalamus. More rostral brain regions, including the telencephalon, are also divided into prosomeric boundaries, the clearest of which are the anatomic boundaries of the developing basal ganglia, the medial and lateral basal ganglia, which arise as bulges along the ventrolateral telencephalon and express the markers Dlx and Arx. The neocortex itself exhibits regionally restricted gene expression. Manipulation of these expression patterns results in shifting of cellular identities

of the neocortex (*FGF8*, *EMX2*). The evidence to date, however, argues against anatomically and regionally restricted boundaries, because cell lineage experiments demonstrate that sibling cells can occupy multiple nuclei throughout the anteroposterior axis.

Prosencephalic Cleavage

Prosencephalic cleavage occurs most actively in the fifth and sixth weeks of gestation and includes three basic cleavages:
1. horizontal, to form the paired optic vesicles, and olfactory bulbs and tracts
2. transverse, to separate the telencephalon from the diencephalons
3. sagittal, to form the paired cerebral hemispheres, lateral ventricles, and the basal ganglia from the telencephalon.

Three crucial thickenings or plates of tissue become apparent around the end of the second month; these are the commissural, the chiasmatic, and the hypothalamic plates. These structures are important in the formation, respectively, of the corpus callosum and septum pellucidum, the optic nerve chiasm, and the hypothalamic structures. The most prominent of these embryologic changes is the formation of the corpus callosum, the earliest component of which appears at 9 weeks. Disorders associated with abnormal development of the prosencephalon are outlined in Table 23-1.

Holoprosencephaly

Holoprosencephaly (HPE) is a complex brain malformation characterized by a failure of the forebrain (prosencephalon) to separate completely into two distinct cerebral hemispheres (i.e., distinct telencephalon and diencephalon). This process is normally completed by the fifth week of gestation [Golden, 1999].

HPE is typically associated with midline facial anomalies.

Historical Background

Individuals with cyclopia have been described for centuries in mythology and in the scientific literature since the late 18th century [Siebert et al., 1990]. In 1882, Kundrat first described the cerebral changes of HPE, including absent olfactory nerves. Believing the absence of olfactory lobes and bulbs was the cardinal feature, he termed the condition "arhinencephaly"

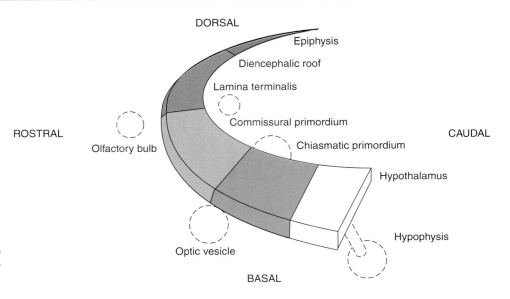

Fig. 23-1 Prosencephalic midline development. The prosencephalic midline is presented by a series of independent but closely related segments. Note particularly the commissural, chiasmatic, and hypothalamic primordia or plates. The proximity of these structures in the developing brain and their derivation from a common primordium explain the spectrum of midline defects associated with septo-optic dysplasia, which include optic nerve hypoplasia and hypothalamic and corpus callosum defects. *(From Leech RW, Shuman RM. Holoprosencephaly and related midline cerebral anomalies: A review. J Child Neurol 1986;1:3.)*

Table 23-1 Disorders of Midline Prosencephalic Development

Region Affected	Disorder
Commissural plate	Agenesis of the corpus callosum and/or septum pellucidum
Commissural and chiasmatic plates	Septo-optic dysplasia
Commissural, chiasmatic, and hypothalamic plates	Septo-optic-hypothalamic dysplasia

[Kundrat, 1882]. Yakovlev recognized involvement of the entire telencephalon and called the single telencephalic ventricle a "holosphere" and the malformation "holotelencephaly" [Yakovlev, 1959]. DeMyer found that the thalamus and other diencephalic structures were also involved and coined the still-favored term "holoprosencephaly" to indicate that the defect involved the entire prosencephalon [DeMyer and Zeman, 1963].

Epidemiology

HPE is the most common developmental defect of the forebrain and midface in humans, and occurs in 1 in 250 pregnancies [Matsunaga and Shiota, 1977], but because only 3 percent of the fetuses with HPE survive to delivery, the incidence in live births is only approximately 1:10,000 [Bullen et al., 2001; Croen et al., 2000; Forrester and Merz, 2000; Rasmussen et al., 1996]. Two-thirds of affected patients have the most severe subtype of HPE [Ming and Muenke, 1998]. However, high-resolution magnetic resonance imaging (MRI) has increased identification of children with less severe forms who are not diagnosed until later in infancy. Therefore, the true live birth prevalence of HPE may be higher than previously estimated, and the proportion of cases with milder subtypes appears to be increasing in more recently reported series [Stashinko et al., 2004]. There also appears to be a slight female preponderance in some case series. A few studies of limited size suggest a higher than average prevalence of HPE in Far East Asians and Filipinos [Forrester and Merz, 2000].

Definition and Subtypes of Holoprosencephaly

The sine qua non of HPE is an incomplete separation of the cerebral hemispheres that results in lack of cleavage (nonseparation) of midline structures involving the telencephalon and diencephalon. HPE typically is divided into three main subtypes, delineated by DeMyer and co-workers [DeMyer, 1987; DeMyer and Zeman, 1963] and distinguished by the degree of separation of the cerebral hemispheres (Figure 23-2).

In the most severe type, alobar HPE, nearly complete lack of separation of the cerebral hemispheres is characteristic, with a single midline ventricle very often communicating with a dorsal cyst. The interhemispheric fissure and corpus callosum are completely absent. In the intermediate form, semilobar HPE, the anterior hemispheres are not separated, but some degree of separation of the posterior hemispheres is seen. Similarly, the genu and body of the corpus callosum are absent, but the splenium is present. The frontal horns of the lateral ventricles are not developed, but the posterior horns are present. The mildest form, lobar HPE, is characterized by lack of separation of the most rostral and ventral aspects of the cerebral hemispheres. The splenium and body of the corpus callosum are present, but the genu is absent. Rudimentary frontal horns may be present.

In addition to DeMyer's classic HPE types, another subtype is identifiable, the middle interhemispheric variant [Simon et al., 2002]. In this variant, the midportion of the cerebral hemispheres is continuous across the midline, with absence

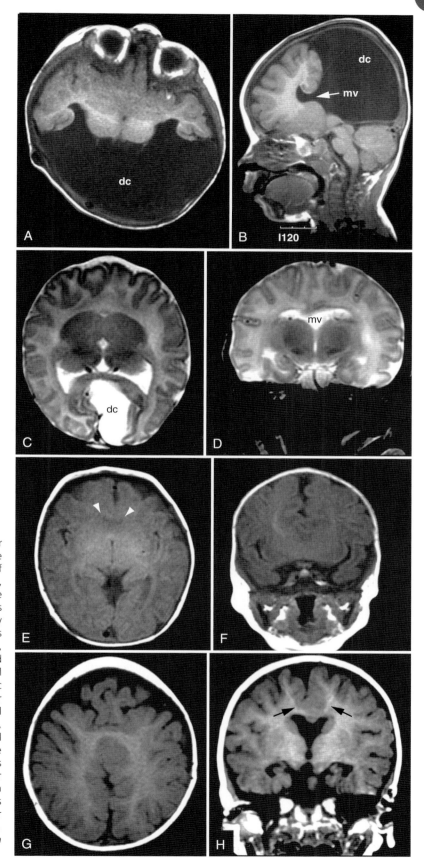

Fig. 23-2 Subtypes of holoprosencephaly. A and **B,** Alobar holoprosencephaly on T1-weighted magnetic resonance imaging (MRI) study. The axial image **(A)** reveals the lack of separation of the cerebral hemispheres and deep gray nuclei, with large dorsal cyst (dc) posteriorly. The sagittal image **(B)** shows the midline monoventricle (mv) that communicates with the dorsal cyst. **C** and **D,** Semilobar holoprosencephaly on T2-weighted MRI study. The axial image **(C)** demonstrates lack of separation of the cerebral hemispheres anteriorly, absence of the anterior horns of the lateral ventricles, and incomplete separation of the basal ganglia. The coronal image **(D)** reveals the absence of the interhemispheric fissure, and the presence of a monoventricle. **E** and **F,** Lobar holoprosencephaly on T1-weighted MRI study. The axial image **(E)** shows the presence of an interhemispheric fissure, both anteriorly and posteriorly, separating the cerebral hemispheres. There are rudimentary frontal horns of the lateral ventricles (arrowheads). The coronal image **(F)** shows the incomplete separation of the inferior frontal lobes near the midline. **G** and **H,** Middle interhemispheric variant on T1-weighted MRI study. The axial **(G)** and coronal **(H)** images demonstrate continuity of the gray matter in the posterior frontal lobes across the midline (arrows). *(From Hahn JS, Plawner LL. Evaluation and management of children with holoprosencephaly. Pediatr Neurol 2004;31:79.)*

of the corpus callosum seen only in this region. There is separation of the anterior frontal lobes, basal forebrain, and occipital lobes. Evidence for this malformation being a subtype of HPE is bolstered by the finding that a mutation in the *ZIC2* gene, which has been implicated in causing the classic forms of HPE, also has been found in patients with the middle interhemispheric variant [Brown et al., 2001; Solomon et al., 2010].

In addition to nonseparation of the cerebral hemispheres, failure of separation also is common in the hypothalamic, caudate, lentiform, and thalamic nuclei. About one-quarter of patients have some degree of midbrain nonseparation [Simon et al., 2000]. Occasionally, isolated neuronal heterotopias are seen, particularly in the middle interhemispheric variant. The gyri often are normally developed, although in alobar and semilobar HPE the gyri may be excessively smooth or broad [Barkovich et al., 2002].

Although HPE is typically divided into these subtypes, the degree of malformation and brain regions involved occur along a spectrum, and individual patients frequently do not fall neatly into any one category [Hahn and Barnes, 2010]. Milder cases are being increasingly identified with use of high-resolution MRI. For example, a mild form of lobar HPE (septo-preoptic type) can be recognized, with minimal cortical fusion restricted to the preoptic regions (involving the suprachiasmic region and anterior hypothalamus) and/or the septal region (subcallosal region) [Hahn et al., 2010].

Neuropathological Findings

Cytoarchitecturally, the brain usually shows normal cortical layering; in some rare cases, the histopathology may show disorganization or abnormal lamination [Golden, 1999]. The defects in cortical organization may represent secondary injury to the cerebral cortex or an abnormality in connections into and out of the cerebral cortex. Periventricular and white-matter glioneuronal heterotopia are also encountered in rare cases. The hippocampus is virtually always present, although it may show incomplete or abnormal development [Golden, 1999]. The cerebellum may show various degrees of cell migration abnormalities, such as misplaced nodules that are aberrantly located in the white matter or within the dentate nuclei [Larroche, 1977].

Etiology

Multiple environmental and genetic factors have been implicated in causing HPE. Prenatal exposures to a variety of toxins, medications, and infections also have been reported. Anecdotal reports suggest viruses, low-calorie diets, hypocholesterolemia, maternal diabetes, and use of salicylates, alcohol, and contraceptives as possible causes [Johnson and Rasmussen, 2010]. The strongest teratogenic evidence exists for maternal diabetes [Barr et al., 1983] and exposure to alcohol [Sulik and Johnston, 1982] and retinoic acid [Croen et al., 2000]. A diabetic mother's risk of having a child with HPE is approximately 1 percent, a greater than 100-fold increase over the general population. A recent population study confirmed the risks of pre-existing maternal diabetes and salicylates (aspirin), but also noted an increased risk with artificial reproductive therapy [Miller et al., 2010]. Some teratogens are thought to produce HPE via interference with the sonic hedgehog gene signaling

pathways, mediated by perturbations of either cholesterol biosynthesis or the ability of target tissue to sense or transduce the sonic hedgehog signal [Cohen and Shiota, 2002].

Approximately 30–50 percent of live births with HPE have chromosomal abnormalities [Bullen et al., 2001; Croen et al., 1996], but this is likely an overestimation based on underreporting of milder cases. HPE can be seen in association with trisomy 13, trisomy 18, or triploidy. HPE can also be seen in several malformation syndromes having normal karyotypes, such as Pallister–Hall syndrome, Rubinstein–Taybi syndrome, and Smith–Lemli–Opitz syndrome [Siebert et al., 1990]. An updated list of genetic disorders associated with HPE can be found on the Online Mendelian Inheritance in Man (OMIM) website (http://www.ncbi.nlm.nih.gov/omim).

In nonsyndromic and nonchromosomal HPE, multiple pedigrees have been described, manifesting various inheritance patterns, most commonly autosomal-dominant and autosomal-recessive inheritance. At least nine genes have been associated with HPE, including *SHH* (7q36), *ZIC2* (13q32), *SIX3* (2p21), *TGIF* (18p11.3), *PATCHED-1* (9q22), *GLI2* (2q14), *DISP1* (1q24), *NODAL* (10q), and *FOXH1* (8q24.3) [Roessler and Muenke, 2010]. Of these genes, the four most commonly affected (*SHH*, *ZIC2*, *SIX3*, and *TGIF*) account for only 25 percent of the cases of HPE with normal chromosomes [Dubourg et al., 2004; Roessler and Muenke, 2010] and approximately 5–10 percent of all HPE patients.

SHH was the first identified HPE-associated mutated gene and has been the most extensively studied [Belloni et al., 1996]. The Shh protein is a secreted intercellular signaling molecule involved in establishing cell fates at several points during development. Shh is expressed early in development in the ventral forebrain and is critical for ventral patterning of the developing neural tube. It also is expressed in the ectoderm of the frontonasal and maxillary processes. Disruption of Shh signaling in several animal models produces the brain and facial malformations seen in HPE.

The SHH signaling network is the common pathway through which multiple environmental and genetic influences interact to cause HPE. Several of the other HPE genes are important components of the SHH signaling network; PTCH is a receptor for SHH and GLI2 is a mediator of SHH target gene transcription. A well-studied example of environmental influences acting through the SHH signaling network is the association of HPE with various causes of hypocholesterolemia [Ming and Muenke, 2002]. SHH is modified by cholesterol, which is felt to be essential for its proper functioning. Maternal hypocholesterolemia has been implicated in causing HPE. The incidence of HPE is also increased in Smith–Lemli–Opitz syndrome, which is due to a defect in 7-dehydrocholesterol reductase, the final enzyme in cholesterol synthesis [Kelley et al., 1996]. In addition, an outbreak of cyclopia (severe midline facial malformation) in sheep was believed to be caused by ingestion of plants containing cyclopamine and jervine, compounds that interfere with sonic hedgehog signaling by binding to and thereby sequestering the protein "smoothened" [Keeler and Binns, 1968].

In addition to the *SHH* gene, the Nodal signaling pathway also appears to be implicated in HPE. This nodal pathway includes TGIF, NODAL, GDF1, TDGF1, and FOXH1. A complex genetic interaction involving these gene products and which causes a reduction in nodal signaling may produce HPE [Roessler and Muenke, 2010; Roessler et al., 2008].

Studies of genotype–phenotype correlation in mutations of *SHH* have found that the same mutation can result in extremely variable phenotypes. Even within the same family, an identical mutation in *SHH* may result in a severe brain malformation, a "mild sign" known as a microform (such as a single median maxillary central incisor), or no phenotypic abnormality. It is estimated that, among carriers of an abnormal gene, 37 percent will have HPE, 27 percent will have a microform, and 36 percent will have no clinical abnormality [Cohen, 1989]. This great phenotypic variability with the same genetic mutation has suggested that, although HPE was thought of as a single-gene disorder, it should be considered a multifactorial disorder, with the specific phenotype being the result of multiple genetic and environmental influences [Ming and Muenke, 2002]. A large majority of HPE cases, therefore, appear likely to be due to a disturbance of a complex network of interacting genes and signaling centers [Roessler and Muenke, 2010]. In addition, the timing of teratogenic exposure appears to be critical to the specific resulting phenotype. An experimental model using cyclopamine, an inhibitor of cholesterol synthesis, has revealed that varying the time of exposure resulted in a continuum of midline facial malformation [Cordero et al., 2004].

Clinical Manifestations and Outcomes

Along with the midline brain malformation seen in HPE, a corresponding midline facial malformation may be present. In its most severe and usually lethal form, cyclopia, with the presence of a single midline eye and a proboscis (rudimentary single-nostril nose) above the eye, can be present. Survivors may have hypotelorism, a flattened nasal bridge, median cleft lip and palate, or a single median maxillary central incisor. The oft-quoted statement "the face predicts the brain" [DeMyer et al., 1964] refers to the observation that the degree of facial malformation frequently reflects the degree of brain malformation. This was amended later to "the face predicts the brain approximately 80 percent of the time," in recognition of individuals with alobar HPE with a normal facial appearance, as well as cases of milder brain malformation associated with abnormal facies [Cohen, 1989].

Previous studies indicated that children with HPE do not survive beyond early infancy. This may have been due to the identification of only the most severe cases. Early death is typical for most cytogenetically abnormal children and those individuals with the most severe facial features (cyclopia or ethmocephaly) [Croen et al., 1996]. In children without these risk factors, more recent studies have indicated that long-term survival is not uncommon. Among cytogenetically normal patients with all types of HPE, more than 50 percent are alive at 12 months [Barr and Cohen, 1999; Olsen et al., 1997]. In one series of 104 HPE patients, the mean age was 4 years, and 15 percent were between 10 and 19 years of age [Hahn and Plawner, 2004]. Even with the most severe type, alobar HPE, children may survive. In an observational study of alobar HPE, 30 percent were alive at 12 months, with long-term survival noted as well [Barr and Cohen, 1999]. When death did occur in the alobar group, causes were associated with brainstem dysfunction, pneumonia, dehydration from diabetes insipidus, and rarely, intractable seizures.

Children with HPE may experience a variety of medical and neurologic problems. A significant proportion develop hydrocephalus. The likelihood of requiring ventriculoperitoneal shunting is much higher in alobar than in semilobar or lobar HPE (60 percent versus 8 percent, respectively) [Plawner et al., 2002]. The risk of developing hydrocephalus also is higher when a dorsal cyst is present [Simon et al., 2001]. The dorsal cyst is thought to form as a result of the thalami being fused across the midline, thereby blocking cerebrospinal fluid egress from the third ventricle and disrupting cerebrospinal fluid. Most children that have HPE without hydrocephalus are microcephalic.

As in children with other midline brain defects, endocrinologic problems are very common. Diabetes insipidus is particularly frequent, and in one series of 68 children, three-quarters of individuals were affected [Plawner et al., 2002]. Diabetes insipidus can be insidious in presentation; serum sodium concentrations of 160 mEq/L or greater have been occasionally detected on routine electrolyte evaluation and were not accompanied by any acute symptoms. Diabetes insipidus also can have a fluctuating course. Growth hormone deficiency, hypocortisolism, and hypothyroidism also may occur. The endocrinopathies may be due to midline defects involving the hypothalamus and are rarely due to a dysgenetic (e.g., hypoplastic or ectopic) pituitary gland.

Approximately half of the children with HPE have epilepsy, and the likelihood of developing seizures does not correlate with the severity of the brain malformation. The most common seizure type is complex partial seizures, with or without secondary generalization. Seizure type, however, can be variable, including generalized tonic-clonic, tonic, atonic, myoclonic seizures or infantile spasms [Hahn and Plawner, 2004]. In 50 percent of affected children, the seizures are relatively easy to control with antiepileptic medication. Having a concurrent area of cortical dysplasia is a risk factor for having difficult-to-control seizures.

Feeding problems and swallowing dysfunction are common in children with HPE, and are correlated with the severity of the brain malformation. Two-thirds of patients with alobar and semilobar HPE require gastrostomy tubes [Plawner et al., 2002]. Abnormalities of muscle tone are also very common in HPE, and the severity correlates with the severity of the brain malformation. Many children have early hypotonia, followed by the development of upper limb and oromotor dystonia, and lower limb spasticity [Hahn and Plawner, 2004].

Developmental disability affects nearly all patients with HPE. The severity of the brain malformation determines the degree of delay and neurological impairments. Severe developmental delay is present in alobar HPE [Barr and Cohen, 1999]. There is no reported case of a child with alobar HPE who is able to sit independently. In lobar HPE, approximately 50 percent of children ambulate (with or without assistance), use their hands functionally, and have some verbal communication [Plawner et al., 2002]. Formal neuropsychologic evaluation in all types of HPE demonstrates relative strengths in receptive language and socialization, and weaknesses in visual reasoning and nonverbal problem skills [Kovar et al., 2001].

In the middle interhemispheric variant, the incidence of endocrinopathies is much lower than has been attributed to the more normally separated hypothalamus seen on MRI. The degree of motor complications (hypotonia evolving into spasticity and dystonia) and developmental dysfunction is similar to that seen in lobar HPE.

Management

Children with alobar HPE, a dorsal cyst, or normo- or macrocephaly should be closely observed for the development of hydrocephalus. Most experts recommend ventriculoperitoneal shunting for hydrocephalus, even in severe HPE, because failure to institute this measure will lead to progressive head enlargement and greater difficulty in caring for the child [Barr and Cohen, 1999; Hahn and Plawner, 2004]. Electrolyte screening should be performed to assess for the subacute development of diabetes insipidus. Screening for other endocrine abnormalities should be considered less frequently, with assays of cortisol, thyroid-stimulating hormone, free thyroxine, and insulin-like growth factor-1 (IGF-1). Because seizures may not develop in half of the children with HPE, prophylactic antiepileptic drugs are not recommended. If seizures do develop, the possibility of acute reactive seizures should be evaluated for and a serum sodium level checked. MRI also should be considered to evaluate for focal heterotopia. Gastrostomy tubes often are necessary to address the complex management issues of ensuring adequate calories related to feeding dysfunction and delivery of adequate free water necessary for management of diabetes insipidus. Motor difficulties and dystonia may be partially responsive to trihexyphenidyl. This agent may improve upper extremity and oromotor function [Hahn and Plawner, 2004]. Motor dysfunction, including hypertonia and dystonia, is common and may require physical, pharmacological, or surgical therapies.

Prenatal Diagnosis and Imaging

The sensitivity of first-trimester ultrasound examination in the detection of HPE remains unclear. It can detect alobar HPE [Filly et al., 1984; Sepulveda et al., 2004], but may be much less sensitive in detecting milder cases. A recent study from Germany reported a series of 51 fetuses (79 percent having a chromosomal abnormality) diagnosed with HPE by ultrasound at a mean age of 22 weeks [Wenghoefer et al., 2010]. The presence of large dorsal cysts, hydrocephalus, or midline craniofacial defects may provide clues that eventually lead to the recognition of the associated HPE.

Fetal MRI has been used to diagnosis various forms of HPE, including alobar, semilobar, lobar [Dill et al., 2009; Wong et al., 2005], and middle interhemispheric variants [Pulitzer et al., 2004] (Figure 23-3). Other midline anomalies, such as agenesis of the corpus callosum (isolated or with interhemispheric cysts), absence of the septum pellucidum, and hydrocephalus with communication of the lateral ventricles, are sometimes misdiagnosed prenatally as HPE [Malinger et al., 2005].

Genetic Counseling and Testing

The recurrence risk of isolated HPE is estimated to be 6 percent [Roach et al., 1975]. Special attention should be given to the family history, to identify "microforms," such as anosmia or a single central incisor. Such a finding would indicate a substantially higher recurrence risk. Genetic testing for *SIX3*, *SHH*, *TGIF*, and *ZIC2* is commercially available and should be considered if familial HPE is suspected. Prenatal testing for these genes is possible by means of amniocentesis or chorionic villus sampling. The gene tests, in conjunction with fetal MRI, have been found to be helpful in prenatal diagnosis and counseling in a series of pregnancies [Mercier et al., 2010].

High-resolution cytogenetic analysis is important in every fetus or newborn with HPE, since abnormalities can be identified in 24–45 percent of all individuals. Newer molecular methods, including subtelomeric multiplex ligation-dependent probe amplification and comparative genomic hybridization microarray testing, have identified chromosomal deletions, duplications, and unbalanced rearrangements in some patients with HPE. These tests may be useful as an addition to the chromosomal and HPE gene mutational analyses [Pineda-Alvarez et al., 2010].

Agenesis of the Corpus Callosum

The corpus callosum forms between the 8th and 14th weeks of fetal development. Nearly 200 million axons course through this structure and innervate each opposing hemisphere in a homotopic manner; that is, each axon innervates structures in the mirror location in the opposing hemisphere. Absence or diminution of this structure is found in over 1 in 3000 live births, and is the most common birth defect of the central nervous system after spina bifida [Glass et al., 2008]. Callosal abnormalities are frequently seen with other malformations of brain development, including polymicrogyria, heterotopia, and midbrain and hindbrain abnormalities, but can present in an isolated manner (Figure 23-4). Many cases are also associated with birth defects in other organ systems, including ophthalmologic, cardiac, and renal defects. Agenesis of the corpus callosum (ACC) can be caused by chromosomal disorders, and there is increasing recognition that subtle copy number variants (CNVs) of particular genes may play a critical role in the etiology of ACC [Sherr et al., 2005; O'Driscoll et al., 2010]. Single-gene mutations and metabolic disorders can also disrupt callosal development. The best-known and most studied environmental cause of ACC, fetal alcohol syndrome, can also result in a significant reduction in white-matter volume. There is a great diversity of clinical outcomes for patients with ACC. Many individuals with ACC have deficits in social cognition, even with a normal IQ. Many of these individuals carry clinical diagnoses that place their phenotype on the autism spectrum. Conversely, individuals with normal IQ and social deficits are often found on MRI to have isolated ACC; no other brain malformations are found. In contrast, in children with ACC and associated brain anomalies, many have seizures and significant developmental impairment, including intellectual disabilities and cerebral palsy. In some individuals with ACC due to chromosomal, metabolic, or single-gene disorders, the outcome can be quite severe, including a significantly shortened life expectancy.

Historical Background

The corpus callosum was mentioned in the literature as early as the 2nd century by Galen, but the first clear description came in 1543 from Vesalius [Barkovich, 1996], who hypothesized that it served mainly as mechanical support for the ventricles and the fornices [Greenblatt and Dagi, 1997]. In addition to this "architectural" function, in the 17th century, Thomas Willis, Giovanni Lancisi, François de la Peyronie, and others thought that the corpus callosum was the "seat of the soul," perhaps analogous to a more recent search for the "seat of consciousness" [Turner, 1955]. In 1908, Liepmann and colleagues reported a patient with unilateral apraxia and agraphia due

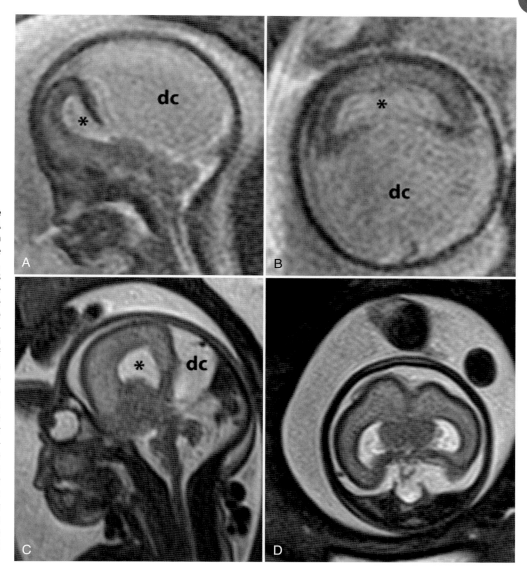

Fig. 23-3 Fetal magnetic resonance imaging in holoprosencephaly. A and B, Fetal MRI (single-shot fast spin echo) of a 21⅚-week gestational age fetus with alobar HPE. The thalami, basal ganglia, and midbrain structures are incompletely delineated on the midline sagittal image **(A)**. A large dorsal cyst (dc) communicates with the monoventricle (asterisk). The hemispheres are not separated, resulting in a holosphere **(B)**. **C** and **D,** Fetal MRI of a 26-week gestational age fetus with trisomy 13 and semilobar HPE. The HASTE fetal sequence in the midsagittal plane **(C)** shows a monoventricle (asterisk), a moderate size dorsal cyst (dc), and inferior cerebellar vermis hypoplasia (Dandy–Walker complex). On the axial image **(D)**, the thalami and basal ganglia appear fused, while the posterior hemispheres are separated. *(From Hahn JS, Barnes PD. Neuroimaging advances in holoprosencephaly: Refining the spectrum of the midline malformation. Am J Med Genet Part* **C** *2010;154C:120–132.)*

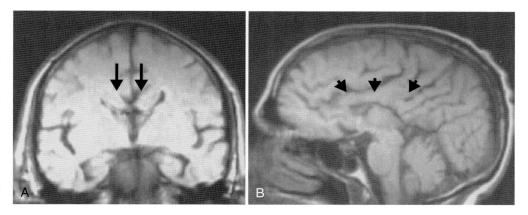

Fig. 23-4 Agenesis of the corpus callosum without other associated central nervous system malformations. A, Coronal image shows Probst bundles (arrows) protruding toward the midline but failing to cross. These are bundles of axons destined to cross at the midline, running rostrocaudally. **B,** Sagittal image shows absence of the characteristic midline corpus callosum (arrows indicate normal location).

to a callosal lesion. This was perhaps the first suggestion that callosal communication was necessary to integrate function of the two cerebral hemispheres. This concept was elegantly investigated by Sperry, Gazzaniga, and others. They demonstrated the concept of the "split brain" in patients who had

undergone a callosotomy for treatment of intractable epilepsy [Gazzaniga, 2000]. These seminal studies presented clear evidence for lateralization and specialization of cerebral function and dependence on integration of the two hemispheres for many cognitive and behavioral tasks [Bloom and Hynd,

2005]. Surprising, however, was the additional observation that severing the corpus callosum, even in a young child, did not necessarily impact development or cognition significantly. None the less, the presence of altered cognitive abilities, even in individuals with ACC having normal IQ, suggests that the corpus callosum plays an important role in brain development, a process that is being better defined by on-going investigation [Paul et al., 2007]. This also underscores the likely significant differences between severing the corpus callosum after birth (and presumably after much of synaptogenesis) and preventing its formation from the onset.

Epidemiology

Agenesis of the corpus callosum is found in 1 in 4000 live births, as assessed by a population-based birth defect study in California [Glass et al., 2008]. This screening method only tracks birth defects (including ACC) that are identified in the first year of life. Because many cases of ACC are detected after the first year, realistic estimates of ACC incidence hover around 1 in 3000. Smaller studies support an incidence ranging from 1 in 1000 to 1 in 7000 [Cockerell et al., 1995; Wang et al., 2004]. In the California cohort, there was a slightly higher prevalence of ACC in African American babies and a lower prevalence in babies of Asian mothers [Glass et al., 2008]. Like many birth defects, the incidence rate of ACC is higher in births from mothers over age 40, with a nearly 3-fold increased risk compared to women in their 20s. There is also a slightly higher prevalence in children born to older fathers, as has also been reported recently for autism [Durkin et al., 2008]. Babies with ACC are nearly four times more likely to be born prematurely than the general population. It should be noted that detection of ACC occurs more commonly with better ultrasound surveillance, and its detection in utero may alert physicians to the increased probability of premature birth [Plasencia et al., 2007]. In addition, knowing about ACC should also alert the clinician to screen for other organ malformations. In infants with non-chromosomal ACC, approximately 20 percent have cardiac malformations, and this has been shown to increase to 61 percent if karyotype-visible cytogenetic abnormalities are present. Musculoskeletal, renal, and gastrointestinal abnormalities were also commonly observed in this series [Glass et al., 2008].

Prenatal Diagnosis and Prediction of Outcomes

The majority of information on the epidemiology of callosal agenesis comes from studies of postnatally diagnosed cases. Because callosal agenesis can be observed only with a brain imaging study, individuals who have a clinical phenotype warranting imaging (ranging from head trauma to epilepsy and global developmental delay) will be diagnosed, while those who are asymptomatic will not be ascertained at the same rate. From these postnatal cases it is unclear what the full spectrum of outcomes is for callosal agenesis. Moreover, there are anecdotal case studies reporting normal outcomes in individuals with callosal agenesis, further underscoring the need to understand outcomes from a perspective free of ascertainment bias [Ramelli et al., 2006]. Routine fetal imaging, particularly as it becomes more common, provides that opportunity. In the studies that investigated all types of ACC in large cohorts, approximately 70 percent of individuals had other associated

anomalies in the central nervous system, including cortical malformations, cysts, and posterior fossa abnormalities [Tang et al., 2009; Glenn et al., 2005; Brisse et al., 1998]. Isolated ACC only accounted for approximately 30 percent of the total number of abnormalities. This distribution also roughly correlates with ratios seen in postnatal cases [Hetts et al., 2006]. The clinical outcomes of these patients have, however, only been studied in case series with a small number of patients, as many of the fetally detected cases result in pregnancy termination [Guillem et al., 2003]. In cases of prenatally detected, isolated ACC, approximately 50 percent show neurological impairment in the first few years of life, but many more show cognitive and behavioral deficits during school years [Moutard et al., 2003]. There is a small subset of individuals who are reportedly normal. These studies also suggest that children with isolated ACC are more likely to have a favorable outcome [Chadie et al., 2008], yet no data are currently available to allow clinicians to stratify prognosis within the isolated ACC group. More studies of large cohorts are needed to address this critical point, and a better understanding of the genetics and other causes of ACC will help in assessing outcomes. Current standard ultrasonography can reliably detect callosal agenesis at 22 weeks' gestation [Bennett et al., 1996]. however, many pregnant women receive a single ultrasound at 18 weeks to evaluate fetal anatomy. There are recommendations within the obstetrical community to perform two ultrasounds, one transvaginally at 14 weeks to assess nuchal translucency and other early visible anatomic changes, and a second study at 20–22 weeks to better visualize later-developing structures, such as the corpus callosum [Timor-Tritsch, 2006].

Development of the Corpus Callosum

The corpus callosum is the largest white-matter tract in the brain, with 190 million axons crossing the midline to innervate homotopic structures. The disproportionate increase in white-matter volume in mammalian, and specifically primate, evolution points to the importance of long-range connectivity (particularly of the frontal lobes) in brain evolution and function [Smaers et al., 2010]. The first callosal fibers can be seen crossing the midline around the 14th week of gestation. The midline is composed of a number of structures that likely assist in guiding these callosal fibers, including the glial wedge, midline zipper glia, glial sling, and indusium griseum glia (Figure 23-5). Some of these structures are known to secrete guidance molecules, such as netrin and Slit2, and the tips of the callosal axons have guidance receptors for these molecules, such as DCC and ROBO [Donahoo and Richards, 2009]. The full complexity of molecular and cellular events necessary for callosal development is not yet known, but these events can be seen within a general framework of developmental steps that include: birth and specification of commissural neurons, guidance of these neurons to the midline, midline fusion and development of key midline structures (as outlined in Figure 23-5), and axonal crossing of the midline with guidance of crossed neurons to final site of connectivity. In patients with ACC, it is difficult to determine which one of these steps is altered, with the exception of patients with microcephaly and absent Probst bundles. These individuals likely have defects in the initial birth and specification of commissural neurons, as found in patients with 1q44 deletions [Boland et al., 2007]. In contrast, it is more likely that patients who have Probst bundles

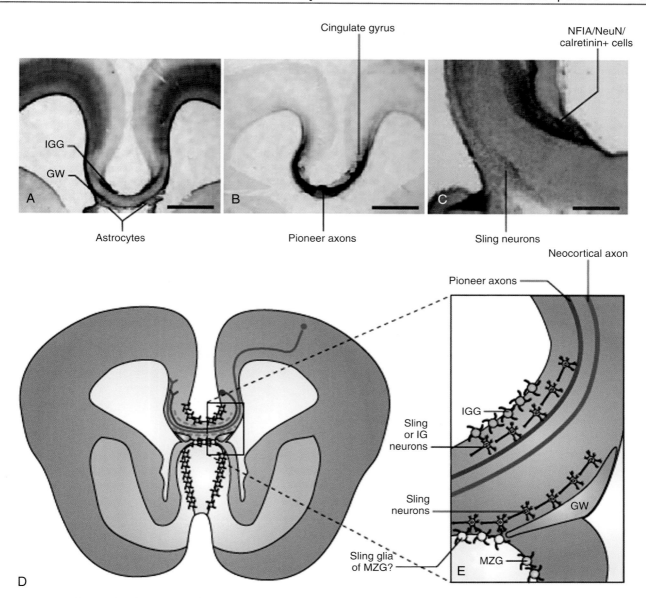

Fig. 23-5 Corpus callosum development. Midline structures support the development of the corpus callosum in the human brain. **A–C,** Coronal sections of human fetal brains at 17 weeks' gestation. Panel **A** is labeled with antiglial fibrillary acidic protein antibody, panel **B** with antineuropilin 1 (NPN1) antibody, and panel **C** with antinuclear factor 1a (NFIA) antibody. **D** and **E,** Schematic drawings of the midline structures that support the development of the corpus callosum. Several midline glial structures are present at the cortical midline, including the glial wedge (GW; panel **A**), the indusium griseum glia (IGG; panel **A**), and the midline zipper glia (MZG; panels **D** and **E**). Pioneer axons, which form an additional potential guidance mechanism, express the guidance receptor NPN1 (panels **B, D,** and **E**) and arise from the cingulate gyrus (panel **B**). In addition, the developing human brain contains subcallosal sling neurons, stained here with an antibody to NFIA (panel **C**). Developing human and mouse brains differ in two significant ways at the midline. First, in humans, differentiating astrocytes are found across the entire width of the midline (panels **A, D,** and **E**). These cells can either be part of the subcallosal sling or an extension of the MZG. Second, a population of NFIA/neuronal-specific nuclear protein (NeuN)/calretinin-positive cells is present above the corpus callosum in humans (panel **C**), but not in mice. It is unclear whether these cells are similar to the subcallosal sling neurons or whether they might form neurons in the IGG (panel **E**). Scale bars: **A** and **B**, 3 mm; **C**, 400 mm. *(Panels **A** and **B** modified, with permission, from Paul LK et al. Agenesis of the corpus callosum: genetic, developmental and functional aspects of connectivity. Nature Neuroscience 2007;8:287–299; © [2006] Wiley and Sons.)*

(and normal or near-normal cerebral white-matter volume) have deficits in axonal guidance or midline fusion.

Imaging and the Corpus Callosum

As outlined above, the initial axons that cross the midline to constitute the corpus callosum do so around 14 weeks of gestation. This cannot reliably be seen by ultrasound until after

20 weeks [Bennett et al., 1996]. Fetal MRI has been used recently as a supplement to ultrasound, and the data suggest that this technology provides greater imaging precision, which may have prognostic implications [Glenn et al., 2005; Malinger et al., 2004]. Imaging of children and adults with ACC has shown that the missing corpus callosum is frequently only one component of the spectrum of brain malformations found in an individual patient. In a retrospective study of 142 cases of

callosal agenesis (82 had agenesis and 60 had hypoplasia), over half of the patients had malformations of cortical development, one-third had cerebellar malformations, and one-quarter had brainstem anomalies. Almost all had reductions in white-matter volume outside of the commissural tracts. Among these 142 patients, only 5 had "isolated" ACC, underscoring the connection between callosal anomalies and other malformations of brain development [Hetts et al., 2006]. It has been observed anecdotally that many patients with ACC have small additional malformations, such as periventricular nodular heterotopia, which are not seen in low-resolution scans and subsequently are only discerned using high-resolution volumetric scans at 3.0 Tesla. Given the high correlation between associated anomalies and seizures, this is clearly important prognostic information to ascertain.

In addition to the knowledge gained from high-resolution conventional structural imaging, new techniques such as diffusion tensor imaging (DTI) have provided novel insights into the full spectrum of changes in callosal agenesis. Evidence suggests that the ventral cingulum bundle (CB) is smaller and has lower fractional anisotropy in ACC patients [Nakata et al.,

2009]. Since the cingulum bundle connects the cingulate cortex with the limbic system, reduction in the CB may explain some of the behavioral deficits observed in patients with ACC. DTI can not only measure the integrity of white-matter tracts but, coupled with tractography, can delineate the anatomical features of major white-matter tracts. This approach has been used in animal models and patients. In experimental studies, conventional dye labeling approaches have shown that the tracts identified by this noninvasive MR technique correlates well with the white-matter histological measurements [Ren et al., 2007]. Because DTI and tractography are noninvasive, these approaches have been applied to many patient populations in the last few years, including patients with partial callosal agenesis (pACC). Two studies have shown that the callosal remnant contains both the normally observed homotopic fibers and aberrant heterotopic fibers. These heterotopic fibers (also called a sigmoid bundle) are fibers that course from the frontal lobe in one hemisphere to the contralateral parietal or occipital lobes [Wahl et al., 2009; Tovar-Moll et al., 2006] (Figure 23-6). Indeed, it appears that many combinations of "rewiring" are observed in these patients. In a few individuals,

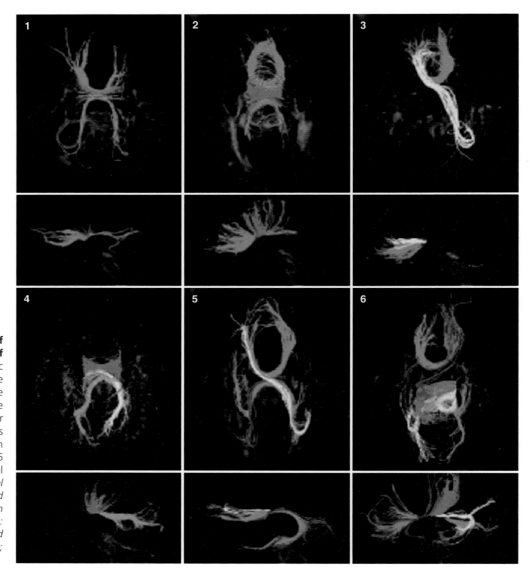

Fig. 23-6 Q-ball tractography of subjects with partial agenesis of the corpus callosum. All homotopic and heterotopic segmented tracts are shown on both axial (top) and midline sagittal (bottom) projections, with the subject number indicated in the upper left corner of the axial images. Fibers are colored as in Figure 23-5, with pink and purple fibers for subject 6 representing anterior frontal-temporal heterotopic connections. *(From Wahl M et al. Variability of homotopic and heterotopic callosal connectivity in partial agenesis of the corpus callosum: A 3T diffusion tensor imaging and Q-ball tractography study. AJNR 2009; 30:282–289.)*

these heterotopic fibers can be visualized by conventional T1 imaging, supporting the benefits of using tractography. The precise significance of these "heterotopic" fibers remains unclear, but they do suggest that aberrant connectivity may be more widespread than just involvement of the corpus callosum. Indeed, an early postmortem pathology study of callosal agenesis cases found evidence for lack of pyramidal tract decussation [Parrish et al., 1979]. Recent investigations in patients with Joubert's syndrome and horizontal gaze palsy with progressive scoliosis lend further support to the notion that DTI coupled with tractography can lead to noninvasive measurements of aberrant axonal tracts [Poretti et al., 2007; Sicotte et al., 2006]. Tractography of patients with a partial corpus callosum also have provided new insight into which regions of the cerebral hemispheres are connected through the residual callosum. The prevailing assumption had been that, if the residual callosum was more anterior, the frontal lobes were likely to be the connected structures. However, data from multiple individuals with pACC appear to contradict this assumption. Rather, tractography data suggest that there is not an obvious correlation between callosal remnant location and the cortical regions innervated (Figure 23-7). These findings suggest that the corpus callosum can be disrupted in more specific ways than previously anticipated and that other white-matter tracts may also be affected, even if none of these findings is detectable on conventional imaging.

Etiology

Genetic

As outlined above, many molecular and cellular processes are necessary for normal callosal formation. Therefore, disruption of any of these processes can lead to callosal agenesis. There are many single-gene recessive disorders that are associated with callosal agenesis (Table 23-2), but it is currently unclear what percentage of cases can be accounted for by single-gene recessive disorders. The rate of familial recurrence has not been studied, but even in large research cohorts the number of multiplex families is small. This suggests that de novo genetic events may play an important role. In the California cohort, 17 percent of ACC patients had a causative chromosomal disorder, ranging from aneuploidies to translocations, deletions, and duplications, which were all cytogenetically visible [Glass et al., 2008]. A recent publication catalogs de novo deletions and duplications at recurrent genetic loci from nearly 400 ACC patients [O'Driscoll et al., 2010]. These include regions in 1p36, 1q4, 6p25, 6q2, 8p, 13q, and 14q. There are also unpublished data demonstrating smaller chromosomal CNVs in ACC patients. Preliminary data from that study suggest that over 15 percent of ACC patients have a large de novo CNV that may be causative. Other modes of inheritance are also likely, such as autosomal-recessive with multiple interacting loci or autosomal-dominant with partial penetrance. Although the initial presumption has been that most cases of

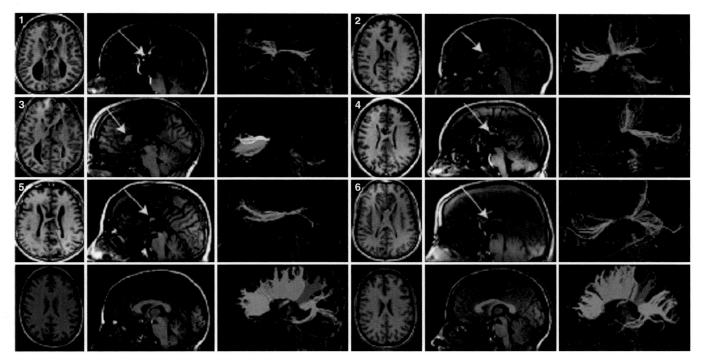

Fig. 23-7 T1-weighted anatomic images and diffusion tensor imaging tractography of six subjects with partial agenesis of the corpus callosum (panels in top three rows) and two representative controls (bottom row of panels). Axial (left) and midline sagittal (middle) T1 sections are shown for each subject. Callosal fragments are identified with yellow arrows, whereas heterotopic fibers visible on T1-weighted images are denoted by red arrows. Midline sagittal diffusion tensor imaging color maps are shown with segmented callosal fibers (right). For subjects with partial agenesis of the corpus callosum, connectivity ranged from anterior frontal connections (subject 3) to only posterior frontal and occipitotemporal connections (subject 4). One individual (subject 5) displayed a discontinuous set of homotopic callosal connections, with anterior frontal and occipitotemporal connectivity but no posterior frontal or parietal connections. All of the control subjects, results from only two of whom are shown, displayed similar callosal morphology and tractography results. Tracts are segmented and colored according to their cortical projections: homotopic anterior frontal, blue; homotopic posterior frontal, orange; homotopic parietal, pink; homotopic occipitotemporal, green; heterotopic left anterior-right posterior, yellow; heterotopic right anterior-left posterior, red. *(From Wahl M et al. Variability of homotopic and heterotopic callosal connectivity in partial agenesis of the corpus callosum: A 3T diffusion tensor imaging and Q-ball tractography study. Am J Neuroradiol 2009;30:282–289.)*

Table 23-2 Disorders Associated with Agenesis of the Corpus Callosum*

Disorder	Salient Features
WITH IDENTIFIED GENES[†]	
Andermann's syndrome (*KCC3*)	ACC, progressive neuropathy and dementia
Donnai–Barrow syndrome (*LRP2*)	Diaphragmatic hernia, exomphalos, ACC, deafness
Frontonasal dysplasia (*ALX1*)	ACC, bilateral extreme microphthalmia, bilateral oblique facial cleft
XLAG (*ARX*)	Lissencephaly, ACC, intractable epilepsy
Microcephaly (*TBR2*)	ACC, polymicrogyria
Microcephaly with simplified gyral pattern and ACC (*WDR62*)	
Mowat–Wilson syndrome (*ZFHX1B*)	Hirschsprung's disease, ACC
Pyridoxine-dependent epilepsy (*ALDH7A1*)	ACC, seizures, other brain malformations
Pyruvate dehydrogenase deficiency (*PDHA1*, *PDHB*, *PDHX*)	ACC with other brain changes
ACC with fatal lactic acidosis (*MRPS16*)	Complex I and IV deficiency, ACC, brain malformations
HSAS/MASA syndromes (*L1CAM*)	Hydrocephalus, adducted thumbs, ACC, MR
ACC SEEN CONSISTENTLY (NO GENE YET IDENTIFIED)	
Acrocallosal syndrome	ACC, polydactyly, craniofacial changes, MR
Aicardi's syndrome	ACC, chorioretinal lacunae, infantile spasms, MR
Chudley–McCullough syndrome	Hearing loss, hydrocephalus, ACC, colpocephaly
FG syndrome	MR, ACC, craniofacial changes, macrocephaly
Genitopatellar syndrome	Absent patellae, urogenital malformations, ACC
Temtamy's syndrome	ACC, optic coloboma, craniofacial changes, MR
Toriello–Carey syndrome	ACC, craniofacial changes, cardiac defects, MR
Vici's syndrome	ACC, albinism, recurrent infections, MR
ACC SEEN OCCASIONALLY (PARTIAL LIST)[‡]	
ACC with spastic paraparesis (*SPG11*; *SPG15*)	Progressive spasticity and neuropathy, thin corpus callosum
Craniofrontonasal syndrome	Coronal craniosynostosis, facial asymmetry, bifid nose
Fryns' syndrome	CDH, pulmonary hypoplasia, craniofacial changes
Marden–Walker syndrome	Blepharophimosis, micrognathia, contractures, ACC
Meckel–Gruber syndrome	Encephalocele, polydactyly, polycystic kidneys
Nonketotic hyperglycinemia (*GLDC*, *GCST*, *GCSH*)	ACC, cerebral and cerebellar atrophy, myoclonus, progressive encephalopathy
Microphthalmia with linear skin defects	Microphthalmia, linear skin markings, seizures
Opitz G syndrome	Pharyngeal cleft, craniofacial changes, ACC, MR
Orofaciodigital syndrome	Tongue hamartoma, microretrognathia, clinodactyly
Pyruvate decarboxylase deficiency	Lactic acidosis, seizures, severe MR and spasticity
Rubinstein–Taybi syndrome	Broad thumbs and great toes, MR, microcephaly
Septo-optic dysplasia (DeMorsier's syndrome)	Hypoplasia of septum pellucidum and optic chiasm
Sotos' syndrome	Physical overgrowth, MR, craniofacial changes
Warburg micro syndrome	Microcephaly, micropthalmia, microgenitalia, MR
Wolf–Hirschhorn syndrome	Microcephaly, seizures, cardiac defects, 4p−

* Reliable incidence data are unavailable for these very rare syndromes.
[†] Gene symbols in brackets.
[‡] Many of these may also consistently have a thin or dysplastic corpus callosum, such as Sotos' syndrome or agenesis of the corpus callosum (ACC) with spastic paraparesis (SPG11). The overlap between ACC and these conditions is still under investigation. Other gene symbols are omitted from this section.
4p−, deletion of the terminal region of the short arm of chromosome 4, defines the genotype for Wolf–Hirschhorn patients; ACC, agenesis of the corpus callosum; ARX, Aristaless-related homeobox gene; CDH, congenital diaphragmatic hernia; HSAS/MASA, X-linked hydrocephalus/mental retardation, aphasia, shuffling gait, and adducted thumbs; KCC3, KCl co-transporter 3; L1CAM, L1 cell adhesion molecule; MR, mental retardation; MRPS16, mitochondrial ribosomal protein S16; SPG11, spastic paraplegia 11; XLAG, X-linked lissencephaly with absent corpus callosum and ambiguous genitalia; ZFHX1B, zinc finger homeobox 1b.

ACC have a genetic etiology, it is possible that nongenetic causes, although less well studied and understood, may play an important etiologic role.

Nongenetic

The best example of environmental causes of ACC is fetal alcohol syndrome. A number of studies report both loss of white-matter volume alone, and callosal agenesis without appreciable white-matter volume loss in fetal alcohol syndrome [Riley et al., 1995; Swayze et al., 1997; Bookstein et al., 2002; Spadoni et al., 2006]. There is clearly variability in the expression of callosal deficits in fetal alcohol syndrome, but it is unclear whether this relates to timing and amount of alcohol consumption or whether genetic factors in the mother or baby may play a role. In mouse models, genetic background does influence severity of brain injury [Wainwright and Gagnon, 1985]. Additionally, the cell surface molecule L1, which is involved in both axon guidance and fasciculation, has been proposed to be a target for alcohol toxicity on the brain by directly inhibiting cell–cell adhesion [Ramanathan et al., 1996]. There are also case reports of herpes simplex virus and cytomegalovirus infections resulting in ACC [Jayaram and Wake, 2010; Chiappini et al., 2007], but these are not well documented. Similarly, there are a few reports of heavy metal toxicity and ACC [Barone et al., 1998], but without many reports, it is difficult to attribute a significant percentage of ACC cases to these causes.

Clinical Manifestations

Association of Agenesis of the Corpus Callosum with Autism and Related Neurodevelopmental Disorders

A wide range of clinical deficits can be seen in individuals with callosal agenesis. Presumably many of these cognitive and behavioral deficits are due to disruption of communication between the cerebral hemispheres associated with ACC.

As in many children with other brain malformations, epilepsy, mental retardation, and cerebral palsy are common [Shevell, 2002]. However, it is difficult to know the precise prevalence of these associated features because most individuals with ACC are evaluated specifically because of their clinical difficulties, introducing ascertainment bias. With that limitation in mind, many studies have reported that patients with ACC have significant cognitive and neuromotor impairment [Lacey, 1985]. Epilepsy is common and is more prevalent in patients who have other associated brain malformations, such as periventricular nodular heterotopia or polymicrogyria. In addition to cognitive impairment, many patients with ACC have behavioral difficulties, such as autism and attention-deficit hyperactivity disorder [Badaruddin et al., 2007]. Autistic features are present in approximately 40 percent of patients with ACC who have normal IQs, and many of these individuals have autism by strict research criteria (i.e., using standardized neuropsychological tests such as the Autism Diagnostic Interview – Revised and the Autism Diagnostic Observation Schedule; see Chapter 48) [Lau et al., 2010]. A more detailed analysis shows that these "high-functioning" individuals with ACC have problems with social cognition, paralinguistic communication, and executive function skills [Paul et al., 2007; Symington et al., 2010; Brown et al., 2005]. These deficits help to explain how individuals with ACC have difficulties holding down jobs, finding partners, and living independently, even though they may have normal intelligence. Indeed, Kim Peek, whose life was fictionalized in the movie *Rain Man*, had callosal agenesis [Ross, 2006]. There is also literature evidence to support the association of schizophrenia with ACC [David, 1994].

Management

Currently, the mainstay of management for patients with ACC includes symptomatic measures similar to those described above for patients with HPE. These may include use of antiepileptic drugs for epilepsy, physical and occupational therapy for hypotonia and cerebral palsy, and speech therapy. Patients with ACC, including apparently high-functioning individuals, often have difficulty with more complex cognitive and behavioral tasks [Paul et al., 2007; Symington et al., 2010; Brown et al., 2005; Brown and Paul, 2000; Paul et al., 2003, Paul et al., 2004]. Anecdotal reports suggest that these individuals do better with therapy targeted at simplifying these tasks, providing repetition, and supporting a slower learning pace. Many individuals with ACC have social deficits, but appear to desire social interactions [Symington et al., 2010]. With recent reports of the potential benefits of intranasal oxytocin treatment for autistic individuals with social deficits, some have hypothesized that similar approaches may have long-lasting benefits in ACC patients. This approach remains to be tested.

Septo-Optic Dysplasia

The constellation of symptoms that comprise septo-optic dysplasia (SOD) is presumed to result from failure of formation of the optic nerves, septum pellucidum, pituitary gland, and all midline structures within the prosencephalon (Figure 23-8). Patients typically present with pituitary hormone abnormalities that can result in hypoglycemia or microphallus at birth,

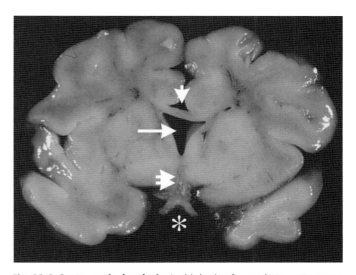

Fig. 23-8 Septo-optic dysplasia. In this brain of a newborn, note corpus callosum thinning (short arrow), absent septum pellucidum (long arrow), hypothalamic hypoplasia (double arrows), and optic nerve hypoplasia (asterisk).

or growth failure and other endocrine manifestations throughout childhood. It is a rare condition, with an estimated incidence of 1–10 in 100,000; known genetic etiologies contribute to only a small percentage of cases. Also, data suggest that young maternal age contributes to the risk of developing SOD. SOD is better viewed as a complex (SOD complex), with variable etiology and clinical presentation.

Definition and Subtypes

There are three cardinal features of SOD: optic nerve hypoplasia, pituitary abnormalities, and midline brain defects (involving primarily the septum pellucidum and, at times, the corpus callosum). The diagnosis of SOD is typically made when two of the three features are present; however, given the heterogeneity intrinsic to this constellation of symptoms, most investigators have initiated their analysis by ascertaining patients with optic nerve hypoplasia (ONH) and then grouping those that had both pituitary dysfunction and absence of the septum pellucidum. From a clinical perspective, those that had ONH and pituitary anomalies but a normal septum pellucidum will have similar management issues. In contrast, those that have ONH and an absent septum pellucidum without pituitary abnormalities often have other brain malformations and likely represent a separate group [Riedl et al., 2008].

Epidemiology

The incidence of SOD has been estimated at between 1 and 10 per 100,000 [Tornqvist et al., 2002 #5096; Patel et al., 2006 #5092; Murray et al., 2005 #5094]. This large range arises from difficulty in fully ascertaining these patients and in utilizing a common definition, as some patients just have bilateral ONH without absence of the septum pellucidum.

Etiology

SOD and ONH have been associated with primiparous birth and young maternal age [Tornqvist et al., 2002; Patel et al., 2006; Murray et al., 2005; Elster and McAnarney, 1979]. Additional risk factors that have been consistently reported include maternal smoking and low socioeconomic status. Other associations, such as in utero exposure to alcohol, cocaine, other drugs of abuse, and antidepressants, have been suggested in case reports but have not been adequately sampled in larger cohort studies. Two genes have been found in association with SOD. The homeobox gene, *HESX1*, was shown to cause anterior prosencephalic disruption in mice and humans, including disruption of anterior pituitary development [Dattani et al., 1998]. Heterozygous mutations in *HESX1* have also been found in approximately 1 percent of SOD patients, although these mutations are inherited and show incomplete penetrance [Thomas et al., 2001; McNay et al., 2007]. Another transcription factor gene, *SOX2*, also has been found to be mutated (mostly de novo single-nucleotide changes) in patients with variable presentations in the SOD spectrum [Kelberman et al., 2006]. Chromosomal changes also have rarely been reported in SOD cases [Singh et al., 2004]. Thus, most patients with SOD are hypothesized to result from a combination of genetic and environmental factors, recognizing that other mechanisms are yet to be discovered.

Clinical Manifestations

SOD can present at birth with manifestations of pituitary insufficiency, including hypoglycemia (with seizures leading to death if not rapidly identified), microphallus and undescended testes (from hypogonadotropic hypogonadism), and midline birth defects, including cleft lip and palate, as well as other brain malformations. Because of disruption in anterior pituitary development, SOD patients are at risk for adrenocorticotropic hormone, thyroid stimulating hormone, and growth hormone deficiency, in addition to lack of gonadotropic hormones. Many patients with SOD have additional central nervous system malformations. In the largest study of MRI findings in SOD, approximately half the patients had brain malformations. These included a thin corpus callosum, hippocampal abnormalities, and other cortical malformations, such as polymicrogyria and schizencephaly. As with HPE and ACC, many patients with SOD have developmental delay and cerebral palsy. This appears to correlate with the involvement of additional brain structures [Riedl et al., 2008].

Management

Symptom management is essential in individuals with SOD and careful attention should be paid to the heterogeneity of this complex disorder. Any child presenting with nystagmus should be evaluated for optic nerve involvement, and if ONH is detected, the patient should be assessed for anterior pituitary hormone deficiency. Additionally, many children with SOD can have developmental delay and seizures, and should be evaluated for these possible concerns [Webb and Dattani, 2010]. Because children are at risk for adrenocorticotropic hormone, thyroid stimulating hormone, and growth hormone deficiency (as well as hypothalamic dysfunction and poor production of the posterior pituitary hormones, antidiuretic hormone and oxytocin), they can present with hypoglycemia, diabetes insipidus, and poor thermoregulation. Multiple case reports of sudden death in SOD patients have described these complications [Brodsky et al., 1997].

Isolated Septum Pellucidum Dysplasias

The septum pellucidum can be divided into two parts: the "true" septum, or septum verum, which is a nerve cell-containing area, and the septum pellucidum [Andy and Stephan, 1968]. The septum pellucidum is a thin translucent plate that forms the medial wall of the lateral ventricle. Its development is linked to the development of the corpus callosum, which accounts for the common association of developmental anomalies of both structures. The two major defects include absence of the septum pellucidum and absence of the cavum septum pellucidum, which are easily differentiated on brain MRI (Figure 23-9).

Absence of the Septum Pellucidum

Absence of the septum pellucidum may be due to primary agenesis or to secondary mechanisms, such as hydrocephalus, with subsequent damage. The prevalence of absence or hypoplasia of the septum pellucidum has been estimated at 2–3 per 100,000 persons, although this is heavily biased by the reason

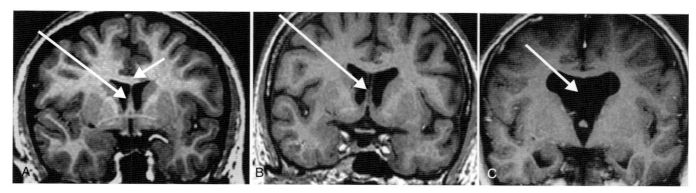

Fig. 23-9 **Septum pellucidum defect. A,** Normal brain, with fused leaflets of the septum pellucidum (long arrow). **B,** Cavum septum pellucidum (arrow) with cerebrospinal fluid between the two leaflets. **C,** Absence of the septum pellucidum. Note the absence of midline structures (arrow), with continuum between the lateral and third ventricles. *(From Born CM et al. The septum pellucidum and its variants. An MRI study. Eur Arch Psychiatry Clin Neurosci 2004;254:295.)*

for imaging and by imaging technique detection rates. Absence nearly always is associated with other central nervous system anomalies, such as SOD, schizencephaly, ACC, hydrocephalus, or encephaloceles [Barkovich and Norman, 1989]. In the rare instance in which no other major central nervous system malformations are identified, then epilepsy and mental retardation are infrequently seen. Absence of the septum pellucidum occasionally is identified on prenatal ultrasound examination, where it may indicate a brain malformation. Most fetuses in which this feature is seen are later found to have a more severe brain malformation, including HPE, hydrocephalus, or SOD [Lepinard et al., 2005; Malinger et al., 2004].

Cavum Septum Pellucidum

Cavum septum pellucidum is identified in approximately 20 percent of normal control subjects [Born et al., 2004]. Controversy exists in the literature over whether this represents a true malformation or just a variant of normal. An elevated prevalence of cavum septum pellucidum has been reported in several psychiatric conditions, including schizophrenia and bipolar disorder. Widely separated pellucidum leaflets greater than 1 cm across occur much less commonly and may be a marker of disturbed brain development, when this finding takes on the same significance as absence of the septum pellucidum. This finding is clearly abnormal only after the neonatal period, because all premature infants exhibit an ultrasonographically demonstrable cavum at up to 34 weeks of gestation. Nevertheless, a large cavum (more than 1 cm in diameter) in a term newborn should be viewed as suggestive of other brain malformations. In one series, all children with such findings had abnormal neurologic outcome [Bodensteiner and Schaefer, 1990].

Disorders of Cerebellar and Brainstem Development

Kathleen J. Millen and Joseph G. Gleeson

A number of newly described syndromes and diseases now allow for careful consideration of cerebellar and brainstem malformations in children. Because computed tomography (CT) scanning offers poor resolving power of the hindbrain due to tight encasement in the posterior fossa, the complete description of these diseases has lagged behind those involving the cerebral cortex. The introduction of magnetic resonance imaging (MRI) in the last 20 years has provided for the delineation of new syndromes, many of which were previously lumped together as "Dandy–Walker variants" (Table 24-1).

Chiari I Malformation

The Chiari I malformation is a disorder of uncertain origin that traditionally has been defined as a downward herniation of the cerebellar tonsils of at least 3–5 mm through the foramen magnum [Tubbs et al., 2007] (Figure 24-1). The anomaly is a leading cause of syringomyelia and occurs in association with osseous abnormalities of the craniovertebral junction. It must be distinguished from the Chiari II malformation (also known as Arnold–Chiari malformation) and the rare Chiari III malformation.

Pathophysiology

Although a number of theories as to the etiology of the Chiari I malformation have been suggested, no clear consensus has emerged. One popular theory that was dispelled was the idea that tethering of the spinal cord causes posterior fossa structures to be pulled into the spinal canal. Another theory gaining favor is that congenital hypoplasia of the posterior fossa occurs due to disrupted mesodermal development [Marin-Padilla and Marin-Padilla, 1981]. There is an increased risk of developing this malformation with growth hormone deficiency and bone defects like rickets. Female patients greatly outnumber male patients, and there is familial clustering, suggesting a genetic predisposition. Gene mutations of chromosomes 9 and 15 may contribute to development of this malformation [Boyles et al., 2006], and it also has recently been linked to Ehlers–Danlos syndrome [Castori et al., 2010]. In about 20 percent of individuals, there is identified trauma that precedes symptom onset.

Clinical Characteristics

Patients with Chiari I malformation may present with a variety of symptoms and signs, ranging from slight headache to severe myelopathy and brainstem compression. The most common presenting feature, in 80 percent of patients, is occipital pain, which increases upon Valsalva maneuver. The headache is described as a heavy, crushing sensation in the back of the head, which radiates to the vertex and to the neck and shoulders, and lacks a pounding quality. The major difference between the childhood and the adult presentation is the increased occurrence of sleep apnea and feeding problems in younger patients. Other common symptoms include pain in the shoulders, back, and limbs, sensory changes, clumsiness, and dysphagia, each observed in 10–50 percent of individuals at the time of presentation.

Initial clinical features largely depend on whether syringomyelia is present, since this defect tends to dominate the clinical picture. Symptoms from syringomyelia, present in 30–70 percent of adult Chiari I patients but in only 12 percent of children, depend on the location and size of the syrinx and can occur as a result of stretching and distention of the cord [Milhorat et al., 1999; Aitken et al., 2009]. Long-tract findings include hyperreflexia, urinary incontinence, muscle wasting, loss of proprioception, and arm numbness/tingling.

Management

Surgical decompression of the posterior fossa with duraplasty is the treatment of choice in selected cases. The purpose of this surgery is to enlarge the bony compartment. It is important to evaluate for coexistent hydrocephalus before any correction is attempted. In patients with a coexistent syrinx, there is a clear indication for surgery, and in a series of 49 children with Chiari-associated syringomyelia, just over half demonstrated clinical and radiographic improvement after hindbrain decompression [Attenello et al., 2008]. In these patients, decompression of the posterior fossa alone is often sufficient to reduce the syringomyelia without directly shunting the fluid collection. In patients without a syrinx but with >5 mm of caudal displacement or with progressive features, surgery may be offered. In some individuals, clinical symptoms and herniation may spontaneously improve, so a conservative approach is generally adopted in minimally affected patients [Novegno et al., 2008] and in those with <3 mm displacement.

Table 24-1 Types of Developmental Cerebellar Disorders

Cerebellar/Brainstem Disorder	Radiographic Hallmark	Clinical Hallmark	Associated Findings	Molecular Findings	Outcome/ Treatment
Chiari I malformation	Herniation of cerebellar tonsils through foramen magnum	Adolescent- to adult-onset headaches and cerebellar symptoms	Cord syringomyelia	None known	Surgical decompression relieves symptoms
Chiari II malformation (Arnold–Chiari malformation)	Herniation of cerebellar tonsils through foramen magnum	Symptoms of hydrocephalus and spinal cord paralysis predominate	Observed in nearly 100% of patients with spina bifida	None known	Surgical repair of neural tube. CSF shunt for hydrocephalus
Cerebellar hypoplasia	Vermis > hemisphere hypoplasia	Neonatal hypotonia and later ataxia	Observed in many genetic and metabolic conditions	Congenital disorders of glycosylation	Hypotonia improves but other features apparent later
Joubert's syndrome and related disorders	Vermis > hemisphere hypoplasia. Molar tooth sign	Neonatal hypotonia, breathing dysregulation	50% with retinal blindness and nephronophthisis	50% with mutations in known "cilia" genes	Stabilization or improvement in most. Cognition may be normal
Dandy–Walker malformation	Cystic dilatation of fourth ventricle with elevated torculum	Mental retardation and ataxia predominate	Hydrocephalus, mental retardation	20% with de novo copy number changes	CSF shunt for hydrocephalus, possible shunt fourth ventricle
Pontocerebellar hypoplasia	Hypoplasia of brainstem with hemisphere > vermis hypoplasia	Severe brainstem defects, as well as hypotonia	Progressive failure to thrive	50% with mutations in mitochondrial tRNA pathway	Patients usually die early in life
Rhombencephalosynapsis	Fusion of cerebellar hemispheres at midline with absent vermis	Ataxia or developmental delay	May be seen with trigeminal anesthesia, scalp alopecia	Occasional chromosomal abnormalities	Highly variable
Lhermitte–Duclos disease	Cerebellar hamartoma	Ataxia, tremor	Cowden's syndrome	*PTEN* mutations	Surgical tumor debulking
Vein of Galen malformation	AVM	Hydrocephalus	Congestive heart failure	None known	Surgical obstruction of AVM
Cerebellar hypoplasia/ atrophy	Vermis > hemisphere hypoplasia	Progressive ataxia		None known	May stabilize over time
Isolated brainstem defects	Morphology may be normal	Ophthalmoplegia	Variable brain defects	*HOX* gene or axon guidance gene defects	Stabilization or improvement in most. Cognition may be normal
Lissencephaly with cerebellar hypoplasia	Cerebral cortical and cerebellar morphology defects	Hypotonia, ataxia, seizures	May be seen with disorder of glycosylation	Basal lamina defects, muscular dystrophy	Highly variable

AVM, arteriovenous malformation; CSF, cerebrospinal fluid.

Cerebellar Hypoplasia

Cerebellar hypoplasia is generally an underappreciated entity until observed on brain MRI, and even then it may be missed, unless specifically looked for based upon symptomatology. Hypoplasia, as opposed to atrophy, excludes conditions in which cerebellar development was normal but then shows progressive degeneration, as in Friedreich's ataxia, vitamin E ataxia, and ataxia with oculomotor apraxia. In patients with cerebellar hypoplasia, psychomotor delay is present in 70–85 percent, and epilepsy in 28 percent [Ventura et al., 2006], although the exact mechanism of the hypoplasia, when identified, can be a better predictor of outcome.

The term "global cerebellar hypoplasia" refers to a cerebellum of reduced volume (Figure 24-2). Typically, the vermis (cerebellar midline) is more severely affected than the hemispheres because the vermis is the last part of the cerebellum to form, and thus, it is probably more sensitive to alterations in genetic programs. The subarachnoid spaces may be passively enlarged. Typical causes include various chromosomal aberrations, such as trisomy 9, 13, and 18, several metabolic disorders including congenital disorders of glycosylation (CDGs) [Vermeer et al., 2007], prenatal teratogenic drugs (e.g., anticonvulsants), fetal infections, or isolated genetic cerebellar hypoplasia, such as that caused by mutations in the

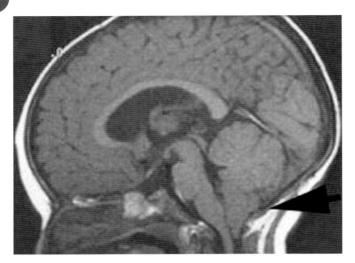

Fig. 24-1 T1 sagittal midline magnetic resonance image of a Chiari I malformation. MRI shows displacement of the cerebellar tonsil below the upper margin of the foramen magnum (arrow).

OPHN1 gene [Tentler et al., 1999]. Cerebellar hypoplasia can also be observed as part of other brain malformation syndromes, such as lissencephaly, pontocerebellar hypoplasia, or those associated with congenital muscular dystrophies.

Pathophysiology

The etiological basis of the cerebellar disorder predicts the pathophysiology, but generally follows some defect in cellular proliferation or differentiation of either the cerebellar Purkinje or granule cells. In the CDGs, as a result of insufficient

protein glycosylation, there is probably an activation of the unfolded protein response, leading to an effect on the cerebellum (see Chapter 35). Likewise, teratogenic exposure to alcohol in animal models can affect neuronal migration by altering established pathways [Jiang et al., 2008].

Clinical Characteristics

An important distinction between the clinical characteristics of cerebellar hypoplasia and atrophy is the striking presence of neonatal hypotonia in the former, and ataxia in the latter. It is important to remember that the cerebellum controls muscle tone in the first few years of life, since the learned motor plans requiring the cerebellum are not in place at that time. After the first few years of life, however, the cerebellum takes on important roles in motor planning, so diseases affecting circuitry predominantly present with prominent features of ataxia, such as tremor and nystagmus, including possible loss of milestones.

Differential Diagnosis

It is critical to evaluate individuals with cerebellar hypoplasia for syndromic forms of this malformation, as well as to consider the various genetic etiologies (Table 24-2). Like most developmental brain anomalies, fetal infections, and toxic exposures, recessive and dominant inherited forms, as well as alterations in genetic copy number (using comparative genomic hybridization), should be considered. Normal transferrin isoelectric focusing can help exclude CDGs. Normal family history may help exclude genetic causes. Baseline laboratory tests, including creatine phosphokinase (CPK), vitamin E levels, and TORCH (toxoplasmosis, other infections, rubella, cytomegalovirus, and herpes simplex virus) titers, looking

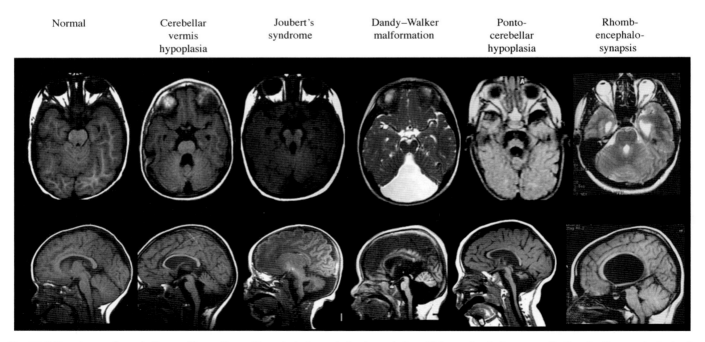

Fig. 24-2 Spectrum of cerebellar malformations. These include cerebellar hypoplasia, which usually displays a predilection for the vermis; Joubert's syndrome, showing the molar tooth sign; Dandy–Walker malformation, showing the cystic dilatation of the fourth ventricle; pontocerebellar hypoplasia, showing involvement of pons and cerebellum; and rhombencephalosynapsis, showing fusion of the two cerebellar hemispheres across the midline and corresponding absence of the vermis. All images are T1 except for fourth image from the left in top row which is a T2 weighted image.

Table 24-2 Causes of Cerebellar Hypoplasia

Cause	Gene	Reference
Cerebellar ataxia, mental retardation and dysequilibrium syndrome	VLDLR, CA8	Boycott et al. [2005]; Turkmen et al. [2009]
Cerebellar hypoplasia with pancytopenia	DKC1	Pearson et al. [2008]
Cerebellar hypoplasia, Norman type (SCAR2) recessive	Unknown	Megarbane et al. [1999]
Cerebellar vermis aplasia (SCA29) dominant	Unknown	Rivier and Echenne [1992]
Cerebellar hypoplasia, mental retardation, distinctive facies	OPHN1	des Portes et al. [2004]
Cerebellar aplasia with diabetes mellitus	PTF1A	Sellick et al. [2004]
Congenital disorders of glycosylation	CDG1 and 2	Jaeken and Matthijs [2007]

for prenatal viral infection, can help exclude muscle-eye-brain disease, vitamin E deficiency, and congenital infections. Mitochondrial disorders should be considered, especially in the setting of features such as growth retardation, hearing loss, acidosis, and respiratory or multi-organ involvement.

Management

The important consideration in individuals with cerebellar hypoplasia is that clinical features usually do not worsen over time. With physiotherapy and nervous system maturation, the clinical features generally diminish. If specific causes can be identified, there is the potential for intervening, e.g., in patients with nutritional deficiencies or specific metabolic disorders.

Joubert's Syndrome and Related Disorders

Joubert's syndrome (JS) and related disorders (JSRDs) are a group of recessive congenital ataxia conditions, usually presenting with neonatal hypotonia, dysregulated breathing rhythms, oculomotor apraxia, and subsequently with mental retardation. JSRDs are the most common inherited congenital cerebellar malformation. The pathognomonic finding in JSRD is the unique molar tooth sign (MTS) on brain imaging (Figure 24-3). There is a tremendously broad spectrum of signs and symptoms, including kidney, retinal, and hepatic involvement, along with polydactyly and facial dysmorphisms.

Clinical Characteristics

The MTS is the result of cerebellar vermis hypoplasia, thick and maloriented superior cerebellar peduncles, and an abnormally deep interpeduncular fossa, which together give the appearance of a tooth. JS is the best-known and probably most common syndrome associated with the MTS. JS is notable for both intrafamilial and interfamilial phenotypic variability. Even in the original pedigree of four affected siblings, two had hypoplasia of the posterior inferior cerebellar vermis and two had complete agenesis of the cerebellar vermis [Joubert et al., 1968].

Clinical features are highly variable for patients with the MTS. Many patients with JS present in the newborn period with an unusual pattern of intermittent respiration, displaying alternating hyperpnea and apnea. In JS, there is no specific lung pathology to explain this respiratory abnormality. Instead, it likely relates to dysfunction of the respiratory centers located in the brainstem or cerebellum [Xu and Fraser, 2002]. Because

some neonates have died from apnea, it is critical to institute careful respiratory care until this feature of JS passes, usually by 1 year of age. Some patients will have relatively mild disease, with congenital ataxia that lessens with age, and a delay in the ability to walk until age 4–5 years, but are otherwise healthy. Other patients will display congenital blindness and renal failure requiring dialysis or renal transplantation. It is important to differentiate the type of JSRD at the time of presentation, and then to monitor the patient periodically for development of any extra-central nervous system signs. If patients do not develop retinal or renal involvement by age 10–15 years, they are unlikely to do so.

The disorders related to JS include cerebellar vermis hypo/aplasia-oligophrenia-ataxia-ocular coloboma-hepatic fibrosis (COACH syndrome), cerebello-oculo-renal syndrome (CORS), and oro-facio-digital syndrome type VI (OFD-VI), all of which share the MTS, but additionally display features that distinguish them from JS [Zaki et al., 2008]. Diagnostic criteria can help distinguish each of the four major clinical entities within the JSRD spectrum.

Pathophysiology

JSRDs fall within the "ciliopathy" spectrum of conditions, which are due to alterations in development or signaling within the cellular primary cilium. Motile cilia are well known for their roles in certain tissues, such as the sperm, where they propel cells, but there is another class of cilia, termed primary cilia, which are nonmotile, typically lacking the central pair of microtubules and outer dynein arms necessary for movement. Several genes associated with JS have now been established, and protein products of these genes are found specifically at the primary cilium in most cells throughout the body. Thus, JS is now included with other ciliopathies, including Bardet–Biedl syndrome, nephronophthisis, Leber congenital amaurosis, congenital hepatic fibrosis, Jeune asphyxiating thoracic dystrophy, and Ellis–van Creveld syndrome, as a disorder of the primary cilium [Tobin and Beales, 2009].

For some of these disorders, like Leber congenital amaurosis (congenital retinal blindness), the relation between primary cilia and pathogenesis is readily apparent, given the fact that the entire photoreceptor outer segment is a modified primary cilium. Within the developing cerebellum, primary cilia have been shown to be essential for reception of the cell signaling ligand sonic hedgehog, which in turn is essential for proliferation of cerebellar granule neurons [Chizhikov et al., 2007; Spassky et al., 2008]. Thus, it is postulated that reduced granule neuron production is the central aspect of the cerebellar hypoplasia.

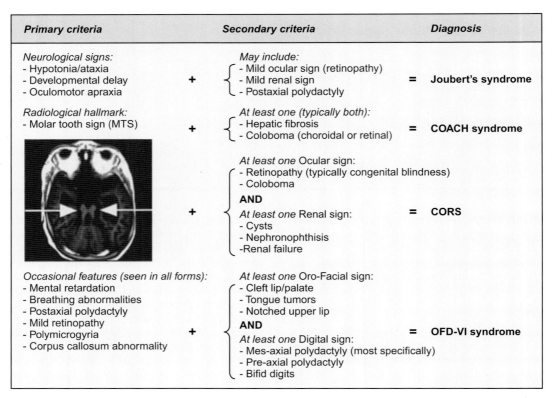

Primary criteria		Secondary criteria		Diagnosis
Neurological signs: - Hypotonia/ataxia - Developmental delay - Oculomotor apraxia	+	*May include:* { - Mild ocular sign (retinopathy) - Mild renal sign - Postaxial polydactyly		= **Joubert's syndrome**
Radiological hallmark: - Molar tooth sign (MTS)	+	*At least one (typically both):* { - Hepatic fibrosis - Coloboma (choroidal or retinal)		= **COACH syndrome**
	+	*At least one* Ocular sign: { - Retinopathy (typically congenital blindness) - Coloboma **AND** *At least one* Renal sign: - Cysts - Nephronophthisis -Renal failure		= **CORS**
Occasional features (seen in all forms): - Mental retardation - Breathing abnormalities - Postaxial polydactyly - Mild retinopathy - Polymicrogyria - Corpus callosum abnormality	+	*At least one* Oro-Facial sign: { - Cleft lip/palate - Tongue tumors - Notched upper lip **AND** *At least one* Digital sign: - Mes-axial polydactyly (most specifically) - Pre-axial polydactyly - Bifid digits		= **OFD-VI syndrome**

Fig. 24-3 Molar tooth sign. T1-weighted axial image through the midbrain–hindbrain junction demonstrates the molar tooth sign (MTS). Note the transformation of the brainstem into a structure with the appearance of a molar tooth (arrows). Primary criteria for Joubert's syndrome-related disease (JSRD) include the presence of neurologic signs, as well as the radiologic hallmark of the MTS. Secondary criteria are used to arrive at a specific diagnosis. The presence of the primary criteria and secondary criteria is used to support the diagnosis of a specific type of JSRD (JS, cerebellar vermis hypo/aplasia-oligophrenia-ataxia-ocular coloboma-hepatic fibrosis [COACH], cerebello-oculo-renal syndrome [CORS], oro-facio-digital syndrome type VI [OFD-VI]).

Differential Diagnosis

JSRDs can be distinguished by the presence of the MTS, which can be detected prenatally and used for diagnosis [Saleem and Zaki, 2010]. In the absence of the MTS, other cerebellar malformations must be considered. In some families, there can be one child with JS and a second child with either a more severe disorder like Meckel–Gruber syndrome, or a less severe disease like Bardet–Biedl syndrome. This heterogeneity cannot be clearly explained by genetics alone, since even identical twins can show divergent severity [Raynes et al., 1999]. It is important to evaluate the whole family to determine if children with such divergent disease might share the same underlying genetic cause.

Management

The management of JSRD can be aided by anticipation of typical problems and the use of genetic testing to help determine prognosis. Patients identified in the neonatal intensive care unit should be monitored closely for apnea. Treatment with caffeine may help promote respiratory drive and an apnea monitor may be required for the first year of life. Because of the heterogeneity of these conditions, it is recommended that

patients be evaluated by a geneticist and undergo screening for coexisting medical problems, including brain MRI, polysomnogram, echocardiogram, careful dysmorphology and retinal evaluation, and annual monitoring with liver function testing and renal ultrasound examinations [Parisi and Dobyns, 2003].

Prenatal diagnosis may be approached in one of several ways. JS is one of the disorders that may be encountered when cerebellar hypoplasia is detected on prenatal ultrasound. In this case, an ultrasonographer may observe nonspecific hypoplasia, and then will seek fetal brain MRI for more specific diagnosis. JS may diagnosed on brain MRI, based on the presence of the MTS [Saleem and Zaki, 2010]. Alternatively, prenatal diagnosis can be made genetically, especially in certain populations with founder mutations [Valente et al., 2010].

Genetic testing can predict disease severity, based upon established genotype–phenotype correlations. Mutations in certain genes for JS, such as *AHI1*, *INPP5E*, *CC2D2A*, and *ARL13B*, can be detected in patients with MTS who do not have involvement of other organs, or they can be detected in patients with MTS together with retinal blindness. Mutations in *TMEM216* and *RPGRIP1L* genes are often encountered in those patients with MTS and renal involvement. Mutations in *CEP290* are encountered in half of patients with MTS together with retinal blindness and renal involvement. Mutations in *TMEM67* are the most common cause of MTS with liver involvement [Brancati et al., 2009]. Thus, the specific gene mutation identified in a patient can help predict the range of organ involvement.

Dandy–Walker Malformation

Dandy–Walker malformation (DWM) is defined by hypoplasia and upward rotation of the cerebellar vermis, accompanied by cystic dilatation of the fourth ventricle and frequently an enlarged posterior skull. It was first described by Dandy and Blackfan in 1914, and is the most common congenital malformation of the cerebellum with an incidence of about 1 in 5000 live births [Parisi and Dobyns, 2003]. Previous definitions of DWM have included features such as the presence of hydrocephalus or the presence of communication between the posterior fossa and the fourth ventricle. Furthermore, the now outdated term, Dandy–Walker variant, used to describe all cerebellar malformations before the routine use of brain MRI, should be replaced using stricter criteria.

Since its original description, additional studies have reported on the various morphological features of the malformation. Studies in the 1970s further defined the characteristic triad of DWM as consisting of:
1. complete or partial agenesis of the vermis
2. cystic dilatation of the fourth ventricle
3. an enlarged posterior fossa with upward displacement of the lateral sinuses, tentorium, and torcular herophili.

This triad can be found in association with supratentorial hydrocephalus, which traditionally has been considered a complication rather than a part of the malformation complex [D'Agostino et al., 1963; Hart et al., 1972]. New data, however, suggest that the hydrocephalus may reflect a common developmental disruption affecting multiple brain regions [Aldinger et al., 2009].

Clinical Characteristics

The clinical spectrum associated with DWM is extremely broad, ranging from asymptomatic to severe mental retardation. Half of the patients have normal cognition, whereas others never achieve normal intellectual function, even when hydrocephalus is treated effectively. The vermis anatomy in DWM is statistically correlated with neurological and intellectual outcome [Klein et al., 2003]. Systemic malformations associated with DWM may include cardiac anomalies (ventriculoseptal defects, patent ductus arteriosus, transposition of the great arteries), urogenital anomalies (hydroceles, vesico-ureteral reflux, abnormal kidney shape), and other abnormalities (duodenal atresia, cleft palate, malformed limbs), and occur collectively in about half of patients [Sasaki-Adams et al., 2008]. Those with isolated DWM can have normal development.

Pathophysiology

An insult that leads to developmental arrest in the formation of the hindbrain, with lack of fusion of the cerebellum in the midline, can be localized temporally between the 7th and 19th gestational weeks. Historically, medial fusion failure was proposed to lead to persistence of the anterior membranous area/roof plate, which could then extend and herniate posteriorly, resulting in a large fourth ventricle. Because DWM represents a fluid accumulation of the fourth ventricle, both Dandy and Walker considered that the defect resulted from atresia of the foramina of Magendie and Luschka, the outflow foramina of the fourth ventricle. However, the finding of normal foramina in DWM, together with new genetic studies, points to defects in the early development of the cerebellum or in the surrounding parenchyma.

The low empiric recurrence risk of approximately 1–2 percent for nonsyndromic DWM suggested that a simple mode of inheritance was unlikely [Murray et al., 1985], and the frequent association with chromosomal anomalies supported this hypothesis. Accumulating evidence suggests that many cases represent de novo alterations in genomic integrity, with focus on chromosome 3q2 and 6p25.3 associated with the Axenfeld–Rieger syndrome [Aldinger et al., 2009]. Additionally, a dominant form has been linked to chromosome 2q36.1 in association with occipital encephalocele.

The genes *ZIC1*, *ZIC4*, and *FOXC1* when deleted can result in DWM. The *ZIC1* [Grinberg et al., 2004; Aldinger et al., 2009] and *ZIC4* genes are produced in cerebellar primordial cells, whereas the *FOXC1* gene is produced by the developing mesenchyme, which gives rise to the meninges and posterior skull, overlying the developing cerebellum. This suggests at least two different mechanisms of disease, one in which some regulatory genes are required in the developing cerebellum itself, and others in the adjacent mesenchyme, with DWM a result of either defect. Because all genes identified to date are transcription factors, DWM is presumably a disorder associated with altered cellular programming during development; however, further research is required to delineate these mechanisms.

Differential Diagnosis

To distinguish DWM from other cerebellar malformations, it is important to acquire both midline sagittal and axial MRIs in order to evaluate for the unique features of DWM. Although some of the older literature attempted to link DWM with Meckel's syndrome, JS, polydactyly, or kidney disease, these previous papers did not specifically evaluate for the MTS. Thus, these patients would probably now better fit within the JS spectrum.

Previous literature also used the term Dandy–Walker variant, which included any of the various cerebellar hypoplasias; this should be dropped in favor of more specific terminology. It is important to consider mega cisterna magna, retrocerebellar cysts, and Blake's pouch cyst in the differential diagnoses [Nelson et al., 2004]. In each of these disorders, there is a fluid collection in the posterior fossa adjacent to the cerebellum, but not within the fourth ventricle, without elevation of the torcula; they thus do not meet the criteria for DWM. Additionally, in these three conditions, which are often found incidentally, the prognosis is usually excellent. In some cases, imaging findings are intermediate between one of these conditions and DWM, and expert review might be necessary to arrive at a precise diagnosis. As mentioned, the association with hydrocephalus, congenital heart disease, urogenital anomalies, and cleft lip/palate can support the diagnosis of DWM.

Management

Hydrocephalus is present in 10–20 percent of patients with DWM and can be treated with placement of a ventriculoperitoneal shunt. In some cases, cystoperitoneal shunting may also be required. Other features are managed symptomatically.

Pontocerebellar Hypoplasia

Pontocerebellar hypoplasia (PCH) is distinguished from other cerebellar and brainstem defects by the presence of hypoplasia of the brainstem structures, as well as of the cerebellum [Barth, 1993]. In the PCH spectrum, reductions in the size of these structures can vary widely, the degree of atrophy being associated with a worse prognosis.

Six forms of PCH have been identified, each with unique clinical and genetic features. In PCH1, there is central and peripheral motor dysfunction from birth, leading to early death, usually before 1 year of age. PCH and gliosis are seen, in association with anterior horn cell degeneration resembling infantile spinal muscular atrophy (SMA) [Rudnik-Schoneborn et al., 2003]. PCH2 is associated with progressive microcephaly from birth, combined with extrapyramidal dyskinesias. Motor and mental development does not progress, and severe chorea and epilepsy are frequent. In contrast to PCH1, signs of anterior horn cell disease are absent. PCH3 is characterized by progressive microcephaly and linkage to chromosome 7q11–q21. PCH4, 5, and 6 are all clinically similar, some with features of mitochondrial encephalopathy.

Clinical Characteristics

Patients typically present at birth with difficulty feeding, with maintaining their airway, or with temperature regulation. Labor may be associated with failure to progress through the birth canal. Patients display global hypotonia with a reduced level of alertness. Brainstem features predominate and include difficulty with coordination of sucking and swallowing and with handling oral secretions. These may be a reflection of defects in brainstem circuitry from development or may represent progressive degeneration of these circuits. There are some clinical features that can help distinguish the various PCH subtypes, but in actuality it is difficult to distinguish precisely between these subtypes solely on clinical grounds, so molecular testing can be helpful (Table 24-3).

Brain MRI shows characteristic involvement of the cerebellum and brainstem, including pontine hypoplasia. PCH is the one structural brain anomaly in which the cerebellar hemispheres may be more severely affected than the midline vermis.

Pathophysiology

The genetic etiologies of several of the PCH subtypes recently have been identified. One of the genes for PCH1 (*VRK1*) encodes for vaccinia-related kinase 1, a serine-threonine kinase required for nuclear envelope formation [Renbaum et al., 2009]. Absence of *VRK1* suggests the presence of a defect in cellular integrity of posterior fossa structures, as well as anterior horn cells, which causes this condition.

Using homozygosity mapping, several of the genes for other forms of PCH have been identified in three of the four subunits of the tRNA splicing endonuclease. These genes, *TSEN2*, *TSEN34*, and *TSEN54*, cause PCH2 and PCH4 when mutated [Budde et al., 2008]. An additional gene mutation in the *RARSL* gene, encoding a mitochondrial arginine tRNA synthase, is mutated in a severe form of PCH, termed PCH6 [Edvardson et al., 2007]. The function of the splicing endonuclease is to remove introns from pre-RNAs, including tRNAs. Since in humans there are several tRNAs that require splicing, these genes presumably help promote maturation of tRNAs that are essential for mitochondrial protein synthesis. These findings suggest that a defect in mitochondrial function underlies some forms of PCH. This has led to the suggestion that PCH represents a form of mitochondrial disorder, although there is yet no evidence of generalized mitochondrial disturbances or accumulation of metabolites typically associated with mitochondrial dysfunction. Furthermore, there is no clear evidence for alterations in muscle integrity or visual or hearing deficits that are often associated with mitochondrial disorders. This raises the possibility of unique functions of these genes in modifying mitochondrial function during brainstem and cerebellar development.

Differential Diagnosis

Diagnosis is based upon MRI review and clinical assessment. It is important to evaluate midline sagittal and axial images to appreciate the reduced size of the cerebellum, as well as the reduction in brainstem volume, best appreciated at the level of the pons, in order to exclude cerebellar hypoplasia from the differential diagnosis. Olivopontocerebellar hypoplasia is a term that recently has fallen out of favor. It was previously used to describe a severe and early lethal form of PCH, and

Table 24-3 Types of Pontocerebellar Hypoplasia

Type	Clinical Feature	Additional Feature	Inheritance	Gene or locus	Function
1	PCH	Anterior horn cell disease	AR	*VRK1*	Serine-threonine kinase involved in nuclear envelope integrity
2	PCH	Progressive microcephaly with dyskinesia and chorea	AR	*TSEN2*, *TSEN34*, *TSEN54*	tRNA splicing endonuclease
3	PCH	Progressive microcephaly, short stature, dysmorphic features	AR	7q11–q21	Unknown
4	PCH	Polyhydramnios, contractures, severe clonus, death in neonatal period	AR	*TSEN2*, *TSEN34*, *TSEN54*	tRNA splicing endonuclease
5	PCH	Fetal-onset olivopontocerebellar hypoplasia	AR	Unknown	Unknown
6	PCH	Fatal infantile encephalopathy with mitochondrial respiratory chain defects	AR	*RARSL*	Mitochondrial tRNA synthetase

AR, autosomal-recessive; PCH, pontocerebellar hypoplasia.

is most similar to type 4 PCH. Certain other genetic mutations can show patterns reminiscent of PCH. For instance, mutations in the *RELN* gene can show reduced brainstem and cerebellar size but without imaging demonstration of progressive atrophy. In addition, the clinical course is not as severe as PCH.

Management

Once a diagnosis of PCH is established, it is important to anticipate life-threatening brainstem dysfunction that may be present at birth or appear later in life. Placement of a gastrostomy tube and airway control can prolong life, but PCH infants are extremely fragile and usually do not survive beyond 1 year of age.

Rhombencephalosynapsis

Rhombencephalosynapsis (Rho) is an exceedingly rare condition of unknown etiology, characterized by midline fusion of the two cerebellar hemispheres. Fusion can be partial or complete, with absence of an identifiable vermis. Brain MRI and neuropathology demonstrate fusion of the cerebellar hemispheres, agenesis or hypogenesis of the vermis, and fusion of the dentate nuclei and the superior cerebellar peduncles.

Clinical Characteristics

The clinical characteristics of Rho are mild and nonspecific, and include signs of developmental delay, hypotonia, and ataxia [Kruer et al., 2009]. Most children can learn to walk and speak, but usually these skills develop between 3 and 6 years of age. There is no evidence of developmental regression and epilepsy is uncommon.

Pathophysiology

The basis of the disease is not established. There are no reported cases with recurrence in family members and there is no increased frequency among families with consanguinity, thus suggesting a sporadic disease. Although a few rare copy number variants have been reported, their pathogenicity remains to be determined.

In one series of 40 cases, Rho was always associated with other brain abnormalities, including Purkinje cell heterotopias, collicular and thalamic fusion, agenesis of the corpus callosum, lobar holoprosencephaly, and neural tube defects [Pasquier et al., 2009].

Differential Diagnosis

Cerebellotrigeminal-dermal dysplasia, also known as Gomez–Lopez–Hernandez (GLH) syndrome, displays Rho, and should be distinguished from isolated forms of this disorder. GLH represents a rare neurocutaneous syndrome of craniosynostosis, ataxia, trigeminal anesthesia, scalp alopecia, cerebellar anomalies, midface hypoplasia, corneal opacities, mental retardation, and short stature. Rho is the most consistent finding in GLH [Poretti et al., 2008a], but most frequently it is seen in isolation from these other findings.

Rho has also been reported in Vacterl-H syndrome [Pasquier et al., 2009], comprising a combination of vertebral, anal, cardiac, tracheoesophageal, renal, limb, and other anomalies, with associated hydrocephalus.

Management

Hydrocephalus occurs infrequently in patients with Rho and, if clinically symptomatic, may require surgical treatment. Affected children also may develop strabismus, and ophthalmological evaluation should be considered.

Lhermitte–Duclos Disease

Lhermitte–Duclos disease (LDD) is a rare condition characterized by a dysplastic gangliocytoma of the cerebellum due to mutations in the phosphatase and tensin homologue (*PTEN*) gene. Whether the lesion represents a malformation, hamartoma, or neoplasm remains controversial because of individual patient heterogeneity. Although the lesion is histopathologically benign, recurrences following surgical resection are not uncommon, suggesting either incomplete resection or independently arising masses.

Clinical Characteristics

Patients with LDD present with ataxia, signs and symptoms of increased intracranial pressure, and seizures [Abel et al., 2005]. LDD is associated with the familial hamartoma-neoplasia syndrome, Cowden's disease (CD), an inherited cancer/hamartoma syndrome involving breast, thyroid, and other organs. Both conditions are linked to germline heterozygous mutations in the *PTEN* gene on chromosome 10 [Backman et al., 2001; Kwon et al., 2001]. LDD is frequently associated with features of CD. In one series of 31 patients with *PTEN* mutations, approximately 10 percent met full criteria for CD; another 30 percent had thyroid disease [Abel et al., 2005].

Brain MRI shows a nonenhancing unilateral lesion in the cerebellum, with mass effect on surrounding structures. The lesion characteristically is hypointense on T1 and hyperintense on T2 images, with alternating parallel hyperintense and isointense stripes that correspond to the inner molecular and granular layers of the cerebellum (Figure 24-4).

Pathophysiology

LDD is believed to be a hamartomatous overgrowth of hypertrophic ganglion cells that replace the granular and Purkinje cell layers of the cerebellum, resulting in global thickening of the cerebellar folia. Histopathologically, there is widening of the molecular layer with abnormal myelination that is occupied by abnormal ganglion cells, absence of the Purkinje cell layer, and hypertrophy of the granular cell layer.

Differential Diagnosis

Since LDD presents in previously healthy children with features of a unilateral cerebellar mass, the main consideration is that of a posterior fossa tumor and secondary hydrocephalus. The unique radiographic appearance of LDD and the association with CD-like features can help distinguish it from tumors.

Management

The typical course consists of an insidious expansion of a posterior fossa mass. Decompressive surgery for symptomatic patients has been successful in improving long-term survival but the lack of clear tumor margins makes resection challenging.

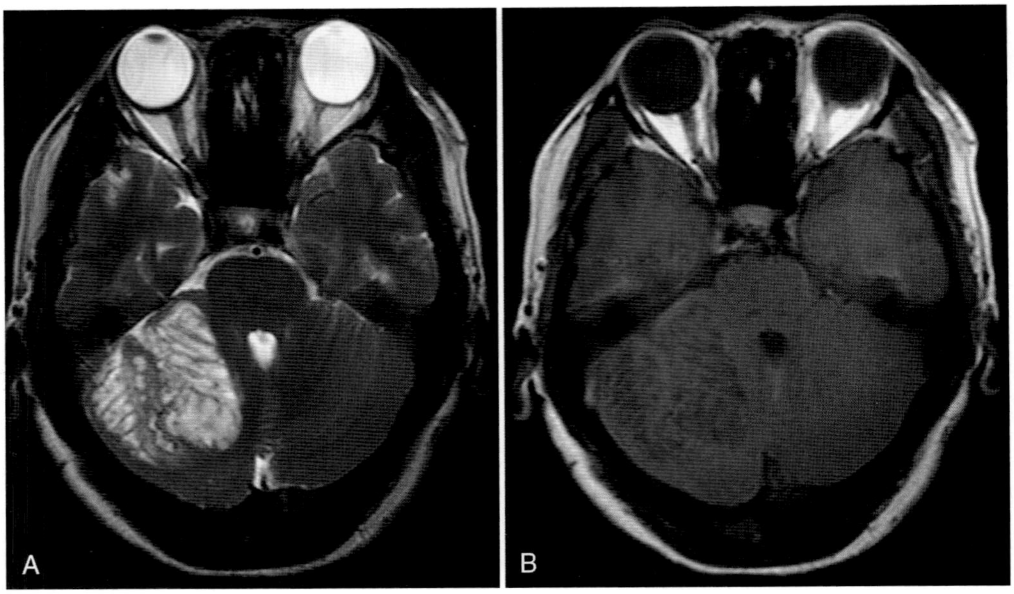

Fig. 24-4 Magnetic resonance imaging appearance of Lhermitte–Duclos disease. **A** and **B**, Right cerebellar hemisphere mass with characteristic striated pattern on T2-(left) and T1-weighted (right) images. *(Used by permission from Qian LJ et al. Neurological picture. Lhermitte–Duclos disease. J Neurol Neurosurg Psychiatry 2010;81:255–256.)*

Chemotherapy is ineffective in treating these hamartomatous-like lesions. Although surgical management and anticipation of other *PTEN*-associated symptoms are the mainstays of treatment, it is possible that use of mammalian target of rapamycin (mTOR) inhibitors (e.g., rapamycin) might be effective, as preliminary studies show hyperactivation of this pathway in LDD [Abel et al., 2005].

Vein of Galen Malformation

Vein of Galen malformations (VGAMs) are rare but clinically significant intracranial arteriovenous shunt lesions that most often present in neonates and infants, classically with enlarging head circumference and heart failure, or at later ages with a combination of central nervous system and cardiac symptoms.

Clinical Characteristics

There are three typical clinical presentations reported within the spectrum of VGAM [Gold et al., 1964]. The neonatal presentation consists of severe cardiorespiratory failure, including hydrops fetalis and renal failure secondary to aortic flow reversal. Of the vast majority of patients presenting in the newborn period, most show high-output cardiac failure with severe pulmonary hypertension, which may be mistaken for congenital heart disease. The infantile form presents with smaller and less hemodynamically apparent cardiac involvement. These patients can present with increasing head circumference due to aqueductal compression by the dilated vein of Galen with resultant hydrocephalus, or can present with nonspecific developmental delay. Other features may include hypothalamic and hypophyseal dysfunction, intracranial or carotid bruit, dilated scalp veins, proptosis, or epistaxis. In the childhood form, the typical presentation is headaches and seizures caused by subarachnoid and intraparenchymal hemorrhages. Such patients usually have insignificant cardiac symptoms [Heuer et al., 2010].

Pathophysiology

The vascular malformation itself is thought to originate around 2–3 months of gestation from the choroidal arteries. The high blood flow, coupled with dural sinus stenosis, causes the anterior segment of the median prosencephalic vein of Markowski (which normally regresses) to progressively enlarge instead, forming the aneurysmal component [Gailloud et al., 2005]. The subsequent left-to-right shunt causes a noncyanotic high-flow state with resultant heart failure and accompanying macrocephaly.

Differential Diagnosis

VGAM should be considered in any newborn evaluated for heart failure, especially in the presence of macrocephaly. Auscultation of a cranial bruit can suggest the diagnosis and brain imaging can confirm it.

Two types of arteriovenous connections have been recognized. The simplest (or "choroidal") type consists of direct, high-flow shunts located within the wall of the venous aneurysm. The second (or "mural") type involves the interposition of an arterial network between arterial feeders and the venous aneurysm itself. This network is usually located in the quadrigeminal cistern and results in less significant blood flow [Gailloud et al., 2005].

Management

Patients with neonatal-onset VGAM historically suffered from a poor prognosis, which has significantly improved with the recent development of standard endovascular embolization. Prenatal ultrasound can detect VGAMs, but MRI and MR angiography can better delineate the anatomic boundaries and blood flow. Conventional angiography is the gold standard for precise evaluation of VGAM architecture, including evaluation of arterial feeders and venous drainage (Figure 24-5). Following radiographic studies, the goal is to stabilize patients with medications until they are old enough to tolerate

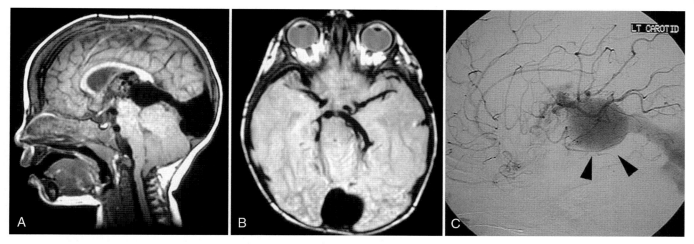

Fig. 24-5 Vein of Galen malformation. A and **B,** Magnetic resonance imaging shows a massively enlarged vein of Galen, straight sinus and torcula, associated with markedly enlarged posterior cerebral arteries on T2 (left) and T1 (right) weighted images. **C,** The angiogram shows a nidus of vessels in the region of the posterior third ventricle, with a large aneurysmal draining venous structure (arrows). *(Courtesy of http://www.med.uc.edu.)*

endovascular surgery. The complete removal of the lesion is rarely achieved because of hemodynamic instability of the infant and location of the lesion. As a result, surgical treatment is now reserved for the evacuation of intracranial hematomas and treatment of hydrocephalus. Embolization is achieved using embolic glue or microcoils. One of the goals is to prevent the development of cerebral venous hypertension, so stepwise embolization to allow for collateral formation is advised [Hoang et al., 2009]. Recently, a 21-point scale was developed to help guide therapy [Lasjaunias et al., 2006], and most children survive, frequently with some neuromotor sequelae.

Cerebellar Atrophy

Cerebellar atrophy (CA) implies the progressive loss of parenchyma following normal development of the cerebellum. The most common presenting features associated with CA are progressive ataxia, tremor, and nystagmus. In practice, it is important, when evaluating a child with such features, to determine if there is associated CA, which can help limit the differential diagnosis.

Clinical and Radiographic Characteristics

In the case of CA, there are few unique MRI findings to establish a specific diagnosis, but clinical features can help differentiate various subtypes. These include those individuals with:

1. pure CA
2. CA with hypomyelination
3. CA with progressive white-matter abnormalities
4. CA with basal ganglion involvement
5. CA with cerebellar cortex hyperintensity [Poretti et al., 2008b].

It can be difficult to separate CA from cerebellar hypoplasia, the former being characterized primarily by the full complement of folia, but with increases in the interfolial cerebrospinal fluid spaces, implying shrinkage of the parenchyma (Figure 24-6). Separation of CA from cerebellar hypoplasia is not always

Fig. 24-6 T1 Magnetic resonance imaging appearance of cerebellar atrophy. This 10-year-old child presented with normal milestones, then progressive ataxia beginning at 6 years of age, without a clear underlying cause. **A,** The sagittal MRI shows normal folia but severe atrophy, with loss of cerebellar parenchyma and wide spaces between the cerebellar folia (arrowhead). The brainstem shows intact structure and appearance. **B,** Axial view shows prominent cerebrospinal fluid spaces between cerebellar folia.

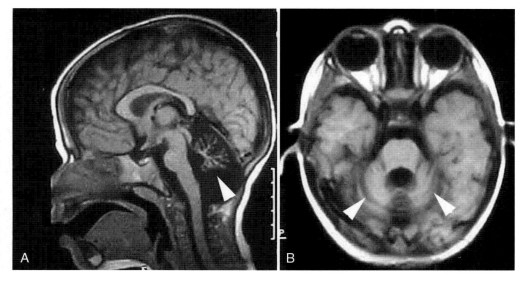

possible and the two can coexist in several different diseases, such as the CDGs.

Pathophysiology

While precise mechanisms are specific to each cause, CA is usually accompanied by some combination of degeneration of the Purkinje and granular cell layer, as well as some involvement of the cerebellar white matter. For instance, ataxia telangiectasia and spinocerebellar ataxias (see Chapter 67) are correlated with Purkinje cell degeneration, whereas in other conditions there is a predilection for the granular layer [Pascual-Castroviejo et al., 1994]. Purkinje cells are extremely vulnerable to various cytotoxic and metabolic derangements, and when these cells are damaged, the whole cerebellum can become atrophic.

Differential Diagnosis

The clinical presentation and appearance of the cerebellum on MRI may suggest the specific etiology of CA (Box 24-1). In some individuals there may be clinical findings to suggest a specific entity, such as the presence of oculocutaneous telangiectasias (e.g., ataxia telangiectasia), cataracts (Marinesco–Sjögren syndrome), progressive myoclonic seizures (neuronal ceroid-lipofuscinosis), or peripheral nerve involvement (infantile neural axonal dystrophy). However, in the majority of patients, such diagnostic findings are usually not present. When they are absent, it is wise to consider a broad differential to include serum albumin and α-fetoprotein (which can be abnormal in ataxia telangiectasia and ataxia-oculomotor apraxia), a lysosomal enzyme panel, liver enzymes, serum copper and ceruloplasmin levels, and a metabolic profile (including a chemistry profile, plasma amino acids, urine organic acids, and serum lactate, pyruvate, and ammonia levels).

Specific considerations for CA include diseases such as toxic exposures to phenytoin or lithium (which are unusual in childhood), postinfectious cerebellar ataxia (usually presents with acute rather than chronic ataxia), and many autosomal-dominant and recessive genetic disorders, as reviewed in Chapter 67. Relatively recently recognized syndromes include cerebellar ataxia with mental retardation, optic atrophy, and skin abnormalities (CAMOS) syndrome, due to mutations in the *ZNF592* gene [Nicolas et al., 2010], and ataxia oculomotor apraxia (AOA) syndrome, which presents very similarly to ataxia telangiectasia (e.g. with progressive ataxia) but backs telangectasias, increased risk for infections, leukemias and lymphomas seen in ataxia telangectasia. Mutations in the *APTX* and *SETX* genes have emerged as the major causes.

CA also may be seen in later stages of Friedreich's ataxia (FA), one of the most common forms of autosomal-recessive ataxia (reviewed in detail in Chapter 67). It usually presents before adolescence with generalized ataxia and absent tendon reflexes, Babinski signs, impaired position and vibration sense, and scoliosis. The triad of hypoactive knee and ankle reflexes and ataxia in childhood is generally sufficient for diagnosis. In FA, it is important to recognize the clinically significant hypertrophic cardiomyopathy and diabetes, as well as the causative trinucleotide expansion in the *FXN* gene, which is involved in mitochondrial function and iron homeostasis. Treatments are emerging for many of the anticipated problems of FA, specifically targeted at underlying pathogenic mechanisms [Schmucker and Puccio, 2010].

Also reviewed in Chapter 67, the various autosomal-dominant forms of spinocerebellar ataxia (SCA) are a cause of CA in children. Although most SCAs present post adolescence, there are a number that can manifest at earlier ages, including SCA13, SCA17, SCA21, SCA25, and the related disorder known as juvenile Huntington's disease. Many of the SCAs are due to CAG trinucleotide repeat expansions within the coding sequence of their respective genes; because the CAG tract encodes for glutamine, such disorders have also been called polyglutamine disorders. Due to the mutability of these expansions, the dominant forms display anticipation, referring to earlier onset and increasing severity of disease in subsequent generations of a family. SCA13 displays childhood onset associated with mild mental retardation and short stature, and is one of the rare dominant SCAs not associated with repeat expansion. SCA17 displays childhood or adult onset associated with mental deterioration, occasional chorea, dystonia, myoclonus, and epilepsy. The other

Box 24-1 Types of Cerebellar Atrophy

Pure Cerebellar Atrophy

- Ataxia telangiectasia
- Ataxia telangiectasia-like disorders
- Late GM$_2$ gangliosidosis
- Ataxia-oculomotor apraxia

Cerebellar Atrophy and Hypomyelination

- Pelizaeus–Merzbacher disease
- Pelizaeus–Merzbacher-like diseases
- Salla disease
- Leukoencephalopathy with ataxia, hypotonia, and hypomyelination
- Hypomyelination and atrophy of basal ganglia and cerebellum

Cerebellar Atrophy and Progressive White-Matter Abnormalities

- Neuronal ceroid-lipofuscinosis

- Niemann–Pick type C disease
- Dentatorubral-pallidoluysian atrophy
- Vanishing white-matter disease

Cerebellar Atrophy and Cerebellar Cortex T2 Hyperintenisty

- Infantile neuroaxonal dystrophy
- Marinesco–Sjögren syndrome
- Mitochondrial disorders

Cerebellar Atrophy and Basal Ganglia Involvement

- Kerns–Sayre and other mitochondrial disorders
- Cockayne's syndrome
- Hypomyelination with atrophy of basal ganglia and cerebellum
- Wilson's disease

forms of SCA listed above have been observed only in single publications.

Management

Except for vitamin E therapy for ataxia with vitamin E deficiency (AVED) (see Chapter 103) and some on-going but as yet inconclusive trials in FA, there are no specific treatments available for the conditions causing CA. Aggravating medications should be avoided. Physical medicine management is helpful (e.g., physical, occupational, and speech therapy; use of canes, walkers, writing instruments, or weights to minimize tremor) and can improve the activities of daily living (see Chapter 105).

Isolated Brainstem Defects

The advent of higher-resolution MRI, as well as diffusion tensor imaging, has allowed for the delineation of a number of developmental brainstem defects [Barkovich et al., 2009]. As the brainstem contains nuclei for oculomotor and facial movements, as well transit and decussation of ascending and descending tracts, the major symptoms of the disorders of brainstem development described to date involve coordination defects, abnormal oculomotor function, and abnormal lateralization of function. The two most important diseases to consider are horizontal gaze palsy with progressive scoliosis (HGPPS) and pontine tegmental cap dysplasia (PTCD) (Figure 24-7). HGPPS patients have congenital horizontal gaze palsy; MRI shows quite characteristic brainstem hypoplasia with absence of the facial colliculi, presence of a deep midline dorsal pontine cleft (split pons sign), and a "butterfly" configuration of the medulla [Rossi et al., 2004]. Neurophysiological studies have demonstrated that there is failure of decussation of the corticospinal and spinocortical tracts [Jen et al., 2004].

PTCD patients display peripheral auditory dysfunction, impaired swallowing, facial palsy, and ataxia. MRI analysis shows a unique protrusion from the dorsal pons into the fourth ventricle, flattened ventral pons, vermis hypoplasia, and absence of the middle cerebellar peduncles [Barth et al., 2007]. Diffusion tensor imaging shows ectopic transverse fiber bundles at the site of the pontine tegmentum and complete absence of transverse fibers in the ventral pons. Because brainstem defects described to date involve unique sets of axonal tracts or brainstem nuclei, clinical characteristics are highly variable. The pathophysiology of some of these diseases has uncovered a role for axon guidance molecules that have been previously identified from mouse genetic studies, including the *ROBO3* and *DCC* genes [Jen et al., 2004; Srour et al., 2010]. The differential

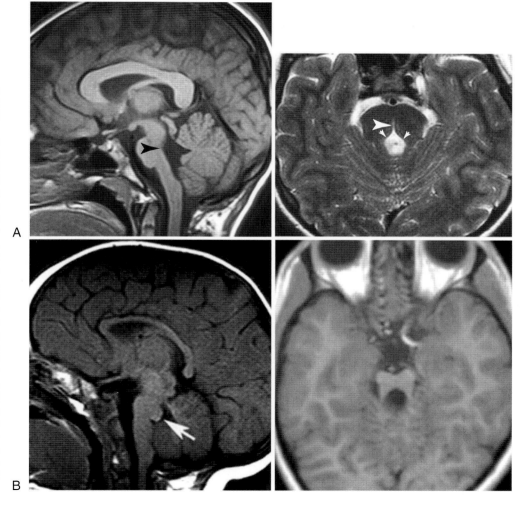

Fig. 24-7 Magnetic resonance imaging analysis of isolated brainstem defects. A, Horizontal gaze palsy with progressive scoliosis. T1 Sagittal MRI (left) shows depression of the floor of the fourth ventricle (arrowhead). The medulla has reduced volume. The T2 axial image (right) shows absence of the colliculi with a "tent"-shaped configuration of the floor of the fourth ventricle and a deep midsagittal cleft extending ventrally from the fourth ventricular floor, producing the split pons sign (arrowhead). **B,** T1 image with pontine Pontine tegmental cap dysplasia, showing the flat profile of the ventral side of the pons, and vaulted structure protruding in the fourth ventricle (arrow). T1 Axial MRI (right) shows an abnormal medullary structure with abnormal orientation of the superior cerebellar peduncles and a "butterfly" configuration. *(Used by permission from Barth PG et al. Pontine tegmental cap dysplasia: a novel brain malformation with a defect in axonal guidance. Brain 2007;130:2258–2266; Rossi A et al. MR imaging of brain-stem hypoplasia in horizontal gaze palsy with progressive scoliosis. AJNR Am J Neuroradiol 2004;25:1046–1048.)*

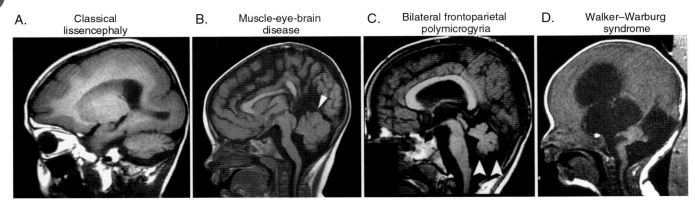

A. Classical lissencephaly   **B.** Muscle-eye-brain disease   **C.** Bilateral frontoparietal polymicrogyria   **D.** Walker–Warburg syndrome

Fig. 24-8 T1 weighted MRI characteristics of lissencephaly with cerebellar hypoplasia. A, Classical lissencephaly (due to *LIS1* mutation) shows mild cerebellar hypoplasia, evident on a parasagittal image. **B,** Muscle-eye-brain disease demonstrates cerebellar hypoplasia and cysts (arrowhead), as well as underdevelopment of the pons. **C,** Bilateral frontoparietal polymicrogyria is characterized by cerebellar hypoplasia with cysts (arrowheads) and underdevelopment of the pons. **D,** Walker–Warburg syndrome reveals characteristic hydrocephalus and severe pontocerebellar hypoplasia.

diagnosis must include the other hindbrain defects discussed in this chapter, and careful review of the structural magnetic resonance, diffusion tensor imaging studies and clinical features can differentiate these from previously described conditions. No known treatment exists for these disorders but rehabilitation medicine management is helpful.

Lissencephaly with Cerebellar Hypoplasia

A number of conditions are connected with cerebellar and brainstem developmental defects associated with cerebral cortical anomalies. These fall into three predominant categories, with unique clinical presentations and imaging anomalies [Jissendi-Tchofo et al., 2009] (Figure 24-8). Many of these conditions are reviewed in other chapters of Part V.

The tubulin pathway defects, associated with mutations in the *LIS1* and *DCX* genes, show predominantly classical lissencephaly with mild cerebellar hypoplasia. The clinical picture is dominated by defects in cerebral cortical lamination, that produce profound mental impairment and intractable epilepsy. The overall cerebellar architecture and brainstem are intact, but they are mildly hypoplastic (see Figure 24-8). Mutation in the tubulin *TUBA1A* shows a wide spectrum of cerebellar and brainstem involvement [Kumar et al., 2010; Lecourtois et al., 2010].

The reelin signaling pathway defects, associated with mutations in *RELN* and *VLDLR*, show cortical pachygyria and severe cerebellar and brainstem hypoplasia. Both the *RELN* and *VLDLR* mutations are associated with unique hindbrain imaging findings, and are discernible with careful review of imaging. The clinical picture of *RELN* is similar to that of classical lissencephaly, with profound mental impairment and intractable epilepsy. Mutations in *VLDLR* have been reported in familial dysequilibrium syndrome and Uner Tan's syndrome (quadripedilism), with variable effects on cognition [Boycott et al., 2005; Ozcelik et al., 2008].

The congenital muscular dystrophies typically show brainstem involvement, although the degree of impairment is highly variable. Walker–Warburg syndrome, due to mutations in *POMT1* and *POMT2* genes, shows the most severe clinical and imaging findings, with hydrocephalus, retinal dysplasia, cataracts, severe cobblestone lissencephaly, diffuse central nervous system white-matter signal abnormalities, and severe brainstem and cerebellar hypoplasia [Beltran-Valero de Bernabe et al., 2002; van Reeuwijk et al., 2005]. Muscle-eye-brain disease, due to mutations in *POMGNT1*, shows intermediate phenotypes with ventriculomegaly, mild cobblestone lissencephaly, and less severe brainstem and cerebellar hypoplasia and cerebellar cysts [Hehr et al., 2007]. Bilateral frontoparietal polymicrogyria, due to mutations in the *GPR56* gene, shows the cobblestone-like appearance of polymicrogyria, as well as cerebellar and brainstem involvement that is similar to that observed in muscle-eye-brain disease [Piao et al., 2002].

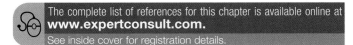

Disorders of Brain Size

Ghayda Mirzaa, Stephen Ashwal, and William B. Dobyns

Introduction

The two obvious disorders of brain size – microcephaly (too small) and macrocephaly (too large) – are very common or relatively common disorders, depending largely on how they are defined. Microcephaly (MIC) and macrocephaly are usually defined as head circumference – or more formally, "occipitofrontal circumference" (OFC) – that is more than 2 standard deviations (SD) below or above the mean for age and gender [Opitz and Holt, 1990; Roche et al., 1987]. However, because this criterion includes many developmentally normal individuals and a host of underlying causes, researchers studying both usually define severe MIC or macrocephaly as OFC more than 3 or 4 SD below or above the mean [Barkovich et al., 1998; Dobyns, 1996; Woods et al., 2005; Jackson et al., 2002].

When defined as OFC smaller than 2 SD below the mean, approximately 2.3 percent of the population would be expected to have MIC if OFC is truly a normally distributed measurement [Ashwal et al., 2009]. The published estimates for OFC below −2 SD at birth are 55.8 per 10,000 [Vargas et al., 2001] and 54 per 10,000 [Dolk, 1991]. Based on 2004 census data of 3.7 million live births in the United States [Dye, 2005], this would predict that 25,000 neonates are born each year with MIC, far less than 2.3 percent of the population, which would be about 85,100 children. The difference may be accounted for by a non-normal distribution of neonatal head size, postnatal MIC, or incomplete ascertainment. If MIC is defined as OFC smaller than 3 SD below the mean, this would be expected to apply to only approximately 0.1 percent of the population, which agrees well with the published estimate of approximately 14 per 10,000 [Dolk, 1991].

The same arguments apply for macrocephaly, but this criterion includes any cause of a large head size, including hydrocephalus, certain bone diseases, and many other causes. When considering specifically increased brain size, the term megalencephaly (MEG), or "large brain," is preferred. Here we will consider the causes of MIC and macrocephaly or MEG separately.

Microcephaly

Microcephaly is a descriptive term that refers to a cranium that is significantly smaller than the standard for the individual's age and sex. It should usually be considered as a neurologic sign rather than a disorder, as it may result from many different causes that affect several different stages of brain development [Ashwal et al., 2009]. MIC is a common neurological sign in isolation, and in association with other abnormalities. Across

the literature and in practice, the definition of MIC and the approach to evaluation of affected individuals are not uniform [Leviton et al., 2002; Opitz and Holt, 1990]. About 1 percent of referrals to child neurologists are specifically for evaluation of MIC [Lalaguna-Mallada et al., 2004], and approximately 15 percent of children referred to child neurologists for evaluation of developmental disabilities have MIC [Watemberg et al., 2002].

Historically, a confusing plethora of terms have been used to describe and classify various types of MIC. When severe congenital MIC is seen without other major brain or somatic malformations it is known as primary microcephaly or microcephalia vera, a term first introduced by Giacomini in 1885 [Giacomini, 1885]. It is likely that primary MIC is not a distinct etiologic category, but a term that describes a group of disorders, many with etiologies not yet known. As MIC can conceivably result from any developmental defect or brain injury that disturbs prenatal or early postnatal brain growth, many different causes are known. Improvements in neuroimaging and genetic technologies have resulted in a better understanding of the types and causes of MIC, suggesting that a reappraisal of schemes for classification and diagnostic testing is warranted. We have chosen to separate MIC into two broad categories, congenital and postnatal onset.

Table 25-1 summarizes some of the common disorders associated with these two groups of microcephaly.

Pathology

The embryology relevant to neuronal proliferation and microcephaly is reviewed in the following chapter describing malformations of cortical development (Chapter 26). The pathological changes described in different types of MIC are diverse, which is not surprising, given the large number of associated conditions. Here we will confine our comments to severe congenital microcephaly. The macroscopic changes described in most pathological reports are subtle, consisting of very small cerebral volume, normal or minimally altered pattern of convolutions, and normal size of the third and lateral ventricles [Robain and Lyon, 1972]. However, our brain imaging experience shows that this is not quite true, as, in many forms, the frontal lobes are disproportionately small, and the number and complexity of the gyri and the depth of sulci are generally reduced.

The microscopic changes, especially those involving the cerebral cortex, are heterogeneous. In one group, the cortex has normal thickness and lamination, but the number of neurons in the brain is dramatically reduced. We suppose these to be the less severely affected individuals, although the available

Table 25-1 Etiologies of Congenital and Postnatal Microcephaly

	Congenital	Postnatal Onset
GENETIC		
Isolated/Inborn errors of metabolism	Autosomal-recessive microcephaly Autosomal-dominant microcephaly X-linked microcephaly (uncertain) Chromosomal (rare: "apparently" balanced rearrangements and ring chromosomes)	Congenital disorders of glycosylation Mitochondrial disorders Peroxisomal disorders Menkes' disease Amino acidopathies and organic acidurias Glucose transporter defect

Syndromic
   Chromosomal
 	
   Contiguous gene deletion
	Trisomy 21, 13, 18
	Unbalanced rearrangements
	4p deletion (Wolf–Hirschhorn syndrome)
	5p deletion (cri du chat syndrome)
	7q11.23 deletion (Williams' syndrome)
	22q11 deletion (velocardiofacial syndrome)
		
		17p13.3 deletion (Miller–Dieker syndrome)

Single-gene defects	Cornelia de Lange syndrome Holoprosencephaly (isolated or syndromic) Smith–Lemli–Opitz syndrome Seckel's syndrome	Rett's syndrome Nijmegen breakage syndrome Ataxia-telangiectasia Cockayne's syndrome Aicardi–Goutières syndrome XLAG syndrome
ACQUIRED		
Disruptive injuries	Fetal death of a twin Ischemic stroke Hemorrhagic stroke	Traumatic brain injury Hypoxic-ischemic encephalopathy Hemorrhagic and ischemic stroke
Infections	TORCHES syndrome and HIV	Meningitis and encephalitis Congenital HIV encephalopathy
Teratogens/Toxins	Alcohol, hydantoin, radiation Maternal phenylketonuria Poorly controlled maternal diabetes	Lead poisoning Chronic renal failure
Deprivation	Maternal hypothyroidism Maternal folate deficiency Maternal malnutrition Placental insufficiency	Hypothyroidism Anemia Malnutrition Congenital heart disease

HIV, human immunodeficiency virus; TORCHES, toxoplasmosis, rubella, cytomegalovirus, herpes simplex, syphilis; XLAG, X-linked lissencephaly with abnormal genitalia.
(Adapted from Ashwal S, et al. Practice parameter: Evaluation of the child with microcephaly [an evidence-based review]: report of the Quality Standards Subcommittee of the American Academy of Neurology and the Practice Committee of the Child Neurology Society, Neurology *73:887–897, 2009.)*

data are not clear on this point. In probably several other types of MIC, the cortex appears abnormally thin, presumably resulting from premature exhaustion of the germinal zone [Barkovich et al., 1992; Evrard et al., 1989].

In the latter, abnormalities of cellular architecture predominate in the first two layers of the cortex, referred to as "type I familial MIC" by Robain [Robain and Lyon, 1972]. Layer two is almost devoid of granule neurons, and may be fragmented into small nests (sometimes called "glomeruli") or small columns that protrude into the molecular layer. In a few individuals, the vertical bands of neurons arising in layer two cross the molecular layer to protrude into the meninges. Neurons may be seen in the molecular layer, either as scattered large pyramidal or stellate neurons, or as persistence of a fetal monolayer of granule neurons found just beneath the pia. The lower cortical layers were less affected, but with abnormal distribution of cells in some areas. In some brains, persistence of fetal wavy or "combed" monocellular bands in the middle of the cortex has been seen [Robain and Lyon, 1972]. In these types of MIC, the cerebellum is typically small but proportionate to the reduced size of the cerebrum or relatively larger.

Severe congenital MIC has been observed in combination with several other types of brain malformations, including holoprosencephaly, disproportionate brainstem and cerebellar hypoplasia, true lissencephaly with widespread malformation of neuronal migration, diffuse periventricular nodular heterotopia, and diffuse polymicrogyria (Table 25-2).

The authors have seen agenesis of the corpus callosum in most different types of MIC, and suspect that, in most, it is a nonspecific feature of slowed brain growth. (The growing cerebral hemispheres must be closely enough apposed for the precallosal sling to cross the gap, which requires growth.) We have therefore not included MIC and agenesis as a classification in its own right at this time, although this may need to be added in the future.

Brain Imaging

In most patients with primary MIC, brain imaging reveals characteristic abnormalities that we designated "microcephaly with simplified gyral pattern" [Barkovich et al., 1998; Dobyns and Barkovich, 1999]. This pattern consists of a reduced

Table 25-2 Severe Congenital Microcephaly Types by Imaging or Pathology

Microcephaly Type	References
MIC WITH SIMPLIFIED GYRAL PATTERN ONLY (PRIMARY MIC)	
MIC with normal six-layer cortex (probably high-functioning)	Barkovich et al. [1992]
MIC with layer two cortical dysplasia	Robain and Lyon [1972]
MIC with simplified gyri and enlarged extra-axial space (may also be associated with postnatal MIC)	Basel-Vanagaite and Dobyns [2010]
MIC WITH DISPROPORTIONATE PONTOCEREBELLAR HYPOPLASIA (MIC-PCH)	
MIC with simplified gyri and pontocerebellar hypoplasia, NOS	Basel-Vanagaite and Dobyns [2010]
MIC with simplified gyri and pontocerebellar hypoplasia and enlarged extra-axial space	Basel-Vanagaite and Dobyns [2010]
Von Monakow type MIC-PCH	Thurel and Gruner [1960]
MICROLISSENCEPHALY (MLIS) WITH TRUE AGYRIA-PACHYGYRIA	
Barth MLIS syndrome	Barth et al. [1982]
Microcephalic osteodysplastic primordial dwarfism type 1 (MOPD1)	Juric-Sekhar et al. [2010]
Norman–Roberts MLIS syndrome	Dobyns et al. [1984]
MIC WITH DIFFUSE PERIVENTRICULAR NODULAR HETEROTOPIA (MIC-PNH)	
MIC-PNH	Robain and Lyon [1972]
MIC WITH DIFFUSE POLYMICROGYRIA (MDP)	
MDP isolated	Barkovich et al. [1992]
MDP with other congenital anomalies (somatic)	Pavone et al. [2000]
MIC WITH OTHER CORTICAL MALFORMATIONS	
MIC with cortical malformations, NOS (not well defined)	

MIC, microcephaly; NOS, not otherwise specified.

number of gyri separated by abnormally shallow sulci. Common associated abnormalities include foreshortened frontal lobes, mildly enlarged lateral ventricles, and sometimes a thin corpus callosum or even partial agenesis of the corpus callosum.

While interpretation of brain imaging studies in MIC would seem to be straightforward, this has proved challenging in practice, primarily for severe congenital MIC. First, scans of children with MIC are often interpreted as normal, other than for the small size, if this is recognized on the imaging study, but close inspection will show the features noted above. While these changes can be subtle, they are not normal. Further, brain imaging in individuals with more severe forms of MIC may show fewer convolutions, with some broader than 2 cm, leading to interpretation as "pachygyria." But imaging in the large majority of these patients shows a normal or an especially thin cortex, while true lissencephaly (agyria and pachygyria) is always associated with an abnormally thick cortex. Clinicians often respond to such reports by ordering tests that are appropriate for children with true lissencephaly, which are always negative. With the rare exception of mutations of *TUBA1A*, no genes associated with microlissencephaly (MLIS) have been reported.

While the first several genes associated with severe congenital MIC were associated with nonspecific brain imaging patterns (as described above), several recently identified MIC genes are associated with recognizable patterns of abnormalities. Focusing on children with severe congenital MIC, the authors recently reviewed brain imaging in approximately 250 children with MIC, most of whom (230 of 247) had MIC without

associated somatic anomalies [Basel-Vanagaite et al., 2010]. Among this group of patients, four relatively common brain imaging patterns were found, which involved abnormalities in the gyral pattern, size of extra-axial space, and relative size of the brainstem and cerebellum in comparison to the cerebrum. The four groups were:

1. microcephaly with simplified gyri only
2. microcephaly with simplified gyri and pontocerebellar hypoplasia
3. microcephaly with simplified gyri and enlarged extra-axial space
4. microcephaly with simplified gyri and both pontocerebellar hypoplasia and enlarged extra-axial space.

Examples are shown in Figure 25-1. Rare forms of severe MIC are associated with additional brain malformations, as listed in Table 25-2.

Clinical Features

The clinical manifestations associated with MIC are remarkably heterogeneous. In most individuals with severe congenital MIC, examination reveals obvious small head size, often with a low, sloping forehead and a flat occiput. The face and ears are normal, but because of the small head size, may appear disproportionately large. Cognitive impairment is moderate in some types, but severe to profound in others. In moderately affected patients, hyperactivity may dominate the patient's behavior, while tone is typically normal. In severely affected children, spasticity and epilepsy predominate. In children with milder forms of MIC, a variety of subtle dysmorphic features may

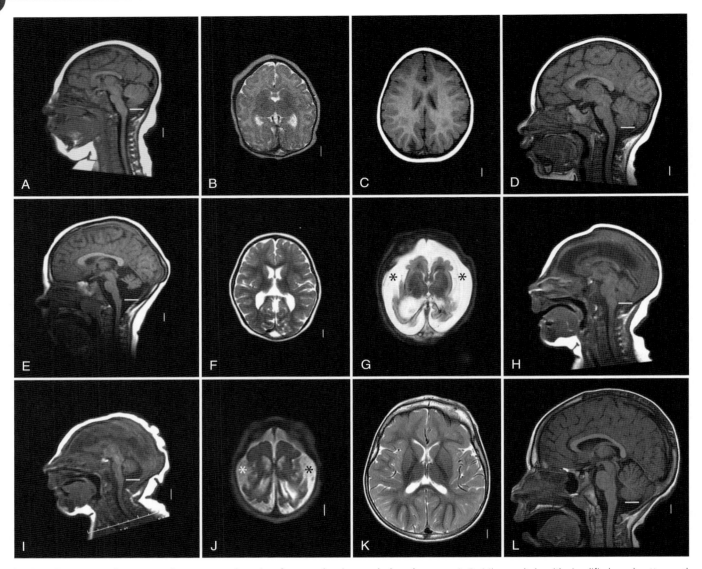

Fig. 25-1 Representative magnetic resonance imaging from each microcephaly subgroup. A–D, Microcephaly with simplified gyral pattern only. **E–F,** Microcephaly with simplified gyri and pontocerebellar hypoplasia. **G–H,** Microcephaly with simplified gyri, enlarged extra-axial space, and proportionate cerebellum. **I–J,** Microcephaly with simplified gyri, enlarged extra-axial space, and marked pontocerebellar hypoplasia. **K–L,** Normal brain magnetic resonance images for comparison purposes. Asterisks indicate enlarged extra-axial space. *(Adapted from Basel-Vanagaite et al., Familial hydrocephalus with normal cognition and distinctive features, 2010.)*

be present and may be helpful in identifying a specific syndrome causing MIC. Features of some of these syndromes are outlined in the different tables in this chapter.

For children with the most common, relatively high-functioning forms of primary MIC, survival far into adult life is typical. For more severely handicapped children unable to walk or feed by mouth, the mortality rate is higher, with survival often limited to 10–20 years, although no formal studies have been done. Children with MIC and other severe brain malformations, especially those with cortical malformations such as lissencephaly, heterotopias, and polymicrogyria, are likely to have much shorter survival.

In general, all forms of MIC are associated with below-average intelligence [Dolk, 1991; Nelson and Deutschberger, 1970]. However, mild MIC with OFC between −2 and −3 SD is not inevitably linked with mental retardation; 7.5 percent of a large group of microcephalic children had normal

intelligence [Martin, 1970; Sells, 1977]. However, some patients with mild MIC have severe or profound mental retardation. Their intellectual disability may be partly explained by associated brain abnormalities, whether developmental or destructive, as brain imaging frequently reveals additional abnormalities [Sugimoto et al., 1993].

Several coexistent conditions, such as varying degrees of cognitive impairment, epilepsy, cerebral palsy, and ophthalmological and audiological disorders, occur commonly in children with microcephaly and are reviewed in the sections below.

Cognitive Impairment

A correlation between MIC and mental retardation has been recognized since studies in the late 1800s, and subsequent research has explored the strength of this correlation in a number of ways, although rarely in a prospective manner among a broad sample of subjects. In reported studies, the incidence of MIC has varied, depending on the population studied. Prevalence estimates of MIC in institutionalized patients have reported a rate of MIC ranging from 6.5 percent [Krishnan et al., 1989] to 53 percent [Roboz, 1973]. In contrast, for children seen in neurodevelopmental clinics, the prevalence of microcephaly averages 24.7 percent (range 6–40.4 percent) [Smith, 1981; Martin, 1970; Desch et al., 1990].

Other studies have looked at the incidence and significance of MIC in children who were functioning normally or had normal intelligence. In one report of 1006 students in mainstream classrooms it was found that 1.9 percent had mild microcephaly (−2–3 SD) and none had severe microcephaly (below −3 SD) [Sells, 1977]. The microcephalic subjects had a similar mean IQ (99.5) to the normocephalic group (105), but lower mean academic achievement scores (49 vs. 70). Another report, looking at the records of 1775 normally intelligent patients aged 11–21 years, followed in adolescent medicine clinics, found 11 (0.6 percent) with severe MIC (below −3 SD) [Barmeyer, 1971]. Among a separate sample of 106 retarded adolescents, the incidence of severe MIC was 11 percent.

A related issue concerns the incidence of developmental disability in individuals with MIC. Several investigations based on the United States National Collaborative Perinatal Project (1959–1974) have data regarding the degree of developmental disability in children with MIC. In an early report, OFC measurements of less than 43 cm (−2.3 SD) for males and 42 cm (−2.4 SD) for females at 1 year of age were associated with IQ <80 at 4 years in half the individuals [Nelson and Deutschberger, 1970]. A second study using these data found congenital MIC (<2 SD) in 1.3 percent that was associated with a greater risk of mental retardation at 7 years (15.3 vs. 7 percent) in selected populations [Camp et al., 1998]. A third study found that, of normocephalic children, 2.6 percent were mentally retarded (IQ ≤70) and 7.4 percent had borderline IQ scores (71–80). Of the 114 (0.4 percent) children with mild microcephaly (2–3 SD), 10.5 percent were mentally retarded and 28 percent had borderline IQ scores [Dolk, 1991]. Severe MIC (below −3 SD) was found in 41 (0.14 percent) children, and 51.2 percent were mentally retarded and 17 percent had borderline IQ scores. These reports have been supported by findings in several other studies [O'Connell et al., 1965; Watemberg et al., 2002].

A number of additional studies of microcephalic children have examined other clinical factors. Available data are conflicting as to whether having proportionate MIC is less predictive of developmental and learning disabilities [Sells, 1977] or not [Nelson and Deutschberger, 1970]. Other studies have shown that early severe medical illness or acquired brain injury can be associated with MIC and a future risk of retardation [Avery et al., 1972]. The pattern of head growth can also be a significant predictor of outcome. Infants whose birth OFCs were normal but who acquired MIC by age 1 year were likely to be severely delayed. On the other hand, when MIC and developmental delay were acquired as a consequence of the combined deprivations of early childhood malnutrition, poverty, and lack of stimulation, as frequently occurs in emerging countries [Grantham-McGregor et al., 2007], significant potential for physical and cognitive recovery exists [Rutter, 1998].

There is also some evidence to support the generally held belief that there is a correlation between the severity of MIC and degree of developmental disability. One study of 212 children with MIC, seen in either a birth defects or a child development clinic, found a significant correlation between the degree of MIC and severity of mental retardation. Among the 113 subjects with mild MIC (2–3 SD below the mean), mental retardation was found in just 11 percent. The mean IQ of the children with the most normal OFC, between 2.0 and 2.1 SD below the mean, was 63. Mental retardation was diagnosed in 50 percent of the 99 subjects with more severe MIC (≥3 SD), and in all of those with an OFC more than 7 SD below the mean. The mean IQ of the children with an OFC between 5 and 7 SD below the mean was 20 [Pryor and Thelander, 1968].

The above studies all underscore the fact that MIC is common in developmentally disabled children, with the incidence greater in those more severely affected. Even in low-risk populations (e.g., children with normal school placements), 1.9 percent have MIC, and in many of these children, subtle cognitive deficits are detected. In addition, there is a 50 percent increased risk for being developmentally delayed in children with MIC compared to children without MIC (e.g., 15.3 vs. 7 percent), and a strong correlation between the severity of MIC and developmental outcome (i.e., mental retardation occurs in 10.5 percent of children with mild MIC [<2 SD] and in 51.2 percent of children with severe microcephaly [below −3 SD]). Because of these observations, it is important for serial developmental screening to be done in children with MIC to detect developmental disorders.

Epilepsy

The relation between MIC and epilepsy is of great clinical importance for several reasons:
1. The incidence of epilepsy is much higher in children with MIC.
2. A greater number of children with epilepsy are likely to be microcephalic.
3. MIC is a significant risk factor for epilepsy being medically refractory.
4. The presence of MIC may help determine the underlying etiology of a child's epilepsy.
5. Epilepsy is a prominent feature of certain MIC syndromes. One study involving 66 children with MIC (<−2 SD) found an overall prevalence of epilepsy of 40.9 percent [Abdel-Salam et al., 2000]. It has also been suggested that epilepsy is more common in postnatal-onset than in congenital MIC. In one study, epilepsy occurred in 50 percent of children with postnatal-onset microcephaly compared to only 35.7 percent of those with congenital MIC [Abdel-Salam et al., 2000]. A second study found that epilepsy was four times more common in postnatal-onset MIC [Qazi and Reed, 1973].

MIC also is a significant risk factor for medically refractory epilepsy [Berg et al., 1996; Chawla et al., 2002; Aneja et al., 2001]. In one study of 30 children, MIC was found in 58 percent of those with medically refractory epilepsy compared to 2 percent in whom seizures were controlled [Chawla et al., 2002].

Although children with MIC are at greater risk for epilepsy, many do not have epilepsy. There are, however, certain MIC syndromes in which epilepsy is a prominent feature. Knowledge

Table 25-3 Severe Epilepsy and Microcephaly Associated Genetic Syndromes*

Disorder	Gene(s) or Locus
STRUCTURAL MALFORMATIONS	
Classic lissencephaly (isolated LIS sequence)	*LIS1, DCX, TUBA1A*
Lissencephaly: X-linked with abnormal genitalia	*ARX*
Lissencephaly: autosomal-recessive with cerebellar hypoplasia	*RELN, VLDLR*
Bilateral frontoparietal polymicrogyria (COB)	*GPR56*
Periventricular heterotopia with microcephaly	*ARFGEF2*
Holoprosencephaly-associated genes	*SHH, SIX3, GLI2, TDGF1, PTCH1, FOXH1, ZIC2, TFIF1, SMAD2*
Holoprosencephaly phenotypes-associated loci	HPE1 21q22.3 HPE2 2p21 HPE3 7q36 HPE4 18p11.3 HPE5 13q32 HPE 6 2q37.1 HPE7 9q22.3 HPE 8 14q13 HPE9 2q14
SYNDROMES	
Wolf–Hirschhorn syndrome	4p16
Angelman's syndrome	*UBE3A*, 15q11–q13
Rett's syndrome	Xp22, Xq28
MEHMO (mental retardation, epilepsy, hypogonadism, microcephaly, obesity)	Xp22.13–p21.1
Mowat–Wilson syndrome (microcephaly, mental retardation, distinct facial features with/without Hirschsprung's disease)	*ZFHX1B*, 2q22

* Adapted from Ashwal S, et al. Practice parameter: Evaluation of the child with microcephaly (an evidence-based review): report of the Quality Standards Subcommittee of the American Academy of Neurology and the Practice Committee of the Child Neurology Society, *Neurology* 73:887–897, 2009. Data extracted from OMIM (http://www.ncbi.nlm.nih.gov/omim); the reader is referred to that source for updated information as new entries are added and data are revised. The reader can also go directly to GeneTests (http://www.genetests.org), to which OMIM links, for updated information regarding the availability of genetic testing on a clinical or research basis.

of these disorders and their genetic basis can help establish a diagnosis and determine prognosis. Some of the more commonly recognized entities are summarized in Table 25-3.

Studies have not examined the role of obtaining a routine electroencephalography (EEG) in children with MIC to determine their risk for developing epilepsy. In one study of children with MIC, EEG abnormalities were found in 51 percent of 39 children who either had no seizures or occasional febrile seizures [Abdel-Salam et al., 2000]. EEG abnormalities (focal, generalized, or mixed epileptiform discharges) were present in 78 percent of 18 children with medically refractory epilepsy.

Overall, it is important to be aware that epilepsy is more common in children with MIC, and when it occurs, it is more difficult to treat. Certain MIC syndromes are associated with a much higher incidence of epilepsy, and increasingly, genetic etiologies defining the relation between MIC and epilepsy are being reported. In addition, there are no systematic studies regarding EEG findings in children with MIC who have or do not have epilepsy.

Cerebral Palsy

Not unexpectedly, many children with MIC are diagnosed later in infancy with cerebral palsy, and likewise, children with cerebral palsy are frequently found to be microcephalic. Data from one study of 216 children with MIC and developmental disabilities found a rate of cerebral palsy of 21.4 percent compared to 8.8 percent in a population of normocephalic developmentally disabled children (p <0.001) [Watemberg et al., 2002]. In contrast, several studies have examined the incidence of MIC in children with cerebral palsy. Three studies of children with cerebral palsy found congenital MIC in 1.8 percent of cases [Croen et al., 2001; Pharoah, 2007; Laisram et al., 1992]. In three other studies, the combined incidence of congenital and postnatal-onset MIC ranged between 32.5 percent and 81 percent, and averaged 47.9 percent [Edebol-Tysk, 1989; Lubis et al., 1990; Suzuki et al., 1999]. In one of these studies, 68 percent were diagnosed with secondary (i.e., acquired microcephaly) and 13 percent had congenital MIC [Edebol-Tysk, 1989]. Others have shown that the yield of determining the etiology of cerebral palsy is improved if MIC is present [Shevell et al., 2003]. These data suggest that it is important for physicians and others caring for children with MIC to monitor for the development of cerebral palsy, so that appropriate physical and occupational therapeutic interventions can be initiated.

Ophthalmological Disorders

No studies have surveyed the incidence of vision loss or specific ophthalmological disorders in children with MIC. One study found an incidence of 145 cases of congenital eye malformations (microphthalmia, anophthalmia, cataracts, coloboma, etc.) in 212,479 consecutive births [Stoll et al., 1997]. MIC was among the malformations in 56 percent of these children. Another study (n = 360) with severe MIC (below −3 SD) found eye abnormalities in 6.4 percent, but in only 0.2 percent of 3600 age-matched normocephalic controls [Kraus et al., 2003]. Other reported eye abnormalities in children with MIC that have been reported when searching the OMIM database for MIC have found associations with anophthalmia, blindness or visual loss, cataracts, colobomas, microphthalmia, nystagmus, optic atrophy, ptosis, and retinal disorders. Table 25-4 lists some of the more common MIC syndromes associated with ophthalmological disorders.

Audiological Disorders

No studies have surveyed the incidence of hearing loss or audiological disorders in children with MIC. One study of 100 children with complex ear anomalies recorded that 85 had neurological involvement and 13 children had MIC [Wiznitzer et al., 1987]. Hearing loss is likely the most common audiological disorder associated with MIC, and Table 25-5 summarizes some of the common MIC syndromes listed in OMIM in which prominent audiological involvement is reported.

Etiology

Mild MIC, which we define as −2 to −3 SD, has been associated with a variety of maternal and other prenatal disorders, prenatal and postnatal brain injuries, familial forms, chromosome disorders, and numerous syndromes with either prenatal- or postnatal-onset MIC. Here we can review only a small selection of the more common causes.

Extrinsic Causes

Extrinsic injuries before birth or early in life can certainly lead to MIC. The developing nervous system is highly vulnerable to infections, including cytomegalovirus, toxoplasmosis, rubella, herpes simplex, and group B coxsackievirus. Intrauterine infections with these can result in MIC [Evrard, 1992; Norman et al., 1995; Volpe, 2000]. MIC also has been reported in infants of women exposed to ionizing radiation, as shown in studies following exposure to atomic bomb radiation or to radium implantation in the cervix during the first trimester [Dekaban, 1968; Wood et al., 1967]. Maternal metabolic disorders during pregnancy, such as diabetes mellitus, uremia, and undiagnosed or inadequately treated phenylketonuria, may result in neonatal MIC [Levy et al., 1996; Rouse et al., 1997]. Malnutrition, hypertension, and placental insufficiency may all result in intrauterine growth retardation and MIC.

Table 25-4 Microcephaly Disorders with Prominent Ophthalmologic Involvement*

Syndrome (OMIM Number)	Ophthalmologic Abnormality
Aicardi–Goutières syndrome (225750)	Visual inattention, abnormal eye movements
Allan–Herndon–Dudley syndrome (300523)	Rotary nystagmus, disconjugate eye movements
Alpers' syndrome (203700)	Blindness, visual disturbances; microcephaly occasional
Borjeson–Forssman–Lehmann syndrome (301900)	Deep-set eyes, nystagmus, ptosis, poor vision, narrow palpebral fissures
Branchial clefts with characteristic facies, growth retardation, imperforate nasolacrimal duct, and premature aging (113620)	Upslanting palpebral fissures, telecanthus, hypertelorism, ptosis, lacrimal duct obstruction, coloboma Coloboma, microphthalmia, cataract
Cerebral dysgenesis, neuropathy, ichthyosis, and palmoplantar keratoderma syndrome (609528)	Downslanting palpebral fissures, hypertelorism, hypoplastic optic discs; described in two families
Cerebro-oculofacioskeletal syndrome (214150)	Cataracts, blepharophimosis Microphthalmia, deep-set eyes, nystagmus
**CHARGE syndrome (214800)	Colobomas, anophthalmia, ptosis, hypertelorism, downslanting palpebral fissures
Cockayne's syndrome (216400)	Pigmentary retinopathy, optic atrophy, corneal opacity, decreased lacrimation, nystagmus, cataracts
Cohen's syndrome (216550)	Downslanting palpebral fissures, chorioretinal dystrophy, myopia, decreased visual acuity, optic atrophy
Down syndrome (190685)	Upslanting palpebral fissures, epicanthal folds, iris Brushfield spots
Fraser's syndrome (219000)	Cryptophthalmos, malformed lacrimal ducts, hypertelorism, blindness
Glucose transport defect (606777)	Abnormal paroxysmal eye movements; eye findings rare
Holoprosencephaly (236100)	Cyclopia, ethmocephaly, cebocephaly, hypotelorism
Incontinentia pigmenti (308300)	Microphthalmia, cataract, optic atrophy, retinal vascular proliferation, retinal fibrosis, retinal detachment, uveitis, keratitis
Jacobsen's syndrome (147791)	Epicanthal folds, hypertelorism Ptosis, strabismus, coloboma, optic atrophy
Kabuki syndrome (147920)	Long palpebral fissures, eversion of lateral third of lower eyelids, ptosis, blue sclerae, broad/arched/sparse eyebrows

Continued

Table 25-4 Microcephaly Disorders with Prominent Ophthalmologic Involvement*—cont'd

Syndrome (OMIM Number)	Ophthalmologic Abnormality
Mental retardation with optic atrophy, deafness, and seizures (309555)	Optic atrophy, severe visual impairment
Mental retardation, microcephaly, growth retardation, and joint contractures (606240)	Ptosis; single case report of two sisters
Microcephaly, hiatus hernia, and nephrotic syndrome (251300)	Absent cleavage of eye anterior chamber; described in one case report
Microphthalmia, syndromic (309800)	Microphthalmia, optic nerve hypoplasia, coloboma, pigmentary retinopathy
Mitochondrial DNA depletion syndrome (251880)	Nystagmus, disconjugate eye movements, optic dysplasia; microcephaly occasional
Mosaic variegated aneuploidy syndrome (257300)	Hypertelorism, upslanting palpebral fissures, epicanthal folds, cataracts, nystagmus
Mucolipidosis IV (252650)	Corneal clouding, corneal opacities, fibrous dysplasia of the cornea, progressive retinal degeneration, optic atrophy, strabismus, decreased electroretinogram
Neuronal ceroid-lipofuscinosis (256730)	Progressive visual loss, optic atrophy, retinal degeneration, macular degeneration, abnormal electroretinogram
Norrie's disease (310600)	Blindness, retinal dysgenesis/dysplasia/detachment, cataracts, optic atrophy, other ocular abnormalities
Oculodentodigital dysplasia (164200)	Microcornea, short palpebral fissures, epicanthal folds, glaucoma, cataract, iris anomalies
Oculopalatocerebral syndrome (257910)	Persistent hypertrophic primary vitreous Microphthalmos, leukocoria, retrolental fibrovascular membrane; rarely reported
Oculopalatoskeletal syndrome (257920)	Blepharophimosis, blepharoptosis, epicanthus inversus, hypertelorism, conjunctival telangiectasia, glaucoma, anterior chamber anomalies, abnormal eye motility; rare
Osteoporosis-pseudoglioma syndrome (259770)	Pseudoglioma, blindness, microphthalmia, vitreoretinal abnormalities, cataract, iris atrophy
Pelizaeus–Merzbacher disease (312080)	Rotary nystagmus, optic atrophy
Peters plus syndrome (261540)	Hypertelorism, Peters anomaly, anterior chamber cleavage disorder, nystagmus, ptosis, glaucoma, cataract, myopia, coloboma
Pyridoxamine 5′-phosphate oxidase deficiency (610090)	Rotary eye movements; rare disorder
Pyruvate decarboxylase deficiency (312170)	Episodic ptosis, abnormal eye movements
Pyruvate dehydrogenase deficiency (312170)	Nystagmus, ptosis, saccade initiation failure, oculomotor apraxia
Rhizomelic chondrodysplasia punctata (215100)	Cataract
Roberts' syndrome (268300)	Hypertelorism, shallow orbits, prominent eyes, bluish sclerae, corneal clouding, microphthalmia, cataract, lid coloboma
Smith–Lemli–Opitz syndrome (270400)	Ptosis, epicanthal folds, cataracts, hypertelorism, strabismus
Spastic paraplegia, optic atrophy, microcephaly, and XY sex reversal (603117)	Optic atrophy and poor vision; single case report
Syndactyly with microcephaly and mental retardation (272440)	One family of several described had optic atrophy and poor vision
Townes–Brocks syndrome (107480)	Chorioretinal coloboma, Duane anomaly; both of these are rare
Velocardiofacial syndrome (192430)	Narrow palpebral fissures, small optic discs, tortuous retinal vessels, posterior embryotoxon
Walker-Warburg syndrome (236670)	Multiple ocular findings including retinal detachment, cataracts, microphthalmia, hyperplastic primary vitreous, optic nerve hypoplasia, colobomata, glaucoma
Warburg micro syndrome (600118)	Multiple ocular findings, including microphthalmia, microcornea, congenital cataracts, optic atrophy, ptosis
Wolf–Hirschhorn syndrome (194190)	Hypertelorism, exophthalmos, ptosis, Rieger anomaly, nystagmus, iris coloboma

* Adapted from Ashwal S, et al. Practice parameter: Evaluation of the child with microcephaly (an evidence-based review): report of the Quality Standards Subcommittee of the American Academy of Neurology and the Practice Committee of the Child Neurology Society, *Neurology* 73:887–897, 2009. From OMIM (http://www.ncbi.nlm.nih.gov/sites/entrez). Gene map loci are listed in each OMIM entry. Disorders are listed alphabetically; prevalence data are not known.
** CHARGE (Coloboma of the eye, Heart defects, Atresia of the choanae, Retardation of growth and/or development, Genital and/or urinary abnormalities, and Ear abnormalities and deafness.

Table 25-5 Microcephaly Syndromes with Prominent Ear or Auditory Impairments*

Syndrome (OMIM Number)	Ear or Audiologic Abnormality
Allan–Herndon–Dudley syndrome (300523)	Large ears, simple ears, pinna modeling anomalies, prominent antihelix, flattened antihelix
Alpha-thalassemia/mental retardation syndrome (309580)	Small ears, low-set ears, posteriorly rotated ears, sensorineural hearing loss
Brachyphalangy, polydactyly, tibial aplasia/hypoplasia (609945)	Overfolded helices, hearing loss, cleft lobules, preauricular tags, cup-shaped ears
Branchial arch syndrome (301950)	Hearing loss and external ear anomalies
Branchial clefts with characteristic facies, growth retardation, imperforate nasolacrimal duct, and premature aging (113610)	Low-set ears, posteriorly rotated ears, hypoplastic superior helix, microtia, ear pits, overfolded ears, supra-auricular sinuses, conductive hearing loss
Camptodactyly, tall stature, and hearing loss syndrome (610474)	Microcephaly occurs occasionally
Cerebrocostomandibular syndrome (117650)	Low-set ears, conductive hearing loss, posteriorly rotated ears
Cerebro-oculofacioskeletal syndrome 1 (214150)	Large ear pinnae
CHARGE syndrome (214800)	Small ears, lop ears, deafness (sensorineural ± conductive), Mondini defect
Chondrodysplasia punctata (215100)	Hearing loss
Chromosome 18 deletion syndrome (601808)	External ear abnormalities
Chromosome 9q subtelomeric deletion syndrome (610253)	Malformed ears, hearing loss
Cockayne's syndrome (216400)	Malformed ears, sensorineural hearing loss
Coffin–Lowry syndrome (303600)	Prominent ears, sensorineural hearing loss
Cornelia de Lange syndrome (122470)	Low-set ears, hearing loss
Cutis verticis gyrate, retinitis pigmentosa, and sensorineural deafness (605685)	Sensorineural hearing loss; only one case report
Deafness, conductive, with malformed external ear (221300)	Conductive hearing loss, malformed external ears, low-set external ears, malformed ossicles
Deafness, congenital, and onychodystrophy (220500)	Sensorineural hearing loss
Dislocated elbows, bowed tibias, scoliosis, deafness, cataracts, microcephaly, and mental retardation (603133)	Single case report of 4 siblings in consanguineous family
Ear, patella, and short stature syndrome (24690)	Bilateral microtia, hearing loss, Mondini malformation, low-set ears, atretic auditory canal
Feingold's syndrome (164280)	"Ear abnormalities" common in one description
Focal dermal hypoplasia (305600)	Protruding, simple ears, low-set ears, narrow auditory canals, mixed hearing loss
Genitopatellar syndrome (606170)	One case report with hearing loss as an associated finding
***GOMBO syndrome (233270)	One case report with conductive hearing loss
Iris coloboma with ptosis, hypertelorism, and mental retardation (243310)	Low-set ears, overfolded helices, sensorineural hearing loss
Johanson–Blizzard syndrome (243800)	Sensorineural hearing loss, cystic dilatation of cochlea and vestibular structures
Kabuki syndrome (147920)	Large prominent ears, recurrent otitis media in infancy, posteriorly rotated ears, hearing loss, preauricular pit
Kearns–Sayre syndrome (530000)	Sensorineural hearing loss
Klippel–Feil syndrome (118100)	One case reported with microcephaly; hearing loss of any type common; external ear abnormalities occasional
Lathosterolosis (607330)	Conductive hearing loss
Mental retardation, with optic atrophy, deafness and seizures (309555)	Hearing loss; described in one family
Mental retardation–hypotonic facies syndrome, X-linked (309580)	Deafness
Microphthalmia, syndromic (601186)	Simple anteverted ears, hearing loss
Monosomy 1p36 syndrome (607872)	Sensorineural hearing loss, external ear abnormalities

Continued

Table 25-5 Microcephaly Syndromes with Prominent Ear or Auditory Impairments*—cont'd

Syndrome (OMIM Number)	Ear or Audiologic Abnormality
Oculodentodigital dysplasia (164200)	Conductive hearing loss
Oculopalatoskeletal syndrome (257920)	Conductive hearing loss
Otopalatodigital syndrome (311300)	Low-set ears, conductive hearing loss, posteriorly rotated ears
POR** deficiency (201750)	Conductive hearing loss, simple ears
Progeroid facial appearance with hand anomalies (602249)	Prominent ears, conductive hearing loss; one case report
Renpenning's syndrome 1 (309500)	Cupped ears
Rubinstein–Taybi syndrome (180849)	Low-set ears, hearing loss
Shprinzten–Goldberg craniosynostosis (182212)	Low-set ears, posteriorly rotated ears, conductive hearing loss (rare)
Townes–Brocks syndrome (107480)	Multiple external ear abnormalities; sensorineural hearing loss
Trichorhinophalangeal syndrome type II (15030)	Hearing loss, large protruding ears
Velocardiofacial syndrome (192430)	Occasional microcephaly and minor auricular abnormalities seen
Waardenburg's syndrome (148820)	Hearing loss
Williams–Beuren syndrome (194050)	Early-onset progressive sensorineural hearing loss
Wolf–Hirschhorn syndrome (194190) (602952)	Preauricular tags, preauricular pits, hearing loss, narrow external auditory canals

* Adapted from Ashwal S, et al. Practice parameter: Evaluation of the child with microcephaly (an evidence-based review): report of the Quality Standards Subcommittee of the American Academy of Neurology and the Practice Committee of the Child Neurology Society, *Neurology* 73:887–897, 2009. From OMIM (http://www.ncbi.nlm.nih.gov/sites/entrez). Gene map loci are listed in each OMIM entry. Disorders are listed alphabetically; prevalence data are not known.
** POR – cytochrome P450 oxido reductase deficiency.
*** GOMBO – Growth retardation, ocular abnormalities, Microcephaly, Brachydactyly and Oligophrenia.

Maternal alcoholism during pregnancy has also been linked with MIC as part of the fetal alcohol syndrome [Clarren et al., 1978; Loebstein and Koren, 1997; Ouellette et al., 1977; Spohr et al., 1993]. The clinical features include growth and mental retardation, midfacial hypoplasia, short palpebral fissures, epicanthal folds, and behavioral disturbances. Neuropathologic findings include MIC, heterotopia, widespread cortical and white-matter dysplasias, and defects of neuronal and glial migration [Wisniewski et al., 1983]. MIC has also been reported with maternal exposure to cocaine [Loebstein and Koren, 1997]. Some other reports are largely anecdotal, so the associations are often not proven.

Familial Mild Microcephaly

Mild MIC may have either complex (polygenic) or autosomal-dominant inheritance. The autosomal-recessive forms typically present with severe primary MIC and many reviews have not clearly separated patients with mild and severe MIC, often making clinical data difficult to interpret. The polygenic or autosomal-dominant forms are generally associated with mild to moderate cognitive problems, with epilepsy being uncommon. The risk of recurrence in siblings may be as high as 50 percent with the assumption of autosomal-dominant inheritance, but is probably lower, considering that polygenic inheritance may be involved. The genetic basis for familial mild MIC is not known, but several genes have been identified that cause mild MIC, as indicated in Table 25-6.

Severe MIC, which we define as birth OFC at or below −3 SD or later OFC at or below −4 SD, is more likely to be associated with a wide variety of genetic disorders, although exceptions are likely (but not well documented).

Patients with primary MIC tend to fall into two further, albeit somewhat heterogeneous, subgroups [Dobyns, 2002]. The first subgroup includes children with severe MIC but only moderate neurologic problems, usually with moderate mental retardation and with no spasticity or epilepsy. The second subgroup consists of severe MIC with a much more severe neurologic phenotype that consists of abnormal neonatal reflexes, generalized spasticity, and epilepsy [Barkovich et al., 1998; Dobyns, 2002; Sztriha et al., 1999; ten Donkelaar et al., 1999]. These children have poor feeding and recurrent vomiting, leading to poor weight gain, profound mental retardation, and severe spastic quadriparesis. Most of these children also have early-onset intractable epilepsy. The wide clinical spectrum suggests pathogenetically heterogeneous conditions, and several syndromes and genes have been identified (see Table 25-6).

Primary Microcephaly

When congenital MIC is the only abnormality on evaluation, the disorder has been designated primary MIC. As discussed previously, this designation becomes much more useful when restricted to children with birth occipitofrontal circumference below −3 SD. Most patients with primary MIC also have mild growth deficiency, with stature typically −2 to −3 SD, which may be part of the syndrome or partly nutritional. This deficiency is much less striking than their head size, which is typically −4 to −8 SD after early childhood. Most affected persons fall into one of two groups described below [Dobyns, 2002].

The first group is composed of children with extreme MIC but only moderate neurologic problems, usually with only moderate mental retardation without spasticity or epilepsy

Table 25-6 Microcephaly Syndromes, Inheritance, and Genes

MIC Types and Syndromes	Inheritance	Gene	Reference
MIC WITH NORMAL TO THIN CORTEX AND RELATIVELY NORMAL GROWTH			
MIC with simplified gyral pattern, normal stature, and relatively high function (primary MIC, autosomal-recessive MIC)	AR	ASPM	Bond et al. [2002]
	AR	CDK5RAP2	Bond et al. [2005]
			Hassan et al. [2007]
	AR	CENPJ	Bond et al. [2005]
	AR	MCPH1	Trimborn et al. [2005]
	AR	STIL	Kumar et al. [2009]
	AR	CEP152	Guernsey et al. [2010]
MIC WITH NORMAL OR MINOR SHORT STATURE AND POOR FUNCTION			
Profound MIC (Amish lethal MIC)	AR	SLC25A19	Rosenberg et al. [2002]
MIC with simplified gyri and poor function	AR	CENPJ	Bond et al. [2005]
	AR	WDR62	Yu et al. [2010]
	AR	PNKP	Shen et al. [2010]
MIC with simplified gyri and enlarged extra-axial space	AR	PNKP	Shen et al. [2010]
Primary MIC (microcephaly vera), NOC	AR	–	
MIC WITH NORMAL OR MINOR SHORT STATURE, POOR FUNCTION, AND ADDITIONAL CONGENITAL (SOMATIC) ANOMALIES			
Extreme MIC with jejunal atresia	Sporadic	–	Strømme and Andersen [1997]
MIC with Disproportionate Pontocerebellar Hypoplasia (MIC-PCH)			
MIC with disproportionate pontocerebellar hypoplasia	AR	–	Basel-Vanagaite and Dobyns [2010]
MIC postnatal with disproportionate pontocerebellar hypoplasia	XL	CASK	Najm et al. [2008]
MIC WITH SEVERE SHORT STATURE			
MLIS with Severe Intrauterine Growth Retardation (IUGR)			
Seckel's syndrome	AR	ATR	O'Driscoll et al. [2003]
	AR	CENPJ	Al-Dosari et al. [2010]
	AR	CEP152	Kalay et al. [2011]
Microcephalic osteodysplastic primordial dwarfism (MOPD) type 1 (unclear if cortex is ever thin, see below)	AR	–	
MOPD type 2	AR	PCNT	Griffith et al. [2008]
MICROCEPHALY WITH (EARLY) FOREBRAIN MALFORMATIONS			
HPE, single maxillary incisor, hypotelorism, learning disabilities	AD	SHH	Roessler et al. [1996]
	AD	ZIC2	Solomon et al. [2010]
	AD	SIX3	Lacbawan et al. [2009]
	AD	TGIF	Dubourg et al. [2004]
MICROCEPHALY WITH (LATER) MALFORMATIONS OF CORTICAL DEVELOPMENT			
Lissencephaly (Most Types of Postnatal MIC)			
Miller–Dieker syndrome due to deletion 17p13.3	AD	LIS1, YWHAE	Dobyns et al. [1991] Nagamani et al. [2009]
Isolated lissencephaly sequence	XL	DCX	Kato and Dobyns [2003]
	AD	LIS1	Kato and Dobyns [2003]
	AD	TUBA1A	Kumar et al. [2010]
Lissencephaly with severe cerebellar hypoplasia	AD	TUBA1A	Kumar et al. [2010]
	AR	RELN	Hong et al. [2000]
	AR	VLDLR	Zhang et al. [2007]
Microlissencephaly (MLIS) with True Agyria-Pachygyria			
Barth MLIS syndrome	AR	–	Kroon et al. [1996]
MOPD type 1	AR	–	Klinge et al. [2002]
Norman–Roberts MLIS syndrome	AR	–	Dobyns et al. [1984]
Lissencephaly with cerebellar hypoplasia, group c-d-f	Sporadic	TUBA1A	Kumar et al. [2010]

Continued

Table 25-6 Microcephaly Syndromes, Inheritance, and Genes—cont'd

MIC Types and Syndromes	Inheritance	Gene	Reference
MIC WITH DIFFUSE PERIVENTRICULAR NODULAR HETEROTOPIA			
MIC (less severe) with diffuse PNH	AR	*ARFGEF2*	de Wit et al. [2009]
MIC WITH DIFFUSE POLYMICROGYRIA (MDP)			
MDP with variable PMG	AR	*WDR62*	Yu et al. [2010] Nicholas et al. [2010]
MDP, NOC			
MIC, ACC and PMG (gene name a.k.a. *EOMES*)	AR	*TBR2*	Baala et al. [2007]
MIC (less severe) with abnormal frontal cortex and thin CC (Warburg micro syndrome)	AR	*RAB3GAP*	Borck et al. [2011]
POSTNATAL MIC WITH DEVELOPMENTAL ENCEPHALOPATHY (RETT'S-LIKE)			
Angelman's syndrome	AD	*UBE3A*	Williams et al. [2010]
Pitt–Hopkins syndrome	Sporadic	*TCF4*	Amiel et al. [2007]
Pitt–Hopkins-like syndrome	AR AR	*NRXN1* *CNTNAP2*	Zweier et al. [2009] Zweier et al. [2009]
Rett's syndrome	XL	*MECP2*	Amir et al. [1999]
MIC, SZ, ataxia (Angelman's-like)	XL	*SLC9A6*	Gilfillan et al. [2008]
FOXG1 syndrome (postnatal MIC, congenital Rett's-like phenotype)	XL	*FOXG1*	Jacob et al. [2009]
MISCELLANEOUS MIC SYNDROMES			
Mowat–Wilson syndrome (congenital or postnatal MIC)	Sporadic	*ZEB2*	Cecconi et al. [2008]
Smith–Lemli–Opitz syndrome (congenital or postnatal MIC)	AR	*DHCR7*	Salen et al. [1996]
Rubinstein–Taybi syndrome	AD	*CREBBP*	Petrij et al. [1995]
Nijmegen breakage syndrome	AR	*NBS1*	Antoccia et al. [2006]
Postnatal MIC, ACC with deletion 1q43q44	–	*AKT3*	Boland et al. [2007]
Congenital MIC, XLMR, MCA (Renpenning's syndrome)	XL	*PQBP1*	Lenski et al. [2004]
MIC, XLMR, short stature	XL	*JARID1C*	Abidi et al. [2009]
XLMR, Fried's syndrome, basal ganglia calcifications	XL	*AP1S2*	Saillour et al. [2007]
XLMR, neuropsychiatric problems	XL	*PAK3*	Peippo et al. [2007]

ACC, agenesis of the corpus callosum; AD, autosomal-dominant; AR, autosomal-recessive; CC, corpus callosum; HPE, holoprosencephaly; LIS, lissencephaly; MCA, multiple congenital anomalies; MIC, microcephaly; MLIS, microlissencephaly; MOPD, microcephalic osteodysplastic primordial dwarfism; NOC, not otherwise characterized; PCH, pontocerebellar hypoplasia; PMG, polymicrogyria; PNH, periventricular nodular heterotopia; SZ, seizures; XL, X-linked; XLMR, X-linked mental retardation.

[Barkovich et al., 1998; Peiffer et al., 1999; Tolmie et al., 1987]. Their neonatal examinations are usually normal, except for MIC, but many children initially have poor feeding and weight gain. They may have normal tone or mild distal spasticity, but do not have moderate or severe spasticity. Seizures are uncommon and are easily controlled. Febrile seizures occur and should be managed as in any other child. Early development is only mildly delayed and many infants progress to walking between 1 and 2 years of age and develop limited language skills. Several genes have been identified from studies of patients with this disorder (see Table 25-6).

The second group consists of primary MIC with a severe neurologic phenotype that includes severe spasticity and epilepsy [Barkovich et al., 1998; Dobyns, 2002; Sztriha et al., 1999; ten Donkelaar et al., 1999; Tolmie et al., 1987]. Neonatal examination demonstrates abnormal neonatal reflexes and generalized spasticity, and these children subsequently develop impaired feeding and recurrent vomiting, leading to poor weight gain, severe developmental delay, profound mental

retardation, and severe spastic quadriparesis. Most of these infants have early-onset intractable epilepsy. In addition to a simplified gyral pattern, brain magnetic resonance imaging (MRI) may demonstrate other abnormalities, as summarized above (see Figure 25-1). Children with Amish lethal microcephaly have this phenotype, except that hypotonia predominates rather than spasticity, and seizures are not prominent [Kelley et al., 2002; Rosenberg et al., 2002].

The term radial microbrain was introduced by Evrard to describe the brain in some patients with severe mental retardation, profound MIC, and early death, describing an abnormally small brain that has a normal gyral pattern, normal cortical thickness, and normal cortical lamination, although the number of cortical neurons was only 30 percent of normal [Evrard et al., 1989; Evrard, 1992]. He hypothesized that a decreased number of radial neuronal-glial units was responsible for this form of MIC. This subgroup fits into the lower-functioning group of patients with primary MIC, rather than comprising an independent syndrome. However, multiple causes with different pathologic changes and clinical courses are likely to emerge from this group.

Severe Microcephaly with Cortical Malformation

Although still incompletely delineated, several syndromes with severe congenital microcephaly and additional severe brain malformations are known. The combination of severe microcephaly and true lissencephaly (with an abnormally thick cortex) has been reported, with at least three different patterns [Barth et al., 1982; Dobyns and Barkovich, 1999; Sztriha et al., 1998]. The most common of these very rare syndromes is probably the Barth microlissencephaly syndrome, which consists of severe microcephaly, diffuse complete agyria, and severe brainstem and cerebellar hypoplasia [Barth et al., 1982; Kroon et al., 1996]. Severe microcephaly with diffuse periventricular nodular heterotopia has been described, and clearly differs from other forms of heterotopia [Robain and Lyon, 1972; Sheen et al., 2004]. Some patients with severe microcephaly also have had diffuse polymicrogyria [Dobyns and Barkovich, 1999].

Severe Microcephaly with Proportionate Growth Deficiency

Several syndromes with severe intrauterine and postnatal growth deficiency and proportionate MIC have been described, although the head size does not keep up with even slow body growth, leading to disproportionate MIC in childhood and later. The best known of these are Seckel syndrome, Majewski syndrome, microcephalic osteodysplastic primordial dwarfism type 1 (MOPD1), also known as Taybi–Linder syndrome and microcephalic osteodysplastic primordial dwarfism type 2 (MOPD2). Several other syndromes with severe growth deficiency and microcephaly have been described in a few patients, however, so it is likely that this group will become a large and complex group of syndromes. In some children, the skeletal changes may be absent or less prominent than in Seckel's syndrome or the MOPD syndromes.

Seckel's syndrome consists of severe intrauterine and postnatal growth deficiency and microcephaly, and abnormal facial features. including large eyes, beaklike protrusion of the nose, narrow face, and receding lower jaw [Majewski and Goecke, 1982; Seckel, 1960]. All affected individuals have severe mental retardation, although the severity varies considerably and some patients live to adulthood. Abnormalities of the brain seen on postmortem examination or brain imaging demonstrate pure microcephaly with deficient production of neurons and other cell types in some patients [Hori et al., 1987], whereas other patients have severe brain malformations, including lissencephaly [Capovilla et al., 2001; Shanske et al., 1997; Sugio et al., 1993]. Some patients have had various hematological disorders, such as pancytopenia or acute myeloid leukemia [Butler et al., 1987; Hayani et al., 1994].

MOPD1, or Taybi–Linder syndrome, consists of similar severe intrauterine and postnatal growth deficiency and microcephaly, combined with abnormal body proportions and short limbs. Typical skeletal changes consist of a low and broad pelvis with poor formation of the acetabulum, short and bowed humerus and femur, dislocated hips and elbows, retarded epiphyseal maturation, cleft vertebral arches, platyspondyly,

horizontal acetabular roofs, and short long bones with enlarged metaphyses. Patients with MOPD1 also may have skin abnormalities, including hyperkeratosis and sparseness of hair and eyebrows [Meinecke et al., 1991; Sigaudy et al., 1998; Taybi, 1992]. Brain malformations, in addition to the severe microcephaly, are common and include lissencephaly, heterotopia, callosal agenesis, and cerebellar vermis hypoplasia [Klinge et al., 2002; Sigaudy et al., 1998].

MOPD2 consists of similar severe intrauterine and postnatal growth deficiency, proportionate microcephaly at birth that progresses to disproportionate microcephaly, shortening of the middle and distal segments of the limbs, a progressive bony dysplasia, abnormal facial appearance, including prominent nose and malformed ears, and a high squeaky voice [Hall et al., 2004; Majewski and Goecke, 1998; Majewski et al., 1982]. These patients may have dilated arteries in the brain that resemble aneurysms or moyamoya disease [Kannu et al., 2004; Young et al., 2004]. Although all affected individuals have severe microcephaly, no other brain malformations have been described [Fukuzawa et al., 2002].

Although these syndromes dominate the literature concerning intrauterine and postnatal growth deficiency and microcephaly, review of many reports suggests an overall substantial causal heterogeneity, with probable confusion among these and other syndromes in this group. In support of this likelihood, several novel syndromes have been reported [Kantaputra, 2002; Okajima et al., 2002].

MLIS MOPD1-TYPE

MLIS occurs in some patients with microcephalic osteodysplastic primordial dwarfism type 1 (MOPD1), a syndrome that is difficult to distinguish from severe forms of Seckel's syndrome [Juric-Sekhar et al., 2010; Klinge et al., 2002; Meinecke et al., 1991; Ozawa et al., 2005]. The phenotype consists of severe prenatal growth deficiency and microcephaly, sparse hair and dry scaling skin, skeletal anomalies such as platyspondyly, slender ribs, short and bowed proximal humeri and femurs, small iliac wings, dysplastic acetabulum and small hands and feet, and profound developmental handicaps. A few have developed aplastic anemia, another overlap with Seckel's syndrome. The neuropathology consists of a variant form of LIS-3L with frontal predominance.

MLIS BARTH-TYPE

The Barth-type of MLIS is possibly the most severe of all the known LIS syndromes. The phenotype consists of polyhydramnios, probably due to poor fetal swallowing, severe congenital microcephaly (birth OFC approximately 28 cm), weak respiratory effort, and survival for only a few hours or days [Barth et al., 1982; Dobyns and Barkovich, 1999; Kroon et al., 1996]. The neuropathology consists of a variant form of LIS-4L with extreme hypoplasia of many structures, as described above.

Genetics

At least five loci for primary microcephaly with mild or moderate phenotype have been mapped to 1q31, 8p22-pter, 9q34, 15q, and 19q13.1–q13.2, and two of these loci (*MCPH1* and *ASPM*) have now been cloned. Two genes causing severe microcephaly with severe phenotype have also been identified, those being the causal genes for Amish lethal microcephaly and microcephaly with periventricular nodular heterotopia. In Seckel's syndrome, defects in DNA repair were suggested by chromosome instability with exposure to mitomycin C [Abou-Zahr et al., 1999; Bobabilla-Morales et al., 2003]. Subsequently, at least three loci for Seckel's syndrome have been confirmed, mapped to chromosomes 3q22.1–q24 and 18p11.31–q11.2, and at least one additional unknown locus [Faivre et al., 2002]. Mutations of the *ATR* gene in 3q2 were recently identified [Alderton et al., 2004; O'Driscoll and Jeggo, 2003]. All of these genes are listed in Table 25-6, with references. Of interest, the two genes associated with microcephaly and mild–moderate phenotype both reveal an evolutionary signature of rapid evolution [Evans et al., 2004a, b].

Antenatal Diagnosis

Microcephaly can often, but not always, be diagnosed by second-trimester fetal ultrasonography [Bromley and Benacerraf, 1995]. This likely is due to variable onset of the deceleration in head growth. When this occurs early, as it often does for severe microcephaly, ultrasound examination should be able to detect the abnormality, but not when it begins in the late second or third trimester.

Genetic Counseling

Some older references cite a 6 percent risk of a family's having a second microcephalic child, but these sources do not consistently address severity of the microcephaly. This percentage may be useful for mild and borderline microcephaly with birth occipitofrontal circumference between −2 and −3 SD below the mean. On the basis of findings in many families with two or more affected siblings with primary microcephaly and other forms of severe microcephaly with birth occipitofrontal circumference below −3 SD, counseling for autosomal-recessive inheritance is appropriate in this group. Thus, most forms of severe congenital MIC (with or without intrauterine growth

retardation) are genetic, most if not all having autosomal-recessive inheritance. Disorders associated with postnatal MIC are much more heterogeneous, with examples of autosomal-dominant (familial or sporadic), autosomal-recessive, and X-linked inheritance (see Table 25-6).

Chromosome Disorders

Many chromosome disorders, including the common trisomies (trisomies 13, 18, and 21), and many structural rearrangements such as cri du chat syndrome (deletion 5p15), are associated with MIC. For most individuals, this presents as a mild congenital form that often is followed by more severe postnatal MIC.

An OMIM search lists more than 400 syndromes with microcephaly, making this an unhelpful search term. Some of the better-known disorders include Angelman's, Cornelia de Lange (Brachmann–de Lange), and Dubowitz's syndromes [Opitz and Holt, 1990].

With potentially hundreds of causes of microcephaly, including prenatal and postnatal onset, as well as genetic and acquired etiologies, diagnostic evaluations may be complex. Investigation of patients with microcephaly includes evaluation for prenatal exposure to teratogens, especially alcohol, drugs, and isotretinoin (a vitamin A analog), and assessment of the family history, birth history, and associated malformations. Laboratory studies should include titers for toxoplasmosis, syphilis, rubella virus, cytomegalovirus, and herpes simplex viruses; neuroimaging [Sugimoto et al., 1993]; evaluation for maternal and childhood metabolic disorders; and genetic testing, including chromosome analysis and testing for small deletions or duplications, which currently is performed by fluorescence in situ hybridization with subtelomeric probes [Knight et al., 2000]. Algorithms for the evaluation of the infant and child with congenital (Figure 25-2) and postnatal (Figure 25-3) microcephaly have recently been published and serve as a generalized approach to the diagnostic evaluation [Ashwal et al., 2009].

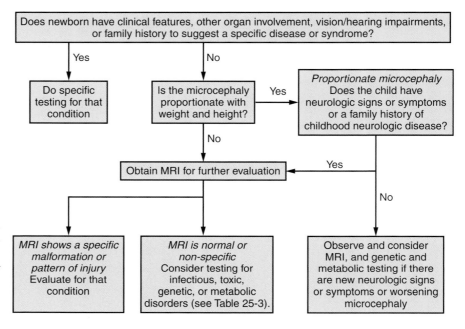

Fig. 25-2 Algorithm for the diagnostic evaluation of the infant or child with congenital microcephaly. *(Adapted from Ashwal S, et al. Practice parameter: Evaluation of the child with microcephaly [an evidence-based review]: report of the Quality Standards Subcommittee of the American Academy of Neurology and the Practice Committee of the Child Neurology Society,* Neurology *73:887–897, 2009.)*

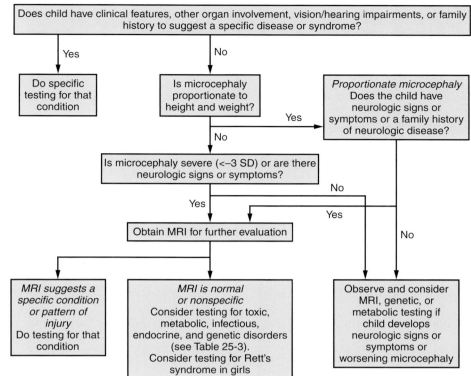

Fig. 25-3 Algorithm for the diagnostic evaluation of the infant or child with postnatal-onset microcephaly. *(Adapted from Ashwal S, et al. Practice parameter: Evaluation of the child with microcephaly [an evidence-based review]: report of the Quality Standards Subcommittee of the American Academy of Neurology and the Practice Committee of the Child Neurology Society. Neurology 73:887–897, 2009.)*

Megalencephaly (and Macrocephaly)

Macrocephaly is defined as an OFC of 2 SDs or more above the mean for age, gender, and gestation, measured over the greatest frontal circumference. It is caused by a myriad of conditions, such as hydrocephalus, cerebral edema, space-occupying lesions, subdural fluid collection, thickening or enlargement of the skull (or hyperostosis), and a truly enlarged brain or megalencephaly (Box 25-1). The classic definition of megalencephaly (MEG) stands as an oversized and overweight brain (or an increased brain mass) that exceeds the mean by 2 SD for age and gender [DeMyer, 1986].

The classification of megalencephaly has been challenging due to its association with a large number of diverse syndromes and etiologies. DeMyer first divided it in 1972 into anatomic and metabolic types [DeMyer, 1972]. Metabolic megalencephalies result from cellular edema or abnormal accumulation of metabolic substrates within the neurons and glia secondary to an underlying biochemical defect (most commonly an enzyme deficiency), without an increase in cell number. The various causes of metabolic megalencephalies are listed in Tables 25-7 and 25-8, and include cerebral organic acid disorders (such as Canavan's disease, glutaric aciduria type I) and lysosomal storage disorders (such generalized, or GM_1, gangliosidosis, Tay–Sachs disease, Krabbe's disease, some mucopolysaccharidoses), among others. A number of these disorders (most notably, Canavan's, Krabbe's, and Alexander's diseases, and megalencephalic leukoencephalopathy with subcortical cysts) are leukoencephalopathies, i.e., demyelinating disorders whereby the underlying biochemical or genetic defect alters myelin formation and function. The metabolic megalencephalies are not true cortical malformations and will not be discussed further in this chapter, but are discussed in other sections of this book.

Anatomic megalencephalies, on the other hand, are secondary to an increase in the size or number of cells, or both, and are disorders of neuronal development, resulting from either overproduction of cells or failure of programmed cell death, or apoptosis. These disorders are quite numerous and will be the focus of the remainder of this chapter. The term "idiopathic megalencephaly" is a clinical term used in the literature for children with abnormally large brains in the absence of disease known to cause an abnormal increase in brain size.

Most of the early literature on megalencephaly predates modern neuroimaging, and earlier diagnoses were based on neuropathology of brain autopsy specimens. Alternatively, and given the difficulty of measuring brain volume accurately, megalencephaly was accepted as the cause of macrocephaly in the absence of other clear etiologies of an enlarged OFC (such as the absence of hydrocephalus or enlarged extra-axial space). Therefore, the terms macrocephaly and megalencephaly have been used somewhat imprecisely in the literature, and clear evidence of true megalencephaly in a number of syndromes is lacking. Furthermore, megalencephaly commonly coexists with variable degrees of ventriculomegaly, hydrocephalus, and/or enlarged extra-axial space, and a correlation between these two conditions and their individual contribution to head size is often absent using earlier neuroimaging methods. The presence of true megalencephaly is better substantiated today, given our improved knowledge of the neuroimaging features of many macrocephaly disorders, as well as the improved use and quality of brain MRIs, and the advent of volumetric analysis of the brain.

With the above-mentioned considerations in mind, Tables 25-9 and 25-10 list the most common syndromes and disorders in which macrocephaly is a defining feature or is of diagnostic significance. The presence of true megalencephaly

Box 25-1 Causes of Macrocephaly

I. Hydrocephalus

- Noncommunicating
  - Arnold–Chiari malformation
  - Aqueductal stenosis
  - X-linked hydrocephalus with stenosis of the aqueduct of Sylvius (HSAS) syndrome (L1CAM)
  - Dandy–Walker malformation
  - Galenic vein aneurysm or malformation
  - Neoplasms, supratentorial and infratentorial
  - Arachnoid cyst, infratentorial
  - Holoprosencephaly with dorsal interhemispheric sac
- Communicating
  - External or extraventricular obstructive hydrocephalus (dilated subarachnoid space)
- Arachnoid cyst, supratentorial
- Meningeal fibrosis/obstruction
  - Postinflammatory
  - Posthemorrhagic
  - Neoplastic infiltration
- Vascular
  - Arteriovenous malformation
  - Intracranial hemorrhage
  - Dural sinus thrombosis
- Choroid plexus papilloma
- Neurocutaneous syndromes
  - Incontinentia pigmenti
- Destructive lesions
  - Hydranencephaly
  - Porencephaly
- Familial, autosomal-dominant, autosomal-recessive, X-linked

II. Subdural Fluid

- Hematoma
- Hygroma
- Empyema

III. Brain Edema (Toxic-Metabolic)

- Intoxication
- Lead
- Vitamin A
- Tetracycline
- Endocrine (hypoparathyroidism, hypoadrenocorticism)
- Galactosemia
- Idiopathic (pseudotumor cerebri)

IV. Thick Skull or Scalp (Hyperostosis)

- Familial variation
- Anemia
- Osteoporosis, severe precocious autosomal-recessive osteoporosis (CLCN7, TCIRG1)
- Pycnodysostosis (CTSK)
- Craniometaphyseal dysplasia (ANKH)
- Craniodiaphyseal dysplasia
- Pyle's dysplasia
- Sclerosteosis (SOST)
- Juvenile Paget's disease
- Idiopathic hyperphosphatasia
- Familial osteoectasia
- Osteogenesis imperfecta
- Rickets
- Cleidocranial dysostosis
- Hyperostosis corticalis generalisata (Van Buchem's disease)
- Proteus' syndrome

V. Megalencephaly and Hemimegalencephaly

- See Tables 25-7 through 25-10

(vs. absolute or relative macrocephaly) is indicated in the second column of Table 25-9.

Unilateral megalencephaly (or hemimegalencephaly) is a rare diffuse enlargement of one cerebral hemisphere, with unique clinical and neuroimaging characteristics and syndromic associations. The most common causes of hemimegalencephaly are outlined in Tables 25-9 and 25-10 as well.

Pathology and Pathogenesis

Numerous animal models of syndromic and nonsyndromic megalencephaly display neuronal and glial hypertrophy. *Pten* (phosphatase and tensin homolog on chromosome ten) mutant mice were found to develop macrocephaly and behavioral abnormalities reminiscent of human autistic spectrum disorder, such as reduced social activity, increased anxiety, and sporadic seizures [Kwon et al., 2001; Kwon et al., 2006; Ogawa et al., 2007], closely resembling the human phenotype of *PTEN*-related disorders that are described later in this chapter. At the cellular level, in vivo effects of loss of *Pten* include loss of neuronal polarity, neuronal hypertrophy, and, in one study, increased astrocyte proliferation and hypertrophy [Kwon et al., 2001; Fraser et al., 2004]. Increasing attention has been paid to the role of the mammalian target of rapamycin (mTOR),

a serine/threonine kinase that has well-known functions in regulation of cellular proliferation and growth, a crucial role in neuronal development and synaptic plasticity [Jaworski and Sheng, 2006], and a contribution to *Pten*-mediated growth regulation in the mammalian nervous system. mTOR inhibition reversed neuronal hypertrophy in *Pten*-deficient mice and also resulted in amelioration of a subset of *Pten*-associated abnormal behaviors, thereby substantiating evidence that the mTOR pathway downstream of *PTEN* is critical for its complex phenotype [Kwon et al., 2003; Zhou et al., 2009].

Loss of *Tsc1* and *Tsc2*, two downstream negative regulators of the mTOR pathway [Inoki et al., 2002; Manning et al., 2002; Potter et al., 2002], has been shown to cause neuronal hypertrophy in vitro and in vivo [Jaworski et al., 2005; Tavazoie et al., 2005; Meikle et al., 2007], supporting a role of *TSC1* and *TSC2* in neuronal growth regulation and synaptic function. Interruptions of *TSC1* and *TSC2* cause tuberous sclerosis complex, known to be associated with megalencephaly, hemimegalencephaly, and focal megalencephaly [Choi et al., 2008]. Zhou et al. suggested that there is a common signal transduction pathway potentially responsible for the autism-like symptoms in individuals bearing *TSC1/2* and/or *PTEN* mutations, and proposed that mTOR inhibitors are potential therapeutic agents for this subset of patients [Meikle et al.,

Table 25-7 Neurometabolic Megalencephaly Syndromes: Inheritance and Genes

Syndrome	Inheritance	Gene	References
CEREBRAL ORGANIC ACID DISORDERS AND DISORDERS OF LYSINE METABOLISM			
N-acetylaspartic aciduria (Canavan's disease)*	AR	ASPA	Fernandez et al. [2006]
Glutaric aciduria (GA) type I*	AR	GCDH	Fernandez et al. [2006]
L-2-Hydroxyglutaric aciduria	AR	L2HGDH	Fernandez et al. [2006]
D-2-Hydroxygylatric aciduria	AR	D2HGDH	Fernandez et al. [2006]
LYSOSOMAL STORAGE DISEASES			
Disorders of Sphingolipid Metabolism			
Generalized gangliosidosis GM$_1$ (early infantile)*	AR	GLB1	Fernandez et al. [2006]

GM$_2$ gangliosidosis
   Tay–Sachs disease (infantile)*
   Sandhoff's disease*
	AR	
		HEXA
		HEXB
			
			Fernandez et al. [2006]
			Fernandez et al. [2006]

Krabbe's disease (globoid cell leukodystrophy) (early infantile)*	AR	GALC	Fernandez et al. [2006]
Mucopolysaccharidoses (MPS)			
Hurler's syndrome (type IH)	AR	IDUA	Fernandez et al. [2006]
Hunter's syndrome (type II)	XL	IDS	Fernandez et al. [2006]
Sanfilippo's syndrome (type III)	AR	SGSH (IIIA) NAGLU (IIIB) HGSNAT (IIIC) GNS (IIID)	Fernandez et al. [2006]
Morquio's syndrome (type IV)	AR	GALNS (IVA) GLB1 (IVB)	Fernandez et al. [2006]
Maroteaux–Lamy syndrome (type VI)	AR	ARSB	Fernandez et al. [2006]
Mucolipidoses[†]			
Mucolipidosis type II (I-cell disease) Mucolipidosis type III	AR AR	GNPTAB GNPTAB (α/β) GNPTG (γ)	Fernandez et al. [2006] Fernandez et al. [2006]
Mannosidosis	AR	MAN2B1 (α) MANBA (β)	Grabb et al. [1995]
LEUKOENCEPHALOPATHIES*			
Alexander's disease (infantile and juvenile forms)	AD	GFAP	Mignot et al. [2004]
Megalencephalic leukoencephalopathy with subcortical cysts	AR	MLC1	Singhal et al. [2003]
MITOCHONDRIAL RESPIRATORY CHAIN DISORDERS			
Complex I and IV deficiency	Maternal/AD/AR	Multiple	Fernandez et al. [2006]

* Other leukoencephalopathies associated with megalencephaly (as indicated in the table): Canavan's disease, glutaric aciduria type I, infantile generalized, or GM$_1$, gangliosidosis, infantile GM$_2$ gangliosidosis (Tay–Sachs and Sandhoff's diseases), infantile Krabbe's disease.
[†] May not be true MAC.
?AD, autosomal-dominant; AR, autosomal-recessive; XL, X-linked.

2008; Zhou et al., 2009]. The *Nf1* knockout mouse was found to have increased neuroglial progenitor/stem cell (NSC) proliferation and gliogenesis in the brainstem, also driven by mTOR-mediated activation [Lee et al., 2010].

Other animal models of megalencephaly include mouse mutants with loss-of-function mutations in genes regulating programmed cell death, or apoptosis, such as *Caspase-3*, *Caspase-9*, and *Apaf-1*, which were found to have gross brain malformations and neuronal hyperplasia. However, these mutations, when germline, are embryonically lethal [Kuida et al., 1996, 1998; Cecconi et al., 1998; Yoshida et al., 1998; Hakem et al., 1998; Marks and Berg, 1999]. Transgenic mice overexpressing insulin-like growth factor (IGF)-I exhibit brain overgrowth characterized by increased numbers of neurons and oligodendrocytes, as well as excessive myelin formation [Carson et al., 1993; Donahue et al., 1996; Petersson et al., 1999; D'Ercole et al., 2002]. IGF-1 stimulates:

1. proliferation of neural progenitors and, possibly, pluripotent neuroglial stem cells (NSC)
2. survival of neurons and oligodendrocytes
3. differentiation of neurons, including neuritic outgrowth and synaptogenesis, and of oligodendrocytes, including expression of myelin gene proteins and myelination.

As a result of these events, brain growth is increased with IGF-I overexpression and reduced with decreased IGF-I signaling. Although much less information is available in humans,

Table 25-8 Neurometabolic Megalencephaly Syndromes: Clinical, Neuroimaging, and Metabolic Features

Disorder	Clinical Features (Other Than MAC)	Neuroimaging Findings	Metabolic Abnormalities
CEREBRAL ORGANIC ACID DISORDERS AND DISORDERS OF LYSINE METABOLISM			
N-acetylaspartic aciduria (Canavan's disease)*	Progressive severe DD, SZ, OA, progressive spasticity, opisthotonus	Diffuse, symmetric WM abnormalities	↓ Aspartoacylase (ASPA) ↑ N-acetylaspartic acid (NAA)
Glutaric aciduria type 1 (GA1*)	Neonatal MAC, dyskinesia, choreoathetosis, dystonia, DD	Frontotemporal atrophy (95%), delayed myelination, high signal intensity in dentate nucleus, subdural effusion/hemorrhage	↓ Glutaryl-CoA dehydrogenase ↑ Glutaryl-CoA ↑ Acylcarnitines:free carnitine ↑ Urinary dicarboxylic acids, 2-oxoglutarate, succinate
L-2-Hydroxyglutaric aciduria	Progressive MAC (50%), DD, SZ, extrapyramidal signs	Swollen subcortical WM, progressive loss of arcuate fibers, severe cerebellar atrophy, signal intensities ↑in dentate nuclei and globi pallidi, and ↓ in thalamus (T2-weighted images)	↓ L-2-hydroxyglutarate dehydrogenase ↑ L-2-hydroxyglutaric acid (CSF > plasma) ↑ hydroxydicarboxylic acid (CSF) ↑ Lysine (CSF, blood)
D-2-Hydroxyglutaric aciduria	Neonatal epileptic encephalopathy with severe DD, hypotonia, CM to mild DD/no symptoms	Delayed and abnormal gyration, myelination, and opercularization, VMEG, cysts over head of caudate nucleus	↓ D-2-hydroxyglutaric acid dehydrogenase ↑ D-2-hydroxyglutaric acid
LYSOSOMAL STORAGE DISEASES			
Disorders of Sphingolipid Metabolism			
Gangliosidosis GM₁(generalized, early infantile)*	DD, HSM, SZ, tone abnormalities, DYS, macular cherry-red spot	Diffuse hypomyelination, mild T2 hyperintensities of caudate nucleus and putamen, normal T2 signal intensity of CC	↓ β-galactosidase ↑ GM₁ ganglioside, asialo-GA₁ (neurons) ↑ Oligosaccharide, minor glycolipids, glycopeptides (visceral organs)
GM₂ gangliosidosis Tay–Sachs disease (infantile)*	Hypotonia, motor weakness, SZ, hyperacusis, macular cherry-red spot, blindness, spasticity, MAC by 18 mo of age	Similar to GM₁	↓ Hexosaminidase A ↑ GM₂-ganglioside (neurons)
Sandhoff's disease*	Organomegaly and bony abnormalities less common	Similar to GM₁	↓ Hexosaminidase A and B ↑ GM₂-ganglioside, asialo-GM₂ (neurons) ↑ Globosides, oligosaccharides (viscera)
Krabbe's disease (globoid cell leukodystrophy) (early infantile)*	PN, opisthotonus, SZ, hyperpyrexia, blindness, loss of bulbar functions, hypotonia	Diffuse WM abnormalities, diffuse cerebral atrophy, calcifications (thalamus, BG, periventricular WM)	↓ Galactosylceramidase ↑ Galactosylceramide (globoid cells) ↑ Galactosylsphingosine (oligodendrocytes, Schwann cells)
Mucopolysaccharidoses (MPS)			
Hurler's syndrome (type IH)	HSM, CNS, DM, DYS, OPH, CAR	WM abnormalities, cerebral atrophy, cervical myelopathy	↓ Iduronidase ↑ Heparan sulfate ↑ Dermatan sulfate
Hunter's syndrome (type II)	HSM, CNS, DM, DYS, OPH, CAR, SK	WM abnormalities, cerebral atrophy, cervical myelopathy	↓ Iduronate-2-sulfatase ↑ Heparin sulfate ↑ Dermatan sulfate
Sanfilippo's syndrome (type III)	CNS, DM (±), DYS (±)	WM abnormalities, cerebral atrophy, cervical myelopathy	↓ Heparan N-sulfatase (IIIA) ↓ N-acetyl-glucosaminidase (IIIB) ↓ Acetyl CoA glucosamine N-acetyl transferase (IIIC) ↓ N-acetyl-glucosamine-6-sulfatase (IIID) ↑ Heparan sulfate
Morquio's syndrome (type IV)	DM, CAR, OPH (±)	WM abnormalities, cerebral atrophy, cervical myelopathy	↓ N-acetylgalactosamine-6-sulfatase (IVA) ↓ β-galactosidase (IVB) ↑ Keratan sulfate
Maroteaux–Lamy syndrome (type VI)	HSM, DM, DYS, OPH, CAR	WM abnormalities, cerebral atrophy, cervical myelopathy	↓ N-acetyl-galactosamine-4-sulfatase ↑ Dermatan sulfate

Table 25-8 Neurometabolic Megalencephaly Syndromes: Clinical, Neuroimaging, and Metabolic Features—cont'd

Disorder	Clinical Features (Other Than MAC)	Neuroimaging Findings	Metabolic Abnormalities
Mucolipidoses[†]			
Mucolipidosis type II (I-cell disease)	HSM, CNS, DM, DYS, OPH, CAR	Cerebral atrophy, WM abnormalities (occasionally)	↓ Transferase[‡]
Mucolipidosis type III	HSM (±), CNS (±), DM, DYS (±), CAR	Cerebral atrophy, WM abnormalities (occasionally)	↓ Transferase[‡]
Mannosidosis	HSM, DM, DYS, CAR, CNS (±)	Partially empty sella turcica, cerebellar atrophy, WM abnormalities (α)	↓ α-Mannosidase (α) ↑ α-Mannosides (α) ↓ β-Mannosidase (β) ↑ β-Mannosides (β)
LEUKOENCEPHALOPATHIES*			
Alexander's disease (infantile and juvenile forms)	DD, SZ, paraparesis, feeding problems	WM abnormalities (frontally predominant), calcification of BG, cerebellar changes, HYD	–
Megalencephalic leukoencephalopathy with subcortical cysts	Progressive spasticity, ataxia	Extensive symmetric WM changes with subcortical cyst	–

* Other leukoencephalopathies associated with megalencephaly (as indicated in the table): Canavan's disease, glutaric aciduria type I, infantile generalized, or GM₁, gangliosidosis, infantile GM₂ gangliosidosis (Tay–Sachs and Sandhoff's diseases), infantile Krabbe's disease.
† May not be true MAC.
‡ Lysosomal UDP-*N*-acetylglucosamine-I-phosphotransferase.
?BG, basal ganglia; CAR, cardiovascular involvement; CC, corpus callosum; CM, cardiomyopathy; CNS, central nervous system regression; CSF, cerebrospinal fluid; DD, developmental delay; DM, dysostosis multiplex; DYS, dysmorphic features; HSM, hepatosplenomegaly; HYD, hydrocephalus; MAC, macrocephaly; OA, optic atrophy; OPH, ocular anomalies (corneal clouding, ophthalmoplegia); PN, peripheral neuropathy; SK, dermatological findings; SZ: seizures; VMEG, ventriculomegaly; WM, white matter.

individuals with IGF-I gene deletions or mutations that result in severe deficits in IGF-1 expression are microcephalic and mentally retarded [Walenkamp and Wit, 2007]. Little evidence supporting comparable actions for IGF-II is available.

The CD81 null mouse has a markedly increased brain size (up to 30 percent larger) due to an increased number of astrocytes and microglia throughout the brain, possibly through regulation of cell proliferation by a contact inhibition-dependent mechanism. CD81 is a member of the tetraspanin family of small membrane proteins associated with the regulation of cell migration and mitotic activity [Geisert et al., 2002]. In yet another animal model, transgenic mice expressing a stabilized β-catenin in neural precursors develop enlarged brains with increased cerebral cortical surface area and folds resembling sulci and gyri of higher mammals [Chenn and Walsh, 2002, 2003]. Brains from these animals have enlarged lateral ventricles lined with neuroepithelial precursor cells that are derived from an expanded precursor population. Compared with the wild type of precursors, a greater proportion of transgenic precursors re-enter the cell cycle after mitosis, which suggests that β-catenin regulates cerebral cortical size by controlling the generation of neural precursor cells.

Among the few models with postnatal progressive megalencephaly are the epileptic megalencephaly BALB/cByJ-Kv1.1^mceph/mceph (called mceph/mceph) mice [Donahue et al., 1996] and the epileptic (epi/epi) chicken [George et al., 1990a]. The mceph/mceph mice carry a spontaneous germline mutation in a gene encoding a potassium ion channel subunit. This mutation makes the channel protein, Kv1.1, non-functional and causes complex partial epilepsy with the limbic system as the major focus (temporal lobe epilepsy [TLE]); interestingly, in parallel to progressive epileptic behavior, the mceph/mceph brains show progressive overgrowth, in the absence of other structural brain abnormalities. This excessive brain enlargement is restricted to the hippocampus and ventral cortical structures, including the piriform/entorhinal cortex and amygdala, whereas the thalamus, olfactory bulb, and cerebellum have wild-type sizes. The volume increase in the mceph/mceph hippocampus is due to a doubling of the number of neurons and astrocytes. In humans, Kv1.1 mutations, where only one amino acid is changed, have been found in patients with epilepsy or episodic ataxia type 1 (EA1). From extensive studies of the mceph/mceph mouse, it has been hypothesized that some human idiopathic megalencephalies with severe early-onset seizures are caused by such severe ion channelopathies [Almgren et al., 2008].

Clinical Features

Nonsyndromic (Idiopathic or Familial) Megalencephaly

The most common and largest group of anatomic megalencephaly is idiopathic megalencephaly that runs in families, the so-called "familial megalencephaly." In one large retrospective series of 557 children referred for macrocephaly, idiopathic megalencephaly was diagnosed in 109, with a familial incidence of at least 50 percent of cases [Lorber and Priestley, 1981]. In a similarly large study, Laubscher et al. observed a familial incidence of 50 out of 71 cases (70 percent) with primary megalencephaly. There are multiple additional reports of familial megalencephaly in the older literature [DeMyer, 1972; Platt and Nash, 1972; Schreier et al., 1974; Asch and Myers, 1976; Day and Schutt, 1979]. This is generally a diagnosis of

Table 25-9 Syndromic and Nonsyndromic Megalencephaly and Hemimegalencephaly: Genes and Inheritance

Disorder (OMIM Number)	MEG/ MAC	Inheritance	Gene (Detection Rate)	References
NONSYNDROMIC MEG				
Familial MEG (153470)	True MEG	AD AR	–	Lorber and Priestley [1981] Laubscher et al. [1990]
SYNDROMIC MEG				
Syndromic MEG with Somatic Overgrowth				
Sotos' syndrome (117550)	MAC	De novo (95%) AD (5%)	NSD1 (90%)	Tatton-Brown et al. [2005] Baujat and Cormier-Daire [2007]
Weaver's syndrome (277590) (genetic overlap with Sotos' syndrome)	MAC	Sporadic (majority) AD (some)	NSD1 (some)	Weaver et al. [1974]
Simpson–Golabi–Behmel (SGB) syndrome type 1 (312870)	MAC	XL	GPC3 (up to 70%)	Simpson et al. [1975] Behmel et al. [1984] DeBaun et al. [2001]
Simpson–Golabi–Behmel (SGB) syndrome type 2 (300209)	MAC	XL	OFD1 (unknown)	Budny et al. [2006]
Nevoid basal cell carcinoma syndrome (NBCCS) (Gorlin S) (109400)	MAC (relative)	AD (70–80%) Sporadic (20–30%)	PTCH1 (up to 90%)	Bale et al. [1991] Kimonis et al. [1997]
Perlman's syndrome (267000)	MAC	Unknown (possibly AR)	–	Perlman et al. [1975]
Duplication 2p24.3 syndrome	MAC (?true MEG)	Sporadic	MYCN	Malan et al. [2010]
Syndromic (Relative) MEG with RASopathies				
Neurofibromatosis type I (162200)	True MEG	AD (505) Sporadic (50%)	NF1 (~97%)	Bale et al. [1991] Said et al. [1996] Cutting et al. [2002]
Legius' syndrome (611431)	MAC	AD	SPRED1 (unknown)	Brems et al. [2007]
Costello's syndrome (218040)	MAC (absolute or relative)	AD Sporadic (majority)	HRAS (80–90%)	Gripp et al. [2010]
Cardio-facio-cutaneous (CFC) syndrome (115150)	MAC	Sporadic (~100%)	BRAF (~80%), MAP2K1, MAP2K2 (~10–15%) KRAS (<5%)	Roberts et al. [2006]
Noonan's syndrome (163950)	MAC (relative)	Sporadic (majority) AD	PTPN11 (50%) SOS1 (10–13%) RAF1 (3–17%) KRAS (<5%)	Allanson [1993–2001]
Syndromic MEG with Partial or No Somatic Overgrowth (Exclude CASK Males)				
M-CM syndrome* (602501) MPPH syndrome* (603387)	True MEG	Sporadic	–	Moore et al. [1997] Mirzaa et al. [2004] Gripp et al. [2009]
Macrocephaly-autism syndrome (605309)	True MEG		PTEN (10–20%)	Butler et al. [2005] Varga et al. [2009] McBride et al. [2010]
Cowden's syndrome (158350)	MAC	Sporadic (majority) AD	PTEN (85%)	Pilarski and Eng [2004]
Bannayan–Riley–Ruvalcaba syndrome (153480)	MAC	AD	PTEN (65%)	Gorlin et al. [1992] Erkek et al. [2005]
Acrocallosal syndrome (ACLS) (200990)	MAC	AR	Unknown	Schinzel [1979] Schinzel and Schmid [1980]
Opitz–Kaveggia (FG) syndrome (305450)	MAC	XL	MED12 (unknown)	Opitz et al. [2008]

Table 25-9 Syndromic and Nonsyndromic Megalencephaly and Hemimegalencephaly: Genes and Inheritance—cont'd

Disorder (OMIM Number)	MEG/ MAC	Inheritance	Gene (Detection Rate)	References
Lujan's (Lujan–Fryns) syndrome (309520) (allelic to FG syndrome)	MAC	XL	MED12 (unknown)	Schwartz et al. [2007]
Polyhydramnios, megalencephaly, and symptomatic epilepsy (PMSE) syndrome (611087)	MEG	AR	LYK5	Puffenberger et al. [2007]
Macrocephaly, megalocornea, motor and mental retardation (MMMM) syndrome[†] (249310)	MAC	Unknown (possibly AR)	–	Frydman et al. [1990]
Macrosomia, obesity, macrocephaly, and ocular abnormalities (MOMO) syndrome[†] (157980)	MAC	Sporadic	–	Moretti-Ferreira et al. [1993]
Clark–Baraitser syndrome[†] (300602)	MAC	XL	–	Clark and Baraitser [1987] Mendicino et al. [2005]
Duplication 1q21.1 syndrome (612475)	MAC (or relative MAC)	–	HYDIN paralog (1a21.1)	Brunetti-Pierri et al. [2008]
MACS (macrocephaly, alopecia, cutis laxa, and scoliosis) syndrome (613075)	MAC	AR	RIN2	Basel-Vanagaite et al. [2009]
XLMR, autism, epilepsy, and MAC	MAC	XL	RAB39	Giannandrea et al. [2010]
Syndromic MEG with Skeletal Involvement				
Achondroplasia (100800)	True MEG	Sporadic (80%) AD (20%)	FGFR3 (~99%)	Dennis et al. [1961] Knisely [1989]
Thanatophoric dysplasia (TDI#187600, TDII#187601)	True MEG	Sporadic (majority) AD	FGFR3 (~99%)	Knisely [1989]
Robinow's syndrome (180700)	MAC (relative)	AD AR	ROR2 (65–100%)	Afzal and Taylor [1993–2005]
Greig's cephalopolysyndactyly syndrome (GCPS) (175700)	MAC	AD	GLI3 (70%)	Biesecker [2008]
NONSYNDROMIC HMEG				
Nonsyndromic HMEG	–	–	–	
SYNDROMIC HMEG				
Syndromic HMEG with Somatic Hemihypertrophy				
Klippel–Trenaunay syndrome (149000)	–	Sporadic	–	Anlar et al. [1988] Matsubara et al. [1983] Torregrosa et al. [2000]
Proteus' syndrome[‡] (176920)	–	Sporadic	PTEN (20%)	Wiedemann et al. [1983] Cohen [1993]
Hypomelanosis of Ito (300337)	–	Possible chromosomal mosaicism	–	Chapman and Cardenas [2008] Sharma et al. [2009]
Syndromic HMEG Without Somatic Hemihypertrophy				
Linear nevus sebaceous syndrome (601359)	–	Sporadic	–	Pavone et al. [1991] Dodge and Dobyns [1995] Flores-Sarnat [2002]
Tuberous sclerosis complex (TSC1 191100; TSC2 613254)	–	AD (33%) Sporadic (67%)	TSC1 (19%) TSC2 (60%)	Griffiths et al. [1998]

* Significant clinical overlap exists between M-CM (macrocephaly-capillary malformation) and MPPH (megalencephaly-polymicrogyria-postaxial polydactyly-hydrocephalus) syndromes; they may represent a single multiple congenital anomalies syndrome [Gripp et al., 2009; unpublished data].
† One and/or few case reports.
‡ Cowden's, Bannayan–Riley–Ruvalcaba, Proteus', and Proteus-like syndromes are PTEN-related disorders and are collectively called the "PTEN hamartoma tumor syndrome."

AD, autosomal-dominant; AR, autosomal-recessive; CASK, calcium/calmodulin-dependant serine protein kinase gene mutation; HMEG, hemimegalencephaly; MAC, macrocephaly; M-CM, macrocephaly-capillary malformation syndrome; MEG, megalencephaly; MPPH, megalencephaly-polymicrogyria-postaxial polydactyly-hydrocephalus syndrome; RAS, "rat sarcoma" oncogene; XL, X-linked; XLMR, X-linked mental retardation.

Table 25-10 Syndromic and Nonsyndromic Megalencephaly and Hemimegalencephaly: Clinical and Neuroimaging Features

Disorder (OMIM Number)	Clinical Features (Besides MAC)	Neurologic Findings	MRI Findings
NONSYNDROMIC MEG			
Familial MEG (153470)	↓ BW/body size (±)	DD, SZ, tone abnormalities (minority)	VMEG/HYD (±) (often mild)
SYNDROMIC MEG			
Syndromic MEG with Somatic Overgrowth			
Sotos' syndrome (117550)	Prenatal and postnatal overgrowth, characteristic facial gestalt, advanced bone age	Hypotonia, DD/behavioral problems (very common), SZ (25%)	Prominent trigone, VMEG/HYD, XAX, CC abnormalities, CSP
Weaver's syndrome (277590) (clinical overlap with Sotos' syndrome)	Characteristic facies (prominent hypertelorism, micrognathia, deep horizontal skin crease), camptodactyly	DD (81%)	Pachygyria, VMEG, cysts of septum pellucidum (rare)
Simpson–Golabi–Behmel (SGB) syndrome type 1 (312870)	Prenatal overgrowth, characteristic facies (macroglossia, macrostomia, central groove of lower lip, ocular hypertelorism), supernumerary nipples	Hypotonia, DD (variable), SZ	HYD, CBTH, ACC (all rare)
Simpson–Golabi–Behmel (SGB) syndrome type 2 (300209)	Ciliary dyskinesia, respiratory problems, DYSM, short fingers	Severe DD, hypotonia	VMEG*
Nevoid basal cell carcinoma syndrome (NBCCS) (Gorlin S) (109400)	Jaw keratocysts, basal cell carcinomas, coarse facial features, facial milia, skeletal anomalies (bifid ribs, wedge-shaped vertebrae)	–	Ectopic calcifications (in falx >90%), medulloblastoma (PNET) (5%)
Perlman's syndrome (267000)	Fetal gigantism, renal hamartomas, nephroblastomatosis, risk for Wilms' tumor	DD (most) (Poor survival)	Abnormalities of CC, HET, WM abnormalities, cerebral atrophy
Duplication 2p24.3 syndrome	Triphalangeal thumb, DYSM (similar to Weaver's syndrome)	DD (mild)	–
Syndromic (Relative) MEG with RASopathies			
Neurofibromatosis type I (162200)	CALs, axillary freckling, cutaneous neurofibromas, short stature	LD (50–75%), severe DD (3%), ADHD, headaches (20%), SZ (10%)	Optic glioma (15%), UBOs on T2-weighted MRI, CC abnormalities, HYD
Legius' syndrome (611431) NF-like phenotype	CALs, freckling, lipomas, MAC, no tumor manifestations	DD, LD, ADHD, headaches, SZ	–
Costello's syndrome (218040)	FTT, short stature, coarse facial features, fine, curly or sparse hair, papillomata, HCM, CHD, malignancy risk (15%)	DD (~100%), hypotonia (most), SZ (20–50%)	CBTH, VMEG/HYD
Cardiofaciocutaneous (CFC) syndrome (115150)	Cardiac abnormalities (VHD, HCM, dysrhythmias), DYSM, multiple cutaneous abnormalities	DD (80%), SZ (50%), hypotonia	HYD/VMEG, cortical atrophy, ACC, NMD
Noonan's syndrome (163950)	Short stature, CHD (PVS, HCM), characteristic facies, webbed neck, coagulation defects, lymphatic dysplasias	DD (variable), language delay	VMEG, CBTH
Syndromic MEG with Partial or No Somatic Overgrowth (Exclude CASK in Males)			
M-CM syndrome† (602501) MPPH syndrome† (603387)	Macrocephaly, capillary malformations, digit anomalies (polydactyly, syndactyly), hemihypertrophy, connective tissue/skin laxity	DD, SZ, hypotonia (variable)	HYD, VMEG, CBTH, PMG, thick CC
Macrocephaly-autism syndrome (605309)	Mild DYSM (frontal bossing, midface hypoplasia, biparietal narrowing), obesity	ASD, DD	–
Cowden's syndrome (158350)	Mucocutaneous lesions, malignancy risk (breast, thyroid, endometrium)	DD (10%)	Cerebellar dysplastic gangliocytoma (Lhermitte–Duclos disease)

Table 25-10 Syndromic and Nonsyndromic Megalencephaly and Hemimegalencephaly: Clinical and Neuroimaging Features—cont'd

Disorder (OMIM Number)	Clinical Features (Besides MAC)	Neurologic Findings	MRI Findings
Bannayan–Riley–Ruvalcaba syndrome (153480)	Overgrowth, hamartomatous intestinal polyposis, lipomas, penile pigmented macules, malignancy risk similar to Cowden's syndrome	Autistic features, DD (70%), SZ (25%), proximal myopathy (60%)	–
Acrocallosal syndrome (ACLS) (200990) (clinical overlap with GCPS)	Polysyndactyly, hypertelorism	SZ, DD (very common)	ACC
Opitz–Kaveggia (FG) syndrome (305450)	Imperforate anus, characteristic facial features, broad thumbs	DD (97%), hypotonia (90%), SZ (70%)	Abnormalities of CC, VMEG, HET
Lujan (Lujan–Fryns) syndrome (309520)	Marfanoid habitus, maxillary hypoplasia, palate and dental problems, long hands, hyperextensible digits	DD (mild–moderate), behavioral abnormalities	Dysgenesis of CC
Polyhydramnios, megalencephaly, and symptomatic epilepsy (PMSE) syndrome (611087)	DYSM, strabismus, skeletal muscle hypoplasia, ASD, nephrocalcinosis	DD, hypotonia, SZ	VMEG (mild), subependymal dysplasia, WM abnormalities
Macrocephaly, megalocornea, motor and mental retardation (MMMM) syndrome* (249310)	Megalocornea, iris hypoplasia, minor facial anomalies	Severe DD, SZ, hypotonia	Abnormalities of CC, delayed myelination
Macrosomia, obesity, macrocephaly, and ocular abnormalities (MOMO) syndrome* (157980)	Macrosomia, obesity, macrocephaly, ocular abnormalities (retinal coloboma, nystagmus), delayed bone age	DD, ASD*	–
Clark–Baraitser syndrome* (300602)	Coarse facial features (prominent forehead), microdontia	DD, SZ	–
Duplication 1q21.1 syndrome (612475)	DYSM	Severe DD, focal SZ, ASD	CVH, pACC
MACS (macrocephaly, alopecia, cutis laxa, and scoliosis) syndrome (613075)	Coarse facial features, gingival hyperplasia, severe joint hypermobility, soft redundant skin, sparse hair, short stature, severe scoliosis	–	–
XLMR, autism, epilepsy, and MAC	MAC	DD/MR, ASD, SZ	–
Syndromic MEG with Skeletal Involvement			
Achondroplasia (100800)	Short stature, rhizomelic limb shortening, characteristic facial features	Hypotonia (neonatal), normal intelligence	HYD, cervicomedullary compression
Thanatophoric dysplasia (TDI#187600, TDII#187601)	Micromelia, characteristic facial features, narrow thorax, short ribs (perinatal-lethal) (types I) Type I: bowed femurs, rare cloverleaf skull deformity	DD, SZ (in long-term survivors)	HYD, NMD
Thanatophoric dysplasia (TDI#187600, TDII#187601)	Micromelia, characteristic facial features, narrow thorax, short ribs (perinatal-lethal) (types II) Type II: straight femurs, uniform moderate to severe cloverleaf skull deformity	DD, SZ (in long-term survivors)	HYD, NMD
Robinow's syndrome (180700)	Mesomelic limb shortening, distinct facial and genital abnormalities	SZ, DD (18%)	Cortical dysplasia*
Greig's cephalopolysyndactyly syndrome (GCPS) (175700)	Polydactyly (preaxial, postaxial, mixed), ocular hypertelorism, craniosynostosis	DD, SZ (<10%)	HYD (uncommon)

Continued

Table 25-10 Syndromic and Nonsyndromic Megalencephaly and Hemimegalencephaly: Clinical and Neuroimaging Features—cont'd

Disorder (OMIM Number)	Clinical Features (Besides MAC)	Neurologic Findings	MRI Findings
NONSYNDROMIC HMEG			
Nonsyndromic HMEG	MAC (asymmetric)	DD (severe), SZ (intractable), hemiparesis	HMEG, VMEG, MCD, WM abnormalities (ipsilateral)
SYNDROMIC HMEG			
Syndromic HMEG with Somatic Hemihypertrophy			
Klippel–Trenaunay syndrome (149000)	Cutaneous VM (capillary, venous, lymphatic), varicose veins, unilateral hypertrophy of bones and soft tissues	DD/SZ (rare)	HYD, calcifications, cerebellar hemihypertrophy
Proteus' syndrome[‡] (176920)	Asymmetric and disproportionate hamartomatous overgrowth of multiple tissues, connective tissue and epidermal nevi, dysregulated adipose tissue, VM, hyperostosis	DD (20%), SZ (13%)	Calcifications, abnormalities of CC, HYD
Hypomelanosis of Ito (300337)	Hypopigmented whorls, streaks, and patches, hemihypertrophy, other anomalies	DD (67%), SZ (35%)	Cerebral atrophy, HET, PMG (all rare)
Syndromic HMEG Without Somatic Hemihypertrophy			
Linear nevus sebaceous syndrome (601359)	Epidermal nevi, ocular anomalies (colobomas), skeletal defects	SZ, DD, tone abnormalities	VMEG, HYD, NMD, ACC, DWM
Tuberous sclerosis complex (TSC1 191100; TSC2 613254)	Skin (hypomelanotic macules, facial angiofibromas, shagreen patches, fibrous facial plaques, ungal fibromas), kidney (angiomyolipomas, cysts), heart (rhabdomyomas, arrhythmias)	SZ (80%), DD (50%), ASD/PDD (40–50%), ADHD	Subependymal nodules, cortical tubers, subependymal giant cell astrocytomas, WM abnormalities, focal MEG

* One or a few case reports.
† Significant clinical overlap exists between M-CM (macrocephaly-capillary malformation) and MPPH (megalencephaly-polymicrogyria-postaxial polydactyly-hydrocephalus) syndromes and they may represent a single multiple congenital anomalies syndrome [Gripp et al., 2009; unpublished data].
‡ Cowden, Bannayan–Riley–Ruvalcaba. Proteus and proteus-like syndromes are PTEN-related disorders and are collectively called the "PTEN hamartoma tumor syndrome".
ACC, agenesis of the corpus callosum; ADHD, attention-deficit hyperactivity disorder; ASD, autistic spectrum disorder; BW, birth weight; CAL, café au lait macules; CBTH, cerebellar tonsillar herniation; CC, corpus callosum; CHD, congenital heart disease; CSP, cavum septum pellucidum; CVH, cerebellar vermis hypoplasia; DD, developmental delay; DWM, Dandy–Walker malformation; DYSM, dysmorphic features; FTT, failure to thrive; HCM, hypertrophic cardiomyopathy; HET, heterotopias; HMEG, hemimegalencephaly; HYD, hydrocephalus; LD, learning disability; MAC, macrocephaly; MEG, megalencephaly; NMD, neuronal migration disorder; PDD, pervasive developmental disorder; PMG, polymicrogyria; PNET, primitive neuroectodermal tumor; PVS, pulmonary valve stenosis; SZ, seizures; UBO, unidentified bright object; VHD, valvular heart disease; VM, vascular malformation; VMEG, ventriculomegaly; WM, white matter; XAX, enlarged extra-axial space; XLMR, X-linked mental retardation.

exclusion following the identification of macrocephaly in a family member, most often a parent, and the absence of an identifiable disorder known to be associated with macrocephaly. Box 25-2 lists the original diagnostic criteria for familial megalencephaly, developed by DeMyer in 1986 [DeMyer, 1986]. The onset of megalencephaly in idiopathic familial and nonfamilial MEG may be congenital or postnatal. OFCs and the progression and velocity of brain growth tend to vary, but the OFC curve generally levels off to parallel the normal one. While most children are neurodevelopmentally normal (and hence the previous designation of "benign" megalencephaly), a wide range of developmental disorders, tone abnormalities, and seizures are present in familial and nonfamilial cases. Clearly, individuals with idiopathic megalencephaly range from those who have fully normal cognitive and motor function to those with substantial neurologic disability [DeMyer, 1972; Schreier et al., 1974; Alvarez et al., 1986; Lewis et al., 1989]. Mild dysmorphic features related to excessive head growth (such as dolichocephaly and frontal bossing) are frequently observed. Neuroradiologically, megalencephaly may be associated with mild or borderline ventriculomegaly, or an enlarged extra-axial space [Alvarez et al., 1986; Laubscher

et al., 1990]. A few familial cases have been complicated by hydrocephalus requiring neurosurgical intervention [Schreier et al., 1974; Day and Schutt, 1979]. Most reported cases of familial megalencephaly appear to be autosomal-dominant, with a strong sex predilection for males; however, very few reports of autosomal-recessive types exist [Gragg, 1971; Härtel et al., 2005].

The clinical features of the most common megalencephaly and hemimegalencephaly syndromes are outlined in Table 25-10, and are discussed briefly below.

Etiology

The most significant macrocephaly (and/or megalencephaly) syndromes are listed in Tables 25-9 and 25-10, with a brief overview of their clinical features, MRI findings, and genetic bases. These include classic overgrowth syndromes, such as Sotos', Weaver's, and Simpson–Golabi–Behmel syndromes; *PTEN*-related disorders, such as Cowden's and Bannayan–Riley–Ruvalcaba syndromes; the macrocephaly-capillary malformation (M-CM) syndrome (previously termed macrocephaly cutis marmorata telangiectatica congenita, or CMTC);

and skeletal dysplasias, such as achondroplasia and thanatophoric dysplasia, as well as a number of chromosomal disorders. By far, the majority of these disorders are inherited as an autosomal-dominant trait. Their clinical features and neurodevelopmental outcome are quite variable and dependent on the ensuing neuronal dysfunction caused by the specific underlying disorder. The most notable megalencephaly/macrocephaly disorders are discussed briefly below.

Overgrowth Syndromes

Macrocephaly frequently occurs in conjunction with body overgrowth (height and weight >2 SD above the mean for age), as in Sotos', Weaver's, and Simpson–Golabi–Behmel syndromes. Many of these overgrowth disorders are characterized by excessive growth in fetal life and infancy, with subsequent decline in growth rate and normalization of growth in adulthood. Partial (or focal) and unilateral overgrowth (or hemihypertrophy) is occasionally seen in other MEG or MAC syndromes, such as M-CM syndrome, *PTEN*-related disorders, and some chromosomal disorders such as Pallister–Killian syndrome. Children who are macrocephalic at birth may become normocephalic or relatively microcephalic when older, if body overgrowth supersedes brain growth, as typically occurs in Beckwith–Wiedemann syndrome.

Sotos' syndrome is an autosomal-dominant disorder due to mutations or deletions of *NSD1* (nuclear receptor-binding SET domain protein-1). Macrocephaly is usually present at all ages in more than 90 percent of children and is considered to be a cardinal feature [Agwu et al., 1999; Rio et al., 2003; Tatton-Brown et al., 2005]. In some series, macrocephaly was present at birth in 50 percent of children, with birth OFCs as high as +4 above the mean, and later OFCs ranging between +2 and +7 SD. Most patients have a nonprogressive neurologic dysfunction characterized by clumsiness and poor coordination [Cole and Hughes, 1994]. Delays in expressive language and motor development during infancy are particularly common and, in some instances, may be followed by attainment of normal or near-normal intelligence. Several patients with Sotos' syndrome and autistic features have been reported [Morrow et al., 1990; Battaglia and Carey, 2006]. Seizures and tone abnormalities are occasionally present [Cohen, 1989, 1999; Cole and Hughes, 1990, 1994]. Brain MRI abnormalities present in patients with Sotos' syndrome and an *NSD1* mutation include enlarged extra-axial fluid and lateral ventricles in 70 percent and 60 percent of patients, respectively, and it has been suggested that these increased CSF spaces are primarily responsible for macrocephaly in Sotos' syndrome, rather than true megalencephaly [Schaefer et al., 1997]. Between 80 and 90 percent of patients have a demonstrable *NSD1* abnormality. *NSD1* is involved in an intricate regulatory network of genes that appear to have a concerted role in various processes, including cell growth and tumorigenesis [Lucio-Eterovic et al., 2010].

NSD1 mutations have also been found in a significant proportion of patients with Weaver's syndrome, a rarer overgrowth disorder characterized by macrocephaly, dysmorphic facial features (especially prominent hypertelorism), metaphyseal flaring of the femurs, camptodactyly, deep-set nails, and hoarse, low-pitched cry. Therefore, significant clinical and genetic overlap exists between these two disorders of macrocephaly and overgrowth [Proud et al., 1998; Rio et al., 2003; Cecconi et al., 2005].

Simpson–Golabi–Behmel syndrome (SGBS) is an X-linked complex congenital overgrowth syndrome characterized by macroglossia, macrosomia, renal and skeletal abnormalities, and an increased risk of embryonal tumors. Macrocephaly is often congenital. Patients may have hypotonia and mild developmental delay, although most have normal intelligence [Neri et al., 1998]. Most cases of SGBS are due to mutations or deletions of the *glypican-3* (*GPC3*) gene at Xq26, a member of a multigene family encoding at least six distinct glycosylphosphatidylinositol-linked cell-surface heparan sulfate proteoglycans (HSPGs); these act as co-receptors for multiple families of growth factors that have been shown to regulate cell proliferation, differentiation, and patterning, including that of the brain. In support of the glypicans' role in development, mice with null mutations in glypican-1 (*Gpc1*) have a severely reduced brain size and an abnormally small-sized cerebellum. Therefore, *Gpc1* may have a role in early neurogenesis, possibly through regulation of fibroblast growth factor (fgf) signaling [Jen et al., 2009].

SGBS type 2 is an X-linked mental retardation syndrome with macrocephaly (OFCs +2 to +6 SD above the mean) and ciliary dysfunction, manifesting as recurrent respiratory tract infections, with abnormal functional studies of the respiratory cilia. Recently, a family with this syndrome co-segregating with a frameshift mutation in the oral-facial-digital type 1 (*OFD1*) gene was reported [Budny et al., 2006].

RASopathies

The Ras/mitogen-activated protein kinase (MAPK) pathway is essential in the regulation of the cell cycle, cell differentiation, growth, and cell senescence, each of which is critical to normal development. The "RASopathies" are a class of developmental disorders caused by germline mutations in genes that encode protein components of the Ras/MAPK pathway, which result in dysregulation of the pathway and profoundly deleterious effects on development. These disorders include neurofibromatosis type 1 (*NF1*), Costello's syndrome (*HRAS*), cardiofaciocutaneous (CFC) syndrome (*KRAS*, *BRAF*, and *MEK1*), and Noonan's syndrome (*PTPN11*, *KRAS*, and *SOS1*), among others. Neurofibromatosis type 1 (NF1) is a disorder of true megalencephaly, whereas Noonan's, Costello's, and CFC syndromes have a high incidence of relative macrocephaly and ventriculomegaly.

NF1 shares features of other overgrowth syndromes, such as the presence of macrocephaly, various types of tumors, and, occasionally, hemihyperplasia of a limb or digit, despite an increased incidence of short stature. Macrocephaly in the absence of hydrocephalus occurs in 50 percent of individuals with NF1 [Tonsgard, 2006]. Quantitative MRI studies have demonstrated the presence of true megalencephaly, largely secondary to increased white-matter volume [Bale et al., 1991; Said et al., 1996; Steen et al., 2001; Cutting et al., 2002]. Learning disabilities have been reported in up to 70 percent of individuals, and 3 percent have severe developmental delay. Their neurocognitive profile may also include easy distractibility, impulsiveness, and deficient visual-motor coordination. Seizures occur in approximately 6–7 percent of patients. Frank hydrocephalus with aqueductal stenosis, as well as asymptomatic ventricular dilatation, has been observed in approximately 4 percent of patients. *NF1* is a tumor suppressor gene, expressed in neurons and glial cells, which encodes neurofibromin, one of the earliest identified regulators of the RAS-MAPK pathway; it thus has important roles in cellular proliferation and differentiation [Daston et al., 1992; Nordlund et al., 1993; Cichowski and Jacks, 2001].

Recently, a dominant condition that overlaps with NF1 clinically (with macrocephaly, café au lait lesions, and axillary freckling) has been described in association with heterozygous mutations in *SPRED1*, a member of the SPROUTY/SPREAD family of proteins that are also regulators of RAS–RAF interaction and MAPK signaling [Brems et al., 2007] (see Legius' syndrome in Tables 25-9 and 25-10).

Costello's syndrome is a unique combination of failure to thrive, cardiac abnormalities, and a predisposition to papillomata and malignant tumors. In a systematic review of 28 patients, absolute or relative macrocephaly was found in 100 percent of patients, and, more specifically an evolving megalencephaly and cerebellar enlargement, overlapping with M-CM syndrome [Gripp et al., 2010]. Neurologic abnormalities include developmental delay/mental retardation, nystagmus, and hypotonia [Quezada and Gripp, 2007; Gripp and Lin, 2009].

Macrocephaly-Capillary Malformation Syndrome

The macrocephaly-capillary malformation (MCAP) syndrome is a distinct syndrome characterized by megalencephaly, vascular malformations (most often cutis marmorata), hemihypertrophy, digit anomalies, and skin and connective tissue laxity. More than 100 patients with M-CM syndrome have been reported [Clayton-Smith et al., 1997; Moore et al., 1997; Vogels et al., 1998; Thong et al., 1999; Franceschini et al., 2000; Robertson et al., 2000; Giuliano et al., 2004; Lapunzina et al., 2004; Canham and Holder, 2008], and its neuroimaging

findings were reviewed by Garavelli et al. [2005] and Conway et al. [2007]. The megalencephaly and perisylvian polymicrogyria with postaxial polydactyly and hydrocephalus (MPPH) syndrome is a more recently described syndrome in an initial cohort of five patients [Mirzaa et al., 2004], and four subsequent single cases [Colombani et al., 2006; Garavelli et al., 2007; Tohyama et al., 2007; Pisano et al., 2008]. Since then, a marked increase in ascertainment of patients with overlapping features of both syndromes has been witnessed, and it is proposed that they represent a single megalencephaly syndrome [Gripp et al., 2009; unpublished data]. MEG is most often congenital, with OFCs ranging from +2 to +4 SD above the mean at birth, and reaching up to +8 SD later in life. Variable degrees of developmental delay, hypotonia, and seizures occur. Vascular anomalies are a characteristic and defining feature and most commonly consist of cutis marmorata, the cutaneous marbled appearance frequently seen in Caucasian newborns that tends to fade with time but often persists. Other vascular anomalies include a midline nevus flammeus, various types of hemangiomas in any location, vascular rings, and telangiectasias. Digit anomalies include the common 2–3 toe syndactyly (>25 percent syndactyly), 2–3–4 finger syndactyly, and postaxial polydactyly. Common MRI abnormalities (Figure 25-4A) include diffuse megalencephaly that is symmetric or mildly asymmetric, a very high rate of hydrocephalus that is often shunted, or ventriculomegaly, progressive posterior fossa crowding with cerebellar tonsillar herniation that may require decompression, polymicrogyria that is by far bilateral perisylvian in distribution, and white-matter abnormalities. A distinct subset of patients has a very thick (or mega-) corpus callosum [Conway et al., 2007; unpublished data]. Serial neuroimaging has demonstrated that, despite shunting procedures, OFCs continue to follow an accelerated growth rate, thereby demonstrating the presence of true megalencephaly. All reported cases to date appear sporadic.

Perhaps as a severe variant of this syndrome, Gohlich-Ratmann et al. reported three sporadic cases with congenital megalencephaly, a greatly hypertrophied corpus callosum, and complete lack of motor development [Gohlich-Ratmann et al., 1998]. Cranial MRI demonstrated bilateral and symmetric megalencephaly and polymicrogyria. Two cases were subsequently reported with similar features, one with minimal motor development (with the ability roll sideways only) [Dagli et al., 2008; Hengst et al., 2010]. Two children from a consanguineous family were similarly reported with mega-corpus callosum, polymicrogyria, and moderate psychomotor retardation, suggestive of autosomal-recessive inheritance. These patients additionally exhibited pontine and cerebellar vermis hypoplasia [Bindu et al., 2010].

PTEN-Related Disorders

PTEN is a tumor suppressor gene, somatic mutations of which have been reported to varying degrees in multiple sporadic malignancies (such as glioblastoma multiforme, among others) [Eng, 2000, 2003]. Germline mutations of *PTEN* have been found in a set of disorders of macrocephaly and hamartomatous overgrowth, namely Cowden's (CS), Bannayan–Riley–Ruvalcaba (BRRS), and Proteus' syndromes, and in a subset of patients with a "Proteus-like" phenotype. CS and BRSS have a high degree of clinical overlap and are believed to constitute a single clinical spectrum (CS-BRRS).

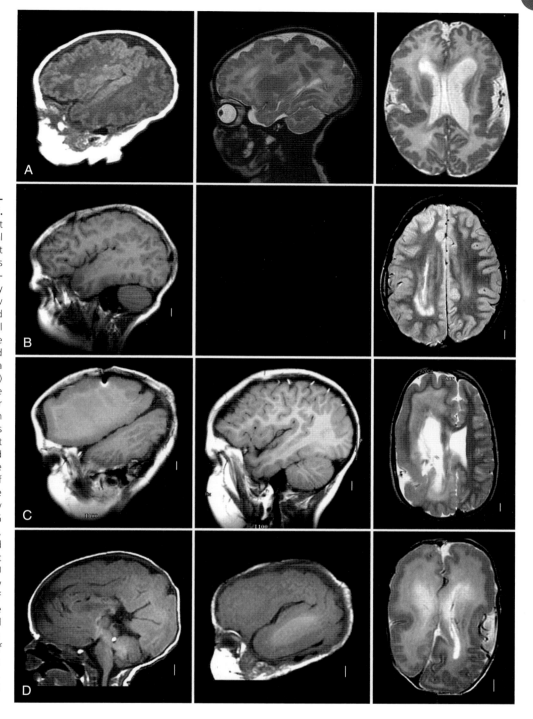

Fig. 25-4 Subtypes of megalencephaly and hemimegalencephaly. Right parasagittal (left column, except midsagittal in D), left parasagittal (middle column), and axial (right column) magnetic resonance images from four patients with megalencephaly (MEG) or hemimegalencephaly (HMEG) variants. **A,** The top row images depict symmetric MEG and perisylvian polymicrogyria with normal white matter. The patient was a female with the originally described "megalencephaly polymicrogyria polydactyly hydrocephalus" (MPPH) syndrome [Mirzaa et al., 2004]. The symmetry and normal white matter distinguish this malformation from HMEG. **B,** The second row images show partial HMEG, with enlargement of the posterior frontal, temporal, and parietal lobes on the right. The abnormal white matter typical of HMEG is seen circling the back of the right lateral ventricle. **C,** The third row images demonstrate severe HMEG involving the entire right hemisphere, but sparing the left. The central and deep white matter has diffusely bright signal, sparing only the superficial U fibers. **D,** The bottom row images show a very rare malformation consisting of bilateral HMEG that is more severe on the left side. The patient survived only a few months. *(Courtesy of Dr. William B Dobyns, University of Washington and Principal Investigator, Center for Integrative Brain Research, Seattle Children's Research Institute, Seattle, WA.)*

Macrocephaly is a prominent and progressive feature, with OFCs typically +4.5 SD or more above the mean, and reaching up to +8 SD. Hypotonia and delayed gross motor skills are common findings. Around 60 percent of patients have a mild proximal myopathy, and 25 percent have seizures. Additional features include hamartomas, lipomas, intestinal polyps, and various types of cutaneous vascular malformations. *PTEN* mutation carriers are at increased risk for various tumors (most notably of the breast, thyroid, and endometrium).

Proteus' syndrome (PS) is a rare and highly variable disorder with relentless asymmetric and disproportionate overgrowth of body parts, vascular malformations, cerebriform connective tissue nevi, epidermal nevi, and dysregulated adipose tissue [Cohen and Hayden, 1979; Wiedemann et al., 1983; Cohen et al., 2002], which has been reported in association with HMEG or unilateral MEG. Given the genetic overlap between these disorders of dysregulated cellular proliferation, the term "*PTEN* hamartoma tumor syndrome" (PHTS) has been coined for this group of distinct conditions [Marsh et al., 1999; Eng,

2000]. *PTEN* mediates cell cycle arrest and/or apoptosis by negatively regulating the phosphinositide-3-kinase-Akt serine/threonine protein kinase (PI3K/Akt) pathway [Furnari et al., 1998; Li et al., 1998; Weng et al., 1999]. Accumulating evidence suggests that *PTEN* also regulates cell survival pathways, such as the MAPK pathway [Gu et al., 1998; Simpson and Parsons, 2001; Weng et al., 2001, 2002]. *PTEN* mutations have recently been identified in patients with isolated macrocephaly and autistic spectrum disorders (ASDs), and/or developmental delay, as discussed below.

Macrocephaly-Autism Syndrome

An increased rate of macrocephaly is a consistent and replicated biological finding in ASD, and appears to be the single most consistent physical characteristic of children with autism. Multiple studies of OFC in persons with ASD have shown that macrocephaly occurs more frequently than expected [Bailey et al., 1993; Bolton et al., 2001; Davidovitch et al., 1996; Woodhouse et al., 1996; Lainhart et al., 1997; Stevenson et al., 1997; Fombonne et al., 1999; Fidler et al., 2000; Miles et al., 2000; Aylward et al., 2002; Gillberg and De Souza, 2002; Deutsch and Joseph, 2003; Dementieva et al., 2005; Lainhart et al., 2006; Courchesne et al., 2010]. These studies show, on average, a rate of macrocephaly of 20 percent in patients with ASD [Fombonne et al., 1999]. Neuroimaging studies of autism have found increased mean total brain volume in children by 2–4 years of age [Courchesne et al., 2001; Sparks et al., 2002; Hazlett et al., 2005]. Furthermore, postmortem studies show increased brain weight in children with autism, with frank megalencephaly in some [Bailey et al., 1998; Kemper and Bauman, 1998]. Causes of macrocephaly other than increased brain volume are rarely found in patients with idiopathic autism [Lainhart et al., 1997; Stevenson et al., 1997; Bailey et al., 1998; Bigler et al., 2003]. Given these data, this common association has been termed the "macrocephaly-autism syndrome."

Butler and colleagues [2005] published the first report directly linking *PTEN* and isolated ASDs, identifying mutations in 3 of 18 individuals. These 3 subjects were boys, 2 of whom had the largest OFCs in the cohort, of +7 SD and +8 SD above the mean [Butler et al., 2005]. A similar study of 71 patients with isolated ASD (57 of whom met the Diagnostic and Statistical Manual of Mental Disorders [DSM]-IV criteria for autism) identified *PTEN* mutations in 2 out of 16 tested individuals who also had macrocephaly [Herman et al., 2007]. Using individuals with ASD and macrocephaly drawn from the Paris Autism Research International Sibpair (PARIS) study, the Autism Genetic Research Exchange [AGRE], and separately recruited patients, Buxbaum et al. found a *PTEN* mutation in 1 of 88 subjects tested [Buxbaum et al., 2007].

Subsequently, *PTEN* mutations were found in 5 of 60 (8.3 percent) individuals with macrocephaly and ASD, and 6 of 49 (12.2 percent) individuals with macrocephaly and developmental delay (DD)/mental retardation (MR) [Varga et al., 2009]; these results were extended by a cohort study whereby *PTEN* mutations were found in 7 of 99 (7.1 percent) individuals with MAC/ASD and 8 of 100 (8 percent) of individuals with MAC/DD [McBride et al., 2010]. Therefore, the estimated *PTEN* mutation frequency in macrocephaly-autism syndrome is approximately 20 percent overall. It is interesting to note that, from a molecular standpoint, mutations in *TSC1/TSC2*, *NF1*, or *PTEN* activate the mTOR/PI3K pathway and lead to syndromic ASD with tuberous sclerosis, neurofibromatosis, or macrocephaly, respectively, as mentioned above.

Disorders of Skeletal Involvement

Achondroplasia and thanatophoric dysplasia are well known to be associated with true megalencephaly from multiple reports in the early literature [Dennis et al., 1961; Cohen et al., 1967; Priestley and Lorber, 1981; Knisely, 1989]. MEG frequently coexists with mild ventriculomegaly, with or without hydrocephalus related to stenosis of the sigmoid sinus at the level of narrowed jugular foramina that rarely requires surgical intervention [Pierre-Kahn et al., 1980]. Robinow's syndrome is a genetically heterogeneous condition characterized by mesomelic limb shortening and facial and genital anomalies. The estimated frequency of MEG (which may be congenital) is up to 64 percent in the dominant form and 25 percent in the recessive form [Mazzeu et al., 2007]. Greig's cephalopolysyndactyly syndrome (GCPS) is a rare pleiotropic, multiple congenital anomaly syndrome characterized by the triad of polysyndactyly, hypertelorism, and macrocephaly, which is not typically associated with other central nervous system anomalies [Biesecker, 2008]. The acrocallosal syndrome resembles GCPS, with the presence of preaxial polysyndactyly and macrocephaly, but is distinguished by agenesis of the corpus callosum, and a much higher incidence of seizures and mental retardation [Johnston et al., 2003].

Chromosomal Abnormalities

Macrocephaly has been reported in several chromosomal disorders, such as trisomy 5p [Leschot and Lim, 1979; Reichenbach et al., 1999], partial duplications of 12p [Rauch et al., 1996], proximal and distal 15q duplications [Hood et al., 1986; Roggenbuck et al., 2004], deletions of 22q13 [Phelan et al., 1992; Tabolacci et al., 2005], and Pallister–Killian syndrome due to mosaic isochromosome 12p [Smigiel et al., 2008]. A number of reciprocal microdeletion and microduplication syndromes are associated with MIC/MAC, such as those involving 1q21.1 [Brunetti-Pierri et al., 2008], 2p24.3 (the locus for the *MYCN* gene) [Malan et al., 2010], and 5q35.3 (the *NSD1* locus) [Lucio-Eterovic et al., 2010]. MEG has also been reported in two patients with Klinefelter's syndrome. One had frank, bilateral, and symmetric MEG, in association with polymicrogyria and neuronal heterotopias [Budka, 1978]; the other had mild, focal, and unilateral MEG, in association with macrogyria [Choi et al., 1980].

Other Megalencephaly/Macrocephaly Syndromes

Relative or absolute macrocephaly occurs in some patients with Opitz–Kaveggia (or FG) syndrome, an X-linked disorder characterized by imperforate anus, broad and flat thumbs, hypotonia, moderate to severe DD, and abnormalities of the corpus callosum, and is due to mutations in *MED12*. Recently, an allelic disorder consisting of macrocephaly, tall, thin (or Marfanoid) habitus, and distinct facial features, called Lujan (or Lujan–Fryns) syndrome, was linked to *MED12* as well.

Other rarer macrocephaly syndromes with few reports in the literature include the macrocephaly, megalocornea, motor and mental retardation (MMMM) syndrome, macrosomia, obesity, macrocephaly, and ocular abnormalities (MOMO) syndrome, and Clark–Baraitser syndrome. A single old report described a patient with ataxia telangiectasia, megalencephaly, and intestinal lymphangiectasia [Scott, 1969].

Unilateral Megalencephaly (or Hemimegalencephaly)

Hemimegalencephaly (HMEG) is a brain malformation characterized by hamartomatous overgrowth of all or part of the cerebral hemisphere, and often associated with ipsilateral cortical malformations. The involved hemisphere is frequently enlarged, with cortical dysgenesis, white-matter hypertrophy, and a dilated and dysmorphic lateral ventricle. There is no clear predilection for the right or left side [Barkovich and Chuang, 1990].

HMEG is most often an isolated congenital abnormality, but is sporadically associated with neurocutaneous and overgrowth syndromes. Overgrowth associations include Proteus' and Klippel–Trenaunay syndromes. Neurocutaneous associations include the linear nevus sebaceous syndrome, tuberous sclerosis, and, occasionally, neurofibromatosis. Hypomelanosis of Ito has both neurocutaneous and overgrowth features.

HMEG traditionally has been regarded as the result of an early disturbance in neuronal proliferation and migration. The known associations of HMEG with other disorders of cellular proliferation (such as tuberous sclerosis complex) support this hypothesis. A relation between epidermal growth factor and excessive proliferation in HMEG has been suggested [Takashima et al., 1991; Kato et al., 1996].

Clinically, macrocephaly is usually apparent at birth, and cranial asymmetry dependent on the degree of HMEG may be evident. OFC may increase rapidly during the first few months, raising the possibility of obstructive hydrocephalus or a space-occupying lesion. However, subsequently, and possibly as a result of intractable seizures, the head size diminishes relative to the normal curve and eventually the patients may become normocephalic or microcephalic. Intractable epilepsy usually begins within the first few months of life, and is the most frequent and severe neurologic manifestation, occurring in up to 93 percent of cases [Vigevano et al., 1989; George et al., 1990b]. Partial, motor, or partial complex seizures are the most frequent types of epilepsy in HMEG, and are associated with infantile spasms in 50 percent of patients. Developmental delay is often early and severe, although in a few cases it can be mild to near normal. Different grades of hemiparesis, ranging from none or mild to overt hemiplegia, are seen contralateral to the HMEG [Flores-Sarnat, 2002].

Neuroimaging shows moderate to marked enlargement of the effected cerebral hemisphere [Fitz et al., 1978; Kalifa et al., 1987], with enlargement of the lateral ventricle. Occasionally, enlargement maybe localized to the frontal or temporoparietal regions. Anomalies of cortical development, including polymicrogyria, pachygyria, and gray-matter heterotopias, are always seen in the affected portions of the hemisphere, but can be seen in the "unaffected" hemisphere as well [Barkovich and Kuzniecky, 1996]. The underlying hemispheric white matter is usually abnormal, with abnormal signal characteristics and/or alteration in volume (increased or decreased) in some individuals. Figure 25-4 (B–D) shows variable degrees of HMEG. EEG abnormalities are often extensive throughout the abnormal hemisphere and a suppression-burst pattern can be observed early on in the most severe cases. Predictors of poor outcome are severity of hemiparesis, the degree of cortical dysplasia on brain MRI, and abnormal EEG activity. Both the epilepsy and the degree of developmental handicap may be improved in selected patients by anatomical or functional hemispherectomy [Delvin et al., 2003; Di Rocco et al., 2006; Kwan et al., 2008].

Malformations of Cortical Development

William B. Dobyns, Renzo Guerrini, and Richard J. Leventer

Development of the human cerebral cortex is a complex and tightly regulated process that can be divided into three broad and overlapping steps, including neural stem cell proliferation and cell type differentiation; neuronal migration; and cortical organization and connectivity. Disruption of any one or more of these processes may result in a wide range of developmental disorders in humans. Many of these are recognized as malformations on brain imaging studies or visual inspection at autopsy, and they collectively comprise a class of disorders that we designate as malformations of cortical development (MCD).

The classification scheme for MCD followed in this chapter (see Box 21-2) is based on enumeration of the developmental step(s) at which the process was first disturbed, the underlying genes and biological pathways disrupted, and – when more objective data are not available – brain imaging features [Barkovich et al., 1996, 2001b, 2005]. This system classifies MCD into three major groups, as noted above: those resulting from abnormalities of cell proliferation; those resulting from abnormalities of neuronal migration; and those resulting from abnormal cortical organization. The large subset of disorders presenting with abnormal brain size – microcephaly and megalencephaly – are reviewed in Chapter 25. The subset of developmental disorders of the cortex in which alterations in brain size are not the dominant feature are reviewed in the present chapter. These include the primary neuronal migration disorders, lissencephaly (including agyria and pachygyria) and subcortical band heterotopia, cobblestone-type cortical malformations, periventricular and subcortical nodular heterotopia, polymicrogyria (including schizencephaly), and other focal cortical dysplasias.

Embryology

A review of normal human cortical development is essential to understanding the pathogenesis of these disorders. The basic pattern of the human brain is established by segmentation to establish an anterior–posterior axis; ventral induction to establish a dorsal–ventral axis; and, in the forebrain, diverticulation of the hemispheres to establish the right–left axis. Formation of the cortex begins at 8 postmenstrual or gestational weeks (GW8, which corresponds to about 6 postconceptual or fetal weeks), and leads to a six-layered cortex by about GW24. The complex pattern of convolutions or gyri that characterizes the mature human brain is not complete until some months

after birth, and from that point onwards, cortical development continues, with myelination of axons, progression of synaptic connectivity, and even generation of new neurons in certain cortical areas, such as the hippocampus.

While the major stages of cortical development have been known for decades [Sidman and Rakic, 1982], several recent discoveries have led to a sea change in our understanding of this complex process. The most important of these include recognition that the primary neural progenitor cells and the classic radial glia cells that guide neuronal migration to the cortical plate are the same cells, that the remarkable expansion of the cerebral cortex in humans results in part from neurogenesis in the subventricular zone, and that an important class of cortical neurons originates from ventral brain regions (Figure 26-1).

Classic Studies

By GW5, the rostral forebrain or telencephalon begins as a single layer of proliferative neuroepithelial cells overlying the newly formed lateral ventricles [Kriegstein et al., 2006; Norman et al., 1995; Sidman and Rakic, 1982]. This primitive layer, known as the ventricular zone (VZ), consists of densely packed and morphologically homogeneous cells that are radially oriented and maintain contact with both the ventricular lumen and the pial surface of the brain. Neural progenitor cells or neuroblasts in the VZ have highly mobile nuclei that move up and down within the cytoplasm of the cell, undergoing division when the nuclei are located near the ventricular surface.

During the next stages of cortical development, several new layers are seen. A marginal layer forms superficial to the VZ as a cell-sparse zone comprised mostly of cytoplasmic processes of cells in the VZ by GW5. Soon thereafter, a new neuronal layer, known as the preplate, forms above the VZ, and then a second proliferative layer of loosely arranged cells, known as the subventricular zone (SVZ) forms between the VZ and preplate. Both the VZ and SVZ contain mitotic cells. As cortical neurogenesis proceeds, newly generated neurons migrate radially out of the proliferative zones by climbing up a scaffold formed by specialized radial glia whose cell bodies are located in the VZ (vzRG)-cells that have long processes that extend up to the cortical surface. The first and smaller wave of neurons is generated in GW8 and migrates into the preplate in GW9, splitting it into a superficial marginal zone and a deeper subplate zone. A second and larger wave begins generating neurons in GW12 and

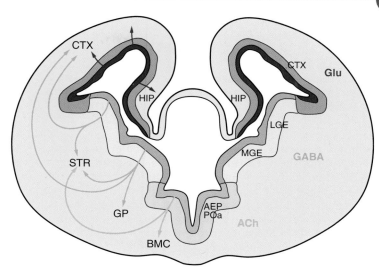

Fig. 26-1 Representation of a coronal section of the brain from an embryonic day 14 mouse (equivalent to a week 15 human embryo). Right half, the major subdivisions of the telencephalic proliferative zones, with the probable regions of origin of neurons expressing specific neurotransmitters, including glutamate (Glu), gamma-aminobutyric acid (GABA), and acetylcholine (ACh). Left half, the migration pathways followed by neurons from the various proliferative zones, with straight arrows representing radial migration in all three major zones and curved arrows representing nonradial migration. Most projection neurons follow radial migration, whereas most interneurons follow nonradial pathways. AEP, anterior entopeduncular area; BMC, basal magnocellular complex; CTX, cortex; GP, globus pallidus; HIP, hippocampus; LGE, lateral ganglionic eminence; MGE, medial ganglionic eminence; POa, anterior preoptic area; STR, striatum. *(Modified from Wilson SW, Rubenstein JLR. Induction and dorsoventral patterning of the telencephalon. Neuron 2000;28:641–651. Reprinted with permission from Elsevier.)*

peaks in GW15-16; these cells begin to migrate outward in GW13 and trail off several weeks after the peak of neurogenesis.

During cortical development, the marginal zone contains pioneer neurons known as Cajal–Retzius cells, which express Reelin and other proteins that regulate neuronal migration, cortical lamination, and later cortical organization [D'arcangelo et al., 1995]. The upper part of the marginal zone persists to form layer one of the mature cortex. Subplate neurons participate in development of critical thalamocortical and corticocortical connections, and also express many regulatory proteins before disappearing late in gestation [Del Rio et al., 2000]. The cortical plate grows rapidly, with newly arriving neurons migrating past earlier-generated cells to form progressively more superficial layers. This process of "inside-out" migration ultimately forms a six-layered cortex in which a neuron's final position is determined primarily by its birth date. The VZ becomes progressively smaller and is eventually replaced by a single layer of ependymal cells that line the lateral ventricles. The SVZ eventually disappears as well, except along the lateral wall of the lateral ventricles, where it persists and continues to provide olfactory and possibly other neurons into adulthood.

Recent Progress

Earlier studies of cortical development suggested that all neurons destined for the cortex are generated in the VZ of the neocortex and climb up radial glia cells to reach the cortical plate, while dividing cells seen in the SVZ were interpreted as the origin of glial cells. However, recent studies have uncovered a far more complex process and overturned several former theories.

Neurogenesis

First, vzRG were found to be primitive multipotential cells that serve as the primary neuronal founder cells, as well as classic radial glia cells [Heins et al., 2002; Malatesta et al., 2000; Miyata et al., 2001; Noctor et al., 2002]. During early stages of cortical development, radial founder cells undergo several sequential symmetric cell divisions to generate additional founder cells. Once some critical number of radial founder cells has been reached – a number that appears to differ between

species – the process changes to a form of asymmetric division that generates one vzRG and one immature neuron. The immature neuron then migrates up the radial glia fiber to reach the cortical plate. The daughter cells generated from each radial founder cell are thought to generate a functional neuronal column or radial unit. The radial unit hypothesis [Rakic, 1995, 2000] proposes that the evolutionary expansion in cortical surface area in primates resulted from an increase in the number of founder cells prior to neurogenesis, with each radial unit generating a column of six layers of neurons. This would have the effect of increasing cortical and ventricular surface area without increasing cortical thickness.

Second, neuronal progenitor cells are found in the SVZ, as well as the VZ. The first type discovered were intermediate progenitor cells (IPCs), which divide symmetrically to produce immature neurons [Haubensak et al., 2004; Miyata et al., 2004; Noctor et al., 2004]. However, the outer portion of the SVZ is also populated with nonepithelial radial glia-like (oRG) cells that are able to self-renew and produce neurons, similar to classic vzRG [Hansen et al., 2010]. Both vzRG and oRG cells undergo asymmetric cell division to produce IPCs, which divide one or a few times to produce immature neurons. The two populations of outer SVZ progenitors – oRG and IPCs (both also called transit amplifying cells) – contribute to a massively expanded outer SVZ in humans and produce a majority of neurons destined for the human cortex [Hansen et al., 2010; Haubensak et al., 2004]. Further, most newborn neurons do not migrate directly to the cortex. Rather, they demonstrate several distinct phases of migration, including a phase of retrograde movement toward the ventricle before migration out to the cortical plate [Noctor et al., 2004].

Specification of neuronal cell type occurs very early in the process, which is regulated by expression of a series of proteins. For example, vzRG and probably oRG progenitors express the paired-class transcription factor Pax6, whereas IPCs express the T-domain transcription factor Tbr2 (also designated EOMES in humans), and immature postmitotic neurons, especially neurons of the preplate and early-generated neurons that reside in cortical layer six, express the related *Tbr1* gene [Englund et al., 2005; Hevner et al., 2001].

Third, the cerebral cortex receives major contributions from both pallial (dorsal neocortical VZ) and subpallial sources.

The latter population consists of neurons that originate in the VZ of the ventral telencephalon, especially the medial ganglionic eminence, and migrate along nonradial pathways through the SVZ and intermediate zone (IZ) to the neocortex, mostly along axonal tracts (see Figure 26-1). These ventral progenitors give rise to inhibitory interneurons that express the neurotransmitter gamma-aminobutyric acid (GABA) [Anderson et al., 1997; Lavdas et al., 1999; Letinic et al., 2002; Wichterle et al., 2001], and constitute 20–30 percent of cortical neurons. This class of neurons modulates cortical output [Cherubini and Conti, 2001; Krimer and Goldman-Rakic, 2001], regulates neuronal proliferation and migration later in corticogenesis [Owens and Kriegstein, 2002], and contributes to postnatal development of cortical circuits [Fagiolini and Hensch, 2000; Huang et al., 1999]. Several distinct subtypes of interneurons have been identified that differ by axonal and dendritic morphology [Lund and Lewis, 1993], chemical markers [Defelipe, 1993; Gonchar and Burkhalter, 1997], connectivity, and physiology [Cauli et al., 1997; Kawaguchi and Kubota, 1996]. The major subtypes of GABAergic interneurons identified by chemical markers include calbindin-, calretinin-, parvalbumin-, somatostatin-, neuropeptide Y- and nitric oxide synthase-positive cells.

Neuronal Migration

Neuroblasts are generated a long distance from their eventual position in the cerebral cortex, a distance that may represent more than a thousand cell body lengths in humans. They undergo a process of movement or migration from either the periventricular zone (glutaminergic neurons) or the ganglionic eminences (GABAergic neurons). Most radial migration occurs by attachment to and locomotion along radial glial fibers, which form an extensive radial lattice that guides radially migrating cells [Gupta et al., 2002; O'Rourke et al., 1992; Rakic, 1971, 1972, 1988]. Radial glia-independent modes of radial migration also occur, particularly by nuclear translocation during the earliest stages while the VZ and cortical plate remain close together [Book and Morest, 1990; Gupta et al., 2002; Morris et al., 1998; Pearlman et al., 1998]. But cells must also receive a polarity signal, adhere to the radial fiber or other extracellular proteins, extend leading processes, translocate their nucleus from the cell body into the leading process to re-establish the cell body in a new location, contract trailing processes, and receive a stop migration signal.

The peak time for neuronal migration is between GW12 and GW20, although migration may continue up to at least GW26 [Evrard et al., 1989; Sidman and Rakic, 1982]. The cortex is formed by an "inside-out" pattern, in which early-generated neurons form the initial cortical plate and later-generated neurons climb past them to progressively more superficial positions. Thus, the earliest neurons to migrate end up in layer six, and the last to migrate in layer two.

Cortical Organization

By approximately 22 weeks, distinctive layers first appear in the cortex. Further maturation consists of additional synaptogenesis, retraction of early axonal collaterals that did not establish appropriate connections, neurotransmitter biosynthesis, and other processes. Most of these processes continue well beyond the perinatal period. The marginal zone of the fetal cortex matures to become layer one, or the molecular layer of mature cortex. The pioneer Cajal–Retzius neurons disappear, leaving a zone of nerve fibers, dendrites, and synapses with only a few cells. The subplate is incorporated into the deep layers of the cerebral cortex. By GW27, all six layers of the mature cortex are visible [Norman et al., 1995]. The cortex also has a columnar or vertical organization that derives from radial (centrifugal) migration of the dominant cell types.

While neuronal identity was specified much earlier in development, migrating neurons only begin the process of differentiation into functional subtypes as their final positions are reached. The critical changes include the appearance of neuronal processes, development of specific neuronal cell membrane properties, and expression of proteins characteristic of a specific type of cell-to-cell transmission. Additional adaptations include further morphologic differentiation, and more complex molecular and physiologic differentiation and synaptic interconnections [Cowan, 1992]. Throughout much of this period, glial cells are dividing and differentiating as well. At least three major types of glial cells are known, including oligodendrocytes, type 1 astrocytes, and type 2 astrocytes. The interactions among these cell types are complex but important in their later role in neuronal migration.

Further Reading

This summary touches on only a few of the advances made over the past decade. Many reviews are available, such as a recent collection of papers in a symposium on "Patterning and Evolving the Vertebrate Forebrain" [Creuzet, 2009; Medina and Abellan, 2009; Merot et al., 2009; Moreno et al., 2009; Saghatelyan, 2009; Subramanian et al., 2009; Suzuki-Hirano and Shimogori, 2009].

Lissencephaly and Subcortical Band Heterotopia

Lissencephaly (LIS), or "smooth brain," and the related malformation known as subcortical band heterotopia (SBH) are the classic malformations associated with deficient neuronal migration. LIS is recognized based on an abnormal gyral pattern consisting of absent or abnormally wide gyri, and an abnormally thick cortex. SBH is less obvious, consisting of a normal or mildly immature or "simplified" gyral pattern associated with a variably thick layer of gray matter replacing the central and upper portions of white matter.

While known from pathological studies for many decades [Culp, 1914; Erhardt, 1914; Matell, 1893], LIS and SBH were brought to modern medical attention between 1963 and 1989 [Barkovich et al., 1989b; Daube and Chou, 1966; Dieker et al., 1969; Miller, 1963]. Their underlying genetic basis first came to light during the same period when several children with LIS and other congenital anomalies associated with deletion of chromosome 17p13.3 were reported, a syndrome now known as Miller–Dieker syndrome [Dobyns et al., 1983; Stratton et al., 1984].

Pathology

LIS is a diffuse brain malformation manifested by a smooth cerebral surface, abnormally thick cortex with four abnormal layers that includes a deep zone of diffuse neuronal heterotopia, and enlarged, dysplastic ventricles [Barkovich et al., 1991; Forman et al., 2005; Norman et al., 1995]. It encompasses the pathologic terms agyria (absent gyri) and pachygyria (broad gyri). SBH consists of symmetric and circumferential bands of gray matter located just beneath the cortex and separated from it by a thin band of white matter. This appearance led to the alternative – although incorrect – term, "double cortex," for this malformation. The overlying cortex appears normal or mildly simplified as a result of abnormally shallow sulci [Barkovich, 2000; Barkovich et al., 1994, 1989b; Dobyns et al., 1996a].

Several different types of LIS have been recognized, based on pathological features. They are most readily distinguished based on the number of cortical layers, and include four-, three-, and two-layered forms [Forman et al., 2005]. In the common four-layered or classic form (LIS-4L), the gyral malformation can be most severe over either anterior or posterior brain regions. The cortex is 12–20 mm thick and composed of a normal marginal layer, a superficial cellular layer that corresponds to the cortical plate, a cell-sparse zone, and a deep cellular layer composed of heterotopic neurons [Forman et al., 2005]. The two major subtypes can also be distinguished by looking at the transition from the deep cellular layer to the underlying white matter. In the posterior predominant (*LIS1* gene) form, the transition is gradual, with no striking features. In the anterior predominant (*DCX* gene) form, the deep cellular layer transitions to multiple small nodules of subcortical heterotopia, and then to white matter. A few patients with classic LIS have mild to moderate cerebellar hypoplasia.

SBH consists of a normal six-layered cortex, a thin zone of white matter underlying the cortex, and then a zone of dense heterotopic neurons that breaks up into nodules at their lower border, closely resembling the X-linked form of LIS described above [Forman et al., 2005]. LIS-4L and SBH comprise a single malformation spectrum, based on observations of rare patients with areas of LIS that merge into SBH, and of many families with LIS in affected males and SBH in affected females [Des Portes et al., 1997; Dobyns et al., 1996a; Pilz et al., 1999].

The rare two-layered form of lissencephaly (LIS-2L) has been seen only in severe LIS variants with complete agyria and severe brainstem and cerebellar hypoplasia [Forman et al., 2005; Lecourtois et al., 2010]. The molecular layer appears normal, and overlies a single thickened and disorganized cortex with randomly arranged and oriented neurons. The three-layered and two-layered forms of LIS have not been seen with SBH.

The rare three-layered form of LIS (LIS-3L), associated with X-linked lissencephaly with abnormal genitalia (XLAG), consists of a hypercellular marginal or molecular layer, a middle zone with a relative increase in pyramidal neurons, and a deep layer that is relatively thick and composed primarily of small and medium sized neurons [Forman et al., 2005]. Other features include an intermediate-thickness (8–12 mm) cortex, disorganization of the basal ganglia with cysts, gliotic and spongy white matter, and agenesis of the corpus callosum [Bonneau et al., 2002; Forman et al., 2005].

Several rare forms of LIS associated with severe congenital microcephaly have been described, currently designated as microlissencephaly (MLIS), based on birth head circumference smaller than −3 standard deviations at birth. This group may overlap with LIS-2L. The first syndrome with MLIS reported, now known as Norman–Roberts syndrome, consists of severe congenital microcephaly, lissencephaly with diffuse agyria,

and several pathological features that differed from classic LIS [Dobyns et al., 1984; Norman et al., 1976]. These included a relatively thin deep cellular layer, no heterotopia of inferior olive or dentate nuclei, and grossly dysplastic cerebellar cortex with reduced granular cells. The authors have seen only one child possibly fitting this syndrome over many years, leading to some doubts regarding its existence. While we believe that this syndrome does exist, several published reports appear to describe different syndromes [Caksen et al., 2004; Iannetti et al., 1993]. In OMIM (number 257320), Norman–Roberts syndrome has been linked to mutations of the *RELN* gene. This entry is egregiously in error, as no pathological data are available from humans with mutations of *RELN* or Reelin pathway genes, and individuals with known *RELN* mutations have normal head size.

Another pathologically distinct three-layered form of LIS (LIS-3L) is associated with microcephalic osteodysplastic primordial dysplasia type 1 (MOPD1). The brain malformation consists of extreme microcephaly, foreshortened frontal lobes, frontal predominant lissencephaly with agyria or pachygyria, agenesis of the corpus callosum, and cerebellar vermis hypoplasia [Juric-Sekhar et al., 2010; Klinge et al., 2002; Meinecke and Passarge, 1991; Ozawa et al., 2005]. The brainstem and cerebellar involvement seems less severe than lissencephaly with cerebellar hypoplasia (LCH). The dysplastic cortex is characterized by extensive but thin glioneuronal heterotopia, a thin superficial layer that appears hyperconvoluted in places (thus somewhat resembling polymicrogyria), a thin second layer of disorganized medium to large neurons, and a thick third layer consisting of mostly small neurons [Juric-Sekhar et al., 2010]. The glioneuronal heterotopia, lack of white-matter cystic changes, the brainstem and cerebellar hypoplasia, and other features distinguish this from the XLAG-type of LIS-3L.

The most severe form of true lissencephaly may be the form reported as "familial lissencephaly with extreme neopallial hypoplasia" that we now designate as Barth-type microlissencephaly [Barth et al., 1982; Dobyns and Barkovich, 1999; Kroon et al., 1996]. The pathological features include extreme congenital microcephaly, severe LIS with diffuse agyria, disorganized cortex with four layers resembling classic LIS-4L, except for a relatively thin deep cellular layer, small collections of cells with scant cytoplasm (possible germinal cells) in the leptomeninges, absent olfactory nerves, severe optic nerve hypoplasia, small thalami resembling streaks, agenesis of the corpus callosum and other commissures, severe brainstem hypoplasia with absent cerebral peduncles, transverse pontine fibers, inferior olives and pyramids, and extreme cerebellar hypoplasia with absent folia.

Finally, use of the old terms "type 1" and "type 2" LIS is strongly discouraged in favor of the new descriptive terms used above. The old "type 1" was first used to refer to the four-layered form, but was later applied to anything that was not "type 2." The old "type 2" form is now designated as cobblestone malformation, discussed in the next section. Only the most severely affected patients have agyria or pachygyria. A few reports have used the term "type 3" LIS to refer to a rare condition with severe fetal akinesia, microcephaly, and undersulcated brain surface [Allias et al., 2004; Encha Razavi et al., 1996]. The cortex in this form appears thin, rather than thick, and has evidence of neuronal cell loss, suggesting a prenatal-onset degenerative disorder that would best not be classified as a form of LIS. In addition, both severe congenital microcephaly and more severe forms of polymicrogyria are commonly misidentified as LIS.

Brain Imaging

Most of the distinguishing features seen on pathological examination can be viewed by brain imaging as well (Figure 26-2). The different types of LIS and SBH may be distinguished by both the pattern and the severity of the malformation. Recognition of these patterns has become essential for syndrome and molecular diagnosis, and for assessing prognosis and genetic risk [Dobyns et al., 1999b; Kato and Dobyns, 2003; Pilz et al., 1998b]. The different patterns of LIS and SBH associated with known syndromes and causal genes are summarized in Table 26-1.

For all forms of true LIS, the brain surface appears smooth with areas of absent gyri (agyria) and abnormally wide gyri (pachygyria), and abnormally thick cerebral cortex [Barkovich et al., 1991; Dobyns and Truwit, 1995]. In normal brains, most gyri are approximately 1–1.5 cm wide and the normal cortex 3–4 mm thick, but thicker in the primary motor cortex and thinner in the primary visual cortex. In all types of LIS, gyri are typically 3 cm wide or more, and the cortex 8–20 mm thick, although this varies with the type (see Figure 26-2A–G, with Figure 26-2H being an exception). Several distinct types of LIS are associated with agenesis of the corpus callosum, moderate to severe cerebellar hypoplasia, designated LCH, or both [Ross et al., 2001].

In SBH (see Figure 26-2I–J), the brain surface appears superficially normal, except that the sulci or crevices between gyri tend to be very shallow (less than 1 cm instead of 1–3 cm), and the cortex is normal and not thick [Barkovich et al., 1994; Dobyns et al., 1996a]. Just beneath the cortex, however, often separated from it by just a few millimeters of white matter, lies a smooth band of neurons that never reached the true cortex. The inner margin of the band is usually smooth, while the outer margin may appear smooth (with thick bands) or follow interdigitations of the overlying cortex (with thin bands).

The most common or classic form of LIS seen on brain imaging corresponds to LIS-4L, and occurs in a continuous series with SBH. The severity varies from complete or nearly complete agyria (grades 1 and 2, see Figure 26-2B); to mixed agyria-pachygyria (grade 3, see Figure 26-2A and C); and then to extensive pachygyria (grade 4, see Figure 26-2D and E); mixed pachygyria and SBH (grade 5, not shown); and finally, SBH alone (grade 6, see Figure 26-2I and J). Both LIS-4L and SBH may be seen with either a frontal or posterior predominant distribution. Thus, the gradient of LIS and SBH can be anterior more severe than posterior (a > p), posterior more severe than anterior (p > a), or anterior equal to posterior (a = p). In LIS-4L, the cortex is usually 12–20 mm thick. Common associated malformations include thick and rounded hippocampi, enlarged posterior portions of the lateral ventricles, and flat anterior portion of the corpus callosum.

Several other types of LCH may be differentiated, based on brain imaging. A few patients with classic LIS have moderate vermis-predominant cerebellar hypoplasia, which corresponds to the previous LCH group a [Ross et al., 2001]. The next consists of intermediate severity LIS with mixed agyria and pachygyria that appears most severe in central (posterior frontal and anterior parietal) regions (see Figure 26-2D). Subtle asymmetry is often seen, as well as hypogenesis or agenesis of the corpus

callosum. Another more severe variant of LCH consists of diffuse agyria with a cortex that appears only moderately thick (not shown). The lower margin of the cortex may be smooth or follow an undulating course. Associated abnormalities include severe hypoplasia of the hippocampus, variable agenesis of the corpus callosum, and severe brainstem and cerebellar hypoplasia. This severe variant corresponds to LIS-2L, and combines the prior LCH groups c, d, and f [Forman et al., 2005; Kumar et al., 2010; Ross et al., 2001].

A less severe LCH variant, which was previously designated as LCH group b [Ross et al., 2001], consists of frontal-predominant lissencephaly consisting of mild to moderate pachygyria, mildly thick 8–10 mm cortex, very small globular hippocampi, mildly small brainstem, and diffuse severe hypoplasia of the cerebellum with absent or nearly absent folia (see Figure 26-2G and H). This pattern has been associated with mutations of Reelin pathway genes.

The LIS variant seen in children with the XLAG syndrome corresponds to LIS-3L [Bonneau et al., 2002; Forman et al., 2005]. It is characterized by mixed agyria and pachygyria that appears most severe over the temporal lobes, next most severe over the parietal and occipital lobes, and least severe over the frontal lobes; the cortex is only moderately thick, usually 8–10 mm (see Figure 26-2F). Associated abnormalities include agenesis of the corpus callosum that is most often complete, abnormal basal ganglia with indistinct borders and cysts, and diffuse abnormal (high T2, low T1) signal of white matter. The brainstem and cerebellum appear normal.

Several rare LIS variants are associated with severe congenital microcephaly. In Norman–Roberts syndrome, the LIS resembles classic LIS by imaging, except for the very small head size [WB Dobyns, unpublished data]. In MOPD1, the LIS appears as frontal-predominant agyria or pachygyria with agenesis of the corpus callosum and probably mild cerebellar vermis hypoplasia. In Barth microlissencephaly syndrome, the LIS is extremely severe with minimal gray–white differentiation seen, absent corpus callosum, pencil-thin brainstem, and extremely small afoliar cerebellum. These syndromes are reviewed in more detail below.

Clinical Features

Children with the most common types of LIS (or SBH) typically appear normal as newborns, although a few have a history of polyhydramnios, apnea, hypotonia, poor feeding, and mildly elevated newborn bilirubin levels that may reflect poor swallowing. With most types of LIS, seizures are uncommon during the first days of life. Most affected children come to medical attention during the first year of life due to:

1. neurological deficits in the first weeks or months, consisting of poor feeding, mild hypotonia, and abnormal arching behavior or opisthotonus
2. delayed motor milestones later in the first year of life
3. onset of seizures during the first year of life, which is by far the most common presentation.

In all affected children, the major medical problems encountered are feeding problems and gastroesophageal reflux, epilepsy of many different types, and recurrent aspiration and pneumonia due to the feeding problems and epilepsy.

A few children feed poorly from the first weeks of life, but this often improves unless they have one of the severe LIS variants. Most feed reasonably well for the first several years,

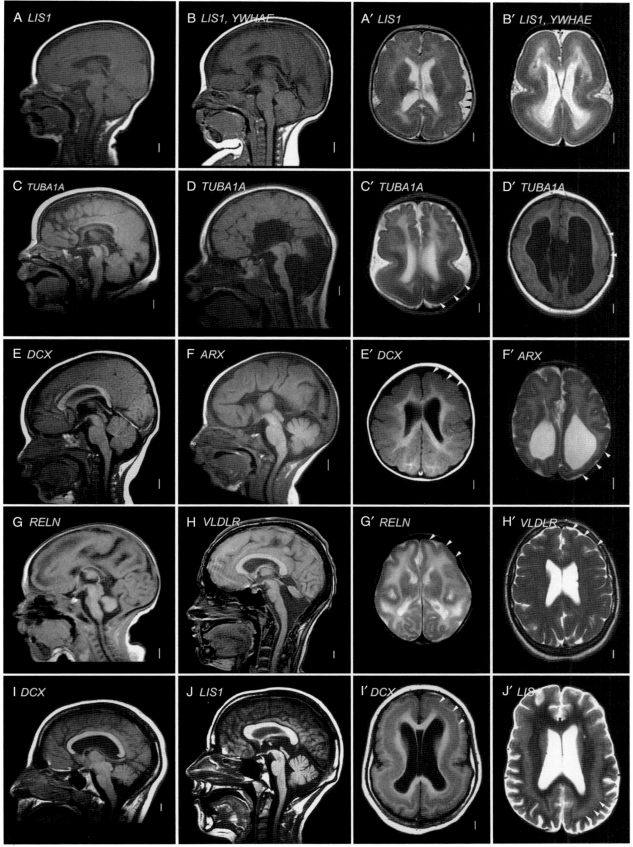

Continued

Fig. 26-2 Subtypes of lissencephaly. Midline sagittal **(A–H)** and high axial **(A′–H′)** magnetic resonance images of lissencephaly (LIS). associated with mutations of seven different genes. The most severely involved brain regions are marked by arrowheads on the axial images. **A–A′,** Classic LIS, with posterior more severe than anterior (p > a) gradient associated with an intragenic mutation of *LIS1*. **B–B′,** Severe classic LIS due to deletion 17p13.3, which results in loss of *LIS1, YWHAE,* and all of the intervening genes in a child with Miller–Dieker syndrome. **C–C′,** Classic LIS with a p > a gradient caused by an intragenic mutation of *TUBA1A*. **D–D′,** Moderate-severity lissencephaly with cerebellar hypoplasia (LCH), with complete agenesis of the corpus callosum, large dysplastic midbrain and tectum, and severe cerebellar hypoplasia associated with another intragenic mutation of *TUBA1A*. **E–E′,** Classic LIS with anterior more severe than posterior (a > p) gradient, caused by intragenic mutation of *DCX*. **F–F′,** Moderate LIS variant with p > a gradient due to mutation of *ARX* in a male patient; lower images (not shown) demonstrate that the temporal lobes are even more severely affected. **G–G′,** LCH with mild frontal pachygyria and severe cerebellar hypoplasia with absent folia due to homozygous mutation of *RELN*. **H–H′,** LCH with very mild frontal pachygyria and severe cerebellar hypoplasia with nearly absent folia due to homozygous deletion of VLDLR. **I–I′,** Diffuse SBH associated with heterozygous mutation of *DCX*. **J–J′,** Posterior predominant SBH associated with mutation of *LIS1*. *(A–H, Reprinted from Dobyns WB. The clinical patterns and molecular genetics of lissencephaly and subcortical band heterotopia. Epilepsia 51[Suppl. 1]:5–9, 2010, with permission from Wiley–Blackwell. I, Courtesy of Dr. William B Dobyns, University of Washington, Departments of Pediatrics and Neurology, Seattle, Washington. These images were selected from patients LR08-316 [A–A′], LR08-401 [B–B′], LR07-008 [C–C′], LR07-244 [D–D′], LR06-020 [E–E′], LR04-245 [F–F′], LP95-137a2 [G–G′], LR08-330 [H–H′], LP94-049 [I–I′], and LP94-051 [J–J′].)*

Table 26-1 **Lissencephaly Syndromes, Inheritance and Genes**

Lissencephaly Type and Syndrome	Inheritance	Genes
LIS-4L SEVERE WITH NO GRADIENT		
Miller–Dieker syndrome (deletion 17p13.3)	SpAD	*LIS1-YWHAE*
Isolated lissencephaly sequence, severe X-linked type	XL	*DCX*
Barth-type microlissencephaly	AR	Unknown
LIS-4L POSTERIOR > ANTERIOR GRADIENT AND VARIANTS		
Isolated lissencephaly sequence with p > a gradient	SpAD	*LIS1, TUBA1A*
Isolated lissencephaly sequence with p > a gradient	AR	Unknown
Subcortical band heterotopia with p > a gradient	SpAD	*LIS1*
Subcortical band heterotopia with p > a gradient	AD	Unknown
Lissencephaly with cerebellar hypoplasia with p > a gradient plus mild cerebellar (vermis) hypoplasia	SpAD	*LIS1*
Lissencephaly with cerebellar hypoplasia with central > posterior > anterior gradient (tubulin-type), moderate cerebellar hypoplasia, and often ACC (group f with central gradient)	SpAD	*TUBA1A*
LIS-4L ANTERIOR > POSTERIOR GRADIENT AND VARIANTS		
Isolated lissencephaly sequence with a > p gradient	XL	*DCX*
Isolated lissencephaly sequence with a > p gradient	AR	Unknown
Subcortical band heterotopia with a > p gradient	XL	*DCX*
Baraitser–Winter syndrome	SpAD	Unknown
LIS-2L SEVERE WITH NO GRADIENT		
Lissencephaly with cerebellar hypoplasia (tubulin-type) with severe cerebellar hypoplasia and ACC (groups c, d, and f with no gradient)	SpAD	*TUBA1A*
LIS-3L POSTERIOR > ANTERIOR GRADIENT VARIANT		
X-linked lissencephaly with abnormal genitalia (XLAG)	XL	*ARX*
XLAG-like syndrome with microphthalmia, and cleft lip and palate	AR?	Unknown
LIS-3L ANTERIOR > POSTERIOR GRADIENT VARIANT		
Microlissencephaly MOPD1-type with cerebellar hypoplasia	AR	Unknown
LIS-RELN ANTERIOR > POSTERIOR GRADIENT		
LCH RELN-type with severe hippocampal and cerebellar hypoplasia (group b, frontal predominance)	AR	*RELN, VLDLR*

ACC, agenesis of the corpus callosum; AD, autosomal-dominant; AR, autosomal-recessive; LCH, lissencephaly with cerebellar hypoplasia; MOPD, microcephalic osteodysplastic primordial dysplasia; SpAD, sporadic with presumed autosomal-dominant inheritance caused by new mutations; XL, X-linked.

except that many have difficulty during intercurrent illnesses. Feeding often worsens later, especially after about 3 years, with increased aspiration, decreased feeding tolerance, and recurrent pneumonia. These problems are frequently related to worsening epilepsy and gastroesophageal reflux, whether obviously symptomatic or not. They lead to placement of gastrostomy tubes and operations to reduce reflux (fundal plications) in many affected children, although the age varies widely within the first decade [Dobyns et al., 1992].

Epilepsy

Most – indeed, probably all – children with LIS have seizures. The onset is usually between 3 and 12 months, but may be later. Between 35 and 85 percent of children with classic LIS develop infantile spasms in the first year of life, although hypsarrhythmia is usually absent. After 1 year, they typically have continued mixed seizure types, including epileptic spasms, typically presenting on awakening, myoclonic, tonic, and tonic-clonic seizures. Many meet criteria for Lennox–Gastaut syndrome, which can be associated with a decline in skills with poor seizure control. In general, the same treatment strategies used for Lennox–Gastaut syndrome generally may be used in patients with LIS or SBH. In children with XLAG, epilepsy is nearly continuous. In both classic LIS and XLAG, studies in mouse mutants have shown deficiencies in cortical interneurons that use GABA as their primary neurotransmitter [Marsh et al., 2009; McManus et al., 2004]. Thus, GABAergic medications have some theoretical basis for use in these children.

Early diagnosis and aggressive attempts to control seizures usually prove helpful in maintaining function. The epilepsy may consist of most types of seizures, and mixed types are common. These seizures may be managed as for those in patients with other causes of Lennox–Gastaut syndrome. Patients often have motor control problems (mixed hypotonia and spasticity), feeding problems, and gastroesophageal reflux, as in children with cerebral palsy, which may be managed similarly.

Prognosis

For children with the most common forms of classic LIS, the mortality rate is greater than 50 percent by 10 years, and few children live past 20 years. Children with severe LIS syndromes, especially Miller–Dieker syndrome, severe forms of LCH, XLAG, MOPD1, or Barth microlissencephaly syndrome have a more severe course and higher mortality rate. However, these data apply to children with severe forms of LIS, and specifically do not apply to children with rare partial forms of LIS, SBH, or Baraitser–Winter syndrome, or to the RELN-associated type of LCH, as all have better cognitive function and much longer survival.

In contrast, most patients with SBH and rare patients with partial forms of LIS have mild to moderate mental retardation, although both normal intelligence and severe mental retardation have been seen. Other clinical features are minimal pyramidal signs and dysarthria [Barkovich et al., 1994; D'Agostino et al., 2002; Dobyns et al., 1996a]. Seizures usually begin in childhood but may appear much later, and multiple types occur that may be difficult to control. Cognitive development may slow after onset of seizures. The frequency and severity vary greatly. EEG investigations usually demonstrate generalized spike-and-wave discharges or multifocal

abnormalities [Battaglia, 1996; D'Agostino et al., 2002; Palmini et al., 1991]. Neurologic outcome usually correlates with the thickness of the subcortical band heterotopia and simplification of the gyral pattern, as seen on magnetic resonance imaging (MRI).

Syndromes, Genetics, and Molecular Basis

While older reports suggested the possibility of extrinsic (nongenetic) causes of LIS, such as prenatal cytomegalovirus exposure or perfusion failure [Dobyns et al., 1992; Norman et al., 1976], clinical experience suggests that all or almost all LIS is genetic. Mutations of the six known LIS genes, including ARX, DCX, LIS1, RELN, TUBA1A, and VLDLR, account for more than 80 percent of patients [Boycott et al., 2005; Gleeson et al., 1998; Hong et al., 2000; Keays et al., 2007; Kitamura et al., 2002; Reiner et al., 1993]. However, several of these are associated with one or more specific LIS or SBH syndromes with different presentations. The contributions of these six genes and the specific mutational mechanisms have been derived from separate studies over many years, making comparisons difficult. An update of the prior results in light of current knowledge is shown in Table 26-2 [Dobyns, 2010]. A review of the major LIS syndromes and their molecular mechanisms is presented in the following sections.

Miller–Dieker Syndrome

Miller–Dieker syndrome is a striking multiple congenital anomaly syndrome, characterized by classic LIS (LIS-4L), typical facial appearance, and variable other birth defects, such as heart malformations. The facial features include prominent forehead, bitemporal hollowing, short nose with upturned nares, protuberant upper lip with thin vermilion border, and small jaw. The brain malformation consists of severe LIS with no apparent gradient (see Figure 26-2B), although rare patients may have the same posterior more severe than anterior gradient seen in patients with isolated lissencephaly sequence with LIS1 mutations [Cardoso et al., 2003; Dobyns et al., 1991]. All patients with Miller–Dieker syndrome have large deletions of chromosomal region 17p13.3 that include LIS1, YWHAE, and all intervening genes, which indicates that the YWHAE gene is an important modifying factor for lissencephaly. Several genes in this region are known oncogenes, and at least two patients with Miller–Dieker syndrome have had childhood cancers [Czuchlewski et al., 2008; Ueda et al., 2006].

Isolated Lissencephaly Sequence

Isolated lissencephaly sequence, which is by far the most common of the LIS syndromes, consists of classic LIS (LIS-4L) with a normal facial appearance, except for mild bitemporal hollowing and small jaw [Dobyns et al., 1992, 1984]. Different patterns of LIS have been found with mutations of the three known causative genes – DCX, LIS1, and TUBA1A. A few patients with mutations of these genes – especially TUBA1A – also have cerebellar hypoplasia. Isolated lissencephaly sequence associated with mutations of the X-linked DCX gene is characterized by either severe lissencephaly with no clear gradient, or lissencephaly with an anterior more severe than posterior gradient (see Figure 26-2E), and normal facial appearance [Dobyns et al., 1999b; Pilz et al., 1998b]. Isolated lissencephaly sequence associated with mutations or deletions

Table 26-2 Mutation Frequencies for Lissencephaly Syndromes with Known Causal Genes

	Full	FISH–	Cohort FISH–SEQ–	FISH–SEQ–MLPA–	Interp	Rec
MDS (CLASSIC LIS)						
17p13 deletion by cytogenetics [Dobyns et al., 1991]	14/21 (66.7%)				66.7%	~67%
17p13 deletion by FISH [Dobyns et al., 1991]	07/21 (33.3%)				33.3%	~33%
ILS (CLASSIC LIS)						
LIS1 deletion by FISH [Pilz et al., 1998a]	47/110 (42.7%)				42.7%	~40%
LIS1 mutation by SEQ [Pilz et al., 1998b]		08/25 (32%)			18.3%	~20%
DCX mutation by SEQ [Pilz et al., 1998b]		05/25 (20%)			11.5%	~10%
LIS1 deletion by MLPA [Haverfield et al., 2009]			18/52 (35%)		9.6%	~10%
TUBA1A mutation by SEQ [Kumar et al., 2010]				05/110 (4.5%)	0.8%	~01%
TOTAL for classic LIS					82.9%	~85%
LCH ± ACC (GROUPS C-D-F)						
TUBA1A mutation by SEQ [Kumar et al., 2010]				10/26 (38.5%)		~40%
LIS-ACC (XLAG PATTERN)						
ARX mutation by SEQ [Kato et al., 2004]	22/23 (95.6%)				95.6%	~95%
SBH IN FEMALES						
DCX mutation by SEQ [Matsumoto et al., 2001]	22/26 (84.6%)				84.6%	~85%
DCX deletion by MLPA [Haverfield et al., 2009]			03/09 (33%)		5.1%	~05%
TOTAL for SBH females					89.7%	~90%
SBH IN MALES						
DCX mutation by SEQ [D'Agostino et al., 2002]	07/24 (29.2%)				29.2%	~30%
LIS1 mutation by SEQ [D'Agostino et al., 2002]	01/24 (4.1%)				04.1%	~04%
TOTAL for SBH males					33.3%	~33%

ACC, agenesis of the corpus callosum; FISH–, negative results for fluorescence in situ hydridization analysis; ILS, isolated lissencephaly sequence; INTERP, interpolated results; LCH, lissencephaly with cerebellar hypoplasia; LIS, lissencephaly; MDS, Miller–Dieker syndrome; MLPA–, negative results for duplication-deletion analysis by Multiplex Ligation-dependent Probe Amplification (MLPA®, MRC-Holland, Amsterdam, The Netherlands); REC, recommended frequency data for clinical uses; SBH, subcortical band heterotopia; SEQ, standard sequencing; SEQ–, negative results for sequencing; XLAG, X-linked lissencephaly with abnormal genitalia.

of the *LIS1* gene or mutations at codon 402 in *TUBA1A* (p.R402C or p.R402H) is characterized by lissencephaly with a posterior more severe than anterior gradient or, less often, an anterior equal to posterior gradient (see Figure 26-2A and C). Facial appearance may be normal, or have subtle dysmorphism similar to that in Miller–Dieker syndrome, but much less severe [Cardoso et al., 2003; Dobyns et al., 1992; Kumar et al., 2010].

For isolated lissencephaly sequence, the parents should be tested whenever mutations of *LIS1* or *TUBA1A* have been found. When the results are normal, the recurrence risk is low, as evidenced by lack of recurrence in more than 100 such families seen. However, the possibility of recurrence exists due to mosaicism in one parent, so that the availability of prenatal diagnosis should be discussed for any future pregnancies. When mutations of *DCX* are found, the rules for X-linked inheritance apply [Dobyns et al., 2004]. Carrier testing in mothers is important, as many are found to be carriers [Gleeson et al., 2000a; Matsumoto et al., 2001], especially when the proband has a less severe phenotype [Guerrini et al., 2003]. The recurrence risk is 50 percent when the mother is found to

be a carrier [Matsumoto et al., 2001]. Testing in fathers of female probands should be considered as well, as one father has been found who is a mosaic carrier of the mutation found in his affected daughter. Recurrence in siblings has been reported in families when results of mutation analysis of the proband are negative [Gleeson et al., 2000b; Kuzniecky, 1994; Ramirez et al., 2004], so counseling for a 10–15 percent recurrence risk is suggested in this situation. When no testing has been done, counseling is difficult.

Subcortical Band Heterotopia

SBH is only rarely associated with other congenital anomalies. Most patients are female because the most common cause is heterozygous mutations of the *DCX* gene on the X chromosome [Dobyns, 2010; Dobyns et al., 1996a; Gleeson et al., 2000a; Matsumoto et al., 2001]. This represents the heterozygous or carrier phenotype found in female relatives of males with *DCX*-related lissencephaly. Many affected males, however, also have been reported [D'Agostino et al., 2002]. Mutations of *DCX* and *LIS1*, the same two genes that cause isolated lissencephaly sequence, have been identified that result in somewhat different patterns of malformation. SBH associated with mutations of *DCX* gene is characterized by diffuse thick bands with no apparent gradient, or by partial frontal thin bands [Gleeson et al., 2000a; Matsumoto et al., 2001]. SBH associated with mutations or deletions of the *LIS1* gene is characterized by partial posterior thin or intermediate bands with an obvious posterior more severe than anterior gradient. This is a rare cause of SBH, and some patients have mosaic mutations of *LIS1* [D'Agostino et al., 2002; Mineyko et al. 2010; Pilz et al., 1999; Sicca et al., 2003] or deletions of 17p13.3 (unpublished data). Several families have been reported with posterior SBH, familial recurrence, and negative testing for both *DCX* and *LIS1* [Deconinck et al., 2003].

Baraitser–Winter Syndrome

The rare Baraitser–Winter syndrome (BWS) consists of facial dysmorphism, typically including trigonocephaly and shallow orbits, colobomas of both iris and retina, and lissencephaly (LIS-4L) with an anterior more severe than posterior gradient [Baraitser and Winter, 1988; Forman et al., 2005; Ramer et al., 1995; Rossi et al., 2003; Verloes, 1993]. The lissencephaly usually is relatively mild, with pachygyria most severe in the mid-frontal region that undergoes transition posteriorly to subcortical band heterotopia and then to a more normal gyral pattern, thus resembling the less severe end of the *DCX* spectrum. Familial recurrence has never been reported, which suggests new-mutation autosomal-dominant inheritance.

LIS Variants

At least seven further types of LIS have been described in rare patients with variant types of LIS, based on neuropathology, brain imaging, or both (see Table 26-1). The key differentiating features in the brain include severe congenital microcephaly (in 2 out of 7), variant cortical histology (2L in 1 of 7 and 3L in 2 of 7), agenesis of the corpus callosum (in 5 of 7), and variable but often severe cerebellar hypoplasia (in 6 of 7). The combination of LIS with severe congenital microcephaly is designated as microlissencephaly (MLIS) only when the cortex is abnormally thick; otherwise, it is classified as "microcephaly with a simplified gyral pattern." The previous classification of LCH into six groups is updated to include several other types [Ross et al., 2001].

Lissencephaly with Cerebellar Hypoplasia RELN-Type

This rare syndrome was first reported as a variant of the so-called dysequilibrium syndrome, and later as "neuronal migration defect, cerebellar hypoplasia, and lymphedema" [Hourihane et al., 1993; Schurig et al., 1981]. The brain malformation consists of moderate frontal-predominant LIS (pachygyria), only moderately thick cortex (8–10 mm), small globular hippocampus, and small, often afoliar, cerebellum, a pattern previously classified as LCH group b (see Figure 26-2G and H) [Ross et al., 2001]. No data on the neuropathology in humans are available, although mouse models have a classic "inverted" cortex [D'Arcangelo et al., 1995; Falconer, 1951]. The phenotype is characterized by moderate to profound mental retardation, delayed ambulation, nonprogressive truncal and peripheral ataxia, and occasional seizures, in addition to the brain malformation [Glass et al., 2005]. Mutations of either *RELN* or *VLDLR* have been found in several patients in this group [Boycott et al., 2009, 2005; Chang et al., 2007; Hong et al., 2000; Ozcelik et al., 2008; Zaki et al., 2007].

Lissencephaly with Cerebellar Hypoplasia Classic-Type

The next, and possibly most common, type resembles isolated lissencephaly sequence (ILS), with the addition of mild cerebellar vermis hypoplasia, which was previously designated as LCH group a [Ross et al., 2001]. The LIS may have either frontal or posterior predominance, and the phenotype closely resembles ILS. As in ILS, the frontal-predominant group is associated with mutations of *DCX*, and the posterior-predominant group with mutations of *LIS1* or *TUBA1A*. Some patients have negative testing for all three genes. The pathology probably consists of LIS-4L.

Lissencephaly with Cerebellar Hypoplasia Tubulin-Type 1

Another phenotype consists of moderate but variable LIS (pachygyria) with central (posterior frontal and anterior parietal) predominance, variable hypogenesis of the corpus callosum, and moderate cerebellar hypoplasia, a phenotype that was previously included in LCH group f (see Figure 26-2D) [Ross et al., 2001]. This subgroup was delineated in a subgroup of children with mutations of *TUBA1A* [Kumar et al., 2010; Morris-Rosendahl et al., 2008; Poirier et al., 2007]. The phenotype is usually severe, similar to isolated LIS, and the pathology probably varies from LIS-4L to more severe changes, based on pathological data from fetal cases [Fallet-Bianco et al., 2008].

Lissencephaly with Cerebellar Hypoplasia Tubulin-Type 2

A more severe but related phenotype consists of severe LIS with diffuse agyria, agenesis or severe hypogenesis of the corpus callosum, and severe diffuse brainstem and cerebellar hypoplasia, a group that had previously been separated into LCH groups c, d, and f [Kumar et al., 2010; Ross et al., 2001]. The phenotype is very severe, with most patients surviving only a few weeks to months. The neuropathology corresponds to the rare two-layered form of LIS [Forman et al., 2005; Lecourtois et al., 2010]. Several have had mutations of *TUBA1A* [Kumar et al., 2010].

Microlissencephaly Microcephalic Osteodysplastic Primordial Dwarfism 1-Type

MLIS occurs in some patients with MOPD1, a syndrome that is difficult to distinguish from severe forms of Seckel's syndrome [Juric-Sekhar et al., 2010; Klinge et al., 2002; Meinecke and Passarge, 1991; Ozawa et al., 2005]. The phenotype consists of severe prenatal growth deficiency and microcephaly, sparse hair and dry scaling skin, skeletal anomalies such as platyspondyly, slender ribs, short and bowed proximal humeri and femurs, small iliac wings, dysplastic acetabulum and small hands and feet, and profound developmental handicaps. A few have developed aplastic anemia, another overlap with Seckel's syndrome. The neuropathology consists of a variant form of LIS-3L with frontal predominance.

Microlissencephaly Barth-Type

The Barth-type of MLIS is possibly the most severe of all the known LIS syndromes. The phenotype consists of polyhydramnios, probably due to poor fetal swallowing, severe congenital microcephaly (birth OFC approximately 28 cm), weak respiratory effort, and survival for only a few hours or days [Barth et al., 1982; Dobyns and Barkovich, 1999; Kroon et al., 1996]. The neuropathology consists of a variant form of LIS-4L with extreme hypoplasia of many structures, as described above.

X-linked Lissencephaly with Abnormal Genitalia

Children with XLAG are almost all males and have severe clinical problems [Berry-Kravis and Israel, 1994; Bonneau et al., 2002; Dobyns et al., 1999a; Kato et al., 2004; Uyanik et al., 2003]. Frequent, and sometimes continuous, seizures are typically seen on the first day of life, often in the delivery room. Other problems include poor temperature regulation leading to persistent hypothermia, hypotonia, very poor feeding, chronic secretory diarrhea, and ambiguous or severely hypoplastic genitalia. The seizures generally do not respond well to therapy, and are accompanied by an infancy-onset dyskinesia that may be difficult to distinguish from seizures. The feeding problems and diarrhea combine to lead to very poor nutrition. Some female relatives, especially sisters and maternal aunts (non-mothers), have isolated agenesis of the corpus callosum [Marsh et al., 2009; Proud et al., 1992]. Mutations of the *ARX* gene have been found in almost all patients [Kato et al., 2004; Kitamura et al., 2002] with this syndrome. The XLAG-associated form of LIS-3L is recognizable on brain imaging, and strongly points to this diagnosis (see Figure 26-2F). However, the same pattern has been seen in two children with a separate syndrome that includes microphthalmia with cleft lip and palate.

Notably, less severe mutations of *ARX* have been found in boys with cryptogenic infantile spasms, infancy-onset dyskinesia, and some less specific mental retardation and epilepsy syndromes [Bienvenu et al., 2002; Kato et al., 2003, 2007; Partington et al., 2004; Scheffer et al., 2002; Stromme et al., 2003; Stromme et al., 2002a, 2002b; Turner et al., 2002]. Studies in a mouse model have found that nonradial migration of inhibitory interneurons from the embryonic ganglionic eminence (the origin of the basal ganglia) to the neocortex is disrupted with loss of *Arx* [Kitamura et al., 2002; Marsh et al., 2009].

Genetic Counseling

All forms of LIS and SBH are genetic, and genetic testing is currently available for more than 80 percent of patients, although this varies with the phenotype (see Table 26-2) [Dobyns, 2010; Haverfield et al., 2009]. When LIS or SBH is suspected but the exact syndrome diagnosis is uncertain, the most productive order of testing begins with analysis for deletions of chromosome 17p13.3 that include the *LIS1* gene, using chromosome microarray or other methods, followed by sequencing of *LIS1*, *DCX*, and *TUBA1A*, and sometimes *ARX* if the phenotype is compatible. However, details of the phenotype can be used by experienced clinicians to change the order of tests, such as testing *DCX* first in females with SBH, or *ARX* first for males with XLAG. Genetic testing for LIS and SBH is important, as several syndromes are associated with high risks of recurrence. This risk is especially great for parents who are carriers of a rearrangement of chromosome 17, and for mothers who carry *ARX* or *DCX* mutations, as both are X-linked. When the causal gene is unknown or unavailable for testing, empiric recurrence risks based on the known or most likely pattern of inheritance are appropriate. These are listed in Table 26-1.

Cobblestone Malformations

Cobblestone malformation or lissencephaly is a severe brain malformation associated with abnormal migration from the brain into the leptomeninges, and frequently with eye anomalies and congenital muscular dystrophy (CMD). The older term, "type 2" lissencephaly, should be abandoned. Cobblestone malformations occur in a graded series of CMDs, with brain involvement associated with reduced glycosylation of α-dystroglycan that, from least to most severe, include CMD with mental retardation and microcephaly without obvious cortical malformation; CMD with mental retardation and isolated cerebellar hypoplasia and dysplasia; Fukuyama congenital muscular dystrophy (FCMD); muscle-eye-brain disease (MEB); and Walker–Warburg syndrome (WWS). While neuropathological confirmation in humans is sparse, cobblestone or cobblestone-like malformations also occur in a growing group of other disorders, including isolated bilateral frontoparietal cobblestone malformation (previously called bilateral frontoparietal polymicrogyria), CEDNIK syndrome (cerebral dysgenesis, neuropathy, ichthyosis and keratoderma), and, so far, two other congenital disorders of glycosylation – Debré-type autosomal-recessive cuts laxa and CHIME-like (colobomas, heart defects, ichthyosiform dermatosis, mental retardation, and either ear defects or epilepsy) syndrome.

Pathology

The brain malformations seen in WWS, MEB, or FCMD consist of poor gyral development, cerebral and cerebellar cortical dysplasia, hydrocephalus, brainstem hypoplasia with dysplasia of the inferior olives and dentate nuclei, and hypoplasia of the corticospinal tracts in brainstem and spinal cord [Bordarier et al., 1984; Dobyns et al., 1985; Towfighi et al., 1984; Williams et al., 1984]. Studies of affected human fetuses demonstrate a striking cerebral and cerebellar cortical dysplasia with discontinuities in the basal lamina at the pial surface (glia limitans) that allow abnormal migration of neurons and glia beyond the cortical plate and into the leptomeninges [Miller et al., 1991; Squier, 1993; Takada et al., 1987]. The same changes are seen in several animal models [Moore et al., 2002; Willer et al., 2004]. The cerebellar cortical cysts result from entrapment of islands of meningeal tissue between adjacent folia [Muntoni et al., 2009].

The postnatal cortical malformation consists of an undersulcated and subtly pebbled surface that includes areas resembling agyria, pachygyria, or polymicrogyria, although the histological appearance is very different. The pebbled surface appearance prompted the name "cobblestone cortex," first proposed by Haltia [Dubowitz, 1996]. The cortex is thick and dysplastic, with no recognizable layers. The original glia limitans is found in the middle of the cortex, which is disrupted by abnormal vascular channels and fibroglial bands throughout that extend into and often obstruct the subarachnoid space. The cortical malformation is most severe with a smooth surface in WWS, and progressively less severe in the other syndromes in this probably continuous series [Dobyns et al., 1985, 1989; Dubowitz, 1994, 1996; Haltia et al., 1997; Takada et al., 1988; Walker, 1942]. The white matter is poorly myelinated, with numerous heterotopic neurons and microscopic cysts. The cerebellum is small and dysplastic, with cerebellar cortical cysts. Other brain abnormalities include obstructive hydrocephalus, brainstem hypoplasia with dysplasia of the inferior olives and dentate nuclei, and hypoplasia of the corticospinal tracts in brainstem and spinal cord. In a few patients, absent septum pellucidum, absent corpus callosum, or occipital cephaloceles may be noted. The brain malformation is frequently associated with eye malformations. Skeletal muscle biopsies show changes of CMD and hypoglycosylated α-dystroglycan [Brockington and Muntoni, 2005; Mercuri et al., 2006; Muntoni et al., 2002].

Only limited human pathological data are available for the cobblestone malformations that are not associated with CMD. Analysis of a Gpr56 knockout mouse shows discontinuities in the pial surface basal lamina and migration of neurons and glia into the leptomeninges, just as in the CMD-associated cobblestone malformations [Li et al., 2008]. The first neuropathology data in humans were recently reported in abstract form, and confirm the cobblestone-type cortical malformation with widespread glioneuronal heterotopia [Fallet-Bianco et al., 2010].

Brain Imaging

The brain imaging changes of CMD-associated cobblestone malformation present a continuous series of malformations that begins with the severe changes of WWS and ends with normal brain imaging. However, most patients cluster into one of the defined syndromes, which consist of WWS, an intermediate group classified as MEB, and progressively less severe forms classified as FCMD, CMD with cerebellar dysplasia and cysts or CMD with microcephaly, and CMD with normal brain imaging. The key imaging features are most easily recognized for WWS, and are collectively pathognomonic for this disorder [Clement et al., 2008; Dobyns et al., 1989; Jissendi-Tchofo et al., 2009; Mercuri et al., 2006; van der Knaap et al., 1997].

The imaging abnormalities seen in WWS begin with macrocephaly and prominent forehead, resulting from existing or prior hydrocephalus, and reduced size and partial obliteration of extra-axial spaces, which is especially prominent between the cerebral hemispheres (Figure 26-3C). The cerebral surface is undersulcated, usually with diffuse agyria. The cerebral cortex is moderately thick, usually about 7–10 mm unless thinned by hydrocephalus. The cortical–white matter border is jagged, with frequent vertical (perpendicular to the cortical–white matter border) striations, which differs from the chaotic striations typical of true polymicrogyria. Just beneath the cortex, streaks of laminar subcortical heterotopia are seen that differ from typical subcortical band heterotopia based on their beaded and discontinuous appearance. The white matter has very abnormal signal (bright on T2 and dark on T1 MRI sequences; dark on computed tomography [CT] scan) and may have small cysts. The white-matter volume may be normal, or thinned by hydrocephalus. The third and lateral ventricles are enlarged and may be very large and rounded, reflecting active hydrocephalus. Very rarely, the ventricles may be small. The corpus callosum is present, although frequently thin.

The brainstem and cerebellum in WWS (see Figure 26-3C) are remarkably dysplastic, with a kink at the midbrain–pons junction in which the midbrain is angled dorsally with respect to the pons [Jissendi-Tchofo et al., 2009]. The lower brainstem appears small, with moderate to severe hypoplasia of the medulla and pons, near-absence of the basis points, and ventral midline clefts of the ventral pons. But the midbrain and especially the tectum are abnormally large. The cerebellum is small, with the vermis more severely involved than the hemispheres, a dysplastic foliar pattern, and often small cysts within or near the cerebellar cortex. The posterior fossa may be enlarged and a few patients have small occipital meningoceles.

The imaging abnormalities in MEB are similar but consistently less severe than in WWS (see Figure 26-3B). The macrocephaly and hydrocephalus are common in MEB as well, while partial obliteration of extra-axial spaces is less extensive. The cerebral surface is again undersulcated, but with frontal-predominant pachygyria rather than agyria; posterior-predominant pachygyria occurs but appears to be rare. Some areas resembling polymicrogyria may be seen. The jagged cortical–white matter border and vertical striations are similar, while fewer streaks of subcortical heterotopia are seen. The white matter has very abnormal signal, similar to WWS in infants, but over time this evolves from diffuse to patchy to minimal signal changes. The frequency of hydrocephalus and thinning of the white matter and corpus callosum is probably similar.

The brainstem and cerebellum in MEB (see Figure 26-3B) are also dysplastic but less severely so than in WWS. The brainstem lacks the kink, but the lower brainstem, especially the pons, appears small while the midbrain and tectum are enlarged. The cerebellar changes are similar but, on average, less severe than in WWS, except that cerebellar cortical cysts may be more common. This may be due to a high frequency of cerebellar cysts in MEB patients with mutations of the *POMGnT1* gene [Muntoni et al., 2009].

The imaging abnormalities in FCMD (see Figure 26-3A) are similar to MEB but less severe. Hydrocephalus is uncommon. The cortical malformation is less severe but still frontal-predominant, although some patients have severe temporal lobe agyria. The brainstem and cerebellum most often appear normal. In contrast, patients with mental retardation and cerebellar cysts have relatively normal forebrain structures and cerebral cortex, although review of some published images shows that the cortex is mildly dysplastic. The cerebellum mimics the appearance seen in MEB.

The brain imaging abnormalities in the cobblestone-like disorders without CMD (see Figure 26-3D) are similar to those in MEB, including the frontal-predominant pachygyria, moderately thick cortex with vertical striations, patchy white-matter abnormalities, hydrocephalus, and brainstem- and vermis-predominant cerebellar hypoplasia and dysplasia [Chang et al., 2003; Van Maldergem et al., 2008]. The brainstem is usually not as thin as is seen in MEB.

Clinical Features

In all of the cobblestone malformation syndromes associated with CMD, the phenotype consists of moderate to profound mental retardation, severe hypotonia, mild distal spasticity, and poor vision. WWS is the most severe, FCMD and mental retardation with cerebellar cysts the least severe, and MEB in

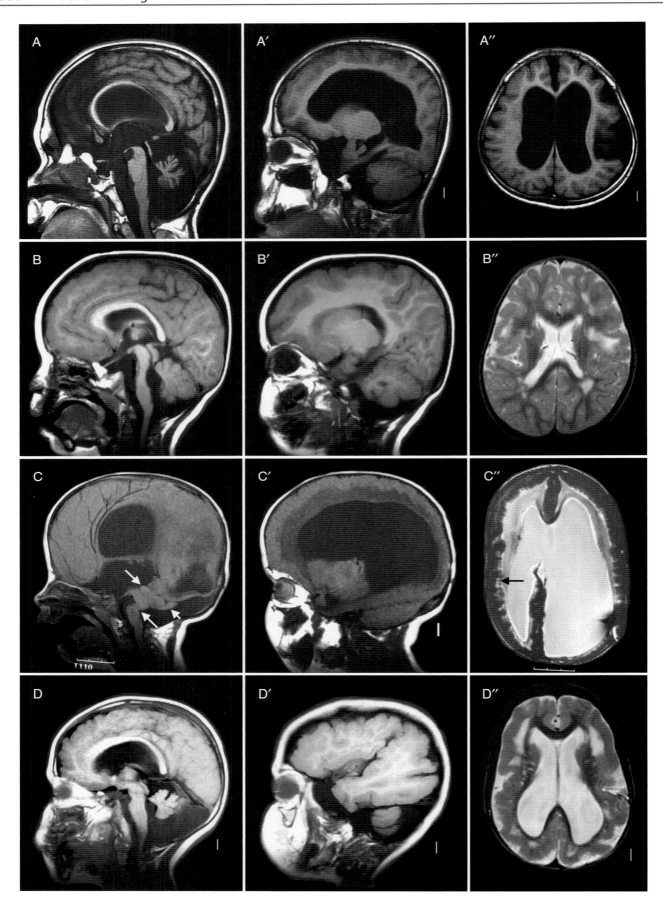

the middle. This is in part a semantic issue, as MEB is the diagnosis used for any intermediate phenotype. Several less severe CMD-associated phenotypes without brain malformations have been associated with different mutations of the same genes. The other (non-CMD) cobblestone syndromes have brain phenotypes that resemble FCMD or MEB, but without the eye or muscle manifestations [Clement et al., 2008; Godfrey et al., 2007; Klein et al., 2008; Muntoni and Voit, 2004].

Prognosis and Management

Children with most of these syndromes have both cobblestone brain malformation and progressive muscle disease, which lead to combined hypotonia (from the brain and muscle disease) and spasticity (from the brain malformation). The combination makes orthopedic and rehabilitation management more difficult. Although the causative genes may be the same, it is important to distinguish among the various clinical syndromes, as the prognosis and thus management differ. WWS is a severe disorder associated with profound mental retardation and congenital hypotonia. Few children with WWS live past the age of 3 years. MEB and FCMD are less severe, with variable survival from later in the first decade into the teens and beyond; some patients have survived into the fifth decade. Some children with WWS reported to live longer than 3 years may be better classified as having MEB.

Optimal management begins with early recognition and accurate counseling regarding the prognosis, as some parents of children with WWS choose to limit life-sustaining interventions, such as ventilation during severe illnesses. Most children with WWS and some with MEB have congenital hydrocephalus that can only be managed with a shunt. Children with WWS who have occipital cephaloceles may not have hydrocephalus at birth, but excision of the cephaloceles is often followed by hydrocephalus. Thus, placement of a shunt should be considered at the time of cephalocele removal. Seizures occur but are rarely as severe as those seen in patients with LIS or SBH. In WWS and MEB, congenital glaucoma and buphthalmos require care by an ophthalmologist. Treatment of other eye anomalies that can interfere with vision, such as retinal nonattachment or detachment, cataracts, and corneal opacity, should be assessed on an individual basis in view of the overall poor prognosis. Children with FCMD have no or only minor eye anomalies.

The muscle disease progresses slowly, so that frequent evaluations to assess orthopedic and other rehabilitation needs are important. Careful seating is essential, owing to severe hypotonia, and contractures need to be managed with physical therapy and splinting when needed. In WWS, the CMD probably progresses slowly over time, but this is not apparent clinically, owing to the severe hypotonia and short survival period. Children with FCMD who learn to walk typically lose this skill several years later.

Syndromes, Genetics, and Molecular Basis

All of the cobblestone malformation syndromes with muscle involvement share the common feature of hypoglycosylated α-dystroglycan on skeletal muscle biopsy, and all of the known genes code for proteins known or suspected to be involved with glycosylation, particularly O-mannosylation of α-dystroglycan, which has led to the general term "dystroglycanopathy" for these and related CMD syndromes with normal brain structure [Brockington and Muntoni, 2005; Hewitt and Grewal, 2003; Muntoni et al., 2002; Ross, 2002]. Alpha- and β-dystroglycan are components of the dystrophin-associated glycoprotein complex that links the actin-associated cytoskeleton and extracellular matrix, and are encoded by the same precursor peptide. Alpha-dystroglycan is a highly glycosylated peripheral membrane protein that binds many extracellular matrix proteins through attached carbohydrate groups. In the dystroglycanopathies, especially the cobblestone-CMD group, glycosyl groups are absent or reduced, resulting in decreased binding of ligands such as laminin-2, agrin and perlecan in skeletal muscle, and neurexin in the brain [Barresi and Campbell, 2006].

Accordingly, all of the genes associated with cobblestone syndromes with muscle involvement code for proteins that

---

Fig. 26-3 **Subtypes of cobblestone cortical malformations.** Midsagittal (left column), parasagittal (middle column), and axial (right column) magnetic resonance images from patients with four different cobblestone malformation syndromes. **A–A″,** The top row demonstrates brain abnormalities in Fukuyama congenital muscular dystrophy. These images show mild frontal pachygyria with 7- to 8-mm-thick cortex, normal to mildly simplified gyral pattern posteriorly, widely open sylvian fissures, especially on the left, moderately enlarged lateral ventricles, intact but stretched corpus callosum, normal brainstem, and moderate cerebellar hypoplasia and atrophy. These images are from a Japanese child with Fukuyama's congenital muscular dystrophy (FCMD), who most likely is homozygous for the Japanese founder mutation consisting of addition of a 3-kb retrotransposon into the 3′ untranslated region of the *FCMD* gene [Kobayashi et al., 1998]. **B–B″,** The second row shows changes in muscle-eye-brain disease. These images show moderate frontal pachygyria with an 8- to 12-mm-thick cortex that extends into the parietal lobe, patches of abnormal white matter with high T2 signal intensity, hypoplastic brainstem, especially in the pons, moderate cerebellar hypoplasia, and a few small cysts in the high white matter. The patient was a boy with a homozygous mutation of *POMGnT1* in exon 20: c.1813delC and H573fs (patient CC described by Yoshida and colleagues [Yoshida et al., 2001] and Taniguchi and associates [Taniguchi et al., 2003]). **C–C″,** The third row shows changes in severe Walker–Warburg syndrome. These images show diffuse agyria with an irregular surface, beaded subcortical heterotopia (black arrow in **C″**), diffuse abnormal signal of white matter with very high T2 signal intensity, very thin corpus callosum, and moderate to severely enlarged lateral ventricles. Posterior fossa abnormalities include severe hypoplasia of the brainstem, enlarged tectum (top white arrow in **C**), classic Walker–Warburg kinking at the junction of the pons and midbrain (bottom long white arrow in **C**), severe cerebellar hypoplasia (bottom short white arrow in **C**), small fluid collection in the posterior fossa, and overall small posterior fossa. No mutation has been identified, although only *POMT1* has been tested. **D–D″,** The bottom row shows the changes in bilateral frontoparietal polymicrogyria, with extensive involvement of the frontal and parietal lobes, extended sylvian fissure, patches of very bright T2 signal of white matter (again, more severe frontally), mildly enlarged lateral ventricles, thin corpus callosum, and hypoplasia of the brainstem and cerebellum. The patient was a girl with a missense mutation of the *GPR56* gene in exon 3: 112C3T and R38W [Piao et al., 2004]. *(Courtesy of Dr. William B Dobyns, University of Washington, Departments of Pediatrics and Neurology, Seattle, Washington. These images were selected from patients LR01-058* **[A]**, *LP95-146* **[B]**, *LR00-181* **[C]**, *and LP93-017* **[D]**).

regulate glycosylation, particularly *O*-mannosylation of α-dystroglycan. At least two of the non-CMD cobblestone syndromes are also congenital disorders of glycosylation [Cantagrel et al., 2010; Morava et al., 2009; Van Maldergem et al., 2008], and another is associated with a heavily glycosylated protein [Jin et al., 2007]. The cobblestone syndromes and associated genes are listed in Table 26-3, with estimated mutation frequencies shown in Table 26-4. Biochemical deficiency has been demonstrated in muscle for some of the proteins involved [Zhang et al., 2003].

Walker–Warburg Syndrome

WWS consists of severe cobblestone malformation with a smooth surface resembling lissencephaly, as well as the most severe brainstem and cerebellar malformations of any of the cobblestone syndromes (see Figure 26-3C). Most patients have hydrocephalus, and approximately 25 percent have occipital cephaloceles [Dobyns et al., 1985, 1989]. All have profound mental retardation, epilepsy, and variable eye abnormalities, such as microphthalmia, congenital glaucoma with or without buphthalmos, Peter anomaly, iris hypoplasia, colobomas, cataracts, persistent hyperplastic primary vitreous, retinal dysplasia, and retinal nonattachment. All have CMD or congenital myopathy, with contractures and elevated serum levels of creatine kinase.

Muscle-Eye-Brain Disease

MEB consists of intermediate-severity cobblestone malformation with severe mental retardation and epilepsy, as well as eye and muscle abnormalities similar to WWS [Godfrey et al., 2007; Klein et al., 2008; Santavuori et al., 1977, 1989; Taniguchi et al., 2003]. The cortical malformation is typically more severe frontally (see Figure 26-3B), and is often confused with polymicrogyria. The white-matter signal changes resolve

Table 26-3 Cobblestone Syndromes, Inheritance and Genes

Cobblestone Type and Syndrome	Inheritance	Genes
CLASSIC COBBLESTONE SYNDROMES WITH CMD		
Walker–Warburg syndrome	AR	*POMT2, POMGnT1, FKRP, FKTN, LARGE*
Muscle-eye-brain disease	AR	*POMT2, POMGnT1, FKRP, LARGE*
Fukuyama CMD	AR	*FKTN*
Mental retardation, microcephaly, and CMD	AR	*POMT1, POMT2*
Mental retardation, cerebellar cysts, and CMD	AR	*FKRP*
VARIANT COBBLESTONE SYNDROMES WITH NORMAL MUSCLE		
Bilateral frontoparietal cobblestone malformation	AR	*GPR56*
Dandy–Walker malformation with CDG*	AR	*B4GALT1*
Debré-type cutis laxa	AR	*ATP6V0A2*
CHIME-like syndrome	AR	*SRD5A3*
CEDNIK syndrome	AR	*SNAP29*

* Cobblestone cortical malformation has not been confirmed for this syndrome.
AR, autosomal-recessive; CDG, congenital disorder of glycosylation; CEDNIK, cerebral dysgenesis, neuropathy, ichthyosis and keratoderma; CHIME, colobomas, heart defects, ichthyosiform dermatosis, mental retardation, and either ear defects or epilesy; CMD, congenital muscular dystrophy.

Table 26-4 Mutation Frequencies for Cobblestone Syndromes with Known Causal Genes*

	POMT1	*POMT2*	*POMGnT1*	*FKTN*	*FKRP*	*LARGE*	Total
BRAIN PHENOTYPES							
FCMD, mild MEB	5					1	6
MEB		7	14		2	1	24
Severe MEB, WWS	25	14	6	9	5	2	61
TOTAL	30	21	20	9	7	4	91
OTHER PHENOTYPES							
CMD			*MDC1C*	*MDC1D*			
LGMD	*LGMD2K*		*LGMD2I*				

* Data combined from several sources [Godfrey et al., 2007; Moore et al., 2006; Muntoni et al., 2009, 2008; van Reeuwijk et al., 2006], with numbers affected by ascertainment differences (severe brain malformations versus all CMD) and by classification of syndromes. The mild MEB group includes mild FCMD-like, CMD or LGMD with mental retardation and microcephaly, and CMD with mental retardation with subtle cortical and cerebellar dysplasia.
CMD, congenital muscular dystrophy; FCMD, Fukuyama congenital muscular dystrophy; LGMD, limb-girdle muscular dystrophy; MEB, muscle-eye-brain disease; WWS, Walker–Warburg syndrome.

over time, and the corpus callosum usually appears normal. The brainstem and cerebellum are hypoplastic, but the brainstem lacks the distinctive kink at the midbrain–pons junction seen in patients with WWS [Jissendi-Tchofo et al., 2009]. The eye anomalies consist of retinal and choroidal hypoplasia, optic nerve pallor, high-grade myopia, anterior chamber-angle abnormalities, glaucoma, iris hypoplasia, cataracts, and rarely colobomas [Santavuori et al., 1989].

Fukuyama Congenital Muscular Dystrophy

FCMD consists of mild cobblestone malformation, moderate to severe mental retardation and epilepsy, and severe CMD with progressive weakness, joint contractures, and elevated serum creatine kinase [Fukuyama and Osawa, 1984; Fukuyama et al., 1981; Osawa et al., 1991]. The brain malformation is less severe than seen in either MEB or WWS (see Figure 26-3A). Typical FCMD is caused by a common founder mutation in the *FKTN* gene in the Japanese population, with rare reports from Korea as well [Kobayashi et al., 1998; Kondo-Iida et al., 1999]. This phenotype has not been associated with any other gene. Less severe syndromes consisting of mental retardation with either microcephaly or cerebellar cysts ("Italian MEB") have been reported in a few patients [Ruggieri et al., 2001; Villanova et al., 2000; Voit et al., 1999].

Cobblestone-Like Syndromes

A growing number of cobblestone-like syndromes with normal muscle have been reported, most with the causal genes also identified (also listed in Table 26-3). Bilateral frontoparietal cobblestone malformation (often described as bilateral frontoparietal polymicrogyria in literature reports) is characterized by global developmental delay, moderate to severe mental retardation, normal head size or mild microcephaly, dysconjugate gaze, spasticity, ataxia, and seizures especially generalized tonic-clonic and myoclonic seizures [Chang et al., 2003, 2004; Dobyns et al., 1996b; Piao et al., 2005; Straussberg et al., 1996]. Mutations of the *GPR56* gene have been found in many affected children.

Similar brain imaging abnormalities have been demonstrated in at least two congenital disorders of glycosylation (CDG). The first is autosomal-recessive Debré-type cutis laxa, which consists of mild to moderate cutis laxa, variable mental retardation, and other features [Kornak et al., 2008; Morava et al., 2009; Van Maldergem et al., 2008]. The second is a syndrome that resembles the rare CHIME syndrome, which includes ocular colobomas, congenital heart disease, early-onset ichthyosiform dermatosis, mental retardation, and ear anomalies or conductive hearing loss [Al-Gazali et al., 2008; Cantagrel et al., 2010]. Another type of CDG has been associated with Dandy–Walker malformation of the cerebellum [Hansske et al., 2002; Peters et al., 2002]. A cobblestone cortical malformation is possible but not proven. Finally, affected individuals with CEDNIK (cerebral dysgenesis, neuropathy, ichthyosis and keratoderma) syndrome have a cobblestone malformation.

Genetic Testing

All of the syndromes associated with the cobblestone malformation, with or without CMD, have autosomal-recessive inheritance. Six genes associated with cobblestone malformations and CMD, and 4–5 associated with cobblestone malformation with normal muscle studies have been identified (see Table 26-3). All have autosomal-recessive inheritance. Testing is available for most of the cobblestone-CMD syndromes and for *GPR56*. Testing serum transferrin isoforms for CDG will detect two (or more) other syndromes.

Antenatal Diagnosis

Several features of the cobblestone syndromes can be detected by prenatal testing. Almost all patients with WWS or MEB have enlarged lateral ventricles, and many have hydrocephalus. Almost all have cerebellar hypoplasia, and a few have gross microphthalmia. Each of these may be detected by prenatal ultrasounds in the mid- to late second trimester. Most fetuses with WWS should be detected, although no large series has been reported. The yield is likely to be lower with less severe syndromes. Molecular genetic testing is possible only when the specific mutation has been identified in the proband.

Neuronal Heterotopia

Neuronal heterotopia consist of groups of neurons in an inappropriate location. The major types include periventricular nodular heterotopia (PNH) that line the lateral ventricles, subcortical nodular heterotopia that tend to form large masses of nodules beneath the cortex, and leptomeningeal or marginal glioneuronal heterotopias found over the surface of the brain. The latter are also known as brain warts. Examples of several types are shown in Figure 26-4.

Periventricular Nodular Heterotopia

PNH consist of nodular masses of gray matter that line the ventricular walls and protrude into the lumen, resulting in an irregular outline (see Figure 26-4). They are recognized as a relatively common malformation that may occur as a single nodule or heterotopion, or as multiple contiguous or noncontiguous nodules or heterotopia [Dobyns et al., 1996a; Dubeau et al., 1995]. When the nodules are single or few in number, they may be associated with seizures or learning problems, but are unlikely to help with diagnosis. When the lesions are bilateral and numerous, a genetic basis is likely. When the nodules are diffuse and contiguous, they may be associated with other brain malformations, especially hypogenesis of the corpus callosum, cerebellar hypoplasia, or polymicrogyria [Parrini et al., 2006; Wieck et al., 2005].

Pathology

On gross examination, periventricular or subependymal heterotopia consist of nodular masses of gray matter that line the walls of the lateral ventricles. Microscopically, the abnormal tissue contains both neurons and glial cells, and forms clusters of rounded, irregular nodules separated by layers of myelinated fibers [Tassi et al., 2005]. An individual nodule or heterotopion may lack any organization or have rudimentary lamination. PNH can be induced in the developing rat by intraperitoneal injection of the cytotoxic agent, methylazoxymethanol acetate, at embryonic day 15. In this model, reciprocal connections between the heterotopia and normal cortex have been found, supporting the hypothesis that neurons within the heterotopia

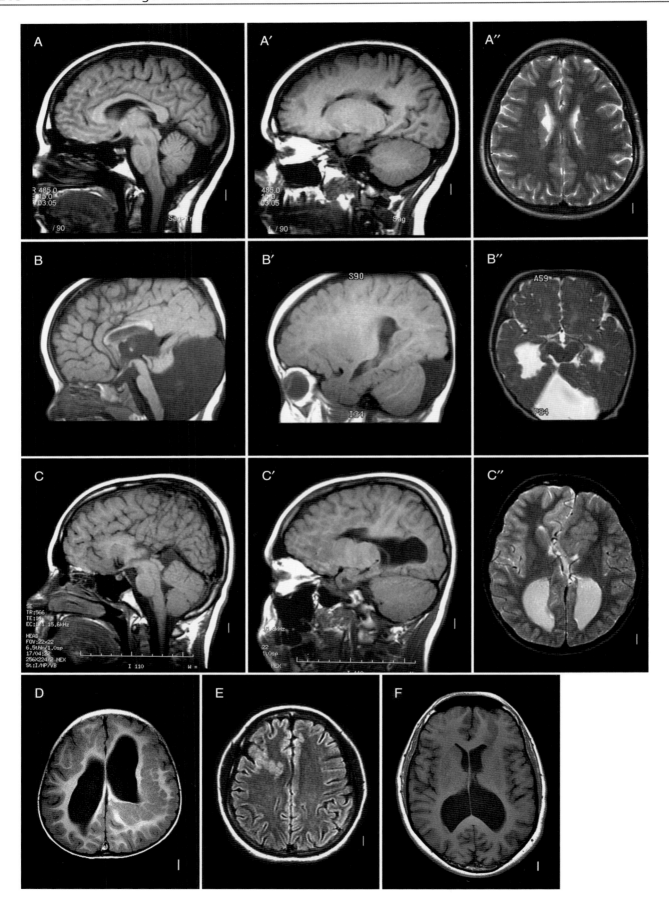

were destined for the cortex before the interruption of their migration [Colacitti et al., 1999].

Brain Imaging

Brain imaging using MRI demonstrates typical nodules along the ventricular walls, with different patterns of involvement that can be used to help to distinguish different syndromes (Table 26-5 and Figure 26-4). Patients with the classic X-linked form (see Figure 26-4A) typically have bilateral contiguous or nearly contiguous PNH that spare the temporal horns, associated with mildly thin corpus callosum, cerebellar vermis hypoplasia, and mega-cisterna magna [Dobyns et al., 1996a; Parrini

et al., 2006; Poussaint et al., 2000]. Patients with autosomal-recessive severe congenital microcephaly and PNH have symmetric nodular heterotopia lining the ventricles, thin overlying cortex with abnormal gyri, mildly enlarged lateral ventricles, and delayed myelination [Sheen et al., 2004a, 2004b]. In the frontal-predominant form, heterotopia are limited to the frontal horns and bodies of the lateral ventricles. They may occur alone, or with overlying polymicrogyria [Wieck et al., 2005]. In the more common and usually syndromic posterior predominant forms (see Figure 26-4B), heterotopia are limited to the trigones and temporal and occipital horns. Posterior heterotopia may be associated with overlying polymicrogyria and cerebellar hypoplasia, hippocampal and

Table 26-5 Types of PNH and Associated Syndromes

Heterotopia Type and Syndrome	Inheritance	Genes
DIFFUSE PNH		
PNH with frontonasal dysplasia	SpAD	Unknown
DIFFUSE PNH SPARING TEMPORAL HORNS		
Classical bilateral PNH (may be unilateral)	XL	*FLNA*
PNH with Ehlers–Danlos syndrome	XL	*FLNA*
PNH with micronodules	SpAD	Unknown
PNH with ambiguous genitalia	SpAD	Unknown
PNH with limb abnormalities	SpAD	Unknown
PNH with severe congenital microcephaly	AR	*ARFGEF2*
ANTERIOR-PREDOMINANT PNH (FRONTAL HORNS TO TRIGONES)		
Frontoperisylvian PNH	SpAD	Unknown
Frontoperisylvian PNH with polymicrogyria	SpAD	Unknown
Posterior-predominant PNH (trigones to temporal and occipital horns)	SpAD	Unknown
Posterior-predominant PNH with polymicrogyria	SpAD	Unknown
Posterior-predominant PNH with hippocampal and cerebellar hypoplasia	SpAD	Unknown
Posterior-predominant PNH with hydrocephalus	SpAD	Unknown
ISOLATED PNH		
Isolated nodules, single or a few (may be unilateral)	Unknown	Unknown
RARE FORMS OF DIFFUSE HETEROTOPIA		
Periventricular laminar heterotopia	SpAD	Unknown
Periventricular ribbonlike heterotopia	SpAD	Unknown

AR, autosomal-recessive; PNH, periventricular nodular heterotopia; SpAD, sporadic with presumed autosomal-dominant inheritance caused by new mutations; XL, X-linked. (Data from several reports [Parrini et al., 2006].)

Fig. 26-4 Subtypes of heterotopia. Midsagittal (left column), parasagittal (middle column), and axial (right column) magnetic resonance images from patients with several different types of heterotopia. **A–A″,** The top row demonstrates bilateral, nearly contiguous periventricular nodular heterotopia (PNH), an overlying normal gyral pattern, and mild cerebellar vermis hypoplasia, with all other structures normal. This is the typical pattern associated with mutations of *FLNA*, although testing has not been performed in this adult woman. **B–B″,** The second row shows hypogenesis of the corpus callosum, thin brainstem, Dandy–Walker malformation, and several PNH adjacent to the trigones and temporal horns. This combination of cerebellar and hippocampal hypoplasia with PNH is a rare malformation syndrome. **C–C″,** The third row depicts a large mass of nodular heterotopia in the left frontal lobe, which compresses the left lateral ventricle and extends upwards to fill much of the subcortical white matter. The overlying cortex appears normal. The mass of heterotopia enlarges the left frontal lobe so that it pushes across the midline to compress the right frontal lobe. This is the characteristic appearance of (giant) subcortical nodular heterotopia. The bottom row shows axial images of typical heterotopia. **D,** Another example of subcortical nodular heterotopia, with prominent infolding of the cortex. **E** and **F,** Transmantle heterotopia, a rare malformation consisting of a column of heterotopic cells that extends from the ventricular surface to the cortex. The lack of a cleft differentiates this condition from schizencephaly. *(Courtesy of Dr. William B Dobyns, University of Washington, Departments of Pediatrics and Neurology, Seattle, Washington. These images were selected from patients LR01-357m, LR06-278, LR03-202, LR09-212, LR04-420m, and LR08-415.)*

cerebellar hypoplasia, or hydrocephalus [Parrini et al., 2006; Wieck et al., 2005].

Clinical Features

The clinical presentation and course found in patients with PNH vary among the recognized syndromes, most of which are listed in Table 26-5. In individuals with PNH but no other brain malformations, seizures and learning problems are common, while more severe developmental problems are not, although exceptions certainly occur. When microcephaly or any other brain malformations are found, the likelihood of mental retardation increases greatly.

Among all forms of PNH, the most common and often the presenting symptom is epilepsy, which has been reported in 80–90 percent of patients, although an ascertainment bias appears likely. The age at seizure onset is variable, but is often delayed until early adulthood [Battaglia et al., 1997]. Most patients have one or more types of partial seizures, which may be easily controlled or refractory. There is no clear relationship between the epilepsy severity and the extent of nodular heterotopia. The associated EEG abnormalities are not specific, consisting of infrequent interictal discharges that may be generalized, multifocal, or focal. Pseudotemporal lobe localization has also been reported [Battaglia et al., 1997; Sisodiya et al., 1999]. Studies using depth electrodes in patients with PNH and epilepsy have found the nodules to be intrinsically epileptogenic [Aghakhani et al., 2005; Kothare et al., 1998; Scherer et al., 2005]. However, seizure onset most often begins within a complex epileptogenic zone that includes both the heterotopia and overlying cortex. Intractable seizures associated with heterotopia should be treated aggressively. Temporal lobe surgery for patients with PNH and associated hippocampal sclerosis generally has not been successful [Li et al., 1997], although selected patients operated on after depth-electrode studies have had a good outcome [Tassi et al., 2005].

Syndromes, Genetics, and Molecular Basis

The most common or classic form of PNH, as well as the linked Ehlers–Danlos form, spares the temporal horns and predominately affects females, which first led to recognition of an X-linked syndrome. The phenotype is generally mild. In addition to seizures, a few patients have had chronic headache or other incidental symptoms, whereas others discovered during family evaluations are asymptomatic. Most patients, especially females, have normal intelligence, although the curve may be shifted slightly to the left, with an average intelligence quotient (IQ) of approximately 85. The phenotype in males varies widely, ranging from the mild female phenotype to prenatal lethality, with mental retardation being more common than in females [Dobyns et al., 1996a; Guerrini et al., 2004; Huttenlocher et al., 1994; Sheen et al., 2001].

Unilateral PNH are less common than the bilateral form. In one large series, 14 patients had bilateral PNH, compared with 6 with unilateral PNH [Dubeau et al., 1995]. The clinical manifestations are similar, including some patients without epilepsy and some with mental retardation. As suggested by anecdotal experience, unilateral PNH may occur as part of other malformation syndromes.

The remaining PNH-associated syndromes (see Table 26-5), including classic PNH in males, have a more severe clinical course that includes global developmental delay, moderate to severe mental retardation, and, more consistently, severe epilepsy, which is often intractable.

PNH, especially when numerous, are most often genetic, but heterotopia can also be acquired due to extrinsic factors, such as infection, injury, or radiation [Ferrer et al., 1993; Montenegro et al., 2002]. The common X-linked form of PNH was first recognized based on observations of a skewed sex ratio toward females among sporadic patients, and reports of several families with multiple affected females and a decreased number of sons born to affected women [Dobyns et al., 1996a; Huttenlocher et al., 1994]. The causative gene was mapped to Xq28, and mutations were identified in the *FLNA* gene [Eksioglu et al., 1996; Fox et al., 1998]. A rare autosomal-recessive form associated with severe microcephaly was later attributed to mutations of the *ARFGEF2* gene on chromosome 20 [Sheen et al., 2004b]. Other forms have been mapped to chromosomes 5p15, 5q14.3, 6q26q27, and 7q11.23 [Backx et al., 2010; Cardoso et al., 2009; Ferland et al., 2006; Sheen et al., 2003], but the causal genes have not been identified.

The pathogenesis of genetic forms of PNH involves actin-binding, vesicle trafficking, and cell adhesion [Pang et al., 2008]. FLNA is a large actin-binding phosphoprotein that stabilizes the cytoskeleton and contributes to formation of focal adhesions along the ventricular epithelium [Lu et al., 2006]. The *ARFGEF2* gene encodes a protein designated BIG2, which converts guanine diphosphate to guanine triphosphate. This activates adenosine diphosphate (ADP)-ribosylation factors, which regulate vesicle trafficking and transport of molecules from the cell interior to cell surface, where they can bind to other molecules or be secreted by the cell. Thus, BIG2 may assist in the transport of FLNA to the cell surface. FLNA may be required for the initial attachment of neurons on to the radial glial scaffolding before migration from the ventricular zone [Lu et al., 2006]. Failure of migrating neurons to attach to radial glia is one likely mechanism leading to formation of heterotopia. Both proteins are highly expressed at the neuroepithelial lining, so deficiency could lead to loss of neuroependymal integrity and reduced cell adhesion.

Genetic Testing

In a large study of 120 patients with PNH, *FLNA* mutations were found in 10 of 10 families with classic X-linked PNH – 8 with classical bilateral PNH, 1 with PNH plus Ehlers–Danlos syndrome and 1 with unilateral PNH – and in 26 percent of sporadic patients with classic bilateral PNH [Parrini et al., 2006]. Overall, mutations were reported in 49 percent of individuals with classic bilateral PNH, irrespective of familial or sporadic occurrence. Not surprisingly, the sex ratio was skewed, with 93 percent of mutations found in females and 7 percent in males. Mutations of *ARFGEF2* have been reported in only two families [Sheen et al., 2004b]. As of 2010, mutation analysis was clinically available for *FLNA* but not *ARFGEF2*. Chromosome microarrays should be considered for patients with PNH and additional developmental abnormalities or congenital anomalies, based on observations of deletions or duplications of several chromosomes.

Antenatal Diagnosis

Periventricular nodular and other heterotopia cannot be visualized reliably at prenatal ultrasound examination, and fetal MRI has not been evaluated for this purpose. When mutations of *FLNA* or *ARFGEF2* have been identified, diagnostic testing for the specific mutation is possible. However, the usefulness of *FLNA* testing is limited, as most hemizygous males are likely miscarried, while heterozygous females usually have normal intelligence.

Subcortical Nodular and other Types of Heterotopia

Although less common and less well recognized, other types of heterotopia are known. Subcortical nodular heterotopia consist of a large mass of nodules expanding a portion of one cerebral hemisphere (see Figure 26-4C and D). This lesion is rarely, if ever, bilateral and may be associated with ipsilateral PNH, agenesis of the corpus callosum, and cerebellar vermis hypoplasia or Dandy–Walker malformation. Overlying cortical dysplasia may be seen [Barkovich, 2000; Barkovich and Kjos, 1992a]. Despite the large size of the heterotopia, development may be normal or only mildly abnormal, and onset of seizures may not occur until the third decade of life. Some patients have overlying cortical dysplasia, which leads to more severe problems, including mental retardation. Transmantle heterotopia, also called transmantle dysplasia, consist of a column of gray matter without nodular features that extends from the ventricular wall upwards to the cortical surface, where it is surrounded by a typically small area of focal cortical dysplasia (see Figure 26-4E–F). Smooth or laminar heterotopia appear to be rare, and/or "ribbon-like", undulating heterotopia even more rare, in the periventricular region. No examples of familial recurrence have been reported with these malformations.

Excessive white-matter neurons have been reported in patients undergoing epilepsy surgery and in postmortem studies. These abnormalities most often are seen in the temporal lobe and less often in the frontal lobes. Isolated heterotopic neurons in the white matter in normal brains also are most numerous in the temporal lobes [Emery et al., 1997; Rojiani et al., 1996]. The clinical correlates of the pathologic disorder are not well understood, although these neurons appear to be increased in patients undergoing temporal lobe resections for seizures [Hardiman et al., 1988]. MRI studies may reveal an abnormal white–gray matter junction if the number of ectopic cells is large. No familial recurrence or specific gender or racial predominance has been observed.

Polymicrogyria and Schizencephaly

The term "polymicrogyria" (PMG) was first used by Bielschowsky in 1916 to describe a cerebral or cerebellar cortex with multiple excessive small convolutions, which may or may not be appreciated macroscopically [Bielschowsky, 1916]. Synonymous terms in the literature include status verrucosus deformis, micropolygyria, and microgyria [Crome, 1952; Crome and France, 1959; Haberland and Brunngraber, 1972]. The definition of PMG does not encompass a specific histological cortical abnormality, but it is generally accepted that PMG is both an abnormality of excessive gyration and a microscopic abnormality of cortical structure and lamination. One specific pattern of PMG occurs in schizencephaly (SCH), a term first used by Yakovlev and Wadsworth to describe full-thickness clefts in the brain [Yakovlev and Wadsworth, 1946a, 1946b]. As part of the definition of

SCH, the clefts must be lined by PMG, and the presence of gray matter lining the cleft is one of the main features distinguishing between SCH and porencephalic cysts, the latter being lined by white matter or gliosis. SCH often occurs in the same central and perisylvian regions as other forms of PMG, and many reports in the imaging and pathology literature have described unilateral SCH and contralateral PMG [Gropman et al., 1997; Hahn and Lewis, 2003]. SCH should be considered a subtype of PMG, and therefore it is presented in this section.

Pathology

Macroscopically, PMG appears as an irregular or pebbled cortical surface. The overfolding and microgyration are easier to see in sections cut perpendicular to the cortical surface [Harding and Copp, 2002], as shown in Figure 26-5. The distribution varies significantly from unilateral forms, to bilateral symmetric and asymmetric forms. The perisylvian cortex is the most frequently affected area and involved sylvian fissures may appear extended and orientated posteriorly, as shown in Figure 26-6C. The midline cortex (e.g., the cingulate gyrus) and hippocampus are usually spared [Harding and Copp, 2002]. The cortex often appears thickened to 8–12 mm, but when viewed microscopically, the cortex is overfolded and not truly thick. PMG may occur at the periphery of many porencephalic or hydranencephalic defects [Friede and Mikolasek, 1978]. While PMG most often occurs as an isolated malformation, it co-occurs with several other brain malformations, including microcephaly and megalencephaly, gray-matter heterotopia, ventriculomegaly, and abnormalities of the septum pellucidum, corpus callosum, brainstem, and cerebellum.

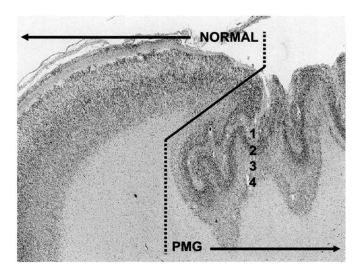

Fig. 26-5 Microscopic features of polymicrogyria. Photomicrograph of a section of cortex of a patient with PMG stained with hematoxylin and eosin. The section is cut perpendicular to the cortex. Note the abrupt transition from the normal six-layered cortex on the left to the abnormal four-layered microgyric cortex on the right. The polymicrogyric area is characterized by overfolding with microgyri and microsulci. There is fusion of the marginal layer between adjacent gyri (1). The remaining layers are composed of two neuron-rich layers (2) and (4), separated by a cell-sparse layer (3). *(Image courtesy of Dr. Jeffrey Golden, University of Pennsylvania.)*

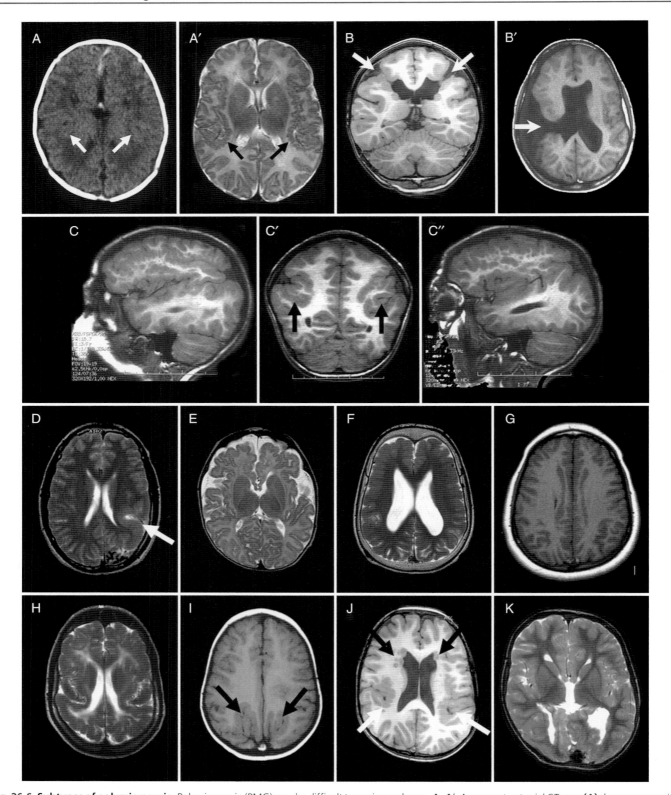

Fig. 26-6 **Subtypes of polymicrogyria.** Polymicrogyria (PMG) may be difficult to see in newborns. **A–A′,** A noncontrast axial CT scan **(A)** shows nonspecific cortical irregularity and possibly deep perisylvian and insular infolding (white arrows), while a T1-weighted axial magnetic resonance imaging (MRI) scan **(A′)** clearly shows bilateral perisylvian PMG. The MRI confirms the abnormal appearance of the insular region, which is lined by overfolded irregular gray matter with stippling of the gray–white junction, typical of PMG (black arrows). The entire insular and perisylvian is affected but the rest of the cortex appears normal. **B–B′,** Classic schizencephaly. Both coronal T1 **(B)** and axial T1 **(B′)**-weighted MRI images show full-thickness clefts lined by irregular gray matter (arrows). Panel **B** shows bilateral closed-lip schizencephaly, while panel **B′** shows right open-lipped schizencephaly and absent septum pellucidum. **C–C″,** Bilateral perisylvian PMG. Right and left parasagittal T1-weighted MRIs **(C and C″)** show abnormal extension of both sylvian fissures, with PMG involving adjacent cortex. The coronal T1-weighted MRI **(C′)** shows that the sylvian fissures are lined by overfolded and irregular gray matter typical of

Continued

The clefts of SCH can be unilateral or bilateral, and "open-lipped" or "closed-lipped," as shown in Figure 26-6B. In open-lipped clefts, the walls of the clefts do not appose each other. In closed-lipped clefts, the walls of the cleft are apposed and often fused, although a line of continuity between the lateral ventricle and subarachnoid space is usually visible; this is known as the "pia ependymal seam" [Yakovlev and Wadsworth, 1946a]. Other brain malformations may accompany SCH. Most are rare, except for absence of the septum pellucidum, which is present in approximately 70 percent of patients, raising the suggestion that SCH and septo-optic dysplasia may be related malformations in the spectrum of "septo-optic dysplasia plus" [Barkovich et al., 1989a; Kuban et al., 1989; Miller et al., 1998].

The extent of PMG visible microscopically may be greater than that suspected by macroscopic inspection, especially if present in the depths of sulci. PMG may show a variety of histological patterns, but all show abnormal cortical lamination, excessive folding, and fusion of adjacent gyri [Harding and Copp, 2002]. Two main forms of PMG are described: unlayered and layered, the latter described as "true" or "structured" PMG [Niewhuijse, 1913]. Controversy remains over which form is the more common [Harding and Copp, 2002]. Both forms may be found in the same patient, suggesting that they may be variations of the same malformation [McBride and Kemper, 1982].

The layered form of PMG shows four layers: a molecular layer and two neuronal layers, separated by an intermediate cell-sparse layer that contains myelinated fibres and few neurons [Harding and Copp, 2002; McBride and Kemper, 1982]. At the boundaries of layered PMG, an abrupt transition to normal cortex may be seen [Kuzniecky et al., 1993]. Layered PMG has been described in association with bilateral perisylvian PMG and in congenital cytomegalovirus infection [Crome and France, 1959; Kuzniecky et al., 1993; Marques Dias et al., 1984].

The unlayered form of PMG contains only a molecular layer and a neuronal layer without true lamination. Although no distinct layers are found, ultrastructural examination reveals different neuronal types positioned at appropriate cortical depths, as well as heterotopic nodules of pyramidal and nonpyramidal neurons in the deeper zones [Ferrer, 1984; Ferrer and Catala, 1991]. The microgyri are fused at the molecular layer, and the neurons often appear immature and contain little cytoplasm. Increased numbers of blood vessels and astrocytes are seen and are described as forming a "scar" [Ferrer and Catala, 1991]. The boundaries of unlayered PMG and normal cortex are not abrupt [Ferrer, 1984]. The unlayered form of PMG is associated with porencephalic cysts, Aicardi's syndrome, and the clefts in SCH [Ferrer et al., 1986; Ohtsuki et al., 1981; Yakovlev and Wadsworth, 1946a, 1946b]. The cortical malformation in Zellweger's syndrome is sometimes referred to as PMG, but is more complex than typical unlayered PMG and commonly involves abnormalities of the brainstem, cerebellum, and white matter, as well [Liu et al., 1976].

Brain Imaging

Using CT (see Figure 26-6A) and low-field-strength MRI, PMG is difficult to discern and may only appear as mildly thickened cortex [Barkovich et al., 1987; Byrd et al., 1989; Kuzniecky and Andermann, 1994]. It is for this reason that PMG is frequently misdiagnosed as pachygyria or lissencephaly. The only role for CT in the evaluation of PMG is to assess for evidence of intracerebral calcifications, which are seen in PMG and result from congenital cytomegalovirus infection or "band-like calcification with simplified gyration and polymicrogyria," also known as "pseudoTORCH" syndrome [Briggs et al., 2008]. Using high-quality MRI at 1.5T or greater with appropriate age-specific protocols, it is now possible to differentiate PMG reliably from other MCDs, provided that the individual interpreting the MRI has knowledge of the imaging features of MCDs [Raybaud et al., 1996]. Sagittal imaging extending laterally to involve the sylvian fissures is of great value, as PMG often affects the opercular regions [Kuzniecky and Andermann, 1994]. In some circumstances, special techniques, such as inversion recovery sequences, volume averaging, focal coils, and curvilinear reformatting, may be required to identify very focal forms of PMG, although these are unusual.

Polymicrogyric cortex often appears mildly thickened (usually 6–10 mm) on imaging, due to cortical overfolding rather than true cortical thickening. This compares with lissencephaly in which the cortex is usually 10–20 mm thick [Thompson et al., 1997]. With thick slices, the cortex may appear mildly thickened, with an irregular or "stippled" gray–white junction; with better imaging (such as inversion recovery) using thin contiguous slices, microgyri and microsulci may be appreciated [Thompson et al., 1997]. In younger children with PMG, the cortex may not appear particularly thickened. This is thought to be due to the immature state of myelination in subcortical and intracortical fibres [Takanashi and Barkovich, 2003]. T2 signal within the cortex is usually normal, although delayed myelination or high T2 signal in the underlying white matter may be seen [Thompson et al., 1997]. Diffusely abnormal white matter signal should raise the question of an in utero infection, such as cytomegalovirus, or a peroxisomal disorder [Barkovich and Lindan, 1994; Barkovich and Peck, 1997; van der Knaap and Valk, 1991; van der Knaap et al., 2004]. The subarachnoid space may be enlarged over PMG, and contain excessive or anomalous venous drainage, especially in the sylvian regions [Thompson et al., 1997]. Other developmental anomalies may include gray-matter heterotopia, ventricular enlargement

---

PMG (arrows). The bottom two rows show several less common PMG variants. **D,** Right unilateral perisylvian PMG, with microgyri surrounding an extended left sylvian fissure (arrow). **E,** Bilateral frontal PMG with subtle irregularity of the cortex throughout the frontal lobes, but not extending beyond the central sulcus. **F,** Bilateral frontoparietal PMG, with PMG maximal in the frontal lobes and extending posteriorly well into the parietal lobes. **G,** Diffuse parasagittal PMG, a very rare pattern. **H,** Bilateral generalized PMG involving all of the brain equally. This scan also shows diffuse high signal throughout the white matter. **I,** Bilateral posterior (parieto-occipital) parasagittal PMG, with microgyri surrounding deep abnormal sulci extending forwards from the occipital poles (arrows). **J,** Bilateral perisylvian PMG (white arrows), with bilateral periventricular nodular heterotopia (black arrows). **K,** Periventricular nodular heterotopia adjacent to the trigones and posterior horns, with overlying PMG. *(Courtesy of Dr. Richard Leventer, Children's Neuroscience Centre and Murdoch Children's Research Institute, Royal Children's Hospital, Melbourne, Australia; and Dr. William B Dobyns, University of Washington, Departments of Pediatrics and Neurology, Seattle, Washington.)*

or dysmorphism, and abnormalities of the corpus callosum and cerebellum [Wieck et al., 2005].

CT or MRI scanning is usually sufficient to diagnose SCH and to determine whether the SCH is associated with an open or closed lip, although MRI is the modality of choice. The gray matter lining the cleft has the imaging appearance of PMG, with apparent mild cortical thickening, an irregular surface, and stippling of the gray–white interface. Subtle SCH may be recognizable by a "puckering" or "dimple" on the outer side of the lateral ventricle, at the point at which the cleft reaches the ventricular margin (seen in Figure 26-6B). By definition, SCH clefts are always lined by gray matter. SCH is frequently asymmetric, and the contralateral hemisphere should be closely evaluated for the presence of a milder SCH or PMG without a cleft. Agenesis of the septum pellucidum and hypoplasia of the optic nerves are common, present in as many as 30 percent of patients [Barkovich et al., 1987, 1989a].

Several types of white-matter abnormalities can be seen with PMG or PMG-like malformations. In typical PMG and SCH, prominent perivascular spaces are common. Extensive white-matter signal changes characteristic of gliosis lining a cleft suggest that the lesion is porencephaly rather than SCH. More extensive white-matter signal changes are seen in cobblestone cortical malformations.

PMG has been described in a number of topographic patterns. Most of these are bilateral and symmetrical, the most common of which is bilateral perisylvian PMG, although the perisylvian form may be asymmetric or unilateral. Other bilateral symmetric forms are generalized, bilateral frontal, and parasagittal parieto-occipital PMG [Barkovich et al., 1999; Guerrini et al., 2000, 1997]. PMG has also been described in association with PNH [Wieck et al., 2005]. The imaging features of these patterns of PMG are shown in Figure 26-6 and described in Table 26-6.

Clinical Features

The clinical sequelae of PMG are highly variable, and depend on several factors. The most consistent predictors of a poor developmental outcome include microcephaly, especially severe microcephaly of −3 SD or smaller; abnormal neurologic examination, especially spasticity; widespread distribution of PMG, especially when bilateral and frontal; and additional brain malformations, such as heterotopia or cerebellar hypoplasia.

PMG is reported as an occasional component in many different conditions, including metabolic disorders, chromosome deletion syndromes, and multiple congenital anomaly syndromes. These patients may have a variety of clinical problems, other than those attributable to the PMG. Some patients with PMG or SCH have fewer clinical problems than would be expected for the location and extent of cortex involved (e.g., perisylvian PMG with deletion 22q11.2), while others

Table 26-6 Clinical and Imaging Features of the Polymicrogyria Syndromes

Syndrome	Clinical Features	Imaging Features
Bilateral perisylvian	Pseudobulbar palsy Speech delay (expressive) Feeding problems Mild intellectual disability Epilepsy (~80%), with onset usually >2 years If PMG extends beyond perisylvian cortex, clinical features may be more severe, including global developmental delay, spastic quadriplegia, and moderate to severe intellectual disability	Bilateral PMG maximal in perisylvian cortex, with severity spectrum ranging from PMG restricted to posterior perisylvian region to PMG extending variable distances anteriorly, posteriorly, and inferiorly from perisylvian region. Sylvian fissures extended posteriorly and often oriented superiorly. Occasional asymmetric forms. Rare forms with periventricular gray-matter heterotopia
Unilateral perisylvian	Congenital hemiparesis Mild or no intellectual disability Epilepsy (~75%), with onset usually >5 years	Unilateral PMG maximal in perisylvian cortex, but may extend beyond into frontal, parietal, and temporal lobes. Sylvian fissures extended posteriorly and often orientated superiorly. Occasional ipsilateral lateral ventricle dilatation, white-matter thinning, prominent subarachnoid space or septum pellucidum agenesis
Generalized	Moderate to severe global developmental delay Microcephaly Feeding problems Spastic quadriplegia Cortical visual impairment Occasional sensorineural hearing loss Epilepsy (~80%), with onset usually in first year	Bilateral symmetric PMG with a generalized or near-generalized distribution, and no gradient or region of maximal severity. White matter occasionally thinned and showing high signal on T2 and FLAIR. Frequent lateral ventricular dilatation or dysmorphism. Frequent corpus callosum abnormalities
Frontal only	Speech delay (expressive) Mild to moderate intellectual disability Mild spastic quadriplegia Occasional visual impairment Epilepsy in ~80%, usually presenting in first year	Bilateral symmetric or asymmetric PMG, with anterior > posterior gradient maximal in frontal lobes and not extending beyond central sulcus. Occasional lateral ventricular dilatation, thinning of frontal white matter, or thinning of anterior corpus callosum. Prominent perivascular spaces
Parasagittal parieto-occipital	Mild global developmental delay Normal intellect or mild intellectual disability Epilepsy in 100%, usually with onset in the second decade	PMG lining mesial occipital and parietal gyri, often with extension anteriorly into deep irregular gyri. May be bilateral symmetric, asymmetric, or unilateral. Occasional mild thinning of adjacent white matter

FLAIR, fluid-attenuated inversion-recovery; PMG, polymicrogyria.

have more severe problems (e.g., perisylvian PMG with deletion 1p36.3). PMG may involve eloquent cortical areas representing language or primary motor functions, yet these functions may occasionally be retained with minimal or no disability. This is especially true with lesions such as unilateral perisylvian PMG [Avellanet et al., 1996; Bisgard and Herning, 1993; Cho et al., 1999]. Also, functional imaging studies have often shown retained activity within polymicrogyric cortex [Araujo et al., 2006].

Perisylvian Polymicrogyria

The most common form of PMG involves the perisylvian regions in a bilateral and relatively symmetric pattern (see Figure 26-6A and C). The combination of bilateral perisylvian PMG (BPP), oromotor dysfunction, and seizure disorder has been called the "congenital bilateral perisylvian syndrome," and is the best-described syndrome of PMG. The first description appeared in the German pathological literature in 1905 [Oekonmakis, 1905], and detailed clinical data have been reported for more than 50 patients with this distribution of PMG [Gropman et al., 1997; Guerrini et al., 1992; Kuzniecky et al., 1993]. Patients with BPP typically have oromotor dysfunction, including difficulties with tongue (tongue protrusion and side-to-side movement), facial and pharyngeal motor function, resulting in problems with speech production, sucking and swallowing, excessive drooling, and facial diplegia. They may also have dysarthria and an expressive dysphasia. More severely affected patients have minimal or no expressive speech, necessitating the use of alternate methods of communication, such as signing or language assistive devices like picture boards or computer-assisted devices. Examination demonstrates facial diplegia, limited tongue movements, brisk jaw jerk, and frequent absence of the gag reflex [Kuzniecky et al., 1993]. Patients presenting in childhood may have other abnormalities, including arthrogryposis, hemiplegia, and hearing loss, although the data available on children are limited [Miller et al., 1998]. Up to 75 percent of affected individuals have mild to moderate intellectual disability [Kuzniecky et al., 1993]. Motor dysfunction may include limb spasticity, although this is rarely severe if present.

A smaller group of patients have unilateral perisylvian PMG, and present with hemiparesis or seizures. Their developmental and neurological deficits are typically less severe.

Other Patterns of Polymicrogyria

Several other patterns of PMG have been described, including bilateral frontal, bilateral parasagittal parieto-occipital, bilateral parieto-occipital, multilobar, and bilateral generalized PMG, as well as PMG associated with periventricular gray-matter heterotopia [Barkovich et al., 1999; Chang et al., 2004; Guerrini et al., 2000, 1997, 1998; Leventer et al., 2010; Sebire et al., 1996; Wieck et al., 2005]. The clinical features of these less common forms of PMG vary from BPP, although epilepsy, developmental delay, and spasticity are common accompaniments. Not surprisingly, spasticity appears to be more frequent when the frontal lobes are involved. The clinical features of the common forms of PMG are shown in Table 26-6. Note that the subtype described elsewhere as "bilateral frontoparietal PMG" [Chang et al., 2003] is probably better classified as bilateral frontoparietal cobblestone malformation, and was discussed in a previous section.

Epilepsy

The data regarding epilepsy in PMG are largely based on the study of patients with BPP. The frequency of epilepsy in these patients is 60–85 percent, although seizure onset may not occur until the second decade, usually between 4 and 12 years of age [Barkovich et al., 1999; Gropman et al., 1997; Kuzniecky et al., 1994a, 1993]. Seizure types include atypical absence (62 percent), atonic and tonic drop attacks (73 percent), generalized tonic-clonic (35 percent), and partial (26 percent). It is rare for the partial seizures to generalize secondarily. Occasionally, patients may develop bilateral facial motor seizures with retained awareness. A small number may present with infantile spasms [Gropman et al., 1997; Kuzniecky et al., 1994a, 1994b], in contrast to patients with lissencephaly, tuberous sclerosis, or focal cortical dysplasia, in which the frequency of spasms is higher. Seizures may occur daily and are intractable in at least 50 percent of patients; the EEG typically shows generalized spike-and-wave or multifocal discharges, with a centro-parietal emphasis [Kuzniecky et al., 1994a]. Polymicrogyria is a frequent cause of epilepsy with continuous spike-and-wave discharges during sleep [Guerrini et al., 1998].

Schizencephaly

Patients with closed-lip SCH typically present with hemiparesis or motor delay, whereas patients with open-lip SCH typically present with hydrocephalus or seizures [Packard et al., 1997]. The same large series reported epilepsy in 57 percent, and moderate to severe developmental delay and cognitive deficits in 83 percent of 47 children with different types of SCH. The median age of seizure onset was 13 months, although those with open-lipped SCH generally had seizure onset at an earlier age than those with closed-lip SCH. The most common seizure type was complex partial, although infantile spasms, and tonic, atonic, and tonic-clonic seizures were also reported. The severity and type of seizures do not appear to correlate with topography of the SCH [Denis et al., 2000; Granata et al., 1996; Packard et al., 1997]. The outcome is worst for those with bilateral open-lipped SCH and best for those with unilateral closed-lip SCH [Barkovich and Kjos, 1992c; Liang et al., 2002]. Many patients have associated brain abnormalities, such as agenesis of the septum pellucidum, that probably contribute to the disability in some patients.

Etiology, Genetics, and Molecular Basis

Few topics in the field have generated as much discussion as the etiology and pathogenesis of PMG. The main points of discussion involve the timing (before or after neuronal migration has completed) and nature of the cause (developmental or destructive). The emerging impression is that several different etiologies contribute to the pathogenesis of PMG, which accordingly may not be a single malformation per se.

Initial theories of PMG suggested that it was the result of vascular defects, such as arterial ischemia or impaired venous drainage [Kundratt, 1882; Marburg and Casamajor, 1944]. The concept of PMG being secondary to a vascular defect has remained a prevalent theme in the literature, with multiple authors relating the observation that PMG often occurs in vascular territories, as in bilateral perisylvian PMG, in which the lesions are in middle cerebral artery territory, or at the peripheries of ischemic porencephalic defects, as evidence of a vascular etiology in the pathogenesis of PMG [De Leon, 1972; Evrard et al., 1989; Ferrer, 1984; Ferrer and Catala, 1991; Yakovlev and Wadsworth, 1946a, 1946b]. The observation of a layer of presumed laminar necrosis in layered PMG supports the theory that PMG is due to postmigratory perfusion failure or hypoxia, as may be seen in other examples of ischemic lesions [Levine et al., 1974; Richman et al., 1974]. In both layered and unlayered PMG, neurons are found in locations that could only be expected if migration had continued to near- or total completion, as appropriate neuronal cell types are often found at the appropriate depth within the cortex in both layered and unlayered PMG.

Numerous causes, both genetic and nongenetic, have since been reported in association with PMG. Nongenetic causes other than hypoxia or hypoperfusion relate mainly to congenital infections, primarily cytomegalovirus, with a few anecdotal reports of toxoplasmosis, syphilis, and varicella zoster virus [Barkovich and Lindan, 1994; Crome and France, 1959; De Leon, 1972; Evrard et al., 1989; Harding and Baumer, 1988]. The pathogenesis of PMG in these infections is uncertain, yet some have suggested that vascular compromise by inflammation or obliteration of the microvasculature may be involved [Gressens et al., 2003; Toti et al., 1998]. No convincing reports of PMG occurring secondary to toxin exposure, radiation, or medications have appeared, other than one report of maternal ergotamine use, in which the PMG was (anecdotally) attributed to placental vasoconstriction [Barkovich et al., 1995].

Numerous reports have described a genetic basis for PMG, based on association with structural chromosome abnormalities, familial recurrence or parental consanguinity, metabolic disorders, other known genetic diseases, or multiple congenital anomaly syndromes. Several chromosome disorders and X-linked forms consistently resemble typical PMG, while some of the other forms appear to have atypical neuropathological or

brain imaging changes. Thus, single-gene inheritance of typical PMG appears to exist but is uncommon, while several "lookalikes" have autosomal-recessive inheritance.

PMG has been described with a growing number of structural chromosomal abnormalities, now including deletion 1p36.3, 4q21.21–q22.1, 6q26–q27, 21q2, and 22q11.2, and duplication 2p16.1–p23.1; the most common of these appears to be deletion 22q11.2 [Dobyns et al., 2008; Jansen and Andermann, 2005; Robin et al., 2006]. All types of single-gene inheritance have been reported. The most common seems to be X-linked perisylvian PMG with three or more genes involved, including the *SRPX2* gene in Xq23 and two putative loci mapped to Xq27 and Xq28 [Borgatti et al., 1999; Guerreiro et al., 2000; Santos et al., 2008; Villard et al., 2002]. Several families with autosomal-dominant inheritance of unilateral perisylvian PMG have been reported [Caraballo et al., 2000; Chang et al., 2006; Guerreiro et al., 2000]. A rare form of autosomal-recessive bilateral posterior PMG has been reported and mapped in one family to 6q16–q22 [Ben Cheikh et al., 2009; Ferrie et al., 1995]. Other reports of autosomal-recessive PMG have appeared but seem to describe several rare heterogeneous forms [Ciardo et al., 2001; De Bleecker et al., 1990; Guerreiro et al., 2000; Hung and Wang, 2003; Sztriha et al., 1998; Sztriha and Nork, 2002]. Several syndromes and genes associated with PMG have been reported but, even collectively, account for a small proportion of patients. These are listed in Table 26-7.

PMG has also been reported with several metabolic diseases with severe phenotypes, including Zellweger's syndrome [Barkovich and Peck, 1997; Kaufmann et al., 1996; van der Knaap and Valk, 1991; Zellweger, 1987], neonatal adrenoleukodystrophy [Van Der Knaap and Valk, 1991; Wanders et al., 1995], fumaric aciduria [Kerrigan et al., 2000], mitochondrial diseases [Keng et al., 2003; Samson et al., 1994], glutaric aciduria type 2

Table 26-7 Polymicrogyria Syndromes, Inheritance and Genes

Polymicrogyria Type and Syndrome	Inheritance	Genes
POLYMICROGYRIA ONLY		
Dyslexia, seizures, perisylvian PMG (in males)	XL	*SRPX2*
POLYMICROGYRIA SYNDROMES		
Band-like calcification with simplified gyration and polymicrogyria	AR	*OCLN*
Microcephaly, diffuse PMG, ACC	SpAD	*EOMES (TBR2)*
Aniridia, absent anterior commissure, temporal PMG	AD, SpAD	*PAX6*
Microcephaly, diffuse PMG, aniridia, microphthalmia, ACC	AR	*PAX6*
Microcephaly, PMG, immunodeficiency	SpAD	*NHEJ1*
Goldberg–Shprintzen syndrome	AR	*KIAA1279*
Warburg micro syndrome	AR	*RAB3GAP*
POLYMICROGYRIA VARIANTS (MOST NOT TYPICAL PMG)		
Microcephaly, frontoparietal PMG (vs. cobblestone variant), ACC, cerebellar hypoplasia	SpAD	*TUBB2B*
Diffuse PMG, ACC, optic nerve hypoplasia	AR	*TUBA8*
Thanatophoric dysplasia	SpAD	*FGFR3*

ACC, agenesis of the corpus callosum; AD, autosomal-dominant; AR, autosomal-recessive; PMG, polymicrogyria; SpAD, sporadic with presumed autosomal-dominant inheritance caused by new mutations; XL, X-linked.
(Data from numerous reports [Abdel-Salam et al., 2008; Abdollahi et al., 2009; Aligianis et al., 2005; Baala et al., 2007; Briggs et al., 2008; Brooks et al., 2005; Brooks et al., 1999; Cantagrel et al., 2007; Glaser et al., 1994; Graham et al., 2004; Hevner, 2005; Ho et al., 1984; Jaglin et al., 2009; Mitchell et al., 2003b; O'Driscoll et al., 2010; Roll et al., 2006; Shigematsu et al., 1985; Sisodiya et al., 2001; Solomon et al., 2009; Warburg et al., 1993; Yamaguchi and Honma, 2001].)

[Bohm et al., 1982], maple syrup urine disease [Martin and Norman, 1967], and histidinemia [Corner et al., 1968]. However, the histopathology differs from classic PMG for several of them, especially the peroxisomal disorders (Zellweger's syndrome and neonatal adrenoleukodystrophy) and glutaric aciduria type 2. Based on a mouse model, it is proposed that the cortical dysplasia in Zellweger's syndrome is secondary to glutamate receptor dysfunction and defective N-methyl-D-aspartate (NMDA) glutamate receptor-mediated calcium mobilization during neuroblast migration [Gressens et al., 2000].

PMG has been attributed to abnormalities during late neuronal migration or early cortical organization, i.e., between 13 and 26 weeks' gestation [Barkovich et al., 2005]. Until recently, there was little molecular evidence to support this assertion. Mutations in the *TUBB2B* gene have, however, recently been identified in four patients with asymmetric PMG with functional studies, suggesting that this gene is required for neuronal migration [Jaglin et al., 2009], although pathological data suggest atypical PMG.

The etiology of SCH has also been controversial; support for nongenetic causes is strong, while genetic forms appear to be very rare and atypical. In SCH, substantial evidence supports an association between PMG and congenital cytomegalovirus infection or in utero ischemic (vascular) injuries, the latter including twin–twin transfusion syndrome [Curry et al., 2005; Iannetti et al., 1998; Landrieu and Lacroix, 1994; Pati and Helmbrecht, 1994; Sener, 1998; Sherer and Salafia, 1996; Van Bogaert et al., 1996]. While very rare, several families with recurrence of SCH have been reported [Granata et al., 1997; Hilburger et al., 1993; Hosley et al., 1992; Tietjen et al., 2005]. A few reports of *EMX2* mutations in SCH were never confirmed, and an association seems doubtful [Granata et al., 1997; Merello et al., 2008; Tietjen et al., 2005].

None the less, genetic causes are likely to account for a significant proportion of patients with PMG, although other causes, such as cytomegalovirus infection and ischemia, may account for significant proportion as well, especially for SCH. PMG undoubtedly has a heterogeneous etiology, with both environmental and genetic causes resulting in a similar phenotypic endpoint: a cortex with excessive folding and abnormal lamination.

Focal Cortical Dysplasia

The term "focal cortical dysplasia" (FCD) was first used in 1971 to describe a histological abnormality seen in surgical specimens from ten patients with epilepsy [Taylor et al., 1971].

Taylor and colleagues described a "malformation," visible by histology and characterized by "congregations of large, bizarre neurons . . . (and) in most . . . cases, grotesque cells . . . present in the depths of affected cortex and in the subjacent white matter." FCD now encompasses a wide spectrum of cortical malformations with variable features, including microscopic neuronal heterotopia, dyslamination, and abnormal cell types: namely, balloon cells and dysmorphic giant or cytomegalic neurons. Here the term FCD is used to describe only those disorders in which a pathological finding of FCD or an MRI appearance highly correlated with FCD has been found. The term FCD is not used to describe HMEG, rare developmental tumors, such as dysembryoplastic neuroepithelial tumors and ganglioglioma, or the tubers of tuberous sclerosis, even though there are similarities among all these lesions. These lesions will be covered in other chapters.

Pathology

FCD shows a wide spectrum of severity in its gross morphology, topography, and microscopic features. The key feature in FCD is the presence of abnormal cortical lamination, although this may be subtle. With more severe forms of FCD, abnormal neuronal and neuroglial cell types are seen. At the mildest end of the spectrum is "microdysgenesis," which is poorly defined. It usually refers to subtle developmental cortical abnormalities, including neuronal heterotopia, undulations of cortical layering, or neuronal clusters among cell-sparse areas [Hardiman et al., 1988]. Microdysgenesis has been found at autopsy more commonly in individuals with epilepsy compared to controls without epilepsy or other neurological disorders, as well as in surgical specimens from patients with medically intractable epilepsy [Hardiman et al., 1988; Meencke and Veith, 1992; Raymond et al., 1995]. Despite this, it is still unclear what degree of "microdysgenesis" may fall within the normal spectrum [Meencke and Veith, 1999].

Several classification systems for FCD have been proposed using neuropathological criteria. Most divide FCD according to both the degree of dysplasia (architectural or cytoarchitectural dysplasia) and the presence or absence of balloon cells, which correspond to FCD types 1 and 2, respectively [Colombo et al., 2003b; Kuzniecky and Andermann, 2003; Tassi et al., 2002]. A proposal to simplify the classification and terminology for FCD suggests that the term "microdysgenesis" be abandoned [Palmini et al., 2004]. The "Palmini classification system" shown in Table 26-8 proposes that subtle cortical abnormalities characterized by ectopic or heterotopic neurons of normal morphology be classified as "mild MCD."

Table 26-8 Proposed Classification System for Focal Cortical Dysplasia

Types	Subtypes	
Type I No dysmorphic neurons or balloon cells	Type IA Isolated architectural abnormalities (dyslamination, accompanied or not by other abnormalities of mild malformations of cortical development)	Type IB Architectural abnormalities, plus giant or immature, but not dysmorphic, neurons
Type II Taylor-type focal cortical dysplasia with dysmorphic neurons; with or without balloon cells	Type IIA Architectural abnormalities with dysmorphic neurons but without balloon cells	Type IIB Architectural abnormalities with dysmorphic neurons and balloon cells

(Summarized from Palmini, et al: Terminology and classification of the cortical dysplasias, Neurology 62[6 Suppl 3]:S2–S8, 2004.)

These authors suggest that the term FCD only be applied to lesions with architectural abnormalities, such as dyslamination or the presence of abnormal cells within the cortex.

But even this more severe end of the FCD spectrum presents difficulties. The pathological features of the tubers of tuberous sclerosis and FCD type IIB have significant overlap. In fact, the term "balloon cells" was first used in the neuropathology literature in the description of the tubers of tuberous sclerosis. Traditionally, however, the tubers of tuberous sclerosis and FCD with balloon cells have been regarded as separate lesions [Kuzniecky and Andermann, 2003].

The extent of FCD is highly variable, ranging from small focal areas involving part of a gyrus to a multilobar distribution in one hemisphere. On macroscopic examination, the cortex may appear normal. Subtle irregularities of the gyral pattern and mildly increased cortical thickness may be localized to the cortex at the depth of a sulcus, a malformation known as "bottom of the sulcus" dysplasia [Barkovich et al., 2005; Besson et al., 2008]. Beginning with these small lesions, a complete series of progressively more extensive forms of FCD has been described, including focal transmantle, sublobar, lobar, posterior quadrantic, and finally hemispheric dysplasias. These demonstrate more obvious abnormalities of cortical morphology, with overlap between hemispheric dysplasia and HMEG [Adamsbaum et al., 1998; Barkovich et al., 1997; Barkovich and Peacock, 1998; D'Agostino et al., 2004].

Given this similarity, the term hemimegalencephaly should perhaps be reserved for patients with significant malformations of noncortical structures, such as enlarged white-matter volume and enlarged, dysmorphic ventricles, although precise criteria to distinguish hemispheric FCD from HMEG have not been developed.

A spectrum of abnormalities may be seen on microscopic examination, including disruption of cortical lamination, neuronal heterotopia within the cortex or subcortical white matter, poor differentiation of neuronal and glial cells, and the presence of abnormal cells, such as balloon cells and large bizarre neurons, examples of which are shown in Figure 26-7A–D and as diagrams in Figure 26-7E [Colombo et al., 2003a, 2003b; Mischel et al., 1995; Prayson et al., 1999, 2002; Tassi et al., 2002; Taylor et al., 1971]. Areas of FCD have been shown to be intrinsically epileptogenic both in vivo, using corticography or depth electrodes, and in vitro, using cortex resected from patients with intractable epilepsy [Avoli et al., 2003; Mattia et al., 1995; Palmini et al., 1995; Tassi et al., 2002]. Single-cell studies have suggested that the dysmorphic or cytomegalic neurons, and not the balloon cells, contribute to epileptogenesis [Cepeda et al., 2005].

Brain Imaging

FCD is rarely visible by CT [Kuzniecky et al., 1995], and may not be visible even with high-quality MRI. Subtle abnormalities in gyration, cortical thickness, and the gray–white junction are best seen using thin-slice T1-weighted images, and may be a clue to underlying FCD [Yagishita et al., 1998]. Some forms of FCD may show increased signal on fluid-attenuated inversion-recovery (FLAIR) and T2-weighted images [Bronen et al., 1997; Colombo et al., 2003a, 2003b; Mackay et al., 2003]. White-matter signal may be abnormal in the region of FCD, producing intractable seizures [Eltze et al., 2005; Palmini et al., 2004], but it is not clear whether this represents dysplastic white matter, or a consequence of abnormal or advanced myelination secondary to frequent seizure activity [Mitchell et al., 2003a].

Mild MCD (microdysgenesis) and FCD type I may not be detectable on MRI. If abnormalities are seen, typical features consist of subtle cortical thickening and irregular sulcation or gyration. FCD type I may also be associated with lobar hypoplasia or atrophy and hippocampal sclerosis. The most striking imaging features of FCD are seen in FCD type II (see Figure 26-7F and G). The lesions in these patients typically show increased cortical thickness, blurring of the gray–white junction, abnormal sulcal and gyral patterns, and high signal at the base of the lesion and in the underlying white matter on T2 and FLAIR sequences.

Several specific named patterns of FCD have been described, based primarily on brain imaging features. FCD has also been shown to occur at the base of a sulcus, with cortical thickening and poor gray–white differentiation, often with a linear band of high signal from the base of the lesion to the lateral ventricle, known as the "transmantle sign," shown for FCD types IB (see Figure 26-7H) and IIB (see Figure 26-7I). In focal transmantle dysplasia, a wedge of dysplastic tissue extends from the lateral ventricle up to the cortical surface (see Figure 26-7J). Histology shows features of FCD with balloon cells plus white-matter astrogliosis, and MRI shows a wedge of disorganized tissue with increased T2 signal [Barkovich et al., 1997]. Sublobar dysplasia is characterized by a deep infolding of the cortex with a thickened cortex and possible poor gray–white differentiation in the malformed region [Barkovich and Peacock, 1998]. Associated brain abnormalities include ventricular dysmorphism and callosal and cerebellar dysgenesis. Tissue has not been available for pathological examination. Another form of FCD affecting one posterior quadrant of the brain has been designated posterior quadrantic dysplasia (see Figure 26-7K) [D'Agostino et al., 2004]. This form of FCD is alternately known by the clumsy term "hemihemimegalencephaly." These lesions have collectively been called "bottom of the sulcus" dysplasias [Barkovich et al., 2005].

Presurgical localization of these lesions often requires advanced MRI techniques and analysis, such as the use of surface coils, volume averaging, curvilinear reformatting, or 3T imaging. Functional studies, including single-photon emission computed tomography (SPECT) and FDG-PET scanning, are also often required to maximize the likelihood of identifying and defining the boundaries of FCD lesions. New MRI methods for lesion detection are being evaluated, including multichannel coils, high field strength (>3T), arterial spin labeling, susceptibility-weighted imaging, and diffusion tensor/spectrum imaging [Madan and Grant, 2009].

Clinical Features

Apart from tuberous sclerosis, no particular dysmorphic, neurocutaneous, or multiple congenital anomaly syndromes have been described in which FCD is a feature. The most common clinical sequelae of FCD are seizures. Developmental delay, cognitive disability, and focal neurological deficits are only observed with extensive dysplasias [Barkovich and Kjos, 1992b; Mackay et al., 2003; Wyllie et al., 1994]. Seizures from FCD may arise at any age from in utero until adulthood, although most patients present in childhood [Du Plessis et al., 1993; Wyllie et al., 1994]. Recent studies have shown consistent

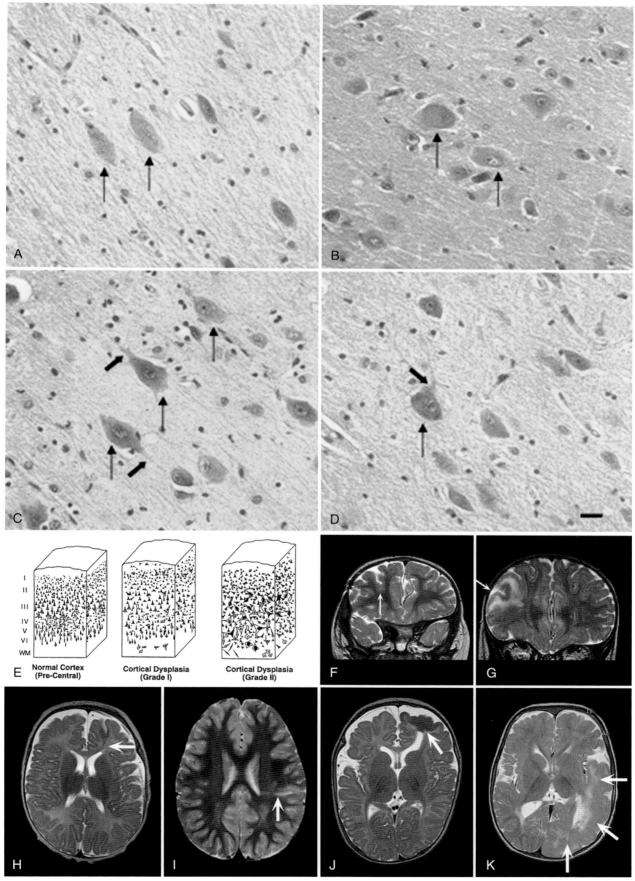

Continued

Fig. 26-7 Microscopic features and subtypes of focal cortical dysplasia. Photomicrographs of cresyl violet (**A, C,** and **D**) and hematoxylin and eosin (**B**) stains of FCD specimens. **A** and **B,** Balloon cells (arrows) with characteristic ovoid shape, enlarged cell soma, and laterally displaced nuclei. **C** and **D,** Dysplastic neurons (thin arrows) have an enlarged cell soma but, in contrast to balloon cells, have a distinctly neuronal morphology with a single apical or basal process (thick arrow) extending from the cell body. Scale bar = 50 μm. **E,** The histologic changes in FCD are demonstrated in a diagram that shows a normally laminated cortex on the left, contrasting with the middle and right images showing increasing severity of cortical dysplasia. The most severe dysplasia is marked by dyslamination, malorientation of neurons, and the presence of large dysmorphic neurons and balloon cells. **F** and **G,** Coronal T2-weighted MRI scans from two unrelated patients with intractable childhood epilepsy show typical FCD. Panel **F** shows areas of irregular gyral formation with deep sulci and mild cortical thickening in the right frontal lobe (arrow). The rest of the right hemisphere also showed mild atrophy and hypoplasia. Histology showed mild dyslamination and the presence of giant neurons consistent with FCDIb. Panel **G** shows an area of gyral irregularity and increased subcortical signal in the right frontal lobe (arrow). Histology showed marked dyslamination and the presence of both dysmorphic neurons and balloon cells consistent with FCDIIB. The bottom row shows T2-weighted images of several less common forms of FCD, including bottom of the sulcus, transmantle, and posterior quadrantic cortical dysplasia. **H,** A deep sulcus in the left frontal lobe with cortical thickening at its base, consistent with "bottom of the sulcus" dysplasia. **I,** A "transmantle sign," consisting of an area of cortical high signal and thickening, plus a line of high signal from the lesion to the lateral ventricle. This is designated focal transmantle dysplasia. **J,** Irregular and thickened cortex with mixed high and low signal in a wedge of tissue radiating out from a dysmorphic left frontal horn consistent with extensive transmantle dysplasia. **K,** A large area of thickened irregular cortex with high signal and blurring of the gray–white junction involving the left temporal, parietal, and occipital regions, consistent with posterior quadrantic dysplasia. (*A–D, reprinted from Lamparello: Developmental lineage of cell types in cortical dysplasia with balloom cells, P. Brain et al 2007;130:2267–2276; E, reprinted from Kuzniecky R, Epilepsia: Magnetic resonance imaging in developmental disorders of the cerebral cortex: 35 Suppl 6:S44–56, 1994. F–K, courtesy of Dr. Richard Leventer, Children's Neuroscience Centre and Murdoch Children's Research Institute, Royal Children's Hospital, Melbourne, Australia.*)

clinical differences between patients with types I and II FCD, respectively. Patients with type II FCD usually have extratemporal lesions, present at a younger age of onset, and have higher seizure frequencies [Fauser et al., 2006; Krsek et al., 2008, 2009b; Lerner et al., 2009]. Seizures may be simple partial, complex partial, or secondarily generalized, depending on the location of the FCD and age of the patient. Younger children may present with asymmetric infantile spasms. The seizure disorder may be intractable and life-threatening [Desbiens et al., 1993], so that surgical resection may be required. Much of the developmental delay and many of the cognitive disabilities associated with FCD may be due to the effects of repeated seizure activity. As complete as possible surgical resection of the FCD is consistently the most important variable for long-term seizure control in epilepsy secondary to FCD unresponsive to anticonvulsants [Kim et al., 2009; Krsek et al., 2009a; Lerner et al., 2009], and accordingly, surgery is being performed at increasingly younger ages in an attempt to protect the child against the deleterious effect of uncontrolled epilepsy and multiple medications [Guerrini et al., 2008; Harvey et al., 2008].

Etiology, Genetics, and Molecular Basis

Apart from FCD due to tuberous sclerosis, the etiology of FCD is largely unknown. No good evidence exists for environmental causes, and no genes or chromosomal loci have been identified for the common patterns of FCD. The highly focal and variable nature of FCD, especially FCD type II, and the close pathological resemblance to tuberous sclerosis led to the hypothesis that somatic mosaic mutations of genes in the mammalian target of rapamycin (mTOR) pathway, which includes the *TSC1* and *TSC2* genes that cause tuberous sclerosis, were involved [Crino, 2007]. In support of this hypothesis, loss of heterozygosity of the *TSC1* gene was found in resected tissue of 11 of 24 patients with FCD, but no changes were found in *TSC2* [Becker et al., 2002]. However, the same *TSC2* mutation was found in nine family members with phenotypes varying from tuberous sclerosis to much milder conditions. Four had classic brain and skin abnormalities consistent with tuberous sclerosis, 3 had seizures and isolated cerebral abnormalities, and 2 had seizures and a normal MRI scan [O'Connor et al., 2003]. Evidence is thus accumulating that the phenotypic spectrum for

patients with mutations in the tuberous sclerosis genes may be wide, and may include some patients not fulfilling current criteria for tuberous sclerosis, who thus have mild expression or a "forme fruste" of tuberous sclerosis.

Further data supporting this link come from human tissue studies of lesions resected from patients with both tuberous sclerosis and FCD. Morphological comparisons between abnormal cells found in FCD and normal cells involved in cortical development have shown that cytomegalic neurons have similarities to subplate cells, while balloon cells have similarities to radial glia. This led to a hypothesis that some forms of FCD may be the consequence of retained prenatal cells and neurons that establish abnormal connections and lead to seizures, a theory the authors termed the "dysmature cerebral developmental hypothesis" [Cepeda et al., 2006]. The mTOR pathway is involved in the control of protein synthesis, cell growth and proliferation, and synaptic plasticity. It has been found to be upregulated in surgical specimens from tuberous sclerosis patients, and its role in other forms of FCD and some developmental tumours is being investigated, including therapeutic trials designed to downregulate the mTOR pathway with the drug rapamycin [Wong, 2010].

One prevailing hypothesis states that balloon cells result from a defect of proliferation or differentiation of primitive neurons or glial cells, as is thought to be the case with those seen in tuberous sclerosis. For this reason, Barkovich and colleagues classify FCD with balloon cells as an MCD secondary to non-neoplastic abnormal cellular proliferation, and FCD without balloon cells as an MCD secondary to abnormal cortical organization [Barkovich et al., 2001a, 2005].

Two autosomal-recessive syndromes with relative or absolute macrocephaly and FCD have been identified in different Amish families. The cortical dysplasia–focal epilepsy syndrome (in which some affected children have pervasive developmental disorder or autism) and a severe developmental encephalopathy that resembles Pitt–Hopkins syndrome have been associated with mutations of *CNTNAP2* [Strauss et al., 2006; Zweier et al., 2009]. Notably, heterozygous deletions of this gene have been associated with epilepsy and schizophrenia [Friedman et al., 2008; Mefford et al., 2010]. Another developmental syndrome, consisting of megalencephaly, severe psychomotor retardation, infancy-onset focal seizures, muscle hypoplasia, and distinctive craniofacial dysmorphism in Amish children, is caused by a homozygous mutation of *LYK5* [Puffenberger et al., 2007]. Several affected children have died, and neuropathological study revealed megalencephaly, ventriculomegaly, cytomegaly, and extensive linear vacuolization and neuronal ectopia within white matter, accompanied by diffuse reactive astrocytosis.

Researchers in the field of human MCD have made assumptions as to the likely timing of the etiologies of different malformations, based on their appearance using both pathological and neuroimaging techniques. For example, heterotopic gray matter is assumed to result from disordered neuronal migration, as the heterotopic neurons appear to have arrested their migration to the cortex prematurely. Assumptions such as these were proposed well before a basic understanding of the genetic and molecular mechanisms of normal cortical development were established. In many instances, these assumptions have proved correct, yet it is now appreciated that many cortical malformations are likely secondary to abnormalities occurring at stages other than that of neuroblast migration. Understanding of the genetic and molecular basis of cortical development is advancing rapidly, with new genes or new roles for known genes being discovered. A more complete understanding of the key genes involved in human cortical development will be required in order to understand the possible timing and molecular basis of many malformations of cortical development.

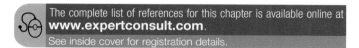

The complete list of references for this chapter is available online at **www.expertconsult.com**. See inside cover for registration details.

Hydrocephalus and Arachnoid Cysts

James M. Drake and Amal Abou-Hamden

Hydrocephalus

Definition

A widely recognized definition for hydrocephalus is lacking. Historically, hydrocephalus is believed to result from an imbalance between cerebrospinal fluid (CSF) production and absorption, with net accumulation of fluid in the cranial cavity, characterized by an increase in the size of the cerebral ventricles and elevation of intracranial pressure, which produces the clinical manifestations of hydrocephalus.

More recently, hydrocephalus has been more broadly defined as a disturbance of formation, flow, or absorption of CSF that leads to an increase in volume occupied by this fluid in the central nervous system (CNS) [Rekate, 2009]. This definition excludes other abnormalities of CSF dynamics, such as benign intracranial hypertension, in which the ventricles are not enlarged. It does not specify the source of production or absorption of CSF nor does it presuppose the mechanisms inherent in ventricular distension.

Conditions such as cerebral atrophy and focal destructive lesions also lead to an abnormal increase of CSF in the CNS. In these situations, ventricular dilatation is not an active process; loss of cerebral tissue leaves a vacant space that is filled passively with CSF. Such conditions are not the result of a hydrodynamic disorder and therefore are not classified as hydrocephalus. An older term used to describe these conditions is hydrocephalus ex vacuo.

Classification

A number of classification systems for hydrocephalus have been suggested [Mori, 1995; Boaz and Edwards-Brown, 1999; Beni-Adani et al., 2006; Oi and Di Rocco, 2006; Rekate, 2009]. These include the following types of hydrocephalus:

- communicating vs. noncommunicating
- obstructive vs. absorptive
- acquired vs. congenital
- genetic or CNS malformation-associated vs. isolated
- intraventricular-obstructive vs. extraventricular
- simple vs. complicated.

The terms compensated and uncompensated hydrocephalus generally refer to whether an increase in ventricular size is associated with evidence of raised intracranial pressure. In compensated, or arrested, hydrocephalus, a gradual increase in ventricular size stabilizes by reaching a new equilibrium and the patient has no symptoms or signs of raised intracranial pressure. In contrast, uncompensated hydrocephalus is associated with clinical symptoms and signs of raised intracranial pressure and usually with progressive dilatation of the ventricles. This is the clinical situation where treatment is indicated. No classification is completely adequate for hydrocephalus at all ages. The classification of hydrocephalus into communicating or noncommunicating dates back to the early 1900s and is based on Walter Dandy's experimental studies into the pathophysiology of hydrocephalus [Richards, 1990].

In communicating hydrocephalus, the flow is not obstructed but CSF is inadequately reabsorbed in the subarachnoid space, whereas in noncommunicating or obstructive hydrocephalus, the flow of CSF from the ventricles to the subarachnoid space is obstructed.

Obstructive is usually synonymous with noncommunicating hydrocephalus and absorptive with communicating hydrocephalus.

Hydrocephalus is also categorized as congenital, which is present at birth and often associated with developmental defects; and acquired, which occurs after development of the brain and ventricles [Mori, 1995; Chahlavi et al., 2001]. Hydrocephalus has also been classified based on the stage of development at the time that the ventricles became dilated [Oi and Di Rocco, 2006]. The various subtypes of fetal hydrocephalus are classified according to the mechanism of obstruction to the flow of CSF to include:

1. primary or simple hydrocephalus with a single point of obstruction to flow
2. dysgenetic hydrocephalus, to include complex abnormalities of the CNS, such as the Arnold–Chiari malformation
3. secondary hydrocephalus from tumor or bleeding.

This classification is cross-referenced to the stage of fetal development (e.g., neuronal maturation, cell migration); it may prove useful in deciding when treatment may be futile if beyond the legal period for terminating a pregnancy, and in identifying potential candidates for early delivery or fetal surgery [Rekate, 2009].

Extraventricular obstructive hydrocephalus is now recognized to represent, almost universally, benign pericerebral collections of infancy that are usually familial, resolve with time, and almost never require treatment [Drake, 2008].

Benign extra-axial collections of infancy involve abnormal enlargement of the head and excessively large subarachnoid space. In infants whose neurological development is normal and in whom the enlargement of the subarachnoid space resolves by 24 months of age, no further work-up or treatment is required. In infants whose neurological development is abnormal or in whom the enlargement of the subarachnoid space does not resolve by 24 months of age, further investigations may be warranted. Several genetic conditions, such as certain mucopolysaccharidoses, achondroplasia, Sotos' syndrome, and glutaric aciduria type I, can feature enlargement of the subarachnoid spaces as either an early or an associated finding on neuroimaging. In the case of the mucopolysaccharidoses, enlargement of the subarachnoid spaces may be a direct consequence of impairment of CSF absorption by the storage material. Thus, enlargement of the subarachnoid spaces may be an important clue to an early genetic diagnosis, which is important, as therapeutic options exist for many forms of mucopolysaccharidosis and for glutaric aciduria type I [Paciorkowski and Greenstein, 2007].

Epidemiology

The overall incidence of hydrocephalus is not known. This is because hydrocephalus not only occurs in isolation, but also can be associated with a large number of conditions, including tumors, infections, trauma, and prematurity. Consequently, epidemiological studies of its incidence, prevalence, and complication rates are difficult to ascertain.

In newborns, the overall incidence of hydrocephalus ranges from 0.3 to 4 per 1000 live births. Occurring as a single congenital disorder, the incidence of hydrocephalus has been reported as 0.9–1.5 per 1000 births [Milhorat, 1972; Serlo et al., 1986; El Awad, 1992; Blackburn and Fineman, 1994; Fernell and Hagberg, 1998]. It is estimated that approximately 125,000 persons are living with ventricular shunts and that 33,000 shunts are placed annually in the United States [Bondurant and Jimenez, 1995].

The incidence of pediatric hydrocephalus has declined in many developed countries [Drake, 2008]. Antenatal screening, genetic testing, and pregnancy termination have reduced the incidence of congenital malformations of the brain that cause hydrocephalus. The incidence of open neural tube defects has also decreased precipitously as a result of maternal folate supplementation, antenatal screening, and termination of pregnancy based on superior antenatal imaging with ultrasound and magnetic resonance imaging (MRI). The incidence of CSF shunting in open neural tube defects, formerly reported to be as high as 90 percent, has also declined, possibly as a result of a general, more conservative approach, and also the selection of lower-grade lesions for delivery with a lower need for shunting [Tulipan et al., 2003; Chakraborty et al., 2008]. The incidence of intraventricular hemorrhage (IVH) has also decreased as a result of better perinatal management of prematurity, and, as such, one of the major complications of posthemorrhagic hydrocephalus (see Chapter 19) [Fernell and Hagberg, 1998].

CSF Production, Circulation, and Absorption

CSF is produced by two mechanisms: Most of the CSF (50–80 percent) is thought to be secreted by the choroid plexus within the cerebral ventricles. Extrachoroidal CSF production in subarachnoid sites and by way of a transependymal route has also

been documented. About 20 percent or more of CSF is derived from brain extracellular fluid created as a byproduct of cerebral metabolism [Bering, 1962; Fishman, 1980; Rekate, 1997]. Normally, rates of production (0.35 mL per minute or approximately 400–500 mL/day) and absorption of CSF are equal. Total CSF volume is 65–140 mL in children, and 90–150 mL in adults. In one study of premature infants born at gestational age 32 ± 1.6 wk, CSF volume was estimated to be 23.33 ± 9.6 mL at birth and 40.66 ± 21.23 mL at term equivalent. Full-term infants have a CSF volume of 32.4 ± 11.1 mL at birth [Zacharia et al., 2006].

The process of CSF formation by the choroid plexus includes plasma ultrafiltration and secretion. Secretion, an energy-dependent process, is initiated by hydrostatic pressure in the choroidal capillaries and by active transport of sodium. The enzymes sodium-potassium adenosine triphosphatase (ATPase) and carbonic anhydrase partly regulate CSF secretion [Fishman, 1980]. CSF production has been reported to remain constant across the normal intracranial pressure range [Pollay, 1977], with CSF production decreasing when intracranial pressure approaches mean arterial pressure. There have been reports, however, of downregulation of CSF production in patients with chronic hydrocephalus [Silverberg et al., 2002].

By contrast, the process of CSF reabsorption is not an energy-dependent process [Rekate, 1997]. After formation, CSF exits from the lateral ventricles through the foramina of Monro into the third ventricle (Figure 27-1). CSF then traverses the aqueduct of Sylvius into the fourth ventricle, leaving though the foramina of Lushka and foramen of Magendie into the cisterna magna, from where it flows through the subarachnoid space around the cerebral hemispheres. Information gained from MRI analysis of CSF movement demonstrates pulsatile to-and-fro motion of CSF within the lateral ventricles, produced from a brain-pumping motion that ejects the CSF and causes a net downward flow [Feinberg and Mark, 1987].

Historically, it has been held that CSF is absorbed into the vascular system mainly through the arachnoid villi within the arachnoid granulations covering the brain and spinal cord leptomeninges [Alksne and Lovings, 1972; Welch, 1975]. This process is thought to be passive and not energy-dependent. A layer of endothelium within the arachnoid villi separates the subarachnoid CSF space from the vascular system. Water and electrolytes pass freely across these arachnoid membranes. There is normally 5–7 mmHg difference in pressure between the dural venous sinuses and the subarachnoid space. This is presumed to be the hydrostatic force behind the absorption of CSF. Larger proteins and macromolecules cannot pass through intercellular junctions but are selectively transported across the cytoplasm of endothelial cells by an active process involving micropinocytosis [Welch, 1975]. Increased absorption through the arachnoid villi protects the brain from transient increases in intracranial pressure [Mann et al., 1978]. Newborn infants do not have visible arachnoid granulations, suggesting that the maximum capacity for reabsorption is less than in the adult, or that CSF is absorbed by different mechanisms in the neonate.

For some time, arachnoid granulations were thought to be the only CSF absorption pathway; however, other mechanisms have been identified, with evidence emerging that arachnoid granulations have only a secondary role. Olfactory nerves, the cribriform plate, and nasal lymphatics have been identified

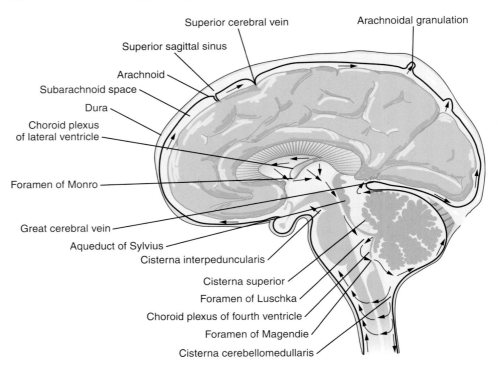

Fig. 27-1 Cerebrospinal fluid pathway. The diagram depicts the structures and spaces through which CSF flows, from its manufacture in and secretion from the choroid plexus in the ventricles, to its ultimate resorption from the subarachnoid space. CSF exits from the lateral ventricles through the foramina of Monro into the third ventricle. It then traverses the aqueduct of Sylvius into the fourth ventricle, leaves though the foramina of Lushka and foramen of Magendie and passes into the cisterna magna, and flows through the subarachnoid space around the cerebral hemispheres.

as important sites for CSF absorption [Johnston and Papaiconomou, 2002; Johnston, 2003; Johnston et al., 2004].

Absorption of CSF across brain tissue into capillaries has also been proposed [Greitz, 2004]. According to this theory, the distending force in the production of chronic hydrocephalus is an increased systolic pulse pressure in the brain tissue, due to decreased intracranial compliance.

Etiology and Pathophysiology

Hydrocephalus can be a symptom of a large number of disorders, and a list of conditions in which it has been reported is summarized in Box 27-1. It is associated with tumors and infections, and may be a complication of prematurity and trauma [Renier et al., 1988; Schrander-Stumpel and Fryns, 1998; Chi et al., 2005]. It is also seen in apparent isolation. High-resolution MRI of postnatal life has provided clues to the etiology of hydrocephalus, which in the past would have been labeled as idiopathic; some of these include IVH (Figure 27-2), aqueductal stenosis (Figure 27-3), and migrational abnormalities [Drake, 2008].

The etiologies of hydrocephalus in one series of pediatric patients are shown in Table 27-1 [Drake et al., 1998]. Hydrocephalus is due to either abnormal CSF reabsorption, or flow, or, rarely, overproduction. The main situation in which CSF production is increased enough to cause hydrocephalus is the presence of a choroid plexus papilloma. These tumors contain functional choroid epithelium and can produce very large amounts of CSF. However, even in the latter case, reabsorption is probably defective, as normal individuals can usually tolerate the elevated CSF production rate of these tumors. CSF accumulation, in turn, leads to raised intracranial pressure.

The etiology of hydrocephalus depends upon the age of the child. During the neonatal to late infancy period (0–2 years),

hydrocephalus is usually caused by a perinatal hemorrhage, meningitis, and developmental abnormalities, the most common being aqueductal stenosis. The hydrocephalus seen in babies with spina bifida usually results from an associated Chiari malformation. In early to late childhood (2–10 years), the most common causes of hydrocephalus are posterior fossa tumors and aqueductal stenosis.

Congenital Causes in Infants and Children

Approximately 55 percent of all cases of hydrocephalus are congenital. Primary aqueductal stenosis accounts for approximately 5 percent of congenital hydrocephalus, whereas aqueductal stenosis secondary to neoplasm, infection, or hemorrhage accounts for another 5 percent [Chi et al., 2005]. Primary aqueductal stenosis usually presents in infancy. Its morphology may be that of "forking" of the aqueduct, an aqueductal septum, "true" narrowing of the aqueduct, or X-linked aqueductal stenosis. Bicker–Adams syndrome is an X-linked hydrocephalus accounting for 7 percent of cases in males. It is characterized by stenosis of the aqueduct of Sylvius, severe mental retardation, and, in 50 percent, an adduction-flexion deformity of the thumb. Secondary aqueductal stenosis is due to gliosis secondary to intrauterine infection or germinal matrix hemorrhage [Hill and Rozdilsky, 1984].

Anatomical malformations frequently observed with idiopathic congenital hydrocephalus are associated with abnormalities of hindbrain development (see Chapter 24), and include Chiari malformations, Dandy–Walker malformation (DWM), and others [Stoll et al., 1992; Schrander-Stumpel and Fryns, 1998]. DWM is associated with atresia of the foramina of Luschka and Magendie, and affects 2–4 percent of newborns with hydrocephalus. About 50 percent of all patients with DWM develop hydrocephalus. The dilated fourth ventricle

Box 27-1 Differential Diagnosis of Hydrocephalus

Congenital Malformations

- Agenesis of the corpus callosum
- Arnold–Chiari malformation
- Autosomal-recessive aqueductal stenosis
- Aqueductal stenosis
- Arachnoid cyst
- Basilar impression
- Cerebellar agenesis
- Dandy–Walker malformation
- Encephalocele
- Peters' anomaly
- Porencephaly

Infectious Causes

- Congenital syphilis
- Cytomegalic inclusion disease
- Elevated cerebrospinal fluid protein content with endocardial fibroelastosis, cataracts
- Mumps
- Postmeningitis
- Postencephalitis
- Toxoplasmosis
- Miscellaneous

Neoplasms

- Brainstem glioma
- Cerebellar astrocytoma
- Choroid plexus papilloma
- Colloid cyst of third ventricle
- Ependymoma
- Histiocytosis X
- Leukemia
- Lymphoma
- Medulloblastoma
- Neuroblastoma
- Pinealoma

Syndromes

- Achondroplasia
- Agyria and retinal dysplasia
- Apert's syndrome
- Cockayne's syndrome
- Coffin–Lowry syndrome
- Crouzon's syndrome
- Biemond's syndrome
- Fryns' syndrome
- Hirschsprung's disease
- Gaucher-like disease
- Glutaric aciduria type I
- Hurler's syndrome
- Incontinentia pigmenti
- Larsen's syndrome
- Klippel–Trenaunay–Weber syndrome
- Knobloch's syndrome
- Krabbe's disease
- Meckel–Gruber syndrome
- Mucopolysaccharidosis VI
- Muscle-eye-brain disease
- Myotonic dystrophy
- Myotubular myopathy
- Neurofibromatosis
- Osteopetrosis
- Ruvalcaba's syndrome
- Thoracic dysplasia
- Shprintzen–Goldberg syndrome
- VACTERL association
- Walker–Warburg syndrome
- X-linked aqueductal stenosis (CRASH syndrome)

Traumatic Causes

- Hemorrhage
- Hypoxic-ischemic encephalopathy
- Posterior fossa surgery

Vascular Causes

- Arteriovenous malformation
- Jugular vein catheterization
- Vein of Galen malformation
- Venous sinus thrombosis

CRASH, corpus callosum agenesis, retardation, adducted thumbs, spastic paraparesis, hydrocephalus; VACTERL, vertebral anomalies, anal atresia, cardiac defect, tracheoesophageal fistula with esophageal atresia, renal abnormalities, limb abnormalities.

does not communicate effectively with the subarachnoid space. In patients with Chiari malformations, hydrocephalus may occur, with fourth ventricle outlet obstruction in Chiari type 1 malformation; it is commonly associated with myelomeningocele in the Chiari type 2 malformation. Hydrocephalus occurs in approximately 80–90 percent of patients with myelomeningocele; of these cases, 50 percent are obvious at birth [Tuli et al., 2003; Tulipan et al., 2003].

Neonatal hydrocephalus can also be part of a major cerebral malformation, such as an encephalocele or holoprosencephaly, or can be associated with inherited metabolic diseases, such as achondroplasia and Hurler's disease. Other causes of congenital hydrocephalus include agenesis of the foramen of Monro, congenital tumors, arachnoid cysts, vascular malformations (vein of Galen), and intrauterine toxoplasmosis.

Acquired Causes in Infants and Children

Infective causes of hydrocephalus include meningitis, especially bacterial, which can lead to hydrocephalus by either inflammatory aqueductal stenosis or leptomeningeal fibrosis. In some geographic areas, parasitic disease, such as intraventricular cysticercosis, can cause hydrocephalus by mechanical obstruction.

Post-hemorrhagic hydrocephalus (PHH) occurs following IVH and can be related to prematurity, head injury, or rupture of a vascular malformation. Communicating hydrocephalus post-subarachnoid hemorrhage is more common in adults and is rarely seen in children. Over the past two decades, there has been remarkable improvement in the survival of extremely low birth weight infants; however, the most immature of these infants remain at increased risk for neonatal complications that

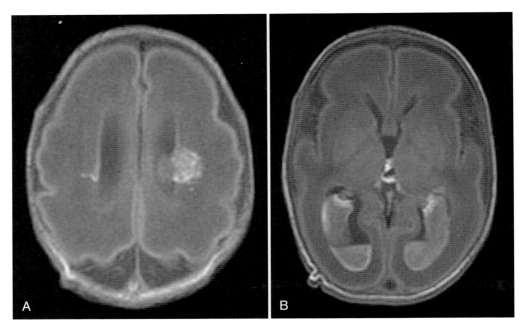

Fig. 27-2 Post-hemorrhagic hydro-cephalus. Hemorrhage into the ventricles and/or subarachnoid space can ultimately result in impairment of CSF flow through the foramina and/or resorption of CSF through the arachnoid villi. Note the intraventricular (**A** and **B**) and periventricular **(A)** hemorrhages with enlargement of the ventricles and subarachnoid space.

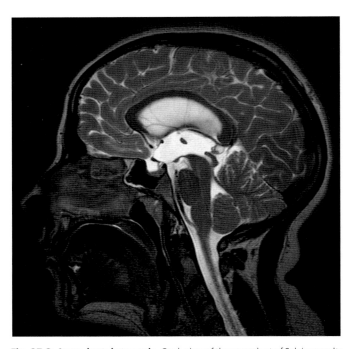

Fig. 27-3 Aqueductal stenosis. Occlusion of the aqueduct of Sylvius results in enlargement of the lateral and third ventricles (proximal to the aqueduct), with relative normalcy of the fourth ventricle (distal to the aqueduct).

Table 27-1 Causes of Hydrocephalus

Causes	Percentage
Intraventricular hemorrhage	24.1
Myelomeningocele	21.2
Tumor	9.0
Aqueductal stenosis	7.0
Infection	5.2
Head injury	1.5
Other	11.3
Unknown	11.0
Two or more causes	8.7

(Modified from Drake JM, et al: Randomized trial of cerebrospinal fluid shunt valve design in pediatric hydrocephalus. Neurosurgery 43[2]:294–303, 1998; discussion 303–295.)

potentially affect long-term neurodevelopmental outcome, including IVH (see Chapter 19). The risk for severe IVH varies inversely with gestational age, with an overall incidence of 7–23 percent [Lemons et al., 2001; Ment et al., 2005; Wilson-Costello et al., 2005]. Approximately one-third of extremely low birth weight infants with an IVH develop PHH, 15 percent of whom will require shunt insertion [Dykes et al., 1989; de Vries et al., 2002; Kazan et al., 2005].

Hydrocephalus after IVH is usually ascribed to fibrosing arachnoiditis, meningeal fibrosis, and subependymal gliosis, which impair flow and resorption of CSF. Recent experimental studies have suggested that acute parenchymal compression and ischemic damage, and increased parenchymal and perivascular deposition of extracellular matrix proteins – probably due, at least partly, to upregulation of transforming growth factor-beta (TGF-β) – are further important contributors to the development of the hydrocephalus. IVH is associated with damage to periventricular white matter and the damage is exacerbated by the development of hydrocephalus; combinations of pressure, distortion, ischemia, inflammation, and free radical-mediated injury are probably responsible [Cherian et al., 2004].

Mass lesions account for 20 percent of all cases of hydrocephalus in children. These are usually tumors, such as medulloblastoma, astrocytoma, and ependymoma, but cysts, abscesses, vascular malformations, or hematomas also can be the cause. Approximately 20 percent of children develop hydrocephalus requiring shunting following posterior fossa tumor removal. This may be delayed up to a year.

Increased venous sinus pressure can also lead to hydrocephalus. This can be related to achondroplasia, some craniosynostosis, or venous sinus thrombosis.

Iatrogenic causes of hydrocephalus include hypervitaminosis A, which can lead to hydrocephalus by increasing secretion of CSF or by increasing permeability of the blood–brain barrier. Hypervitaminosis A is a more common cause of idiopathic intracranial hypertension.

Clinical Characteristics

The clinical features of hydrocephalus depend on the age of the child at presentation and the time of onset in relation to closure of the cranial sutures. With the current advances in antenatal monitoring, the majority of congenital cases of hydrocephalus are diagnosed early (Figure 27-4), allowing for planned cesarian delivery in the moderate to severe cases where cephalopelvic disproportion is expected.

Symptoms and Signs in Infants

Hydrocephalus can present as acute raised intracranial pressure but, because of the relative distensibility of the infant skull, the presentation may be more subtle, with symptoms of failure to thrive or delayed development. Infants with hydrocephalus may be drowsy and irritable. Poor feeding and vomiting are common. These infants may have apneic spells, episodes of bradycardia, and a bulging, tense anterior fontanel. Head circumference increases abnormally across centiles and the head circumference is at or above the 98th percentile for age. Scalp veins may be distended, scalp skin thin and shiny, and cranial sutures splayed. In the minority of individuals, an abnormally large head is present at birth. In most children, however, the hydrocephalus only gradually becomes obvious. In advanced cases, clinical examination reveals a significant craniofacial disproportion, with expansion of the dome and low-set ears and eyes. Percussion over the skull may produce a "cracked-pot"

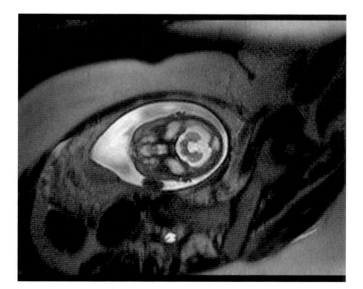

Fig. 27-4 Antenatal MRI showing fetal hydrocephalus. Symmetrical enlargement of the ventricular system is readily seen in the brain of this fetus.

percussion note (McEwen's sign). In very severe cases, where the cerebral cortex is thinned, transillumination of the cranial cavity may be possible. Epileptic seizures are rarely seen as a result of hydrocephalus alone.

Papilledema is rare in this age group, although funduscopy may reveal retinal venous engorgement. Oculomotor abnormalities may include abducens nerve palsy. Upgaze palsy, from third ventricular pressure on the midbrain tectum producing a "setting-sun" sign, can be observed, although this is usually absent in premature infants. In infants over the age of 6 months, limb tone may be increased, with spasticity preferentially affecting the lower limbs. However, some infants with definite hydrocephalus exhibit no such signs, as hydrocephalus may have developed slowly and the splaying of the sutures may have prevented the intracranial pressure from increasing considerably. Some infants with hydrocephalus after IVH may show hypotonia.

Symptoms and Signs in Older Children

In children older than 2 years, the head circumference is usually within normal limits if hydrocephalus develops after closure of the cranial sutures, or may be increased in children with preexisting (infantile) but unrecognized progressive hydrocephalus.

Learning problems and reduced intellectual function are common, and neurological development may be delayed. School-age children may have deteriorating school performance as a result of headaches, failing mental function, memory loss, or behavioral disturbances. More acutely, these children present with symptoms and signs of increased intracranial pressure, such as headache, nausea, vomiting, drowsiness, gait changes, papilledema, or impaired upward or lateral gaze. Failure of upward gaze is due to pressure on the tectal plate through the suprapineal recess. The limitation of upward gaze is of supranuclear origin. When intracranial pressure is significantly increased, other elements of the dorsal midbrain syndrome (Parinaud's syndrome) may be observed, such as light-near dissociation, convergence-retraction nystagmus, and eyelid retraction (Collier sign).

Abnormal hypothalamic functions (e.g., short stature, gigantism, obesity, delayed puberty, primary amenorrhea, menstrual irregularity, and diabetes insipidus) may occur secondary to increased intracranial pressure or dilatation of the third ventricle. Difficulty in walking may develop secondary to truncal and limb ataxia or limb spasticity. This affects the lower limbs preferentially because the periventricular pyramidal tracts are stretched by the enlarged ventricles. Neck pain may indicate associated tonsillar herniation; blurred vision may be present as a consequence of papilledema, which, if untreated, may cause optic atrophy.

Genetics

Although commonly considered a single disorder, hydrocephalus is a collection of heterogeneous complex and multifactorial disorders. A growing body of evidence suggests that genetic factors play a major role in its pathogenesis [Zhang et al., 2006].

Congenital hydrocephalus may occur alone (nonsyndromic) or as part of a syndrome with other anomalies (syndromic). It is estimated that about 40 percent of individuals with hydrocephalus have a genetic etiology [Haverkamp et al., 1999]. The isolated (nonsyndromic) form of congenital hydrocephalus is a primary and major phenotype caused by a specific faulty gene. In syndromic forms, it is difficult to define the defective gene because of the association with other anomalies. A discussion of the genetics of all syndromic forms of hydrocephalus is beyond the scope of this chapter and is reviewed elsewhere in this section on developmental malformations. This chapter will focus mainly on the genetic disorders associated with isolated forms of hydrocephalus.

Autosomal-recessive, autosomal-dominant, X-linked recessive [Castro-Gago et al., 1996] and X-linked dominant [Ferlini et al., 1995] forms of hydrocephalus are recognized (Table 27-2).

At least 43 gene mutations linked to hereditary hydrocephalus have been identified in animal models and humans. To date, nine genes associated with hydrocephalus have been identified in animal models, whereas only one such gene has been identified in humans: the hydrocephalus (X-linked) gene [Haverkamp et al., 1999]. X-linked hydrocephalus (HSAS1, OMIM) occurs in approximately 5–15 percent of congenital cases in which a genetic etiology is determined [Halliday et al., 1986; Haverkamp et al., 1999]. The gene responsible for X-linked human congenital hydrocephalus is at Xq28, encoding for L1CAM (L1 cell adhesion molecule) [Jouet et al., 1993]. Mutations are distributed over the functional protein domains. The exact mechanisms by which these mutations cause a loss of L1 protein function are still under investigation. L1CAM belongs to the immunoglobulin superfamily of neural cell adhesion molecules that is expressed in neurons and Schwann cells and appears to be essential for brain development and function. It plays a role in cell adhesion, axon growth and path-finding, and neuronal migration and myelination [Wong et al., 1995]. One of the possible mechanisms leading to the pathogenesis of hydrocephalus is the disruption of neural cell membrane proteins that play an important function during brain development.

The L1 disorders were initially described as different entities:
1. X-linked hydrocephalus with stenosis of the aqueduct of Sylvius (HSAS)
2. spastic paraparesis type 1
3. X-linked agenesis of the corpus callosum
4. mental retardation, aphasia, shuffling gait, and adducted thumbs (MASA) syndrome.

During the 1990s, it became clear that these disorders resulted from a mutation in a single gene, *L1CAM* [Fransen et al., 1995]. Some investigators have suggested that these separately named conditions be combined under the acronym CRASH (corpus callosum agenesis, retardation, adducted thumbs, shuffling gait, and hydrocephalus). The clinical phenotype is variable, even within a single family, but some genotype–phenotype correlations have been made [Fransen et al., 1998]. Hirschsprung's disease (HSCR) is characterized by the absence of ganglion cells and the presence of hypertrophic nerve trunks in the distal bowel. There have been several reports of patients with X-linked hydrocephalus and HSCR with a mutation in the *L1CAM* gene. Decreased L1CAM may therefore be a modifying factor in the development of HSCR [Okamoto et al., 2004]. Congenital aqueductal stenosis can also be inherited as an autosomal-recessive disorder (OMIM 236635) [Lapunzina et al., 2002].

In general, the recurrence risk for congenital hydrocephalus excluding X-linked hydrocephalus is low. Empiric risk rates range from <1 to 4 percent [Burton, 1979], indicating the rarity of autosomal-recessive congenital hydrocephalus [Halliday et al., 1986; Chow et al., 1990; Haverkamp et al., 1999]. However, multiple human kindreds have been reported [Halliday et al., 1986; Teebi and Naguib, 1988; Haverkamp et al., 1999; Zhang et al., 2006]. The loci or genes for human autosomal-recessive congenital hydrocephalus have not yet been identified, but there is at least one locus for this trait. Furthermore, since there is heterogeneity among clinical phenotypes, there may be more genetic loci in human autosomal-recessive congenital hydrocephalus.

Two kindreds in which congenital hydrocephalus was transmitted in an autosomal-dominant fashion have been reported. One was associated with aqueductal stenosis but was not associated with mental retardation or pyramidal tract dysfunction, which is in contrast to X-linked or recessive congenital hydrocephalus with HSAS, in which these abnormalities are common [Verhagen et al., 1998]. The other kindred in which hydrocephalus developed had an 8q12.2–q21.2 microdeletion. This trait was also transmitted in an autosomal-dominant pattern [Vincent et al., 1994].

Hydrocephalus has been observed in many mammals [Zhang et al., 2006]. Animal hydrocephalus models have many histopathological similarities to humans and can be used to understand the genetics and pathogenesis of these disorders. It has been well documented that the majority of cases of congenital hydrocephalus in animal models occur on a genetic basis with specific mapping and identification of different loci. The development and progression of congenital hydrocephalus constitute a dynamic process that is not yet well understood. It is probably the consequence of abnormal brain development and perturbed cellular function, which emphasizes the important roles that congenital hydrocephalus

Table 27-2 **Summary of Current Known Loci of Hydrocephalus in Humans**

Clinical Form	Trait	Locus	Chromosome	Human Gene
Congenital	AR	Unknown	Unknown	
Congenital	AD	Unknown	8q12.2–21.2 or unknown	
Adult-onset	AD	NPH	Unknown	
Congenital	XL	L1cam	X	*L1CAM*
Adult-onset	XL	Unknown	X	

AD, autosomal-dominant; AR, autosomal-recessive; NPH, normal pressure hydrocephalus; XL, X-linked.
(Adapted from Zhang J, et al: Genetics of human hydrocephalus. J Neurol 253:1255–1266, 2006.)

genes play during brain development. It is thought that it may develop at an important and specific embryonic time period of neural stem-cell proliferation and differentiation [Zhang et al., 2006].

Although advances have been made in determining the genetic basis of congenital hydrocephalus in animal models, there are much fewer genetic data regarding this condition in humans. The histopathological similarities of animal models can be used to help understand the pathogenesis and genetic underpinnings of human hydrocephalus. Such knowledge will hopefully lead to better diagnostic tools and more effective therapeutic modalities.

The current molecular genetic evidence from animal models indicates that, in the early stages of development, impaired and abnormal brain development, caused by abnormal cell signaling and functioning, eventually lead to the congenital hydrocephalus. However, it is not certain whether these data can be extrapolated to infants and children. The known hydrocephalus genes mostly code for important cytokines, growth factors, or related molecules in cell signaling pathways during early brain development. It is likely that perturbation of almost any molecule that plays a crucial role in early brain development and regulation of CSF dynamics potentially could cause congenital hydrocephalus.

Hydrocephalus may also be caused by alterations in ependymal cell function [Takano et al., 1993; Wagner et al., 2003]. The protein of the axonemal heavy chain 5 gene (*Mdnah5*), dynein, is specifically expressed in ependymal cells, and is essential for ultrastructural and functional integrity of ependymal cilia. In *Mdnah5*-mutant mice, lack of ependymal flow causes closure of the aqueduct and subsequent formation of triventricular hydrocephalus during early postnatal brain development. The higher incidence of aqueductal stenosis and hydrocephalus formation in patients with disorders associated with ciliary defects supports the relevance of this novel mechanism in humans [Ibanez-Tallon et al., 2004].

Hydrocephalus may be caused by changes in the development and function of mesenchymal cells. In murine embryonic brain, the *Msx1* gene is expressed along the dorsal midline. This regulatory gene is involved in epithelio-mesenchymal interactions in limb formation and organogenesis. In homozygous *Msx1* mutants, there is absence or malformation of the posterior commissure and of the subcommissural organ, collapse of the cerebral aqueduct, and hydrocephalus. About one-third of the heterozygous mutants also develop hydrocephalus, suggesting that the phenotype may be determined by the *Msx1* gene dosage during a critical developmental period [Ramos et al., 2004]. An example of this is the autosomal-recessive congenital hydrocephalus mouse model in which a truncated protein lacking the DNA-binding domain of the forkhead/winged helix gene, *Mf1*, was generated. Mesenchymal cells from Mf1lacZ embryos differentiate poorly into cartilage in micromass culture, and the differentiation of arachnoid cells in meninges of the mutant mice also was abnormal. Human patients with deletions in the region containing human Mf1 homolog FREAC3 were also found to develop multiple developmental disorders, including hydrocephalus [Kume et al., 1998].

Another mechanism for development of hydrocephalus may be associated with changes in growth factor signaling [Fukumitsu et al., 2000]. In mouse models, severe hydrocephalus has been observed in transgenic mice overexpressing TGF-β1, an important cytokine and growth-signaling molecule, in astrocytes [Galbreath et al., 1995]. In mouse models, fibroblast growth factor-2 (FGF-2) seems to play a predominant role in the proliferation of neuronal precursors and in neuronal differentiation in the developing cerebral cortex, even at relatively late stages of brain neurogenesis [Ohmiya et al., 2001].

Hydrocephalus may also be caused by disruption of the extracellular matrix (ECM). In the TGF-β1 overexpression mouse model, the changing expressions of a remodeling protein, matrix metalloproteinase-9 (MMP-9), and its specific inhibitor, tissue inhibitor of metalloproteinases-1 (TIMP-1), were found to be important factors in the spontaneous development of hydrocephalus by altering the ECM environment [Crews et al., 2004]. Furthermore, increased expression of cytokines such as TGF-β1 might reciprocally play an important role by disrupting vascular ECM remodeling, promoting hemorrhage and altering reabsorption of CSF. In another mouse model, ablation of the non-muscle myosin heavy chain II-B (NMHC-B) results in severe hydrocephalus with enlargement of the lateral and third ventricles. These defects may be caused by abnormalities in the cell adhesive properties of neuroepithelial cells, and suggest that NMHC-B is essential for early and late developmental processes in the mammalian brain [Tullio et al., 2001].

Other genetic mutations identified in animal models of hydrocephalus include those coding α-SNAP protein, which is essential for apical protein localization and cell fate determination in neuroepithelial cells [Chae et al., 2004]. α-SNAP plays a key role in a wide variety of membrane fusion events in eukaryotic cells, a function which is required for transport of molecules to inter- and intracellular compartments and for intercellular communication.

Neuroimaging

Cranial Ultrasound

In the presence of an open anterior fontanel in neonates and infants, transfontanellar ultrasound can visualize ventricular anatomy. This is by far the quickest, least expensive, and most convenient method to demonstrate ventricular enlargement. Ultrasonography is useful for the diagnosis of intrauterine hydrocephalus and communicating and noncommunicating PHH. Serial imaging after injury or in children with developmental malformations can be used to follow the evolution and possible development or progression of hydrocephalus (see Chapter 11).

Ventricular width measured from the midline to the lateral border of the lateral ventricle in the midcoronal view is the measurement with the least interobserver variability, and centiles for gestational age have been compiled [Levene, 1981]. Sedation is not required during acquisition of ultrasound images, and the procedure can be repeated frequently without any adverse effects. Limitations of cranial ultrasonography (see Chapter 11) are that it requires operator experience and often cannot establish a cause for the hydrocephalus.

Computed Tomography

Computed tomography (CT) demonstrates ventricular size and morphology, and presence of periventricular lucencies, and can reveal underlying pathologies, such as hemorrhage or posterior fossa tumors. Imaging of asymptomatic patients (especially after shunt revision) may serve as a reliable baseline study for comparison with subsequent imaging studies when patients become symptomatic. CT is widely available in many facilities and often does not require sedation of the child. The limitations of CT are exposure to radiation, particularly with serial CT imaging, and the fact that it may not always reveal the underlying cause of hydrocephalus.

Magnetic Resonance Imaging

MRI provides better morphological definition and etiological diagnosis, such as the presence of low-grade gliomas or colloid cysts, which may not be demonstrated on CT. MRI is better for evaluating Chiari malformations or cerebellar or periaqueductal tumors. It also affords better imaging of the posterior fossa than CT. Cine MRI is am MRI technique to measure CSF stroke volume in the cerebral aqueduct; it can be used for demonstrating patency of third ventriculostomy fenestration. Limitations of MRI are that children often require general anesthesia for the MRI to be acquired, and programmable shunt valves require reprogramming after MRI.

There are no reliable measurement values that can confirm or exclude the presence of hydrocephalus in a single series. Serial imaging demonstrating an increase in ventricular size may be required in equivocal cases. Conversely, an apparently normal ventricular size cannot exclude active hydrocephalus in a patient with a pre-existing shunt. A number of methods have been used to attempt to define hydrocephalus quantitatively on CT or MRI studies [leMay and Hochberg, 1979]. Hydrostatic hydrocephalus is suggested when either:

1. the size of both temporal horns is ≥2 mm in width, and the sylvian and interhemispheric fissures are not visible, or
2. both temporal horns are ≥2 mm, and the ratio of the largest width of the frontal horns to the internal diameter from inner table to inner table at this level is >0.5.

Other features suggestive of hydrostatic hydrocephalus include ballooning of the frontal horns of the lateral and third ventricles, periventricular hypoattenuation on CT, and periventricular high-intensity signal on T2-weighted images and fluid-attenuated inversion recovery (FLAIR) sequences on MRI, suggesting transependymal exudate or migration of CSF, compression of sulci and basal cisterns, upward bowing of the corpus callosum, and downward displacement of the floor of the third ventricle on sagittal MRI. The Evans ratio is the ratio of largest width of the frontal horns to the maximal biparietal diameter. A ratio greater than 30 percent is suggestive of hydrostatic hydrocephalus.

Radiologic criteria for chronic hydrocephalus include the following. Skull radiographs may depict erosion of the sella turcica, or "beaten copper cranium." The latter can also be seen in craniosynostosis. Temporal horns may be less prominent than in acute hydrocephalus and the third ventricle may herniate into the sella turcica. The corpus callosum may be atrophied; this is best appreciated on sagittal MRI. In infants with chronic hydrocephalus, sutural diastasis and delayed closure of fontanels may be seen. In communicating hydrocephalus, all ventricles are dilated. If the lateral and third ventricles are dilated and the fourth ventricle is small, it is likely that the obstruction is at the level of the aqueduct of Sylvius. An enhanced CT or MRI will help determine the cause, such as defining the presence of an obstructing tumor.

Radiography

Shunt X-ray series constitute the mainstay of the evaluation of the integrity of ventricular drainage systems. Anteroposterior and lateral skull, anteroposterior chest, and anteroposterior abdominal radiographs are required.

Diagnosis

Modern ultrasonography and, since the late 1980s, fetal MRI have significantly improved the ability to detect ventricular enlargement as a result of hydrocephalus in utero. Antenatal ultrasound and MRI provide reasonably detailed fetal brain anatomy and can detect malformations (at 17–21 weeks) and fetal ventriculomegaly (at 8–21 weeks) [Benacerraf and Birnholz, 1987; Oi et al., 1998]. Normative data for ventricular size allow serial investigation during gestation [Rich et al., 2007].

Anatomical ventriculomegaly is not sufficient to diagnose hydrocephalus. When diagnosing hydrocephalus in neonates or infants, it is essential to establish that there is a truly abnormal rate of skull growth. Records of head circumference (HC) measurements and its comparison with body weight and length centile charts are an integral part of postnatal follow-up of any child. Head circumference must be recorded and plotted on an accepted growth curve chart, with the patient's exact age (see Chapter 4 for standardized charts). In the presence of hydrocephalus, any of the following may be observed: HC more than 2 SD above normal or disproportionate to body length or weight, accelerated growth crossing centile curves, or continued head growth of more than 1.25 cm per week.

Evaluation of the patient with an enlarged head entails consideration of the many causes of macrocephaly, including hydrocephalus. Evaluation should include a history of trauma or CNS infection. The family history may demonstrate X-linked hydrocephalus caused by stenosis of the aqueduct of Sylvius or may reveal familial macrocephaly.

After a full review of the pregnancy, delivery, and neonatal history, as well as the clinical examination, and ultrasound examination, it is usually possible to classify hydrocephalus into an etiological group. If no obvious explanation can be determined, then the possibility of an intrauterine infection should be investigated. Coagulation factor deficiencies, as well as thrombocytopenia, should be excluded, as isoimmune thrombocytopenia and coagulation factor V deficiency can present as congenital hydrocephalus resulting from congenital IVH.

Differential Diagnosis

Besides hydrocephalus, causes of increasing head size include chronic subdural effusions or hematomas, pseudotumor cerebri, neurofibromatosis, metabolic abnormalities of bone or brain, cerebral gigantism (Sotos' syndrome), and benign familial forms.

Benign extracranial hydrocephalus is a condition in infants and children with enlarged subarachnoid spaces accompanied by increasing head circumference with normal or mildly dilated ventricles. This condition is also known as "benign subdural collections of infancy" or "pericerebral CSF collections." This disorder has been postulated by some to be a variant of communicating hydrocephalus, but tends to run a benign course and stabilize by 12–18 months of age [Ment et al., 1981; Barlow, 1984; Alvarez et al., 1986]. Close serial monitoring of head circumference and serial imaging with CT or MRI are recommended to monitor for ventriculomegaly. Shunting is rarely, if ever, required.

A rare but striking condition that can mimic hydrocephalus is hydranencephaly or anencephaly, a postneurulation defect that results in total or near-total absence of the cerebral tissue, with the intracranial cavity being filled with CSF. This is usually due to fetal bilateral internal carotid artery infarction or infection. Other brain malformations, such as agenesis of the corpus callosum and alobar holoprosencephaly, may also be associated with hydrocephalus, but more often represent expansion of the third ventricle and separation of the lateral ventricles. These are described in other chapters of this section.

Other conditions may present as hydrocephalus. Hydrocephalus ex vacuo is due to atrophy rather than altered CSF dynamics. Certain metabolic and degenerative disorders, such as glycogen storage and Alexander's disease, can cause macrocephaly. Brain tumors of infancy may reach an enormous size, producing a large head, whether there is associated hydrocephalus or not. Finally, there may be a family history of large heads. In these instances, there is often no increase in intracranial pressure or developmental abnormality, and both the brain and the cerebral ventricles are larger than normal.

Pathology

The precise pathologic features of hydrocephalus vary, depending on the age of onset, the rate of ventricular enlargement, and the degree of ventriculomegaly. Typically, elevated CSF pressure initially enlarges the frontal horns of the lateral ventricles, followed by enlargement of the entire ventricular system above the site of obstruction. Hydrocephalus is associated with flattening and destruction of the ventricular ependymal lining, as well as edema and necrosis of the periventricular white matter [Weller and Shulman, 1972]. Periventricular glial cells proliferate, resulting in a layer of reactive gliosis. The pathologic findings may be a result of reduced blood flow to the white matter, causing hypoxic injury or toxicity to the white matter due to build-up of waste products not removed appropriately because of changes in the extracellular matrix [Del Bigio, 2004]. In PHH, high concentrations of proinflammatory cytokines [Savman et al., 2002], free iron, and hypoxanthine [Bejar et al., 1983; Savman et al., 2001], which can generate highly reactive radicals, have been measured in the CSF.

Separation of the ependymal lining of the ventricles enhances permeability, which increases edema formation in adjacent white matter (transependymal fluid absorption). The expanding ventricles flatten the cerebral gyri and obliterate the sulci over the cortical surface. Unless the acute obstruction is relieved, increasing pressure may hinder cerebral blood flow, cause cerebral herniation and compromising brainstem function.

Increasing pressure and ventricular enlargement are associated with necrosis of brain parenchyma. Cerebral white matter is more vulnerable to destruction than gray matter in the presence of progressive hydrocephalus [Rubin et al., 1972]. The corpus callosum may also be preferentially affected, with evidence of transcallosal swelling, thickening, or demyelination [Spreer et al., 1996; Suh et al., 1997]. These effects do not appear to be associated with cognitive changes nor neuropsychologic evidence of callosal disconnection.

Management

Management of hydrocephalus is the most common problem in pediatric neurosurgery. In infants and children with symptomatic or progressive ventriculomegaly, the decision to treat with a CSF diversion procedure poses no therapeutic dilemma. However, not all patients with enlarged ventricles require treatment.

In patients with obstructive hydrocephalus secondary to a mass that is surgically accessible, resection of the mass may lead to resolution of the hydrocephalus and a shunt might not be necessary. This situation occurs infrequently in comparison with communicating hydrocephalus. If no documented obstruction or operable lesion is present and the hydrocephalus is mild and slowly progressive, a trial period of observation or medical management may be indicated, especially in preterm infants.

Another situation where observation is reasonable is arrested hydrocephalus, which is an uncommon state of chronic hydrocephalus in which the CSF pressure has returned to normal and there is no pressure gradient between the cerebral ventricles and the brain parenchyma. Patients should be followed carefully, with neurological examinations, neuropsychological assessments, and careful assessment of their development. A shunt will be necessary if there is any deterioration of those parameters.

Rapid-onset hydrocephalus with increased intracranial pressure is an emergency. Depending on the specific patient, any of the following procedures can be performed:
1. ventricular tap in infants
2. external ventricular drainage
3. lumbar puncture in post-hemorrhagic and post-meningitic hydrocephalus
4. placement of a ventriculoperitoneal shunt.

Shunts

Patients with hydrocephalus are most commonly treated with placement of an extracranial shunt. The principle of shunting is to establish a communication between the CSF (ventricular or lumbar) and a drainage site, such as the peritoneal or pleural cavity.

Ventriculoperitoneal (VP) shunting is the most accepted and most commonly used initial procedure. The lateral ventricle is the usual proximal location. The advantage of this shunt is that the need to lengthen the catheter with growth may be obviated by using a long peritoneal catheter. In patients with contraindications to ventriculoperitoneal shunting, such as the presence of peritonitis or peritoneal adhesions following abdominal surgery, ventriculopleural or ventriculoatrial shunts can be used. The latter is also called a "vascular shunt," and shunts the cerebral ventricles through the jugular vein and superior vena cava into the right cardiac atrium. This shunt requires repeated lengthening in a growing child [Vernet et al., 1995].

Shunts cause CSF to flow unidirectionally under the aegis of a valve system. Pressures required to overcome valve resistance are preset and can be used in patients with different pressure requirements. The first spring, ball, and diaphragm valves were superseded by a number of innovative valve designs, including antisiphon devices [Portnoy et al., 1973], horizontal–vertical valves [Drake and Sainte-Rose, 1995], flow-controlled valves [Sainte-Rose et al., 1987], adjustable valves [Black et al.,

1994], and others, developed with the hope that they would decrease shunt malfunction. Although each new valve was heralded as a significant advance that, functionally, was more physiological, with improved results in uncontrolled studies, prospective and randomized trials were all negative. Use of an antisiphon device developed in the 1970s improved the success rate of shunting by reducing overdrainage of CSF but was also associated with complications [Portnoy et al., 1973; DaSilva and Drake, 1991]. Orbis-Sigma valves or Delta valves have flow/pressure characteristics that reduce overdrainage [Drake and Kestle, 1996]. However, use of these systems did not reduce time to first shunt failure [Kestle et al., 2000]. When standard valves, a novel flow-controlled valve (Orbis Sigma, Cordis, Miami, Florida), and an updated antisiphon valve (Delta Valve; Medtronic PS Medical, Goleta, California) were compared in a prospective, randomized trial, there was no difference [Drake et al., 1998; Kestle et al., 2000]. Programmable valves are an alternative system that allows multiple pressure settings to adjust the valve for over- or underdrainage, avoiding a shunt revision for that reason; as the child grows, adjustments in flow can be made. Study of the time to shunt failure with these valves, however, did not show any difference from standard valves [Pollack et al., 1999]. A single-arm prospective study of an adjustable Delta valve, the Strata valve, suggested its failure rate was no different than any other previously studied valves [Kestle and Walker, 2005]. Furthermore, when ventricular size was measured pre- and postoperatively, comparing three very different valves, there was no difference over time, which indicates that the valves were not performing as the engineers had predicted [Tuli et al., 1999]. Studies on varying ventricular catheter position and endoscope-assisted catheter placement also did not demonstrate any improvement in outcome [Kestle et al., 2003].

Endoscopic Third Ventriculostomy

Endoscopic third ventriculostomy is an alternative to CSF shunting in appropriate patients [Drake, 2007; Jones et al., 1996; Barlow and Ching, 1997]. This creates an outlet in the floor of the third ventricle. A ventriculoscope is introduced into the lateral ventricle via a frontal horn approach, passed into the third ventricle through the foramen of Monro, and the floor of the third ventricle is then fenestrated just anterior to the mamillary bodies, allowing CSF to bypass any obstruction in the CSF pathway and be reabsorbed by the arachnoid villi.

Ventriculostomy is particularly useful in patients with congenital aqueductal stenosis that requires CSF diversion, and in selected patients with intracranial cysts or loculated cystic ventricular CSF collections [Drake, 2007]. The ventricles do not decrease in size to the degree they do with a ventriculoperitoneal shunt, so determining the function of a ventriculostomy by neuroimaging can be difficult [Kestle, 2003].

Complications of endoscopic third ventriculostomy are not infrequent and may be serious; they include as perforation of the basilar artery [McLaughlin et al., 1997]. CSF leak, meningitis, hypothalamic injury, and cranial nerve injury have all been reported [Teo et al., 1996]. The overall surgical complication rate appears to be approximately 10–15 percent. A rare and initially unrecognized complication is late rapid clinical deterioration. When this happens, patients initially appear to be doing well after the procedure, but begin to complain of headache and then rapidly deteriorate. Without immediate access to neurosurgery, they lapse into unconsciousness, and most die. A recent report compiled 15 such cases from the literature and around the world [Drake et al., 2006]. Thirteen patients died and, in all who had an autopsy or repeat endoscopic third ventriculostomy performed, the opening in the floor of the third ventricle was closed.

Management of Hydrocephalus in Preterm Infants

Hydrocephalus in preterm infants presents a therapeutic dilemma. In such infants, hydrocephalus may develop as a result of IVH originating from the periventricular germinal matrix. The IVH may lead to hydrocephalus by occlusion of the arachnoid granulations by breakdown products of the hemorrhage, although this theory remains unproven.

Shunting of these infants frequently is unnecessary and hazardous [Brockmeyer et al., 1989]. The course of the ventricular dilatation is variable; patients may demonstrate an arrest or reduction in ventriculomegaly with no treatment. Complications of shunting in this age group include a collapsed cortical mantle, subdural hemorrhage, marked cerebral conformational changes, intraparenchymal hemorrhage, or hardware erosion through the skin [Bass et al., 1995].

In view of the high morbidity for shunt placement in premature infants, multiple other interventions have been used. Studying the effectiveness of these interventions is challenging because of the variable course of post-hemorrhagic ventricular dilatation and the multiple other insults that occur in these infants. Acetazolamide and furosemide have been used in the past to reduce CSF output. Results of a larger, multicenter, randomized controlled trial, however, did not support the use of diuretics [Kennedy et al., 2001]. The principal secondary outcome measure of death in the first year of life or neurodevelopmental disability was significantly higher in infants receiving diuretic therapy. In addition, nephrocalcinosis developed in 25 percent of infants in the diuretic treatment group.

Repeated lumbar punctures to remove CSF are a common method of attempting to prevent ventricular dilatation after IVH, and as a therapy to manage symptomatic hydrocephalus. The theory is that removal of CSF containing blood and protein might allow the normal resorption of CSF to be restored. There have been two trials of repeated lumbar punctures in preventing development of hydrocephalus [Mantovani et al., 1980; Anwar et al., 1985], and two trials of infants with IVH and progressive ventricular dilatation that examined the effect of lumbar punctures [Dykes et al., 1989], or lumbar punctures or ventricular tapping [Ventriculomegaly Trial Group, 1990]. None of the studies demonstrated that CSF tapping decreased the need for shunting or decreased the likelihood of death or disability. The Ventriculomegaly Trial found a higher incidence of CSF infections in those infants who received CSF taps. A Cochrane review of this topic [Whitelaw, 2005] concluded that CSF tapping for infants at risk of or having developed PHH could not be recommended. However, the reviewers additionally stated that, despite the lack of evidence, CSF tapping should still be considered for symptomatic raised intracranial pressure. Likewise, despite the lack of evidence, some experts continue to recommend the use of CSF tapping in specific situations.

Intraventricular fibrinolytic agents to prevent the development of hydrocephalus after IVH have been found to be ineffective [Whitelaw, 2001]. Other options in patients with rapidly progressive ventriculomegaly who are too small for ventriculoperitoneal shunt placement include placement of an external ventricular drain, a subgaleal ventricular reservoir, or a subgaleal shunt. These devices can be used until the infant is large enough for permanent shunt placement. In addition, 25 percent of patients with these devices have arrest of their hydrocephalus, and do not require permanent shunt placement [Garton and Piatt, 2004].

Complications

The overall failure rate of shunts is 40 percent in the first year after placement [Drake et al., 1998; Pollack et al., 1999; Kestle et al., 2000]. Common reasons for failure are obstruction, infection, mechanical failure, overdrainage, loculated ventricles, and abdominal complications. Shunt malfunction caused by disconnection, kinking, or obstruction of the tubing results in typical signs and symptoms of increased intracranial pressure, or may present with more subtle symptoms. Fever may occur if infection is present, but shunt infection occasionally can be asymptomatic. In neonates, shunt malfunction manifests as alteration of feeding, irritability, vomiting, fever, lethargy, somnolence, and a bulging fontanel. Older children and adults present with headache, fever, vomiting, and meningismus. With VP shunts, abdominal pain may occur. *Staphylococcus epidermidis* and *Staphylococcus aureus* are the most common causes of shunt-related infection, which usually occurs within 2 months of shunt placement.

The infection rate varies but can be up to 10 percent [Drake, 2008]. Organisms that ordinarily are nonpathogenic may cause infection in the presence of shunt tubing in the ventricles, body cavities, or circulation. Whenever suppurative infection is suspected, appropriate blood and CSF specimens for culture must be obtained, the organism isolated, and sensitivities determined to facilitate effective antimicrobial therapy. Most shunts can be tapped to obtain CSF specimens and to assess CSF dynamics. If infection leads to impairment of the shunt mechanism, removal and replacement usually are required; temporary insertion of an external ventriculostomy may be necessary until the infection is controlled. In one series of patients whose shunts were tapped, normal CSF values correlated with an overall incidence of complications of 39.2 percent, whereas abnormal CSF values were correlated with a complication rate of 90.9 percent [Caldarelli et al., 1996]. Rates of infective complications were 2.7 percent in the patients with normal CSF and 77.3 percent in patients with abnormal CSF.

Other complications of VP shunts include peritonitis, CSF ascites, inguinal hernia, intra-abdominal cysts, intracranial granulomas, gastrointestinal obstruction, migration of the shunt within the peritoneal cavity, headache, and perforation of abdominal viscera [Sgouros et al., 1995; Caldarelli et al., 1996]. Abdominal pseudocysts manifest with nausea, vomiting, and abdominal distention and pain; abdominal ultrasonography may demonstrate the cysts [Hann et al., 1985]. Thromboembolic phenomena, cardiac dysrhythmias, cardiovascular perforation, endocarditis, catheter embolization, pulmonary hypertension and thromboembolism, and immune complex shunt nephritis are special complications of ventriculoatrial shunts [Lam and Villemure, 1997]. Correction of longstanding hydrocephalus may cause subdural hematomas.

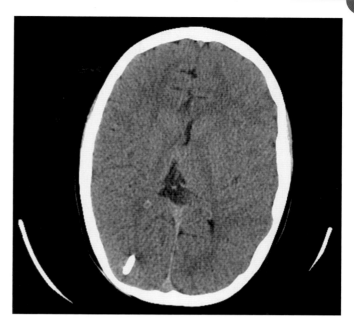

Fig. 27-5 Slit ventricle syndrome. Patients who have undergone ventricular shunting for hydrocephalus and develop severe headache may have normal or small (as seen in this figure) ventricles on imaging studies. The etiology of this syndrome is best determined in the individual patient by intracranial pressure measurement and can include severe intracranial hypotension analogous to spinal headaches, intermittent obstruction of the ventricular catheter, intracranial hypertension with small ventricles and a failed shunt (normal-volume hydrocephalus), intracranial hypertension with a working shunt (cephalocranial hypertension), or shunt-related migraine.

The "slit ventricle syndrome" (SVS; Figure 27-5) is defined as severe, life-modifying headaches in patients with shunts for the treatment of hydrocephalus and normal or smaller than normal ventricles [Rekate, 2008]. There are five potential pathophysiologies that may be involved in this condition. These pathologies are defined by intracranial pressure measurement as severe intracranial hypotension analogous to spinal headaches, intermittent obstruction of the ventricular catheter, intracranial hypertension with small ventricles and a failed shunt (normal-volume hydrocephalus), intracranial hypertension with a working shunt (cephalocranial hypertension), and shunt-related migraine [Rekate, 2008]. Management of SVS requires an understanding of the specific pathogenesis of the problem in individual patients, whether based on monitoring of intracranial pressure or observation at the time of shunt failure or symptoms. Overdrainage syndromes are managed with valve upgrades and the addition of devices that retard siphoning. Other management options used for this condition are subtemporal decompression, calvarial expansion or shunting devices that access the cortical subarachnoid space, such as lumboperitoneal shunts, or shunts involving the cisterna magna.

Prognosis

Before the 1950s, the outlook of untreated hydrocephalus was extremely poor. Some 49 percent of patients had died by the end of the 20-year observation period and only 38 percent of survivors had an IQ greater than 85 [Laurence and Coates, 1962]. The development of satisfactory shunting substantially improved the outlook of children with hydrocephalus but brought its own set of problems and complications. Most children with hydrocephalus will require multiple shunt revisions. Shunt dependence carries a 1 percent per year mortality [Sainte-Rose et al., 1991; Iskandar et al., 1998]. Another series of 907 patients reported a mortality rate of 12 percent at 10 years from the time of initial shunt insertion [Tuli et al., 2004], with the main risk factor for death being a history of shunt infection. Shunt-related complications, including death, have been reported to be greater in patients with myelomeningocele than in those who required shunt placement for the treatment of other conditions [Iskandar et al., 1998; Tuli et al., 2003].

The neurologic and intellectual disabilities among patients with hydrocephalus depend on many factors, including etiology and degree of hydrocephalus, thickness of the cortical mantle and corpus callosum [Fletcher et al., 1992], requirement for a shunt, and presence of other brain anomalies [Dennis et al., 1981]. Associated conditions, such as IVH, CNS infection [Tuli et al., 2004], and hypoxia, may dictate the ultimate prognosis more than the hydrocephalus.

A series of 233 patients with congenital hydrocephalus evaluated for longer than 20 years reported a mortality rate of 13.7 percent [Lumenta and Skotarczak, 1995]. The average number of shunt revisions was 2.7. In this series, 115 patients underwent psychological evaluation; approximately 63 percent showed normal performance, whereas 30 percent had mild retardation, and 7 percent had severe retardation. Another study found that children with congenital hydrocephalus were less likely to require special education placement (29 percent) than those in whom hydrocephalus was due to meningitis (52 percent) or IVH (60 percent) [Casey et al., 1997].

Epilepsy also is more prevalent in patients with hydrocephalus, and complications of shunt surgery appear to play a relatively minor role in its development [Piatt and Carlson, 1996].

Intellectual sequelae include significant scatter among Wechsler Intelligence Scale for Children-Revised (WISC-R) subtest scores, often with greater impairment of performance and motor tasks, as well as of nonverbal compared with verbal skills [Brookshire et al., 1995]. Normal intellectual function is present in 40–65 percent of patients who received appropriate treatment [Dennis et al., 1981]. The probability of normal intelligence is enhanced if shunts are placed early and proper function is maintained. A study of 99 children ranging in age from 6 to 13 years with shunted or arrested hydrocephalus demonstrated a close correlation between the area of the corpus callosum and nonverbal cognitive skills and motor abilities [Fletcher et al., 1996]. Behavioral problems also are more common in children with hydrocephalus, irrespective of etiology [Fletcher et al., 1995].

Intracranial Arachnoid Cysts

Definition

Intracranial arachnoid cysts are benign, nongenetic developmental cysts that contain spinal fluid and occur within the arachnoid membrane [Gosalakkal, 2002]. The mechanism of formation during embryogenesis is uncertain [Hirano and Hirano, 2004; Naidich et al., 1985–1986]. Several mechanisms could account for the enlargement of these cysts, including

Table 27-3 Distribution of Arachnoid Cysts

Location	Percentage of Cysts
Sylvian fissure	49
Cerebellopontine angle	11
Quadrigeminal area	10
Vermian area and sellar-suprasellar area	9
Interhemispheric fissure	5
Cerebral convexity	4
Clival area	3

(Modified from Rengachary SS, Watanabe I. Ultrastructure and pathogenesis of intracranial cysts. J Neuropathol Exp Neurol 40:61, 1981.)

secretion by the cells forming the cyst walls, a unidirectional valve, or liquid movements secondary to pulsations of the veins [Gosalakkal, 2002]. The cysts occur in proximity to arachnoid cisterns, most often in the sylvian fissure (Table 27-3). Common neurologic features are headache, seizures, hydrocephalus, focal enlargement of the skull, and signs and symptoms of elevated intracranial pressure and developmental delay, as well as specific signs or symptoms resulting from neural compression. Some arachnoid cysts remain asymptomatic [Mason et al., 1997]. Progressive enlargement and intracystic or subdural hemorrhage are potential complications. Suprasellar arachnoid cysts may produce neuroendocrine dysfunction, hydrocephalus, and optic nerve compression. Posterior fossa cysts are now more frequently recognized with the use of MRI and CT, and frequently require surgical treatment [Domingo and Peter, 1996].

In a series of 61 children with arachnoid cysts, about 53 percent of cases were diagnosed before age 1 year; 42 percent were supratentorial and 46 percent infratentorial [Pascual-Castroviejo et al., 1991]. Macrocephaly was the presenting symptom in 72 percent, and associated features included cranial asymmetry in 39 percent, aqueductal stenosis in 16 percent, and agenesis of the corpus callosum in 13 percent. Developmental delay was a common finding. Skull radiographs may suggest the diagnosis; CT or MRI is the definitive diagnostic procedure [Weiner et al., 1987] (Figure 27-6). Injection of contrast medium into the cyst to document communication with the ventricular system is seldom necessary.

Clinical Characteristics

Symptoms vary, depending on the size of the cyst and its location. Several common locations have been well described in the literature.

Sylvian Fissure/Middle Cranial Fossa

Nearly two-thirds of pediatric arachnoid cysts are located in the sylvian fissure/middle cranial fossa [Gosalakkal, 2002]. They may increase in volume, opening the fissure and exposing the middle cerebral artery. This exposure may result in compression and underdevelopment of the anterior superior surface of the temporal lobe. The origins of these cysts have been the subject of debate since they were first described. Controversy remains concerning whether they originate directly from the meninges adjacent to the temporal pole, or whether

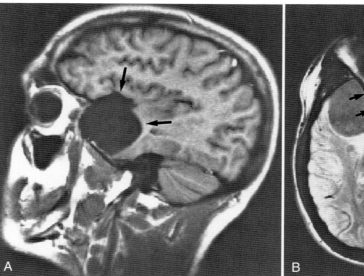
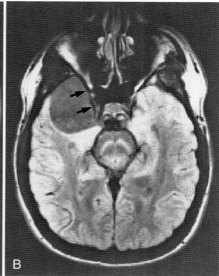

Fig. 27-6 Arachnoid cyst. A, A cystic mass with signal intensity suggestive of cerebrospinal fluid is seen to deform the right temporal lobe (arrows) on this parasagittal image from a T1-weighted magnetic resonance imaging (MRI) study. **B,** Note the eroded appearance of the greater sphenoid wing (arrows) from the arachnoid cyst on this axial image from a spin density-weighted MRI study. *(Courtesy of Joseph R Thompson, Department of Radiation Sciences, Loma Linda University School of Medicine, Loma Linda, California.)*

partial agenesis of the temporal lobe favors secondary formation of the cyst. Headaches are the most common presenting symptom; proptosis, contralateral motor weakness, and seizures also may occur. In 10 percent of children, developmental delay may be present. Treatment, as discussed later, depends on clinical symptoms. Recent studies have suggested some cognitive improvement after surgical treatment [Raeder et al., 2005]. Children with bitemporal arachnoid cysts also should be evaluated for the possibility of glutaricaciduria type 1 [Lutcherath et al., 2000]. Bitemporal arachnoid cysts also have been reported in children with neurofibromatosis [Martinez-Lage et al., 1993].

Sellar Region

Both suprasellar and intrasellar cysts can occur in children. Suprasellar cysts can cause third ventricular obstructive hydrocephalus at the level of the foramen of Monro, and may be associated with visual impairment and endocrine dysfunction [Mohn et al., 1999]. Progressive head enlargement, growth retardation, developmental delay, and bitemporal hemianopsia have all been described [Gosalakkal, 2002]. A bobble-head doll syndrome, with involuntary head movements secondary to increased pressure on the third ventricle and dorsomedial thalamic nuclei, is responsible [Fioravanti et al., 2004]. Endoscopic surgical approaches are now preferred.

Posterior Fossa

Arachnoid cysts of the posterior fossa are uncommon and must be differentiated from other cystic malformations of the posterior fossa, such as the Dandy–Walker malformation [Gosalakkal, 2002]. Macrocrania and raised intracranial pressure are frequently observed. Cerebellar cysts demonstrate nystagmus and other cerebellar signs. Other rare manifestations reported include cervical spinal cord compression, which may improve after posterior fossa cystoperitoneal shunting or endoscopic surgery. In such patients, gait disturbances and headache are commonly seen. Posterior fossa cysts may be very large [Lancon and Ellis, 2004] and also can occur in families [Sinha and Brown, 2004].

Complications

Several clinical complications are believed to be associated with arachnoid cysts, although the relation between cyst presence and development of symptoms remains controversial; thus, the decision to operate is difficult and must be made on a patient-by-patient basis. Surgery is indicated when the cyst is causing obstructive hydrocephalus or if neuroimaging demonstrates mass effect, with compression of normal brain or brainstem structures. The relation between symptoms such as attention-deficit disorder, aphasia, or migraine-like headaches is uncertain, and correlation between cyst location and specific symptoms or congruent electroencephalogram (EEG) abnormalities is necessary before symptoms can be attributed to the cyst.

Epilepsy

Anecdotal studies suggest a relation between seizure reduction and removal of arachnoid cysts [D'Angelo et al., 1999]. The relation between the presence of arachnoid cysts and occurrence of seizures when the intracranial pressure is normal is uncertain, however, and differences in outcomes, whether patients are managed medically or surgically, are similar [Koch et al., 1995]. In addition, interictal and ictal EEG may not correspond to the site of the arachnoid cyst, raising the question of whether the presence of an EEG abnormality is incidental.

Subdural Hematoma and Hygroma

Subdural hematomas and hygromas are infrequently encountered complications of arachnoid cysts of the middle cranial fossa and are particularly rare with cysts in other regions [Donaldson et al., 2000]. Minor head trauma has been suggested to be a precipitating factor. Arachnoid cysts of the middle cranial fossa were found in 2.43 percent of patients with chronic subdural hematomas or hygromas in one report [Parsch et al., 1997].

Neuropsychiatric Disorders

Attention-deficit hyperactivity disorder, speech delay, and developmental delay have been found in association with arachnoid cysts, particularly in the temporal lobe, but a causal relation remains uncertain [Millichap, 1997]. Mental impairment and developmental delay have been associated with large arachnoid cysts [Gosalakkal, 2002], and the presence of cysts and developmental delay may be part of a common developmental process. Recent studies have suggested improvements in cognition after surgical treatment [Raeder et al., 2005]. The increased incidence of arachnoid cysts in conditions such as Down syndrome, mucopolysaccharidosis, schizencephaly, and neurofibromatosis suggests a higher incidence in children with underlying abnormalities of the brain [Gosalakkal, 2002]. Aphasia, including that of Landau–Kleffner syndrome, also has been associated with the presence of left sylvian arachnoid cysts. Even in patients in whom CT and MRI failed to reveal mass effect, positron emission tomography (PET) has demonstrated hypometabolism in speech areas. Postoperative improvement in PET studies corresponded to improvement in vocabulary [De Volder et al., 1994].

Management

When symptoms warrant, surgical intervention to decompress the cyst, including endoscopic management or shunting procedures, is required [Abbott, 2004; Germano et al., 2003; Godano et al., 2004; Raffel and McComb, 1988]. Arachnoid cysts may occur with or without hydrocephalus. The success rate of fenestration is higher in those patients without hydrocephalus (i.e., 73 percent required no additional treatment) than in hydrocephalus patients (32 percent) [Fewel et al., 1996]. About 12 percent of patients with hydrocephalus treated with fenestration alone may require a cystoperitoneal shunt. In general, cyst fenestration should be the primary procedure in patients without hydrocephalus. If hydrocephalus is present, cyst fenestration is still recommended, but a VP shunt should be placed if hydrocephalus is marked or after fenestration if the hydrocephalus is progressive [Fewel et al., 1996]. Congenital intraspinal cysts also can occur and require surgical evaluation [Chang, 2004].

Conclusion

Pediatric hydrocephalus, arachnoid cysts, and benign extra-axial collections are common, complex, and, in many ways, poorly understood disorders. While persistent efforts over the last century to improve understanding and, where required, treatment of these disorders have had modest success, recent advances in imaging, neurophysiology, and molecular biology have led to important discoveries, suggesting that significant advances are imminent.

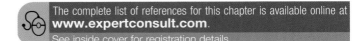

Congenital Anomalies of the Skull

Pedro A. Sanchez-Lara and John M. Graham, Jr.

Introduction

Congenital anomalies of the skull can arise any time during gestation and must be distinguished from anomalies that arise after birth. During the first 4–6 weeks of development from conception, neural crest cells in the fetal head region migrate and differentiate into mesenchymal cells that form the bones of the face, while the cranial base and base of the skull are derived from the occipital somitomeres. Within the flat cranial bones, the mesenchyme differentiates directly into bone through membranous ossification. The neurocranium is the portion surrounding the brain, and it develops directly from mesenchyme derived from the occipital somitomeres. The viscerocranium is derived from neural crest and it forms the cartilaginous bones of the face [Sadler and Langman, 2009]. The neurocranium is divided into the membranous part, forming the flat bones of the cranial vault, and the chondrocranium, forming the cartilaginous bones of the base of the skull. The chondrocranium develops by fusion of a number of cartilaginous structures, which ossify by endochondral ossification to form the base of the skull. Posteriorly, the base of the occipital bone is formed from parachordal cartilage and three occipital sclerotomes. Anteriorly, the sphenoid and ethmoid bones are formed from the hypophyseal cartilages and trabeculae cranii. On either side of the medial plate, the ala orbicularis and ala temporalis form the sphenoid bones, and the periotic capsule forms the temporal bones. The membranous neurocranium (dura mater) ossifies to form the cranial vault through bone spicules, which progressively radiate from primary ossification centers near the center of each bony plate toward the periphery, where the sutures develop. Membranous bones enlarge during fetal and postnatal life by the apposition of new layers to the outer surface of the skull (ectocranial bone deposition), while endocranial osteoclastic bone resorption occurs on the inner surface. Growth of the cranial bones is directly related to brain growth, and premature fusion of cranial sutures can be related to the cessation of brain growth (e.g., primary microcephaly).

There are six fibrous areas where two or more cranial bones meet (fontanels). The five major sutures are the metopic, sagittal, coronal, squamosal, and lambdoid sutures; the six fontanels are the anterior (1), anteriolateral (sphenoidal) (2), posterolateral (2), and posterior (1) fontanels (Figure 28-1). The presence of the sutures and fontanels allows the bones of the skull to overlap each other (termed molding) during the birth process. Different sutures become ossified at different times, with the metopic suture being the first to ossify at 4–7 months and the remaining sutures not completely ossifying until adulthood.

Craniosynostosis versus Deformational Plagiocephaly

The term craniostenosis (literally "cranial narrowing") is used to describe an abnormal head shape that results from premature fusion of one or more sutures, while craniosynostosis is the process of premature sutural fusion that results in craniostenosis. In clinical usage, the term craniosynostosis is used more widely, perhaps in an effort to distinguish deformational nonsynostotic head shapes from those caused by underlying sutural synostosis, but the two terms are often used interchangeably. Plagiocephaly is a nonspecific term used to describe an asymmetric head shape, which can result from either craniosynostosis or cranial deformation, and differentiation between these two causes is critical to determining the proper mode of treatment (i.e., surgery vs. physical or molding techniques). Craniosynostosis is usually treated with a neurosurgical procedure involving partial calvariectomy, while deformational plagiocephaly usually responds to early physical therapy, repositioning, and/or cranial orthotic therapy if those measures are unsuccessful [Graham and Smith, 2007; Graham et al., 2005].

In an otherwise normal fetus, prenatal relaxation of normal growth-stretch tensile forces in the underlying dura across a suture for a significant period of time during late fetal life can result in craniosynostosis [Graham et al., 1979, 1980; Higginbottom et al., 1980; Graham and Smith, 1980; Koskinen-Moffett et al., 1982]. This may also occur when the lack of growth stretch is caused by a deficit in brain growth, as in severe primary microcephaly. Experimental prolongation of gestation in pregnant mice, resulting in fetal crowding after installation of a cervical clip, has been shown to result in craniosynostosis [Koskinen-Moffett and Moffet, 1989]. The degree of craniosynostosis was greatest among those fetuses located more proximally in the uterine horns, where the crowding was most severe. The most common cause of craniosynostosis in otherwise normal infants is constraint of the fetal head in utero [Graham et al., 1979, 1980; Higginbottom et al., 1980; Graham and Smith, 1980; Koskinen-Moffett et al., 1982; Koskinen-Moffett and Moffet, 1989; Sanchez-Lara et al., 2010]. When external fetal head constraint

FONTANELS   SUTURES

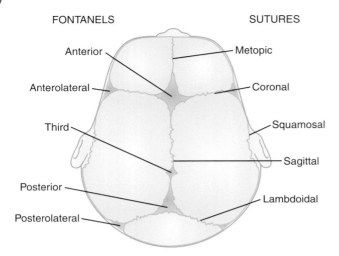

Fig. 28-1 Schematic showing name and location of cranial sutures and fontanels.

limits growth stretch parallel to a cranial suture, it may lead to craniosynostosis of an intervening suture between the constraining points. Sagittal craniosynostosis (the most common type of craniosynostosis) usually is isolated and occurs in an otherwise normal child. The constrained suture tends to develop a bony ridge, especially at the point of maximal constraint between the biparietal eminences. Such ridging can easily be palpated or visualized on skull radiographs, and three-dimensional cranial computed tomography (3D-CT) allows the ridge to be seen even more clearly (Figure 28-2).

Craniosynostosis is usually recognized shortly after birth from the abnormal shape of the head and lack of molding resolving to normal. Early closure of a fontanel, head asymmetry, and/or palpable ridging along a closed suture can be presenting features. With synostosis, cranial radiographs may reveal sclerosis of the suture with no apparent intervening sutural ligament, but it may be difficult to distinguish an overlapping suture from synostosis. On cross-sectional images, dense ridging over the suture may be evident, particularly with sagittal and metopic synostosis. If there is uncertainty as to whether sutures are truly synostotic, 3D-CT can provide a more accurate appraisal (see Figure 28-2).

In general, craniosynostosis begins at one point and then spreads along a suture [Koskinen-Moffett and Moffet, 1989; Cohen and MacLean, 2000]. At the fused location, there is complete sutural obliteration, with nonlamellar bone extending completely across the sutural space, while further away from the initial site of fusion, the sutural margins are closely approximated with ossifying connective tissue. As age increases, there is a tendency for more of the suture to become synostotic, with synostosis usually beginning at only one location in most cases [Koskinen-Moffett and Moffet, 1989]. Synostosis prevents future expansion at that site, and the rapidly growing brain then distorts the calvarium into an aberrant shape, depending upon which sutures have become synostotic (see Figure 28-2). The earlier the synostosis takes place, the greater the effect on skull shape. Craniosynostosis may be caused by many different mechanisms, such as mutant genes, chromosome disorders, storage disorders, hyperthyroidism, or failure of normal brain growth The entire topic of craniosynostosis has been comprehensively reviewed by Cohen [Cohen and MacLean, 2000].

Sutural Anatomy and Head Shape

Different terms have been used to describe the different head shape alterations caused by craniosynostosis, with the resultant head shape dependent on the suture involved. A long, keel-shaped skull with prominent forehead and occiput is termed dolichocephaly or scaphocephaly. This head shape is usually

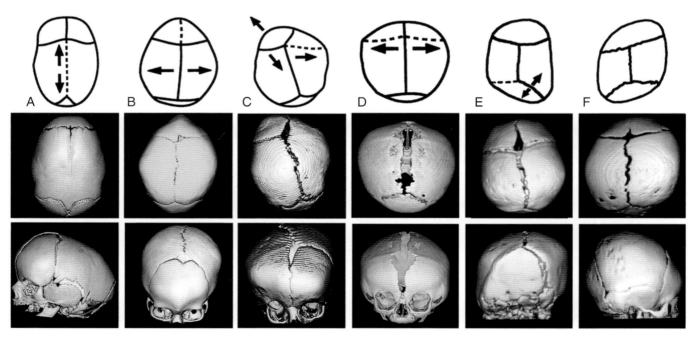

Fig. 28-2 Schematic drawing and three-dimensional computed tomography reconstructions of synostosis and plagiocephaly. A, Sagittal synostosis with dolichocephaly. **B,** Metopic synostosis. **C,** Right coronal synostosis. **D,** Bilateral coronal synostosis. **E,** Left lambdoid synostosis. **F,** Right occipital deformational plagiocephaly.

associated with premature sagittal suture closure and a palpable ridge toward the posterior end of the suture (see Figure 28-2A). Sagittal synostosis must be distinguished from deformation of the infant cranium due to persistently sleeping on the side of the head (more common in prematurely born infants) or breech-head deformation sequence. Individuals with scaphocephaly and dolichocephaly have a decreased cephalic index (CI) of less than 76 percent (CI = head width/head length × 100 percent).

Premature fusion of both coronal sutures produces a high, wide forehead with a short skull, resulting in brachycephaly (see Figure 28-2), while fusion of one coronal suture produces an asymmetric head shape termed plagiocephaly. When coronal craniosynostosis occurs, it is important to examine the patient carefully for associated anomalies that might suggest a recognizable genetic syndrome. Evaluation of the limbs, ears, and cardiovascular system is quite helpful in diagnosing syndromes associated with coronal craniosynostosis. Limb defects, such as syndactyly, brachydactyly, carpal coalition, or broad, deviated thumbs and/or halluces, can suggest an associated genetic syndrome and indicate what types of molecular analysis to pursue. It is also important to examine both parents for similar anomalies, carpal coalition, and/or facial asymmetry, since these findings may represent variable expression of an altered gene in a parent.

Premature fusion of both the coronal and sagittal sutures generally leads to a tall, tower-like skull (turricephaly), with more severe synostosis of multiple sutures producing a tall, pointed skull (acrocephaly or oxycephaly). In this condition, the limitations of calvarial expansion are so extreme that there may be limited room for brain growth (Figure 28-3a). Synostosis of multiple cranial sutures is more likely to result in elevated intracranial pressure and to require shunting for hydrocephalus. In extreme cases, a cloverleaf head shape can result from multiple suture synostosis, usually with signs of increased intracranial pressure and a "beaten copper" radiographic appearance of the inner table of the skull (see Figure 28-3b). There may also be optic atrophy, proptosis, and loss of vision. Combinations of sutural synostosis, such as sagittal plus coronal, are also referred to as compound craniosynostosis, and multiple suture synostosis usually has a genetic basis.

A triangle-shaped skull (trigonocephaly) is caused by premature fusion of the metopic suture (see Figure 28-2). The similarity in epidemiological features between sagittal and metopic craniosynostosis suggests that prenatal lateral constraint of the frontal part of the head may be a frequent cause of metopic craniosynostosis. Examples of constraint-induced metopic synostosis have included a monozygotic triplet whose forehead was wedged between the buttocks of her two co-triplets, and an infant whose head was compressed within one horn of his mother's bicornuate uterus [Graham and Smith, 1980]. Syndromic metopic synostosis can also occur, and trigonocephaly is seen in a variety of syndromes, some of which are associated with mental retardation or chromosome anomalies.

Unilateral lambdoid synostosis results in trapezoidal plagiocephaly, which differs from deformational posterior plagiocephaly due to supine positioning and torticollis, and from synostotic anterior plagiocephaly due to unicoronal synostosis (see Figure 28-2). Unlike coronal synostosis, facial structures and orbits are usually not affected by lambdoid synostosis. Radiographic signs include trapezoidal cranial asymmetry,

small posterior fossa, and sutural sclerosis with ridging; however, sole reliance on skull radiographs and clinical signs can lead to misdiagnosis, so it is best to confirm the diagnosis of suspected lambdoid synostosis with a 3D-CT scan, which clearly images the involved suture(s) and permits secure diagnosis. Among 232 patients referred for either deformational posterior plagiocephaly or craniosynostosis, only 4 patients (3.1 percent) manifested clinical, imaging, and operative features of true unilambdoidal craniosynostosis [Huang et al., 1996]. These features included a thick bony ridge over the fused suture, with contralateral parietal and frontal bulging, and an ipsilateral occipitomastoid bulge, leading to tilting of the ipsilateral skull base and a downward/posterior displacement of the ear on the synostotic side. In contrast, infants with deformational, nonsynostotic posterior plagiocephaly had a parallelogram-shaped head, with forward displacement of the ear and frontal bossing on the side ipsilateral to the occipitoparietal flattening, accompanied by contralateral occipital bossing [Graham et al., 2005].

When craniosynostosis occurs secondary to decreased brain growth associated with severe microcephaly, the head shape tends to be normal, but quite small.

Brachycephaly, turricephaly, and acrocephaly associated with exophthalmos, shallow orbits, low-set ears, broad nasal bridge, a narrow, highly arched palate, and malocclusion may suggest a syndromic form of craniosynostosis, especially when there are associated distal limb anomalies (broad deviated halluces or thumbs, total or partial 3–4 syndactyly, and/or clinodactyly). Syndromic craniosynostosis can be associated with mental retardation, hydrocephalus, and/or optic atrophy secondary to increased intracranial pressure. Craniosynostosis has also occurred with numerous chromosomal abnormalities, and may arise secondarily when there is reduced brain growth, or metabolic/hematological alterations of cranial bone.

Plagiocephaly (which translates literally from the Greek term *plagio kephale* as "oblique head") is a term used to describe asymmetry of the head shape, when viewed from the top [Graham and Smith, 2007]. The term deformational plagiocephaly should suffice to distinguish this type of defect and its proper type of management. The side of the plagiocephaly is usually indicated by the bone that has been most flattened by the deforming forces (usually the occiput for infants who sleep on their backs). Deformational plagiocephaly is usually not associated with premature closure of a cranial suture, but since craniosynostosis can also be caused by fetal head constraint, when both deformational plagiocephaly and craniosynostosis occur together, the diagnosis can be difficult, requiring complex management.

By definition, this anomaly involves deformation or reshaping of normal structures; thus, the growth and development of the brain are usually normal. However, infants with limited mobility due to hypotonia, hydrocephalus, macrocephaly, or limb anomalies are also more likely to develop deformational plagiocephaly, so this anomaly can complicate syndromes with these features. Predisposing factors resulting in excessive or asymmetric head deformation include: restrictive intrauterine environments, poor muscle tone, torticollis, clavicular fracture, cervical-vertebral abnormalities, sleeping position, multiple gestation, and incomplete bone mineralization. The development of excessive positional brachycephaly, with or without plagiocephaly, can be an early indication that parents are not providing their infants with adequate "tummy time." It is important to distinguish deformational plagiocephaly from

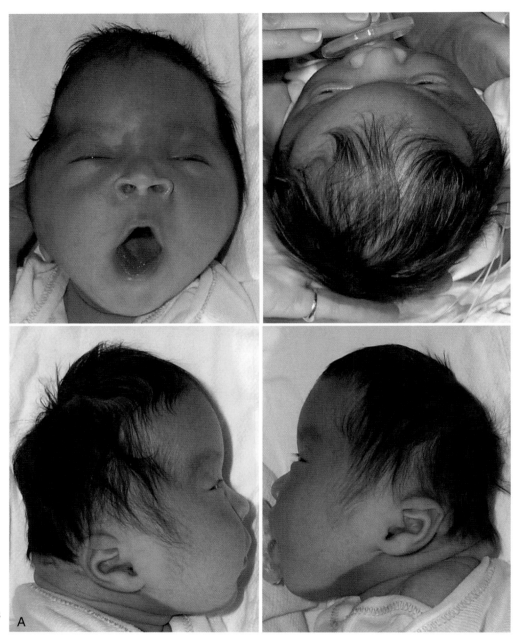

Fig. 28-3A Multiple suture synostosis resulting in a cloverleaf skull.

A

that which results from craniosynostosis, because therapy and management differ.

Epidemiology of Craniosynostosis

The incidence of craniosynostosis is 3.4 per 10,000 births, and it is usually an isolated, sporadic anomaly in an otherwise normal child. About 8 percent of all craniosynostosis cases are familial. Familial types of craniosynostosis are most frequent in coronal synostosis, accounting for 14.4 percent of coronal synostosis, 6 percent of sagittal synostosis, and 5.6 percent of metopic synostosis [Lajeunie et al., 1995, 1996, 1998], while lambdoidal synostosis is almost never familial. The frequency of associated twinning is increased, and most twin pairs are

discordant, especially with sagittal and metopic synostosis, which would tend to support fetal crowding as a cause for these types of synostosis; concordance for coronal synostosis is much higher for monozygotic twins than for dizygotic twins, suggesting that many cases of coronal synostosis have a genetic basis [Lajeunie et al., 1995].

Sagittal synostosis is the most common type of craniosynostosis, accounting for 50–60 percent of cases and occurring in 1.9 per 10,000 births, with a 3.5:1 male:female sex ratio [Lajeunie et al., 1996]. Only 6 percent of cases are familial, with 72 percent of cases sporadic and no paternal or maternal age effects noted. Twinning occurred in 4.8 percent of 366 cases, with only one monozygotic twin pair being concordant [Lajeunie et al., 1996].

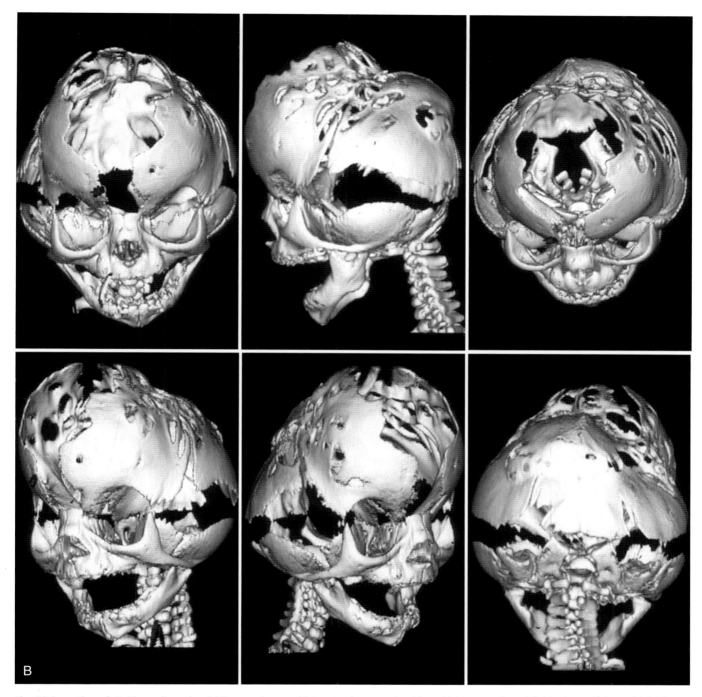

Fig. 28.3 continued. B, Three-dimensional CT scans show multiple sutural synostosis with multiple areas of cranial thinning, which would yield a "beaten copper" appearance on skull radiographs.

Coronal craniosynostosis is the second most frequent type of craniosynostosis (accounting for 20–30 percent of cases). Unilateral coronal craniosynostosis can be either genetic or due to fetal head constraint from an aberrant fetal lie, multiple gestation, or small uterine cavity [Graham et al., 1980; Higginbottom et al., 1980]. Approximately 71 percent of unilateral coronal craniosynostosis is right-sided, and 67 percent of vertex presentations are in the left occiput transverse position, possibly explaining the prevalence of right-sided, unilateral, coronal craniostenosis [Graham et al., 1980]. Non-syndromic coronal craniosynostosis occurs 0.94 per 10,000 births, with 61 percent of cases sporadic, and 14.4 percent of 180 pedigrees familial. Bilateral cases occur much more frequently than unilateral cases, and coronal synostosis is more frequent in females (male to female ratio 1:2). The paternal age is statistically older than average (32.7 years), and these data have been interpreted as being consistent with fresh dominant mutation and autosomal-dominant inheritance with 60 percent penetrance, when the synostosis has a genetic basis [Lajeunie et al., 1995].

Metopic synostosis occurs in about 0.67 per 10,000 births, making it the third most frequent type of craniosynostosis (accounting for 10–20 percent of patients). Like sagittal synostosis, metopic synostosis is more frequent in males (3.3:1 male: female ratio) and seldom familial (5.6 percent of cases) [Lajeunie et al., 1998]. There is no maternal or paternal age effect, and the frequency of associated twinning was 7.8 percent of 179 pedigrees studied, with only 2 twin monozygotic pairs concordant [Lajeunie et al., 1998].

Familial craniosynostosis is usually transmitted as an autosomal-dominant trait with incomplete penetrance and variable expressivity. A wide variety of chromosomal anomalies have also been associated with craniosynostosis. This emphasizes the importance of chromosomal analysis for patients with syndromic craniosynostosis in whom a recognizable monogenic syndrome is not apparent, particularly when there is associated developmental delay and growth deficiency. As comparative genomic hybridization becomes more widely utilized, this will be even more useful than standard cytogenetics for many such cases. In addition, craniosynostosis can also occur as a component of numerous syndromes, many of which manifest phenotypic overlap and genetic heterogeneity [Cohen and MacLean, 2000] Craniosynostosis syndromes with a demonstrated mutational basis include Apert's syndrome, Crouzon's syndrome, Pfeiffer's syndrome, Saethre–Chotzen syndrome, Jackson–Weiss syndrome, Boston craniosynostosis, Beare–Stevenson cutis gyrata syndrome, and fibroblast growth factor receptor 3 (FGFR3)-associated coronal synostosis; however, the efficiency of actually detecting a mutation for a given syndrome varies from about 60 percent for Crouzon's syndrome to 98 percent for Apert's syndrome [Cohen and MacLean, 2000].

Secondary craniosynostosis can occur with certain primary metabolic disorders (e.g., hyperthyroidism, rickets), storage disorders (e.g., mucopolysaccharidosis), hematological disorders (thalassemia, sickle cell anemia, polycythemia vera, congenital hemolytic icterus), brain malformations (e.g., holoprosencephaly, microcephaly, encephalocele, or overshunted hydrocephalus), and selected teratogenic exposures (e.g., diphenylhydantoin, retinoic acid, valproic acid, aminopterin, fluconazole, cyclophosphamide) [Cohen and MacLean, 2000].

Inability to demonstrate a mutation does not rule out a genetic basis for the craniosynostosis, and not every person with a pathogenic mutation manifests craniosynostosis. Bilateral coronal synostosis often lacks sutural ridging and usually has a genetic pathogenesis, suggesting that all such patients should be screened for mutations. Among 57 patients with bilateral coronal synostosis, mutations in FGFR genes were found for all 38 patients with a syndromic form of craniosynostosis. Among 19 patients with nonsyndromic bilateral craniosynostosis, mutations were found in or near exon 9 of FGFR2 in 4 patients, as well as the common Pro250Arg mutation being found in exon 7 of FGFR3 in 10 patients; only 5 patients (9 percent) lacked a detectable mutation in FGFR 1, 2, or 3 [Mulliken et al., 1999]. This study suggests that mutation analysis should be considered in most patients with bilateral coronal synostosis.

Kleeblattschadel (Cloverleaf Skull)

Kleeblattschadel is a term used to describe a cloverleaf skull configuration consisting of protrusion of each of the cranial bones, with broadening of the temporal region and face. These cranial protrusions are separated into focal bulges by furrows along the suture lines. The eyes often protrude, leading to corneal ulceration, scarring, and subsequent blindness, if the corneal surface remains unprotected [Stevenson, 1986]. Occipital encephaloceles can occur, and associated hydrocephalus is common. The palate is usually highly arched, but clefting is rare. The presence of Kleeblattschadel indicates that multiple sutural fusions occurred during early prenatal life. Increased thickening of the base of the occipital bone prevents lengthening of the skull, thus yielding the typical shape [Dambrain et al., 1987]. One child has also been described who had a cloverleaf skull without craniosynostosis (in which the primary defect was thought to be a cranial bone dysplasia that allowed for eventration of the brain and resultant cloverleaf configuration) [DR, 1988].

Multiple sutural synostosis is much more likely to result from genetic mutations in FGFR genes, TWIST, or MSX2, all of which result in syndromes which can present with cloverleaf skull [Cohen and MacLean, 2000]. The most common syndrome associated with cloverleaf skull is thanatophoric dysplasia type 2, which is due to mutations in *FGFR3*. Type 2 Pfeiffer's syndrome, due to mutations in *FGFR2*, can result in cloverleaf skull, as can Crouzon's syndrome and Apert's syndrome, which are also due to mutations in *FGFR2*. Other syndromes, like FGFR3-associated coronal synostosis, rarely result in cloverleaf skull, but some rare syndromes like Boston craniosynostosis and Crouzon's syndrome with acanthosis nigricans can sometimes manifest cloverleaf skull. In Boston craniosynostosis, the mutant MSX2 product has enhanced affinity for binding to its DNA target sequence, resulting in activated osteoblastic activity and aggressive cranial ossification [Warman et al., 1993; Jabs et al., 1993; Ma et al., 1996]. In Crouzon's syndrome with acanthosis nigricans, a specific *FGFR3* mutation (Ala391Glu), leads to early onset of acanthosis nigricans during childhood, often with associated choanal atresia and hydrocephalus [Schweitzer et al., 2001].

Eighty-five percent of children with Kleeblattschadel will have other anomalies, and the pattern is often consistent with a syndrome diagnosis. The prognosis is usually syndrome-dependent and can be quite poor, with early death due to respiratory difficulties or progressive brain damage from hydrocephalus being common [Frank et al., 1985]. However, subtotal craniectomy within the first 3 weeks of life in individuals with mild Kleeblattschadel may result in normal or near-normal development [Frank et al., 1985; Kroczek et al., 1986; Turner and Reynolds, 1980]. Early extensive calvariectomy is merited to preserve brain function and development, as well as to allow reformation of the craniofacial skeletal features. Many craniofacial surgeons prefer to begin with a posterior skull release in the early months of life (mean age 4 months), followed by fronto-orbital advancement around the end of the first year (mean age 14 months), with insertion of a ventriculo-peritoneal shunt at the time of the first procedure if there is associated hydrocephalus [Sgouros et al., 1996]. The use of postoperative orthotic molding can help to channel brain growth into a more normal form, leading to improved postoperative results over those obtained via surgery alone [Schweitzer et al., 2001]. When lambdoid synostosis occurs as part of a syndrome with multiple suture involvement, there is often bilateral involvement, and early posterior release may alleviate some associated increased intracranial pressure. Patients with Kleeblattschadel need to be followed carefully for hydrocephalus, which may be part of the syndrome, rather than due to the multiple suture synostosis. Restricted growth of the posterior fossa is particularly common in severe craniofacial dysostosis syndromes. The purpose of surgery should be to decompress the brain, expand the bony orbits to accommodate the globes, and open airway passages [Kroczek et al., 1986].

Treatment and Outcomes of Craniosynostosis

Mild degrees of craniosynostosis may not always require surgery; however, in moderately severe cases, early surgery is usually warranted. The usual indication for surgery is to restore normal craniofacial shape and growth. When both the coronal and sagittal sutures are synostotic, impairing brain growth early in infancy, surgery is indicated to help prevent neurological and ophthalmologic complications associated with increased intracranial pressure and inadequate orbital volume. A variety of neurosurgical techniques have been developed for the treatment of craniosynostosis [Cohen and MacLean, 2000]. Most of these techniques involve removing the aberrant portion of the bony calvarium from its underlying dura, including the area surrounding the synostotic suture(s). If this is done within the first few months after birth, a new bony calvarium will usually develop within the remaining dura mater under the same principles that guide normal prenatal calvarial morphogenesis. As long as there is continued growth stretch from the expanding brain, the sites over the dural reflections remain unossified, thereby maintaining the sutures in a fibrous, open state. Thus, the calvarium and its sutures usually re-form normally after a partial calvariectomy for craniosynostosis. The new bony calvarium begins to develop within 2–3 weeks after surgery, and is usually firm by 5–8 weeks after surgery. If the procedure is done after 3–4 months of age, the approach is similar, with the exception that pieces of the calvarium are usually replaced in a mosaic pattern over the dura mater to act as niduses for the mineralization of new calvarium. Newer endoscopic repair techniques have been developed, followed by postoperative orthotic molding. Such procedures are most effective if done relatively early in infancy. These techniques are most effective in normal infants without a syndromic type of craniosynostosis.

Following early surgery for isolated craniosynostosis (primarily fronto-orbital advancement and/or calvarial vault remodeling at a mean age of 8 months), only 13 percent of 104 patients (10 bilateral coronal, 57 unilateral coronal, 29 metopic, and 8 sagittal) required a second cranial vault operation for residual defects at a mean age of 23 months. Perioperative complications were minimal (5 percent), with 87.5 percent of patients considered to have satisfactory craniofacial form, and low rates of hydrocephalus (3.8 percent), shunt placement (1 percent), and seizures (2.9 percent). Among such cases of isolated craniosynostosis, unilateral coronal synostosis was the most problematic type due to vertical orbital dystopia, nasal tip deviation, and altered craniofacial growth problems with residual craniofacial asymmetry [McCarthy et al., 1995]. In a second study of 167 children with both

nonsyndromal (isolated) and syndromal craniosynostosis (12 bilateral coronal, 18 unilateral coronal, 39 metopic, and 46 sagittal), repeat operations were necessary in only 7 percent. Repeat operations were more common in syndromic cases (27.3 percent) than in nonsyndromic craniosynostosis (5.6 percent) [Williams et al., 1997].

Even though intracranial pressure can be elevated in patients with nonsyndromic craniosynostosis, they may not have decreased cranial volumes either before or after surgical repair, and as a group show slightly larger intracranial volumes when compared with normal controls. This could reflect the impact of fetal head constraint on fetuses with larger heads, or it might relate to the known association of macrocephaly with nonsyndromic coronal craniosynostosis due to the common Pro250Arg mutation in *FGFR3* (which was not analyzed in these studies) [Polley et al., 1998]. Hydrocephalus occurs in 4–10 percent of patients with craniosynostosis and is more frequent with syndromic and multiple sutural craniosynostosis. In nonsyndromic patients, the rate of cerebral ventricular dilatation is the same as that observed in the general population, and it appears to be related to venous hypertension induced by jugular foramen stenosis. Such dilatation usually stabilizes spontaneously and rarely requires shunting. Some cases of progressive hydrocephalus in syndromic craniosynostosis cases were related to multiple sutural involvement, thereby constricting cranial volume, constricting the skull base, crowding the posterior fossa, and causing jugular foraminal stenosis [Cinalli et al., 1998]. These findings were most frequent among patients with Crouzon's, Pfeiffer's, and Apert's syndrome, especially in association with cloverleaf skull abnormalities. A diffuse beaten copper pattern on skull radiographs, along with obliteration of anterior sulci or narrowing of basal cisterns in children under the age of 18 months, is predictive of increased intracranial pressure in over 95 percent of cases [Tuite and Lindquist, 1996].

Nonsyndromic Craniosynostosis Neurocognitive Development

When considering neurocognitive outcomes in craniosynostosis, it is important to exclude primary defects of brain, such as the holoprosencephaly malformation complex, and syndromes, such as Opitz C trigonocephaly syndrome. Metopic craniosynostosis can also result from various chromosomal abnormalities, such as deletions of chromosome 9p22–p24 and 11q23–q24 (Jacobsen's syndrome). Since some of these chromosome abnormalities can be quite subtle, high-resolution chromosome studies or comparative genomic hybridization studies are indicated in children with associated malformations and neurodevelopmental problems.

There is a growing body of evidence that single-suture craniosynostosis is associated with neurobehavioral problems [Kapp-Simon, 1998; Magge et al., 2002]. In the 2004 manuscript, Speltz et al. nicely summarized all of the published neurobehavioral studies conducted on children with single suture craniosynostosis [Speltz et al., 2004].

Few studies have documented actual rates of mental retardation (typically defined as standardized test scores below 70). Several older studies reported slightly increased rates of mental retardation (from 6.5 to 12 percent) in comparison to an expected rate of about 2.2 percent in the population [Kapp-Simon, 1998; Hunter and Rudd, 1976, 1977; Sidoti et al., 1996].

Syndromes with multiple-suture fusions have more commonly been associated with elevated rates of mental retardation and learning disabilities [Cohen, 1991]. Most studies have found adverse neurocognitive outcomes in about 35–40 percent of assessed cases [Bottero et al., 1998; Shimoji et al., 2002; Shipster et al., 2003], with an occasional study finding this number to be as high as 50 percent [Kapp-Simon, 1998; Magge et al., 2002]. A few studies have reported a 3–5 times higher than average risk of poor neurobehavioral outcome. In studies that directly measured the IQs of children with sagittal synostosis, a discrepancy of greater than 20 standard score points between language and nonverbal IQ scores was found [Magge et al., 2002; Shipster et al., 2003]. In 2002, Magge et al. reported a 50 percent incidence of learning disability and found that verbal IQ was significantly higher than nonverbal IQ.

Sagittal synostosis has not been found to affect the neurological function of the infant or toddler significantly [Kapp-Simon et al., 1993]. However, older children may demonstrate moderately severe speech and language difficulties in up to 37 percent of cases, and the tendency toward such problems is associated with a positive family history for such difficulties and later age of surgical correction [Shipster et al., 2003; Virtanen et al., 1999; Panchal et al., 1999]. In a study of 30 older untreated children (average age 9.25 years) with sagittal synostosis, almost all patients and parents were pleased with their decision and patients demonstrated normal cognitive and school performance, as well as normal behavior and psychological adjustment on standardized testing [Boltshauser et al., 2003].

In a long-term neurodevelopmental outcome study of non-syndromic cases, a correlation was found between outcomes and timing of surgery, with 22.6 percent of those operated on before 12 months showing impaired mental development, versus 52.2 percent impaired mental development in those operated on after age 12 months. Overall, 31 percent of trigonocephaly cases had delayed development, and this appeared to be related to the severity of the problem and the presence of associated malformations [Bottero et al., 1998].

Wide Cranial Sutures

Cranial sutures are considered to be widened when the sutural separation is more than 2 SD above the mean sutural width for age. Diagnosis is confirmed radiographically, although it may also be appreciated on palpation of the skull. Criteria for determining suture width in infants up to 45 days old have been published by Erasmie and Ringertz [Erasmie and Ringertz, 1976]. Wide cranial sutures in themselves cause no impairment, but they can be an indication of increased intracranial pressure or caused by craniosynostosis in another part of the skull. Wide cranial sutures are a feature of numerous syndromes (e.g., cleidocranial dysostosis, Hajdu–Cheney syndrome, or pycnodysostosis) with several proposed causes including increased intracranial pressure, delayed maturation of bone, or resorption of bone. The younger the child, the earlier sutural diastasis will appear after acutely increased intracranial pressure. The prognosis depends on the underlying cause.

Anomalies of Fontanels

A fontanel whose size is either 2 SD above or 2 SD below the mean for age is termed large or small, respectively. Closure of the anterior fontanel before 6 months is considered early, whereas closure after 18 months is late. The other fontanels are normally closed at birth.

The anterior fontanel is the largest of the fontanels, is diamond-shaped, and normally closes by 18 months. The posterior fontanel is triangular in shape and is usually closed at birth. Fontanel size may be measured in several different ways. Measurement of the anterior fontanel may be expressed as width (measurement along the coronal suture), length (measurement along the sagittal suture), area (width × length), or diagonal diameter. Standard curves are available for measurements taken by each method [Hall, 2007]. The posterior fontanel is usually measured only in length (measurement along the sagittal suture), but may also be measured along the lambdoid suture (width) and the area calculated (length × width).

Depending on the cause, a small or absent anterior fontanel may be noted at birth by palpation and confirmed by measurement and comparison with normal values for length and width [Hall, 2007]. A small or absent anterior fontanel usually indicates some type of underlying pathology, with the most common etiologies including any cause of congenital microcephaly, craniosynostosis (particularly involving the metopic suture), or accelerated bone maturation such as occurs in hyperthyroidism [Popich and Smith, 1972].

Large fontanels may be noted at birth by palpation and confirmed by measurement. Causes of both large fontanels and delayed closure include increased intracranial pressure or delayed ossification of the cranium [Popich and Smith, 1972]. Cleidocranial dysplasia is a common genetic syndrome that results in delayed closure of the anterior fontanel with widened cranial sutures and hypoplastic clavicles.

Occasionally, the anterior fontanel will ossify into a bony plate, which may be slightly elevated in relation to the rest of the cranium. This may relate to decreased growth-stretch tensile forces across the anterior fontanel, and is sometimes seen in cases of craniosynostosis, but it can also occur in otherwise normal infants, in which case, it is considered a normal variant [Keats and Anderson, 2001]. Instead of the usual flat, uncalcified, diamond-shaped anterior fontanel, there is a slightly raised diamond-shaped plate of bone in its place.

A small or absent anterior fontanel may be secondary to microcephaly (because of decreased brain growth), craniosynostosis affecting the metopic, sagittal, and/or coronal suture, or accelerated osseous maturation. There have also been reports of normal infants with absent anterior fontanels at birth. The shape of the anterior fontanel bone often remains visible on skull radiographs throughout childhood and on into adulthood, with a characteristic appearance on Towne projection. The appearance of the fusing anterior fontanel bone can be confused with a depressed skull fracture in the lateral projection [Girdany and Blank, 1965]. Occasionally, children thought to have a small or absent anterior fontanel will be found to have an anterior intrafontanel bone, which is of no significance. Causes of large or late-closing fontanels include increased intracranial pressure or delayed ossification of the skull [Popich and Smith, 1972].

Anterior fontanel closure occurs in 1 percent of normal infants by age 3 months, in 38 percent by 12 months, in

70 percent by 18 months, and in 97 percent by 24 months [Duc and Largo, 1986]. Therefore, early or late closure is reasonably common, but care must be taken to rule out underlying pathology. In normal infants, there is no sex difference in the size and age of closure of the anterior fontanel; nor is there any correlation with gestational age at delivery, head circumference, or bone age. The size of the fontanel at birth does not predict time of closure [Duc and Largo, 1986].

Extra fontanels are inconsistently occurring bony defects situated along the suture lines or at the junction of major bone plates of the skull. One such extra fontanel occurs along the sagittal suture about 2 cm anterior to the posterior fontanel. This fontanel is called the obeliac, interparietal, or sagittal fontanel, as well as the fontanel of Gerdy. Being midline, it is distinct from the parietal foramen, but parietal foramina may involve the lateral extremes of a large sagittal fontanel. Glabellar, metopic, or cerebellar fontanels also exhibit extra fontanels [Sidoti et al., 1996]. Diagnosis of an extra fontanel is made by palpation or radiography. It is often an isolated malformation, but may sometimes be associated with rare syndromes. In all cases, prognosis is dependent on the underlying cause. If the anomaly is isolated, there is no ill effect.

A sagittal fontanel is found in 6.3 percent of all newborns and is caused by a lack of union at the medial edge of junction of the two parietal ossification centers. This union normally occurs by the seventh month of gestation, but may occur 2–3 months after birth [Cohen, 1991]. In one study of infants with a sagittal fontanel diameter of greater than 13 mm, 5 percent had major anomalies and 35 percent had minor anomalies. In those with a diameter less than 13 mm, 2 of 45 infants studied had Down's syndrome and 1 had a major anomaly. The latter group accounted for two-thirds of all children with this third fontanel [Keats and Anderson, 2001]. Although it is unknown whether there is ethnic variability in the prevalence of sagittal fontanels, the majority of individuals with this feature are male [Cohen, 1991]. Individuals with Down syndrome commonly have large fontanels that close late, along with a sagittal fontanel and persistence of the metopic suture [Cohen, 1991].

Cranial Dermal Sinus

A cranial dermal sinus is a midline depression or tract lined by stratified squamous epithelium that extends from the skin toward the central nervous system or its coverings. Cranial dermal sinuses are associated with bony defects in 80 percent of cases [Shackelf et al., 1974]. Diagnosis is best achieved radiographically via CT scan, which reveals a low-density lesion that may be surrounded by an enhancing ring [Starinsky et al., 1988]. Cranial dermal sinuses are most common in the occipital region, but can be found anywhere. Size can vary from a very small defect to a large, expanding mass. Clinical presentation is often as a cutaneous localized swelling that presents an infection or cystic expansion of the sinus tract beneath the skin surface, occasionally with drainage. There is often an abnormal distribution of hair along the defect. Occasionally, cystic expansion occurs within the cranial cavity, which obstructs cerebrospinal fluid flow, compresses the adjacent neural structures, and/or ruptures to cause sterile meningitis, which can be recurrent [Shackelf et al., 1974; Starinsky et al., 1988]. Cranial dermal sinuses are thought to be the result of faulty separation of neuroectoderm from cutaneous ectoderm during early gestation [Shackelf et al., 1974]. The recommended treatment is surgery; prognosis is good if treatment is done prior to the development of complications.

In the facial region, the most frequent congenital midline mass is a nasal dermoid sinus cyst, which can have intracranial extension and be associated with other anomalies [Posnick et al., 1994; Wardinsky et al., 1991]. Nasal dermoid sinus cysts constitute 11–12 percent of dermoids found in the head and neck [Wardinsky et al., 1991], and usually arise sporadically, although reports of familial occurrence have been documented [Posnick et al., 1994; Wardinsky et al., 1991]. At 50–60 days gestation, the nasal and frontal bones develop through intramembranous ossification, remaining separated by a space termed the fonticulus nasofrontalis. During growth, the nasal process of the frontal bone separates the skin from the dura, which maintains a connection between the base of the skull and the nasal tip via a dural projection, which ends at an opening in the frontal bones termed the foramen cecum. The foramen cecum eventually fuses with the fonticulus nasofrontalis in the area of the future cribriform plate, thereby obliterating this previous neuroectodermal connection. If this process remains incomplete, dermal connections (termed nasal dermoid sinus cysts) may occur anywhere from the nasal tip to the intracranial space through the foramen cecum [Posnick et al., 1994]. Such dermoid sinus cysts contain both ectodermal and mesodermal derivatives, and are composed of a stratified squamous epithelial lining, hair follicles, pilosebaceous glands, and smooth muscle [Posnick et al., 1994]. Nasal pits are present in 50 percent of patients with nasal dermoids [Mccaffrey et al., 1979]. often with hairs protruding from the pit, and they can appear anywhere along the nose, with intracranial extension noted in 36–45 percent of cases [Posnick et al., 1994; Wardinsky et al., 1991]. Associated anomalies were present in 41 percent of one series examined by a multidisciplinary team, and they were associated with many different syndromes, including hemifacial microsomia, oral-facial-digital (OFD) syndrome (type 1), frontonasal dysplasia, VATER (vertebral anomalies, anal anomalies, tracheoesophageal fistulae, esophageal atresia, renal and/or radial anomalies) association, and chromosome anomalies [Wardinsky et al., 1991]. Complications can result from enlargement of the cyst, skeletal distortion, and recurrent infection, so surgical excision is recommended after CT scanning to identify intracranial extension and plan the surgical approach.

Parietal Foramina (Includes Cranium Bifidum)

Parietal foramina are small defects in the superoposterior angles of the parietal bones via which emissary veins may pass through the calvarium (Figure 28-4). Usually, parietal foramina present as symmetrical oval defects situated on each side of the sagittal suture, and their size diminishes with age. They are covered with normal scalp and hair, and are detected through palpation and radiography. Occasionally, brain covered by dura and intact scalp can bulge through extensive lesions, suggesting the possibility of an encephalocele, but the location of these lesions off the midline differentiates them from neural tube closure defects.

Parietal foramina are usually small, with 60 percent being less than 1 mm. Such small defects are only detectable radiographically; however, 10 percent are 5 mm or more and can

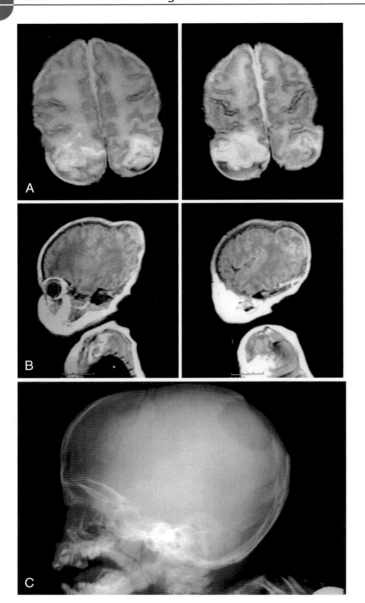

Fig. 28-4 Parietal foramina. A and **B,** Large parietal defects at birth detected by MRI. **C,** Partial closure by age 16 months on skull radiograph.

be as large as 50 mm in diameter. Reported individuals have had defects as large as 57 mm in diameter, with seizures apparently secondary to venous obstruction [Epstein and Epstein, 1967]. Small parietal foramina are found in 60–70 percent of all adults, whereas large parietal foramina are present in less than 1 percent of adults [O'Rahilly and Twohig, 1952; Little et al., 1990; Currarino, 1976]. Small unilateral defects are more common than bilateral defects. When the defect is unilateral, it more often involves the right side, and males are more commonly affected than females, with a ratio of 5:3 [O'Rahilly and Twohig, 1952]. Parietal foramina themselves cause no impairment, usually manifest autosomal-dominant inheritance with variable expression, and can occur as part of the phenotype in a few syndromes [Little et al., 1990].

Wilkie et al. [2000] described heterozygous *MSX2* mutations in three unrelated families with enlarged parietal foramina, suggesting that loss of *MSX2* activity results in calvarial defects

[Wilkie et al., 2000]. A second gene has been implicated in those families who do not link to 5q34–q35, where *MSX2* is located, and mutations or deletions of *ALX4* on 11p11.2 can also result in parietal foramina [Wu et al., 2000]. Parietal foramina can occur as an isolated trait due to mutations in or haploinsufficiency of *MSX2* or *ALX4*, or as a component of a multiple congenital anomaly syndrome, such as Saethre–Chotzen syndrome, cleidocranial dysplasia, or Rubinstein–Taybi syndrome. The combination of parietal foramina with multiple exostoses is now known to be a contiguous gene deletion of *ALX4* and *EXT2* on chromosome 11p11–p12 (also termed DEFECT11 syndrome).

Surgery is usually unnecessary, since the lesions tend to ossify in on their own, but occasionally a protective helmet is used for extensive defects. Care must be exercised during delivery to avoid trauma to the brain underlying such extensive parietal foraminal defects. Location and intact scalp tissue help to differentiate parietal foramina from encephaloceles. This lesion must also be differentiated from scalp vertex aplasia, which is also inherited in an autosomal-dominant fashion, when it is an isolated trait. There is usually denuded scalp over such lesions, which can include both scalp and calvarium, but their location in the midline near the hair whorl sets these lesions apart from parietal foramina. Finally, vertex craniotabes can present as an extensive area of incomplete calvarial ossification over the vertex in the midline, but the edges are not sharp and demarcated like parietal foramina, and vertex craniotabes ossifies quite rapidly within the first few months after birth.

Cranium bifidum literally means "cleft skull," and presents as a wide opening between the frontal and parietal bones, which normally begin their process of intramembranous ossification in the center of each bone and then spread towards the sutures. During mid-childhood, these areas ossify, leaving only symmetric openings in the frontal and parietal bones. One reported family included individuals with both cranium bifidum and parietal foramina, confirming the fact that cranium bifidum in infancy and early childhood can evolve into large parietal foramina in later childhood and adulthood [Little et al., 1990].

Wormian Bones

Wormian bones were named after Dr. Worm, who initially described them as accessory bones that occur within cranial suture lines or fontanels [Gooding, 1971; Pryles and Khan, 1979]. They can occur singly, or in large numbers, and are diagnosed radiographically. Although they can occur within any suture, they are rare in coronal or sagittal sutures (Figure 28-5). Although they do not cause any impairment themselves, their significance is variable. In one study, the majority of children with an "excessive" number of Wormian bones had some abnormality of the central nervous system [Pryles and Khan, 1979]. These abnormalities ranged from gross malformations to minimal brain dysfunction, though this study may have been biased since it arose from a hospital-based population. Thus, some individuals with many Wormian bones may have other anomalies and/or central nervous system dysfunction.

The pathogenesis of Wormian bones is thought to be related to intracranial strain along with open sutures causing ossification

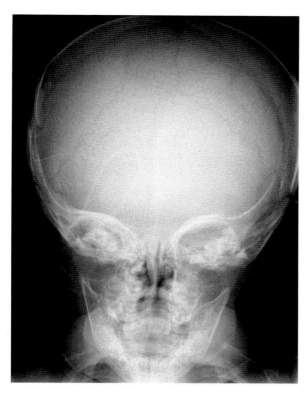

Fig. 28-5 **Osteogenesis type IV with marked osteopenia of the skull and spine, and multiple Wormian bones.** The patient also had a history of multiple fractures with minimal trauma.

defects [Sanchez-Lara et al., 2007]. Such sutural bones persist and are not incorporated into the adjacent bone during mineralization and maturation [Gooding, 1971]. Although the prevalence of Wormian bones in the general population is 17 percent, the prevalence varies with age. Males are more often affected than females, and differences between ethnic groups have been noted. Wormian bones are commonly seen in osteogenesis imperfecta and other disorders resulting in defective cranial bone mineralization. The more severe the defective mineralization, the more numerous the Wormian bones, and such infants can also become quite brachycephalic as a consequence of postnatal supine positioning with soft cranial bones [Graham et al., 2005]. The increased frequency of Wormian bones in Chinese infants might relate to traditional supine sleep positioning practices in this population, and their resultant brachycephaly. If so, an increased frequency of Wormian bones may soon be noted in other cultures that now follow recommendations for supine sleep positioning to prevent sudden infant death syndrome (SIDS).

Scalp Vertex Aplasia

Scalp vertex aplasia, or aplasia cutis congenita (ACC), is a relatively common congenital defect resulting in localized absence of skin, usually occurring on the scalp as an isolated finding not associated with other abnormalities. Scalp vertex aplasia begins as multiple or solitary, sharply marginated, raw areas with absence of skin. These lesions mature into atrophic scars devoid of adnexal structures, usually in the vertex area or midline superior occipital region (Figure 28-6) [Tann and Tay, 1997]. The cause of these lesions is heterogeneous and includes vascular disruption, trauma, teratogens, and genetic factors [Evers et al.,

1995]. Because vascular disruption and placental infarcts are seen in antiphospholipid antibody syndrome, some cases of extensive scalp vertex aplasia may be related to the effects of this maternal disease state or some other type of thrombophilia during pregnancy [Evers et al., 1995; Roll et al., 1999]. The frequency is 1 per 3000 live births, and a classification system of subtypes for ACC has been suggested by Frieden.

Lesions may be ulcerated, bullous, cicatricial, or covered with a tough, translucent membrane, and they occasionally extend to the bone or dura [Tann and Tay, 1997]. They may be circular, elongated, stellate, or triangular in shape, and of variable depth [Rudolph et al., 1974], with 86 percent of the solitary lesions occurring on the scalp, most often near the parietal hair whorl [Demmel, 1975; Stephan et al., 1982]. Type 1 ACC manifests scalp involvement without other abnormalities, and when familial, it manifests autosomal-dominant inheritance [Fimiani et al., 1999; Itin and Pletscher, 1988]. Less frequently, other parts of the body may be involved, with or without associated defects. When the lesions are midline and overlying the spine or midcranium, they can be associated with occult spinal dysraphism or tiny encephaloceles (ACC type 4). When there are multiple areas of ACC involving primarily the lower extremities, particularly the flank, thighs, and knees, a careful examination of the placenta may reveal a fetus papyraceus, which occurs 1 in 12,000 live births and affects 1 in 200 twin pregnancies [Leaute-Labreze et al., 1998; Daw, 1983; Mannino et al., 1977].

Larger defects can be complicated by hemorrhage, venous thrombosis, and rarely meningitis. With extensive ACC and other vasculodisruptive defects, survival during the neonatal period can be severely compromised [Lane and Zanol, 2000]. ACC can be associated with teratogenic or genetic disorders, and it is important to search for associated malformations in order to counsel parents concerning prognosis and recurrence risks in relation to the underlying disorder. ACC associated with epidermal nevus or nevus sebaceus syndrome (or ACC type 3) is the association of a sebaceous nevus (a linear yellow verrucous nevus) on the head and neck with variable ocular, cerebral, neurological, skeletal, cardiac, and other abnormalities, usually on a sporadic basis [Shields et al., 1997; Hogler et al., 1999]. Epidermolysis bullosa (EB) is a term applied to a group of hereditary skin disorders that result in the formation of blisters after minor skin trauma. EB can be associated with pyloric atresia and/or ACC; it manifests autosomal-recessive inheritance and histopathology is usually of the junctional type [Maman et al., 1998]. These findings suggest that when ACC occurs with EB, it is most likely to be autosomal-recessive, and some cases of junctional EB with pyloric atresia have demonstrated mutations in integrin beta 4 [Maman et al., 1998]. Finally, ACC has been associated with numerous cytogenetic and genetic malformation syndromes as ACC type 9 [Evers et al., 1995; Fimiani et al., 1999; Zvulunov et al., 1998; Edwards et al., 1994].

Wound treatment in cases of superficial ulceration is conservative, with antibacterial dressings, but extensive or deep lesions may require reconstruction of the scalp. Small hairless areas can be excised and covered with a neighboring flap from the scalp [Kruk-Jeromin et al., 1998]. This approach works for the most common scalp ACC lesions, which are frequently round, punched-out lesions in the vertex region, or less frequently triangular lesions in the temporal region (termed temporal triangular alopecia) [Kruk-Jeromin et al., 1998; Trakimas et al., 1994]. With extensive scalp lesions (over 6 cm in diameter), it is especially important to avoid eschar

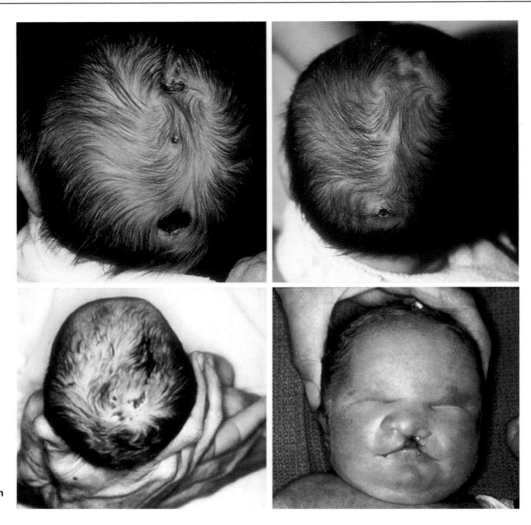

Fig. 28-6 Aplasia cutis congenita in association with trisomy 13.

formation immediately after birth by covering exposed dura with split-thickness skin grafts from adjacent healthy scalp and moist dressings. Prompt closure is important because of the high risk of fatal hemorrhage from the sagittal sinus when the eschar becomes dry and separated, causing the underlying dura to become damaged and to tear [Yang and Yang, 2000]. Once the superficial defect is completely healed, the subsequent scar alopecia may be treated by tissue-expanded local flaps, pericranial flaps, or free vascularized flaps when the child is older. With prompt closure and a healthy underlying dura, cranial bone growth will occur after prompt early wound closure, and the risk of fatal hemorrhage or meningitis is greatly lessened [Yang and Yang, 2000].

Thin Cranial Bones

Thin cranial bones are those that appear thinner than average and have little or no diploe. The diagnosis of thin cranial bones is made radiographically and is usually subjective [Ethier, 1971]. Thin calvarial bones can be secondary to craniosynostosis (particularly adjacent to the ridging in sagittal synostosis) and hydrocephalus, or can occur as part of several syndromes in which undermineralization is a feature [Hodges, 1989]. Areas of radiolucency are called craniolacunae (luckenschadel) and are often secondary to spinal dysraphism. These generally disappear by

age 1 year [McRae, 1971]. Regionally thinned areas can also occur in association with porencephaly, subdural hygroma, arachnoid cyst, and some tumors [Hodges, 1989]. Generalized thinning of cranial bones also results from increased dural distension, when expansion of the brain outpaces the growth of the skull. In other instances, undermineralization is the cause. As with thickened cranial bones, it is unknown whether thin cranial bones can occur as an isolated trait. Craniolacunae probably represent defective membranous bone formation, particularly along the inner periosteum of the cranial vault [McRae, 1971]. Craniolacunae probably do not occur as isolated traits. Prognosis is dependent on the underlying cause of this condition, and lacunar skull defects themselves have no direct effects on the infant.

Undermineralization of the Skull

Undermineralization of the skull results in increased radiolucency of the cranial bones and is attributable to decreased calcium deposition. Congenital undermineralization occurs in a number of syndromes, particularly osteogenesis imperfecta and hypophosphatasia (see Figure 28-5). Hypophosphatasia occurs in at least three forms, including infantile, childhood, and adult forms. Undermineralization is most pronounced in the infantile form and least evident in the adult form. The infantile form can usually be diagnosed by fetal ultrasound, whereas the other forms are often diagnosed after birth by radiographs and measurement of serum alkaline phosphatase levels [Goodman and Gorlin, 1983; Wynne-Davies et al., 1985]. Fluorosis and vitamin D-dependent rickets can also produce postnatal undermineralization of the skull, but areas of sclerosis are also present in fluorosis. The incidence of undermineralization is low, and prognosis is dependent on cause, varying widely from stillbirth or death during infancy to little effect at all.

Craniotabes

Prolonged forceful pressure on the fetal vertex may result in diminished cranial mineralization affecting the superior portions of the parietal bones. Such craniotabes is more likely to occur in first-born infants, especially with early fetal head descent into a vertex presentation for a prolonged period of time. Mild degrees of craniotabes occur in about 2 percent of newborn babies, and more extensive degrees of craniotabes are less common [Fox and Maier, 1984]. Craniotabes was first described in congenital syphilis, and it can also be seen with subclinical rickets due to vitamin D deficiency [Kokkonen et al., 1983]. Rickets should be considered in any infant with a nonvertex presentation, whose mother might be at risk for nutritional deficiency, and such infants usually manifest generalized craniotabes with osteomalacia.

With compression-related craniotabes, the superior parieto-occipital region tends to be soft to palpation, and often indents upon finger compression. In extreme cases, the entire top of the head can be involved. The presence of normally firm bone along the sides of the calvarium and in the mastoid regions readily differentiates this benign form of craniotabes from more generalized problems of decreased mineralization, such as hypophosphatasia, osteogenesis imperfecta, or infantile rickets. Within the affected region of the calvarium, the sutures and fontanels may also feel wider than usual. Accentuated vertex molding can be an associated feature in a fetus with prolonged vertex engagement. Benign vertex craniotabes has not been reported in babies in breech presentation, and radiolucency of the parietal bones in the vertex of the skull is considered to be a normal anatomic variant on neonatal head CT scans [Pastakia and Herdt, 1984].

With compression-related craniotabes, the prognosis is excellent, and the calvarium usually mineralizes in a normal fashion within 1–2 months after birth [Graham and Smith, 2007]. If the mother has vitamin D-deficient rickets and there is more generalized craniotabes and osteomalacia, this condition usually manifests a prompt response to vitamin D therapy over the next few months. Vitamin D-deficient rickets generally is accompanied by metaphyseal changes at the wrist and low 25-hydroxyvitamin D concentrations (less than 12 ng/mL), with a variably elevated alkaline phosphatase level. As in other defects of skeletal mineralization, such as osteogenesis imperfecta and hypophosphatasia, initial care must be taken to avoid fractures. Infants with osteogenesis imperfecta or hypophosphatasia usually show generalized osteomalacia, brittle bones, and Wormian bones.

Thick Cranial Bones

Increased thickness of cranial bones is detected on radiographic examination, and there may be normal or increased cranial density. The calvarium has three tables; the inner and outer tables are composed of compact bone, while the middle table (diploe) consists of cancellous bone. In general, the thickness of the normal skull is proportionate to the width of the middle table. The diagnosis of a thickened cranium is made radiographically, although no formal criteria have been established for determining whether cranial bones are thick. Although there is wide variability among different individuals, the thickest part of a normal cranium is not, in general, any greater than 1 cm. There are both ethnic- and sex-related variations in skull thickness. Women have thicker skulls than men, and blacks have thicker skulls than whites.

Numerous syndromes with thick calvarial bones have been described. It is unknown whether thick cranial bones can occur as an isolated trait, and the prognosis depends on the underlying condition. Thickening of the middle table is usually a manifestation of overproliferation of bone marrow in hemolytic disease or bone diseases. In hemolytic diseases, such as thalassemia, vertical striations ("hair-on-end" appearance) occur, whereas in bone diseases such as osteopetrosis, sclerosis occurs [Hodges, 1989]. Overgrowth of the middle table can also occur in microcephaly. In situations in which a shunt has been placed to relieve hydrocephalus, thickening of both inner and middle tables can occur.

Sclerosis and Hyperostosis of the Skull

Increased density or overmineralization of the cranial bones can be generalized or localized, and this is termed sclerosis or hyperostosis of the skull. Sclerosis generally refers to an increase in bone density without an alteration in width, while hyperostosis is caused by bone overgrowth that leads to an increase in density and width, though not all cases fit cleanly into one category or the other [Kozlowski and Beighton, 1995]. Hyperostosis is distinct from thick cranial bones, although hyperostosis and occasionally sclerosis can also cause thick cranial bones [Ethier, 1971]. Most of the sclerosing bone dysplasias manifest generalized changes, which are classified on the basis of the distribution and configuration of these abnormalities. One subclassification divides these disorders into osteosclerosis, craniotubular dysplasis, and craniotubular hyperostoses. In such conditions, basal sclerosis may be present without significant calvarial involvement, but the converse rarely occurs [Kozlowski and Beighton, 1995].

The presence of sclerosis or hyperostosis can be diagnosed radiographically or by CT, and scintigraphy may provide information on disease progression (Figure 28-7) [Kumar et al., 1981]. Radiologic changes are age-related, and definitive diagnosis may be difficult in early childhood [Kozlowski and Beighton, 1995]. All conditions that cause generalized osteosclerosis affect the skull [Kozlowski and Beighton, 1995]. Localized sclerosis of the base of the skull can occur in fibrous dysplasia, Jansen-type metaphyseal dysplasia, severe anemia, hypercalciuria, and Paget's disease. It may also be seen with a meningioma or inflammation [Kozlowski and Beighton, 1995]. Symptoms include narrowing of cranial nerve foramina, which in turn can cause nerve palsy, deafness, or vision defects [Beighton et al., 1976]. Increased intracranial pressure is not uncommon, and papilledema can also occur as a complication. Craniosynostosis also occurs in some cases, perhaps related to overstimulation of bone

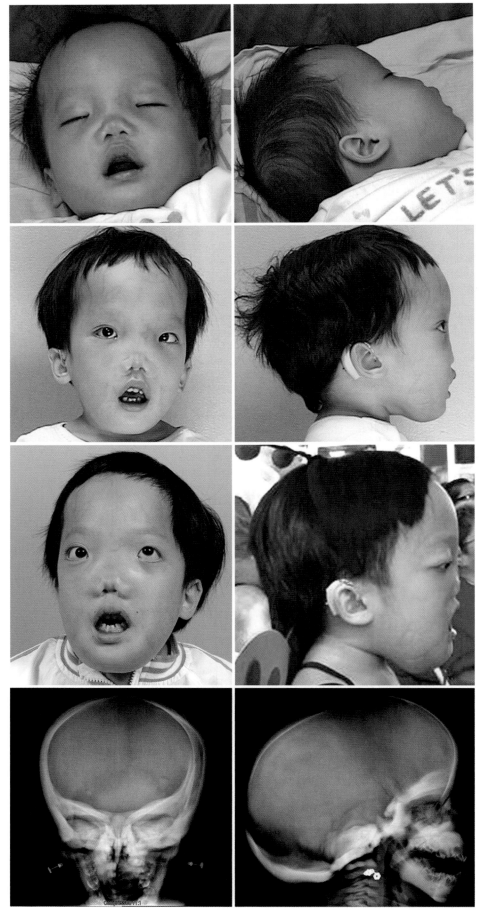

Fig. 28-7 Craniometaphyseal dysplasia presenting with progressive craniofacial changes and hearing loss.

growth along suture edges. Several syndromes have sclerosis as a feature.

Two primary pathologic processes can lead to sclerosis: overproduction of bone and/or failure of osteoclastic absorption of bone [Ethier, 1971]. The prognosis depends on the underlying cause and varies from individuals being asymptomatic to sudden death from medullary compression. In addition, facial palsy, as well as hearing and vision loss, may occur due to cranial nerve compression within stenotic foramina, which may require surgical decompression [Kumar et al., 1981; Beighton et al., 1976]. Craniotomy to relieve increased intracranial pressure may also be indicated.

Anomalies of the Sella Turcica

Anomalies include abnormal size and/or shape of the sella turcica, which is the central depression within the sphenoid bone that contains the pituitary gland. Assessment of the sella turcica can best be done radiographically or by CT [Pribam, 1971]. Measurements of normal sella turcica size have been published, with considerable overlap between normal and abnormal ranges [Fisher and Dichiro, 1964; Oon, 1963]. Small sellas have been described in patients with hypopituitarism and myotonic dystrophy, whereas large sellas occur in patients with storage disorders, pituitary tumors, empty sella syndrome, craniopharyngioma, intrasellar aneurysm, untreated hypogonadism, and hypothyroidism.

A J-shaped sella describes the lateral profile of the sella turcica, in which the sella resembles a "J" lying on its side. A J-shaped sella can occur as a normal variant, but may also occur in individuals with calvarial enlargement or optic nerve gliomas [Swischuk, 1972]. Bridged sella is caused by bony bridging between anterior and posterior clinoids and can be a normal variant. It can also be seen in nevoid basal cell carcinoma syndrome (Gorlin's syndrome).

The sphenoid bone consists of two main cartilaginous parts (hypophyseal cartilage) until the seventh or eighth month of gestation. The presphenoid will contribute to the anterior part of the sella turcica, while the postsphenoid forms the remainder. At birth, the sella is only a small depression; it begins to ossify soon after birth. Since 80 percent of the sella is occupied by the pituitary gland, it is not unusual for pituitary anomalies to cause abnormalities in the sella. In individuals with optic nerve gliomas, the chiasmatic groove will appear scalloped, whereas in cases of calvarial enlargement it will appear elongated [Swischuk, 1972]. Sellar abnormalities do not themselves require treatment. However, they are usually indicative of an underlying pathologic process that may require treatment. Prognosis, therefore, is dependent on the underlying cause.

Anomalies of Foramen Magnum

The foramen magnum is normally an oval-shaped opening in the occipital bone bounded anteriorly by the basiocciput, laterally by the occipital condyles, and posteriorly by the supraocciput [McRae, 1971]. These bones are separated by two anterior and two posterior synchondroses that begin to fuse at 12 months and completely fuse by 3–4 years and 7 years, respectively [Hecht et al., 1985]. If enchondral ossification is abnormal, or suture fusion premature, or both, a small foramen magnum is the result. Anomalies include either small

or large size, or a keyhole shape. MRI best achieves diagnostic assessment of foramen magnum size or shape, although radiography or CT may also be used. Tables have been published indicating normal foramen magnum size [Hecht et al., 1985]. Effects of a small foramen magnum vary from producing no symptoms to being associated with weakness, apneic spells, hyperreflexia, hydrocephalus, and abnormal somatosensory-evoked potentials and/or polysomnograms [Hecht et al., 1985]. Achondroplasia is the most common syndrome in which a small foramen magnum occurs, but other skeletal dysplasias and disorders associated with sclerosis of the skull can also lead to a small foramen magnum. Patients with achondroplasia usually do not experience neurological complications until the foramen magnum is 4 SD or more below the mean [Hecht et al., 1985], and 96 percent of achondroplastic patients with neurological manifestations have foramen magnum sizes more than 3 SD below the mean [Wang et al., 1987]. A small foramen magnum can be accompanied by a short cranial base, and anterior herniation of the brain through an open metopic suture has been known to occur in such cases [McRae, 1971]. Premature synostosis of one or two sutures may cause asymmetry [Coin, 1971]. A large foramen magnum usually results from chronic increased intracranial pressure or from direct effects of an expanding process within the foramen magnum (syringomyelia, Arnold–Chiari malformation) [Wang et al., 1987; Coin, 1971; Salonen et al., 1981]. Asymmetry of the foramen magnum occurs with craniovertebral anomalies or premature synostosis of one or more of the occipital synchondroses [Coin, 1971]. Children with the latter may tend to hold their heads obliquely. A keyhole-shaped foramen magnum has been described in the hydrolethalus syndrome [Salonen et al., 1981].

Prognosis for a small foramen magnum is variable, but the most serious outcome of brainstem compression may be sudden death. Recommended treatment is suboccipital craniectomy [Hecht et al., 1985]. The prognosis for a large or abnormally shaped foramen magnum is dependent on the underlying cause.

Anomalies of the Other Basal Foramena and Canals

Anomalies of other basal foramina can include abnormal configuration or size of openings in the basal part of the skull that transmit nerves, blood vessels, or both. There are at least 11 foramina and canals in the base of the cranium through which blood vessels and nerves enter or leave the intracranial space. Increased intracranial pressure, aneurysms, tumors, and arteriovenous malformations can all cause pathologic enlargement of these foramina. Congenital anomalies include asymmetry of paired foramina, communication with other foramina, and absence if the transmitted structure is absent. Diagnosis of these anomalies is achieved radiographically or by using basal tomography, although they are usually incidental findings.

Basilar Impression

Basilar impression is a malformation or deformation of the cranial base consisting of indentation of the base of the skull at the craniospinal junction. Primary basilar impression is a malformation in which the base of the skull and the upper two cervical vertebrae fail to segment and exist as a bony mass within which the posterior fossa, brainstem, and upper cervical spinal cord may become compressed. Some degree of basilar impression may occur with platybasia, defined as a craniocervical angle of greater than 140°. Basilar impression may be suspected when there is limited movement and shortening of the neck, but definitive diagnosis requires radiography, CT scan, or MRI scan [Sondheimer, 1971]. In basilar impression, the odontoid moves cephalad and can protrude into the foramen magnum, thus compromising function of the spinal cord, brainstem, and cerebellum, as well as impeding the flow of cerebrospinal fluid. Symptoms include pain, limitation of movement, increased intracranial pressure, hydrocephalus, and cranial nerve symptoms [Teodori and Painter, 1984; Roger et al., 1948]. Symptoms may appear suddenly or develop over several months.

Primary basilar impression is caused by a congenital defect of osseous structures in the cervico-occipital region, and can occur as an autosomal-dominant trait [Bull et al., 1955]. Secondary basilar impression is related to disease of the skull. It has been reported in association with Paget's disease, histiocytosis X, rheumatoid arthritis, rickets, and hypoparathyroidism. It also occurs in several skeletal dysplasias and malformation syndromes. The incidence in the general population is 1 in 3300, although it may be more common in Eskimos, and in cultures where carrying heavy loads on the top of the head is practiced [Teodori and Painter, 1984].

The prognosis is quite variable. Affected individuals may be asymptomatic, develop sudden or progressive symptoms, or die suddenly. Most patients present with symptoms in late childhood or early adulthood, which corresponds to the time of closure of the anterior synchondroses (6 years) and spheno-occipital synchondrosis (25 years) of the occipital bone [Adam, 1987]. Treatment consists of immobilization or, in severe cases, decompression of the foramen magnum, laminectomy of the first and second cervical vertebrae, and cervico-occipital fusion [Rush et al., 1989]. Shunting for hydrocephalus may also be indicated.

Miscellaneous Anomalies of the Skull

Paracondylar Process

A paracondylar process is an asymptomatic anatomic variant that is visible only on CT; it consists of a process of bone that arises from the lateral aspect of the condyloid process and extends toward the transverse process of the atlas. It is generally of no significance, but has been reported in children with hemifacial microsomia. It is present in 7–8 percent of all human skulls [Silverman et al., 1993].

Bathrocephaly

Bathrocephaly is a skull deformation that appears as a steplike deformity at the back of the skull, and it is also termed an occipital shelf. It is not associated with craniosynostosis, but can occur secondary to breech position in utero. When associated with breech presentation, the head is usually also dolichocephalic in shape. When associated with other abnormal fetal positions, such as a transverse lie, face presentation, or brow presentation, the forehead may be compressed. Hence, any constraining fetal position that retroflexes the head against the posterior neck and shoulders can result in bathrocephaly. Other anomalies related to breech presentation are often present, and these include dislocated hips, congenital muscular torticollis, clubfoot, or uplifted earlobes. In general, this anomaly is of no significance, and spontaneous improvement usually occurs. Prognosis is poor only if breech position is secondary to malformation or neurological dysfunction [Silverman et al., 1993].

Occipital Horns

Occipital horns are bony protuberances situated on both sides of the foramen magnum and pointing caudad. They have only been described in individuals with an X-linked syndrome that also includes obstructive uropathy, joint laxity, and other features of Ehlers–Danlos type IX [Lazoff et al., 1975].

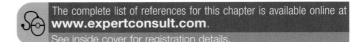

The complete list of references for this chapter is available online at **www.expertconsult.com**. See inside cover for registration details.

Prenatal Diagnosis of Structural Brain Anomalies

Tally Lerman-Sagie, Gustavo Malinger, and Liat Ben-Sira

Introduction

The fetal brain develops during the course of pregnancy, from its primitive three-vesicle stage into a complex structure with an array of sulci and gyri resembling the adult brain by the end of gestation [Nadich et al., 1994]. Fetal brain development is characterized by well-defined, genetically programmed, morphological and maturational changes, including neuronal migration, sulcation, and myelination that can be studied by ultrasound, starting from gestational week 6–7 until delivery [Ertl-Wagner et al., 2002]. Fetal magnetic resonance imaging (MRI) enables good demonstration of anatomy, particularly of cortical development and diagnosis of diverse anomalies, starting at around 18–20 weeks of pregnancy.

Sonography is the most important imaging method for prenatal malformation screening. It is noninvasive, widely available, and safe for both mother and child. The ultrasonographic approach to the evaluation of the fetal brain is based on the transabdominal visualization of three different axial planes: the transventricular, the transthalamic, and the transcerebellar (Figure 29-1). The use of these three planes enables good visualization of the lateral ventricles but is not sufficient for depiction of malformations of the cortex and of midline brain structures, mainly the corpus callosum, the third ventricle, and the cerebellar vermis [Malinger et al., 2007]. The use of a more comprehensive, multiplanar approach, in which coronal and sagittal planes are added to the classical axial planes, and addition of a transvaginal or transfundal approach overcome these limitations [Malinger et al., 1993] (Figure 29-2 and Figure 29-3).

Fetal MRI is used primarily to confirm and characterize brain abnormalities detected by routine prenatal sonography. More than 25 years after its introduction into fetal imaging, MRI is considered a valuable complementary tool in the imaging of structural anomalies of the fetal brain [Guibaud, 2009; Sonigo et al., 1998].

Implementation of fast and ultrafast sequences has allowed reduction of acquisition time, which has subsequently decreased artifacts resulting from fetal movement and allowed one to obtain good-quality images. Fetal MRI has higher contrast resolution than prenatal sonography and may allow better differentiation of normal from abnormal tissue.

Fetal MRI is performed primarily using ultrafast MRI techniques known as single-shot, fast spin-echo (SS-FSE) or half-Fourier acquired single-shot turbo spin-echo (HASTE). Using these rapid-pulse sequences, a single T2-weighted image can be acquired in less than 1 second, reducing the likelihood of fetal motion during image acquisition [Brugger et al., 2006; Glenn and Barkovich, 2006]. When the fetal brain is being evaluated, images are obtained with a section thickness of 3 mm with no gap, in axial, sagittal, and coronal planes. Good orthogonal planes may not always be obtainable.

T1-weighted imaging and fast multiplanar gradient recalled-echo techniques, such as FMPSPGR (fast multiplanar spoiled gradient recalled acquisition in the steady state), are primarily used to detect hemorrhage or calcification [Glenn and Barkovich, 2006].

With the recent application of advanced MRI techniques, an opportunity to investigate the developing brain is available beyond the qualitative morphologic evaluation [Limperopoulos and Clouchoux, 2009; Glenn, 2009]. Diffusion-weighted imaging (DWI) and diffusion tensor imaging (DTI) are used to evaluate maturation-dependent microstructural changes associated with brain growth and development of cerebral white matter. DWI provides quantitative information about water motion and tissue microstructure, and provides additional applications for destructive brain processes. DTI allows the visualization and quantification of white-matter fiber direction. Advanced postprocessing techniques, such as the formation of high-resolution three-dimensional structural images, can be used to study morphometry [Glenn, 2009]. MR spectroscopy can be applied in the third trimester for the study of cerebral metabolism in vivo, since metabolites such as N-acetyl aspartate, creatine, and choline can be detected [Limperopoulos and Clouchoux, 2009].

The dynamic stages of fetal brain development can be imaged accurately with ultrasound and fetal MRI. An understanding of embryologic aspects of brain development and their correlative appearance on ultrasound and MRI is critical in order to be able to diagnose structural brain defects prenatally.

Prenatal Assessment of Normal Brain Development in the First Trimester

Brain development in the embryonic phase is only assessed by ultrasound. Blaas and Eik-Nes [2009] describe the milestones of normal brain development between 7 and 12 weeks' gestation based on longitudinal two-dimensional and three-dimensional ultrasound studies. Cortical development starts at about 7 weeks' gestation and other brain structures develop synchronously with the cortex, including the commissures and

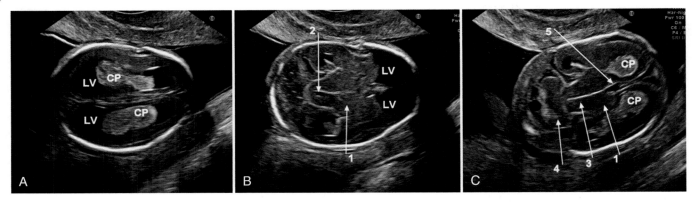

Fig. 29-1 Ultrasound: axial sections of the fetal brain at 16 weeks of gestation. A, Transventricular plane. **B,** Transthalamic plane. **C,** Transcerebellar plane. CP, choroid plexus; LV, lateral ventricle; 1, thalamus; 2, aqueduct of Sylvius; 3, middle cerebellar peduncles; 4, cerebellum; 5, cavum septi pellucidi.

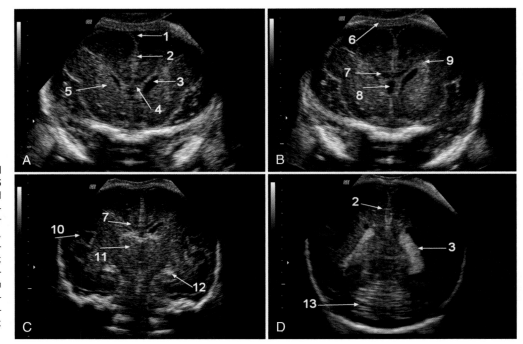

Fig. 29-2 Ultrasound: coronal sections of the fetal brain at 25 weeks of gestation. A, Transfrontal plane. **B,** Transcaudate plane. **C,** Transthalamic plane. **D,** Transcerebellar planes. 1, superior sagittal sinus; 2, interhemispheric fissure; 3, lateral ventricle; 4, genu of the corpus callosum; 5, head of the caudate; 6, anterior fontanel; 7, corpus callosum; 8, cavum septi pellucidi; 9, periventricular vascular hyperechogenicities; 10, sylvian fissure; 11, thalamus; 12, hippocampus; 13, cerebellum.

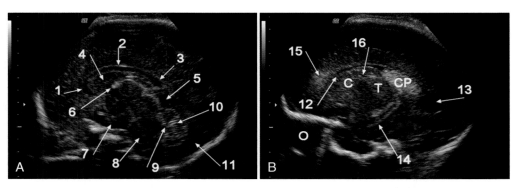

Fig. 29-3 Ultrasound: sagittal sections of the fetal brain at 25 weeks of gestation. A, Midsagittal plane. **B,** Parasagittal plane. **C,** caudate; CP, choroid plexus; O, orbit; T, thalamus; 1, genu of the corpus callosum; 2, body of the corpus callosum; 3, splenium of the corpus callosum; 4, cavum septi pellucidi; 5, cavum interpositi; 6, choroid plexus of the third ventricle; 7, basal cistern; 8, pons; 9, fourth ventricle; 10, vermis; 11, cisterna magna; 12, anterior horn of the lateral ventricle; 13, occipital horn of the lateral ventricle; 14, temporal horn of the lateral ventricle; 15, periventricular vascular hyperechogenicities; 16, caudothalamic groove.

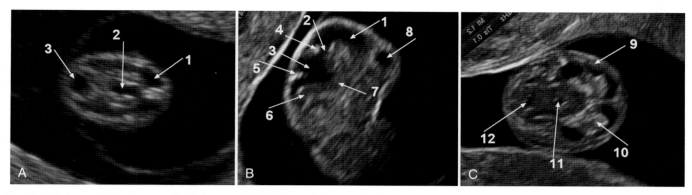

Fig. 29-4 High-resolution transvaginal ultrasound (12 MHz probe). A. Axial plane at 8 weeks of gestation. **B,** Sagittal plane at 8 weeks of gestation. **C,** Axial plane at 13 weeks of gestation. 1, telencephalic supraventricle; 2, aqueduct; 3, rhombencephalon; 4, tectum; 5, rhomboencephalon choroid plexus; 6, upper medulla; 7, pontine flexure; 8, eye; 9, cortical rim; 10, lateral ventricle choroid plexus; 11, third ventricle; 12, fourth ventricle.

the cerebellum. At 7–8 weeks, the lateral ventricles are seen as separated, small, round hypoechogenic brain cavities, and the future third ventricle runs posteriorly. The curved tube-like mesencephalic cavity (future sylvian aqueduct) lies anteriorly, and the broad and shallow rhombencephalic cavity is in the cranial pole of the embryo (Figure 29-4).

By the end of the first trimester (weeks 10–12), the cortex is about 1–2 mm thick and the crescent hemispheres fill the anterior part of the head and conceal the diencephalic cavity. The lateral ventricles are large and filled by the echogenic choroid plexuses. The insula appears as a slight depression on the lateral surface of the hemispheres. The diencephalon lies between the hemispheres, and the mesencephalon gradually moves towards the center of the head. The width of the third ventricle narrows. The corpus callosum is not yet visible. The cerebellar hemispheres seem to meet in the midline [Blaas and Eik-Nes, 2009].

Major structural defects, particularly malformations of dorsal induction and prosencephalic development that are usually severe or lethal, can be identified in first-trimester studies. Examples of these anomalies include acrania, anencephaly, craniorachischisis, iniencephaly, holoprosencephaly, and encephalocele.

Prenatal Assessment of Normal Development of the Cortex

Initially, the brain surface is smooth. Gyration can be observed by the second month of intrauterine life. It continues to the end of the pregnancy and even later after birth. The primary sulci appear as shallow grooves on the surface of the brain that become progressively more deeply infolded and then develop side branches, designated secondary sulci. Gyration proceeds with the formation of other side branches of the secondary sulci, referred to as tertiary sulci [Nadich et al., 1994]. The major fissures and sulci develop in predictable patterns, starting at about 16 weeks [Dorovini-Zis and Dolman, 1997], and therefore the timing of their appearance is a reliable estimate of gestational age. Anatomical changes precede ultrasound and MRI detection by about 2 weeks [Levine and Barnes, 1999] (Table 29-1).

Several studies [Toi et al., 2004; Cohen-Sacher et al., 2006] have assessed the development of the fetal cortex by ultrasound. Major sulci can be discerned, starting at about 18–19 weeks'

gestation. At 18–20 weeks, the brain surface is almost completely smooth, with only the major fissures present. The callosal sulcus is observed between 18 and 20 weeks. Between 22 and 26 weeks, the calcarine fissure, the cingulate sulcus, and the central sulcus gradually appear. The most active period of cortical development, as demonstrated by ultrasound, is between 28 and 30 weeks. During this time, most sulci become detectable. After 32 weeks, all structures, other than the insular and olfactory sulci, are present. During the last 4 weeks of pregnancy, the sulci over the convexity are best demonstrated using sagittal planes [Cohen-Sacher et al., 2006] (see Table 29-1). Early sulci are easier to evaluate by ultrasound than later-developing complex secondary and tertiary patterns [Malinger et al., 2006].

MRI after about 20 weeks of gestation provides excellent information unimpeded by calvarial calcification. Similar to ultrasound, it shows age-related predictable patterns of development, but, in addition, brain parenchyma and myelination can be evaluated [Garel et al., 2001].

Brain MRI can depict the walls of the ventricles, which are critical to normal brain development. They are lined by the ventricular zone (germinal matrix), which is very thick earlier in gestation, and appears as a smooth band of dark T2 signal and bright T1 signal lining the lateral ventricles. The cerebral mantle is seen on fetal MRI until about 28 weeks of gestation in a multilayered pattern [Kostovic and Vasung, 2009]. When viewed from the ventricular margin to the pial surface of the brain, five layers can be demonstrated (Figure 29-5).

The development of the cortex can be visualized from mid-pregnancy. On MRI, gyration starts with the appearance of a shallow indentation of the fetal brain in the temporal regions at the 18th gestational week. At the same time, the anterior cingular fissure and the parieto-occipital fissure occur. The central sulcus begins to be visible at 24 weeks' gestation. Fissures then become deeper and tighter, and gyri bulge into the subarachnoid space. Until the 35th gestational week, all primary and most of the secondary sulci are present, with secondary sulci appearing from the 24th gestational week, and tertiary after the 28th gestational week [Garel et al., 2001; Prayer et al., 2006] (see Table 29-1; Figure 29-6).

The development of the sylvian fissure is one of the major brain maturational processes occurring in fetal life, and abnormalities in this process are frequent in children with developmental delay. The appearance and shape of the sylvian fissure

Table 29-1 Chronology of Sulcation According to Neuropathological, Sonographic, and Magnetic Resonance Imaging Studies

	Anatomic Appearance [Chi et al., 1977]	Detectable in 25–75% of Brains by MRI [Garel et al., 2001]	Detectable in 25–75% of Brains by Ultrasound [Cohen-Sacher et al., 2006]	Present in >75% of Brains by MRI [Garel et al., 2001]	Present in >75% of Brains by Ultrasound [Cohen-Sacher et al., 2006]
Interhemispheric fissure	10			22–23	18
Sylvian fissure	14	24–25		29	18
Parieto-occipital fissure	16		18	22–23	20
Hippocampal fissure				22–23	18
Callosal sulcus	14			22–23	18
Calcarine fissure	16	22–23	20	24–25	22
Cingular sulcus	18	22–23	20	24–25	24
Central sulcus	20	24–25	26	27	28
Postcentral sulcus	25	27	28	28	30
Precentral sulcus	24	26	28	27	30
Superior temporal sulcus	23	26	28	27	30
Inferior temporal sulcus	30	30	28	33	30
Superior frontal sulcus	25	24–25	28	29	30
Inferior frontal sulcus	28	26	28	29	30
Secondary cingular sulcus	32	31	30	33	32
Insular sulcus	34–35	33	30	34	32
Secondary occipital sulcus	34	32	26	34	30
Olfactory sulcus	16		24		30
Marginal sulcus		22–23	26	27	30

can be evaluated both by ultrasound and MRI [Lerman-Sagie and Malinger, 2008; Garel et al., 2001; Chen et al., 1995]. It is observed in all fetuses at 22–23 weeks' gestation as a shallow depression at the surface of the brain, and the insula is wide open at this time. The temporal lobe folds over to engulf the insula, and the progressive closure begins posteriorly and extends anteriorly. By 33 weeks' gestation, insular sulci are recognizable and the surface of the Sylvian fissure becomes more and more indented [Garel et al., 2001; Quarello et al., 2008].

Prenatal Assessment of Normal Development of the Corpus Callosum

The corpus callosum develops between gestational weeks 8 and 20 as axons from the developing cerebral hemispheres navigate to and through the hemispheres and interhemispheric fissure. The corpus callosum is difficult to visualize by ultrasound during the performance of routine transabdominal evaluations using axial planes. For a complete demonstration of this structure, it is necessary to obtain sagittal planes through the anterior or posterior fontanels or the sagittal suture with the transvaginal or transfundal approach. Coronal planes are useful for studying the relationship between the corpus callosum and neighboring structures. The completely formed corpus callosum may be depicted using high-resolution transducers by 18–20 weeks of gestation, as an arched hypoechogenic structure delimited by the more echogenic callosal sulcus cranially and

the anechogenic cavum septi pelucidi caudally. At this age, its shape is already very similar to that of the mature corpus callosum, and the genu, body, and splenium can be well demonstrated (see Figures 29-2 and 29-3). The corpus callosum develops in a linear pattern during pregnancy, its length progressively increasing from 20 mm at 20 weeks to 40 mm close to term. Nomograms of callosal growth during pregnancy, including length and thickness, can be used to assess normal development [Malinger et al., 1993].

The corpus callosum can be depicted by MRI on midline sagittal T2 images by gestational week 20 as a band of low signal intensity superior to the fornix (Figure 29-7). It can also be seen on coronal T2 images. It has fairly uniform thickness [Toi et al., 2009].

Prenatal Assessment of Normal Development of the Posterior Fossa

Both ultrasound [Malinger et al., 2001] and MRI [Glenn, 2009; Adamsbaum et al., 2005] can evaluate the development of the fetal cerebellum.

The ultrasonographic evaluation should include multiplanar images of the cerebellum. The axial plane is useful for determining the transcerebellar diameter, cisterna magna size, and the cerebellar peduncle's thickness. The coronal plane enables differentiation between the cerebellar hemispheres and the vermis. The midsagittal plane is the most important plane to

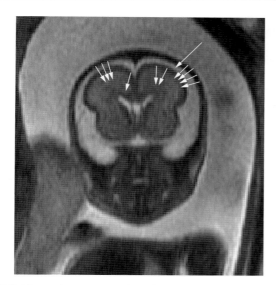

Fig. 29-5 Magnetic resonance imaging at 23 weeks demonstrates five layers. 1, Ventricular zone – the innermost layer of the cerebral mantle, lining the lateral ventricles; it appears dark on T2-weighted images (short single arrow). 2, Periventricular fiber-rich zone – this is located just superficial to the ventricular zone and is a thin area of increased T2 (two arrows). 3, Subventricular and intermediate zones – the subventricular zone and intermediate zone (site of the fetal white matter) lie superficial to the periventricular zone and appear as a fairly homogeneous band of slightly hypointense T2 (three arrows). 4, Subplate zone – this appears as a band of hyperintense T2 (four arrows). 5, Cortical plate – the developing cortex appears dark on T2-weighted images, and is similar in signal intensity to the germinal matrix (long single arrow).

be investigated, since it allows depiction of the vermian lobules, fissures, and shape of the fastigium; measurements of the vermian diameter and surface; and calculation of the ratio between the superior and inferior parts. This plane also permits evaluation of the size and shape of the pons, cisterna magna, and tentorium [Malinger et al., 2001].

The cerebellar vermis can be detected in the midsagittal plane as early as 18 weeks of gestation. The midsagittal anterior–posterior diameters increase in a linear fashion, from nearly 10 mm at 20–21 weeks' gestation to 24 mm at term.

The cerebellar vermis measurements and calculations (midsagittal anterior–posterior and craniocaudal diameters, circumference, and surface area) correlate linearly with gestational age, biparietal diameter, head circumference, and transverse cerebellar diameter.

The primary fissure is observed between 27 and 30 weeks of pregnancy. Some degree of differentiation between lobules is possible, starting from 30–32 weeks of gestation.

The fourth ventricle is uniformly observed as a triangular structure anterocaudal to the vermis. The inferior lobe of the vermis and the nodulus separate the fourth ventricle and the cistern magna [Malinger et al., 2001].

MRI is highly accurate in illustrating the morphologic MRI biometry of cerebellar development [Adamsbaum et al., 2005; Triulzi et al., 2005]. The cerebellar vermis is best assessed by MRI on direct midline sagittal images and on coronal images; the measurements should be compared with established norms. The cerebellar hemispheres are best assessed on non-oblique axial and coronal views.

Fetal MRI shows gestational age-specific changes in signal intensity in the normal development and maturation of the cerebellar hemispheres and brainstem [Huisman et al., 2002]. The cerebellar cortex, dentate nucleus, tectum, dorsal pons, and medulla are T1-hyperintense and T2-hypointense. The changes in signal intensity in the brainstem and cerebellum are not encountered until 20–23 weeks of gestation. By 26–27 weeks of gestation, a three-layered pattern is noted in the cerebellar hemispheres, corresponding to the cerebellar cortex, cerebellar white matter, and dentate nucleus. Fetal brain MRI can show the fissures of the cerebellum, depending on the gestational age. The primary fissure is identified on sagittal images at 22 weeks but the cerebellar surface is smooth. From 24 to 29 weeks, foliation of the vermis and posterior lobes of the cerebellum is seen on sagittal images. The cerebellar surface is smooth, with the appearance of some indentations corresponding to the horizontal and secondary fissures on axial images. The convoluted pattern of the cerebellum is well identified from 30 weeks on and is always seen beyond 33 weeks. [Fogliarini et al., 2005a].

Posterior fossa anatomy is sufficiently well defined in order to diagnose most cerebellar abnormalities prenatally; however, there may be many pitfalls in the differentiation of normal and abnormal cerebellar development [Malinger et al., 2009; Limperopoulos et al., 2008].

Prenatal Diagnosis of Ventriculomegaly

Assessment of the width of the atria of the lateral cerebral ventricles is recommended as part of the routine anomaly scan. Enlargement of the fetal lateral ventricles is the most common indication for referral for dedicated neurosonography and MRI, since it may be a sign of a possible brain anomaly.

The lateral ventricle should be measured by ultrasound in the axial plane, at the level of the frontal horns and cavum septi pellucidi, with the calipers positioned at the level of the internal margin of the medial and lateral wall of the atria, at the level of the glomus of the choroid plexus, on an axis perpendicular to the long axis of the lateral ventricle [ISUOG guidelines, 2007].

Ventriculomegaly is defined as a lateral ventricular width equal to or larger than 10 mm [ISUOG guidelines, 2007]. Fetal ventriculomegaly may be classified as mild when the lateral ventricular width is between 10 and 15 mm, and severe when larger than 15 mm; it may be unilateral or bilateral (Figure 29-8).

Ventriculomegaly is defined as isolated if there is no sonographic evidence of associated malformations or markers of aneuploidy at the time of the initial presentation. Isolated mild ventriculomegaly represents a diagnostic and counseling difficulty, as it can be an apparently benign finding, but can also be associated with chromosomal abnormalities, congenital infection, cerebral vascular accidents or hemorrhage, and other fetal cerebral and extracerebral abnormalities; it may also have implications regarding long-term neurodevelopmental outcome [Melchiorre et al., 2009]. Therefore, upon confirmation of ventriculomegal, a complete search for associated central nervous system and non-central nervous system anomalies should be attempted, including a study of the brain in a multiplanar approach with particular attention to the shape of the ventricles, periventricular white matter, sulcation, corpus callosum,

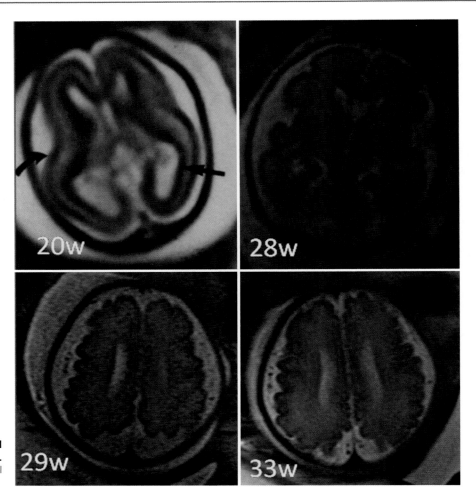

Fig. 29-6 Magnetic resonance imaging: axial images at different weeks of gestation. Normal development of sulcation and normal "closure" of the insula are demonstrated.

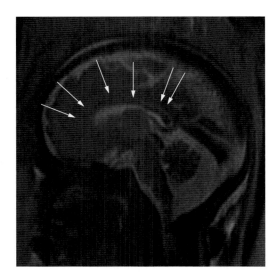

Fig. 29-7 Magnetic resonance imaging: midsagittal image of normal corpus callosum. Note the very sharp posterior border (splenium) relative to the indistinct anterior corpus (genu).

and posterior fossa [Malinger et al., 2006]. The investigation should also include screening for in utero infection, amniocentesis, and fetal echocardiography. Many studies have indicated that MRI may add important information to that obtained by

ultrasound imaging [Ouahba et al., 2006]. Information relevant enough to modify obstetric management can be obtained in 6–9 percent of cases, including cortical malformations, absence of the septum pellucidum, partial agenesis of the corpus callosum, and agenesis of the cerebellar vermis [Salomon et al., 2006; Valsky et al., 2004].

Follow-up examinations at 3–4-week intervals are indicated to assess progressive enlargement of ventricles or to diagnose associated pathologies not previously detected [Ouahba et al., 2006].

When mild ventriculomegaly is isolated, the outcome is usually good [Ouahba et al., 2006; Melchiorre et al., 2009]. However, the risk for abnormal outcome increases when there are associated anomalies, the ventriculomegaly is asymmetric, the atrial width is greater than 12 mm, or there is a progressive increase of the lateral ventricular width [Pilu et al., 1999; Sadan et al., 2007; Falip et al., 2007]. A false-negative diagnosis of associated anomalies is possible in up to 12.8 percent of cases [Melchiorre et al., 2009].

The outcome of severe ventriculomegaly depends mainly on the presence of associated pathologies. When associated pathologies are diagnosed, the prognosis is usually very poor. Even when isolated, the risk of perinatal death or severe neurologic sequelae is in the range of 50 percent of survivors [Kennelly et al., 2009].

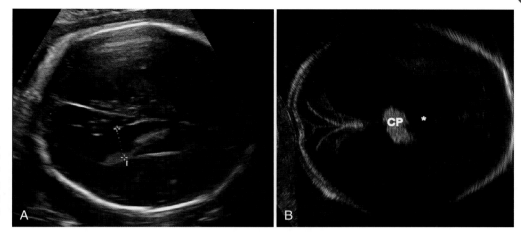

Fig. 29-8 Ultrasound: ventriculomegaly. A, Mild at 34 weeks of gestation. **B,** Severe at 22 weeks of gestation. Note that the choroid plexus (CP) of the proximal ventricle has moved into the distal ventricle due to disruption of the septi pellucidi (*).

Prenatal Diagnosis of Abnormalities of the Corpus Callosum

Developmental abnormalities of the corpus callosum include agenesis, hypogenesis (or partial agenesis), dysgenesis, hypoplasia, and secondary destruction [Glenn and Barkovich, 2006]. Agenesis of the corpus callosum (ACC) can be detected prenatally by routine sonography, for which the important signs include absence of the cavum septum pellucidum, colpocephaly, high-riding third ventricle, widening of the interhemispheric fissure, and radiating medial hemispheric sulci. Ultrasound can also depict an abnormally thick corpus callosum, which usually signifies a poor prognosis [Lerman-Sagie et al., 2009].

Fetal MRI is clinically helpful in suspected cases of ACC because it can confirm the absence of the corpus callosum and diagnose associated anomalies. Since the corpus callosum is not myelinated in utero, it can often be very difficult to distinguish on sagittal images, so agenesis of the corpus callosum can often be concluded from an altered shape of the lateral ventricles with straight anterior horns and colpocephalic posterior horns (Figure 29-9).

ACC is rarely isolated. Additional abnormalities occur frequently (93 percent). The most common findings are sulcation and posterior fossa abnormalities. Abnormal sulcal morphology can be detected as early as 19 gestational weeks. The gyral abnormalities include polymicrogyria, lissencephaly, pachygyria, schizencephaly, and other nonclassified abnormalities [Tang et al., 2009].

Interestingly, in 10 percent of fetuses with ACC, there may be evidence of destructive changes in the brain parenchyma, suggesting either an acquired etiology or a genetic/metabolic abnormality [Prasad et al., 2009].

Prenatal Diagnosis of Malformations of Cortical Development

Although the migration process terminates around the end of the first half of pregnancy, malformations of cortical development are seldom diagnosed in utero, possibly because the time of appearance of significant morphological changes is beyond the recommended time of the anatomic scan (19–23 weeks), and because ultrasound evaluation of the brain is often limited to visualization of the lateral ventricles and cerebellum [Malinger et al., 2004].

Abnormal sulcation landmarks can be observed as early as the 22nd week of gestation in fetuses suffering from Miller–Dicker and Walker–Warburg lissencephaly [Fong et al., 2004]. In patients with migration disorders, the ultrasound usually demonstrates one of the following patterns: delayed or premature appearance of sulcation; a thin and irregular cortical mantle; wide abnormal overdeveloped gyri; wide opening of isolated sulci, nodular bulging into the lateral ventricles,

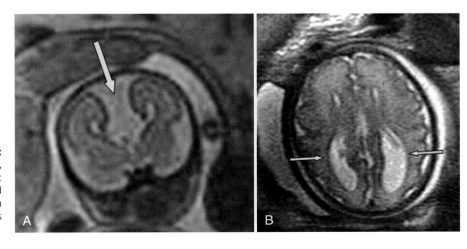

Fig. 29-9 Magnetic resonance imaging: complete agenesis of the corpus callosum. A, Coronal image at 26 weeks, with multicystic dysplasia of the interhemispheric meninges and overriding third ventricle. **B,** Axial image of a different fetus at 30 weeks demonstrates colpocephaly with parallel ventricles.

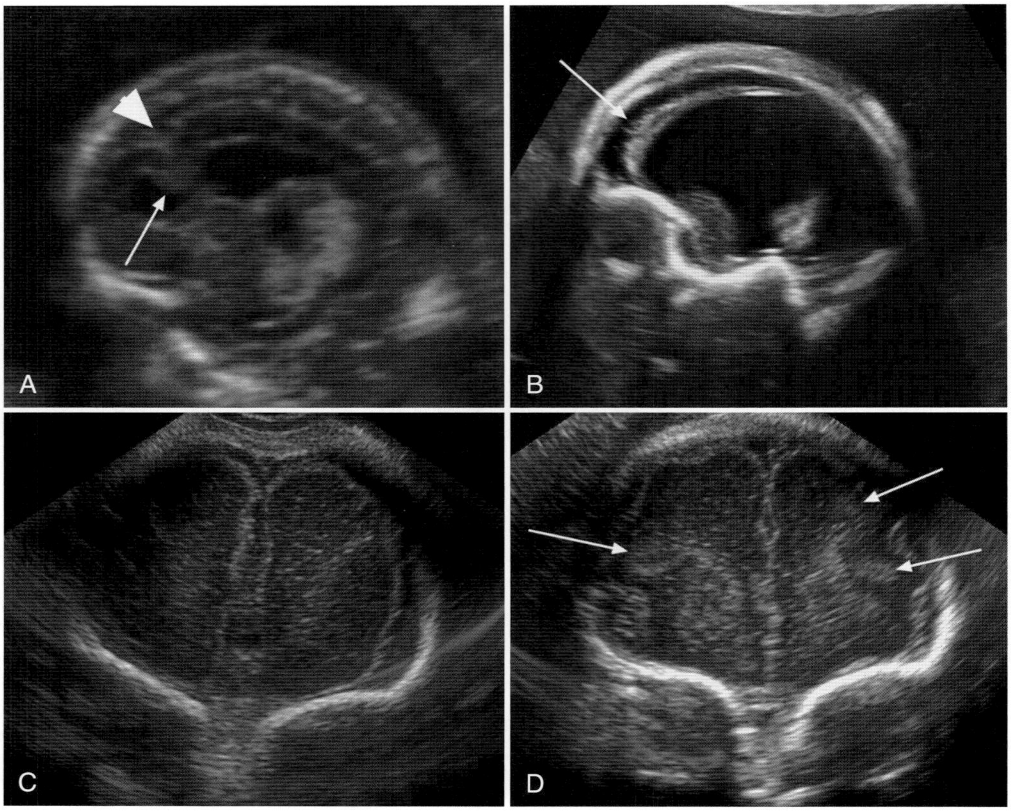

Fig. 29-10 Ultrasound findings in fetuses with malformations of cortical development. Transvaginal parasagittal views. **A,** Ultrasound at 16 weeks of gestation shows the presence of an abnormal gyrus (arrowhead) and brain tissue bulging into the lateral ventricle (arrow). **B,** Ultrasound at 25 weeks of gestation shows thin cortical mantle with irregular surface (arrow) consistent with cobblestone lissencephaly. Transvaginal frontal coronal views. **C,** Ultrasound at 34 weeks of gestation shows lack of normal sulcation in a fetus with type 1 lissencephaly. **D,** Ultrasound at 26 weeks of gestation in a fetus with tuberous sclerosis presenting with multiple cardiac rhabdomyomata and discrete parenchymal nodules (arrows).

cortical clefts, and intraparenchymal echogenic nodules [Malinger et al., 2007; Malinger et al., 2006] (Figure 29-10).

A definitive diagnosis is hard to reach prenatally; ultrasound can identify abnormal migration but cannot definitively differentiate between different pathologies.

MRI may identify cortical malformations more accurately, particularly late in pregnancy. The imaging signs suggestive of abnormal sulcation are mild ventriculomegaly associated with delayed cortical development, dysgenesis of the sylvian fissure, delayed sulcal appearance, callosal abnormality, cortical thickening, heterotopias, absence or abnormal appearance of fissure, irregular, abnormal, asymmetric gyri, and noncontinuous cortex in schizencephaly [Guibaud et al., 2008; Fong et al., 2004].

Chen et al. [1995] defined abnormal patterns of operculization and divided them into five types. Further studies [Quarello et al., 2008] have proven that, when the operculum is unformed or abnormally formed, the prognosis is usually poor and an underlying malformation of cortical development may be detected. When the operculum is underdeveloped for gestational age, it is usually associated with an abnormal head circumference or other brain anomalies. When it is an isolated finding, it may represent a metabolic disease, chromosomal anomaly, or benign delayed maturation of the operculum, usually associated with macrocephaly and enlargement of the subarachnoid spaces.

Prenatal Diagnosis of Lissencephaly Type I

Fetuses with lissencephaly type 1 or Miller–Dieker syndrome can be diagnosed after 27–30 weeks' gestation when most of the primary sulci are already present, either by detailed

neurosonography or MRI, by demonstration of dysgenesis of the sylvian fissure, delayed sulcal appearance, callosal abnormality, and cortical thickening [Saltzman et al., 1991; Greco et al., 1991] (see Figure 29-10C and Figure 29-11). Sometimes, zones of normal cortex and zones of pachygyric or agyric cortex alternate. The bilateral opercular dysplasia is responsible for a figure-eight-shaped brain [Fong et al., 2004].

Mild ventriculomegaly and delayed sulcal development are the earliest signs and can be diagnosed by 23 weeks' gestation in fetuses at risk [Malinger et al., 2004]. Fetuses with Miller–Dieker syndrome have abnormal parieto-occipital and sylvian fissures by the time of the second-trimester ultrasound examination [Malinger et al., 2004]. Fluorescence in situ hybridization (FISH) or mutation analysis for 17p13.3 abnormalities helps confirm the diagnosis.

Prenatal Diagnosis of Cobblestone Complex/ Lissencephaly Type 2

The prenatal diagnosis of Walker–Warburg syndrome has been reported in families at risk [Crowe et al., 1985; Rodgers et al., 1994]. An early diagnosis in the first trimester may be made if there is a cephalocele [Crowe et al., 1985]. Other findings suggestive of lissencephaly type 2 are early enlargement of the lateral ventricles, abnormal vermis, retinal detachment [Farrell et al., 1987], cataract, and abnormal sulcation [Monteagudo et al., 2001].

The presence of abnormal sulcation may only be demonstrated during the third trimester. MRI can better visualize the posterior fossa and gyration [Gasser et al., 1998; Kojima et al., 2002], and can demonstrate a kinked brainstem and bifid pons [Strigini et al., 2009; Mitchell et al., 2000] (see Figure 29-10B and Figure 29-12).

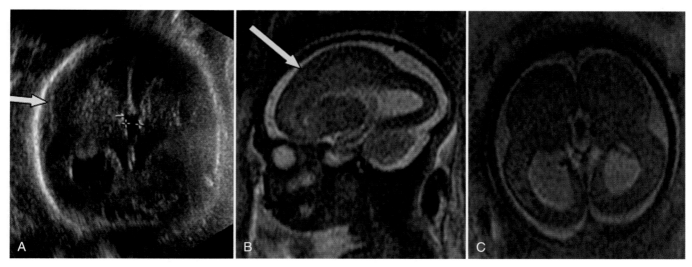

Fig. 29-11 Magnetic resonance imaging: lissencephaly type 1 at 33 weeks of gestation. A, Axial ultrasound with agyria and thick cortex (arrow). **B,** Parasagittal MRI confirming thick featureless cortex (arrow). **C,** Axial MRI demonstrating "figure of eight" configuration.

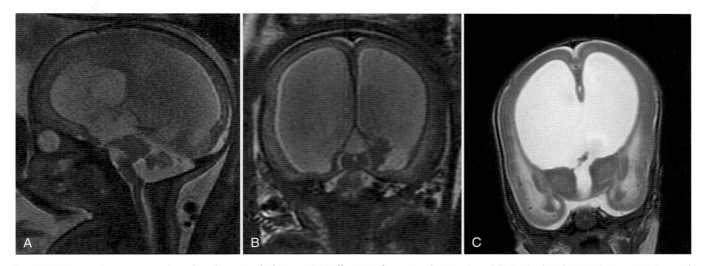

Fig. 29-12 Magnetic resonance imaging: lissencephaly type 2/Walker–Warburg syndrome. A and **B,** Sagittal and coronal images at 34 weeks demonstrate pathognomonic "z"-shaped (kinked) brainstem with severe ventricular dilatation and abnormal sulcation. **C.** Coronal postnatal MRI confirming a typical cobblestone cortex. Note abnormal white matter. *(Courtesy of Dr. Chen Hoffman.)*

Prenatal Diagnosis of Periventricular Nodular Heterotopia

Periventricular nodular heterotopia should be considered when ultrasound depicts an irregular lateral ventricular wall with indentations of periventricular tissue and a signal similar to that of the cortex (see Figure 29-10A). The sonographic diagnosis is difficult, particularly when the lateral ventricle width is normal. MRI demonstrates multiple small nodular subependymal foci of low signal intensity, isointense to the germinal matrix, similar to that of the gray matter, located in the margins of the lateral ventricles (Figure 29-13). They cannot be distinguished reliably from the subependymal nodules seen in tuberous sclerosis; therefore, it is important to search for other manifestations of tuberous sclerosis, such as cortical hamartomas (which are hypointense compared with normal unmyelinated white matter) and cardiac rhabdomyomas [Glenn and Barkovich, 2006] A mega cisterna magna, which can be seen in females with filamin A mutations, may be the initial abnormality and, in association with periventricular nodules, may suggest the prenatal diagnosis of periventricular nodular heterotopia [Mitchell et al., 2000; Bargallo et al., 2002].

Heterotopia may be not recognized when the nodules are small or subcortical. Large nodules may be confused with tumoral or hemorrhagic masses [Onyeije et al., 1998].

Prenatal Diagnosis of Polymicrogyria

The cortical changes of polymicrogyria take place late in pregnancy and appear as localized and/or generalized absence of normal sulcation with multiple abnormal infoldings of the affected cortex [Glenn and Barkovich, 2006]. It is more apparent on MRI than ultrasound. In young fetuses (24 weeks), the identification of the cortical malformation is quite difficult and the manifestations in both ultrasound and MRI are subtle. They include presence of sulci that are not as expected, according to the gestational age; an irregular surface of the brain;

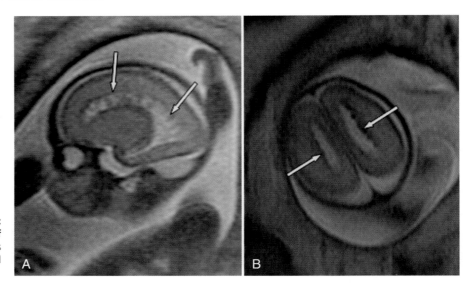

Fig. 29-13 Magnetic resonance imaging: periventricular heterotopias at 25 weeks of gestation. A and **B,** Parasagittal and axial images demonstrate multiple hypointense, subependymal nodules bulging into ventricles.

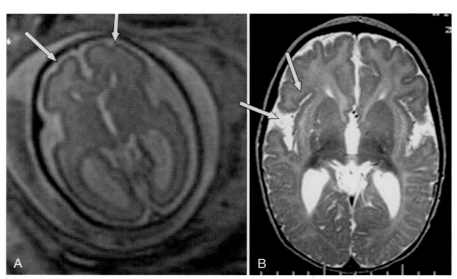

Fig. 29-14 Magnetic resonance imaging: bilateral frontal polymicrogyria. A, Fetal MRI at 28 weeks demonstrates subtle irregularity of the frontal cortex with subtle abnormal operculum bilaterally. **B,** Postnatal axial T2 MRI demonstrates diffuse, mildly thickened, irregular, frontal cortex extending into the insula.

and absence of the normal signal of the cortical ribbon (Figure 29-14). Late in pregnancy, the MRI features are similar to what is known in the postnatal period: packed and serrated microgyri, irregular cortex–white-matter junction, and an aberrant and asymmetrical sulcal pattern [Fogliarini et al., 2005a]. The most frequent MRI presentation diagnosed in utero demonstrates mild ventricular dilatation associated with numerous sulci in the perisylvian area, with irregular cortex–white-matter junction and a prominent subarachnoid space overlying the cortical malformation. Since the MRI pattern of polymicrogyria changes with increasing gestational age, it is important to follow young fetuses and repeat the ultrasound and MRI examinations in order to confirm the diagnosis.

Prenatal Diagnosis of Schizencephaly

Prenatal ultrasound enables diagnosis of schizencephaly, although prenatal MRI is more specific in detection of the gray matter lining the defect, communication with the ventricle, and other associated structural abnormalities [Oh et al., 2005]. The prenatal diagnosis of schizencephaly depends on the extent of cleft separation; closed-lip and open-lip variants with a very

small gap remain undiagnosed. The prenatal diagnosis of schizencephaly has been described as early as 21 weeks. Fetuses are usually diagnosed after a routine ultrasound examination demonstrates enlarged lateral ventricles, fluid-filled cavities, or absence of the cavum septum pellucidum [Malinger et al., 2007]. Neurosonography demonstrates bilateral or unilateral open-lip wedge-shaped defects, usually in the parietotemporal regions, frequently accompanied by absence of the cavum septum pellucidum. Fetal MRI shows schizencephalic clefts extending from the pial surface to the ventricle lined with gray matter, which is seen as a low-signal-intensity line covering the edge of the remaining brain parenchyma (Figure 29-15). This finding allows differentiation of the defect from porencephaly [Oh et al., 2005; Denis et al., 2001].

Prenatal Diagnosis of Posterior Fossa Anomalies

Infratentorial anomalies are usually diagnosed in utero when associated with an enlarged cisterna magna, with or without an abnormal fourth ventricle. The suspicion of abnormal

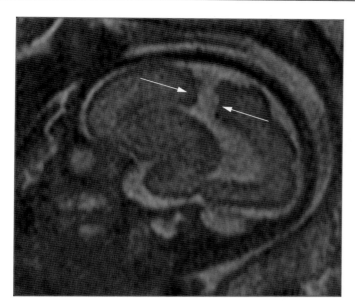

Fig. 29-15 Magnetic resonance imaging: open-lip schizencephaly. Wide gray matter-lined cavity connecting the ventricle with the extra-axial space.

cerebellar development is usually raised following the visualization of a small cerebellum or a large communication between the fourth ventricle and the cisterna magna, using the transcerebellar axial plane [Malinger et al., 2006]. Severe anomalies, such as Arnold–Chiari malformation type 2, Dandy–Walker malformation [Oh et al., 2005; Denis et al., 2001], and cerebellar hypoplasia, are usually detected during routine second-trimester ultrasound examinations. However, prenatal diagnosis of isolated cerebellar and/or vermian anomalies may be difficult because of the complexity of normal development of these structures.

A systematic approach to the posterior fossa is recommended in order to enable differentiation between normal and abnormal development [Guibaud and des Portes, 2006; Adamsbaum et al., 2005]. Understanding the anatomy is vital to avoid misdiagnosis and to characterize the abnormalities accurately. Confirmation of the diagnosis necessitates the visualization of the cerebellum in the coronal planes, and a true midline sagittal picture of the vermis, brainstem, and fourth ventricle. Particular care should be taken in order to differentiate between the vermis and the cerebellar hemisphere in cases of suspected vermian agenesis or hypoplasia. Visualization of the normal triangular shape of the fourth ventricle, and of the primary vermian fissure, facilitates exclusion of vermian pathologies [Denis et al., 2001]. Vermian agenesis may also be part of the molar tooth-associated syndromes.

The in utero diagnosis of the pontocerebellar hypoplasias [Klein et al., 2003] necessitates measurements of the pons circumference in addition to the cerebellar dimensions.

In cases of diagnostic uncertainties, a follow-up examination is pertinent, since a false positive diagnosis of vermian agenesis may be made before 24 weeks of pregnancy, due to delayed closure of the fourth ventricle owing to a persistent Blake pouch cyst [Robinson and Goldstein, 2007], and cerebellar hypoplasia may be missed early in pregnancy because the arrest of growth occurs later [Malinger et al., 2009].

A dysplastic cerebellum, which refers to disorganized development, such as an abnormal folial pattern or the presence of heterotopic nodules of gray matter, is rarely diagnosed in utero, even by MRI, since it does not produce signal abnormalities [Tilea et al., 2007]. However, in most cases of posterior fossa anomalies, there is good agreement between fetal MRI and fetopathological results.

Prenatal Diagnosis of Chiari Type II

The posterior fossa is relatively small in Chiari II, and spinal neural tube defects are present with variable hindbrain herniation. The Chiari II malformation may be associated with callosal anomalies, fenestration of the falx, and cortical malformations. The cisterna magna is often obliterated with a low-lying torcula, vermian herniation through the foramen magnum, and a small slitlike fourth ventricle. The herniated cerebellum often degenerates and may be virtually absent in severe cases [Boltshauser et al., 2002]. When visible, the cerebellum is banana-shaped due to the herniation and small posterior fossa. The fetus may demonstrate a lemon-shaped skull [Van den Hof et al., 1990]. The lemon sign is created by the flattened frontal bones and, in most cases, is seen with an open myelomeningocele before 24 weeks' gestation. Ultrasound is sensitive and specific for detection of the Chiari II malformation [Oh et al., 2007].

Prenatal Diagnosis of Dandy–Walker Malformation

Prenatal diagnosis of Dandy–Walker malformation is usually possible during the second trimester; midsagittal planes enable visualization of the abnormal vermis, the communication between the fourth ventricle and the enlarged cisterna magna, and the elevated torcula (Figure 29-16C). It should not be confused with partial vermian agenesis, in which there is a large communication between the fourth ventricle and the cisterna magna without elevation of the torcula (Figure 29-17B and Figure 29-17C). Dandy–Walker malformation may be associated with other central nervous system anomalies, such as callosal dysgenesis, occipital encephalocele, polymicrogyria, or heterotopias, so these should be sought. Hydrocephalus may only develop late in pregnancy or postnatally.

The prognosis following a prenatal diagnosis of Dandy–Walker malformation is variable; however, the presence of a normally lobulated vermis and the absence of associated brain anomalies are associated with a more favorable outcome [Bolduc and Limperopoulos, 2009].

Prenatal Diagnosis of Mega Cisterna Magna, Posterior Fossa Arachnoid Cyst, Blake's Pouch Cyst

Isolated enlargement of the posterior fossa is frequently diagnosed by fetal ultrasound or MRI. It may be seen in three situations: mega cisterna magna, posterior fossa arachnoid cyst, and Blake's pouch cyst. The prognosis in all three entities is usually good [Dror et al., 2009].

In mega cisterna magna, the posterior fossa depth is greater than 10 mm, but the vermis and torcula location are normal. The term has been loosely applied to a large-appearing retro-cerebellar cerebrospinal fluid space with a normal vermis and

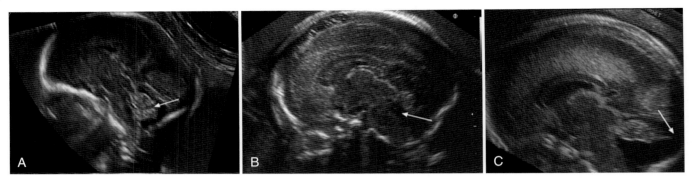

Fig. 29-16 Ultrasound of cerebellar pathologies, midsagittal planes. A, Ultrasound of normal vermis at 23 weeks of gestation; the arrow indicates the primary fissure. **B,** Ultrasound at 22 weeks of gestation; fetus with a small vermis and large fourth ventricle (arrow). **C,** Ultrasound at 22 weeks of a fetus with classical Dandy–Walker malformation; the arrow shows the elevated tentorium.

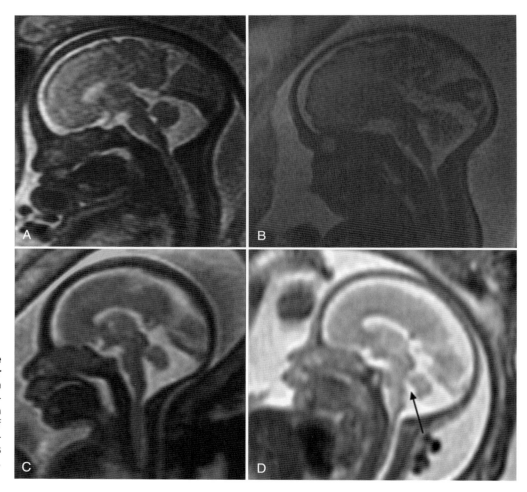

Fig. 29-17 Magnetic resonance imaging of various cerebellar pathologies. A, Mega cisterna magna, 31 weeks. **B,** Joubert's syndrome, 32 weeks. **C,** Partial vermian agenesis, 24 weeks. **D,** Rotation of a normal vermis in a fetus with persistent Blake's pouch; the arrow shows the apparently large fourth ventricle, 24 weeks.

cerebellar hemispheres. It is usually an incidental finding, but it can be associated with other anomalies. Mega cisterna magna can be difficult to distinguish from an arachnoid cyst, as both are anechoic fluid spaces and may result in mild scalloping of the skull (see Figure 29-17A). Some authors [Nelson et al., 2004] claim that mega cisterna magna is not a true diagnosis since, when such spaces are carefully examined at autopsy, delicate membranes of a retrocerebellar cyst become apparent and histologically they are usually of the arachnoid or Blake's pouch variety.

Congenital arachnoid cysts are extra-axial, and 10–45 percent occur in the posterior fossa. They present on ultrasound as anechoic avascular cysts with mass effect on the cerebellum or internal table of the skull. Associated congenital anomalies are rare.

Doppler ultrasound should be used to exclude any internal vascularity, which would be seen in a vascular malformation or cystic tumor [Oh et al., 2007].

Blake's pouches have the same radiographic appearance as do arachnoidal cysts, with the exception that, in some cases, the choroid plexus may be identified, as it extends through the median aperture along the superior cyst wall, carrying the anterior lip of the median aperture far up the vallecula. Blake's pouches usually communicate with the fourth ventricle and may or may not produce mass effect on the cerebellum. The falx cerebelli is usually present and the torcula is usually in a normal position, but may be elevated. There may be pressure erosion of the occipital bone. Occasionally, there is the appearance of compression or absence of the inferior vermis (see Figure 29-17D). Other central nervous system malformations are rarely associated with Blake's pouches [Nelson et al., 2004]. It may be hard to differentiate between inferior vermis hypoplasia and a Blake's pouch cyst [Limperopoulos et al., 2006].

Cysts of the posterior fossa must be differentiated from Dandy–Walker malformation. The classic malformation consists of a huge posterior cyst, which is the fourth ventricle, with absent or markedly hypoplastic vermis and cerebellar hemispheres, and elevated lateral and straight sinuses and torcula herophili with identifiable choroid plexus; but on the other end of the spectrum is a mildly hypoplastic vermis with a large fourth ventricle filling a normal-sized posterior fossa with a torcula herophili in normal position. The falx cerebelli is usually absent. However, the identification of a normal fourth ventricular choroid plexus in the inferior medullary velum rules out a Dandy–Walker malformation.

Prenatal Diagnosis of Vermis Hypoplasia/Agenesis

The term Dandy–Walker variant has been used to describe a heterogeneous group of disorders with different degrees of cerebellar vermis agenesis, slight or absent upward rotation of the vermis, and variably sized posterior fossa fluid collections, but without enlargement of the posterior fossa. However, in recent years, it has been strongly advocated that the term Dandy–Walker variant be abandoned altogether, given its multiple and variable definitions [Parisi and Dobyns, 2003]. The terms hypoplasia and agenesis are used interchangeably in the literature on fetal vermian abnormalities, but actually the definitions of these entities are completely different [Guibaud and des Portes, 2006]. Vermian agenesis means either complete or partial absence of the vermis. In partial vermian agenesis, part of the vermis is absent and the remaining part is anatomically of normal volume. Due to the craniocaudal development of the vermis, partial agenesis involves its inferior part (see Figure 29-17C). Vermian hypoplasia means a small but complete vermis with congenital volume diminution.

Vermis agenesis is associated with central nervous system and non-central nervous system anomalies in up to 71 percent of children, with the most common being ventriculomegaly and agenesis of corpus callosum. Extra-central nervous system anomalies have also been reported in up to 65 percent, with cardiac, renal, extremity, and facial anomalies occurring most frequently [Bolduc and Limperopoulos, 2009].

Vermian development is assessed in the midline sagittal view from the caudal extent of the inferior vermis over the fourth ventricle. The diagnosis of inferior vermis agenesis (still referred to in the literature as hypoplasia) is made when there is partial absence of the inferior portion of the cerebellar vermis with normal- or near-normal-shaped cerebellar hemispheres,

a normal-sized posterior fossa without obvious cystic lesions, and normal supratentorial structures. The normal proportion of anterior vermis to posterior vermis (1:2) is lost. A correct diagnosis of inferior vermian agenesis is difficult and, even with MRI, there is a false-positive rate of 32 percent [Limperopoulos et al., 2006].

In cases of sonographically suspected vermian hypoplasia or agenesis, fetal MRI is helpful in determining the shape and size of the vermis, and the relationship between a posterior fossa cyst and the fourth ventricle [Glenn and Barkovich, 2006]. The identification of an intact vermis can help to differentiate it from a mega cisterna magna. However, even when apparently isolated vermian hypoplasia/agenesis is detected, it is difficult to be certain of the diagnosis, and therefore it warrants subsequent fetal MRI studies or postnatal MRI confirmation [Triulzi et al., 2006].

Inferior vermian agenesis should be differentiated from failure of "closure" of the vermis with normal morphology and biometry, and without any associated fetal abnormalities, this probably represents isolated elevation or rotation of the vermis due to a persistent Blake's pouch [Robinson et al., 2007] and does not necessarily indicate an adverse outcome. Failure of "closure" seems to result from two potential processes: arrest of vermian development so that it does not cover the fourth ventricle at its inferior extent, or failure of adequate fenestration of the fourth ventricular outflow foramina, leading to a secondary elevation of an otherwise normal vermis. The prognosis in these situations is completely different.

Prenatal Diagnosis of Cerebellar Hypoplasia

Cerebellar hypoplasia implies abnormal development rather than atrophy. When a small-appearing cerebellum is seen, either the cerebellum is truly small or the posterior fossa is relatively large. Diagnosis is made by measurement of the transverse cerebellar diameter in millimeters, which should be about equal to the gestational age in weeks [Oh et al., 2007]. Many fetuses with cerebellar hypoplasia or agenesis do not present with an enlarged cisterna magna [Tilea et al., 2007].

Severe cerebellar hypoplasia is easily identified in utero after 22 weeks as a very small cerebellum associated with a shallow brainstem and absence of the anterior bulging of the pons, resulting in pontocerebellar atrophy/hypoplasia of extremely poor prognosis. The cerebellum resembles an arrested brain at the embryonic period with a persistent pontine flexure.

Isolated cerebellar hypoplasia with a normal bulge of the pons is more challenging and difficulty in distinguishing malformation from necrosis can occur, especially in unilateral hypoplasia. An intact cerebellar cortex, whether irregular or not, is most likely seen in cerebellar hypoplasia, as opposed to cerebellar necrosis, in which the cortical ribbon is usually absent [Fogliarini et al., 2005b].

Prenatal Diagnosis of Rhombencephalosynapsis

Ultrasound diagnosis of rhombencephalosynapsis is generally suspected after 22 weeks of gestation, and usually the abnormality is suggested by ventriculomegaly [Pasquier et al., 2009]. The diagnosis is raised, following demonstration of a small

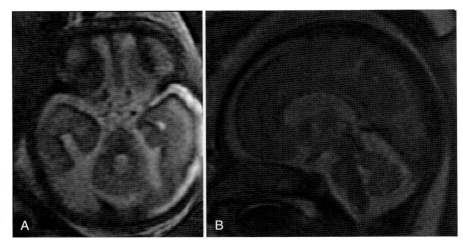

Fig. 29-18 Magnetic resonance imaging: rhombencephalosynapsis. A, Axial view at 31 weeks demonstrates small continuous folia of the cerebellum, "diamond-shaped." **B,** Sagittal view shows lack of the normal primary fissure and fastigium.

transcerebellar diameter. Ultrasound and MRI both demonstrate a hypoplastic, single-lobed cerebellum with fused cerebellar hemispheres, no vermis, and transverse folia (Figure 29-18). Associated cerebral abnormalities are usually found and include additional midline defects, such as aqueductal stenosis leading to hydrocephalus, holoprosencephaly, corpus callosum dysgenesis, and septo-optic dysplasia. Extracranial anomalies include segmentation and fusion anomalies of the spine, musculoskeletal anomalies, and cardiovascular, respiratory, and urinary tract defects. Rhombencephalosynapsis may be frequently associated with VACTERL-H (vertebral anomalies, anal atresia, cardiac defects, tracheoesophageal fistula, esophageal atresia, renal anomalies, hydrocephalus) syndrome [Pasquier et al., 2009].

It is important to emphasize that coronal and axial planes are superior for diagnosis of rhombencephalosynapsis, since a midline sagittal cut through the cerebellum can be mistaken for a vermis. A narrow diamond-shaped fourth ventricle and a fused horseshoe-shaped dentate nucleus are the features seen on axial MRI planes. Sagittal views, when carefully interpreted, can demonstrate the lack of visualization of the primary vermian fissure and lack of a normal fastigial point of the fourth ventricle [McAuliffe et al., 2008].

Prenatal Diagnosis of Molar Tooth-Related Syndromes

The diagnosis of the molar tooth (deep interpeduncular fossa, thick and elongated superior cerebellar peduncles, vermis agenesis) is difficult to visualize in utero. However, the prenatal diagnosis of Joubert's syndrome or related disorders has been described in the literature, usually following a positive family history and the finding of abnormal posterior fossa anatomy on fetal ultrasonography or the presence of associated suggestive features, such as kidney anomalies, polydactyly, or an abnormal fetal breathing pattern [Doherty et al., 2005; Fluss et al., 2006]. Ultrasound and MRI demonstrate an enlarged fourth ventricle with an abnormal fastigium, and the vermis is not clearly observed in the coronal and sagittal planes (see Figure 29-17B). The molar tooth features may be visualized in the axial plane, including the interpeduncular fossa, cerebellar peduncles, and brainstem.

The complete list of references for this chapter is available online at **www.expertconsult.com**.
See inside cover for registration details.

Introduction to Genetics

William B. Dobyns, Susan L. Christian, and Soma Das

In the broadest sense, genes are simply units of hereditary information; the genome is the totality of all the hereditary information in a cell or organism; and genetics may be defined as the study of genes and genomes. With the advent of modern molecular biology and the Human Genome Project, all aspects of genetics have come to play a more prominent role in the day-to-day evaluation and management of children with neurologic diseases, most of which have a genetic basis. This chapter presents a brief synopsis of the most important principles of genetics, to serve as background for information presented elsewhere in this text. More detailed information on genetics is available in many excellent textbooks, such as *Genetics in Medicine* [Nussbaum et al., 2007], *Genes IX* [Lewin, 2007], and *Human Molecular Genetics* [Strachan and Read, 2010]. Other resources are available from the National Center for Biotechnology Information website (Table 30-1).

Molecular Basis of Heredity

Modern theories of molecular biology hold that all information needed for function of cells and organisms is contained in macromolecules composed of simple repeating units. The flow of genetic information is (almost) exclusively unidirectional: DNA to RNA to protein. That is, the sequence of deoxyribonucleic acid (DNA) specifies the synthesis and sequence of ribonucleic acid (RNA) by a process known as transcription. Messenger RNA in turn specifies the synthesis and sequence of polypeptides, which are the building blocks of proteins, by a process known as translation. Other forms of RNA function independently. This theory is the central dogma of molecular biology. Accordingly, we begin with a review of the structure and function of these three macromolecules, and continue with reviews of the processes involved in gene and protein expression, including gene structure and organization, RNA processing, and epigenetics. Epigenetics refers to modification of genes other than changes in the DNA sequence, especially by addition of methyl groups to DNA, which alters gene expression. The two most important epigenetic changes found to be relevant to clinical disorders to date are imprinting and X-inactivation.

Structure and Function of DNA

DNA is a large polymer or macromolecule composed of linear sequences of simple repeating units. The specific sequence of these units contains all of the genetic information of an individual cell or organism. The structure of DNA in its native state was deduced by Watson and Crick in 1953 [Watson and Crick, 1953]. The basic repeating unit of DNA is the nucleotide, which consists of a five-carbon sugar known as deoxyribose; a phosphate group; and a nitrogen-containing base, which may be either a purine or a pyrimidine (Figure 30-1A). In DNA, the purine base may be either adenine (A) or guanine (G), and the pyrimidine base may be either thymine (T) or cytosine (C). Nucleotides polymerize into long chains by formation of phosphodiester bonds between the 5′ carbon position of one deoxyribose molecule and the 3′ carbon of the preceding deoxyribose molecule (Figure 30-1B).

Each DNA molecule consists of two strands of nucleotides that are held together by weak hydrogen bonds between pairs of bases: A pairs only with T, and G pairs only with C. These paired units are known as basepairs (bp). In the native state, the two strands wind around each other to form a double helix that resembles a right-hand spiral staircase, with two unequal grooves known as the major and minor grooves (Figure 30-2). A single turn of the helix measures 3.4 nm and contains ten nucleotides. Each strand has a directionality imparted by the deoxyribose sugar backbone. Adjacent nucleotides are linked by phosphodiester bonds between the 5′ and 3′ carbon atoms of the sugar residues, so that one end of the DNA strand has an unlinked 5′ carbon (the 5′ end) and the other end of the strand has an unlinked 3′ carbon atom (the 3′ end). The two strands are antiparallel – that is, they run in opposite directions so that the 5′ end of one strand is paired with the 3′ end of the other. Within living cells, DNA is associated with proteins and supercoiled into more complex structures known as chromosomes, which are described later in the chapter.

Thus, when the sequence of one DNA strand is known, the sequence of the opposite or complementary strand may be predicted. Precise replication of DNA is therefore possible, a process that involves initiation, elongation, and termination stages. The process begins with recognition of an "origin of replication." Such points of origin are specific DNA sequences, recognized by a protein complex known as the primosome, that occur every 50–300 kilobases (kb) of DNA; the unit kb refers to 1000 sequential nucleotides. The two parental DNA strands must first be separated by helicase, an enzyme that unwinds the supercoiled DNA helix to create a replication fork. The process of elongation occurs at the site of the replication fork or replisome. Synthesis of new strands begins with the addition of approximately ten RNA bases by a protein complex known as primase, and then continues with chain elongation using the original strands as templates. This process is known as semiconservative replication. Both initiation or RNA priming and chain elongation involve large protein complexes that include several DNA polymerases.

Table 30-1 Genetic Information Websites

Site	Internet Address
NCBI[1] GENETIC DISEASE WEBSITES	
GeneTests, GeneReviews[2]	http://www.ncbi.nlm.nih.gov/sites/GeneTests/
OMIM[3]	http://www.ncbi.nlm.nih.gov/omim/
NCBI[1] GENOME DATA WEBSITES	
NCBI[1] homepage (Entrez)	http://www.ncbi.nlm.nih.gov/
dbGaP Genotypes and Phenotypes	http://www.ncbi.nlm.nih.gov/gap
dbSNP (SNP database)	http://www.ncbi.nlm.nih.gov/snp/
OTHER GENOME DATA WEBSITES	
Ensembl Human Genome Browser	http://uswest.ensembl.org/index.html
HUGO[4]	http://www.genenames.org/index.html
DOE[5] Genomics Websites, includes Human Genome Project	http://genomics.energy.gov/
UCSC Genome Bioinformatics[6]	http://genome.ucsc.edu/

[1] National Center for Biotechnology Information.
[2] Disease summaries in GeneReviews are authored by experts and peer-reviewed, and so are typically highly accurate and up to date.
[3] Disease summaries in OMIM (Online Mendelian Inheritance in Man) are done by staff with oversight and contain both dated and new data; all information from OMIM should be confirmed from a second source.
[4] The HUGO Gene Nomenclature Committee website established accepted names for human genes.
[5] U.S. Department of Energy Office of Science websites, which include the Human Genome Project website.
[6] University of California–Santa Clara Genome Bioinformatics site, which contains the most widely used human genome browser, sometimes called "Golden Path."

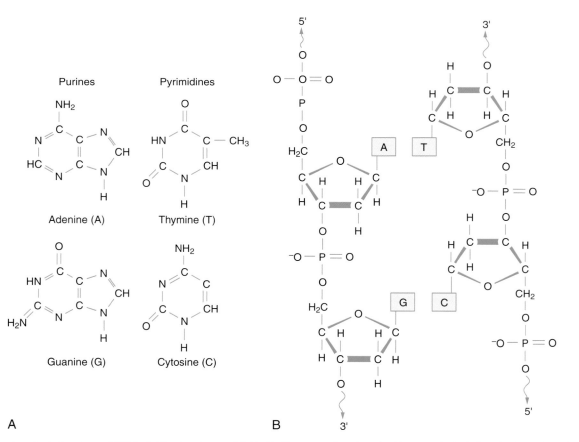

Fig. 30-1 The chemical structure of DNA. A, The four bases of DNA. **B,** The sugar-phosphate backbone and 3′–5′ phosphodiester bonds.

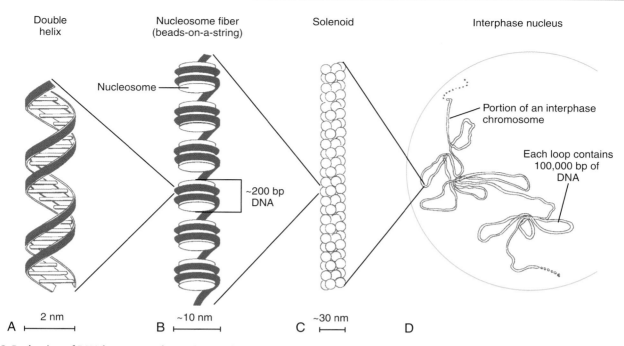

Fig. 30-2 Packaging of DNA by structural proteins. A, The right-handed double helix of DNA. **B,** This wraps around a histone core to form nucleosomes. **C,** The nucleosomes are packed into a solenoid structure. **D,** Loops of solenoids compose an interphase chromosome. *(Modified from Thompson MR et al. Genetics in medicine, 5th edn. Philadelphia: WB Saunders, 1991.)*

Table 30-2 DNA Polymerases in Mammalian Systems

Polymerase	Location	Function	3′ to 5′ Exonuclease
α(I)	Nuclear	Priming, especially of lagging strand	No
β	Nuclear	DNA repair	No
γ	Mitochondrial	Replication of mitochondrial DNA	Yes
δ(III)	Nuclear	Synthesis or elongation	Yes
ε(II)	Nuclear	DNA repair	Yes

Five distinct DNA polymerases have been isolated in mammalian systems, including human cell cultures (Table 30-2). They are able to copy DNA only by adding nucleotides to the 3′ end of the growing chain, so DNA can elongate only in the 5′ to 3′ direction. Thus, the template DNA can be read only in the reverse, or 3′ to 5′, direction. As DNA is unwound, the replication fork necessarily unwinds one strand in the 3′ to 5′ direction and the other in the 5′ to 3′ direction. The 3′ to 5′ or leading strand is replicated in a continuous fashion at the replication fork by DNA polymerases α(I), which primes the reaction, and δ(III), which synthesizes the DNA chain. The new strand is complementary and so elongates in the opposite, or 5′ to 3′, direction.

The 5′ to 3′, or lagging, strand cannot be copied continuously because this would require synthesis of the complementary new strand in a 3′ to 5′ direction, which is not possible, because DNA polymerases are able to synthesize DNA only in the 5′ to 3′ direction. Thus, the lagging strand must be copied by DNA polymerases α(I) and δ(III) in small segments of 100–1000 bp in the opposite direction from the replication fork. These small DNA molecules are known as Okazaki fragments. DNA replication is described as semidiscontinuous because of the continuous replication of the leading strand and the discontinuous replication of the lagging strand. The Okazaki fragments are then joined by another enzyme, DNA ligase. DNA replication is a long process, requiring about 8 hours in most human cells in culture. Thus, the function of DNA is reliably to encode and store the genetic information needed for the cell and organism to function. It has no direct functions itself but rather acts by directing synthesis of both RNA and protein.

Structure and Function of RNA

RNA differs chemically from DNA in the substitution of ribose for deoxyribose in the sugar backbone of the molecule, and of uridine (U) for thymine as one of the pyrimidine bases. Also, RNA normally exists as a single-stranded rather than double-stranded molecule. Recent advances have demonstrated far more diverse functions for RNA than were previously appreciated, particularly involving genes that produce functional RNA products that do not code for proteins. These probably represent at least 5 percent of all human genes, as suggested by current knowledge [Strachan and Read, 2010]. Several distinct classes of RNA molecules have been recognized, most of which are involved with regulating or assisting gene expression.

Ribosomal RNA

Ribosomal RNAs (rRNAs) are functional RNA transcripts that constitute one of the main components of cytoplasmic ribosomes. The genes coding for the major form of cytoplasmic rRNA are located in multiple copies on the short arms of the acrocentric chromosomes: 13, 14, 15, 21, and 22. They code for a single large 45S primary transcript that is cleaved into 28S, 18S, and 5.8S rRNA classes, designated by their separation in centrifugation gradients and by several associated proteins. Multiple copies of another gene on chromosome 1 produce 5S rRNA.

Transfer RNA

Transfer RNAs (tRNAs) are small RNA transcripts that bind specific amino acids and transport them to ribosomes for use during protein synthesis. More than 40 subfamilies of tRNA genes are known, dispersed across the genome. The mitochondrial genome uses a separate set of tRNAs.

Messenger RNA

Messenger RNAs (mRNAs) are the RNA transcripts of all genes that encode polypeptides and some other genes that encode unprocessed functional RNA molecules. Most are large. All mRNA transcripts undergo further processing, including excision of large segments of noncoding RNA known as introns, the addition of 7-methylguanosine to the first 5′ nucleotide, forming a CAP structure, cleavage of the 3′ end at a specific point downstream from the end of the coding sequence, and addition of the polyA tail at a site specified in part by the sequence AAUAAA, which is located in the 3′ untranslated region (3′ UTR) of the gene. The polyA tail appears to increase the stability of mRNA. The fully processed mRNA is transported to the cytoplasm, where translation occurs.

Small Nuclear RNA

Small nuclear RNA (snRNA) transcripts are small, uridine-rich RNA transcripts that associate with specific proteins to form ribonucleoprotein particles (RNPs). Some of them function in RNA splicing (removing introns from mRNA). They comprise a large family of genes dispersed across the genome.

Small Nucleolar RNA

Small nucleolar RNAs (snoRNAs) are small RNA transcripts that are present in the nucleolus and have important roles in specific cleavage reactions and base-specific modifications during maturation of ribosomal RNA. About 200 snoRNA genes have been identified.

MicroRNA

MicroRNAs (miRNAs) are another class of small noncoding genes that regulate the expression of protein-encoding genes at the post-transcriptional RNA level [Denli et al., 2004]. The process begins with transcription (synthesis) of primary RNA transcripts that range in size from several hundred to several thousand kb. These transcripts are recognized and cut into precursor miRNAs in the nucleus by a protein known as Dicer, moved to the cytoplasm, and processed into mature miRNAs. The mature miRNAs join the RNA-induced silencing complex (RISC), which recognizes and cleaves (or otherwise silences) a target gene. This process has been demonstrated in many organisms, including mammals, and appears likely to play a key role in regulation of many genes.

Structure and Function of Polypeptides and Proteins

Proteins are composed of one or more polypeptide chains. Polypeptides are large polymers or macromolecules composed of linear sequences of repeating units known as amino acids, which are more complex than the repeating units of DNA or RNA. Amino acids consist of a three-carbon backbone, with an amino group attached to carbon 1 and a carboxyl group to carbon 3. They differ in the composition of a side chain attached to carbon 2. With rare exceptions, all polypeptides and proteins in nature are built from different sequences of 20 amino acids (Table 30-3). The side chains may be neutral and hydrophobic, neutral and polar, basic, or acidic. The simplest amino acid is valine, which has a hydrogen ion as the side chain.

The process of information transfer from RNA polypeptides to proteins is known as translation. It relies on the genetic code, the system by which the nucleotide sequence of mRNA specifies the amino acid sequence of a polypeptide chain. In this nearly universal code, each set of three adjacent bases in the mRNA transcript constitutes a codon, and different

Table 30-3 Classification of Amino Acids by Side Chain

Amino Acid	3-letter Code	1-letter Code
NEUTRAL AND HYDROPHOBIC		
Alanine	Ala	A
Isoleucine	Ile	I
Leucine	Leu	L
Methionine	Met	M
Phenylalanine	Phe	F
Proline	Pro	P
Tryptophan	Trp	W
Valine	Val	V
NEUTRAL AND POLAR		
Asparagine	Asn	N
Cysteine	Cys	C
Glutamine	Glu	Q
Glycine	Gly	G
Serine	Ser	S
Threonine	Thr	T
Tyrosine	Tyr	Y
ACIDIC		
Aspartic acid	Asp	D
Glutamic acid	Glu	E
BASIC		
Arginine	Arg	R
Histidine	His	H
Lysine	Lys	K

Table 30-4 The Nuclear Genetic Code

	U		C		A		G	
U	UUU	Phe	UCU	Ser	UAU	Tyr	UGU	Cys
	UUC	Phe	UCC	Ser	UAC	Tyr	UGC	Cys
	UUA	Leu	UCG	Ser	UAA	Stop	UGA	Stop
	UUG	Leu	UCG	Ser	UAG	Stop	UGG	Trp
C	CUU	Leu	CCU	Pro	CAU	His	CGU	Arg
	CUC	Leu	CCC	Pro	CAC	His	CGC	Arg
	CUA	Leu	CCA	Pro	CAA	Gln	CGA	Arg
	CUG	Leu	CCG	Pro	CAG	Gln	CGG	Arg
A	AUU	Ile	ACU	Thr	AAU	Asn	AGU	Ser
	AUC	Ile	ACC	Thr	AAC	Asn	AGC	Ser
	AUA	Ile	ACA	Thr	AAA	Lys	AGA	Arg
	AUG	Met	ACG	Thr	AAG	Lys	AGG	Arg
G	GUU	Val	GCU	Ala	GAU	Asp	GGU	Gly
	GUC	Val	GCC	Ala	GAC	Asp	GGC	Gly
	GUA	Val	GCA	Ala	GAA	Glu	GGA	Gly
	GUG	Val	GCG	Ala	GAG	Glu	GGG	Gly

combinations of bases within the codon specify the individual amino acids (Table 30-4). The small tRNA molecules serve as the molecular link between mRNA codons and amino acids. One segment of each tRNA transcript contains a three-base anticodon that is complementary to a specific codon on the mRNA, whereas another segment contains a binding site for one of the 20 amino acids.

With a total of only 20 amino acids and 64 possible codons, most amino acids are specified by more than one codon. For some of the different amino acids, the base in the third position in the triplet may be either of the purines, either of the pyrimidines, or sometimes any of the four bases. For this reason, the third position in the codon sometimes is called the wobble position. Arginine and leucine are each specified by six codons, whereas only methionine and tryptophan are specified by a single codon. Three codons signal termination of translation and accordingly are called stop codons.

Transcription

The process of information transfer from DNA to RNA is known as transcription. Synthesis of RNA begins at a specific transcription start site and continues in a 5′ to 3′ direction with regard to the RNA product. The DNA strand that corresponds to the RNA sequence is known as the coding or sense strand. This strand, however, is not used as the template for synthesis of an RNA molecule. Rather, the complementary DNA strand, known as the noncoding or antisense strand, actually serves as the template and is read in the 3′ to 5′ direction. The RNA product is known as a transcript.

Translation

The process of information transfer from RNA to polypeptide or protein is known as translation. This process takes place in the cytoplasm on small structures known as ribosomes, macromolecules composed of the four species of rRNA noted earlier. They function like small migrating factories that travel along an mRNA template, engaging in rapid cycles of peptide bond synthesis. The process consists of initiation, elongation, and termination stages.

The ribosome contains a large site that binds about 35 bp of mRNA, and two adjacent sites for binding the smaller aminoacyl-tRNA molecules. The first is the acceptor or A site, which holds the incoming aminoacyl-tRNA. The second is the donor or P site, which is occupied by a tRNA carrying the growing polypeptide chain. Translation begins with mRNA binding to the ribosome at the site of the first AUG base triplet, which specifies the amino acid methionine, and also serves as the start signal for synthesis of the polypeptide chain and establishes the reading frame of the mRNA.

The mRNA and tRNA then move in the same direction along the ribosome, with the tRNA moving from the "A" site to the "P" site, and the mRNA sliding over three bases, allowing recognition of the next codon. Bonding between the mRNA codon and tRNA anticodon brings the appropriate amino acid into position on the ribosome to form a new peptide bond to the carboxyl end of the growing polypeptide chain. As part of this reaction, the polypeptide chain is released from the tRNA at the "P" site, but remains bonded to the tRNA at the "A" site. The tRNA and mRNA then move another 3 bp along the chain, and the process is repeated. This reaction continues until one of the stop codons is reached. Thus, proteins are synthesized from the amino to the carboxyl terminus, which corresponds to translation from the 5′ to the 3′ end of the mRNA molecule, and methionine is always the first amino acid of each polypeptide chain, although it usually is removed before protein synthesis is completed.

Gene Structure and Organization

As noted earlier, a gene traditionally has been defined as a unit of genetic information. This concept has gradually progressed to a more useful definition, which states that a gene is a sequence of DNA on a chromosome that is required for production of a functional product, which can be either a protein or a functional RNA molecule [Nussbaum et al., 2007]. By convention, genetic information is always read in the 5′ to 3′ direction, whether encoded in DNA or RNA – in an upstream to downstream direction. The nomenclature regarding the 5′ and 3′ positions of the sugar backbone can be confusing. The 5′ carbon of the first nucleotide of a sequence is joined by a phosphodiester bond to a nucleotide not involved in the sequence, whereas its 3′ carbon is joined to the 5′ carbon of the second nucleotide, and so on. The last nucleotide of the sequence has a 3′ carbon, which joins another uninvolved nucleotide.

Genes

Genes are composed of a continuous length of DNA with definable start and end points, which include the sequence that codes for the RNA or polypeptide product and is thus known as the coding region. It has become clear, however, that the structure of a gene is complex and includes much more than the coding sequence of the protein. All genes include additional sequences on either end of the coding region – designated the 5′ and 3′ UTRs – that do not code for an RNA product or polypeptide. These regions function to regulate transcription and RNA stability. The gene is considered to include the entire sequence represented in the RNA product because some mutations within noncoding regions can impair gene function.

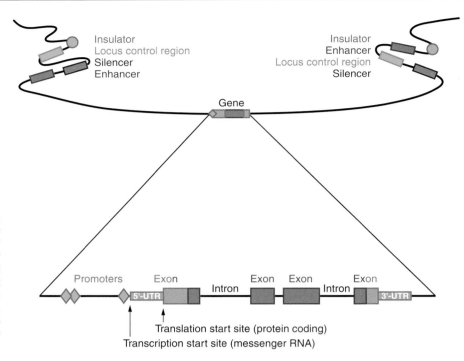

Fig. 30-3 The structure of a typical human gene. The gene includes a primary regulatory region known as the promoter just upstream of the transcription start site that is required for binding of both DNA and RNA polymerases (red diamonds), as well as several types of distant regulatory elements that protect the gene from regulation of other nearby genes (insulator), increase or decrease gene expression (enhancers and silencers), or regulate several genes in the region (locus control region).

A model of a typical human gene is shown in Figure 30-3. Promoter sequences required for regulation and initiation of RNA transcription (red diamonds in Figure 30-3) are present at the 5′ end of the gene, such as the CAT and TATA boxes whose sequences are tightly conserved among many different genes and species. Downstream from the promoter sequences is a specific sequence that signals the start of transcription. A short way further downstream is an initiator codon, AUG, which codes for methionine. This triplet is the translation start site, which signals the start of the coding sequence for the polypeptide product. The region between the transcription and translation start sites is the 5′ UTR.

The next segment of the gene is the coding region. The coding regions of most genes in prokaryotes and lower eukaryotes are colinear, which means that the coding sequence corresponds exactly to the sequence of amino acids in the polypeptide. By contrast, most higher eukaryotic genes, including human genes, contain additional sequences that lie within the coding region, interrupting the sequence that represents the polypeptide. The regions that code for the final polypeptide (or functional RNA) product are known as exons, whereas the regions that are missing from the final mRNA product are introns. The removal of introns from the final mRNA product is known as splicing, a complex process that is regulated by a large number of proteins and functional RNA transcripts.

The coding sequence ends at one of three specific stop codons: UAA, UAG, or UGA. The last segment of the gene is the 3′ UTR, which contains a polyadenylation signal and presumably a signal to end transcription, although no transcription stop sequence has been identified. The length of a gene may vary, ranging from less than 1 kb to several hundred kb. The longest gene known, which codes for dystrophin, spans more than 2000 kb of genomic sequence, although this is not the largest protein produced in the cell.

Regulatory Regions

Many genes have highly conserved sequences, a longer distance upstream and downstream of the transcribed gene, that are involved in regulating expression, including enhancers, silencers, locus control regions, and insulators (see Figure 30-3). Enhancer elements function to increase gene expression, while silencers reduce gene expression. Locus control regions may regulate expression of several genes within a chromosome region, while insulators prevent co-regulation of more distant genes and gene regions. All of these are sequences that bind proteins called transcription factors, which can be ubiquitous, tissue-specific, and/or temporally expressed. Promoters are located immediately 5′ of the gene and bind to RNA polymerase II, a necessary step for transcription. Other transcription factors bind upstream of the promoter and activate transcription. Enhancers and silencers are often located at a distance from the promoter, and increase or decrease transcription in a tissue-specific or temporal manner. Overall, the transcription of each gene is tightly regulated, with multiple transcription factors involved.

RNA Processing

Transcription of DNA gives rise to a precursor RNA that corresponds exactly to the genome sequence but must be modified in several ways to become functional, especially for mRNA. The first modification to mRNA is the addition of a CAP structure to the 5′ end and this is followed by the removal or splicing of introns. The mechanism of mRNA splicing depends on the specific nucleotide sequences at the exon/intron boundaries called splice junctions (Figure 30-4). The most important of these is the GT-AG rule: introns almost always start with GT (actually GU, because this occurs in RNA), which is therefore called the splice-donor site, and end with AG, which is called the splice-acceptor site. Several additional specific sequences are also

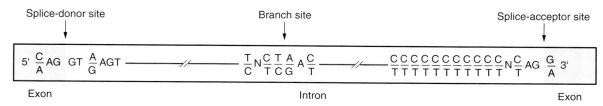

Fig. 30-4 Consensus sequences at the splice-donor, branch, and splice-acceptor sites in introns of higher eukaryotes. The GT dinucleotide at the start of the intron, the A near the end of the branch site, and the AG dinucleotide that ends the intron are invariant, whereas most others represent only the most common nucleotide. When two nucleotides are depicted at a single position, no preference is shown as to which is listed on the top or on the bottom. Abbreviations: A, adenine; C, cytosine; G, guanine; N, any nucleotide; T, thymine. *(Modified from Strachan T, Read AP. Human molecular genetics. New York: Wiley-Liss, 1996.)*

needed, including sequences within the intron just after the GT splice-donor site, at a highly conserved branch site located about 40 bp before the end of the intron and just before the AG splice-acceptor site. The splicing mechanism produces the following:

1. cleavage at the 5′ donor site splice junction just before the invariant G
2. nucleolytic attack by the terminal G of the splice-donor site at the invariant A of the branch site to form a "lariat"-shaped structure
3. cleavage at the 3′ splice-acceptor site at the 3′ splice junction, leading to release of the intronic RNA as a lariat or loop, and splicing of the two exons.

These reactions are catalyzed by large complexes composed of snRNA and specific proteins. The snRNAs involved have specific sequences that allow binding with conserved intronic sequences or the recognition sites of other snRNAs. The snRNA–protein–target RNA complexes form large particles known as spliceosomes. Once a 5′ splice site is recognized, the complex scans the RNA sequence until it encounters a branch site, which aids in identifying the nearby 3′ splice-acceptor site. This process does not necessarily happen in linear order along the RNA. Rather, the order likely is determined by the vagaries of RNA folding. The last steps involve cleavage of part of the 3′ UTR, which occurs at a specific point downstream from the end of the coding sequence, and addition of a long sequence of adenosine nucleotides that is called the polyA tail. The site of the polyA tail is specified in part by the sequence AAUAAA, which is located within the 3′ UTR.

Imprinting and X-Inactivation

Several regions of the genome are subject to inactivation under special circumstances, with no changes to the DNA sequence. The processes involved thus represent a form of "epigenetic" modification. The two processes reviewed here, imprinting and X-chromosome inactivation, both can result in a phenotype when disrupted.

Imprinting

The process by which certain genes in specific chromosomal regions are expressed from only one chromosome, depending on the parental origin of the chromosome, is known as "imprinting." Although the mechanism is only partly understood, a key component involves allele-specific DNA methylation, found predominantly at the carbon 5 position of about 80 percent of all cytosines that are part of symmetrical cytosine-guanine

(CpG) dinucleotides [Jiang et al., 2004; Strachan and Read, 2010; Weksberg et al., 2003].

This process is controlled by regulatory imprinting "centers," located nearby on the same chromosome as that of the silenced or "imprinted" gene. In effect, then, two alleles of the same gene that are identical in nucleotide sequence but derived from opposite parents are regulated differently in the same nucleus. This process is reversible, so that the silent, imprinted allele can be reactivated and the active allele silenced when passed through the germline of the opposite-sex parent. Most imprinted genes are found in large clusters of greater than 1 Mb (megabase pairs) in length. Imprinted clusters have been identified in chromosomes 6q24, 7p11.2, 11p15.5, 14q32, 15q11–q13, and 20q13.2, and others may exist as well [Cavaille et al., 2002; Gardner et al., 2000; Hall, 1990; Jiang et al., 2004; Weksberg et al., 2003; Wylie et al., 2000]. Imprinted regions share several common characteristics, including differential DNA methylation, allele-specific RNA transcription, antisense transcripts, histone modifications, and differences in timing of replication.

X-Inactivation

In mammalian cells with two (or more) X chromosomes, all but one undergo widespread gene silencing by methylation. This phenomenon, known as X-chromosome inactivation (Xi), causes one of the two X chromosomes in cells of female mammals to become transcriptionally inactive early in embryonic development, a phenomenon known as the Lyon hypothesis [Lyon, 1961, 2002]. In mutant cells with more than two X chromosomes, all but one become inactivated. This has the effect of balancing gene dosage of X-linked genes between male and female cells. The process of Xi is random, so that on average the maternally and paternally derived X chromosomes are each inactivated in approximately 50 percent of cells. Changes in this pattern are seen in female carriers of some X-linked diseases, resulting in skewing of Xi. This alteration can be favorable, with decreased severity of the phenotype, or unfavorable, with increased severity of the phenotype [Dobyns et al., 2004].

Cell Cycle and Chromosomal Basis of Heredity

Current knowledge regarding the chromosomal basis of heredity and that concerning the cell cycle are inextricably linked because the intracellular structures now known as chromosomes were first seen in cells undergoing cell division. The existence of chromosomes was foreshadowed by Gregor Mendel's work. For years after he described independent sorting of genetic traits, occasional exceptions to Mendel's law of segregation were discovered. Certain traits were found that were typically inherited as a group. These observations were eventually explained by the discovery of chromosomes. The nuclear material of a cell, or chromatin, appears homogeneous during most of the cell cycle, but condenses into distinct rod-shaped organelles during cell division. These tiny structures were called chromosomes because they stain darkly with various biologic dyes.

Cell Cycle

Humans begin life as a single diploid cell or zygote, which gives rise to all of the cells of the body by a combination of cell growth and cell division, with the latter including both asexual (mitosis) and sexual (meiosis) cell division. The life cycle of somatic cells is divided into four stages. After cell division, the cell enters the G_1 (gap 1) resting phase, during which DNA synthesis does not occur. Some differentiated cells, such as neurons, stop growth in a modified G_1 phase known as G_0. Late in G_1, the cell passes a critical point, after which it proceeds through the rest of the cell cycle at a standard rate. G_1 is followed by the S phase, during which DNA synthesis or replication occurs. The genetic material is duplicated in the form of two chromatids (future chromosomes), joined by attachment to a single centromere. The cell then enters the G_2 (gap 2) resting phase, which is much shorter than G_1. The G_1, S, and G_2 phases together constitute interphase.

Mitosis

Somatic cell division, or mitosis, is an elaborate mechanism that distributes one chromatid of each duplicated chromosome to each of the two daughter cells. The process is continuous but has been divided into the following five stages: prophase, prometaphase, metaphase, anaphase, and telophase (Figure 30-5).

In prophase, the chromatin begins to condense, the nucleolus disappears, and the mitotic spindle begins to form. Prophase is followed by prometaphase, during which the nuclear membrane disappears, allowing the chromosomes to disperse in the cell and attach to the spindle by paired kinetochores located at the centromere. In metaphase, the chromosomes are maximally contracted and arranged at the equatorial plane of the cell. In anaphase, the replicated chromosomes separate at the centromere, allowing the two chromatids to become daughter chromosomes, which move to opposite ends of the cell. In telophase, the chromosomes decondense, the nuclear membrane reforms, and the nucleus returns to the interphase appearance. Shortly afterward, the cytoplasm divides to form two daughter cells. For routine studies, chromosomes are examined during metaphase. For high-resolution studies, they are examined before the point of maximal contraction, during prophase or prometaphase.

Meiosis

Reproductive cell division, or meiosis, is an even more complex mechanism in which two successive cell divisions, known as meiosis 1 and meiosis 2, give rise to the haploid germ cells (Figure 30-6). Meiosis is of critical importance in

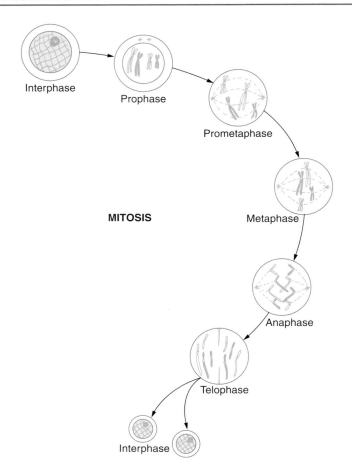

MITOSIS

Fig. 30-5 Diagram of mitosis demonstrating two chromosome pairs.

understanding many of the methods of modern molecular genetics and the pathogenesis of many genetic diseases.

In meiosis 1, the chromosome number is reduced from the diploid to the haploid number. The key step consists of close pairing of homologous chromosomes during prophase 1, which is further divided into several stages. During leptotene, the chromosomes first become visible, with homologs located close together. During zygotene, the homologs begin to pair closely along their entire length, held together by a thin protein-containing structure known as a synaptonemal complex. During pachytene, synapsis or pairing is completed, and the homologs appear as a bivalent. Pachytene is the stage during which exchange of homologous segments between nonsister chromatids occurs, which is known as recombination or crossing over. The remaining steps are similar to mitosis, except that it is the paired homologs that are pulled apart rather than the centromeres. In meiosis 2, which closely resembles mitosis, the chromatids separate at the centromere to form daughter chromosomes. Ova and sperm have remarkably different timing, but the sequence of meiosis is the same.

Chromosomal Basis of Heredity

Chromosome Structure

In humans, the nuclear DNA is dispersed among 46 separate linear structures or chromosomes, each of which consists of a single, uninterrupted double helix that contains 50–250Mb

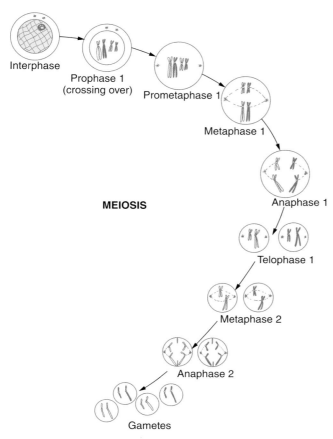

Fig. 30-6 Diagram of meiosis depicting two chromosome pairs.

of DNA, and a group of associated proteins that form the support structure or scaffolding. The scaffolding consists of five basic proteins called histones and several more acidic nonhistone proteins. Two copies of each of four histones – H2A, H2B, H3, and H4 – join to form an octamer. The DNA double helix wraps almost twice around the octamer, which involves about 140 bp. Adjacent octamers are separated by a short spacer segment of 20–60bp that is associated with histone H1. The complex of DNA and core histones is known as a nucleosome (see Figure 30-2).

Strings of nucleosomes are further compacted into a secondary helical structure known as a solenoid. These structures have a diameter of about 30 nm (see Figure 30-2) and contain six nucleosomes per turn. The solenoids are packed into large loops of 10–100 kb of DNA, which are attached to a nonhistone protein scaffolding. These loops pack together loosely to form interphase chromosomes. During early prophase, they pack together more closely to form knoblike thickenings known as chromomeres, which then coalesce further to form the bands observed in prometaphase and metaphase chromosomes when stained with appropriate dyes.

The alternating light and dark bands that characterize all nuclear chromosomes with a variety of staining methods likely reflect the compartmentalization of the genome into isochores, defined as large regions with variation in base composition or variable spacing of scaffold attachment regions. The dark bands observed with Giemsa staining are AT-rich, replicate late in the DNA synthesis phase of the cell cycle, and contain relatively few genes. The light bands observed with Giemsa are

GC-rich, replicate early, and contain many genes. Some are greatly enriched for GC and contain high concentrations of genes. Most, although not all, such bands are located near the ends or telomeres of chromosomes and therefore are known as T bands.

Specialized Regions

All nuclear chromosomes have specialized regions that are required for chromosome integrity and function, including centromeres, telomeres, and origins of replication. Centromeres are DNA sequences that act in *cis*. That is, they act on the chromosome on which they are located and are responsible for the segregation of chromosomes during cell division. Centromeres contain extensive repeats of an approximately 171-bp unit known as alpha-satellite DNA, the sequence of which differs slightly between each chromosome. Fragments of chromosomes that lack a centromere, known as acentric fragments, are lost during cell division.

The two ends of a chromosome are called telomeres and also are required for chromosome stability. In humans, they consist of long arrays of tandem repeats of the sequence TTAGGG, which extend about 5–20 kb. DNA polymerases are unable to replicate the telomeres because of the lack of a template. This problem is resolved by the enzyme telomerase, which contains an RNA component to serve as a template to prime further synthesis on the leading strand. Further extension of the leading strand provides the needed template for the lagging strand.

Origins of replication are specialized sequences where DNA replication begins, and thus are important in maintaining chromosome number and integrity. They consist of autonomously replicating sequence elements that contain a core consensus sequence and some imperfect copies with a length of about 50 nucleotides. A consensus human autonomously replicating sequence has been identified [Strachan and Read, 2010].

Regions of variable staining known as heterochromatin consist of long arrays of repeat sequences as short as 5 bp. These regions are located primarily in the pericentromeric regions of chromosomes 1, 9, and 16, and in distal Yq. The five human acrocentric chromosomes have small satellites attached to the short arm by short stalks or secondary constrictions that contain the rRNA genes.

Chromosome Number

Each human somatic cell contains 46 chromosomes that consist of 22 matched pairs known as autosomes and two sex chromosomes: XX in females and XY in males (Figure 30-7). In contrast, human germ cells contain only 23 chromosomes, consisting of 22 unpaired autosomes and a single sex chromosome. The former is known as the diploid or 2n number, and the latter is known as the haploid or 1n number. The autosomes were numbered according to length, with chromosome 1 the longest and chromosome 22 thought to be the shortest. Although chromosome 21 later proved to be shorter than chromosome 22, the numbers were retained for historical reasons. The two members of each pair of autosomes and the two X chromosomes in females carry the same genes and are known as homologous chromosomes, or homologs. Although they appear similar under the microscope, homologs are not strictly identical. They contain the same genes, but the nucleotide sequence differs at thousands of positions.

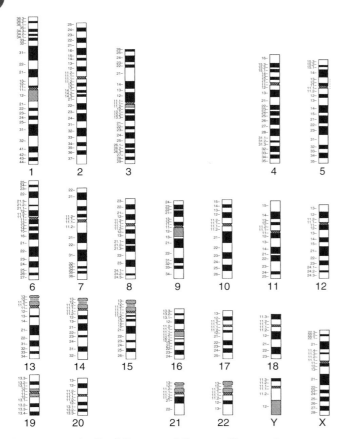

Fig. 30-7 Standardized diagram or idiogram of human chromosomes at the 400-band stage.

Chromosome Identification

Individual chromosomes may be seen only when tightly contracted during cell division. Since DNA replication is complete, each chromosome consists of two chromatids that are joined at the primary constriction or centromere. In standard cytogenetic nomenclature, the centromere divides the chromosome into two arms, with the shorter designated the "p" arm and the longer the "q" arm. The tip of each arm is the telomere. Human chromosomes are classified into three types according to the position of the centromere:

1. metacentric, in which the centromere is centrally placed and the two arms are of about equal length
2. submetacentric, in which the centromere is off center and the arms are of unequal length
3. acrocentric, in which the centromere is near one end.

Organization of the Human Genome

The human genome comprises the total of all genetic information in the cell. It is divided into two separate compartments – a large and complex nuclear genome and a much smaller and simpler mitochondrial genome. The mitochondrial genome consists of a single circular DNA molecule that is present in many copies in each mitochondrion, while the nuclear genome is distributed among the 46 nuclear chromosomes. The available data regarding the genome have become much more extensive and accurate with completion of the Human Genome

Project. A few of the most useful Human Genome Project-related websites are listed in Table 30-1.

The Nuclear Genome

The human nuclear genome consists of approximately 3×10^9 bp, or 3000 Mb of DNA. About 75 percent of this represents unique or single-copy DNA, which includes genes and some important regulatory elements. The remaining 25 percent consists of several classes of repetitive DNA [Lander et al., 2001; Nussbaum et al., 2007; Venter et al., 2001].

Genes and Conserved Noncoding DNA

Somewhat surprisingly, recent estimates predict that the human genome contains less than 30,000 protein-coding genes (possibly closer to 20,000) and an uncertain number of other genes producing functional RNA products. This is far fewer than earlier estimates, and accounts for only about 1.2 percent of nuclear DNA [Lander et al., 2001; Venter et al., 2001]. Another 5 percent of the human genome is more conserved than would be expected from estimates of neutral evolution, which suggests that many of these regions have specific, regulatory functions [Chiaromonte et al., 2003; Waterston et al., 2002]. Studies of these highly conserved regions of DNA have used different thresholds, such as stretches of more than 100 bp with 70–80 percent conservation between mouse and human. Some of these regions have been found to contain important noncoding elements [Dermitzakis et al., 2002, 2003; Frazer et al., 2004; Hardison, 2000]. More stringent analysis demonstrates that the human genome contains 481 sequences of 200 or more bp that are 100 percent conserved among human, mouse, and rat [Bejerano et al., 2004]. These segments were designated "ultra-conserved elements," and are preferentially located near genes involved in RNA processing or regulation of transcription and development. Similarly, about 5000 sequences of 100 bp or more are conserved among these three species, which emphasizes that noncoding sequences are common and important.

Repetitive DNA

Repetitive DNA in the human genome consists of several classes of DNA whose nucleotide sequence is repeated, either exactly or with minor variations, hundreds to millions of times. Some classes are clustered, whereas others are dispersed throughout the genome. Clustered, repeated sequences constitute 10–15 percent of the genome and are collectively called satellite DNA because of their separation from other DNA on density centrifugation. Satellite DNA consists of head-to-tail or tandem arrayed repeat sequences that can extend for several thousand kb. Dispersed, repeat sequences constitute 6–10 percent of the genome and belong to several different classes. Minisatellite or variable number of tandem repeat (VNTR) sequences are dispersed, intermediate-length (15–65 bp) repeats that usually span only several kb. The Alu family of DNA repeats includes about 500,000 related sequences that are each about 300 bp in length and together make up about 3 percent of the genome. The L1 family of repeats includes about 10,000 related sequences that extend up to 6 kb in length and make up another 3 percent of the genome. Although the origin of these sequences is not known, no functions have been identified, and it appears likely that they simply exploit cellular processes to propagate themselves. Several classes have been useful as polymorphic DNA markers.

Low Copy Repeats

Segmental duplications, also known as low copy repeats (LCRs), are DNA sequences of 10–250 kb, present in multiple copies with greater than 95 percent sequence identity, that make up approximately 5 percent of the human genome [Babcock et al., 2003; Bailey et al., 2002; Cheung et al., 2001; Stankiewicz and Lupski, 2002]. LCRs are dynamic regions of the genome because specific repeats tend to cluster within the same genomic regions, where they mediate unequal nonhomologous recombination events, producing segmental deletions and duplications that are collectively designated "copy number variants" (CNVs). Several of these have been associated with well-known developmental disorders in humans, such as Williams' syndrome in 7q11.23, Angelman's syndrome and Prader–Willi syndrome in 15q12, hereditary neuropathy with predisposition to pressure palsies and Charcot–Marie–Tooth neuropathy type 1A in 17p12, Smith–Magenis syndrome in 17p11.2, and DiGeorge's syndrome in 22q11.2 [Babcock et al., 2003]. Many new CNV-associated devlopmental brain disorders have been described over the past few years.

Polymorphisms

A mutation is a permanent change in the DNA of an individual organism, specifically a change in the nucleotide sequence anywhere in the genome [Nussbaum et al., 2007]. Genetic diseases and many cancers are caused by mutations that adversely affect function of one or more genes, although most mutations have little or no effect on gene function and therefore do not change the survival or reproductive fitness of an individual. Some of these persist in the population as morphologic variants known as polymorphisms. Sequence changes that have frequencies of less than 1 percent are known as rare variants, whereas those with frequencies of 1 percent or more are known as polymorphisms. By convention, a genetic polymorphism is defined as the occurrence of two or more variants or alleles in a region of DNA where at least two alleles appear with frequencies greater than 1 percent. Several different classes of polymorphisms occur in the genome, and several methods in molecular biology take advantage of the normal variation between individuals.

Minisatellites

One of the most useful classes of polymorphisms in the genome is that of the minisatellite or VNTR DNA sequences. These are intermediate-length (15–65 bp) DNA sequences that are repeated one to several dozen times in tandem and usually span several kb in total length. They are highly polymorphic, and their extreme polymorphic nature, coupled with the complexity of multilocus minisatellites, makes them valuable for DNA fingerprinting applications, such as forensic, paternity, and zygosity testing and linkage mapping. They also are inherently unstable and susceptible to mutation at a higher rate than observed for other sequences of DNA.

Microsatellites

Microsatellites, also known as satellite DNA or short tandem repeats, are segments of DNA 2–5 nucleotides in length (dinucleotide, trinucleotide, tetranucleotide, or pentanucleotide repeats) that are scattered throughout the genome in noncoding regions between genes or within genes (in introns). They often are used as markers for linkage analysis because of the naturally occurring high variability in repeat number between individuals. These regions are inherently unstable and susceptible to mutations.

The most common microsatellite family consists of 50,000–100,000 cytosine-adenine (CA) repeats, which consist of short tandem repeats of the dinucleotide CA on one strand and guanine-thymine on the complementary strand. They thus take the form $(CA)n/(GT)n$, with n in the range of 6–30 [Weber and May, 1989]. The number of repeats within a $(CA)n$ block varies greatly among different members of a species, producing a set of alleles that always differ in size by multiples of two bases. About 70 percent of the human population is heterozygous at any given $(CA)n$ repeat locus, making these highly polymorphic. The human genome contains about 50,000–100,000 interspersed $(CA)n$ blocks, which is enough to place 1 block every 30–60 kb, if evenly spaced.

For both VNTR and CA repeat sequences, the combination of high frequency in the genome and a high rate of polymorphism has made them very useful for genetic mapping and association studies. Some microsatellite repeats, most often trinucleotide repeats, present within coding regions of genes or, less often, the $5'$ or $3'$ UTR, can expand to an abnormal length and are the basis of triplet repeat diseases such as Huntington's disease, some forms of spinocerebellar ataxia, and fragile X syndrome.

Single-Nucleotide Polymorphisms

Single-nucleotide polymorphisms (SNPs, pronounced "snips") are DNA sequence variations that occur when a single nucleotide (A, T, C, or G) in the genome sequence is changed. For example, a SNP might change the DNA sequence TCACG to TTACG. The most common sequence change involves replacement of cytosine (C) with thymidine (T), which accounts for about two-thirds of all SNPs. As with other types of sequence variation, a SNP must occur in at least 1 percent of the population to be classified as a polymorphism. SNPs occur in both unique-sequence (coding and noncoding) and repetitive DNA, and are responsible for about 90 percent of human genetic variation. On average, SNPs are found approximately every 100–300 bases along the entire human genome. Although most SNPs likely have no function, some are known to influence disease predisposition or responses to drugs, and thus are proving to be very valuable in studying the causes of common human diseases. The current inventory of known SNPs can be found in the Human SNP database (dbSNP) on the NCBI Entrez website (see Table 30-1).

Restriction enzymes are DNA-cutting enzymes or endonucleases derived from bacteria that cut DNA at specific short sequences found at locations across the entire genome. SNPs can alter the sequences recognized by restriction enzymes, thus adding or removing a cutting site. This is the biological basis for restriction enzyme fragment length polymorphisms (RFLPs). Depending on the location of restriction enzyme sites, specific DNA fragment lengths are obtained on digestion with restriction endonucleases. The presence of a SNP at one of these restriction enzyme sites will affect cleavage and produce two DNA fragments of different sizes that is the RFLP. RFLPs also can be produced by any change that alters the size of the DNA fragment on which the restriction site is located, such as deletions or duplications. RFLPs are a measure of naturally occurring variations or polymorphisms of normal DNA, and are inherited according to mendelian principles. RFLPs have been useful for gene mapping.

Mitochondrial Genome

Mitochondria are cellular organelles that are primarily responsible for cellular respiration and production of adenosine triphosphate. Each cell contains numerous mitochondria, and each mitochondrion contains many copies of a small 16.5-kb circular chromosome, adding up to thousands per cell. The mitochondrial chromosome contains 37 genes that code for two types of rRNA, 22 types of tRNA, and 13 polypeptides. The two DNA strands differ significantly in base composition, with a heavy strand rich in guanines that codes for 28 genes, and a light strand rich in cytosines that codes for 9 genes. It is very densely packed, with 93 percent comprising coding sequence [Strachan and Read, 2010].

All of the genes coded by the mitochondrial chromosome are expressed only in the mitochondria. The rRNA genes differ in size from those in nuclear DNA. The genetic code by which tRNAs decipher mRNAs differs slightly from nuclear DNA. The 13 polypeptides function as subunits of the mitochondrial oxidative phosphorylation system. The nuclear genome encodes the remaining 80 or more subunits and also encodes all mitochondrial ribosomal proteins and many other essential genes, such as mitochondrial DNA and RNA polymerases.

Human Genome Project

The importance of DNA, including both genes and noncoding regions, became increasingly apparent during the 1970s and 1980s, leading to one of the most ambitious scientific research projects ever undertaken – a plan to sequence the entire human genome. This project, which was begun in 1990, came to be known as the Human Genome Project. The goals of the project, as taken from the Human Genome Project website (see Table 30-1), were as follows:

- to identify all of the approximately 20,000–25,000 genes in human DNA
- to determine the sequences of the 3 billion chemical bp that make up human DNA
- to store this information in databases
- to improve tools for data analysis
- to transfer related technologies to the private sector
- to address the ethical, legal, and social issues (ELSIs) that may arise from the project.

The successful completion of the Human Genome Project has had the effect of changing genetic research from "bottom up" to "top down" research. That is, a major goal of research before completion of the Human Genome Project was to determine the nucleotide sequence of genes associated with the disease under study. Following completion of the project, research now typically begins with the nucleotide sequence. Although the Human Genome Project has been officially completed, numerous difficult regions of duplicated DNA remain to be sequenced correctly, and data analysis of the entire project is on-going. The effects of the Human Genome Project have already been enormous. Research projects that once required several years now can be done in several weeks or months.

Technology of Cytogenetics

The modern field of cytogenetics began in the 1950s, when methods for arresting cells during mitosis were developed. This is a stage of the cell cycle when chromosomes are maximally contracted and can be visualized under the microscope with various stains. The human diploid chromosome number of 46 was discovered, and many different defects in chromosome number and structure were found, such as Down syndrome. The field has expanded, with development of new computerized image recognition systems for chromosome identification and a variety of methods that make use of molecular genetics methodologies. Thus, the distinction between cytogenetics and molecular genetics has become blurred. In general, cytogenetics tests examine large regions of the genome, such as chromosomes or regions of chromosomes, whereas standard molecular genetics methods focus on smaller regions of the genome, from single nucleotides to genes and gene regions.

Chromosome Analysis

When methods for examining chromosomes under the microscope were first developed, individual chromosomes could not be identified because of solid staining. Instead, they were separated into seven groups (A to G), based on their length and centromere position. It is now possible to identify all 24 human chromosomes individually, using several different staining techniques that take advantage of differences in chromatin structure and composition to produce a recognizable pattern of bands, as shown in the diagram in Figure 30-7. These methods are now used to examine the entire chromosome complement of an individual, which is known as the karyotype. The same term is used to describe the normal chromosome complement of a species.

The three most commonly used staining methods are G-banding, R-banding, and Q-banding. For Giemsa or G-banding, the chromosomes are treated with trypsin and then Giemsa stain to produce the alternating light and dark bands known as G bands. For reverse or R-banding, the chromosomes are pretreated with heat and then stained with Giemsa. The resulting R bands are the exact reverse of those produced by G-banding. For quinacrine or Q-banding, chromosomes are stained with quinacrine mustard and examined under fluorescent light. A specific pattern of bright and dim Q bands is seen, with the bright Q bands corresponding to the dark G bands.

For standard chromosome analysis, cell division is arrested in metaphase, when 400–550 bands per haploid set can be seen. Analysis should be performed on cells with at least 550-band resolution. For high-resolution chromosome analysis, cell division is arrested in prophase before full contraction has occurred, when 550–850 bands per haploid set can be seen. This technique is labor-intensive but may be useful for finding very small chromosome rearrangements.

A uniform system of human chromosome classification and nomenclature was developed at a series of international conferences, and most recently revised in 2009 [ISCN, 2009]. In this system, the chromosomes are separated into regions and subregions, based on the banding pattern. For example, band 17p13.3 (read as "17-p-one-three-point-three") is found near the telomere of the short arm of chromosome 17. During the past decade, computer image analysis systems have been developed that can locate chromosome spreads on the slide, recognize and automatically sort chromosomes, and help with analysis. However, review by trained cytogenetic technicians is still required.

Fluorescence In Situ Hybridization

Fluorescence in situ hybridization (FISH) is a technique used to detect specific chromosomes or chromosomal regions through hybridization (attachment) of fluorescently labeled DNA probes to denatured chromosomal DNA. Examination under fluorescent lighting detects the presence or absence of the hybridized fluorescent signal (and hence presence or absence of the chromosome material).

This study usually is performed on metaphase chromosomes (Figure 30-8) but also can be used on cells in interphase. Interphase FISH often is used for rapid detection of specific types of aneuploidy in fetal cells and for detection of certain deletions, duplications, and other abnormalities in tumor cells. In contrast with metaphase FISH, interphase FISH does not permit visualization of the actual chromosomes, so that most types of structural rearrangements cannot be detected. FISH can be used to examine a small set of chromosomal regions at once, usually 1 or 2, although study of 8–10 is possible with special fluorescent markers. Telomere-specific FISH analysis is an example of hybridization with multiple probes simultaneously. Telomere-specific probes that correspond to the telomeres of

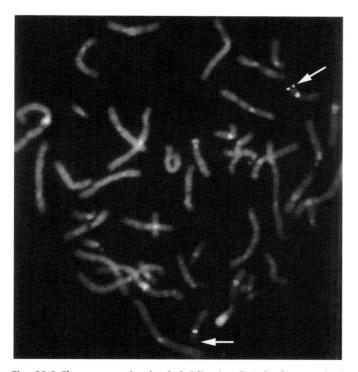

Fig. 30-8 Fluorescence in situ hybridization (FISH) of a standard metaphase spread using a set of three overlapping cosmids at D17S379. The top arrow points to two distinct D17S379 probe signals on the two chromatids of one chromosome 17 homolog. The bottom arrow points to the tip of the other chromosome 17 homolog, which lacks the normal signal and is thus deleted for this probe. The chromosome 17 centromeres are marked by a larger signal just below (top) or above (bottom) the arrows. Different colors are used for the D17S379 and 17 centromere probes so that they can be differentiated easily under the microscope. *(Courtesy of David H. Ledbetter, Emory University, Atlanta, GA.)*

all of the chromosomes are hybridized to metaphase chromosomes in groups and used to detect abnormalities at the ends of chromosomes that are not visible by routine chromosome analysis.

Chromosome Microarrays

Several new methods have been developed to test for loss or gain of DNA sequence that have much higher resolution than chromosome analysis. These include comparative genomic hybridization (CGH) using either bacterial artificial chromosomes or short DNA molecules called oligonucleotides or "oligos," or SNP arrays modified to detect dosage of individual markers.

CGH is a molecular cytogenetics method developed to detect changes in copy number between two genomes, typically those of a control and an experimental subject. The alterations are classified as DNA gains (duplications) and losses (deletions), and reveal a characteristic pattern that includes mutations at chromosomal and subchromosomal levels. Equal amounts of DNA from two different sources (control and experimental) are labeled with two different fluorescent labels and hybridized to normal metaphase chromosome spreads. For example, control DNA may be labeled with red, and experimental subject DNA with green. When the control and the subject samples both contain a DNA fragment of interest, both labels are seen; this produces yellow fluorescence on the metaphase chromosome spread. When a given DNA fragment is deleted in the experimental subject, only the red control label is seen. When a given DNA fragment is duplicated in the subject, only the green subject label is seen.

Array formats for CGH have been developed that have increased the resolution of this technique for detecting smaller deletions and duplications. Instead of hybridizing on to metaphase chromosome spreads, a set of DNA probes across the entire genome is used. The probes are placed on microarrays that can detect DNA fragments with the same sequence as for the probe. Several different methods have been developed using different probes, such as bacterial artificial chromosome (BAC) DNA, complementary DNA (cDNA), or DNA fragments produced by cleavage of genomic DNA by the restriction enzyme BglII [Ishkanian et al., 2004; Lucito et al., 2003; Sebat et al., 2004]. These offer different resolution, with probes every 15–100 kb approximately. The total number of probes has increased from approximately 40,000 to 1 million on commercially available arrays. CGH technology has numerous advantages over FISH, including coverage of the entire genome, finer resolution, and lower cost per probe tested. Thus, clinical tests based on CGH technology have begun to replace FISH technology.

DNA gains and losses may also be detected using the same SNP-based microarrays in common use for genotyping. They are used to measure intensity differences and ratios of alleles at up to 1 million single nucleotides across the genome, detecting many CNVs, as well as detecting intercellular mosaicism and copy-neutral loss of heterozygosity, as occurs with uniparental disomy and other rare mechanisms. In general, the cost per probe is lower with SNP-based microarrays than for CGH-based microarrays, but the results are easier to interpret for CGH-based arrays due to more favorable signal-to-noise ratio. An example of a 14-Mb deletion of human chromosome 1 is shown in Figure 30-9.

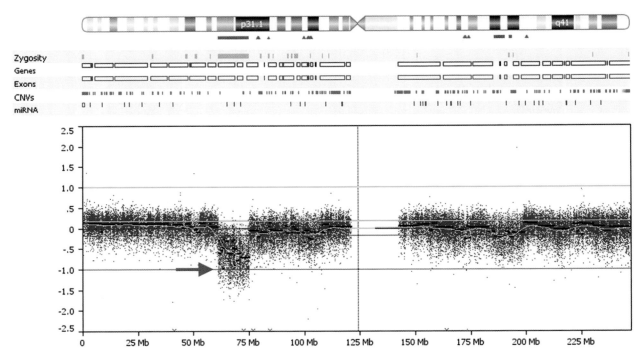

Fig. 30-9 Data from a SNP-based chromosome microarray shows a 14-Mb deletion of human chromosome 1p31. The copy number loss is shown here by reduced dosage (red arrow). These SNP data were generated from a Human660W-Quad v1 DNA Analysis BeadChip® from Illumina, Inc., and the figure generated from Nexus Copy Number® software from Biodiscovery, Inc.

Technology of Molecular Genetics

Molecular genetics is that branch of genetics concerned with the structure and function of genes at the molecular DNA level. The rapid gains in this field during the past decade have resulted from discovery of several new techniques that have made detailed analysis of both normal and abnormal genes possible. These discoveries have in turn led to better understanding of many important biologic processes, as well as the molecular basis for many genetic diseases. Several of these methods have proved to be of particular importance and are commonly used in research studies. Some familiarity with these procedures is helpful in understanding the nature and significance of new discoveries in this area. This section presents a brief introduction to some of the more important procedures. More detailed information can be found in several laboratory manuals, especially *Current Protocols in Human Genetics* [Haines et al., 2010].

DNA Clones

A vector is a DNA molecule that can replicate itself in a host cell, such as a bacterium or yeast. Integration of DNA fragments into the vector with restriction endonucleases and DNA ligase results in propagation of the DNA fragment along with the vector, producing large quantities of the fragment of interest. Vectors with inserted recombinant DNA fragments of interest are known as clones, and the methods used to generate them are collectively known as cloning. Clones are chosen at random from clone libraries, which are large collections of clones originating from a specific source, such as the total genomic DNA or chromosome-specific DNA of a human or other organism.

Several common types of vectors have been used, including phage (bacterial virus) (up to 20-kb insert DNA), plasmids (accessory circular bacterial chromosomes, used to clone several kb of DNA), cosmids (approximately 35–45 kb), BACs (approximately 100–150 kb), P1 plasmid artificial chromosomes (PACs, approximately 100–150 kb), and yeast artificial chromosomes (YACs, up to 1000 kb). The most commonly used at present are BACs and PACs [Stein, 1997], which have proved to be useful for FISH, CGH, and many other technologies. Creation of chromosome-specific DNA libraries by cloning followed by mapping and sequencing is the basis of the information obtained through the efforts of the Human Genome Project.

Restriction Enzymes

Restriction enzymes or endonucleases are bacterial enzymes that recognize short, double-stranded DNA sequences and cut the DNA molecule at or near the recognition site [Lewin, 2007]. When a mutation occurs that changes as few as one of the basepairs in the sequence, it is no longer recognized and cut by the enzyme. Several hundred restriction endonucleases have been isolated. Most of the recognition sites are palindromes, which means that they read the same in the $5'$ to $3'$ direction on both strands, and most of the enzymes leave short overhangs of single-stranded DNA that are known as sticky ends. For example, the enzyme BamHI recognizes the sequence GGATCC and cuts it between the two G bases, leaving the following 4-base overhang:

$$5'-GGATCC-3' \rightarrow 5'-G \qquad\qquad GATCC-3'$$
$$3'-CCTAGG-5' \rightarrow 3'-CCTAG \qquad\qquad G-5'$$

Restriction endonucleases have several important uses in molecular biology. First, they are used to cut or "digest" large

DNA molecules into a reproducible collection of a million or more smaller and more manageable DNA fragments that can be identified on the basis of their size. Second, a mutation at any of the recognition sites that changes the sequence, or a mutation elsewhere that creates a new recognition site, can potentially be detected. Finally, DNA molecules cut with the same restriction endonuclease all have the same sticky ends and may be joined using the enzyme DNA ligase. This condition allows specific DNA sequences of interest to be inserted into vectors and introduced into cells such as the bacterium *Escherichia coli* or the yeast *Saccharomyces cerevisiae* (common bakers' yeast), which then can be propagated to produce large amounts of the sequence of interest. DNA sequences inserted into a vector are known as recombinant DNA. This is the basis of DNA cloning.

Polymerase Chain Reaction

The polymerase chain reaction (PCR) technique has revolutionized the field of molecular genetics. It is a simple but elegant method to amplify a small amount of DNA greater than a million-fold within a matter of hours. PCR results in the enrichment and amplification of a particular DNA region of interest from the total genome, making it more amenable to study, without the use of cloning or Southern blots (described later). The region of DNA with known base sequence to be amplified, such as part of a gene, is selected, and two short DNA sequences flanking the region of interest are synthesized to serve as primers for amplification.

To construct the primers, a short sequence of about 20–25 bp just upstream or 5′ of the target sequence on the DNA "sense" strand is chosen as a starting site, and an oligonucleotide (or primer) that is complementary to this short upstream sequence is synthesized. Another short sequence upstream or 5′ of the target sequence on the complementary (or "antisense") strand also is chosen, and a second complementary oligonucleotide is synthesized. The two primers thus flank the region of interest on opposite strands. The DNA is denatured to separate the strands, after which the oligonucleotides are hybridized to the complementary sequences. The short oligonucleotides then serve as primers for synthesis of a complete complementary DNA strand with appropriate deoxynucleotide triphosphate molecules (adenosine, cytosine, guanosine, and thymidine triphosphate [dATP, dCTP, dGTP, and dTTP]) being added; this is mediated by the enzyme DNA polymerase. Because both strands are copied, one round of amplification results in a complete second copy of the original target sequence. Repeated cycles of heat denaturation, hybridization of the primers, and DNA synthesis result in the exponential amplification of the target sequence. Within a few hours, more than a million copies of the sequence may be made (Figure 30-10).

Methods of General Mutation Detection

DNA Sequence Analysis

SANGER SEQUENCING

DNA sequence analysis is the most sensitive and direct method to detect mutations at the level of individual nucleotides [Haines et al., 2010]. The most widely used method of DNA sequencing is the Sanger method, also known as dideoxy sequencing or chain termination. It is based on the use of

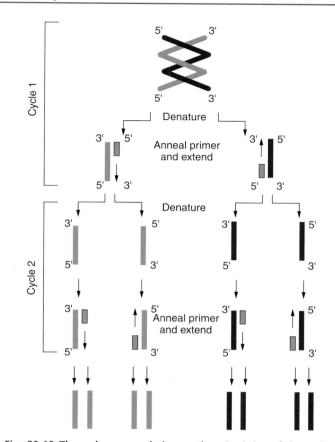

Fig. 30-10 The polymerase chain reaction. Depiction of the cycling process of denaturation, annealing, and extension that results in the exponential amplification of DNA.

synthetic nucleotide analogs – 2,3-dideoxynucleoside triphosphates (ddNTPs). Dideoxy NTPs differ from nucleotides found in natural DNA in that they lack the 3′-hydroxyl group. When integrated into a sequence, they prevent the addition of further nucleotides as phosphodiester bonds cannot form between a dideoxynucleotide and the next incoming nucleotide. Thus, the DNA chain is terminated.

DNA sequencing most commonly is performed by the method of cycle sequencing, in which the DNA region to be sequenced (which is first generated by PCR) is denatured and a short oligonucleotide is annealed to one of the template strands. DNA synthesis occurs in the presence of DNA polymerase, ddNTPs, and nucleotides and starts from the 3′ end of the annealed oligonucleotide. As the DNA is synthesized, nucleotides are added on to the growing chain by the DNA polymerase; however, on occasion, a ddNTP is incorporated into the chain in place of a normal nucleotide, resulting in a chain-terminating event. At the end of the sequencing reaction, multiple DNA molecules are present such that, at each nucleotide position, a proportion of molecules are terminated owing to the incorporation of a ddNTP. These products are separated by size on capillary or polyacrylamide gel electrophoresis systems, and the fluorescently labeled ddNTPs are detected. Each ddNTP is labeled with a different fluorophore. Shorter DNA molecules migrate faster than longer molecules on electrophoresis, and by analyzing the different fluorescent signal of all of the different-sized molecules, the DNA sequence can be determined. For example, ddCTP is labeled with a blue fluorophore.

Everywhere a G residue exists in the template DNA, either a dCTP or a ddCTP will be incorporated into the synthesized strand. For every G residue in the template DNA, a proportion of molecules with a ddCTP at that site will be present. Each of these molecules will be of a different size, depending on where a G residue resides in the sequence, and will be distinguished by electrophoresis. The same applies for the other ddNTPs. Specialized DNA sequencing software exists that can convert the different fluorescent signal to different-color peaks that constitute a DNA sequence chromatogram.

HIGH-THROUGHPUT SEQUENCING

High-throughput sequencing, also known as next-generation or second-generation sequencing, is a much more high-throughput form of DNA sequencing that is revolutionizing the field of genetics and resulting in the ability to sequence entire genomes at a fraction of the cost and time compared to Sanger-based sequencing [Haines et al., 2010]. The basis of second-generation sequencing is cyclic-array sequencing, which is the sequencing of a dense array of DNA features by repetitive cycles of enzymatic reactions and imaging-based data collection. At the time of writing, there are three main commercially available platforms for second-generation sequencing, which include: Solexa technology (used by Illumina), 454 sequencing (used by Roche Applied Science), and the SOLiD platform (used by Life Technologies). While each of these platforms differs with regard to the biochemistry of the sequencing reaction and the generation of the array, the overall concept is similar. This is as follows:

1. DNA is randomly fragmented and common adaptor sequences are ligated to the ends to form "libraries."
2. Each library is clonally amplified by approaches such as emulsion PCR or bridge PCR to form clusters/colonies of sequence features.
3. Each clonally amplified product is spatially clustered or arrayed on a solid surface.
4. Sequencing by synthesis of the clonally amplified products is performed by alternating cycles of enzyme-mediated nucleotide extension and imaging.

Specialized software present for each of the platforms converts the images obtained into DNA sequence. The array-based format of second-generation sequencing, as compared to the capillary-based format of Sanger sequencing, allows for a much higher degree of parallel processing in second-generation sequencing; this results in a throughput ranging from hundreds of megabases to gigabases of sequence per run at a dramatic reduction in cost per base sequenced.

Second-generation sequencing produces short reads of DNA sequence ranging from approximately 36 bp to approximately 400 bp, depending on the platform used. The huge amount of sequence information generated requires intensive bioinformatics and computational approaches for mapping and aligning the sequence data generated to the appropriate genomic reference sequence. Several different computational pipelines are currently used for mapping, aligning, and base-calling of second-generation sequencing data. The accuracy per base of second-generation sequencing is still of relative low quality; therefore, the more times a base is sequenced, or the "deeper" the coverage at that base, the higher the accuracy of the base call. Currently, $8\times$ coverage per base is considered the minimum requirement for base calling; however, for accurate base-calling comparable to Sanger-based sequencing, a coverage of $20–30\times$ per base is probably required.

Second-generation sequencing can be used for the sequencing of whole genomes, exomes (coding exons in the genome), or targeted subsets of genes. For targeted sequencing of exomes or a subset of genes, an enrichment/amplification of this sequence prior to sequencing is necessary. Enrichment can be performed using oligo capture platforms that are available in solution or solid phase. Exome capture kits are commercially available that contain oligos specific to the human exome. Custom oligo kits can be manufactured for specific genes of interest. Targeted amplification of select genes for second-generation sequencing can also be performed by standard PCR; however, the number of genes sequenced by this approach will be limited to the number of genes amplifiable. Newer methods of droplet-based PCR are available that increase the throughput of the number of genes that can be amplified per reaction.

Mutation Scanning

Mutation scanning refers to methods used to determine the presence of a sequence change in a region of DNA (such as an exon of a gene). These methods need to be followed up by DNA sequencing, however, to determine the exact nature of the sequence change. Mutation scanning generally is less labor-intensive, faster, and more cost-effective to perform than DNA sequencing and may be the method of choice when a large gene needs to be analyzed for the presence of mutations. The exons of the entire gene are subjected to mutation scanning, and only those exons that demonstrate the presence of a sequence change need to be sequenced to determine the precise nature of the sequence change.

Various methods of mutation scanning exist that differ in their sensitivities of mutation detection [Cotton, 1997; Eng and Vijg, 1997; Grompe, 1993]. The general basis of most mutation scanning methods is the abnormal migration of a DNA fragment that contains a sequence change from a normal "wild-type" sequence. All are PCR-based methods – the DNA region to be studied is amplified by PCR before the different mutation scanning methods are performed.

SINGLE-STRANDED CONFORMATIONAL POLYMORPHISM

With the single-stranded conformational polymorphism (SSCP) technique, DNA fragments are denatured and made single-stranded. The single-stranded DNA takes on a specific conformation, depending on its sequence. A change in the DNA sequence will result in a change in the single-stranded conformation structure. Denatured fragments are separated on polyacrylamide gels under a series of differing conditions, and fragments with different conformation structures will migrate differently and can be detected. This method has an approximate sensitivity of 80 percent for detecting DNA sequence changes.

DENATURING GRADIENT GEL ELECTROPHORESIS

With denaturing gradient gel electrophoresis (DGGE), DNA fragments are denatured and allowed to re-anneal slowly. In the absence of a sequence change, the only DNA molecules that will be formed are homoduplexes (i.e., with no mismatch of DNA sequence between the complementary strands). In the presence of a sequence change, molecules representing both homoduplexes and heteroduplexes (i.e., a normal-sense strand binds to a mutant antisense strand, or vice versa, to create a mismatch of DNA sequence at the position of the mutation) will be formed. These products are allowed to migrate on a polyacrylamide gel with an increasing gradient, and at a particular gradient, the structure of the heteroduplex molecules changes significantly and affects its migration, compared with that of the homoduplex molecules. For this technique it is important to have specialized GC clamps at the ends of the DNA fragment that enhance the difference between the heteroduplex and homoduplex molecules, and these are included in the PCR primers used to generate the DNA fragment. This method has a high sensitivity, approximately 98–100 percent.

DENATURING HIGH-PERFORMANCE LIQUID CHROMATOGRAPHY

Denaturing high-performance liquid chromatography (DHPLC) also is based on the separation of DNA homoduplex from heteroduplex molecules. The medium of separation is a column composed of a polystyrene-divinylbenzene copolymer to which DNA binds and is released through interaction with specific buffers. At increased temperatures, heteroduplex molecules are released from the column faster than are homoduplex molecules, and therefore can be detected. This method does not require the sophisticated GC clamps of DGGE and has a high sensitivity, close to 100 percent.

PROTEIN TRUNCATION TEST

As the name suggests, the protein truncation test (PTT) is used for the detection of mutations that result in a protein truncation, such as a frameshift or nonsense mutation. The starting material is generally RNA that is converted to cDNA by reverse transcription PCR. In vitro transcription and translation are performed, and the protein products are labeled and separated by sodium dodecyl sulfate (SDS) polyacrylamide gel electrophoresis. A DNA fragment that contains a truncation mutation will result in a protein product that will be shorter in length than a normal product, and therefore can be detected. This technique will not detect mutations that do not result in protein truncation, such as missense mutations.

SOUTHERN BLOT ANALYSIS

Southern blot analysis, named after its inventor, EM Southern, has been used extensively for DNA analysis, particularly for the detection of DNA abnormalities. With the advent of PCR techniques, the use of this analytic method is decreasing. It still remains useful, however, for the detection of large deletions or duplications that affect a part or the whole of a gene.

Genomic DNA is digested with a restriction enzyme, which results in the production of different-sized DNA fragments that are separated on an agarose gel by electrophoresis. The separated DNA fragments are made single-stranded by treatment with an acid and then transferred and fixed on to a nylon membrane. The single-stranded fixed DNA is hybridized with a radioactively labeled probe specific for a certain gene. A probe can be a cloned fragment of a gene or a PCR product of a gene. The probe will hybridize to that region of the DNA where it finds its complementary sequence. Excess probe is washed off, and the nylon membrane is exposed to an x-ray film to reveal where the probe has bonded. When a large deletion,

duplication, or other form of DNA rearrangement occurs, either deletion or creation of restriction enzyme sites can result. Using a probe that binds to the deleted, duplicated, or rearranged area will reveal a different pattern of hybridization, based on what restriction enzymes have been affected. The presence of a different hybridization pattern, compared with a normal control, is indicative of a change in the DNA structure.

Methods for Detecting Specific Sequence Changes (Genotyping)

Different methods exist for the detection of specific mutations in genes, especially point mutations or insertions and deletions of a few basepairs. These methods are useful for the detection of the common mutations present in diseases such as sickle cell anemia, cystic fibrosis, and hereditary hemochromatosis. These techniques are possible only when the base sequence and precise point mutation responsible for the disease phenotype are known.

Allele-Specific Oligonucleotide Hybridization

For allele-specific oligonucleotide (ASO) hybridization, separate ASO probes complementary to either the normal or a specific mutant allele are synthesized. The probes consist of the point mutation or its normal counterpart and 9–12 bp flanking it on either side, for a total length of 19–25 bp. The probes then are hybridized to the DNA source under stringent conditions. Because the probes are short, they are highly sensitive to sequence changes at even a single nucleotide. A probe complementary to the normal allele will hybridize to the normal allele but not to the mutant allele, and vice versa. Thus, DNA from a person homozygous for the normal gene will hybridize to the ASO probe complementary to the normal DNA sequence, but not to the probe complementary to the point mutation. DNA from persons homozygous for the mutation will hybridize to the ASO probe complementary to the mutation, but not to the normal probe. Only DNA from heterozygotes will hybridize to both probes. It is important to remember that DNA from persons who are heterozygous for different mutations in the same gene – compound heterozygotes – also will hybridize to the normal probe. Several different formats have been developed to detect ASO probes, ranging from radioactivity to chemiluminescence to fluorescence, and can be performed in both solid and liquid phases.

Single-Base Extension

Oligonucleotide primers of approximately 20 bp are designed to hybridize just upstream or downstream of the nucleotide to be genotyped, and an extension reaction – more specifically, a single-base extension (SBE) reaction – is performed in the presence of ddNTPs. In the case of a normal sequence, a ddNTP corresponding to the complementary normal nucleotide is added to the primer; in the case of a mutation, a ddNTP corresponding to the complementary mutant nucleotide is added to the primer. The ddNTPs generally are labeled with different fluorochromes, allowing their detection. In a person homozygous for a normal gene, extension will occur only with the ddNTP corresponding to the normal allele, whereas in a person homozygous for a mutated gene, extension will occur only with the ddNTP corresponding to the mutated allele.

A heterozygous person will have both normal and mutated extension products. Several different formats have been developed to detect SBE products and can be performed in both solid and liquid phases.

DNA Arrays

In DNA arrays, hundreds to thousands of DNA targets are arranged (arrayed) on a solid medium such as a glass slide or microchip. DNA arrays are of two main types – genotyping arrays and sequencing arrays. Genotyping arrays consist of hundreds to thousands of different ASO probes or SBE primers arrayed on a chip that allows the genotyping of a large number of different loci simultaneously. DNA sequencing arrays consist of a series of hundreds of thousands of approximately 20-bp oligonucleotides, spanning the length of a gene, that are arranged with equal spacing, or "tiled," across the microchip. For each nucleotide to be sequenced, four oligonucleotides are present that differ only at the central position and have an A, C, G, or T. Digested DNA is fluorescently labeled and hybridized to the tiled oligonucleotide chip under stringent conditions. The DNA hybridizes to those oligonucleotides that correspond to the correct sequence and the fluorescent signal read from which the DNA sequence is deciphered. DNA sequencing and genotyping arrays are available for several genes and are still largely used for research, although some clinical applications have been developed. Expression arrays are different and refer to cDNA arrays to which RNA is hybridized and are used to determine the expression profile of hundreds of genes simultaneously. This technique is currently used only in the research setting.

Restriction Enzyme Analysis

Some mutations result in the destruction or creation of a restriction enzyme site in the DNA sequence. PCR amplification of the region of interest, followed by digestion of the genomic DNA with the appropriate restriction enzyme and gel electrophoresis, can be performed to determine the presence or absence of a mutation that affects a restriction enzyme site. Destruction or creation of a restriction enzyme site will result in a different-sized DNA fragment compared with a normal control fragment. The sickle cell anemia mutation and the hereditary hemochromatosis mutation both affect restriction enzyme sites.

DNA Methylation Analysis

DNA methylation analysis can be performed for the detection of abnormalities in imprinted genes. Of the two alleles of an imprinted gene, one allele is methylated at the promoter (silenced allele), and the other is unmethylated (expressed). Any aberration that affects the imprinting status (e.g., deletion or uniparental disomy) will affect the methylation pattern. Methylation can be assayed with the use of methylation-sensitive restriction enzymes, followed by Southern blot analysis or by methylation-specific PCR techniques. For methylation-specific PCR assays, genomic DNA is treated with the chemical sodium bisulfite, which converts all cytosine molecules to thymidine, except if methylated. The methylated cytosine molecules are left unchanged. As a result, a methylated sequence will be changed in its nucleotide content, as compared with an unmethylated sequence after bisulfite treatment,

and can be distinguished by the use of specific PCR primers. Genes subject to X-inactivation also are methylated and can be detected using the same method.

Clinical Cytogenetics

Chromosome abnormalities may involve either the number or the structure of chromosomes. The former are considered genome mutations, and the latter, chromosome mutations. The mechanisms involved in the two major types of mutations are quite different, but both may result in loss or gain of DNA in the nucleus. Both types may involve all of the cells of an organism or only a proportion. When only a proportion of cells are involved, the abnormality is termed mosaic, discussed in detail later in this section.

Abnormalities of Chromosome Number

For germ and somatic cells, the normal chromosome complement consists of the haploid and the diploid number, respectively. Any deviation from these numbers is associated with significant abnormalities. The most common types result from abnormal segregation of chromosomes in germ cells; epidemiologic studies have estimated a rate of abnormal segregation of approximately 1 per 25–50 meiotic cell divisions.

Triploidy and Tetraploidy

Occasionally, fetuses with three or four times the normal haploid number of chromosomes have been observed. These abnormal chromosome complements are called triploidy (3n) and tetraploidy (4n). The few children who are liveborn survive only briefly after birth, unless the abnormality is mosaic (i.e., involves only a proportion of their cells). Failure of a maturational division in either egg or sperm results in triploidy, whereas failure of completion of an early division of the zygote causes tetraploidy.

Aneuploidy

Aneuploidy is defined as any chromosome complement that deviates from a multiple of the haploid number. In most cases, it consists of either monosomy, which is defined as loss of an entire chromosome, or trisomy, which refers to gain of an entire chromosome. Aneuploidy is the most common and clinically significant type of chromosome disorder, occurring in 3–4 percent of all recognized pregnancies.

Both monosomy and trisomy of autosomes are lethal during early pregnancy in a large majority of affected fetuses. Autosomal monosomy is uniformly lethal, except for a few reports of liveborn children with monosomy 21. Monosomy X is prenatally lethal in most affected fetuses, but many survive and will have the phenotype of Turner's syndrome. The effects of trisomy vary, depending on the chromosome involved. Trisomy 16 is the most frequent autosomal trisomy at conception but is uniformly lethal before birth. The most common type of trisomy in liveborn infants is trisomy 21, which is the chromosome abnormality observed in 95 percent of children with Down syndrome. The only other autosomal trisomies observed at appreciable frequencies are trisomy 13 and trisomy 18, although trisomy 8 may be observed in mosaic form.

The most common mechanism is nondisjunction, which is the failure of a pair of chromosomes to separate correctly during one of the two stages of meiosis, usually meiosis 1. The consequences of nondisjunction during meiosis 1 and 2 are somewhat different. If the error occurs during meiosis 1, the unbalanced gamete with 24 chromosomes contains both the maternal and the paternal members of the pair. If the error occurs during meiosis 2, the unbalanced gamete will contain either the maternally or the paternally derived chromosome, but not both.

Abnormalities of Chromosome Structure

Structural chromosome rearrangements consist of loss, gain, or altered position of segments of chromosomes, and many different types have been recognized. The estimated frequency is about 1 per 1700 cell divisions, making them much less frequent than aneuploidy. Rearrangements are termed balanced if the chromosome complement has a normal amount of genetic information, regardless of its location. They are termed unbalanced if there has been either loss or gain of DNA sequence. The phenotypic effects often are severe. The chromosomes involved in the reconfiguration are known as derivative chromosomes. Many different types of rearrangements have been reported, as described in the following sections. Only those derivative chromosomes that contain a functioning centromere and telomeres, however, are stable and capable of being transmitted unaltered to daughter cells during mitosis or meiosis. Derivatives lacking a centromere or telomere are unstable and are lost during cell division. Some regions of the genome, such as 8p, contain a noncentromeric sequence that is sufficiently similar to function as a "neocentromere" during cell division [Giglio et al., 2001].

Mechanisms

Some progress has been made recently in current understanding of the mechanisms causing or at least predisposing to structural chromosome rearrangements. Many appear to occur randomly, with no evidence of recurrent breakpoints. For example, no consistent breakpoints have been found for the interstitial deletions and reciprocal translocations involving chromosome band 17p13.3 [Cardoso et al., 2003]. In many other locations, the small duplicated regions known as LCRs can mediate several different types of rearrangements. These were first identified as the cause of common deletion or microdeletion syndromes, such as deletion (del) 2q13 with juvenile nephronophthisis and Joubert's syndrome-related disorder [Parisi et al., 2004; Saunier et al., 2000], 7q11.23 in Williams' syndrome [Osborne et al., 2001; Urban et al., 1996], del 15q11.2–q13 in Angelman's syndrome and Prader–Willi syndrome [Amos-Landgraf et al., 1999], del17p12 in hereditary neuropathy with predisposition to pressure palsies [Chance et al., 1994], del17p11.2 in Smith–Magenis syndrome [Chen et al., 1997], and del22q11.2 in DiGeorge's syndrome/velocardiofacial syndrome [McDermid and Morrow, 2002]. The same LCRs are associated with duplications of the same regions, including duplication 15q11.2–q13 [Mohandas et al., 1999], 17p12 [Pentao et al., 1992], and 17p11.2 [Potocki et al., 2000]. A simple diagram of this mechanism is shown in Figure 30-11.

Many of the LCRs are inverted with respect to each other, which can lead to very complex combinations of deletions and duplications. This can occur for LCRs on the same

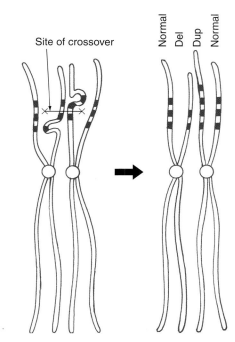

Fig. 30-11 Drawing of a recombination event mediated by low copy repeats. The black boxes represent low copy repeats and the long four-armed linear structures represent chromosomes with two chromatids each during meiosis 1. In the drawing on the left, the outermost chromatids have paired correctly, while the inner two chromatids have paired incorrectly (long arrow pointing to site of crossover). In the drawing on the left, the outermost chromatids appear normal. But in the innermost pair, the crossover event within the mispaired region results in one daughter chromosome with a duplication and another with a deletion. The dark squares represent the low copy repeats.

chromosome, as seen with Williams' syndrome and some X chromosome rearrangements [Giglio et al., 2000; Osborne et al., 2001], or between homologous chromosomes. The latter appears to be more common when two matching LCRs on homologous chromosomes are inverted with respect to each other, a novel type of polymorphism [Giglio et al., 2001]. Similar mechanisms also can predispose to structural rearrangements between completely different chromosomes involving either an LCR or a gene cluster, such as olfactory receptor clusters [Giglio et al., 2002; Spiteri et al., 2003].

Balanced and Unbalanced Chromosomal Rearrangements

As noted previously, structural chromosome rearrangements that result in no net loss or gain of genomic sequence are balanced, whereas those that do result in a net loss or gain of material are unbalanced. Persons with balanced rearrangements usually are normal, unless one of the chromosomal breaks disrupts an important gene. More recent studies, however, have found that chromosome rearrangements that appear balanced often have submicroscopic loss or gain of material and so are actually unbalanced [Astbury et al., 2004b], and some chromosome rearrangements are more complex than standard chromosome analysis suggests [Astbury et al., 2004a].

Specific Types of Chromosome Rearrangements

The most common structural rearrangements include terminal and interstitial deletions and duplications, reciprocal and robertsonian translocations, inversions, and rings. Examples of most of these are shown in Figure 30-12.

Deletions and Duplications

A deletion consists of loss or gain of a chromosome segment. Deletions may be either interstitial or terminal, with terminal deletions including the telomere (see Figure 30-8 and Figure 30-12D), whereas most duplications are interstitial. Most interstitial deletions and duplications result from unequal crossing over in LCRs (see Figure 30-11). Terminal deletions are more likely to result from simple chromosome breakage, although some apparently terminal deletions prove to be interstitial deletions in which one breakpoint happens to be close to the telomere. Any carrier of a deletion is hemizygous for the information on the corresponding segment of the normal homolog. Thus, small but cytogenetically visible deletions involving critical genes occasionally produce single-gene phenotypes, such as lissencephaly or retinoblastoma.

Duplicated segments usually are adjacent to each other and may be in the same orientation (direct dup), or inverted (inverted dup) with respect to one another. In general, the phenotypic effects of duplications are less severe than the effects of deletion of a similar segment. Small duplications also can result in single-gene phenotypes, such as Charcot–Marie–Tooth neuropathy [Chance et al., 1994], although this is recognized less often than with deletions.

Inversions

Inversions are segments within a chromosome that are inverted with respect to the normal orientation; they result from crossovers within existing duplicated segments (LCRs) or from two breaks within a single chromosome, followed by inversion of the intervening segment and repair of the breaks. When the inverted segment includes the centrosome, the rearrangement is described as a pericentric inversion (see Figure 30-12A), whereas rearrangements in which the inverted segment does not include the centrosome are designated as paracentric inversions. Both types of inversions may result in production of unbalanced gametes because of the effects of recombination within the inverted segment. With pericentric inversions, a loop is formed between the inverted chromosome and its homolog during meiosis 1 (Figure 30-13). Recombination is somewhat, but not completely, suppressed within inversion loops, so crossovers are common in larger loops.

Recombination within a pericentric inversion loop produces derivative chromosomes in which segments distal to the breaks are either duplicated or deleted (see Figure 30-13C). The effects on the phenotype are inversely proportional to the size of the inversion. Thus, the distal segments typically are large with small pericentric inversions, and most unbalanced offspring are spontaneously aborted. Liveborn children with birth defects are more likely with larger inversions that lead to relatively small distal segments.

Crossovers within a paracentric inversion loop, which commonly result from crossovers within LCRs, result in acrocentric or dicentric chromosomes. Acrocentric chromosomes are quickly lost during subsequent rounds of cell division. Dicentric chromosomes inactivate one of the two centromeres and are retained. For both, the loss or gain of chromosomal

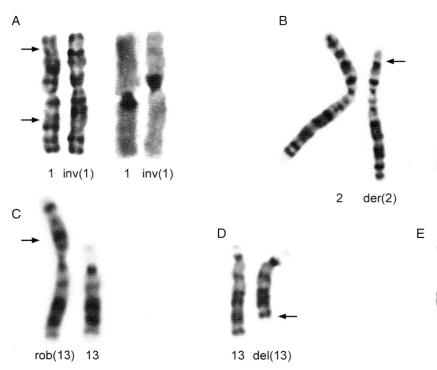

Fig. 30-12 Partial karyotypes of structural chromosome rearrangements. A, Pericentric inversion: 46, XX,inv(1)(p36.1q32). The pair on the left are stained for G bands, and the pair on the right for C bands (centromere bands). **B,** Reciprocal translocation: 6,XX,t(2;4)(p22.2;q35.2). **C,** Robertsonian translocation: 45,XX,t (13q14q). **D,** Interstitial deletion: 46, XY,del(13)(q21.3q31). **E,** Ring: 46,XY, r(17)(p13.3q25.3). *(Karyotypes in **A** from Johnson DD et al. Hum Genet 1988;78:315; those in **B, C,** and **D** courtesy of BA Hirsch, Department of Laboratory Medicine and Pathology, University of Minnesota Medical School; karyotype in **E** from Dobyns WB et al. J Pediatr 1983;102:552.)*

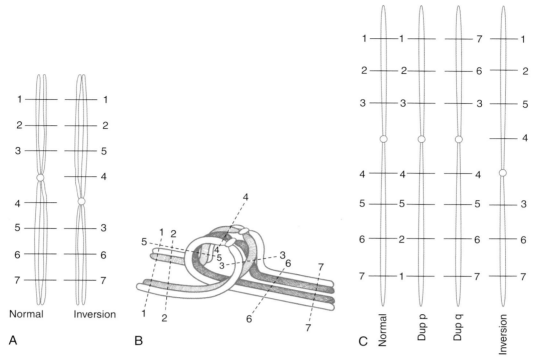

Fig. 30-13 The effect of recombination within the loop of a pericentric inversion. A, A normal chromosome is depicted on the left, with loci 1 to 7 in order and the centromere located between loci 3 and 4. A pericentric inversion is depicted on the right, with the segment containing loci 3–5 and the centromere inverted. **B,** Pairing of the normal and inverted chromosomes during meiosis 1, with a crossover occurring within the inversion loop in the middle two chromatids. **C,** The four types of gametes produced after completion of meiosis include a normal chromosome, a derivative chromosome with duplication of the distal short arm and deletion of the distal long arm (dup p), the reverse derivative chromosome with duplication of the distal long arm and deletion of the distal short arm (dup q), and a balanced pericentric inversion.

material and genes is so great that almost all affected embryos are spontaneously aborted, unless a large part of the derivative chromosome happens to break off and become lost. This mechanism has been proved and may be more common than appreciated [Giglio et al., 2002].

Reciprocal Translocations

Reciprocal translocations consist of breaks in nonhomologous chromosomes, with a reciprocal exchange of the broken segments (see Figure 30-12B). Usually, only two chromosomes are involved, but complex translocations involving three or more chromosomes have been described and likely are more common than standard chromosome analysis has suggested [Astbury et al., 2004a]. Population studies have detected reciprocal or robertsonian translocations in about 1 in 500 newborns.

Reciprocal translocations often result in the production of unbalanced gametes. During meiosis 1, the derivative chromosomes and their normal homologs form a quadriradial shape that may separate into pairs in one of three ways: alternate, adjacent 1, and adjacent 2 segregation. Alternate segregation produces balanced gametes that have either normal chromosomes or both derivatives, which are therefore balanced. Adjacent 1 segregation produces unbalanced gametes in which homologous centromeres separate into different daughter cells. It results in duplication of the distal segment of one derivative chromosome and deletion of the distal tip of the other. In most translocation carriers, alternate and adjacent 1 segregation account for a large majority of the gametes (Figure 30-14). Adjacent 2 segregation also produces unbalanced gametes. In this

uncommon mechanism, homologous centromeres pass to the same daughter cell. The resulting nondisjunction produces 3:1 and even a 4:0 segregation.

Reciprocal translocations often are detected in normal adults evaluated because of repeat fetal loss, or after the birth of a child with multiple congenital anomalies caused by transmission of the translocation in unbalanced form. Apparently balanced reciprocal translocations sometimes are found in children with birth defects or abnormal development. In these instances, the abnormal phenotype usually results from either submicroscopic loss of genetic material or disruption of a gene at one of the breakpoints [Astbury et al., 2004b].

Robertsonian Translocations

Robertsonian translocations involve two acrocentric chromosomes that fuse in or near the centromere region, with loss of the short arms (see Figure 30-12C). Because the short arms contain repetitive DNA elements, especially rRNA, no phenotypic effects result. Carriers of a robertsonian translocation on chromosome 21 have a high risk of producing a child with translocation Down syndrome.

Insertions

Insertions occur when a small segment of a chromosome is removed and inserted into a different region on the same or another chromosome. If the segment is inserted with the same orientation with respect to the centromere, it is known as a direct insertion. If it is inserted with the reverse orientation,

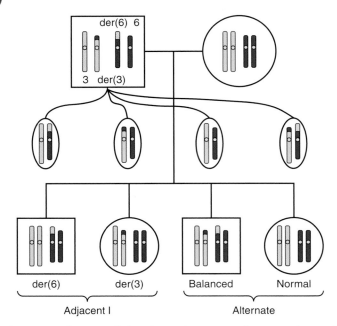

der(6) 6

3 der(3)

der(6)   der(3)   Balanced   Normal

Adjacent I   Alternate

Fig. 30-14 Diagram of the alternative types of segregation and gametes produced in the carrier of a reciprocal translocation between the short arms of chromosomes 3 (light purple) and 6 (dark purple). The top line represents the parental chromosome pairs, the middle line represents the four types of gametes produced by the father, and the bottom line represents four possible chromosome combinations that may be observed in offspring. Alternate segregation (depicted on the right) produces offspring with either normal chromosomes or the balanced translocation. Adjacent 1 segregation (depicted on the left) produces offspring with unbalanced karyotypes. Children with the derivative 6 karyotype (der[6]) have deletion of the distal segment of 6p and duplication of the distal segment of 3p. Children with the derivative 3 karyotype (der[3]) have deletion of 3p and duplication of 6p. In both alternate and adjacent 1 segregation, homologous centromeres pass to different daughter cells. In adjacent 2 segregation (not depicted), homologous centromeres pass to the same daughter cells, leading to even greater chromosomal imbalance.

Table 30-5 Examples of Chromosomal Abnormalities Using Standard Nomenclature (Short System)

Rearrangement	Karyotype
GENOME MUTATIONS	
Triploidy	69,XXX
Monosomy	45,X (Turner's syndrome)
Trisomy	47,XX,+21 (Down syndrome)
DELETION	
Terminal	46,XY,del(8)(p21.1)
Interstitial	46,XX,del(17)(p11.2p11.2)
Ring	46,XY,r(17)(p13.3q22.3)
DUPLICATION	
Direct	46,XY,dir dup (2)(p14p23)
Inverted	46,XX,inv dup (11)(p12p15)
PARACENTRIC INVERSION	
Balanced	46,XX,inv(1)(p32p36.1)
Unbalanced	46,XX, dup q, inv(1)(p32p36.1)
PERICENTRIC INVERSION	
Balanced	46,XX,inv(1)(p36.1q32)
Unbalanced	46,XY,dup(q),inv(1)(p36.1q32)mat
RECIPROCAL TRANSLOCATION	
Balanced	46,XY,t(−17,+der(17),t(7;17)(p22.3;p13.3)pat
ROBERTSONIAN TRANSLOCATION	
Balanced	46,XX,rob(13;21)
Unbalanced	46,XY, −13,+der(13),rob(13;21)mat

del, deletion; der, derivative; dir, direct; dup, duplication; inv, inversion; mat, maternal; pat, paternal; r, ring; rob, robertsonian translocation; t, translocation.

it is called an inverted insertion. Insertions are rare because three separate chromosomal breaks are required. Segregation during meiosis can produce either abnormal offspring, with duplication or deletion of the inserted segment, or normal offspring and balanced carriers.

Rings

Rings – ring chromosomes – are formed when a chromosome undergoes two breaks, usually one in each arm, and the broken ends are rejoined (see Figure 30-12E). The two segments distal to the breaks are lost, resulting in deletion of both telomeres and adjacent regions of both the short and the long arms of the chromosome. Rings may not segregate properly during mitosis and meiosis, especially if a crossover occurs. Crossover often results in breakage followed by fusion, which may produce larger or smaller rings.

Isochromosomes and Dicentrics

Isochromosomes are chromosomes in which one arm is missing and the other is duplicated as the result of misdivision of the centromere during meiosis 2. Isochromosomes also can result from translocation of an entire arm to its homolog with a

breakpoint adjacent to the centromere. The most commonly observed isochromosome involves Xq. Dicentrics are rare chromosomes in which two segments, each containing a centromere, fuse end to end. They tend to break during mitosis because of the double centromeres.

Cytogenetic Nomenclature

Detailed rules regarding nomenclature of chromosomes and chromosomal abnormalities have been published [ISCN, 2009]. Examples of most of the major types of abnormalities are listed in Table 30-5 using standard nomenclature. Note that breakpoints on the same chromosome are not separated by any punctuation, whereas breakpoints on different chromosomes are separated by a semicolon.

Mutations and Genetic Diseases

The number of genetic changes causing disease, including neurologic disorders, is far too great to cover here, although many of these are reviewed in other chapters of this book. Here we review the general mechanisms that lead to genetic diseases, starting with a definition of mutation.

As a very basic definition, a mutation is simply a permanent change in the DNA of an individual. The change most often is a change in the nucleotide sequence anywhere in the genome, although some chemical modifications of DNA can result in mutations as well. Such modifications are known as epigenetic mechanisms. Genetic diseases are caused by mutations that adversely affect function of one or more genes. The same is true for many types of cancer.

Classes of Mutations

Mutations have been subdivided into three main types: genome, chromosome, and gene mutations. They may occur in either somatic or germ cells, although only germ cell mutations can be transmitted to offspring. All three occur often enough for affected individuals to be observed in clinical practice.

Genome and Chromosome Mutations

Abnormalities of chromosome number, including triploidy, tetraploidy, and aneuploidy, are classified as genome mutations. Similarly, structural rearrangements are classified as chromosome mutations. Both of these were reviewed in the preceding section. Genome and chromosome mutations are rarely perpetuated to the next generation because most result in spontaneous abortions. Thus, the frequencies cited are probably underestimates.

Gene Mutations

Gene mutations differ from genome and chromosome mutations because the segment of DNA involved is much smaller and the mechanisms are different. The most common types are basepair substitutions and small deletions or insertions that can be caused by an error during DNA replication or by base changes induced by extrinsic agents referred to as mutagens. Because genome and chromosome mutations usually are lethal, most significant heritable mutations are gene mutations.

DNA Replication Errors

DNA replication normally is an accurate process. The DNA polymerases (see Table 30-2) insert an incorrect base only once in every 10 million bp. A series of DNA repair enzymes exist that are able to recognize and replace noncomplementary bases, correcting more than 99.9 percent of errors. The overall mutation rate is therefore only 10^{-10} per basepair per cell division. The human genome consists of about 6×10^9 bp, so this mutation rate results in less than 1 bp mutation per cell division. Nevertheless, an estimated 10^{15} cell divisions occur during the lifetime of an adult human. Thus, thousands of new mutations occur at virtually every position in the genome. Not surprisingly, inherited defects in DNA replication and repair enzymes lead to a striking increase in the frequencies of all types of mutations.

Most of the mutations occur in somatic cells, where they may cause cancer or a genetic disease affecting only part of the body, such as segmental neurofibromatosis. Fewer mutations occur in germ cells. During oogenesis, female germ cells undergo mitosis approximately 22 times and begin meiosis only once during fetal life. The cells are suspended in meiosis from fetal life till shortly before ovulation during the reproductive years. Spermatogenesis consists of approximately 30 mitoses from conception until puberty and approximately 20–5 per year

thereafter. Thus, the opportunity for mutations is expected to be far greater for sperm than for ova. This phenomenon has been confirmed in several genetic disorders, such as neurofibromatosis type 1, achondroplasia, and hemophilia A. It has been estimated that as many as 1 in 10 sperm in healthy males may carry a new deleterious mutation. Most are recessive or lethal, and therefore not apparent in liveborn children.

Mutation Rate

The mutation rate for any given gene or other DNA segment depends on both its size and its location. The location may be important because certain areas of the genome are known to be "hot spots" for recombination. The average mutation rate is about 1×10^{-6} mutation per locus per generation, but the rate varies by more than a thousand-fold for different genes. For example, the number of new mutations per 10^6 gametes is 40–100 for Duchenne muscular dystrophy and neurofibromatosis 1, but only 2–5 for aniridia and hemophilia B. These statistics include only mutations causing genetic diseases. The rate of change of protein polymorphisms suggests a rate as high as 6×10^{-6} per locus per generation. (A locus is the position of a gene on a chromosome.)

Specific Types of Gene Mutations

The development and widespread use of modern molecular techniques have led to the discovery of specific mutations at many different loci. From among these, many different types of mutations have been recognized, all of which have the potential for causing genetic diseases. They may be divided by size into single- and multiple-base changes. The latter may involve only one or a few bases or may involve millions of basepairs. In any specific gene, mutations are almost always heterogeneous, although some types may be more common than others. Thus, the specific mutations in unrelated persons with the same genetic disease often are different. A few notable exceptions to this rule have been identified, such as achondroplasia, which almost always is caused by a specific single-base change in the fibroblast growth factor receptor 3 gene [Bellus et al., 1995].

Nucleotide Substitutions

Point mutations or single-base substitutions represent one of the most common types of mutation. Most are related to an error in DNA synthesis by the enzyme DNA polymerase that was not corrected by DNA repair enzymes. Some combinations of nucleotides are mutation-prone, however. More than 30 percent of point mutations found in some genetic diseases are the result of cytosine to thymine transitions, which are caused by methylation of cytosine residues to 5-methylcytosine, especially cytosine residues occurring as the first base in a 5′-CG-3′ dinucleotide pair. The latter then undergoes spontaneous deamination to thymidine. Thus, the 5′-CG-3′ doublet represents a "hot spot" for mutation in the human genome.

Deletions, Duplications, and Insertions

The remainder of mutations consist of loss or gain of nucleotide bases somewhere in the genome; a variety of mechanisms for such changes are known. A deletion consists of any loss of DNA sequence, whereas a duplication consists of a second copy of a DNA sequence that is usually located immediately adjacent to the first copy. An insertion consists of a DNA sequence that has been removed or copied from one location and moved to a nonhomologous region elsewhere on the same chromosome or to a different chromosome. Deletions, duplications, and insertions that involve one or a few basepairs can be detected only by nucleotide sequencing. Larger deletions and duplications may be detected by several of the methods described earlier, including direct sequencing, Southern blot analysis, FISH, and CGH.

Effects of Mutations on Gene Function

The effect of mutations on gene function depends as much or more on the specific location of the mutation as on the size. Mutations that occur in DNA outside functioning genes usually have no consequences. Mutations within the boundaries of a gene may inactivate it or have little or no effect, depending on the nature of the change.

Missense Mutations

A point mutation within the coding region of a gene can alter the genetic code by changing the nucleotide triplet and cause the replacement of one amino acid by another in the gene product, thus altering function of the gene product. Such mutations are called missense mutations and do not change the reading frame of the DNA sequence. The best-known example is the A to T substitution in the sixth codon of the β-globin gene, which causes sickle cell anemia, by substituting valine for glutamic acid in the β-globin protein chain. Not all mutations within coding regions of a gene result in a missense mutation, however. All but 2 of the 20 amino acids are specified by more than one codon, most often differing in the third or "wobble" position of the triplet. The gene product will be identical if the new triplet codes for the same amino acid.

Nonsense (Chain Termination) Mutations

Mutations that generate one of the three stop codons result in premature termination of translation, whereas those that alter a stop codon allow translation to continue until the next stop codon is reached. Those mutations that result in a premature stop codon are called nonsense mutations. In general, these mutations have no effect on transcription (DNA to RNA), but the shortened polypeptide may have lost critical functional domains of the protein, or the mRNA may be so unstable that it is rapidly degraded in the cell. The latter process is known as nonsense-mediated mRNA decay, a process by which mRNA species containing premature termination codons are recognized and degraded before translation, although this typically spares truncation mutations in the last coding exon [Frischmeyer and Dietz, 1999]. Both base substitutions and nucleotide loss or gain mutations may result in nonsense mutations.

RNA Splicing Mutations

The sequence surrounding intron splice sites is highly conserved, and mutations of key nucleotides frequently prevent or reduce efficiency of splicing. The key nucleotide sequences at most splice junctions are shown in Figure 30-4.

Splicing mutations may either inactivate existing splice sites or create new ones. In the first type, the mutation alters the splice-donor, branch, or splice-acceptor site, resulting in failure to splice the intron correctly at that site. This failure results in a large insertion of nucleotides that normally are not translated into the processed mRNA. This insertion is almost certain to introduce a stop codon within the next hundred or so codons, because 3 of the possible 64 triplet combinations are stop codons. In the second type, mutations within the intron create alternative splice-donor or acceptor sites that compete with the normal splice sites during mRNA processing. Thus, a proportion of the mature mRNA will contain incorrectly spliced intron sequences. Both base substitutions and nucleotide loss or gain mutations may result in splicing mutations.

One example of the first type is a G to C transition in the first position of the intron at the donor splice site in the hexosaminidase A gene found in many Ashkenazi Jewish patients with Tay–Sachs disease [Nussbaum et al., 2007]. In this example, the bases in the exon are capitalized, whereas those in the intron are not, and the mutation is underlined.

Normal allele:	5′–CCAGGCTCTGgtaagggt–3′
Tay–Sachs allele:	5′–CCAGGCTCTGctaagggt–3′

Frameshift Mutations

Small nucleotide loss or gain mutations may alter the reading frame of the mRNA product from the point of the mutation on, which results in a completely different amino acid sequence at the carboxyl end of the protein product, or premature chain termination if a stop codon is encountered in the new reading frame. Any loss or gain mutation that involves a multiple of three bases maintains the reading frame, whereas a mutation that does not involve a multiple of three nucleotides changes the reading frame. Larger deletions that include one or more introns also may cause a frameshift mutation, because exon/intron splice sites may occur at any point in the reading frame, thereby splitting codons. If the exon just downstream from the deletion normally begins at a different position in the triplet than the deleted intron, the reading frame will be changed. By contrast, base substitutions do not cause frameshift mutations. Deletions and insertions cause dysfunction of the gene more often than point mutations because of the possibility of a frameshift.

One of the best-known frameshift mutations is a single-base deletion in the ABO blood group locus that results in the nonfunctional O allele. The deletion alters the reading frame at codon 86 until a premature stop codon is reached 30 codons later. The stop codon is normally out of frame and is therefore not read.

With some intermediate-size deletions of approximately 1 kb to 1 Mb, one or more exons of a gene may be duplicated or deleted. About two-thirds of these will change the reading frame and result in a frameshift mutation. Those that maintain the reading frame produce truncated products that may or may not retain function. These relatively small deletions and duplications are too small to be seen with chromosome analysis or FISH and cannot be found by sequencing, which is not sensitive to dosage (recall that all autosomal genes and X-linked genes in females have two copies of each gene). These may be rare or common mechanisms of mutation. For example, small deletions and duplications are the most common mutational types for Duchenne muscular dystrophy and Becker muscular dystrophy, both caused by mutations of the dystrophin or *DMD* gene. These are simple to detect for X-linked diseases in males, because only one gene copy is present. When any autosome of the X chromosome in a female is involved, the mutation can be detected by other methods, such as quantitative PCR assay.

Transcriptional Control Mutations

Mutations involving promoter sequences in the 5′ UTR or other regulatory sequences in the 3′ UTR of a gene may result in a significant decrease in the amount of mature, processed mRNA produced. Both base substitutions and nucleotide loss or gain mutations may result in transcriptional control abnormalities.

Principles of Medical Genetics

Several principles of genetics derived from the chromosomal and molecular basis of heredity form the basis for the different patterns of inheritance observed in genetic diseases. A working understanding of the principles of inheritance is important for understanding the genetic diseases encountered in pediatric neurology clinics, for formulating an optimal management approach to patients with these diseases, and for providing accurate genetic counseling. The simplest and best-known patterns of inheritance involve mutations of single genes; however, more complex patterns of inheritance likely are more common. Here we review some of these principles and examine the basis for genetic counseling.

Patterns of Inheritance

A discussion of inheritance requires familiarity with a special vocabulary. As reviewed previously, a gene is a sequence of DNA that is required for production of a functional product. The position of a gene on a chromosome is known as its locus. The alternative forms of a gene that may occupy a given locus are known as alleles. Different alleles typically result from one or more minor differences in nucleotide sequence. When both alleles at a given locus are identical, the person is said to be homozygous for that trait. When the alleles are different, the person is described as heterozygous. When only one allele is present, the person is hemizygous.

The genetic constitution of an individual is the genotype. At any given locus, the normal genotype consists of either a single allele or a pair of alleles. Only a single allele is present for most genes on the X chromosome in males, who have only one X chromosome. A pair of alleles is present for all genes on the autosomes, and for a subset of genes on the X chromosome located in "pseudoautosomal" regions, which have functional homologs on the Y chromosome. The observable expression of the genotype is the phenotype. Penetrance has been defined as the percentage of persons with a particular genotype who have the expected phenotype; this is an all-or-none phenomenon. Expressivity is defined as the extent to which a genetic trait or disease is expressed and may vary greatly between affected persons. The proband is the affected family member through whom a family is identified; the consultand is the person in the family who seeks advice, regardless of whether affected or not. A pedigree is a diagram of the family history that shows the family members, their relationships to the proband, and their status with regard to the hereditary condition. Some of the symbols used for pedigrees in medical genetics are illustrated in Figure 30-15. A more detailed standardized nomenclature has been proposed for publication of pedigrees [Bennet et al., 1995].

The most widely recognized patterns of inheritance are single-gene or "mendelian" patterns, which include autosomal-dominant, autosomal-recessive, and X-linked modes of inheritance; example pedigrees are shown in Figure 30-16. All of these result from mutations in a single gene. The disorder or trait is autosomal if located on human chromosomes 1–22, and X-linked when located on the X chromosome.

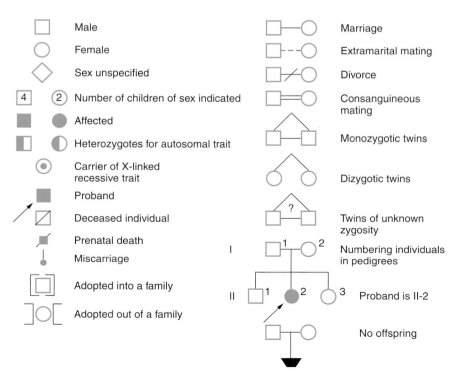

Fig. 30-15 Common symbols used in pedigrees.

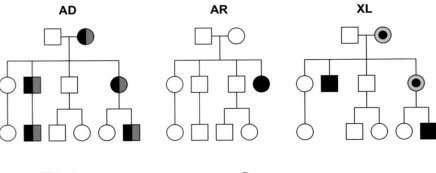

Fig. 30-16 Examples of autosomal-dominant (AD), autosomal-recessive (AR), and X-linked (XL) pedigrees.

The only true Y-linked trait is male sex determination (the *SRY* gene). Autosomal traits are considered dominant when expressed in both heterozygotes and homozygotes, and recessive when expressed only in homozygotes; neither of these terms really fits with X-linked inheritance, as reviewed later on. The pattern of single-gene inheritance is modified in special cases in which mutations involve genes subject to imprinting or X-inactivation, or involve only a proportion of cells in the body or affected tissue. Finally, many diseases have more complicated inheritance.

Autosomal-Dominant Inheritance

The most important attributes of autosomal-dominant inheritance are expression of the trait in heterozygotes and male-to-male transmission (see Figure 30-16). The autosomal-dominant pattern may be recognized because:

1. The trait or disease typically appears in every generation, except that it may arise by new mutation in the first affected family member.
2. Any child of an affected person has a 50 percent risk of inheriting the trait.
3. The offspring of unaffected family members also are unaffected.
4. The trait may be transmitted by a parent of either sex to a child of either sex, and specifically may be transmitted from father to son, which distinguishes it from X-linked inheritance.

Autosomal-dominant inheritance is readily identified in most families but may be difficult to discern in others. When the disease occurs as a result of a new mutation, no relatives are affected. With reduced penetrance, low expressivity, and late age at onset, other affected family members may go unrecognized. Among the best examples for each of these characteristics are myotonic dystrophy and Huntington's disease. Finally, incorrect information regarding family relationships, such as false paternity, may complicate interpretation of the pedigree.

Most persons affected by a disorder of autosomal-dominant inheritance are heterozygous, but rarely a homozygous person is encountered. Generally, the phenotype in homozygous persons is significantly more severe than in heterozygous persons. For example, one child born to parents who each had hereditary motor and sensory neuropathy type I had a much more severe neuropathy consistent with Dejerine–Sottas disease, or hereditary motor and sensory neuropathy type III [Killian and Kloepfer, 1979]. The best-known exception to this rule is Huntington's disease, in which persons heterozygous for this trait cannot be distinguished from homozygotes.

Autosomal-Recessive Inheritance

The most important attributes of autosomal-recessive inheritance are expression in homozygotes and equal gender distribution (see Figure 30-16). This pattern may be recognized by the following four characteristics:

1. The trait or disease may affect multiple siblings but not parents, children, or other relatives, except in highly inbred populations.
2. Each full sibling of an affected person has a 25 percent chance of inheriting the trait.
3. The parents are more likely than usual to be related.
4. With rare exceptions, males and females are equally likely to be affected.

In Western societies, a child with a disorder of autosomal-recessive inheritance may be the only affected person in the family, owing to small family size and a tendency for parents of affected children to have fewer children after the birth of a child with a genetic disease. This practice does not hold true in many other cultures, especially those with inbred populations.

When the frequency of a rare recessive allele is relatively high within a family or population, the disease may appear in more than one generation. This pattern is known as pseudodominant inheritance. Some genes on the X chromosome have functional homologs on the Y chromosome, and traits or diseases associated with these genes will behave in the same manner as for autosomal loci. This pattern is known as pseudoautosomal inheritance.

The risk of bearing a child with an autosomal-recessive disease or trait is increased when the parents are consanguineous or related by descent. More formally, the probability that a homozygote has received both alleles of a pair from an identical ancestral source is known as the coefficient of inbreeding. It also is the proportion of loci at which a person is homozygous by descent. For example, any child born to first cousins is homozygous at 1/16 of all loci. Although the relative risk of abnormal offspring is higher for first cousins than for unrelated parents, it is still low, at about 5 percent.

X-Linked Inheritance

The inheritance of diseases and traits associated with genes located on the X chromosome differs markedly from autosomal forms of inheritance because females have two

X chromosomes, whereas males have only one. Thus, when mutations of an X-linked gene occur in males, no genetic "backup" is available. The situation in heterozygous (carrier) females is more complicated, owing to the phenomenon of X chromosome inactivation (Xi), which ensures that dosage for X-linked genes is the same in male and in female cells. Because Xi is random in most females, the maternally derived and paternally derived X chromosomes usually are active in about half of the cells in a female organism. Thus, mutation of one gene should cause no more than a 50 percent loss of function of the protein or other gene product. With this background, several mechanisms have been described that lead to disease expression in female carriers of X-linked mutations. First, some genes are dosage-sensitive, so that 50 percent expression is not enough for normal function. Next, by chance or because of cell selection (usually favoring the normal allele), some females have skewing of X-inactivation, such that one X chromosome is inactivated in a high proportion (80–100 percent) of cells. Unfavorable skewing will cause or worsen disease, whereas favorable skewing will prevent or reduce disease expression. Finally, skewing of X-inactivation also may result from mutations of the genes that actually control inactivation, especially the *XIST* gene, which is responsible for inactivation of one of the two X chromosomes. Not surprisingly, affected females usually have a less severe phenotype than that seen in affected males.

The important characteristics of X-linked inheritance result from differential segregation of the X and Y chromosomes in males and females, and the differences in gene dosage. The most consistent characteristics include more severe phenotype in males than in females, transmission of disease through carrier females who are unaffected or less affected than males, and lack of male-to-male transmission (see Figure 30-16). The last is explained by transmission of the Y chromosome from fathers to sons, whereas the disease genes are located on the X chromosome. X-linked disorders traditionally have been divided into dominant and recessive subtypes, just as for autosomal single-gene disorders. This distinction was first made in fruit flies under experimental conditions but has never worked very well for human disorders. In a recent survey of more than 30 X-linked diseases, a remarkably wide range of penetrance was found, with many disorders intermediate between so-called X-linked dominant and recessive patterns [Dobyns et al., 2004]. On the basis of these and other arguments, use of these subtypes should be discontinued. The rules for X-linked inheritance have been modified to reflect this change (Box 30-1).

In many instances, children with X-linked diseases present primarily or frequently to pediatric neurologists, including those with adrenoleukodystrophy, the Duchenne and Becker forms of muscular dystrophy, fragile X syndrome, many X-linked mental retardation syndromes, two forms of X-linked lissencephaly, and many others. These diseases all result in more severe phenotypes in males than in females. Another class of X-linked disorders, "X-linked, male lethal," have proved to be particularly important in pediatric neurology. These diseases are observed almost exclusively in females and are thought to cause prenatal lethality in males or to cause a much more severe phenotype that is not recognized as the same disorder. Examples are Aicardi's, Goltz's, and Rett's syndromes and orofaciodigital syndrome type I.

Box 30-1 Rules for X-Linked Inheritance in Humans

Rules Related to Segregation of the X and Y Chromosomes

Hemizygous males transmit X chromosomes to daughters and Y chromosomes to sons

- Male-to-male transmission of X–linked disorders cannot occur
- Sons of hemizygous males never inherit the disorder
- Daughters of affected males all are heterozygous (carriers or affected)
- All affected males in a family are related through heterozygous females

Heterozygous females transmit X chromosomes to both sons and daughters

- Fifty percent of sons of heterozygous females will be hemizygous males
- Fifty percent of daughters of heterozygous females also will be heterozygous females

Rules Related to Penetrance, Expressivity, and Sex Ratio

Penetrance and Expressivity

- In general, penetrance is higher and expressivity more severe in hemizygous males than in heterozygous females

Sex Ratio of Affected Persons

- Males are predominantly affected when female penetrance is low
- Female to male ratio is close to 2:1 when female penetrance and male survival are high
- Females are predominantly affected, with prenatal lethality in males

---

Genomic Imprinting

In most single-gene disorders, the expression of a trait or disease is expected to be the same, regardless of whether the gene was inherited from the mother or the father. Significant differences in expression based on the gender of the transmitting parent, however, have been observed in several disorders. This phenomenon is known as imprinting and reflects differences in the state of the maternal and paternal contributions to the genome, especially differential methylation of the maternally and paternally derived chromosomes. An imprinted gene can be imprinted or differentially methylated (i.e., differentially silenced) in all cells of the body, or only in selected tissues, such as brain.

This differential silencing means that imprinted genes will be expressed from the maternally derived gene or from the paternally derived gene, but not from both. So if the functioning copy of an imprinted gene is lost owing to a deletion or mutation, the affected person is left with no functioning gene, and a disease phenotype will result. The underlying mechanisms are under study but still are not well understood [Hall, 1990; Jiang et al., 2004]. Imprinting disorders result from deletions or other types of mutations of genes within imprinted regions (or in the imprinting control regions). The most common of these result in infantile developmental disorders relevant for pediatric neurologists, such as Beckwith–Wiedemann syndrome due to defects of imprinted genes on 11p15.5 [Weksberg et al., 2003], and Angelman's and Prader–Willi syndromes due to defects of imprinted genes on 15q11.2–q13 [Amos-Landgraf et al., 2006]. These disorders are reviewed elsewhere in this book.

Uniparental Disomy

Defects of imprinted genes also may result from a rare mutation type known as uniparental disomy (UPD). UPD is defined as the presence of a diploid cell line containing two chromosome homologs inherited from the same parent. It is believed to result from nondisjunction, which produces trisomy for a particular chromosome. Trisomy is followed by loss of one of the three homologs, reducing the chromosome number back to normal. This mutation is known as uniparental isodisomy when the two homologs are identical, and uniparental heterodisomy when they are different (as a result of crossing over, different regions of the affected chromosomes usually are involved).

When UPD involves a chromosome with an imprinted region, problems occur. For example, a child may inherit two paternally derived chromosomes, in which case no maternally derived chromosome will be present. Any genes that are normally expressed only from the maternally derived gene will not be expressed at all. This is one cause of Angelman's syndrome. The same type of problem occurs in reverse if the child inherits two maternally inherited chromosomes. No paternally derived genes will be present, and a disease will occur. This is one cause of Prader–Willi syndrome [Amos-Landgraf et al., 2006].

Very rarely, UPD can result in a genetic disease by causing homozygosity of a recessive disease gene. Because the two chromosomes are identical, they are homologous at all loci. If the involved chromosome contains any recessive disease loci, the person with the mutation will be homozygous and therefore affected.

Mosaicism

Mosaic is a term used to refer to an individual organism or tissue that contains two or more cell lines that differ in DNA sequence, although they are derived from a single zygote. All organisms begin with a specific DNA sequence in the cell of origin or zygote. As cell division proceeds, some mutations occur that produce small differences among different cell lines. The presence of two or more cell lines differing in their DNA sequence but derived from a single zygote is known as mosaicism. Mosaicism is clinically important in many disorders and probably explains some unusual diseases in which only part of the body appears to be affected with a birth defect or genetic disease. A good example is segmental neurofibromatosis.

This phenomenon can involve any tissue or group of tissues in the body. When mosaicism is found in lymphocytes, fibroblasts, or other somatic cells of the body, it is designated somatic mosaicism. The mosaic individual typically demonstrates at least mild signs of disease. When mosaicism is found only in germ cells (egg, sperm), it is known as gonadal mosaicism. The mosaic individual usually is identified as the parent of two or more children with a genetic disease, despite having no signs of the disease clinically or on mutation analysis. Mosaicism may begin with a somatic mutation in the germline

of the affected person, which then persists in the clonal descendants of that cell, including a proportion of the ova or sperm. When the mutation exists only in the germline, the parent has no signs of the disease but may conceive multiple affected children. This phenomenon has been seen frequently in Duchenne muscular dystrophy due to mutations of the *DMD* gene, the autosomal-dominant form of osteogenesis imperfecta associated with mutations of the *COL1A1* or *COL1A2* gene, and X-linked lissencephaly due to mutations of the *DCX* gene. The distinction between somatic and germline mosaicism is most likely artificial, however, because standard evaluations examine very few tissues.

Complex Inheritance

The most important attributes of complex or multifactorial inheritance are lack of a clear pattern of inheritance in single families, although more than one relative may be affected, and a relatively low risk for first-degree relatives (approximately the square root of the population risk), typically in the range of 1–5 percent. This form of inheritance results from variation at two or more loci with two or more alleles each, often with a prominent environmental influence. This pattern also is referred to as polygenic (we prefer oligogenic) or multifactorial inheritance. Examples of traits inherited in this pattern are head circumference, autism, neural tube defects, and common forms of epilepsy. Some are continuous traits that can be measured, such as head circumference, whereas others fall into non-overlapping groups, such as autism and epilepsy. For continuous traits, such as head circumference, children are likely to be intermediate between their parents, or closer to the mean than either parent (so-called regression to the mean).

Mitochondrial Inheritance

Mitochondria are the cellular organelles that are primarily responsible for cellular respiration and production of adenosine triphosphate, both essential for cellular energy management. Each mitochondrion contains multiple copies of a small 16.5-kb circular chromosome that codes for 13 proteins and many rRNA and tRNA genes that differ in sequence from the nuclear rRNA and tRNA genes. The proteins all are components of the respiratory chain, and the remainder of the respiratory pathway enzymes are encoded by nuclear genes.

The mitochondria in any one person are derived almost exclusively from the mother through the ovum. Each ovum contains hundreds of mitochondria, and each mitochondrion contains many copies of the circular mitochondrial chromosome. Sperm contain a few mitochondria, most of which are degraded rapidly by the proteasome-dependent protein degradation pathway of the ubiquitin system within the ovum after fertilization [Sutovsky et al., 2003]. A small paternal contribution of mitochondria, however, has been demonstrated in several species, such as sheep [Zhao et al., 2004]. The same likely is true for humans, as suggested by one example of paternal inheritance of a mitochondrial disorder [Schwartz and Vissing, 2002]. This must be very rare, however, owing to the small proportion of paternal compared with maternal mitochondria, and as indicated by studies in humans with mitochondrial diseases [Filosto et al., 2003].

In patients with mutations of mitochondrial genes, a variable proportion of the mitochondrial chromosomes carry the mutation. Thus, diseases caused by mutations in mitochondrial DNA exhibit strict maternal inheritance (with very rare exceptions) and usually will exhibit phenotypic variation within a family owing to variation in the proportion of mutant and normal mitochondria between individuals [Zeviani et al., 1989].

Maternal inheritance may be recognized because:

1. The incidence of the disease is equal in males and females.
2. The disease is transmitted from mother to offspring of both genders, but never from father to offspring.
3. Variable expression is common.

These criteria have been met for several diseases associated with mitochondrial DNA mutations, including Kearns–Sayre syndrome, Leber's hereditary optic neuropathy, MELAS (mitochondrial encephalomyopathy, lactic acidosis, and strokelike episodes), and MERRF (myoclonic epilepsy with ragged-red fibers).

Genetic Counseling

Medical genetics differs from other specialties because family members other than the patient may be at high risk for a disease first recognized in the patient, who then becomes the proband. The person or persons actually seeking advice may not themselves be affected. Ideally, the patient or the parents or guardians of minor children or incompetent adults, and all other family members at risk, should be made aware of both the clinical and the reproductive consequences of a genetic disease. Genetic counseling is the process of providing this information. Although any physician may provide genetic counseling as part of overall patient management, it is more commonly conducted in genetics clinics.

Standard of Care

All physicians have a professional responsibility to make certain that genetic counseling has been provided in appropriate situations and to ensure that the counseling meets current standards of practice [Directors and Directors, 1995; Parker, 2010]. Failure to provide this information may have tragic results. Perhaps the best example for pediatric neurologists is the birth of a second or even a third male with Duchenne muscular dystrophy in a family. Courts have upheld the principle of physician responsibility to provide accurate counseling on several occasions. For example, the parents of a child with Down syndrome claimed negligence because the mother had not been referred for prenatal diagnosis. In another case, parents who were tested for Tay–Sachs disease carrier status both were told that they were not carriers. They later had an affected child and filed a claim. Cases of this type are known as wrongful life claims.

Responsibility to Relatives

The responsibility to provide genetic counseling does not formally extend beyond the consultand, or person seeking genetic advice. People with genetic disorders are entitled to the same confidentiality as for persons with any other type of disease. Nevertheless, the need for confidentiality does not mean that no effort should be made to inform relatives of a common risk. Whenever the genetic evaluation suggests that other family members or their future children may be at risk, the consultand should be encouraged to contact those persons or ask the physician (or designee) to contact them and advise them to seek genetic evaluation.

A majority of people act responsibly in this regard, but exceptions do arise that may present an ethical dilemma for health-care practitioners providing the counseling.

Relevance for Pediatric Neurology

The obligation to provide accurate genetic counseling is particularly important for pediatric neurologists. Many neurologic and neuromuscular diseases in children have a genetic basis or a genetic component, including some of the most common problems seen in clinics. For disorders such as Duchenne muscular dystrophy, neurofibromatosis type 1, and tuberous sclerosis, the genetic basis and need for genetic counseling are well known. For others, the genetic basis or contribution is not widely recognized. Febrile seizures, benign rolandic epilepsy, and some types of primary generalized epilepsy may affect many persons in a family and appear to have autosomal-dominant inheritance, although penetrance is not complete. Mental retardation, microcephaly, and cerebral palsy have a significant genetic component, with recurrence risks of 5–10 percent. Most brain malformations are sporadic, but familial recurrence of almost every known type of brain malformation has been described.

Because of the possibility of recurrence in relatives, pediatric neurologists should take a genetic history and advise patients and parents of their genetic risks. Referrals from pediatric neurology clinics to genetics clinics should occur frequently. Even for single-gene disorders with a known risk of recurrence, referral usually is needed to provide an accurate presentation of methods of prevention, such as prenatal diagnosis when this is available, artificial insemination by donor, contraception, sterilization, and adoption. If the parents decide to terminate a pregnancy, continued professional support is an appropriate and important part of genetic counseling.

Genetic Risk

One of the most crucial steps in offering accurate genetic counseling is to estimate the risk of recurrence of a genetic disorder in other family members. Estimation is not difficult for most diseases with a single-gene pattern of inheritance, but even these may be complex because of late age at onset or incomplete penetrance. For many other disorders, empirical recurrence risk estimates are used. These risk figures are derived from previous experience with the same disorder. Although such figures generally are accurate, exceptions occur because of causal heterogeneity and lack of knowledge regarding many rare disorders. The recurrence risks for some of the more common diseases seen in pediatric neurology clinics were reviewed by Baraitser [Baraitser, 1997]. In any given family, the recurrence risk may be different; consultation with a geneticist or genetic counselor may be helpful in providing this information.

Prenatal Diagnosis

Prenatal diagnosis can now be performed for hundreds of genetic disorders, including many of those discussed in this chapter. The major methods used include chromosome analysis, enzyme assays and other biochemical tests, molecular genetic tests, and direct examination of the fetus by ultrasonography. The last is a far more rigorous procedure than routine prenatal ultrasonography and usually is referred to as high-resolution, level 2, or genetic ultrasonography. The purposes of prenatal diagnosis are to provide:

1. a range of informed choices for parents at risk for having a child with an abnormality
2. reassurance to reduce anxiety, especially among parents at high risk
3. an opportunity for parents, who otherwise would choose not to have children, to conceive and bear healthy children.

The results of prenatal tests are normal in more than 98 percent of pregnancies evaluated, and parents are reassured that the infant will be unaffected by the condition in question. Of course, the infant remains at risk for other disorders, just as do children born to any other parents. In a small proportion of cases, the fetus is indeed found to have a serious defect. Because effective prenatal therapy is not possible for most disorders, the parents then have the option of terminating the pregnancy.

Genetics and Medicine

Genetics has become one of the most rapidly expanding fields in all of biology, and it is likely that this trend will continue. The past few years have seen completion of the Human Genome Project and identification of many genes relevant to neurologic disorders of childhood. The next few years will see the isolation of new genes responsible for common and complex diseases and many more single-gene disorders.

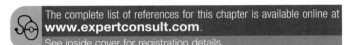

The complete list of references for this chapter is available online at **www.expertconsult.com**.
See inside cover for registration details.

Chromosomes and Chromosomal Abnormalities

Maria Descartes, Bruce R. Korf and Fady M. Mikhail

The development and maintenance of the human body is directed by an estimated 20,000 genes, consisting of some 3 billion basepairs (bp) of DNA. These genes encode the structure of proteins and noncoding RNAs, which together are responsible for the orderly unfolding of human development, beginning with the fertilized egg (zygote), and for the maintenance of body structure and function. The entire pool of genetic information must be replicated with each cell division and a complete set of information apportioned to the two daughter cells. In addition, the full complement of genes must be transmitted from generation to generation through the germ cells.

Genes do not exist as isolated entities within the cell nucleus but rather are arranged on structural units called chromosomes. Each chromosome contains hundreds or thousands of genes arranged in a linear order. This order is reproducible from cell to cell within an individual organism, and from individual to individual in the population. The normal human chromosome complement consists of 46 chromosomes, including 22 pairs of nonsex chromosomes (autosomes), and either two X chromosomes in females or an X and a Y in males. Each of these chromosomes has a characteristic structure and includes a specific set of genes arranged in a specific order. The chromosomes are units that ensure the orderly distribution of a complete set of genetic information during cell division.

Chromosome number and structure are tightly regulated, and deviations from the norm usually are associated with clinical problems. Multiple genes are simultaneously disrupted as a consequence of chromosomal abnormalities; accordingly, the phenotypic consequences usually are complex. Because of the complexity of the nervous system and its dependence on multiple genes, neurologic problems accompany most of the chromosomal disorders.

Chromosomal abnormalities were among the first genetic disorders to be studied in the laboratory. From the late 1950s on, with the advent of reliable techniques for chromosomal analysis, a set of syndromes resulting from changes in chromosome number or structure were described. Initially, these were syndromes associated with loss or gain of entire chromosomes or large chromosome segments, such as Down syndrome, resulting from trisomy 21. Refinements in analytic technology have gradually improved the resolution of chromosomal analysis, permitting progressively smaller changes to be detected. Current techniques are bridging the gap between chromosomal anomalies visible with the light microscope and changes in individual genes at a submicroscopic level. At the same time, techniques have been developed that permit chromosomal analysis in nondividing cells and in various tissues that can be sampled prenatally.

This chapter focuses on the approach to chromosomal disorders in pediatric neurology. The various methods of chromosomal analyses are considered first, followed by a description of the various types of chromosomal abnormalities. This discussion is followed by an overview of the clinical approach to chromosomal abnormalities, and then a brief clinical description of chromosomal syndromes relevant to the practice of pediatric neurology. The chapter closes with a look at the future of cytogenetic analysis (see also chapter 30).

Methods of Chromosome Analysis

Chromosome Prepraration

The history of clinical cytogenetics can be characterized as a series of technical advances, each of which has led to the recognition of new clinical syndromes due to chromosomal abnormalities. The modern era in human cytogenetics began with the discovery of methods to permit individual chromosomes to be identified in dividing cells. The key breakthrough was the use of hypotonic treatment to spread the chromosomes apart, thereby avoiding overlaps. This advance led, in 1956, to the discovery that the normal human chromosome number is 46, rather than 48, as had been previously thought. The second major advance was the discovery that the kidney bean extract, phytohemagglutinin, can stimulate lymphocytes to divide in culture, providing an easily obtained source of dividing cells for analysis. The first golden age of discovery of chromosomal abnormalities began with the recognition of trisomy 21 in persons with Down syndrome in 1959, and continued through the early 1960s with the identification of other aneuploidy syndromes.

Chromosome structure is most easily appreciated during mitosis, when the chromatin fiber is condensed and coiled into a characteristic structure. Spontaneously dividing cells are rarely available, except in tumors or chorionic villus tissue used in prenatal diagnosis. Rather, cells are grown in short-term culture. For routine analysis, peripheral blood lymphocytes most commonly are used, although skin fibroblasts also may be cultured and analyzed. Phytohemagglutinin-stimulated peripheral blood usually is grown in culture for 3 days. Blocking the mitotic spindle with a drug such as colchicine leads to accumulation of dividing cells, which then are induced to swell by treatment with hypotonic saline, fixed, and spread on to a microscope slide.

Chromosome Banding

Until the 1970s chromosomes were identified on the basis of their size and the position of the centromeres. This allowed chromosomes to be classified into groups labeled A to G (A: chromosomes 1–3, B: chromosomes 4–5, C: chromosomes 6–12 and X, D: chromosomes 13–15, E: chromosomes 16–18, F: chromosomes 19–20, G: chromosomes 21–22 and Y), but not unambiguously identified. The introduction of banding techniques finally allowed each chromosome to be identified, as well as permitted the identification of chromosome regions, bands, and sub-bands. Most laboratories use Giemsa stain banding (G-banding), which involves treatment of the metaphase chromosomes with a protease (i.e., trypsin), followed by Giemsa staining for routine analysis. The advent of chromosome banding stimulated a second wave of discovery of structural chromosomal abnormalities during the 1970s.

Chromosomes are displayed as a karyotype (Figure 31-1), which is prepared by arranging homologous chromosomes in an orderly fashion, starting from chromosome 1 and ending with chromosome 22, as well as the sex chromosomes. Subsequent developments in laboratory cytogenetics have gradually improved the resolution of chromosomal analysis. As the cell proceeds through mitosis, the chromosome gradually contracts, until anaphase, when the chromatids separate. If cells are collected during early prophase, chromosomes are highly extended, revealing a fine, highly detailed banding pattern. This banding pattern has facilitated recognition of subtle chromosome rearrangements involving small chromosome segments. Even with this approach, however, the resolution is limited to 3–5 million bp (Mb) of DNA, which may include dozens of genes.

Molecular Cytogenetics

The gap between light microscope resolution of chromosome structure and the gene was bridged by the introduction of several molecular cytogenetic techniques. Fluorescence in situ hybridization (FISH) involves hybridizing a fluorescently labeled single-stranded DNA probe to denatured chromosomal DNA on a microscope slide preparation of metaphase chromosomes and/or interphase nuclei prepared from the patient's sample. After overnight hybridization, the slide is washed and counterstained with a nucleic acid dye (e.g., DAPI, or 4′,6-diamidino-2-phenylindole), allowing the region where

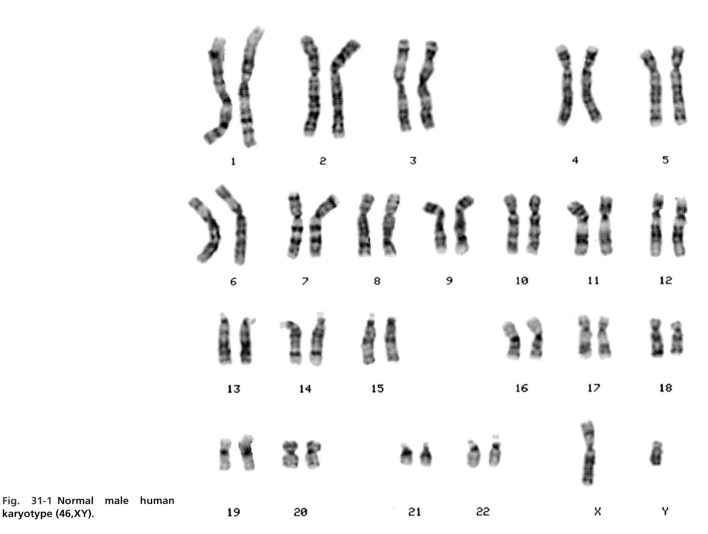

Fig. 31-1 Normal male human karyotype (46,XY).

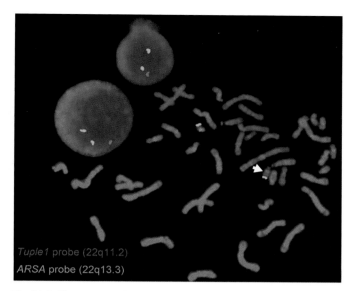

Fig. 31-2 Fluorescence in situ hybridization (FISH) analysis using the DiGeorge/VCF syndrome probe. Note the deleted *Tuple1* (22q11.2) red probe on one chromosome 22 (arrow). The *ARSA* (22q13.3) green probe is included as an internal control.

hybridization has occurred to be visualized using a fluorescence microscope. FISH is now widely used for clinical diagnostic purposes. There are different types of FISH probes, including locus-specific probes, centromeric probes, and whole-chromosome paint probes. Locus-specific probes are specific for a particular single locus. They are especially useful for identifying subtle submicroscopic deletions and duplications (Figure 31-2). Centromeric probes are specific for unique repetitive DNA sequences (e.g., alpha-satellite sequences) in the centromere of a specific chromosome. They are suitable for making a rapid diagnosis of one of the common aneuploidy syndromes (trisomies 13, 18, and 21, and sex chromosome aneuploidies) using nondividing interphase nuclei. This is particularly useful in a prenatal setting using amniotic fluid or chorionic villi samples (CVS). Whole-chromosome paint probes consist of a cocktail of probes obtained from different regions of a particular chromosome. When this cocktail mixture is used in a single hybridization, the entire relevant chromosome fluoresces (is "painted"). Whole-chromosome paints are useful for characterizing complex chromosomal rearrangements, and for identifying the origin of additional chromosomal material, such as small marker or ring chromosomes.

FISH using locus-specific probes has been extremely useful in the detection of "microdeletion syndromes" resulting from deletions of multiple contiguous genes. These are subtle submicroscopic deletions that are below the resolution of the routine G-banded chromosome analysis. Also, two-color and three-color FISH applications are routinely used to diagnose specific deletions, duplications, or other rearrangements, both in metaphase chromosomes and in interphase nuclei. Use of FISH usually requires that the patient either exhibits features consistent with a well-defined syndrome with known chromosomal etiology, or demonstrates an abnormal karyotype. This is because single FISH probes reveal rearrangements only of the segments being interrogated, but do not provide information about the rest of the genome. Another limitation of FISH is the number of probes that can be applied in a simultaneous assay. FISH

techniques have been developed utilizing pools of whole-chromosome paint probes for every chromosome to provide a multicolor human karyotype in which each pair of homologous chromosomes can be identified on the basis of its unique color when studied using special computer-based image analysis software (spectral karyotyping and multicolor or M-FISH) [Liehr et al., 2004].

One type of FISH that has the potential to reveal chromosomal imbalances across the genome is comparative genomic hybridization (CGH). In CGH, DNA specimens from the patient and a normal control are differentially labeled with two different fluorescent dyes and hybridized to normal metaphase chromosome spreads. Difference between the fluorescent intensities of the two dyes along the length of any given chromosome will reveal gains and losses of genomic segments [Levy et al., 1998]. The limitations of this technology include many of the same limitations of G-banded chromosome analysis. Thus, like G bands, the resolution of CGH is limited to that of metaphase chromosomes, which is approximately 5 Mb for most clinical applications [Liehr et al., 2004].

The latest addition to molecular cytogenetic techniques is array CGH, where CGH is applied to an array of DNA targets (probes), each representing a part of the human genome and fixed to a solid support (usually a glass slide). Like CGH, array CGH directly compares DNA content between two differentially labeled DNA specimens (a test or patient, and a reference or normal control), which are labeled and co-hybridized on to the array. Arrays have been constructed with a variety of DNA targets, ranging from bacterial artificial chromosomes (BACs), which are 80–250 thousand bp (kb) long [Shaffer and Bejjani, 2006] to oligonucleotides (oligos), which are 25–80 bp long [Lucito et al., 2003; Ylstra et al., 2006]. Following hybridization and washing to remove unbound DNA, the array is scanned and analyzed using special computer software to measure the relative ratios of fluorescence of the two dyes, and detect gains/losses of genomic regions represented on the array (Figure 31-3). The resolution of array CGH is dependent on the type of probes used (BACs or oligos) and the distance between them. In the past few years, high-resolution whole-genome coverage array CGH platforms have been increasingly used in clinical molecular cytogenetic labs. These provide a relatively quick method of scanning the entire genome for gains and/or losses with significantly higher resolution and greater clinical abnormality yield than was previously possible. This led to the identification of novel genomic disorders in patients with autistic spectrum disorders (ASD), developmental delay (DD), mental retardation (MR), and/or multiple congenital anomalies (MCAs) [Edelmann and Hirschhorn, 2009].

Chromosomal Abnormalities

Most chromosomal abnormalities exert their phenotypic effects by increasing or decreasing the quantity of genetic material. Chromosomal abnormalities can be divided into numerical and structural abnormalities.

Numerical Abnormalities

The most straightforward of chromosomal abnormalities are alterations of chromosome number. Deviation from the normal diploid complement of 46 chromosomes is referred to as "aneuploidy"; an extra chromosome results in "trisomy,"

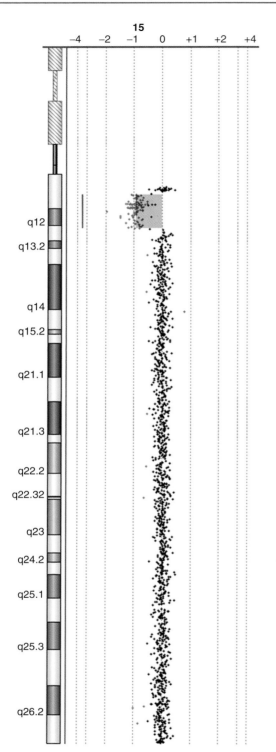

Fig. 31-3 Array comparative genomic hybridization (array CGH) analysis using a whole-genome coverage oligo-array. A chromosome 15 plot is shown with a one copy loss (heterozygous deletion) in the Prader–Willi/Angelman region at 15q11.2q13.1.

only viable monosomy involves the X chromosome (45,X, resulting in Turner's syndrome).

Aneuploidy results from an error in cell division referred to as "nondisjunction," in which two copies of a chromosome go to the same daughter cell during meiosis or mitosis. Nondisjunction occurs most often in the first meiotic division in the maternal germline. Mitotic nondisjunction results in the presence of an aneuploid and a normal cell line – a condition referred to as "mosaicism." The causes of nondisjunction are unknown. The only well-documented risk factor is advanced maternal age.

The term "polyploidy," on the other hand, refers to presence of a complete extra set of chromosomes; "triploidy" represents three sets with 69 chromosomes, whereas "tetraploidy" represents four sets with 92 chromosomes. Rarely, a triploid fetus will be liveborn, but in general polyploidy is lethal. In a few instances, however, mosaicism for a diploid and a triploid cell line producing congenital anomalies has been compatible with long-term survival.

Structural Abnormalities

Structural chromosomal rearrangements result from chromosome breakage, with subsequent reunion in a different configuration. They can be balanced or unbalanced. In balanced rearrangements the chromosome complement is complete, with no loss or gain of genetic material. Consequently, balanced rearrangements are generally harmless, with the exception of rare cases in which one of the breakpoints disrupts an important functional gene. Carriers of balanced rearrangements are often at risk of having children with an unbalanced chromosome complement. When a chromosome rearrangement is unbalanced, the chromosome complement contains an incorrect amount of genetic material, usually with serious clinical effects.

Deletions and Duplications

A deletion involves loss of part of a chromosome and results in monosomy for that segment of the chromosome, whereas duplication represents the doubling of part of a chromosome, resulting in trisomy for that segment. The result is either decrease (in a deletion) or increase (in a duplication) in gene dosage. In general, duplications appear to be less harmful than deletions. Very large deletions usually are incompatible with survival to term. Deletions or duplications larger than approximately 5 Mb in size can be visualized under the microscope using G-banded chromosome analysis. Clinical syndromes resulting from submicroscopic deletions or duplications (i.e., microdeletions/microduplications) with a size <5 Mb have been identified with the help of molecular cytogenetic techniques, including FISH and array CGH. In these syndromes, groups of contiguous genes are either deleted or duplicated, resulting in a defined set of congenital anomalies. The molecular mechanisms responsible for these microdeletions/microduplications have been extensively studied and are well documented [Gu et al., 2008]. Specific microdeletion/microduplication syndromes of neurologic interest are described later in this chapter.

Translocations

Translocations involve the exchange of genetic material between chromosomes. In a balanced reciprocal translocation the exchange is equal, with no loss or gain of genetic material,

whereas a missing chromosome results in "monosomy." Although all the possible chromosomal trisomies have been observed in spontaneous abortions, trisomies 13, 18, and 21 are the only autosomal trisomies to be observed in a nonmosaic state in liveborns. All autosomal monosomies are lethal. The though it is possible for a gene to be disrupted at one of the breakpoints. More often, the carrier of a balanced translocation is free of clinical signs or symptoms but is at risk for having offspring with unbalanced chromosomes. The risk for production of unbalanced gametes from a balanced translocation carrier depends on the chromosomes involved, the specific breakpoints of the translocation, and the sex of the carrier. Empirical data are available for some specific translocations [Daniel et al., 1989]. Risks include miscarriage and birth of a liveborn child with congenital anomalies, resulting from chromosome imbalance. The phenotype usually is a complex mixture of the results of loss or gain of at least two chromosome segments and therefore can be difficult to predict.

One specific type of translocation that is relatively common is the "robertsonian translocation." This results from a fusion of two acrocentric chromosomes (chromosomes 13, 14, 15, 21, or 22) at the centromere. Carriers of a robertsonian translocation have 45 chromosomes and are clinically unaffected. The most common clinically significant outcome is trisomy 21, in which a carrier for a robertsonian translocation involving chromosome 21 produces a gamete with both the translocation chromosome and a normal 21, resulting in trisomy 21 after fertilization.

Inversions

Inversions occur when there are two breaks in a chromosome and the intervening material flips 180 degrees. Inversions that span the centromere are referred to as "pericentric," whereas those that do not are called "paracentric." Inversions generally do not result in added or lost genetic material, and therefore usually are viewed as neutral changes. Disruption of a gene at one of the breakpoints, however, could change the function of that gene. Also, alteration of gene order at the borders of the inversion could affect the function of blocks of genes that are coordinately regulated ("position effect"). If a crossover occurs in the inverted segment of a pericentric inversion during meiosis, two recombinant chromosomes result, one with duplication of one end and deletion of the other end, and the other having the opposite arrangement. Such a crossover event in a paracentric inversion results in dicentric or acentric chromosomes that tend to be unstable.

Insertions

An insertion occurs when a segment of one chromosome becomes inserted into another chromosome. Because these changes require three chromosomal breakpoints, they are relatively rare. Abnormal segregation in a balanced insertion carrier can produce offspring with either duplication or deletion of the inserted segment, as well as balanced carriers and normal offspring.

Marker and Ring Chromosomes

A "marker" chromosome is a rearranged chromosome whose genetic origin is unknown based on its G-banded chromosome morphology. Usually, these chromosomes are present in addition to the normal chromosome complement and are thus called supernumerary marker chromosomes (SMCs). The birth prevalence of SMCs is in the range of 2–7 per 10,000, and 30–50 percent originate from chromosome 15 [Gardner

and Sutherland, 2004]. Two-thirds of de novo marker chromosomes can be associated with an abnormal outcome, whereas inherited ones can be passed from generation to generation without apparent clinical effects. Larger markers with more genetically active material are more likely to be of clinical significance. FISH and array CGH have proved very helpful in the precise identification of the genetic origin of SMCs.

Ring chromosomes are formed when a chromosome undergoes two breaks and the broken ends reunite in a ring structure. Rings encounter difficulties in mitosis and are unstable, resulting in some cells that lose the ring and are therefore monosomic for the chromosome, and others that have multiple copies of the ring.

Isochromosomes

An "isochromosome" is a chromosome in which one arm is missing and the other duplicated in a mirror-image fashion. The most probable mechanism for the formation of an isochromosome is the misdivision through the centromere in meiosis II, wherein the centromere divides transversely rather than longitudinally. The most commonly encountered isochromosome is that which consists of two long arms of the X chromosome. This accounts for approximately 15 percent of all cases of Turner's syndrome [Gardner and Sutherland, 2004].

Cytogenetic Nomenclature

By convention, each chromosome arm is divided into regions, and each region is subdivided into bands and sub-bands, numbered from the centromere outwards. Cytogeneticists describe findings of chromosomal analysis using a standardized system of nomenclature (International System for Human Cytogenetic Nomenclature). Detailed description of this system is beyond the scope of this chapter, but major terms with examples are listed in Table 31-1. The normal male karyotype is designated 46,XY and the normal female karyotype is 46,XX. Any chromosomal abnormality is described after the sex chromosome constitution.

Incidence of Chromosomal Abnormalities

Estimates of the incidence of chromosomal abnormalities vary with the mode of ascertainment and the technology used for chromosome analysis. In general, the incidence falls rapidly from conception to birth. The highest rates have been observed among products of conception from first-trimester spontaneous abortions. Approximately 50 percent of these spontaneous miscarriages have a chromosomal abnormality [Boue et al., 1973]. By birth, the rate of chromosomal abnormalities declines to approximately 0.5–1 percent in liveborn infants, although the rate is much higher (5–10 percent) in stillborn infants [Jacobs et al., 1992].

Clinical Indications for Cytogenetic Analysis

Chromosome analysis has been incorporated in the routine battery of tests available to the clinician. This section considers some of the more common indications for chromosome analysis.

Table 31-1 **Abbreviations Used to Describe Chromosomes and their Abnormalities, and Representative Examples**

Abbreviation	Meaning	Example	Interpretation
		46,XX	Normal female karyotype
		46,XY	Normal male karyotype
		69,XXY	Triploid karyotype with XXY sex chromosome complement
+	Additional chromosome	47,XX,+21	Female karyotype with trisomy 21
−	Missing chromosome	45,XX, −22	Female karyotype with monosomy 22
add	Additional material of unknown origin	46,XX,add(19)(p13)	Female karyotype with additional material of unknown origin attached to chromosome 19 at band p13
arr	Microarray	arr 15q11.2q13.1 (21,258,345–26, 194,049)x1	Microarray analysis demonstrating an interstitial deletion on the long arm of chromosome 15 between linear genomic positions 21,258,345 and 26,194,049 bp in the Prader–Willi/Angelman region
del	Deletion	46,XX,del(5)(p14)	Male karyotype with a terminal deletion on the short arm of chromosome 5, with breakpoint at band p14
der	Derivative chromosome	46,XX,der(1)t(1;3)(p22; q13)	Female karyotype with a "derivative" chromosome 1, resulting from segregation of a balanced translocation between chromosomes 1 and 3, with breakpoints at bands 1p22 and 3q13, respectively
dup	Duplication	46,XX,dup(1)(q22q25)	Female karyotype with a duplication on the long arm of chromosome 1, with breakpoints at bands q22 and q25
i	Isochromosome	46,X,i(X)(q10)	Female karyotype with one normal X chromosome and an isochromosome for the long arm of X chromosome
ins	Insertion	46,XY,ins(5;2)(p14; q22q32)	Male karyotype with a segment of the long arm of chromosome 2 between bands 2q22 and 2q32 inserted into the short arm of chromosome 5 at band 5p14
inv	Inversion	46,XY,inv(2)(p21q31)	Male karyotype with an inversion on chromosome 2, with breakpoints at band p21 on the short arm and band q31 on the long arm (pericentric inversion)
ish	In situ hybridization	46,XX.ish del(22) (q11.2q11.2)(*Tuple1* −)	Normal female karyotype by G-banded chromosome analysis, but with microdeletion on chromosome 22 at band q11.2 (DiGeorge region) detected by metaphase FISH analysis using the *Tuple1* probe
mar	Marker chromosome	47,XY,+mar	Male karyotype with an additional unidentified marker chromosome
mos	Mosaic karyotype	mos 47,XY,+21[12]/46, XY[18]	Mosaic karyotype with trisomy 21 cell line in 12 cells and normal male cell line in 18 cells
p	Short arm of chromosome		
q	Long arm of chromosome		
r	Ring chromosome	46,XX,r(7)(p22q36)	Female karyotype with a ring chromosome 7, with breakpoints at band p22 on the short arm and band q36 on the long arm
rob	Robertsonian translocation	45,XX,rob(13;21)(q10; q10) 46,XX,rob(13;21)(q10; q10),+21	Female karyotype with a robertsonian translocation representing fusion of chromosomes 13 and 21; balanced karyotype Female karyotype with a robertsonian translocation but with additional chromosome 21, resulting in trisomy 21
t	Translocation	46,XY,t(2;5)(q21;q31)	Male karyotype with a balanced reciprocal translocation involving chromosomes 2 and 5, with breakpoints at bands 2q21 and 5q31, respectively

Abbreviations summarized from the International System for Human Cytogenetic Nomenclature (ISCN) 2009.

Multiple Congenital Anomalies

Genetic imbalance resulting from a chromosomal abnormality usually leads to aberrant embryonic development. Most commonly, this abnormal development involves multiple tissues, including the brain. Many specific syndromes can be recognized from a constellation of dysmorphic physical features and specific congenital anomalies. The clinician should be familiar with the most common syndromes, especially those resulting from trisomies 13, 18, and 21, as well as the sex chromosome aneuploidies (47,XXX, 47,XXY, and 45,X).

Phenotypes resulting from duplication or deletion of smaller amounts of genetic material can be more difficult to identify clinically. Some of the more important syndromes are described in the next section. Some clues to the occurrence of a chromosomal abnormality are provided in Box 31-1. As a rule, chromosomal studies should be performed in a patient who exhibits congenital anomalies involving two or more tissues, in whom a specific alternative diagnosis cannot be established, and if the anomalies are not related to one another as cause and effect (e.g., hydrocephalus resulting from spina bifida).

Developmental Delay and/or Mental Retardation

In some chromosomal abnormalities, the phenotype is primarily that of developmental delay (DD) and/or mental retardation (MR), with few or no congenital anomalies. Sometimes, minor dysmorphic features are present, but these often are not noticed on routine examination. G-banded chromosome analysis and array CGH testing therefore should be considered in the evaluation of a child with unexplained DD/MR. MR is a common condition that affects 1–3 percent of the population, and the cause is established in only 50 percent of the cases [Anderlid et al., 2002; Kriek et al., 2004] (also see chapter 43).

The use of array CGH to analyze the genomes of normal humans led to the discovery of extensive genomic copy number variations (CNVs), both gains and losses, ranging in size from kb to Mb, and not recognized by high-resolution G-banded chromosome analysis [Iafrate et al., 2004; Sebat et al., 2004]. CNVs have been proposed to be a major factor responsible for human diversity [Lupski, 2006]. Through genomic rearrangement of rearrangement-prone regions as a result of the genomic architecture, CNVs can cause genomic disorders due to gains and/or losses of dosage-sensitive gene(s), resulting in a clinical phenotype [Stankiewicz and Beaudet, 2007]. Using array CGH technologies, clinically significant pathogenic CNVs have been reported in up to 17 percent of patients with ASD, DD, MR, and/or MCAs [Stankiewicz and Beaudet, 2007; Edelmann and Hirschhorn, 2009].

Fertility Problems

Chromosomal imbalance most often leads to miscarriage rather than to live birth. Carriers of balanced rearrangements, including translocations or inversions, may therefore come to attention through recurrent miscarriage [Flint and Gibb, 1996; Hook and Cross, 1989]. It is recommended that couples who have experienced two or more unexplained first-trimester miscarriages be offered chromosomal analysis. Finding a balanced rearrangement permits genetic counseling of the couple, including offering prenatal diagnosis for future pregnancies. Other members of the family also may carry the balanced rearrangement and should be offered counseling and testing. Unexplained infertility should prompt a request for chromosome studies, especially for women presenting with primary amenorrhea, and for men presenting with azoospermia.

Unexplained Stillbirth/Neonatal Death

Chromosome abnormalities account for approximately 5–10 percent of all stillbirths and neonatal deaths, and not all of these babies have multiple abnormalities that would immediately suggest a chromosomal cause.

Prenatal diagnosis

Chromosomal analysis of a developing fetus can be achieved through collection of fetal cells by CVS, amniocentesis, or peripheral umbilical blood sampling (PUBS) [D'Alton and DeCherney, 1993]. CVS involves sampling part of the fetal placenta using a biopsy device either passed through the cervix or inserted by a needle through the mother's abdomen [Pijpers et al., 1988; Smidt-Jensen and Hahnemann, 1988]. It is performed at 10–12 weeks of gestation. CVS offers the advantage of early testing. Amniocentesis involves sampling amniotic fluid at 16–18 weeks of gestation. Fetal cells in the fluid are cultured and can be used for chromosomal analysis. PUBS is offered after 20 weeks of gestation and involves sampling fetal blood by nicking the umbilical vein under ultrasound guidance [Sermon et al., 2004].

Indications for prenatal testing are listed in Box 31-2. General practice is to offer prenatal testing for pregnancies in which the risk of a chromosomal abnormality exceeds the risk of a complication of the procedure. For couples in which one partner carries a chromosome rearrangement, prenatal testing to detect unbalanced chromosomes can be offered. The actual risk of unbalanced chromosomes in the pregnancy depends on the nature of the rearrangement but generally is greater than 1 percent. The laboratory performing the prenatal testing must be informed of the details of the rearrangement, to ensure that subtle changes are detected. The recurrence risk for future trisomy for a couple who have had one pregnancy affected with trisomy is approximately 1 percent [Lister and Frota-Pessoa, 1980]. This risk is irrespective of the particular chromosome involved in the trisomy. Pregnancies are increasingly being monitored for fetal anomalies by ultrasound or maternal serum screening, with findings indicative of increased risk followed up by prenatal diagnostic testing.

Malignancy

Genetic studies have revealed that cancer cells acquire their oncogenic properties through a series of changes in the genetic information. These changes include gene mutations and chromosome rearrangements. The chromosome rearrangements result in abnormal gene dosage because of deletion or duplication, or in juxtapositions of genetic material that alter gene regulation. Consideration of the various genes that are involved in malignancy, many of which are oncogenes and tumor suppressor genes, is beyond the scope of this chapter. In several instances, however, specific chromosomal rearrangements have been associated with particular cancers. Chromosomal analysis can be helpful in these disorders to provide diagnostic information, to assess appropriate treatment and prognosis, and to follow response to therapy.

Specific Cytogenetic Syndromes

Polyploidy

Cytogenetics

Tetraploidy is an infrequent chromosomal abnormality, but triploidy occurs fairly often. Most triploid embryos miscarry in the first trimester. In approximately 20 percent of first-trimester spontaneous abortions the conceptus is found to have a triploid karyotype. Liveborn infants with triploidy exhibit multiple congenital anomalies and rarely survive the newborn period. Those that do usually are mosaics for a diploid and a triploid cell line (sometimes referred to as "mixoploids," because diploid and triploid cell lines may arise from separate fertilizations).

Clinical Features

The triploid phenotype is distinct and easily recognized. Polyhydramnios or pre-eclampsia may complicate the pregnancy. The placenta may be large, and hydatidiform changes may be seen. Birth weight usually is low. Syndactyly involving the third and fourth digits is characteristic. Craniofacial features include low-set, malformed ears, hypertelorism, and micrognathia. Cardiac, renal, and central nervous system malformations are common. Males may have dysplastic external genitalia. Studies of the parental origin of the three chromosome sets in triploidy have revealed that a majority of affected persons have two maternal sets, perhaps because of more frequent survival to term of triploid fetuses with two maternal sets of chromosomes (digynic triploids) [McFadden et al., 1993]. Long-term survivors often are mosaics and may have less obvious phenotypic features. Body asymmetry and pigmentary dysplasia may be clues to chromosomal mosaicism in general, including, in some cases, triploidy [Woods et al., 1994].

Management

Most triploid fetuses are spontaneously aborted or are still-born. Most liveborn infants with full triploidy die in the early days of life. Survivors require supportive care for their congenital anomalies and developmental impairment.

Aneuploidy

Only a minority of aneuploid embryos survive to term; the rest miscarry, usually in the first trimester. Only the most common trisomy and monosomy syndromes compatible with live birth are considered in the following discussion.

Trisomy 13 (Patau Syndrome)

Cytogenetics

Trisomy 13 occurs in approximately 1 in 7000 live births [Savva et al., 2010]. A majority of affected persons have 47 chromosomes, with an extra copy of chromosome 13. Approximately 5–10 percent have trisomy because of translocation between 13 and another acrocentric chromosome, usually chromosome 14 (robertsonian translocation). Mosaicism occurs in a small proportion of cases and may ameliorate the phenotype. Duplication of part of chromosome 13 resulting from unbalanced translocation can result in abnormal phenotypic features, although not necessarily similar to those seen in full trisomy 13. Advanced maternal age has been a factor in the occurrence of this aneuploidy syndrome.

Clinical Features

Trisomy 13 is associated with congenital anomalies involving most major organ systems (Figure 31-4). Holoprosencephaly is the hallmark central nervous system anomaly [Moerman et al., 1988], occurring in about 80 percent of cases. Infants with trisomy 13 who demonstrate holoprosencephaly usually have accompanying craniofacial anomalies. The eyes may be set closely together (hypotelorism) or even fused in a single orbit (cyclopia). Other ocular anomalies include microphthalmia, iris colobomata, cataracts, and retinal dysplasia. Premaxillary agenesis and cleft lip or palate also may be present. Ulcer-like defects in scalp skin (cutis aplasia) occur commonly. Limb anomalies include postaxial polydactyly in two-thirds of patients and rocker-bottom foot. Congenital heart defects, especially ventricular septal defect (VSD), are common, as are renal anomalies, including cystic dysplasia. The phenotype overlaps to some degree with that of Meckel–Gruber syndrome (encephalocele, polydactyly, polycystic kidney), inherited as an autosomal-recessive trait due to mutation of the *MKS1* gene. This overlap underlines the importance of confirming the clinical diagnosis of trisomy 13 by chromosomal analysis.

Management

Few infants with trisomy 13 survive the newborn period, with apnea being the most common cause of death [Rasmussen et al., 2003]. Often the anomalies are too numerous and severe to be corrected. In the absence of life-threatening malformations, however, long-term survival has been well documented, albeit usually with severely impaired cognitive function. Baty

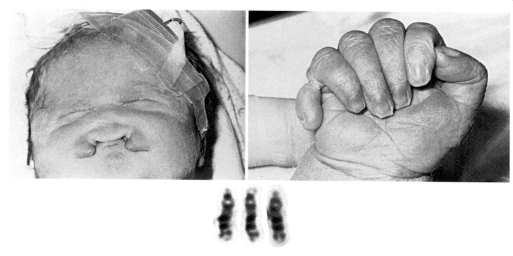

Fig. 31-4 A newborn with trisomy 13. *(Karyotype courtesy of M Rochon, Sherbrooke, Quebec, Canada.)*

47, XX, +13

and co-workers documented the natural history of this disorder [Baty et al., 1994; Baty et al., 1994a & b].

Trisomy 18 (Edwards' Syndrome)

Trisomy 18 affects approximately 1 in 4000 live births. It is virtually always associated with a 47-chromosome karyotype, although a small proportion of affected newborns have a mosaic karyotype. Segregation of a parental balanced translocation may result in trisomy for part of the short or long arm of chromosome 18. Molecular analysis has revealed that most

nondisjunction events that lead to trisomy 18 occur in maternal meiosis, which is most likely to occur at older maternal age.

Clinical Features

Infants with trisomy 18 have low birth weight and microcephaly. Other common features include a prominent occiput, low-set "simple" ears, and a small mouth (Figure 31-5). Hands usually are tightly clenched in a characteristic configuration, with the fourth and fifth fingers overlapping the first and second. Terminal phalanges often are hypoplastic, and rocker-bottom foot may

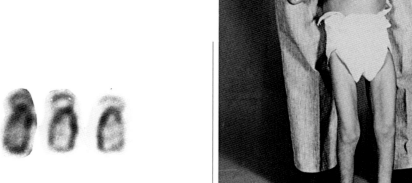

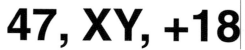

Fig. 31-5 A patient with trisomy 18 at 7 years of age. *(Karyotype courtesy of M Rochon, Sherbrooke, Quebec, Canada.)*

47, XY, +18

be present. Congenital heart defects and renal anomalies also are common. Brain malformations include heterotopias, agenesis of the corpus callosum, Dandy–Walker malformation, and Arnold–Chiari malformation. Infants commonly are jittery and hypertonic, and have apnea and seizures.

Management

No definitive treatment exists for trisomy 18. Most affected infants die in the neonatal period [Rasmussen et al., 2003; Hsiao et al., 2009]. Long-term survivors have developmental impairment and require supportive care.

Trisomy 21 (Down Syndrome)

Trisomy 21 is the most common and widely recognized of the autosomal trisomy syndromes. It occurs in approximately 1 in 800 live births, with a striking increase in frequency with advanced maternal age. The frequency of Down syndrome at birth may be lower in areas in which prenatal screening and testing are offered. Full trisomy 21 occurs in about 95 percent of cases. Translocation, usually between chromosome 21 and another acrocentric chromosome, most often chromosome 14, is identified in approximately 4 percent. A parent who carries such a translocation may be at risk for recurrence of Down syndrome. Rarely, patients with clinical Down syndrome have only a partial trisomy of 21. The remaining 1 percent of affected persons have a mosaic karyotype. The pathogenesis of the features of Down syndrome is attributed to increased dosage of genes on chromosome 21. The levels of gene expression apparently are tightly regulated, with increased levels of expression leading to aberrant development. Efforts are under way to identify specific genes responsible for specific components of the Down syndrome phenotype.

Clinical Features

Down syndrome consists of a set of characteristic physical features and developmental impairment (Figure 31-6). Short stature and brachycephaly are characteristic, and mild microcephaly may be noted. Down syndrome growth charts are available and should be used to monitor growth in affected children [Cronk et al., 1988]. Craniofacial features include upslanted palpebral fissures, epicanthal folds, flat facial profile, and small, low-set ears with narrow ear canals. White speckles (Brushfield spots) may be seen on the iris. A common finding is redundant folds of nuchal skin, which is one of the markers used for prenatal diagnosis by ultrasound examination [Gray and Crane, 1994]. Fingers are short, with incurving of the fifth finger (clinodactyly) and, often, a single transverse palmar crease. A wide space between the first and second toes is a frequent finding. The hallmark neurologic feature of Down syndrome is hypotonia. No gross central nervous system malformation is consistently seen, although lack of normal growth of the brain is typical. Microscopic analysis has revealed impaired myelination, reduced density of neurons, malformed dendritic trees and spines, defective lamination of the cortex, and abnormality of synaptic density [Wisniewski et al., 1990]. Impaired neurologic development is a universal feature

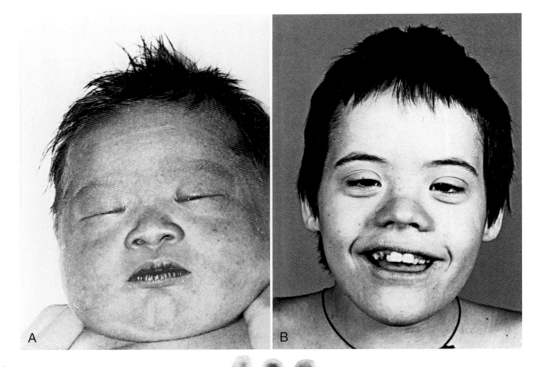

Fig. 31-6 Patients with trisomy 21 (Down syndrome). A, A newborn with trisomy 21 (Down syndrome). **B,** A boy with Down syndrome at 12 years of age. *(Karyotype courtesy of M Rochon, Sherbrooke, Quebec, Canada.)*

44, XX, +21

[Silverman, 2007], but the degree of impairment varies widely. Children with Down syndrome benefit from early intervention [Fidler and Nadel, 2007; Feeley and Jones, 2008], physical therapy, and being reared in a family setting. An increased frequency of psychiatric problems, such as depression and behavioral problems, including hyperactivity, disruptive behaviors, and repetitive behaviors, have been documented [Visootsak Sherman, 2007; Dykens, 2007], as have sleep problems [Carter et al., 2009]. Linguistic ability may be impaired out of proportion to cognitive impairment. Seizures, including infantile spasms, may be seen with increased frequency [Smigielska-Kuzia et al., 2009]. An increased frequency of dementia, associated with pathologic changes of Alzheimer's disease, has been described in patients with Down syndrome [Nieuwenhuis-Mark, 2009; Waldman et al., 2008; Deb et al., 2007]. Congenital anomalies commonly associated with Down syndrome include heart and gastrointestinal defects. The most typical heart defect is common atrioventricular (AV) canal, although other anomalies, such as VSD or tetralogy of Fallot, may be seen. Gastrointestinal malformations include duodenal atresia and Hirschsprung's disease.

Management

The American Academy of Pediatrics has published guidelines for management of children with Down syndrome [American Academy of Pediatrics: Health supervision for children with Down syndrome, 2001]. Children with Down syndrome frequently require surgery for correction of congenital anomalies, such as heart defects or gastrointestinal malformations. They have a markedly increased risk of respiratory infection and sleep-related upper airway obstruction. often requiring antibiotic treatment. The frequency of leukemia is increased in children with Down syndrome. Transient leukemoid reactions also may occur.

Children with Down syndrome are at risk for atlantoaxial dislocation. Whether screening for dislocation should be offered for children with Down syndrome, particularly those who will participate in sports activities, has been the subject of controversy [Atlantoaxial instability in Down syndrome: subject review. American Academy of Pediatrics Committee on Sports Medicine and Fitness, 1995]. All children with Down syndrome should be monitored for neurologic signs of cervical cord compression. Parents of children with Down syndrome should be counseled regarding the natural history of the disorder, opportunities for intervention, and genetic recurrence risks, and should be provided emotional support. Life expectancy for persons with Down syndrome has improved with advances in surgery and medical treatment of complications of the disorder.

Trisomy 8 (Warkany's Syndrome)

The only other autosomal trisomy compatible with live birth is trisomy 8. This trisomy is lethal in utero, except as a mosaic karyotype. Phenotypic features include hypertelorism; camptodactyly and other joint contractures; long, slender habitus; absence of patellae; and deep creases of the palms and soles (Figure 31-7). Asymmetric growth, presumably due to chromosomal mosaicism, also may be a feature.

Turner's Syndrome

Cytogenetics

Turner's syndrome is associated with a 45,X karyotype, with a single X chromosome. Mosaicism is not uncommon, however, with a separate cell line containing either a normal 46,XX or XY karyotype, or 46 chromosomes including a structurally rearranged X or Y [Crocker, 1992]. Turner's syndrome occurs in about 1 in 4000 female live births worldwide but it is much more common in stillbirths and miscarriages. Unlike other aneuploidy syndromes, the frequency of Turner's syndrome does not increase with advancing maternal age.

Clinical Features

Patients with Turner's syndrome typically have a female phenotype, although those with a cell line including a Y chromosome may have some degree of virilization, often with ambiguous genitalia. At birth, infants may manifest pedal edema or diffuse edema (Figure 31-8). Facial features include small mandible, narrow maxilla, and epicanthal folds.

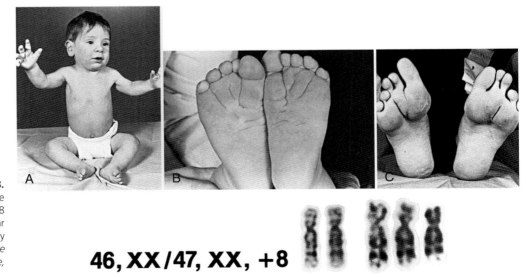

Fig. 31-7 A patient with trisomy 8. A and **B,** At 18 months of age. **C,** The same patient with trisomy 8 at 18 years of age. Note the deep palmar and plantar creases that are commonly seen in these patients. *(Karyotype courtesy of M Rochon, Sherbrooke, Quebec, Canada.)*

46, XX / 47, XX, +8

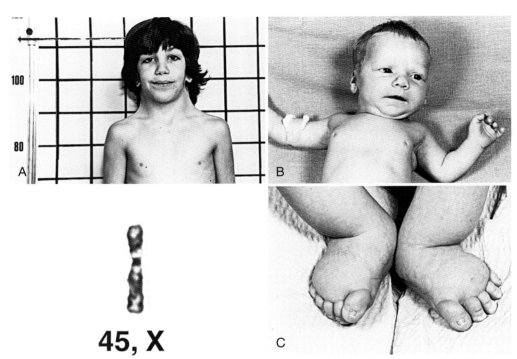

Fig. 31-8 A girl with Turner's syndrome. A, At 9 years of age. **B,** At 1 month of age. **C,** At birth. *(Courtesy of K Khoury; karyotype courtesy of M Rochon, Sherbrooke, Quebec, Canada.)*

45, X

In older children and adults with Turner's syndrome, short stature and webbing of the neck are seen commonly. The thorax is broad, with increased distance between the nipples. Congenital anomalies include abnormalities of the lymphatic system, cardiac defects, especially coarctation of the aorta and bicuspid aortic valve, and renal anomalies, such as horseshoe kidney.

Although mental retardation is rare, delays in both gross and fine motor development are common in females with Turner's syndrome [Nijhuis-van der Sanden et al., 2003]. Some patients display cognitive problems, but difficulties with visuospatial perception are most common [Pennington et al., 1982]. Hearing impairment occurs frequently and children should be monitored for deficits or progression of impairment.

Management

Recommendations for diagnosis and management of Turner's syndrome have been published [Frias and Davenport, 2003; Health supervision for children with Turner syndrome. American Academy of Pediatrics. Committee on Genetics, 1995]. Newborns should be evaluated for renal and cardiac defects, and monitored if these are found. An increased risk for dissection of the aorta has been reported in affected adults [Elsheikh et al., 2002]. Thyroid autoimmunity may be a feature, so monitoring of thyroid function is recommended. Although not all children with Turner's syndrome are growth hormone-deficient, significant growth hormone-induced improvement has been demonstrated in affected individuals.

Turner's syndrome typically is associated with the presence of a streak gonad, lack of secondary sexual development, and infertility. Referral to an endocrinologist for hormonal induction of puberty should be done at an appropriate age. Intra-abdominal gonads in patients with Turner's syndrome who have a Y chromosome are at risk of transformation into gonadoblastoma and therefore should be removed.

Klinefelter's Syndrome

Cytogenetics

Klinefelter's syndrome occurs in about 1 in 1000 males and is associated with a 47,XXY karyotype. The incidence increases as a function of maternal age in half of the cases. Rare patients may have multiple X chromosomes (e.g., 48,XXXY or 49, XXXXY). Usually the presence of multiple X chromosomes in such persons is associated with more severe cognitive impairment.

Clinical Features

The diagnosis of Klinefelter's syndrome usually is not suspected at birth. Affected males tend to be tall, with long limbs (Figure 31-9). They display hypogonadism, and virilization may be incomplete at puberty; gynecomastia develops in some patients. Azoospermia and infertility are characteristic. Breast cancer is 20 times more common in Klinefelter's syndrome than in the normal male population. As in Turner's syndrome, mental retardation is not a typical feature of Klinefelter's syndrome. Learning disabilities, language delay, and behavior problems are reported [Boada et al., 2009; Ross et al., 2009].

Management

Children with Klinefelter's syndrome require support at home and school for learning and behavioral problems. Testosterone is administered, beginning in adolescence, to improve secondary sexual development.

Other Sex Chromosome Aneuploidies

Two other major sex chromosome aneuploidies are 47,XXX and 47,XYY. The XXX aneuploidy is associated with a female phenotype and tall stature; usually other major physical stigmata are absent. XYY is associated with a male phenotype

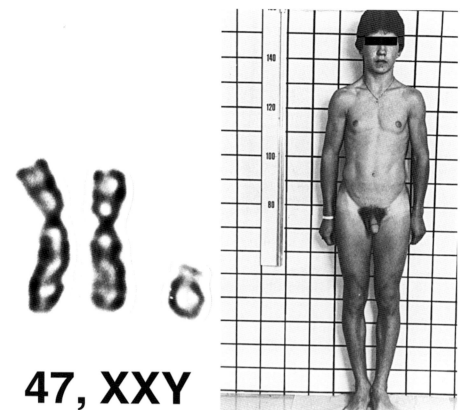

Fig. 31-9 A boy with Klinefelter's syndrome at age 13 years. *(Courtesy of K Khoury; karyotype courtesy of M Rochon, Sherbrooke, Quebec, Canada.)*

47, XXY

and tall stature but no other physical features. Learning disabilities and neuromotor impairment occur commonly in 47,XXX females [Bender et al., 2001]. The behavioral phenotype of XYY syndrome has been a source of some controversy because of reports associating the karyotype with criminal behavior. The frequency of learning disabilities and behavioral problems is increased among affected males, although a wide range of cognitive outcomes have been reported [Ross et al., 2009].

Structural Abnormalities

Structural abnormalties of chromosomes cause phenotypic effects resulting from loss and/or gain of genetic material. In some cases, these occur sporadically as a result of de novo chromosome rearrangements, whereas in others, they may be inherited as a consequence of segregation of a familial balanced chromosomal rearrangement. Some deletion or duplication syndromes are fairly well characterized in terms of phenotypic effects and may be recognized clinically. Clinical diagnosis often is complicated, however, by a number of factors. First, most of these syndromes are much less common than the trisomy syndromes. Second, the exact extent of deleted or duplicated material may differ from one affected child to another, leading to subtle but important variation in clinical manifestations. Third, many of these syndromes are seen as a consequence of malsegregation of a familial balanced chromosomal rearrangement. The usual consequence is imbalance of two or more distinct chromosome regions, resulting in a set of anomalies that combine the phenotypic effects of both segments.

Microdeletion/microduplication syndromes constitute a relatively recent addition to the list of disorders caused by

chromosomal imbalance. The clinical phenotypes of these syndromes may be explained in two ways. First, many of these are "contiguous deletion syndromes"; that is, a cluster of closely linked genes are simultaneously deleted, leading to a complex phenotype that reflects the contributions of multiple genes. Specific components of the phenotype may be present or absent in any given case, depending on the extent of deletion. This mechanism is operative, for example, in the WAGR (Wilms tumor, aniridia, genitourinary dysplasia, and mental retardation) association, occurring with deletion of a region on the short arm of chromosome 11. Depending on the extent of deletion, features may include Wilms tumor, aniridia, genitourinary anomalies, and developmental impairment, or some combination of these features. The second mechanism is that a deletion can result in altered or absent expression of one critical gene in the region that itself leads to a complex phenotype. Deletion is likely to be one of many mechanisms of mutation of the gene; thus, FISH and/or array CGH analysis will not reveal the deletion in all affected persons. This mechanism accounts for Rubinstein–Taybi syndrome, Angelman's syndrome, and Alagille's syndrome. These two mechanisms, of course, are not mutually exclusive. Deletion of a major gene may account for much of a particular phenotype, but deletion of contiguous genes may contribute additional phenotypic features in some patients.

To date, most genomic imbalances have been classified as either benign or pathogenic, and most microdeletion/microduplication syndromes are presumed to be well-defined clinical conditions. Well-known genomic disorders can be phenotypically heterogeneous and variable, however, owing to incomplete penetrance or variable expression. Clinical variability could also be explained in part by other genetic or environmental determinants, modifying factors of other genes, multigenic inheritance, imprinting, and unmasking of recessive genes. Array CGH and genomic copy-number analysis using single-nucleotide polymorphism (SNP) genotyping arrays are proving particularly effective for the investigation of patients with developmental delay, learning disabilities, mental retardation, dysmorphic features, and/or multiple congenital anomalies, and are identifying the probable underlying cause of the disease phenotype in approximately 17 percent of previously undiagnosed cases [Stankiewicz and Beaudet, 2007; Edelmann and Hirschhorn, 2009]. Moreover, a genomic basis to several late-onset disorders, e.g., early-onset Alzheimer's disease with amyloid angiopathy (EOAD), and adult-onset autosomal-dominant leukodystrophy, has now been defined [Firth et al., 2009]. Table 31-2 lists the microdeletion/microduplication syndromes reported to date, as shown in the DECIPHER database (https://decipher.sanger.ac.uk/application/). In the following section, some of these syndromes that are clinically relevant to the practice of pediatric neurology are discussed.

22q11.2 Deletion Syndrome

The 22q11.2 deletion syndrome includes the phenotypes previously called DiGeorge's syndrome (DGS), velocardiofacial syndrome (VCFS, Shprintzen's syndrome), conotruncal anomaly face syndrome, many cases of autosomal-dominant Opitz G/BBB syndrome, and Cayler's cardiofacial syndrome (asymmetric crying facies) [McDonald-McGinn et al., 1997]. The condition is clinically heterogeneous. Congenital heart defects are present in most affected individuals (74 percent), particularly conotruncal malformation. Additional findings include palatal abnormalities and velopharyngeal incompetence

Table 31-2 Microdeletion/Microduplication Syndromes Listed in the DECIPHER Database

Syndrome	OMIM Number
12q14 microdeletion syndrome	166700
15q13.3 microdeletion syndrome	612001
15q24 recurrent microdeletion syndrome	–
15q26 overgrowth syndrome	–
16p11.2 autism susceptibility locus	611913
16p11.2–p12.2 microdeletion syndrome	–
16p13.11 recurrent microdeletion (MR/MCA susceptibility locus)	–
16p13.11 recurrent microduplication (uncertain significance)	–
17q21.3 recurrent microdeletion syndrome	610443
1p36 microdeletion syndrome	607872
1q21.1 recurrent microdeletion (susceptibility locus for neurodevelopmental disorders)	612474
1q21.1 recurrent microduplication (possible susceptibility locus for neurodevelopmental disorders)	612475
1q21.1 susceptibility locus for thrombocytopenia-absent radius (TAR) syndrome	274000
22q11.2 deletion syndrome (velocardiofacial/DiGeorge's syndrome)	192430, 188400
22q11.2 duplication syndrome	608363
22q11.2 distal deletion syndrome	611867
22q13 deletion syndrome (Phelan–McDermid syndrome)	606232
2p15-16.1 microdeletion syndrome	612513
2q33.1 deletion syndrome	–
2q37 monosomy	600430
3q29 microdeletion syndrome	609425
3q29 microduplication syndrome	611936
6p deletion syndrome	612582
7q11.23 duplication syndrome	609757
8p23.1 deletion syndrome	222400
9q subtelomeric deletion syndrome	610253
ATR-16 syndrome	141750
AZF a, b, and c	415000
Adult-onset autosomal-dominant leukodystrophy (ADLD)	169500
Angelman's syndrome (types 1 and 2)	105830
Cat-eye syndrome (type I)	115470

Table 31-2 Microdeletion/Microduplication Syndromes Listed in the DECIPHER Database—cont'd

Syndrome	OMIM Number
Charcot–Marie–Tooth syndrome type 1A (CMT1A)	118220
Cri du chat syndrome (5p deletion)	123450
Early-onset Alzheimer's disease with cerebral amyloid angiopathy	605714
Familial adenomatous polyposis	175100
Hereditary liability to pressure palsies (HNPP)	162500
Leri–Weill dyschondrostosis (LWD) – SHOX deletion	127300
Miller–Dieker syndrome (MDS)	247200
NF1-microdeletion syndrome	162200
Pelizaeus–Merzbacher disease	312080
Potocki–Lupski syndrome (17p11.2 duplication syndrome)	610883
Potocki–Shaffer syndrome	601224
Prader–Willi syndrome (types 1 and 2)	176270
RCAD (renal cysts and diabetes)	137920
Rubinstein–Taybi syndrome	180849
Smith–Magenis syndrome	182290
Sotos' syndrome	117550
Split hand/foot malformation 1 (SHFM1)	183600
Steroid sulphatase deficiency (STS)	300747
WAGR 11p13 deletion syndrome	194072
Williams–Beuren syndrome (WBS)	194050
Wolf–Hirschhorn syndrome	194190
Xq28 (MECP2) duplication	300260

ATR, alpha thalassemia/mental retardation syndrome; AZF, azoospermic factors; MCA, multiple congenital anomalies; MR, mental retardation; WAGR, Wilms tumor, aniridia, genitourinary dysplasia, and mental retardation.

(VPI), learning disabilities, immune deficiencies, hypocalcemia, and characteristic facies. Also reported are hearing loss, seizures without hypocalcemia, speech delays, and behavioral difficulties. The 22q11.2 deletion affects an estimated 1:2000 to 1:4000 live births. The deletion occurs in 2 percent of patients with isolated conotruncal heart defects and in 5–8 percent of individuals with isolated cleft palate. Most cases are de novo and approximately 6 percent are familial. The inheritance is autosomal-dominant. Some cases with deletion 10p13p14 have a deletion 22q11.2-like phenotype. The phenotype of the reciprocal microduplication of the 22q11.2 region is mild and highly variable, with familial transmission frequently observed.

Prader–Willi and Angelman's Syndromes

The recognition of the phenomenon of genomic imprinting has led to the discovery of a new class of genetic disorders associated with aberrations of imprinted genes. The prototype disorders are Prader–Willi and Angelman's syndromes (Figure 31-10 and Figure 31-11) [Gurrieri and Accadia, 2009]. The features of these syndromes are described in Table 31-3. Prader–Willi syndrome (PWS) is characterized by hypotonia and feeding difficulties in early life, hyperphagia and obesity later, short stature, hypogonadism, and acromicria. Behavior problems are common and psychomotor development is mildy affected. PWS affects 1:5000 to 1:10,000

individuals. Approximately 70–75 percent of the individuals with PWS have a deletion of the paternally contributed 15q11.2q13.1 region, while in Angelman's syndrome (AS), 70 percent of affected individuals have a deletion of the maternally contributed region. The AS phenotype is completely different and it is characterized by severe mental retardation, absent speech, autistic behavior, unique behavior (inappropriate happy demeanor), gait ataxia, epilepsy, electroencephalogram (EEG) abnormalities (2–3-Hz, large-amplitude slow-wave bursts), microcephaly, and dysmorphic features. The EEG may be abnormal, even in the absence of seizures, however; a normal EEG and/or absence of seizures do not exclude the diagnosis. Approximately 1:40,000 children are affected with AS. Most patients with PWS who do not have the 15q11.2q13.1 deletions have uniparental disomy for chromosome 15, with two maternal copies and no paternal copies. Either mechanism – deletion or uniparental disomy – leads to deficiency of a gene or genes on chromosome 15 that are expressed in the paternal but not the maternal homolog. Paternal uniparental disomy accounts for a low percentage of cases of AS. Mutations in the UBE3A gene (a ubiquitin ligase gene involved in early brain development), located at 15q11.2, have been found in some patients with AS [Kishino et al., 1997]. This gene is imprinted in the brain [Albrecht et al., 1997; Rougeulle et al., 1997], and is the gene responsible for the AS phenotype. Deletion of the paternally

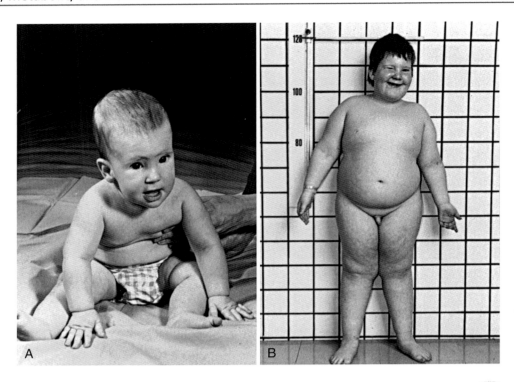

Fig. 31-10 A boy with Prader–Willi syndrome. A, At 7 months of age. **B,** At 6 years of age. *(Karyotype courtesy of MG Mattei, Marseilles, France.)*

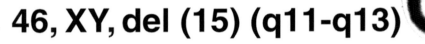

46, XY, del (15) (q11-q13)

expressed HBII-85 C/D box small nucleolar RNA cluster has been implicated in PWS [Sahoo et al., 2008]. A small proportion of patients with PW or AS may have a small deletion or other mutation that leads to aberrant imprinting of the region [Buiting et al., 1995]. These findings have led to major advances in genetic diagnosis of PW and AS. Chromosome 15 deletions usually are submicroscopic but are easily detected by FISH and/or array CGH. Defects in imprinting or uniparental disomy can be identified by studies of patterns of DNA methylation in the region. One particular cloned segment of DNA is methylated in the maternal, but not the paternal, genome. Failure to identify the methylated or nonmethylated copy of the sequence is indicative of deletion, uniparental disomy, or a mutation that alters the imprinting mechanism.

Imprinted genes are expressed only from one of the two parental alleles (gene pair). In mammals, genomic imprinting is an event in which particular genes are expressed differentially, depending on the parent of origin. Genomic imprints are reversible and lead to differential expression in the course of development. Genomic imprinting is an epigenetic process that involves methylation and histone modifications in order to achieve monoallelic gene expression without altering the genetic sequence. Genome-wide research for imprinted genes

in the human genome has identified over 150 candidate imprinted genes [Luedi et al., 2007]. Other examples of human disorders of genomic imprinting include Silver–Russell syndrome, Beckwith–Wiedemann syndrome, Albright hereditary osteodystrophy, and uniparental disomy 14 (maternal and paternal forms).

William–Beuren Syndrome

The William–Beuren syndrome (WBS) is a microdeletion syndrome of chromosome 7 at band q11.23, and occurs in 1:10,000 live births [Tassabehji, 2003]. Cardiovascular disease is present in 80 percent of affected individuals, mostly in the form of supravalvular aortic stenosis (SVAS), peripheral pulmonary stenosis, elastin arteriopathy, and hypertension. The 7q11.23 microdeletion encompasses the elastin gene (*ELN*), which is also mutated in isolated SVAS. Characteristic facial features include periorbital fullness, long philtrum, wide mouth, full lips, full cheeks, and small, wide-spaced teeth. Affected individuals have mild to moderate MR, specific cognitive profile/learning disabilities, and unique or distinctive behavior/personality characteristics. Growth and endocrine abnormalities (hypercalcemia, hypothyroidism, hypercalciuria), and feeding difficulties in infancy are also common.

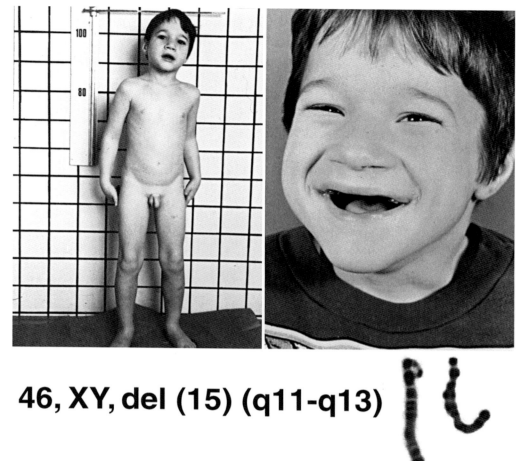

46, XY, del (15) (q11-q13)

Fig. 31-11 **A boy with Angelman's syndrome at 6 years of age.** *(Karyotype courtesy of M Rochon, Sherbrooke, Quebec, Canada.)*

1p36 Deletion Syndrome

1p36 deletion syndrome is considered to be the most common subtelomeric microdeletion syndrome with an estimated incidence of 1 in 5000 to 1 in 10,000. It accounts for 0.5–1.2 percent of idiopathic MR [Battaglia et al., 2008]. Clinical findings include a characteristic craniofacial appearance: microbrachycephaly, large and late-closing anterior fontanel, straight eyebrows, deep-set eyes, epicanthic folds, broad nasal bridge, midface hypoplasia, abnormally formed low-set ears, and limb and skeletal defects. DD and MR with absent/poor expressive language are constant features. Affected individuals often face serious physical disabilities that include congenital heart defects (70 percent), cardiomyopathy (25 percent), brain abnormalities (88 percent), seizures (44 percent), and EEG abnormalities (100 percent). Ocular malformations or vision problems and hearing loss are observed approximately 50 percent of affected individuals.

Wolf–Hirschhorn Syndrome

Wolf–Hirschhorn syndrome (WHS) results from a variable-sized deletion on the terminal end of the short arm of chromosome 4 [Bahi-Buisson et al., 2005]. It is characterized by distinctive facial appearance, growth delay, psychomotor retardation, and seizures, and is confirmed by detection of a deletion of the Wolf–Hirschhorn critical region (WHCR) (chromosome 4p16.3). The syndrome has clinical and cytogenetic variability. In some, the deletion is visible by G-banded chromosome analysis; in others, it is cryptic, and molecular cytogenetic analysis is required to make the diagnosis. Characteristic facial features include the "Greek warrior helmet" appearance of the nose (the broad bridge of the nose continuing to the forehead), microcephaly, high forehead with prominent glabella, ocular hypertelorism, epicanthus, highly arched eyebrows, short philtrum, downturned mouth, micrognathia, and poorly formed ears with pits/tags. MR ranges from mild to severe. Other birth defects have been reported in individuals with WHS. One-third of the patients have structural central nervous system defects, and seizures occur in 50–100 percent of affected children. In 75 percent of patients with WHS, the deletion is de novo, and in about 13 percent of patients the deletion results from the unbalanced segregation of a parental balanced translocation. It is now recognized that WHS and Pitt–Rogers–Danks syndrome (PRDS) represent the clinical spectrum associated with a single syndrome [Moretti et al., 2001].

Cri du Chat Syndrome

Cri du chat syndrome is a genetic syndrome resulting from a variable-sized deletion on the terminal end of the short arm of chromosome 5. The first description was made by Lejeune et al., in 1964 [Lejeune et al., 1964]. The incidence ranges from 1:15,000 to 1:50,000. A high-pitched, cat-like cry is among the main clinical features; hence the name of the syndrome. Other frequently described features are microcephaly, broad nasal bridge, epicanthic folds, micrognathia, impaired growth, and severe psychomotor and mental retardation. The syndrome

Table 31-3 Comparison of Features of Prader–Willi and Angelman's Syndromes

	Prader–Willi Syndrome*	Angelman's Syndrome[†]
Diagnostic criteria	Major clinical criteria 　Neonatal hypotonia 　Feeding problems in infancy 　Rapid weight gain between 1 and 　6 years of age 　Characteristic facies 　Hypogonadism 　Developmental delay 　Hyperphagia Minor criteria 　Decreased fetal movement 　Characteristic behaviors 　Sleep disturbances 　Short stature 　Small hands 　Narrow hands 　Esotropia/myopia 　Thick, viscous saliva 　Speech articulation defects 　Skin picking Supportive findings 　High pain threshold 　Decreased vomiting	Consistent features (100%) 　Developmental delay 　Speech impairment 　Movement disorder (ataxia of gait, tremulous movement of limbs) 　Behavioral features: frequent laughter or smiling, hand flapping Frequent features (80%) 　Acquired microcephaly 　Seizures (usually in patients younger than 3 years) 　Abnormal EEG (high-amplitude 2- to 3-Hz spike-wave discharge) Associated features (20–80%) 　Flat occiput, occipital groove 　Protruding tongue 　Prognathism 　Wide mouth and widely spaced teeth 　Drooling, chewing, mouthing movements 　Strabismus 　Hypopigmentation 　Brisk lower limb deep tendon reflexes 　Sleep disturbance
Cytogenetics	70–75% paternal 15q11.2q13.1 deletion	70% maternal 15q11.2q13.1 deletion
Uniparental disomy	20–25% maternal disomy	2% paternal disomy
Imprinting defect	1–3%	2–5%
Gene mutation	Unknown	5–10% *UBE3A* gene mutation

EEG, electroencephalogram.
* Data from Holm V et al. 1993. Prader–Willi syndrome: consensus diagnostic criteria. Pediatrics 1993;91(8424017):398–402.
[†] Data from Williams CA et al. Angelman syndrome: consensus for diagnostic criteria. Angelman Syndrome Foundation. Am J Med Genet 1995;56(2):237–238.
(Mutation analysis data from Buiting K et al. Epimutations in Prader-Willi and Angelman syndromes: a molecular study of 136 patients with an imprinting defect. Am J Hum Genet 2003;72[12545427]:571–577; Jiang Y et al. Genetics of Angelman syndrome. Am J Hum Genet 1999;65[10364509]:1–6.)

has significant clinical and cytogenetic variability. Clinical analysis of affected individuals and detailed molecular cytogenetic analysis suggest the existence of two critical regions, one on 5p15.2 for facial dysmorphism, microcephaly, and MR, and another on 5p15.3 for the typical cry [Zhang et al., 2005]. Eighty percent of affected individuals are the result of a de novo deletion, and 10 percent are the result of the unbalanced segregation of a parental balanced translocation.

Deletions Involving Distal 6p

Deletions involving distal 6p are relatively rare. These deletions can be divided into two groups: interstitial with breakpoints within the 6p22p24 region, and terminal deletions with breakpoints within the 6p24pter region. The terminal deletion of 6p results in a distinct phenotype, including hypertelorism, downslanting palpebral fissures, flat nasal bridge, Dandy–Walker malformation, congenital heart defect, anterior eye chamber abnormalities, hearing loss, and DD [Lin et al., 2005]. Hydrocephalus has been seen in patients with terminal 6p deletions but the majority has been associated with Dandy–Walker malformation [Murray et al., 1985].

Chromosome 9q Subtelomeric Deletion

The chromosome 9q subtelomeric deletion represents one of the most common subtelomeric deletions (6 percent) [Ravnan et al., 2006]. The syndrome can be caused either by a submicroscopic 9q34.3 deletion, or by mutations in the

EHMT1 gene, which is involved in histone methylation. Affected individuals invariably have severe hypotonia, with speech and gross motor delay. Facial features include micro-/brachycephaly, hypertelorism, synophrys, arched eyebrows, midface hypoplasia, short nose with upturned nares, protruding tongue, everted lower lip, and downturned corners of the mouth. Congenital heart defects have been reported in approximately 50 percent of affected individuals. Epilepsy and behavior and sleep disturbances have also been reported in some (10–20 percent) [Kleefstra et al., 2009].

Langer–Giedion Syndrome

Patients with the Langer–Giedion syndrome (LGS), also called tricho-rhino-phalangeal syndrome type II (TRPSII), have a de novo deletion on chromosome 8 at band q24.11, comprising a contiguous deletion of the *TPRS* and *EXT1* genes [Shanske et al., 2008]. The syndrome is characterized by short stature, sparse scalp hair, long nose with a bulbous tip, notched alae nasi, long, flat philtrum, thin lips, cone-shaped epiphyses, and multiple cartilaginous exostoses.

WAGR 11p13 Deletion Syndrome

The cardinal features of the WAGR 11p13 deletion syndrome include Wilms tumor, aniridia, genitourinary abnormalities, and growth and mental retardation. The size of the deletion varies but always includes *WT1* and *PAX6* genes, which accounts for the oncogenic, ocular, and genitourinary features, respectively. Approximately 30 percent of infants with sporadic aniridia will be positive for the characteristic deletion [Robinson et al., 2008]. The majority of patients have MR, and more than 20 percent of patients also have features of autism [Xu et al., 2008].

Jacobsen's Syndrome

Jacobsen's syndrome is a contiguous gene deletion syndrome caused by partial deletion of the long arm of chromosome 11 (11q23.3qter). Typical features include DD, MR, short stature, congenital heart defects, thrombocytopenia, and characteristic dysmorphic facial features. Malformation of heart, kidney, gastrointestinal tract, central nervous system, and skeleton is common. Some of the facial dysmorphism described includes skull deformities, hypertelorism, epicanthic folds, ptosis, broad nasal bridge, and small ears. The deletion is de novo in 85 percent of cases, and in the remaining patients it results from the unbalanced segregation of a parental balanced chromosome rearrangement [Mattina et al., 2009].

Charcot–Marie–Tooth Neuropathy Type 1A and Hereditary Neuropathy with Liability to Pressure Palsies

Charcot–Marie–Tooth neuropathy type 1A (CMT1A) represents 70–80 percent of all CMT1 and results from an approximately 1.5-Mb duplication at 17p11.2, which encompasses the *PMP22* gene (peripheral myelin protein 22) [Szigeti et al., 2006]. This protein is predominantly produced by Schwann cells and is a major component of the peripheral nervous system. Reciprocal deletion of the same region results in the milder phenotype of hereditary neuropathy with liability to pressure palsies (HNPP). The duplication is inherited in around two-thirds of individuals and is de novo in the remaining third. Please see Chapter 89 for more details.

Smith–Magenis Syndrome and Potocki–Lupski Syndrome

Approximately 90 percent of individuals with the Smith–Magenis syndrome (SMS) have a deletion on chromosome 17 at band p11.2 that encompasses the *RAI1* gene. The remaining 5–10 percent of cases carry a mutation in the *RAI1* gene. Physical features include short stature, obesity, craniofacial dysmorphism, and small hands and feet. Behavior disturbances, especially sleep problems and self-injurious behavior, are frequently reported. The self-injurious behavior includes self-hitting, self-biting and/or skin picking, inserting foreign objects in body orifices (polyembolokoilamania), and pulling nails (onchotillomania). Self-hug or spasmodic upper-body squeeze, hand licking, and page flipping ("lick and flip") constitute stereotypic behavior that appears to be specific for SMS. All the affected individuals have mild to severe learning disabilities [Elsea and Girirajan, 2008]. The phenotypic features may be subtle in infancy and early childhood. The facial appearance is characterized by a broad, square-shaped face, brachycephaly, prominent forehead, synophrys, mildly upslanting palpebral fissures, deep-set eyes, broad nasal bridge, midfacial hypoplasia, short, full-tipped nose, flat nasal bridge, micrognathia in infancy changing to relative prognathia with age, and fleshy, everted upper lip. With progressing age, the facial appearance becomes more distinctive and coarse.

The reciprocal duplication of this 17p11.2 region has been reported (Potocki–Lupski syndrome). The most frequent features of this syndrome are hypotonia in infancy, DD, language and cognitive impairment, autistic features, poor feeding and failure to thrive in infancy, oral-pharyngeal dysphagia, obstructive and central sleep apnea, structural cardiovascular abnormalities, EEG abnormalities, and hypermetropia. Most have short stature and mild to normal facies [Potocki et al., 2007]. Variability in the phenotype is observed. It is expected that persons with large duplications that encompass the more distal CMT1A region will have a more severe phenotype, including peripheral neuropathy.

Miller–Dieker Syndrome

Miller–Dieker syndrome represents a microdeletion syndrome spanning the *LIS1* gene at 17p13.3, which results in severe lissencephaly with characteristic facial changes, other more variable malformations, and severe neurologic and developmental abnormalities. The facial features consist of high and prominent forehead, bitemporal hollowing, short nose with upturned nares, protuberant upper lip with downturned vermillion border, and small jaw [Cardoso et al., 2002]. The reciprocal duplication results in DD, hypotonia, and facial dysmorphism. In contrast to the patients with the deletion, those with the duplication have neither gross brain malformations nor lissencephaly [Roos et al., 2009].

Neurofibromatosis Type 1

Approximately 5 percent of patients with neurofibromatosis type 1 (NF1) have deletions of the entire *NF1* gene and contiguous genes at 17q11.2, resulting in the NF1 microdeletion syndrome. NF1 with large deletions is more likely to have dysmorphic features, cardiac anomalies, connective tissue dysplasia, and MR [Mensink et al., 2006]. Patients with reciprocal microduplications have been reported.

Alagille's Syndrome

Alagille's syndrome (AGS) is a complex multisystem disorder involving primarily the liver, heart, eyes, face, and skeleton. The clinical features are highly variable, even within families. The major clinical manifestations of AGS are cholestasis, congenital cardiac defects, posterior embryotoxon in the eye, typical facial features, and butterfly vertebrae. Renal and central nervous abnormalities also occur. The two genes associated with AGS are *JAG1* and *NOTCH2* [Krantz et al., 1999; McDaniell et al., 2006]. Sequence analysis of *JAG1* detects mutations in over 88 percent of individuals who meet clinical diagnostic criteria, whereas FISH and/or array CGH analyses detect a microdeletion encompassing *JAG1* at 20p12.2 in approximately 7 percent of affected individuals.

Potocki–Shaffer Syndrome

Potocki–Shaffer syndrome (PSS) is a contiguous gene deletion syndrome that results from a deletion of the 11p11.2p12 region [Wu et al., 2000]. The clinical features can include DD, MR, multiple exostoses, parietal foramina, enlarged anterior fontanel, minor craniofacial anomalies, ophthalmologic anomalies, and genital anomalies in males. Parietal foramina and multiple exostoses are the primary characteristic of this syndrome. Larger deletions of proximal 11p may result in features of PSS and WAGR.

X-Linked Ichthyosis Due to Steroid Sulphatase Enzyme Deficiency

Males with X-linked ichthyosis due to steroid sulphatase enzyme deficiency have generalized scaling that usually starts shortly after birth. In 90 percent of cases, it is caused by a microdeletion encompassing the *STS* gene (Xp22.31). In 5 percent of cases, the deletion is extensive enough to involve adjacent genes, resulting in learning disabilities, autism, and epilepsy in some of the affected boys [Gohlke et al., 2000].

Loss of Function of the MECP2 Gene/ Duplication of the MECP2 Region (Xq28)

Loss of function of the *MECP2* gene results in Rett's syndrome in females, and both syndromic and nonsyndromic forms of MR in males. Duplication of the *MECP2* region (Xq28) in males is associated with severe MR and progressive spasticity. This duplication spans the *L1CAM* and *MECP2* genes [Van Esch et al., 2005].

Autistic Spectrum Disorders

About 5–10 percent of patients with ASDs are associated with chromosomal abnormalities or monogenic disorders [Folstein and Rosen-Sheidley, 2001; Jacquemont et al., 2006]. They are also the most frequently identified cause of DD and/or MR, and are often seen in conjunction with growth retardation, dysmorphic features, and various congenital anomalies [Aradhya et al., 2007]. According to Fernandez et al., ASDs are etiologically heterogeneous [Fernandez et al., 2009]. About 10 percent are associated with a mendelian syndrome. Another 5–7 percent are associated with the maternal 15q11.2q13.1 duplication. Teratogens have also been implicated. The remainder of affected individuals are presumed to have multifactorial forms of ASD. More recently, de novo CNVs have been observed in 7–10 percent of sporadic ASD, and in 2–3 percent of affected individuals from multiplex families. The most frequent are 15q11.2q13.1 duplication, and 2q37 and 22q13.3 deletions [Folstein and Rosen-Sheidley, 2001]. The following are some of the recently reported genomic disorders described as clinically significant CNVs sometimes associated with ASDs.

MATERNAL DUPLICATION OF THE 15q11.2q13.1 REGION

Chromosome 15q11.2q13.1 contains a cluster of imprinted genes essential for normal development. Deficiencies in paternal or maternal 15q11.2q13.1 result in PWS or AS, respectively, as previously discussed. Maternal duplication of the 15q11.2q13.1 region leads to a distinct condition that often includes autism. Despite incomplete penetrance of autism in this syndrome, this duplication is the leading cytogenetic cause of autism [Hogart et al., 2009]. Recently, the 15q11.2q13.1 duplication has been associated with a distinct pattern of mitochondrial abnormalities that include a deficiency of complex III [Frye, 2009].

15q13.3 MICRODELETION

Manifestations of the 15q13.3 microdeletion include idiopathic generalized epilepsy, autism, intellectual disability, and schizophrenia. The condition has highly variable intra- and interfamilial phenotypic heterogeneity, with some carriers having no clinical manifestations [Mulley and Dibbens, 2009]. Cardiac defects have also been reported. Patients with the reciprocal duplication do not share a recognizable phenotype [van Bon et al., 2009].

15q24 MICRODELETION SYNDROME

The 15q24 microdeletion syndrome has a distinct clinical phenotype with specific facial features, DD, microcephaly, and digital and genital anomalies. Facial features include hypertelorism, strabismus, downslanted palpebral fissures, epicanthic folds, full lower lip, high frontal hairline, broad medial eyebrows, long/smooth philtrum, and palate and ear anomalies. Umbilical and inguinal hernias, genital anomalies in males, and musculoskeletal anomalies have also been reported [Klopocki et al., 2008].

RECURRENT 16p11.2 MICRODELETIONS AND MICRODUPLICATIONS

Recurrent 16p11.2 microdeletions and microduplications appear to be associated with approximately 1 percent of unexplained, idiopathic, and nonsyndromic autism [Weiss et al., 2008]. The phenotypic spectrum probably also includes MR, DD, variable nonspecific dysmorphism, and/or possibly other primary psychiatric disorders.

16p11.2p12.2 MICRODELETION

The 16p11.2p12.2 microdeletion should be distinguished from the 16p11.2 microdeletion. All reported patients with the 16p11.2p12.2 microdeletion have shared a common distal breakpoint at 16p12.2, but the proximal breakpoint varies [Ballif et al., 2007; Hempel et al., 2009]. Common features of this microdeletion syndrome include facial dysmorphism, orofacial clefting, heart defects, frequent ear infections, short stature, feeding difficulties, hypotonia, and DD. The facial features include flat face, deep and low-set eyes, and posteriorly rotated ears.

DELETIONS AND RECIPROCAL DUPLICATIONS OF THE CHROMOSOME 16p13.11 REGION

Deletions and reciprocal duplications of the chromosome 16p13.11 region have recently been reported in several cases of autism and MR. Current clinical data indicate that deletions that are either de novo or inherited from clinically normal parents are likely to be pathogenic, whereas the clinical significance of the duplications is still uncertain [Hannes et al., 2009].

22q13 MICRODELETION SYNDROME (PHELAN–MCDERMID SYNDROME)

The 22q13 microdeletion syndrome (Phelan–McDermid syndrome) is a chromosome microdeletion characterized by neonatal hypotonia, global DD, normal to accelerated growth, absent to severely delayed speech, and dysmorphic features [Phelan, 2008]. Reported features include dolicocephaly, long eyelashes, large or unusual ears, large hands, dysplastic toe nails, full cheeks, bulbous nose, and pointed chin. Behavior tends to be autistic-like.

17q21.31 MICRODELETION SYNDROME

17q21.31 is a new microdeletion syndrome with recognizable clinical phenotype of MR, hypotonia, and characteristic facies, including long hypotonic face, tubular nose with bulbous nasal tip, large low-set ears, and blepharophimosis. The prevalence of this new syndrome has been estimated to be between 1 in 13,000 and 1 in 20,000. The reciprocal microduplication appears to have unspecific features, such as hypotonia and feeding difficulties in the newborn period [Sharp et al., 2006; Kirchhoff et al., 2007].

INTERSTITIAL MICRODELETION AT 2p15p16.1

The clinical phenotype of the interstitial microdeletion at 2p15p16.1 includes moderate to severe intellectual disability, autistic features, poor motor and speech development, microcephaly, structural brain anomalies, renal anomalies, digital anomalies, vision impairment, and a distinctive pattern of craniofacial features. The reported structural brain anomalies include cortical dysplasia/pachygyria. Dysmorphic craniofacial features include microcephaly, bitemporal narrowing, wide inner canthal distance, short downslanted palpebral fissures, epicanthic folds, prominent nasal tip, long straight eyelashes, smooth philtrum, and everted lower lip [Rajcan-Separovic et al., 2007].

TERMINAL DELETIONS OF THE LONG ARM OF CHROMOSOME 2 (2q37)

Terminal deletions of the long arm of chromosome 2 (2q37) have a recognizable clinical phenotype, including MR (mild to severe), seizure disorder, autistic features, a recognizable pattern of dysmorphism, major malformations, and a pattern of findings described as Albright hereditary osteodystrophy-like (AHO) metacarpal/metatarsal shortening phenotype. Other phenotypes associated with 2q37 deletions include Wilms tumor and urogenital anomalies, epilepsy, and eczema [Falk and Casas, 2007].

7q11.23 MICRODUPLICATION

The 7q11.23 microduplication is the exact reciprocal of the common WBS deletion with an estimated incidence of 1:13,000 to 1:20,000. The main clinical feature is variable speech/language delay with cognitive disabilities ranging from normal to moderate MR. Autism has been reported in some patients. Specific dysmorphic features noted include high and broad nose, short philtrum, thin lips and straight eyebrows. Triplications of this region have a similar phenotype but are more severe than observed in patients with the duplication of the same region [Depienne et al., 2007].

The Future of Clinical Cytogenetics

Clinical cytogenetics began with the cytological analysis of chromosomes in the 1950s, but has steadily moved towards an increasingly molecular approach. This began with the advent of FISH, and has accelerated since the introduction of array CGH. In the cytological era, chromosomal analysis could be viewed as a crude form of whole-genome analysis. It was not necessary to have a preconceived notion of where in the genome to look, since any rearrangement large enough to be evident with the light microscope could be seen. Nonetheless, the resolution was very limited. FISH analysis increased the resolution, but it was necessary to specify in advance the areas of interest, since it was not practical to explore all possible deletions or duplications, given that each required use of a different DNA probe. Array CGH is moving us back towards a whole-genome approach with no need to know in advance where to look. This is raising questions about whether array CGH should be used prior to a comprehensive dysmorphology evaluation, since many of the deletions or duplications detected are not associated with well-delineated syndromes. A caution in use of this approach, however, is that some gene-dosage changes are not known to be associated with an abnormal phenotype and are likely to be benign variants of no clinical significance. Therefore, correct interpretation of dosage changes still requires a high level of sophistication and care in counseling the patient/family. It is likely that the resolution of genomic analysis will continue to increase, converging ultimately with DNA sequence analysis, which is also rapidly increasing in power. This will undoubtedly reveal an increasing number of genomic changes that underlie neurological disorders, increasing the power and precision of genetic diagnosis.

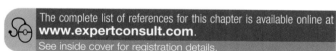
The complete list of references for this chapter is available online at **www.expertconsult.com**. See inside cover for registration details.

Aminoacidemias and Organic Acidemias

Gregory M. Enns, Tina M. Cowan, Ophir Klein, and Seymour Packman

Approximately 4 percent of individuals born in the United States have a genetic or partly genetic disorder. Inborn errors of metabolism contribute significantly to this total. Although individually rare, the aggregate incidence of metabolic disease is relatively high and may be greater than 1 in 1000 newborns. Newborn screening programs using tandem mass spectrometry, which can detect approximately 20 inborn errors of metabolism, typically have reported an incidence of 1 in 2000 to 1 in 4000. Because there are hundreds of known metabolic conditions, the aggregate estimate seems reasonable.

Metabolic diseases infrequently produce symptoms immediately at birth, and they can manifest with slowly progressive encephalopathies. In this setting, histologic or biochemical abnormalities may be present in the fetal central nervous system (CNS) by 4–5 months' gestation. Inborn errors of metabolism also can manifest with rapid clinical deterioration in the newborn period or after an interval period of good health. Presenting clinical features are often nonspecific, and they may be misdiagnosed as infection, cardiovascular compromise, other causes of hypoxemia, trauma, primary brain anomalies, or the effects of a toxin. Recognition of patterns of clinical presentation and rapid implementation of laboratory investigations are essential for the initiation of appropriate therapy without delay. Unless appropriate therapy is initiated with dispatch, there is a high risk of morbidity or mortality, regardless of the cause of the acute illness.

This chapter provides an overview of concepts of diagnosis and treatment for two categories of inborn errors: aminoacidopathies and organic acidemias. The general approaches described are broadly applicable to other heritable metabolic disorders, such as disorders of fatty acid oxidation, urea cycle disorders, and lactic acidosis syndromes. Descriptions of selected disorders of amino acid and organic acid metabolism are provided to illustrate and emphasize the approaches to diagnosis, treatment, and genetic counseling in this area of genetic medicine.

Signs and Symptoms

Any infant, child, or adult who presents with neurodevelopmental delays, lethargy, feeding difficulties, vomiting, jaundice, failure to thrive, apnea or tachypnea, hypotonia or hypertonia, ataxia, movement disorders, seizures, or coma should be considered to suffer from diseases in one of two broad categories: disorders resulting from causes such as infection, cardiopulmonary dysfunction, other causes of hypoxemia, toxins, or trauma, or from primary brain abnormalities or disorders caused by an inborn error of metabolism. Because metabolic diseases are individually rare, there is a tendency to consider them only after excluding more common causes of acute or chronic illness or distress. However, the clinician must consider the possibility of an inborn error on initial presentation. In many cases, only rapid diagnosis and management can prevent death or significant morbidity. Appropriate laboratory investigations should be obtained immediately. Even conventional clinical laboratory tests, such as those for blood gases, blood glucose, electrolytes, lactate, ammonia, liver function, hematologic counts and indices, and urinalysis (including pH, ketones, mellituria, and concentration) may provide valuable clues to the underlying diagnosis.

The onset of symptoms of metabolic disease is generally postnatal, often appearing after an interval of apparent good health. This interval may be as short as a few hours or may last several days to years. An affected individual may fare well until subjected to a catabolic insult (e.g., infection, fasting, dehydration) or an excessive protein or carbohydrate load, after which the infant, child, or adult may suddenly become strikingly ill. In a neonate, the absence of a normal period of apparent good health does not exclude an inborn error from diagnostic consideration. Neonatal distress from asphyxia or pregnancy complications may be the environmental stress that unmasks an underlying metabolic disease.

Irritability and feeding difficulties may be associated with uncoordinated sucking or swallowing or with abnormal muscle tone. Persistent and severe vomiting and seizures may occur. In mildly affected patients, symptoms can disappear, only to recur in days or weeks. More severely affected infants and children have inexorable progression from lethargy to coma, episodic apnea, and death.

More limited symptoms, often in the form of generalized or partial seizures, may occur in some instances. These can include staring spells, eye rolling or myoclonus, and various combinations of tone abnormalities, tremulousness, lethargy, and a weak cry. The electroencephalogram (EEG) may suggest nonspecific, diffuse encephalopathy. Unless an inborn error is suspected, the child may be misdiagnosed as having hypoxic-ischemic encephalopathy, intraventricular hemorrhage, sepsis, heart failure, or gastrointestinal illness (e.g., pyloric stenosis, intestinal obstruction).

Physical Findings

A paucity of abnormal physical findings is the general rule in heritable metabolic diseases. Nevertheless, certain components of the physical examination should be emphasized. A detailed ocular examination is essential. Corneal clouding, cataracts, optic nerve abnormalities, and macular or retinal pigmentary changes may be helpful in establishing a diagnosis. Hepatomegaly can occur with organic acidemias that may have a Reye's syndrome-like presentation. Alopecia, abnormal hair, or nonspecific eczematoid dermatitis may be seen in some aminoacidopathies and organic acidemias. An unusual odor to the child's body or urine has been associated with several organic acidemias and disorders of amino acid metabolism. Ketosis accompanies many of these conditions, and ketone bodies in the urine cause its sweet odor. Although dysmorphic features suggest the diagnosis of a congenital developmental disorder rather than a heritable metabolic disorder, craniofacial and structural abnormalities of organ systems are being recognized in an increasing number of inborn errors of intermediary metabolism.

Laboratory Approaches to Diagnosis

Because the clinical presentation of patients with metabolic disorders is often nonspecific and suggests a wide variety of conditions, a rational and systematic laboratory approach is imperative for rapid and accurate diagnosis to implement early and appropriate treatment. It is rarely possible to base a precise diagnosis on clinical findings or results of routine laboratory tests.

Laboratory testing for the symptomatic patient can proceed at many levels, including metabolic screening tests, quantitative metabolite profiles, specific enzyme or other functional assays, and DNA mutation analysis. The specific laboratory approach is often dictated by the clinical and family history and by results of routine laboratory investigations. An extensive description of diagnostic algorithms for the laboratory evaluation of patients suspected of having a metabolic disease has been published [Saudubray and Charpentier, 2001].

For the acutely ill patient, a comprehensive evaluation should include quantitative assessment of plasma amino acids, urine organic acid analyses, plasma carnitine (free and total) levels, and identification and quantitation of acylcarnitines in plasma or serum. These tests should be ordered in conjunction with other basic tests, including hematologic cell counts, electrolytes, blood glucose, blood gases, uric acid, liver transaminases, ammonia, and lactic and pyruvic acid levels. This approach can identify many cases of amino acid disorders and organic acidemias. The interpretation of metabolic tests is greatly enhanced when the laboratory is made aware of the clinical, medication, and dietary history of the patient because these factors can significantly influence results. Depending on the clinical evaluation and results of basic chemistry studies, additional testing may be warranted; this may include levels of urine orotic acid (e.g., elevated in certain urea cycle defects) (see Chapter 33), cerebrospinal fluid glycine (together with the plasma glycine level, which is elevated in glycine encephalopathy), cerebrospinal fluid neurotransmitters (see Chapter 39), and urine S-sulfocysteine (elevated in sulfite oxidase deficiency or molybdenum co-factor deficiency).

Laboratory investigations are most useful when samples are collected during an acute episode, because metabolic abnormalities are most pronounced at that time. However, subtle abnormalities can often be appreciated even between episodes, particularly if the laboratory is made aware of the clinical evaluation at the time of testing. However, normal results, particularly if obtained when the patient is well, do not exclude a metabolic disorder and should be followed by repeat testing of specimens obtained during an acute illness if possible.

Metabolic screening tests in urine can be useful in certain situations, particularly in the assessment of older patients with a nonspecific history of developmental delay or mental retardation. Such testing includes qualitative amino acid screening by thin-layer chromatography or paper chromatography, the ferric chloride test for phenylketones (for identification of phenylketonuria and tyrosinemia), the cyanide-nitroprusside test for sulfur-containing amino acids (for identification of homocystinuria), and other colorimetric or flocculation tests. When taken in conjunction with clinical and other laboratory finding, these tests can give an inexpensive and rapid indication of an abnormality, and they can be useful in determining the direction of more specific testing. These tests are not appropriate in the evaluation of an acutely ill patient, for whom specific, quantitative metabolic studies are essential.

Depending on the results of initial metabolic studies, confirmation of the diagnosis or delineation of specific disease subtypes may be established by specific enzyme assays. If the expression of enzyme activity is tissue-specific, a biopsy (e.g., skin, muscle, liver) may be required. After a precise biochemical diagnosis has been established, molecular studies for the specific gene mutation may be possible. In many cases, delineation of the specific mutations can provide important prognostic information and can be used in the testing of other family members and in prenatal diagnosis.

Treatment

For all inborn errors, acute symptoms must be treated immediately, regardless of the cause, and often before the results of screening and specialized laboratory tests become available. The success of treatment is a function of time; the longer the neurologic derangements persist before treatment, the poorer the prognosis. Because acidosis (or alkalosis) is observed in these disorders, acid–base status must be corrected immediately, along with necessary adjustments in electrolyte balance and hydration. Glucose infusions should be used as a source of calories and to control hypoglycemia, if present. Hemodialysis can improve a number of disorders of amino acid and organic acid metabolism, and it should be instituted if the evidence suggests such a disorder.

Selective avoidance of a particular nutrient or class of nutrients is specific and crucial. This generally means avoidance of one or more specific micronutrients that can accumulate proximal to the metabolic block. Protein should be avoided in the acute phase of treatment of any child presenting with neurologic dysfunction; continuation of dietary protein in a child with an aminoacidopathy or organic acidemia can be lethal. The response to protein avoidance may be of diagnostic help. When specific nutritional restrictions are instituted for a known or suspected inborn error, attention must be paid to adequate total caloric intake – by parenteral or oral administration – to prevent catabolism and to avoid iatrogenic nutritional deficiencies.

Specific supplements may be invaluable as treatment adjuncts under the general strategy designed to remove toxic metabolites by alternative or minor pathways. In selected disorders, glycine supplementation promotes the formation of rapidly excreted and nontoxic acylglycine conjugates. Carnitine administration favors the formation and excretion of acetylcarnitine and other acylcarnitines, thereby ameliorating ketosis and the accumulation of toxic organic acid metabolites in organic acidemias. A number of inborn errors respond favorably and, in some instances, dramatically to the administration of vitamins, which stabilize or otherwise increase the catalytic activity of incompletely defective enzymes. Vitamins such as cobalamin (B_{12}), pyridoxine, thiamine, biotin, riboflavin, lipoate, folate, and niacin, administered in pharmacologic doses, may be lifesaving. In a child who is gravely ill and whose course has been one of inexorable decline, it is appropriate to administer a battery of rationally chosen co-factors and supplements in the hope that the child's biochemical lesion will respond to one of the pharmacologic agents.

Inheritance and Genetic Counseling

Treatment of heritable metabolic disorders involves considerations beyond the acute phase of the illness and even beyond the prognosis of the proband. Because of the importance of genetic counseling to the family, the physician has an obligation to try to arrive at a diagnosis, however poor the prognosis for the proband. Identifying a specific entity enables the family to be counseled about recurrence risks. Most inborn errors of metabolism are inherited as autosomal-recessive traits. There are a few disorders, such as the urea cycle defect of ornithine transcarbamylase deficiency, that are inherited as X-linked disorders. In the case of an autosomal-recessive condition, the affected relative is a sibling of either gender. In X-linked disorders, the affected relative may be a maternal uncle, a brother, or a mildly affected mother or other female relative. Some disorders are caused by mitochondrial DNA mutations (see Chapter 37), and maternal transmission to all children in a sibship is observed. In all circumstances, a detailed family history may reveal an affected relative who has a similar illness, and this can be of diagnostic importance. Special attention should be given to a family history of stillbirths, unexplained deaths, and neurologic diseases or delayed development of any degree or severity.

The therapeutic repertory for inborn errors is expanding beyond nutritional manipulations and restrictions of micronutrient precursors proximal to a metabolic block. Modalities being used or clinically investigated include co-factors as pharmacologic agents in vitamin-responsive inborn errors; enzyme inhibitors to prevent the synthesis of a toxic metabolite; enzyme-stabilizing agents; organ transplantation (e.g., liver, bone marrow); enzyme replacement therapy; and gene therapy. Such therapies may be intrusive and expensive. Genetic counseling for inborn errors must include a discussion of recurrence risk and address issues related to therapeutic options, prognosis, prenatal management, and the emotional, psychologic, and financial burdens of the birth and long-term treatment of children with such chronic disorders. Many of the inborn errors discussed in this chapter and elsewhere can be diagnosed prenatally, giving

families a number of reproductive options. The successful prenatal treatment of co-factor-responsive disorders and the expanding repertory of other novel postnatal treatment approaches augur an increasing focus on unique therapeutic opportunities in inborn errors.

Aminoacidemias

Phenylketonuria

Phenylketonuria, described by Asbørn Følling in 1934 [Følling, 1994], is caused by deficient activity of phenylalanine hydroxylase (PAH), a hepatic enzyme that converts phenylalanine to tyrosine (Figure 32-1). The biochemical block results in the accumulation of phenylalanine, which is then converted to phenylpyruvic acid and phenyllactic acid, phenylketones that are excreted in the urine. Tetrahydrobiopterin is a necessary co-factor in the PAH reaction, and elevated phenylalanine levels rarely may be caused by inherited disorders of tetrahydrobiopterin synthesis, including guanosine triphosphate (GTP) cyclohydrolase I, 6-pyruvoyltetrahydrobiopterin synthase, pterin-4α-carbinolamine dehydratase, and dihydropteridine reductase deficiencies (see Figure 32-1). Phenylalanine is neurotoxic, and untreated patients with classic phenylketonuria are typically mentally retarded. In the 1950s, a diet in which phenylalanine intake was restricted was shown to normalize plasma phenylalanine levels and stop urinary excretion of phenylpyruvic acid [Bickel et al., 1953]. Selective restriction of phenylalanine intake by using phenylalanine-free medical formulas and foods (and tyrosine supplementation), which provides enough additional protein and nutrients to support normal growth, remains the mainstay of phenylketonuria therapy.

Mandatory population newborn screening for phenylketonuria, in combination with postnatal presymptomatic therapy, was begun in the 1960s using the Guthrie bacterial inhibition assay [Guthrie and Susi, 1963; Koch, 1997]. Modern newborn screening programs have switched to techniques that directly assay phenylalanine and tyrosine levels; the most recent innovation is tandem mass spectrometry. The presymptomatic institution of and continued adherence to specific dietary therapy prevents mental retardation. Phenylketonuria is a paradigmatic and landmark success story in biochemical genetics, and it is reviewed in some detail.

Classification

A blood phenylalanine level above the normal range (30–110 μM) is referred to as hyperphenylalaninemia. Patients have been classified as having nonphenylketonuria hyperphenylalaninemia if their blood phenylalanine levels without dietary therapy are 360–600 μM. Classic phenylketonuria is characterized by untreated phenylalanine levels of more than 1000 μM [Scriver and Kaufman, 2001]. A range of reduced PAH-specific activity correlates broadly with the severity of the phenotype. When it has been measured directly (i.e., liver biopsy) or indirectly (i.e., L-[1-^{13}C]phenylalanine breath test), residual liver PAH-specific activity is relatively high in milder hyperphenylalaninemic patients, whereas enzyme activity is zero to low in the more severe cases of classic phenylketonuria [Bartholome et al., 1975]. Measured PAH activity also correlates to some degree with tolerance for dietary protein [Güttler et al., 1996]. Patients with classic phenylketonuria can tolerate very little

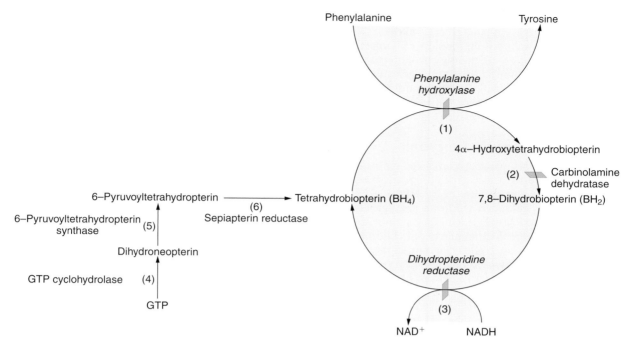

Fig. 32-1 Regulation of phenylalanine hydroxylase activity. Phenylalanine is converted to tyrosine (1) by the holoenzyme phenylalanine hydroxylase (PAH). PAH requires tetrahydrobiopterin (BH₄) as an active co-factor, and is recycled by the sequential actions of carbinolamine dehydratase (2) and dihydropteridine reductase (3). BH₄ is synthesized in vivo through a complex series of steps that involve guanosine triphosphate (GTP) cyclohydrolase (4), 6-pyruvoyltetrahydropterin synthase (5), and sepiapterin reductase (6). Genetic defects at any of these steps may be associated with hyperphenylalaninemia. *(From Wilcox WR, Cederbaum SD. Amino acid metabolism. In: Rimoin D, Connor J, Pyeritz R, Korf B, eds. Principles and practice of medical genetics, 4th edn. Philadelphia: Churchill Livingstone, 2002:2406.)*

phenylalanine in the diet (<500 mg/day). The classification of phenylketonuria into subtypes based on blood phenylalanine levels is arbitrary, and some patients (i.e., mild, variant, or atypical phenylketonuria) fall between the two extreme biochemical phenotypes. Because environmental (phenylalanine intake) and genetic (modifier genes) factors alter the biochemical and neurodevelopmental phenotypes in this single-gene disorder, phenylketonuria in many ways behaves more like a complex trait than a monogenic disorder [Kayaalp et al., 1997].

Clinical Manifestations

Profound mental retardation is the most significant clinical finding in untreated or poorly treated phenylketonuria. Acute metabolic encephalopathy, a common feature of many inborn errors of metabolism, does not occur in phenylketonuria. Children with phenylketonuria appear normal at birth and have normal early development, even if untreated. Neurologic manifestations appear insidiously and include reduced rate of growth of head circumference, developmental delay, abnormalities in muscle tone, and hyperactive deep tendon reflexes. Affected children may have lighter pigmentation than other family members (i.e., reduced melanin synthesis) and a musty odor attributed to phenylacetic acid. Eczema and decreased bone mineral density may occur [Zeman et al., 1999]. Patients exposed to chronically elevated phenylalanine levels ultimately develop microcephaly, seizures (e.g., tonic-clonic, myoclonic, infantile spasms), tremors, athetosis, and spasticity, and they may be misdiagnosed as having cerebral palsy. Psychiatric and behavior problems, including autistic behavior and

attention-deficit hyperactivity disorder, are common [Pietz et al., 1997; Smith and Knowles, 2000].

Brain magnetic resonance imaging (MRI) may detect dysmyelination, especially T2 enhancement in the periventricular white matter, a finding that is potentially reversible with the initiation of dietary therapy [Cleary et al., 1995]. Abnormal areas of white matter demonstrate restricted diffusion of water, possibly indicating increased myelin turnover [Phillips et al., 2001].

In the past, most untreated phenylketonuria patients were institutionalized, and many born before universal newborn screening remain so. An eloquent and inspiring description of the life of a child with untreated phenylketonuria is given in a short monograph by Pearl S. Buck [Buck, 1950].

As a rule, well-treated classic phenylketonuria patients have normal IQs. However, recent studies have found that children and adults with phenylketonuria may experience cognitive symptoms, such as problems in executive functioning, as well as disturbance in emotional and behavioral functioning despite early and continuous treatment [Enns et al., 2010]. Dietary control of the blood phenylalanine level appears to be the best predictor of ultimate IQ [Waisbren et al., 1987], but careful psychometric testing of well-treated individuals has detected instances and degrees of impairment in visual-motor skills, abstract reasoning, problem solving, specific aspects of executive control, attention, verbal memory, expressive naming, and verbal fluency [Fishler et al., 1987]. Such neuropsychologic impairments may be a consequence of mid-dorsolateral prefrontal cortex dysfunction caused by abnormal catecholamine levels [Huijbregts et al., 2002]. Abnormal EEG patterns, including general slowing and generalized paroxysmal activity with or without spikes, may be demonstrated for children with phenyl-ketonuria, even if they are well treated [Pietz et al., 1988]. Emotional disorders (e.g., depression, anxiety, phobias) and hyperactive behavior are more frequently encountered in persons with classic phenylketonuria than in the general population [Smith and Knowles, 2000]. However, untreated mild hyperphenylalaninemic patients are not at risk for developing neuropsychologic impairment [Weglage et al., 1996].

Maternal Phenylketonuria Syndrome

Elevated maternal blood phenylalanine levels can cross the placenta and cause fetal birth defects, including microcephaly, dysmorphic features, and congenital heart defects. Children with the maternal phenylketonuria syndrome are typically heterozygous for the mutant PAH allele, and they are not affected with phenylketonuria. More than 90 percent of children born to women with untreated classic phenylketonuria have mental retardation; 70 percent have microcephaly, 40 percent have intrauterine growth retardation, and 12 percent have congenital heart disease [Lenke and Levy, 1980]. The risk to the fetus is greatest with increasing phenylalanine levels in maternal blood. Dietary control should ideally be achieved before 3 months prior to conception, and mothers with phenylketonuria should be monitored carefully by an experienced center throughout pregnancy [ACOG, 2009]. Optimal birth outcomes occur when blood phenylalanine levels between 120 and 360 μM are achieved by 8–10 weeks' gestation [Widaman and Azen, 2003]. Mothers with phenylketonuria can safely breastfeed their children.

Diagnosis

The Guthrie bacterial inhibition assay was a technical breakthrough, allowing newborn screening of large populations. The growth inhibition of *Bacillus subtilis* by β-2-thienylalanine is prevented by phenylalanine, phenylpyruvic acid, and phenyllactic acid, and this forms the basis of the Guthrie test. Fluorometric assays or tandem mass spectrometry is used in screening and monitoring [Chace et al., 1993]. False-positive results may be seen in neonates with low birth weight or liver disease, or in infants on parenteral alimentation. False-negative results may occur if the newborn screen is performed too early (especially less than 12 hours after birth) [Hanley et al., 1997]. Confirmation of the diagnosis is made by analysis of blood phenylalanine and tyrosine concentrations by means of high-performance liquid chromatography, fluorescent methods, or tandem mass spectrometry. Without the introduction of a phenylalanine-restricted diet, maximal elevation in plasma phenylalanine is typically reached within or soon after the first week of life in patients with classic phenylketonuria. Urine phenylpyruvic acid causes the appearance of a deep green color when ferric chloride is added. This ferric chloride test is sometimes performed as part of a metabolic screening panel for the evaluation of patients suspected of having an inborn error of metabolism, but it should not be used to confirm a diagnosis of phenylketonuria because of a lack of sensitivity and specificity. All patients with confirmed hyperphenylalaninemia must have urine pterins analyzed for defects in tetrahydrobiopterin metabolism. Phenylketonuria may be suspected in a child or adult and should reasonably be included in the differential diagnosis of a given patient of any age presenting with neurodevelopmental delay of unknown origin. In such settings, diagnostic testing for phenylketonuria (i.e., serum phenylalanine levels) must be done, even if there is a history or a record of a normal newborn screen.

Genetics

Phenylketonuria is an autosomal-recessive disorder with an incidence of 1 case per 10,000 people in the general white population of northern European ancestry [Eisensmith and Woo, 1994]. Phenylketonuria is more common in Turkey, Scotland, and Czechoslovakia, and among Arabic populations and Yemenite Jews (1 case per 2500–5000 persons). It is relatively uncommon in Japan and Finland, and among African Americans (1 case per 100,000–200,000 persons) [Scriver and Kaufman, 2001]. Nonphenylketonuria hyperphenylalaninemia has an overall incidence of 1 case per 50,000 persons.

The *PAH* gene on chromosome 12q24.1 spans 90 kb and contains 13 exons [Kwok et al., 1985]. Almost 500 mutations have been reported throughout all exons and flanking sequences. A detailed account of *PAH* mutant alleles and other DNA variations is maintained at the PAH Mutation Analysis Consortium website (http://www.pahdb.mcgill.ca/) [Waters and Scriver, 1998]. Most DNA alterations are missense mutations, although splice, nonsense, and frameshift mutations and large deletions and insertions have been identified. Most patients are compound heterozygotes, carrying a different mutant allele on each chromosome. Prevalences of specific mutant alleles differ from population to population [Eisensmith and Woo, 1994]. For example, R408W, IVS12nt1, and IVS10nt11 are severe mutations that account for about 50 percent of mutant alleles in Europeans, but they are rare in Asians. Conversely, mutant alleles R243Q, R413P, and Y204C are common in Asians, but they are rare in Europeans [Eisensmith and Woo, 1994].

Pathogenesis

Although PAH is a hepatic enzyme, the major effect of its deficiency is brain dysfunction. Elevated phenylalanine appears to be the cause of neurotoxicity. However, the precise cause of the mental retardation observed in untreated phenylketonuria is not understood. Defective brain myelination may be related to decreased biosynthesis of myelin proteins, because brain protein synthesis is inhibited by excessive phenylalanine [Huether et al., 1982]. CNS effects may be ascribable to more global amino acid imbalances; elevated phenylalanine may affect the CNS concentrations of neutral amino acids by competitive inhibition of a shared amino acid transporter, with relative brain deprivation of tyrosine, tryptophan, and branched-chain amino acids [Huttenlocher, 2000]. Decreased brain tyrosine and tryptophan may lead to decreased neurotransmitter synthesis. The cause of abnormal brain myelination is also unclear. In a phenylketonuria mouse model (i.e., enu2 mouse), there is evidence that oligodendrocytes overexpress glial fibrillary acid protein and become nonmyelinating [Dyer et al., 1996]. Increased myelin turnover has also been observed in the enu2 mouse [Hommes and Moss, 1992]. In phenylketonuria patients studied by positron emission tomography (PET), brain protein synthesis appears to be impaired, which could also affect the myelination process [Paans et al., 1996]. Brain pathology in untreated classic phenylketonuria includes abnormalities in width of the cortical plate, cell density and organization, dendritic arborization and number of synaptic spines, and abnormal myelination [Bauman and Kemper, 1982].

Genotype-Phenotype Correlations

Mutations in the *PAH* gene cause phenylketonuria and non-phenylketonuria hyperphenylalaninemia. However, the final biochemical phenotype (i.e., blood phenylalanine level and dietary phenylalanine tolerance) and clinical phenotype (i.e., IQ) depend on the severity of the mutations, and are influenced by patient adherence to a strict diet, the effects of modifying genetic factors, and other environmental factors. Potential modifier genes may encode proteins mediating interindividual rates of protein synthesis (and phenylalanine use) or basal metabolism; synthesis and degradation of the PAH enzyme protein; gastrointestinal absorption of phenylalanine; hepatic uptake of circulating phenylalanine; metabolism of the tetrahydrobiopterin co-factor; and rate of phenylalanine transport across the blood–brain barrier [Dipple and McCabe, 2000; Treacy et al., 1997]. Because patients – including sibling patients – with identical mutations can have divergent neurodevelopmental progress, mutation identification may not predict the severity of the disease with certainty in a given patient [DiSilvestre et al., 1991; Enns et al., 1999b].

Genes encoding proteins responsible for transport of amino acids across the blood–brain barrier are especially attractive candidates for modifying factors in phenylketonuria. In a study of two siblings with identical genotypes but widely different IQ, in vivo nuclear MR spectroscopy documented lower peak brain phenylalanine levels and more rapid decreases in brain phenylalanine concentration in the less severely affected sibling after a phenylalanine load [Weglage et al., 1998]. Subsequent studies have confirmed the wide interindividual variation of brain to blood phenylalanine concentrations in classic phenylketonuria patients with divergent cognitive phenotypes [Moller et al., 2003].

Despite these considerations, trends can be identified in whole populations. In general, individuals with classic phenylketonuria and poor dietary control have mental retardation, although exceptions exist. If patients with severe mutations are started on strict dietary therapy in the neonatal period and maintained on such treatment throughout life, cognition will be normal. Using in vitro expression analysis in cultured cells transfected with mutant cDNAs, specific mutant alleles (i.e., genotype) can be categorized as severe or mild; such categorization correlates with biochemical or clinical severity (i.e., phenotype) in most patients in relatively homogenous populations. In a study of German and Dutch subjects, the predicted level of PAH activity correlated strongly with neonatal pretreatment levels of blood phenylalanine and dietary phenylalanine tolerance in both populations [Okano et al., 1991]. In relatively homogeneous German, Swedish, and southeastern U.S. populations, similar genotype-phenotype correlations were observed [Eisensmith et al., 1996; Kayaalp et al., 1997; Trefz et al., 1993]. However, when populations with high ethnic diversity are studied in this way, a clear genotype-phenotype correlation may not be apparent [Enns et al., 1999b; Treacy et al., 1997], and the genotype-phenotype correlation is not straightforward in some patients. Although phenylketonuria is a single-gene mendelian disorder, the observed clinical spectrum is more in keeping with a complex multifactorial trait [Scriver and Waters, 1999].

Genetic Counseling

After the diagnosis of phenylketonuria and once the newborn screening process has confirmed the diagnosis, a family is likely to be first seen by the medical care team. The initial emphasis is on the institution of nutritional therapy, the support of the family, and the conveying of information on the broadly favorable prognosis. Genetic counseling in phenylketonuria cases is a continuing process. Understanding on the part of the parents and patients of the nature of the disorder, the genetics of the disorder, and the complexities of the phenotype and prognosis occurs over time during the course of multiple clinic visits. Mutation analysis, with characterization of both parental alleles, is possible, and it may facilitate detection of carrier status in other family members and subsequent prenatal diagnosis. Genotyping may eventually prove valuable in predicting a patient's phenotype, helping to optimize therapy, and aiding determination of long-term prognosis. However, because phenylketonuria behaves in many ways like a complex trait, care is needed when interpreting genotypic data.

In the instance of a child with milder hyperphenylalaninemia or atypical phenylketonuria, recurrence risk counseling must consider the possibility that such mild hyperphenylalaninemia may not be the only outcome in a subsequent homozygous affected child. If one parent is a compound heterozygote for a mild and a severe mutation, but the other parent is a heterozygote for a severe mutation, their child may be born with classic phenylketonuria. Accordingly, after ascertainment of a child with milder hyperphenylalaninemia or atypical phenylketonuria, measuring the blood phenylalanine levels of the parents and characterizing both parents' mutations are important studies to obtain.

Patients who are diagnosed in the neonatal period and who adhere to the phenylalanine-restricted diet have normal intelligence. However, learning problems can occur in well-treated patients and include problems in basic spelling, reading, and mathematical calculation skills. Patients may also be more prone to depression, anxiety, phobic tendencies, and isolation from their peers [Smith and Knowles, 2000; Welsh et al., 1990]. Such potential adverse and unpredictable manifestations should be brought to the attention of parents and carefully explained, with care and support, during the on-going genetic counseling process.

Treatment

Medical nutrition therapy consists of using modified low-phenylalanine and low-protein products, supplemented by a small amount of natural protein to provide required amounts of phenylalanine. After an initial positive newborn screen, a confirmatory determination of blood phenylalanine level must be obtained without delay. Dietary restriction of phenylalanine is begun only after a diagnosis of phenylketonuria has been established or if the initial phenylalanine level is highly elevated in a term infant not being supplemented with total parenteral nutrition as anticipatory management with the advice and collaboration of a metabolic center skilled in the management of phenylketonuria patients. Total elimination of phenylalanine from the diet is not done for longer than 1–2 days, because phenylalanine deficiency leads to tissue catabolism and rebound elevation of blood phenylalanine levels. It is important to screen for the presence of disorders affecting tetrahydrobiopterin metabolism if confirmatory testing corroborates persistent hyperphenylalaninemia. If the low-phenylalanine diet is initiated in the neonatal period (between 7 and 14 days) and maintained throughout life, the underlying biochemical toxicity is ameliorated, and mental retardation is prevented. In the neonatal period, breastfeeding is possible and should be encouraged in any mother who desires to do so. Breast milk contains a lower protein (and lower phenylalanine) concentration than commercial formulas, and it can be used in conjunction with the special phenylketonuria formulas required to provide the infant with appropriate calories, nutrients, and protein for sustained, normal growth.

Significant restriction of dietary phenylalanine is required for treatment, but the exact level of daily phenylalanine intake varies from patient to patient, and varies with age in an individual patient. Because phenylalanine is an essential amino acid, detrimental effects on growth and development may occur if restriction of phenylalanine intake is too severe and the blood level drops to below normal. Although there is no worldwide consensus about optimal plasma phenylalanine levels, most clinics in the United States strive to maintain levels between 120 and 360 μM in children younger than 12 years and between 120 and 600 μM in individuals older than 12 years [Phenylketonuria, 2000]. Phenylalanine levels in unaffected individuals are usually below 120 μM. In general, phenylketonuria patients who harbor severe mutations require a greater limitation of phenylalanine intake to maintain acceptable blood phenylalanine levels. However, individual variations of phenylalanine tolerance may occur, even in patients with identical genotypes. Blood phenylalanine levels therefore are monitored frequently, especially in the first year of life, and the diet is adjusted with care for each individual patient. The regimen must be initiated and overseen by experts in phenylketonuria at a specialized center, and referral of the patient to such a specialized center is mandatory. An expert, coordinated team approach is clearly the most effective way of managing phenylketonuria; stricter management improves developmental outcome [Camfield et al., 2004].

In earlier therapeutic protocols, phenylalanine restriction was continued only through the first few years of life, theoretically corresponding to the age at which brain myelination is complete. As developmental data accumulated, it became evident that treatment throughout childhood and adolescence was the best course to preserve IQ [Smith et al., 1991]. In later studies, it has been found that characteristic periventricular T2 white matter signal abnormalities on conventional MRI, restricted white matter diffusion in diffusion-weighted imaging, and electrophysiologic testing abnormalities referable to the CNS are observed in adults who are on unrestricted phenylalanine intake or poorly compliant with dietary therapy [Phillips et al., 2001]. There is evidence that MRI changes in cases of phenylketonuria are at least partially reversible if patients return to a low-phenylalanine diet [Cleary et al., 1995]. Accordingly, it is reasonable to continue therapy into adulthood, and most centers recommend lifelong treatment. Reassessment of adult phenylalanine tolerance may be necessary as body mass changes with age [MacLeod et al., 2009].

A variety of medical food products is available as special formulas for the treatment of phenylketonuria. These special formulas are low in phenylalanine or do not contain any phenylalanine, and they typically contain supplemental tyrosine and a balanced mixture of the additional amino acids, carbohydrates, essential fatty acids, vitamins, and minerals, including zinc, selenium, and molybdenum. The metabolic medical foods provide a variable amount of calories (up to 70 percent of daily requirement) in the form of starch (e.g., dextrose, cornstarch, dextromaltose, Polycose) and fat (i.e., corn or other oils), and they constitute a major source of nutrition for the lifetime of the patient. The special formula or medical food, containing no phenylalanine, is continued even after solid food is introduced. The special formula or medical food is ingested together with regular food during the same meal, providing the phenylalanine in food plus the amino acids, vitamins, and nutrients in the special formula in a complementary, beneficial manner. The medical and regular foods therefore should be given in a calculated proportion together in intervals throughout the day. Overall, the targeted total amino acid intake for children younger than 2 years is approximately 3 g/kg/day, and it is about 2 g/kg/day for older children [Cockburn and Clark, 1996]. If the medical food is ingested in a single sitting, the supply of amino acids may induce hyperinsulinism and hypoglycemia.

Medical food products continue to be modified to increase palatability and optimize the treatment of phenylketonuria. Amino acid powders and gels with added carbohydrate and with or without fats, vitamins, and minerals are examples of commonly used protein substitutes. Newer protein substitutes include amino acid tablets and capsules, which do not contain carbohydrate, vitamins, or minerals. Special amino acid bars and a protein that is almost phenylalanine-free (glycomacropeptide) are also available [van Spronsen and Enns, 2010]. Phenylketonuria dietary research has focused on making the medical food products more palatable. Although low-phenylalanine flour, pastas, cookies, and nutrition bars are available, the phenylketonuria diet remains very bland, and poor dietary compliance can be a major problem, especially after childhood. Early efforts to make a more palatable amino acid mixture have met with preliminary success, with some patients preferring the new products to traditional medical foods.

It is important to monitor complete blood cell counts and serum vitamin B_{12} levels periodically, because clinical and subclinical B_{12} deficiency has been reported in adolescents and adults with classic phenylketonuria, even in those poorly compliant with the restricted diet [Hanley et al., 1996].

In contrast to the strict dietary control required in the treatment of classic phenylketonuria, patients with nonphenylketonuria hyperphenylalaninemia (i.e., untreated blood phenylalanine levels of 360–600 μM) are not necessarily placed on the special diet as long as their phenylalanine levels are in treatment range; many of these patients are able to maintain acceptable blood phenylalanine levels with protein restriction alone. These patients have normal intelligence, and they do not have the psychologic findings or head MRI changes that have been documented in classic phenylketonuria [Weglage et al., 1996]. Dietary therapy may be recommended in some instances for pregnant women with nonphenylketonuria hyperphenylalaninemia to minimize the risk of maternal phenylketonuria syndrome.

Additional and Novel Therapies

A complementary therapeutic approach has received U.S. Food and Drug Administration approval: administration of dietary supplementation of large, neutral amino acids. Large, neutral amino acids compete with phenylalanine for transport across the blood–brain barrier by the L-type amino acid carrier and consequently decrease the level of phenylalanine in the CNS [Matalon et al., 2003; van Spronsen and Enns, 2010]. In a study of six adult subjects with classic phenylketonuria, large, neutral amino acid supplementation resulted in increased blood concentrations of tyrosine and tryptophan (the respective precursors for dopamine and serotonin) and decreased brain phenylalanine concentration, as measured by ^{1}H-MR spectroscopy, toward the carrier range. All patients reported improvements in well-being and energy levels [Koch et al., 2003].

Deficiencies of carnitine and long-chain polyunsaturated fatty acids (i.e., arachidonic and docosahexaenoic acids) may contribute to CNS toxicity in uncontrolled phenylketonuria. Dietary supplementation of these fatty acids and of carnitine may benefit phenylketonuria patients who have low plasma levels of these essential metabolites [Infante and Huszagh, 2001]. Supplementation with omega-3, long-chain, polyunsaturated fatty acids resulted in improvement in visual-evoked potential latencies in 36 children with early-treated phenylketonuria [Beblo et al., 2001].

A novel therapeutic approach uses the nonmammalian enzyme phenylalanine lyase [van Spronsen and Enns, 2010]. This enzyme converts phenylalanine to trans-cinnamic acid, a harmless compound, and it has been found to reduce hyperphenylalaninemia in phenylketonuria rat and mouse models [Bourget and Chang, 1986; Sarkissian et al., 1999]. Enteral phenylalanine lyase therapy has the theoretic potential to increase dietary phenylalanine tolerance substantially, but significant practical hurdles need to be overcome; phenylalanine lyase is destroyed by gastric acidic pH and intestinal proteolysis. Alternative approaches being considered include the use of polyethylene glycol derivatization to produce protected forms of PAH for potential enzyme replacement therapy [Gamez et al., 2004; Kang et al., 2010].

Oral administration of tetrahydrobiopterin, the naturally occurring co-factor for the PAH reaction, reduces serum phenylalanine concentrations, especially in patients with mild hyperphenylalaninemia [Muntau et al., 2002]. However, response to tetrahydrobiopterin has also been documented in patients with classic or variant phenylketonuria [Matalon et al., 2004; van Spronsen and Enns, 2010]. These patients have mutations in the *PAH* gene, not in one of the genes encoding enzymes involved in tetrahydrobiopterin biosynthesis (see the section on biopterin disorders below). It has been suggested that the *PAH* mutations in such patients affect the structure of domains that are involved in the binding of tetrahydrobiopterin to the PAH enzyme. Tetrahydrobiopterin also may act as a chemical chaperone, preventing the PAH enzyme from misfolding or protecting PAH from inactivation [Pey et al., 2004]. If these observations and hypotheses are borne out, it may be possible to define by mutation analysis a subset of patients who would predictably benefit from co-factor supplementation. Tetrahydrobiopterin may prove useful in the treatment of maternal phenylketonuria [Trefz and Blau, 2003]. These, and other, novel therapies are under close investigation, especially given recent findings of suboptimal outcomes in phenylketonuria patients who have been continuously treated from the neonatal period [Enns et al., 2010].

Biopterin Disorders

Neonatal hyperphenylalaninemia may rarely be caused by defects in the synthesis or recycling of tetrahydrobiopterin, an essential co-factor in the PAH reaction (see Figure 32-1). Worldwide, it has been estimated that approximately 2 percent of patients with hyperphenylalaninemia have a defect in one of the four enzymes responsible for maintaining tetrahydrobiopterin levels [Blau et al., 1996]. Guanosine triphosphate

cyclohydrolase (GTPCH) I and 6-pyruvoyltetrahydrobiopterin synthase (PTPS) are essential enzymes for tetrahydrobiopterin biosynthesis, whereas pterin-4α-carbinolamine dehydratase (PCD) and dihydropteridine reductase (DHPR) are responsible for tetrahydrobiopterin recycling [Blau et al., 2001]. All forms of tetrahydrobiopterin disorders that cause hyperphenylalaninemia are inherited as autosomal-recessive traits. An autosomal-dominant form of GTPCH deficiency (e.g., dopa-responsive dystonia, Segawa's disease, hereditary progressive dystonia) manifests with dystonia, but it is not associated with elevated phenylalanine levels (see Chapter 39).

Because the tyrosine and tryptophan hydroxylases also require tetrahydrobiopterin for proper functioning, these disorders also result in deficiencies of the neurotransmitters L-DOPA and 5-hydroxytryptophan. Hyperphenylalaninemia in association with neurotransmitter deficits causes the neurologic manifestations associated with the defects in tetrahydrobiopterin synthesis and recycling.

More than 600 patients with tetrahydrobiopterin disorders have been identified (BIODEF database, http://www.bh4.org/). PTPS deficiency is the most common of these disorders, occurring in 54 percent of cases of reported tetrahydrobiopterin disorders. DHPR deficiency is seen in 32 percent, whereas PCD and GTPCH deficiencies are rare, each reported in 4 percent of cases (BIODEF database, http://www.bh4.org/).

Clinical Manifestations

Most patients with GTPCH, DHPR, and PTPS deficiencies have severe forms of disease, although mild forms of DHPR and PTPS deficiencies exist, and some forms of PTPS deficiency may be transient [Blau et al., 2001]. PCD deficiency is usually not associated with significant abnormalities other than transient tone abnormalities. Untreated patients with typical severe disorders of tetrahydrobiopterin synthesis or recycling usually develop neurologic manifestations by 4 months, although symptoms can appear in the neonatal period. Clinical manifestations include microcephaly, progressive neurologic deterioration, movement disorders, delayed motor development, seizures, tone disturbances, oculogyric spasms, swallowing difficulties, hypersalivation, and hyperthermia [Blau et al., 1996, 2001; Dhondt, 1993]. Diurnal fluctuation of dystonia may occur. The clinical course is similar in severe untreated tetrahydrobiopterin deficiency, regardless of the enzymatic defect. Head MRI findings have only rarely been reported [Pietz et al., 1996]. However, in DHPR deficiency, brain abnormalities such as diffuse demyelination, atrophy, spongy vacuolation of brainstem long tracts, and basal ganglia calcification may occur. Abnormal vascular proliferation in the cortex, white matter, and basal ganglia may also be detected [Gudinchet et al., 1992; Schmidt et al., 1988].

Diagnosis

Patients with tetrahydrobiopterin defects are often identified by mandatory newborn screening programs because of hyperphenylalaninemia. All children with persistent hyperphenylalaninemia must be screened for aberrations in the levels of pterin metabolites (i.e., neopterin and biopterin). Patients with GTPCH deficiency have decreased urinary excretion of neopterin and biopterin. In PTPS deficiency, neopterin is increased and biopterin decreased, resulting in a greatly elevated neopterin to biopterin ratio (normally, the ratio is about 1:1).

The neopterin to biopterin ratio in PCD deficiency is also increased but not to the same extent as in PTPS deficiency. In PCD deficiency, the characteristic feature is the presence of primapterin (7-biopterin) in the urine [Ayling et al., 2000]. In DHPR deficiency, the percentage of biopterin is elevated (>80 percent in most cases), but urine screening may miss it in some patients [Dhondt, 1984]. The measurement of DHPR activity in neonatal dried blood spots using a spectrophotometric assay is an effective method for diagnosis of DHPR deficiency. Urine pterin analysis and DHPR activity screening should be performed early in the management of a new patient with persistent hyperphenylalaninemia, or these disorders may be missed. Mutation analysis has yet to identify clear genotype-phenotype correlations [Blau et al., 1996].

Treatment

The goals of therapy are to decrease the level of phenylalanine to an acceptable range (120–360 µM) and correct the neurotransmitter deficiencies with exogenous supplementation. The diet is similar to that used to treat classic phenylketonuria, but patients tend to have a higher phenylalanine tolerance (300–700 mg/day) [Blau et al., 2001]. Tetrahydrobiopterin supplementation (2–20 mg/kg/day) is also used to help control blood phenylalanine levels. Lower tetrahydrobiopterin doses (2–5 mg/kg/day) may be effective in GTPCH and PTPS deficiencies, whereas higher doses (up to 20 mg/kg/day) may be required in DHPR deficiency. L-DOPA and 5-hydroxytryptophan are administered in a dose of 1–10 mg/kg/day. Carbidopa, an inhibitor of peripheral aromatic amino acid decarboxylase, decreases the conversion rates of L-DOPA to dopamine and 5-hydroxytryptophan to serotonin, allowing for the use of lower doses of these compounds; these therapeutic adjuncts may be especially helpful in severe forms of tetrahydrobiopterin deficiency. The optimal dose of each medication must be determined for each patient. Mild forms of disease may respond to tetrahydrobiopterin supplementation alone. Measuring levels of cerebrospinal fluid neurotransmitter metabolites (i.e., homovanillic acid and 5-hydroxyindolacetic acid) is useful in monitoring the efficacy of treatment [Blau et al., 2001; Shintaku, 2002].

Side effects of therapy include choreoathetosis, dystonia, and on-off phenomena, which are also features of the underlying disorders [Tanaka et al., 1989]. Tachycardia, diarrhea, and anorexia are associated with 5-hydroxytryptophan administration [Dhondt, 1993]. L-Deprenyl, a monoamine oxidase inhibitor, has been useful in decreasing catabolism of L-DOPA and 5-hydroxytryptophan, allowing lower dosing [Schuler et al., 1995; Spada et al., 1995, 1996]. A low concentration of cerebrospinal fluid folate is typical in DHPR deficiency, and it is treated by folinic acid supplementation (10–20 mg/day) [Shintaku, 2002]. Trimethoprim-sulfamethoxazole and methotrexate are DHPR inhibitors, and they may cause serious side effects in patients with tetrahydrobiopterin deficiency [Millot et al., 1995; Woody and Brewster, 1990]. Neurologic function may improve with therapy, but the overall prognosis for these disorders is largely unknown.

Hepatorenal Tyrosinemia

Hepatorenal tyrosinemia (i.e., tyrosinemia type I) is characterized principally by liver, kidney, and peripheral nerve involvement. The clinical spectrum ranges from severe hepatic failure in early infancy to later presentations of chronic liver disease and rickets in an older child. The overall incidence is 1 case per 100,000 births. In Quebec the incidence is quite high, at 1 in 16,700 births [Bergeron et al., 1974].

Pathophysiology

Hepatorenal tyrosinemia is caused by a deficiency of fumarylacetoacetate hydrolase, a distal enzymatic step in the processing of the amino acid tyrosine (Figure 32-2). Some investigations suggest that metabolites of tyrosine accumulating proximal to the blocked reaction step are toxic to liver and kidney, acting as alkylating agents or by disruption of sulfhydryl metabolism [Russo et al., 2001]. One of the accumulating metabolites, succinylacetone, has been implicated in the peripheral neuropathy of tyrosinemia [Sassa and Kappas, 1983; Sassa et al., 1983].

Clinical Manifestations

In states and countries that include tyrosinemia in newborn screening panels, infants are detected within the first weeks of life. Onset of disease manifestations may be sudden and may occur in the first month of life; a more gradual clinical course may also be seen. Children often manifest failure to thrive, and vomiting, diarrhea, and hepatosplenomegaly are common.

Traditional classifications of acute and chronic disease have been replaced by assessment of disease status in target organs (e.g., peripheral nerve, liver, and kidney). Liver disease can include acute decompensations and cirrhosis. There is a high incidence of progression to hepatocellular carcinoma, likely caused by accumulation of mutagenic metabolites. Renal dysfunction ranges from mild tubular dysfunction to frank renal failure. Vitamin D-resistant renal rickets is a common feature.

Neurologic involvement can include paresthesias, opisthotonic-like posture, bruxism and tongue biting, and in some cases, motor paralysis leading to respiratory failure and death [Mitchell et al., 1990]. Neurologic crises occur in up to 42 percent of individuals with tyrosinemia [Kvittingen, 1991].

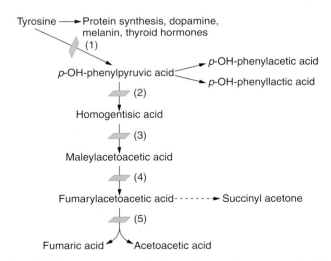

Fig. 32-2 The tyrosine metabolic pathway. The pathway involves several enzymes: tyrosine aminotransferase (1); p-OH-phenylpyruvic acid dioxygenase (2); homogentisic acid oxidase (3); maleylacetoacetic acid isomerase (4); and fumarylacetoacetic acid hydrolase (5). (*From Wilcox WR, Cederbaum SD. Amino acid metabolism. In: Rimoin D, Connor J, Pyeritz R, Korf B, eds. Principles and practice of medical genetics, 4th edn. Philadelphia: Churchill Livingstone, 2002:2411.*)

These crises are biphasic, with an active period of pain, autonomic dysfunction, and sometimes paralysis lasting 1–7 days, followed by a period of recuperation. Succinylacetone blocks the heme biosynthetic pathway, and the neurologic crises – a major source of morbidity – therefore have a physiologic basis similar to those in porphyria [Russo et al., 2001].

Laboratory Tests

Plasma amino acid analysis will reveal moderate elevations of tyrosine, often together with methionine and phenylalanine, reflecting generalized liver damage. The presence of succinylacetone in the urine is pathognomonic for tyrosinemia type I. Other findings include diminished serum phosphorus and elevated urinary excretion of phosphate, due to reduced tubular phosphorus reabsorption. Glucosuria and hyperaminoaciduria result from renal tubular impairment. Liver dysfunction leads to hyperbilirubinemia and hypoproteinemia. Patients usually have leukopenia, anemia, and thrombocytopenia.

Management

2-[2-Nitro-4-trifluoromethylbenzoyl]-1,3-cyclohexanedione (NTBC) is an inhibitor of 4-hydroxyphenylpyruvate dioxygenase (4-HPD), a proximal step in tyrosine catabolism. Inhibition thereby prevents the synthesis of succinylacetone and related metabolites, which accumulate because of the enzymatic block at fumarylacetoacetate hydrolase, a distal step in the pathway. Treatment with this compound is effective within hours and dramatically reduces the risk of neurologic and hepatic crises [Holme and Lindstedt, 2000; McKiernan, 2006]. Dietary restriction of phenylalanine and tyrosine is used in combination with NTBC. Liver transplantation is curative for hepatic and nervous system disease, and it is used in those who are refractory to nonsurgical treatment.

Acute management of neurologic crises includes analgesia, glucose (which inhibits ALA synthetase), and symptomatic treatment of hypertension. Repletion of sodium, potassium, and phosphate is necessary. The use of barbiturates and other medications that aggravate porphyria should be avoided before stabilization on NTBC [Kang and Gerald, 1970].

Other Categories of Tyrosinemia

Several causes of hypertyrosinemia exist in addition to fumarylacetoacetate hydrolase deficiency (see Figure 32-2). Deficiency of tyrosine aminotransferase causes tyrosinemia type II (oculocutaneous tyrosinemia) [Hunziker, 1980]. In type II disease, developmental delay, corneal thickening, and hyperkeratosis of palms and soles occur, but there is usually no hepatorenal involvement. Type III disease is caused by deficiency of 4-HPD and has a spectrum of manifestations, ranging from clinically normal to severe mental retardation and neurologic anomalies, including ataxia [Cerone et al., 1997; Ruetschi et al., 2000]. A 4-HPD dysfunction can also cause hawkinsinuria, a rare condition that can manifest with failure to thrive and metabolic acidosis, but it usually resolves as the patient's metabolism matures [Borden et al., 1992].

Liver failure can lead to elevated tyrosine levels [Mitchell et al., 2001], as can postprandial testing and diseases such as vitamin C deficiency and hyperthyroidism. Premature infants may manifest transient tyrosinemia of the newborn because of temporary immaturity in the function of 4-HPD. This condition resolves spontaneously, but mild developmental delay has been reported [Nyhan, 1984].

Maple Syrup Urine Disease

In 1954, Menkes and colleagues described four siblings who died in early infancy from a cerebral degenerative disease, with onset occurring when they were 3–5 days old. Symptoms included feeding difficulty, irregular respiratory pattern, hypertonia, opisthotonus, and failure to thrive. All had urine with the smell of maple syrup [Menkes et al., 1954]. Soon thereafter, another patient with a similar history was found to have elevated levels of branched-chain amino acids in urine and blood, and the syndrome was initially referred to as maple sugar urine disease [Westall et al., 1957]. Maple syrup urine disease is caused by mitochondrial branched-chain α-ketoacid dehydrogenase complex deficiency (compared with the composite branched-chain amino acid pathways in Figure 32-6 below). The enzymatic defect leads to accumulation of branched-chain amino acids and branched-chain α-ketoacids. Five forms of maple syrup urine disease (i.e., classic, intermediate, intermittent, thiamine-responsive, and dihydrolipoyl dehydrogenase [E3] deficiency) have been delineated based on clinical presentation, level of enzyme activity, and response to thiamine administration [Chuang and Shih, 2001].

Clinical Manifestations

CLASSIC MAPLE SYRUP URINE DISEASE

In the classic form, the clinical phenotype is one of severe neonatal encephalopathy, unless presymptomatic therapy is initiated because of abnormal newborn screening, prenatal diagnosis, or positive family history. Untreated neonates typically develop symptoms by the end of the first week of life. Feeding difficulties, alternating hypertonia and hypotonia, opisthotonic posturing, abnormal movements ("fencing" or "bicycling"), and seizures commonly occur. The characteristic urine smell develops on day 5–7 of life [Strauss and Morton, 2003a]. Unless an underlying inborn error of metabolism is suspected, affected children may be misdiagnosed as having sepsis and progress to coma and death. Ketosis is often found, and hypoglycemia may occur, but severe metabolic acidosis tends not to occur. Plasma amino acid analysis reveals elevated levels of branched-chain amino acids and the diagnostic presence of alloisoleucine in plasma [Schadewaldt et al., 1999]. Urine organic acid analysis demonstrates excretion of branched-chain α-ketoacids. Hyponatremia and cerebral edema are frequent sequelae during acute metabolic decompensation [Morton et al., 2002]. Other complications include pseudotumor cerebri, pancreatitis, and eye abnormalities [Burke et al., 1991; Kahler et al., 1994]. Ocular findings in untreated or late-diagnosed patients include optic atrophy, gray optic papilla, nystagmus, ophthalmoplegia, strabismus, and cortical blindness [Burke et al., 1991]. Children who survive the initial metabolic crisis typically have significant neurodevelopmental delays and spasticity [Chuang and Shih, 2001]. Although motor, visual, and learning deficits may occur, rapid identification of affected infants and careful institution of appropriate therapy can result in normal development [Kaplan et al., 1991; Morton et al., 2002].

Neuroimaging studies (Figure 32-3) are typically abnormal in patients with untreated classic maple syrup urine disease

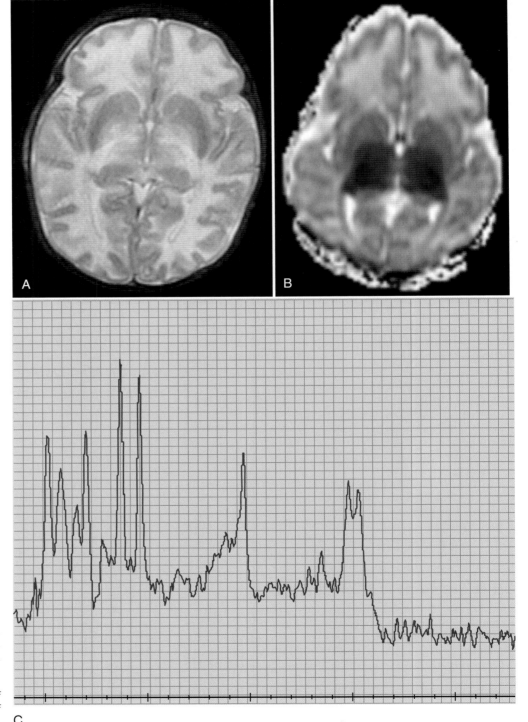

Fig. 32-3 Maple syrup urine disease. A, Axial view, T2-weighted image shows edema in the internal capsules, lateral thalami, and globus pallidi. **B,** Axial view, calculated apparent diffusion coefficient image at the same level shows hypointensity, indicated by reduced water diffusion, in the affected areas. **C,** Proton MR spectroscopy (echo time of 26 msec) shows a large peak at 0.9 ppm, believed to represent resonances of methyl protons from branched-chain amino acids and branched-chain α-ketoacids that accumulate as a result of defective oxidative decarboxylation of leucine, isoleucine, and valine. (*Courtesy of Dr. A James Barkovich, University of California, San Francisco, CA.*)

who are in crisis. Computed tomographic (CT) scans appear normal in the first few days of life, but they reveal progression to marked generalized cerebral edema if the patient remains untreated [Brismar et al., 1990]. An unusual pattern of edema may occur, characterized by involvement of the cerebellar deep white matter, posterior brainstem, cerebral peduncles, posterior limb of the internal capsule, and posterior aspect of the centrum semiovale. Edema tends to subside in the second

month of life [Brismar et al., 1990]. Patients with classic maple syrup urine disease in metabolic crisis with associated hyponatremia demonstrate a prominently increased T2 signal on brain MRI in the brainstem reticular formation, dentate nucleus, red nucleus, globus pallidus, hypothalamus, septal nuclei, and amygdala [Morton et al., 2002]. One report observed that brain MRI abnormalities were absent or only slight in sick patients with maple syrup urine disease in the absence of hyponatremia

[Morton et al., 2002]. Cranial ultrasonography of neonates in acute metabolic crisis reveals symmetrically increased echogenicity of the periventricular white matter, basal ganglia, and thalami [Fariello et al., 1996]. Chronic changes, including hypomyelination of the cerebral hemispheres, cerebellum, and basal ganglia and cerebral atrophy, may supervene in poorly controlled patients. CT- and MRI-defined abnormalities and the clinical phenotype may improve after implementation of appropriate dietary therapy [Taccone et al., 1992]. Diffusion-weighted imaging and spectroscopy have also documented abnormalities during the acute phase of disease [Cavalleri et al., 2002]. Markedly restricted proton diffusion, suggestive of cytotoxic or intramyelinic sheath edema, was demonstrated in the brainstem, basal ganglia, thalami, cerebellar and periventricular white matter, and cerebral cortex in six patients with maple syrup urine disease. MR spectroscopy demonstrated abnormal elevations of branched-chain amino acids, branched-chain α-ketoacids, and lactate in the four patients. All of these changes were reversed after the institution of appropriate nutritional and antibiotic therapy to treat intercurrent illness [Jan et al., 2003].

A characteristic comblike EEG pattern may be demonstrated for some patients with classic maple syrup urine disease between the second and third weeks of life [Tharp, 1992]. This unusual rhythm pattern resolves with the institution of dietary therapy [Tharp, 1992].

INTERMEDIATE MAPLE SYRUP URINE DISEASE

Children who have the intermediate form of maple syrup urine disease do not present in the neonatal period, despite having persistently elevated plasma levels of branched-chain amino acids. Developmental delay and failure to thrive are common. Severe neurologic impairment is absent; episodes of metabolic decompensation may occur, although severe ketoacidosis episodes are variable [Gonzalez-Rios et al., 1985a]. These children have a higher tolerance for dietary protein than those who have the classic form [Gonzalez-Rios et al., 1985a]. Rarely, patients with intermediate-type maple syrup urine disease respond to thiamine administration.

INTERMITTENT MAPLE SYRUP URINE DISEASE

Patients with intermittent maple syrup urine disease typically come to medical attention when they are 5 months to 2 years old and after stress induced by infection or high protein intake; some have been detected as late as the fifth decade of life [Chuang and Shih, 2001]. The intermittent form of maple syrup urine disease can be particularly difficult to diagnose, because affected individuals have normal levels of branched-chain amino acids and no odor between episodes of metabolic decompensation. Episodic decompensation is characterized by ataxia, disorientation, and altered behavior, which may progress to seizures, coma, and even death unless therapy is instituted. Early development and intellect are usually normal.

THIAMINE-RESPONSIVE MAPLE SYRUP URINE DISEASE

The clinical course of patients with the thiamine-responsive variant of maple syrup urine disease is similar to that of the intermediate form of disease. Plasma levels of branched-chain amino acid and urine excretion of branched-chain α-ketoacids decline days to weeks after thiamine administration (10–1000 mg/day)

is started [Scriver and Kaufman, 2001]. Patients are also treated with nutritional regimens similar to those used in other forms of maple syrup urine disease. Developmental delay may be present, but normal intelligence has also been documented [Scriver et al., 1971].

DIHYDROLIPOYL DEHYDROGENASE-DEFICIENT MAPLE SYRUP URINE DISEASE

The dihydrolipoyl dehydrogenase (E3)-deficient form of maple syrup urine disease is characterized by ketoacidotic crises in infancy. There is also lactic acidemia because the E3 subunit of the branched-chain α-ketoacid dehydrogenase complex is also required for catalytic function of pyruvate dehydrogenase and α-ketoglutarate dehydrogenase. In addition to the typical maple syrup urine disease metabolites, urine organic acid analysis reveals the presence of lactate, pyruvate, and α-ketoglutarate. The neonatal period is usually uneventful, but progressive neurologic deterioration, characterized by developmental delay, hypotonia or hypertonia, and dystonia, supervenes. Death in early childhood is common. Attempts at therapy have had limited success [Chuang and Shih, 2001; Sakaguchi et al., 1986].

Laboratory Tests

Maple syrup urine disease can be detected easily and accurately by tandem mass spectrometry analysis of the newborn blood spot [Chace et al., 1995]. Tandem mass spectrometry used in newborn screening is effective in identifying maple syrup urine disease, and is performed in all states in the U.S. (see http://genes-r-us.uthscsa.edu/nbsdisorders.htm) and many countries worldwide. Urine screening tests for the presence of α-ketoacids (i.e., ferric chloride and 2,4-dinitrophenylhydrazine [DNPH]) may be positive, but are nonspecific and insensitive. Plasma amino acid analysis demonstrates elevations of leucine, isoleucine, and valine (5- to 10-fold greater than normal) [Strauss and Morton, 2003a], as well as the pathognomonic finding of elevated alloisoleucine [Schadewaldt et al., 1999]. Levels of branched-chain amino acids are greatly elevated in urine and cerebrospinal fluid [Chuang and Shih, 2001]. The branched-chain α-ketoacids 2-oxoisocaproic acid, 2-oxo-3-methylvaleric acid, and 2-oxoisovaleric acid, derived from the branched-chain amino acids leucine, isoleucine, and valine, respectively, are found to be elevated on urine organic acid analysis during metabolic crises. Branched-chain amino acids levels and excretion of branched-chain α-ketoacids may be normal between episodes of decompensation in the intermittent form of disease.

The branched-chain α-ketoacid dehydrogenase complex consists of three catalytic components – a thiamine pyrophosphate-dependent carboxylase (E1) with an $\alpha_2\beta_2$ structure, a transacylase (E2), and a dehydrogenase (E3) – as well as two regulatory enzymes (a kinase and a phosphatase) [Chuang and Shih, 2001]. Deficient activity of this complex leads to the accumulation of leucine, isoleucine, and valine and their corresponding α-ketoacids. The decarboxylation activity can be measured in leukocytes, lymphoblasts, or fibroblasts, and it is loosely related to the clinical phenotype: 0–2 percent of normal activity in classic maple syrup urine disease, 3–30 percent activity in intermediate, 5–20 percent in intermittent, 2–40 percent in thiamine-responsive, and 0–25 percent in E3 deficiency [Chuang and Shih, 2001; Scriver et al., 1971]. Because significant overlap exists between measured enzyme activity and clinical phenotype, enzymatic activity cannot be used to predict the clinical course with certainty.

Genetics

Maple syrup urine disease is a pan-ethnic, autosomal-recessive condition that can be caused by mutations in any of the components of the mitochondrial branched-chain α-ketoacid dehydrogenase complex. In a study of 63 individuals, E1β subunit mutations were most common (38 percent), followed by E1α (33 percent), and E2 (19 percent) mutations [Nellis and Danner, 2001]. Branched-chain α-ketoacid dehydrogenase phosphatase or kinase mutations are also predicted to cause maple syrup urine disease, but such abnormalities have not yet been detected. The overall incidence is approximately 1 case per 150,000 people in the general population, but maple syrup urine disease is more common in Old Order Mennonites in southeastern Pennsylvania (1 in 176 births) [Danner and Doering, 1998]. A novel founder mutation in the E1β subunit has been reported in the Ashkenazi Jewish population [Edelmann et al., 2001]. In general, increased residual branched-chain α-ketoacid dehydrogenase activity should convey some advantage, but there is a wide overlap between measured enzymatic activities and clinical outcome. Given the complexity of the molecular genetics, the potential for modifier gene and environmental interactions, and the multiple clinical phenotypes associated with maple syrup urine disease, a lack of definitive genotype-phenotype relationships is not surprising.

Treatment

Chronic care of the child with maple syrup urine disease includes regular visits to an integrated metabolic clinic for medical and nutritional assessment. Adequate calories (100–120 kcal/kg/day) and protein (2–3 g/kg/day) are needed for growth. Chronic valine or isoleucine deficiency may cause an exfoliative dermatitis, and supplementation of these amino acids is often needed [Koch et al., 1993]. Thiamine supplementation is administered to patients with thiamine-responsive forms of maple syrup urine disease. Because patients on restricted diets are at risk for micronutrient and essential fatty acid deficiencies, patients should be periodically monitored for such deficits and supplementation given as needed.

Because significant metabolic intoxication may occur rapidly, even in patients with apparently well-controlled disease, it is crucial to have carefully considered home and hospital emergency protocols in place for each child [Morton et al., 2002; Strauss and Morton, 2003a]. Acute metabolic decompensation (e.g., fasting or illness severe enough to cause catabolism) is a medical emergency that requires prompt intervention. Initial intervention is aimed at correcting dehydration, starting high-dose intravenous thiamine, and providing adequate calories (approximately 120–140 kcal/kg/day) to prevent further protein catabolism and higher rise in plasma leucine levels. To this end, high-dextrose intravenous fluids (to provide approximately 10 mg/kg/min) and intralipid are often administered. Branched-chain amino acid-free parenteral nutrition or enteral formula, delivered by continuous nasogastric drip, can also be used [Nyhan et al., 1998; Parini et al., 1993]. The rate of decrease of leucine is slowed in the face of valine and isoleucine levels inadequate to stimulate protein synthesis. Acute valine and isoleucine deficiency can be avoided by careful supplementation of these amino acids [Parini et al., 1993]. Leucine is reintroduced to the diet after therapeutic levels are achieved [Morton et al., 2002].

In a study of 36 maple syrup urine disease patients, plasma leucine levels fell to less than 400 μM 2–4 days after the initiation of therapy with enteral and parenteral nutrition. Initial leucine levels ranged from 233 to 778 μM in a group diagnosed on the first day of life (n = 18) and 1489 to 3359 μM in a group diagnosed between days 3 and 16 (n = 18). Over an 11-year period, neurologic examinations, gross motor development, and speech were normal in 34 of 36 children [Morton et al., 2002]. Enteral nutrition was also found to be beneficial when instituted within the first 20 days of life. Four patients receiving nasogastric drip feeding as the only treatment of neonatal classic maple syrup urine disease had normal development when 3–5 years old [Parini et al., 1993]. Hemodialysis and continuous venovenous extracorporeal removal therapies result in more rapid fall in plasma levels of branched-chain amino acids, but these modalities typically have been described in single case reports or small series with relatively short follow-up, and it is difficult to ascertain the long-term outcome of such intervention [Gouyon et al., 1996; Puliyanda et al., 2002]. Nevertheless, normal development has been reported for 8 of 12 children after continuous venovenous extracorporeal removal therapy [Jouvet et al., 2001]. Branched-chain amino acids levels often rebound after initial dialysis in cases of severe metabolic imbalance characterized by extremely high leucine levels, and dialysis may need to be repeated in such cases. Peritoneal dialysis is no longer routinely used; there is a tendency for leucine levels to plateau between 1000 and 1500 μM after 24 hours, limiting the utility of this therapeutic modality [Gortner et al., 1989]. Levels of branched-chain amino acids and branched-chain α-ketoacids tend to plateau with exchange transfusion therapy [Nyhan et al., 1998; Wendel et al., 1982].

Although enteral and intravenous therapy may be sufficient to manage many patients with maple syrup urine disease in acute crisis, various dialysis methods are commonly used and should be considered, especially when clearance of branched-chain amino acids by nutritional support is not effective or when other considerations, such as life-threatening cerebral edema, renal imbalance, or cardiovascular abnormalities, exist [Jouvet et al., 2001; Nyhan et al., 1998]. Liver transplantation has been performed rarely for maple syrup urine disease. Three patients who underwent successful transplantation were able to resume normal diets and were no longer at risk for metabolic decompensation [Wendel et al., 1999]. More recently, domino hepatic transplantion for maple syrup urine disease was successfully performed [Barshop and Khanna, 2005].

Because hyponatremia and subsequent brain edema are serious and relatively common complications, it is important to monitor serum sodium and serum and urine osmolalities closely and to replace urinary losses with saline [Morton et al., 2002]. Critical brain swelling and abnormal brainstem function may develop with only a moderate reduction in serum sodium level (by only 8–10 mEq/L) [Morton et al., 2002]. Low-dose diuretics may also be used to prevent water retention [Strauss and Morton, 2003a]. Mannitol is reserved for life-threatening episodes of increased intracranial pressure [Morton et al., 2002].

Glycine Encephalopathy

Glycine encephalopathy, also known as nonketotic hyperglycinemia, is an autosomal-recessive disorder caused by defective function of the multimeric glycine cleavage enzyme system,

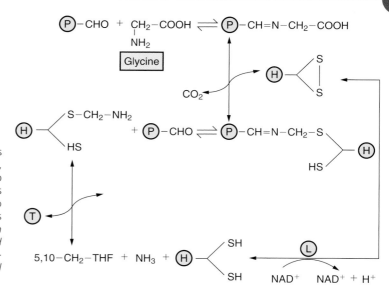

Fig. 32-4 The glycine cleavage system. Circles designate proteins with the active group shown. In the presence of P and H proteins, glycine is decarboxylated, and the remaining aminoethyl group binds to the reduced lipoic acid on the H protein. T protein is required to release ammonia and transfer the x carbon of glycine to tetrahydrofolate (THF), forming 5,10-CH$_2$-THF. The L protein is necessary to regenerate the correct form of the H protein. *(From Scriver C, Beudet A, Sly W, Valle D, eds. The metabolic and molecular basis of inherited disease, 8th edn. New York: McGraw-Hill, 2001:2066. Reprinted with permission from The McGraw-Hill Companies.)*

leading to accumulation of glycine in all body tissues, including the CNS (Figure 32-4). Gerritsen et al., 1965 described the initial patient in 1965. The glycine cleavage enzyme system has four components: the P protein (a pyridoxal phosphate-dependent glycine decarboxylase), the T protein (a tetrahydrofolate-dependent protein), the H protein (a hydrogen carrier protein), and the L protein (lipoamide dehydrogenase). Infants with classic disease present in the first week of life with apnea, lethargy, severe hypotonia, and feeding difficulties [Hoover-Fong et al., 2004]. Respiratory failure, hiccups, and intractable seizures develop, and most infants die unless assisted ventilatory support is provided. Intermittent ophthalmoplegia is a relatively frequent finding [MacDonald and Sher, 1977]. The EEG commonly has a burst suppression pattern, but hypsarrhythmia has been reported rarely [Hoover-Fong et al., 2004].

Brain imaging results are normal for about one-half of the neonatal-onset cases [Hoover-Fong et al., 2004]. Relatively common brain abnormalities include agenesis of the corpus callosum, progressive atrophy, and delayed myelination [Hoover-Fong et al., 2004]. Acute hydrocephalus, requiring shunting, may occur and is a poor prognostic sign [Van Hove et al., 2000]. [1]H-MR spectroscopy detects increased intracerebral levels of glycine, lactate, and creatine [Viola et al., 2002]. The lethal form of glycine encephalopathy appears to be associated with elevated levels of brain myo-inositol glycine, creatine, and *N*-acetylaspartate. Diffusion-weighted imaging has shown high-signal-intensity lesions in the pyramidal tracts, middle cerebellar pedicles, and dentate nuclei, likely reflecting myelin spongiosis [Sener, 2003].

Atypical and transient variants of glycine encephalopathy have also been reported in patients with cerebrospinal fluid to plasma glycine ratios of more than 0.08. Atypical forms manifest in infancy or early childhood after an uneventful pregnancy and neonatal period. Clinical features include seizures (in most cases) and relatively mild developmental delay. Atypical glycine encephalopathy documented by liver enzymology has also been reported in siblings with normal cerebrospinal fluid glycine levels and cerebrospinal fluid to plasma glycine ratios [Jackson et al., 1999]. Transient glycine encephalopathy is characterized by the same initial clinical and biochemical findings as the classic form, but it has only rarely been reported.

In the transient form, cerebrospinal fluid and plasma glycine levels partially or completely resolve, and most patients have normal development [Aliefendioglu et al., 2003; Korman et al., 2004; Lang et al., 2008]. Transient elevations of cerebrospinal fluid glycine and the cerebrospinal fluid to plasma glycine ratio occurred in an asphyxiated patient with pyridoxine-dependent seizures [Maeda et al., 2000].

Diagnosis of glycine encephalopathy is established by detecting an elevated cerebrospinal fluid glycine concentration, typically 15–30 times normal, in association with an increased cerebrospinal fluid to plasma glycine ratio (normal <0.02) [Applegarth and Toone, 2001; Hamosh and Johnston, 2001]. Classic neonatal-onset patients often have ratios higher than 0.2, whereas atypical patients have ratios of approximately 0.09 [Hamosh and Johnston, 2001]. A ratio higher than 0.08 is usually considered diagnostic for glycine encephalopathy. The plasma and cerebrospinal fluid samples should be obtained as closely as possible to one another, and the presence of blood in the cerebrospinal fluid invalidates the amino acid results [Applegarth and Toone, 2001]. Other causes of increased cerebrospinal fluid glycine levels include valproate therapy, brain trauma, and hypoxic-ischemic encephalopathy. Secondary elevations of plasma glycine, associated with ketosis, are often encountered in organic acidemias (e.g., methylmalonic, propionic, and isovaleric acidemias and β-ketothiolase deficiency) [Applegarth and Toone, 2001; Korman and Gutman, 2002]. Because sulfite oxidase deficiency (isolated or as part of molybdenum co-factor deficiency), folinic acid-responsive seizures, and disorders of neurotransmitters may have presentations similar to that of glycine encephalopathy, an aliquot of cerebrospinal fluid should also be frozen and saved for appropriate analyses in the event that the result of amino acid analysis is normal.

Definitive confirmation of the diagnosis may be accomplished by assaying glycine cleavage enzyme in liver. In practice, molecular testing of the genes encoding glycine cleavage system subunits is less invasive and more widely available [Hamosh et al., 2009]. Between 60 and 80 percent of patients with the classic neonatal form have defects in the P protein. T protein deficiency occurs in 5–20 percent of cases, whereas H protein and L protein defects are rarely reported [Tada and Kure,

1993]. Prenatal diagnosis by glycine cleavage enzyme system measurement in uncultured chorionic villus samples has resulted in false-negative and false-positive results in at least 1 percent of cases studied [Applegarth et al., 2000]. DNA analysis, when mutations are known, remains the most reliable form of prenatal diagnosis [Kure et al., 1999].

Comprehensive mutation analysis in 68 families with glycine encephalopathy detected *GLDC* (P protein gene) or *AMT* (T protein gene) mutations in 68 percent of neonatal and 60 percent of infantile types, respectively. No *GCSH* (H protein gene) mutations were identified [Kure et al., 2003]. The L protein is a component of pyruvate dehydrogenase and branched-chain ketoacid dehydrogenase, as well as the glycine cleavage enzyme system. However, L protein deficiency leads to a variant form of maple syrup urine disease or pyruvate dehydrogenase deficiency, rather than glycine encephalopathy [Applegarth and Toone, 2001]. Few glycine encephalopathy patients have been identified who carry the same mutations, making genotype-phenotype correlations problematic, although some possible correlations have been found [Applegarth and Toone, 2004]. Three of four patients with transient glycine encephalopathy and homozygosity for a novel *GLDC* mutation (A802V) had a normal outcome after intensive therapy as neonates. High residual activity of the mutant enzyme and therapeutic intervention during a critical period of brain sensitivity may have contributed to the good outcome in some cases of transient or mild glycine encephalopathy. The three-dimensional structures of the T protein, H protein, and L protein have been determined, which can aid in understanding the molecular mechanisms underlying the effects of missense mutations on glycine cleavage enzyme system activity [Lee et al., 2004].

In postmortem examination specimens from infants who died because of glycine encephalopathy, brain glycine concentrations are elevated 2–8-fold [Perry et al., 1977]. Neuropathology has demonstrated deficient myelination, abnormal cortical neuron morphology, and spongiosis of the white matter with associated astrocytic gliosis [Brun et al., 1979].

Treatment of glycine encephalopathy has not improved the overall dismal prognosis in the classic form of disease [Chien et al., 2004]. Therapy is focused on controlling seizures with antiepileptic drugs, decreasing tissue glycine levels, and administering *N*-methyl-D-aspartate (NMDA) receptor antagonists to diminish glycine-induced neuronal excitotoxicity. Valproate is contraindicated because it can inhibit the glycine cleavage enzyme system, and can cause hyperglycinemia in patients without glycine encephalopathy [Jaeken et al., 1977]. Sodium benzoate is given because of its ability to conjugate to glycine to form hippurate, which can then be excreted in the urine. A glycine-specific mitochondrial enzyme, benzoyl-coenzyme A (CoA):glycine acyltransferase, catalyzes the condensation of benzoate and glycine to form hippurate [Webster et al., 1976]. Sodium benzoate therapy can reduce plasma levels of glycine to the normal range and may have a mild effect on cerebrospinal fluid glycine levels, but it does not affect the dismal prognosis. Because high-dose sodium benzoate therapy can result in carnitine deficiency, plasma carnitine levels should be monitored closely and appropriate supplementation provided [Van Hove et al., 1995]. Dextromethorphan, an antagonist of the NMDA receptor, is also commonly used in therapy. Treatment with dextromethorphan may lead to improved seizure control and level of interaction in some patients. Ketamine has been used rarely, but it may provide benefit in controlling seizures and improving overall level of interaction [Boneh et al., 1996]. A low-protein diet has no proven efficacy and may result in severe protein malnutrition, micronutrient deficiency, and exfoliative dermatitis if not monitored carefully [Samady et al., 2000]. Sodium benzoate, alone or combined with imipramine, has been effective in improving clinical manifestations in milder forms of glycine encephalopathy [Neuberger et al., 2000; Wiltshire et al., 2000].

Sulfur Amino Acid Metabolism and the Homocystinurias

Homocysteine lies at a critical juncture between the trans-sulfuration and remethylation pathways of methionine metabolism, at which point homocysteine can be converted to cystathionine or methionine. The malfunctioning of three enzymes is known to cause homocystinuria: cystathionine β-synthase, methylene tetrahydrofolate reductase, and methionine synthase. The β-synthase enzyme is involved in the trans-sulfuration pathway (Figure 32-5), and the latter two enzymes are involved in the sulfur conservation pathway. Several of the mutations that cause methylmalonic acidemia also cause homocystinuria, and these are discussed in the section on cobalamin complementation groups. A transport abnormality, selective intestinal malabsorption of vitamin B_{12}, can also cause homocystinuria. The overall incidence of homocystinuria is approximately 1 case in 335,000 persons, but it varies from 1 in 65,000 in Ireland to 1 in 900,000 in Japan [Naughten et al., 1998].

Cystathionine β-Synthase Deficiency

Cystathionine β-synthase deficiency is characterized by multisystem involvement, including mental retardation, lens dislocations, occlusive vascular events, and skeletal deformities.

PATHOPHYSIOLOGY

The trans-sulfuration pathway converts methionine into cysteine. In cystathionine β-synthase deficiency, methionine, homocysteine, and homocystine accumulate in the blood and are excreted in large quantities in the urine [Christensen et al., 1991; Mudd et al., 1964]. Two major categories of cystathionine β-synthase deficiency have been described, one responsive to pyridoxine and the other nonresponsive [Barber and Spaeth, 1969]. One-half of patients with cystathionine β-synthase deficiency respond to pyridoxine therapy, and only modest restriction of methionine in their diet is required [Mudd et al., 1985].

Biochemical abnormalities in the CNS are thought to account for the occurrence of mental retardation and neurologic abnormalities. Synthesis of cystathionine, an important free amino acid in the brain [Brenton et al., 1965], is impaired, and this compound is virtually absent from the brain in affected individuals. Abnormalities in homocysteine, methionine, and other metabolites probably contribute to central nervous disease as well.

Arterial and venous thromboses are prominent in many organs, including the brain. Large and medium-sized blood vessels (i.e., arteries, veins, and dural sinuses) are compromised. Fibrous thickening of the intima occurs, the vessel lumen may be compromised, and the media is also involved, with increased deposition of collagen and frayed, split smooth muscle

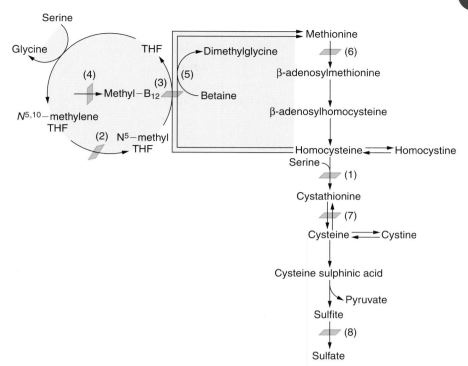

Fig. 32-5 Abbreviated diagram for the trans-sulfuration pathway. The known genetic defects that cause homocystinuria are a deficiency of cystathionine β-synthase (1), $N^{5,10}$-methylenetetrahydrofolate reductase (2), methionine synthase or methionine synthase reductase (3), and deficient synthesis of methylcobalamin (4). Other defects in the pathway are cystathioninuria caused by γ-cystathionase deficiency (7), sulfite oxidase and molybdenum cofactor synthesis deficiencies (8), and hypermethioninemia from methionine adenosyltransferase deficiency (6). Betaine can be given therapeutically to treat homocystinuria by increasing remethylation of homocysteine by betaine-homocysteine methyltransferase (5). THF, tetrahydrofolate. *(From Wilcox WR, Cederbaum SD. Amino acid metabolism. In: Rimoin D, Connor J, Pyeritz R, Korf B, eds. Principles and practice of medical genetics, 4th edn. Philadelphia: Churchill Livingstone, 2002:2419.)*

fibers. A clotting diathesis is also involved [D'Angelo and Selhub, 1997]. An increased tendency of intravascular thrombosis may be related to abnormal adhesiveness of platelets. However, no single mechanism has been demonstrated to cause the vascular complications. Homocysteine elevation is an independent risk factor for arteriosclerotic vascular disease. This factor has been demonstrated for affected patients and for individuals in the general population who may have modest elevations in homocysteine concentrations.

Degenerative changes in the fibers that hold the optic lens likely are caused by interference with fibrillin function [Sakai et al., 1986]. The bone disease likely results from abnormalities in connective tissue, such as defective fibrillin function or perhaps abnormal collagen cross-linking [Harris and Sjoerdsma, 1966].

CLINICAL MANIFESTATIONS

Four organ systems demonstrate major involvement: the central nervous, skeletal, ocular, and vascular systems [Mudd et al., 1985]. Other organs, such as the liver, hair, muscles, blood, and skin (e.g., hypopigmentation), may be involved.

When the CNS is involved, the most frequent finding is mental retardation, which can manifest as developmental delay during the first year of life. There is a spectrum of cognitive function in untreated patients, with IQ scores ranging from 10 to 138. Intelligence in B_6-responsive patients tends to be higher than in B_6 nonresponders. Psychiatric disturbances are common, and seizures and extrapyramidal signs occasionally are seen. Focal neurologic signs point to a cerebrovascular occlusion. Patients identified on newborn screening who receive early treatment have normal cognitive function [Yap et al., 2001].

Skeletal abnormalities include osteoporosis, scoliosis, increased length of long bones, metaphyseal and epiphyseal anomalies, biconcave vertebrae, arachnodactyly, pes planus,

and genu valgum. The skeletal and ocular findings may lead to confusion with Marfan's syndrome.

Involvement of the eye is manifested by ectopic lenses (i.e., dislocated downward) and myopia. Involvement occasionally is manifested by glaucoma, retinal changes, cataracts, and corneal changes.

Thromboembolic events (arterial and venous), livedo reticularis, and malar flush are some of the vascular findings. Patients have suffered from pulmonary, cerebral, and renal infarction. Cerebral venous sinus thrombosis has been documented with scanning studies. An increased risk of myocardial infarction exists in patients with homocystinuria and in hyperhomocysteinemic members of the general population [Stampfer et al., 1992]. One-half of patients will have a vascular event before age 30 years.

LABORATORY TESTS

Homocystinuria occurs in all untreated patients [Isherwood, 1996], but this is not sufficient to establish the diagnosis because it may occur in patients with other conditions. Serum amino acid analysis reveals elevated methionine and free homocysteine, with variably low levels of cysteine. Plasma total homocysteine levels are abnormally elevated. Direct assays are used to confirm the enzymatic deficiency, and these can be performed on skin fibroblasts, liver, or leukocytes.

TREATMENT

The goals of treatment are to reduce the severe hyperhomocysteinemia and other biochemical abnormalities. Supportive treatment of complications is essential. Treatment of patients who are B_{12}-responsive consists of pyridoxine in combination with folic acid and vitamin B_{12} [Wilcken and Wilcken, 1997]. For vitamin B_{12} nonresponders, treatment is achieved with a methionine-restricted, cystine-supplemented diet [Komrower et al., 1966; Perry et al., 1966]. Pyridoxine, folic acid, and vitamin B_{12} have been used in pyridoxine nonresponders as co-factors of methionine metabolism to promote homocysteine conversions partially to other metabolites. Betaine, a methyl donor that remethylates homocysteine to methionine, is also an effective component of treatment [Wilcken et al., 1985].

Methionine Synthase Deficiency

Methionine synthase lies at the intersection of folate, cobalamin, and sulfur-containing amino acid metabolism. Patients with defects in this enzyme have homocystinuria and low (or normal) methionine levels, but they do not have methylmalonic acidemia.

PATHOPHYSIOLOGY

Two complementation groups (CblE and CblG) have very similar clinical and laboratory presentations, and they are discussed together. These patients have isolated defects in methionine synthase function caused by mutations in the enzyme itself or abnormalities in the synthesis of the methylcobalamin co-factor.

CLINICAL MANIFESTATIONS

Most patients present in early infancy with poor feeding, emesis, lethargy, hypotonia, seizures, and developmental delay [Watkins and Rosenblatt, 1989]. There is usually a neurologic presentation, but this can vary and can include gait disturbances and multiple sclerosis-like features [Carmel et al., 1988]. There is a strong association with megaloblastic anemia.

LABORATORY TESTS

Serum cobalamin and folate levels are normal or high, and methylmalonic aciduria is generally not seen [Tuchman et al., 1988]. Homocystinuria is a consistent feature, and CblE and CblG can be differentiated from other causes of homocystinuria by biochemical studies of cultured cells.

TREATMENT

Administration of hydroxocobalamin in pharmacologic doses (with intramuscular administration at initial treatment stages) should begin as soon as the diagnosis is made. This typically leads to rapid biochemical improvement. Some patients also have improvement of anemia on folinic acid [Harding et al., 1997]. Prenatal therapy has been used for early diagnoses with success [Rosenblatt et al., 1985].

Methylene Tetrahydrofolate Reductase Deficiency

In methylene tetrahydrofolate reductase deficiency, the degree of clinical severity varies with enzyme activity. In addition to the severe and moderate cases discussed later, the common $677C \rightarrow T$ polymorphism – which can cause mild elevations in homocysteine levels – appears to be a risk factor for hypercoagulable states in the population at large.

PATHOPHYSIOLOGY

Major findings are demyelination and vascular changes, such as those seen in cystathionine β-synthase deficiency [Beckman et al., 1987]. Other changes include dilated cerebral ventricles, hydrocephalus, and microgyria [Kanwar et al., 1976;

Wong et al., 1977]. Methylene tetrahydrofolate reductase deficiency is thought to result in low levels of brain folate [Levitt et al., 1971].

CLINICAL MANIFESTATIONS

Clinical findings vary with enzyme function and include developmental delay, motor and gait abnormalities, seizures, and psychiatric disease such as psychosis and schizophrenia [Haan et al., 1985; Mudd et al., 1972]. Patients rarely have megaloblastic anemia. Severe disease is often lethal. Age at presentation ranges from birth in severe cases to adulthood in milder ones.

LABORATORY TESTS

Moderate hyperhomocysteinemia and homocystinuria are seen, with low or normal methionine levels. The homocysteine excretion is significantly lower than in cystathionine β-synthase deficiency [Fowler and Jakobs, 1998].

TREATMENT

Severe disease is refractory to treatment, and, although several treatments have been tried (i.e., folate, methionine, pyridoxine, cobalamin, and carnitine), none has been particularly effective [Fowler, 1998]. Betaine has somewhat improved the prognosis [Al Tawari et al., 2002; Sakura et al., 1998].

Sulfite Oxidase Deficiency

Deficiency of sulfite oxidase function may occur as an isolated enzyme defect or as part of a combined deficiency (see Figure 32-5). This rare disorder results in abnormalities of metabolism of sulfated amino acids. The cardinal feature of this condition is severe seizures in the neonatal period. Although some therapies lead to mild improvements, there is no effective treatment.

Pathophysiology

The molybdenum co-factor is composed of the metal and a small pterin group [Johnson et al., 1980a]. This prosthetic group is required for the function of three enzymes: sulfite oxidase, xanthine dehydrogenase, and aldehyde oxidase [Johnson et al., 1980b]. Most patients have mutations in one of several enzymes of the co-factor synthetic chain, whereas a minority has mutations in the sulfite oxidase gene. Postmortem examination of patients with sulfite oxidase or co-factor deficiencies has found encephalopathy with loss of neurons and myelin, attributable largely to deficiency of sulfite oxidase function and accumulation of sulfite in the brain [Roth et al., 1985]. Absence of sulfite oxidase leads to alternate metabolic pathways for sulfites, including formation of S-sulfocysteine and thiosulfate [Mudd et al., 1967]. S-sulfocysteine may substitute for cysteine in connective tissue, leading to ocular lens dislocation.

Clinical Manifestations

The clinical picture includes severe neurologic abnormalities, dislocated ocular lenses, and mental retardation [Mudd et al., 1967]. This presentation is similar in isolated sulfite oxidase deficiency cases and in patients in whom the co-factor is absent. Although some variability is seen among patients, the key feature is neonatal seizures. It is recommended that all patients with neonatal seizures have metabolic testing. Other neurologic signs can include opisthotonus, axial hypotonia with peripheral hypertonia, regression, and loss of milestones. Ophthalmologic abnormalities can include nystagmus, coloboma, and cortical blindness [Lueder and Steiner, 1995]. Craniofacial dysmorphology includes bitemporal narrowing with deep-set eyes, long palpebral fissures, thick lips, elongated philtrum, and a small nose. Heterozygote carriers are unaffected.

Laboratory Tests

Positive sulfite test results are usually observed on urine dipstick, although false-negative results can occur [van der Klei-van Moorsel et al., 1991]. The cysteine metabolite *S*-sulfocysteine is characteristically elevated in urine and plasma, and plasma total homocysteine may be low [Johnson and Rajagopalan, 1995; Tan et al., 2005]. Low levels of urinary urothion, a degradation product of molybdopterin, are essentially diagnostic of molybdenum co-factor deficiency, and an elevated urinary thiosulfate level is diagnostic of sulfite oxidase deficiency or molybdenum co-factor deficiency.

Treatment

Management for this condition is largely supportive because therapies are often ineffective. Molybdenum co-factor is too unstable to be used therapeutically. Patients with milder forms of isolated sulfite oxidase deficiency may respond to a diet low in sulfur-containing amino acids [Touati et al., 2000].

Hartnup's Disease

Hartnup's disease is an aminoaciduria that is usually clinically silent, but it can manifest with episodes of cerebellar ataxia and a pellagra-like rash. Incidence has been estimated at 1 case in 33,000 persons [Wilcken et al., 1977].

Pathophysiology

The metabolic aberration in Hartnup's disease results from an error in the transport of monoamino-monocarboxylic (neutral) amino acids that affects renal tubular reabsorption and intestinal absorption [Baron et al., 1956; Mahon and Levy, 1986; Scriver et al., 1987]. There is deficient transport of neutral amino acids, including glutamine, histidine, valine, phenylalanine, tyrosine, tryptophan, alanine, asparagine, citrulline, isoleucine, leucine, serine, and threonine. Large amounts of the amino acids and of the amides of glutamate and aspartate are excreted in the urine [Bonetti and Dent, 1954]. The disorder arises from mutations in *SLC6A19*, the gene encoding the amino acid transporter B^0AT1, involved in co-transport of Na^+ and neutral amino acids from the luminal compartment into the cells [Kleta et al., 2004; Seow et al., 2004; Cheon et al., 2010]. Two tissue-specific forms of Hartnup's disease are recognized: renal plus intestinal involvement, and renal involvement alone.

Amino acids, such as tryptophan, remain in the intestinal lumen [Milne et al., 1960], where they are converted to indolic compounds by bacteria and then absorbed [Asatoor et al., 1963]; these compounds are toxic to the CNS. Urinary excretion of large amounts of indican (a tryptophan metabolite) is characteristic of the disease. Large quantities of neutral amino acids are excreted in the feces [Scriver, 1965]. The lack

of tryptophan absorption leads to niacin deficiency, which results in the pellagra-like symptoms and photosensitivity.

Clinical Manifestations

Patients who have been detected by population screening usually have been clinically normal, and Hartnup's disease is usually benign [Scriver et al., 1987]. Nevertheless, some patients are affected, suggesting a monogenic trait with strong polygenic influence [Scriver, 1988]. The most prominent neurologic feature in affected individuals is attacks of cerebellar ataxia, which vary in intensity. These episodes may persist for as long as 2 weeks before improvement is evident. Less common neurologic disabilities include spasticity, wide-based gait, double vision, nystagmus, dystonia, and tremulousness. Psychiatric disturbances consisting of fear, anxiety, and mood swings may occur, as may constant headaches.

Clinical involvement varies considerably among symptomatic individuals. Neurologic symptoms are often accompanied by a rash on areas of sun-exposed skin [Baron et al., 1956]. The skin is dry and reddened, resembling pellagra (i.e., nicotinamide deficiency). Sun exposure usually exacerbates the lesions, as does sulfonamide administration. Skin may become hyperpigmented.

Laboratory Tests

Urine has strikingly elevated levels of neutral amino acids, but basic and acidic amino acids in urine are relatively normal [Tada et al., 1967]. Serum levels of amino acids are normal or low [Cusworth and Dent, 1960].

Treatment

In the rare symptomatic patient, increasing amino acid intake in the form of a high-protein diet can overcome the deficient transport and loss of neutral amino acids [Scriver et al., 1987]. Conversely, poor nutrition can lead to attacks in patients who would otherwise be asymptomatic. Symptomatic patients should protect themselves from sunlight and other aggravating agents, such as photosensitizing drugs. Administration of nicotinic acid offsets deficiency in nicotinamide synthesis [Halvorsen and Halvorsen, 1963].

Histidinemia

Histidinemia is benign in almost all affected individuals, although in rare cases, this condition may lead to CNS disease. The benign nature makes treatment unnecessary in almost all cases. Overall incidence has been estimated at between 1 in 8000 in Japan and 1 in 37,000 in Sweden [Virmani and Widhalm, 1993].

Pathophysiology

Histidinemia results from deficiency of L-histidase (L-histidine ammonia lyase) [Auerbach et al., 1962], resulting in accumulation of histidine and its metabolites in blood, urine, and cerebrospinal fluid, and in a deficiency of urocanic acid [Levy et al., 1974]. Enzyme activity is essentially undetectable in liver and other tissues of patients, but may be normal in skin [Woody et al., 1965].

Clinical Manifestations

The initial patients identified with histidinemia were mentally retarded and had speech abnormalities; the group identified was likely a result of ascertainment bias. Prospective follow-up of newborns with histidinemia detected by newborn screening did not provide evidence of disease in affected individuals [Levy et al., 1974; Tada et al., 1982]. Although it is clear that histidinemia does not produce severe disease, there is still debate about possible minor effects on speech and intelligence.

Laboratory Tests

The diagnosis is based on elevated plasma and urine levels of histidine.

Treatment

Low-histidine diets have been successfully used to reduce blood histidine concentration; however, studies of mean IQ and general level of functioning revealed no statistical advantage of therapy. Therapy is not indicated for most patients who remain asymptomatic [Scriver and Levy, 1983]. If concern exists that elevated histidine is contributing to findings, consultation with a biochemical specialist is recommended.

Organic Acidemias

Propionic Acidemia

Propionic acidemia is caused by deficiency of propionyl-CoA carboxylase (PCC), a biotin-requiring enzyme that catalyzes the conversion of propionyl-CoA to methylmalonyl-CoA in the metabolic pathways of valine, isoleucine, methionine, threonine, and odd-chain fatty acids (Figure 32-6). This condition is estimated to occur in 1 of 50,000 to 100,000 livebirths.

Propionyl-CoA carboxylase is a multimer consisting of six α subunits (PCCA) and six β subunits (PCCB), encoded by genes on chromosomes 13q22 and 3q21–q22, respectively. Biotin, the required co-factor, is bound to the α subunit to form the fully functional enzyme. More than 40 mutations in each of the PCC-subunit genes have been described in propionic acidemia patients. There is growing evidence for genotype-phenotype correlations, with null mutations often associated with the most severe clinical outcomes [Clavero et al., 2002; Perez-Cerda et al., 2003].

A deficiency of PCC activity also results from mutations in two other genetic loci encoding enzymes in the biotin use and recycling pathway: holocarboxylase synthase and biotinidase. Primary defects in either enzyme lead to functional deficiencies of all four biotin-requiring carboxylases, including PCC, and are discussed elsewhere in this chapter (see the section on multiple carboxylase deficiencies).

Clinical Manifestations

The clinical presentation of propionic acidemia resembles that of the other so-called ketotic hyperglycinemias, including methylmalonic acidemia and isovaleric acidemia. More than 80 percent of propionic acidemia patients experience acute onset of symptoms within the first 3 months of life [Fenton et al., 2001; Sass et al., 2004a]. Symptoms of severe metabolic decompensation include vomiting, lethargy, and coma, accompanied by severe ketoacidosis, hyperammonemia, hyperglycinemia, and decreased serum carnitine. The disease is often fatal,

particularly if diagnosis and implementation of treatment are delayed. Patients with onset in childhood or in adulthood have been described with episodes of neurologic decompensation associated with periods of ketoacidosis. Even for patients presenting later in life, the metabolic decompensation can be fatal [Lucke et al., 2004]. Patients with late-onset disease have been described with developmental delay or mental retardation but without a history of episodic ketoacidosis or hyperammonemia.

Diagnosis

Urine organic acid analysis reveals a characteristic pattern of metabolite excretion, including 3-hydroxypropionic acid, propionylglycine, methylcitrate, and tiglylglycine. Samples collected during an acute episode can also have massive elevations of lactic, β-hydroxybutyric, and acetoacetic acids. Plasma acylcarnitine profile has markedly elevated propionylcarnitine, with elevations of acetylcarnitine in acute samples, reflecting ketosis. There is often a significant deficiency of free and total carnitine, with an elevated ratio of acylcarnitine to free carnitine. The diagnosis is confirmed by demonstration of deficient PCC activity in cultured fibroblasts. Assays of other carboxylases, including 3-methylcrotonyl-CoA carboxylase and pyruvate carboxylase, can be performed to exclude multiple carboxylase deficiency. Molecular studies for mutations in the PCCA and PCCB genes are available in a limited number of laboratories worldwide.

Because abnormal elevations of propionylcarnitine are readily detected by tandem mass spectrometry, presymptomatic patients with propionic acidemia are identified in states in which expanded newborn screening by tandem mass spectrometry has been implemented. Early diagnosis of these patients, ideally before the onset of symptoms, allows initiation of specific therapies designed to reduce the risk of metabolic decompensation. The long-term outcome of propionic acidemia patients identified in this way has not been established [Leonard et al., 2003]. Some patients with propionic acidemia, particularly those with milder variant forms, have been missed by newborn screening. It is therefore important to maintain a high index of suspicion for patients presenting with symptoms compatible with this or any other organic acidemia, even in the face of normal newborn screening results.

Treatment

Management of propionic acidemia patients during acute episodes is aimed at correcting the acidosis and hyperammonemia, and limiting catabolism of propionate precursors by restricting protein and providing fluids and glucose. If hyperammonemia is severe and persistent, dialysis and ammonia-scavenging medications (e.g., sodium benzoate, sodium phenylacetate) may be necessary.

Long-term management of propionic acidemia consists of carnitine supplementation and a protein-restricted diet that includes supplementation with a special formula. Biotin supplementation has not been demonstrated to be effective [Fenton et al., 2001]. Liver transplantation has been performed in a small number of propionic acidemia patients, with preliminary results indicating a dramatic reduction in the risk for metabolic decompensation with less strict dietary restrictions. The long-term outcome of these patients is unknown [Yorifuji et al., 2004].

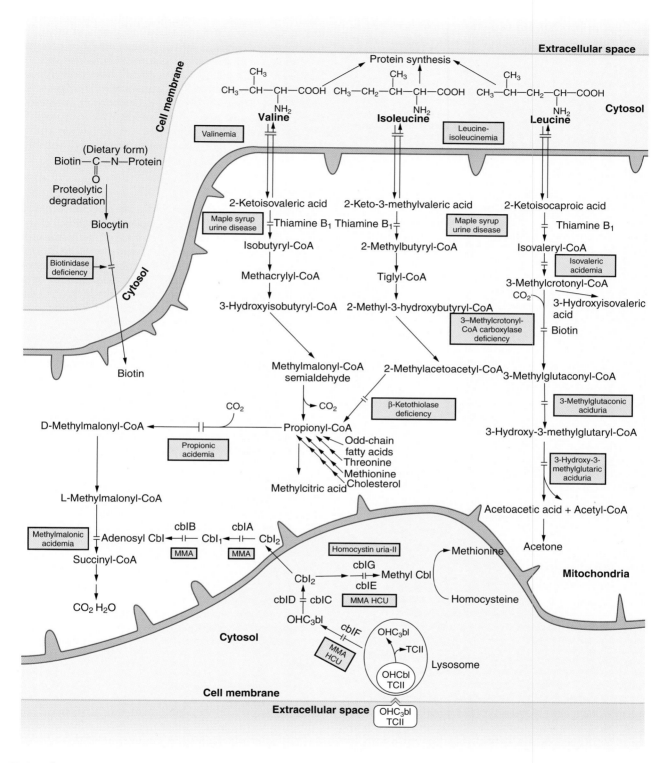

Fig. 32-6 Pathways in the metabolism of the branched-chain amino acids, biotin, and vitamin B₁₂ (cobalamin). Cbl, cobalamin; cbl, defect in metabolism of cobalamin; HCU, homocystinuria; MMA, methylmalonic acidemia; OHCbl, hydroxycobalamin; TC, transcobalamin. *(From Rezvani I. Defects in metabolism of amino acids. In: Behrman R, Kliegman R, Jenson H, eds. Nelson textbook of pediatrics, 16th edn. Philadelphia: WB Saunders, 2000:355.)*

Methylmalonic Acidemias

Several genetic defects can lead to methylmalonic acidemia, in which methylmalonic acid and its derivatives accumulate in physiologic fluids. These conditions are caused by deficiencies in transport and metabolism of vitamin B_{12}, or cobalamin (Cbl), and by mutations in enzymes requiring this co-factor (see Figure 32-6). Because of the variety of causative defects, this group of conditions has significant clinical heterogeneity and differences in response to therapy. Incidence is estimated at 1 case per 50,000 persons [Coulombe et al., 1981].

Pathophysiology

The methylmalonic acidemias can be caused by defects in adenosylcobalamin-dependent methylmalonyl-CoA mutase, intracellular cobalamin metabolism, transcobalamin II deficiency, and intrinsic factor, or by dietary cobalamin deficiency [Fowler, 1998]. Methylmalonyl-CoA mutase isomerizes methylmalonyl-CoA to succinyl-CoA, which then enters the tricarboxylic acid cycle and is converted to pyruvate. Methylmalonyl-CoA is a derivative of propionyl-CoA, which is a metabolite derived from isoleucine, valine, threonine, methionine, thymine, uracil, cholesterol, and odd-chain fatty acids.

The major causes of methylmalonic academia are divided into several different complementation groups: mut0, mut-, CblA, CblB, CblC, CblD, CblF, and CblH [Rosenblatt and Cooper, 1990]. Mutase activity is completely and partially abolished in the mut0 and mut- groups, respectively. Defective adenosylcobalamin synthesis is responsible for CblA, CblB, and CblH. CblC and CblD cause methylmalonic acidemia and homocystinuria because of cobalamin reduction abnormalities that interfere with formation of adenosylcobalamin and methylcobalamin biosynthesis. Abnormal lysosomal transport of cobalamin leads to CblF disease, which also leads to combined methylmalonic acidemia and homocystinuria. CblE and CblG diseases involve defects in homocysteine metabolism; they are discussed in the section on homocystinuria (see "Sulfur Amino Acid Metabolism and the Homocystinurias").

Clinical Manifestations

There is significant variability in presentation, depending on the particular enzymatic deficiency, although several complementation groups share the general characteristics of failure to thrive, developmental delay, megaloblastic anemia, and neurologic dysfunction [Cooper and Rosenblatt, 1987]. Mut0, mut-, CblA, and CblB patients often present in the first few weeks of life with poor feeding, dehydration, increasing lethargy, emesis, and hypotonia [Lindblad et al., 1968; Matsui et al., 1983; Rosenberg et al., 1968]. These patients exhibit a short interval of apparent good health before presentation with symptoms. Metabolic acidosis may be catastrophic. Mild mut- or other forms of methylmalonic acidemia decompensate later in infancy or in childhood with hypoglycemia, acidosis, seizures, and lethargy. A CblC patient can present early in infancy or in later childhood with myopathy, lower-extremity paresthesias, and thrombosis due to homocystinuria [Enns et al., 1999a]. Severely affected children with CblC methylmalonic acidemia can also have ocular abnormalities, such as retinopathy, nystagmus, and worsening vision, as well as hydrocephalus and microcephaly [Rosenblatt et al., 1997]. Cranial imaging usually reveals pathology of the basal ganglia and white matter.

The two initial cases reported with CblD presented in later childhood with mental retardation and behavioral problems, although subsequent reports have documented infantile onset with hypotonia and seizures, and early childhood presentations with ataxia and gait abnormalities [Goodman et al., 1970; Suormala et al., 2004]. CblF patients have been reported to have minor facial anomalies and hematologic defects [Shih et al., 1989]. Transcobalamin II deficiency can manifest as failure to thrive in the first months of life, with neurologic disease and mental retardation [Hall, 1992]. A benign form of methylmalonic acidemia has been reported in otherwise healthy children [Ledley et al., 1984].

Laboratory Tests

Methylmalonic acidemia can clinically resemble other organic acidemias, necessitating analysis of urine organic acids for diagnosis. This test reveals large amounts of methylmalonic acid, as well as methylcitrate, propionic acid, and 3-hydroxypropionic acid [Barness et al., 1963; Rosenberg et al., 1968]. Serum amino acids sometimes demonstrate elevation of glycine and hyperhomocysteinemia in the groups in which methylcobalamin metabolism is affected. Ketosis and hyperammonemia are common. Total plasma homocysteine levels are elevated in CblC, CblD, and CblF diseases. Total and free carnitine levels tend to be low, and acylcarnitine profiles reveal increased propionylcarnitine. The cobalamin transport deficiencies are assessed by measuring serum cobalamin levels and absorption by the Schilling test [Cooper and Rosenblatt, 1987]. Determination of complementation group may be approached by complementation studies in fibroblasts or, in some cases, by direct DNA analysis of genes involved in intracellular cobalamin or methylmalonate metabolism [Adams and Venditti, 2008].

Treatment

During acute metabolic crises, treatment is directed toward limiting catabolism and restricting protein intake. The usual protein intake is stopped, and fluid and glucose are given intravenously. Pharmacologic treatment includes carnitine, intramuscular hydroxocobalamin, metronidazole, or neomycin to decrease intestinal propionate production, betaine, and folate [Ogier de Baulny et al., 1998; Roe and Bohan, 1982; Rosenblatt and Cooper, 1987; Thompson et al., 1990]. Improved growth and enhanced nutrition status are seen in patients with methylmalonic acidemia fed an elemental medical food [Yannicelli et al., 2003]. Patients should consume a diet low in the micronutrient precursors proximal to the metabolic block and with adequate calories and total protein to enable growth. Plasma methylmalonic acid levels are followed for metabolic control [Nyhan et al., 1973].

Several transplantations of liver and kidneys in infants and children with methylmalonic acidemia have been reported. Although this approach seems to protect against metabolic crises, it does not lead to complete biochemical correction [Leonard et al., 2001].

Isovaleric Acidemia

Isovaleric acidemia is a clinically variable disorder that can manifest with early metabolic crises, often leading to coma, or it can result in a later, chronic condition. Patients may be developmentally normal, but mild to severe mental retardation has been reported. Supportive care during crises, and specific treatments such as glycine and carnitine, have helped to improve outcomes. Overall incidence is estimated at less than 1 case per 200,000 persons.

Pathophysiology

Deficiency of the mitochondrial enzyme isovaleryl-CoA dehydrogenase, part of the leucine catabolic pathway (see Figure 32-6), leads to accumulation of several metabolites [Rhead and Tanaka, 1980]. Although the toxicity of individual metabolites is not well understood, isovaleric acid is an inhibitor of the tricarboxylic acid cycle and of hematopoiesis in cultured cells [Bergen et al., 1982; Hutchinson et al., 1985].

Clinical Manifestations

Historically, approximately one-half of reported patients present with an acute neonatal metabolic crisis, and the remainder have chronic, intermittent illness. Both forms result from the same inborn error, and the differences in presentation may reflect the timing of catabolic insults or genetic background. The phenotypes of isovaleric acidemia have more recently been described along a continuum of severity ranging from severely affected to mild or even asymptomatic [Vockley and Ensenauer, 2006].

The acute form occurs in infants who are clinically well at birth but who, within the first several days of life, begin to vomit, refuse feeding, and become listless, dehydrated, and lethargic [Mendiola et al., 1984]. They may have seizures, and the odor of sweaty feet often is detected. Untreated patients progress to coma and often to death, which can be caused by metabolic acidosis or attendant features such as infection [Wilson et al., 1984]. Patients who survive have the chronic, intermittent form of the disease, and they may have normal development. In the chronic form, the first episode occurs during the first year of life after a trigger such as a mild infection or protein load. Recurrent episodes involve vomiting, acidosis with ketonuria, lethargy that can progress to coma, and the cheesy or sweaty feet odor. Most patients with isovaleric acidemia who survive crises intact have normal development, but some have mild delay or even severe mental retardation.

Laboratory Tests

Because clinical features of isovaleric academia can resemble several other conditions, analysis of urine organic acids is necessary. During crises, significant elevations of isovalerylglycine and 3-hydroxyisovaleric acid are seen in urine [Tanaka et al., 1968]. Other laboratory abnormalities include metabolic acidosis with mild to moderate ketonuria and lactic acidemia, and sometimes include hyperammonemia. Hematologic abnormalities, such as thrombocytopenia, neutropenia, and pancytopenia, are common [Kelleher et al., 1980]. Hypocalcemia and hyperglycemia often occur.

Treatment

During crises, treatment should ideally be administered by a metabolic specialist. It is similar to that for other organic acidemias: protein restriction and glucose infusion to decrease protein catabolism. Management during intervening episodes includes protein restriction and supplementation with leucine-free foods. Two targeted treatment options, glycine

and carnitine, conjugate with isovaleryl-CoA and lead to excretion of the nontoxic products [Cohn et al., 1978; Mayatepek et al., 1991].

3-Methylcrotonyl-CoA Carboxylase Deficiency

3-Methylcrotonyl-CoA carboxylase (MCC) deficiency, also known as 3-methylcrotonylglycinuria, is an autosomal-recessive disorder in the catabolic pathway of leucine (see Figure 32-6). MCC is a biotin-requiring enzyme consisting of two nonidentical subunits, α (MCCA) and β (MCCB), with the biotin-binding site located on the α subunit. Mutations have been identified in both subunits in patients with MCC deficiency, defining two complementation groups for this disorder [Baumgartner et al., 2001]. Although isolated MCC deficiency was once thought to be rare, an unexpectedly large number of patients have been identified in tandem mass spectrometry-based newborn screening programs, and the frequency is estimated at 1 case per 50,000 livebirths [Baumgartner et al., 2001]. Like propionyl-CoA carboxylase deficiency, MCC deficiency can arise from defects in the enzymes of the biotin use and recycling pathway: holocarboxylase synthase and biotinidase (see the section on multiple carboxylase deficiencies).

Clinical Manifestations

The clinical presentation of MCC deficiency is highly variable and ranges from apparently benign to severe and life-threatening. The classic presentation is in infancy or childhood, with rare cases occurring in the neonatal period [Bannwart et al., 1992]. Episodes are often associated with a mild infection or other stress, and they involve vomiting, feeding difficulties, lethargy, hypotonia, hyperreflexia, hypoglycemia, metabolic acidosis, and ketosis. Investigations of family members of affected patients have revealed a number of individuals with MCC deficiency with a normal clinical phenotype. MCC deficiency has been described in healthy mothers of infants identified by expanded newborn screening programs with elevated metabolites suggestive of MCC deficiency [Gibson et al., 1998]. Clinical severity, or lack thereof, is not predicted by the severity of MCC mutation or amount of residual MCC activity, in that most mutations identified in patients are associated with absent or severely diminished MCC activity [Desviat et al., 2003].

Diagnosis

The diagnosis of MCC deficiency is established through studies of urine organic acids and plasma acylcarnitine profile, and enzyme assays for MCC in cultured fibroblasts. Abnormalities include the characteristic excretion of 3-hydroxyisovaleric acid and methylcrotonylglycine in urine, and elevation of 3-hydroxyisovalerylcarnitine in plasma. Free carnitine is often significantly decreased, with an elevated ratio of acylcarnitine to free carnitine. Urine acylglycine analysis also reveals elevated excretion of 3-methylcrotonylglycine and is a useful adjunct test. In addition to assays of MCC activity, assays of other carboxylases, including propionyl-CoA carboxylase and pyruvate carboxylase, can be performed to exclude multiple carboxylase deficiency.

Asymptomatic or presymptomatic patients with MCC deficiency are also detected in expanded newborn screening programs as having elevated 3-hydroxyisovalerylcarnitine in dried blood spots [Koeberl et al., 2003]. This finding should be followed with urine organic acid and acylcarnitine studies for the patient and the mother [Gibson et al., 1998].

Treatment

Treatment of acute episodes is aimed at restoring glucose homeostasis and correcting acidosis [Arnold et al., 2008]. Long-term treatment with carnitine supplementation and dietary restriction of leucine has been found to result in normal growth and development [Sweetman and Williams, 2001]. Responsiveness to biotin has been demonstrated in a small number of cases [Baumgartner et al., 2004].

Multiple Carboxylase Deficiencies

The biotin-responsive multiple carboxylase deficiencies include at least two autosomal-recessive disorders with somewhat distinct but overlapping clinical manifestations, referable to enzymopathies affecting the biotinylation of the four mammalian carboxylases. The carboxylases all require biotin for catalytic activity, and include cytosolic acetyl-CoA carboxylase, the rate-limiting step for the de novo synthesis of fatty acids; mitochondrial pyruvate carboxylase, catalyzing the conversion of pyruvate to oxaloacetate, a tricarboxylic acid cycle intermediate and a precursor for gluconeogenesis; mitochondrial methylcrotonyl-CoA carboxylase, catalyzing an intermediate reaction step in leucine catabolism; and mitochondrial propionyl-CoA carboxylase, which catalyzes an intermediate step in the conversion of isoleucine, valine, and other precursors to succinic acid (see Figure 32-6). In each of these enzymes, the biotin is linked to the epsilon amino group of a lysine residue, situated within the highly conserved amino acid sequence of the biotin-binding site. The clinical presentations and metabolic derangements in the multiple carboxylase deficiencies mirror those of primary deficiencies of each of the carboxylases and the clinical features of acquired nutritional biotin deficiency.

The first patient was described in 1971 and was originally reported as having biotin-responsive β-methylcrotonylglycinuria [Gompertz et al., 1971]. A little more than a decade later, two different disorders – biotinidase deficiency, a defect in the recycling of biotin, and holocarboxylase synthase deficiency, a defect in the biotinylation of carboxylases – were characterized.

Biotinidase Deficiency

CLINICAL MANIFESTATIONS

Patients with biotinidase deficiency usually present in early to middle infancy, but they may come to medical attention in very early infancy or in later childhood. Because of the usual age of presentation, biotinidase deficiency was delineated as late-onset or infantile-onset multiple carboxylase deficiency [Packman et al., 1981b; Thoene et al., 1981]. Symptoms may be insidious or acute, and can include lethargy, hypotonia, anorexia or vomiting, developmental delays, ataxia, seizures, and coma. Dermatologic manifestations are a frequent feature and can include alopecia, rashes, and mucocutaneous candidiasis. The rash bears a resemblance to that seen in essential fatty acid deficiency or acrodermatitis enteropathica [Williams et al., 1983]. Hearing loss and optic atrophy can be significant long-term complications that do not uniformly respond to therapy. Patients presenting in later childhood or adolescence can come

to medical attention because of motor weakness and spastic paresis or because of loss of visual acuity [Wolf, 2007]. When studied, neuropathologic findings in biotinidase deficiency have included changes suggestive of Leigh's disease and Wernicke's encephalopathy [Sander et al., 1980]. Such findings are consonant with the notion that neurologic sequelae may result from abnormal intracerebral lactate concentrations [Schurmann et al., 1997].

LABORATORY TESTS

In patients presenting clinically, the aberrant clinical chemistries include metabolic acidosis, with ketosis and lactic acidosis; hypoglycemia; hyperammonemia; and a distinct organic acid pattern that represents the combination of individual carboxylase deficiencies. The organic academia includes propionic acid, 3-hydroxypropionate, methylcitrate, and tiglylglycine, referable to propionyl-CoA carboxylase deficiency; lactic acid (and pyruvic acid and alanine), referable to pyruvate carboxylase deficiency; and 3-methylcrotonate, 3-methylcrotonylglycine, and 3-hydroxyisovaleric acid, referable to the derangement in the methylcrotonyl-CoA carboxylase step. Serum biotinidase activity is markedly deficient, or <10 percent of mean normal activity.

ETIOLOGY

The defect in the infantile-onset form of biotin-responsive multiple carboxylase deficiency was determined by Wolf et al., 1983 to reside in a deficiency of biotinidase activity. Biotinidase is required in the recycling of biotin from carboxylases after the proteolytic degradative turnover of these enzymes (see Figure 32-6). When a carboxylase is hydrolyzed, biotinyl lysine is released, with the biotin remaining bound to the lysine as a compound called biocytin. The release of biotin from biocytin requires the extracellular catalytic activity of biotinidase. In the absence of biotinidase, the cleavage of biocytin does not occur, and biotin is not released for reuse. Biotinidase may also be required for the release of biotin bound to dietary protein, resulting in reduced availability of dietary biotin. The failure to recycle biotin gradually leads to biotin deficiency, a secondary deficiency of biotin-dependent carboxylase activity, and the symptoms of biotinidase deficiency.

Although the focus has been on the consequences of deficiency of the mitochondrial carboxylases, the contribution of acetyl-CoA carboxylase to the clinical manifestations also has been investigated [Gonzalez-Rios et al., 1985b; Packman et al., 1984, 1989; Proud et al., 1990]. Cells deficient in acetyl-CoA carboxylase cannot synthesize malonyl-CoA, required for de novo fatty acid synthesis and fatty acid elongation reactions. In such cells, the fatty acid pattern and composition of membranes and structural elements is abnormal, leading to speculation that such alterations may contribute to the dermatitis [Munnich et al., 1980], to the immunologic derangements reported in a number of patients [Cowan et al., 1979], and to some components of the neurologic manifestations.

DIAGNOSIS

A small but significant fraction of cases ascertained because of clinical symptoms may not demonstrate the characteristic organic aciduria. Accordingly, serum biotinidase activity should be measured in any patient with features – especially cutaneous and neurologic features – that are consistent with biotinidase deficiency. Assay of serum biotinidase is a test with wide clinical availability.

All states in the U.S. and many countries worldwide have incorporated biotinidase testing on filter paper blood spots in state-sponsored newborn screening programs. Ascertainment of biotinidase deficiency in such newborn screening programs has led to the identification of two broad clinical cohorts of patients: those with profound biotinidase deficiency (less than 10 percent of control subjects) and children with partial biotinidase deficiency (10–30 percent of control subjects) [Wolf, 1991]. The combined incidence of profound and partial deficiency is estimated at 1 in 60,000, with the two forms each having approximately equal incidences. The natural history of partial deficiency is not entirely known. Because there are reports of patients with partial deficiency who have become symptomatic, it has been suggested that treatment for partial deficiency might be indicated [McVoy et al., 1990; Wolf, 2010].

TREATMENT

Patients with biotinidase deficiency can be treated with pharmacologic dosages of biotin of 5–20 mg/day. Children with partial biotinidase deficiency have been treated with somewhat lower dosages of 1–5 mg/day. With treatment, the biochemical derangements (including the lactic acidosis) resolve, the dermatologic manifestations rapidly resolve, developmental delays are ameliorated or reversed, and there is often resolution of seizures and ataxia. Hearing loss and visual loss may remain as long-term complications and be refractory to treatment. The presymptomatic treatment of patients identified by newborn screening prevents the onset of symptoms.

Holocarboxylase Synthase Deficiency

CLINICAL MANIFESTATIONS

Children with holocarboxylase synthase deficiency generally present in the first several days or weeks of life with severe and life-threatening metabolic encephalopathy. The clinical course is variably marked by irritability, lethargy, feeding problems, vomiting, tachypnea, hypertonia or hypotonia, and progression to seizures and coma. The timing of the acute presentation led to the initial characterization of patients as representing a neonatal-onset form of multiple carboxylase deficiency [Packman et al., 1981a, 1984]. Patients with milder forms of holocarboxylase synthase deficiency present later or have a more protracted clinical course [Packman et al., 1984]. These children may have alopecia, rash, ataxia, and developmental delays, a clinical presentation that overlaps that of biotinidase deficiency.

LABORATORY TESTS

Abnormal clinical laboratory findings include metabolic acidosis (e.g., lactic acidosis, ketosis), hyperammonemia, evidence of the bone marrow toxicity of organic acidemias (e.g., thrombocytopenia), and the characteristic organic aciduria of multiple carboxylase deficiencies: 3-methylcrotonylglycine, 3-hydroxyisovalerate, lactate, 3-hydroxypropionate, methylcitrate, and tiglylglycine.

ETIOLOGY

The basic defect is in the activity of the enzyme holocarboxylase synthase [Burri et al., 1981], which catalyzes a two-step reaction that results in the covalent binding of biotin to apocarboxylases. All patients with deficient holocarboxylase synthase activity have shown detectable residual activity. Multiple mutations have been identified, with most resulting in the synthesis of an enzyme with an elevated Michaelis–Menten dissociation constant (K_M) for biotin. Some patients have mutations that result in a normal K_M for biotin but a reduced value for maximum velocity of enzyme-catalyzed reactions (V_{max}). These observations have led to speculation that a complete absence of holocarboxylase synthase activity might be lethal [Wolf, 2007].

DIAGNOSIS

Holocarboxylase synthase assay can be performed in cultured fibroblasts or lymphocytes and in amniotic fluid cells [Packman et al., 1982]. A more widespread clinical approach involves measurements of individual carboxylase activities in fibroblasts cultured in low-biotin medium and in high-biotin medium. If the cells are grown in low-biotin medium, individual carboxylase activities will be low, but the activities will be normal or approach normal levels if the cells are grown in high-biotin medium. This assay result contrasts with that for biotinidase deficiency fibroblasts, which demonstrates normal activities, whether grown in high- or low-biotin culture medium [Packman et al., 1984].

Prenatal diagnosis is performed by assay of carboxylases in amniocytes or chorionic villi [Packman et al., 1982; Thuy et al., 1999a], or by molecular identification of mutations in the *HLCS* gene [Malvagia et al., 2005]. As an adjunct to enzymatic assay and to achieve a rapid result, it is possible to measure the concentration of accumulating analytes (e.g., 3-hydroxyisovalerate, methylcitrate) in amniotic fluid, by stable isotope dilution analysis [Jakobs et al., 1984], but such studies may not be conclusive [Thuy et al., 1999b]. In two pregnancies, prenatal treatment by administration of biotin to the mother during pregnancy [Packman et al., 1982; Roth et al., 1982] was successfully performed in paradigmatic studies of the application and efficacy of co-factor therapy in such settings.

TREATMENT

Patients respond well to oral biotin in pharmacologic doses. Generally, the starting dose is 10 mg/day. However, the K_M for biotin can range from 3 to 70 times normal [Wolf, 2007]. Some patients may require a higher dose, because the mutant enzyme has a higher K_M for biotin. There is also a suggestion that patients with mutant holocarboxylase synthase enzymes exhibiting a reduced V_{max} may have a poorer response to biotin therapy than those with K_M values for biotin mutations [Sakamoto et al., 1999]. Accordingly, careful monitoring of clinical status (including neurologic and cutaneous manifestations), of organic acid levels (including lactate), and of conventional clinical chemistries (i.e., ammonia, electrolytes, and ketones) is mandatory to arrive at optimal dosing of biotin. After treatment levels have been achieved, no dietary restrictions are required.

3-Methylglutaconic Aciduria

At least four different conditions have the common feature of abnormal urinary excretion of 3-methylglutaconic acid, and they are designated as 3-methyglutaconic aciduria types I, II,

III, and IV. The metabolite 3-methylglutaconic acid occurs in the leucine catabolic pathway and is converted by 3-methylglu-taconyl-CoA hydratase to 3-hydroxy-3-methylglutaric acid, leading ultimately to ketone body formation and the production of cholesterol precursors. The clinical features, diagnosis, and treatment approaches for each type of 3-methylglutaconic aciduria are discussed in the following sections.

Type I: Primary 3-Methylglutaconyl-CoA Hydratase Deficiency

Primary 3-methylglutaconyl-CoA hydratase deficiency is a rare, autosomal-recessive disorder caused by mutations in the 3-methylglutaconyl-CoA hydratase gene (*AUH*) and characterized by abnormal urinary excretion of 3-methylglutaconic and 3-hydroxyisovaleric acids. The 3-hydroxyisovaleric acid levels are not elevated in the other three types of 3-methylglutaconylaciduria. In the small number of patients reported with this disorder, the spectrum of clinical abnormalities ranges from mild to extremely severe. Although the presentation varies, many patients have had retardation, acidosis, hypoglycemia, hypotonia, and seizures. Suspicion of the diagnosis is raised by the characteristic pattern of urine organic acid excretion, and it is confirmed by assays for the 3-methylglutaconyl-CoA hydratase activity in cultured fibroblasts. Molecular studies to identify mutations in the *AUH* gene are available in only a limited number of laboratories. Treatment with leucine restriction or L-carnitine supplementation may be effective in some patients [Sweetman and Williams, 2001].

Type II: Barth Syndrome

Barth's syndrome, also known as X-linked cardioskeletal myopathy and neutropenia, is characterized by mitochondrial abnormalities and abnormal excretion of 3-methylglutaconic acid. Barth's syndrome is caused by mutations in the G4.5 gene (*TAZ*), which produces, through alternate splicing, a class of proteins called the tafazzins. Tafazzins are mitochondrial proteins thought to play a role in the structure and function of cardiolipin, a membrane lipid required for proper functioning of the mitochondrial electron transport chain. Clinically, cardiomyopathy and skeletal muscle weakness are usually apparent in affected males in the first year of life. Neutropenia can vary from mild to severe, even within the same patient. Many patients die before they are 4 years old, although some reports suggest an improvement in survival rates due to increased awareness of the diagnosis and more aggressive management of cardiomyopathy and infections [Barth et al., 2004]. No specific symptoms have been identified in heterozygous females, and there is no effective treatment for Barth's syndrome.

Type III: Costeff Optic Atrophy Syndrome

Costeff's syndrome is a rare, autosomal-recessive disorder characterized by early-onset bilateral optic atrophy and choreiform movement disorder, and by variable later-onset spasticity and mental retardation. Excretion of 3-methylglutaconic and 3-methylglutaric acids is moderately elevated, and the activity of 3-methylglutaconyl-CoA hydratase is normal. This disorder was once thought to be confined to patients of Iraqi Jewish background, but it has been described in non-Iraqi Jews [Kleta et al., 2002]. Linkage studies of large Iraqi Jewish families have identified mutations in the *OPA3* gene, which encodes a protein of unknown function, as being the underlying cause of the disorder [Anikster et al., 2001]. Suspicion of the diagnosis is raised on clinical grounds and confirmed by urine organic acid analysis. No effective treatment is available [Sweetman and Williams, 2001].

Type IV: Unclassified

The type IV 3-methyglutaconic acidurias constitute a heterogeneous group of disorders. Patients share the common features of abnormal excretion and normal 3-methylglutaconyl-CoA hydratase activity. The abnormal 3-methylglutaconic aciduria may result from a variety of causes, possibly affecting energy metabolism. The varied clinical features include severe psychomotor retardation, cerebellar dysgenesis, neonatal hypotonia, absent reflexes, and optic atrophy. No specific treatment is available [Sweetman and Williams, 2001].

Beta-Ketothiolase Deficiency

Inherited β-ketothiolase deficiency, also known as mitochondrial acetoacetyl-CoA thiolase deficiency, is a rare autosomal-recessive disorder caused by defects in mitochondrial acetoacetyl-CoA thiolase, also known as β-ketothiolase, T2, or 3-oxothiolase (see Figure 32-6). This enzyme participates in the pathways of ketone body and isoleucine metabolism. It is related to, but distinct from, four other β-ketothiolase enzymes that participate in reactions of mitochondrial β-oxidation of short- and medium-chain fatty acids, cholesterol synthesis, and peroxisomal β-oxidation. Numerous mutations in the mitochondrial acetoacetyl-CoA thiolase gene (*ACAT1*) have been described in patients, with some completely abolishing β-ketothiolase activity and others associated with significant residual activity. The degree of clinical severity does not appear to be associated with the molecular severity of mutation nor the degree of residual activity [Fukao et al., 2001, 2003].

Clinical Manifestations

There is wide clinical variability associated with β-ketothiolase deficiency, with most patients presenting with acute ketoacidosis between 5 and 24 months. Attacks are often accompanied by moderate hyperammonemia and hyperglycinemia. Patients are typically well between episodes, with attacks often precipitated by an intercurrent illness or other stress. A small number of patients have been reported with dystonia, which reflects basal ganglia damage, and with mental retardation [Mitchell and Fukao, 2001]. A β-ketothiolase deficiency has been described in asymptomatic siblings of affected patients.

Diagnosis

Urine organic acid analysis of patients with β-ketothiolase deficiency reveals a characteristic pattern of 2-methyl-3-hydroxybutyric and 2-methylacetoacetic acids, with variable excretion of 2-butanone and tiglylglycine. The diagnosis is confirmed by assays for β-ketothiolase activity in lymphocytes or cultured fibroblasts [Mitchell and Fukao, 2001].

Treatment

Treatment of acute episodes is aimed at correcting ketoacidosis with fluids, glucose, and carnitine supplementation, and includes careful monitoring of plasma ammonia, glucose, and electrolytes. Patients are managed long-term with normal or slightly reduced protein intake and with careful monitoring of urine ketones during mild intercurrent illnesses. With appropriate treatment, the long-term prognosis is excellent for those patients in whom neurologic damage has not occurred before diagnosis [Mitchell and Fukao, 2001].

Canavan's Disease

Canavan's disease, also known as spongy degeneration of the brain, is an autosomal-recessive disorder caused by a deficiency of aspartoacylase (or *N*-acyl-L-aspartate amidohydrolase). This enzyme catalyzes the hydrolysis of *N*-acetyl-L-aspartic acid (NAA) to aspartic acid and acetic acid, and is particularly abundant in white matter of the brain. NAA itself is found only in the CNS, and its function is largely unknown [Beaudet, 2001]. Although the disorder is pan-ethnic, it occurs more frequently among patients of Ashkenazi Jewish descent, for whom the carrier frequency is estimated at 1 case per 40 persons. Two specific aspartoacylase mutations, E285A and Y231X, account for most of the disease alleles.

Clinical Manifestations

Patients with Canavan's disease are typically normal for the first 1–2 months of life, but then develop hypotonia, poor head control, poor contact, and seizures, as well as macrocephaly and loss of early milestones. In most patients, neurologic abnormalities and macrocephaly are apparent by 6 months of age. Imaging studies demonstrate severe changes in the subcortical white matter and the lower layers of the gray matter, with relative sparing of the central white matter. Later features of the disorder may include spasticity, opisthotonus, and decerebrate or decorticate posturing. Most patients die within the first 3 years of life, although a small number of cases have been reported with later onset and a milder or more variable course [Beaudet, 2001].

Diagnosis

The diagnosis of Canavan's disease is suspected on the basis of clinical evaluation and neuroimaging studies (Figure 32-7), and confirmed by urine organic acid analysis and the demonstration of abnormal excretion of NAA. Enzyme assays for aspartoacylase activity are available in only a small number of laboratories worldwide and are typically unnecessary to establish a diagnosis. Molecular analysis for common aspartoacylase mutations in the Jewish and European populations can be used for confirmation of the diagnosis and carrier testing of family members. Prenatal diagnosis can be performed by DNA analysis in cases where parental mutations are known. Prenatal diagnosis has also been performed through assays of aspartoacylase activity in chorionic villi or amniocytes, or NAA levels in amniotic fluid, but these approaches have been shown to be unreliable in a number of cases [Beaudet, 2001].

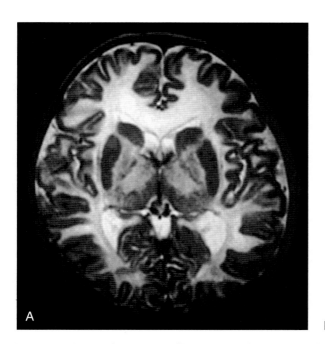

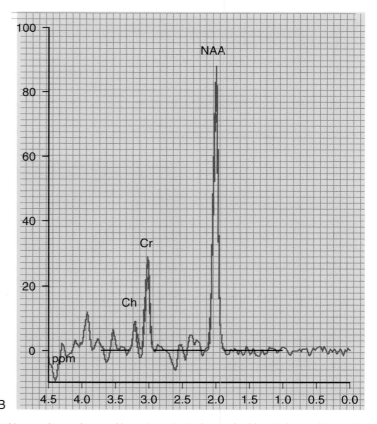

Fig. 32-7 Patient with Canavan's disease. A, Axial view, T2-weighted image shows abnormal hyperintensity in the cerebral hemispheric white matter, globus pallidi, and thalami. **B,** Proton MR spectroscopy (echo time of 288 msec) shows a markedly increased *N*-acetyl-L-aspartic acid (NAA) peak. *(From Barkovich AJ. Pediatric neuroimaging, 4th edn. Philadelphia: Lippincott Williams & Wilkins, 2005.)*

Treatment

There is no known treatment for Canavan's disease. The American College of Obstetrics and Gynecology (ACOG) has recommended that molecular carrier testing for Canavan's disease be offered to all Ashkenazi Jewish patients [American College of Obstetrics and Gynecology, 2004]. Such carrier screening programs are aimed at disease prevention through the identification of couples at risk of having an affected child. As with similar screening programs for Tay–Sachs disease, this is expected to reduce the occurrence of infants with Canavan's disease born in this population dramatically.

Glutaric Aciduria Type 1

In 1975, Goodman et al., 1975 described glutaric acidemia and aciduria in siblings with a neurodegenerative disorder beginning in infancy and characterized by opisthotonus, dystonia, and athetosis. Glutaric acidemia type 1, also known as glutaryl-CoA dehydrogenase deficiency, is an autosomal-recessive condition caused by deficiency of glutaryl-CoA dehydrogenase activity and has an estimated prevalence of approximately 1 case per 100,000 persons [Lindner et al., 2004]. Glutaric acidemia type 1 is relatively common in the Old Order Amish in Lancaster County, Pennsylvania. Glutaric acidemia type 2 (i.e., multiple acyl-CoA dehydrogenase deficiency) is associated with defects in mitochondrial electron transfer flavoprotein or electron transfer flavoprotein dehydrogenase, and is discussed further in Chapter 37. Glutaryl-CoA dehydrogenase is a key enzyme in the degradation pathway for lysine, hydroxylysine, and tryptophan. Deficiency results in accumulation of glutarate and, to a lesser extent, of 3-hydroxyglutarate and glutaconate in body tissues, blood, cerebrospinal fluid, and urine.

Glutaric acidemia type 1 is characterized by irreversible focal striatal necrosis after an acute illness, most often between the ages of 3 and 18 months. Affected children often have macrocephaly, dystonia, and dyskinesia [Strauss et al., 2003]. Macrocephaly may not be present at birth, but head growth velocity is increased [Hoffmann et al., 1996]. Intraretinal hemorrhages and subdural effusions may be mistaken for nonaccidental injury [Morris et al., 1999]. In some cases, the presentation is insidious, with gradual appearance of symptoms [Hoffmann et al., 1996]. Systemic manifestations typical of many other organic acidemias, such as pronounced metabolic ketoacidosis, hypoglycemia, and hyperammonemia, do not occur [Hoffmann et al., 1996; Kyllerman et al., 2004; Strauss et al., 2003]. There appears to be a window of neurologic susceptibility to damage during the first years of life. Striatal injury is rarely encountered after age 3 years, although initial presentation as late as age 19 years has been described [Bahr et al., 2002; Strauss and Morton, 2003b].

The most characteristic head MRI finding in symptomatic children is symmetric widening of the sylvian fissure with poor operculization ("bat wing" appearance) caused by frontotemporal atrophy or hypoplasia (Figure 32-8). Other features include basal ganglia injury, subdural effusions, ventriculomegaly, and delayed myelination [Neumaier-Probst et al., 2004]. Diffusion-weighted imaging may be more sensitive in demonstrating brain lesions than CT or MRI [Elster, 2004].

Urine organic acid analysis often documents highly elevated glutarate and lesser elevations of 3-hydroxyglutarate and glutaconate, but some children with a classic phenotype have low or undetectable levels of these metabolites (so-called low excretors) [Baric et al., 1999]. Newborn screening using tandem mass spectrometry has the potential for presymptomatic detection of glutaric acidemia type 1, although the existence of a low-excretor phenotype will undoubtedly result in missed cases [Lindner et al., 2004; Gallagher et al., 2005]]. In a study of 215 patients, complete absence of glutaryl-CoA dehydrogenase activity was found in more than 50 percent, whereas 34 percent had residual activity up to 5 percent, and a few had residual activity between 5 and 15 percent [Christensen et al., 2004]. Some correlations between severity of mutation and biochemical parameters have been established (e.g., patients with at least one mild mutation frequently have a low-excretor phenotype). However, no correlation between clinical outcome and genotype or biochemical phenotype has been established [Christensen et al., 2004].

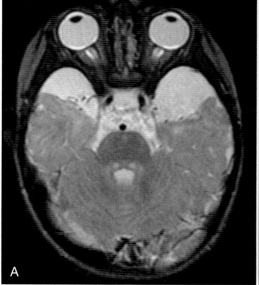 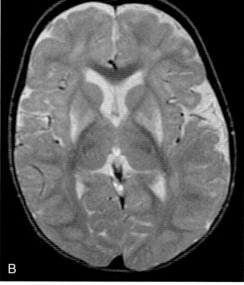

Fig. 32-8 MRI in glutaric acidemia. A, Axial view, T2-weighted image shows markedly enlarged sylvian fissures bilaterally and abnormal hyperintensity of the central tegmental tract. **B,** Axial view, T2-weighted image at a slightly higher level shows abnormal hyperintensity of the lentiform nuclei bilaterally. *(Courtesy of Dr. A James Barkovich, University of California, San Francisco, CA.)*

Increased glutarate and 3-hydroxyglutarate levels may induce an imbalance in glutamatergic and GABAergic neurotransmission by inhibiting glutamate decarboxylase, the key enzyme in gamma-aminobutyric acid (GABA) synthesis, or through direct damage to striatal GABAergic neurons [Kolker et al., 2004]. 3-Hydroxyglutarate may mimic the excitatory neurotransmitter glutamate and thereby cause excitotoxic cell damage mediated through activation of NMDA receptors [Kolker et al., 2004]. Glutarate inhibits synaptosomal uptake of glutamic acid and produces striatal lesions when injected directly into rat brain [Goodman, 2004]. Other potential contributors to neurotoxicity include cytokine-induced cell damage, mitochondrial dysfunction, increased production of reactive oxygen species, and production of toxic quinolinic acid, an intermediate in tryptophan metabolism in brain [Goodman, 2004; Strauss and Morton, 2003b]. Other reports have emphasized the relatively weak neurotoxicity of glutarate and 3-hydroxyglutarate in animal models and primary neuronal cell cultures. The pathogenesis of striatal necrosis and brain lesions in glutaric acidemia type 1 remains the subject of intensive investigation [Freudenberg et al., 2004; Lund et al., 2004]. Animal models may help resolve these conflicting results.

Treatment of glutaric acidemia type 1 is based on restriction of protein and lysine intake, carnitine and riboflavin supplementation, and rapid intervention in times of intercurrent illness [Muhlhausen et al., 2004]. Antioxidants and creatine have theoretical therapeutic advantages, but such compounds are not routinely used [Muhlhausen et al., 2004; Strauss et al., 2003]. Despite early identification and aggressive management, permanent neurologic damage occurs in approximately one-third of patients [Strauss and Morton, 2003b]. Anticholinergic drugs, such as trihexyphenidyl, and botulinum toxin are beneficial in treating generalized or focal dystonia in patients with glutaric acidemia type 1 [Burlina et al., 2004]. Stereotactic pallidotomy has been performed in three children, with one improving only slightly [Muhlhausen et al., 2004; Rakocevic et al., 2004].

5-Oxoprolinuria

Glutathione (L-γ-glutamyl-L-cysteinylglycine) is a key component in cellular protection from oxidant damage. 5-Oxoprolinuria (i.e., pyroglutamic aciduria) may be caused by defects in enzymes involved in the synthesis and degradation of glutathione, including glutathione synthetase and 5-oxoprolinase, or as a secondary finding in a variety of conditions that are associated with glutathione depletion, including inborn errors of metabolism unrelated to the glutathione cycle (e.g., methylmalonic acidemia, propionic acidemia, urea cycle defects, hepatorenal tyrosinemia, mitochondrial disorders), certain medication exposure (e.g., vigabatrin, acetaminophen, antibiotics), severe burns, multi-organ failure, and malnutrition [Mayatepek, 1999].

Glutathione synthetase deficiency is an autosomal-recessive condition that features massive urine excretion of 5-oxoproline. Clinical manifestations include metabolic acidosis, mental retardation, ataxia, spasticity, seizures, psychiatric disturbances, recurrent bacterial infections, and hemolytic anemia [Ristoff et al., 2001]. Ophthalmologic findings, consisting of minor lens opacities, granular retinal hyperpigmentation, and abnormal electroretinography, were found in two sisters with glutathione synthetase deficiency [Larsson et al., 1985]. Head imaging may reveal brain atrophy [Al-Jishi et al., 1999]. Mild, moderate, and severe phenotypes have been described [Ristoff et al., 2001]. Postmortem examination has revealed generalized cerebellar atrophy, caused by a diffuse loss of granule cells, and ventriculomegaly, especially of the fourth ventricle [Skullerud et al., 1980]. Although patients with 5-oxoprolinase deficiency also excrete large amounts of 5-oxoproline, they are typically asymptomatic. The detection of developmental delay in some patients with 5-oxoprolinase deficiency may reflect ascertainment bias.

The excessive urinary excretion of 5-oxoproline should be detected easily on urine organic acid analysis. 5-Oxoproline is derived from increased synthesis of γ-glutamylcysteine, and it is present in amounts that exceed the normal capacity of 5-oxoprolinase to convert it to glutamate [Wellner et al., 1974]. Definitive diagnosis is made by measuring erythrocyte glutathione synthetase activity or DNA analysis, or both. Varieties of missense and splice site mutations have been found in the *GSS* gene [Shi et al., 1996].

Treatment of glutathione synthetase deficiency includes correction of metabolic acidosis and high-dose supplementation with vitamins C and E [Ristoff et al., 2001]. Supplementation with *N*-acetylcysteine may also increase levels of plasma and leukocyte glutathione and may be of therapeutic benefit [Jain et al., 1994; Martensson et al., 1989]. Patients with glutathione synthetase deficiency should avoid medications associated with hemolytic crises in glucose-6-phosphate dehydrogenase deficiency.

Isobutyryl-CoA Dehydrogenase Deficiency

Isobutyryl-CoA dehydrogenase deficiency is an autosomal-recessive disorder of valine metabolism that was first described by Roe et al., 1998. Defective enzyme activity results in impairment of the conversion of isobutyryl-CoA to methylacrylyl-CoA. The initial patient was a developmentally normal 2-year-old girl who developed a dilated cardiomyopathy at age 11 months. She had profound carnitine deficiency, and after carnitine supplementation, acylcarnitine analysis detected markedly increased levels of butyrylcarnitine and isobutyrylcarnitine. Urine organic acids were normal [Roe et al., 1998]. Mutations in the *ACAD8* gene were later identified in this patient [Nguyen et al., 2002]. Tandem mass spectrometry newborn screening has identified asymptomatic children [Sass et al., 2004b]. It is uncertain whether children are at risk for serious clinical sequelae or whether therapy is needed.

3-Hydroxyisobutyric Aciduria

3-Hydroxyisobutyric aciduria is a rare autosomal-recessive disorder of valine metabolism; the deficient enzyme has not been identified. The initial patient had repeated episodes of ketoacidosis, failure to thrive, and chronic lactic acidemia [Ko et al., 1991]. Microcephaly, dysmorphic facial features (i.e., short, sloped forehead; telecanthus; down-slanting palpebral fissures; long, prominent philtrum; and micrognathia), seizures, cerebral dysgenesis, brain atrophy, focal white matter abnormalities, and intracerebral calcification have also been described [Chitayat et al., 1992; Sasaki et al., 2001]. This condition has been misdiagnosed as cerebral palsy [Sasaki et al., 2001]. Although most patients have had prominent mental retardation, mild disease and normal intelligence have been reported [Boulat et al., 1995]. Treatment with carnitine and dietary valine and protein restriction appear to be beneficial [Ko et al., 1991; Sasaki et al., 2001].

2-Methylbutyryl-CoA Dehydrogenase Deficiency

2-Methylbutyryl-CoA dehydrogenase deficiency is also known as short- or branched-chain acyl-CoA dehydrogenase deficiency. 2-Methylbutyryl-CoA dehydrogenase catalyzes the conversion of 2-methylbutyryl-CoA to tiglyl-CoA in the isoleucine degradative pathway [Korman, 2006]. Deficiency of this enzyme leads to increased 2-methylbutyrylglycine and 2-methylbutyrlycarnitine in physiologic fluids. A neonate with metabolic acidosis, hypoglycemia, and apnea was the initial reported case. MRI demonstrates ischemic changes bilaterally in parietal and occipital lobes, with increased signal intensity in the lentiform nuclei [Gibson et al., 2000]. Motor delay, strabismus, and generalized muscular atrophy developed during the second year of life in another patient [Andresen et al., 2000]. Tandem mass spectrometry newborn screening identified elevated 5-carbon-saturated acylcarnitine species in eight children of Hmong ancestry. All were treated with a low-protein diet and carnitine supplementation. All patients remained asymptomatic at ages 3–14 months, except for one who developed mild hypotonia [Matern et al., 2003].

Mevalonate Kinase Deficiency

Deficiency of mevalonate kinase, an essential enzyme in cholesterol and nonsterol isoprenoid biosynthesis, leads to two distinct clinical phenotypes:
1. mevalonic aciduria and hyperimmunoglobulinemia D
2. periodic fever syndrome (HIDS).

Both disorders are inherited as autosomal-recessive traits. As abnormal isoprenoid synthesis can lead to fever and inflammation, these conditions are classified as autoinflammatory disorders [Houten et al., 2003].

Mevalonic aciduria is characterized by psychomotor retardation, failure to thrive, dysmorphic features (i.e., dolichocephaly, frontal bossing, down-slanting palpebral fissures, and low-set, posteriorly rotated ears), and intercurrent episodes of crisis that feature high fever, vomiting, and diarrhea. Severe cerebellar atrophy and associated ataxia are common. Ocular involvement (e.g., cataracts, retinal dystrophy), hypotonia, mild hepatosplenomegaly, and cholestatic liver disease also occur [Hoffmann et al., 1993]. Recurrent febrile crises tend to decrease with advancing age and are not present in all cases.

Patients with HIDS have lifelong recurrent febrile episodes, lymphadenopathy, splenomegaly, arthralgias, and rashes that begin in infancy. HIDS is not associated with neurologic impairment, and patients are typically asymptomatic in between episodes of fever. Because phenotypic overlap between mevalonic aciduria and HIDS exists, these conditions most likely represent a continuous spectrum of disease, rather than two distinct entities [Simon et al., 2004].

Mevalonic aciduria is diagnosed by detecting elevated mevalonic acid on urine organic acid analysis. Standard clinical chemical investigations find normal or slightly reduced cholesterol and elevated creatine kinase levels, especially during crises [Hoffmann et al., 1993]. Although the level of serum immunoglobulin D may be elevated in mevalonic aciduria, this finding is not invariable. An elevated serum IgD level is a marker for HIDS. Mild elevations of urine mevalonic acid may occur in HIDS during attacks [Cuisset et al., 2001]. Analyzing mevalonate kinase activity in lymphoblasts or using direct DNA analysis can confirm the diagnosis. Most patients are compound heterozygotes for mutant alleles. Some mutations are common to mevalonic aciduria and HIDS [Cuisset et al., 2001].

Treatment for both conditions is largely supportive. Oral cholesterol supplementation, alone or with various combinations of ursodeoxycholic acid, ubiquinone, and vitamin E, did not result in improvement of clinical or biochemical parameters. Lovastatin administration has resulted in the development of severe clinical crises, but some patients have responded dramatically to corticosteroid therapy during acute clinical crises [Hoffmann et al., 1993].

Inborn Errors of Urea Synthesis

Uta Lichter-Konecki and Mark L. Batshaw

Inherited urea cycle disorders represent a devastating group of inborn errors of metabolism that are associated with hyperammonemic encephalopathy and high mortality and morbidity rates. They comprise deficiencies in any of the six enzymes and two amino acid transporters involved in urea synthesis (Figure 33-1). Accordingly, these disorders are named as follows (estimated prevalence rates are given) [Brusilow and Maestri, 1996; Tuchman, 1992; Yamanouchi et al., 2002]:

- *N*-acetylglutamate synthase (NAGS) deficiency (prevalence unknown)
- carbamyl phosphate synthetase I (CPS I) deficiency (1 case per 62,000 population)
- ornithine transcarbamylase (OTC) deficiency (1 per 14,000)
- citrullinemia type II (mitochondrial aspartate/glutamate transport carrier [citrin] deficiency) (1 per 21,000 in Japan)
- argininosuccinate synthetase (ASS) deficiency (citrullinemia) (1 per 57,000)
- argininosuccinate lyase (ASL) deficiency (argininosuccinicaciduria) (1 per 70,000)
- arginase (ARG) deficiency (hyperargininemia) (1 per 353,000)
- hyperornithinemia-hyperammonemia-homocitrullinuria (HHH) syndrome (mitochondrial ornithine carrier deficiency) (prevalence unknown).

These disorders are inherited as autosomal-recessive traits, except for ornithine transcarbamylase deficiency, which is X-linked. Because of the absence of mass newborn screening for these disorders, the true incidence of urea cycle disorders is unknown. Based on case reports and questionnaires about referred patients, the combined prevalence of all urea cycle disorders is estimated to be 1 per 8200 [Brusilow and Maestri, 1996].

Other than in arginase deficiency, infants with a complete deficiency of a urea cycle enzyme (*N*-acetylglutamate synthase, CPS I, ornithine transcarbamylase, argininosuccinate synthetase, or argininosuccinate lyase) commonly present in the newborn period with hyperammonemic coma. Despite aggressive treatment that relies primarily on hemodialysis, the mortality rate in infancy has been reported to approximate 50 percent [Maestri et al., 1999], and as demonstrated by our previous studies, virtually all of the survivors are left with developmental disabilities [Msall et al., 1984; Krivitzky et al., 2009]. Patients with late-onset disease (those with partial enzyme deficiencies, including ornithine transcarbamylase-deficient female heterozygotes) may present at any age with hyperammonemic crises that carry a 10 percent mortality rate and a significant risk of intellectual disabilities [Batshaw et al., 1986]. Even asymptomatic ornithine transcarbamylase-deficient heterozygotes have been shown to have mild cognitive deficits [Batshaw et al., 1980; Gyato et al., 2004].

The Urea Cycle

Dietary protein, on average, contains approximately 16 percent nitrogen. More than 90 percent of the nitrogen that is not used for anabolic processes normally is metabolized and excreted as urea. Therefore, substantial urea synthesis capacity (approximately 16 g per day in adults) is required [Linder, 1985]. With a deficiency of one of the urea cycle enzymes, an insufficient amount of urea will be formed, and nitrogen in the form of ammonia will accumulate. Accumulation in brain causes altered mental status and encephalopathy.

The urea cycle was proposed by Hans Krebs and Kurt Henseleit in 1932, and was the first cyclic pathway elucidated. Six enzymes, one co-factor, and two transporters are necessary for optimal urea cycle activity (see Figure 33-1). The clinically most important co-factor is *N*-acetylglutamate, which is formed from acetyl coenzyme A (acetyl-CoA) and glutamate in a reaction catalyzed by *N*-acetylglutamate synthase. *N*-acetylglutamate activates the first enzyme of the urea cycle, carbamyl phosphate synthetase I, which uses adenosine triphosphate, bicarbonate, and glutamine or ammonia to synthesize carbamyl phosphate, contributing the first atom of waste nitrogen to the cycle. Carbamyl phosphate synthetase I is expressed in periportal hepatocytes and intestinal mucosa epithelial cells [Ryall et al., 1985]. It is the most abundant protein in liver mitochondria, accounting for 20 percent of the mitochondrial matrix protein [Lusty, 1978]. The enzyme consists of a single polypeptide with a molecular weight of 165,000 and approximately 1500 amino acid residues [Haraguchi et al., 1991].

The second enzyme in the urea cycle, ornithine transcarbamylase, like CPS I, is mitochondrial. Citrulline is formed by the action of ornithine transcarbamylase on carbamyl phosphate and ornithine. Once formed, citrulline is actively moved, by means of the ornithine transporter, out of the mitochondrion and into the cytosol, where it is conjugated with aspartate to form argininosuccinic acid by argininosuccinate synthetase. Here the second atom of waste nitrogen is contributed to the cycle by aspartate. A defect in argininosuccinate synthetase leads to citrullinemia, the accumulation of citrulline in blood. A second form of citrullinemia called type II or citrin deficiency is caused by deficient activity of the mitochondrial aspartate/glutamate carrier, citrin, which facilitates the exchange of aspartate for glutamate and a proton across the inner mitochondrial membrane. Argininosuccinic acid subsequently is cleaved to yield fumarate and arginine by the enzyme argininosuccinate lyase. A deficiency of this enzyme is called argininosuccinicaciduria, characterized by marked urinary excretion (and accumulation in blood) of argininosuccinic acid.

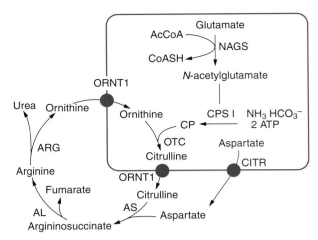

Fig. 33-1 The urea cycle. AcCoA, acetyl coenzyme A; AL, argininosuccinate lyase; ARG, arginase; AS, argininosuccinate synthetase; CITR, citrin; CoASH, uncombined acetyl coenzyme A; CPS I, carbamyl phosphate synthetase I; NAGS, N-acetylglutamate synthase; ORNT1, ornithine transporter 1; OTC, ornithine transcarbamylase.

The final step in the urea cycle involves cleavage of arginine to form urea and ornithine by arginase. A deficiency of this enzyme results in elevated arginine levels and argininemia or hyperargininemia. Once formed, ornithine is transported back into the mitochondrion by the ornithine transporter. A defect in this transporter leads to the marked accumulation of ornithine in blood, resulting in hyperornithinemia-hyperammonemia-homocitrullinuria syndrome. The complete urea cycle is found only in hepatocytes.

Clinical Description of Urea Cycle Disorders

N-Acetylglutamate Synthase Deficiency

Inherited N-acetylglutamate synthase (NAGS) deficiency leads to hyperammonemia by causing a secondary deficiency of CPS I. This disorder has been reported in approximately two dozen patients to date [Bachmann et al., 1982; Elpeleg et al., 2002; Caldovic et al. 2007], but is likely to be underdiagnosed because of the lack of specific biochemical markers and the physiologically low abundance of NAGS in the liver. NAGS deficiency is inherited as an autosomal-recessive disorder and has a phenotype that is similar to that found in CPS I deficiency. It is characterized by hyperammonemia in the newborn period or later in life, and can be fatal or lead to mental retardation and other developmental disabilities. Plasma amino acid analysis usually demonstrates an increased level of glutamine and reduced or absent levels of citrulline. Urinary orotic acid level is normal or low. NAGS activity in the liver has a variable degree of deficiency (ranging from undetectable to normal residual activity) that is unresponsive to L-arginine. Because enzyme analysis requires large amounts of liver tissue and may not be entirely reliable, analysis of genomic DNA for mutations in the N-acetylglutamate synthase gene is the best diagnostic method [Morizono et al., 2004]. Treatment of NAGS deficiency used to consist of a low-protein diet and use of ammonia-scavenging drugs (Table 33-1). A more specific therapy using N-carbamyl-L-glutamate is now possible because N-carbamyl-L-glutamate has been approved for the treatment of NAGS deficiency. N-carbamyl-L-glutamate is a stable structural analog of N-acetylglutamate and can substitute for it in the activation of CPS I.

Carbamyl Phosphate Synthetase I Deficiency

CPS I deficiency was first reported in 1969 [Hommes et al., 1969]. This mitochondrial urea cycle enzyme should be distinguished from a similar cytosolic enzyme, carbamyl phosphate synthetase 2, which is involved in de novo pyridine synthesis. This disorder can manifest with hyperammonemic coma in the newborn period or later in childhood. Biochemically, the principal findings are hyperammonemia, an increased level of plasma glutamine, and reduced level or absence of citrulline on plasma amino acid analysis. Urinary orotic acid level is normal or low. Patients with neonatal-onset disease generally demonstrate less than 5 percent normal CPS I activity in liver, whereas those with late-onset disease have higher residual activity [Qureshi et al., 1986]. Like most of the other urea cycle disorders, CPS I deficiency does not arise from a common mutation [Funghini et al., 2003; Summar, 1998]. Therapy consists of dialysis and/or intravenous alternate pathway therapy

Table 33-1 Long-Term Alternative Pathway Treatment of Urea Cycle Disorders (UCDs)*

Disorder	L-Citrulline	L-Arginine Free Base	Sodium Phenylbutyrate	N-Carbamylglutamate
NAGS deficiency	–	–	–	0.10 g/kg/d if <25 kg 2.2 g/m²/d in larger patients
CPS I or OTC deficiency	0.17 g/kg/d or 3.8 g/m²/d	–	0.45–0.60 g/kg if <25 kg 9.9–13.0 g/m²/d in larger patients	–
Citrullinemia	–	0.40–0.50 g/kg/d or 8.8–11.0 g/m²/d	0.45–0.60 g/kg if <25 kg 9.9–13.0 g/m²/d in larger patients	–
Argininosuccinic acidemia	–	0.40–0.50 g/kg/d or 8.8–15.4 g/m²/d	0.45–0.60 g/kg if <25 kg 9.9–13.0 g/m²/d in larger patients	–
Argininemia	–	–	0.45–0.60 g/kg/d if <25 kg 9.9–13.0 g/m²/d in larger patients	

* Drugs and dose ranges are those commonly used in patients with UCD; however, doses can vary and need to be adjusted based on the severity of the disorder. While using doses at the upper recommended range or above, consideration should be given to increased risk of drug toxicity.
CPS I, carbamyl phosphate synthetase I; NAGS, N-acetylglutamate synthase; OTC, ornithine transcarbamylase.

during severe hyperammonemic episodes, and low-protein diet and oral alternate pathway therapy for chronic treatment (see Table 33-1). Patients with the neonatal-onset form who survive the initial crisis generally require liver transplantation for long-term survival.

Ornithine Transcarbamylase Deficiency

Ornithine transcarbamylase deficiency was first reported in 1962 in two girls, aged 20 months and 6 years, who were found to have hyperammonemia associated with episodic vomiting, delirium, stupor, failure to thrive, and mental retardation [Russell et al., 1962]. The mothers of the children were sisters, and both demonstrated evidence of a similar but less marked metabolic disorder. Both girls died before the age of 8 years.

Several years later, this disorder also was identified in males. The delayed recognition in males was attributable to the almost total lack of enzyme activity and rare survival of affected males beyond the newborn period. The reason for this difference between males and females subsequently was determined to be related to its X-linked inheritance pattern, with the occurrence of symptomatic females explained by skewed X chromosome inactivation [Ricciuti et al., 1976]. The classic presentation of OTC deficiency in hemizygous males is as a catastrophic illness in the first week of life. In symptomatic female heterozygotes and in males with partial OTC deficiency, symptoms rarely present in the newborn period. Only one case of lethal OTC deficiency in a female neonate has been reported [Klosowski et al., 1998]. In partial deficiencies, age at presentation after the newborn period covers a wide spectrum, with development of hyperammonemic episodes in infancy in some patients, in later childhood in others, and not until adulthood in still others [Ahrens et al., 1996; Ausems et al., 1997; McCullough et al., 2000]. These patients generally have 5–30 percent of normal OTC activity in liver on in vitro measurement. Biochemically, the principal findings are hyperammonemia, hyperglutaminemia, reduced levels or complete absence of citrulline in plasma, and increased urinary orotic acid level.

More than 340 different point mutations and polymorphisms have been found in OTC-deficient patients, and no mutations are prevalent [McCullough et al., 2000; Tuchman et al., 2002]. In about 80 percent of affected families, prenatal diagnosis using DNA techniques is possible [Grompe et al., 1991]. When the mutation has been identified, carrier testing and prenatal diagnosis can be offered to the family. With severe OTC deficiency being an X-linked lethal disease, the calculated probability for the mother of an affected male to be a carrier is 2/3 or 66 percent, and the probability that the patient has a de novo mutation is 1/3 or 33 percent. The identification of common intragenic polymorphisms allows tracking of the mutant allele, even when the deleterious mutation is unknown [Plante and Tuchman, 1998]. Although most families have point mutations, 8 percent of families have large deletions of one or more exons, 10 percent have small deletions or insertions of a few basepairs, 18 percent have splice site mutations, and in about 20 percent no mutation can be found. In about half of those where no mutation could be found, large deletions involving the OTC locus were detected using microarray technology [Shchelochkov et al., 2009]. There are several disease genes very close to the OTC locus, including the Duchenne muscular dystrophy gene and the chronic granulomatous disease gene. Patients with these large deletions may thus have other severe genetic diseases at the same time, making them extremely difficult to manage [Deardorff et al., 2008]. Amongst those patients with point mutations, mutations causing neonatal disease affect amino acid residues that are in the interior of the enzyme, especially around the active site, whereas those associated with late-onset and milder phenotypes tend to be located on the surface of the protein [Tuchman et al., 1998].

Heterozygote detection of OTC deficiency is important both to identify at-risk family members and to offer prenatal diagnosis. It can be accomplished by either molecular studies or, in cases where no mutation was found, by provocation testing. The best provocation testing is an allopurinol load [Hauser et al., 1990]. This test has replaced the protein loading test, which can precipitate a hyperammonemic episode. The allopurinol load (300 mg given orally to adults) leads to increased excretion of orotic acid, reaching 10–20 times control values in 90 percent of OTC heterozygotes [Hauser et al., 1990]. Approximately 15 percent of OTC-deficient heterozygous females will become symptomatic during their lifetime [Batshaw et al., 1986]. (Heterozygotes for other urea cycle disorders are asymptomatic.) Therapy for the neonatal-onset form of OTC deficiency consists of dialysis and administration of intravenous ammonia scavenger drugs, followed by maintenance on a low-protein diet and long-term alternative pathway therapy (see Table 33-1). Patients with the neonatal-onset form who survive the initial crisis generally require liver transplantation.

Citrullinemia

Citrullinemia was first reported in 1962 [McMurray et al., 1962]. Its name derives from the marked elevation of citrulline in blood of affected persons. This disorder also has been called citrullinuria because of the increased excretion of citrulline in urine, and argininosuccinic acid (argininosuccinate) synthetase deficiency to denote its enzyme deficit. Heterogeneity is seen clinically, biochemically, and at the molecular level. Two distinct forms have been reported: neonatal/childhood-onset citrullinemia (type I; with diminished levels of argininosuccinate synthetase in all organs) and citrullinemia type II or citrin deficiency, an adult-onset citrullinemia that is in some but not all cases preceeded by neonatal cholestasis and decreased synthetic function of the liver (caused by a defect in citrin) [Saheki et al., 1987].

Biochemically, the principal findings are hyperammonemia, citrullinemia, and citrullinuria. Citrulline levels generally are elevated 50–100-fold [normal levels less than 50 μmol/L] [Batshaw et al., 1981]. Urinary orotic acid levels also may be increased but less so than in OTC deficiency or argininemia. Citrullinemia is inherited as an autosomal-recessive trait. The gene has been localized to the q34 region of chromosome 9, and the nucleotide coding sequence and deduced amino acid sequence for the enzyme are known [Gao et al., 2003]. To date, more than 50 mutations have been identified; some involve single base changes in the coding sequence, and others involve skipping of an exon in the messenger RNA (mRNA) due to abnormal splicing. Most patients appear to be compound heterozygotes of two different mutations. In neonatal-onset cases, argininosuccinate synthetase activity in liver is less than 5 percent of normal, whereas in childhood-onset cases, 10–25 percent residual activity is seen [Brusilow and Horwich, 2001].

Therapy for citrullinemia (type I) consists of dialysis during severe hyperammonemic crises, followed by low-protein diet and long-term alternative pathway therapy (see Table 33-1). After the initial crisis, patients are in general more stable and easier to manage than patients with more proximal defects (CPS I and OTC deficiencies).

Citrullinemia Type II or Citrin Deficiency

Citrullinemia type II was identified first in Japan but the mutation has been traced back to China. Citrin deficiency is caused by mutations in a gene encoding a previously unknown calcium-dependent mitochondrial membrane protein named citrin (*SLC25A13*) [Kobayashi et al., 2003]. This inner mitochondrial membrane carrier enables the exchange of matrix aspartate for cytosolic glutamate across the inner mitochondrial membrane [Palmieri et al., 2001]. Plasma ammonia levels are less severely elevated during acute episodes than in other urea cycle disorders, and citrulline levels are elevated up to 20-fold [Kobayashi et al., 1993]. It has been noted that serum pancreatic secretory trypsin inhibitor also is increased and may be useful as a diagnostic marker for the disorder [Kobayashi et al., 1993].

Citrullinemia type II, citrin deficiency, manifests in adulthood with cyclical bizarre behavior patterns (aggression, irritability, hyperactivity), dysarthria, seizures, motor weakness, and coma. Dementia and hepatomegaly eventually develop. Cases of hepatocellular carcinoma also have been reported in affected persons [Hagiwara et al., 2003]. In retrospect, many of the patients have had symptoms since childhood that suggested hyperammonemia, including recurrent episodes of vomiting, lethargy, and irritability [Okeda et al., 1989]. Treatment generally relies on alternate pathway therapy (arginine and phenylbutyrate) [Imamura et al., 2003]; however, liver transplantation is becoming a more common practice in the treatment of this disorder because of the possible liver complications [Ikeda et al., 2001; Yazaki et al., 2004].

More recently, a neonatal-onset form of citrin deficiency has been identified; this form is associated with intrahepatic cholestasis [Tamamori et al., 2002; Tazawa et al., 2001]. Affected infants have multiple metabolic abnormalities, including aminoacidemia, galactosemia, hypoproteinemia, hypoglycemia, and cholestasis. Treatment usually is by high-protein/low-carbohydrate diet, and symptoms often disappear within a year [Saheki et al., 2004]. A few children, however, have a severe form of the disorder with liver damage and tyrosinemia that necessitate liver transplantation. Hyperammonemia is not a major component of this disorder.

Argininosuccinicacidemia

Argininosuccinicacidemia was first described in 1958 by Allan et al. [1958]. Its name derives from the marked elevation of argininosuccinic acid in blood of affected persons. This disorder also has been called argininosuccinicaciduria (ASA) because of the increased excretion of argininosuccinic acid in urine, and argininosuccinate lyase deficiency to denote the underlying enzyme deficiency. In addition to hyperammonemic coma in the newborn period and recurrent hyperammonemic episodes later in childhood, a specific abnormality of the hair termed trichorrhexis nodosa develops in affected children. Nodules appear on the hair shaft, and the hair is friable. A

generalized erythematous maculopapular skin rash also may appear in this disorder. Both conditions are associated with arginine deficiency and respond to arginine supplementation [Brusilow and Horwich, 2001].

Chronic marked hepatomegaly has been reported in patients managed with protein restriction and in those receiving arginine supplementation, but this finding is not universal. Pathologic examination reveals modest fatty infiltration and fibrosis. Results of liver function tests frequently are abnormal, especially during hyperammonemic crises, and patients may develop cirrhosis [Zimmermann et al., 1986]. Why some patients with ASA develop cirrhosis and others do not is not understood.

The gene for ASL has been localized to the long arm of chromosome 7 [Kleijer et al., 2002]. The deficient enzyme, a homotetramer of 50-kilodalton (kDa) subunits, is expressed in multiple tissues, including the brain. Evidence of multiple allelic mutations and intragenic complementation, indicating extensive genetic heterogeneity, is characteristic of this disorder [Yu et al., 2001]. The frequency of some mutations, however, is higher than that of others; such mutations may occur at "hot spots" with higher susceptibility for alteration [Linnebank et al., 2002]. The multiple mutations may account for some of the observed heterogeneity in this disease at the clinical level.

Biochemically, the principal findings are elevated citrulline level, hyperammonemia, argininosuccinicacidemia, and argininosuccinicaciduria. The plasma argininosuccinic acid peak is large (normally it is undetectable) [Batshaw et al., 1981]. Of note, this peak may be missed, because it can overlie the peak for leucine or isoleucine. The presence of the two anhydrides of argininosuccinic acid, however, in areas of the chromatogram where homocystine and gamma-aminobutyric acid (GABA) normally are found, aids in the diagnosis. Markedly increased levels of argininosuccinic acid also are readily identifiable in the urine. Additionally, citrulline levels are increased 3–10-fold (to 100 to 300 μmol/L).

The diagnosis can be confirmed by measuring ASL in erythrocytes or fibroblasts, although this is rarely needed. In cerebrospinal fluid, elevated concentrations of argininosuccinic acid and its anhydrides, as well as pyrimidines (pseudouridine and uridine), have been found [Gerrits et al., 1993]. After the initial hyperammonemic crisis and establishment of the diagnosis, recommended treatment for argininosuccinicacidemia consists of a low-protein diet and L-arginine supplementation (see Table 33-1). Many metabolic physicians are also using ammonia scavengers in their treatment regimen.

Argininemia

Argininemia, or hyperargininemia, was first described in 1969 by Terheggen and colleagues [Terheggen et al., 1969]; it is caused by a deficiency of arginase 1. Its name derives from the marked elevation of arginine in the blood of affected persons. Argininemia presents differently from all of the other congenital urea cycle disorders. It usually appears as a progressive neurologic disorder, rather than as an acute encephalopathy [Cederbaum et al., 1979; Prasad et al., 1997].

Clinical symptoms do not classically start with hyperammonemic coma in infancy. In one report, however, a 2-month-old child with recurrent vomiting, persistent jaundice, and hepatomegaly (with associated cirrhosis) was diagnosed as having hyperargininemia [Braga et al., 1997]. Another patient presented with cerebral edema and growth retardation [Harrington et al., 2000]. More commonly, development for the first few years of life appears to be normal, although a detailed history often reveals evidence of protein aversion (often with anorexia, vomiting, and irritability) and some developmental delay. The disease runs a chronic course, but with acute episodes of ataxia, behavioral disturbances, vomiting, lethargy, and seizures. Such episodes often are precipitated by intercurrent viral illnesses [Grody et al., 1993]. Associated biochemical abnormalities usually include moderately elevated plasma ammonia levels of 3–4 times normal and plasma arginine levels of greater than 5 times normal, often exceeding 1000 μmol/L (normal is less than 120 μmol/L).

The unique feature of this disorder is the development of progressive muscle weakness, tremor, and spasticity (diplegia or quadriplegia) [Prasad et al., 1997; Scheuerle et al., 1993]. Mental retardation and growth failure also commonly are evident by childhood, and glaucoma has been reported [Sacca et al., 1996]. Affected children generally do not succumb to hyperammonemic coma and therefore have a longer life span than those affected by proximal urea cycle disorders.

Arginase 1 is found in liver and red blood cells. By contrast, renal arginase (arginase 2) is found in the mitochondrial matrix and differs from the liver type of enzyme in biochemical, molecular, and antigenic properties [Cederbaum et al., 2004]. Arginase 2 also is found in the small intestine and the brain, and its levels have been found to be elevated in patients with argininemia [Iyer et al., 1998]. It is possible that the presence of arginase 2 in hyperargininemia provides some degree of protection from nitrogen accumulation, resulting in less severe hyperammonemic episodes than in other urea cycle disorders. The gene for liver arginase has been localized to chromosome band 6q23 [Sparkes et al., 1986]. Available evidence suggests multiple point mutations and microdeletions in this disorder, indicating extensive genetic heterogeneity [Vockley et al., 1996], and many affected persons are compound heterozygotes. Correlation between the severity of the mutation and the degree of clinical symptoms has been shown [Uchino et al., 1998].

The principal biochemical finding is markedly elevated plasma levels of arginine. Arginine plus ornithine, aspartate, threonine, glycine, and methionine levels are elevated in cerebrospinal fluid [Cederbaum et al., 1982]. In addition, a generalized dibasic aminoaciduria (argininuria, lysinuria, cystinuria, ornithinuria) is present. Urinary excretion of orotic acid and guanidine compounds also is markedly increased [Marescau et al., 1990]. The diagnosis can be confirmed by measuring arginase 1 activity in erythrocytes.

The mechanism responsible for the spasticity and cognitive deficits in argininemia is unknown but is unlikely to be the result of the generally moderate hyperammonemia. Arginine, its guanidine metabolites, and altered biogenic amines are candidate neurotoxins [Marescau et al., 1990]. Arginine is the substrate for nitric oxide synthetase, so overproduction of nitric oxide may play a role in neuropathology [Iyer et al., 1998]. It is theoretically possible that pharmacologic inhibitors of nitric oxide synthetase may be beneficial. Treatment with alternate pathway therapy appears to halt the progression of the spasticity, and botulinum toxin (Botox) and surgical tendon release may improve function.

Hyperornithinemia-Hyperammonemia-Homocitrullinuria Syndrome

HHH syndrome was first described in 1969 [Shih et al., 1969], and only about 50 cases have been reported in the literature, most being in the French-Canadian population in Quebec [Gjessing et al., 1986]. Clinical symptoms are similar to those in other urea cycle disorders but rarely develop in infancy [Zammarchi et al., 1997]. Spastic paraparesis also has been noted and occasionally coagulation disorders occur [Gallagher et al., 2001; Lemay et al., 1992; Salvi et al., 2001a, b]. Plasma ornithine concentrations are elevated, ranging from 400 to 600 mmol/L. Plasma lysine level typically is low, and urinary excretion of homocitrulline is increased. The high blood levels and urinary excretion of homocitrulline likely are the result of conversion of lysine to homocitrulline by ornithine transcarbamylase, in the absence of ornithine in mitochondria. The etiology of HHH syndrome begins with a mutation in the ornithine transporter gene, ORNT1, also called SLC25A15, whose product is a member of the solute mitrochondrial carrier protein family [Camacho et al., 1999]. This leads to decreased ornithine levels in mitochondria and secondary impairment of urea synthesis. The expression of ORNT2, an intronless gene or processed pseudogene, encoding a protein about 90 percent identical to OTNT 1, may explain the milder clinical signs and symptoms compared with those in CPS I and OTC deficiencies [Camacho et al., 2003]. Treatment of HHH syndrome involves protein restriction, phenylbutyrate, and citrulline supplementation.

Common Clinical Presentations of Urea Cycle Disorders

The classic presentation of a complete defect in the urea cycle (other than arginase) is as a catastrophic illness in the first week of life. Clinical manifestations appear between 24 and 72 hours of age, starting as a poor suck, hypotonia, vomiting, lethargy, and hyperventilation with rapid progression to coma and seizures. The electroencephalographic (EEG) pattern during hyperammonemic coma is one of low voltage with slow waves and asymmetric delta and theta waves. The tracing may demonstrate a burst suppression pattern, and the duration of the interburst interval may correlate with the height of ammonia levels [Clancy and Chung, 1991]. Neuroimaging studies reveal cerebral edema with small ventricles, flattening of cerebral gyri, and diffuse low density of white matter; evidence of intracranial hemorrhage also may be seen [Kendall et al., 1983].

Partial urea cycle enzyme deficiencies have a spectrum of presentations, with hyperammonemic episodes developing in infancy in some patients, in later childhood in others, and not until adulthood in still others. Symptoms may be delayed in onset with a mild deficiency or by dietary self-restriction – specifically, avoidance of meats, fish, eggs, milk, and other high-protein foods. Signs and symptoms in childhood include anorexia, ataxia, and behavioral abnormalities such as episodes of erratic behavior, acting out of character, irritability, cloudedness to frank mental status change, nocturnal restlessness, and attention-deficit and hyperactivity [Rowe et al., 1986]. In adults, signs and symptoms may mimic those of psychiatric or neurologic disorders, and include migraine-like headache, nausea, dysarthria, ataxia, confusion, hallucinations, and visual impairment (blurred vision, scotomas, lost vision) [Arn et al., 1990]. In a case report of late-onset OTC deficiency, the patient was a heterozygote who presented with a syndrome mimicking complex partial status epilepticus [Bogdanovic et al., 2000]. Neurologic findings may include increased deep tendon reflexes, papilledema, and decorticate/decerebrate posturing. Seizures generally are a late complication; the seizure episode typically is preceded by alteration in consciousness. There are indications that patients with urea cycle disorders may also be prone to seizures outside of hyperammonemic episodes, as seizures seemed to be observed more often in this patient group than in the general population in one clinic [Zecavati et al., 2008]. Analysis of data collected longitudinally from patients with urea cycle disorders [Tuchman et al., 2008; Seminara et al., 2010] will allow further investigation of this impression. A possible explanation for increased frequency of seizures in hyperammonemic coma and chronic hyperammonemia in urea cycle disorder patients could be increased extracellular potassium levels [Lichter-Konecki et al., 2008a; Lichter-Konecki, 2008b], which lower the seizure threshold.

In affected persons, hyperammonemic episodes have been precipitated by high-protein meals, infection, medication, trauma, surgery, and delivery/postpartum period. It is not uncommon for the initial hyperammonemic episode in a child with a partial deficiency to occur after weaning, when low-protein breast milk is replaced by formula or cow's milk with a higher protein content. This is also the time when protein avoidance/self-restriction may first be observed. The puerperium in OTC-deficient heterozygotes and valproate therapy in partial CPS, OTC, and ASL deficiencies also has been associated with hyperammonemic crises [Arn et al., 1990; Batshaw et al., 1981; Honeycutt et al., 1992; Morgan et al., 1987]. The posited mechanism of valproate-induced hyperammonemia is through accumulation of the branched short-chain fatty acyl-CoA metabolites of valproate, which inhibit *N*-acetylglutamate formation, the co-factor of the first enzyme in the urea cycle, CPS I. This also has been the proposed explanation for hyperammonemia in the organic acidemias where propionyl-CoA was found to competitively inhibit *N*-acetylglutamate synthase. In a case report of haloperidol-induced hyperammonemia in a patient with partial OTC deficiency, a similar mechanism is likely [Rubenstein et al., 1990].

Associated Medical Conditions

A number of medical conditions have been associated with urea cycle disorders. For example, it is recognized that chronic liver dysfunction develops in patients with argininosuccinicacidemia. Other examples are anecdotal observations of a propensity for hypertension, electrolyte abnormalities (hypokalemia and hypomagnesemia), gastrointestinal abnormalities, including anorexia, stunted growth, microcytic anemia, and nutritional deficiencies [Brusilow and Horwich, 2001]. Pancreatitis has also been described, although the etiology is unclear [Anadiotis et al., 2001]. In addition, metabolic stroke-like episodes have been described in CPS and OTC deficiencies involving the caudate and putamen, with resultant extrapyramidal syndromes [Keegan et al., 2003].

Histopathologic Features of Urea Cycle Disorders

Histopathologic examination of liver in urea cycle disorders may be normal but often demonstrates diffuse microvesicular steatosis, marked increased glycogen in periportal cells, and

variable portal fibrosis [Badizadegan and Perez-Atayde, 1997]. Cirrhosis has been identified in some patients with argininosuccinicaciduria (ASA), citrullinemia type II, and arginase deficiency [Zimmermann et al., 1986]. Why some patients with ASA develop cirrhosis is not known at this point but nitric oxide metabolism may play a role [Brunetti-Pierri et al., 2009].

Neuropathologic findings in urea cycle disorders are similar to those following hepatic encephalopathy and hypoxic-ischemic insults. They depend both on the duration of hyperammonemic coma, and on the interval between coma and death. Neonates dying in hyperammonemic coma have prominent cerebral edema and generalized neuronal cell loss on postmortem examination [Crome and France, 1971]. Histologically, astrocyte swelling was one of the first observations made in an animal model for hepatic encephalopathy [Norenberg, 1977], leading to the hypothesis that swollen astrocytes may be the cellular correlate of the brain edema in acute hyperammonemia. The central role of astrocytes in hyperammonemic encephalopathy was felt to be underscored by the finding of Alzheimer type II astrocytes in the brains of patients in whom coma had taken an irreversible course. In survivors of prolonged coma, changes observed on neuroimaging studies obtained months later include ventriculomegaly with increased sulcal markings, bilateral symmetric low-density white matter defects, cystic degeneration, injury to the bilateral lentiform nuclei, and diffuse atrophy with sparing of the cerebellum [Kendall et al., 1983; Majoie et al., 2004; Takanashi et al., 2003; Yamanouchi et al., 2002]. Neuropathologic findings in those children who subsequently died were consistent with the neuroimaging findings and included ulegyria, cortical atrophy with ventriculomegaly, prominent cortical neuronal loss, gliosis (often with Alzheimer type II astrocytes), and spongiform changes at the gray–white matter interface and in the basal ganglia and thalamus [Dolman et al., 1988].

Mechanism of Neuropathology

The mechanism of the ammonia-induced neuropathology remains unclear [Bachmann et al., 2004]. Ammonia normally is detoxified in astrocytes by glutamate dehydrogenase and glutamine synthase. Accumulation of ammonia and glutamine in brain has a number of potentially toxic effects.

Downregulation of Astrocytic Glutamate Transporters

Astrocytic glutamate transporters were shown to be downregulated [Desjardin et al., 2001] and extracellular glutamate levels to be elevated [Felipo and Butterworth, 2002] in hyperammonemia. This led to the hypothesis that the brain damage in hyperammonemic coma is caused by overstimulation of neurons by elevated extracellular glutamate levels, a mechanism of brain damage called excitotoxicity. However, only a limited amount of neuronal cell death and little indication of excitotoxicity were observed in the animal models studied [Butterworth, 2007].

Elevated Glutamine Levels

A negative correlation between the height of brain glutamine levels and brain myoinositol levels has been observed, suggesting depletion of the osmolyte myoinositol by high glutamine levels [Takanashi et al 2002; Gropman et al., 2008]. High brain glutamine levels may have an osmotic effect and cause brain swelling. Inhibition of glutamine synthase by methionine sulfoximine was reported to prevent astrocyte swelling in experimental hyperammonemia [Willard-Mack et al., 1996].

Altered Water Transport Through Aquaporin 4 Water Channels

Water transport at blood–brain and brain–cerebrospinal fluid interfaces is facilitated by channel proteins called aquaporins. Aquaporin 4 (Aqp4) is the main astrocytic water channel and is expressed in astrocytic endfeet at the brain vasculature. While upregulation of Aqp4 expression in astrocytes exposed to ammonia in culture was reported [Rama Rao et al., 2003b], downregulation of this channel was found in the brains of hyperammonemic animals. The regulation of Aqp4 expression was shown to depend on the type of brain injury and type of edema.

Altered Glucose Metabolism/Disturbed Energy Metabolism

Ammonia stimulates phosphofructokinase, the key enzyme of glycolysis. Ammonium may play a significant role in regulating glycolysis in astrocytes under physiological conditions in vivo [Tsacopoulos and Magistretti, 1996]. Increased ammonia levels, on the other hand, inhibit α-ketoglutarate dehydrogenase in brain [Lai and Cooper, 1986]. Increased α-ketoglutarate levels were measured in the brain of hyperammonemic mice [Ratnakumari et al., 1994]. Stimulation of phosphofructokinase, as well as inhibition of α-ketoglutarate dehydrogenase, the key enzyme of the tricarboxylic cycle, will cause increased formation of lactate in brain. A block in the tricarboxylic cycle will lead to compromised brain energy metabolism.

Interference with the Normal Flux of Potassium Ions

The consideration that ammonia could interfere with potassium homeostasis is due to the fact that NH^{4+} has properties similar to those of the potassium ion. An important astrocytic function is the maintenance of potassium homeostasis. NH^{4+} can cross cell membranes through ion channels or membrane transporters, and can replace K^+ on different transporters. In cultured mouse astrocytes, ammonium was shown to enter the cell through inward rectifying K^+ channels [Marcaggi and Coles, 2001]. Ammonia may thus interfere with potassium channel or potassium transporter function. An elevated extracellular K^+ concentration was measured in the parietal cortex of healthy rats infused with ammonium acetate to cause hyperammonemia [Sugimoto et al., 1997]. Lichter-Konecki et al. [2008a] found downregulation of the major astrocytic water, gap-junction, and potassium channels in hyperammonemia in an animal model for urea cycle disorders, and concluded a possible disturbance of potassium and water homeostasis in brain during hyperammonemia.

Oxidative and Nitrosative Stress

An increase in free radical production and nitric oxide synthesis causes oxidative/nitrosative (O/N) stress. Ammonia causes free radical production and a decrease in antioxidant enzyme activity, while antioxidants prevented astrocyte swelling after ammonia exposure. In addition to oxidative stress, there is also nitrosative stress in hyperammonemic encephalopathy, as an upregulation of nitric oxide synthase (NOS) activity and expression was detected in animal models for hepatic encephalopathy [Rao et al., 1997]. Increased amounts of nitric oxide were found in the brains of such animals, and NOS inhibitors prevented astrocyte swelling in vivo and in vitro. How O/N stress would cause astrocyte swelling is not known but a mechanism under consideration is induction of mitochondrial permeability transition (MPT). In this scenario, oxidative stress would cause opening of the permeability transition pore (PTP) of the inner mitochondrial membrane and ions would flow, changing the membrane potential. This would lead to mitochondrial dysfunction and more free radical production, causing cell damage.

In summary, downregulation of astrocytic glutamate transporters may lead to elevated extracellular glutamate levels, which could cause excitotoxicity. Elevated glutamine levels may have an osmotic effect and cause astrocyte swelling. Astrocyte swelling may also be caused by altered water transport through Aqp4 water channels. Altered glucose metabolism may lead to disturbed energy metabolism, and interference with the normal flux of potassium ions may disturb the electrophysiology of neurons. Oxidative and nitrosative stress through increased free radical production and increased nitric oxide synthesis may further contribute to the damage.

Besides the amino acid glutamine, tryptophan and serotonin also are increased in the brain of the spf/Y mouse, an animal model for OTC deficiency, and in cerebrospinal fluid of children with urea cycle disorders [Bachmann et al., 1982; Batshaw et al., 1993; Inoue et al., 1987]. This finding led to the hypothesis that high glutamine levels also may cause other amino acid imbalances in the brain. Increased tryptophan levels result in increased levels of its metabolite, quinolinate, [Robinson et al., 1995], an excitotoxin at the N-methyl-D-aspartate receptor.

Differential Diagnosis

In the newborn period, hyperammonemia is similar in presentation to a number of acquired conditions, including sepsis, intracranial hemorrhage, and cardiorespiratory disorders. The measurement of plasma ammonia levels is critical to distinguish between these conditions. The acquired disorders generally are not associated with significant elevations in ammonia levels, whereas the inborn errors are. As a consequence, plasma ammonia levels should be measured as part of the routine evaluation for serious illness in the newborn period. Apart from urea cycle disorders, a number of other inborn errors of metabolism can cause hyperammonemia. These include organic acidemias, nonketotic hyperglycinemia, congenital lactic acidoses, lysinuric protein intolerance, and defects in fatty acid oxidation. An algorithm for distinguishing between these disorders is presented in Figure 33-2.

In the organic acidemias (e.g., methylmalonicacidemia, propionicacidemia, isovaleicacidemia, glutaricacidemia type II,

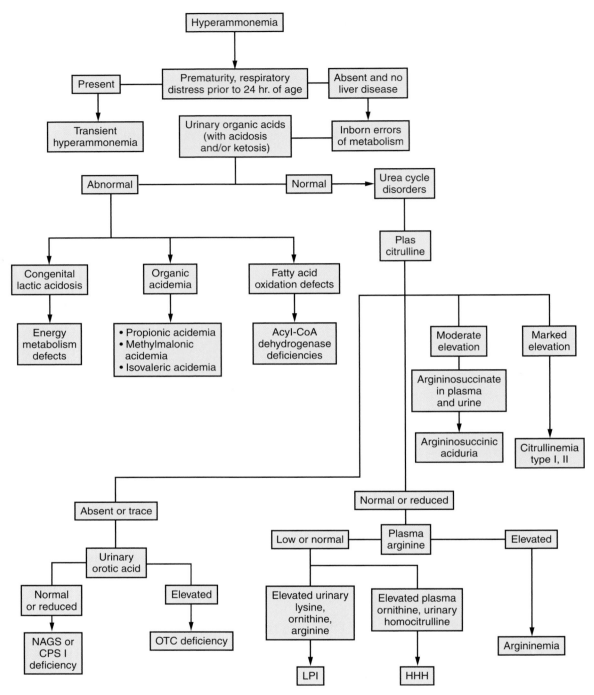

Fig. 33-2 Algorithm for differential diagnosis of hyperammonemia. Plasma amino acids, serum lactate, and urinary excretion of orotic acid and organic acids are measured. Acyl-CoA, acyl coenzyme A; CPS I, carbamyl phosphate synthetase I; HHH, hyperammonemia-hyperornithinemia-homocitrullinuria syndrome; LPI, lysinuric protein intolerance; NAGS, *N*-acetylglutamate synthase; OTC, ornithine transcarbamylase.

multiple carboxylase deficiency), the usual findings include a marked metabolic acidosis, ketosis, and increased anion gap. Hypoglycemia and pancytopenia also may be present. Mass spectrometry of urine organic acids or acylcarnitine analysis in blood will make the specific diagnosis. In propionic acidemia/organic acidurias, plasma (but not cerebrospinal fluid) will have an elevated glycine level – whence came the initial name, ketotic hyperglycinemia. By contrast, with nonketotic

hyperglycinemia, ketosis is absent, glycine levels in both plasma and cerebrospinal fluid are markedly elevated, and cerebrospinal fluid glycine to plasma glycine ratio is increased [Tada and Hayasaka, 1987].

Fatty acid oxidation defects, caused by different-chain-length acyl-CoA dehydrogenase deficiencies, manifest in the neonatal period with hypoglycemia and decreased ketones, as well as liver and heart disease. Analysis of urinary organic acids shows a dicarboxylic aciduria; plasma carnitine levels may be low; and abnormal acylcarnitine species are found [Roe and Ding, 2001].

Congenital lactic acidosis can be the result of a primary deficiency of pyruvate carboxylase or pyruvate dehydrogenase, or secondary to a defect within the mitochondrial respiratory chain [McCormick et al., 1985]. The principal biochemical finding is lactic acidosis. In pyruvate dehydrogenase deficiency and mild pyruvate carboxylase deficiency, the ratio of lactate to pyruvate remains normal. In severe pyruvate carboxylase deficiency, mitochondrial respiratory chain defects, and secondary lactic acidosis, however, this ratio is significantly increased [Zeviani et al., 1989]. In oxidative phosphorylation defects and other mitochondrial diseases the 3-hydroxybutyrate to acetoacetate ratio also is elevated. These findings are in contrast with those in inborn errors of urea synthesis, in which the urinary organic acid profile is normal and plasma lactate level is normal or mildly increased. Although peak plasma ammonia levels generally are in the range of 150 to 500 μM (normal 15 to 40 μM) in these disorders, they are likely to be above 500 μM in neonatal-onset urea cycle disorders.

Plasma amino acid patterns also are distinct in urea cycle disorders, with low levels of arginine and ornithine and either low or high levels of citrulline. Citrulline is the product of CPS I and OTC, and the substrate for ASS and ASL. Thus, it either is absent, or is present only in trace amounts, in NAGS, CPS I, and OTC deficiencies, and levels are markedly elevated in ASS and ASL deficiencies [Hudak et al., 1985]. Differentiation of ASS from ASL deficiencies depends on finding argininosuccinic acid in plasma and urine in ASL deficiency. In HHH syndrome, biochemical findings include accumulation of ornithine in blood and of homocitrulline in the urine.

Differentiation of CPS I from OTC deficiency depends on detecting excessive urinary orotic acid excretion in OTC deficiency and decreased excretion in CPS I deficiency. A deficiency of NAGS is associated with low to normal orotic acid excretion.

In summary, it is likely that measurement of ammonia, amino acids, and lactate in blood and of amino acids, organic acids, and orotic acid in urine will identify virtually all genetic causes of hyperammonemia. Confirmation of the diagnosis may require specific enzymatic or DNA analyses in a few instances (CPS I and NAGS deficiencies) but is not necessary to begin treatment.

In older children and adults, identification of partial-defect urea cycle disorders often has been delayed by misdiagnoses that have included migraine, cyclical vomiting, viral encephalitis, stroke, Reye's syndrome, drug toxicity, child abuse, psychosis, postpartum depression, seizure disorder, and cerebral palsy [Christodoulou et al., 1993; de Bruijn et al., 1976; DiMagno et al., 1986; Drogari and Leonard, 1988; Finkelstein et al., 1990]. Studies have found a mean delay of 8–16 months between the onset of symptoms and diagnosis of late-onset urea cycle disorders in children [Rowe et al., 1986]. During this time, progressive abnormalities in growth and cognitive/motor development may be noted.

Diagnosis of late-onset urea cycle disorders may be less clear-cut than in neonatal cases. Plasma ammonia levels may be in the range of 150–250 μM during symptomatic episodes and normal when the patient is clinically stable. Serum (blood) urea nitrogen, which clearly is subnormal in neonatal-onset deficiencies, may be normal. Plasma citrulline levels often are low to normal in partial OTC and CPS I deficiencies, rather

than absent or trace, as in complete defects. Yet, as noted previously, oroticaciduria can be provoked by an allopurinol load to detect partial OTC deficiencies, and marked elevations of argininosuccinic acid in blood and urine are characteristic in ASL deficiency (up to 1500 μM in plasma, normally undetected), of citrulline in ASS deficiency (range 1000–5000 μM in plasma, normal 6–50 μM), and of arginine in arginase deficiency (up to 1500 μM, normal less than 100 μM) [Batshaw et al., 1981]. In HHH syndrome, marked elevations of homocitrulline in urine and of ornithine in blood are seen.

Apart from urea cycle disorders, other inborn errors of metabolism that manifest with symptomatic hyperammonemia in later childhood/adulthood include the organic acidemias and lysinuric protein intolerance [Simell et al., 1975]. These disorders can be distinguished by specific patterns of urinary organic acids, urinary amino acids, plasma amino acids, and plasma carnitine/acylcarnitine levels. A number of acquired disorders also can manifest with hyperammonemia, including hepatic encephalopathy, Reye's syndrome, drug toxicity, and hepatotoxins. The medical history, prothrombin time, a urinary toxin screen, and analysis of plasma amino acid pattern (low branched-chain amino acids, high aromatic amino acids in chronic liver disease, elevated lysine in Reye's syndrome) should help differentiate these disorders.

Treatment

Therapy of urea cycle disorders consisted of only protein restriction and dialysis during acute hyperammonemic crises until the advent of ammonia-scavenging agents – sodium benzoate, sodium phenylacetate, sodium phenylbutyrate, and L-arginine. In the United States, standardized medical treatment with sodium phenylbutyrate (Buphenyl, Ucyclyd Pharma, Scottsdale, AZ) became available in 1996. These scavenging compounds decrease ammonia levels by stimulating alternative pathways for waste nitrogen excretion. The long-term treatment of urea cycle disorders now consists of a low-protein diet combined with this alternative pathway therapy. Use of ammonia-scavenging drugs also is first-line therapy during hyperammonemic crisis in patients with urea cycle disorders. Liver transplantation is being used with increasing frequency for definitive treatment of severe cases.

In the newborn period, treatment of urea cycle disorders may be reactive or anticipatory. In families who have had a previously affected child or in OTC-deficient kindreds, the birth of an at-risk or prenatally diagnosed infant provides the opportunity for prospective management. Within hours of birth, the child can be placed on oral alternate pathway therapy before the development of hyperammonemia (see Table 33-1). Of 15 infants with urea cycle disorders treated in this fashion, all but 3 survived the newborn period without hyperammonemic coma [Maestri et al., 1991].

Hemodialysis

In infants who are diagnosed during hyperammonemic coma, hemodialysis should be started immediately [McBryde et al., 2004; Tuchman, 1992]. In addition, L-arginine HCl (except in hyperargininemia), sodium benzoate, and sodium phenylacetate (Ammonul, Ucyclyd Pharma) should be given intravenously at the same doses used to treat intercurrent hyperammonemia.

Liver Transplantation

Long-term treatment of urea cycle disorders depends on the severity of the disease. For neonatal-onset CPS I and OTC deficiencies, current clinical guidelines recommend that liver transplantation be considered as a form of enzyme replacement therapy [Leonard and McKiernan, 2004]. This procedure usually is performed at 6–12 months of age, with use of alternate pathway therapy before surgery [Leonard and McKiernan, 2004; Saudubray et al., 1999]. More recently, and as a result of favorable outcome with liver transplantation, other neonatal-onset urea cycle and poorly controlled late-onset disorders also have been considered for this treatment.

The Studies in Pediatric Liver Transplantation (SPLIT) reported that 114 children with urea cycle disorders (UCDs) received a liver transplant between December of 1995 and June 2008 [Arnon et al., 2010]. The 1-year survival rate for patients with UCDs was 95.2 percent and the 1-year survival rate of their grafts was 91.8 percent. The 5-year patient survival rate was 88.7 percent, and the 5-year graft survival rate 83.7 percent. Living donors provided the liver in 7.9 percent of cases, and some form of cadaveric liver (whole, split, reduced) was used in 87.8 percent of cases. SPLIT is a cooperative research consortium that was established in 1995 to assess transplanted patients, their grafts, and management practices. SPLIT registers about 60 percent of liver transplants performed in children in the United States.

A number of case reports have been published concerning the results of liver transplantation with regard to correction of the metabolic defects in urea cycle disorders [Leonard and McKiernan, 2004; Saudubray et al., 1999]. These reports suggest that transplantation corrects most of the metabolic abnormalities (although citrulline levels remain low in OTC and CPS I deficiencies) and prevents future hyperammonemic episodes. In terms of morbidity, concerns have included neurodevelopmental lags, and frequent and prolonged hospitalizations for treatment of infections and regulation of immunosuppressing drugs. Overall, however, the reported quality of life has been much improved with normalization of diet and a decreased frequency of hospital admissions [Leonard and McKiernan, 2004].

Protein Restriction

In all urea cycle disorders other than citrullinemia type II, a protein-restricted diet should be combined with alternate pathway therapy unless liver transplantation has been performed. In general, using the minimum daily protein requirement for the child's age is recommended. For neonatal-onset disease, this generally is given half as an essential amino acid supplement (e.g., Cyclinex, Ross Pharmeuticals) and half as natural protein. For mild late-onset disease, protein restriction alone may be sufficient. In children receiving sodium phenylbutyrate, monitoring branched-chain amino acid levels and supplementing these as needed also has been suggested [Scaglia et al., 2004]. Additional calories can be provided via nonprotein formulas, such as Prophree or MJ80056. The diet should be supplemented with vitamins, minerals, and trace elements. Also recommended is routine monitoring of weight, growth, hair, skin, nails, and biochemical indices of nutritional status.

Alternative Pathway Therapy

For late-onset CPS I and OTC deficiencies, as well as for the other urea cycle disorders, long-term therapy generally involves nitrogen restriction combined with alternative pathway therapy (see Table 33-1) [Batshaw et al., 2001; Berry and Steiner, 2001]. Approaches to stimulating alternative pathways of waste nitrogen excretion vary with the site of the enzymatic block. In the case of ASS and ASL deficiencies (including citrullinemia type II), arginine can stimulate waste nitrogen excretion through enhanced production and excretion of citrulline and argininosuccinic acid [Imamura et al., 2003]. In CPS I and OTC deficiencies, sodium phenylbutyrate has been used to provide an alternative pathway. It initially is converted to sodium phenylacetate, which then conjugates with glutamine to form phenylacetylglutamine, which is excreted by the kidney [Burlina et al., 2001; MacArthur et al., 2004]. Arginase deficiency has been managed with an arginine-restricted diet supplemented with sodium phenylbutyrate.

N-Carbamyl-L-Glutamate

In NAGS deficiency, administration of *N*-carbamyl-L-glutamate (Carbaglu, Orphan Europe, Paris, France) may be an effective therapy. *N*-carbamyl-L-glutamate is a stable structural analog of N-acetylglutamate and theoretically could substitute for it in the activation of CPS I [Hall et al., 1958]. Although the affinity of *N*-carbamyl-L-glutamate for CPS I is lower than that of *N*-acetylglutamate ($K_M = 2$ and $0.15 \ \mu M$, respectively) [Rubio and Grisolia, 1981], it is much more resistant to degradation by aminoacylase [Kim et al., 1972]. *N*-carbamyl-L-glutamate is therefore attractive for therapy of *N*-acetylglutamate synthase deficiency. Moreover, unlike *N*-acetylglutamate, *N*-carbamyl-L-glutamate can cross the mitochondrial membrane into the mitochondrion, where *N*-acetylglutamate synthase resides [Kim et al., 1972]. Several patients with *N*-acetylglutamate synthase deficiency have been reported to respond clinically to treatment with *N*-carbamyl-L-glutamate [Guffon et al., 1995; Hinnie et al., 1997; Morris et al., 1998; Schubiger et al., 1991]. One homozygous affected subject underwent a 15N-tracer study of ureagenesis rate before and after 3-day treatment with oral *N*-carbamyl-L-glutamate, it completely restored normal urea cycle function [Caldovic et al., 2003].

Management of Intercurrent Hyperammonemic Crises

If vomiting occurs or if lethargy becomes evident, and ammonia levels are above 3–5 times normal, more aggressive treatment is needed. This approach involves hospitalization, with temporary complete elimination of protein and institution of intravenous administration of sodium benzoate, sodium phenylacetate, and L-arginine. (Caution: arginine HCl may cause metabolic acidosis, and extravasation may lead to tissue necrosis.) Although these medications are not associated with severe adverse events when they are given at therapeutic doses, severe toxicity and death have resulted from dosing errors [Praphanphoj et al., 2000]. Therefore, double-checking of drug administration orders is essential, and monitoring plasma levels is recommended.

In the event that ammonia levels do not respond to this conservative management approach and biochemical abnormalities or clinical signs and symptoms worsen, hemodialysis should be initiated. The relative effectiveness of peritoneal dialysis, exchange transfusion, hemodialysis, and continuous arteriovenous hemofiltration has been the subject of some controversy. Yet nitrogen balance studies clearly demonstrate the advantage of hemodialysis, with continuous arteriovenous hemodiafiltration being second best if hemodialysis is unavailable [McBryde et al., 2004]. Hemodialysis should be continued until ammonia levels fall to less than five times normal; peritoneal dialysis or continuous hemofiltration may then be initiated if needed. Hemodialysis using an extracorporeal membrane oxygenation pump has been reported to be effective for rapidly removing ammonia [Summar et al., 1996].

Outcome

Before the development of alternative pathway therapy, few children with a complete urea cycle defect survived infancy [Shih, 1976]. Most died in the newborn period, and the remainder succumbed to intercurrent hyperammonemic episodes or protein malnutrition later in infancy or early childhood. Long-term survival, however, has improved with the introduction of alternative pathway therapy and liver transplantation [Brusilow and Horwich, 2001]. The mortality and morbidity rates currently cited for urea cycle disorders were obtained in the 1980s, when the index of suspicion for these disorders was low, leading to significant delays in diagnosis. In addition, no standardized treatment regimen was in use. At that time, the 5-year survival rate for a small prospective cohort of patients with neonatal-onset disease was reported to be approximately 25 percent, and the morbidity (e.g., mental retardation, seizure disorders, cerebral palsy) was found to be virtually universal for infants rescued from hyperammonemic coma [Batshaw et al., 1982; Msall et al., 1984]. In a retrospective study of mortality among infants with neonatal-onset urea cycle disorders referred to one major metabolic center during that period [Maestri et al., 1999], 34 of 74 infants (46 percent) died during their neonatal hyperammonemic episode, and among the 40 infants surviving the initial hyperammonemic episode, the median survival period was 3.8 years. More recently, with the general availability of plasma ammonia assays at most hospitals, an increased index of suspicion for metabolic disorders, and standardized alternative pathway therapy, it is likely that the outcome has improved.

Although mortality has decreased, morbidity remains high among survivors of neonatal hyperammonemic coma. More than three-quarters of these children have mental retardation, and frequent comorbid conditions include cerebral palsy, seizure disorder, and visual deficits [Msall et al., 1984]. A correlation between intellectual function and duration of hyperammonemic coma has been noted. Children in coma for less than 3 days had a far better outcome than those in coma for longer periods [Msall et al., 1984]. Cognitive outcome also was better in infants with complete defects who received prospective treatment and in children with partial defects. Of interest, even OTC-deficient women with subtle clinical signs or symptoms (e.g., protein aversion) have been found to have mild cognitive impairments suggestive of a nonverbal learning disability [Gropman and Batshaw, 2004; Maestri et al., 1991; Nagata et al., 1991; Widhalm et al., 1992].

Acknowledgment

Work on which this chapter is based was supported by the following NIH grants: 5P30HD040677, U54RR019453, and M01RR013297.

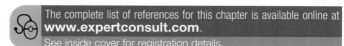

The complete list of references for this chapter is available online at **www.expertconsult.com**. See inside cover for registration details.

Diseases Associated with Primary Abnormalities in Carbohydrate Metabolism

Marc C. Patterson and Kenneth F. Swaiman

Introduction

Carbohydrates are essential elements in the cellular energy economy, and the inability to activate sugars ingested in the diet for use as metabolic fuels, as in the galactosemias, to mobilize glucose from glycogen, as occurs in the glycogen storage diseases, or to oxidize glucose in the glycolytic pathway, leads to a variety of phenotypes. The more frequent features of derangements in these pathways include symptoms and signs referable to the liver and musculature predominantly, and include hepatomegaly, altered volume of skeletal muscle (both increases and decreases), decompensation in the face of stress (manifest as weakness, cramping, and myoglobinuria), and nonspecific manifestations of hypoglycemia. This chapter surveys the primary diseases of carbohydrate metabolism, particularly as they affect the developing nervous system.

Abnormalities of Galactose Metabolism

Galactosemia

Galactosemia describes a family of autosomal-recessive disorders characterized by increased blood levels of galactose. Galactose cannot be used directly for glycolysis, and must be converted to glucose-1-phosphate. Five enzymes are involved in this interconversion in most species: galactose mutarotase, galactokinase, galactose-1-phosphate uridyltransferase, uridine diphosphogalactose-4-epimerase, and phosphoglucomutase [Sellick et al., 2008]. Mutations in the *GALK*, *GALT*, and *GALE* genes that encode the second, third, and fourth enzymes, respectively, cause deficiency or absence of these enzymes, with consequent galactosemia [Fridovich-Keil, 2006]. These enzymes comprise the Leloir pathway. Human galactose mutarotase deficiency has not been described.

Galactose-1-Phosphate Uridyltransferase Deficiency

Galactose-1-phosphate uridyltransferase (GALT) deficiency is by far the most common cause of galactosemia. The incidence of galactosemia in Western Europe varies between 1:23,000 and 1:44,000 [Bosch, 2006]. Neonatal screening programs have found population incidence rates as high as 1 in 19,700 in Estonia [Ounap et al., 2010].

PATHOLOGY

The precise link between the metabolic abnormality and the neuropathologic condition remains unknown. Galactose-1-phosphate uridyltransferase is present in the brain in low concentrations. Studies of rat brain reveal no significant site-specific differences in enzyme activity [Rogers et al., 1992]. Hypoglycemia may contribute significantly to the pathologic findings in many cases. The toxic effect of galactitol accumulation is not fully understood but is clearly relevant to adverse outcomes in the brain and lens. Animal data suggest that osmotic and oxidative stress in the lens activates the unfolded protein response [Mulhern et al., 2006]. Great variety and widespread distribution of the accompanying lesions have been documented.

Only two autopsy reports have been published; these were reviewed by Ridel et al. [2005]. The two patients were severely impaired and died at 8 and 25 years, respectively. In both cases, there was diffuse white matter gliosis, with focal areas of infarction. There was marked depletion of cerebellar Purkinje cells, with sparing of the granular layer and neuronal loss in the dentate nuclei and inferior olives. Cortical neuronal degeneration depleted the entire cerebral cortex, including Ammon's horn, albeit to a variable extent and in different patterns. Spongiform changes are pronounced in some areas. Other findings included mild pigmentary changes in the surviving neurons, perineuronal satellitosis, and mild, diffuse microglial activation. Sclerotic and atrophic white matter were evident, as were dense accumulations of iron-containing and non-iron-containing pigment material in the reticular zone of the substantia nigra and the globus pallidus. Histochemical staining of the pigment indicated the presence of lipoprotein and polysaccharides. Pigment accumulation was accompanied by neuronal degeneration in the substantia nigra and dysmyelination in the globus pallidus. Bright pink eosinophilic hyaline-like bodies resembling axonal spheroids were present in the thalamus.

BIOCHEMISTRY

The primary abnormality in galactosemia is the deficiency of activity of galactose-1-phosphate uridyltransferase (Figure 34-1) that leads to accumulation of galactose-1-phosphate in red blood cells, liver, and brain [Lai et al., 2009].

Galactose is metabolized through the following four possible pathways [Fridovich-Keil, 2006]:
1. the reduction of galactose to galactitol
2. oxidation of galactose to galactono-γ-lactone
3. the reaction of galactose-1-phosphate with uridine triphosphate to form uridine diphosphate galactose and eventually glucose-1-phosphate
4. the reaction of galactose-1-phosphate with uridine diphosphate-glucose to form uridine diphosphate-galactose and glucose-1-phosphate.

In classic galactosemia, the fourth pathway is obstructed; the other pathways function normally.

Shih and colleagues assigned the *GALT* locus to 9p13 by gene dosage [Shih et al., 1984]. A number of mutations produce abnormal enzymes with little or no galactose-1-phosphate uridyltransferase activity [Reichardt, 1991; Reichardt et al., 1992]. It is therefore not surprising that various genetic forms of galactosemia result from the presence of inefficient isoenzymes of galactose-1-phosphate uridyltransferase (Table 34-1). Most patients are compound heterozygotes, not true molecular homozygotes [Elsas et al., 1995].

The isoenzymes are separated and identified by electrophoresis. Cross-reactivity patterns for the enzyme variants have been studied using rabbit antibodies to purify human placental galactose-1-phosphate uridyltransferase [Andersen et al., 1984]. Transferase activity is absent in homozygous classic galactosemia (Q188R – the most common mutation in the United States, arising in Western Europe about 20,000 years ago [Flanagan et al., 2010]) and the African American variant (S135L – accounting for 8.4 percent of U.S. cases [Lai and Elsas, 2001]), virtually absent in the Rennes variant [Schapira and Kaplan, 1969], and abnormally low in the Chicago, Indiana, and Duarte (N314D) variants [Beutler et al., 1965; Lai et al., 1998; Levy et al., 1978]. Activity is normal in the Los Angeles

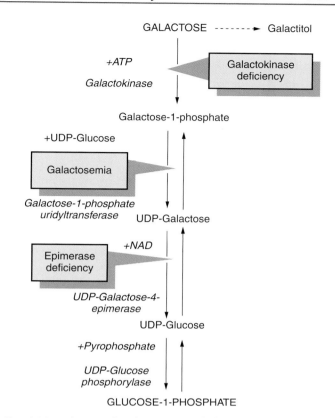

Fig. 34-1 Pathway of galactose metabolism depicting sites of metabolic block that lead to galactosemia. ATP, adenosine triphosphate; NAD, nicotinamide adenine dinucleotide; UDP, uridine diphosphate.

variant (L218L) [Applegarth et al., 1976; Ng et al., 1973]. A screening method utilizing a standard newborn screening blood spot has been described that detects the four most common *GALT* alleles (Q188R, S135L, K285N, and L195P) and the N314D Duarte variant with a turnaround time of less than 2 hours [Dobrowolski et al., 2003]. By January 2010, 239

Table 34-1 Biochemical Criteria for Assigning Phenotypes of Galactosemia*

Activity[†]	Mobility[†]	Galactose-1-Phosphate Uridyltransferase Phenotype	Zygosity
Normal	Normal	Normal	–
Absent	None	Galactosemic (classic form)	Homozygous
Decreased	Duarte (fast)	Duarte variant	Homozygous
Absent	None	African American variant	Homozygous
Decreased	Normal	Galactosemic (classic form)	Heterozygous
Decreased	Slower	Indiana variant	Heterozygous
Much less	Slower	Rennes variant	Heterozygous
Increased	Faster	Los Angeles variant	Heterozygous
Decreased	Fast	Chicago variant	Heterozygous
Decreased	Normal	Munster variant	Heterozygous

* Characteristics of galactose-1-phosphate uridyltransferase.
† Compared with normal.

sequence variants had been described in the GALT mutation database [Calderon et al., 2007], most of which were missense mutations. The precise molecular mechanisms of galactosemia are not yet known, but a computational biology approach has yielded insights into the structure–function relationships of many mutations [Facchiano and Marabotti, 2010].

The precise mechanisms of central nervous system dysfunction and developmental aberrations remain unexplained. Hypoglycemia associated with galactosemia may be responsible for some of the neurologic (including higher cortical function) abnormalities observed in these patients, but the accumulation of unusual metabolites also may contribute to the pathogenesis of the disorder. Hypoglycemia may be the result of inhibition of phosphoglucomutase and accompanying failure of hepatic glycogenesis. The high concentration of galactose may increase both insulin production and release, and the increased galactose also may compete with glucose for transport sites and carrier mechanisms across the blood–brain barrier.

Galactose-1-phosphate accumulates in erythrocytes, liver, lenses, and kidneys, and may be influential in disruption of both tissue structure and function, but galactitol accumulation likely is a more important factor in cataract development and perhaps other tissue disruptions and cerebral dysfunction.

Galactokinase or transferase activity appears to be lower than expected in many women who give birth to nongalactosemic children with cataracts [Harley et al., 1974].

CLINICAL CHARACTERISTICS

Infants usually are normal at birth, except for a slight decrease in birth weight [Hsia and Walker, 1961]. Symptoms become apparent when milk feedings begin. Jaundice usually develops between 4 and 10 days of age and persists for a longer period than does physiologic jaundice [Donnell et al., 1967]. Progressive hepatic involvement in the first several weeks causes edema, hepatomegaly, and hypoprothrombinemia. Renal dysfunction is accompanied by generalized aminoaciduria, proteinuria, and acidosis. *Escherichia coli* sepsis is a common complication [Levy et al., 1977]. Mild hypoglycemia also is common [Donnell et al., 1967]. Cataracts appear between 4 and 8 weeks, reflecting the accumulation of galactose-1-phosphate or galactitol. Studies in animals show that apoptosis of lens epithelial cells and cataract formation are directly related to galactitol accumulation and are prevented by aldose reductase inhibitors [Murata et al., 2001]. Apoptosis may be triggered by altered p53 expression secondary to the accumulating metabolites [Takamura et al., 2003].

Central nervous system impairment is manifested by lethargy and hypotonia, often associated with cerebral edema [Huttenlocher et al., 1970; Welch and Milligan, 1987], and may be documented by computed tomography (CT) scanning [Belman et al., 1986]. Cerebral edema in an encephalopathic neonate with galactose-1-phosphate uridyltransferase deficiency has been correlated with increased brain galactitol on magnetic resonance (MR) spectroscopy [Berry et al., 2001]. A subgroup of patients may develop marked ataxia and tremor, which does not correlate with cognitive abilities or dietary restriction [Ridel et al., 2005]. Seizures have been reported in two siblings with galactosemia [Ridel et al., 2005], and chorea in a single case [Shah et al., 2009]. After the appearance of neurologic symptoms, the patient may experience anorexia, vomiting, or diarrhea.

Galactosemia may prove fatal at any time. Cirrhosis progresses inexorably in patients who do not receive treatment. If the disease progresses more slowly and therapy is not optimal, mild gastrointestinal symptoms and failure to thrive persist.

Gonadal function in women with galactosemia is abnormal and usually manifests as primary ovarian failure. Both hypergonadotropic hypogonadism and abnormal response to gonadotropin-releasing hormone may be present. The mechanisms of ovarian failure are not yet fully understood, but likely include direct toxicity of galactose and its metabolites, incomplete galactosylation of glycoconjugates, oxidative stress and activation of apoptosis [Forges et al., 2006]. Some women with galactosemia do become pregnant; neither they nor their offspring seem to be affected by elevated levels of galactose, at least in the short term [Gubbels et al., 2008].

If treatment is not instituted, moderate to severe intellectual and motor retardation ensue in a majority of cases. Even in patients who are treated adequately, cognitive disability is common, but usually does not progress over time [Schadewaldt et al., 2010]. Language impairment is prominent [Hansen et al., 1996], and takes the form of verbal dyspraxia in about 50 percent of patients with galactose-1-phosphate uridyltransferase deficiency [Webb et al., 2003]. The risk of dyspraxia is associated with elevated mean galactose-6-phosphate and urinary galactitol concentrations, and with impaired total body galactose metabolism, as assessed by a carbon dioxide breath test [Hansen et al., 1996; Webb et al., 2003]. The characteristics of retardation resulting from untreated galactosemia are nonspecific. Pregnant women at risk of giving birth to galactosemic infants require strict restriction of galactose intake and close metabolic monitoring to prevent congenital cataracts in offspring. One study of 33 subjects aged 4–16 years found that children with galactosemia and speech disorders had a 4–6 times greater risk for language impairment than children with early speech disorders of unknown origin. Notwithstanding a negative effect of early dietary lactose exposure, the data suggested an antenatal origin of language disorder in most cases [Potter et al., 2008]. The incidence of speech and language disorders also appears to be increased in children with Duarte galactosemia, in whom galactose was restricted in the first 12 months [Powell et al., 2009].

Prenatal diagnosis is possible by means of galactose-1-phosphate uridyltransferase assay using cultured amniotic fluid cells or chorionic villus biopsy specimens, and by galactitol estimation in amniotic fluid supernatant [Holton et al., 1989]. When both mutations in an index case have been identified, direct molecular analysis is the preferred method of prenatal diagnosis [Elsas, 2001].

Occasional patients with genotypes and residual enzyme activity usually associated with severe phenotypes present with mild manifestations despite lack of dietary restriction. In one such case, the patient's markedly reduced galactitol production, presumably reflecting limited aldose reductase activity, was identified as a major factor in preventing neurologic injury despite her classic Q188R missense mutations [Lee et al., 2003; Segal, 2004].

CLINICAL LABORATORY TESTS

Biochemical tests for galactosemia screen for elevated levels of small molecules and directly assay the enzymes in the Leloir pathway. Detailed protocols have been published outlining the methods, including their rationale and interpretation [Cuthbert et al., 2008].

A fluorescent spot test for erythrocyte transferase activity (the Beutler test) is quite sensitive [Beutler and Baluda, 1966], but can yield false-negative results if the subject has received a blood transfusion up to 120 days earlier, because of residual galactose-1-phosphate uridyltransferase activity in the transfused blood. Enzyme activity is relatively low in heterozygous persons; this phenomenon aids in identifying carriers.

Galactose tolerance testing is potentially dangerous and should be undertaken only for well-planned investigational purposes [Donnell et al., 1967]. Bedside urine testing is positive for reducing substances (Benedict's test) but negative for glucose by the glucose oxidase method. Chromatography definitively identifies galactose as the abnormal metabolite.

Antibiotics may interfere with neonatal screening [Clemens et al., 1986]. Urinary galactose may be present in neonates with hepatic dysfunction in disorders other than galactosemia. Repeated attempts at detecting the reducing substance must be made because galactosuria may be inconstant as a result of fluctuating galactose or lactose ingestion. Generalized aminoaciduria, proteinuria, and abnormalities on liver function tests are common.

Screening tests that use *E. coli* bacteriophage assay of galactose and galactose-1-phosphate in dried blood samples are available and are useful for large-volume applications [Jinks et al., 1987; Schulpis et al., 1997].

Magnetic resonance imaging (MRI) in 67 transferase-deficient galactosemic patients revealed that 22 had mild cerebral atrophy, 8 had cerebellar atrophy, and 11 had multiple small hyperintense lesions in the cerebral white matter on T2-weighted images. The patients with classic galactosemia (those without measurable transferase activity) older than 1 year of age did not manifest the expected maturational decrease in peripheral white matter signal intensity on intermediate- and T2-weighted images. Interference with normal galactocerebroside formation may explain these findings [Nelson et al., 1992]. A study of MRI and MR spectroscopy in 14 sibling pairs found that delayed or absent myelination of the deep white matter was the most common finding; some individuals showed cerebellar atrophy, others ventricular dilatation [Hughes et al., 2009]. There was no correlation between dietary control or clinical status and the imaging findings. An infant was studied with MRI and MR spectroscopy, and was found to have increased signal in the cerebral white matter associated with increased diffusion. MR spectroscopy showed a peak at 3.7 ppm, consistent with galactitol. NAA/Cr, Cho/Cr, mI/Cr ratios were also decreased [Cakmakci et al., 2009].

MANAGEMENT

Because galactose is a nonessential nutrient, exclusion from the diet is relatively easy and without complication. Milk, the primary galactose-containing fluid, can be avoided by the use of vegetable product substitutes [Hansen, 1969]. Unfortunately, certain fruits and vegetables contain relatively high concentrations of galactose, including bell peppers, dates, tomatoes, papaya, and watermelon [Gross and Acosta, 1991]. Appropriate diets are available. The widespread use of cow's milk in the newborn diet makes early diagnosis essential. Intellectual and personality impairment is most successfully prevented with early treatment [Fishler et al., 1972]. Studies

of the long-term outcome of therapy have been relatively disappointing, particularly in regard to central nervous system and ovarian dysfunction [Widhalm et al., 1997]. A report based on a German cross-sectional study was more encouraging, suggesting that infants given appropriate treatment by 5 days of age achieved better outcomes than did those in whom treatment was begun later [Schweitzer-Krantz, 2003].

Most acute sequelae of the disease, including cirrhosis, are ameliorated with therapy, even if briefly delayed [Donnell et al., 1967]. Cataracts also may recede or disappear. Cataract formation in severely galactosemic rats has been prevented by inhibitors of aldose reductase. Signs or symptoms of sepsis should be investigated with blood, urine, and cerebrospinal fluid cultures to detect *E. coli*.

Because dietary therapy does not uniformly alleviate many of the sequelae of the disease, new strategies for therapy are necessary. The use of folic acid has been advocated as a supplement to galactose restriction to enhance transferase activity [Segal and Rogers, 1990]. Uridine administration demonstrated some promise in enhancing galactose transformation [Holton, 1990], but a trial of oral uridine did not reveal any evidence of benefit to neurocognitive functioning in treated versus untreated cases [Manis et al., 1997]. Neurologic complications may occur as late as the fourth decade of life [Friedman et al., 1989].

Unfortunately, galactose-1-phosphate appears to accumulate in the galactosemic fetus in spite of maternal milk restriction [Irons et al., 1985].

Uridine Diphosphogalactose Epimerase Deficiency

Uridine diphosphogalactose epimerase (GALE) deficiency has conventionally been separated into peripheral and generalized forms, implying a dichotomy between levels of enzyme activity in blood and other tissues. Ten children in a study were diagnosed with peripheral GALE deficiency as neonates were found to have a range of GALE activity in lymphoblasts (i.e., nonperipheral tissue), that was correlated with metabolic abnormalities in some patients, implying that this is a spectrum disorder, and not a binary condition as suggested in the older literature [Openo et al., 2006]. Children previously recognized with generalized (severe) deficiency of GALE (see Figure 34-1) [Bowling et al., 1986; Garibaldi et al., 1986; Sardharwalla et al., 1988; Walter et al., 1999] had manifestations resembling those in classic galactosemia. Most survivors were dysmorphic and deaf. The GALE locus is at 1p36–p35; the human *GALE* gene is about 4 kilobases (kb) in length and contains 11 exons [Maceratesi et al., 1998]. The coding sequence of the *GALE* gene and screening for mutations in epimerase-deficient persons have been reported by the same investigators. The patients are either homozygotes or compound heterozygotes for mutations. Two forms of enzyme deficiency were originally described, one type benign (with expression restricted to the lens) and the other severe [Quimby et al., 1997], but an intermediate form is now recognized [Openo et al., 2006]. Three mutations (S81R, T150M, and P293L) have been reported in children with this intermediate form of GALE deficiency [Chhay et al., 2008]. Patients with GALE deficiency require exogenous galactose for the synthesis of glycolipids and glycoproteins.

Galactokinase Deficiency

Galactokinase deficiency was first detected in the Bulgarian gypsy (Romany) population. Its birth incidence varies, ranging from a high of 1 in 52,000 in Bulgaria to 1 in 2,200,000 in Switzerland [Kalaydjieva et al., 1999]. Deficiency of galactokinase activity causes a clinical condition similar to that in classic galactosemia. Patients have cataracts and accumulation of galactose. As in galactosemia, galactitol, a reduction metabolite of galactose, is found in the urine and tissues [Egan and Wells, 1966]. The existence of two *GALK* genes is likely. The *GALK1* gene is located at 17q24 [Bergsma et al., 1996]. *GALK2* may reside on chromosome 15 [Lee et al., 1992]; its metabolic role is unknown, but it does not appear to be necessary for galactose metabolism. No mutations in *GALK2* have been described. The structure of *GALK1* has been solved and its relationship to other members of the GHMP kinase superfamily defined, as well as its role as an essential componenet of the 'switch' permitting expression of the Leloir pathway genes in the presence of galactose [Holden et al., 2004]. More than 20 mutations in *GALK1* have been described, most in compound heterozygotes for private mutations [Sangiuolo et al., 2004]. Only one common mutation, P28T, has been recognized in the Romany population [Kalaydjieva et al., 1999].

BIOCHEMISTRY

Galactokinase deficiency causes the accumulation of galactose, which eventually is metabolized to galactitol (see Figure 34-1). Enzyme activity is reduced rather than absent in erythrocytes [Xu et al., 1989]. Galactose-1-phosphate does not accumulate. Large amounts of circulating galactose result in urinary excretion of galactose, which causes positive results on copper sulfate screening tests for urinary reducing substances. Specific assays for galactose-1-phosphate or galactose-1-phosphate uridyltransferase are necessary to differentiate between deficiency of galactose-1-phosphate uridyltransferase and deficiency of galactokinase.

CLINICAL CHARACTERISTICS

The clinical manifestations of 55 patients reported in the literature were reviewed in 2002 [Bosch et al., 2002]. Cataract was present in all cases, except for those detected by newborn screening. Thirty-five percent of the patients had other manifestations; only mental retardation and pseudotumor occurred in more than one patient in this series. The mental retardation was thought to be unrelated to the *GALK* deficiency. Forty percent of the patients were of Roma ancestry and 26 percent were the product of consanguineous unions. One child deteriorated following the onset of epilepsy at 17 years.

Cataracts, the only consistent manifestation of galactokinase deficiency, form in the first months of life. Cataract formation is likely related to the production and accumulation of the osmotically active sugar alcohol galactitol from galactose through the activity of aldose reductase (see earlier).

MANAGEMENT

Treatment consists of elimination of galactose from the diet, as is the case for classic galactosemia.

Abnormalities of Fructose Metabolism

Hereditary Fructose Intolerance

Biochemistry

Fructose is rapidly absorbed from the gut, facilitated by the glucose transporters GLUT 2 and GLUT5, and is metabolized in the liver by the fructokinase pathway, through which it is linked to glycolysis, gluconeogenesis, glycogenolysis, and lipid metabolism. Fructose can also be synthesized endogenously from sorbitol, an important point in management [Bouteldja and Timson, 2010]. Hereditary fructose intolerance was first described by Chambers and Pratt [1956]. This condition results from a deficiency of hepatic fructose-1-phosphate aldolase B [Hers and Joassin, 1961]. (Isoenzyme A is found in most vertebrate tissues and isoenzyme C in brain.) The gene encoding this enzyme maps to 9q22 [Henry et al., 1985]. Normal fructokinase activity results in the accumulation of large amounts of fructose-1-phosphate in the liver and kidneys. Fibroblasts from patients with hereditary fructose intolerance consume less glucose, produce less lactate, and contain less glycogen compared with control cells [Lemonnier et al., 1987]. A radioisotopic method for fructose-1-phosphate assay is available [Shin et al., 1983]. The enzyme deficiency is inherited as an autosomal-recessive trait and has an estimated prevalence in central Europe of 1:26,100 (95 percent confidence interval 1: 12,600–79,000) [Santer et al., 2005].

Urinary fructose excretion also is present in a harmless metabolic variant resulting from fructokinase deficiency that should not be confused with hereditary fructose intolerance.

Clinical Characteristics and Differential Diagnosis

Patients with hereditary fructose intolerance who ingest fructose experience nausea and vomiting; with continued exposure, weight gain is poor. Hypoglycemia begins immediately and reaches its low point 30–90 minutes after ingestion [Froesch et al., 1963]. Subsequent clinical and neuropathologic alterations result primarily from the hypoglycemia. Immoderate fructose feedings lead to albuminuria, jaundice, and a generalized aminoaciduria. Examination reveals jaundice and hepatomegaly.

Neurologic impairment is relatively uncommon but may result from hypoglycemia, cardiovascular collapse, or liver failure. Central nervous system complications include seizures with subsequent epilepsy, increased intracranial pressure, mental retardation, quadriplegia, and deafness [Labrune et al., 1990; Rennert and Greer, 1970]. Imaging findings include cortical atrophy, hydrocephalus, and parenchymal hemorrhage [Labrune et al., 1990].

Microscopic examination of the brain demonstrates neuronal loss and decreased myelination, attributed to hypoglycemia. Cirrhosis of the liver usually is marked.

Clinical Laboratory Tests and Diagnosis

The diagnosis may be corroborated by intravenous fructose challenge (0.1–0.2 g/kg, with adequate precautions to manage hypoglycemia). A positive response includes hypoglycemia, hypomagnesemia, hypouricemia, and hyperphosphatemia.

Assay of fructose-1-phosphate aldolase B in liver tissue permits definitive diagnosis, but liver biopsy may be avoided by direct genotyping in most patients. Although more than 20 mutations of the aldolase B gene have been described, two alleles (A149P and A174D) account for 70 percent or more of cases in Western Europe and North America, and may be readily detected in leukocytes by restriction fragment length polymorphism (RFLP) analysis [Kullberg-Lindh et al., 2002]. Fructosemia causes abnormal glycosylation of transferrin, leading to misdiagnosis of CDG1x on occasion [Quintana et al., 2009].

Management

Fructose elimination from the diet is accomplished by limited selection of vegetables and cereal products. Sorbitol should also be avoided, as it is an endogenous source of fructose. Dietary counseling is required for proper therapy [Bell and Sherwood, 1987].

Fructose-1,6-Diphosphatase Deficiency

Another inborn error of metabolism, fructose-1,6-diphosphatase (i.e., fructose-1,6-bisphosphatase [FBPase]) deficiency, also is characterized by hypoglycemia after fructose ingestion [Baker and Winegrad, 1970; Hulsmann and Fernandes, 1971]. About half of the cases manifest in infants, with life-threatening episodes of hypoglycemia and metabolic acidosis. The causal relationship between the enzyme deficiency and hypoglycemia in this abnormality is not fully explained. Some data, however, suggest that α-glycerol phosphate, fructose-1-phosphate, and fructose-1,6-diphosphate all inhibit phosphorylase a activity [Kaufmann and Froesch, 1973]. This relationship may explain the hypoglycemic episodes in both hereditary fructose intolerance and fructose-1,6-diphosphatase deficiency. The role of the enzyme deficiency in glycolysis and gluconeogenesis requires further clarification [Adams et al., 1990].

The diagnosis can be established by measuring FBPase activity and mutational analysis in cultured monocytes, without the necessity for liver biopsy [Kikawa et al., 2002]. A retrospective study of Japanese patients with FBPase deficiency treated with intravenous glycerol, which contains fructose in Asian countries, found a relationship between the infusion of glycerol and the onset of cerebral edema in some patients [Hasegawa et al., 2003]. In one case FBPase deficiency was associated with a prolonged prothrombin time, which corrected with intravenous glucose and bicarbonate [Nitzan et al., 2004]. Another patient gave birth to normal children after three uncomplicated pregnancies, but developed subsequent hearing loss and cognitive impairments despite careful metabolic monitoring [Krishnamurthy et al., 2007].

Glycogen Storage Diseases

The biochemistry of the glycogen storage diseases (GSDs) illustrates the diverse effects of genetically determined enzymatic deficiencies along a single metabolic pathway. In spite of a few inconsistencies and a number of unexplained conditions, a logical approach to these diseases is practical. The GSDs are a family of diseases sui generis, with the exception of at least two disorders that can be included under the rubric of lysosomal storage diseases – Pompe's disease and Danon's disease. Indeed, the first lysosomal storage disease defined as such was Pompe's disease [Hers, 1963]. General characteristics of this disease family are discussed in Chapter 36. Patients have also been described who accumulate glycogen in autophagic vacuoles but who do not appear to have an enzymatic deficiency [Danon et al., 1981]. This phenotype, named Danon's disease, is known to result from deficiency of lysosomal-associated membrane protein 2 [Nishino et al., 2000]. This X-linked dominant disorder has multisystem effects, most consistently involving the heart and skeletal muscle [Sugie et al., 2002].

There is general agreement on the numeric designations of GSDs I to VI, but the nomenclature beyond that is confusing. For example, GSD types VIII and X were originally considered distinct conditions, but are now classified with GSD VI by many authors.

Clinical manifestations of GSD often result from glucose deficiency, with ensuing hypoglycemia occurring separately or in association with increased glycogen storage. The location of the enzymatic block in the pathway determines whether the configuration of the glycogen is normal or abnormal.

GSDs result in the accumulation in various tissues of increased concentrations of glycogen of normal or abnormal configuration (Table 34-2). These diseases result from a deficiency or absence of specific enzyme activity in the metabolic pathway of glycogen.

The glucose molecule is the prime building block in the multistep synthesis of glycogen (Figure 34-2; see also Table 34-2). Glycogen synthesis occurs in many tissues, predominantly in liver, kidney, and muscle. Glucose transported in the blood enters the cell, facilitated by a glucose transporter [Scheepers et al., 2004], is phosphorylated in a reaction catalyzed by the enzyme hexokinase, and becomes glucose-6-phosphate. In the next step, the enzyme phosphoglucomutase mediates the transformation to glucose-1-phosphate. Glucose-1-phosphate, in association with uridine triphosphate, is transformed to uridine diphosphate-glucose with the participation of uridine diphosphate glucose pyrophosphorylase. The glucose portion of this molecule is then attached by a 1,4 linkage to a terminal glucosyl unit. This reaction is facilitated by the active form of the enzyme glycogen synthase (uridine diphosphate–glucose-glycogen glucosyl transferase). Glycogenin is a protein primer that initiates glycogen synthesis by covalently attaching individual glucose residues to tyrosine 194. This process occurs by autoglycosylation to form a short priming chain of glucose residues that are a substrate for glycogen synthase [Hurley et al., 2006]. When the glucosyl chain becomes 6–12 units long, this section is transferred and affixed to another glucosyl chain by a 1,6-linkage as a result of the action of the branching enzyme α-1,4-glucan: α-1,4-glucan-6-glucosyl transferase. A 1,6 linkage constitutes the branch point, a final stage in glycogen formation. Glycogen exists in the cell in association with proteins (including the enzymes described above) as organelles known as glycosomes. Glycosomes may occur free in the cytosol (lyoglycosomes) or in association with other structures (desmoglycosomes), including myofibers, mitochondria, and sarcoplasmic reticulum cisterna.

During the degradation process, the phosphorylase enzymes split the 1,4 linkages, which results in formation of free glucose-1-phosphate molecules. Both muscle and hepatic phosphorylase isoenzymes exist. Activation of phosphorylase takes place

Table 34-2 Glycogen Storage Diseases (GSDs)

Name*	Clinical Manifestations	Glycogen Structure	Enzyme Defect
1. Glucose-6-phosphatase deficiency (von Gierke's disease, Cori type I GSD)	Enlarged liver and kidneys; hyperlipidemia; hypoglycemia; ketoacidosis; seizures	Normal	Glucose-6-phosphatase
2. Infantile acid maltase deficiency (Pompe's disease, Cori type II GSD)	Cardiomegaly; death in infancy; progressive hypotonia and weakness; swallowing and respiratory difficulty	Normal	Acid maltase
3. Late infantile acid maltase deficiency, adult acid maltase deficiency	Atonic anal sphincter; calf muscle hypertrophy; hip weakness (Gowers' sign); slow or regressing motor development, contractures of Achilles tendons	(?)Abnormal – short outer chains	Acid maltase
4. Debrancher deficiency (Forbes limit dextrinosis, Cori type III GSD)	Hepatomegaly; hypoglycemia; late-onset weakness; mild growth failure; early, severe weakness with myopathy rare	Abnormal – short outer chains, increased branch points	Amylo-1,6-glucosidase
5. Brancher deficiency (Andersen's disease, Cori type IV GSD)	Cirrhosis; growth failure; hepatosplenomegaly; hypotonia; muscle wasting in lower extremities; slow motor development; weakness	Abnormal	Amylo-1,4→1,6-transglucosidase
6. Myophosphorylase deficiency (McArdle's disease, Cori type IV GSD)	Atrophy in older patients; myoglobinuria; poor stamina; severe muscle cramps with exercise	Normal	Muscle phosphorylase
7. Hepatophosphorylase deficiency (Hers' disease, Cori type VI GSD)	Growth retardation; hepatomegaly; hypoglycemia; mild ketosis	Normal	Muscle phosphorylase
8. Phosphorylase kinase deficiency (also deficiency of activation sequence including loss of activity of 3',5'-AMP-dependent kinase in muscle and probably liver)	Marked hepatomegaly, with glycogen storage; no hypoglycemia; no skeletal muscle disease; normal mental development	Normal	Phosphorylase kinase or 3',5'-AMP-dependent kinase
9. Phosphoglucomutase deficiency	Calf hypertrophy; mild generalized weakness; regression in motor development; toe-walking	Normal	Phosphoglucomutase
10. Phosphohexose isomerase deficiency	Late-onset myopathy; muscle cramps; poor stamina	Normal	Phosphohexose isomerase
11. Phosphofructokinase deficiency plus other defects of terminal glucolysis, including deficiency of phosphoglycerate kinase and lactate dehydrogenase	Similar to those in myophosphorylase deficiency	Normal	Phosphofructokinase
12. Glycogen synthetase deficiency	Hypoglycemia; mental retardation; seizures	Normal	Glycogen synthetase

* The accompanying numerals identify these abnormalities in the pathway of glycogen metabolism shown in Figures 34-2 and 34-3.

through a cascade of reactions ultimately involving phosphorylase b kinase (Figure 34-3). As the cleavage of 1,4 bonds moves near the 1,6 branching point, "three-glucose" residues are removed in a block by oligo-1,4 alpha 1,4-glucan transferase, and the 1,6 linkage is disrupted by the debranching enzyme (amylo-1,6 glucosidase), with the resultant release of a free glucose molecule. Approximately 8 percent of glucose in glycogen is involved at 1,6 branch points and may be released in this free form. This process continues along the branches of the glycogen molecule. Therefore, both glucose-1-phosphate and free glucose molecules result from this series of degradation reactions.

The glucose-1-phosphate molecules subsequently are converted to glucose-6-phosphate by the action of the enzyme phosphoglucomutase. Phosphate is released from glucose-6-phosphate in liver and kidney by glucose-6-phosphatase, and free glucose molecules result. (Glucose-6-phosphatase activity is absent in skeletal muscle.) The free glucose is transported by the circulation to other organs, where it is used. In other organs and in muscle the glucose-6-phosphate formed on entry is phosphorylated to fructose-1,6-diphosphate, which is transformed by the metabolic steps in the Embden–Meyerhof pathway that leads eventually to the formation of pyruvic acid and lactic acid.

Glucose-6-Phosphatase Deficiency (Von Gierke's Disease, Glycogen Storage Disease Type I, Hepatorenal Glycogenosis)

Pathology

In 1929, Von Gierke described the pathology of "hepato-nephromegalia glycogenica," and in 1952 the Coris described glucose-6-phosphatase deficiency as its cause (and established an enzyme deficiency as the cause of an inborn error of metabolism for the first time) [Moses 2002]. Patients with von Gierke's disease, now known as glycogen storage disease type I, have hepatomegaly and renomegaly. Light microscopy

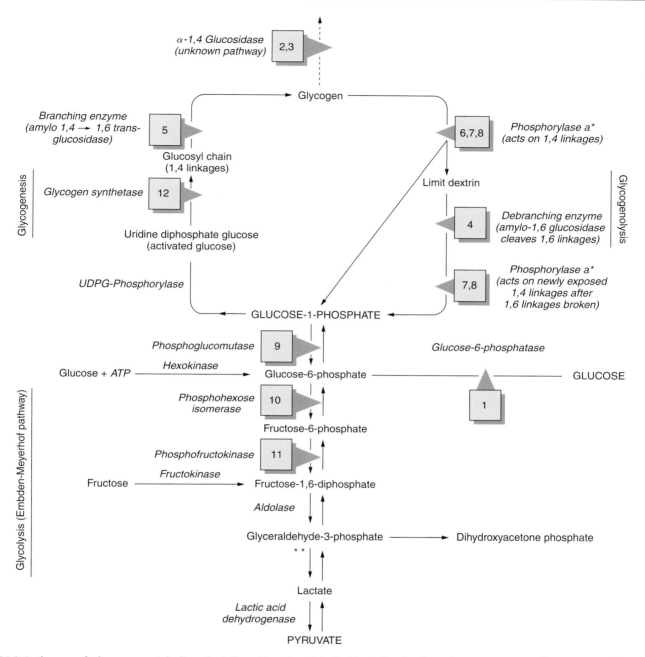

Fig. 34-2 Pathways of glycogen metabolism depicting sites of metabolic block that lead to glycogen storage disease. See Table 34-2 for description of abnormalities denoted by Arabic numerals enclosed in boxes. *See Figure 34-3 for phosphorylase activation sequence. **Other defects of terminal glycolysis.

reveals enormous amounts of glycogen in liver cells and in the cells of the renal convoluted tubules. No increase in the concentration of glycogen is found in skeletal muscle, tongue, or heart. Best's stain marks the presence of glycogen. Tissue must be fixed in a nonaqueous medium such as absolute alcohol; otherwise, the glycogen dissolves, and only vacuolar spaces will remain to mark the areas of deposit.

Electron microscopy of glycogen storage disease type I liver reveals loss of microvilli of the membranes lining Disse's spaces and bile canaliculi. Changes in endoplasmic reticulum include the development of doubly contoured vesicles that appear to help ribosomes only on the innermost surface of the inner

membrane. Glucose-6-phosphatase is located in or on the membranes of endoplasmic reticulum, and these findings parallel a disturbance of the phospholipid environment of the enzyme as a consequence of the mutation that affects enzyme activity [Spycher and Gitzelmann, 1971].

Biochemistry

Two distinct subgroups of glycogen storage disease type I have been identified: those with primary glucose-6-phosphatase deficiency (type Ia) and those phenocopies with additional features of immune impairment (neutropenia and neutrophil

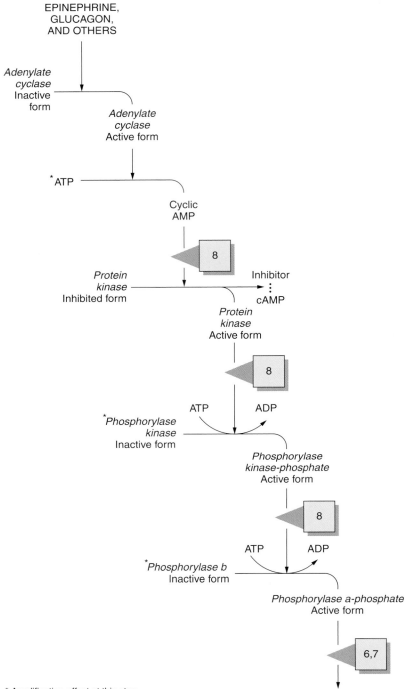

Fig. 34-3 Activation sequence of phosphorylase. See Table 34-2 for description of abnormalities denoted by the Arabic numerals enclosed in boxes. ADP, adenosine diphosphate; ATP, adenosine triphosphate; cAMP, cyclic adenosine monophosphate. (*Modified from Goldberg NB. Vigilance against pathogens. Hosp Pract 1974;9:127.*)

* Amplification effect at this step.

adherence defects), now designated as glycogen storage disease type I non-a [Moses, 2002]. Glycogen storage disease type I non-a disorders originally were thought to result from defects in a multicomponent translocase system responsible for transporting glucose-6-phosphatase into microsomes [Annabi et al., 1998]. This model postulated three transport proteins, T1, T2, and T3, to chaperone glucose, glucose-6-phosphatase, phosphate, and pyrophosphate across the endoplasmic reticulum membrane. Cloning of the glucose-6-phosphatase translocase gene (*G6PT*) demonstrated that the previously proposed subtypes b, c, and d all were associated with mutations in

G6PT, producing different kinetic variants [Matern et al., 2002; Moses and Parvari, 2002]. The *G6PC* gene that codes for glucose-6-phosphatase is located at 17q21 [Brody et al., 1995]. A number of allelic variants have been described. Glucose-6-phosphatase comprises at least five different polypeptides. The *G6P* locus is at 11q23 [Annabi et al., 1998]; several mutations have been characterized [Matern et al., 2002].

All forms share common clinical manifestations that are attributable to abnormal metabolism of glucose-6-phosphate. In type Ia, glucose-6-phosphatase deficiency results in storage of glycogen of normal configuration in the liver and kidneys. The glycogen concentration usually exceeds 4 percent by weight. The enzyme activity frequently is absent or extremely low [Cori and Cori, 1952]. Glucose-6-phosphatase is important in regulating the entry of free glucose into the circulation from the liver. Because of this pivotal role, deficiency of the enzyme produces hypoglycemia.

Ethanol causes decreased blood lactate and pyruvate content, presumably by diverting carbon to triglyceride formation [Sadeghi-Nejad et al., 1975]. A study of insulin secretion in five adult patients with glucose-6-phosphatase deficiency found that their capacity to increase blood insulin was significantly less than normal. As patients with this condition mature, they become normoglycemic and characteristically have abnormal glucose tolerance curves. These studies suggest that the increasing clinical stability noted with age and the associated tendency toward normoglycemia reflect a decrease in insulin responsiveness that may develop as an adaptive process [Lockwood et al., 1969]. Diabetes mellitus has been reported in GSD type 1 [Spiegel et al., 2005]. The intricacies of the glucose-6-phosphatase system and its role in glucose metabolism have been reviewed [Foster and Nordlie, 2002].

Clinical Characteristics

Hypoglycemia causes much of the morbidity during the first year of life. Seizures are frequent and almost invariably are the presenting complaint of affected children. Hypoglycemia may result in severe, chronic neurologic impairment, including hemiplegia [Fine et al., 1969]. Hepatomegaly and the failure to thrive syndrome are commonly present. An association with moyamoya disease has been described [Goutières et al., 1997]. A study of 19 patients with glycogen storage disease type I (median age 11 years) in one center found prevalence rates for epilepsy, deafness, and neuroradiologic abnormalities of 10.5 percent, 15 percent, and 57 percent, respectively, far in excess of the rates in the general population, or in children with other causes of neonatal hypoglycemia. MRI abnormalities included dilatation of occipital horns and/or hyperintensity of subcortical white matter in the occipital lobes in all patients [Melis et al., 2004]. Subcutaneous fat often is increased, especially over the buttocks, breasts, and cheeks. Xanthomas of the skin occur over the extensor surfaces of the limbs and at times over the buttocks [Hou et al., 1996; Hou and Wang, 2003]. Affected children frequently have a protuberant abdomen because of massive enlargement of the liver. Hepatomegaly may be present at birth. The liver edge is hard and not tender. Careful palpation may reveal enlarged kidneys. Hepatic adenomas develop in between one-half and three-quarters of adults with glycogen storage disease I; about 10 percent undergo malignant transformation. Some data suggest that lower frequencies are associated with better dietary control [Lee, 2002]. Hepatocellular carcinoma has been reported as complicating hepatic adenomas, and may reflect poor metabolic control [Franco et al., 2005]. Patients carrying mutations that cause relatively mild expression of the disease in childhood, often without hypoglycemia (such as 727 G>T), are associated with adult presentation of hepatocellular carcinoma [Matern et al., 2002].

Type I non-a patients typically have recurrent stomatitis, frequent infections, and chronic inflammatory bowel disease secondary to neutropenia and neutrophil dysfunction [de Parscau et al., 1988]. The neutropenia seen in GSD1b has been attributed to endoplasmic reticulum and oxidative stress secondary to the G6PT deficiency [Chou et al., 2010]. Seventy-five percent of 36 GSD type I non-a patients had chronic gastrointestinal complaints, and 28 percent had proven inflammatory bowel disease. A further 22 percent had a highly suggestive history [Dieckgraefe et al., 2002].

Clinical Laboratory Tests

The diagnosis can be made by assaying the enzyme activity in liver and peripheral white blood cells [Maire et al., 1991]. Direct assay of hepatic glucose-6-phosphatase activity in liver remains the definitive diagnostic procedure but can be replaced by mutational analysis in many patients. Just five mutant alleles account for almost 70 percent of cases of glucose-6-phosphatase deficiency, so that mutation screening is a reasonable initial diagnostic approach, avoiding the risks and discomfort of liver biopsy [Matern et al., 2002]. Molecular analysis of the *G6P* and *G6PT* genes permits rapid confirmation of the diagnosis in most cases [Janecke et al., 2001].

Severe hypoglycemia frequently occurs because of the failure of glucose formation from glucose-6-phosphate. Postprandial blood glucose concentration may be exceedingly high. Severe acidosis, which may vary in degree but usually is associated with lacticacidemia and pyruvicacidemia, and hyperuricemia are frequent. The presence of ketoacidosis has been unduly stressed.

Hyperuricemia has often been documented, but is poorly understood. Adenosine triphosphate depletion has been postulated as a causative factor [Greene et al., 1978]. Ketoacidosis and hyperthermia during anesthesia in a child with GSD type I has been described [Edelstein and Hirshman, 1980]. Blood cholesterol, fatty acids, and triglycerides are elevated; overt lipemia may be present.

Decreased bone density documented by radiography may be related to chronic metabolic acidosis. Serum inorganic phosphate may be decreased in the presence of normal alkaline phosphatase activity.

Provocation with epinephrine or glucagon demonstrates failure of the patient's blood glucose concentration to increase within 10–20 minutes, although intracellular glucose-6-phosphate is formed quickly after the induced activation of liver phosphorylase.

Management

The goal of therapy is to provide sufficient free glucose to maintain a normal blood glucose concentration. Continuous nocturnal intragastric infusion of glucose has been relatively successful [Greene et al., 1976]. Subsequently, the use of cornstarch suspensions given during the day obviated the need for nocturnal infusion in some children [Chen et al., 1984; Wolfsdorf et al., 1990]. The dietary carbohydrate must be monitored because excess glucose leads to glycogen storage in the liver and kidneys. Frequent small feedings of carbohydrates are provided. Severity of the disease reaches a plateau after the fourth or fifth year of life. Vigorous treatment is, therefore, worthwhile until the plateau is reached. A long-term study of 15 children with GSD type I, beginning in infancy, found that careful metabolic control, aiming for high to normal plasma glucose levels and normal urine lactate, was associated with normal growth and lowering, but not normalization, of plasma lipids. Hepatic adenomas or renal impairment developed in none of the patients who reached adolescence [Daublin et al., 2002; Weinstein et al., 2002].

Dietary substitution of medium-chain triglycerides for long-chain triglycerides was attempted in glucose-6-phosphatase deficiency, to alter the hyperlipemic state by means of the unique absorptive and metabolic properties of medium-chain triglycerides. The results suggested that substitution of medium-chain triglycerides for long-chain triglycerides in the diet, along with normal carbohydrate consumption, leads to significant decrease in serum lipid levels, disappearance of eruptive xanthomas, and decrease in liver mass [Cuttino et al., 1970].

The hyperglycemic agent diazoxide has been beneficial [Rennert and Mukhopadhyay, 1968]. The drug's action is not well understood, but normal blood glucose concentration has been maintained with this drug. Phenytoin also has been used [Jubiz and Rallison, 1974].

Surgical treatment for glucose-6-phosphatase deficiency involves creation of a portacaval shunt, which increases the peripheral blood glucose by allowing portal blood to bypass the liver after absorption of glucose from the gut; excellent metabolic control can be achieved over the long term, and the operation does not preclude subsequent liver transplantation [Corbeel et al., 2000]. The postoperative course has been complicated by severe hypoglycemia, hypocalcemia, acidosis, and respiratory impairment, the last primarily because of hepatomegaly. Preoperative intravenous hyperalimentation appears to eliminate these metabolic problems, reduce the size of the liver, and provide a smoother and shorter postoperative course [Folkman et al., 1972]. Liver transplantation was reported to produce beneficial results [Malatack et al., 1983]. One report suggested that this procedure, usually indicated for management of multiple hepatic adenomas, does not itself benefit metabolic control, and indeed, careful systemic management is essential to prevent graft complications [Labrune, 2002]. A more recent report of living donor liver transplantation in four children with GSD1b described markedly improved quality of life [Kasahara et al., 2009]. Another case report described a 47-year-old woman with GSD1a, whose fasting tolerance was significantly improved after infusion of hepatocytes [Muraca et al., 2002].

Chronic inflammatory bowel disease similar to Crohn's disease has been associated with GSD type I non-a [Dieckgraefe et al., 2002]. Initial studies suggested benefit from therapy with colony-stimulating factors [Roe et al., 1992]. A retrospective study of 57 patients with GSD type I non-a found evidence of less frequent infections and diminished severity of inflammatory bowel disease in those who received granulocyte colony-stimulating factor [Visser et al., 2002]. Splenomegaly was associated with granulocyte colony-stimulating factor therapy in this group. Renal disease also may ensue in older patients [Chen, 1991].

Brain abscess has been reported in a patient with type I non-a disease [Park et al., 1991]. Renal transplantation has been used for terminal renal failure, and occasionally, combined hepatic and renal grafting has been used. In both circumstances, meticulous systemic metabolic management is essential to successful outcome [Labrune, 2002].

Acid α-Glucosidase (GAA, Acid Maltase) Deficiency, Infantile Type (Pompe's Disease, Idiopathic Generalized Glycogenosis, Glycogen Storage Disease Type II)

Pathology

Infants with GSD type II have a severe vacuolar myopathy, with accumulation of large amounts of periodic acid–Schiff-positive material within cardiac, skeletal, and smooth muscle fibers and in liver, renal tubules, lymphocytes, glial cells, anterior horn cells, and brainstem nuclei, in infantile cases. Storage in later-onset cases is largely restricted to skeletal muscle. Large amounts of metachromatic material are found within the muscle fibers in the infantile cases. Metachromasia is not seen as often in the adult cases. The metachromasia reflects glycolipid or glycoprotein accumulation. Glycogen also accumulates in anterior horn cells. Scattered, sparse, perivascular lymphocytic infiltrates are seen in the interstitial tissue [Hudgson and Fulthorpe, 1975].

Biochemistry

Hers [1963] first reported the deficiency of activity of the lysosomal enzyme acid maltase (α-1,4-glucosidase), located at 17q25.2–q25.3 [Kuo et al., 1996; Martiniuk et al., 1985]. Glycogen structure has consistently been normal, and its accumulation is restricted primarily to lysosomes, although lysosomal breakdown and cytoplasmic accumulation with disruption of muscle fibers occur in severe cases. Although direct injury of muscle fibers by glycogen leaking from lysosomes was thought to be the major cause of contractile dysfunction, experimental and pathological evidence suggests that the accumulation of autophagosomes is the major culprit, and that these pathologic orgenelles impair the effectiveness of enzyme replacement therapy by acting as a sink for infused enzyme [Shea and Raben, 2009; Raben et al., 2009]. Hypoglycemia is not a feature of this condition, but increased protein turnover with increased leucine flux and oxidation and increased resting energy expenditure has been found in late-onset cases [Bodamer et al., 2000].

Attempts have been made to differentiate biochemically among the infantile, late infantile, and adult-onset forms of acid maltase deficiency. Activity of α-1,4-glucosidase (acid maltase) at various pH values in infants, children, and adults with acid maltase deficiency has been studied. Only traces of neutral maltase are found in the heart, and significantly decreased neutral maltase activity was measured in the skeletal muscle and liver of an affected infant. In the late infantile form, neutral acid maltase activity is decreased only in the liver; in the adult form, neutral maltase is not deficient in any tissue. An absolute decrease of leukocyte acid maltase was found in four adults and a relative decrease in 1 of 5 adults with acid maltase deficiency. Decrease in the pH ratio of acid to neural maltase activity in leukocytes may be of diagnostic importance in adult acid maltase deficiency [Angelini and Engel, 1972].

A number of allelic variations have been described and may explain the differences in age at onset. The theoretical abnormalities that could result in a deficiency of α-glucosidase include synthesis of catalytically inactive protein, absence of messenger RNA (mRNA) for the enzyme, decreased synthesis of the precursor, lack of phosphorylation of the precursor, impaired conversion of the precursor to the mature enzyme, and synthesis of unstable precursor [Tager et al., 1987; Zhong et al., 1991]. In general, the location and nature of mutations predict the phenotype, but exceptional cases are described in which relatively mild phenotypes occur despite low levels of α-glucosidase expression in cultured cells and in the patient's tissues [Hermans et al., 2004; Kroos et al., 2004]. Thus far, unidentified genetic modifiers and environmental factors are presumed to account for such variability.

Unexplained storage of increased neutral lipid is coupled with low carnitine concentration and reduced β-hydroxyacyl-CoA dehydrogenase in muscle [Verity, 1991].

Clinical Characteristics

Development usually is normal for several weeks to several months; then the affected infant presents with feeding difficulties, weakness, or respiratory impairment. The median age at presentation was 1.6 and 1.9 months, respectively, in 20 Dutch patients and 133 patients described in the literature [Van den Hout et al., 2003] (Figure 34-4). Little spontaneous movement occurs, and the cry is short-lived and weak. Swallowing is grossly limited, and secretions pool in the posterior oropharynx. Respiratory difficulty reflects weakness of the accessory muscles of respiration [Tanaka et al., 1979]. Massive cardiomegaly develops, and a soft systolic murmur is often heard along the left sternal border [Pompe, 1932]. Obstruction to ventricular outflow and impairment of inflow may develop [Seifert et al., 1992], and serial echocardiography reveals progressive left ventricular posterior wall diastolic thickening [Van den Hout et al., 2003]. Hepatomegaly is almost universally present. The liver has a sharp edge and a firm consistency on palpation. Subcutaneous fat over all areas of the body is sparse, and the muscles are small and firm. The tongue often is enlarged and may protrude. Intermittent cyanosis reflects respiratory

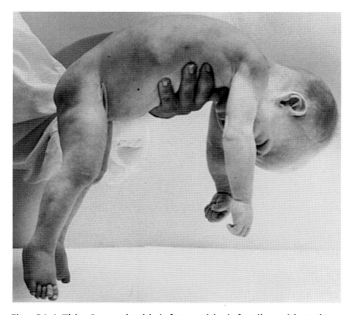

Fig. 34-4 This 8-month-old infant with infantile acid maltase deficiency (Pompe's disease) is profoundly hypotonic and weak. The child is draped over the examiner's hand while the infant's arms and legs are immobile against gravity. *(From Swaiman KF, Wright FS. Pediatric neuromuscular diseases. St. Louis: Mosby, 1979.)*

and cardiac embarrassment. Deep tendon reflexes are lost by the age of 6 months. Affected infants undergo progressive debilitation, and most die, at median ages of 6 and 7.7 months in the literature cases and Dutch series, respectively. Fewer than 10 percent survive beyond 1 year; only two patients have been described who survived 18 months [Van den Hout et al., 2003], and almost all die by 2 years. A subgroup of children has been described who present later in infancy, with lesser degrees of weakness and cardiac impairment, who have survived for periods as long as 13 years with ventilatory and nutritional support [Slonim et al., 2000].

Clinical Laboratory Tests

The quantity of glycogen storage and activity of the enzyme involved in glycogen metabolism can be monitored by using skin removed with a vacuum skin-blistering technique or fibroblasts grown from skin biopsy material. Among the enzymes in skin are phosphorylase, acid maltase, and the debranching enzyme amylo-1,6-glucosidase. No glucose-6-phosphatase activity is present in skin.

Both skin fibroblasts and amniotic fluid cells can be used for assay of acid maltase (α-1,4-glucosidase) activity [Butterworth and Broadhead, 1977; Leathwood and Ryman, 1971]. Prenatal diagnosis by biochemical study of uncultured amniotic fluid cells and chorionic villus biopsy material using maltose as a substrate have been reported [Hug et al., 1984; Park et al., 1992]. Mutational analysis has superseded these techniques in some cases, and complemented enzyme analysis and ultrasound examinations in others, as in a report of a fetus with this deficiency diagnosed in the second trimester, in which glycogen accumulation was detectable in muscle, as well as a visibly enlarged tongue on prenatal ultrasound examination [Chen et al., 2004].

A simple differential immunoprecipitation assay of urinary acid and neutral α-glucosidases has been developed [Tsuji et al., 1987].

The chest x-ray reveals massive cardiomegaly [Ruttenberg et al., 1964]. The electrocardiogram contains depressed ST segments, inverted T waves, and a shortened P-R interval. These changes may be confused with those of myocarditis. Electromyography (EMG) shows myopathic changes; polyphasic potentials and a reduced interference pattern with low voltage are the usual findings. Unusual high-frequency discharges, best described as myotonic-like, are very common [Gutman et al., 1967; Hogan et al., 1969]. Muscle and liver biopsy specimens contain large amounts of structurally normal glycogen when studied by both light and electron microscopy. Changes in peripheral nerve also have been reported [Araoz et al., 1974].

Genetics

GAA deficiency is inherited as an autosomal-recessive trait. The gene for human acid α-glucosidase is contained on chromosome 17 (segment q21–q23) [Martiniuk et al., 1986]. The structural gene for human acid α-glucosidase is undergoing intensive study; it is approximately 28 kb in length and contains 20 exons [Martiniuk et al., 1991]. Various mutations may result in the phenotype; missense mutations and failure of an allele to manifest mRNA expression have been reported [Zhong et al., 1991]. Prenatal diagnosis has been available since the 1970s [Hug et al., 1974]. The use of chorionic villus assay allows first-trimester diagnosis [Chowers et al., 1986].

Both adult-onset and infantile glycogenosis type II have been detected in one family. Two types of mutant alleles were identified; one leads to complete deficiency of the enzyme, and the other results in reduced net production of active α-glucosidase, resulting in partial enzyme deficiency [Hoefsloot et al., 1990].

Management

Before the advent of enzyme replacement therapy (ERT), no practical treatment was available. Therapies previously studied included epinephrine administration, which reduced liver, but not muscle, glycogen content to normal [Hug, 1974]. Dietary supplementation with L-alanine, designed to reduce the elevated protein turnover characteristic of acid maltase deficiency, has apparently slowed progression of weakness and even reversed cardiomyopathy in some patients with late infantile and juvenile forms [Bodamer et al., 1997, 2000, 2002].

Attempts to replace the deficient enzyme date back to 1964, but effective ERT was not possible until suitable sources of receptor-targeted human recombinant acid glucosidase became available in the late 1990s. This substance was derived from both rabbit milk and Chinese hamster ovary (CHO) cells. The first clinical trial began in 1998 [Reuser et al., 2002; Winkel et al., 2004], and in 2006, ERT received Food and Drug Administration (FDA) approval for treatment of acid maltase deficiency [Koeberl et al., 2007]. Infants who received treatment early in the course of their illness demonstrated improved strength and cardiac function, with survival now extending over several years. It has become apparent that ERT is most effective at reversing cardiomyopathy and extending the life span of infants, but that skeletal muscle disease is relatively resistant to this modality [Schoser et al., 2008]. The follow-up interval has been too short to determine if anterior horn cell and glial storage of glycogen will lead to chronic weakness and impairment of cerebral function in long-term survivors.

Late Infantile GAA Deficiency

A number of children have been reported who are deficient in acid maltase activity but without the phenotype of Pompe's disease [Smith et al., 1966, 1967]. These children usually are asymptomatic during the first year of life and live beyond the age of 2 years. Most have slowly progressive weakness but no gross signs of overt deposits of glycogen in skeletal or heart muscle or in visceral organs.

Symptoms and signs may mimic those of Duchenne muscular dystrophy. In this condition, the gastrocnemius and deltoid muscles may be firm and rubbery, with accompanying hypertrophy of the gastrocnemius muscle. Waddling gait, increased lumbar lordosis, and Gowers' sign (Figure 34-5) are frequently present. Achilles tendon contractures result in equinus gait. Cardiomegaly is absent, and an intermittent soft, systolic murmur may be heard. Two patients had a patulous anal sphincter.

Clinical Laboratory Tests

Light and electron microscopy of muscle biopsy material displays moderate glycogen storage (Figure 34-6). In muscles stained with hematoxylin and eosin, the glycogen-containing areas appear vacuolated. In one report, only type I fibers were involved [Papapetropoulos et al., 1984]. A few patients with glycogen storage in lysosomes have been described who

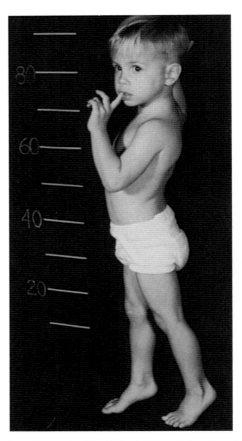

Fig. 34-5 This 22-month-old child with late infantile acid maltase deficiency has increased lumbar lordosis, pseudohypertrophy of the calf muscles, and contractures of the Achilles tendons. *(From Swaiman KF, Wright FS. Pediatric neuromuscular diseases. St. Louis: Mosby, 1979.)*

appear to have normal acid maltase enzyme activity [Tachi et al., 1989].

Electron microscopy depicts monogranular and multigranular deposits of glycogen free in the sarcoplasm, as well as membrane bound in lysosomes. EMG documents polyphasic potentials and a reduced, low-voltage interference pattern. The bizarre, myotonic-type potentials described in early infantile acid maltase deficiency also occur in the late infantile form.

Biochemistry

Aside from the accumulation of glycogen and its possible abnormal architecture, the most prominent abnormality described is a deficiency of acid maltase activity. Quantitation of glycogen reveals increased content. The liver may or may not contain increased glycogen stores [Smith et al., 1966, 1967]. Two patients have been described who had glycogen of abnormal configuration because of shortened outer chains.

Management

Attempts to manage patients by dietary means enjoyed modest success after initially disappointing results (see earlier) [Bodamer et al., 1997, 2000, 2002].

At present, ERT appears to offer the best hope for definitive treatment in this group of patients [Reuser et al., 2002]. Investigational studies are on-going.

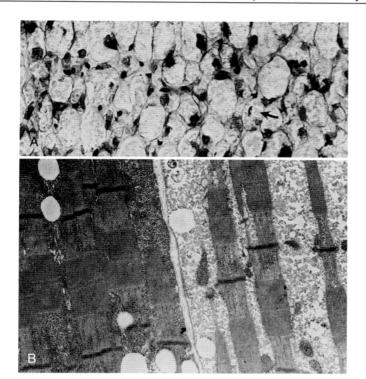

Fig. 34-6 Infantile acid maltase deficiency. A, Ballooned muscle cells with dispersed myofibrils (arrow) resulting from glycogen appearing as clear areas. (Verhoeff–van Gieson stain; × 170.) **B,** Ultrastructure showing excessive glycogen beneath the sarcolemma and between myofibrillar bundles. (× 10,050.) *(A and B, Courtesy of Dr. Stephen A Smith.)*

Juvenile and Adult GAA Deficiency

A slowly progressive myopathy characterizes juvenile and adult GAA deficiency. The literature has been reviewed and consensus criteria for diagnosis established [AANEM, 2009]. Limb girdle weakness is the most common presentation, but muscle pain is underappreciated and relatively common. Most patients complain of fatigue. Ventilatory failure may be the presenting complaint in as many as one-third of adults, sometimes with predominantly nocturnal symptoms.

Laboratory abnormalities include increased serum enzyme activity of creatine kinase (normal to as much as 15-fold elevated [AANEM, 2009]), aspartate aminotransferase, and lactate dehydrogenase. Adult cases cannot be delineated from infantile and late infantile cases on the basis of muscle GAA activity. The enzymatic deficiency is demonstrable in adult patients [Wokke et al., 1995].

Neutral maltase activity appears to be normal in adult cases but may be decreased in infantile and late infantile cases. Glycogen content of muscles in adult patients does not differ from that in patients with deficiency of infantile and late infantile onset and ranges from 1.8 to 5.8 percent.

In both the juvenile and adult forms, weakness associated with acid maltase deficiency develops during the second through the sixth decades of life. Weakness is greater proximally than distally, and is more prominent in the pelvis than in the shoulder girdle. Weakness varies from muscle to muscle. Intercostal and diaphragmatic muscles are involved in many patients. Adult patients do not have enlargement of the liver, heart, or tongue. There is a broad differential diagnosis that includes muscular dystrophies, other metabolic myopathies,

congenital myopathies, inflammatory myopathies, anterior horn cell diseases, and disorders of the neuromuscular junction [AANEM, 2009].

In one series, 16 patients with adult-onset acid maltase deficiency were compound heterozygotes. Patients presented with proximal weakness of the legs or fatigue. The patients manifested progressive symptoms [Wokke et al., 1995]. Some diminution of α-glucosidase activity was identified in muscle [Wokke et al., 1995].

EMG changes and histologic and electron microscopic findings in muscle biopsy specimens in adult cases are similar to changes in infantile and late infantile cases. In general, histologic findings in muscle biopsies also are the same in adults. Diastase digestion of fresh frozen sections confirms that the stored material is glycogen. Electron microscopy demonstrates no differences among infantile, late infantile, and adult cases.

Replacement therapy with rabbit-derived recombinant human α-glucosidase in patients aged 11, 16, and 32 years over a 3-year period produced stabilization of pulmonary function and strength in the older patients, and sufficient improvement in strength that the youngest patient was able to dispense with his wheelchair and walk unassisted [Winkel et al., 2004].

Amylo-1,6-Glucosidase Deficiency (Debrancher Deficiency, Cori's Disease, Forbes' Disease, Limit Dextrinosis, Glycogen Storage Disease Type III)

Pathology

Electron microscopy of skeletal muscle of persons with glycogenoses has demonstrated glycogen deposits just inside the sarcolemmal membrane and between the filaments of the I and A bands, as well as between the myofibrils. These abnormalities are not pathognomonic for this glycogenosis [Neustein, 1969], now classified as glycogen storage disease type III. Glycogen storage in liver is indistinguishable from glycogen storage in other glycogenoses that involve the liver.

Biochemistry

A complementary DNA encoding the human muscle glycogen debranching enzyme *(AGL)* was used to localize the gene to 1p21 by somatic cell hybrid analysis and in situ hybridization [Yang-Feng et al., 1992]. The *AGL* gene was cloned and found to encode six isoforms that manifested tissue-specific distribution and two distinct functions, both as a debranching enzyme and as a transferase [Bao et al., 1996]. Polymorphic markers within the gene can be used for linkage analysis for prenatal diagnosis and carrier detection [Shen et al., 1997], although direct mutational analysis is frequently used. GSD type III has marked genetic heterogeneity, with almost 70 mutations described by 2004 [Lam et al., 2004; HGMD, 2010]. Although genotype–phenotype correlations are difficult in rare recessive phenotypes such as GSD type III, in which most patients are compound heterozygotes for private mutations, it appears that GSD type IIIa is associated with mutations downstream to exon 3, whereas GSD type IIIb is associated with mutations in exon 3 [Lucchiari et al., 2002, 2003]. There is considerable allelic heterogeneity in different ethnic groups harboring mutations in this gene [Endo et al., 2006; Aoyama et al., 2009].

Several designated biochemical categories of type III glycogenosis have been identified. In type IIIa deficiency (both transferase and glucosidase deficiency), debranching enzyme activity is either absent or greatly reduced in liver and muscle. When the enzyme activity is deficient in liver alone, the condition is designated type IIIb. Type IIIc patients have deficient glucosidase but not transferase activity. A 12-year-old girl homozygous for p.R1147G has been diagnosed with isolated glucosidase deficiency [Aoyama et al., 2009]. Some patients have the reverse: that is, isolated transferase deficiency with retention of glucosidase activity (type IIId disease) [Ding et al., 1990]. The likelihood of myopathy and cardiomyopathy can be determined from assay of debranching enzyme and debranching enzyme transferase activity [Coleman et al., 1992]. Approximately 70 percent of the patients have no activity in all tissues studied. In another 10 percent of patients, enzyme activity is absent in liver but present to a small degree in muscle tissue. In yet another group, some activity of the debranching enzyme is present in either or both liver and skeletal muscle. The use of skin fibroblasts for study of debrancher enzyme activity is the usual initial approach to enzyme studies [Brown et al., 1978]. Oligo-1,4 α1,4-transglucosylase (transferase) activity may be present in muscle and liver of patients with type III glycogenosis but absent in their leukocytes. Electron microscopy of skin indicates glycogen storage in eccrine sweat glands [Sancho et al., 1990].

Characterization of the enzyme indicates immunochemical similarity of debranching enzyme in liver and in muscle. The evidence also suggests that deficiency of debranching enzyme activity in GSD type III is the result of the absence of debrancher protein [Chen et al., 1987].

Assay of liver tissue of a patient with debrancher enzyme deficiency revealed increased activity of fructose-1,6-diphosphatase. Lack of enzymatic activity limits the breakdown of glycogen, and during fasting, the release of glucose from the liver stems from gluconeogenesis. The increase in fructose-1,6-diphosphatase activity likely reflects increased gluconeogenesis. Administration of galactose [Hers, 1959], dihydroxyacetone [Brombacher et al., 1964], fructose [Hers, 1959], casein [Fernandes and van de Kamer, 1968], and glycerol [Senior and Loridan, 1968] has resulted in increased blood glucose concentrations; these findings support the critical compensatory role of gluconeogenesis in this condition [Sadeghi-Nejad et al., 1970]. In patients with deficient muscle enzyme activity, incorporation of uridine-^{14}C-glucose into red cell glycogen is either very low or absent.

Myogenic hyperuricemia is common in this condition but is not unique; hyperuricemia also accompanies glycogenosis type V and type VII [Mineo et al., 1987].

Clinical Characteristics

INFANTILE TYPE

Patients with debrancher enzyme deficiency may have muscle or liver involvement, or both. The infantile type usually manifests in the first few months of life and is associated with hypoglycemia, failure to thrive, and hepatomegaly [Forbes, 1953]. Affected infants are hypotonic and weak, and have poor head control. Glycogen deposition in cardiac muscle rarely is sufficient to create clinical disturbances; however, gross cardiac involvement with glycogen accumulation was reported in a 3-month-old patient, who died suddenly [Miller et al., 1972].

Association of debranching disease with profound cardiac muscle and skeletal muscle involvement accompanied by thyroid insufficiency also has been reported. The simultaneous presence of these two conditions is unexplained [Goutières and Aicardi, 1971].

The presence in infancy of hypoglycemia and hepatomegaly in this enzyme deficiency parallels abnormalities found in Von Gierke's disease (glucose-6-phosphatase deficiency), but the abnormalities are less pronounced.

One infant with both GSD type IIIa and Costello's syndrome has been described [Kaji et al., 2002]. The significance of this association is unclear.

CHILDHOOD TYPE

Abnormal findings in a 7-year-old female with GSD type III included exercise intolerance and heart failure. Cardiac and skeletal muscle contained increased stores of glycogen. Branching enzyme deficiency was confirmed with further studies [Servidei et al., 1987]. Hyperlipidemia appears to be common in children with GSD III, particularly those under 3 years [Bernier et al., 2008]. Hypertriglyceridemia correlates negatively with age; it may reflect more severe hypoglycemia in younger children. Children may also have reduced bone density, although this cannot be reliably determined by serum or urine markers [Cabrera-Abreu et al., 2004].

ADULT TYPE

Debrancher enzyme deficiency also has been reported in older children and adults [Brunberg et al., 1971]. Adult patients with GSD type III manifesting as chronic progressive myopathy in middle age have been described [DiMauro et al., 1978; Momoi et al., 1992]. Patients with debrancher deficiency should be monitored for cardiac involvement [Moses et al., 1989]. A 52-year-old woman was reported from Korea, who presented with symptomatic hypertrophic cardiomyopathy, severe general weakness, and hepatomegaly [Kim et al., 2008]. An adult with GSD type IIIa presented with diabetes mellitus, complicating hepatic failure. He was successfully managed with an α-glucosidase inhibitor, which delays carbohydrate glycolysis in the gut, thus blunting postprandial hyperglycemia and the consequent risk of hypoglycemia [Oki et al., 2000]. Progressive cirrhosis may be more common in adult GSD type III than was previously recognized, and occasionally is complicated by hepatocellular carcinoma [Siciliano et al., 2000]. One study of 45 patients aged 20 months to 67 years with GSD III identified two cases of hepatocellular carcinoma. Both arose on a background of cirrhosis. There are no reliable biomarkers for malignant transformation, and vigilant follow-up is essential for early diagnosis [Demo et al., 2007].

Debrancher deficiency has been associated with flaccidity, as reported in a 13-year-old patient [Forbes, 1953; Pearson, 1968], and with "weak tone," described in a 3-year-old patient [van Creveld and Huijing, 1965]. A history of a protuberant abdomen during childhood often is present. Patients complain of muscle fatigue without tenderness, cramping, or associated hematuria. Persistent diffuse weakness is present, and wasting of the hand and forearm muscles with loss of body weight ensues. Sugar-containing foods are of no clinical benefit, and symptoms of hypoglycemia are absent. The family history may include death of siblings in late childhood from a similar illness.

Clinical Laboratory Tests

Pseudomyotonic discharges are present on EMG. Serum creatine kinase activity may increase before and after exercise. Blood studies demonstrate mild fasting hypoglycemia, hyperlipidemia, fasting ketonuria, and diabetic glucose tolerance curves. Blood glucose concentration usually is not responsive to epinephrine or glucagon, but at times a mild response may occur. Results on galactose, fructose, and glycerol tolerance testing are normal. Blood lactic acid does not increase on ischemic exercise. Abnormally structured glycogen containing short outer chains has been demonstrated in liver, skeletal muscle, and red and white cells [Brandt and DeLuca, 1966; Van Hoof, 1967; Van Hoof and Hers, 1967].

Genetics

GSD type III is inherited as an autosomal-recessive trait. The use of cultured amniotic fluid cells and chorionic villus assay allows first-trimester diagnosis [Chowers et al., 1986; Yang et al., 1990]. Heterozygotes cannot be diagnosed with certainty using enzyme analysis [Cohn et al., 1975], but mutational analysis can accurately identify both affected persons and carriers when two mutant alleles have been detected in a proband.

Management

Patients with growth failure and hepatic dysfunction, including hypoglycemia, appear to benefit from the administration of oral cornstarch [Borowitz and Greene, 1987; Gremse et al., 1990]. It may be important to avoid overtreatment with carbohydrate; cardiomyopathy was reversed in a 16-year-old patient by increasing the protein content of the diet from 20 to 30 percent of caloric intake, with corresponding reduction of cornstarch to the minimum level required to avoid hypoglycemia [Dagli et al., 2009].

Amylo-1,4 →1,6 Transglucosidase Deficiency (Brancher Enzyme Deficiency, Glycogen Storage Disease Type IV)

GSD type IV (Andersen's disease) results from a deficiency of glycogen branching enzyme (GBE), leading to the accumulation of abnormal glycogen resembling amylopectin in affected tissues. The reported phenotypes are highly varied but for the most part have been marked primarily by liver involvement. GSD type IV has been characterized as the most heterogeneous of the glycogen storage diseases [Moses and Parvari, 2002].

A few infants with severe congenital hypotonia and cardiomyopathy have been described [Nambu et al., 2003; Janecke et al., 2004]. A mild, predominantly myopathic variant has been reported in older children [Reusche et al., 1992]. Adults with polyglucosan body disease who manifest late-onset pyramidal quadriparesis, micturition difficulties, peripheral neuropathy, and mild cognitive impairment have been described. Diagnosis in those cases was made initially by sural nerve biopsy. MRI revealed marked white matter alterations. Branching enzyme activity in leukocytes was about 15 percent of control values [Lossos et al., 1991], although some affected persons identified subsequently have normal enzyme activity. Five Jewish families with adults with polyglucosan body disease have been described in which affected persons were homozygous for a Tyr329Ser mutation in *GBE1*. Not all such patients

have recognized *GBE* mutations or impaired GBE activity, suggesting both phenotypic and genotypic heterogeneity [Klein et al., 2004].

Pathology

Glycogen may accumulate disproportionately in the tongue and diaphragm in comparison with other striated muscle groups. The characteristic lesion is the polyglucosan body, a periodic acid–Schiff-positive inclusion that also is seen in phosphofructokinase deficiency, Lafora body disease, double athetosis (Bielschowsky bodies), and aging (corpora amylacea) [Cavanagh, 1999]. Electron microscopy of the deposits reveals branched filaments, osmiophilic granules, and electron-dense amorphous material. Autopsy of a neonate who died at 1 month of life of cardiorespiratory failure showed vacuoles filled with periodic acid–Schiff-positive diastase-resistant materials in cells including neurons. Electron microscopy demonstrated polyglucosan bodies in all tissues examined. *GBE1* activity was markedly reduced in muscle and fibroblasts, and absent in liver and heart, as well as glycogen synthase activity. The patient was homozygous for p.E152X in *GBE1* [Lamperti et al., 2009].

Biochemistry

The first patient described with deficiency of brancher enzyme activity manifested cirrhosis of the liver and glycogen accumulation [Anderson, 1956], but patients with normal [Holleman et al., 1966] and decreased muscle glycogen concentrations [Sidbury et al., 1962] also have been described. Brancher enzyme deficiency results in the synthesis of unbranched glycogen composed of elongated chains of glucose molecules joined together in 1,4 linkages. As a result, the glycogen is composed of long outer chains, has few branch points, and resembles the pattern of starch also known as amylopectin.

The glycogen brancher enzyme has been purified beyond 3000-fold from rabbit skeletal muscle. The enzyme appears to have a molecular weight of 92–103 kilodaltons (kDa), depending on the choice of reference protein. Amylopectin polysaccharide isolated from the liver of a patient with branching deficiency is branched in the presence of the purified enzyme and α-D-glucose-1-phosphate at pH 7 [Gibson et al., 1971].

Study of the fine structure of glycogen from a patient with brancher enzyme deficiency found that the similarity of abnormal glycogen to amylopectin is in some ways superficial. The abnormal glycogen contains a significant number of short branches. This finding is consistent with the hypothesis that a normal debranching enzyme system in these patients can participate in a reverse reaction, with a resultant small degree of branching activity. The short chains are explained further by the supposition that the glycogen debranching enzyme system would form branch points by the apposition of 1→6 bonded α-glucose units by amylo-1,6-glucosidase. Further elongation of this chain would occur by transfer of oligosaccharide by the oligo-1,4→1,4-transferase component of the debranching system. The transferase favors transfer of maltotriosyl residue, which creates a four-unit branch. Brancher enzyme from muscle or liver ordinarily transfers glucose units containing seven glucose molecules. The shorter branches formed by a reversal of the debranching enzyme system are not as readily extended by glycogen synthetase. If the units are shorter than four glucose units, it may be impossible for them to be extended by synthetase [Mercier and Whelan, 1970]. The presence of short branches suggests that reversal of the debranching mechanism is operative.

Clinical Characteristics

Manifestations of the disease – failure to thrive, hepatosplenomegaly, and liver failure with cirrhosis – usually appear in the first 6 months of life. Affected infants exhibit delayed motor and social development, hypotonia, weakness, and muscle atrophy, accompanied by absent or decreased deep tendon reflexes [McMaster et al., 1979; Zellweger et al., 1972]. The most severe phenotype presents in the fetus. Manifestations of this lethal disorder include cervical cystic hygroma, fetal hydrops, and fetal akinesia in differing combinations [L'Hermine-Coulomb et al., 2005]. A more benign form with clinical onset at the age of 2 years manifested as hepatomegaly and elevated liver enzyme activity. The patient had no neurologic abnormalities, and the liver disease was not progressive [Greene et al., 1988]. Another patient, a 3-year-old male, had mild glycogen storage, as well as dicarboxylicaciduria and secondary carnitine deficiency. Notable clinical improvement occurred with administration of oral L-carnitine [Maaswinkel-Moody et al., 1987]. Yet another patient had mild clinical symptoms at 8 years of age despite profound deficiency of glycogen branching enzyme [Guerra et al., 1986]. Adult myopathic variants have been described [Bornemann et al., 1996].

Clinical Laboratory Tests

Diagnosis of brancher deficiency by assay of peripheral white blood cells, skin fibroblasts, and amniotic cell activity is feasible [Howell et al., 1971]. Confirmation of the diagnosis by mutational analysis is now possible, and is often preferable, given that enzyme analysis may sometimes be difficult to interpret [Li et al., 2010].

Genetics

Early studies confirmed an autosomal-recessive mode of inheritance [Legum and Nitowsky, 1969]. Enzyme activity in cultured fibroblasts is less than control levels in patients and both parents, corroborating the presence of an autosomal-recessive mode of inheritance. Prenatal testing using cultured amniocytes and chorionic villi is feasible [Brown and Brown, 1989] but has been superseded by molecular analysis when available. The gene encoding brancher enzyme, GBE1, was identified in 1993 [Thon et al., 1993]. By 2010, 34 mutations had been described [Li et al., 2010]. Most are missense, but nonsense, intronic donor and acceptor splice-site mutations, small deletion frameshift mutations, small insertion frameshift mutations, and large deletions have all been reported. Although genotype–phenotype correlations are imperfect, missense mutations are more likely to be associated with milder phenotypes, and truncating mutations or large deletions with severe forms of the disease.

Management

Treatment with a combination of zinc-glucagon and α-glucosidase decreased liver glycogen concentration, but the infant died at 11 months of age from an infection [Fernandes and Huijing, 1968]. Liver transplantation has been successful in a number of patients [Selby et al., 1991]. Orthotopic liver transplantation has been attempted with varied success [Selby et al., 1991]. In one report, cardiac amylopectinosis occurred 9 months after successful transplantation [Sokal et al., 1992].

McArdle's Disease (Myophosphorylase Deficiency, Glycogen Storage Disease Type V)

In 1951, McArdle reported a condition characterized by weakness, fatigue, and severe muscle cramping with pain after exercise. He subsequently noted the lack of normal lactate production in the affected muscles after ischemic work [McArdle, 1951; Pearson et al., 1961; Schmid and Mahler, 1959]. McArdle's disease is classified as glycogen storage disease type V (GSD V).

Pathology

Light microscopic studies of muscle reveal moderately increased stores of glycogen beneath the sarcolemmal membrane. Electron microscopy demonstrates disorganization of the I band region and distortion of the myofibrils secondary to glycogen deposition [Rowland et al., 1963]. Histochemical study of muscle suggests the absence of myophosphorylase activity, but only quantitative biochemical studies are reliable to confirm the diagnosis. Critical and definitive diagnosis depends on assay for the enzymatic deficiency in the affected muscle tissue.

Biochemistry

Glycogen breakdown to lactate begins with the initial disruption of the 1,4 linkage between glucosyl units. The enzyme myophosphorylase facilitates this reaction in skeletal muscle. After this linkage is cleaved, glucose-1-phosphate is freed and metabolized to lactate through the Embden–Meyerhof pathway. The myophosphorylase enzyme is regenerated in a complex reaction involving a number of other enzymes, including phosphorylase kinase (see Figure 34-3).

Absence of myophosphorylase activity results in decreased glucose-1-phosphate production; as a result, lactic acid is not formed in exercised muscle, and serum lactic acid concentration is not appropriately elevated (Figure 34-7). Structure of the excess glycogen stored is normal. Mitochondrial metabolism is normal [Argov et al., 1987].

Histochemical stains of fresh frozen sections of skeletal fibers demonstrate absence of phosphorylase. Studies of early multinucleated fibers and striated myofibers grown in vitro from these tissues reveal definite evidence of phosphorylase activity. Genetic coding for developing a form of myophosphorylase activity must be present in the precursor cells of regenerating skeletal muscle. The observation suggests the presence of a mechanism for loss of activity during maturation of tissues. Feasible explanations include the following possibilities: muscle maturation may result in loss of an enzyme that maintains phosphorylase production, survival, or activity; an abnormal specific protease may develop with maturity and inactivate myophosphorylase; a normally repressed myophosphorylase repressor gene may be "de-repressed"; and a normally present but inactive myophosphorylase-inhibiting or destroying enzyme may be activated and inhibit myophosphorylase enzyme

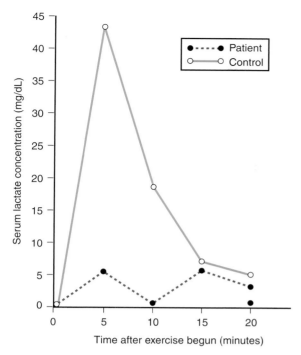

Fig. 34-7 This line graph reflects the failure of increase in blood lactic acid concentration during ischemic exercise of the arm in a patient with McArdle's disease.

activity or survival [DiMauro et al., 1978; Roelofs et al., 1972]. Occasionally, patients are found to have no immunologic cross-reactive material to normal myophosphorylase [Koster et al., 1979].

Clinical Characteristics

Affected children have decreased stamina and tire easily. Fatigue may be mediated in part by ammonia accumulation [Coakley et al., 1992]. Severe cramping pain after minimal exercise is noted in the involved skeletal muscles and primarily affects distal muscles. Cardiac symptoms have not been reported, but cardiac muscle is involved [Ratinov et al., 1965]. Myoglobinuria occurs with moderate or strenuous exercise. In adolescence and adulthood, persistent weakness may develop, with moderate loss of muscle bulk [Schmid and Hammaker, 1961]. A "second wind" phenomenon has been described in which the patient appears to recover after a 15-minute period of weakness and fatigue [Braakhekke et al., 1986]. This phenomenon has been attributed to improved energy production when metabolic dependence switches from glycogen stores to blood-borne fuels, including glucose and fatty acids, and is consistently seen in GSD type V but not in GSD type VII, whose phenotype is otherwise indistinguishable [Haller and Vissing, 2004]. Prolonged or frequent repetitive episodes of myoglobinuria should be avoided because they may result in both acute and chronic renal failure.

Renal failure occurs primarily in men, especially those who perform unusually vigorous exercise, thereby inducing myoglobinuria. These men generally are aware that they are exceeding their usual exercise tolerance. Acute renal failure may not be reversible in these patients [Bank et al., 1972]. One patient with recurrent myoglobinuria and renal failure was found to have had previously unrecognized convulsive seizures as the precipitating events for his episodes [Walker et al., 2003]. In another case, the presence of sickle cell trait and bulimia were likely significant stressors [Pillarisetti and Ahmed, 2007].

Onset usually is in childhood; neonatal onset has been reported [Milstein et al., 1989]. Adult-onset McArdle's disease also has been reported. One patient had onset at 60 years of age [Felice et al., 1992]. Frequent ingestion of glucose or fructose has had little therapeutic effect. Muscle damage after prolonged exercise may be demonstrated by means of radionuclide scanning techniques [Swift and Brown, 1978].

A 4-week-old female manifested diffuse, progressive muscle weakness and died at 13 weeks of age. She subsequently was demonstrated to have myophosphorylase deficiency and glycogen storage in the muscles. A female sibling died at 4 months of age from the same condition [Miranda et al., 1979]. A very severe phenotype, lethal in infancy, was reported in a child born to consanguineous parents with mutations in both *PYGM* and *dGK*, the gene encoding deoxyguanosine kinase, whose deficiency causes the hepatic form of mitochondrial depletion syndrome [Mancuso et al., 2003].

Clinical Laboratory Tests

Exercise results in elevated serum creatine kinase activity and increase in activity of other serum enzymes released from muscle, ostensibly a result of loss of sarcolemmal membrane integrity. The EKG may demonstrate an increased QRS amplitude, a prolonged R-S interval, T wave inversion, and bradycardia [Ratinov et al., 1965].

Electromyographic study of contracted muscles after exercise reveals a decreased interference pattern; after ischemic exercise, the contracted muscles may demonstrate no electrical activity.

Ischemic exercise effects may be studied using two blood pressure cuffs, one at the wrist and one just above the elbow. The cuffs are inflated to above systolic pressure, and the pressure is maintained for 3 minutes. Blood is removed from the antecubital vein at 0, 3, 5, 10, 15, and 20 minutes. After the initial blood specimen is drawn (at time 0), the patient is asked to contract and extend the fingers over a rubber ball or rod while the cuff pressure is maintained. A patient with McArdle's disease, or with any of the glycolytic abnormalities that interfere with lactate production, will experience severe contractures and complain bitterly of pain within 30 seconds after the initiation of ischemic exercise. The contracture phenomenon may be related to delayed reaccumulation of calcium ions in the sarcoplasmic reticulum [Gruener et al., 1968]. The exercise test may not identify patients with low levels of myophosphorylase, in contradistinction to those patients with absence of the enzyme [Taylor et al., 1987].

A test in which subjects cycle with moderate intensity for 15 minutes revealed a consistent decrease in heart rate from 7 to 15 minutes in GSD type V patients, in contrast with an elevation in heart rate in control subjects and patients with other glycogen storage diseases. The test appears specific and sensitive in this population [Vissing and Haller, 2003a]. Near-infrared spectroscopy (NIRS) is another noninvasive approach to screening for GSD V. This technique involves measurement of deoxyhemoglobin and deoxymyoglobin levels in the vastus lateralis muscle as surrogates for oxygen extraction. Patients with GSD V show reduced oxygen extraction compared to controls [Grassi et al., 2007]. Pulmonary oxygen uptake kinetics are negatively correlated with NIRS findings in these patients [Grassi et al., 2009].

Relaxing factor (which controls accumulation of calcium ions by the sarcoplasmic reticulum) appears to be normal in patients with McArdle's disease [Brody et al., 1970]. Spectroscopy studies are useful in the detection of excessive muscle glycogen [deKerviler et al., 1991; Jehenson et al., 1991].

Genetics

The gene encoding synthesizing myophosphorylase, *PYGM*, is located at 11q13 [Lebo et al., 1990]. A number of mutations have been described [Vorgerd et al., 1998] but do not appear to explain the clinical heterogeneity of GSD type V. A study of potential genetic modifiers found a strong association between angiotensin-converting enzyme genotype and clinical phenotype, suggesting that angiotensin-converting enzyme is a modifier of *PYGM* [Martinuzzi et al., 2003]. A further study of 99 Spanish patients confirmed this relationship, and also found that female gender conferred a more severe phenotype [Rubio et al., 2007]. GSD V is transmitted as an autosomal-recessive trait and may manifest in a heterozygote [Schmidt et al., 1987]. Study of muscle biopsy material demonstrates molecular heterogeneity, including near-normal expression of phosphorylase mRNA concentration and size in some patients [McConchie et al., 1990].

Management

A fat-rich diet was administered to a 21-year-old male patient; he subsequently had a shortened recovery period from the acute physical load and suffered no induration of the deltoid muscle after sustained abduction to 90°. Maximal strength did not appear to be improved by the fat-rich diet, but tolerance of submaximal loads appeared to be increased, and recovery from muscle discomfort was accelerated [Viskoper et al., 1975]. The interrelationship of pyridoxal phosphate and glycogen phosphorylase offered some hope for nutritional therapy [Beynon et al., 1996], but this has not been supported by more recent studies. A controlled trial of oral sucrose loading showed improved exercise tolerance and stable glucose levels in 12 adults with GSD type V [Vissing and Haller, 2003b]. Although not suitable for continuous use owing to its tendency to induce weight gain, this regimen, combined with aerobic conditioning, appears likely to be useful in improving performance under stressful conditions and may protect against acute rhabdomyolysis [Amato, 2003]. A review of published trials cited this study and one other in which oral creatine improved ischemic performance, suggesting these as the only therapies with evidence of benefit [Quinlivan and Beynon, 2004]. A more recent review noted that, while low doses of creatine monohydrate improved performance, higher doses could produce worsening of function [Tarnopolsky, 2007]. A trial of aerobic conditioning in eight adults led to increased exercise capacity without adverse effects [Haller et al., 2006]. A short-term

trial of gentamicin as "read through" therapy in four patients with stop mutations showed no evidence of benefit [Schroers et al., 2006].

Hepatophosphorylase Deficiency (Hers' Disease, Glycogen Storage Disease Type VI)

Biochemistry

GSD type VI was described by Hers in 1959, and is characterized by increased glycogen stores of normal configuration in the liver. Hepatic phosphorylase (hepatophosphorylase) activity is diminished or absent.

Because of the possibility of abnormalities in the complex activating mechanism of hepatophosphorylase, systematic study of enzyme activity in suspected hepatophosphorylase deficiency is necessary to exclude phosphorylase kinase deficiency and other metabolic errors in the activating sequence. One patient had hepatomegaly with increased glycogen content and low activity of hepatophosphorylase. No abnormalities of muscle tissue enzymes or glycogen configuration were noted. A liver homogenate prepared from the patient's biopsy specimen converted rabbit muscle phosphorylase b to phosphorylase a. Hepatic homogenate from the patient manifested no phosphorylase activity under the same conditions in which control human liver homogenate demonstrated phosphorylase activity through activation procedures. No activity was observed in the patient's hepatic homogenate after the addition of phosphorylase kinase [Hug and Schubert, 1970].

GSD VI could only be diagnosed by enzymology of liver tissue [Hug et al., 1974] until the gene was identified. This identification was accomplished in a Mennonite kindred, whose affected members harbored a single base pair change in a splice donor site of intron 13 in the *PYGL* gene [Chang et al., 1998]. The technique is particularly helpful in distinguishing patients with relatively high residual enzyme activity from heterozygotes [Tang et al., 2003]. A series of eight patients with GSD VI from seven families were studied, and found to harbor 11 novel mutations, most of which were missense [Beauchamp et al., 2007b]. The patients' symptoms ranged from hepatomegaly and subclinical hypoglycemia, to severe hepatomegaly with recurrent severe hypoglycemia and postprandial lactic acidosis.

Clinical Characteristics

The patients display various degrees of growth retardation, hypoglycemia, ketosis, and hepatomegaly. Specific neurologic findings are absent. Muscle and cardiovascular tissues are not primarily involved.

Genetics

The gene coding for the enzyme liver glycogen phosphorylase is located on chromosome 14 [Newgard et al., 1987] at 14q21–22. The condition is transmitted as an autosomal-recessive trait [Wallis et al., 1966]. Most mutations are missense; there are no common mutations [Beauchamp et al., 2007b].

Management

Symptoms can be controlled with frequent small carbohydrate meals. No other forms of therapy have been necessary or recommended.

Muscle Phosphofructokinase Deficiency (Tarui's Disease, Glycogen Storage Disease Type VII)

Biochemistry

The enzyme phosphofructokinase transforms fructose-6-phosphate to fructose-1,6-diphosphate. Decreased activity of this enzyme results in increased muscle glycogen stores of normal structure and increased concentration of glucose-6-phosphate and fructose-6-phosphate [Tarui et al., 1965; Layzer et al., 1967; Thomson et al., 1963; Vora et al., 1987]. The history of GSD type VII, since its discovery as the first enzymatic disorder of glycolysis in 1965, has been reviewed [Nakajima et al., 2002]. Phosphofructokinase exists in five different isoforms with tissue-specific distribution. The gene consists of varying combinations of liver (L), muscle (M), and platelet (P) subunits. Muscle phosphofructokinase is a homotetramer of M subunits [Vora et al., 1980].

Clinical Characteristics

Motor development is normal during the first decade. Nevertheless, patients experience decreased exercise tolerance and easy fatigability during childhood. They perform poorly in games requiring physical stamina and complain of muscle stiffness and weakness, and occasionally of muscle cramps. Myoglobinuria may follow moderate to strenuous exercise and has precipitated acute renal failure [Exantus et al., 2004]. The clinical pattern is reminiscent of McArdle's disease, except for the absence of a "second wind" phenomenon in GSD type VII [Haller and Vissing, 2004]. One patient with hyperuricemia and gout has been described [Agamanolis et al., 1980].

An unusual infantile syndrome characterized by limb weakness, seizures, cortical blindness, and corneal opacifications has been reported. The infant died at 7 months of age. Microscopic studies of the brain revealed typical features of neuroaxonal dystrophy [Servidei et al., 1986]. Another infant has been reported with infantile seizures and a relatively mild course; two of his sisters died in infancy with hypotonia, delayed milestones, and epilepsy [Al-Hassnan et al., 2007]. A 70-year-old male with progressive weakness of the legs has also been described [Vora et al., 1987]. An Ashkenazi kindred with GSD type VII has been described whose members had clinical manifestations of diabetes in addition to abnormal results on glucose tolerance testing, confirming that *PFKM* mutations can cause impaired glucose responses to insulin [Ristow et al., 1997]. Affected persons in this family had first become symptomatic in childhood, with easy fatigability after exercise.

A 66-year-old female with epilepsy and cardiac disease attributed to GSD type VII manifested slow progression of symptoms over an 8-year period, but showed marked improvement after effective treatment of her seizures and cardiac disease [Finsterer et al., 2002]. This report emphasizes the importance of meticulously treating (or preferably preventing) complications, rather than adopting a nihilistic approach.

Physical examination in patients with GSD type VII is unremarkable, except for variable weakness and loss of skeletal muscle bulk.

Clinical Laboratory Tests

After exercise, serum creatine kinase and other serum enzymes released from muscle may be elevated. EMG findings may be normal. Ischemic exercise testing, as described earlier for McArdle's disease, results in muscle contracture and decreased lactic acid production. The definitive diagnosis is made by enzymatic assay of muscle tissue.

Phosphofructokinase activity is about 50 percent of the expected value in the erythrocytes of these patients. A decrease from normal levels of activity also is noted in other patients [Sivakumar et al., 1996]. Immunologic study suggests that half of the total activity of erythrocyte phosphofructokinase is derived from an enzyme form identical to phosphofructokinase. One patient with phosphofructokinase deficiency was found to have (incidental) Gilbert's syndrome (hepatic glucuronyltransferase deficiency) [Fogelfeld et al., 1990].

Genetics

The phosphofructokinase gene (*PFKM*) is encoded at 12q13.3 [Howard et al., 1996]. GSD type VII is prevalent in Ashkenazim; 68 percent of mutant alleles in this population are accounted for by a splicing mutation in exon 5 [Raben and Sherman, 1995]. About 20 disease-causing mutations in *PFKM* have been described [Toscano et al., 2007].

Hepatic Phosphorylase Kinase Deficiency and Activation Abnormalities

Some patients with glycogen storage disease have defects in control of the phosphorylase system at the phosphorylase kinase level, rather than a deficiency of the phosphorylase enzyme (see Figure 34-3). Although they appear to have hepatic phosphorylase deficiency disease, further studies identify the presence of the enzyme when activation cycle materials are added in vitro. Hug et al. [1969] described five children with hepatomegaly and increased liver stores of glycogen of normal configuration. An additional three patients, who were siblings, had a mild form of the disease [Gray et al., 1983]. Hepatomegaly, attacks of ketonuria with fasting, and intermittent diarrhea may be prominent. Other patients with the same enzymatic deficiency have involvement of muscle with accompanying weakness [Madlom et al., 1989].

Phosphorylase kinase has a hexadecameric structure: (α, β, γ, δ)4. The δ subunit is calmodulin, which interacts with calcium. The α subunit is encoded by *PHKA2* (at Xp22), the β subunit by *PHKB*, and the γ subunit by *PHKG2*. Mutations in these three genes have been associated with phosphorylase kinase deficiency and a GSD phenotype [Ban et al., 2003]. The analysis of the responsible genes confirms the prior clinical recognition of both autosomal-recessive and X-linked inheritance [Huijing and Fernandes, 1969; Schimke et al., 1973]. The classification of phosphorylase kinase system disorders into GSD subtypes is highly confusing; various deficiencies have been designated as GSD VIa, VIII, and IX by different workers [Ozen, 2007]. We will simply describe the enzyme defects here, without invoking GSD nomenclature.

One patient with deficiency of phosphorylase kinase activity had normal phosphorylase activity in leukocytes, with deficiency in liver. Three siblings with the condition exhibited a deficiency in red cell and leukocyte phosphorylase b kinase. Specific therapy may not be necessary [Gray et al., 1983]. Treatment with diazoxide may be beneficial, because fasting hypoglycemia is curtailed. Diazoxide inhibits insulin release, increases adrenal medullary secretion of epinephrine, and inhibits the cyclic adenosine monophosphate phosphodiesterase activity. Together these actions should increase intracellular cyclic adenosine monophosphate. Neither insulin suppression nor associated decrease in hepatomegaly occurred in this patient [Ludwig et al., 1972].

In another patient, findings included evidence of central nervous system dysfunction and associated incomplete activation of brain phosphorylase [Hug et al., 1966]. Glucagon appeared to reverse the deficiency.

Glucagon administration does not lead to clinical improvement in all patients with decreased hepatic phosphorylase kinase activity. Hug and Schubert [1970] described a 3-year-old child with marked hepatomegaly and no splenomegaly. A slight tendency to develop hypoglycemia without acidosis was noted. Mental development was normal. Administration of either glucagon or epinephrine did not stimulate phosphorylase activity. Phosphorylase activity was reinstituted by in vitro methods employing addition of cyclic adenosine monophosphate or its substituted derivatives.

Reduced hepatophosphorylase activity may result from several separate defects in the phosphorylase activating system [Hug, 1972]. Hepatic tissue removed from a patient may fail to activate either endogenous or exogenous phosphorylase. Purified exogenous phosphorylase kinase may restore the phosphorylase activity, which establishes a deficiency of liver phosphorylase kinase. There may be no abnormalities in the cyclic adenosine monophosphate-dependent protein kinase cycle [Hug, 1972].

A 5-year-old male with phosphorylase kinase deficiency manifested improved growth, stabilization of blood glucose, and improvement in laboratory measures with uncooked cornstarch supplementation [Nakai et al., 1994].

A study of 15 patients from 12 families emphasized the importance of molecular diagnosis in this condition, since enzymology is often uninformative [Beauchamp et al., 2007]. Most patients (13 of 15) were boys, with onset of symptoms between 6 months and 7 years. They presented with varying combinations of hypoglycemia, hepatosplenomegaly, short stature, liver disease, and muscular symptoms, including weakness, fatigue, and motor delay. Laboratory abnormalities included elevated lactate, urate, and lipids. Mutations were identified in the *PHKA2*, *PHKG2*, and *PHKB* genes. Patients with *PHKG2* mutations had severe manifestations, whereas those with *PHKB* mutations were mildly affected. There was a range of manifestations associated with *PHKA2* mutations.

Phosphohexose Isomerase Deficiency (Satoyoshi's Disease)

Phosphohexose isomerase is also known as glucose phosphate isomerase and phosphoglucose isomerase. This enzyme catalyzes the interconversion of glucose-6-phosphate and fructose-6-phosphate in the Embden–Meyerhof pathway. Most reported cases of deficiency of this enzyme have been manifested as hemolytic anemia, but a few kindreds have been reported with skeletal muscle dysfunction.

Satoyoshi and Kowa [1967] described a family whose members experienced muscle pain and stiffness with exercise, beginning in childhood. The symptoms become more prominent in later life. Muscle contractures do not occur after ischemic exercise. Routine examination is normal. Heavy exercise leads to stiffness and tenderness of the muscles without apparent weakness. Lactic acid does not increase during ischemic exercise and serum creatine kinase is increased, but findings on EMG remain normal.

Schroter and co-workers [1985] described a male with severe hemolytic anemia requiring splenectomy at 5 years. Eight years later he had mild hemolytic anemia, gallstones, and jaundice; neurologic findings included weakness, mixed sensory and cerebellar ataxia, and mental retardation. He was found to have a unique mutation (glucose phosphate isomerase Homburg) that produced severe enzyme deficiency.

GPI has been assigned to 19cen–q12. It consists of 18 exons and is 40 kb in length [Walker et al., 1995]. The gene codes for two proteins in addition to hexosephosphate isomerase: neuroleukin, a chemokine, and autocrine motility factor [Niinaka et al., 1998]. Antibodies to glucose phosphate isomerase have been shown to sustain a rheumatoid arthritis-like condition in experimental animals [Schaller et al., 2001]. A Japanese report summarized the expanded phenotype of Satoyoshi's disease, which includes painful muscle cramps, alopecia, intractable diarrhea, bone and joint deformity, and endocrine disturbances. The authors postulated that antibody-induced inhibition of spinal interneurons and excitation of anterior horn cells might explain the cramps, based on the reaction of patients' sera with an 85 kDa protein derived from human brain lysate [Arimura, 2004].

Phosphoglucomutase Deficiency (Thomson's Disease)

The phosphoglucomutases are a family of enzymes catalyzing the interconversion of glucose-1-phosphate and fructose-1-phosphate. In early infancy, a male experienced numerous episodes of supraventricular tachycardia, requiring digitoxin treatment; development then proceeded normally until the age of 2 years, when he began to walk on his toes [Thomson et al., 1963]. Examination revealed mild weakness and poor muscle development. His calf muscles were bulky and firm, and shortening of the Achilles tendons was noted. No clinical history of exercise intolerance, muscle pain, or myoglobinuria was elicited. Serum enzyme activities, including creatine kinase, aldolase, glutamic-oxaloacetic transaminase, and glutamic-pyruvic transaminase, were elevated. Examination by EMG showed myopathic changes.

In vitro study of biopsy tissue indicated a number of relative enzymatic deficiencies, but phosphoglucomutase deficiency was most pronounced. Glycogen structure appeared normal. Also evident was extensive replacement of muscle tissue by glycogen.

Another patient, a 5-month-old male, presented with recurrent vomiting, lethargy, and poor weight gain. Metabolic acidosis was profound. In addition to the expected enzyme deficiency, he had decreased muscle and serum carnitine levels [Sugie et al., 1988]. The carnitine changes most likely were a secondary phenomenon.

A 38-year-old male presented with a history of easy fatigability and exercise-induced weakness of the extremities since he was 20. He had weakness, wasting of extremities, bilateral clubbed fingers, and hypoesthesia of the distal portion of extremities. Fasting plasma glucose was low (58 mg/dL), and no rise in lactate occurred after ischemic exercise. Phosphoglucomutase activity was 15 percent of control, and muscle biopsy depicted a small amount of glycogen storage [Nakashima et al., 1992]. A 35-year-old man with exercise-induced cramps, mild limb girdle weakness, episodes of rhabdomyolysis, normal elevation of lactate, and hyperammonemia on a forearm-exercise test has also been reported the investigators suggested that this disorder should be designated glycogenosis type XIV. Given the confusion surrounding the numeric designation of glycogenoses, we suggest referring to the disorder by its enzyme deficiency.

Other Defects of Glycolysis Causing Glycogen Storage

Three enzyme defects affecting the terminal glycolysis pathway have been reported, involving phosphoglycerate kinase, phosphoglycerate mutase, and lactate dehydrogenase [Bresolin et al., 1983; Tsujino et al., 1993; Toscano et al., 2007]. Phosphoglycerate kinase deficiency is an X-linked disorder manifesting with varying combinations of hemolytic anemia, seizures, mental retardation, and exercise intolerance with myoglobinuria [Bresolin et al., 1984]. Up to 1990, 33 patients had been reported. Of these, 11 of the 33 had hemolytic anemia and central nervous system involvement (seizures, mental retardation, strokes); 9 of the 33 had a purely myopathic form. This phenotype features recurrent episodes of exercise-induced cramps and myoglobinuria, and may be indistinguishable clinically from deficiencies of phosphorylase b kinase (PHK), myophosphorylase (GSD V, McArdle's disease), phosphofructokinase (PFK, GSD VII, Tarui's disease), phosphoglycerate mutase (PGAM), and lactate dehydrogenase. Phosphoglycerate mutase deficiency (PGAMD) has been associated in adults with

myalgia, cramps, and myoglobinuria after exercise [Tonin et al., 1993]. Twelve well-verified patients had been described by 2009, 9 of whom were African American [Naini et al., 2009]. Tubular aggregates, an expression of sarcoplasmic reticulum proliferation, are seen in about one-third of patients with this disease; the pathogenic mechanism is unclear [Naini et al., 2009]. A patient with PGAMD who experienced muscle cramps on forearm ischemic exercise testing was protected from cramps by dantrolene, suggesting that cramps in this disease reflect excessive calcium release from the sarcoplasmic reticulum relative to calcium reuptake capacity [Vissing et al., 1999]. The *PGAMD* gene has been cloned, and molecular diagnosis is feasible [Tsujino et al., 1993.] Lactate dehydrogenase M subunit deficiency has been reported in three families with exertional myoglobinuria [Kanno et al., 1988]. Additional cases have been identified, and a number of mutations identified in the responsible gene [Maekawa et al., 1994; Tsujino et al., 1994]. Successful pregnancy in an affected female has been described [Anai et al., 2002].

Conclusions

The disorders of carbohydrate metabolism are a large, heterogenous group, which are most likely to present to the child neurologist with manifestations of a metabolic myopathy. The presence of cardiac, hepatic, or hematologic abnormalities is often helpful in guiding the practitioner to the correct diagnosis. Although molecular testing is increasingly available to diagnose these disorders, many still require sophisticated biochemical investigation, electrodiagnostic testing and tissue biopsy – guided, as always, by a complete and accurate history and careful physical examination.

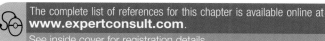

The complete list of references for this chapter is available online at **www.expertconsult.com**.
See inside cover for registration details.

Disorders of Glycosylation

Hudson H. Freeze and Marc C. Patterson

Eukaryotic cells synthesize hundreds of types of sugar chains called glycans, which function within the cell, at the cell surface, and beyond. Within the cell, glycans influence protein folding, stability, turnover, and intracellular trafficking [Varki et al., 2009]. At the cell surface, they influence or determine cell-cell binding, receptor-ligand interactions, assembly of signaling complexes, binding to the extracellular matrix, tissue pattern formation, trafficking of lymphocytes, and much more [Varki et al., 2009]. The same glycan can function differently on different proteins or in different settings. This three-dimensional complexity makes understanding the roles of glycans challenging but provides the body with an extraordinarily sensitive fine-tuning mechanism for many physiologic functions. It is not surprising that disrupting normal glycosylation causes moderate to severe pathology in multiple human organ systems.

More than 40 rare inherited disorders of glycan biosynthesis have been identified [Jaeken et al., 2008; Grunewald, 2007; Freeze, 2007; Marquardt and Denecke, 2003]. Most of these are the newly defined congenital disorders of glycosylation (previously called carbohydrate-deficient glycoprotein syndrome and disialotransferrin developmental deficiency syndrome). Others, such as muscle-eye-brain disease and Walker–Warburg syndrome, were well known, but elucidation of their relation to glycosylation has provided new insights into their pathophysiology and opens possibilities for therapy.

Defining Types of Glycosylation

Glycans are named according to their linkage to proteins, which defines the biosynthetic pathways, and suggests their usual location in the cell and the typical functions they serve. Most of the congenital disorders of glycosylation defects occur in the N-linked pathway, which is defined by asparagine (Asn) to N-acetylglucosamine (GlcNAc) couplings. O-linked glycans come in several forms. Lesions in the biosynthesis of threonine/serine (Thr/Ser) to mannose (Man), or O-Man glycans, cause muscle-eye-brain disease and some cases of Walker–Warburg syndrome. A rare form of progeria results from defects in xylose (Xyl)-based glycans, O-Xyl, which initiates the synthesis of glycosaminoglycans such as chondroitin sulfate, dermatan sulfate, and heparan sulfate. A few disorders are caused by mutations impairing the synthesis of glycosphingolipids and glycophosphatidylinositol anchors. A growing set of disorders results from defects in the maintenance of Golgi homeostasis and intracellular trafficking.

N-Linked Glycosylation

Overview
Sugar chains are added to newly synthesized proteins in the lumen of the endoplasmic reticulum; they are quickly and extensively remodeled there, and later in the Golgi apparatus. All eukaryotic cells make a 14-sugar lipid-linked oligosaccharide in the endoplasmic reticulum membrane that is composed of Man, GlcNAc, and glucose (Glc). This entire chain is transferred to Asn within an Asn-X-Thr/Ser/Cys [Zielinska et al., 2010] consensus sequence (X is any amino acid except proline) as newly made proteins emerge from the ribosome into the endoplasmic reticulum lumen. Forty or more genes are required to synthesize and transfer this glycan to proteins [Freeze, 2001b].

Extensive remodeling begins soon after sugar chain transfer. Up to two-thirds of the original lipid-linked oligosaccharide glycan is discarded, and 6–15 other sugar units are added back to create a dazzling array of sugar chains. Why generate this complex process? The initial glycan helps proteins fold and also provides important checkpoints for monitoring of proper protein folding in the endoplasmic reticulum [Parodi, 2000]. The addition of more sugars in the Golgi usually imparts greater specificity to the sugar chain function. Understanding the biosynthetic pathways is important for appreciating the nature of the defects.

Biosynthesis
Individual monosaccharides are synthesized from glucose, derived from the diet, or salvaged from degraded glycans, and must be activated to their nucleotide sugar derivatives [Freeze, 1999]. Figure 35-1 depicts an abbreviated version of the known monosaccharide pathways. We employ widely used standard symbols to denote the different sugars [Varki et al., 2009]. Note that phosphorylation of the monosaccharide is the first step, and some pathways interconvert phosphorylated forms, such as Man-6-P→Man-1-P. Also, several alternative routes generate uridine diphosphate (UDP)-GlcNAc, UDP-galactose (Gal), and guanosine diphosphate (GDP)-fucose (Fuc). For some types of glycosylation, the nucleotide sugar donates the sugar to a lipid carrier derived from the polyprenol, dolichol phosphate (P-Dol) [Schenk et al., 2001a]. These products include Man-P-Dol and Glc-P-Dol. Dolichol itself is made from polyprenols using a specific reductase [Cantagrel et al., 2010].

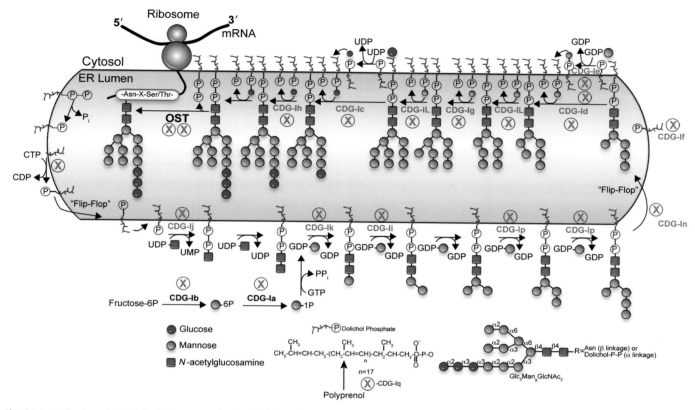

Fig. 35-1 Early steps in *N*-linked glycan synthesis. The biosynthesis and assembly of the lipid-linked oligosaccharide precursor (LLO), and its transfer to Asn-X-Thr/Ser/Cys sequences in the endoplasmic reticulum (ER) lumen. The first steps involve the activation and interconversion of monosaccharides (sugars) to their donors, the nucleotide sugars or phosphoryldolichols. Some congenital disorders of glycosylation (CDGs) result from defects (indicated by a circled "X") in some of these steps. Dolichol phosphate serves as the lipid carrier for the sugar chain, which is synthesized in a series of precisely ordered steps that involve addition of *N*-acetylglucosamine, mannose, and glucose. The completed glycan is transferred to proteins. Twenty-one CDG defects are caused by mutations in genes serving this portion of the pathway. Following transfer to proteins, oligosaccharide processing begins by removing all three glucose units and a mannose unit (bottom left). CMP, cytidine monophosphate; CTP, cytidine triphosphate; ER, endoplasmic reticulum; GDP, guanosine diphosphate; OST, oligosaccharyl transferase; UDP, uridine diphosphate.

N-*linked Glycan Biosynthesis*

Biosynthesis of the lipid precursor oligosaccharide involves a series of steps and enzymes that add sugars in specific linkages and in a specific order [Freeze, 2001a]. It begins with P-Dol + UDP-GlcNAc forming GlcNAc-P-P-Dol on the cytosolic face of the endoplasmic reticulum. Another UDP-GlcNAc donates a second GlcNAc using a different GlcNAc transferase, and this is followed by the addition of five Man units derived from GDP-Man. At this point, a "flippase" reorients the entire molecule from the cytosolic face into the endoplasmic reticulum lumen. A series of Man transferases use Man-P-Dol to add four more Man units, making a three-branched structure. Three glucosyltransferases sequentially add Glc from Glc-P-Dol to one branch to complete the sugar chain. This 14-sugar unit molecule is the optimal substrate for the multisubunit oligosaccharyl transferase (OST) complex that recognizes the Asn-X-Thr/Ser consensus sequence on the protein and adds the sugar chain to Asn. Recent studies indicate that some Asn-X-Cys sites can also be glycosylated [Zielinska et al., 2010; Ostasiewicz et al., 2010]. Truncated glycans are poorly transferred and sometimes fail to occupy normal glycosylation sites. Following glycan transfer, P-P-Dol is converted back to P-Dol and then to Dol. Recycling of these carriers is extensive.

Within a few minutes of transfer to protein, the sugar chain is processed (Figure 35-2; see also Figure 35-1). A set of two glucosidases removes the Glc units. For some proteins, processing stops here, but for the great majority, a mannosidase in the endoplasmic reticulum removes a single Man unit. The proteins are carried to the Golgi, where another mannosidase called Golgi mannosidase I removes up to three more Man units. At this point, processing starts to add sugars. UDP-GlcNAc donates a GlcNAc to one branch, making the sugar chain an acceptable substrate for Golgi mannosidase II, which removes an additional two Man units. This process clears the way for the addition of a second GlcNAc to a Man on the remaining branch. Depending on the protein, up to three more GlcNAc transferases add GlcNAc units to the Man residues in a specific order to initiate up to five branches. These branches are then extended with Gal, derived from UDP-Gal, and sialic acid (Sia), derived from cytidine monophosphate (CMP)-Sia. In some cases, GDP-Fuc donates a Fuc to one or more of the branches or to the GlcNAc linked to the protein. In other cases, sulfates, phosphates, or glucuronic acids are added to selected sugars. Individual branches may accumulate several repeating units of Galβ1,4GlcNAc before being capped by Sia. These reactions occur in selected cisternae of the Golgi, and each

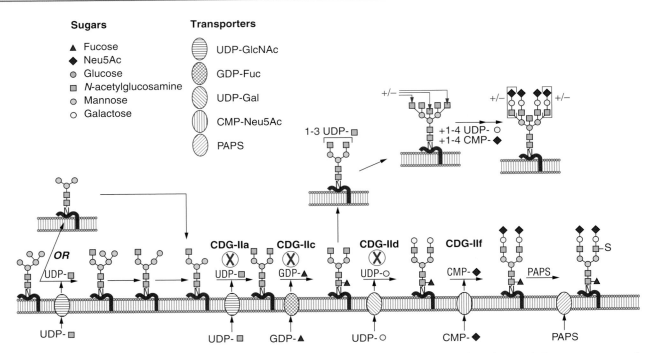

Fig. 35-2 Processing of *N*-linked glycans in the Golgi membrane. Mannose trimming of the protein-bound sugar chains may stop or continue, as shown at the extreme left. Addition of a single *N*-acetylglucosamine or continued mannose trimming next leads to the build-up of sugar chains with 2–5 branches containing *N*-acetylglucosamine, galactose, and sialic acid. Fucose may be added to some chains, and sulfate may be attached to several other sugars using specific transferases. All of these reactions require delivery of the nucleotide sugar into the Golgi by specific transporters. Congenital disorder of glycosylation (CDG) defects (indicated by a circled "X") occur in one of the trimming glycosidases, in a glycosyltransferase, and in two transporters. A series of mutations in 6 of the 8 COG subunits and a vacuolar H^+/ATPase disturb *N*-glycan processing and other biosynthetic pathways by disrupting Golgi homeostasis. CMP, cytidine monophosphate; GDP, guanosine diphosphate; PAPS, 3'-phosphoadenosine–5'-phosphosulfate; UDP, uridine diphosphate.

nucleotide sugar donor must be translocated from its origin in the cytoplasm or nucleus to the Golgi by a substrate-selective transporter [Gerardy-Schahn et al., 2001].

Enzymes and Cell Biology

The sugar-activating enzymes reside in either the cytoplasm or the nucleus. The *N*-linked biosynthetic enzymes all are in the endoplasmic reticulum or Golgi, with their active sites situated in the expected orientation. Most of the glycosyltransferases used for building the lipid-linked oligosaccharide and the Golgi transporters span the membrane many times [Ishida and Kawakita, 2004]. Most enzymes participating in glycan processing are attached to the membrane by a single membrane span. The transferases and nucleotide sugar transporters are constantly recycled in the dynamic Golgi to maintain their correct relationship to the maturing glycoproteins as they pass through the Golgi. Therefore, correct trafficking of the biosynthetic machinery is essential for optimal function.

Congenital Disorders of Glycosylation

Glycosylation is complex, and its disorders do not always lend themselves to phenotypic or symptomatic pigeonholing. Congenital disorders of glycosylation (CDG) nomenclature is still evolving as attempts are made to design a systematic, clinically useful system based on biochemical origins. Until 2008, CDGs resulting from defects in lipid-linked oligosaccharide

biosynthesis and transfer to protein were defined as group I. The remaining CDGs that affect the biosynthesis and processing of the protein-bound sugar chains constituted group II. Individual disorders in group I or II were assigned lower-case letters (designating types, as noted earlier) when the genetic defect is proved. Several reviews provide comprehensive and up-to-date perspectives [Vodopiutz and Bodamer, 2008; Jaeken and Matthijs, 2007; Grunewald, 2007; Freeze, 2007; Marquardt and Denecke, 2003]. In 2008 a simplification of the nomenclature was proposed, as the growth in the number of disorders had produced a confusing series of letters and numbers that did not help the clinician or researcher. In the new system, diseases will be grouped in four categories: disorders of protein *N*-glycosylation, disorders of protein *O*-glycosylation, disorders of glycosphingolipid and glycosyl-phosphatidylinositol anchor glycosylation, and disorders of multiple glycosylation pathways. Individual disorders will be listed by the gene involved and, in parallel, its protein product. The authors suggest that the previous CDG designation may be listed in parentheses during the transitional period as the new nomenclature is adopted [Jaeken et al., 2008].

Diagnosis

In most patients with CDGs the diagnosis is straightforward and is based on the analysis of serum transferrin isoforms. Several methods are suitable and commercially available. These include isoelectric focusing [Freeze, 2001a; Jaeken and Matthijs, 2001], mass spectrometry [Wada, 2007; Kleinert et al., 2003; Lacey et al., 2001], zone electrophoresis, and high-pressure liquid chromatography [Quintana et al., 2009]. Electrospray ionization-mass spectrometry [Babovic and O'Brien, 2007] is the most informative because it easily distinguishes the absence of entire sugar chains, which characterizes group I CDGs, from the absence of one or more individual monosaccharide units typical of group II CDGs. The predominant isoform in normal transferrin has two sugar chains, each containing two negatively charged Sia molecules, designated tetrasialotransferrin. In group I disorders, isoelectric focusing analysis demonstrates loss of one or both entire glycan chains, producing "disialotransferrin" or "asialotransferrin," respectively, but clearly this is an incomplete description. By contrast, electrospray ionization-mass spectrometry demonstrates that the loss of one or two chains reduces the mass by about 2200 or 4400 mass units, respectively. In group II disorders, isoelectric focusing may distinguish among "tri-," "di-," "mono-," and "asialo" forms, reflecting variable loss of Sia, whereas electrospray ionization-mass spectrometry can indicate specific loss of Sia alone or combinations of Sia with additional sugars. This distinction is essential for determining assignment to group I or group II, and provides a signpost for specific identification of the defect. The single-step electrospray ionization-mass spectrometry technique can be accomplished using less than 5 mL of blood in less than 30 minutes [Lacey et al., 2001; Babovic and O'Brien, 2007]. This technique is therefore suitable for large-scale population screening for CDGs.

Transferrin isoform analysis produces few false-positive results. Uncontrolled fructose and galactose intolerance and recent heavy alcohol consumption produce a pattern typical of group I disorders [Kleinert et al., 2003]. In apparently rare instances, patients with genetically confirmed CDGs exhibited normal transferrin isoelectric focusing profiles, and in some patients, previously abnormal patterns normalized in preadolescence [Dupre et al., 2001; Fletcher et al., 2000]. Thus, a normal transferrin pattern should not exclude follow-up testing. Healthy neonates sometimes have a slightly abnormal transferrin pattern, which normalizes within a few weeks. Suspicious results in neonates should be repeated.

Until recently, specific diagnosis of the defect usually involved enzymatic, biochemical, and genetic analysis of the patient's fibroblasts or leukocytes. Relatively few laboratories performed these analyses. With routine gene sequencing becoming more cost-effective, some genetic centers and commercial laboratories now offer various CDG gene diagnostic panels. In the coming years, decreasing costs, improved sequencing technology, and better informatics are likely to make this approach the first option. Prenatal testing is available for confirmed at-risk families [Matthijs et al., 1998, 2004].

General Clinical Features

About 1000 CDG patients have been identified, presenting with multiple organ dysfunction [Haeuptle and Hennet, 2009]. Patients with CDGs have protean presentations that, in some cases, may mimic mitochondrial (oxidative phosphorylation) disorders [Briones et al., 2001], but lack a history of maternal inheritance. An informal survey of CDG-affected families indicated that earlier nonspecific diagnoses frequently included a metabolic defect or cerebral palsy. Most patients first present to pediatric neurology or metabolic clinics. They frequently have combinations of liver, gastrointestinal, and coagulation disturbances [Jaeken and Matthijs, 2001; Marquardt and Denecke, 2003]. The possibility of a CDG should be investigated in any child presenting with developmental delay, seizures, hearing loss [Jaeken et al., 2009] or strabismus, particularly if any of these manifestations is accompanied by abnormal coagulation, liver dysfunction, or a gastrointestinal disorder. Most affected children are hypotonic and demonstrate failure to thrive.

Specific Disorders

Table 35-1 summarizes the known CDG defects, utilizing the classification scheme proposed in 2008. This includes the mutated genes and major signs and symptoms. The known defects cover every aspect of the *N*-linked biosynthetic pathway. Activation or presentation of precursors (PMM2, PMI, DPM1, DPM3 MPDU1 [CDG-Ia, Ib, Ie, If]), glycosyltransferases for lipid-linked oligosaccharide biosynthesis (ALG6, NOT56L, ALG12, ALG8, ALG2, DPAGT1, HMT1, DOBD1 [CDG-Ic, Id, Ig, Ih, Ii, Ij, Ik, Il]), glycosidases that trim the protein-bound sugar chain (GLS1 [CDG-IIb]), Golgi-localized nucleotide sugar transporters (SLC35C1, SLC35A1 [CDG-IIc and IIf]), and glycosyltransferases that extend the trimmed chain (MGAT2, BG4ALT1 [CDG-IIa and IId]). DK1 (CDG-Im) impairs dolichol kinase function and impairs the final step of the de novo synthesis of dolichol phosphate [Denecke and Kranz, 2009]. SRD5A3 encodes the α-reductase that converts various polyprenols to dolichols [Cantagrel et al., 2010]. The conserved eight-subunit oligomeric Golgi (COG) complex that binds to the cytoplasmic face of the Golgi is needed for intra-Golgi or Golgi to endoplasmic reticulum retro-trafficking of multiple resident glycosyltransferases and nucleotide sugar transporters. Disorganized trafficking impairs multiple glycosylation pathways [Ungar et al., 2002]. Defects have now been identified in COG7, COG1, COG4 [CDG-IIe, IIg, IIj], COG8, COG5 and COG6 [Lübbehusen et al., 2010; Foulquier, 2009]. Appreciation of the importance of Golgi homeostasis in glycosylation led to the discovery of another disorder caused by mutations in a subunit of a vacuolar H^+/ATPase that maintains appropriate pH of various organelles within the endocytic and exocytic pathways [Marshansky and Futai, 2008; Kornak et al., 2008; Guillard et al., 2009]. The intravesicular pH progressively decreases from the endoplasmic reticulum to Golgi, endosomes, and, finally, lysosomes.

The remainder of this chapter will focus on CDGs with significant neurologic manifestations.

Defects in Protein *N*-glycosylation

PMM2 (CDG-Ia)

PMM2 (CDG-Ia) is the best-known and most frequently recognized form of CDGs, first reported by Jaeken and co-workers in 1980 [Jaeken et al., 1980]. The defective gene was identified in 1995 as *PMM2*, which encodes the phosphomannomutase (PMM) that converts Man-6-P $\rightarrow$ Man-1-P. This defect results in insufficient production of lipid-linked oligosaccharide, leading to empty glycosylation sites. More than 800 patients are known worldwide, and more than 100 mutations have been cataloged [Barone et al., 2008; Jaeken, 2003; Matthijs et al., 2000; Haeuptle and Hennet, 2009].

Table 35-1 **Inherited Glycosylation Disorders**

Disorder	Gene	Enzyme	OMIM No.	Key Features
CDG-Ia	*PMM2*	Phosphomannomutase II	212065	MR, hypotonia, esotropia, lipodystrophy, cerebellar hypoplasia, strokelike episodes, seizures
CDG-Ib	*MPI*	Phosphomannose isomerase	602579	Hepatic fibrosis, protein-losing enteropathy, coagulopathy, hypoglycemia
CDG-Ic	*ALG6*	Glucosyltransferase IGlc-P-Dol: $Man_9GlcNAc_2$-P-P-Dol glucosyltransferase	603147	Moderate MR, hypotonia, esotropia, epilepsy
CDG-Id	*ALG3*	Man-P-Dol:$Man_5GlcNAc_2$-P-P-Dol mannosyltransferase	601110	Profound psychomotor delay, optic atrophy, acquired microcephaly, iris colobomas, hypsarrhythmia
CDG-Ie	*DPM1*	Man-P-Dol synthase I GDP-Man: Dol-P-mannosyltransferase	603503	Severe MR, epilepsy, hypotonia, mild dysmorphism, coagulopathy
CDG-If	*MPDU1*	MPDU1/Lec35	608799	Short stature, ichthyosis, psychomotor retardation, pigmentary retinopathy
CDG-Ig	*ALG12*	Man-P-Dol:$Man_7GlcNAc_2$P-P-Dol mannosyltransferase	607143	Hypotonia, facial dysmorphism, psychomotor retardation, acquired microcephaly Frequent infections
CDG-Ih	*ALG8*	Glucosyltransferase II Glc-P-Dol:Glc_1 $Man_9GlcNAc_2$-P-P-Dol glucosyltransferase	608104	Hepatomegaly, protein-losing enteropathy, renal failure, hypoalbuminemia, edema, ascites
CDG-Ii	*ALG2*	Mannosyltransferase II GDP-Man: $Man_1GlcNAc_2$-P-P-Dol mannosyltransferase	607906	Normal at birth; mental retardation, hypomyelination, intractable seizures, iris colobomas, hepatomegaly, coagulopathy
CDG-Ij	*DPAGT1*	UDP-GlcNAc:dolichol phosphate *N*-acetylglucosamine 1-phosphate transferase	608093	Severe MR, hypotonia, seizures, microcephaly, exotropia
CDG-Ik	*ALG1*	Mannosyltransferase I GDP-Man: $GlcNAc_2$-P-P-Dol mannosyltransferase	608540	Severe psychomotor retardation, hypotonia, acquired microcephaly, intractable seizures, fever, coagulopathy, nephrotic syndrome, early death
CDG-IL	*ALG9 mannosyltransferase*	Mannosyltransferase Man-P-Dol:Man_6 and $Man_8GlcNAc_2$-P-P-Dol	608776	Severe microcephaly, hypotonia, seizures, hepatomegaly
CDG-IIa	*MGAT2*	GlcNAc-transferase 2 (GnT II)	212066	MR, dysmorphism, stereotypies, seizures
CDG-IIb	*GLS1*	Glucosidase I	606056	Dysmorphism, hypotonia, seizures, hepatomegaly, hepatic fibrosis (death at 2.5 months)
CDG-IIc	*SLC35C1/FUCT1*	GDP-fucose transporter	266265	Recurrent infections, persistent neutrophilia, MR, microcephaly, hypotonia (normal Tf)
CDG-IId	*B4GALT1*	β-1,4,-Galactosyltransferase	607091	Hypotonia (myopathy), spontaneous hemorrhage, Dandy–Walker malformation
CDG-IIe	*COG7*	Conserved oligomeric Golgi complex subunit 7	608779	Fatal in early infancy; dysmorphism, hypotonia, intractable seizures, hepatomegaly, progressive jaundice, recurrent infections, cardiac failure
CDG-IIf	*SLC35A1*	CMP-sialic acid transporter	–	Thrombocytopenia, no neurologic symptoms, normal Tf, abnormal platelet glycoproteins
Mucolipidoses II and III	*GNPTA*	UDP-GlcNAc: lysosomal enzyme, GlcNAc-1 phosphotransferase	252500	Coarsening, organomegaly, joint stiffness, dysostosis, median neuropathy at wrist; type III less severe than type II, which manifests in infancy

Table 35-1 Inherited Glycosylation Disorders—cont'd

Disorder	Gene	Enzyme	OMIM No.	Key Features
Walker–Warburg syndrome	POMT1	O-mannosyltransferase 1	236670	Type II lissencephaly, cerebellar malformations, ventriculomegaly, anterior chamber malformations, severe delay; death in infancy
Muscle-eye-brain disease	POMTGNT1	O-mannosyl-β-1,2-N-acetyl-glucosaminyltransferase 1	253280	Type II lissencephaly, progressive myopia, developmental delay, weakness, hypotonia; resembles but is less severe than Walker–Warburg syndrome
Fukuyama's muscular dystrophy	FCMD	Fukutin, a putative glycosyltransferase	253800	Cortical dysgenesis, myopia, weakness and hypotonia; 40 percent have seizures
Ehlers–Danlos syndrome	B4GALT7	β-1,4-Galactosyltransferase	130070	Progeroid Ehlers–Danlos syndrome; macrocephaly, joint hyperextensibility
Hereditary multiple exostosis	EXT1/EXT2	Glucuronyltransferase/N-acetylglucosaminyltransferase	133700	Multiple exostoses (diaphyseal, juxtaepiphyseal)
Chondrodysplasias	DTDST/ SLC26A2	Sulfate anion transporter	222600	Diastrophic dysplasia: scoliosis, talipes equinovarus, "hitchhiker thumb," malformed ears; airway collapse and early death in severe cases; adult survival reported
			600972	Achondrogenesis Ib: short-limbed dwarfism, thin ribs with fractures and respiratory failure; usually stillborn or die in early infancy
			256050	Atelosteogenesis II: severe skeletal malformations with small chest and pulmonary hypoplasia; typically fatal in infancy

CMP, cytidine monophosphate; GDP, guanosine diphosphate; GlcNAc, N-acetylglucosamine; Man, mannose; MR, mental retardation; OMIM, Online Mendelian Inheritance in Man; P-Dol, dolichol phosphate; Tf, transferrin; UDP, uridine diphosphate.

Hagberg and associates described four stages of the typical (severe) phenotype [Hagberg et al., 1993]. The first is the infantile phase, marked by various combinations of dysmorphism, abnormal fat distribution (supragluteal and vulval fat pads, focal lipoatrophy), inverted nipples, cryptorchidism, esotropia, recurrent infections, cardiomyopathy or pericardial effusions, coagulopathies, nephrotic syndrome, hypothyroidism, life-threatening episodes of hepatic failure, and unexplained coma. As many as 20 percent of infants with CDG-Ia succumb in this phase [Jaeken and Matthijs, 2001]. In the second phase (comprising the remainder of the first decade), children experience seizures and strokelike episodes, often precipitated by intercurrent infections. The third phase (in the second decade of life) is marked by slowly progressive cerebellar ataxia and limb wasting, and by progressive visual loss secondary to pigmentary retinopathy. Adult survivors have moderate mental retardation with severe ataxia and hypogonadism, with or without skeletal deformities. Presentations are highly variable. In one girl with CDG-Ia, findings on computed tomography (CT) of the head were normal at 9 months, but subsequent imaging studies demonstrated progressive atrophy [Mader et al., 2002]. The investigators concluded that the cerebellar hypoplasia reported in infancy in most children with CDG-Ia likely reflects atrophy of antenatal onset, rather than hypoplasia.

More extensive testing for CDGs has led to the identification of milder CDG-Ia phenotypes [Briones et al., 2002; de Lonlay et al., 2001; Grünewald, 2009]. The patients often have high residual levels of PMM2 activity [Drouin-Garraud et al., 2001; Grünewald et al., 2001; Westphal et al., 2001b]. Some patients have only borderline cognitive impairment, but strabismus persists in these very mild cases. Few adult CDG-Ia patients are employed. A longitudinal study of eight Spanish patients confirmed the wide range of clinical manifestations, ranging from neonatal hemorrhage, non-immune hydrops, and death, through mental retardation and motor impairment without acute decompensation in patients in their 20s, to one individual with normal development and only gastrointestinal dysfunction in childhood [Perez-Duenas et al., 2009].

The carrier frequency of the most common mutant allele is about 1 in 70 in the northern European population [Schollen et al., 2000]. It is believed to be lethal in the homozygous state. Genotype-phenotype correlations have not been informative, but some evidence suggests that frequent polymorphisms in other glycosylation-related genes may influence the severity of the phenotype. No effective specific therapy for CDG-Ia exists. Experiments using CDG-Ia cells suggested that increasing dietary mannose might improve glycosylation in patients, but clinical trials demonstrated no benefit [Kjaergaard et al., 1998; Marquardt et al., 1997; Mayatepek et al., 1997].

Population studies find the risk of having a second child with CDG-Ia to be close to 1 in 3, rather than the expected mendelian ratio of 1 in 4, suggesting that reduced glycosylation may have some selective advantage [Schollen et al., 2004b]. At-risk couples should be counseled appropriately.

MPI-CDG (Ib)

MPI-CDG (Ib) is caused by mutations in *MPI*, the gene encoding phosphomannose isomerase, which interconverts Man-6-P and Fructose (Frc)-6-P. This reaction produces most of the mannose for glycoprotein synthesis [de Koning et al., 1998; Niehues et al., 1998]. About 25 patients have been identified since its discovery in 1998 [de Lonlay and Seta, 2009]. This phenotype is not associated with any primary neurologic symptoms. Gastrointestinal and hepatic pathology, with hypoglycemia, coagulopathy, and protein-losing enteropathy, is characteristic.

MPI-CDG (Ib) is unique in that simple dietary mannose therapy corrects the abnormalities, except for liver fibrosis [de Lonlay and Seta, 2009; Durand et al., 2003; Niehues et al., 1998]. The dietary mannose is taken up through transporters and converted to Man-6-P, thereby bypassing the metabolic block. Mannose has no known side effects at the concentrations used. Nonenzymatic protein glycation occurs at high concentrations of mannose, which is considerably more reactive than glucose, and can raise hemoglobin A1c (HbA1c) levels [Harms et al., 2002]. Some patients have received such treatment for longer than 10 years without complications [Westphal et al., 2001a; de Lonlay and Seta, 2009]. Twenty percent of the patients who were subsequently confirmed to have phosphomannose isomerase deficiency, however, died before discovery of the disorder [Freeze, 2001a]. The potentially fatal outcome and availability of simple, effective treatment mandate investigation for CDGs in suspected cases. One adult patient with MPI deficiency was not able to tolerate oral mannose, but her protein-losing enteropathy appeared to respond to heparin therapy [Liem et al., 2008].

ALG6-CDG (Ic)

ALG6-CDG (Ic) resembles, but is less severe than PMM2-CDG. It is characterized by moderate psychomotor retardation, hypotonia, esotropia, seizures, and ataxia. Nevertheless, at least five children have died of CDG-related complications [Marquardt and Denecke, 2003; Newell et al., 2003; Westphal et al., 2000]. The defect is in a glycosyltransferase, hALG6, that results in production of a truncated lipid-linked oligosaccharide sugar chain, which is inefficiently transferred to proteins. Patients sometimes experience life-threatening protein-losing enteropathy during bouts of gastroenteritis [Westphal et al., 2000]. Skeletal dysplasia, including a unique form associated with brachytelephalangy has been described in a compound heterozygote for ALG6 [Drijvers et al., 2010]. An adult woman has been identified in whom ALG6 deficiency was associated with mental retardation, skeletal anomalies, virilization, and deep vein thrombosis [Sun et al., 2005]. ALG6 deficiency was first identified in 1998 and subsequently in more than 35 patients [Haeuptle and Hennet, 2009; Burda et al., 1998; Grünewald et al., 2000; Imbach et al., 2000a], making it the second most common form of CDG.

NOT56L-CDG (Id)

Patients with NOT56L-CDG have mutations in *NOT56L* (ALG3), which encodes the mannosyltransferase used to synthesize $Man_6GlcNAc_2$ [Körner et al., 1999]. The index patient had microcephaly, optic nerve atrophy, iris colobomas, epilepsy, spastic quadriparesis, and profound psychomotor delay. Another patient had similar features plus Dandy–Walker malformation, with agenesis of the cerebellar vermis and corpus callosum. She also had recurrent hypoglycemia, thrombocytopenia, hypoalbuminemia, and coagulopathy. A total of eight children with NOT56L-CDG have now been described; all have a severe phenotype, with 7 of the 8 manifesting neurological impairments, including seizures, visual impairment, psychomotor retardation, and cerebral or cerebellar hypoplasia; there were varying combinations of hepatic, hematologic, endocrine, and dysmorphic manifestations, as well [Kranz et al., 2007b].

ALG12-CDG (Ig)

Eight cases of ALG12-CDG (Ig) have been reported [Chantret et al., 2002; Grubenmann et al., 2002; Thiel et al., 2002; Eklund et al., 2005; Kranz et al., 2007c]. The patients had typical CDG abnormalities, including hypotonia, generalized developmental delay, cerebellar hypoplasia, and decreased coagulation factors. Dysmorphic features included a long thin face, flat nasal bridge, and epicanthal folds. Frequent infections probably reflect reduced immunoglobulin G (IgG) concentrations. Affected males have genital hypoplasia, a feature not reported in other types of CDGs. More recent reports have emphasized features of skeletal dysplasia. These patients have mutations in *hALG12*, which encodes dolichol-P-mannose: $Man_7GlcNAc_2$-PP-dolichyl mannosyltransferase. Patients accumulate the truncated lipid-linked oligosaccharide, which is inefficiently transferred to proteins.

ALG8-CDG (Ih)

Eight patients have been described with ALG8-CDG (Ih), caused by a deficiency in *hALG8*, the gene encoding the second glucosyltransferase in lipid-linked oligosaccharide synthesis [Chantret et al., 2003; Schollen et al., 2004a; Stolting et al., 2009; Vesela et al., 2009]. Three patients had mild clinical presentations, including two siblings with pseudogynecomastia, epicanthus, hypotonia [Stolting et al., 2009], mental retardation, and ataxia, whereas the others all had severe multi-organ failure. Most died within a few months, but one patient with severe developmental delay survived a year before succumbing to renal failure. The others experienced hepatointestinal symptoms; one girl had cortical, cerebellar, and optic atrophy and intractable seizures before her death from systemic complications at 2 months [Vesela et al., 2009].

ALG2-CDG (Ii)

The only child with ALG2-CDG (Ii) recognized to date was normal at birth, except for an iris coloboma. Seizures, hepatomegaly, and coagulation abnormalities emerged in the first year. Imaging studies revealed cerebral hypomyelination. Pathologic mutations were found in hALG2, the enzyme that adds the second mannose to the growing lipid-linked oligosaccharide sugar chain [Thiel et al., 2003].

DPAGT1-CDG (Ij)

DPAGT1-CDG (Ij) is caused by a deficiency in UDP-GlcNAc: dolichol phosphate *N*-acetylglucosamine-1 phosphate transferase (GPT) activity encoded by *DPAGT1*. Two patients had severe hypotonia, intractable seizures, mental retardation, microcephaly, and exotropia [Wu et al., 2003].

ALG1/HMT1-CDG (Ik)

Ten children with HMT1-CDG (Ik) have been described [Kranz et al., 2004; Schwarz et al., 2004; Dupre et al., 2010]. Fifty percent had complications during pregnancy, and several had postnatal complications. Eighty percent were hypotonic, and all had at least one seizure, most being intractable; 8 of the 10 were dysmorphic, 7 of the 10 had visual impairment, and 5 of the 10 were microcephalic. Fifty percent had a fatal outcome. Patients with HMT1-CDG are deficient in GDP-Man:GlcNAc$_2$-P-P-dolichol mannosyltransferase, encoded by the *hALG1* gene, which adds the first Man to the lipid-linked oligosaccharide chain.

ALG9/DIBD1-CDG (Il)

Two patients with ALG9/DIBD1-CDG (Il) have been described. Abnormalities in the first case included severe microcephaly, central hypotonia, seizures, developmental delay, hepatomegaly, and bronchial asthma. This patient was found to carry a homozygous point mutation in human *hALG9*, whose product catalyzes the addition of both the seventh and ninth mannose units to the lipid-linked oligosaccharide chain [Frank et al., 2004]. The second patient was a girl with delayed development, epilepsy, hypotonia, failure to thrive, pericardial effusion, cystic renal disease, hepatosplenomegaly, esotropia, and inverted nipples. Neither lipodystrophy nor dysmorphic facial features were present. Magnetic resonance imaging (MRI) of the brain reflected cerebral and cerebellar atrophy and delayed myelination. Antithrombin III, factor XI, and cholesterol levels were low [Weinstein et al., 2005].

RFT1-CDG (In)

Six children have been described with RFT1-CDG (In) [Haeuptle et al., 2008; Clayton and Grunewald, 2009; Vleugels et al., 2009; Jaeken et al., 2009]. Most children have typical manifestations of the CDG spectrum: feeding problems, failure to thrive, severe developmental delay, poor to absent visual contact, epilepsy, and hypotonia, and variable respiratory, gastrointestinal, and coagulation abnormalities. All, however, have sensorineural deafness, which has only rarely been reported in other forms of CDG, and which is an important clue to this diagnosis. RFT1 is thought (but not absolutely proven) to be the flippase that transfers Man$_5$GlcNAc$_2$-PP-Dol from the cytoplasmic to the luminal face of the endoplasmic reticulum membrane.

MGAT2-CDG (IIa)

Three children with MGAT2-CDG (IIa) have been described [Cormier-Daire et al., 2000; Jaeken et al., 1994; Tan et al., 1996]. They were of Belgian, Iranian, and French descent, respectively, and all had severe psychomotor delay, acquired microcephaly and growth retardation, and variable combinations of hypotonia, ventricular septal defects, craniofacial dysmorphism (thin lips, hooked nose, large ears, hypertrophied gums, short neck), stereotypies, and coagulation defects. All were found to have impaired activity of the processing enzyme N-acetylglucosaminyltransferase II (MGAT2), which decreases the formation of multibranched N-linked glycans. A targeted disruption of this gene in the mouse faithfully recapitulates the human disorder [Wang et al., 2001].

GLS1-CDG (IIb)

Only one patient with GLS1-CDG (IIb) has been described [De Praeter et al., 2000]. Her parents were consanguineous. She had dysmorphic features, hypotonia, reduced nerve conduction velocity, seizures, and hepatomegaly with abnormal bile duct proliferation and fibrosis. The patient died at 2.5 months. This disorder was caused by mutations in α-glucosidase I, which trims the outermost glucose from oligosaccharides just after their transfer to nascent proteins. Although activity of the enzyme was severely decreased in this patient's fibroblasts, transferrin glycosylation remained normal. This patient would be missed by the standard diagnostic assays. An endo-α-mannosidase apparently bypasses the glucosidase defect to permit normal oligosaccharide processing. Abnormal accumulation of fully glycosylated sugar chains may overwhelm the capacity of endoplasmic reticulum chaperone lectins.

TUSC3-CDG

Nine patients have been described with TUSC3-CDG. Seven were members of four sibships in a large consanguinous Iranian kindred, and all had nonsyndromic, moderate to severe mental retardation [Garshasbi et al., 2008]. Two were sibs from a small French family [Molinari et al., 2008]. *TUSC3* codes for a subunit of the oligosaccharyltransferase complex (OST). It is not clear why these patients have no other systemic manifestations of hypoglycosylation, but it is theorized that differential tissue expression of another subunit associated with the OST (IAP) might compensate for TUSC3 deficiency in non-neurologic tissues [Garshasbi et al., 2008].

IAP-CDG

Screening of samples from 250 families with X-linked nonsyndromic mental retardation led to the identification of one patient who carried a c.932T/G, p.V311G mutation in the *IAP* gene [Molinari et al., 2008]. IAP (implantation-associated protein) is an ortholog to yeast Ost 6p. Like *TUSC3*, IAP is expressed in all tissues, including adult and fetal brain.

ALG11-CDG (Ip)

A brother and sister born to consanguineous Turkish parents were found to carry homozygous c.T257C mutations in the *hALG11* gene; this disorder was designated ALG11-CDG, or CDG-Ip [Rind et al., 2010]. The proband was a girl who presented in the neonatal period with dysmorphism, vomiting, and hypotonia. She had visual and hearing impairment, intractable seizures, lipodystrophy, and elevated lactate without another metabolic explanation. She died at 2 years. Subsequently, a brother was born, who presented with hypotonia and vomiting at 6 weeks, and who was found to carry the same mutation. ALG11 encodes GDP-Man:Man$_3$GlcNAc$_2$-PP-dolichol mannosyltransferase. Deficiency of this enzyme impairs the elongation of lipid-linked oligosaccharides at the outer leaflet of the endoplasmic reticulum.

Defects in Protein *O*-Glycosylation
O-Xylosylglycan Synthesis

Glycosaminoglycans are very large glycan chains that usually are built on selected core proteins [Esko, 1999]. These molecules are located in the extracellular matrix, where they provide mechanical support and help to organize the matrix. At the cell surface, they bind growth factors and act as signaling molecules that enhance or inhibit cell proliferation. They are the most diverse and complex glycans. The protein-bound glycosaminoglycan molecules include heparan sulfate, chondroitin sulfate, dermatan sulfate, and keratan sulfate. All but the last are linked to protein through *O*-xylose, which is extended with two galactose units and a glucuronic acid. Each of these glycosaminoglycan chains is extended by one of several alternating disaccharides composed of GlcNAcα1,4GlcAβ1,4) (heparan sulfate) or GalNAcβ1,3GlcAβ1,3 (chondroitin sulfate and dermatan sulfate) or GlcNAcβ1,3Galβ1,4 (keratan sulfate). All of these glycosaminoglycans are partially sulfated. Hyaluronon, GlcNAcβ1,4GlcAβ1,3, is the only glycosaminoglycan that exists as a free glycan chain and is not sulfated.

Three known defects in glycosaminoglycan synthesis cause clinical disorders, but none has neurologic manifestations. Mutations in the gene *B4GALT7* cause abnormal synthesis of dermatan sulfate and are associated with the progeroid variant of Ehlers–Danlos syndrome [Quentin et al., 1990; Faiyaz-Ul-Haque et al., 2004]. This gene encodes an enzyme, xylosylprotein 4-β-galactosyltransferase, that adds the first galactose residue to xylose in the core of glycosaminoglycan chains. Patients exhibit multiple abnormalities in connective tissue, leading to short stature, diffuse osteopenia, loose but elastic skin, hypermobile joints, and hypotonia. Cognitive impairment has not been reported.

The condition multiple hereditary exostoses is inherited as an autosomal-dominant trait and characteristically affects the metaphyses of long bones [Zak et al., 2002]. Patients with multiple hereditary exostoses have mutations in the genes *EXT1* and *EXT2*, both of which encode co-polymerase components that participate in the assembly of alternating residues of GlcNAc and GluA that form the backbone of the heparan sulfate glycosaminoglycan chains. Because heparan sulfate binds to many types of growth factors, a partial decrease in heparan sulfate is thought to upset the delicate regulation of chondrocyte proliferation. This situation in turn leads to enhanced chondrocyte growth and the formation of exostoses. Surprisingly, a significant proportion of patients fall within the autistic spectrum. Rigorous experiments in Ext-deficient mouse models indicate molecular alterations corresponding to dramatic behavioral changes that correlate with reduced heparan sulfate content of selected tissues.

Macular corneal dystrophy (types I and II) is caused by a deficiency in a specific sulfotransferase (CHST6) called corneal *N*-acetylglucosamine-6-sulfotransferase (GlcNAc6ST), which is responsible for the sulfation of corneal keratan sulfate [Akama et al., 2000]. The unsulfated keratan chains are poorly soluble, and their eventual precipitation disrupts the collagen network, leading to thinning and loss of transparency of the corneal stroma. This progressive disorder manifests between ages 5 and 9 with very small, punctate corneal opacities. Erosions, painful photophobia, and sensation of an ocular foreign body develop subsequently.

O-N-*acetylgalactosamine Synthesis*

These mucinous types of molecules are located at the surface of epithelial cells or in their secretions, and typically subserve barrier functions [Marth, 1999]. They usually are composed of large clusters of *O*-galactose *N*-acetylglucosamine

(*O*-GalNAc)-linked sugar chains, each containing 2–10 sugars. Only a few are known to serve specific functions: for example, in lymphocyte recirculation and leukocyte extravasation [Lowe, 2003]. Few biosynthetic defects are known, and none has obvious neurologic manifestations.

O-mannosylglycan Synthesis: Congenital Muscular Dystrophy and Limb-Girdle Spectrum

OVERVIEW

The dystrophin glycoprotein complex assembles on the sarcolemma of skeletal muscle cells. Mutations that affect the integrity of this complex cause congenital muscular dystrophies by compromising the integrity of the basement membrane [Martin, 2003]. Alpha-dystroglycan is a major component of this complex and contains *O*-mannose-linked glycans (i.e., those with an *O* linkage between Ser/Thr and mannose residues). Mutations in genes encoding enzymes involved in this *O*-linked glycosylation cause a group of rare congenital muscular dystrophies with an autosomal-recessive inheritance pattern and a variable degree of brain involvement [Martin and Freeze, 2003]. Additional types of congenital muscular dystrophy likely will be found to result from as yet unrecognized defects in this glycosylation pathway (Figure 35-3).

BIOSYNTHESIS OF *O*-MANNOSE GLYCANS

POMT1 (protein-*O*-mannosyltransferase 1) and POMT2 (protein-*O*-mannosyltransferase 2) form a complex and use Man-P-Dol to form the Man-O-Ser/Thr linkage, in the endoplasmic reticulum lumen. This linkage is extended by addition of β1,2-GlcNAc through a pathway-specific GlcNAc transferase (POMGnT1). Both POMT1/2 and POMGnT1 have proven enzymatic activities [Endo, 2004]. In α-dystroglycan, this disaccharide can be extended with β1,4-Gal and capped by α-2,3-Sia. Alternatively, the GlcNAc is extended by GalNAc, Man is converted to Man-6-P and further to an undefined Man-6-P-diester. The presence of Man-6-P diester is considered essential for normal binding of α-dystroglycan to the matrix [Yoshida et al., 2010]. The biosynthetic pathway and specific structures are unknown, but it is clear that this pathway is not the same one as that used for lysosomal enzyme targeting. More complex branched glycans with glucuronic acid (GlcA) or sulfate can be found in the brain, suggesting that this pathway is much more complex [Yuen et al., 1997]. About one-third of all *O*-linked chains in the brain are built on O-Man, and α-dystroglycan is clearly not the only protein with these glycans, since brain-specific deletion of α-dystroglycan does not significantly change the amount of O-Man glycans [Yoshida et al., 2010].

Functional Defects

Defects in this pathway are depicted in Table 35-1. Deficiencies in POMT1 and POMT2 impair the addition of the linkage Man unit to the protein, preventing further elongations at that site. These mutations account for about 30 percent of the diagnosed cases of Walker–Warburg syndrome [Beltran-Valero de Bernabe et al., 2002; Muntoni et al., 2004]. Defects in POMGNT1 impair addition of GlcNAc to Man and cause muscle-eye-brain disease [Zhang et al., 2003].

Other congenital muscular dystrophies also have been linked to glycosylation abnormalities, but the specific molecular

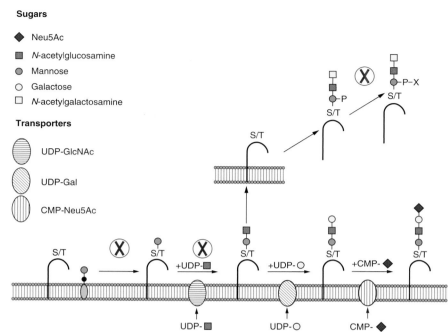

Fig. 35-3 O-mannose glycan biosynthesis. Biosynthesis of O-mannose-linked glycans on molecules such as α-dystroglycan begins with the addition of mannose from Man-P-Dol in the lumen of the endoplasmic reticulum. Defects in its addition are responsible for some cases of Walker–Warburg syndrome. An N-acetylglucosamine is added to the O-linked mannose using a specific transferase and a transporter-delivered UDP donor. Mutations in this transferase cause muscle-eye-brain disease. Extension can occur using GalNAc or by galactose and followed by sialic acid. All of these require transporter-delivered donors. A novel pathway converts O-Man to O-Man-6-P, and then an additional reaction involving LARGE forms a phosphodiester of unknown composition on GalNAc-GlcNAc-Man-Ser/Thr glycans. CMP, cytidine monophosphate; S/T, serine/threonine; UDP, uridine diphosphate.

mechanisms are not known. These proteins include fukutin, fukutin-related protein, and LARGE. Mutations in *FCMD* cause Fukuyama congenital muscular dystrophy, common in Japan. Mutations in the fukutin-related protein gene, *FKRP*, cause CMD1C and limb-girdle muscular dystrophy [Muntoni et al., 2004]. The *LARGE* gene causes a form of murine muscular dystrophy, and mutations in its human homolog were found in a patient with a congenital muscular dystrophy and mental retardation [Longman et al., 2003]. The clinical presentations of congenital muscular dystrophies reflect the manifestations associated with specific mutations and may overlap. Mutations in *POMT1*, *FKRP*, and *FCMD* all have been associated with a Walker–Warburg syndrome phenotype [Muntoni et al., 2004]. *FCMD*, *FKRP*, and *LARGE* all have glycosyltransferase-like domains and characteristic catalytic residues, but transferase activity has not been demonstrated. Sequence homologies usually are insufficient to predict the specific transferase reactions because sugar-specific signatures are few, and the acceptor substrate may require both peptide and glycan recognition. Overexpression of *LARGE* can functionally bypass multiple glycosylation defects in α-dystroglycan, offering a potentially broad therapeutic approach [Barresi et al., 2004].

Clinical Features

The European Neuromuscular Center proposed a set of diagnostic criteria for congenital muscular dystrophies. These include hypotonia beginning in the first 6 months, early multiple contractures, diffuse weakness and muscular atrophy with sparing of extraocular muscles, normal mental development (in many), variable course, early elevation of serum creatine kinase, myopathic changes on electromyography (EMG), and necrotic-regenerative changes on muscle biopsy [Dubowitz, 1997].

The three forms of congenital muscular dystrophy associated with impaired O-glycosylation have considerable phenotypic overlap, as mentioned earlier. Fukuyama congenital muscular dystrophy is characterized by cortical dysgenesis and simple myopia. Affected children have global developmental delay, with regression in motor skills in the latter half of the first decade and death in adolescence [Messina et al., 2010]. Almost all of the patients with Fukuyama congenital muscular dystrophy have seizures. Fukuyama congenital muscular dystrophy is the most common form of congenital muscular dystrophy in Japan, in contrast with Western populations, in which merosin deficiency predominates.

Muscle-eye-brain disease is characterized by more severe pathologic changes than in Fukuyama congenital muscular dystrophy, including cobblestone lissencephaly, midline defects, and brainstem flattening associated with progressive myopia, retinal degeneration, and cataracts.

Walker–Warburg syndrome also features type II lissencephaly, in combination with ventriculomegaly, cerebellar malformations, retinal and anterior chamber malformations, and congenital cataracts. Walker–Warburg syndrome represents the most severe congenital muscular dystrophy phenotype, with congenital blindness, hypotonia, profound developmental delay, and failure to thrive. Most affected children die in the first 6 months of life [Messina et al., 2010].

Biochemical and Genetic Tests

Several monoclonal antibodies recognize some feature of the O-Man chain on α-dystroglycan, and their binding is greatly reduced or eliminated in all of these disorders [Michele et al., 2002]. Antibody against the peptide portion binds normally, but the loss of the glycan chains reduces the apparent size of the protein. Specific enzymatic assays can be used to diagnose muscle-eye-brain disease [Zhang et al., 2003], and for POMT1 [Lommel et al., 2010]. Sequencing of the genes is needed to identify specific mutations. It is likely that additional biosynthetic genes will be identified soon.

Defects in Glycosphingolipid and Glycosylphosphatidylinositol Glycosylation

Developmental delay, seizures, and blindness are found in autosomal-recessive Amish infantile epilepsy. A large Amish family was identified with a nonsense mutation in *SIAT9* that truncated protein [Simpson et al., 2004]. SIAT9 is a sialyltransferase needed for synthesis of gangliosides GM3 (Siaα2-3Galβ1-4Glc-ceramide) from lactosylceramide (Galβ1-4Glc-ceramide). Patients accumulate nonsialylated plasma glycosphingolipids, such as GM3, and also lack downstream GM3-dependent molecules.

Only one defect in glycophosphatidylinositol anchor synthesis with neurological features is known, and has been reported as Mabry's syndrome [Thompson et al., 2010]. Genetic mapping demonstrated that patients with mental retardation, hyperphosphatasia, unusual facial features, hypotonia, and seizures have mutations in *PIGV*. The gene encodes the second mannosyltransferase used for GPI-anchor synthesis. Total surface anchors are reduced, including glycophosphatidylinositol-anchored alkaline phosphatase, which is instead found at very high levels in the plasma [Krawitz et al., 2010].

Defects in Multiple Glycosylation and Other Pathways

DPM1-CDG (Ie)

DPM1-CDG is another severe phenotype, characterized by psychomotor delay, profound hypotonia, microcephaly, cortical blindness, and intractable seizures [Imbach et al., 2000b; Kim et al., 2000]. Laboratory testing revealed elevated creatine kinase and depressed antithrombin III. Some children have dysmorphic features, including downslanting palpebral fissures, flat occiput and nasal bridge, hemangiomas of the occiput and sacrum, a high narrow palate, and mild limb shortening. Dolichol phosphate mannose synthase (DPM1) activity is markedly diminished in all reported cases.

DPM3-CDG (Io)

A 27-year-old woman has been reported with DPM3 deficiency, whose phenotype includes short stature, dilated cardiomyopathy, a strokelike episode, and a myopathy characterized by mild proximal weakness and absent glycosylated α-dystroglycan on muscle biopsy [Lefeber et al., 2009]. DPM activity is required to provide Man-P-Dol precursors for N-, C-, and O-linked glycosylation and for glycophosphatidylinositol anchor biosynthesis. In this case, a primary defect in the N-glycosylation pathway has led to an O-linked disorder – an α-dystroglycanopathy.

MPDU1-CDG (If)

Four children with MPDU1-CDG have been described. Abnormalities included severe psychomotor retardation and variable features, including growth retardation, optic nerve atrophy, icthyosis, dysmorphism (parietal bossing, thin lips), hypo- or hypertonia, enlarged extra-axial spaces, thrombocytopenia, transient deficiency of growth hormone and insulin-like growth factor 1, and mild elevations of creatine kinase [Kranz et al., 2001; Schenk et al., 2001b]. All have mutations in *MPDU1/Lec35*, leading to deficient function of the Lec35 protein. Lec35 may act as a chaperone for P-Dol in the

endoplasmic reticulum membrane, ensuring appropriate lateral spacing of Man-P-Dol and Glc-P-Dol. In the absence of such spacing, these compounds may form rafts that alter local concentration gradients, impairing synthesis of the lipid-linked oligosaccharide and its accessibility to the oligosaccharyltransferase complex.

B4GALT1-CDG (IId)

A single patient with B4GALT1-CDG (IId) has been described. Abnormalities included psychomotor retardation, a Dandy–Walker malformation, progressive hydrocephalus, hypotonia, and myopathy [Hansske et al., 2002]. CDG-IId was caused by mutations in *B4GALT1*, encoding one of the isozymes that add β-1,4-galactose units to N-linked glycans during processing. The other isozymes do not compensate for this transferase deficiency.

GNE-CDG

Mutations in *GNE*, which encodes UDP-N-acetylglucosamine 2-epimerase/N-acetylmannosamine kinase, cause both hereditary inclusion body myopathy (IBM2) and distal myopathy with rimmed vacuoles [Grandis et al., 2010]. IBM2 presents with a distal myopathy that later spreads proximally, but characteristically spares the quadriceps. Creatine kinase is mildly elevated. The disorder is most frequent among Iranian Jews, who carry an M712 T mutation in *GNE*. Nonaka myopathy, or distal myopathy with rimmed vacuoles, has a similar presentation, but is usually associated with different mutations.

SLC35A1-CDG (IIf)

The sole reported patient with SLC35A1-CDG (IIf) had severe thrombocytopenia and complete loss of the sialyl-Lewis-X antigen on leukocytes [Willig et al., 2001; Martinez-Duncker et al., 2005]. This disorder was associated with mutations in the gene encoding the Golgi cytidine monophosphate (CMP)-sialic acid transporter [Martinez-Duncker et al., 2005]. Although platelet membrane proteins exhibited altered glycosylation, transferrin and other serum glycoproteins were normal. This finding underscores the limitations of transferrin analysis.

SLC35A1-CDG (IIc)

SLC35A1-CDG (IIc) was originally described as leukocyte adhesion deficiency II and is characterized by moderate to severe mental retardation, rhizomelic short stature, a broad flat nasal bridge, microcephaly, elevated leukocytes, frequent infections, persistent marked neutrophilia, and periodontitis. The disorder is caused by mutations in the GDP-fucose transporter, which limits the synthesis of fucosylated glycans [Lübke et al., 2001; Lühn et al., 2001]. One of these is sialyl Lewis-X (sLeX), a glycan essential for leukocyte rolling before extravasation. Oral fucose supplements effectively reduced leukocytosis in two patients by allowing synthesis of sufficient sLeX [Hidalgo et al., 2003; Marquardt et al., 1999]. These patients also lack fucosylated H-antigen, the precursor for the ABO blood group. Fucose supplements have not provoked antigen synthesis or immunologic reactions. Transferrin glycosylation is normal in this type.

COG complex

COG7-CDG (IIE)

The first report of COG7-CDG (IIe) described two siblings. Manifestations included perinatal asphyxia and dysmorphic features, including low-set dysplastic ears, micrognathia, short neck, and loose wrinkled skin [Wu et al., 2004]. They had generalized hypotonia, hepatosplenomegaly, and progressive jaundice that appeared shortly after birth. A CT scan revealed an enlarged cisterna cerebelli superior in one patient; severe epilepsy developed in both. They both died by 10 weeks from recurrent infections and cardiac insufficiency. A total of 8 patients are now known, most with similar presentations, although one [Zeevaert et al., 2009] was less severely affected. This type is caused by a mutation in *COG7*, which encodes one of the eight subunits of the COG complex [Oka et al., 2004; Ungar et al., 2002]. This cytoplasmic complex associates with the cytoplasmic face of the Golgi, and is involved in the shuttling of glycosyltransferases and nucleotide sugar transporters between the Golgi and other intracellular compartments. The mutation destabilizes the complex and slows the trafficking of these molecules, presumably leading to their degradation or mislocalization.

COG1-CDG (IIG)

The sole COG1-CDG (IIg) patient described to date is a girl with hypotonia, rhizomelic short stature and acquired microcephaly [Foulquier et al., 2006]. She had mild dysmorphic features, subtle hepatosplenomegaly, mild developmental delay at 21 months, and slight cerebral and cerebellar atrophy. Transferrin isoelectric focusing demonstrated a type II pattern; ApoC-III isoelectric focusing also demonstrated a hypoglycosylated pattern, confirming abnormal *O*-linked glycosylation. The patient was found to have a homozygous insertion (c.2659–2660insC) in the *hCOG1* gene, which would predict a truncated COG1 protein.

COG8-CDG (IIH)

Two patients have been described with COG8-CDG (IIh). The first had a severe phenotype, characterized by delayed development and hypotonia, first appreciated in the latter half of the first year, with the subsequent evolution of myoclonic seizures and growth failure, with a height and weight below the first percentile for age [Kranz et al., 2007a]. At last follow-up at 8.5 years, the child suffered from severe retardation, double incontinence, intolerance of wheat and dairy products, markedly reduced muscle mass, mild spasticity and contractures of the lower extremities, and esotropia. Laboratory studies had demonstrated evidence of chronic axonal neuropathy. This child was heterozygous for two *COG8* mutations: IVS3+1G>A and 1687–1688 del TT. Both mutations produce a truncated protein. The second case was a girl who presented at 6 months with an acute encephalopathy after initial normal development [Foulquier et al., 2007]. The child regressed, and manifested hypotonia and alternating esotropia and pseudoptosis. She subsequently developed a progressive cerebellar syndrome, accompanied by action myoclonus. Over time, the deep tendon reflexes disappeared, and oculomotor apraxia has emerged. Laboratory abnormalities have included abnormal levels of coagulation factors, transaminases, and creatine kinase. In both cases, transferrin isoelectric focusing documented a type II pattern, and Apo C-III was hypoglycosylated. This child was homozygous for a nonsense mutation (C to G) at position c.1611 in the COG8 cDNA.

COG4-CDG (IIJ)

There is a single report of a child with COG4-CDG (IIj) [Reynders et al., 2009]. This child became symptomatic around 4 months of age, following immunization, when he experienced fever, irritability, and the onset of complex partial seizures. He had dysmorphic features, including thick hair and unusual facies, axial hypotonia, and mild limb spasticity and hyperreflexia. From 12 months, he experienced frequent infections, and by 3 years was microcephalic, with ataxia, delayed milestones (including absent speech), and frontotemporal atrophy on imaging studies. Laboratory investigations indicated elevated transaminases, alkaline phosphatase, LDL cholesterol, and low levels of coagulation factors and platelets. Studies of the *COG4* gene identified a point mutation of the paternal allele (C2185T) and a microdeletion of the maternal allele.

COG5-CDG

The sole patient described with COG5 deficiency was a girl who presented at 8 years with mild mental retardation (IQ 50–55), mild dysarthria, truncal and appendicular ataxia, and hypotonia [Paesold-Burda et al., 2009]. She had no systemic abnormalities and extensive metabolic investigation was negative. MRI documented diffuse cerebellar and brainstem atrophy. Subsequently, she made slow developmental progress. Investigation at 12 years revealed evidence of abnormal *N*-linked and *O*-linked glycosylation. Sequencing of the *COG5* gene identified a homozygous mutation (c.1669–15T>C), which explained the observed altered splicing of the transcript.

COG6-CDG

An infant with an early lethal phenotype was found to be homozygous for mutations (c.G1646T) in the *COG6* gene [Lübbehusen et al., 2010]. The child experienced vomiting, intractable partial seizures, and intracranial hemorrhage, associated with vitamin K deficiency.

When to Suspect and Test for Congenital Disorders of Glycosylation

A congenital disorder of glycosylation should be suspected in any child presenting with an unexplained syndrome, particularly those characterized by developmental delay, hearing loss, hypotonia, and seizures, especially in combination with lipodystrophy, skeletal dysplasia, or gastrointestinal, hepatic, or coagulation abnormalities. However, nonsyndromic mental retardation or "pure" neurologic syndromes do occur, including dramatic episodes of regression, apparently provoked by intercurrent illness or immunization. Testing for an abnormal transferrin should be considered. Not all types will demonstrate abnormal transferrin, and some confirmed patients may normalize transferrin in time. Therefore, it is best to test patients early (1–18 months of age). Patients with CDGs may have phenotypes resembling mitochondrial disorders, Joubert syndrome, or Dandy–Walker malformation. Even with abnormal transferrin, extensive genetic testing will be needed to identify the defect. Some commercial laboratories now offer various CDG gene panel analyses. As technology improves and costs decrease in the coming years, genome or exome sequencing will indicate the specific defects, but additional biochemical and physiological analysis will be needed to provide therapeutic hopes.

Summary

Glycosylated molecules are present on the surface and in the interior of all cells. The biosynthesis of sugar chains is complex, with the potential to produce thousands of different structures at different times in response to endogenous and exogenous signals. At least 2 percent of the known genes encode proteins that either synthesize or bind to sugar chains, often with exquisite specificity. Disrupting glycan biosynthesis leads to a multitude of downstream effects that may involve every aspect of central nervous system development and function. The analysis of transferrin glycosylation status can point to glycosylation abnormalities in many patients. A few patients respond to simple dietary supplements of sugars. Although glycosylation disorders appear to be rare, their recent discovery makes it likely that the true frequency is unknown. As for all inborn errors of metabolism, many patients with mild or atypical manifestations will be found and new disorders will be recognized as diagnostic testing, including gene sequencing, becomes more widely available and applied.

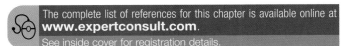

Lysosomal Storage Diseases

Gregory M. Pastores

Overview and General Concepts

The lysosomal storage diseases are a clinically heterogeneous group of inborn errors of metabolism that have traditionally been classified according to the biochemical nature of the incompletely degraded macromolecules that accumulate in various tissues. The lysosomal storage diseases are represented by about 50 different clinical entities (Table 36-1). Most of the individual conditions also have an eponymous designation in recognition of the investigator who provided seminal descriptions of the typical manifestations and clinical course of specific variants, often before elucidation of their biochemical or molecular bases.

As a central compartment in the endosomal-lysosomal pathway, the lysosome maintains an acidified milieu enriched with catabolic enzymes to facilitate the degradation of various byproducts of cellular turnover, which are mainly delivered to the lysosome through endocytosis. Phagocytosis and autophagy provide alternative points of substrate entry into the lysosome [Falguières et al., 2009]. These complex substrates may include sphingolipids, glycoproteins, and glycosaminoglycans (mucopolysaccharides). The particular metabolite that builds up (and the ensuing pattern and severity of the associated diseases) is primarily dependent on the substrate tissue-source and the relevant metabolic pathway and transport systems that are compromised. For instance, keratan sulfate is a major constituent of cartilage and the cornea; abnormalities in the turnover of keratan sulfate partly explain the characteristic features of skeletal dysplasia and the corneal opacities associated with the mucopolysaccharidoses [Wegrzyn et al., 2004]. Analysis (through a combination of immune quantification assays and tandem mass spectrometry) of the glycosphingolipid and oligosaccharide profiles in the blood and urine of affected patients may prove useful; as surrogate markers of disease activity, they may enable early diagnosis and the monitoring of clinical responses with directed therapies (such as enzyme replacement or substrate synthesis inhibition) [Parkinson-Lawrence et al., 2006].

The enzymes and transport or integral membrane proteins that are responsible for facilitating the intralysosomal metabolism of these substrates are formed within the endoplasmic reticulum and subsequently refined (through distinct post-translational mechanisms) by the Golgi apparatus [Eskelinen et al., 2003]. The uptake of newly synthesized enzymes by the lysosome, as opposed to other cellular organelles such as the peroxisome or mitochondria, is achieved largely through the mannose 6-phosphate (M6P) receptor pathway. Thus, phosphorylation of the mannose residues of the complex carbohydrate side-chains of the various relevant proteins is an essential step in its maturational processing [Urayama

et al., 2004]. Elucidation of this pathway of lysosomal protein delivery, including uptake by the mannose receptors, was critical in the development of enzyme therapy for the lysosomal storage diseases [Grabowski and Hopkin, 2003].

Absent or defective hydrolytic activity within the lysosome, which can come about as a consequence of mutations within the specific encoding gene (for the functional enzyme or its activator or co-factor), is the most common cause of disease (Table 36-2) [Ballabio and Gieselmann, 2009]. For example, deficient glucocerebrosidase activity, as in Gaucher's disease, results in the accumulation of its substrate, the glycosphingolipid glucosylceramide. Sphingolipid co-factors called saposins facilitate the interaction between the water-soluble glycoprotein enzymes and their lipid-soluble substrates [Matsuda et al., 2007]. Mutation of the saposin C gene is associated with the incomplete metabolism of glucosylceramide in vivo and a rare condition that has clinical features that overlap with the chronic neuropathic form of Gaucher's disease (type 3 disease). Unlike other lysosomal hydrolases, which rely on the M6P receptor pathway, glucocerebrosidase is targeted to the lysosome via LIMP-2 [Reczek et al., 2007]; mutations of the encoding gene for LIMP-2 have been associated with a progressive myoclonic epilepsy and nephrotic syndrome [Balreira et al., 2008].

Other proteins (e.g., cathepsin A) serve as a constituent of a multienzyme complex and play a protective role, preventing the intralysosomal degradation of its component enzymes (i.e., β-galactosidase and sialidase). Deficiency of cathepsin A leads to the clinical entity known as galactosialidosis, which combines the clinical features encountered in the two different primary enzyme deficiency disorders: namely, GM_1-gangliosidosis and sialidosis. Alternatively, a flaw in the processing of certain newly synthesized enzymes (e.g., because of a failure in generating M6P residues) leads to their functional loss by keeping the enzyme from assuming its operational conformation or denying access to the lysosome. This flaw is one type of post-translational defect that can lead to the loss of activity of multiple lysosomal enzymes (as in mucolipidosis II and III).

Other lysosomal disorders result from a defective protein involved in substrate transport (e.g., Niemann–Pick disease type C) or vesicle fusion (e.g., Danon's disease) [Dierks et al., 2009; Ruivo et al., 2009]. Additional defects of lysosomal transport (e.g., cystinosis, sialic acid storage disorders) involve a dysfunction of intracellular membrane transporters that mediate the movements of the hydrolyzed products outside of the lysosome for their final excretion [Ruivo et al., 2009]. With respect to pathogenesis, cellular toxicity is hypothesized to occur when the lysosomal substrate burden has reached a critical threshold and presumptively triggers a cascade of downstream events that ultimately lead to cell death and the development of

Table 36-1 **The Lysosomal Storage Disorders Classified According to Relevant Substrate Involved**

Stored Substrate	Disease	Enzyme/Protein Deficiency	Gene Locus
SPHINGOLIPIDS			
GM$_2$ gangliosides, glycolipids, globoside oligosaccharides	Tay–Sachs disease	α Subunit of β-hexosaminidase	15q23–24
	GM$_2$ gangliosidosis (three types) Sandhoff's disease GM$_2$ gangliosidosis	β Subunit of β-hexosaminidase	5q13
	GM$_2$ gangliosidosis, AB variant	GM$_2$ activator	5q32–33
GM$_1$ gangliosides, oligosaccharides, keratan sulfate, glycolipids	GM$_1$ gangliosidosis (three types)*	β-Galactosidase	3p21–3pter
Sulfatides	Metachromatic leukodystrophy	Arylsulfatase A (galactose-3-sulfatase)	22q13.31–qter
GM$_1$ gangliosides, sphingomyelin, glycolipids, sulfatide	Metachromatic leukodystrophy variant	Saposin B activator	10q21
Galactosylceramides	Krabbe's disease	Galactocerebrosidase	14q31
α-Galactosylsphingolipids, oligosaccharides	Fabry's disease	α-Galactosidase A	Xq22
Glucosylceramide, globosides	Gaucher's disease (three types)*	β-Glucosidase	1q21
Glucosylceramide, globosides	Gaucher's disease (variant)	Saposin C	10q21
Ceramide	Farber's disease (seven types)	Acid ceramidase	8p22–21.2
Sphingomyelin	Niemann–Pick disease types A and B	Sphingomyelinase	11p15.1–15.4
MUCOPOLYSACCHARIDES (GLYCOSAMINOGLYCANS)			
Dermatan sulfate and heparan sulfate	MPS I, Hurler–Scheie	α-L-Iduronidase	4p16.3
	MPS II, Hunter	Iduronate-2-sulfatase	Xq27.3–28
Heparan sulfate	MPS IIIA, Sanfilippo A MPS IIIB, Sanfilippo B MPS IIIC, Sanfilippo C	Sulfamidase α-N-Acetylglucosaminidase Acetyl-CoA: α-glucosaminide-N-acetyltransferase	17q25.3 17q21.1 14
	MPS IIID, Sanfilippo D	N-Acetylglucosamine-6-sulfatase	12q14
Keratan sulfate	MPS IVA, Morquio A MPS IVB, Morquio B	Galactosamine-6-sulfatase β-D-Galactosidase	16q24.3 3p21.33
Dermatan sulfate	MPS VI, Maroteaux–Lamy	N-Acetylgalactosamine-4-sulfatase	5q13–14
Dermatan sulfate and heparan sulfate	MPS VII, Sly	Hyaluronidase	7q21.1–22
Hyaluronan	MPS IX	β-D-Glucuronidase	3p21.3
GLYCOGEN			
Glycogen	Pompe's disease, glycogen storage disease type IIA	α-D-Glucosidase	17q25
Glycogen	Danon's disease	Lysosomal associated membrane protein-2 (LAMP-2)	Xq24
OLIGOSACCHARIDES/GLYCOPEPTIDES			
α-Mannoside	α-Mannosidosis	α-Mannosidase	19p13.2–q12
β-Mannoside	β-Mannosidosis	β-Mannosidase	4q22–25
α-Fucosides, glycolipids	α-Fucosidosis	α-Fucosidase	1p34.1–36.1
α-N-Acetylgalactosaminide	Schindler–Kanzaki disease	α-N-Acetylgalactosaminidase	22q13.1–13.
Sialyloligosaccharides	Sialidosis	α-Neuraminidase	6p21.3
Aspartylglucosamine	Aspartylglucosaminuria	Aspartylglucosaminidase	4q34–35

Table 36-1 The Lysosomal Storage Disorders Classified According to Relevant Substrate Involved—cont'd

Stored Substrate	Disease	Enzyme/Protein Deficiency	Gene Locus
MULTIPLE ENZYME DEFICIENCIES			
Glycolipids, oligosaccharides	Mucolipidosis II (I-cell disease); mucolipidosis III (pseudo-Hurler polydystrophy) three – complementation groups	N-Acetylglucosamine-1-phosphotransferase	4q21–q23 Mucolipidosis III subtype C: γ subunit mutations on 16p; α/β subunit on 12q23.3
	Galactosialidosis	Protective protein/cathepsin A	20
Sulfatides, glycolipids, glycosaminoglycans	Multiple sulfatases	SUMF-1	3p26
LIPIDS			
Cholesterol esters	Wolman's disease, cholesteryl ester storage disease	Acid lipase	10q23.2–q23.3
Cholesterol, sphingomyelin	Niemann–Pick disease type C	NPC1; HE1	18q11–12; 14q24.3
MONOSACCHARIDES/AMINO ACID MONOMERS			
Sialic acid, glucuronic acid	Salla disease, infantile free sialic acid storage disease	Sialin	6q14–15
Cystine	Cystinosis	Cystinosis	17p13
PEPTIDES			
Bone proteins	Pyknodysostosis	Cathepsin K	1q21
S-ACYLATED PROTEINS			
Palmitoylated proteins	Infantile neuronal ceroid lipofuscinosis	Palmitoyl-protein thioesterase	1p32
Pepstatin-insensitive lysosomal peptidase	Late infantile neuronal ceroid lipofuscinosis	Pepstatin-insensitive lysosomal peptidase	11p15

* Three types imply infantile, childhood, and adulthood presentations.

Table 36-2 Illustrative List of Underlying Causes

Etiology	Disease (Examples)
Single hydrolytic enzyme deficiency	Gaucher's disease Tay–Sachs disease Niemann–Pick disease
Single protease enzyme deficiency	Late infantile neuronal ceroid lipofuscinosis (pepinase)
Co-factor/activator protein deficiency	Gaucher's disease variant (saposin) Tay–Sachs disease (GM$_2$ activator)
Multiple enzyme deficiencies	Galactosialidosis (protective protein/cathepsin A) Multiple sulfatase deficiency (SUMF-1) I-cell disease (mucolipidosis II)
Membrane protein defect	Juvenile neuronal ceroid lipofuscinosis (battenin)
Small-molecule transport protein	Cystinosis Sialic acid storage disorders
Endocytosis, membrane-vesicle trafficking defect	Mucolipidosis IV Danon's disease (LAMP-2) Niemann–Pick disease type C

disease-specific complications. These consequent mechanisms of disease for most of the individual lysosomal storage diseases remain to be fully clarified.

There is increasing recognition that, besides mechanical forces, other pathologic factors (e.g., inflammation and apoptosis) may play contributory roles in the evolution of the disease phenotype. For instance, in the GM$_2$-gangliosidoses, several markers of an inflammatory response have been found to be elevated and may partly explain the neurodegenerative features encountered in this group of diseases [Jeyakumar et al., 2002, 2003]. Studies have also suggested that certain lysosomal proteases may play active roles in the apoptotic execution process and can act as mediators of programmed cell death [Tardy et al., 2004]. Defects of autophagy are also being recognized as having a role in the pathogenesis of several lysosomal storage diseases [Settembre et al., 2008]. Oxidative damage and cytotoxic cell involvement has been suggested as a factor in the neuronal pathogenesis of mucopolysaccharidosis (MPS) type III [Villani et al., 2009]. Recent studies involving the animal model of mucopolysaccharidosis type I suggest that the absence of recycled precursors results in major shifts in the energy utilization of the cells [Woloszynek et al., 2009]. This finding susggests that lysosomal storage disease may be characterized as diseases of deficiency as well as overabundance (lysosomal storage).

The majority of genes that encode lysosomal proteins are ubiquitously expressed, and each of the various lysosomal storage disease subtypes is characterized by multisystemic involvement. There is wide heterogeneity in the clinical presentation of each entity among individually affected patients, and the concordance between genotype and phenotype is often imperfect even among siblings [Wilcox, 2004]. Disease manifestations may be evident prenatally or at any time from birth to adulthood. Certain lysosomal storage diseases present with nonimmune hydrops fetalis, and the failure to establish causality before the child's death can lead to potential recurrence in future pregnancies among couples at risk [Staretz-Chacham et al., 2009]. On the other hand, Gaucher's and Fabry's diseases may not be associated with prominent symptoms during childhood, and the diagnosis can be missed because the patients have either a mild or an atypical course. This is true especially when the family history is uninformative. To some extent, the variable disease severity encountered between the individual patients has been attributed to different mutations that produce a protein with either no functional activity (in severe cases) or some residual enzyme activity (as observed in those with later onset of clinical expression). Because most lysosomal storage diseases are autosomal-recessive disorders, heterozygotes (or carrier individuals with a single defective gene copy) often have sufficient enzyme activity generated by their other (normal) allele. Carriers for these conditions do not exhibit evidence of tissue storage or suffer from the relevant disease that segregates in the family.

There are at least three disorders, Fabry's and Danon's diseases and Hunter's syndrome (MPS II), that are transmitted as X-linked traits. Although females who are carriers of the trait for Hunter's syndrome do not appear to develop clinical problems related to the presence of a mutant protein, a proportion of females who are carriers of Fabry's disease or Danon's disease may experience disease-related complications, which in a few cases can be as severe as those found in classically affected males. The variable expression in these carrier females has been partly attributed to lyonization (i.e., the random inactivation during early embryogenesis of one of the two X chromosomes). Lyonization results in varying proportions of the mutant gene product in different organ systems [Orstavik, 2009]. Skewed lyonization may be seen in females with an X:autosome translocation. In these cases, there is inactivation of the intact X chromosome. If the X chromosome that is attached to an autosome remains functional and if it happens to bear a gene mutation, disease expression may be unmasked. In addition, rare cases have been reported of females with Hunter's syndrome who also happen to have Turner's syndrome (45,X), wherein the single X chromosome that is present bears a mutation of the gene leading to the enzyme (iduronate-2-sulfatase) deficiency.

Although the individual disorders are infrequent to rare and considered orphan disorders by drug regulatory agencies, the lysosomal storage diseases have a combined prevalence of about 1 in 5000 to 8000 [Pinto et al., 2004]. This relatively high occurrence has prompted investigations of the feasibility of targeted screening [Meikle et al., 2004; Zhang et al., 2008]. The rationales given for these programs include:

1. the high frequency of certain disorders among a defined ethnic group (e.g., Tay–Sachs, Gaucher's, and Niemann–Pick A diseases among the Ashkenazi Jewish population) [Slatkin, 2004]

2. the potential to intervene before the development of significant neurologic sequelae in cases that are diagnosed early and are potentially treatable (e.g., bone marrow transplantation for juvenile Krabbe's disease [globoid cell leukodystrophy])

3. the opportunity for prevention during subsequent pregnancies in at-risk families (Table 36-3).

Several advances in the understanding of lysosomal storage diseases have resulted from investigations of animal disease models, which either have arisen spontaneously or have been generated by the application of recombinant genetic techniques (primarily involving mice) [Suzuki et al., 2003]. Numerous insights into the role of certain metabolites in embryonic and fetal development and their functions in various organs have been obtained from experiments involving these different animal models, which have also been useful in the development and preclinical testing of new putative therapies [Desmaris et al., 2004; Haskins, 2009]. Although most mouse disease models are genetically authentic and mimic the human phenotype, several reproduce only some aspects or may have no clinical manifestations at all (e.g., the Tay–Sachs disease knockout mouse) [Elsea and Lucas, 2002].

On the therapeutic front, industrial-scale production of recombinant human enzymes (through manipulation of mammalian cells in culture) has enabled the introduction of enzyme replacement therapy for several disorders, including Gaucher's, Fabry's, and Pompe's (glycogen storage disease II) diseases, and Hurler–Scheie (MPS I H/S), Hunter's (MPS II) and Maroteaux–Lamy (MPS VI) syndrome [Pastores, 2003; Pastores and Barnett, 2005]. In diseases primarily associated with central nervous system (CNS) degeneration (e.g., Tay–Sachs disease and Niemann–Pick disease type C) and for which protein delivery across the blood–brain barrier represents a major obstacle, trials with substrate reduction therapy have been undertaken [Platt and Lachmann, 2009]. The rationale for this approach is based on the following: in cases wherein mutant cells express residual enzyme activity, metabolic homeostasis may be restored or maintained by limiting the amount of intralysosomal substrate accumulation through inhibition of the amount of precursor material that is synthesized [Pastores and Barnett, 2003; Platt and Jeyakumar, 2008]. In Gaucher's disease, substrate reduction therapy is feasible with the use of the imino sugar miglustat (which inhibits the activity of ceramide-specific glucosyltransferase, the rate-limiting enzyme involved in the biosynthesis of glycosphingolipids).

Before enzyme replacement therapy and substrate reduction therapy, bone marrow transplantation was undertaken in selected cases (see Table 36-3) [Prasad and Kurtzberg, 2008]. The high procedure-related morbidity and mortality risks associated with bone marrow transplantation (e.g., from graft-versus-host disease or infections) preclude its general application, even in cases in which clear therapeutic gains could be established in the successfully engrafted patients. The use of hematopoietic or mesenchymal stem cells and less intensive (i.e., nonmyeloablative) conditioning regimens is being examined as a means to improve clinical outcome and to minimize procedural risks [Prasad and Kurtzberg, 2008].

Another novel approach, termed enzyme enhancement therapy, is also under investigation. Enzyme enhancement therapy is a potential treatment strategy for diseases resulting from a defective enzyme associated with a mutation that leads to its misfolding and rapid degradation [Desnick, 2004]. In these

Table 36-3 **Diagnosis and Therapeutic Options for the Lysosomal Storage Disorders**

Disease*	Diagnostic Method†	Treatment‡
Tay–Sachs disease (B variant)	Enz; Mol; Prenat (Enz/Mol)	SRT (in clinical trials)
GM₂ gangliosidosis (three types)		
Sandhoff's disease (O variant)	Urine oligo; Enz; Mol; Prenat (Enz)	Palliative
GM₂ gangliosidosis		
GM₂ gangliosidosis, AB variant	Func; Mol; Prenat (Mol)	Palliative
GM₁ gangliosidosis (three types)	Enz; Mol; Prenat (Enz)	Palliative
Metachromatic leukodystrophy	Enz; Mol; Prenat (Enz)	HSCT/BMT
Metachromatic leukodystrophy variant (saposin B deficiency)	Func/Subs; Mol; Prenat (Mol)	Palliative
Krabbe's disease	Enz; Mol; Prenat (Enz)	HSCT/BMT
Fabry's disease	Enz/Subs; Mol; Prenat (Enz/Mol)	ERT
Gaucher's disease types 1, 2, and 3	Enz; Mol; Prenat (Enz)	ERT, primarily for types 1 and 3; SRT
Gaucher's disease (saposin C variant)	Func/Subs; Mol; Prenat (Mol)	Palliative
Farber's disease (seven types)	Enz; Mol; Prenat (Enz)	Palliative
Niemann–Pick disease types A and B	Enz; Mol; Prenat (Enz)	ERT (in clinical trials primarily for type B)
MPS I, Hurler–Scheie	Urine GAG; Enz; Mol; Prenat (Enz)	ERT; HSCT/BMT
MPS II, Hunter	Urine GAG; Enz; Mol; Prenat (Enz)	ERT (in clinical trials)
MPS IIIA-D, Sanfilippo A to D	Urine GAG; Enz; Mol; Prenat (Enz)	Palliative
MPS IVA, Morquio A	Urine GAG; Enz; Mol; Prenat (Enz)	Palliative
MPS IVB, Morquio B	Urine GAG; Enz; Mol; Prenat (Enz)	Palliative
MPS VI, Maroteaux–Lamy	Urine GAG; Enz; Mol; Prenat (Enz)	ERT (in clinical trials)
MPS VII, Sly	Urine GAG; Enz; Mol; Prenat (Enz)	Palliative
MPS IX	Enz; Mol; Prenat (none reported)	Palliative
Pompe's disease, glycogen storage disease IIA	Urine oligo; Enz; Mol; Prenat (Enz)	ERT (in clinical trials)
Danon's disease	Mol; Prenat (Mol)	Palliative
α-Mannosidosis	Urine oligo; Enz; Mol; Prenat (Subs)	HSCT/BMT
β-Mannosidosis	Urine oligo; Enz; Mol; Prenat (Enz)	HSCT/BMT
α-Fucosidosis	Mol; Prenat (Mol)	HSCT/BMT
Schindler–Kanzaki disease	Urine oligo; Enz; Mol; Prenat (Enz)	Palliative
Sialidosis (mucolipidosis I)	Enz; Mol; Prenat (Enz)	Palliative
Aspartylglucosaminuria	Urine oligo; Enz; Mol; Prenat (Enz)	Palliative
Mucolipidosis II (I-cell disease)	Urine oligo; Mul Enz; Mol; Prenat (Enz)	Palliative; BMT (1 case)
Mucolipidosis IV	Mol; Prenat (Mol)	Palliative
Galactosialidosis (protective protein/cathepsin A deficiency)	Urine oligo; Mul Enz; Mol; Prenat (Mul Enz)	Palliative
Multiple sulfatases	Urine GAG; Mul Enz; Mol; Prenat (Enz)	Palliative
Wolman's disease, cholesteryl ester storage disease (acid lipase deficiency)	Enz; Mol; Prenat (Enz)	Palliative
Niemann–Pick disease type C	Func/Subs; Mol; Prenat (Func/Subs)	SRT (in clinical trials)
Salla disease, infantile free sialic acid storage disease	Subs; Mol; Prenat (Subs)	Palliative
Cystinosis	Func/Subs; Mol; Prenat (Func/Subs)	Cysteamine
Pyknodysostosis	Enz; Mol; Prenat (none reported)	Palliative
Neuronal ceroid lipofuscinosis	Enz; Mol; Prenat (Enz/Mol for certain subtypes)	Palliative

* As listed in Table 36-1.
† Enz, enzyme assay; Func, functional assay (see text); GAG, glycosaminoglycans; Mol, molecular/DNA/gene defect analysis; Mul Enz, multiple enzyme in either cultured cells/amniotic fluid or serum media; Oligo, oligosaccharides; Prenat, prenatal diagnosis available; Subs, substrate analysis (see text).
‡ BMT, bone marrow transplantation; ERT, enzyme replacement therapy; HSCT, hematopoietic stem cell transplantation; SRT, substrate reduction therapy.

instances, the use of an agent that acts as a chaperone to stabilize the mutant enzyme may help restore its function. Proof of principle for this strategy has been demonstrated in Fabry's disease, for which the regular intravenous administration of galactose has led to the resolution of cardiomyopathy and improvement in the associated hemodynamic changes in one patient [Frustaci et al., 2001]. Currently, clinical trials with a pharmacologic chaperone are being undertaken in Gaucher's and Fabry's diseases [Pastores and Sathe, 2006].

Gene therapy is also being explored as an option, although most studies to date have only been with animal (primarily mouse) models, except for Gaucher's disease, for which clinical trials have been performed [Caillaud and Poenaru, 2000; Ellinwood et al., 2004; Eto et al., 2004; Gieselmann et al., 2003b; Shen et al., 2004; Sly and Vogler, 2002]. Unfortunately, gene therapy performed in the patients with Gaucher's disease resulted in only transient expression of the functional enzyme [Cabrera-Salazar et al., 2002]. Although experiments in animal models provide a foundation for translational studies in humans, the increased size and complexity of the human brain present particular challenges that may not be clarified by studies in the mouse models. Thus, studies in large animal models are increasingly preferred [Haskins, 2009]. Additionally, immunological rejection of the vector and viral products may lead to adverse outcome; ways to address these problems will be needed, to reduce procedure-related risks and promote long-term gene expression. Furthermore, the CNS and synovial joints are sites that can be challenging to treat with systemic gene therapy, and may require direct approaches for delivery of the relevant gene. For most lysosomal storage diseases, the mainstay of treatment has been palliative or supportive care. Treatment of the secondary disabilities (e.g., seizures, sensory impairment, and behavioral, sleep–wake cycle, or communication problems) can have a positive impact on the patient's quality of life and may help address some sources of parental frustration. Genetic counseling of affected individuals and their relatives is also an important component of comprehensive care of the patient and family.

Sphingolipidoses

The sphingolipidoses are several disorders characterized by abnormalities in the metabolism of multiple glycolipid substrates that form a component of myelin or of lipid rafts within membranes (Figure 36-1). Most of the clinical variants in this group are associated with neurodegenerative features.

The myelin sheath is an extended, modified plasma membrane that, in the CNS, represents an extension of oligodendroglial cell processes. Examination of normal myelin with polarized microscopy and radiographic diffraction has exhibited a protein-lipid-protein-lipid-protein structure. Chemical investigations have determined that the lipid layers are composed of a bimolecular layer of hydrocarbon chains, cholesterol, phospholipids, and glycolipids (primarily galactocerebroside and sulfatide). The glycolipids are amphiphilic and have a hydrophobic ceramide moiety that acts as a membrane anchor and a hydrophilic, extracellularly oriented oligosaccharide chain. Rather than diffuse distribution in the cell membrane, current studies support the localization of glycosphingolipids, cholesterol, and certain proteins in specialized patches of membranes referred to as lipid rafts. Lipid rafts play key roles in intracellular transport, protein-sorting, and signal-transduction processes. Disturbed distribution of raft lipids and consequently protein subcellular localization due to a gridlock in the endocytic pathway, as seen in certain lysosomal storage diseases, is believed to lead to cell and organ functional impairments [Saravanan et al., 2004; Walkley and Vanier, 2009]. In addition, abnormalities of myelin membrane lipid composition result in the loss of membrane stability and its degeneration.

The degradation of glycosphingolipids takes place in the lysosomes through a stepwise action of specific acid hydrolases. Several of these enzymes (such as β-glucosidase, β-galactocerebrosidase, arylsulfatase A, and acid ceramidase) also require the assistance of nonenzymatic glycoprotein co-factors, the so-called sphingolipid activator proteins (or saposins). Examination of tissue sections obtained from affected individuals with glycosphingolipid storage disease typically reveals

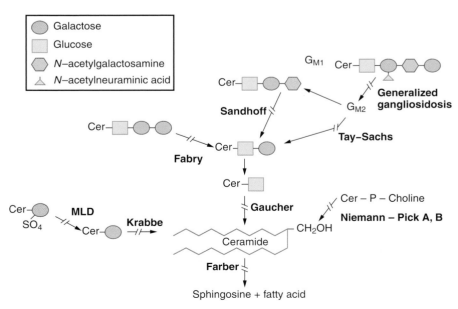

Fig. 36-1 Metabolic pathway and the sites of disruption in sphingolipid catabolism. MLD, metachromatic leukodystrophy.

membranous cytoplasmic bodies, which represent lipid material enclosed by the lysosomal membranes [Abramovich et al., 2001].

Studies in animal models of Sandhoff's disease and Niemann–Pick disease type A revealed elevated levels of phosphatidylcholine surfactant in lung tissue [Buccoliero et al., 2004]. Subsequent studies have confirmed these findings in human patients with Sandhoff disease, Gaucher disease type I, and sialidosis type I [Buccoliero et al., 2007]. These observations suggest that changes in phospholipid levels and composition in lung surfactant might be a general feature of sphingolipid storage diseases and may in part be responsible for the increased susceptibility of these patients to respiratory infections and lung disease.

Gangliosidoses

The gangliosides are complex lipids (with a ceramide backbone on which hexoses and sialic acids are attached); they are found predominantly in brain gray matter. Disorders of ganglioside metabolism are identified on the basis of the specific underlying enzyme deficiency and the resultant accumulation of its substrates (named by L. Svennerholm according to the presence of a sialic acid group [M, D, T, and Q] and their distinct chromatographic mobility [1, 2, and 3]). Within each disease category, there are several variants that are distinguished on the basis of the age at onset, including a classic (early or late) infantile and later-onset (juvenile or adult) form. These delineations are artificial; in practice, most of the affected patients actually fall within the broad spectrum of disease expression, partly influenced by the absence or the presence of residual enzyme activity.

Ganglioside (primarily GM_2 and GM_3) accumulation has also been found to occur secondarily in other disorders, such as the mucopolysaccharidoses [Walkley and Vanier, 2009]. In the mucopolysaccharidoses, the primary storage of glycosaminoglycans is believed to lead to inhibition of the activity of several ganglioside-degrading lysosomal enzymes. In other disorders (e.g., Niemann–Pick disease type C), secondary ganglioside accumulation is believed to result from a disruption in retroendocytic movement of the substrate and does not appear to reflect simply the nonspecific changes in tissue cellularity (arising from neuronal loss and gliosis) [Walkley and Vanier, 2009].

Neuronal cells that have GM_2 ganglioside storage exhibit meganeurite formation (i.e., axonal hillock enlargement) and ectopic dendritogenesis (i.e., the sprouting of new synapse-covered dendritic neurites at the axon hillock) [Walkley and Vanier, 2009]. Axonal spheroid formation (or neuroaxonal dystrophy) is also often noted. The spheroids occur as focal enlargements of various sizes scattered along myelinated and unmyelinated axons in the gray and white matter. In contrast to neuronal cell bodies, which contain characteristic storage material, spheroids consist of collections of multivesicular and dense bodies, mitochondria, and other organelles that would normally be found being transported along axons [Walkley and Vanier, 2009]. These observations suggest that the development of spheroids may involve defective endocytic trafficking within axons.

GM₁ Gangliosidoses

Generalized gangliosidosis or GM_1 gangliosidosis is associated with the neuronal storage of the monosialoganglioside GM_1, which normally constitutes approximately 20 percent of all gangliosides found in the brain and 80 percent of ganglioside in myelin. This disorder results from a deficiency of the enzyme β-galactosidase, which is responsible for the cleavage of the terminal galactose of GM_1. The same enzyme is also defective in another disorder, Morquio's syndrome type B. Apart from mutations within its encoding gene, the activity of the enzyme β-galactosidase (combined with deficiency of sialidase [also known as neuraminidase]) can be compromised secondarily as a result of a deficiency of the protective protein/cathepsin A. This condition, called galactosialidosis, is a separate disorder. The gene encoding β-galactosidase also gives rise, after alternative splicing, to the elastin-binding protein that is involved in elastic fiber deposition.

Deficient β-galactosidase activity leads to the incomplete metabolism of several other substrates, including galactose-containing glycoproteins, N-acetylgalactosamine, lactose, and keratan sulfate (a glycosaminoglycan). Phenotypic differences likely result from varying activities of the mutant β-galactosidase enzyme against its various substrates, which may explain the dysmorphic facial features reminiscent of the mucopolysaccharidoses in the early infantile form of GM_1 gangliosidosis and the predominance of skeletal disease in Morquio's syndrome type B (due to allelic mutations) [Brunetti-Pierri and Scaglia, 2008]. Allelic mutations involve distinct sequence alterations of the same gene; the phenotype encountered may be different because the specific underlying gene defects involve distinct domains of the protein that subserve different functions. Studies in the mouse model of GM_1 gangliosidosis have found that GM_1 storage leads to several cellular changes (including activation of the unfolded protein response pathway), the upregulation of BiP and CHOP (C/EBP homologous transcription factor), and the activation of JNK2 and caspase 12, which lead to neuronal apoptosis [Tessitore et al., 2004].

In the early infantile form, dysmorphic facial features (i.e., frontal bossing; wide, depressed nasal bridge; gingival hypertrophy or thickened alveolar ridges) may be present at birth or become more apparent with time. In the first few months of life, hepatosplenomegaly is also usually noted, and lateral spine radiographs reveal hypoplasia and anterior beaking of the thoracolumbar vertebrae. An additional skeletal radiographic finding is widening of the diaphysis (the midshaft) of long bones. These bone deformities (referred to as dysostosis multiplex) are similar to those found in the mucopolysaccharidoses. In affected individuals, the heart may be enlarged, and cardiac failure may develop as a consequence of endocardial fibroelastosis and valvular incompetence (secondary to thickening of the heart valves). The distinctive facies and visceromegaly observed in these patients, also seen with mucolipidosis II (I-cell disease), are unusual characteristics for most of the other neurovisceral lipidoses.

Hypotonia, feeding difficulties, and failure to thrive may be evident in the first weeks of life in patients with early infantile GM_1 gangliosidosis. A macular cherry-red spot is found in about 50 percent of cases, and there is hyperacusis (or exaggerated acousticomotor response); these features are also typical of Tay–Sachs disease. In these diseases, substrate accumulation in the ganglion cells produces a white ring or halo of lipid-laden neurons encircling the red, ganglion cell-free region of the fovea, which is observed as the characteristic cherry-red spot. Ultimately, patients with infantile GM_1 gangliosidosis develop spasticity, tonic spasms, and pyramidal signs. Affected infants who survive beyond 12 months usually exhibit decerebrate rigidity. Seizures can occur, generally during the later stages of disease. Death usually occurs by 2 years of age from respiratory failure and bronchopneumonia.

Histologic examination of the brain of two infants with GM_1 gangliosidosis revealed a marked decrease in the number of oligodendrocytes and myelin sheaths [van der Voorn et al., 2004]. An immunohistochemical decrease in proteolipid protein and a more profound deficiency of myelin basic protein were also found; these observations indicate that the brain lesions may not simply result from a delay or arrest in myelination, but are due to a "dying-back" oligopathy. In addition, amyloid precursor protein–immunoreactive aggregates were observed in proximal axons and meganeurites, as well as in white matter axons. These data suggest that the myelin deficit results from a loss of oligodendrocytes and abnormal axoplasmic transport, consequent to the massive neuronal storage of GM_1 gangliosides.

The late infantile form (with onset usually between 12 and 18 months of life) often manifests with gait disturbances and frequent falls. There is usually no distinctive facial dysmorphism, and the liver and spleen are not enlarged. Skeletal deformities, such as hypoplasia of the acetabula and proximal deformity of the metacarpal bones, may be found on radiographic examination but are usually milder than those noted in the early infantile form of GM_1 gangliosidosis. Patients develop seizures and spastic quadriparesis, with prominent pseudobulbar signs (i.e., drooling and dysphagia) (Figure 36-2). Death is usual between

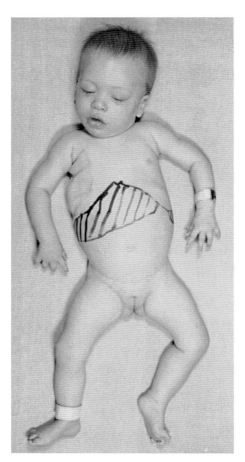

Fig. 36-2 A 6-month-old girl with generalized GM₁ gangliosidosis. The facies are dull, and there is nonpitting edema of the face. Hepatomegaly and less obvious splenomegaly are present.

the ages of 3 and 10 years. The absence of peripheral nerve involvement (i.e., normal conduction velocities) and normal cerebrospinal fluid findings help distinguish this condition from metachromatic leukodystrophy and Krabbe's disease.

In the juvenile or late-onset form, disease symptoms usually develop in late childhood or adolescence but may also occur as late as the third or fourth decade of life. Delayed onset is partly related to the presence of residual enzyme activity, which in one patient was reported to be associated with homozygosity for R521C mutation in the β-galactosidase gene [Silva et al., 1999]. This clinical variant has been observed in different ethnic groups but appears to be prevalent among the Japanese. Affected individuals have a protracted clinical course characterized by dysarthria and extrapyramidal signs (especially dystonia). Pathologic studies have revealed marked GM_1 ganglioside storage in the basal ganglia. Intellectual impairment is slight to moderate.

Laboratory findings in patients with GM_1 gangliosidosis include vacuolization of peripheral blood lymphocytes and the presence of galactose-containing oligosaccharides and keratan sulfate in urine. These urinary findings help distinguish GM_1 gangliosidosis from mucolipidosis II (I-cell disease). For diagnostic purposes, deficient β-galactosidase activity can be demonstrated in peripheral blood leukocytes and cultured skin fibroblasts, or prenatally by use of cultured chorionic villi or amniocytes.

Mutation analyses have revealed broad heterogeneity, with 102 β-galactosidase gene defects described to date [Brunetti-Pierri and Scaglia, 2008]. Certain gene defects tend to be common in particular subtypes; for instance, the R482H and R208C are often seen in infantile cases, R201C in the late infantile/juvenile patients, and I51T among rare adult/chronic cases. In contrast to the first two mutations, the last two defects are associated with moderate catalytic activity, consistent with expectations for the resultant phenotype. The R59H has been reported to be prevalent among Brazilians, Iberian, and Roma patients with GM_1 gangliosidosis.

Only symptomatic treatment is available. In preclinical studies, substrate reduction therapy using two related imino sugars revealed that *N*B-DGJ led to an optimal response (in terms of survival and fewer side effects in a mouse model of GM_1 gangliosidosis), when compared to treatment with *N*B-DNJ (miglustat). However, functional improvement was greater with *N*B-DNJ, probably due to the greater impact of *N*B-DNJ on CNS inflammation [Elliot-Smith et al., 2008].

GM₂ Gangliosidoses

The GM_2 gangliosidoses include several variants, all of which are associated with the neuronal storage of the monosialoganglioside GM_2, resulting in the formation of meganeurites (i.e., distorted and ballooned neurons) and ectopic dendritogenesis. Primary accumulation of GM_2 gangliosides occurs with mutations involving the genes encoding the α (Tay–Sachs disease) or β (Sandhoff's disease) subunit of hexosaminidase A or the GM_2 activator protein (in the AB variant) [Fernandes Filho and Shapiro, 2004]. The hexosaminidase A enzyme (with a molecular mass of approximately 100 kDa) is a trimer consisting of one α and two β subunits, encoded by structural genes on different chromosomes (see Table 36-1). Mutations of the β subunit also lead to deficiency of hexosaminidase B (a tetrameric homopolymer of β subunits).

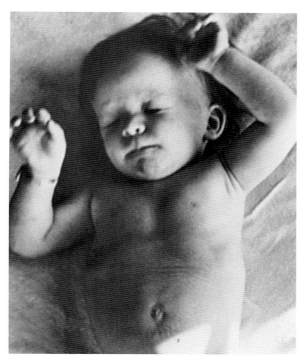

Fig. 36-3 A patient with Tay–Sachs disease demonstrating a massive startle response to a relatively subtle sound stimulus. *(From Swaiman KF. In: Baker AB, ed. Clinical Neurology. New York: Harper & Row, 1985.)*

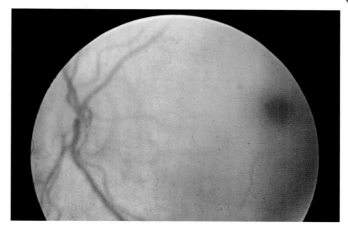

Fig. 36-4 Macular cherry-red spot, a characteristic of Tay–Sachs disease and a few other lysosomal storage diseases.

GM$_2$ ganglioside storage is also seen in the so-called B1 variant, resulting from an altered substrate specificity of hexosaminidase A, wherein the mutated enzyme retains the ability to degrade the artificial substrate (used in most diagnostic assays), but not the sulfated or natural substrate in vivo. Clinical and imaging findings are congruent with those reported for Tay–Sachs and Sandhoff's diseases [Grosso et al., 2003]. The highest incidence (approximately 3.1 per 100,000 live births) for the B1 variant of GM$_2$ gangliosidoses has been described in Portugal, which has been suggested as the point of origin of a founder mutation (R178H) seen in Brazilian patients [Tutor, 2004].

The "classic" infantile form of Tay–Sachs disease is named after a British ophthalmologist (Warren Tay) and an American neurologist (Bernard Sachs); both provided initial descriptions (in the 1880s) of the typical disease manifestations. Affected infants with Tay–Sachs disease have psychomotor deterioration and hyperacusis together with axial hypotonia, bilateral pyramidal signs, and blindness (associated with persistent pupillary responses) (Figure 36-3). The macular cherry-red spot is a characteristic hallmark of the disease (Figure 36-4). Head control is poor, and the size of the head increases markedly in the second year of life from enlargement of the brain (megalencephaly) and not because of tension hydrocephalus. Ultimately, with loss of the neurons and further gliosis, the ventricles may appear enlarged. Affected children become spastic and cachectic. Death usually occurs between 3 and 5 years of age. As patients approach the terminal stages, generalized tonic-clonic and minor motor seizures can occur. The patients do not have any of the following signs: dysmorphic features, visceromegaly, skeletal deformities, and signs of peripheral nerve involvement. These observations are useful in the delineation of Tay–Sachs

disease from other lysosomal storage diseases associated with neurodegenerative features (Box 36-1).

In the general population, the incidence of Tay–Sachs disease has been estimated at 1 in 112,000 live births. Tay–Sachs disease used to be prevalent (1 in 3900 live births) among Ashkenazi Jews, but this situation has been addressed successfully through targeted screening programs. The success of targeted screening has prompted extension of the program to other disorders that are also common in Ashkenazi Jewish individuals, such as Gaucher's disease, Niemann–Pick disease, and mucolipidosis IV. These particular disorders were chosen because they are found with increased carrier frequency among the Ashkenazi Jews, in whom causality has been attributed to a limited number of "common" mutations [Zhang et al., 2004].

The later-onset forms of GM$_2$ gangliosidosis (referred to as LOTS, which stands for late-onset Tay–Sachs disease) can manifest in childhood, adolescence, or even adulthood. In contrast to the infantile-onset form, patients with juvenile- or adult-onset disease follow a more protracted course and show no ethnic predilection. Affected individuals develop dysarthria and walking problems, primarily resulting from spastic paraparesis (in the childhood-onset form, between the ages of 3 and 6 years) or proximal muscle weakness (in the adult form, with symptom onset in the teens). Differences in the age at onset and disease course have led to distinction of the childhood-onset form (usually referred to as chronic GM$_2$ gangliosidosis) from the adult-onset variant (or late-onset Tay–Sachs disease) [Maegawa et al., 2006]. The phenotype associated with the B1 variant is similar to that encountered in the childhood-onset form.

Ataxia with cerebellar atrophy is also a prominent disease sign in the later-onset forms, and peripheral neuropathy has been described in a subset of patients [Shapiro et al., 2008]. Tonic-clonic or myoclonic seizures are encountered in some children; psychiatric disturbances (i.e., bouts of psychosis and episodes of depression) are present and may be the initial manifestation of disease, particularly among adult-onset patients [Zaroff et al., 2004]. Consideration of late-onset GM$_2$ gangliosidosis should be made in the differential diagnosis of patients with signs of lower motor neuron and spinocerebellar dysfunction. Vision is not impaired and optic fundi are normal, although intellectual deterioration is frequent. The rate of progression and disease severity usually correlate with the age at onset (presumably determined by the severity of

Box 36-1 Clinical Manifestations Reported in Patients with Lysosomal Storage Disorders

Nonimmune hydrops fetalis

- Disseminated lipogranulomatosis (Farber's disease)
- Galactosialidosis (neuraminidase deficiency)
- Gaucher's disease
- GM_1 gangliosidosis
- Infantile free sialic acid storage disease
- MPS IV and VII
- Mucolipidosis II (I-cell disease)
- Niemann–Pick disease type C
- Sialidosis type I
- Wolman's disease

Myoclonic seizures

- Galactosialidosis
- Gaucher's disease type 3I
- GM_2 gangliosidosis
- Neuronal ceroid lipofuscinosis
- Niemann–Pick C
- Oligosaccharidosis (α-N-acetylgalactosaminidase deficiency, fucosidosis, sialidosis type 1)

Ataxia

- Galactosialidosis
- Gaucher's disease type 3
- GM_1 gangliosidosis
- Krabbe's disease
- Late-onset GM_2 gangliosidosis (cerebellar hypoplasia)
- Metachromatic leukodystrophy
- Neuronal ceroid lipofuscinosis
- Niemann–Pick C
- Salla disease

Extrapyramidal signs

- Gaucher's disease type 3
- GM_1 gangliosidosis (adult form)
- Late-onset GM_2 gangliosidosis
- Krabbe's disease
- Niemann–Pick C
- Oligosaccharidosis

Cortical atrophy

- I-cell disease
- Late stage of GM_1 and GM_2 gangliosidosis (cerebellar atrophy)
- Metachromatic leukodystrophy
- Neuronal ceroid lipofuscinosis

Cytopenia (anemia, thrombocytopenia)

- Gaucher's disease
- Niemann–Pick disease
- Wolman's disease (acanthocytosis)

Vacuolated lymphocytes

- GM_1 gangliosidosis (Landing's disease)
- I-cell disease
- Multiple sulfatase deficiency (Austin's disease)
- Neuronal ceroid lipofuscinosis
- Niemann–Pick disease
- Oligosaccharidosis (aspartylglucosaminuria, sialidosis)
- Pompe's disease (glycogen storage disease type II)

Cerebrovascular or strokelike episodes and other vascular events (e.g., Raynaud's phenomenon)

- Fabry's disease

Dementia, psychosis

- Fabry's disease
- Gaucher's disease type 3
- GM_1 gangliosidosis
- Late-onset GM_2 gangliosidosis
- Krabbe's disease
- Metachromatic leukodystrophy
- MPS III (Sanfilippo's disease)
- Neuronal ceroid lipofuscinosis
- Niemann–Pick C

Macrocephaly

- Krabbe's disease
- Sandhoff's disease
- Tay–Sachs disease

Peripheral neuropathy

- Krabbe's disease
- Metachromatic leukodystrophy (spastic paraplegia)
- Multiple sulfatase deficiency

Deafness*

- Fabry's disease
- Galactosialidosis
- Gaucher's disease type 2
- I-cell disease
- Infantile Pompe's disease
- Metachromatic leukodystrophy
- MPS I, II, IV
- Oligosaccharidosis (α- and β-mannosidosis)

Interstitial lung disease

- Gaucher's disease
- Niemann–Pick disease

Obstructive airway disease

- Fabry's disease
- Mucopolysaccharidoses

Cardiomyopathy

- Fabry's disease (arrhythmia, conduction abnormalities)
- Mucopolysaccharidoses (valvular disease)
- Pompe's disease (hypotonia)

Cherry-red spot,[†] optic atrophy, visual loss

- Galactosialidosis
- GM_1 gangliosidosis
- Infantile free sialic acid storage disease
- MPS IV and MPS VII
- Mucolipidosis II (I-cell disease)
- Neuronal ceroid lipofuscinosis

---

[*] Conductive, sensorineural, or a combination, with involvement of cochlear and CNS dysfunction.

[†] Describes the normal red macula surrounded by a pale retina, reflecting storage material in the perifoveal ganglion cells.

Box 36-1 Clinical Manifestations Reported in Patients with Lysosomal Storage Disorders—cont'd.

- Niemann–Pick disease type A
- Sialidosis type I
- Sandhoff's disease
- Tay–Sachs disease

Retinitis pigmentosa

- Fabry's disease
- I-cell disease (mucolipidosis II)
- MPS I, IV, VI
- Mucolipidosis IV
- Neuronal ceroid lipofuscinosis
- Oligosaccharidosis (late-onset α-mannosidosis)

Lenticular opacities (cataracts)

- Fabry's disease
- Oligosaccharidoses (sialidosis, α-mannosidosis)

Ophthalmoplegia (abnormal eye movements)

- Gaucher's disease type 3
- Niemann–Pick C and D
- Nystagmus

Hepatosplenomegaly

- Danon's disease (8–36 percent of cases)
- Gaucher's disease
- Mucopolysaccharidoses
- Niemann–Pick disease A and B
- Niemann–Pick C (cholestatic jaundice)
- Oligosaccharidoses
- Pompe's disease (hepatomegaly)
- Wolman's disease and cholesteryl ester storage disease

Nephrolithiasis

- Cystinuria

Proteinuria

- Cystinosis (aminoaciduria, Fanconi's syndrome)
- Fabry's disease

Osteopenia

- Gaucher's disease
- I-cell disease

Punctate epiphyseal calcifications

- β-Glucuronidase deficiency

Degenerative arthritis, bone infarcts

- Fabry's disease
- Farber's disease
- Gaucher's disease
- I-cell disease
- MPS I
- Mucolipidosis III

Pain crises

- Gaucher's disease types 1 and 3 (bone)
- Krabbe's disease
- Metachromatic leukodystrophy

Dysostosis multiplex[‡]

- Mucopolysaccharidoses (coarse facies)
- Oligosaccharidoses

Angiokeratoma

- Fabry's disease
- Oligosaccharidosis (aspartylglucosaminuria, fucosidosis, galacto-sialidosis, β-mannosidosis, sialidosis)

[‡] Refers to constellation of radiologic findings, including macrocephaly, thickened calvaria, J-shaped sella turcica, spatulate ribs, bullet-shaped phalanges that are shortened, rounding and anterior beaking of the vertebral bodies (especially in the lumbar region), and flaring of the iliac wings.

---

the underlying mutation). Childhood-onset disease often leads to death by 15 years of age, preceded by a period characterized by progressive spasticity, rigidity, and dementia, and ending in the vegetative state. Adult-onset patients may live into their 50s or early 60s. Mutation analyses performed in patients with late-onset Tay–Sachs disease have identified a high prevalence of the G269S gene defect, which is associated with residual hexosaminidase A activity, usually in combination with a null allele typical of classic Tay–Sachs disease [Neudorfer et al., 2005].

The AB variant due to a deficiency of the GM_2 activator, which is necessary for the hydrolysis of GM_2 gangliosides by hexosaminidase A in vivo, has a clinical phenotype that is indistinguishable from the infantile form of Tay–Sachs disease [Li et al., 2003; Sakuraba et al., 1999]. It is a rare condition associated with normal laboratory test results in assays of hexosaminidase A and B enzyme activity with use of the artificial substrates. Diagnostic confirmation requires highly specialized methods, available only through a few laboratories.

Sandhoff's disease (O variant), due to mutations of the β subunit of hexosaminidase A, has an age at onset and clinical course characterized by neurologic and ophthalmologic

findings that are similar to Tay–Sachs disease. Sandhoff's disease is a pan-ethnic disorder. A distinguishing feature is hepatosplenomegaly and the presence of N-acetylglucosamine–containing oligosaccharides in urine (as only hexosaminidase B, which is also deficient in Sandhoff's disease but not in Tay–Sachs disease, is responsible for cleaving the N-acetylglucosamine moiety of globosides) [Sakuraba et al., 2002]. Cardiomyopathy has also been noted occasionally. Death usually occurs between 2 and 4 years of age. There are extremely rare cases of patients with juvenile- or late-onset Sandhoff's disease [Hendriksz et al., 2004].

The enzymatic basis of GM_2 gangliosidosis can be ascertained by assays of total hexosaminidase and hexosaminidase A activity, which can be measured in leukocytes and cultured skin fibroblasts. The biochemical tests can be complemented by analysis of the underlying hexosaminidase A gene mutations. Among the Ashkenazi Jewish population, two null hexosaminidase A mutations (a four-base pair insertion [TATC1278] in exon 11 and a splice site gene defect [IVS12]) account for 96 percent of disease alleles among cases of Tay–Sachs disease [Frisch et al., 2004]. In this same population of patients, an allelic glycine to serine substitution at position 269 of the hexosaminidase A gene (G269S) represents the most common mutation among the adult-onset cases of GM_2 gangliosidosis. Among non-Jewish patients, one mutation (IVS9) accounts for 14 percent of disease alleles [Cordeiro et al., 2000]. Pseudodeficiency for hexosaminidase A activity associated with decreased enzyme activity in vitro exists and can be clarified by DNA testing or analysis of enzyme activity with use of the natural rather than the artificial substrate. Two mutations (i.e., R247W and R249W) have been associated with pseudodeficient hexosaminidase A activity [Cordeiro et al., 2000].

Investigations have proved that the infantile cases of Tay–Sachs disease are usually due to a combination of severe deleterious mutations, whereas patients with the later-onset forms often have a combination of one deleterious mutation and a second "milder" mutation associated with residual enzyme activity (based on in vitro mutagenesis and protein expression studies). The most frequent mutation responsible for the B1 variant of GM_2 gangliosidosis is R178H [Matsuzawa et al., 2003].

Pathologic brain studies reveal widespread neuronal GM_2 ganglioside storage throughout the cortex and central nuclear structures, the spinal cord, and the autonomic ganglia. Evidence of neuronal storage has been established in fetuses as early as 12–22 weeks of gestation. GM_2 gangliosides are implicated in synaptogenesis, and it has been speculated that an altered pattern of cellular gangliosides may interfere with normal synaptic transmission [Zhao et al., 2004].

Lyso-derivatives of GM_2 gangliosides, which are cytotoxic and may be responsible for inducing the neuronal degeneration, are found to be increased in tissues of patients with GM_2 gangliosidoses. When they were initially described, the lysolipids were believed to exert their toxicity through inhibition of protein kinase C. More recently, studies in animal models have found that progressive CNS inflammation (as evident from the expression pattern of several inflammatory markers and cytokines) and an alteration in the integrity of the blood–brain barrier occurred coincidentally with the onset of clinical disease signs [Jeyakumar et al., 2003].

Prenatal diagnosis for the various types of GM_2 gangliosidoses is available through biochemical and molecular testing of cultured cells obtained by chorionic villus sampling or amniocentesis.

Definitive therapy for GM_2 gangliosidoses is not available. Substrate reduction therapy is currently under investigation. This approach is based on the inhibition of glucosylceramide synthesis by the imino sugar miglustat (*NB-DNJ*), and more recently by the galacto-derivative [Andersson et al., 2004]. Preclinical studies have found that animal models of GM_2 gangliosidosis (primarily the Sandhoff mouse) given miglustat had a reduction in tissue storage of GM_2 ganglioside, with delayed symptom onset and extended survival [Jeyakumar et al., 1999]. Treatment with *NB-DGJ* demonstrated greater therapeutic efficacy (specifically, extended life expectancy and increased delay in symptom onset) than *NB-DNJ*, with none of the side effects, such as weight loss and gastrointestinal tract distress, reported with *NB-DNJ* [Andersson et al., 2004]. Unfortunately, clinical trials using miglustat did not alter ultimate neurologic prognosis in pediatric and adult patients with GM_2 gangliosidosis [Maegawa et al., 2009; Shapiro et al., 2009]. Salutary changes noted in the animal models subjected to bone marrow transplantation have generated renewed interest in cellular approaches to treatment of the GM_2 gangliosidoses; potentially in combination with substrate reduction therapy [Jeyakumar et al., 2001].

Fabry's Disease

Fabry's disease is an X-linked disorder, first described independently in 1898 by Johanes Fabry (from Germany) and William Anderson (from the UK). It is caused by a deficiency of the lysosomal hydrolase α-galactosidase A and the accumulation of glycosphingolipids (predominantly globotriaosylceramide [ceramide trihexoside] and galabiosylceramide) [Schiffmann, 2009]. As a consequence, lipid deposits can be found in the epithelial cells of the cornea, glomeruli and tubules of the kidneys, cardiac myocytes, and endothelial and smooth muscle cells of blood vessels. In the nervous system, lipid deposits are evident in ganglion cells of the dorsal root and autonomic nervous system, and in specific cortical and brainstem structures. The distribution pattern of the storage material determines the associated clinical findings, including corneal and lenticular opacities, acroparesthesias, angiokeratomas, and anhidrosis or hypohidrosis (abnormal sweating) [MacDermot et al., 2001a]. Major morbidity in Fabry's disease derives from renal, cardiac, and brain involvement.

Although the disease primarily affects males, a significant proportion of females may also develop disease-related complications; however, onset among carrier females may be delayed [MacDermot et al., 2001b]. Disease incidence has been estimated at 1 in 117,000 males; however, this is likely an underestimate as certain patients may have atypical features (including later onset of cardiac complications) and not be properly identified. Most estimates also do not include females who may be missed because they remain asymptomatic. Recent studies have led to identification of cases of Fabry's disease among patients with cryptogenic stroke, and those with hypertrophic cardiomyopathy or on dialysis or post-kidney transplant [Rolfs et al., 2005; Monserrat et al., 2007; Kleinert et al., 2009]. In the absence of a positive family history, the diagnosis of Fabry's disease is often delayed (by as much as a decade).

In late childhood or adolescence, affected individuals may experience recurrent attacks of burning or lancinating pains in the distal extremities (acroparesthesias), often associated temporally with physical activity and fever [MacDermot and MacDermot, 2001]. The pains may last for days or weeks, and edema of the hands and feet may occur. Physical examination often reveals angiokeratomas (telangiectatic skin lesions) distributed over the "bathing trunk" area between the nipple line and above the knees, in the umbilical region, and, in males, over the penis and scrotum (Figure 36-5). Corneal opacities, noted as a diffuse haze or in a verticillate or whorl-like pattern on slit-lamp examination, are typical; they are usually also seen among females and used to identify potential carriers before the availability of genetic test results. These eye findings do not interfere with vision, although central retinal artery occlusion can rarely occur and may lead to acute blindness [Orssaud et al., 2003]. Unilateral or bilateral hearing loss may develop [Germain et al., 2002]. Most patients also experience abdominal pains and bouts of diarrhea. The vasomotor, sweating, and gastrointestinal problems may reflect a dysfunction of the autonomic nervous system [Kolodny and Pastores, 2002].

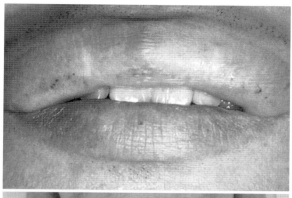

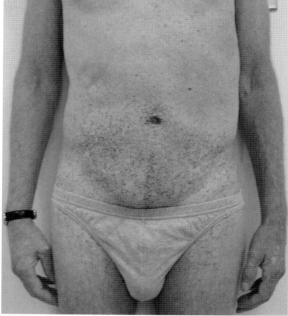

Fig. 36-5 Angiokeratoma in a patient with Fabry's disease.

In classically affected males, the condition leads to chronic renal insufficiency and eventually renal failure (usually between the ages of 35 and 45 years), often preceded by proteinuria (mostly in the non-nephrotic range) and hyposthenuria [Thadhani et al., 2002]. In early or middle adulthood, patients may develop cardiac conduction problems or arrhythmia together with hypertrophic cardiomyopathy and ultimately heart failure [Glass et al., 2004]. Obstructive airway disease may contribute to limitations in exercise tolerance. Patients are also at risk for transient ischemic events or stroke, related to ischemic or thrombotic events [Kolodny and Pastores, 2002]. Cerebral imaging and blood flow studies have paradoxically revealed hyperperfusion attributed to altered vascular reactivity rather than arterial occlusive disease [Moore et al., 2003]. There is increased tortuosity of the blood vessels (predominantly in the posterior circulation) and white matter signal abnormalities. Studies have also found that patients with Fabry's disease have evidence of endothelial dysfunction and leukocyte activation consistent with a prothrombotic state, which may explain the risk for focal cerebral signs such as aphasia and hemiplegia [Altarescu et al., 2001]. Median cumulative survival in untreated males (50 years) and females (70 years) is reduced [MacDermot et al., 2001a, b].

The diagnosis of Fabry's disease can be established in males (hemizygotes) on the basis of reduced α-galactosidase A activity in plasma, or more reliably in leukocytes and cultured skin fibroblasts. A significant proportion of carrier females (heterozygotes) may have residual enzyme activity that overlaps with measurements obtained for the general population. Mutation analysis is a more reliable means for assignment of female carrier status, although this approach necessitates sequence characterization to identify the causal gene defect because most affected individuals tend to have a "private" mutation (i.e., unique or limited to few affected families). Lyonization may partly explain the wide variability in clinical presentation among carrier females. In addition, certain mutations may be associated with significant residual enzyme activity and may explain the delayed onset of symptoms or atypical disease course observed in some patients [Garman and Garboczi, 2002]. Affected individuals have elevated urinary excretion of ceramide trihexoside, although this requires demonstration with specialized testing (by high-performance liquid chromatography or tandem mass spectrometry). Biochemical or molecular genetic testing can be performed for prenatal diagnosis.

Before the introduction of enzyme therapy with agalsidase alfa (Replagal) or agalsidase beta (Fabrazyme), treatment was primarily symptomatic. Analgesics and often opiate-type medications are given for acroparesthesia. The frequency and severity of the pain episodes may be reduced or eliminated by chronic low-dose phenytoin (Dilantin) or carbamazepine (Tegretol) treatment. Patients are usually also given low-dose aspirin or antiplatelet aggregating agents for stroke prophylaxis and angiotensin-converting enzyme inhibitors (e.g., enalapril [Vasotec]) for renal protection in those with proteinuria. Dialysis or kidney transplantation is introduced after renal failure, and patients may require a pacemaker or defibrillator for cardiac conduction abnormalities or arrhythmias. Patients with severe heart valve problems may need a mechanical or tissue heart valve replacement, and cardiac transplantation has been performed in patients with cardiomyopathy and heart failure [Karras et al., 2008].

Enzyme therapy for Fabry's disease is safe and effective in reducing the amount of tissue lipid storage. Associated benefits include the reduction of both pain episodes and the use of chronic pain medications, stabilization or improvement of renal function in patients with normal or mildly reduced kidney function (glomerular filtration rate of 60 mL/min or higher), and a reduction of excess cardiac mass among those so affected [Pastores and Thadhani, 2002; Lidove et al., 2007]. Gastrointestinal complaints and abnormal sweating have also improved with enzyme therapy [Hoffmann et al., 2004; Schiffmann et al., 2003]. Cerebrovascular studies have demonstrated reversibility of the functional abnormalities with treatment, although patients remain at risk for stroke [Moore et al., 2002; Schiffmann, 2009]. Long-term studies will be required to ascertain the effectiveness of therapy in altering the natural history of the disease and improving survival. Additional studies will also be necessary to ascertain the determinants of therapeutic response, which is likely influenced by the presence of preexisting pathologic processes (e.g., glomerulosclerosis, calcified and stenotic heart valves). A significant proportion of enzyme-treated patients form antibodies against the administered protein, which results in neutralization of enzyme activity [Linthorst et al., 2004]. The long-term implications of antibody formation will need to be carefully assessed, although serial measurements indicate immunotolerance (i.e., a decrease in antibody titers over time) [Pastores, 2004]. Substrate reduction therapy and the use of pharmacologic chaperones, which remain investigational, are potential alternative or adjunctive strategies in the treatment of Fabry disease [Heare et al., 2007; Benjamin et al., 2009]. Gene therapy experiments currently being undertaken in the mouse model of Fabry's disease appear to suggest promising results [Ziegler et al., 2004].

Gaucher's Disease

The disease described by PCE Gaucher (in 1882) as an epithelioma of the spleen is known to be a lipid storage disorder resulting from a deficiency of the lysosomal enzyme glucocerebrosidase (acid β-glucosidase) [Butters, 2007]. The accumulation of its incompletely metabolized substrate, glucocerebroside (glucosylceramide), is confined to cells of monocyte-macrophage lineage. Glucocerebroside in the peripheral system is derived primarily from the breakdown of senescent red and white blood cell membranes. In the CNS, glucocerebroside is a byproduct of the catabolism of globosides and gangliosides.

There are three major clinical subtypes, delineated on the basis of the presence or absence of neurologic involvement. Assignment of clinical subtype is based on observations of the age at onset, evolution of the disease, and, when it is present, the rate and severity of psychomotor deterioration [Goker-Alpan et al., 2003].

Type 1 Gaucher's disease encompasses the non-neuropathic type associated with hepatosplenomegaly, anemia and thrombocytopenia, pulmonary involvement, and bone disease. Although type 1 Gaucher's disease has been referred to as the adult type, this designation is misleading as onset of disease may be evident from childhood. There is wide heterogeneity in clinical presentation. A small proportion of patients remain asymptomatic for most of their adult lives; others may develop significant disease progression earlier. Although the patients do not have a primary neurodegenerative disease, there can be secondary neurologic complications (e.g., local nerve injury due to hemorrhage and entrapment, or from spinal cord compression with collapse of a vertebral body) [Pastores et al., 2003].

There are several reports of adult patients with type 1 Gaucher's disease who have developed Parkinson's disease [Lwin et al., 2004]. Neuropathologic studies of brains obtained from patients with type 1 Gaucher's disease have revealed focal regions of gliosis (especially in the hippocampal CA2–CA4 region and calcarine cortex) and the presence of α-synuclein–immunoreactive cortical and brainstem-type Lewy bodies [Wong et al., 2004]. These observations suggest a potential causal relationship that requires further investigation [Mata et al., 2008].

Type 1 Gaucher's disease is a pan-ethnic disorder that has been noted as prevalent among individuals of Ashkenazi Jewish descent (carrier frequency of approximately 1 in 20) [Colombo, 2000]. In most populations, type 1 Gaucher's disease represents the most common lysosomal storage disorder with an estimated frequency of about 1 in 50,000 [Applegarth et al., 2000]. The hematologic and visceral findings that typify type 1 Gaucher's disease are also encountered in the neuropathic subtypes (Figure 36-6).

Type 2 Gaucher's disease represents the acute neuropathic form, associated with disease onset before the age of 12 months. Patients develop spasticity with head retraction, dysphagia, and a rapidly fatal course (with death usually between 2 and 3 years of age). Laryngeal stridor and trismus (due to bulbar spasticity) are added problems, and aspiration pneumonia is a frequent complication. Patients do not have dysmorphic features or the cherry-red spot that is typical of infantile Tay–Sachs disease and Niemann–Pick disease.

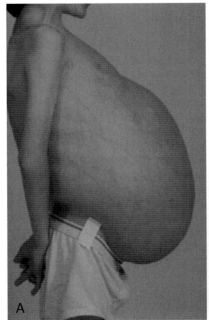
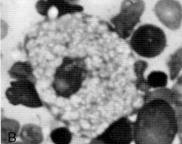
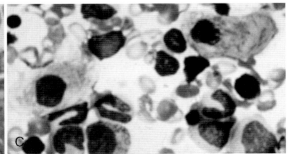

Fig. 36-6 Effects of storage material accumulation. A, Hepatosplenomegaly in a child with Gaucher's disease type 1, a presentation also typical for patients with Niemann–Pick disease type B. Examination of bone marrow cells demonstrates differences in the appearance of the storage material within histiocytes. B, Foamy histiocyte seen in patients with Niemann–Pick disease. C, Wrinkled silk appearance of the cytoplasm with eccentric nucleus in lipid-engorged histiocytes seen in a patient with Gaucher's disease.

However, the most severely affected patients can present with congenital ichthyosiform-collodion skin abnormalities or nonimmune hydrops fetalis [Staretz-Chacham et al., 2009]. The latter phenotype is characterized by an aggressive course, with death in the first few weeks of life. Similar findings were noted in the animal (mouse) model for Gaucher's disease in association with an alteration of the glucocerebroside to ceramide ratio and a disruption in the lipid membranes at the level of the stratum corneum [Eblan et al., 2005]. Bone involvement, characteristically found in patients with types 1 and 3 Gaucher's disease, is not seen in type 2 Gaucher's disease, perhaps because there is insufficient time for the skeletal disease process to evolve.

Type 3 Gaucher's disease, which may manifest before the age of 2 years, is associated with chronic neurologic problems including tonic-clonic and myoclonic seizures, ataxia, and extrapyramidal rigidity, often complicated by severe pulmonary involvement (including interstitial lung disease) [Campbell et al., 2003]. Paralytic strabismus with oculomotor apraxia (i.e., saccadic initiation failure) is a characteristic finding in patients with primary neuropathic Gaucher's disease. Brainstem auditory-evoked response testing often reveals diverse results, including prolonged peak and interpeak latencies for waves I–V and generally dysmorphic wave formation [Bamiou et al., 2001].

The clinical expression of type 3 Gaucher's disease can be complex, but neurologic problems can occasionally be restricted to supranuclear horizontal gaze palsy despite significant extraneurologic systemic problems. An increased number of cases have been identified in the Norrbottnian region of Sweden, attributed to a founder effect (for the L444P mutation) [Dahl et al., 1993]. The founder effect refers to the phenomenon wherein the increased frequency of a certain gene defect within a defined population is explained by common ancestry (i.e., a shared identity by descent) [Slatkin, 2004].

The basis of primary neurologic involvement in certain Gaucher's disease subtypes has not been fully elucidated. In contrast to the amount of lipid storage material measured in the liver and spleen, levels of glucocerebroside are not significantly elevated in brain tissue. Glucosylsphingosine (psychosine), an alternative metabolic byproduct of severely deficient glucocerebrosidase deficiency, is believed to play a contributory role [Schueler et al., 2003]. Evidence of neuronal apoptosis has been demonstrated in type 2 Gaucher's disease, and lipid-filled cells can be found in the perivascular Virchow–Robin spaces. Neuronophagic microglial nodules can also be found in several regions of the brain (e.g., cortex, thalamus, basal ganglia, brainstem, and cerebellum) and in the spinal cord (Figure 36-7). Elevation of glucocerebroside in neurons, possibly involving endoplasmic reticulum membranes, leads to increased calcium stores (possibly secondary to modulation of the ryanodine receptors) [Lloyd-Evans et al., 2003]. These cellular changes may be added factors that promote neuropathic forms of Gaucher's disease. Analysis of gene expression profiles in brains of the Gaucher's disease mouse model revealed downregulation of the *bcl-2* gene in the brainstem and cerebellum, but not in cortex [Hong et al., 2004a]. In situ labeling of DNA fragmentation by the terminal transferase-mediated dUTP nick-end labeling (TUNEL) assay confirmed that apoptosis occurred at these sites. These observations suggest that the accumulation of either glucocerebroside or glucosylsphingosine affects the expression of apoptosis mediators and could be responsible for

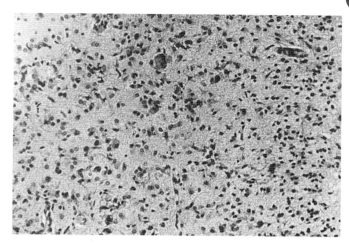

Fig. 36-7 Section of occipital cortex in an infant with Gaucher's disease. Marked neuronal loss and associated astrogliosis are revealed, and occasional neurons are distended with lipid. *(Courtesy Joo Ho Sung, Minneapolis, MN.)*

neuronal cell death. Reduced expression of brain-derived neurotrophic factor and nerve growth factor has also been observed in the cerebral cortex, brainstem, and cerebellum of the Gaucher's mouse, compared with that in wild-type mouse, and extracellular signal-regulated kinase (ERK) 1/2 expression was downregulated in neurons and correlated with a decreased number of neurons [Kim et al., 2006].

An atypical rare variant characterized predominantly by cardiac problems, such as aortic and mitral valve calcification, appears to be restricted to patients with a unique genotype (i.e., homozygosity for the D409H mutation) [George et al., 2001]. These findings were first reported among Arab patients with Gaucher's disease from the Jenin area, but this phenotype has since been reported among other ethnic groups.

Rare patients with evidence of glucocerebroside storage and normal glucocerebrosidase activity in vitro have been described; careful investigations have revealed a deficiency of saposin [Elleder et al., 2005]. Patients with saposin C or prosaposin deficiency usually present with symptoms characteristic of subacute neuropathic Gaucher's disease (i.e., progressive horizontal ophthalmoplegia, pyramidal and cerebellar signs, myoclonic jerks, and generalized seizures). Saposin C, which is derived from the proteolytic cleavage of a precursor molecule (prosaposin), is a co-factor required by glucocerebrosidase in the hydrolysis of glucocerebroside. In biochemical assays to measure glucocerebrosidase activity, the role of saposin C is replaced by the use of detergents. This replacement explains the normal results obtained when the activity of glucocerebrosidase is measured in vitro. Prosaposin, through activation of mitogen-activated protein kinases, may act as an apoptosis suppressor [Misasi et al., 2004]. Thus, a prosaposin deficiency could promote neuronal cell loss.

Several markers, readily measured in the plasma or serum of patients with Gaucher's disease, are often elevated. Testing often reveals elevated measures of tartrate-resistant acid phosphatase, angiotensin-converting enzyme, ferritin, CCL18/PARC, and chitotriosidase activity [Wajner et al., 2004; Aerts et al., 2005]. Although these findings have not been associated with a specific pathologic mechanism, the alterations have been taken to reflect the systemic burden of disease. Polyclonal hypergammaglobulinemia is also a frequent finding, particularly in the elderly, and the risk for multiple myeloma in these patients is increased [Taddei et al., 2009].

Bone involvement (e.g., severe osteopenia and osteonecrosis of major joints including the humeral and femoral heads) can be a major source of morbidity for patients with types 1 and 3 Gaucher's disease. The indicators of bone turnover (e.g., osteocalcin, bone-specific alkaline phosphatase, N-telopeptides) have not been consistently abnormal, even when significant bone disease exists, suggesting the dominance of local (possibly vascular) over systemic factors [Ciana et al., 2003; Pastores and Meere, 2005].

Cardiopulmonary complications can occur, and severe interstitial lung diseases and alveolar consolidation have been described. Rare cases of patients with pulmonary hypertension, which has been found primarily among splenectomized adult patients, have also been reported [Mistry et al., 2002].

The diagnosis of Gaucher's disease, regardless of clinical subtype, is based on deficient glucocerebrosidase activity, which can be measured in peripheral blood leukocytes or cultured skin fibroblasts. Prenatal diagnosis for Gaucher's disease is based on analysis of glucocerebrosidase activity in cultured chorionic villi or amniocytes.

Biochemical testing is often complemented by analysis of the common mutations (specifically, N370S, L444P, IVS2+1, 84insG, and R496H). Carrier assignment can also be performed more reliably through mutation analysis. The five gene defects noted account for approximately 96 percent of disease alleles among Ashkenazi Jewish individuals, but for only about 40–60 percent of mutations among the non-Jewish patients (wherein the 55-base pair deletion is frequent) [Wallerstein et al., 2001]. Correlation studies have revealed genotype–phenotype concordance to be imperfect, with isolated exceptions. For instance, the presence of at least one N370S (1226G) allele precludes development of primary CNS involvement. In general, patients homozygous for the N370S mutation tend to have milder disease compared with other patients who are compound heterozygotes for the other more deleterious alleles. Patients homozygous for the L444P mutation tend to have severe disease, often (but not invariably) associated with primary neurologic manifestations.

Examination of bone marrow tissue (not the preferred method of diagnosis) reveals clumps of lipid-engorged macrophages (Gaucher cells). Magnetic resonance imaging (MRI) of the spine (sagittal views) and femurs (coronal views) has been useful in assessment of the degree of bone marrow infiltrative disease in Gaucher's disease [Maas et al., 2003]. On occasion, Gaucher-like cells (or pseudo-Gaucher cells) in isolation may be detected in other disorders, such as chronic myelocytic leukemia, and in disease states associated with increased cell turnover [Saito et al., 2007]. True Gaucher cells are periodic acid–Schiff-positive, and their cytoplasm has an irregular wrinkled appearance (see Figure 36-6B). Studies have revealed that Gaucher cells are alternative activated macrophage-like cells that express acid phosphatase, CD68, CD14, and HLA class II, but not CD11b, CD40, or dendritic cell markers [Boven et al., 2004]. Furthermore, Gaucher cells exhibited infrequent immunoreactivity for mannose receptor and did not express proinflammatory cytokines such as tumor necrosis factor-α and monocyte chemoattractant protein 1, but they did express the markers CD163, CCL18, and interleukin-1 receptor antagonist.

Before the introduction of enzyme therapy, the care of affected individuals was primarily palliative and included analgesics for bone pain, blood transfusions for severe anemia and thrombocytopenia, and splenectomy for severe hypersplenism. In addition, supplemental agents (such as bisphosphonates, calcium, and vitamin D) have been administered to patients (primarily adults) with Gaucher's disease and severe osteopenia. Pregnancy in affected women requires careful monitoring and attention to risk reduction for bleeding and other problems, especially around labor and delivery in those who are severely thrombocytopenic [Elstein et al., 2004].

Enzyme replacement therapy is based on the regular intravenous administration of glucocerebrosidase, initially purified from human placenta (alglucerase [Ceredase]), and more recently by use of the recombinant enzyme (imiglucerase [Cerezyme]) and generated from overexpression in cultured mammalian cells [Charrow, 2009]. The therapeutic protein is modified from its native form by sequential deglycosylation to expose the mannose residues necessary for targeted cellular uptake through the mannose receptor.

Enzyme therapy reverses the hematologic and visceral manifestations of Gaucher's disease and leads to the stabilization or improvement of bone involvement [Charrow et al., 2004; Pastores et al., 2004]. Enzyme therapy does not influence the ultimate progression of neurologic complications in patients with type 2 Gaucher's disease, and thus its use for this subgroup of patients is deemed inappropriate. Although intravenously administered enzyme does not lead to delivery of significant amounts of the protein across the blood–brain barrier, its use in patients with type 3 Gaucher's disease leads to improved quality of life (as a consequence of the reversal of the extraneurologic disease manifestations). Abnormal brainstem auditory-evoked response findings noted at baseline in eight children with type 3 Gaucher's disease continued to deteriorate with high-dose enzyme replacement therapy [Campbell et al., 2004]. Thus, patients with type 3 Gaucher's disease and their parents should be counseled appropriately about long-term outcome and the possibility that certain aspects of the disease may continue to progress. Enzyme therapy alone appears to improve bone density in patients with significant osteopenia, but only after years of treatment; thus, it is not uncommon for these patients to be prescribed supplemental treatment with bisphosphonates [Wenstrup et al., 2004; Sims et al., 2008].

Substrate reduction therapy (with miglustat [Zavesca]) has been shown to lead to improvements in several key clinical features of Gaucher's disease. This approach, when it is used alone (i.e., monotherapy), is based on the partial reduction of the synthesis of the substrate (to meet the metabolic capacity of the mutant enzyme) [Cox et al., 2000; Pastores and Barnett, 2003]. Studies have proved that a significant proportion of the orally administered agent (miglustat) can be found in cerebrospinal fluid [Platt and Butters, 2000]. Unfortunately, clinical trials with this drug in patients with type 3 Gaucher's disease on concomitant enzyme therapy has not been shown to alter ultimate neurologic prognosis [Schiffmann et al., 2008].

A minority of patients (about 10–15 percent) receiving enzyme replacement therapy have developed antibodies (primarily immunoglobulin G) against the infused glucocerebrosidase, although only a few have developed overt adverse events (mainly pruritus and hives), which respond readily to oral premedications (such as antihistamines) [Charrow, 2009]. This safety profile has led to consideration of enzyme therapy as the preferred treatment for patients with Gaucher's disease, including those with type 3 disease. In patients with type 3 Gaucher's disease and progressive CNS manifestations, bone marrow transplantation has been performed with favorable outcomes. However, the procedural risks associated with bone marrow transplantation and the prospect of graft-versus-host disease have limited its indication to carefully selected cases. The feasibility of gene therapy for Gaucher's disease remains to be re-examined [Hong et al., 2004b]. Meanwhile, alternative treatment options, including the use of a pharmacologic chaperone (isofagomine), are being explored [Yu et al., 2007].

Niemann–Pick Disease, Including Types A and B

Niemann–Pick disease is the eponymous designation for the storage disorders characterized by a primary deficiency of acid sphingomyelinase (ASM), associated with the progressive storage of sphingomyelin (phosphorylcholine) in the reticuloendothelial system. Impaired formation of ceramide within the lysosome or in the plasma membrane and its role as an apoptosis inducer are being actively examined as a potential added mechanism of disease [Jenkins et al., 2009]. In the acid sphingomyelinase "knockout" mouse, which develops a phenotype largely mimicking that of the neuronopathic form of Niemann–Pick disease (type A), the observed myelin deficiency has been attributed to reduced oligodendrocyte metabolic activity [Buccinnà et al., 2009].

The original patient described by A. Niemann (1914), an 18-month-old girl with hepatosplenomegaly, presented with progressive intellectual and motor deterioration. These clinical features were reminiscent of type 2 Gaucher's disease, but eventually Ludwig Pick (1927) provided further clinical and pathologic descriptions that helped in the delineation of these two disorders. The causal enzyme defect was first isolated by R. O. Brady and colleagues at the National Institutes of Health (in 1966).

Currently, Niemann–Pick disease types A and B are the terms used to refer to the infantile neuropathic and later-onset non-neuropathic forms of the disease, respectively. In actuality, both Niemann–Pick disease types A and B are allelic disorders (i.e., involving different mutations of the same gene) that result in primary deficiency of acid sphingomyelinase and represent the spectrum of phenotypes associated with mutations of the acid sphingomyelinase gene. Additional subtypes, referred to as Niemann–Pick disease types C and D in a classification scheme proposed by A. Crocker (1961), have clinical features that overlap with the classic Niemann–Pick disease types A and B. Eventually, Niemann–Pick disease types C and D were recognized as being associated with secondary and not primary acid sphingomyelinase deficiency. Indeed, a different cause for Niemann–Pick disease type C had been suggested by studies involving the fusion of cells (or formation of heterokaryons) from type A or B disease with type C cells. More recent investigations have found that Niemann–Pick disease types C and D are also allelic disorders due to mutations of one of two different genes (designated *NPC1* and *NPC2*) leading to disruption in the trafficking or metabolism of cholesterol and sphingolipids [Walkley and Suzuki, 2004]. These various Niemann–Pick disease subtypes are all inherited as autosomal-recessive traits.

Patients with early infantile Niemann–Pick disease (type A) present with failure to thrive and hepatomegaly in the first few weeks or months of life, usually before evident neurologic regression and the appearance of the macular cherry-red spot. The disorder is prevalent among individuals of Ashkenazi Jewish ancestry (carrier frequency of 1 in 90). In contrast to Gaucher's disease, there is marked abdominal distention due to hepatosplenomegaly and liver dysfunction. Serum levels of acid phosphatase are normal. Affected infants do not have dysmorphic facial features or skeletal deformities. Respiratory problems develop, and chest radiographs often reveal a fine miliary infiltration of the lungs [Minai et al., 2000]. There is developmental delay, with head lag and the inability to sit, and eventual regression with reduction in spontaneous movements and loss of interest in the surroundings. Unlike in Tay–Sachs disease, an exaggerated acousticomotor response cannot be elicited, and head circumference is either normal or moderately reduced. With disease progression, there is rigidity and opisthotonos. The findings on cerebrospinal fluid examination are normal. Death occurs in the second or third year of life.

Niemann–Pick disease type B is associated with visceral involvement (and by convention no neurologic problems) [Kolodny, 2000; Wasserstein et al., 2004]. The absence of significant brain involvement may be a consequence of the underlying mutation's association with residual enzyme activity. Hepatosplenomegaly and pulmonary infiltrative disease may be detected in late infancy or early childhood. Progressive pulmonary infiltration is generally the major disease complication. On high-resolution chest computed tomography (CT), the main abnormalities consist of thickening of the interlobular septa and patchy areas of ground-glass attenuation [Minai et al., 2000]. These changes correspond to the reticular or reticulonodular pattern of abnormalities, involving mainly the lower lung zones, that can be seen on chest radiographs. Abnormal linear growth and delayed skeletal maturation are also common in children and adolescents with Niemann–Pick disease type B [Wasserstein et al., 2003].

An intermediate phenotype may be encountered, with retinal degeneration and other neurologic signs (including slowed nerve conduction velocities) appearing in late childhood, adolescence, or adulthood (Figure 36-8). A study involving 45 patients (23 males and 22 females, ranging in age from 3 to 65 years) with Niemann–Pick disease type B revealed the presence of macular halos or cherry-red spots that incidentally were found not to be an absolute predictor of neurodegeneration [McGovern et al., 2004a]. The course of disease in patients with a phenotype intermediate between type A and type B is similar to that observed in type 3 Gaucher's disease, although the latter condition is often characterized by oculomotor apraxia and the absence of the cherry-red spot. In addition, there are differences found in the levels of chitotriosidase activity between patients with Gaucher's disease (600-fold increase) and those with Niemann–Pick disease (30-fold increase) [Wajner et al., 2004].

Investigations of lipid abnormalities in ten patients with Niemann–Pick disease type A and 30 additional patients with Niemann–Pick disease type B revealed that all had low (<35 mg/dL) high-density lipoprotein cholesterol [McGovern et al., 2004b]. Also noted were hypertriglyceridemia and increased low-density lipoprotein cholesterol in 25 of 40 (62 percent) and 27 of 40 (67 percent) of the patients, respectively. Coronary artery calcium scores were positive (>1.0) in 10 of 18 type B patients studied, which suggests that Niemann–Pick disease may be associated with a risk for early atherosclerotic heart disease.

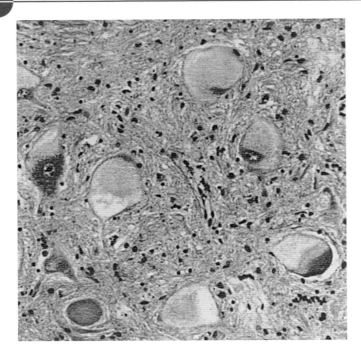

Fig. 36-8 Ballooned anterior horn cells of the spinal cord in a 5-year-old boy with late infantile Niemann–Pick disease. Hematoxylin and eosin stain.

The diagnosis of Niemann–Pick disease types A and B can be established on the basis of deficient acid sphingomyelinase activity, demonstrable in leukocytes or cultured skin fibroblasts. It has been reported that the biochemical assay to measure acid sphingomyelinase activity by use of the artificial substrate 2-*N*-(hexadecanoyl)-amino-4-nitrophenyl phosphorylcholine can occasionally lead to a missed diagnosis [Harzer et al., 2003]. In this particular study, four patients had the Q292K mutation on at least one allele. Thus, when the diagnosis of Niemann–Pick disease remains strongly suspected and a negative result is obtained on enzyme testing, it is important to determine whether the assay was performed with the artificial substrate (as is the custom in most laboratories). Another approach in these cases may entail examination of bone marrow (see Figure 36-6B).

Bone marrow examination (not the preferred initial means of diagnosis) reveals lipid-laden "foamy" histiocytes (with a soap bubble appearance), also evident in tissue sections obtained from the liver. The accumulated material is sudanophilic and periodic acid–Schiff-negative. On occasion, the atypical storage cells in bone marrow have been designated sea-blue histiocytes [Candoni et al., 2001].

Three acid sphingomyelinase gene mutations (specifically, two missense defects, R496L and L302P, and one frameshift mutation, fsP330) represent the most common Niemann–Pick disease gene defects, accounting for approximately 95 percent of disease alleles among Ashkenazi Jewish patients with Niemann–Pick disease type A [Schuchman and Miranda, 1997]. Among Niemann–Pick disease type B cases from North Africa, a three-base in-frame deletion of exon 6 (R608del) is frequent (87 percent of mutant alleles). This mutation was also found to be prevalent among patients with Niemann–Pick disease type B from the Canary Islands of Spain, located on the northwest coast of Africa [Fernandez-Burriel et al., 2003]. Among patients with Niemann–Pick disease type B,

homozygosity for the R608del mutation tends to be associated with a relatively milder phenotype compared with other combinations of acid sphingomyelinase gene mutations [Simonaro et al., 2002]. Several mutations in patients (primarily of Italian ancestry) with Niemann–Pick disease type B have been identified; in these studies, no correlation was found between onset of pulmonary symptoms and genotypes [Pittis et al., 2004]. Information about the causal mutation for specific families enables accurate carrier assignment. Niemann–Pick disease types A and B are pan-ethnic disorders, but the mutations that lead to disease outside of the populations just described tend to be private and require analysis of the acid sphingomyelinase gene sequence for identification. Prenatal diagnosis can be made by assay of acid sphingomyelinase activity in cultured chorionic villi or amniocytes [Vanier, 2002]. Preimplantation genetic diagnosis for Niemann–Pick disease type B has been reported [Hellani et al., 2004].

Only symptomatic treatment is available for Niemann–Pick disease types A and B, although enzyme therapy is under consideration for subtype B. In the murine model of Niemann–Pick disease, pulmonary delivery of recombinant acid sphingomyelinase improved clearance of lysosomal sphingomyelin from the lungs [Ziegler et al., 2009]. Repeated subcutaneous implantation of amniotic epithelial cells has not been shown to influence the ultimate disease course in prior therapeutic studies [Bembi et al., 1992]. Niemann–Pick disease type A is not amenable to hematopoietic stem cell transplantation because of its rapid progression, but limited experience suggests that hematopoietic stem cell transplantation may have some beneficial effects for Niemann–Pick disease type B. Report of a 16-year follow-up of allogeneic bone marrow transplantation carried out on a 3-year-old girl with Niemann–Pick disease type B revealed severe neurologic involvement (including bilateral cherry-red spots), despite normal findings on neurologic examination at the time of transplantation [Victor et al., 2003]. However, baseline pulmonary infiltration regressed after bone marrow transplantation, although there was no clinical evidence of pulmonary insufficiency. Her post-transplant course was complicated by severe graft-versus-host disease and respiratory arrest, factors that may have had an adverse influence on the neurologic outcome.

Niemann–Pick Disease, Including Types C and D

Niemann–Pick disease type C is a neurovisceral lipid storage disorder associated with a wide spectrum of clinical phenotypes. It is characterized neuropathologically by the widespread appearance of axonal spheroids, an accumulation of intraneuronal cytoplasmic inclusions, and neuronal loss [Vanier and Millat, 2003]. The disease incidence has been estimated at 1 in 150,000. Approximately 95 percent of cases have mutations in a gene (designated *NPC1*) that encodes a large transmembrane glycoprotein, localized primarily in the endosomes [Sturley et al., 2004]. A smaller group of patients who are clinically and biochemically indistinguishable from individuals with *NPC1* mutations have a defect of the *NPC2* gene, which encodes a small soluble lysosomal protein with cholesterol-binding properties (previously identified as epididymal secretory glycoprotein 1 [HE1]) [Vanier and Millat, 2004]. It is likely that both protein products (i.e., NPC1 and NPC2) function in a coordinated fashion, as studies performed on skin fibroblasts obtained from patients with either mutation reveal the accumulation of unesterified cholesterol and glycolipids in the lysosome–late endosome. Furthermore, the mating of mice genetically deficient for each protein (i.e., NPC1 or NPC2) results in the generation of double-deficient mice that resemble the single-disease mutants [Pentchev, 2004]. A consequence of cholesterol sequestration is a reduction in its availability, and an impairment of cholesterol-mediated homeostatic responses in the endoplasmic reticulum [Karten et al., 2009]. An abnormality of autophagy has also been demonstrated in cells obtained from the Niemann–Pick disease type C mouse model [Ishibashi et al., 2009], and other studies have shown an impairment of neurosteroidogenesis [Griffin et al., 2004].

Immunohistochemical studies involving the HE1/NPC2 protein revealed its localization in pyramidal or projection neurons in the cerebral cortex and amygdala, and in the Purkinje neurons of the cerebellum [Ong et al., 2004]. This regional pattern of expression is similar to the findings with NPC1, with a low level of expression of both proteins in regions derived from the diencephalon (such as the thalamus and hypothalamus). In contrast to NPC1, which is found predominantly in astrocytes, HE1/NPC2 has been observed mainly in neurons. The HE1/NPC2 protein has also been found in the cytosol of dendrites and on postsynaptic densities. These results suggest that NPC1 and HE1/NPC2 are differentially enriched in astrocytes and neurons, respectively, and that HE1/NPC2 may function in supporting the integrity of the postsynaptic densities of neurons [Ong et al., 2004].

The classically affected patients (accounting for 50–60 percent of cases) often have a benign, self-limited jaundice in early infancy and an unremarkable childhood [Vanier and Millat, 2003]. Eventually, between the ages of 3 and 8 years (less often after the 10th year of life), they are noted to be clumsy, have a tendency to fall, and develop ataxia. Hepatosplenomegaly may be noted, and supranuclear (vertical) gaze palsy, which may be accompanied by blinking or head thrusting, is evident on examination. With disease progression, patients experience dysarthria, dysphagia, and dementia. Additional neurologic manifestations include dystonia, choreoathetosis, and seizures (of the generalized tonic-clonic and myoclonic type). A proportion of patients with Niemann–Pick disease type C may present at birth with ascites or develop neonatal (cholestatic) jaundice and a rapidly fatal disease.

Cataplexy also occurs late in the disease but rarely may be the presenting feature of Niemann–Pick disease type C [Vankova et al., 2003]. Typically, the loss of postural tone is evoked by a humorous stimulus (gelastic cataplexy). Examination of cerebrospinal fluid has revealed reduced hypocretin-1 levels in two patients with Niemann–Pick disease type C, which suggests that the storage abnormalities may have an impact on the hypothalamus and, more specifically, hypocretin-containing cells [Kanbayashi et al., 2003]. These changes may be partially responsible for the sleep abnormalities and cataplexy seen in these patients.

Psychiatric disturbances, including psychosis, have been reported to occur in patients with Niemann–Pick disease type C, usually coinciding with the onset of puberty [Josephs et al., 2003]. Most patients develop spasticity and rigidity, and die of pulmonary complications in their teens or early adulthood. Pertinent negative findings include the absence of retinal changes, visual failure, and signs of lower motor neuron disease; cerebrospinal fluid examination findings are also normal.

A clinical severity scale has been developed to characterize and quantify disease progression in patients with Niemann–Pick disease type C. A linear increase in severity scores over time has been observed, independent of age of onset [Yanjanin et al., 2009]. In addition to neuronal storage, studies involving the mouse model of Niemann–Pick disease type C have revealed conspicuous hypomyelination in the cerebral white matter and corpus callosum. In brains from patients with Niemann–Pick disease type C, studies have found neuropathologic abnormalities (e.g., formation of tauopathies and neurofibrillary tangles) similar to those found in Alzheimer's disease [Nixon, 2004]. Furthermore, the aggregated amyloid precursor protein cleavage product amyloid beta accumulates in late endosomes. In addition, presenilins (normally localized in the endoplasmic reticulum and endoplasmic reticulum–Golgi intermediate compartment) were distributed to late endosomes. These observations suggest that endosome dysfunction and the disruption of cholesterol homeostasis may promote mechanisms common to both Niemann–Pick disease type C and Alzheimer's disease. In the mouse model, intracerebroventricular administration of two potent inhibitors (roscovitine and olomoucine) of the cyclin-dependent kinases attenuated the hyperphosphorylation of the neurofilament tau and mitotic proteins [Zhang et al., 2004]. These observations were associated with a reduction in the number of spheroids, the modulation of Purkinje neuron death, and the amelioration of the motor defects in these mice. The diagnosis of Niemann–Pick disease type C is based on demonstration in cultured skin fibroblasts of impaired cholesterol esterification and intralysosomal storage of unesterified cholesterol (which gives off an intense perinuclear fluorescence with filipin staining) (Figure 36-9). Identification of the causal NPC1 or NPC2 mutations requires specialized studies because of the existence of genetic heterogeneity (i.e., similar clinical disorder or phenotype resulting from two different gene defects) and private mutations in most of the patients (outside defined populations). In one study involving 143 unrelated patients with Niemann–Pick disease type C, mutation analysis led to identification of 251 of 286 (88 percent) disease alleles [Park et al., 2003]. The most common NPC1 mutation, I1061T, was detected in 18 percent of NPC alleles.

The designation Niemann–Pick disease type D was used to describe affected individuals among the French Acadians in

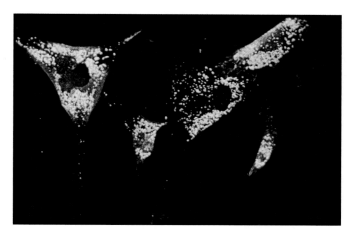

Fig. 36-9 Filipin-stained fibroblasts viewed under fluorescent light from a patient with Niemann–Pick disease type C.

Nova Scotia (Canada) [Greer et al., 1999]. In these patients, disease onset is usually between the ages of 2 and 4 years. After characterization of the *NPC1* gene, studies revealed a common founder mutation (G309T) in this population of patients. Similarly, a specific gene defect (I106T) has been identified among Spanish American cases of Niemann–Pick disease type C in the Upper Rio Grande Valley (Colorado) attributed to a founder effect [Millat et al., 1999].

The management of patients with Niemann–Pick disease type C is primarily symptomatic. A therapeutic trial involving dietary restriction of cholesterol and the administration of cholesterol-lowering agents (i.e., statins) has resulted in the reduction of hepatic and plasma cholesterol levels but no effect on neurologic outcome [Patterson and Platt, 2004].

Secondary accumulation of GM_2 ganglioside in the brains of patients with Niemann–Pick disease type C, and as also shown in the mouse model, is believed to contribute to the neuronal degeneration. Preclinical studies in the knockout mouse model treated with miglustat have led to delayed onset of symptoms and increased survival. Outcome in the affected mice was enhanced when substrate reduction therapy was given in combination with bone marrow transplantation [Jeyakumar et al., 2001]. Miglustat given to one patient with Niemann–Pick disease type C reduced pathologic lipid storage, improved the endosomal uptake, and returned lipid trafficking to normal in peripheral blood B lymphocytes [Lachmann et al., 2004]. Demonstration that treatment with miglustat, which has no direct effect on cholesterol metabolism, corrects the abnormal lipid trafficking suggests that glycosphingolipid accumulation is the primary pathogenetic event. In a randomized controlled study, miglustat treatment was shown to improve or stabilize several clinically relevant markers, such as horizontal saccadic eye movement (which is impaired in affected individuals), improved swallowing capacity and auditory acuity, and led to a slower deterioration in ambulatory index [Patterson et al., 2010].

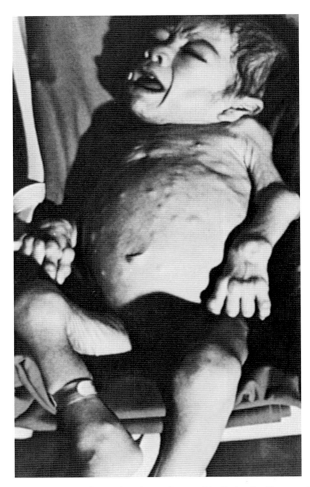

Fig. 36-10 A severely cachectic patient with Farber's disease. The patient exhibits multiple subcutaneous lymphogranulomas and periarticular swelling. *(From Gellis S, Feingold M. Contributed by TRC Sisson. Am J Dis Child 1971;122:573.)*

Farber's Disease (Lipogranulomatosis)

Farber's disease, initially described by S. Farber and colleagues (1957), is characterized by widespread granulomatous tissue infiltration by ceramide-containing foamy macrophages resulting from a deficiency of lysosomal acid ceramidase [Park and Schuchman, 2006]. Examination of the lysosomal degradation of sphingomyelin-derived ceramide in situ with use of the affected patient's skin fibroblasts has found a significant correlation between the ceramide accumulation and the severity of Farber's disease [Levade et al., 1995]. Insertional mutagenesis of the mouse acid ceramidase gene has been shown to lead to early embryonic lethality in homozygotes and progressive lipid storage disease in heterozygotes [Li et al., 2002]. Recent studies suggest that acid ceramidase is an essential factor required for embryo survival, and functions by removing ceramide from the newly formed embryos and inhibiting the default apoptosis pathway [Eliyahu et al., 2007].

Clinical features include painful swollen and deformed joints and dysphonia (hoarse cry), with onset usually before the age of 4 months [Mondal et al., 2009; Sana et al., 2009] (Figure 36-10). Dyspnea due to infiltration of the peribronchial and perialveolar spaces is common. Firm subcutaneous nodules may be found on the fingers, wrist, elbows, and spine. Hand radiographs reveal destructive juxta-articular bone

lesions [Toppet et al., 1978]. Although lipid storage is present in neurons and glial cells (mainly in the brainstem nuclei, basal ganglia and ganglion cells of the retina, and anterior horn cells), neurologic signs are usually not prominent (Figure 36-11). Formal evaluation of any developmental problem is complicated by the severe inanition and fixed joints [Jameson et al., 1987]. Some patients have progressive mental deterioration and visual loss. Cerebrospinal fluid protein levels are increased. Anorexia, vomiting, and swallowing difficulties lead to cachexia. Cholestatic jaundice and rapidly evolving liver failure have been described in two siblings [Willis et al., 2008]. Severe muscle atrophy, in part a consequence of immobilization of the joints, is also seen. Death generally occurs within the first 2 years of life, although there are rare cases of patients with an attenuated form of the disease and more prolonged clinical course [Pavone et al., 1980].

The diagnosis is often based on quantification of ceramide (a fatty acylsphingosine) accumulation in tissues or cultured skin fibroblasts [Mitsuo et al., 1988]. Analysis of ceramidase activity in vivo can also be performed on the same tissues; however, residual ceramidase activity has not been found to correlate with disease severity. Several mutations in the gene encoding lysosomal acid ceramidase have been identified [Bar et al., 2001].

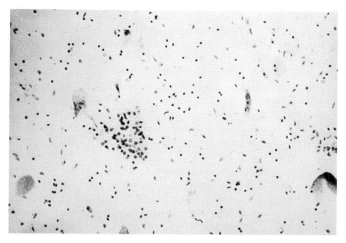

Fig. 36-11 Section of spinal cord from a patient with Farber's disease. The section exhibits swollen neurons, neuronophagia, and loss of neurons in the anterior horn area. *(Courtesy Hugo W. Moser, Baltimore, MD.)*

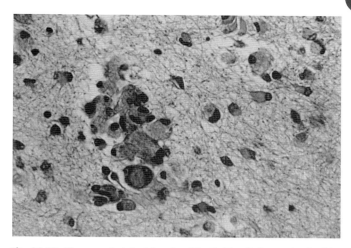

Fig. 36-12 Clumps of globoid and epithelioid cells in cerebral white matter in Krabbe's disease. The background area demonstrates demyelination and gliosis. *(Courtesy Joo Ho Sung, Minneapolis, MN.)*

There is no specific treatment, although affected individuals may obtain relief from joint pains with analgesics. In a 9-year-old girl with occasional painful locking of the metacarpophalangeal (MCP) joints of the middle fingers and severe tenderness of the dorsal aspect of the wrists, resection of several nodules within the MCP joint and of a nodule that was firmly attached to the extensor pollicis longus tendon beneath the extensor retinaculum relieved pain and enabled the patient to perform daily activities [Moritomo et al., 2002]. Supportive care may be required for laryngeal and respiratory symptoms. Gene therapy is under investigation; one study has evaluated in vivo delivery of human acid ceramidase via cord blood transplantation and direct injection of lentivirus as treatment approaches [Ramsubir et al., 2008].

Krabbe's Disease (Globoid Cell Leukodystrophy)

In 1916, K. Krabbe, a Danish neurologist, described two siblings with an acute infantile diffuse "sclerosis" of the brain (characterized by unusual cells in the white matter termed globoid cells by Collier and Greenfield) (Figure 36-12). The condition has since been attributed to a deficiency of galactocerebroside β-galactosidase (β-galactosidase C, galactosylceramidase), which normally cleaves the bond between ceramide and the galactose moiety of galactosylceramide [Suzuki, 2003]. Disease incidence in the general population is estimated at 1 in 201,000, although an increased prevalence (1 in 25,000) of the early infantile form has been reported in Sweden [Arvidsson et al., 1995]. An authentic animal model (the twitcher mouse, which is galactosylceramidase-deficient) has been described [Yagi et al., 2004].

The majority of cases are an early infantile form (with onset between 3 and 6 months of life) (Figure 36-13). Patients demonstrate irritability and develop rapidly progressive generalized rigidity and tonic spasms [Korn-Lubetzki and Nevo, 2003]. Affected infants often have a clenched fist and develop myoclonic jerks. Blindness and optic atrophy appear later, along with pendular nystagmus. Abnormalities of the brainstem auditory-evoked responses are among the first objective indications of

CNS disease; visual-evoked potential abnormalities also occur. Brain MRI shows signs of leukodystrophy, with symmetric signal abnormalities usually noted in the periventricular region of the posterior cerebral hemispheres. Diffusion tensor imaging has been shown to detect significant differences in the corticospinal tracts of asymptomatic neonates [Escolar et al., 2009]. Fluorine 18-labeled 2-fluoro-2-deoxyglucose positron emission tomography (PET) in one 2½-year-old male revealed a marked decrease in the metabolism of the left cerebral cortex and no uptake in the caudate heads [Al-Essa et al., 2000]. However, normal glucose uptake was observed in the thalami, lentiform nuclei, and cerebellum.

Cerebrospinal fluid protein is elevated in Krabbe's disease, and examination of the peripheral nervous system reveals markedly reduced nerve conduction velocities [Husain et al., 2004]. There is no visceromegaly or skeletal abnormalities. Death, usually due to respiratory difficulties and bronchopneumonia, occurs between the ages of 1 and 2 years. A clinical disease staging system for affected infants has been developed, which is based solely on signs and symptoms of disease. The index was found to be useful in predicting outcomes after umbilical cord blood transplantation, whereas standard neurophysiological and neuroimaging tests were not useful in the staging algorithm [Escolar et al., 2006].

In a small proportion (about 10–15 percent) of patients, onset is in the late infantile or juvenile period. Several such cases have been identified in southern Italy (and Sicily). These patients exhibit signs of progressive walking problems, spastic paraparesis, and cerebellar ataxia, mostly before the age of 5 years [Lyon et al., 1991]. With disease progression, patients may develop dystonia and visual failure (due to optic atrophy and demyelination of the optic radiation). In one report, a 48-year-old man presented with asymmetric upper and lower motor neuron signs initially attributed to a motor neuron disease [Henderson et al., 2003]. In this patient, nerve conduction studies and neuroimaging provided important signs leading to the correct diagnosis. In another report, which described three affected brothers with disease onset in the fifth decade, the neurologic examination found features of asymmetric peripheral neuropathy associated with pyramidal signs [Sabatelli et al., 2002]. Two of the patients in this family died at 59 and 61 years

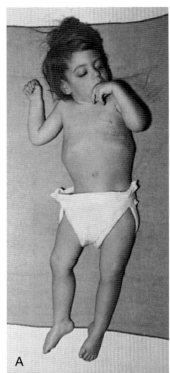

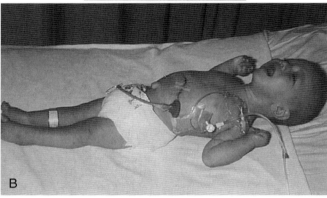

Fig. 36-13 Krabbe's disease. A, This female first manifested signs and symptoms of Krabbe's disease at 2 years of age. She underwent a progressive course thereafter. There is fisting of the right hand, folding of the thumb, and spasticity of both legs. She experiences frequent episodes of myoclonic and generalized tonic-clonic seizures. B, A 9-month-old male with Krabbe's disease manifesting opisthotonos, flexion of the arms, cortical thumb positioning, extension of the legs, spontaneous extensor toe signs, and extreme irritability.

of age of respiratory failure. Other cases have been described with presentations consistent with spastic paraplegia [Bajaj et al., 2002]. Behavioral changes and intellectual impairment have also been reported, and these problems may be the initial complaints, particularly in juvenile-onset patients before recognition of the other features of Krabbe's disease.

A study examined the results of testing involving 26 children with Krabbe's disease, 20 with the early infantile disease (range of ages at onset, 0.5–6 months), and 6 with the late-onset disease (range of ages at onset, 10–60 months) [Aldosari et al., 2004]. The results revealed that patients with early infantile disease had abnormal flash visual-evoked potentials (53 percent),

abnormal brainstem auditory-evoked response (88 percent), and abnormal electroencephalograms (65 percent). Nerve conduction studies were abnormal in all of these patients. Among the late-onset patients, none had abnormal visual-evoked potentials, whereas brainstem auditory-evoked responses and electroencephalograms were abnormal in 40 percent and 33 percent of the children. Only 20 percent of the late-onset patients had abnormal nerve conduction studies. Abnormal neurophysiologic studies were found to correlate with more extensive disease as measured by MRI scans [Korn-Lubetzki et al., 2003].

Brain magnetic resonance spectroscopy (MRS) performed in patients with infantile Krabbe's disease has revealed elevation of myo-inositol and choline-containing compounds in affected white matter, consistent with demyelination and glial proliferation [Brockmann et al., 2003; Zarifi et al., 2001]. The accompanying decrease of N-acetylaspartate points to neuroaxonal loss. In juvenile-onset cases, MRS indicated astrocytosis with minor neuroaxonal damage in white matter [Farina et al., 2000]. Spinal involvement may be evident on MRI as abnormal contrast enhancement of the lumbosacral nerve roots [Given et al., 2001].

Pathologic studies of brains from patients with Krabbe's disease reveal a rapid disappearance of myelin and myelin-forming cells (i.e., oligodendrocytes in the CNS and Schwann cells in the peripheral nervous system). In addition, there is reactive astrocytic gliosis and tissue infiltration by multinucleated macrophages (globoid cells) filled with materials that are periodic acid–Schiff-positive [Itoh et al., 2002]. These findings are considered to reflect a reaction to psychosine (galactosylsphingosine), a toxic metabolite that accumulates in the tissues of patients with Krabbe's disease [Haq et al., 2003]. Exposure of an immortalized human oligodendroglial cell line (MO3.13) to exogenous psychosine results in the concurrent upregulation of JNK AP-1 (a pro-apoptotic pathway mediator) and downregulation of the NF-κB pathway (an anti-apoptotic pathway factor) [Haq et al., 2003]. Another study, which examined a mouse-derived oligodendrocyte progenitor cell line (OLP-II), revealed that psychosine caused cytotoxic effects in a dose-dependent manner [Zaka and Wenger, 2004]. Moreover, psychosine treatment resulted in the activation or cleavage of initiator caspases 8 and 9, and effector caspase 3. These results provide further support for a role for psychosine in cell death through an apoptotic mechanism. Recently, psychosine has been shown to accumulate specifically in lipid rafts in the twitcher mouse brain and sciatic nerve, and in samples from brains of human Krabbe's disease patients. The psychosine accumulation was accompanied by an increase in cholesterol in these domains and changes in the distribution of the lipid raft markers flotillin-2 and caveolin-1, potentially leading to a disruption of multiple signaling pathways [White et al., 2009a, b].

In a separate study that examined brain obtained from three patients with Krabbe's disease, white matter lesions were found (in the corona radiata, corpus callosum, and cerebellar peduncles) in addition to the neuronal loss in the thalamus, cerebellum, and inferior olivary nucleus [Itoh et al., 2002]. Ramified microglia was immunoreactive for ferritin and HLA-DR α chain, and both the small and large globoid cells exhibited immunoreactivity for ferritin KP-1 and neural cell adhesion molecule. T lymphocytes immunoreactive for leukocyte common antigen, ubiquitin carboxyl-terminal esterase L1, and CD3 were increased around the vessels in the white matter.

These data suggest that immunoreactive changes may partly be involved in the myelin breakdown and glial pathologic changes in Krabbe's disease.

The diagnosis of Krabbe's disease is based on demonstration of decreased galactosylceramidase activity in peripheral leukocytes or cultured skin fibroblasts [Randell et al., 2000]. Mutation analysis has led to identification of more than 40 gene defects responsible for Krabbe's disease [Fu et al., 1999]. A deletion mutation (502del) has been reported as common, accounting for up to 40 percent of disease alleles. Homozygosity for this mutation is associated with the severe infantile form of the disease. Mutation analysis in a patient with late-onset disease revealed compound heterozygosity for the 809GÆA (G270D) and 1609GÆA (G537R) mutations [De Gasperi et al., 1999]. The relatively mild clinical phenotype observed in this patient was attributed to the 809GÆA allele, based on the presence of residual galactosylceramidase activity in vitro. Indeed, this mutation has been found in several other patients with late-onset Krabbe's disease.

There is no specific treatment for the infantile form of Krabbe's disease. However, the irritability encountered in the infantile form of Krabbe's disease has been successfully controlled with low-dose morphine [Stewart et al., 2001]. Bone marrow transplantation with appropriate timing in the later-onset forms has returned cerebrospinal fluid protein to normal levels and stabilized the neurologic findings, neuropsychologic function, and extent of demyelination on MRI [Caniglia et al., 2002]. Newborn screening has been recommended for early detection and early intervention by hematopoietic stem cell transplantation to improve outcome [Galvin-Parton, 2003; Li et al., 2004]. Transplantation of umbilical cord blood from unrelated donors in newborns with infantile Krabbe's disease has been reported to alter the natural history of the disease favorably, but only when initiated before the onset of symptoms [Escolar et al., 2005]. However, a longer period of follow-up has indicated that over 80 percent of the transplanted infants have gross motor problems, and in some instances required assistance with ambulation [Prasad and Kurtzberg, 2008]. These observations and other considerations have raised several concerns regarding the newborn screening program for Krabbe's disease initiated in New York State and planned to be introduced in the state of Illinois [Steiner, 2009]. Enzyme replacement therapy, which may necessitate intracerebroventricular administration of galactocerebrosidase to bypass the blood–brain barrier, is under investigation [Lee et al., 2005, 2007]. Stem cell-based strategies, using glial progenitor cells and other cell types, are also being explored [Goldman et al., 2008]. Experimental studies in the twitcher mouse model with vascular endothelial growth factor (VEGF), an endothelial cell mitogen and permeability factor, given intravenously at the time of birth, led to increased blood–brain barrier permeability [Young et al., 2004]. Systemic treatment with VEGF before bone marrow transplantation or the administration of recombinant lentivirus resulted in increased numbers of either donor cells or virus-transduced cells in the recipient brain. This approach may prove to be useful in future studies of cellular or enzyme replacement therapies for Krabbe's disease and other lysosomal storage diseases with primary CNS involvement.

Deficiency of saposin A was demonstrated to cause late-onset, slowly progressive globoid cell leukodystrophy in the mouse [Matsuda et al., 2001b]. The saposin A-null mouse developed slowly progressive hind-limb paralysis, with onset at 2.5 months of age. Tremors and shaking, prominent in other myelin mutants, were not obvious until the terminal stage. Pathologic and analytic biochemistry revealed findings that were qualitatively identical to but generally much milder than those seen in the typical human infantile Krabbe's disease. Interestingly, in affected female mice that became pregnant, neurologic symptoms greatly improved, compared with affected nulliparous female mice or affected male mice. Immune-related gene (monocyte chemoattractant protein 1, tumor necrosis factor-α) expression was found to be significantly down-regulated in the brain of pregnant saposin A-null mice. In addition, there was intense expression of the estrogen receptors (alpha and beta) on the globoid cells, activated astrocytes, and microglia in the demyelinating area [Matsuda et al., 2001a]. When these mice were subcutaneously implanted with timed-release 17β-estradiol pellets, the pathologic process was vastly improved. These findings suggest that the higher levels of estrogen during pregnancy may have a protective effect. Saposin A deficiency has not been described in human patients but might be anticipated as a cause of late-onset chronic leukodystrophy without primary galactosylceramidase deficiency.

Metachromatic Leukodystrophy (Sulfatide Lipidosis)

Deficiency of arylsulfatase A activity leads to the accumulation of its incompletely metabolized substrate, galactosylsulfatide (cerebroside sulfate), in the white matter of the central and peripheral nervous system [Gieselmann, 2003]. The associated clinical condition derives its name from the brownish or reddish birefringent (metachromatic) color of the sulfatide deposits, noted when involved tissues are stained with cresyl violet or toluidine blue [Gieselmann et al., 2003a]. Sulfatides are a component of myelin, and their increased concentration in tissues of the patients with metachromatic leukodystrophy may lead to instability and myelin breakdown (Figure 36-14). It has also been hypothesized that lysosulfatide (a deacylated form of sulfatide) may be cytotoxic and promote the

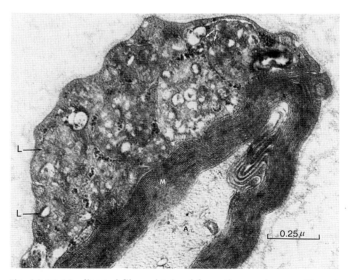

Fig. 36-14 Myelinated fiber obtained from the sural nerve. There is accumulation of lysosomal sulfatide in the Schwann cell cytoplasm of this 2-year-old child. L, lamellar inclusion; M, myelin; A, axon. (×132,000.) *(Courtesy Stephen A. Smith, Minneapolis, MN.)*

dissolution of myelin. Lysosulfatide has been shown to regulate the motility of a neural precursor cell line (B35 neuroblastoma cells) via calcium-mediated process collapse (by rapidly promoting process retraction and cell rounding) [Hans et al., 2009].

The overall incidence of metachromatic leukodystrophy has been estimated at 1 in 121,000. The relatively high frequency (1 in 2520 live births, with an estimated carrier frequency of 1 in 25 to 1 in 50) in the Navajo Indians of the southwestern United States has been attributed to a "genetic bottleneck" that occurred in the mid-19th century [Holve et al., 2001]. Genetic bottleneck refers to an evolutionary event leading to a drastic reduction in population size. The same phenomenon explains the increased frequency (1 in 75 live births) of metachromatic leukodystrophy in a small Jewish community that lived in Habban (Yemen), isolated from the other Jewish populations [Zlotogora et al., 1995]. There have been rare patients with saposin B deficiency who are unable to catabolize sulfatide and other glycosphingolipids in vivo, leading to their accumulation and a neurodegenerative disease that is viewed as a variant of metachromatic leukodystrophy [Wrobe et al., 2000; Deconinck et al., 2008]. Saposin B (also known as sphingolipid activator protein 1) is a small glycoprotein that acts as an activator of arylsulfatase A and is required for the hydrolysis of galactosylsulfatide [Whitelegge et al., 2003]. Patients with saposin B deficiency have clinical features that overlap with the juvenile-onset form of metachromatic leukodystrophy [Wrobe et al., 2000]. These individuals have evidence of tissue sulfatide storage with normal arylsulfatase A activity in vitro; their diagnosis can be confirmed by tests using specific antibodies against saposin B or identification of the causal saposin B gene mutation.

Late infantile-onset metachromatic leukodystrophy represents the most common clinical form of the disease, accounting for 60–70 percent of all cases (Figure 36-15). Later-onset forms of the disease, developing in childhood or adolescence and even during adulthood, have been described.

In late infantile metachromatic leukodystrophy, affected children usually present with progressive gait problems, manifesting between the ages of 14 and 16 months. Examination of the lower extremities may initially reveal a mixed picture, with flaccid paralysis or more commonly with pyramidal signs (e.g., spasticity and bilateral Babinski signs) and depressed or hyperactive deep tendon reflexes. Electrophysiologic testing reveals evidence of peripheral nerve involvement, with marked slowing of the motor and sensory nerve conduction velocities. The cerebrospinal fluid protein level is elevated. Brain MRI reveals leukodystrophy, with a hyperintense signal in the periventricular and central white matter on T2-weighted images, which may initially be limited to the parieto-occipital region [Sener, 2003]. In one 17-month-old male with metachromatic leukodystrophy, an echo-planar diffusion magnetic resonance sequence revealed a restricted diffusion pattern in the deep white matter [Sener, 2002]. Proton MRS revealed a marked decrease in choline, a metabolite related to myelin turnover [Sener, 2003]. These observations likely represent dysmyelination.

The disease is progressive, and affected patients with metachromatic leukodystrophy are eventually unable to stand or sit up. Additional findings include dysarthria, drooling, and dysphagia. There may be visual failure. Seizures occur in a small proportion of patients in the terminal stages of their disease, by which time the children are rigid and assume decerebrate

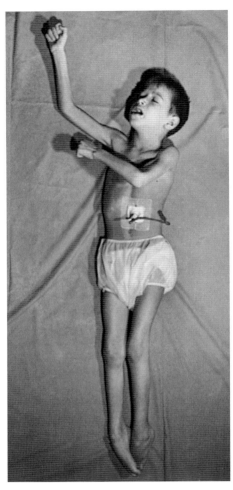

Fig. 36-15 An 11-year-old boy with the juvenile form of metachromatic leukodystrophy. The patient is in a vegetative state. Marked spasticity and contractures are present. The patient has gross impairment of bulbar function and is fed through a gastric feeding tube.

or decorticate postures [Cameron et al., 2004]. Deposition of sulfatides in the gallbladder can cause the formation of papillomatous changes and lead to cholecystitis [Vettoretto et al., 2001]. Death in patients with late infantile metachromatic leukodystrophy usually occurs between the ages of 3 and 7 years.

Metachromatic leukodystrophy may manifest in later life, from early childhood (3–8 years of age) to adolescence or even adulthood [Ito et al., 2009]. Behavioral abnormalities, cognitive deficits, and dementia may be more prominent in the later-onset forms [Baumann et al., 2002; Black et al., 2003; Mihaljevic-Peles et al., 2001]. Abnormalities of nerve conduction and cerebrospinal fluid protein elevation may be minimal. Brain white matter alterations on MRI may also be less pronounced. The variability in clinical presentation can often lead to a missed diagnosis, and metachromatic leukodystrophy should be considered in cases characterized by deterioration in behavioral or mental capacities, a progressive disorder of gait or coordination, or a progressive polyneuropathy. It is important to exclude arylsulfatase A pseudodeficiency in these patients. The course of disease in the late-onset forms of metachromatic leukodystrophy can be protracted, with survival of more than 5–10 years not unusual. However, disease may evolve more rapidly in some patients.

Impaired cortical glucose metabolism (especially of the medial temporal and frontal cortices) was observed with PET and fluorine 18-labeled fluorodeoxyglucose in a 41-year-old male patient with late-onset metachromatic leukodystrophy [Johannsen et al., 2001]. In addition, brain MRI displayed confluent hyperintensities of periventricular and subcortical white matter. Neuropsychologic assessment demonstrated that he had mild amnesia, visuospatial dysfunction, and attention deficits with a slow psychomotor speed. The neuropsychologic deficits in this individual were related to the location of deficits in glucose metabolism.

To a certain extent, the clinical course of metachromatic leukodystrophy is associated with the nature of the causal mutation [Biffi et al., 2008]. Patients with a combination of deleterious alleles for this autosomal-recessive condition have a late infantile onset, whereas those with a combination of a severe and mild mutation or two mild mutant alleles have delayed onset and follow a subacute or chronic disease course. Two gene defects – namely, 459+1G to A and 1277C to T (Pro426Leu) – account for almost 50 percent of metachromatic leukodystrophy mutations; the remaining alleles are rare or private [Eng et al., 2003, 2004]. In a study of 12 adult metachromatic leukodystrophy patients with primary motor signs (pyramidal, cerebellar, and less often dystonia) and a peripheral neuropathy, the major adult arylsulfatase A mutation P426L [Lugowska et al., 2002]. In contrast, patients with the psychocognitive forms (associated with modifications of mood, peculiar social reactions, and a progressive mental deterioration) were often noted to be compound heterozygotes, with the I179S mutation on one allele [Lugowska et al., 2002]. In a separate study, screening for the mutations in 34 unrelated patients with metachromatic leukodystrophy from Poland revealed that the I179S mutation accounted for 17 percent of examined alleles (2 of 12) in adults and as much as 42 percent (5 of 12 alleles) in patients with late juvenile metachromatic leukodystrophy [Berger et al., 1997]. The I179S mutation has not been found in the late infantile or early juvenile cases.

The diagnosis of metachromatic leukodystrophy is based on demonstration of deficient arylsulfatase A activity in leukocytes or cultured skin fibroblasts. Peripheral nerve biopsy, which is often unnecessary, reveals the typical prismatic and tuffstone inclusions in Schwann cells. Polymorphisms that give rise to arylsulfatase A pseudodeficiency (associated with decreased arylsulfatase A activity in vitro) are common in the general population (approximately 10 percent) [Rafi et al., 2003]. Biochemical assays for the enzyme with the artificial 4-methylumbelliferyl substrate may lead to an erroneous diagnosis of affected and carrier status in these individuals. Increased urinary sulfatide excretion (detected by thin-layer chromatography) is found only in affected patients with metachromatic leukodystrophy who have a true deficiency of arylsulfatase A activity [Whitfield et al., 2001]. Sulfatide loading tests performed with tissues in culture can help distinguish arylsulfatase A pseudodeficiency from a true carrier or affected status, but these methods require specialized expertise and have generally been replaced by a combination of biochemical and molecular assays.

The sequence variation leading to arylsulfatase A deficiency has been characterized, and most laboratories offering the biochemical test can check for these mutations. In families in which the causal arylsulfatase A gene defects are known, true carrier status can be assigned reliably by mutation analysis. In families at risk for having an affected child, the presence of the arylsulfatase A pseudodeficiency allele should be ascertained in both parents to avoid mistakes in prenatal diagnosis. One study reported a higher incidence of evident or possible microorganic brain damage in metachromatic leukodystrophy–pseudodeficiency and metachromatic leukodystrophy heterozygotes, although none of these carriers had overt clinical problems [Tylki-Szymanska et al., 2002b]. On the other hand, there is a separate report that describes the neuropsychologic profiles and brain MRI findings of eight family members of a 7-year-old female with metachromatic leukodystrophy [Weber Byars et al., 2001]. All eight relatives were heterozygous carriers, including five who were also carriers of the arylsulfatase A pseudodeficiency gene. The patient's younger sister had features of nonverbal learning disability despite a normal MRI study, whereas two members with minor white matter findings did not [Weber Byars et al., 2001]. Thus, the findings in this family do not support the concept of a syndrome of nonverbal learning disability in heterozygous carriers of the gene for metachromatic leukodystrophy, even in association with the metachromatic leukodystrophy pseudodeficiency gene.

There is no effective treatment for metachromatic leukodystrophy. In a child with metachromatic leukodystrophy who required surgery for gastroesophageal reflux, general anesthesia was performed with a lumbar epidural technique [Hernandez-Palazon, 2003]. In this patient, the epidural catheter enabled the delivery of analgesia postoperatively, avoiding the risk of respiratory depression associated with the use of opioids in these high-risk patients.

Bone marrow transplantation, when it is undertaken early, may slow or halt the progression of the disease, but not when neuropsychologic signs are advanced. Bone marrow transplantation may be a reasonable option for presymptomatic patients, or while neuropsychologic function and independence in activities of daily living remain intact. Recently, the outcome of umbilical cord blood transplantation in three siblings with juvenile metachromatic leukodystrophy at different stages of disease has been described [Pierson et al., 2008]. After transplant, the oldest sibling experienced disease progression, whereas his two siblings had near- or total resolution of signal abnormalities on neuroimaging. Neuropsychological testing has remained stable, and nerve conduction studies have shown improvement.

Investigators are currently examining the role of mesenchymal stem cell infusion. In a study of four patients with metachromatic leukodystrophy, there were significant improvements in nerve conduction velocities after mesenchymal stem cell infusion [Koc et al., 2002]. Bone mineral density was either maintained or slightly improved in all the patients. However, there was no clinically apparent change in the patients' overall health and mental and physical development after mesenchymal stem cell infusion. Enzyme replacement therapy is also being evaluated as a potential therapeutic option. Repeated intravenous injection of the cognate enzyme in a mouse model of metachromatic leukodystrophy improved ataxic gait and CNS histopathology [Matzner et al., 2009]. Sulfatide accumulation in oligodendroglia and neurons has been described in the arylsulfatase A-null mouse model of metachromatic leukodystrophy [D'Hooge et al., 2001]. Neuronal sulfatide storage was most prominent in many nuclei of the medulla oblongata and pons, and in several nuclei of the midbrain and forebrain.

In the mouse studies, sulfatide storage did not affect the overall composition of most myelin proteins but specifically caused a severe reduction of myelin and lymphocyte (MAL) protein, indicating the existence of a regulatory mechanism between lipid and myelin protein synthesis in oligodendrocytes [Wittke et al., 2004]. MAL is a myelin proteolipid protein with four transmembrane domains that tightly binds glycosphingolipids with particular sulfatides. MAL is developmentally regulated in differentiated cultured oligodendrocytes, and its expression level peaks in the nervous system during myelin formation. The specific reduction and mistargeting of MAL protein may contribute to the pathogenic mechanisms in metachromatic leukodystrophy. Interestingly, there was no obvious sign of widespread demyelination in the arylsulfatase A-null mice, except for loss of neurons in two nuclei of the auditory pathway of aged mice, specifically in the ventral cochlear nucleus and nucleus of the trapezoid body. Several observations in the arylsulfatase A-null mice, such as hyperactivity, motor incoordination and slowing, and age-related learning and memory deficits, may relate to the decline of neuromotor and cognitive functions seen in patients with metachromatic leukodystrophy. These findings could be used as correlative or outcome measures in preclinical investigations of prospective therapies before their introduction in human trials.

Multiple Sulfatase Deficiency (Austin's Disease)

A defect of post-translational modification of several sulfatases leads to a neurovisceral disorder characterized by tissue accumulation of sulfatides, glycosaminoglycans (mucopolysaccharides), and cholesteryl sulfate [Dierks et al., 2009]. The gene mutated in this disease is *SUMF1*, which encodes a protein, the human C(α)-formylglycine generating enzyme, which activates sulfatases by modifying a key cysteine residue within their catalytic domains [Cosma et al., 2003; Dierks et al., 2003]. The particular clinical picture encountered in the individual patient depends on the pattern of enzyme deficiencies [Macaulay et al., 1998]. An accumulation of autophagosomes resulting from defective autophagosome–lysosome fusion has also been observed in the mouse model, which is hypothesized to play a contributory role in disease resulting from multiple sulfatase deficiency [Settembre et al., 2008]. Activated microglia have been detected in the cerebellum and brain cortex of the mutant mouse model, associated with remarkable astrogliosis and neuronal cell loss. An increase in the expression levels of inflammatory cytokines and of apoptotic markers in both the CNS and liver suggests that inflammation and apoptosis may occur during the late stage of the disease process [Settembre et al., 2007].

The clinical features of multiple sulfatase deficiency represent a combination of the neurologic findings noted in patients with early infantile metachromatic leukodystrophy and the dysmorphic facial features and skeletal deformities (i.e., dysostosis multiplex) seen with mucopolysaccharidosis [Schlotawa et al., 2008]. Patients have ichthyosis (dry, scaly skin), usually evident in the first few weeks of life [Busche et al., 2009; Castano Suarez et al., 1997]. Inclusions (Alder–Reilly granules) may be seen in peripheral blood leukocytes [Soong et al., 1988]. Associated findings include retarded psychomotor development, hepatosplenomegaly, deafness, and peripheral neuropathy [Guerra et al., 1990]. Brain MRI has been reported to demonstrate extensive diffuse symmetrical high signal in the deep white matter of both cerebral hemispheres and brainstem, with enlargement of sulci and subdural spaces and mild brain atrophy [Zafeiriou et al., 2008]. Nerve conduction velocities are decreased, and cerebrospinal fluid protein is elevated. Urine analysis reveals increased excretion of sulfatides, heparan sulfate, and dermatan sulfate.

Two unusual cases of multiple sulfatase deficiency with variable enzymatic deficiency of arylsulfatases A, B, and C have been reported. Both patients had ichthyosis, broad thumbs and index fingers, and an unusually slow progression of their neurologic symptoms [Blanco-Aguirre et al., 2001]. In addition, they lacked the hepatosplenomegaly that is typical of multiple sulfatase deficiency. Olivopontocerebellar atrophy was present, and one of the patients had a large retrocerebellar cyst. Mucopolysaccharides were not detected in the urine from either subject. Another patient has also been reported to develop early, severe visual impairment associated with prominent pigmentary retinopathy.

Analysis of the lipid composition of the brain obtained from two patients with multiple sulfatase deficiency revealed sulfatide concentration in the white matter that was 3–4 times that of normal brains [Eto et al., 1976]. The ganglioside pattern in the gray and white matter was abnormal, with a higher proportion of GM_3, GM_2, and GD_3 gangliosides. Increased amounts of glucocerebroside, ceramide lactoside, and ceramide trihexoside were also present. The fatty acid compositions of myelin sulfatide and sphingomyelin were almost normal, whereas the nonhydroxy fatty acids of cerebroside contained fewer long-chain fatty acids.

A variant of multiple sulfatase deficiency described in Saudi Arabian children presented with corneal clouding, macrocephaly, and dysostosis multiplex [al Aqeel et al., 1992]. Ichthyosis was absent, and steroid sulfatase activity was normal. Mental retardation was reported to be mild. This Saudi variant of multiple sulfatase deficiency accounts for 5 percent of all lysosomal storage disease cases in the Cell Repository Registry of the Inborn Errors of Metabolism Laboratory at the King Faisal Specialist Hospital and Research Centre in Riyadh, Saudi Arabia.

The diagnosis of multiple sulfatase deficiency can be made on the basis of characteristic clinical manifestations in conjunction with variable deficiencies of the arylsulfatases A, B (*N*-acetylgalactosamine-4-sulfate sulfatase), and C (steroid sulfatase), and four other sulfatases involved in the degradation of specific glycosaminoglycans [Mancini et al., 2001]. The identification of the responsible gene has led to characterization of several different mutations associated with variable clinical expression, including milder disease variants [Cosma et al., 2004].

There is no effective treatment. Simple emollients or those containing α-hydroxy acids (e.g., glycolic acid, lactic acid) or urea may be soothing and provide relief for ichthyosis.

Wolman's Disease and Cholesteryl Ester Storage Disorder

The enzyme lysosomal acid lipase is normally involved in the hydrolysis of cholesteryl esters and triglycerides that have been internalized by receptor-mediated endocytosis of lipoprotein particles [Wolman, 1995]. Deficiency of lysosomal acid lipase leads to the massive accumulation of exogenous cholesteryl esters throughout most organ systems, giving rise to one of two phenotypes: the severe Wolman's disease or the more benign cholesteryl ester storage disease. The observed differences in clinical disease course are likely due to expression of genetic mutations that either abolish lysosomal acid lipase enzyme activity in the more severe Wolman's disease phenotype or lead to some residual activity as in cholesteryl ester storage disease [Hooper et al., 2008; Zschenker et al., 2001].

Wolman's disease was first described in 1956 by Abramov and colleagues, who referred to it as a generalized xanthomatosis with calcified adrenals. The condition is clinically characterized by vomiting, diarrhea, malabsorption, and failure to thrive, with onset in infancy [Browne et al., 2003]. Patients are hypotonic and develop anemia and massive hepatosplenomegaly. Liver tissue sections reveal microsteatosis and macrosteatosis, and cholesterol crystals in hepatocyte cytoplasm. The adrenal glands are enlarged and calcified, features detectable on CT scans. Bone marrow aspiration demonstrates a marked increase in foamy macrophages. Death occurs within the first year of life as a consequence of liver failure, coagulopathy, and pancytopenia.

Cholesteryl ester storage disease has a more variable phenotype; it may be benign and remain undetected into adulthood [D'Agostino et al., 1988]. Lipid deposition is widespread, but hepatomegaly is the principal and sometimes the only sign of the disease, even when it is noted from birth or in early childhood. Patients develop early atherosclerosis and hepatic fibrosis, with possible evolution to cirrhosis. Atypical combined hyperlipidaemia in a patient with "fatty liver disease," in the absence of overweight, should lead to consideration of cholesteryl ester storage disease as a potential diagnosis [Decarlis et al., 2009].

The diagnosis of Wolman's disease and cholesteryl ester storage disease is based on demonstration of deficient lysosomal acid lipase activity in cultured skin fibroblasts and blood lymphocytes. Bone marrow transplantation has been reported to lead to normalization of peripheral leukocyte lysosomal acid lipase activity in a patient (6.5 months of age) with Wolman's disease and to result in the resolution of diarrhea and return of liver function to normal [Krivit et al., 2000]. At the age of 4 years, the patient was noted to be gaining developmental milestones. Follow-up data have revealed that the patient has required treatment for seizures, severe short stature, and hyperthyroidism [Tolar et al., 2009]. Treatment of Wolman's disease with hematopoietic stem cell transplantation is deemed to be extremely challenging, with the majority of attempts resulting in death because of liver failure from progressive disease or sinusoidal obstruction syndrome, as well as other transplant-related complications including infection, graft-versus-host disease, and failure to engraft [Gramatges et al., 2009].

Enzyme therapy and gene therapy experiments have been performed in the mouse model of Wolman's disease [Du et al., 2002, 2008], establishing preclinical proof of concept for these therapeutic strategies.

Mucopolysaccharidoses

The mucopolysaccharidoses are an etiologically heterogeneous group of disorders resulting from various individual deficiencies of the lysosomal enzymes (i.e., glycosidases and sulfatases) involved in the sequential degradation of glycosaminoglycans [Clarke, 2008; Muenzer, 2004] (Figure 36-16). The glycosaminoglycans consist of polysaccharide chains that are attached to a polypeptide core through a xylose link; their incomplete hydrolysis leads to tissue deposition and increased urinary excretion of the substrates dermatan sulfate, heparan sulfate, keratan sulfate, and chondroitin sulfate. The pattern of substrate storage and corresponding urinary excretion profile are influenced by the specific underlying enzyme deficiency [Hochuli et al., 2003].

Glycosaminoglycans (GAG) are engaged in the trafficking of molecules through the endosomal network, maintenance of steady state levels of intracellular and extracellular oligosaccharides and proteoglycans, the activity of lysosomal enzyme, and the regulation of GAG-dependent inhibitors (serpins, serine proteinase inhibitors and cathepsins) [Clarke, 2008]. Thus, defects in the lysosomal degradation of substrates likely influence diverse biochemical and physiological processes. Tissue deposits, when examined under the electron microscope, reveal different types of intralysosomal inclusion bodies, the most characteristic of which have been designated zebra bodies. Testing for the presence and pattern of urinary glycosaminoglycan excretion is often used to screen for the diagnosis of mucopolysaccharidosis (MPS) in suspected cases. However, this test often yields a false-negative result [Mabe et al., 2004]. Definitive diagnosis of a particular mucopolysaccharidosis subtype is ultimately based on the specific assay for a particular enzyme with use of plasma, leukocytes, or cultured skin fibroblasts.

The mucopolysaccharidoses are infrequent, with a collective incidence of about 1 in 25,000 to 1 in 50,000 [Nelson et al., 2003]. The individual disorders are assigned a number (based on the sequence of their historical description), and each has an eponymous designation. However, the former classification of MPS V and VIII as separate disorders has been dropped, after the recognition that these entities represent an attenuated form of other previously designated mucopolysaccharidosis subtypes. The relatively milder form of disease expression in certain variants has been partly attributed to residual enzyme activity associated with less deleterious mutations. The absence of perfect concordance between residual enzyme activity and the clinical disease severity is hypothesized to result from the failure to account for the efficiency of substrate synthesis.

Although each MPS subtype is due to a distinct enzyme deficiency, there is significant overlap in the non-neurologic manifestations across the individual diagnostic entities. The two most characteristic manifestations are coarse facial features and dysostosis multiplex. Coarsening of the facial features is a consequence of the storage of glycosaminoglycans in the soft tissues of the orofacial region and the underlying facial bone dysostosis. The term dysostosis multiplex refers to the typical skeletal changes and constellation of radiographic findings (e.g., bullet-shaped phalanges, flattening of the vertebral bodies and their anterior beaking) (Figure 36-17). These changes, in conjunction with deposition and thickening of the skin, lead to joint contractures and limitations in the range of neck and limb movements. Increased apoptosis has been described in chondrocytes from animals affected with MPS VI (Maroteaux–Lamy syndrome), and may be a common pathologic mechanism for this group of disorders [Simonaro et al., 2001]. Recent studies suggest that the accumulation of GAG in murine MPS I bone has an inhibitory effect on cathepsin K activity, resulting in impaired osteoclast activity and decreased cartilage resorption, changes that may contribute

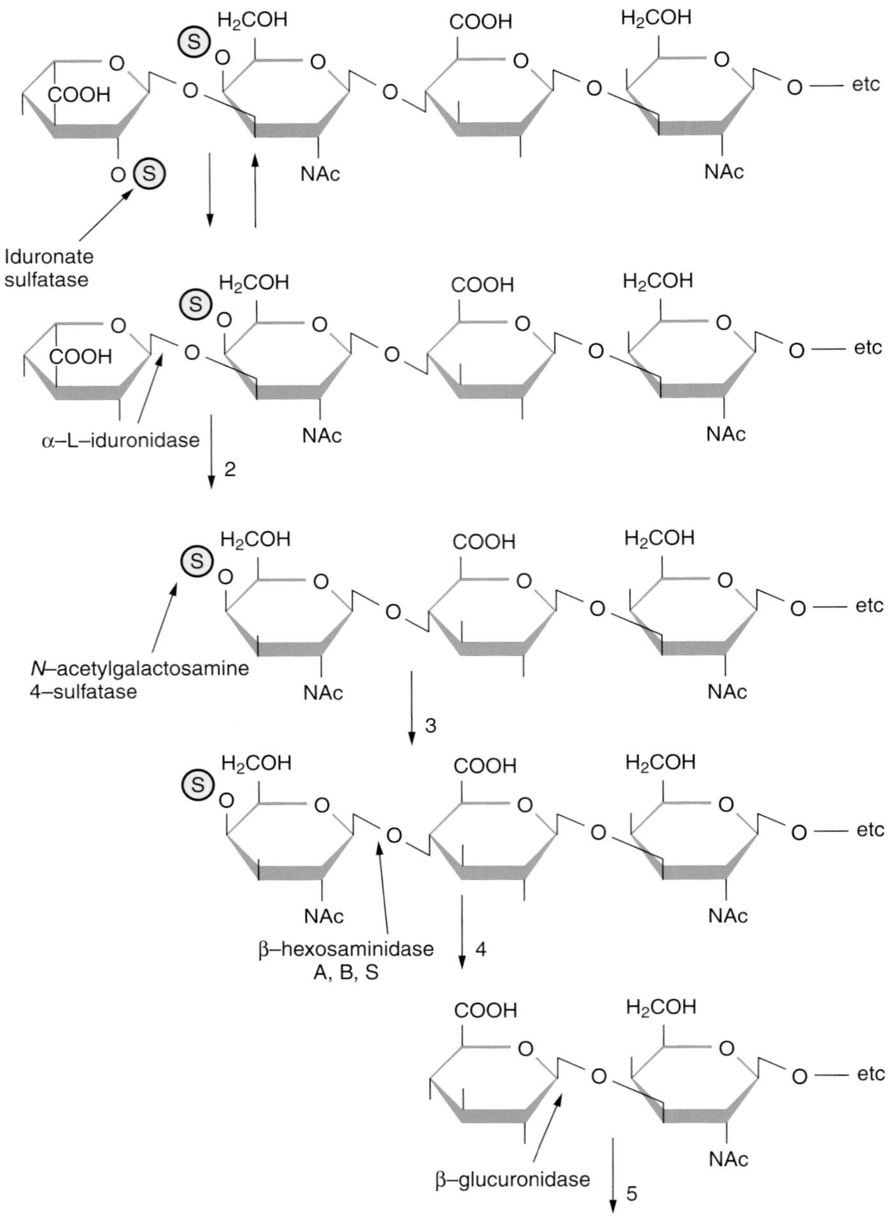

Fig. 36-16 Metabolic block in the sequential degradation of glycosaminoglycans.

to the skeletal dysplasia seen in the mucopolysaccharidoses [Wilson et al., 2009].

Ophthalmologic complications, such as corneal stromal opacity, pigmentary retinal degeneration, optic nerve atrophy, and glaucoma, are also common in patients with mucopolysaccharidoses. Membrane-bound vacuoles in the nonpigmented epithelium of the ciliary processes have been observed by electron microscopy. Multiple iridociliary cysts have also been reported in patients with MPS I S (Scheie's syndrome) and MPS VI [Sato et al., 2002]. Other abnormalities of diagnostic importance include deafness, hepatosplenomegaly, obstructive airway problems, and umbilical and inguinal hernia [Shih et al., 2002].

Recurrent upper respiratory tract and ear infections are prominent complaints in infancy, and cardiovascular abnormalities are frequent. In a study of 39 patients (aged 4–22 years) with various mucopolysaccharidoses, valvular lesions, and

different forms of cardiac involvement were detected [Mohan et al., 2002]. The most common finding, regardless of the MPS type, was thickening of the mitral valve with regurgitation or stenosis [Rigante and Segni, 2002].

Developmental regression is a feature of most but not all MPS subtypes, each of which constitutes a spectrum of disorders associated with variable expression of the skeletal and somatic anomalies noted before. The accumulation of heparan sulfate and the secondary storage of gangliosides in neurons may be partly responsible for the cerebral dysfunction. In one study, two patients with MPS IIIA with signs of CNS degeneration but only mild somatic features excreted a highly sulfated variant of heparan sulfate, whereas a patient with MPS I S and two patients with MPS II who presented primarily with coarse facial features, joint contractures, and skeletal deformities excreted a different type of heparan sulfate with lower sulfation [Perkins et al., 2001]. In the most severely involved cases,

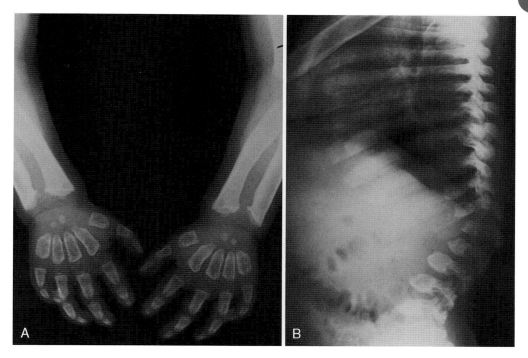

Fig. 36-17 Bone changes of dysostosis multiplex. A, Widened tubular bones and expanded metacarpal bones. B, Beaking of vertebrae and widening of the ribs. *(Courtesy Robert Gorlin, Minneapolis, MN.)*

the storage problem can be compounded by tension hydrocephalus due to the deposition of glycosaminoglycans (which leads to impairment of cerebrospinal fluid absorption) and the histiocytic infiltration and collagen proliferation in the meninges (pachymeningitis) [Paulson et al., 1974]. Progressive glycosaminoglycan storage at various sites may lead to compartment syndromes (e.g., carpal tunnel syndrome) and secondary focal neurologic deficits due to spinal cord or nerve root compression. Brain imaging studies involving 20 patients with different forms of MPS (with mental retardation in 11 individuals and normal cognitive function in 9) indicated a significant correlation between white matter alterations and mental retardation [Gabrielli et al., 2004].

The mucopolysaccharidoses are inherited in an autosomal-recessive manner, with one exception (MPS II, or Hunter's syndrome, which is transmitted as an X-linked trait). Most forms are associated with significant morbidity as a consequence of skeletal and visceral complications; application of palliative care can have a positive influence on the patient's health-related and functional quality of life [Dumas et al., 2004]. Attention to obstructive airway problems and consideration of continuous positive airway pressure or tracheostomy, when appropriate, can lead to significant relief [Khan and Khan, 2002; Shinhar et al., 2004]. Anterior instrumented correction and fusion of the spine is effective in treating the thoracolumbar kyphosis associated with MPS [Dalvie et al., 2001a].

Bone marrow transplantation has altered the course of disease in certain subtypes of MPS, and enzyme therapy has become available for MPS I, II, and VI. There have also been several studies involving different animal models (of various MPS subtypes) that have examined the potential safety and effectiveness of gene therapy for these disorders [Bosch and Heard, 2003; Haskins et al., 2002]. Substrate reduction therapy may also be a potential therapeutic option. Genistein (4′,5,7-trihydroxyisoflavone), a small-molecule nutripharmaceutical, has been shown to inhibit the synthesis of GAGs (mediated

through an epidermal growth factor-dependent pathway) in cultures of fibroblasts of MPS patients, thereby reducing tissue storage [Jakóbkiewicz-Banecka et al., 2009]. The availability of enzyme therapy for MPS I, II, and VI and its consideration in the other mucopolysaccharidoses necessitate a sensitive and reliable method not only for early diagnosis but also for serial quantitative monitoring of therapeutic responses, if any [Kakkis, 2002]. In one study, examination of urine samples from 68 patients with MPS (by electrospray ionization–tandem mass spectrometry) led to identification of an oligosaccharide profile for each group of patients [Fuller et al., 2004; Ramsay et al., 2003]. Each of the urine oligosaccharide profiles enabled the identification of all patients and their subtypes, with the exception of MPS IIIB and IIIC. In three individuals with different MPS disorders (specifically, MPS I, IVA, and VI) who underwent bone marrow transplantation, a substantial reduction in the level of diagnostic oligosaccharides was observed after transplantation. These observations provide a disease-specific fingerprint that can be used in targeted screening and the biochemical monitoring of current and proposed therapies. Two other factors have been recently identified: heparin co-factor II–thrombin complex and dipeptidyl peptidase IV (DPP-IV; CD26), which may be used as surrogate marker of disease stage and in the monitoring of treatment [Beesley et al., 2009; Randall et al., 2008].

Prenatal diagnosis is available for all MPS subtypes.

Mucopolysaccharidosis Type I (MPS I)

This disorder is caused by a deficiency of α-L-iduronidase (IDUA) in association with the accumulation in tissues and increased urinary excretion of dermatan and heparan sulfate. The phenotypic spectrum has been arbitrarily divided into three clinical forms on the basis of the age at onset and severity of disease expression. Hurler's syndrome (MPS IH) is named after G. Hurler, who (in 1919) described infants with a gibbus deformity, corneal clouding, and mental retardation. This subtype constitutes the most severe end of the clinical spectrum. Scheie's syndrome (MPS IS), formerly classified under MPS V, includes patients initially described by Scheie and colleagues in 1962. Affected individuals with MPS IS have normal intelligence, but suffer from restricted movements of their joints and develop the clawhand deformity. They may have normal or more often short stature. The intermediate form has been designated the Hurler–Scheie syndrome (MPS I H/S).

Children with Hurler's syndrome appear normal at birth but gradually develop a distinctive facies typical of the mucopolysaccharidoses (Figure 36-18). Affected infants have a large scaphocephalic head, depressed nasal bridge, frontal bossing, and thickened skin, scalp hair, and eyebrows. These findings, including developmental delay, may not be apparent even to the parents until the age of 12–15 months, particularly when the affected infant is the first-born child. A review of the past medical history often reveals recurrent upper respiratory tract and ear infections. Additional clues to the diagnosis include the presence of clawhands with stubby digits, kyphosis, enlarged tongue, hepatosplenomegaly, umbilical and inguinal hernias, and corneal opacities. The eye findings may initially be mild and detectable only by slit-lamp examination. Body hair is also often increased, and the skin has a leathery (thickened) texture.

Brain MRI in patients with MPS I reveals several abnormalities, including abnormal signal intensity in the white matter, widening of the cortical sulci and the size of the supratentorial

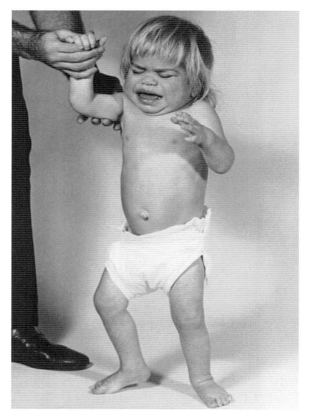

Fig. 36-18 Hurler's syndrome. This 18-month-old female with Hurler's syndrome has a protuberant abdomen, umbilical hernia, and flexion contractures of the elbows and knees. There is a widened and flattened nasal bridge and thick eyebrows.

ventricles, dilatation of the perivascular spaces, and enlargement of the subarachnoid spaces. In one study of six patients with MPS I, no relationship was found between the brain MRI findings and clinical manifestations of the disease [Matheus et al., 2004].

Skeletal radiographs in a child with Hurler's syndrome reveal a dolichocephalic skull with synostosis of the sutures, widening of the diaphyses of the metacarpals and long bones, and hypoplastic vertebrae with anterior beaking.

Complications that often develop in affected children include upper airway obstruction, coronary artery occlusion, cardiomegaly, and heart valve problems. A study involving 99 patients (aged 1–24 years; median age, 10.3 years) with MPS I found that increasing age and abnormalities of the cardiac ejection fraction were significant risk factors for death [Mohan et al., 2002]. Pulmonary complications, such as sleep apnea, develop because of airway obstruction due to a combination of factors, including enlarged tonsils and adenoids, narrowing of the trachea, and thickening of the mucosal lining of the airways. These airway problems are aggravated by a small chest and an enlarged liver and spleen pushing up against the diaphragm.

Increased intracranial pressure from communicating hydrocephalus can be a major source of morbidity if it is unrecognized. Neurosensory and conductive hearing difficulties develop as a consequence of recurrent middle ear infections, deformities of the ossicles, narrowing of the skull foramina, and pressure applied on the auditory nerve. Open-angle glaucoma, retinal pigmentary degeneration, and optic atrophy have been reported to lead to loss of vision. Death in patients with Hurler's syndrome often ensues in the first decade of life.

Children with the intermediate phenotype, Hurler–Scheie syndrome, have normal or nearly normal intellectual development. Disease manifestations, including the skeletal and other somatic features typical of Hurler's syndrome, are usually evident later (between 3 and 8 years of age). However, the clinical findings are initially less severe, and the condition tends to progress at a slower rate. Some patients reach adulthood, often with several complications as described for the patients with Hurler's syndrome, although the prognosis may be modified by the current availability of enzyme therapy.

Individuals with the attenuated form, Scheie's syndrome, are often missed because they have normal intelligence and may achieve normal adult stature. Characteristic findings on close inspection may reveal corneal clouding, short neck, stiff joints, and cardiac valvular disease. in vivo confocal microscopy images of the cornea in a 13-year-old male with MPS I S revealed brighter intercellular spaces than those of normal corneas [Grupcheva et al., 2003]. Cicatrization of the anterior stroma was identified, and the keratocytes of the middle and posterior stroma exhibited markedly altered morphologic shape, often round or elliptic, and with clearly demarcated, hyporeflective centers. In addition, the nerve fibers of the sub-basal plexus were somewhat more irregular and difficult to distinguish, possibly because of underlying fibrosis.

Radiographic studies in patients with MPS I S reveal subtle skeletal changes. These individuals often seek consultation with an orthopedic surgeon or rheumatologist because of increasing limitation in joint range of motion and development of the clawhand deformity or the carpal tunnel syndrome. As with other forms of MPS I, urinary glycosaminoglycan excretion is increased.

Molecular characterization of MPS I patients has resulted in the identification of more than 70 distinct mutations in the *IDUA* gene [Matte et al., 2003; Yogalingam et al., 2004]. Mutation analyses have indicated that, to a certain extent, the wide variability in clinical presentation of patients with MPS I is a reflection of the high degree of genetic heterogeneity [Terlato and Cox, 2003]. Two mutations, W402X and Q70X, that are prevalent among individuals of European extraction (and account for up to 70 percent of MPS I disease alleles) tend to be associated with the severe MPS I H when they are found in homozygosity or in combination with another deleterious allele. On the other hand, two other less common mutations, R89Q and R89W, tend to be found in patients with the attenuated phenotypes MPS I H/S and MPS I S [Hein et al., 2003]. Additional common mutations in the *IDUA* gene include P533R (among Moroccan and Sicilian Italian patients with MPS I) and R383H; these two mutations are associated with residual enzyme activity. In a survey of 29 Brazilian patients with MPS I, the frequency of common mutations identified was as follows: W402X, 37 percent; P533R, 11.6 percent; and R383H, 3.3 percent [Matte et al., 2003].

Palliative care, including measures to relieve signs of upper airway obstruction (e.g., continuous positive airway pressure, tracheostomy) and shunting for hydrocephalus (as indicated), is an important component of the overall management [Chan et al., 2003; Muenzer et al., 2009]. The patients also are at increased risk for complications during administration of anesthesia, and appropriate precautions must be taken before any elective surgical procedure [Ard et al., 2005; Walker et al., 2003b].

The routine follow-up care of affected individuals, including those with attenuated disease subtypes, must include a thorough neurologic examination because motor and sensory deficits (e.g., carpal tunnel syndrome, spinal cord compression) may develop, necessitating appropriate intervention to eliminate or to minimize long-term neurologic deficits. Carpal tunnel syndrome may be under-recognized because its onset is insidious and may be associated with few or none of the typical symptoms of numbness and tingling, except for thenar atrophy [Yuen et al., 2007]. The diagnosis of carpal tunnel syndrome often requires testing of nerve conduction velocities. Congenital umbilical hernias in MPS I are generally treated conservatively because complications such as incarceration or perforation are rare [Hulsebos et al., 2004].

Bone marrow transplantation in infants with Hurler's syndrome, by providing an endogenous source of the enzyme, leads to clinical improvements such as the resolution of hepatosplenomegaly and obstructive airway disease [Souillet et al., 2003]. These positive changes mostly occur in the early years after bone marrow transplantation, and clinical benefit is greatest in the patients who received their transplant before the age of 2 years. Neuropsychologic responses to bone marrow transplantation are variable and related to the patient's age and intellectual capacity at the time of engraftment [Staba et al., 2004]. Certain disease features, such as skeletal problems, have a much poorer response, likely because of the poor penetration of the enzyme into the relevant tissues [Weisstein et al., 2004]. Unfortunately, most children who successfully undergo transplantation ultimately require major orthopedic surgery for genu valgum, hip dysplasia, kyphoscoliosis, carpal tunnel syndrome, and trigger digits. Intellectual and developmental deterioration may occur, and cardiac valvular deformities

persist. A proportion of patients undergoing transplantation also experience graft failure, and life-threatening pulmonary hemorrhage has been encountered after the procedure [Gassas et al., 2003].

Enzyme therapy for MPS I has been approved on the basis of clinical trials primarily involving patients with the Hurler–Scheie phenotype. The studies proved that enzyme replacement therapy leads to improved pulmonary function (based on increased forced expiratory volume in 1 second) and increased exercise capacity (based on the 6-minute walk test, wherein distance traveled over time is measured) [Wraith et al., 2004]. Added observations noted in the treated patients include increased range of joint motion, reduction in sleep apnea or hypopnea, resolution of hepatosplenomegaly, and decreased urinary excretion of glycosaminoglycans. Weekly infusions of the recombinant enzyme (laronidase [Aldurazyme]) given to patients orally premedicated (with acetaminophen and diphenhydramine) were relatively well tolerated, despite the high incidence of antibody formation. Antibody formation was not associated with loss of therapeutic benefit, perhaps because of a decrease in antibody titers with time [Kakavanos et al., 2003]. The recombinant enzyme formulation has also been prescribed to infants not subjected to or just before bone marrow transplantation and until engraftment has been established [Wraith et al., 2007; Wynn et al., 2009]. The benefit of enzyme therapy in these clinical settings remains to be established. Reversal of somatic and visceral problems, commonly encountered in all clinical forms, is anticipated to improve the treated patient's quality of life.

Intrathecally administered recombinant human α-iduronidase given to MPS I-affected dogs penetrates the brain and reaches tissues in deep brain sections lacking cerebrospinal fluid contact [Kakkis et al., 2004]. These findings suggest that intrathecal enzyme administration may be an effective way to treat the CNS disease in MPS I. Intrathecal enzyme adminstration in a patient with symptomatic spinal cord compression has been reported to be beneficial; however, additional studies are required before this approach can be generally recommended [Munoz-Rojas et al., 2008].

Mucopolysaccharidosis Type II (MPS II)

Deficiency of iduronate-2-sulfatase is the cause of MPS II (Hunter's syndrome), the only X-linked disorder among the mucopolysaccharidoses. The clinical manifestations evident among affected males are akin to the findings in patients with MPS I, except for the absence of corneal opacities. Rarely, females with iduronate-2-sulfatase deficiency have been described, primarily carriers with inactivation of the X chromosome bearing the normal iduronate-2-sulfatase gene sequence, from nonrandom lyonization (in the presence of an X:autosome translocation) or the Turner (45,X) genotype, wherein the extant X chromosome happens to bear a mutant iduronate-2-sulfatase gene.

There are two clinical MPS II variants, which have similar somatic features but vary in degree [Wraith et al., 2008]. The MPS II subtypes are distinguished on the basis of intellectual development and rate of disease progression. In the severe form, there is mental retardation and neurologic involvement (as noted in patients with Hurler's syndrome) (Figure 36-19). In the attenuated form, intelligence is preserved or mildly impaired. Median age at death was significantly lower in patients

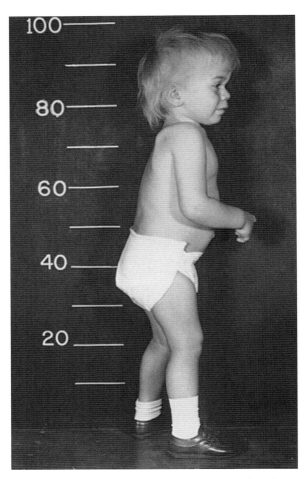

Fig. 36-19 Hunter's syndrome. This 16-month-old male with Hunter's syndrome has many similarities with the patient in Figure 36-18. Flexion contractures of the knees and elbows are prominent. The facial features are also characteristic.

An Alu-mediated recombination has been implicated in a patient with MPS II who showed the skipping of exon 8 at the cDNA level and the generation of a new large rearrangement [Ricci et al., 2003]. Laboratory studies have revealed that evaluation of residual iduronate-2-sulfatase activity by gene analysis, expression studies, and transcript analysis does not always allow prediction of a patient's phenotype.

Bone marrow transplantation ameliorates the systemic manifestions of Hunter's syndrome, but reported neuropsychological outcomes have been variable and appeared to be related to the severity. A recent report describes the outcome in eight boys who received bone marrow transplanted between the ages of 3 and 16 years [Guffon et al., 2009]. On follow-up, from 7 to 17 years post-transplant, cardiovascular abnormalities were stabilized, hepatosplenomegaly was resolved, and joint stiffness improved. Perceptual hearing defects remained stable, while transmission hearing defects improved. Only one child required subsequent surgery to correct kyphosis. Enzyme therapy (idursulfase) for MPS II has been shown to lead to a marked decrease in urinary GAG as well as reduced GAG accumulation in several tissues [Muenzer et al., 2006]. Associated clinical findings in treated patients include improvement in soft-tissue joint contractures, increased physical endurance as measured by the distance that they can achieve in the 6-minute walk test, and stabilization or improvement in pulmonary function tests [Muenzer et al., 2006]. Somatic gene therapy, with viral and nonviral (i.e., encapsulated heterologous cells and muscle electrogene transfer) approaches, is under investigation with use of MPS II primary fibroblasts [Tomanin et al., 2002].

Mucopolysaccharidosis Type III (MPS III)

The Sanfilippo syndrome (or MPS III) includes a group of patients with a similar phenotype resulting from a defect of heparan sulfate degradation on account of four different enzyme deficiencies (see Table 36-1) [Valstar et al., 2008]. Diagnosis of the individual subtypes is based on the specific enzyme deficiency, as measured in biochemical assays performed on leukocytes or cultured skin fibroblasts. Each disorder is further classified by alphabetical letters into MPS III A, B, C, and D. MPS IIIA is the most common variant, and its expression tends to be more severe. The protein that is deficient in patients with MPSIIIC has been characterized as a lysosomal membrane enzyme, heparan sulfate acetyl-CoA (AcCoA): alpha-glucosaminide N-acetyltransferase. This protein catalyzes transmembrane acetylation of the terminal glucosamine residues of heparan sulfate prior to their hydrolysis by alpha-N-acetylglucosaminidase. Several mutations have been reported among patients with MPS IIIA and IIIB [Beesley et al., 2005; Esposito et al., 2000; Yogalingam and Hopwood, 2001]; mutations in MPS IIIC and IIID are just beginning to be identified [Beesley et al., 2003; Feldhammer et al., 2009].

Unlike the other MPS subtypes that are associated with prominent skeletal and somatic features, the Sanfilippo syndrome has clinical features dominated by early and marked behavioral problems (Figure 36-20). Hyperactivity and aggressive behavior, which become apparent between the ages of 2 and 6 years, represent common initial concerns, followed by signs of arrest in intellectual development and speech delay. Altered sleep–wake cycles and insomnia are also frequent sources of parental frustration [Fraser et al., 2002]. Examination of the brain of the mouse model of MPS IIIB (alpha-N-acetylglucosaminidase deficiency) revealed P-tau in the medial entorhinal cortex

with cognitive involvement (11.7 years) compared with those without cognitive involvement (14.1 years) [Jones et al., 2009]. Neurological complications encountered in patients with Hunter syndrome include hydrocephalus, spinal cord compression, cervical myelopathy, optic nerve compression, and hearing impairment [Al Sawaf et al., 2008]. Chronic diarrhea is also a common problem in these patients, whose serial evaluations require careful attention to the potential for pulmonary and cardiac complications. Some patients have whitish macular skin lesions over the back, shoulders, and thighs; this is a distinctive dermatologic feature of Hunter's syndrome and is useful in its differential diagnosis.

The diagnosis of MPS II is based on demonstration of deficient iduronate-2-sulfatase activity in leukocytes and cultured skin fibroblasts. Prenatal diagnosis is feasible on the basis of enzyme assay. A new method for diagnosis with a novel fluorigenic 4-methylumbelliferyl substrate has been described [Keulemans et al., 2002]. Mutation analyses in patients with MPS II indicate that most have unique gene defects [Froissart et al., 2007]. However, more than 35 percent of independent point mutations at the iduronate-2-sulfatase gene locus are found at CpG sites [Tomatsu et al., 2004b]. Large deletions of the gene encoding iduronate-2-sulfatase tend to correlate with more severe degrees of mental retardation.

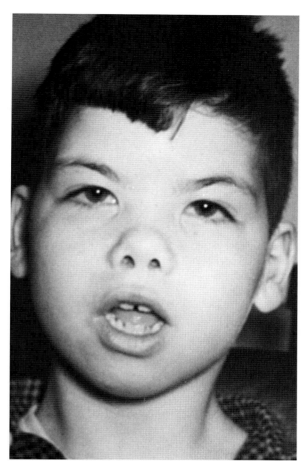

Fig. 36-20 Sanfilippo syndrome. This patient with Sanfilippo syndrome has coarse facial features, but they are not of the same degree as those seen in Hunter's and Hurler's syndromes. *(Courtesy Robert Gorlin, Minneapolis, MN.)*

[Ohmi et al., 2009]. Electron microscopy of dentate gyrus neurons showed cytoplasmic inclusions of paired helical filaments, P-tau aggregates characteristic of tauopathies. Separate studies in the mouse model have also shown that heparan sulfate oligosaccharides, which accumulate in MPS IIB, activate the degradation of synaptophysin by the proteasome with consequences on synaptic vesicle components [Vitry et al., 2009].

The disease is progressive, and the patients become severely demented and often are bedridden by the end of the first decade. An exceptional report has described two sisters with MPS IIIC with adult-onset dementia and retinitis pigmentosa [Berger-Plantinga et al., 2004]. Another report also provides a description of an adult patient with MPS IIIA who presented at the age of 45 years with hypertension [Van Hove et al., 2003]. At the age of 53 years, she was found to have severe concentric hypertrophic nonobstructive cardiomyopathy. There was no coarsening of facial features. In addition, her neurologic function, skeleton, cornea, liver, and spleen were normal.

As the somatic and skeletal features of MPS III may be subtle and the diagnosis often missed, inclusion of this disorder in the differential diagnosis of children presenting with behavioral problems is important. Studies of bone turnover and bone mineral density in three patients with MPS III revealed low serum vitamin D concentration and greatly reduced bone mineral density at lumbar and femoral sites [Rigante and Caradonna, 2004]. Screening for excessive urinary excretion of heparan sulfate may enable detection of MPS III. As testing of the urine alone may give false-negative results, in circumstances when the diagnosis remains strongly suspected, analysis for the putative enzyme deficiency should be performed [Chih-Kuang et al., 2002].

There is no specific treatment for MPS III. Investigations suggest that the sleep disruption in patients with MPS III consists of an irregular sleep–wake pattern, which at its onset might appear to be a disorder of initiating or maintaining sleep [Mariotti et al., 2003]. This finding could explain why some patients do not respond to conventional hypnotics. Therapies aimed at resynchronization (such as behavioral treatment, light therapy, or melatonin) have been recommended. Behavior modification and medications to control aggressive behavior may be required, although these approaches only work modestly at best. The use of antipsychotic medications has been reported to lead potentially to increased incidence of extrapyramidal syndrome in affected individuals [Tchan and Sillence, 2009]. Several gene therapy experiments conducted in various mouse models for MPS IIIA and IIIB provide a rationale for this approach in human patients [Fu et al., 2007; McIntyre et al., 2008]. Pathologic studies in the caprine (goat) model indicate that prenatal therapeutic intervention is likely to be necessary to prevent or to ameliorate substantive CNS and systemic lesions [Jones et al., 2004].

Mucopolysaccharidosis Type IV (MPS IV)

This subtype, also referred to as Morquio's syndrome, includes two genetically distinct enzyme deficiency disorders (identified as MPS IVA and B) [Haas, 2002]. Both subtypes are phenotypically similar or have overlapping clinical features. Intellect is usually normal, but secondary neurologic complications are frequent and related to the skeletal abnormalities and increased joint laxity [Ebara et al., 2003]. Affected patients have a high risk for cervical cord compression because of severe hypoplasia of the odontoid process and laxity of the cervical ligaments. The potential for atlantoaxial subluxation during anesthesia and while engaged in sports necessitates appropriate precautions [Dalvie et al., 2001b; Morgan et al., 2002]. Lower leg paresis due to kyphoscoliosis was reported in a 65-year-old woman who developed compression of the spinal cord around T12 to L2 [Ebara et al., 2003]. In these patients, surgery to stabilize the cervical spine is usually necessary as a preventive measure [White et al., 2009a]. With increased survival, there is a risk for respiratory failure secondary to abnormalities of the thoracic cage.

Keratan sulfate is increased in urine among affected individuals with MPS IV from deficiency of either *N*-acetylgalactosamine-6-sulfate (MPS IVA) or β-galactosidase (MPS IVB). Histological analysis, performed on bone, cartilage, and fibroblasts obtained from two unrelated patients with MPS IVA, showed that the collagen of bone and the collagen deposited by fibroblasts were normal, whereas the extracellular matrix of cartilage was abnormal and prone to degeneration [Bank et al., 2009].

Mutation analysis performed on MPS IVA patients from Latin America revealed 12 different gene defects, with R386C accounting for 32.5 percent of the unrelated mutant alleles

[Tomatsu et al., 2004a]. One mutation (R380S) was associated with an attenuated disease form.

The underlying enzyme deficiencies for MPS IVB and GM$_1$ gangliosidosis are identical; the variable disease expression has been attributed to distinct allelic mutations in the gene encoding β-galactosidase. An imbalanced substrate specificity of the mutant β-galactosidase that induces predominant accumulation of keratan sulfate has been demonstrated in skin fibroblasts of patients with MPS IVB and may be useful in differential diagnostic analysis and prognostication [Hinek et al., 2000]. Most mutations in MPS IVB are associated with homozygosity or heterozygosity for the W273L mutation, which expresses residual enzyme activity [Paschke et al., 2001].

There is no specific treatment. The anesthetic care of these patients, before any elective surgical procedures, should take into consideration increased risks resulting from the respiratory, craniofacial, cardiac, skeletal, ocular, and hepatic abnormalities [Walker et al., 2003a]. Because intellect is normal and skeletal deformities associated with the lysosomal storage diseases are not significantly modified by bone marrow transplantation, there is no role for this procedure in the management of patients with MPS IV A or B. Enzyme therapy in the mouse model for MPS IVA resulted in reduction of keratan sulfate storage in visceral organs, sinus lining cells in bone marrow, heart valves, ligaments, and connective tissues, providing a rationale for this therapeutic approach in human patients [Tomatsu et al., 2008].

Mucopolysaccharidosis Type VI (MPS VI)

Maroteaux–Lamy syndrome (MPS VI) results from a deficiency of *N*-acetylgalactosamine-4-sulfate (arylsulfatase B) in association with the excessive urinary excretion of dermatan sulfate. Investigations in fibroblasts from MPS VI patients has revealed lysosomal storage of dermatan sulfate to be associated with impaired autophagy, accumulation of polyubiquitinated proteins, and mitochondrial dysfunction [Tessitore et al., 2009].

There is a wide variability in clinical expression, including mild and severe phenotypes, with skeletal and somatic features that are typical for the mucopolysaccharidoses. Corneal opacities result from deposition of keratan sulfate and other proteoglycans in lysosomes, causing the death of keratocytes and an abnormal build-up of proteoglycans in the stroma [Akhtar et al., 2002]. These changes are believed to be responsible for the lateral aggregation of collagen fibrils and impaired fibrillogenesis in MPS VI. Degenerate swollen keratocytes, together with gross changes in epithelial, stromal, and endothelial cells, would be expected to increase light scattering significantly in these involved corneas.

Affected individuals with MPS VI usually have normal intelligence. Myelopathy secondary to thickening of the dura in the cervical region has been described. Hydrocephalus is another complication that, if unrecognized, may contribute to mental decline. The recognition of precocious excessive growth in two patients with MPS VI facilitated an early diagnosis [Heron et al., 2004]. A study involving Brazilian patients with MPS VI found no significant correlation between clinical manifestations and the levels of urinary glycosaminoglycans or the residual arylsulfatase B activity [Azevedo et al., 2004]. In this population of patients, a 23-base pair deletion causing a shift in reading frame has been found to be relatively common

[Petry et al., 2003]. Molecular characterization of the gene encoding arylsulfatase B among other groups of patients has revealed broad heterogeneity in underlying gene defects [Garrido et al., 2008].

Bone marrow transplantation in patients with MPS VI has resulted in the resolution of hepatomegaly and splenomegaly, stabilization of cardiopulmonary function, and improvement of visual acuity and joint mobility [Wang et al., 2008]. Corneal transplantation performed in a female who underwent bone marrow transplantation at the age of 13 years has been reported to help maintain clear corneal grafts [Ucakhan et al., 2001]. In clinical trials involving 39 patients (ranging in age from 5 to 29 years), enzyme therapy (galsulfase) for MPS VI led to improvements in physical endurance, as measured by the distance walked in 12 minutes and the number of steps taken during the 3-minute stair climb test [Harmatz et al., 2006a]. In treated patients, as opposed to patients receiving placebo, these findings were associated with significant reductions in urinary excretion of glycosaminoglycans. Infusions of the recombinant investigational enzyme (Aryplase [BioMarin Pharmaceutical Inc.] at 1 mg/kg weekly) were generally well tolerated. Longer-term follow-up of treated patients indicated that the clinical improvements were sustained, except in those with advanced skeletal disease who were at high risk for progression of hip disease and cervical spinal cord compression [Harmatz et al., 2008]. Enzyme therapy studies in the feline model indicate overall improvement in the disease (from a physical, neurologic, and skeletal perspective) that was most pronounced for cats treated from birth compared with those treated at a later age. These findings support the arguments for early intervention [Auclair et al., 2003].

Mucopolysaccharidosis Type VII (MPS VII)

Sly's syndrome (MPS VII) results from a deficiency of β-glucuronidase. There are about 40 cases reported in the medical literature. The disease is characterized by a wide spectrum of clinical manifestations. A severe neonatal form is associated with nonimmune hydrops fetalis [Cheng et al., 2003]. Craniovertebral instability and spinal cord compression have also been reported to occur in MPS VII [Dickerman et al., 2004].

Studies in the mouse model to elucidate the basis of the skeletal disease in MPS VII revealed that the growth plates had reduced tyrosine phosphorylation of STAT3 (a pro-proliferative transcription factor), decreased expression of leukemia inhibitory factor (LIF) and other interleukin-6 family cytokines, and reduced phosphorylated tyrosine kinase 2 (TYK2), Janus kinase 1 (JAK1), and JAK2 (known activators of STAT3 phosphorylation) [Metcalf et al., 2009]. These observations are consistent with reduced chondrocyte proliferation and ultimately shortened bones. Using brain tissue obtained from the mouse model, gene expression profile studies have indicated roles for microglial activation and induction of apoptotic pathways in the neurodegenerative process associated with MPS VII [Richard et al., 2008].

Bone marrow transplantation has been performed in a 12-year-old female homozygous for the A619V mutation in the β-glucuronidase gene [Yamada et al., 1998]. The donor cells were obtained from an HLA-identical unrelated female donor. Reported improvements included almost normal β-glucuronidase activity in circulating lymphocytes and greatly diminished urinary excretion of glycosaminoglycans. These observations were associated with improved motor function (including independent ambulation), and decreased frequency of upper respiratory tract and middle ear infections. Previous problems that the patient had experienced, such as dyspnea on exertion and vertigo, also improved.

The diagnosis of MPS VII is based on demonstration of decreased β-glucuronidase activity. Several mutations have been described in the β-glucuronidase gene [Tomatsu et al., 2009]. In the longest known survivor (a patient who died at the age of 37 years), mutation analysis revealed two novel missense mutations, K350N and R577L [Storch et al., 2003]. Expression studies revealed that the K350N gene defect was associated with residual enzyme activity, whereas the mutant protein resulting from the R577L transcript was rapidly degraded. Prenatal diagnosis of MPS VII can be made reliably by analysis of enzyme activity in amniotic fluid or cultured chorionic villi or amniocytes [Natowicz et al., 2003].

Several studies, including investigations of gene therapy, are taking place in the animal model of MPS VII [Sferra et al., 2004]. A report noted that peripheral administration of a recombinant adeno-associated virus type 2 vector in adult MPS VII mice led to transgene expression levels sufficient for improvements in both the peripheral and central manifestations of this disease [Sakurai et al., 2004]. These results correlate with findings in another study, which revealed that enzyme transport into brain parenchyma in early postnatal life in the mice was mediated by the mannose 6-phosphate/insulin-like growth factor-2 receptor, which was not observed in the adult mice [Urayama et al., 2004]. The transplantation of genetically modified bone marrow stromal cells to the lateral ventricle of newborn MPS VII mice has been found to reduce the brain content of glycosaminoglycans, with marked improvement in cognitive function compared with the untreated mice [Shen et al., 2004]. In a separate study, β-glucuronidase gene transfer led to a reversal of storage lesions in neurons that project to the gene expression site, but not in nearby structures that would have been corrected if the effect had been mediated by diffusion [Frisella et al., 2001]. In addition, transduction of cells in the subventricular zone resulted in the uptake of β-glucuronidase by cells entering the rostral migratory stream. These findings suggest that gene transfer to specific neuronal circuits or cells in the migratory pathways may facilitate delivery to the global brain lesions found in these disorders [Shen et al., 2004]. Interestingly, chemical modification of the human β-glucuronidase enzyme to eliminate its uptake by mannose 6-phosphate and mannose receptors in cultured cells, resulted in slowed plasma clearance and improved effectiveness in clearing CNS storage, compared with changes observed using the native enzyme at the same dose [Grubb et al., 2008].

Mucopolysaccharidosis Type IX (MPS IX)

The first patient subsequently classified as having MPS IX (Natowicz syndrome) had a relatively mild phenotype (compared with patients with other forms of MPS). Clinical characteristics included periarticular soft tissue masses, mild short stature, and acetabular erosions of the joints [Natowicz et al., 1996]. The patient also did not have signs of neurologic or visceral involvement. Histologic examination of affected tissues revealed macrophages with hyaluronan-filled lysosomes. Serum hyaluronidase activity was noted to be deficient, and the concentration of hyaluronan in the serum was elevated

38- to 90-fold above normal [Natowicz et al., 2003]. Hyaluronan is an important structural and functional component of the extracellular matrix. Changes in hyaluronan turnover have been associated with many processes involving cell proliferation, migration, and differentiation, and with embryogenesis, inflammation, wound healing, and metastasis. Histological studies of the knee joint in the mouse model of MPS IX showed a loss of proteoglycans occurring as early as 3 months and which progressed with age [Martin et al., 2008]. An increased number of chondrocytes displaying intense pericellular and/or cytoplasmic hyaluronic acid staining were detected in the epiphyseal and articular cartilage.

Two mutations (as expected for an autosomal-recessive trait) have been identified in the lysosomal hyaluronidase 1 gene. A 1412G to A mutation introduces a nonconservative amino acid substitution [Glu268Lys] in a putative active site residue [Triggs-Raine et al., 1999]. The second mutation is a complex intragenic rearrangement [1361del37ins14] that results in a premature termination codon. Subsequent studies have revealed that additional enzymes (hyaluronidase 2 and 3) are encoded by genes found to cluster on human chromosome 3p21.3 [Csoka et al., 2001]. The three enzymatic forms of hyaluronidase have markedly different tissue expression patterns, consistent with their differing roles in hyaluronan metabolism.

There is no specific treatment.

Glycoproteinoses

The glycoproteins are composed of oligosaccharide chains covalently attached to a peptide backbone. They consist of at least two forms, including the *N*-glycosidic asparagine-linked type, which serves as a substrate for several lysosomal enzymes. Most of the lysosomal enzymes involved in the hydrolysis of the glycoprotein carbohydrate side-chains are exoglycosidases, which sequentially remove terminal monosaccharides [Michalski and Klein, 1999]. Deficiencies involving these enzymes lead to disorders of glycoprotein degradation, referred to as the glycoproteinoses. These diseases are distinct from the carbohydrate-deficient glycoprotein syndromes associated with defective *N*-glycan synthesis and *O*-glycosylation [Marquardt and Denecke, 2003].

The clinical features of patients with a glycoproteinosis are similar to those found in the mucopolysaccharidoses, including the coarsening of facial features, some degree of dysostosis multiplex, and mental retardation. Other shared signs include hearing loss, macroglossia, and hepatosplenomegaly.

Patients with glycoproteinoses have excessive urinary excretion of oligosaccharides, the pattern of which can be discerned by thin-layer chromatography. More recently, electrospray ionization–tandem mass spectrometry has been used to identify characteristic oligosaccharide profiles from small samples of urine, plasma, or whole blood spotted on to filter paper [Ramsay et al., 2003]. However, the diagnosis of the particular underlying enzyme deficiency still requires the performance of relevant biochemical assays on leukocytes or cultured skin fibroblasts.

Mannosidosis

Mannosidosis results from a deficiency of either α- or β-mannosidase. Two clinical forms of the α-mannosidosis have been distinguished, delineated on the basis of disease onset and severity [Sun and Wolfe, 2001]. Alpha-mannosidosis has been described in humans, cattle, cats, mice, and guinea pigs. Analysis of the neurodegenerative processes relative to clinical disease in the α-mannosidosis guinea pigs has revealed widespread neuronal lysosomal vacuolation, including secondary accumulation of GM_3 ganglioside, widespread axonal spheroids, and reduced myelination of white matter; these findings were present prior to the onset of obvious neurologic abnormalities at 2 months [Crawley and Walkley, 2007]. Subsequently, additional abnormalities including accumulation of GM_2 ganglioside and cholesterol, astrogliosis, neuron loss, particularly in the cerebellum, and activation and infiltration of the CNS with microglia/macrophages were noted.

The infantile form (type I) is associated with severe mental deterioration; facial dysmorphism, dysostosis multiplex, and hepatosplenomegaly are obvious features. Disease course in these patients is brief, with death occurring usually between the ages of 3 and 10 years. In the relatively milder form (type II), mental retardation may not be evident until 2 or 3 years of life. Speech is characteristically delayed and may remain imperfect. Motor performance is poor. The examination of the eyes reveals superficial corneal opacities and spokelike posterior lens opacities. This attenuated clinical subtype follows a protracted course, extending into adulthood, and most patients become wheelchair-dependent [Malm and Nilssen, 2008]. Additional features include deafness, subtle facial dysmorphism (with prominent jaw and gum hyperplasia), and skeletal abnormalities on radiographic examination. Hydrocephalus and spastic quadriplegia may develop. Brain MRI has revealed widening of the diploic space with underdevelopment of the sinuses, prominent periventricular Virchow–Robin spaces, and perioptic cerebrospinal fluid spaces [Patlas et al., 2001]. Storage of oligosaccharides in the joints can lead to their destruction in children and young adults [DeFriend et al., 2000; Gerards et al., 2004]. Prosthetic hip replacement might be successful in some of these patients, although diminished bone quality increases the risk of loosening of the prosthesis. A report delineates the phenotype in three siblings (aged 38–47 years) with the rare adult variant of α-mannosidosis [Gutschalk et al., 2004]. All had late-onset ataxia and retinal degeneration in addition to hearing loss, cognitive impairment, and dysostosis multiplex. One sibling also had psychosis. MRI revealed cerebellar atrophy and predominantly parieto-occipital white matter changes. MRS revealed no evidence of demyelination.

Mutation analysis involving 43 patients (from 39 families of European ancestry) revealed 21 novel α-mannosidase gene defects [Berg et al., 1999]. Most of the mutations identified were private or occurred in only two or three families, except for a missense mutation resulting in an R750W substitution, which was found in 13 patients and accounted for 21 percent of the disease alleles. There was no correlation between the types of mutations found and the observed clinical manifestations.

Patients with β-mannosidosis develop severe psychomotor retardation, behavioral problems, hearing loss, and seizures. Clinical manifestations can be widely variable, even among affected individuals from the same family [Bedilu et al., 2002]. Angiokeratoma and tortuosity of retinal vessels have been observed. Serial brain MRI in a patient followed for up to 14 years showed generalized cortical and subcortical atrophy in the absence of white matter changes [Labauge et al., 2009]. Electron microscopic examination of skin biopsy specimens has demonstrated cytoplasmic vacuolization of lysosomes in the blood and lymph vessels, endothelial cells, fibroblasts, secretory portions of the eccrine sweat glands, neural cells, and basal keratinocytes in the epidermis. A few mutations in the β-mannosidase gene have been described [Riise Stensland et al., 2008; Uchino et al., 2003]. Disease presentation, even among patients with null mutations, can be variable, ranging from mild to severe.

Several patients with α-mannosidosis have undergone bone marrow transplantation. The risk of pulmonary complications is increased during the first several months after the procedure. Follow-up studies suggest that neurocognitive and cardiopulmonary function is often preserved [Grewal et al., 2004]. In addition, improvements in adaptive skills and verbal memory have been reported, with improvement in hearing to normal or nearly normal for speech frequencies.

Axonal polyneuropathy was reported to develop in a 23-year-old woman with juvenile-onset α-mannosidosis after bone marrow transplantation, complicated by chronic graft-versus-host disease [Mulrooney et al., 2003]. Progressive muscle weakness and paresthesias developed during at least 4 months and made her nonambulatory. in vitro studies involving microglia derived from the feline model reveal significant secretion of α-mannosidase (compared with the other lysosomal enzymes) [Sun and Wolfe, 2001]. This observation may explain why the disease response to bone marrow transplantation has been better. Enzyme therapy has also been administered to the mouse model for α-mannosidosis, resulting in the clearance of neutral oligosaccharide from the liver, kidney, and heart [Roces et al., 2004]. More recently, treated mice showed reversal of peripheral and central neural storage and ataxia [Blanz et al., 2008]. Interestingly, inhibition of L-type calcium channels, using either diltiazem or verapamil, partially restored mutant α-mannosidosis homeostasis in fibroblasts from affected individuals [Mu et al., 2008].

Fucosidosis

Fucosidosis results from deficient α-fucosidase activity and the accumulation of fucose-containing oligosaccharides, glycopeptides, and glycolipids in tissues, with their excessive urinary excretion. The storage material consists largely of glycoasparagines (glycoproteins) and, to a lesser extent, oligosaccharides, mucopolysaccharides, and glycolipids. There is wide variability in clinical expression, but neurologic dysfunction is a prominent feature in all [Kanitakis et al., 2005; Willems et al., 1991].

There is an early-onset form, with neurologic deterioration evident between 6 and 18 months of age and rapid progression to a state of decerebrate rigidity [Cragg et al., 1997]. In the later-onset form, neurologic regression may not be appreciable until the second or third year of life, and the disease proceeds at a slower pace [Inui et al., 2000]. In both subtypes, death usually ensues between the ages of 4 and 6 years. A third group of patients may have signs of neurologic involvement in the first few years of life, but disease progression henceforth occurs slowly and extends into adolescence or adulthood [Fleming et al., 1998]. The presence of angiokeratoma can often serve as a clue to the diagnosis of fucosidosis, and examination of the eyes may reveal tortuosity of the conjunctival vessels and a pigmentary degeneration of the retina [Fleming et al., 1997; Kanitakis et al., 2005].

The clinical distinction between the different forms of fucosidosis is artificial; the variable presentations result from allelic mutations of the gene encoding the enzyme α-fucosidase [Cragg et al., 1997]. Indeed, clear-cut differentiation of subtypes may be complicated by their overlapping occurrence in members of the same family. A survey of 77 affected individuals revealed that most have a slower disease course; death before the age of 5 years was observed in only 7 (9 percent), whereas 36 patients (64 percent) reached the second decade of life [Willems et al., 1991]. In this study, the investigators noted wide clinical heterogeneity that bore no relationship to either residual fucosidase activity or cross-reacting immunoreactive material. Mutation analyses have revealed at least 22 gene defects, including 4 missense and 17 nonsense mutations consisting of 7 stop codon mutations, 6 small and 2 large deletions, 1 duplication, 1 small insertion, and 1 splice site mutation [Willems et al., 1999]. All these mutations led to nearly absent enzyme activity and severely reduced cross-reacting immunoreactive material.

Brain MRI in affected patients with fucosidosis indicates extensive and progressive changes in the signal intensity of the white matter, including the following areas: the corpus medullare; the periventricular, lobar, and subcortical supratentorial areas; the internal and external capsules; and the internal medullary laminae of the thalami [Galluzzi et al., 2001; Oner et al., 2007]. The globus pallidus and substantia nigra may demonstrate high signal intensity on T1-weighted images and low signal intensity on T2-weighted and FLAIR images. Brain MRS findings showed a decreased N-acetylaspartate/choline ratio together with an abnormal peak at 3.8 ppm, presumably caused by accumulating macromolecules [Oner et al., 2007]. Cerebral and cerebellar atrophy have also been described in older patients with fucosidosis [Terespolsky et al., 1996].

The diagnosis is based on demonstration of decreased α-fucosidase activity in leukocytes or cultured skin fibroblasts. Serum and plasma are not suitable for enzymatic diagnosis of fucosidosis because a proportion of individuals in the general population who are otherwise healthy may have markedly decreased enzyme activity in these body fluids. Thin-layer chromatography analysis of urine may reveal an excess amount of fucose-containing oligosaccharides and glycolipids. Analysis of urine may help with diagnostic confirmation as some patients may have a relatively high residual enzyme activity. Mutation analysis is available only on a research basis.

Hematopoietic stem cell transplantation for fucosidosis has been reported in only a few patients [Sauer et al., 2004]. One report describes a 4-year post-hematopoietic stem cell transplantation follow-up in an asymptomatic female diagnosed at the age of 5 months as a result of family screening studies (performed after fucosidosis was detected in an older sister) [Miano et al., 2001]. The younger patient was 11 months old at the time of the transplant; clinical assessments a month earlier had revealed moderate hepatomegaly and mild psychomotor delay. Brain MRI revealed diffuse hypomyelination, and brainstem and somatosensory-evoked responses were altered. Thirty-two months after hematopoietic stem cell transplantation, the brain MRI revealed good myelination with small residual areas of hypomyelination and slight cerebellar atrophy. Follow-up brain scans at 38 and 46 months were reported to be nearly normal. Development was delayed but noted as better than that of the untreated sibling (who died at the age of 7 years, after a long period of paraplegia and a vegetative state). At 42 months of age, evaluations (by the Brunet–Lezine test) revealed that the child who had undergone hematopoietic stem cell transplantation had the posture and coordination of a 27-month-old and the social skills of a 24-month-old. The child was also reported to walk independently, starting at the age of 30 months.

Aspartylglycosaminuria

Aspartylglycosaminuria results from a deficiency of aspartylglucosaminidase, which is normally responsible for cleaving the bond between asparagine and N-acetylglucosamine during the degradation of N-linked glycoproteins [Saito et al., 2008]. The majority of cases have been found in Finland [Valkonen et al., 1999]. Randomized urine samples from 151 of 178 retarded children in eastern Finland identified three affected individuals with aspartylglycosaminuria (incidence of 1 in 3643), consistent with an estimated carrier frequency of 1 in 30 [Mononen et al., 1991]. In this study, aspartylglycosaminuria was, after trisomy 21 (n = 19) and the fragile X syndrome (n = 6), the most common genetic cause of mental retardation.

Affected individuals with aspartylglycosaminuria have speech problems and severe behavioral abnormalities, with alternating periods of hyperactivity and apathy [Arvio and Arvio, 2002]. Recurrent infections and diarrhea may dominate the clinical picture in the early months and years of life. Gradual deterioration in motor and mental functions develops insidiously between the ages of 5 and 15 years. Mild coarsening of the facial features and skeletal abnormalities (i.e., deformities of the thoracolumbar vertebrae, periosteal thickening of the long bones, and thickening of the calvaria) are usually evident by adolescence [Arvio et al., 2002a]. An analysis of facial photographs of 76 patients with aspartylglycosaminuria revealed a consistent dysmorphic gestalt with hypertelorism, short and broad nose with round nares, simple and often small ears with small or missing lobule and modest folding of the helices, thick lips, and square-shaped face [Arvio et al., 2004]. Additional findings in affected individuals include short stature and joint laxity. Epilepsy and sleep-related nonepileptic problems are common in patients [Lindblom et al., 2006]. Macrocephalia in childhood, followed in adulthood by reduced brain volume, reflected by a decrease in head size, is evident in patients with aspartylglycosaminuria [Arvio et al., 2005].

In a 21-year-old man with aspartylglycosaminuria, who had progressive severe gait disturbance with frequent falls and generalized epileptic seizures triggered by unexpected stimuli, treatment with a combination of clonazepam, valproate, and phenobarbital led to a dramatic improvement in his abnormal startle and seizures, enabling him to walk alone unaided [Labate et al., 2004]. This entity in aspartylglycosaminuria is important; progressive gait disorder with frequent falls could easily be misinterpreted as an additional irreversible manifestation of the anticipated ongoing neurologic deterioration (rather than poor seizure control).

The diagnosis is based on demonstration of increased aspartylglucosamine in urine and decreased aspartylglucosaminidase activity in plasma, leukocytes, or cultured skin fibroblasts. Interestingly, examination of a group of 131 aspartylglycosaminuria carriers (the parents of patients) revealed that 3 (2.3 percent) had chronic arthritis and 17 (13 percent) were rheumatoid factor-positive, higher than the percentages among Finns (in general, approximately 1.4 percent and 5 percent, respectively) [Arvio et al., 2002b].

Several aspartylglucosaminidase gene defects have been identified, including missense mutations (65 percent) and deletions (27 percent) [Saarela et al., 2001]. Many of these are predicted to interfere with the complex intracellular maturation and processing of the aspartylglucosaminidase polypeptide. Proper initial folding of aspartylglucosaminidase in the endoplasmic reticulum is dependent on intramolecular disulfide bridge formation and dimerization of two precursor polypeptides [Saarela et al., 2004]. One mutation, identified as the AGUFinn major, is responsible for 98 percent of disease alleles among Finnish patients; this observation permits facile screening of the population.

Hematopoietic stem cell transplantation has been performed in two siblings with aspartylglycosaminuria with use of unrelated HLA A, B, and DR identical donors at the ages of 10 years 5 months and 5 years 10 months [Malm et al., 2004]. During a 5-year follow-up, no neuropsychologic or clinical deterioration was noted in the children, who had a stable enzyme expression. The spinal fluid concentration of tau protein, a marker of neuronal and axonal degeneration and damage, peaked at approximately 12 months after hematopoietic stem cell transplantation and then declined to almost normal levels after 5 years. By MRI, an improvement of myelination in the younger sibling and an arrest of demyelination in the older one were observed [Autti et al., 1999]. Another study involving two patients who received transplants found them to be more severely mentally retarded than the patients with aspartylglycosaminuria who did not receive transplants after 7 and 5 years of follow-up [Arvio et al., 2001]. The poorer outcome in these patients may have been related to post-transplantation complications. Additional experience should clarify the appropriate counseling of families with affected children who may be deemed potential candidates for hematopoietic stem cell transplantation. Studies involving bone marrow transplantation in the mouse model showed improved clearance of the storage material in the brain by use of wild-type compared with heterozygote donors [Laine et al., 2004]. This observation underscores the need for careful selection of potential bone marrow donors.

Cellular gene therapy experiments incorporating the aspartylglucosaminidase promoter resulted in higher specific enzyme activity in glia than in neurons [Harkke et al., 2003]. The use of glial fibrillary acidic protein and neuron-specific enolase promoters also produced a clear overexpression of the enzyme in glial cells and neurons, respectively. The amount of exocytosed enzyme was significantly higher in glial cells than in neurons, and glial cells were also found to have a greater capacity to endocytose the enzyme. These data indicate the importance of glial cells in the expression and transport of aspartylglucosaminidase.

Sialidosis

Deficiency of α-neuraminidase (sialidase) is associated with at least two clinical variants (known as sialidosis types I and II). Affected patients with either form have increased urinary excretion of sialyloligosaccharides. Human α-neuraminidase occurs in a high-molecular-mass complex with several other proteins, including cathepsin A and β-galactosidase [Achyuthan and Achyuthan, 2001]. Multiprotein complexation is important for the in vivo integrity and catalytic activity of α-neuraminidase [Lukong et al., 2000].

In sialidosis type I, progressive visual loss, polymyoclonus, and seizures develop in late childhood or adolescence [Naganawa et al., 2000]. Multiple, irregular myoclonic jerks may be precipitated by action (movement), sensory stimuli, and emotional upset, and also by menstruation and smoking [Palmeri et al., 2000]. Evaluation performed in 12 patients with sialidosis type I revealed abnormal cortical excitability with preserved brainstem and spinal reflexes [Huang et al., 2008] The clinical problems that affected patients experience are often progressive and can eventually interfere with their speech, walking, and feeding. Eye examination reveals a macular cherry-red spot and, in some patients, punctate lenticular opacities [Federico et al., 1991]. Blindness and optic atrophy occur, and there is intellectual deterioration. Cerebral and cerebellar atrophy are evident on brain CT or MRI scans. In one report, a brain CT scan performed at 21 years of age in one patient revealed enlargement of the fourth ventricle [Palmeri et al., 2000]. Brain MRI performed at the age of 40 years in the same patient found severe atrophy of the cerebellum and pontine region, cerebral hemispheres, and corpus callosum.

Affected patients with sialidosis type I do not have dysmorphic facial features, bone and joint abnormalities, or hepatosplenomegaly. There is a report of an unusual case of α-neuraminidase deficiency associated with acute onset and fulminant nephrotic syndrome and with complications that led to the patient's death [Roth et al., 1988]. Pathologic examination of the kidneys revealed renal epithelial cell damage, most marked in the membranes of the glomeruli and proximal tubules.

An autopsy of a patient with sialidosis type I, whose genotype was V217M/G243R, revealed perikaryal expansion of cytoplasm, mostly in motor neurons (in the anterior horn and the brainstem), dorsal root ganglia, cerebellar dentate neurons, and some neurons in the thalamus and nucleus basalis of Meynert [Uchihara et al., 2009]. Neuronal loss in these nuclei, however, was not frequent in spite of frequent and massive cytoplasmic expansion. Neocortex exhibited a mild spongiosis with some swelling of neurons, which contained lipofuscin-like granules and a small amount of lamellar structures in lysosomes. In the cerebellar vermis, dysplastic features, such as abnormal layering of Purkinje cells, thinning and rarefaction of the granule cell layer, incomplete formation of synapse, and disordered proliferation of Bergmann's glia, were focally accentuated, suggesting some developmental abnormality not secondary to the storage process.

In sialidosis type II, there are neurologic, visceral, and skeletal abnormalities similar to those found in galactosialidosis (a distinct condition resulting from deficiency of cathepsin A). Sialidosis type II is also known as mucolipidosis type I. Affected individuals have dysostosis multiplex, Hurler-like phenotype, mental retardation, and hepatosplenomegaly.

Occasional cases in newborns with hepatosplenomegaly and ascites have been described [Sergi et al., 1999]. Further details about this disorder can be found in the section on the mucolipidoses.

The diagnosis is based on deficient α-neuraminidase activity in leukocytes and cultured skin fibroblasts (the preferred clinical material for enzyme testing). Analysis of α-neuraminidase gene mutations has revealed considerable heterogeneity [Bonten et al., 2000]. Patients who are compound heterozygotes, with a combination of a mild and severe mutation, usually have a milder disease [Itoh et al., 2002]. Patients with the severe form mainly have frameshifts or other mutations resulting in premature protein truncation [Seyrantepe et al., 2003]. Some mutations may disrupt α-neuraminidase binding with lysosomal cathepsin A or β-galactosidase in the multienzyme lysosomal complex [Ostrowska et al., 2003].

There is no specific treatment. Airway assessment and management are particularly crucial in patients with sialidosis who require elective surgery [Tran et al., 2001].

Studies in the sialidase knockout mouse have revealed progressive deformity of the spine, high incidence of premature death, age-related extramedullary hematopoiesis, and lack of early degeneration of cerebellar Purkinje cells. These observations were unique to the sialidase knockout mice and not found in the galactosialidosis mouse model [de Geest et al., 2002]. Administrations of the recombinant sialidase enzyme alone or in combination with protective protein/cathepsin A (PPCA) resulted in uptake by resident macrophages in many tissues [Wang et al., 2005]. Restored sialidase activity persisted for up to 4 days, depending on the tissue, and resulted in a significant reduction of lysosomal storage.

Galactosialidosis

Galactosialidosis results from the combined deficiency of α-neuraminidase and β-galactosidase, arising from defects of PPCA. This multienzyme complex formation allows its correct compartmentalization in lysosomes and offers the protection required against rapid proteolytic degradation [Pshezhetsky and Ashmarina, 2001]. Studies also suggest that PPCA is present in a second complex, including the elastin-binding protein receptor, the major component of the nonintegrin cell surface receptor that is involved in elastogenesis [Malvagia et al., 2004].

Galactosialidosis is characterized clinically by cerebellar ataxia, myoclonus, and visual failure, features that are usually evident in late childhood or adolescence [Friedhoff et al., 2003]. Additional findings include the cherry-red macular spot, dysmorphic facial features, hepatomegaly, and skeletal changes [Nobeyama et al., 2003]. Recurrent neuropathic pain associated with hyperesthesia, starting at 1.5 years of age, has been described in a patient with juvenile galactosialidosis [Darin et al., 2008]. Patients with juvenile onset may survive into adulthood. Early and late infantile forms have also been described. A report of a 14-year-old male patient of Middle Eastern descent described cardiac valvular abnormalities (i.e., mitral regurgitation and aortic stenosis) similar to those found in patents with mucopolysaccharidoses [Bursi et al., 2003]. The majority of reported cases have been from Japan [Kawachi et al., 1998].

The diagnosis of galactosialidosis is based on demonstration of combined deficiency of α-neuraminidase and β-galactosidase activity in leukocytes or cultured skin fibroblasts, or mutations in the gene encoding PPCA. Electron microscopic examination of skin tissue reveals membrane-limited vacuoles in the cytoplasm of the endothelial cells, pericytes, and fibroblasts. The material found in the cytoplasmic vacuoles appears to be glycoproteins with sialic acid, stained by the *Limax flavus* agglutinin (a lectin that binds specifically with sialic acid) [Nobeyama et al., 2003].

A few mutations in the gene encoding PPCA have been described. In an Italian patient with galactosialidosis and hydrops fetalis, two *PPCA* gene mutations, c60delG and IVS2+1GÆT, were detected and found to lead to a frameshift and a

premature stop codon, respectively [Groener et al., 2003]. The deleterious effect of such mutations was confirmed by the complete absence of the PPCA protein on Western blots. Molecular studies in two Dutch patients with the early infantile form revealed that one patient was a compound heterozygote, with a single missense mutation (Gly57Ser) and a single C insertion at nucleotide position 899, which gave rise to a frameshift and premature termination codon, respectively [Groener et al., 2003]. The second patient was found to be homozygous for the C899 insertion. Both patients presented with nonimmune hydrops fetalis.

There is no specific treatment. In studies involving macrophages isolated from the PPCA-null (-/-) mouse, recombinant proteins (produced by baculovirus expression in insect cells) were readily taken up [Bonten et al., 2004]. Subsequently, intravenously injected recombinant PPCA given to affected mice has been shown to be efficiently internalized in resident macrophages of many organs and leads to clearance of the lysosomal storage deposits. These findings suggest that enzyme therapy may be an effective treatment for the extraneurologic manifestations of galactosialidosis. Bone marrow transplantation in mutant animals, with use of transgenic bone marrow overexpressing the corrective enzyme in either erythroid cells or monocytes-macrophages, was effective in modifying the phenotype [Leimig et al., 2002].

Schindler–Kanzaki Disease (α-N-Acetylgalactosaminidase Deficiency)

This rare condition is a form of neuroaxonal dystrophy that results from deficiency of the lysosomal enzyme α-N-acetylgalactosaminidase, a glycosyl hydrolase [Herrmann et al., 1998]. The disorder was initially described by D. Schindler (1987) in two German brothers with progressive motor and mental deterioration who were bedridden by the age of 4 years. Additional findings included myoclonic seizures, pyramidal signs with hyperreflexia, hypotonia, and optic atrophy. Brain atrophy was noted on MRI. Cerebrospinal fluid protein level was not elevated, and nerve conduction velocity studies were normal. Subsequent investigations revealed that these patients had an E325K mutation in the gene encoding α-N-acetylgalactosaminidase (*NAGA*), which has also been found in two Moroccan siblings with α-N-acetylgalactosaminidase deficiency. The index patient in the latter family was a 3-year-old male with congenital cataracts and slight motor retardation; however, his older sibling, who was also enzyme-deficient, had no clinical or neurologic symptoms on examination at the age of 7 years [Bakker et al., 2001]. PET and administration of 2-[^{18}F]fluoro-2-deoxy-D-glucose in another 4.8-year-old male with α-N-acetylgalactosaminidase deficiency revealed that overall cerebral glucose metabolism was reduced in proportion to the degree of cerebral atrophy [Rudolf et al., 1999].

In 1989, Kanzaki and colleagues described a group of adult Japanese patients without overt neurologic manifestations but who had diffuse angiokeratoma, α-N-acetylgalactosaminidase deficiency, and increased urinary excretion of several glycopeptides [Kanda et al., 2002]. Molecular studies revealed an R329W/Q mutation in the *NAGA* gene. Immunocytochemical analysis revealed that the main lysosomal storage material in cultured fibroblasts from these patients (whom they referred to as having Kanzaki's disease) is the Tn antigen, a glycoprotein that forms the core of O-linked glycoconjugates and a substrate for α-*N*-acetylgalactosaminidase [Sakuraba et al., 2004]. In two other Japanese cases, analysis of the composition of the storage material by immunoelectron microscopy with mouse antibodies revealed GalNAc(α)1-*O*-Ser/Thr (Tn) in vacuolated lysosomes of vascular endothelial cells, eccrine sweat gland cells, fibroblasts, and pericytes [Kanda et al., 2002].

A more recent report presented another patient (aged 59 years) with α-*N*-acetylgalactosaminidase deficiency who developed sensorimotor polyneuropathy [Umehara et al., 2004]. The patient had mildly impaired intellectual function and suffered from repeated episodes of vertigo. Sural nerve biopsy revealed decreased density of myelinated fibers with axonal degeneration. Additional investigations revealed abnormal brain MRI findings (specifically, cerebral atrophy, predominantly in the parieto-occipital region, high-intensity areas in the posterior periventricular white matter, and some high-intensity spots in the centrum semiovale on T2-weighted images) and sensorineural hearing impairment.

Additional patients with Schindler–Kanzaki disease have since been described, including altogether 12 individuals from eight different families [Keulemans et al., 1996; Kodama et al., 2001]. Broad heterogeneity in clinical presentation and disease course has been noted [Chabas et al., 1994]. Investigations to date suggest that disease expression consistent with Kanzaki's disease may be due to a single enzyme (α-*N*-acetylgalactosaminidase) deficiency, and that other factors (which remain to be defined) in addition to a defect of α-*N*-acetylgalactosaminidase may contribute to the severe neurologic features encountered in Schindler's disease. The corresponding *NAGA* gene in the mouse has been described [Wang et al., 1998]. Three-dimensional structural studies of the mutant α-*N*-acetylgalactosaminidase have shown that two different gene mutations (R329W or R329Q) cause structural changes in enzyme, resulting in different substrate specificities and clinical phenotypes [Kanekura et al., 2005]. Generation of a mouse model of α-*N*-acetylgalactosaminidase deficiency may further clarify the essential pathologic mechanisms leading to variable clinical expression in Schindler–Kanzaki disease [Keulemans et al., 1996].

The diagnosis of Schindler–Kanzaki disease is based on demonstrated α-*N*-acetylgalactosaminidase deficiency in leukocytes and cultured skin fibroblasts [Prence et al., 1996]. Thin-layer chromatography can be performed to analyze abnormally excreted oligosaccharides in urine. Labeling the oligosaccharides with a tag, such as 8-aminonaphthalene-1,3,6-trisulfonic acid, also allows easy identification of the excreted compounds by matrix-assisted laser desorption/ionization time-of-flight mass spectrometry [Horiuchi et al., 2002].

Mucolipidoses

The mucolipidoses represent a cluster of disorders with clinical features that resemble those encountered in the mucopolysaccharidoses, except for the absence of increased urinary excretion of glycosaminoglycans [Spranger and Wiedemann, 1970]. Van Hoff and Hers, and Spranger and Wiedemann were among the first to draw attention to the mucolipidoses. The name for the group is derived from the combined tissue storage of glycosaminoglycans and sphingolipids, noted as concentric membranous cytoplasmic bodies. The classification can actually be misleading because each of the clinical disorders that belong to the group displays considerable biochemical and clinical differences.

Mucolipidosis Type I (Sialidosis Type II)

Affected patients have Hurler-like dysmorphic features and skeletal abnormalities. Clinical variants are delineated on the basis of age at onset. In the congenital form, nonimmune hydrops, hepatomegaly, and skeletal dysplasia are evident. Affected infants are usually stillborn or die within a few weeks [Godra et al., 2003]. In the early infantile form, hepatosplenomegaly and ascites may be evident in the neonatal period or may develop a few weeks later. The macular cherry-red spot and punctate lenticular opacities are usually demonstrable on eye examinations. Neurologic development is severely impaired, and death occurs in most patients after a few months or by the second year of life.

Some children may live longer with severe mental retardation, seizures, and motor difficulties. A subgroup of patients manifests with severe renal dysfunction and proteinuria, with survival into adolescence [Toyooka et al., 1993; Tylki-Szymanska et al., 1996]. Pathologic examination of the kidneys reveals renal epithelial cell damage, most marked in the membranes of the glomeruli and proximal tubules, findings that are consistent with the high sialic acid content of the membrane in these areas of the nephron. Chemical analyses indicate that the bulk of the stored material is in the form of polar sialyloligosaccharides of high molecular weight. In the late infantile and juvenile forms, patients exhibit mild developmental delay and signs of dysmorphic facial features and dysostosis multiplex. Patients experience progressive problems, including seizures and myoclonus, and eventually become severely disabled. Death often occurs in the second or third decade.

The diagnosis of mucolipidosis type I or sialidosis type II is based on increased urinary excretion of sialyloligosaccharides and decreased α-neuraminidase activity in leukocytes or cultured skin fibroblasts. The distinction between normal (unaffected) and affected ranges of enzyme activity in leukocytes can be quite small, and when the index of suspicion for this condition remains high, analysis of α-neuraminidase activity in freshly cultured skin fibroblasts should be performed. In addition, the overlap in clinical expression with galactosialidosis necessitates the differentiation of this diagnosis from sialidosis type II based on the added demonstration of decreased β-galactosidase activity or mutations of the *PPCA* gene.

Mutation analysis performed in three patients (including two siblings) with sialidosis type II revealed homozygosity for the C808T mutation in the neuraminidase gene [Rodriguez Criado et al., 2003]. The patients were from a small area to the east of the city of Seville (Spain), suggesting the existence of a founder mutation. Another study reported five novel gene defects, including four missense mutations and one nonsense mutation [Pattison et al., 2004]. None of the mutant alleles expressed significant enzyme activity, which likely explains the severe phenotypes of the patients.

Mucolipidosis Type II (I-Cell Disease) and Type III (Pseudo-Hurler Polydystrophy)

These disorders result from an abnormality of the intracellular transport of newly synthesized enzymes to the lysosome and the associated deficiency in the metabolism of the relevant substrates. Defects in the synthesis of mannose 6-phosphate, the recognition marker for the lysosomal targeting of several enzymes, explain the underlying biochemical abnormalities

[Dierks et al., 2009]. In mucolipidosis types II and III, UDP-*N*-acetylglucosamine-1-phosphotransferase (NAGPT) enzyme activity is defective. Studies involving patients with mucolipidosis type III have shown three complementation groups (namely, A, B, and C), suggesting genetic heterogeneity. Mutation analysis in patients with mucolipidosis type III subtype C has revealed defects in the NAGPT γ subunit gene located on chromosome 16p [Raas-Rothschild et al., 2004]. A missense mutation in the phosphotransferase alpha/beta subunit gene, which is located on chromosome 12q23.3 and encodes the catalytic portion of the enzyme, has been described in a patient with mucolipidosis III and a mild clinical phenotype [Tiede et al., 2005].

Patients with I-cell disease manifest with dysmorphic facial features, gingival hypertrophy, dysostosis multiplex, and progressive severe psychomotor retardation (Figure 36-21). Impaired cathepsin-L activity has been suggested to have a key role in the establishment of the skin and gingival abnormalities in I-cell disease [Nishimura et al., 2002]. Renal proximal tubular dysfunction has also been documented and is characterized by increased excretion of low-molecular-weight proteins, aminoaciduria, hyperphosphaturia, and high or slightly increased urinary calcium concentration [Bocca and Monnens, 2003]. In these patients, the serum level of 1,25-dihydroxycalciferol is increased, and rickets is evident on skeletal radiographs. A case of I-cell disease with neonatal cholestasis has also been described [Hochman et al., 2001]. Death usually ensues by the age of 5–8 years, usually from congestive heart failure and recurrent pulmonary infections. The clinical observation made in human patients with I-cell disease is mimicked by the feline model [Mazrier et al., 2003].

Patients with mucolipidosis type III have similar (but more variable severity of) clinical manifestations, including stiffness of the fingers (with the clawhand deformity) and shoulders, short stature, and scoliosis [Song et al., 2003] (Figure 36-22). Mild coarsening of the face with corneal clouding, mild retinopathy, astigmatism, and cardiac valve involvement are also commonly seen [Pourjavan et al., 2002]. The condition can progress into adulthood. Bone involvement is slowly progressive, and bone pain and disability due to destruction of hip joints are the most frequent source of debilitation [Tylki-Szymanska et al., 2002a].

The diagnosis of mucolipidosis types II and III is based on a combination of biochemical studies involving plasma, leukocytes, and cultured skin fibroblasts. Affected individuals usually have markedly increased lysosomal enzyme activities (such as those of hexosaminidase and arylsulfatase A) in plasma; the corresponding activities in cultured skin fibroblasts are markedly decreased (except for β-glucosidase). Increased rates of lysosomal enzyme activities (found in the culture medium) are noted with increasing incubation time, usually to a greater extent among affected patients than in normal control subjects.

Examination of peripheral blood lymphocytes obtained from affected individuals reveals vacuole-like inclusions that are negative for periodic acid–Schiff and Sudan black B staining [van der Meer et al., 2001].

Prenatal diagnosis is feasible, using cultured chorionic villi or amniocytes and the same enzyme assays applied to cultured

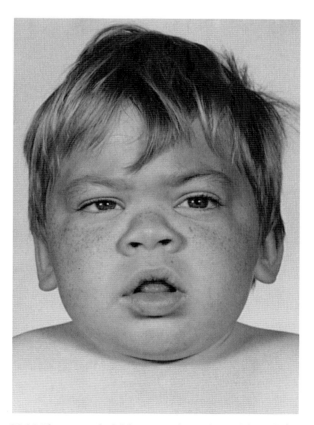

Fig. 36-21 The coarse facial features of a patient with I-cell disease, These are reminiscent of Hurler's disease, along with the flattened bridge of the nose and widened alae nasi.

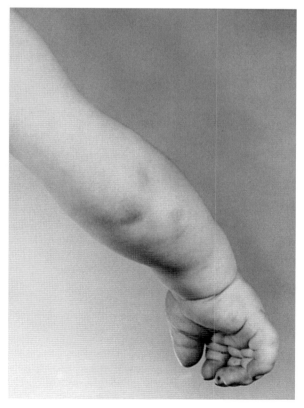

Fig. 36-22 This patient with I-cell disease has a characteristic contracture of the elbow. The widened hand with stubby, puffy fingers is also found in I-cell disease.

skin fibroblasts. Molecular analysis has also been performed, in a large Bedouin–Moslem family in which an affected individual was homozygous for the founder haplotype and the mutational single-stranded conformational polymorphism pattern of mucolipidosis type IIIC [Falik-Zaccai et al., 2003].

There is no specific treatment for mucolipidosis types II and III, although bone marrow transplantation performed in a 19-month-old female with I-cell disease revealed no new problems. Respiratory infections have diminished and cardiac function was noted to be normal at the age of 7 years (i.e., 5 years after transplantation) [Grewal et al., 2003]. The patient is also reported to continue to gain neurodevelopmental milestones, although at a very slow rate. However, musculoskeletal deformities have worsened despite bone marrow transplantation. In two siblings with mucolipidosis type III, intravenous pamidronate treatment given monthly for a year resulted in a reduction in bone pain and consequent improvement in mobility, despite the incomplete suppression of bone resorption as assessed on biochemical, radiographic, and histologic criteria [Robinson et al., 2002].

Mucolipidosis Type IV

Mucolipidosis type IV is characterized by the combination of corneal clouding, retinal degeneration, and mental and motor retardation in the absence of dysmorphic facial features [Altarescu et al., 2002]. Patients with mucolipidosis type IV do not have signs of hepatosplenomegaly or skeletal abnormalities. The responsible gene (*MCOLN1* mapped to chromosome 19p13.3–13.2) has been characterized and found to encode a protein called mucolipin, which normally functions as a calcium-permeable cation channel that is also involved in lysosomal biogenesis and membrane trafficking [LaPlante et al., 2002; Sun et al., 2000]. Fusion between late endosomes and lysosomes is a calcium-dependent process, related to signaling pathways involved in the regulation of intracellular calcium homeostasis [LaPlante et al., 2004; Raychowdhury et al., 2004]. Examination of cells from patients with mucolipidosis type IV reveals enlarged lysosomes, attributed to abnormal sorting and trafficking of these and related organelles. More recently, abnormalities in lysosomal pH have been found in fibroblasts obtained from patients with mucolipidosis type IV, which suggests that an alteration of the lysosomal microenvironment may be the basis for the storage of various substrates [Soyombo et al., 2006]. Yeast two-hybrid and co-immunoprecipitation experiments identified interactions between TRPML1 and Hsc70 and Hsp40, members of a molecular chaperone complex required for protein transport into the lysosome during chaperone-mediated autophagy [Venugopal et al., 2009]. These findings implicate defects in autophagy as a putatitve disease mechanism.

Studies in the mouse model of mucolipidosis type IV revealed ganglioside accumulation, including increases in GM_2, GM_3, and GD_3, and redistribution of GM_1, throughout the CNS, independent of significant cholesterol accumulation [Micsenyi et al., 2009]. In addition, P62/Sequestosome 1 (P62/SQSTM1) inclusions were identified, suggesting deficiencies in protein degradation. Glial cell activation was increased in brain, and there was evidence of reduced myelination in cerebral and cerebellar white matter tracts. Moreover, axonal spheroids were prevalent in white matter tracts and Purkinje cell axons.

Affected individuals usually present with arrested neurologic development and visual impairment between 3 and 8 months of age. There also is severe impairment in motor development, and most patients eventually lose the ability to walk independently. Speech is generally lacking. Corneal opacity may be observed, and retinal degeneration with amblyopia and an "extinction" (electronegative) pattern on electroretinography is usually demonstrable [Pradhan et al., 2002]. Ophthalmologic findings in patients with mucolipidosis type IV have been extensively characterized [Smith et al., 2002]. In this study, all patients were found to have some degree of corneal epithelial haze, optic nerve pallor, retinal vascular attenuation, and retinal pigment epithelial changes. The eye findings were noted to be age-related. Conjunctival cytologic studies reported characteristic lysosomal inclusions on light and electron microscopy.

Variability in the clinical expression of mucolipidosis type IV has been described [Chitayat et al., 1991; Reis et al., 1993]. The disease usually runs a protracted course, extending well into adolescence and early adulthood. Correlation of the genotype with the neurologic handicap and corpus callosum dysplasia has been described [Frei et al., 1998].

Brain imaging studies involving 14 patients with mucolipidosis type IV (including 11 children and 3 adults) have revealed significant reductions in the ratios of *N*-acetylaspartate/creatine-phosphocreatine and *N*-acetylaspartate/choline-containing compounds [Bonavita et al., 2003]. No difference was found for the ratio of *N*-acetylaspartate/creatine-phosphocreatine between younger and older patients, suggesting that mucolipidosis type IV may be a largely static developmental encephalopathy associated with diffuse neuronal and axonal damage or dysfunction.

The diagnosis of mucolipidosis type IV was previously based on demonstration by electron microscopy of lysosomal inclusions in conjunctival and skin biopsy specimens. In skin there are several types of lysosomal residual bodies, membrane-bound vacuoles, and avacuolar lamellar bodies resembling membranous cytoplasmic bodies, containing a diverse spectrum of lipopigments including curvilinear and fingerprint profiles [Bargal et al., 2002] (Figure 36-23). For prenatal diagnosis, demonstration of the storage bodies in cultured

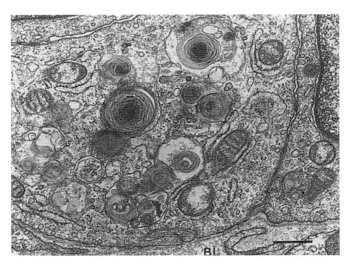

Fig. 36-23 Biopsy specimen of skin from a patient with mucolipidosis type IV.

amniocytes was used. These methods, which require considerable expertise, have been replaced by molecular genetic analysis.

Mucolipidosis type IV is prevalent among individuals of Ashkenazi Jewish ancestry, but it has also been reported in other ethnic groups. The two most common mutations among the Ashkenazi Jewish patients are an A to G transition in the acceptor splice site of the third intron (IVS3-1A to G) and a partial gene deletion [Bargal et al., 2001]. Together, these two mutations account for approximately 95 percent of the Ashkenazi Jewish mucolipidosis type IV alleles, enabling targeted population screening to identify carrier couples at risk of having an affected child [Edelmann et al., 2002]. Non-Jewish patients with mucolipidosis type IV are usually compound heterozygotes for rare disease-causing alleles [Bargal et al., 2001].

There is no specific treatment for mucolipidosis type IV, although the corneal clouding can be decreased by the regular use of artificial tears.

Glycogen Storage Disease Type II (Pompe's Disease)

This disorder of glycogen metabolism is due to a deficiency of the lysosomal hydrolase α-glucosidase (also known as acid maltase). There is a range of phenotypes resulting from α-glucosidase deficiency, from the most severe presentation known as classic infantile-onset Pompe's disease to the later-onset (proximal-type) myopathy [Kishnani and Howell, 2004]. The prevalence of Pompe disease has been estimated to be 1 in 146,000, although it is found to be higher in certain populations, such as the Chinese (1:50,000) [Ko et al., 1999].

In Pompe's disease, affected infants usually present with cardiomegaly and hypotonia during the first 6 months of life, with death due to cardiorespiratory failure usually before 2 years of age. The chances of survival beyond 1 year of life were better when signs of disease were not manifest until after 6 months of age, and when residual α-glucosidase activity was present [Kishnani et al., 2006]. An age-related increase in the diastolic thickness of the left ventricular posterior wall and the cardiac weight (at postmortem examination) has been noted [van den Hout et al., 2003].The physiologic effects of severe myocardial hypertrophy and existing or potential ventricular dysfunction in patients with glycogen storage disease type II necessitate careful monitoring, attention to intravascular volume, and selection of appropriate anesthetic induction agents before any elective procedures requiring sedation [Ing et al., 2004].

Patients with the juvenile- or adult-onset form develop progressive proximal myopathy and ultimately impairment in respiratory function. The adult form manifests itself at different ages but usually begins in the third or fourth decade as a myopathic disorder, resembling polymyositis or limb-girdle muscular dystrophy [Bosone et al., 2004]. A questionnaire-based study of 225 children and adults revealed that disease severity was associated with disease duration and not with age, although patients under the age of 15 years included a subgroup with a more severe and rapid disease course [Winkel et al., 2005]. The study also found that the odds for wheelchair use and respiratory support increased by 13 percent and by 8 percent, respectively, per year following diagnosis. Death usually occurred secondary to respiratory failure by 6 years of age (range 0.9–24) for patients who presented before age 1 year,

and by 25 years (6.5-40.5) in those who presented between 1 and 18 years of age. Mean age at death among patients who presented after 18 years was 44.9 years (25–66).

Sarcoplasmic accumulation of sarcolemmal proteins, including dystrophin and sarcoglycans, has been demonstrated around some of the glycogen vacuoles and within nonvacuolated fibers. Utrophin has also been discovered to be upregulated and found at extrajunctional sarcolemmal locations of many fibers. These results demonstrate a close association of dystrophin and sarcoglycans during sarcoplasmic processing, and may suggest a mechanism for the myopathy found in patients with α-glucosidase deficiency [Radojevic et al., 2003]. A combination of disuse atrophy and lipofuscin-mediated apoptosis of myocytes is also thought to contribute to the gradual loss of muscle mass. The presence of α-glucosidase deficiency has also been noted to affect the homeostasis of receptors (e.g., glucose transporter 4) cycling through the endosomes-lysosomes [Radojevic et al., 2003]. This disorder is further reviewed in Chapters 35 and 94.

A few cases of acid maltase deficiency with onset in the sixth and seventh decades have been described [Swash et al., 1985]. In these later-onset cases, deep tendon reflexes may be normal, diminished, or absent. Serum creatine kinase and liver transaminase levels may be moderately elevated (or even normal in the later-onset cases). Electrocardiogram abnormalities and arrhythmias may be present, although cardiac enlargement generally does not occur in the juvenile- or adult-onset form (in contrast to the infantile form). Intracranial aneurysms, especially of the basilar district, have also been reported as an associated feature.

Electromyography in patients with glycogen storage disease type II reveals variable pseudomyotonic discharges and irritability. Muscle MRI has demonstrated a selective progressive pattern of muscle involvement, with a constant involvement of the adductor magnus and semimembranous muscles at the early stage of disease and a later fatty infiltration of the long head of the biceps femoris, semitendinosus, and anterior thigh muscles [Pichiecchio et al., 2004]. In advanced cases, a selective sparing of the sartorius, rectus, and gracilis muscles and peripheral portions of the vastus lateralis is also evident. Muscle strength and MRI findings are positively correlated, which suggests that muscle MRI may prove to be of value in the diagnosis and assessment of accurate muscle involvement in acid maltase deficiency and in monitoring of the progression of the disorder or its response to therapy (if any).

Sleep-disordered breathing and respiratory failure are major complications in patients with later-onset glycogen storage disease type II, attributed to diaphragm weakness. Vital capacity correlates with respiratory muscle function [Mellies et al., 2001]. Sleep studies have demonstrated that respiratory insufficiency occurs most severely during rapid eye movement sleep. Patients have benefited clinically from the institution of nocturnal noninvasive bilevel positive airway pressure [Puruckherr et al., 2004].

Assessment of the health-related quality of life of patients with late-onset Pompe's disease has revealed scores that are markedly decreased for physical health domains [Hagemans et al., 2004]. However, scores for the mental health domains were only slightly lower than in the general population. Not surprisingly, the use of a wheelchair and artificial ventilation were both noted to be associated with lower physical and social functioning scores.

The diagnosis of glycogen storage disease type II is based on demonstration of decreased α-glucosidase in lymphocytes and cultured skin fibroblasts (the preferred clinical material for analysis) [Whitaker et al., 2004]. Testing with use of rehydrated dried blood spots (on filter paper) incubated with the enzyme substrates is feasible [Chamoles et al., 2004]. In this assay, acarbose is used as an inhibitor of an interfering acid α-glucosidase present in neutrophils. This technique has been adapted for multiplex screening, with use of the relevant substrates for the diagnosis of the following additional lysosomal storage diseases: Gaucher's disease, Niemann–Pick disease types A and B, Fabry's disease, and Krabbe's disease. Thus, this diagnostic approach may prove to be useful in targeted populations or newborn screening programs. In countries where the enzyme assay may not be available for prenatal diagnosis, electron microscopy for the detection of fibrocytes with the typical glycogen-filled vacuoles has been performed [Phupong et al., 2005].

Several mutations in the α-glucosidase gene have been identified, including missense, nonsense, and frameshift mutations [Fernandez-Hojas et al., 2002; Lam et al., 2003; Montalvo et al., 2004]. Patients with an attenuated phenotype usually have α-glucosidase gene mutations associated with residual enzyme activity [Hermans et al., 2004; Kroos et al., 2004]. Most adult-onset patients (up to 70 percent) share the same defect: namely, a splicing out of exon 2 caused by a 13 T to G transversion in intron 1 [Laforet et al., 2000].

Enzyme therapy for Pompe's disease decreases left ventricular mass and posterior wall thickness [Reuser et al., 2002]. Life span was also increased in the treated patients, beyond the expected length of survival for untreated patients. Improved skeletal muscle (i.e., gross motor) strength has been seen in some but not all patients [Van den Hout et al., 2004]. Relatively high doses of recombinant human α-glucosidase may be required to reduce the abnormal glycogen storage in cardiac and skeletal muscles because of the inefficient cation-independent mannose 6-phosphate receptor-mediated endocytosis of the enzyme by the affected target cells [Zhu et al., 2004]. The recombinant enzyme formulation that has been used in the different trials was isolated from Chinese hamster ovary cells in culture or the milk of transgenic rabbits.

Reversible nephrotic syndrome during prolonged, high-dose, experimental enzyme therapy with recombinant human α-glucosidase has been observed in one patient [Hunley et al., 2004]. Histologic evaluation of kidney tissue revealed glomerular deposition of immune complexes containing recombinant human α-glucosidase itself, in a pattern of membranous nephropathy. The nephrotic syndrome gradually resolved after the dose of recombinant human α-glucosidase was decreased, indicating that decrease of the antigenic load can ameliorate glomerular immune complex deposition associated with enzyme replacement in a highly sensitized patient. Antibody formation may potentially limit the extent and duration of clinical benefit derived from enzyme therapy, and may necessitate the use of immunomodulation in certain cases to enable an optimal response [Sun et al., 2007]. Early treatment with enzyme therapy may have a positive influence on long-term outcome, prompting the suggestion of adding testing for Pompe's disease to an expanded newborn screening program to enable early detection [Kishnani et al., 2009].

A 30- to 90-dB hearing loss was discovered in four infants with Pompe's disease who participated in a separate trial of enzyme therapy [Kamphoven et al., 2004]. Auditory brainstem response thresholds, but not the interpeak latency times, were increased, which pointed to a middle or inner ear disease rather than to involvement of the central auditory nervous system. The possible occurrence of cochlear disease was supported by the absence of otoacoustic emissions. Investigations in the mouse model revealed glycogen storage in the inner and outer hair cells of the cochlea, the supporting cells, the stria vascularis, and the spiral ganglion cells. These observations suggest that cochlear disease is the most likely cause of hearing loss, not an adverse reaction to the infused recombinant human α-glucosidase.

Oral alanine supplementation in a patient with the late infantile form has been found to result in slower progression of the skeletal myopathy and almost complete resolution of the patient's cardiomyopathy [Bodamer et al., 2002]. Gene therapy for Pompe's disease is also under investigation. Hepatic targeting of a modified adenovirus vector expressing human α-glucosidase corrects the glycogen accumulation in multiple affected muscles in the α-glucosidase knockout mice [Raben et al., 2002]. In experiments involving transgenic expression of human α-glucosidase (in skeletal and cardiac muscle of α-glucosidase knockout mice) that could be turned on at different stages of disease progression by use of a tetracycline-controllable system, it has been demonstrated that α-glucosidase levels of approximately 20–30 percent of normal activity were sufficient to clear glycogen in the heart of the young mice, but not in older mice with a considerably higher glycogen load [Xu et al., 2004]. However, in skeletal muscle, the induction of α-glucosidase expression in young mice to levels greatly exceeding wild-type values did not result in full phenotypic correction, and some muscle fibers exhibited little or no glycogen clearance. These results may have implications for the treatment of later-onset cases of glycogen storage disease type II.

There also is interest in the use of pharmacologic chaperones. Two imino sugars, deoxynojirimycin (DNJ) and N-butyldeoxynojirimycin (NB-DNJ), have been shown to increase α-glucosidase activity (1.3–7.5-fold) in fibroblasts obtained from patients carrying certain mutations (L552P and G549R) [Parenti et al., 2007]. In these experiments, NB-DNJ promoted α-glucosidase export from the endoplasmic reticulum to the lysosomes, wherein its activity was stabilized. However, the effect appears to be restricted to certain mutations and thus it is likely that this approach would only be applicable to patients with residual enzyme activity and later-onset forms of the disease.

Danon's Disease

Danon's disease (also termed X-linked vacuolar myopathy and cardiomyopathy) is due to a defect in LAMP-2, a lysosomal-associated membrane protein [Horvath et al., 2003]. LAMP-2 is thought to protect the lysosomal membrane from proteolytic digestion and to act as a receptor for proteins that are imported into the lysosome [Ruivo et al., 2009]. Defects in endosomal-lysosomal trafficking and the accumulation of autophagic vacuoles have been described among affected patients [Nishino et al., 2000]. The reason for the primary involvement of muscle cells in this condition remains to be determined, but it may be partly explained by the predominant expression of one LAMP-2 isoform (LAMP-2b) in the heart and skeletal muscles. Studies in the mouse model, which recapitulates the human disease, show that the autophagosome accumulation associated with disruption of the *LAMP-2* gene is a result of slower maturation rather than increased formation [Eskelinen et al., 2002]. Impaired recycling of 46-kDa mannose 6-phosphate receptors and partial mistargeting of lysosomal enzymes may be contributory disease mechanisms [Eskelinen et al., 2002].

Affected individuals develop abnormalities of the heart (e.g., cardiomyopathy and conduction defects) and skeletal muscles (e.g., mild proximal limb and neck weakness) [Sugie et al., 2002]. Variable degrees of mental retardation also occur. Retina and liver defects are also observed. Although it is an X-linked trait, carrier (heterozygous) females may develop disease-related symptoms. However, the incidence of disease complications is higher among affected male patients, with findings evident before the age of 20 years and in the majority during childhood (between 5 and 10 years of age) [Sugie et al., 2002].

Electrocardiography and echocardiography reveal hypertrophic or dilated cardiomyopathy and cardiac conduction problems, including the Wolff–Parkinson–White syndrome (seen in 35 percent of cases) [Charron et al., 2004]. In one survey, mean age at death from cardiac failure or sudden cardiac arrest was 19 years (range, 12–29 years) among males (n = 20) and 40 years (±7 years) among symptomatic females (n = 14) [Sugie et al., 2002]. Heart transplantation has been performed in patients with Danon's disease who have developed cardiomyopathy and heart failure, and those with heart block have undergone pacemaker insertion [Maron et al., 2009].

The diagnosis of Danon's disease can be based on demonstration of LAMP-2 deficiency through immunohistochemistry or Western blot analysis [Usuki et al., 1994]. Muscle biopsy reveals basophilic vacuoles filled with glycogen but normal α-glucosidase activity. Sarcolemmal proteins and basal lamina are associated with the vacuolar membranes. Serum levels of creatine kinase and aldolase are increased.

Several *LAMP-2* mutations resulting in splicing defects or protein truncation have been identified; mutation analysis is available commercially, obviating the need for tissue biopsy. In one report, a novel *LAMP-2* mutation of the exon 8 splice acceptor site (IVS7-1G to A), which predicts abnormal splicing, has been identified; the two affected individuals presented solely with hypertrophic cardiomyopathy [Horvath et al., 2003]. In a population survey of 197 cases with cardiomyopathy, two different *LAMP-2* mutations (leading to premature stop codons) were found in patients who evolved toward severe heart failure (<25 years old) [Charron et al., 2004]. Germline mosaicism in Danon's disease has been identified in a family wherein a son and daughter were affected and carried the same mutation that was not detected in their mother's peripheral blood or buccal cells [Takahashi et al., 2002]. This observation has important implications for genetic counseling.

Sialic Acid Storage Disorders

The sialic acid storage disorders include the allelic disorders infantile free sialic acid storage disease (ISSD) and Salla disease (or the Finnish variant). These disorders result from mutations of the sialin (*SLC17A5*) gene, which normally encodes a lysosomal membrane protein involved in the transport of sialic acid (*N*-acetylneuraminic acid), a negatively charged monosaccharide [Aula et al., 2002; Ruivo et al., 2009]. Investigation

performed in the mouse model of sialic acid storage disorders revealed that sialin is predominantly expressed in neurons of the CNS, wherein it is suspected to play a role in the secretory processes of neuronal cells [Aula et al., 2004]. Sialin is a bifunctional transporter able to import aspartate and glutamate into acidic organelles in addition to its well-established sialic acid export activity [Miyaji et al., 2008]. Thus, impaired aspartatergic neurotransmission may contribute to some neurological symptoms in patients with sialic acid storage disorders.

Another inborn error of metabolism named sialuria, which is a nonlysosomal disorder, has been described with increased sialic acid excretion [Enns et al., 2001]. In this condition, there is a defect in the feedback inhibition of UDP-*N*-acetylglucosamine (UDP-GlcNAc) 2-epimerase by the endproduct (CMP-NeuAc) of the sialic acid synthetic pathway. Recent evidence suggests that sialuria is an autosomal-dominant disorder. Only a few patients (<10) have been documented to have such an enzyme defect. A boy with sialuria monitored to age 11 years has been described. He had coarse features and massive hepatomegaly, but showed normal growth and relatively normal development [Krasnewich et al., 1993]. Similar findings were noted in a more recently described case [Ferreira et al., 1999].

Elevated free sialic acid in the cerebrospinal fluid of five adult patients, including two sisters, with cerebellar ataxia, peripheral neuropathy, and cognitive decline or behavioural changes has been described [Mochel et al., 2009]. Cerebral MRI showed mild to moderate cerebellar atrophy, as well as white matter abnormalities in the cerebellum. Two-dimensional gel analyses revealed significant hyposialylation of transferrin in cerebrospinal fluid, a finding not present in the cerebrospinal fluid of patients with Salla disease. Analysis of four candidate genes in the free sialic acid biosynthetic pathway did not reveal any mutation. The condition, for which the term CAFSA (cerebellar ataxia with free sialic acid) is suggested, represents a distinct diorder.

The sialic acid storage disorders are autosomal-recessive traits. The severe infantile form (infantile free sialic acid storage disease) presents with nonimmune hydrops, hypertrophic cardiomyopathy, ascites, hepatosplenomegaly, and inguinal hernias [Kleta et al., 2003]. A protein-losing form of gastroenteropathy has also been described [Kirchner et al., 2003]. Coarse facies (large forehead, broad depressed nasal bridge, puffed eyelids, and long upper lip) and dysostosis multiplex may also be evident. Death often ensues within the first 2 years of life.

The rare juvenile form is characterized by mild coarsening of the facial features, hepatomegaly, and psychomotor retardation [Strehle, 2003]. Lateral spine radiographs reveal mild beaking of the vertebrae. Developmental delays and growth retardation are seen in early childhood.

A third phenotype called Salla disease is named after a region in northeastern Finland, where most of the cases can be found [Varho et al., 2002]. Affected children manifest with hypotonia, ataxia, and mental retardation during the first year of life. Exotropia (squint) and truncal ataxia are also frequently noted. Walking is delayed or never achieved, and speech is usually absent or reduced. There may be mild coarsening of the facial features, but there is no visceromegaly or skeletal abnormalities. Combined growth hormone and gonadotropin deficiencies of hypothalamic pituitary origin have been described [Grosso et al., 2001]. The life span of patients with Salla disease is nearly normal.

Brain MRI reveals central hypomyelination with thinning of the corpus callosum and cerebellar atrophy in patients with ISSD and Salla disease [Parazzini et al., 2003; Varho et al., 2000]. Nerve conduction studies revealed abnormalities in nearly half of the patients with Salla disease (10 of 21) examined [Varho et al., 2000]. Four severely disabled patients and the oldest patient in the group had greatly reduced nerve conduction velocity and prolonged distal latencies compatible with demyelinating polyneuropathy. In addition, somatosensory-evoked potential was abnormal in the majority of the patients, but visual-evoked potential and brainstem auditory-evoked potential were abnormal in only a few cases. Brain MRS revealed higher N-acetyl and phosphocreatine concentrations in parietal white matter but lower concentrations of choline-containing compounds compared with the age-matched control subjects [Varho et al., 2000]. In this study, peripheral nervous system involvement was clearly associated with both the phenotypic severity and brain MRI findings.

On the basis of neurologic and neurocognitive evaluation of patients with Salla disease (n = 41, ranging in age from 11 months to 63 years), the phenotype could be classified into two main categories [Alajoki et al., 2004]. The majority of patients (90 percent) with the so-called conventional phenotype have relatively mild symptoms. Their cognitive profile consisted of better verbal ability, especially speech comprehension, compared with nonverbal functioning. All but two patients with the conventional phenotype were homozygous for the Finnish founder mutation (R39C). Four patients (aged 15–28 years) were severely disabled and profoundly mentally retarded, likely reflecting an underlying compound heterozygous genotype (with deleterious mutation) [Aula et al., 2000].

The diagnosis of sialic acid storage disorders is based on demonstration of increased amounts of free sialic acid in serum and urine [Kleta et al., 2004b]. The high-performance liquid chromatography–tandem mass spectrometry method for free sialic acid quantitation in urine is a rapid, accurate, sensitive, and selective test [Valianpour et al., 2004]. Intracellular accumulations of free sialic acid can also be demonstrated in cultured skin fibroblasts and several tissues, including the brain [Schleutker et al., 1995].

Ninety-five percent of the Finnish patients with Salla disease have a missense mutation (R39C) in the sialin gene [Aula et al., 2002]. The high prevalence of one founder mutation in this population enables targeted screening and appropriate counseling of carrier couples at risk for having an affected child.

Prenatal diagnosis of sialic acid storage disorders can be performed through sialic acid assays and genetic linkage or mutation detection analyses with use of cultured chorionic villi or amniocytes [Salomaki et al., 2001]. Currently, only symptomatic therapy is available.

Cystinosis

Cystinosis is a lysosomal transport disorder characterized by an intralysosomal accumulation of cystine, the disulfide component of the amino acid cysteine. It is the most common inherited cause of the renal Fanconi's syndrome, which manifests with acidosis, electrolyte imbalance, and hypophosphatemic rickets and failure to thrive in the first year of life. There are various clinical forms, including an infantile and juvenile variant, delineated on the basis of age at onset and severity of symptoms. Infantile nephropathic cystinosis is estimated to occur in approximately 1 per 100,000–200,000 live births [Middleton et al., 2003].

The major clinical manifestation is renal failure, which typically sets in between the ages of 9 and 10 years [Marx et al., 2004]. Affected individuals tend to have relatively fair (lighter) skin and hair pigmentation. Long-term complications that develop in a significant number of post-kidney transplant patients include retinal blindness and corneal erosions, diabetes mellitus, pancreatic insufficiency, and primary hypogonadism (in males) [Kalatzis and Antignac, 2003; Quinn et al., 2004]. Affected individuals have normal intelligence, but some adults have signs of neurologic deterioration, such as swallowing difficulties and distal myopathy [Geelen et al., 2002]. Diffusion tensor imaging (DTI) in 24 children with cystinosis (age 3–7 years) revealed bilaterally decreased fractional anisotropy (FA) and increased mean diffusivity (MD) in the inferior and superior parietal lobules, implicating a dissociation of the dorsal and ventral visual pathways [Bava et al., 2009]. The causative gene, CTNS, encodes a novel seven-transmembrane domain lysosomal protein called cystinosin, identified as an H^+-driven cystine transporter [Kalatzis et al., 2004]. Approximately 40 percent of patients with cystinosis from northern Europe are homozygous for the 57-kilobase deletion, which removes the promoter region and the first 10 exon of the CTNS gene [Mason et al., 2003]. Free (i.e., not protein-bound) cystine accumulates and forms crystals within the lysosome of most tissues of affected patients. Cystinotic cells exhibit increased sensitivity to apoptosis that might be connected to their thiol-related redox status [Park et al., 2002]. In addition, cystinotic cell lines have been demonstrated to have decreased glutathione content during the exponential growth phase, resulting in increased solicitation of oxidative defenses of the cell, as denoted by concurrent superoxide dismutase induction [Chol et al., 2004].

The diagnosis of cystinosis is based on demonstration of elevated cystine content in leukocytes or cultured fibroblasts. Serial measurement of cystine in peripheral mononuclear cells has been recommended for the monitoring of cysteamine treatment [Levtchenko et al., 2004]. Slit-lamp examination of the eyes reveals corneal crystals. Prenatal diagnosis can be done through measurement of cystine in cultured chorionic villi or amniocytes.

The symptomatic management of cystinosis includes the initiation of dialysis or kidney transplantation after renal failure and hormone replacement therapy as needed for hypothyroidism, pancreatic insufficiency, and hypogonadism [Kleta et al., 2004a; Schneider, 2004]. The angiotensin-converting enzyme inhibitor enalapril given to patients with cystinosis diminishes albuminuria and thus may slow the progression of renal insufficiency attributed to proteinuria [Levtchenko et al., 2003]. Erythropoietin has also been given to anemic patients with renal failure. Cysteamine eye drops can dissolve corneal crystals [Dureau et al., 2003; Khan and Latimer, 2004].

Chronic oral administration of the aminothiol cysteamine significantly lowers leukocyte and tissue cystine levels, resulting in growth improvement and obviating the need for thyroid hormone replacement [Gahl, 2003]. Oral cysteamine, if it is given in the first 2 years of life, often enables an increase in glomerular filtration rate. Side effects of cysteamine include nausea and vomiting [Dohil et al., 2003].

The perioperative care of a cystinotic patient requires attention to potential problems related to renal insufficiency, Fanconi's syndrome, and photophobia [Ray and Tobias, 2004]. Hematopoietic stem cell transplantation in the mouse model of cystinosis prevented the natural progression of renal dysfunction and deposition of corneal cystine crystals, suggesting a role for this approach in the management of affected patients [Syres et al., 2009].

Neuronal Ceroid Lipofuscinoses

The neuronal ceroid lipofuscinoses are a group of neurodegenerative disorders characterized by the intralysosomal aggregation of proteinaceous material (i.e., ceroid and lipofuscin) [Cooper, 2003]. These so-called aging pigments have the unique property of autofluorescence by light microscopy [Sinha et al., 2004]. Recent studies suggest that disruptions in microtubule assembly and non-muscle myosin II function may be responsible for the accumulation of lysosomal autofluorescent storage material [Seehafer and Pearce, 2009].

The term neuronal ceroid lipofuscinosis was coined by Zeman and colleagues to distinguish "familial cerebromacular degeneration" clinically and pathologically from the gangliosidoses. The nature of the responsible biochemical defect has been identified for several subtypes (Table 36-4). The abnormal products synthesized by the underlying causal genes have been demonstrated to be either a soluble lysosomal enzyme or a membrane protein that is localized to either the lysosome or endoplasmic reticulum; their functional role is not completely known [Mole, 2004a]. These disorders are also further reviewed in Chapter 41.

As a group, the neuronal ceroid lipofuscinoses represent a common inherited neurodegenerative disorder in childhood, with a combined prevalence of approximately 1 in 12,500 births [Mole, 2004b]. There are ten major subtypes that are delineated on the basis of age at onset, clinical symptoms, neurophysiologic abnormalities, and pathologic findings [Jalanko and Braulke, 2009]. Characteristic features include seizures, myoclonus, ataxia, arrest of cognitive and motor development, and retinal degeneration leading to blindness (Table 36-5) [Santavuori et al., 2000]. In the congenital form (NCL10), there is primary microcephaly, neonatal epilepsy, and death in early infancy [Siintola et al., 2006]. The various subtypes of neuronal ceroid lipofuscinoses are further reviewed in Chapter 41.

Studies in cultured fibroblasts have found that overexpression of human CLN3 (the mutant protein in Batten's disease) induces the aggregation of another protein called Hook1, potentially by mediating its dissociation from the microtubules [Luiro et al., 2004]. An associated defect in receptor-mediated endocytosis and endocytic membrane trafficking has also been found. In a newly described variant referred to as NCL9, CLN9-deficient cells were found to have altered cell adhesion and

Table 36-5 Neuronal Ceroid Lipofuscinosis: Clinical Features

Clinical Form	Onset	Typical Presenting Features	Life Expectancy
Infantile	<2 years of age	Seizures and visual loss	Usually 8–11 years
Late infantile	Between 2 and 4 years of age	Seizures	6–30 years
Juvenile	Between 4 and 10 years of age	Visual loss	Late teens to the 30s
Adult disease	Around 30 years of age	Seizures or behavioral abnormalities	Usually within a decade of onset of disease

Table 36-4 Neuronal Ceroid Lipofuscinosis

Clinical Form	Gene	Locus	Gene Product and Localization	Electron Microscopy of Storage Material
Congenital	CLN10	11p15	Cathepsin D	Lysosome
Late infantile and juvenile variant	CLN1	1p32	Lysosomal palmitoyl-protein thioesterase	Granular osmiophilic deposits
Classic, late infantile and juvenile variant	CLN2	11p15	Lysosomal tripeptidyl peptidase	Curvilinear/mixed
Late infantile, Finnish variant	CLN5	13q22	Novel 407 AA lysosomal membrane protein	Fingerprint, curvilinear, rectilinear complex
Late infantile, Costa Rican variant	CLN6	15q21–23	Novel 311 AA endoplasmic reticulum membrane protein	Curvilinear, fingerprint, rectilinear
Late infantile, Turkish variant	CLN7	4q28	Membrane protein	Fingerprint/mixed
Classic, juvenile	CLN3	16p12.1	Lysosomal membrane protein (438 AA)	Fingerprint/mixed
Epilepsy with mental retardation, Northern epilepsy	CLN8	8p23	286 AA endoplasmic reticulum membrane protein	Curvilinear or osmiophilic granular-like
Juvenile variant	CLN1	1p32	–	–
Juvenile variant	CLN2	11p15	–	–
Juvenile variant	CLN9	?	–	–
Kufs' disease	CLN4	?	–	–

apoptosis [Schulz et al., 2003]. Sphingolipid metabolism is also perturbed, and the cells have decreased levels of ceramide, sphingomyelin, lactosylceramide, ceramide trihexoside, and globoside, with an increased activity of serine palmitoyl transferase. In NCL10, there is a defect of cathepsin D, a lysosomal enzyme believed to be important for neuronal stability [Siintola et al., 2006].

The mechanism involved in cell death in the neuronal ceroid lipofuscinoses has not been conclusively determined. It has been hypothesized that the progressive neuronal loss may be related to augmented apoptosis, based on elevated concentrations of the pro-apoptotic lipid mediator ceramide in the brains of affected individuals [Mitchison et al., 2004].

Several mutations for each of the relevant genes have been identified. In the most frequently identified subtype, juvenile-onset neuronal ceroid lipofuscinosis (Batten's disease), a 1-kilobase deletion in the *CLN3* gene is the most common mutation (accounting for approximately 80–85 percent of disease alleles) [Rothberg et al., 2004]. Molecular genetic studies have also revealed that, in a few cases, defects in the same gene (i.e., allelic mutations) may give rise to more than one subtype (e.g., *CLN1* mutations may give rise to the infantile or juvenile forms) [Steinfeld et al., 2004]. In a series of 620 patients with neuronal ceroid lipofuscinosis in the Batten Disease Registry at the Institute for Basic Research in Developmental Disabilities in New York, juvenile neuronal ceroid lipofuscinosis accounted for 43.2 percent of cases; late infantile disease represented 40.6 percent, infantile neuronal ceroid lipofuscinosis 7 percent, and Kufs' disease 9.2 percent [Goebel and Wisniewski, 2004]. These various neuronal ceroid lipofuscinosis subtypes are inherited in an autosomal-recessive manner, except for some rare families with the adult form, in which the mode of inheritance appears to be autosomal-dominant [Nijssen et al., 2003]. Patients with childhood- or juvenile-onset disease experience premature death.

Brain proton MRS performed in eight cases with the infantile form (*CLN1*) revealed cortical hypoperfusion and the loss of cortical benzodiazepine receptor ligand [Vanhanen et al., 2004]. Electroretinographic studies in patients with the infantile form of neuronal ceroid lipofuscinosis document normal scotopic bright flash a-wave amplitudes with severe loss of b wave (i.e., electronegative electroretinogram), indicating dysfunction at or proximal to the photoreceptor inner segments [Weleber et al., 2004]. Histopathologic studies revealed reduced cell numbers in all retinal layers, including the inner nuclear layer, and a central epiretinal membrane. Autofluorescent lipofuscin granules have been found in all neuronal cell types in the retina.

Adult-onset (Kufs') disease is distinguished from the other subtypes by the absence of visual failure and delayed disease onset (at around 30 years of age) [Vadlamudi et al., 2003]. Two siblings of Irish descent have been described, one of whom was a 38-year-old woman with intractable seizures, delusions, and hallucinations followed by ataxia, declining cognitive function, and death [Callagy et al., 2000]. At postmortem examination, there was widespread cerebral neuronal accumulation of autofluorescent pigment, in which fingerprint profiles were demonstrated. Systemic involvement was not demonstrated. In her older brother (aged 43 years), who developed slowly progressive cerebellar ataxia, similar neuronal autofluorescent pigment was found on brain biopsy [Callagy et al., 2000].

Electroencephalographic findings in five patients with biopsy-proven Kufs' disease revealed that one patient had generalized atypical spike and slow-wave complexes and marked photoparoxysmal responses, particularly at low flash frequencies [Sinha et al., 2004]. Three patients had generalized slowing. One other patient had focal sharp and spike waves and quasi-periodic slow waves maximal over anterior regions of the head.

The specificity of the various intralysosomal inclusions (described as osmiophilic granular deposits, curvilinear bodies, or fingerprint deposits) has been the subject of much discussion, particularly the justification for using them as markers of the different neuronal ceroid lipofuscinoses (see Table 36-4) [Topcu et al., 2004] (Figure 36-24). Although the intralysosomal inclusions are somewhat pleomorphic, especially in older patients, one type of deposit predominates in each form of neuronal ceroid lipofuscinosis in biopsy specimens of skin cells, examined by electron microscopy [Goebel and Wisniewski et al., 2004]. Mitochondrial ATP synthase C protein is stored in neurons for most subtypes except NCL1, which is uniquely associated with the predominant accumulation of the sphingolipid activator proteins A and D. The storage material is widely distributed, but cell death appears to be specific to CNS neurons and the neural retina. Selective glial activation is also seen and may precede obvious neurodegeneration.

There are no current specific therapies for the neuronal ceroid lipofuscinoses, but palliative care may be helpful. Long-term antioxidant supplementation with vitamin E and sodium selenite has been given to patients with the infantile- and juvenile-onset neuronal ceroid lipofuscinoses (Batten–Spielmeyer–Vogt disease) with no clear improvement in the clinical course of the disease [Jarvela and Glueck, 2002]. Hematopoietic stem cell transplantation has been tried as a treatment for the infantile form of neuronal ceroid lipofuscinosis (PPT1 enzyme deficiency) with only transient amelioration of the classic symptoms of the disease [Lonnqvist et al., 2001]. Further studies are needed for a better understanding of the function of the defective

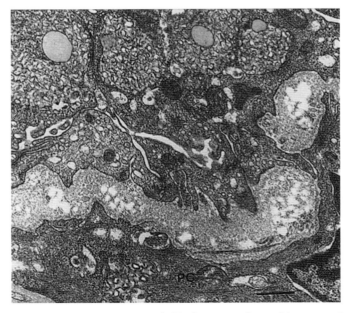

Fig. 36-24 Biopsy specimen of skin from a patient with neuronal ceroid lipofuscinosis.

proteins underlying neuronal ceroid lipofuscinosis to establish the rationale for clinical drug trials.

The management of patients with neuronal ceroid lipofuscinosis centers on seizure control and attention to other concerns, such as insomnia, malnutrition, gastroesophageal reflux, pneumonia, sialorrhea, hyperactivity and behavior problems, depression, spasticity, and dystonia [Mitchison and Mole, 2001]. Careful selection of antiepileptic drugs is important. Studies suggest that carbamazepine and phenytoin may increase seizure activity and lead to clinical deterioration [Aberg et al., 2000]. A significant proportion of patients with juvenile neuronal ceroid lipofuscinosis receiving valproic acid had sleep disturbances or excessive sedation; patients receiving clonazepam had increased salivation and respiratory secretions, which, together with gastroesophageal reflux, may increase the risk for pneumonia (particularly among bedridden individuals). Lamotrigine appears to be better tolerated and leads to relative seizure control. Low-dose risperidone, an atypical neuroleptic medication with usually few extrapyramidal side effects, given to a patient with juvenile neuronal ceroid lipofuscinosis for hallucinations, triggered a neuroleptic malignant syndrome [Vercammen et al., 2003]. It has been hypothesized that the loss of dopaminergic neurons in this condition may make these patients more vulnerable to this severe adverse effect. Benzodiazepine, particularly clorazepate, improves weight and helps control myoclonus and spasticity. Trihexyphenidyl improves dystonia and sialorrhea. Doxepin improves sleep, mood, and gastric emptying. Careful monitoring of patients undergoing surgery and anesthesia is required, with particular emphasis given to avoidance of intraoperative hypothermia [Yamada et al., 2002].

The availability of murine animal models is enabling the investigation of directed therapeutic strategies, such as gene therapy and neuronal stem cell transplantation [Guillaume et al., 2008; Haskell et al., 2003; Pierret et al., 2008; Zhong and Wisniewski, 2001]. In subtypes due to a soluble lysosomal protein deficiency, enzyme therapy may also prove to be an option, although there are potential limitations related to the presence of the blood–brain barrier and the paucity of mannose 6-phosphate receptors in neurons.

Prenatal diagnosis for the neuronal ceroid lipofuscinoses may be considered in the subtypes in which the mutant gene or enzyme deficiency has been established [Young et al., 2001].

Mitochondrial Diseases

Darryl C. De Vivo and Salvatore DiMauro

Introduction

Mitochondrial diseases represent one of the most exciting chapters of modern medicine. Knowledge of mitochondria and the relationship of mitochondrial dysfunction to human diseases has evolved during the past century, with an explosion of new information in the last decade [DiMauro and Bonilla, 2004]. During the last half of the 19th century, scientists gradually recognized the presence of subcellular organelles, and Benda coined the term mitochondrion in 1898 [Benda, 1898]. Benda was aware of threadlike granules within the cell that were barely detectable by existing methods. After this seminal observation, the metabolic role of mitochondria in cellular function was defined by a series of observations during the early part of the 20th century. The cytochrome system was described in 1925 [Keilin, 1925], and oxidation–reduction processes were described 4 years later [Warburg and Negelein, 1929]. The Krebs cycle was conceptualized in 1937, and later the phosphorylation of adenosine diphosphate (ADP) to adenosine triphosphate (ATP) was documented, together with the dependence of phosphorylation on oxygen consumption [Krebs and Kornberg, 1957]. By the middle of the 20th century, it was clear that the mitochondrion represented the intracellular domain for intermediary metabolism. In 1961, the chemiosmotic theory was proposed to explain the proton motive force that facilitates the synthesis of adenosine triphosphate [Mitchell, 1961]. In parallel with these biochemical observations, a series of studies described the ultrastructural characteristics of the mitochondrion [Palade, 1953]. The four components of the organelle were characterized, including the outer and inner membranes, the intermembranous space, and the inner matrix compartment. Subsequent studies have demonstrated that the inner mitochondrial membrane is largely impermeable to molecules of all sizes, and special adaptive mechanisms are necessary for the translocation of metabolites and proteins from the intermembranous space to the matrix. The protein importation process is energy-dependent, and requires the macromolecules to be unfolded before traversing the mitochondrial membranes and then refolded after entering the mitochondrial matrix [Bolender et al., 2008]. Surprisingly, only a handful of mitochondrial diseases have been attributed to defects of mitochondrial protein importation, and possible reasons for this are described later in this chapter.

Two important observations were made in 1963. Each observation is central to the understanding of mitochondrial diseases. The first observation recognized the presence of intramitochondrial fibers with DNA characteristics [Nass and Nass, 1963]. This observation was the first of many reports documenting DNA in mitochondria. It is realized that many human diseases are the result of mitochondrial DNA (mtDNA) mutations. The second observation was the description of ragged red fibers in biopsy specimens of skeletal muscle [Engel and Cunningham, 1963].

Because all mtDNA is derived from the ovum, mtDNA characteristics are inherited exclusively from the mother – hence the terms mitochondrial inheritance, maternal inheritance, and cytoplasmic inheritance [Fine, 1978; Giles et al., 1980]. These interchangeable terms describe a non-mendelian pattern of inheritance that characterizes human diseases resulting from mtDNA mutations. Each mitochondrion contains 2–10 copies of the mtDNA genome. Because cells have hundreds or thousands of mitochondria, more than 10,000 copies of mtDNA may exist in each cell. This genome is a small, double-stranded circular molecule containing 16,569 basepairs (bp) [Anderson et al., 1981]. The circular molecule contains a heavy and a light strand, and each strand contains its own origin of replication (Figure 37-1). Clear differences exist between the mitochondrial genome and the nuclear genome (Table 37-1). The mitochondrial genome contains no introns. The only noncoding region in mtDNA is the displacement loop (D-loop). The D-loop region contains 1000 basepairs and is the site of origin for replication of the heavy strand and the promoter regions for both light and heavy strand transcription. Because the universal genetic code does not apply to mtDNA, the mitochondrial genome requires its own transcriptional and translational factors for synthesis of mitochondrial proteins. The mitochondrial genome contains 37 genes. Thirteen genes encode structural proteins in the respiratory chain. The mitochondrial genome also contains 24 genes for protein synthesis. These genes include 2 ribosomal RNAs and 22 transfer RNAs. The mtDNA genes code for 13 messenger RNAs, and all 13 gene products are located in the respiratory chain (Table 37-2).

The mitochondrial genotype is homoplasmic if all mtDNA genomes are identical. Conversely, the genotype is heteroplasmic if the genomes represent a mixture of wild-type mtDNAs and mutated mtDNAs. The phenotype is determined by the proportion of mutated genomes; when this proportion exceeds a threshold, the biologic behavior of the cell, the tissue, and indeed the individual changes, reflecting the impaired energy state. The threshold effect is a relative concept influenced by several factors, such as the age of the patient and the energy demands of any specific tissue or organ. For example, brain and muscle cells have high energy demands, as do the tissues of the developing child. In these situations, the threshold for phenotypic expression of a pathogenic mutation is lower. The threshold may vary from 60 to 70 percent in chronic progressive external ophthalmoplegia due to single large-scale

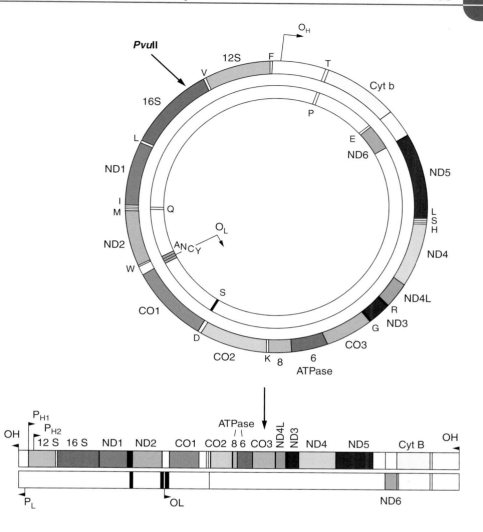

Fig. 37-1 Mitochondrial DNA contains 16,569 basepairs and 37 genes. These genes include 2 ribosomal RNA, 22 transfer RNA, and 13 structural reading frames. Digestion of human mtDNA with a single endonuclease (*Pvu*II) cleaves the circular molecule in one place and produces a linearized version. CO, cytochrome-*c* oxidase; Cyt, cytochrome; ND, NADH-CoQ reductase; O_L and O_H, origin of replication for L and H strands; P_{H1}, P_{H2}, primary transcripts of the H strand starting at H1, H2; P_L, light (l-strand promoter). *(From DeVivo DC: The expanding clinical spectrum of mitochondrial diseases. Brain and Development. 15;1–22, 1993. Elsevier Science Publishers, 1993.)*

Table 37-1 Comparison of the Human Nuclear and Mitochondrial Genomes

Nuclear DNA	Mitochondrial DNA
Located in nucleus	Located in cytoplasmic organelle
3×10^9 bp/haploid genome	1.6×10^4 bp/genome
Many introns	No introns
Diploid in somatic cells	Polyploid in somatic cells
23 linear chromosomes	One circular chromosome
23,000 genes	37 genes (rRNAs, tRNAs, mRNAs)
mRNAs encode all cellular functions	Only respiratory chain mRNAs
Universal genetic code	Modified genetic code
Exon/intron gene organization	No intron in any gene
Many symmetric replication origins	One asymmetric replication origin
Monocistronic transcription	Polycistronic transcription

Table 37-2 Structural (Mit) Gene Products Encoded by Mitochondrial DNA

Respiratory Chain Complex	Structural Protein
I	1, 2, 3, 4, 4L, 5, 6
II	None
III	Apocytochrome b
IV	I, II, III
V	6, 8

mtDNA deletions, to 90–95 percent in the syndromes of mitochondrial encephalomyopathy with lactic acidosis and stroke-like episodes (MELAS) and myoclonus epilepsy and ragged red fibers (MERRF).

Replicative segregation is a biologic concept that refers to the stochastic redistribution of the mtDNA genomes during mitochondrial and cell divisions. The random segregation of the mitochondrial genomes during replication influences the oxidative capability of the cellular progeny. The concepts of threshold effect and replicative segregation have provided some explanations for the variable phenotypic expression of maternally transmitted human diseases.

Inheritance Patterns

One of the many exciting features of mitochondrial diseases is the pattern of inheritance of these diverse conditions. The unique dual influence of the nuclear and mitochondrial genomes on the respiratory chain has captivated students of mitochondrial diseases. A biochemical defect involving the respiratory chain may be transmitted either by mendelian or by nonmendelian patterns. The strictly maternal inheritance of mitochondria determines the pattern of vertical transmission of mtDNA mutations. Clinical conditions related to mtDNA point mutations are transmitted from the mother to all her male and female progeny, but only daughters pass the condition to succeeding generations (Figure 37-2). This genetic profile is reminiscent of mendelian inheritance, including autosomal-dominant and X-linked patterns, but both genders are equally affected and there is no father-to-son transmission. Expression of the maternally inherited genetic defect is determined by replicative segregation and by the threshold effect. These biologic principles are demonstrated in several neurologic diseases associated with mtDNA mutations, including Leber's hereditary optic neuropathy (LHON), MERRF, MELAS, and the syndrome of neuropathy, ataxia, retinitis pigmentosa/maternally inherited Leigh's syndrome (NARP/MILS).

Single deletions of mtDNA generally occur sporadically, as is the case with Kearns–Sayre syndrome, progressive external ophthalmoplegia, and Pearson's syndrome.

However, the pattern of inheritance for most mitochondrial diseases is not maternal. Rather, classic mendelian inheritance patterns apply to all disorders affecting biochemical pathways other than the respiratory chain, including defects of fatty acid oxidation, pyruvate utilization, and the Krebs cycle. Also, not surprisingly, several defects of the respiratory chain are inherited by mendelian inheritance because most subunits of respiratory chain complexes are encoded by nuclear DNA (nDNA) genes. Interestingly, many abnormalities of mtDNA are also due to mutations in nDNA genes; these mendelian diseases associated with mtDNA defects are due to faulty communications between the two genomes and are usually called defects of intergenomic signaling. For example, syndromes of progressive external ophthalmoplegia with multiple deletions of mtDNA are inherited as autosomal-dominant or, more rarely, autosomal-recessive traits. Another defect of intergenomic signaling is due to a quantitative defect of mtDNA (mtDNA depletion). The nuclear gene defects in these cases alter the biologic integrity or the replication of the mitochondrial genome and predispose the patient to multiple mtDNA deletions or mtDNA depletion that characterize these clinical syndromes [Spinazzola and Zeviani, 2009].

Metabolic Disturbances

The principal function of mitochondria is the oxidation of substrates and the synthesis of ATP. The primary oxidizable substrates include pyruvate, fatty acids, ketone bodies, and amino acids. Mitochondria also play a role in the intracellular sequestration of calcium and in the detoxification of ammonia in the urea cycle. Biochemical defects involving these

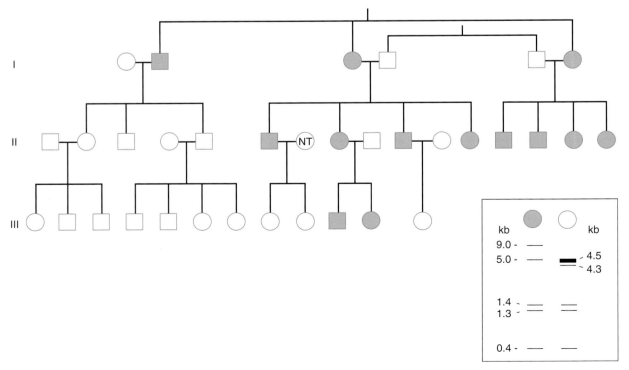

Fig. 37-2 Inheritance of a mitochondrial DNA HaeII polymorphism in a 33-member three-generation family. The typical mitochondrial DNA cleavage pattern is depicted in the open symbols, and the atypical cleavage pattern is depicted in the black symbols. NT, not tested. *(From Giles RE, Blanc H, Cann HM, et al. Proc Natl Acad Sci USA 1980;77:6715.)*

pathways are associated with distinctive metabolic disturbances. A biochemical defect altering pyruvate metabolism directly or indirectly causes an elevation of pyruvic acid. Pyruvate is in equilibrium with lactate and alanine. As a result, there is lactic acidosis that is proportionate or disproportionate to the elevation of pyruvate, depending on the associated effect of the biochemical defect on the oxidation-reduction potential. If the oxidation–reduction potential is unaffected by the biochemical defect, the lactate and pyruvate elevations are proportional and the lactate/pyruvate ratio is normal (<20). In contrast, if the oxidation–reduction potential is disturbed by a primary defect involving the respiratory chain, the lactate values are disproportionately elevated and the lactate/pyruvate ratio is increased (>20). Patients with pyruvate dehydrogenase (PDH) deficiency typically have elevated lactate, pyruvate, and alanine concentrations and a normal lactate/pyruvate ratio. In contrast, patients with cytochrome-c oxidase (COX) deficiency have elevated lactate, pyruvate, and alanine concentrations, but the lactate/pyruvate ratio is increased. These metabolic observations serve as clues to the underlying biochemical defect and may be helpful when all other clinical and metabolic factors are considered simultaneously.

Defects of fatty acid metabolism may be associated with elevated free fatty acids, hypoketonemia, hypocarnitinemia, and dicarboxylic aciduria. Patients with biochemical defects involving beta oxidation typically have hypoketotic hypoglycemia, dicarboxylic aciduria, and secondary carnitine deficiency. Medium-chain acyl coenzyme A dehydrogenase (MCAD) deficiency is the classic example. The hypocarnitinemia associated with defects of beta oxidation typically is accompanied by a disturbance of the ratio of free carnitine to esterified carnitine. The disproportionately high esterified carnitine fraction is characteristic of the secondary carnitine deficiency states [Tein, 1995, 2003]. Defects of the carnitine cycle produce a different metabolic profile. As with defects of beta oxidation, affected patients may have hypoketotic hypoglycemia during fasting. However, carnitine cycle defects are not associated with dicarboxylic aciduria as a rule. The disturbances of carnitine also are more variable. Defects of the membrane carnitine transporter system and the carnitine-acylcarnitine translocase system are typically associated with low serum and tissue carnitine concentrations, whereas defects of carnitine palmitoyltransferase II (adult form) and carnitine palmitoyltransferase I are associated with normal or high serum and tissue carnitine concentrations. In contrast, the infantile multiorgan form of carnitine palmitoyltransferase II deficiency is associated with low serum and tissue carnitine concentrations [Tein, 2003; Ohkuma et al., 2009].

Equally important observations can be made by measuring circulating ketone body concentrations. Ketone bodies normally are negligible in the fed state and elevated in the fasting state. Ketone bodies are formed primarily in the liver from the metabolism of fatty acids and are exported to extrahepatic tissues that are capable of metabolizing these substrates. Classically, hypoketotic hypoglycemia develops in patients with defects of fatty acid metabolism during fasting. Serum ketone body values also are helpful in distinguishing the biochemical defects associated with congenital lactic acidosis. The serum ketone body concentrations in these various defects reflect the intracellular concentration of acetyl coenzyme A. Acetyl coenzyme A is the pivotal metabolite in mitochondrial metabolism. Acetyl coenzyme A may be formed from the decarboxylation of pyruvate, fatty acids, or ketone bodies. A fraction of the acetyl coenzyme A pool may be shunted into the β-hydroxy-β-methylglutaryl coenzyme A cycle in the liver to form ketone bodies. Defects involving the pyruvate dehydrogenase complex prevent the conversion of pyruvate to acetyl coenzyme A. Therefore, ketone bodies cannot be formed, and the increased pyruvate concentrations are shunted disproportionately into the gluconeogenic pathway. As a result, patients with pyruvate dehydrogenase deficiency have elevated pyruvate, lactate, and alanine concentrations, relative resistance to hypoglycemia during fasting, and a disproportionately low serum ketone body concentration, particularly during fasting. In contrast, patients with pyruvate carboxylase deficiency fail to convert pyruvate to oxaloacetate. As a result, acetyl coenzyme A concentrations increase, and there is a paradoxical formation of ketone bodies in the setting of the lactic acidosis. The deficiency of oxaloacetate and the secondary decrease in tissue aspartate concentrations also cause a paradoxical increase in the cytoplasmic oxidation–reduction potential and a decrease in the intramitochondrial oxidation–reduction potential. Therefore, patients with pyruvate carboxylase deficiency have an increased lactate/pyruvate ratio and a decreased β-hydroxybutyrate/acetoacetate ratio [De Vivo et al., 1977; Wang and De Vivo, 2009]. This metabolic profile is distinctive for pyruvate carboxylase deficiency. Similar, although less striking, observations may be seen with defects of the Krebs cycle or the respiratory chain as it relates to the paradoxical presence of ketosis in the setting of lactic acidosis.

Biochemical defects involving the urea cycle, specifically ornithine transcarbamoylase deficiency and carbamoyl phosphate synthetase deficiency, are associated with hyperammonemia. The urine orotic acid concentrations are increased in ornithine transcarbamoylase deficiency and decreased in carbamoyl phosphate synthetase deficiency.

Combinations of metabolic abnormalities also may exist. For example, defects involving the metabolism of long-chain fatty acids may be associated with the distinctive patterns of free fatty acidemia, dicarboxylicaciduria, hypocarnitinemia, hyperammonemia, and lactic acidosis. This profile is particularly evident in defects of the trifunctional enzyme protein and very-long-chain acyl coenzyme A dehydrogenase that are located in the inner membrane of the mitochondrion [Di Donato and Taroni, 2003]. These patients also have increased tissue concentrations of long-chain acylcarnitine, which may explain the organ toxicity associated with the defects of long-chain fatty acids.

Histopathologic Disturbances

The tissue reactions in mitochondrial diseases may be informative and direct the clinician's attention to the primary metabolic defect, or they may be modest or absent. A normal muscle biopsy result does not rule out a mitochondrial disease. The skeletal muscle biopsy specimen often looks normal in defects of pyruvate carboxylase, pyruvate dehydrogenase, the Krebs cycle, and the urea cycle. The biopsy tissue may appear normal, with some defects involving fatty acid metabolism, including the adult form of carnitine palmitoyltransferase II, and several defects involving the respiratory chain. A lipid storage myopathy signifies a defect in fatty acid metabolism. Lipid accumulation is common in defects of beta oxidation, including glutaric aciduria type II and the infantile multiorgan form of carnitine palmitoyltransferase II deficiency. This tissue abnormality may be particularly striking in patients with the tissue-specific form of short-chain acyl coenzyme A dehydrogenase deficiency. In fact, several patients previously described with the myopathic carnitine deficiency syndrome [Engel and Angelini, 1973] later proved to have muscle-specific short-chain acyl coenzyme A dehydrogenase deficiency. Lipid storage in muscle is massive in two conditions due to defects of neutral triglyceride lipases. The first, also known as neutral lipid storage disease with ichthyosis (NLSDI), or Chanarin–Dorfman syndrome, characterized by weakness, hepatopathy, steatorrhea, and ichthyosis, is due to mutations in the *GCI-58* gene. The second, known as neutral lipid storage disease with myopathy (NLSDM), is characterized by juvenile- or adult-onset myopathy, sometimes associated with cardiopathy, and is due to mutations in the *PNPLA2* gene [Ohkuma et al., 2009].

Ragged red fibers are present in many respiratory chain diseases, including many nDNA defects. Ragged red fibers represent the morphologic counterpart of large-scale rearrangements of mtDNA or point mutations affecting transfer RNA (tRNA) genes and some, but not all, protein-coding genes.

The pathologic process in the brain is distinctive in many mitochondrial diseases. Three patterns are common. The first is a widespread insult to the brain tissue, with resulting microcephaly and ventricular dilatation. This pattern is seen in defects of the urea cycle, several defects associated with congenital lactic acidosis, and some of the defects associated with fatty acid metabolism. Malformations also may be seen, including agenesis of the corpus callosum, ectopic displacement of the olivary nuclei, and cystic destruction of the basal ganglia. This pattern is particularly striking in infants with pyruvate dehydrogenase E1 alpha-subunit deficiency. The second pattern is best typified by the neuropathologic changes associated with Leigh's syndrome [Leigh, 1951]. These patients have a symmetric subcortical distribution of tissue injury, with a particular predilection for the basal ganglia, thalamus, brainstem, and cerebellar roof nuclei. Microscopic features include loss of brain cells, proportionate loss of myelin, reactive astrocytosis, and proliferation of the cerebral microvessels. In some patients, particularly those with MELAS, multifocal encephalomalacia develops. This pathologic condition typically is located in the posterior aspect of the cerebral hemisphere. The third pattern is a spongy encephalopathy with loosening and rarefaction of the neuropil. The spongy encephalopathy is the histopathologic counterpart of a defect in cerebral energy metabolism and is commonly seen in patients with Kearns–Sayre syndrome. Magnetic resonance imaging (MRI) may reflect these patterns of brain-tissue injury with a hyperintense signal of the central white matter on the T2-weighted image (Figure 37-3). Stroke-like lesions in the posterior cerebral hemisphere are typical of MELAS. Signal hyperintensities involving the putamen, globus pallidus, and caudate nuclei are characteristic of Leigh's syndrome. A diffuse signal abnormality involving the central white matter is typical of Kearns–Sayre syndrome. Intracranial calcifications also are seen in these conditions. Basal ganglia calcifications are most commonly associated with Kearns–Sayre syndrome and MELAS.

Classification of Mitochondrial Diseases

Several classification schemes of mitochondrial diseases are based on different criteria [DiMauro et al., 1985; Moraes et al., 1991; Shoffner et al., 1990]. The original attempts to classify mitochondrial diseases by clinical or morphologic criteria were unsatisfactory. The phenotypic heterogeneity of mitochondrial diseases complicated the clinical classification efforts. Similarly, the lack of histopathologic uniformity undermined the morphologic classification efforts. A biochemical classification of mitochondrial diseases was introduced in 1985 [DiMauro et al., 1985]. The clinical conditions were subclassified according to the primary site of the biochemical defect. In 1988, primary mutations of the mitochondrial genome were first recognized [Holt et al., 1988; Wallace et al., 1988]. These findings were particularly relevant to respiratory chain defects because this metabolic pathway is under the dual genetic influence of the mitochondrial and nuclear genomes. In recent times, the term mitochondrial diseases has been increasingly restricted to defects of one biochemical pathway, the respiratory chain [DiMauro and Schon, 2003], and further subgrouped as nuclear DNA defects and mtDNA defects (Box 37-1). However, in this review, the more general, biochemical classification for defects resulting from mutations in nuclear DNA is used, whereas for defects of the respiratory chain, a genetic classification is used.

General Clinical Features

From the clinical perspective, mitochondrial diseases can be divided into the following three major categories: defects of fatty acid oxidation, defects of pyruvate metabolism, and defects of the respiratory chain. Most mitochondrial diseases can be subsumed under these major categories.

Defects of Fatty Acid Oxidation

These conditions have specific clinical and metabolic signatures [Tein, 2003; DiDonato and Taroni, 2004]. Patients with defects of fatty acid oxidation experience metabolic decompensation during fasting. Organs that depend on fatty acid oxidation are primarily affected, including skeletal and cardiac musculature. Fatty acids accumulate in the liver in most of these defects and are shunted into auxiliary pathways, including omega oxidation. Omega oxidation occurs in the cytoplasm and accounts for the formation of dicarboxylic acids. Dicarboxylicaciduria is particularly evident in defects of beta oxidation (Figure 37-4). Acylglycine and acylcarnitine esters also accumulate in patients with defects of beta oxidation, offsetting the sequestration of coenzyme A that occurs with accumulating acyl coenzyme A thioesters. Depletion of serum and tissue carnitine stores may result. Increased bound carnitine fractions are characteristic of mitochondrial beta-oxidation defects. Absolute decreases of free and total carnitine fractions are particularly distinctive in carnitine cycle defects (see Figure 37-4). Defects of fatty acid oxidation result in the underproduction of acetyl coenzyme A and the resulting impairment of Krebs cycle activity and hepatic ketogenesis. As a result, many patients with defects of fatty acid oxidation have hypoketotic hypoglycemia. This metabolic state is associated with neurologic symptoms of altered consciousness. The precise mechanism of the cerebral

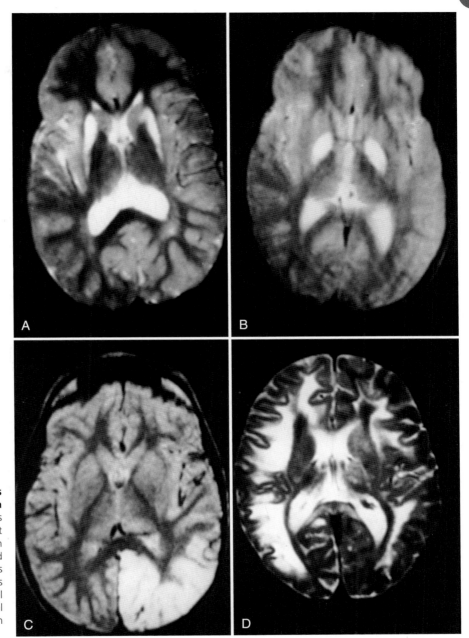

Fig. 37-3 Characteristic cranial abnormalities in mitochondrial encephalomyopathies on magnetic resonance imaging. The images represent T2-weighted images from four different patients. **A,** Bilateral putaminal hyperintensities in a child with cytochrome-c oxidase-associated Leigh's syndrome. **B,** Bilateral globus pallidus hyperintensities in a child with a familial Leigh's syndrome phenotype. **C,** A left posterior cerebral hyperintensity in a child with MELAS. **D,** Bilateral white-matter hyperintensities in a child with Kearns–Sayre syndrome.

Box 37-1 Biochemical Genetics Classification of Mitochondrial Diseases

Inherited Conditions

Nuclear DNA Defects

- Defects of substrate transport
- Defects of substrate utilization
- Defects of the Krebs cycle
- Defects of oxidation–phosphorylation coupling
- Defects of the respiratory chain
- Defects of protein importation
- Defects of intergenomic signaling

Mitochondrial DNA Defects

- Sporadic large-scale rearrangements
- Transmitted large-scale rearrangements
- Point mutations affecting structural genes
- Point mutations affecting synthetic genes

Acquired Conditions

- Infectious (e.g., Reye's syndrome)
- Toxic (e.g., MPTP (mitochondrial permeability transition pore))
- Drugs (e.g., zidovudine)
- Aging

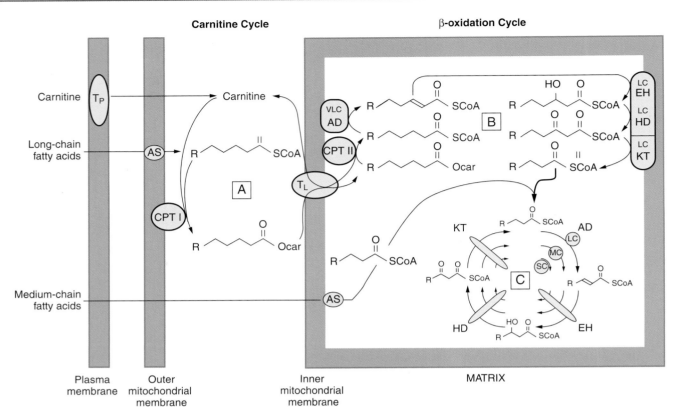

Fig. 37-4 Schematic representation of fatty acid oxidation. This metabolic pathway is divided into the carnitine cycle (A), the inner mitochondrial membrane system (B), and the mitochondrial matrix system (C). The carnitine cycle includes the plasma membrane transporter, carnitine palmitoyltransferase I, carnitine-acylcarnitine translocase system, and carnitine palmitoyltransferase II. The inner mitochondrial membrane system includes the very-long-chain acyl-CoA dehydrogenase and the trifunctional protein with three catalytically active sites. Long-chain acylcarnitines enter the mitochondrial matrix by the action of the carnitine palmitoyltransferase II to yield long-chain acyl-CoAs. These thioesters undergo one or more cycles of chain shortening, catalyzed by the membrane-bound system. Chain-shortened acyl-CoAs are degraded further by the matrix beta oxidation system. Medium-chain fatty acids enter the mitochondrial matrix directly and are activated to the medium-chain acyl-CoAs before degradation by the matrix beta oxidation system. AD, acyl-CoA dehydrogenase; CoA, coenzyme A; CPT, carnitine palmitoyltransferase; EH, 2-enoyl-CoA hydratase; HD, 3-hydroxyacyl-CoA dehydrogenase; KT, 3-ketoacyl-CoA thiolase; LC, long chain; MC, medium chain; SC, short chain; T_L, carnitine-acylcarnitine translocase; T_P, carnitine transporter; VLC, very long chain. *(Modified from Pons R, De Vivo DC: Primary and secondary carnitine deficiency syndromes. J Child Neurol 1995;10:1. With the kind assistance of Dr. Horst Schulz.)*

dysfunction that is associated with defects of fatty acid oxidation is unknown. Decreased availability of ketone bodies and glucose deprives the brain of its two principal metabolic fuels. Fatty acids may enter the brain, but they are poorly metabolized. The accumulation of fatty acid intermediates in brain tissue also may have deleterious effects on cellular function.

Many patients with specific defects of fatty acid oxidation have been described since 1973, when the adult form of carnitine palmitoyltransferase type II and the myopathic form of carnitine deficiency were described [DiMauro and DiMauro, 1973; Engel and Angelini, 1973]. About half of all cases involve medium-chain acyl coenzyme A dehydrogenase deficiency. In 1975, the first patient with systemic carnitine deficiency was described [Karpati et al., 1975]. Many patients with systemic carnitine deficiency have been restudied and found to have medium-chain acyl coenzyme A dehydrogenase deficiency [DiDonato and Taroni, 2004]. The fatty acid oxidation defects can be subdivided into defects of the carnitine cycle, defects of the inner mitochondrial membrane, and defects of beta oxidation (see Figure 37-4). The specific clinical conditions are discussed later in this chapter.

Defects of Pyruvate Metabolism

Pyruvate is the end product of glycolysis. This metabolite can be reduced to lactate or transaminated to alanine in the cytoplasm. Otherwise, pyruvate is translocated across the mitochondrial membrane (Figure 37-5). In the mitochondrial matrix, pyruvate is carboxylated to oxaloacetate, or decarboxylated and activated to acetyl coenzyme A. The first reaction is catalyzed by pyruvate carboxylase, and the second is catalyzed by the pyruvate dehydrogenase complex. The two reaction products – oxaloacetate and acetyl coenzyme A – condense to form citrate as the primary reactant in the Krebs cycle. Defects of pyruvate metabolism involve the pyruvate dehydrogenase complex, pyruvate carboxylase, or several enzymes in the Krebs cycle [De Meirleir, 2002; De Vivo et al., 2002]. These defects are associated with elevated serum and tissue concentrations of pyruvate, lactate, and alanine. The lactate/pyruvate ratio is relatively preserved because the oxidation–reduction potential is maintained. This generalization, although not absolute, is helpful in attempts to distinguish defects of pyruvate metabolism from defects of the respiratory chain (discussed later). The Krebs cycle is central

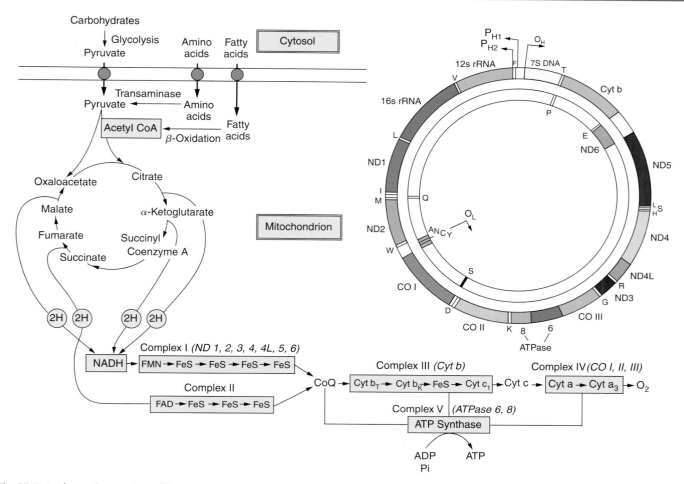

Fig. 37-5 A schematic overview of intermediary metabolism. Fatty acid oxidation is illustrated in detail in Figure 37-4. Pyruvate metabolism involves two reactions: pyruvate carboxylase and pyruvate dehydrogenase. Condensation of these two reaction products produces citrate at entry point of the Krebs cycle. Reducing equivalents are generated in the Krebs cycle and reoxidized by the respiratory chain. The five respiratory chain complexes contain approximately 80 polypeptides. Thirteen polypeptides are encoded by mitochondrial DNA, as illustrated in the upper right. The 13 mitochondrial DNA gene products are noted in parentheses above complexes I, III, IV, and V. ADP, adenosine diphosphate; ATP, adenosine triphospate; CO, cytochrome-c oxidase; CoA, coenzyme A; Cyt, cytochrome; ND, NADH-CoQ reductase; O_L and O_H, origin of replication for L and H strands; P_{H1}, P_{H2}, primary transcripts of the H strand starting at H1, H2. *(From De Vivo DC. The expanding clinical spectrum of mitochondrial diseases. Brain and Development. 15;1–22, 1993. Elsevier Science Publishers, 1993.)*

to intermediary metabolism. Complete biochemical defects of this pathway are probably incompatible with life. Four partial defects of the Krebs cycle have been described and are discussed later in this chapter.

Defects of the Respiratory Chain

The respiratory chain contains five functional units or complexes that are embedded in the inner mitochondrial membrane (see Figure 37-5). The five complexes contain approximately 80 polypeptides, 13 of which are encoded by mtDNA (see Figure 37-5 and Table 37-2). Complex II, unlike the other four complexes, is solely under the control of the nuclear genome. The function of the respiratory chain is the transfer of electrons from the reduced pyridine nucleotides and flavoproteins to molecular oxygen, with the resulting oxidation of reduced nicotinamide adenine dinucleotide phosphate and flavin adenine dinucleotide and the production of water. Biochemical defects of the respiratory chain are associated with lactic acidosis. However, unlike defects of pyruvate metabolism, respiratory chain defects are associated with a

disturbed cellular oxidation–reduction potential manifested by an elevated lactate/pyruvate ratio (>20).

Clinical presentation of defects involving the respiratory chain should include failure of organs that have a high oxidative metabolic demand. This conclusion is confirmed by the frequent involvement of brain, muscle, heart, retina, renal tubule, and organ of Corti in these clinical syndromes. However, the expression of the biomolecular defect is modified by various factors, including selective alteration of tissue-specific isoforms and the degree of completeness of the generalized defect. Many of the earlier case reports describing patients with respiratory chain defects were published before the importance of mitochondrial genetics was understood. As a result, it is difficult to classify many of the earlier cases from the molecular point of view. Respiratory chain defects also are complicated by the diversity of clinical presentations. Some of the patients have neurologic or neuromuscular symptoms and are grouped together in the neurologic literature reports as examples of mitochondrial encephalomyopathies. Other patients may have non-neurologic symptoms, including dysfunction of the liver, heart, kidney, bone marrow, pancreas, or gastrointestinal tract. The specific clinical syndromes associated with the five respiratory chain complexes are discussed later in the chapter.

Clinical Features of Mitochondrial Diseases

Inherited Conditions Associated with Nuclear DNA Defects

Defects of Substrate Transport

Several genetically determined defects of substrate transport have been described. Perhaps the best examples are the defects involving the carnitine cycle. There are four such defects, involving:

1. the carnitine transporter
2. carnitine palmitoyltransferase I
3. the carnitine–acylcarnitine translocase
4. carnitine palmitoyltransferase II.

The carnitine cycle is illustrated in Figure 37-4. Carnitine is actively transported from the blood across the plasma membrane. Approximately 90 percent of carnitine body stores reside in skeletal muscle, with skeletal muscle concentration of carnitine being about 60-fold higher than the plasma concentration. Long-chain fatty acids are translocated across the inner mitochondrial membrane as the carnitine ester. Medium-chain fatty acids enter the mitochondrial matrix directly before being activated to the thioester (see Figure 37-4).

A common defect in this cycle involves the carnitine transporter system [Tein, 2003]. This condition is inherited as an autosomal-recessive trait, and is clinically manifested in infancy or early childhood as a carnitine-responsive cardiomyopathy, associated with hypotonia, weakness, failure to thrive, hypoketotic hypoglycemia, and altered consciousness or coma. The defect is generalized, with involvement of skeletal muscle, heart, and kidney. Studies of cultured skin fibroblasts define the condition and identify the heterozygote asymptomatic carriers. Molecular genetic studies have identified pathogenic mutations in the gene (*OCTN2*) encoding the sodium-dependent, high-affinity carnitine transporter, OCN2 [Lamhonwah et al., 2009]. Oral carnitine supplementation is life-saving, with resolution of clinical symptoms and restoration of normal cardiac function.

Carnitine palmitoyltransferase I deficiency is a clinical condition of infancy manifested by nonketotic hypoglycemic coma [DiDonato and Taroni, 2003; Tein, 2003]. The patients have marked hepatomegaly and hypertriglyceridemia, even when they are clinically asymptomatic. The clinical syndrome mimics Reye's syndrome, but dicarboxylicaciduria is absent and the serum carnitine values are normal or high. Hyperammonemia, disturbed liver function test results, and marked hepatomegaly are distinctive; persistent renal tubular acidosis may be present. Medium-chain triglycerides may be used to document a ketotic response and as treatment for this autosomal-recessive condition. Muscle from these patients has normal activities for both carnitine palmitoyltransferase I and carnitine palmitoyltransferase II, suggesting the existence of tissue-specific isoenzymes for carnitine palmitoyltransferase I. This finding has been confirmed by molecular studies, demonstrating that there are two distinct genes for carnitine

palmitoyltransferase I. One encodes the muscle–heart isoform; the other encodes the liver–fibroblast isoform.

Several infants with carnitine–acylcarnitine translocase deficiency have been described, combining hypoketotic hypoglycemia, hepatomegaly, cardiomyopathy, seizures, lethargy, and coma [DiDonato and Taroni, 2003; Tein, 2003]. The gene for carnitine–acylcarnitine translocase is located on chromosome 3p21.31, and several mutations have been identified in patients.

Carnitine palmitoyltransferase II was the first primary biochemical defect of fatty acid oxidation to be described [DiMauro and DiMauro, 1973]. The adult form is relatively benign and consistent with a normal life expectancy. A disproportionate number of affected males have been reported, despite the fact that it is an autosomal-recessive trait. The clinical picture is that of a metabolic myopathy, with recurrent muscle pain and myoglobinuria. Symptoms are provoked by fasting, prolonged exercise, cold exposure, infection, or emotional stress. Fixed limb weakness develops in about 10 percent of patients at an older age, and a similar percentage have evidence of a lipid storage myopathy [DiDonato and Taroni, 2003; Tein, 2003]. Carnitine concentrations are normal in this clinical syndrome. Several mutations compatible with some residual activity ("leaky mutations") in the *CPT2* gene have been associated with the myopathic form. A common mutation (Ser113Leu) has been identified in at least 50 percent of patients and may be used for diagnostic screening in genomic DNA isolated from blood.

Carnitine palmitoyltransferase II deficiency in newborns is a generalized lethal disease, with reduced enzyme activity in multiple organs and corresponding signs of liver failure, cardiomyopathy, hypoketotic hypoglycemia, and mild myopathy. There are reduced concentrations of free and total carnitine and increased concentrations of lipids and long-chain acylcarnitines. It remains unclear what distinguishes the relatively benign adult, myopathic form of carnitine palmitoyltransferase II deficiency from the lethal infantile form. The residual enzyme activity is similar in these two phenotypes, but oxidation of long-chain fatty acids may be more severely impaired in the infantile form [DiDonato and Taroni, 2003].

Some patients with the mild form of multiple acyl coenzyme A dehydrogenase deficiency have a riboflavin-responsive syndrome, suggesting a genetic defect in flavin adenine nucleotide biosynthesis or transport [DiDonato and Taroni, 2003, 2004]. Riboflavin supplementation, together with L-carnitine and a low-protein, low-fat diet, represents effective treatment in this subgroup of patients with the glutaricaciduria type II phenotype. A mostly myopathic presentation of glutaricaciduria type II, due to mutations in the gene (*ETFDH*) encoding the electron-transferring flavoprotein dehydrogenase, is associated with coenzyme Q_{10} (CoQ_{10}) deficiency in muscle, and responds to CoQ_{10} and flavoprotein administration [Gempel et al., 2007].

Defects of Substrate Utilization

Pyruvate carboxylase deficiency, pyruvate dehydrogenase complex deficiency, and defects of beta oxidation are examples of substrate utilization defects. The sites of these biochemical defects are illustrated in Figure 37-4 (beta-oxidation defects) and Figure 37-5.

Classic pyruvate carboxylase deficiency, an autosomal-recessive condition, is life-threatening in infancy and is associated with hypotonia, psychomotor retardation, failure to thrive, and metabolic acidosis [De Vivo et al., 1977; Wang and De Vivo, 2009; Wang et al., 2008]. Approximately 50 patients with pyruvate carboxylase deficiency have been described. The severe French phenotype is associated with absence of the enzyme protein. These patients die in early infancy and have lactic acidosis, ketoacidosis, citrullinemia, hyperlysinemia, hyperammonemia, and aspartate depletion. The less severe, although equally fatal, North American phenotype is associated with severe mental and motor developmental delay, and death in late infancy or early childhood. A mutated protein is present in tissue with some residual enzyme activity. Three patients have had the laboratory features of the North American phenotype but were clinically spared, with normal mental and motor development between recurrent attacks of metabolic crisis. Consanguinity and mosaicism are quite evident in this group of patients, and mosaicism may mute the severity of the clinical phenotype [Wang et al., 2008].

Biotin deficiency affects pyruvate carboxylase, together with the other three biotin-dependent carboxylase reactions: propionyl-coenzyme A carboxylase, β-methylcrotonyl-coenzyme A carboxylase, and acetyl coenzyme A carboxylase. All carboxylation reactions occur in the mitochondria, except for the carboxylation of acetyl coenzyme A. Multiple carboxylase deficiency, an autosomal-recessive trait in all of its clinical presentations, is seen in early infancy as a result of holocarboxylase synthetase deficiency, or later in infancy as the result of biotinidase deficiency. These patients may have irregular breathing patterns, failure to thrive, alopecia, rash, immunologic disturbances, optic atrophy, hearing loss, seizures, and metabolic acidosis; they respond to high-dose biotin supplementation, particularly if they are treated early in the disease course.

Several hundred patients with defects involving the pyruvate dehydrogenase complex have been described [De Meirleir, 2002]. Most patients have a defect involving the E1 alpha subunit, and a male predominance is expected because the gene is located on the X chromosome. Two patients had mutations in the E1 beta subunit, inherited as an autosomal-recessive trait [Brown et al., 2004]. The neonatal presentation includes hypotonia, episodic apnea, convulsions, weak suck, dysmorphic features, lethargy, low birth weight, failure to thrive, and coma. Dysmorphic features include broad nasal bridge, upturned nose, micrognathia, low-set and posteriorly rotated ears, short fingers, short arms, simian creases, hypospadias, and anteriorly placed anus. The infantile phenotype has been described in about 100 patients, and usually is seen between 3 and 6 months of age, with psychomotor retardation, hypotonia, convulsions, episodic apnea, ataxia, pyramidal tract signs, lethargy, dysmorphic features, deceleration of head growth, ophthalmoplegia, optic atrophy, peripheral neuropathy, ptosis, dysphagia, deceleration of somatic growth, extrapyramidal signs, and cranial nerve palsies. Postmortem examinations were performed in 21 cases of the infantile form; of these, 81 percent were consistent with Leigh's syndrome [DeVivo and Van Coster, 1991]. Seven male children had a benign phenotype, with fluctuating ataxia, post-exercise fatigue, transient paraparesis, and thiamine responsiveness. These children had normal mental and motor development between episodes. A high-fat diet has been recommended as an alternative source of acetyl coenzyme A in patients with pyruvate dehydrogenase deficiency [Wexler et al., 1997]. Thiamine, lipoic acid, and ʟ-carnitine supplementation may be helpful in selected cases.

Seven genetically determined conditions have been described involving enzyme deficiencies in the beta-oxidation pathway (see Figure 37-4) [DiDonato and Taroni, 2004; Tein, 2003]. All are transmitted as autosomal-recessive traits. Five of the genetic defects (deficiencies of medium-chain acyl coenzyme A, short-chain acyl coenzyme A, long-chain acyl coenzyme A, electron transfer flavoprotein, and electron transfer flavoprotein-coenzyme Q oxidoreductase) involve the first step in beta oxidation. The other two conditions (long-chain 3-hydroxyacyl-CoA dehydrogenase deficiency and short-chain 3-hydroxyacyl-CoA dehydrogenase deficiency) involve the third step in beta oxidation. Two more enzyme defects involve the two membrane-bound enzymes of beta oxidation, very-long-chain acyl-CoA dehydrogenase (VLCAD), and the trifunctional enzyme protein. VLCAD deficiency, as carnitine palmitoyltransferase II deficiency, can present in infancy with hypoketotic hypoglycemia, hepatopathy, and cardiomyopathy, or in adult life as recurrent myoglobinuria [DiDonato and Taroni, 2003]. The gene (*ACADVL*) for VLCAD has been mapped to chromosome 17p12, and a relatively good genotype–phenotype relationship is emerging. The severe infantile form is associated with nonsense mutations, whereas the benign adult form is due to missense mutations compatible with some residual VLCAD activity.

Trifunctional enzyme protein is a hetero-octamer composed of four alpha subunits catalyzing the long-chain ʟ-3-hydroxyacyl-CoA dehydrogenase (LCHAD) and the long-chain 2-enoyl-CoA hydratase (LCEH) activities, and four beta subunits catalyzing the long-chain 3-ketoacyl-CoA thiolase (LCKT) activity. Trifunctional enzyme protein deficiency had been diagnosed as LCHAD deficiency until more careful biochemical analysis revealed combined defects of LCHAD, LCEH, and LCKT activities. In fact, most patients with mitochondrial trifunctional protein deficiency have isolated LCHAD deficiency, with relative sparing of LCEH and LCKT activities. In infancy and early childhood, clinical features include recurrent attacks of hypoketotic hypoglycemia, cardiomyopathy, limb weakness, sensory neuropathy, pigmentary retinopathy, and hepatic dysfunction. Later in childhood, recurrent attacks of myoglobinuria are common. Two syndromes associated with LCHAD deficiency have been labeled HELLP (hemolysis, elevated liver enzymes, low platelets) and AFLP (acute fatty liver of pregnancy). The latter condition occurs in pregnant women carrying an affected fetus. A common mutation (G1528C) has been identified in the LCHAD domain of the alpha subunit. Full mitochondrial trifunctional protein deficiency, that is, combined severe deficiency of LCHAD, LCEH, and LCKT, is much rarer, and symptoms are similar but more severe than in isolated LCHAD deficiency. The molecular basis of full mitochondrial trifunctional protein deficiency is heterogeneous, with mutations in both alpha and beta subunits. Mutations have been identified in the *HADHA* and the *HADHB* genes, both located on chromosome 2p23 [DiDonato and Taroni, 2003].

Medium-chain acyl coenzyme A dehydrogenase deficiency commonly develops before 2 years of age and represents about 50 percent of the described cases associated with beta oxidation defects [Roe and Coates, 1989]. The metabolic crisis in medium-chain acyl coenzyme A dehydrogenase deficiency is provoked by fasting or intercurrent infection. The classic picture is that of episodic vomiting, hypotonia, obtundation, or coma. The patient is healthy between attacks. This condition may masquerade as systemic carnitine deficiency, recurrent Reye's syndrome, or sudden infant death syndrome. Developmental disabilities, chronic seizure disorder, and proximal limb weakness represent long-term consequences of this condition. The molecular defect involves a gene on chromosome 1p31. In multiple studies of white patients, one mutation, A985G, was found in 90 percent of mutant medium-chain acyl coenzyme A dehydrogenase alleles. This mutation alters protein stability and assembly of the subunits into the holoenzyme tetramer.

The phenotypes of the other six defects resemble medium-chain acyl coenzyme A dehydrogenase deficiency, but there are some clinical caveats. Long-chain acyl coenzyme A dehydrogenase deficiency tends to be more severe in infancy, with a worse prognosis. Cardiac involvement is prominent, and patients may develop microcephaly, hypotonia, and pigmentary retinopathy. Limb weakness may be seen with all beta-oxidation defects except medium-chain acyl coenzyme A dehydrogenase deficiency. Short-chain acyl coenzyme A dehydrogenase deficiency may present in infancy with vomiting, hypoglycemia, developmental delay, limb weakness, muscle carnitine deficiency, and a lipid storage myopathy, or it may present in adulthood with progressive limb weakness and lipid storage myopathy [Turnbull et al., 1984]. Electron transfer flavoprotein or electron transfer flavoprotein-coenzyme Q oxidoreductase deficiency states may present the clinical picture of multiple acyl coenzyme A dehydrogenase deficiency (glutaricaciduria type II). The neonatal presentation may be associated with congenital anomalies, including facial dysmorphism with low-set ears, hypertelorism, high forehead, hypoplastic midface, rocker-bottom feet, muscle defects of the anterior abdominal wall, and anomalies of the external genitalia. These patients usually die during the first week of life. The neonatal presentation may occur without congenital anomalies, and these patients have hypotonia, tachypnea, metabolic acidosis, hepatomegaly, hypoglycemia, and a peculiar odor reminiscent of isovaleric acidemia. An adult phenotype may exhibit episodic vomiting, hypoglycemia, hepatomegaly, and limb weakness. Some patients with the milder form of multiple acyl coenzyme A dehydrogenase deficiency respond to riboflavin. Patients with LCHAD deficiency have persistent hepatic dysfunction, low serum carnitine concentrations, and a neuropathy or myopathy with recurrent myoglobinuria [Dionisi-Vici et al., 1991]. The short-chain 3-hydroxyacyl-CoA dehydrogenase phenotype appears to be similar to the LCHAD phenotype, but only three cases have been described [Tein et al., 1991].

Defects of the Krebs Cycle

Several partial defects of this cycle have been described. The first patient, described with dihydrolipoyl dehydrogenase deficiency, died at the age of 6 months with persistent metabolic acidosis and progressive neurologic symptoms, including respiratory difficulties, lethargy, hypotonia alternating with irritability, optic atrophy, and hyperreflexia [Robinson et al., 1977]. The organic acid profile includes elevations of α-ketoglutarate, branched-chain α-keto acids, pyruvate, and lactate. A few cases of α-ketoglutarate dehydrogenase deficiency have been described [Bonnefont et al., 1992]. This condition is devastating in infancy.

Fumarase deficiency is a progressive infantile encephalopathy with failure to thrive, hypotonia, microcephaly, and fumaric aciduria. This condition may be associated with enlarged cerebral ventricles and polyhydramnios in utero [De Meirleir, 2002; Zinn et al., 1986].

Succinate dehydrogenase is a critical step in the Krebs cycle and the first component of complex II in the respiratory chain (see Figure 37-5). Before the molecular era, several patients were described with defects of complex II and progressive encephalomyopathy. A mutation in the flavoprotein subunit of succinate dehydrogenase was identified in two sisters with Leigh's syndrome [Bourgeron et al., 1995], the first example of a nuclear DNA mutation resulting in a respiratory chain disorder. A few more cases of Leigh's syndrome were later associated with mutations in the same gene [DiMauro and Bonilla, 2004].

Defects of Oxidation–Phosphorylation Coupling

Luft's disease (nonthyroidal hypermetabolism) is the singular example of a defect in this pathway. Only two cases have been reported, both sporadic and with negative family histories [Luft et al., 1962; DiMauro et al., 1976]. Onset is in adolescence, with fever, heat intolerance, profuse perspiration, polyphagia, polydipsia, resting tachycardia, and exercise intolerance. Both women died in middle age. Numerous ragged red fibers were present in skeletal muscle, but the underlying biochemical defect has not yet been elucidated.

Defects of the Respiratory Chain

The respiratory chain contains five functional units or complexes that are embedded in the inner mitochondrial membrane (see Figure 37-5). The respiratory chain is unique in that it is controlled by the nuclear and mitochondrial genomes. Complex II, unlike the other four complexes, is under the control of the nuclear genome only. As a result, any defects involving this complex are inherited as mendelian traits. Box 37-1 represents a molecular classification of defects of the respiratory chain. However, patients studied before the "molecular era" (1988) cannot be classified by these criteria. Classification is also complicated by the diversity of clinical presentations. Some patients with neurologic or neuromuscular symptoms are grouped together in the neurologic literature as examples of mitochondrial encephalomyopathies. Other patients have non-neurologic symptoms resulting from primary involvement of other organs, such as the liver, heart, kidney, bone marrow, pancreas, or gastrointestinal tract [DiMauro and Schon, 2003].

Complex I (reduced nicotinamide adenine dinucleotide phosphate-coenzyme Q reductase) is the largest complex of the respiratory chain, containing about 46 polypeptides and several nonprotein components. Seven of the polypeptides are encoded by mtDNA. Patients with complex I deficiency can be subclassified as examples of a myopathy or a multisystem disorder. The myopathy may develop in childhood or early adult life, and is manifested by exercise intolerance and limb weakness. The weakness may become prevalent as the disease progresses. These patients are often sporadic and harbor "somatic mutations" in mtDNA-encoded genes of complex I – that is, spontaneous de novo mutations in the mitochondrial genome occurring in the oocyte or in the embryo, but affecting myoblasts after germ-layer differentiation [DiMauro et al., 2003].

Patients with multisystem involvement of complex I deficiency can be subdivided into three clinical conditions. The first is manifested by a fatal infantile disorder with congenital lactic acidosis, weakness and hypotonia, developmental delay, and death resulting from cardiopulmonary failure [Hoppel et al., 1987; Moreadith et al., 1984; Robinson et al., 1986]. The molecular basis of this rapidly fatal infantile presentation is not known but may relate to mutations in nuclear genes (see later). The second presentation is associated with the clinical and neuroradiologic features of Leigh's syndrome. In fact, complex I deficiency is one of the major causes of Leigh's syndrome, although it may be overlooked because of the difficulty of documenting the biochemical defect in frozen tissues. This concept seems confirmed by studies of nuclear genes, revealing a number of mutations in children with Leigh's syndrome or leukodystrophy [Smeitink and van den Heuvel, 1999; Triepels et al., 2001; Distelmaier et al., 2009]. Attention has recently been drawn to mutations in mtDNA-encoded complex I (ND) subunits, especially mutations in the *ND5* gene, which appears to be a hotspot. These mutations have been associated with maternally inherited MELAS, MERRF, and Leigh's syndrome phenotypes, or various overlap syndromes of these phenotypes [Liolitsa et al., 2003; Naini et al., 2005; Shanske et al., 2008].

Complex II (succinate-coenzyme Q reductase) contains only polypeptides encoded by the nuclear genome. There are few examples of complex II deficiency, and again, the clinical picture is that of an encephalomyopathy. Haller and colleagues [1991] and Schapira and associates [1990] described two patients with lack of succinate dehydrogenase stain in muscle biopsy specimens. One was a 22-year-old man with exercise intolerance and recurrent myoglobinuria; the other was a 14-year-old girl with exercise intolerance but no myoglobinuria. The complex II deficiency in these patients was accompanied by partial defects of complex I, complex III, and aconitase, and was attributed to defective importation of nonheme iron–sulfur clusters into mitochondria. As mentioned before, a few patients with Leigh's syndrome and complex II deficiency had mutations in the gene encoding the flavoprotein subunit of the complex [Bourgeron et al., 1995; Parfait et al., 2000; Taylor et al., 1996]. The first defect in an assembly factor of complex II, a LYR-motif protein, has been associated with infantile leukoencephalopathy characterized by progressive psychomotor delay starting at 6–12 months of age, spastic quadriparesis, and dystonia. Proton nuclear MR spectroscopy reveals lactate peaks in the white matter [Ghezzi et al., 2009].

Coenzyme Q_{10} serves as an electron shuttle between complexes I and II and complex III. There are three clinical presentations of what appears to be primary, autosomal-recessive coenzyme Q_{10} deficiency. The myopathic form, first described in 1989 in two sisters [Ogasahara et al., 1989], has been reported in three more patients [DiGiovanni et al., 2001; Sobreira et al., 1997]. It is characterized by the triad:

1. myopathy with recurrent myoglobinuria
2. muscle biopsy with ragged red fibers and lipid storage
3. central nervous system dysfunction, with seizures, ataxia, or mental retardation.

The ataxic form is dominated by cerebellar ataxia and cerebellar atrophy, inconsistently accompanied by seizures, pyramidal signs, and mental retardation [Gironi et al., 2004; Lamperti et al., 2003; Musumeci et al., 2001]. Some of these patients have mutations in a gene involved in CoQ_{10} biosynthesis and should be considered primary CoQ_{10} defects [Lagier-Tourenne et al., 2008; Mollet et al., 2008]. Several primary infantile encephalomyopathic forms have been attributed to mutations in biosynthetic genes (*COQ1*, *COQ2*, and *COQ9*) and are often accompanied by nephrosis [Quinzii et al.,

2006; López et al., 2006; Mollet et al., 2007; Duncan et al., 2009]. It is important to consider these syndromes because all patients, but especially those with the myopathic and the infantile forms, often respond dramatically to oral supplementation with coenzyme Q_{10}.

Complex III (coenzyme Q-cytochrome-*c* oxidoreductase) contains 11 subunits, one of which is encoded by mtDNA. Defects involving complex III are subdivided into generalized multisystem disorders manifested by limb weakness, exercise intolerance, and various neurologic signs, or a tissue-specific syndrome manifested either as a pure myopathy with onset in childhood or adolescence or as a pure cardiopathy ("histiocytoid cardiomyopathy") manifested in early infancy. Some patients with the myopathic phenotype and without apparent maternal inheritance have mutations ("somatic" mutations; see earlier) in the cytochrome-*b* gene of mtDNA [Andreu et al., 1999; DiMauro and Bonilla, 2004]. A rapidly fatal infantile disorder, observed in Finland and dubbed GRACILE (growth retardation, aminoaciduria, cholestasis, iron overload, lactacidosis, and early death), was associated with mutations in an assembly protein (BCS1L) needed for the correct synthesis and function of complex III [Visapaa et al., 2002]. Mutations in the same nuclear gene (*BCS1L*) have also been found in children with Leigh's syndrome [de Lonlay et al., 2001].

Complex IV (cytochrome-*c* oxidase, COX) contains 13 subunits, three of which are encoded by mtDNA. In keeping with the clinical presentations of respiratory chain defects, complex IV deficiency can be divided into a myopathic form and a multisystemic form [DiMauro and Bonilla, 2004].

There are two infantile myopathic presentations, a fatal infantile syndrome and a "benign" (reversible) infantile syndrome. The fatal infantile syndrome may be restricted to skeletal muscle and manifested by congenital lactic acidosis and progressive respiratory insufficiency [Bresolin et al., 1985]. These patients die before 1 year of age. Some of these patients may have kidney dysfunction with the de Toni–Fanconi syndrome, whereas others may have abnormalities of cardiac function. The cause of this condition is still unclear but some cases may be due to unrecognized mtDNA depletion. The reversible infantile myopathy is virtually indistinguishable from the fatal infantile form in the newborn period [DiMauro et al., 1983]. These patients also have respiratory insufficiency and severe lactic acidosis. Patients with the benign syndrome, however, spontaneously improve during subsequent months and are essentially normal by 1–3 years of age. The reversible COX-deficient myopathy has been clearly associated with a homoplasmic mtDNA mutation (m.14674T>C in tRNA^{Glu}), but it is clear that the phenotype is conditioned by a modifier nuclear gene [Horvath et al., 2009]. On the other hand, somatic mutations in mtDNA genes encoding COX I or COX III can cause exercise intolerance and recurrent myoglobinuria [Karadimas et al., 2000; Keightley et al., 1996].

The most common clinical presentation for the partial generalized defect of complex IV is Leigh's syndrome [DiMauro and De Vivo, 1996; Van Coster et al., 1991]. These patients are clinically asymptomatic during early infancy. Somatic and neurologic symptoms subsequently develop after 6 months of age, and patients die around 4–5 years of age. This syndrome is inherited as an autosomal-recessive trait. Cytochrome-*c* oxidase-associated Leigh's syndrome can be distinguished clinically from pyruvate dehydrogenase complex-associated Leigh's syndrome and from maternally inherited Leigh's syndrome due to mutations in the ATPase 6 gene of mtDNA [Santorelli et al., 1993]. Patients with cytochrome-*c* oxidase deficiency are clinically symptomatic in the neonatal or early infantile period, and die within 6–12 months of life. Patients with pyruvate dehydrogenase complex-associated Leigh's syndrome or maternally inherited Leigh's syndrome commonly have seizures and recurrent apnea; in addition, patients with maternally inherited Leigh's syndrome may have retinitis pigmentosa, which – when present – is pathognomonic. Patients with cytochrome-*c* oxidase-associated Leigh's syndrome have a slower clinical course, deceleration of head growth, and peripheral neuropathy. Seizures are uncommon in patients with cytochrome-*c* oxidase-associated Leigh's syndrome. In 1998, two groups discovered that most cases of cytochrome-*c* oxidase-associated Leigh's syndrome were due to mutations in a cytochrome-*c* oxidase assembly gene, *SURF1* [Tiranti et al., 1998; Zhu et al., 1998]. This finding has greatly improved genetic counseling and has made prenatal diagnosis possible. Mutations in several other ancillary proteins needed for cytochrome-*c* oxidase assembly have been found in children with Leigh-like encephalopathy and involvement of one other tissue, liver, heart, or kidney. Thus, mutations in the *SCO2* gene cause cardioencephalopathy [Papadopoulou et al., 1999]; in general, the cardiopathy predominates and causes early death, but a few cases presented as spinal muscular atrophy with cardiopathy [Salviati et al., 2001]. Mutations in *COX15* also cause cardioencephalopathy [Antonicka et al., 2003], whereas mutations in *SCO1* cause hepatoencephalopathy [Valnot et al., 1999], and mutations in *COX10* cause nephroencephalopathy [Valnot et al., 2000]. The reasons for the selective involvement of specific tissues besides brain remain unclear.

Alpers' disease [Alpers, 1931] has been associated with complex IV deficiency, but it is now clear that typical cases of Alpers–Huttenlocher syndrome with hepatocerebral presentation are due to mtDNA depletion due to mutations in the *POLG* gene, which encodes the mitochondrial polymerase-γ [Naviaux et al., 1999; Kurt et al., 2010].

Complex V (mitochondrial ATP synthase) is composed of 12–14 subunits, two of which are encoded by mtDNA. The most important causes of complex V deficiency seem to be mutations affecting the ATPase 6 gene of mtDNA. Two mutations at the same nucleotide, G8993T and G8993C, cause syndromes of different severity. Depending on the abundance of mutant mtDNAs (mutation load), the T8993G mutation can cause maternally inherited Leigh's syndrome in infants (mutation load around 90 percent), or a milder encephalomyopathy called neuropathy, ataxia, and retinitis pigmentosa in young adults. (The two conditions can coexist in the same family.) The T8993C mutation causes milder symptoms in both children and adults, often associated with familial bilateral striatal necrosis. In accordance with the more severe presentation, there is biochemical evidence of severely impaired ATP production in cells harboring the T8993G mutation, whereas ATP production is essentially normal in cells harboring the T8993C mutation (whose pathogenic mechanism remains unclear) [Schon et al., 2002]. A few mutations elsewhere in the ATPase 6 gene have been associated with encephalomyopathy and familial bilateral striatal necrosis [DiMauro and Schon, 2003].

The first nuclear defect impairing complex V function has been described. It involves a gene (ATP12) encoding an assembly protein, and it is accompanied by congenital lactic acidosis and a fatal infantile multisystemic disease [De Meirleir et al., 2004]. Mutations in another nuclear gene (*TMEM70*) have been associated with complex V deficiency in children of Roma ethnic origin, with multisystem involvement, lactic acidosis, and 3-methylglutaconic aciduria [Cizkova et al., 2008].

Defects of Protein Importation

The protein importation process is energy-dependent and needs the proteins to be unfolded before traversing the mitochondrial membranes, then refolded before reaching their final destination. This process requires a complex machinery involving leader peptides, chaperonins, translocases in the outer and inner membranes, and proteases [Bolender et al., 2008]. Relatively few human diseases have been attributed to dysfunction of mitochondrial protein import, possibly because of the devastating consequences that disruption of the general import machinery would have. Most of these mutations involve leader peptides. One affected the enzyme methylmalonyl-CoA mutase and accounted for one form of methylmalonicaciduria [Ledley et al., 1990]. Another affected the leader sequence of the E1 alpha subunit of the pyruvate dehydrogenase complex in a child with pyruvate dehydrogenase deficiency and Leigh's syndrome [Takakubo et al., 1995]. One cause of primary hyperoxaluria type I was associated with the misdirecting of a mutated alanine glyoxylate aminotransferase enzyme protein to the mitochondrial matrix rather than to the peroxisome [Purdue et al., 1990]. The enzyme, although catalytically intact, was unable to perform its biologic function because it had been misdirected to the wrong intracellular compartment. Some defects of ornithine transcarbamoylase and carbamylphosphate synthetase I, the two urea cycle enzymes located in the mitochondrion, may be additional examples of mitochondrial protein importation defects. Two children have been described with a defect of heat-shock protein 60, a chaperonin needed for the correct folding and assembly of imported proteins. One infant female, the product of a consanguineous marriage, presented at birth with dysmorphic features, hypotonia, respiratory insufficiency, and severe lactic acidosis, and died 2 days later [Agsteribbe et al., 1993]. The second child also had dysmorphic facial features, congenital hypotonia, and failure to thrive, and she died at 4.5 years of age [Briones et al., 1997]. The molecular bases of these biochemical defects were not established. However, two disorders have been associated with mutations in components of the transport machinery. The first is an X-linked disease called deafness-dystonia syndrome (Mohr–Tranebjaerg syndrome), characterized by neurosensory hearing loss, dystonia, cortical blindness, and psychiatric symptoms; it is due to mutations in the *TIMM8A* gene, which encodes the deafness-dystonia protein (DDP1), a component of the transport machinery [Roesch et al., 2002]. The second is an autosomal-dominant form of hereditary spastic paraplegia due to mutations in the chaperonin heat-shock protein 60 [Hansen et al., 2002].

Defects of Intergenomic Signaling

Two clinical syndromes result from primary molecular defects involving the nuclear genome but affecting either the quality or the quantity of mtDNA. The first condition is associated with multiple deletions of mtDNA and was first described by Zeviani and colleagues [1989]. Patients with multiple mtDNA deletions have progressive external ophthalmoplegia, which can be the dominating feature or can be associated with multisystemic involvement. Patients with autosomal-dominant progressive external ophthalmoplegia usually become symptomatic in the third decade of life, with ophthalmoplegia, progressive limb weakness, bilateral cataracts, depression, parkinsonism, and precocious death. At least four genes affect mtDNA maintenance and have been associated with multiple mtDNA deletions:

- *ANT1*, encoding the adenine nucleotide translocator
- *PEO1* (*Twinkle*), encoding an mtDNA helicase
- *POLG*, encoding the mtDNA polymerase γ
- *OPA1*, encoding a protein involved in mitochondrial fusion [Kaukonen et al., 2000; Spelbrink et al., 2001; Van Goethem et al., 2001; Hudson et al., 2008].

A special form of autosomal-recessive progressive external ophthalmoplegia is the mitochondrial neurogastrointestinal encephalomyopathy syndrome, in which gastrointestinal dysfunction (chronic diarrhea, intestinal pseudo-obstruction), peripheral neuropathy, and leukodystrophy are prominent [Nishino et al., 2000]. In both conditions, there are ragged red fibers in the muscle biopsy specimen. The molecular bases of these conditions are being understood at a rapid pace. Mutations in the gene for thymidine phosphorylase (TP) are responsible for mitochondrial neurogastrointestinal encephalomyopathy [Nishino et al., 1999].

The second example of an intergenomic signaling defect is the mtDNA depletion syndrome with variable tissue expression. This condition was first described by Moraes and colleagues [1991] as an autosomal-recessive trait associated with a quantitative reduction of mtDNA copy number. Two major phenotypes have emerged, one dominated by myopathy, the other by liver and brain involvement. The myopathic form of mtDNA depletion syndrome may present as a congenital and rapidly fatal myopathy (generally associated with very low residual mtDNA in muscle) or as a childhood progressive myopathy (associated with higher residual amounts of mtDNA). The "hepatocerebral" form can present as fulminant hepatopathy of infancy or as a multisystem disorder affecting predominantly brain and liver (not unlike Alpers' syndrome). However, symptoms overlap; for example, infants with the "myopathic" phenotype sometimes mimic spinal muscular atrophy, and mtDNA depletion should be considered in children with spinal muscular atrophy but without mutations in the *SMN* gene. Mutations in nine nuclear genes, all but one involved in mitochondrial nucleotide homeostasis, have been associated with mtDNA depletion syndrome, although they do not explain all cases [Poulton et al., 2009]. Mutations in the gene encoding thymidine kinase (*TK2*) are more common in patients with the myopathic presentation [Saada et al., 2001], whereas mutations in the gene encoding deoxyguanosine kinase (*dGK*) predominate in patients with the hepatocerebral presentation [Mandel et al., 2001].

Defects of the Lipid Milieu of the Inner Mitochondrial Membrane

This pathogenetic mechanism is illustrated by Barth's syndrome, an X-linked recessive disorder characterized by mitochondrial myopathy, cardiopathy, and leukopenia [Barth et al., 1999]. Mutations in the tafazzin (*TAZ*) gene are responsible for Barth's syndrome, and *TAZ* encodes a family of proteins, named tafazzins, that are homologous to phospholipid acyltransferases [Bione et al., 1996]. Analysis of phospholipids

in target tissues from patients with genetically proven Barth's syndrome found markedly decreased levels of cardiolipin, as well as altered cardiolipin composition [Schlame et al., 2002, 2003]. Cardiolipin is the main phospholipid component of the inner mitochondrial membrane, where it not only functions as a "scaffold" but also interacts with respiratory chain complexes. Thus, alterations of cardiolipin amount and composition can affect respiratory function.

Defects of Mitochondrial Motility, Fusion, and Fission

Mitochondria are dynamic organelles forming complex tubular structures in many cells, which requires constant fusion of the mitochondrial tubules, balanced by fission. Also, individual mitochondria move in the cell – sometimes covering considerable distances, as in axons – propelled by energy-requiring dynamins along cytoskeletal microtubular rails [Chan, 2006].

Mutations in a gene (*OPA1*) encoding a dynamin-related guanosine triphosphatase have been associated with an autosomal-dominant form of optic atrophy (DOA) resulting in young-onset blindness, similar to Leber's hereditary optic neuropathy [Alexander et al., 2000; Delettre et al., 2002], as well as with progressive external ophthalmoplegia and multiple mtDNA deletions (see above).

Mutations in the gene (*MFN2*) encoding mitofusin 2, an outer membrane fusion protein, cause Charcot–Marie–Tooth 2A, a severe and early-onset form of axonal neuropathy [Zuchner et al., 2004; DiMauro and Schon, 2008].

Inherited Conditions Associated with Mitochondrial DNA Defects

Since 1988, numerous clinical syndromes have been associated with defects of the mitochondrial genome. These conditions can be subdivided into disorders associated with large-scale rearrangements of mtDNA, syndromes associated with point mutations affecting mtDNA genes, and syndromes associated with intergenomic signaling defects resulting from mutations of the nuclear genome. This latter category is discussed above in the section covering nuclear DNA defects.

Large-scale rearrangements of mtDNA can be sporadic or genetically transmitted. Sporadic syndromes include Kearns–Sayre syndrome, sporadic progressive external ophthalmoplegia, and Pearson's syndrome [DiMauro and Bonilla, 2004; Schon et al., 2002]. A genetically transmitted condition is diabetes mellitus and deafness [Ballinger et al., 1992].

Sporadic Large-Scale Rearrangements

Kearns–Sayre syndrome is the prototype of this group of diseases [Moraes et al., 1989; Zeviani et al., 1988]. Males and females are affected in roughly equal numbers, and the risk of maternal transmission is exceedingly small [Chinnery et al., 2004]. The dominant clinical features include progressive eye signs, such as ptosis, restricted eye movements, and pigmentary retinopathy. Neurologic symptoms include cerebellar ataxia, mental retardation, and episodic coma. Seizures are infrequent and are usually associated with hypoparathyroidism. Complete heart block may lead to sudden death. Insertion of a pacemaker is life-saving. Short stature and hearing loss are common. Endocrine disturbances include diabetes mellitus, hypoparathyroidism, and isolated growth hormone deficiency.

Ragged red fibers are found in almost all affected patients. Calcification of the basal ganglia usually occurs in the setting of hypoparathyroidism. The surprisingly rare incomplete forms of Kearns–Sayre syndrome demonstrate progressive external ophthalmoparesis as an invariant clinical sign. Some cases have unusual clinical presentations, such as renal tubular acidosis, whereas others may overlap with clinically distinct syndromes, such as MELAS [Eviatar et al., 1990; Zupanc et al., 1991].

Pearson's syndrome is a non-neurologic disorder of infancy characterized by pancytopenia, disturbed pancreatic exocrine function, and liver abnormalities [Pearson et al., 1979; Rötig et al., 1990]. The few survivors of this infantile condition may later develop clinical features of Kearns–Sayre syndrome [Blaw and Mize, 1990; Larsson et al., 1990; McShane et al., 1991]. The phenotypic transformation from Pearson's syndrome to Kearns–Sayre syndrome is an example of tissue-specific modifications of mitochondrial heteroplasmy (mitotic segregation).

Point Mutations Affecting Protein-Coding Genes

There are six clinical conditions that are maternally inherited and associated with point mutations in mtDNA protein-coding genes. Two of these, Leber's hereditary optic neuropathy (LHON) and the syndrome of neuropathy, ataxia, and retinitis pigmentosa (NARP), affect structural genes in the mitochondrial genome. Lactic acidosis is usually absent in LHON and may be absent in NARP; ragged red fibers are conspicuously absent in the skeletal muscle biopsy specimens from patients with both conditions.

LHON is dominated clinically by the sudden onset of visual loss in a young adult and is more common in men [Carelli et al., 2006]. The peak age at onset is between 20 and 24 years, although children as young as 5 years have been described. Visual loss is bilateral in the majority of cases, although the condition may first develop in one eye, followed by involvement of the second eye in weeks or months. The presentation is that of a retrobulbar neuropathy, often associated with disc edema and subtle alterations of retinal vessels. The male predominance suggests an X-linked factor that modulates the expression of the mtDNA point mutation [Hudson et al., 2005; Shankar et al., 2008]. The condition is relatively static after the subacute visual loss. Other neurologic and psychiatric symptoms have been described in patients and their family members, signifying the global nature of the molecular defect. Variable findings have included hyperreflexia, Babinski signs, incoordination, peripheral neuropathy, and cardiac conduction abnormalities. Three mutations, all of them in genes encoding subunits of complex I (G3460A in *ND1*, G11778A in *ND4*, and T14484C in *ND6*) are considered "primary": that is, capable of causing LHON in and by themselves.

The second point mutation affecting an mtDNA structural gene results in NARP (see earlier). Holt and associates [1990] described four family members of three successive generations with a variable combination of retinitis pigmentosa, ataxia, developmental delay, dementia, seizures, proximal limb weakness, and sensory neuropathy. This maternally transmitted condition was associated with an mtDNA point mutation involving the gene for subunit 6 of mitochondrial H^+-ATPase. The most severely affected member was 3 years old. She had exhibited reduced fetal movements. Development was delayed, and a pigmentary retinopathy was noted. She had increased limb tone, hyperreflexia, bilateral Babinski signs, and generalized ataxia.

As already mentioned, the T8993G mutation in the ATPase 6 gene of mtDNA has been recognized as one important cause of Leigh's syndrome [DiMauro and Schon, 2003]. Curiously, a different mutation at the very same nucleotide (T8993C) causes a milder clinical phenotype and a less severe impairment of ATP synthesis in mitochondria isolated from cultured fibroblasts [Santorelli et al., 1996]. Mutations in the ATPase 6 gene of mtDNA appear to be associated with various syndromes characterized by the neuroradiologic features of Leigh's syndrome or bilateral striatal necrosis [DiMauro and Schon, 2003].

Point Mutations Affecting Synthetic Genes

There are more than 200 pathogenic point mutations but the two most common clinical conditions that are maternally inherited and associated with mtDNA point mutations affecting transfer RNA genes are mitochondrial encephalopathy with lactic acidosis and strokelike episodes (MELAS), and myoclonus epilepsy and ragged red fibers (MERRF). MELAS was first described in 1984 [Pavlakis et al., 1984] and appears to be the most common mtDNA-related disease. Most patients become symptomatic before the age of 40 years, and 90–100 percent of patients have normal early development, followed by the onset of exercise intolerance, strokelike episodes, seizures, and dementia. Almost all patients have lactic acidosis and had ragged red fibers in skeletal muscle biopsy specimens [Kaufmann et al., 2009]. Recurrent migraine-like headaches preceded by nausea and vomiting are common, as are hearing loss, short stature, learning difficulties, hemiparesis and hemianopia, and limb weakness. The cerebrospinal fluid protein concentration is normal in half of the patients and only mildly elevated in the other half. One-third of patients have basal ganglia calcifications. Seizures are common and often precede the strokelike events. Progressive external ophthalmoparesis was noted in approximately 10 percent of cases. The A3243G mutation in the tRNA$^{\text{leu(uur)}}$ gene of mtDNA is responsible for about 80 percent of MELAS cases worldwide [Goto et al., 1990]. Several other mutations in the same gene have been associated with MELAS [Kaufmann et al., 2004], as well as increasing numbers of mutations in structural genes of mtDNA [Liolitsa et al., 2003; Manfredi et al., 1995; Naini et al., 2005; Shanske et al., 2008].

MERRF was first described in 1980 [Fukuhara et al., 1980]. The major clinical features include cerebellar syndrome, generalized convulsions, myoclonus, dementia, hearing loss, impaired deep sensation, and a positive family history consistent with maternal inheritance. Other findings may include optic atrophy and short stature [DiMauro et al., 2002]. In 1990, Shoffner and colleagues [1990] described a point mutation (A8344G) involving the mtDNA gene for tRNA^{lys}. Two more mutations in the same gene (T8356C and G8363A) are less frequent causes of typical MERRF. Only one mutation in a different gene (G611A in the tRNAPhe gene) has been reported to cause typical MERRF [Mancuso et al., 2004].

Acquired Conditions Associated with Mitochondrial Dysfunction

The inherited conditions causing mitochondrial diseases have dominated medical news in recent years. However, a number of acquired conditions associated with mitochondrial dysfunction have emerged. Reye's syndrome has been viewed as the prototype of an acquired illness associated with generalized mitochondrial dysfunction [De Vivo, 1978; Pranzatelli and

De Vivo, 1987]. This clinical condition typically develops in the wake of a childhood infection, commonly influenza or varicella. The syndrome is dominated clinically by a diffuse encephalopathy with brain swelling. The laboratory abnormalities reflect a generalized disturbance of liver function with elevated serum transaminases, hyperammonemia, and a complex coagulopathy. A statistical association exists between the ingestion of aspirin-containing products and the development of Reye's syndrome [Hurwitz et al., 1987], and the frequency of this condition has declined dramatically with the discontinuation of aspirin.

Toxic mechanisms also have been implicated as a cause of acquired mitochondrial dysfunction. Exposure to 1-methyl-4-phenyl-1,2,3,6-tetrahydropyridine causes an impairment of brain complex I activity and results in a parkinsonian syndrome [Langston et al., 1983; Nicklas et al., 1985]. Parkinsonism, but not typical Parkinson's disease, is seen in patients with multiple mtDNA deletions and mutations in the *POLG* gene. The best evidence of mitochondrial involvement in Parkinson's disease comes from the documentation of mutations in a gene (*PINK1*) encoding a mitochondrial kinase (PTEN-induced kinase 1), which may phosphorylate – and protect – mitochondrial proteins in situations of stress [DiMauro and Schon, 2008].

Drug treatment also may produce mitochondrial dysfunction. Mitochondrial DNA depletion may be acquired via chronic exposure to zidovudine. The depletion in this setting is reversible when zidovudine is discontinued. Zidovudine is incorporated into mtDNA by polymerase γ. As a result, this incorporation inhibits mtDNA replication [Arnaudo et al., 1991; Dalakas et al., 1990]. Another example of drug-induced mitochondrial damage is aminoglycoside-induced deafness, a form of deafness induced by aminoglycoside drugs, such as gentamicin, kanamycin, and streptomycin, in persons harboring a homoplasmic A1555G mutation in the 12s rRNA gene of mtDNA [Schon et al., 2002].

Finally, there is intriguing evidence to suggest that mtDNA damage may accumulate during oxidative stress. Mitochondrial DNA damage has been described in hypoxic hearts that were removed at transplantation [Corral-Debrinski et al., 1991]. Mitochondrial DNA deletions also have been described during the natural aging process, with particular predilection for the corpus striatum [DiMauro et al., 2002]. The clinical significance of these observations awaits further investigation.

Summary

The clinical manifestations of mitochondrial diseases result from dysfunction of organ systems that are highly dependent on aerobic metabolism. These systems include the brain, skeletal muscle, heart, liver, and kidney. Presentation in infancy causes a delay in psychomotor development. The rate of brain growth is compromised, with resulting deceleration of head growth and acquisition of microcephaly. Impairment of vision and hearing is common, and convulsions may occur. Peripheral neuropathy also may be present and has been described with defects of long-chain fatty acid metabolism, generalized cytochrome-*c* oxidase deficiency, and the NARP mutation. The respiratory pattern may be affected and cause central hypoventilation or apnea. Incoordination and hypotonia are common, and Babinski signs are present. Eye findings may include optic atrophy, retinal pigmentary degeneration, ptosis, and ophthalmoparesis. Limb weakness is common, and muscle atrophy

frequently occurs. Cardiomyopathy develops in many patients with mitochondrial diseases. Conduction defects may coexist and predispose the patient to dysrhythmias or complete heart block. Kidney involvement produces tubular dysfunction with a generalized aminoaciduria, hypophosphaturia, and acidosis. This multisystemic involvement may be associated with somatic growth failure characterized by short stature and poor weight gain. Endocrinopathies are increasingly recognized in patients with mitochondrial diseases. Diabetes mellitus, hypothyroidism, hypoparathyroidism, and isolated growth hormone deficiency have been described.

Distinctive laboratory abnormalities represent the metabolic signatures of mitochondrial diseases. The abnormalities reflect the metabolic pathway that is disturbed. Lactate, pyruvate, and alanine concentrations typically are elevated in the blood, urine, and cerebrospinal fluid when the defect involves pyruvate metabolism, the Krebs cycle, or the respiratory chain. Elevated serum free fatty acids, hypoketonemia, primary or secondary carnitine deficiency, and dicarboxylicaciduria commonly are associated with fatty acid oxidation defects. Elevated ammonia concentrations are expected with urea cycle defects. Hypoglycemia results from defects involving gluconeogenesis or fatty acid oxidation. The lactate/pyruvate ratio may be normal when the oxidation–reduction potential is preserved, or elevated when the primary defect involves the respiratory chain. Citric acid cycle intermediates, such as fumaric acid and α-ketoglutarate, may be elevated in the urine with specific biochemical defects involving the Krebs cycle.

Effective treatment for mitochondrial diseases is limited. Biotin supplementation is of value in biotinidase deficiency and in the Km mutant of holocarboxylase synthetase deficiency. Thiamine and lipoic acid have been recommended in deficiencies affecting the pyruvate dehydrogenase complex. A ketogenic diet also may help patients with pyruvate dehydrogenase deficiency, and medium-chain triglycerides may bypass the fatty acid oxidation defect when the defect involves the metabolism of long-chain fatty acids. Treatment of the lactic acidosis has been relatively unsuccessful. Sodium bicarbonate may exacerbate the cerebral symptoms in patients with mitochondrial diseases. Dichloroacetate, an experimental agent, may prove to be beneficial due to its direct action on the pyruvate dehydrogenase complex, lowering the serum lactate concentrations, but it causes disabling peripheral neuropathy as a toxic side effect [Kaufmann et al., 2006]. Folic acid concentrations are low in the cerebrospinal fluid of patients with Kearns–Sayre syndrome, and oral replacement is recommended. Similarly, coenzyme Q_{10} has been recommended as a treatment for many mitochondrial diseases. L-Carnitine is also recommended because a secondary carnitine deficiency syndrome develops in many of these patients. L-Carnitine is life-saving in patients with the primary carnitine-responsive cardiomyopathy of infancy. A cardiac pacemaker is important in Kearns–Sayre syndrome, and naltrexone may be helpful in treating some patients with central hypoventilation. Nutritional supplements, nasogastric tube feedings, and gastrostomies should be considered early in the management of infants and children with mitochondrial diseases to maintain adequate calorie intake.

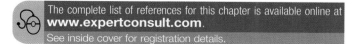

Peroxisomal Disorders

Gerald V. Raymond, Kristin W. Baranano, and S. Ali Fatemi

Disorders of the peroxisome – organelles found in all eukaryotic cells – are characterized by alterations in their unique metabolic functions in the cell and tissues. The pervasive presence of the peroxisome leads to far-reaching consequences of these genetic disorders. Peroxisomal disorders are divided into two major categories. In the first, the organelle fails to develop normally, leading to disruption of multiple peroxisomal enzymes. The second category consists of those disorders in which the peroxisome structure is normal but functioning of a single peroxisomal enzyme is defective. Box 38-1 lists the known peroxisomal disorders; their combined incidence is estimated at 1 in 25,000 or higher [Heymans, 1984]. Because peroxisomal disorders are genetically determined, with a majority readily identifiable by biochemical means, including prenatal testing, and nearly all affecting the nervous system, knowledge of these diseases is important. As the pathophysiology of these disorders is better understood, novel therapeutic strategies may be developed, which gives new hope for advances not only in the diagnosis but also in the management and outcome of peroxisomal disorders.

Historical Overview

The organelle was identified in 1954 by Rhodin and named the "microbody" [Rhodin, 1954]. In 1960, it was found that this structure contained urate, D-amino acid oxidase, and catalase; it was named the peroxisome by de Duve and Baudhuin [1966]. Recognition of its function in active cellular processes came with the demonstration of its role in the β-oxidation of fatty acids (Figure 38-1) [Lazarow, 1978] and plasmalogen synthesis [Hajra and Bishop, 1982]. That change in peroxisome function results in disease was not evident until 1973, when Goldfischer and colleagues determined its absence in Zellweger's syndrome [Goldfischer et al., 1973]. The link between peroxisomes and human disease was not made until that time, even though peroxisomal disorders had been described much earlier, including X-linked adrenoleukodystrophy in 1923 [Siemerling and Creutzfeldt, 1923], acatalasemia in 1948 [Takahara and Migamoto, 1948], and Zellweger's syndrome in 1964 [Bowen et al., 1964]. From the initial three enzymes identified, more than 40 enzymes have been localized to the peroxisomes [Tolbert, 1981].

Structure and Function of Peroxisomes

The peroxisome is bound by a single membrane and contains a fine granular matrix. Histologically, these organelles are identified by the presence of catalase, are present in all human tissues except mature erythrocytes, and demonstrate variation in size and number. In liver and kidney, where they are abundant, the average diameter is 500 nm, whereas in the nervous system, fibroblasts, and amniocytes, they measure 100–250 nm [Hruban and Rechcigl, 1969]. They do not contain DNA and appear to be devoid of glycoproteins. The membrane is 6.5–7 nm thick and has a trilaminar appearance and a unique protein composition. Peroxisome membrane proteins with molecular masses of 22, 26, 27, 41, 57, 68, and 70 kDa have been identified [Hashimoto et al., 1986; Imanaka et al., 1991]. The peroxisomal membrane also contains four ATP binding cassette (ABC) proteins. Although the precise role of these proteins in the peroxisomal membrane is still under investigation, it is known that this family of proteins has important intracellular roles in transport and other functions. As discussed later on, the ABC protein, ABCD1, is defective in X-linked adrenoleukodystrophy, the most prevalent peroxisomal disorder [Wanders et al., 2007].

The process of peroxisomal biogenesis is highly conserved in all eukaryotic organisms, which has permitted the study of yeast to identify the cellular mechanism for the assembly of the organelle and targeting of proteins to the developing vesicle [Weller et al., 2003]. The early concept of peroxisome biogenesis by budding of the endoplasmic reticulum has undergone significant revision. Peroxisomal proteins are encoded by nuclear genes, synthesized on free polyribosomes, and discharged into the cytosol in the mature form. Work in yeast has identified more than 20 genes labeled *PEX* whose products, peroxins, are required for the incorporation of peroxisome membrane proteins and matrix protein importation. Peroxins are required for the proper importation and have roles in receptor docking, stability, and translocation across the membrane [Weller et al., 2003; Ma and Subramani, 2009].

Targeting information directing matrix proteins into the peroxisomes is inherent in the mature polypeptide. A majority of proteins destined for the peroxisome use peroxisome targeting sequence 1 (PTS1), which consists of a terminal tripeptide of serine-lysine-leucine (-SKL) that is recognized by the soluble receptor Pex5p [Gould et al., 1987, 1988, 1990; Keller et al., 1991; Miyazawa et al., 1989]. Not all matrix proteins contain the carboxyl-terminal PTS1 signal. Peroxisomal 3-ketoacyl-coenzyme A (CoA) thiolase and phytanoyl-CoA hydroxylase have a different peroxisomal targeting sequence (PTS2). PTS2 consists of a nine-residue signal located at the amino terminus. It directs the import of a smaller number of proteins using the soluble receptor Pex7p [Swinkels et al., 1991].

Both Pex5p and Pex7p receptors bind their targeted proteins in the cytoplasm outside the peroxisome. The present model has the receptor-peptide complex dock at the peroxisome surface by means of membrane-associated complexes containing

Box 38-1 Peroxisomal Disorders

Disorders of Peroxisome Biogenesis

Zellweger's spectrum

- Zellweger's syndrome
- Neonatal adrenoleukodystrophy
- Infantile Refsum's disease

Rhizomelic chondrodysplasia punctata (RCDP)

- Refsum's disease secondary to *PEX7* mutation

Disorders of Single Peroxisomal Enzymes

X-linked adrenoleukodystrophy

- CADDS
- Acyl CoA-oxidase deficiency
- Bifunctional enzyme deficiency
- DHAP acyltransferase deficiency
- Alkyl DHAP synthase deficiency
- Hyperoxaluria type 1
- Adult Refsum's disease
- Acatalasemia
- Mulibrey nanism

CADDS, contiguous ABCD1 DXS1357E deletion syndrome; CoA, coenzyme A; DHAP, dihydroxyacetone phosphate.

other peroxisome assembly proteins including Pex3p, Pex13p, Pex14p, and Pex17p. Other peroxins appear to function later in the process of translocation. Several are zinc-binding proteins acting downstream of the docking complex and are postulated to constitute the translocation complex involved in matrix protein import. Recent evidence has demonstrated that Pex5p is translocated into the peroxisome and is capable of returning to the cytoplasm – an extended shuttle model [Dammai and Subramani, 2001].

This import method has no parallel with any other organelle. Walton and colleagues demonstrated that peroxisome import allows the uptake of folded, oligomerized proteins and even the import of non-PTS-containing substances, so long as it was with PTS-containing cargo [Walton et al., 1995]. This mechanism is in contrast with that in the mitochondria and lysosome, which have a translocon mechanism with structural modification occurring within the targeted organelle [Lanyon-Hogg et al., 2010].

In contrast with the proteins targeted for the matrix, the proteins used in the membrane utilize another mechanism. Jones and associates examined PMP34 and found that it contained at least two targeting regions. Examining another peroxisomal membrane protein, Pex13, these investigators again found that it had multiple nonoverlapping targeting signals [Jones et al., 2001]. These and other peroxisomal membrane proteins did not share targeting regions. Regions were relatively long and contained at least one membrane-spanning domain.

Peroxisomal number and division appear to be under metabolic control. Hypolipidemic agents, such as clofibrate and industrial phthalate plasticizers, result in the proliferation of liver peroxisomes [Hess et al., 1965; Lazarow et al., 1985]. These agents induce a 20- to 30-fold increase in the activity of the fatty acid β-oxidation system by the rapid coordinated increase of peroxisomal acyl coenzyme A (acyl-CoA) oxidase and bifunctional enzyme [Reddy et al., 1986]. This effect is mediated by activation of peroxisome proliferator-activated receptorα (PPARα), a binding protein related to the steroid hormone receptor superfamily [Issemann and Green, 1990; Lalwani et al., 1987]. Activated PPARα heterodimerizes with a second member of the nuclear receptor superfamily, retinoid X receptor, to form an active transcription factor [Weller et al., 2003]. Peroxisomes also are induced by high-fat diets [Neat et al., 1980], by adrenocorticotropic hormone [Black and Russo, 1980], by thyroid hormone [Fringes and Reith, 1982], and by the agent 4-phenylbutyrate [Wei et al., 2000].

PEROXISOMAL β-OXIDATION PATHWAYS

L-SPECIFIC PATHWAY	D-SPECIFIC PATHWAY	
Substrates: Straight, long chain, and very long chain fatty acids	Substrates: Branched-chain fatty acids	Substrates: Bile acid intermediates
Lignoceryl-CoA (C24) ↓ Acyl-CoA-oxidase	Methyl-palmitoyl-CoA ↓ BC-oxidase	Trihydroxy-coprostanoyl-CoA ↓ BC-oxidase
Lignocerenoyl-CoA ↓ MFP-1	Methy-hexadecanoyl-CoA ↓ MFP-2	Trihydroxy-coprostanoyl-CoA ↓ MFP-2
Hydroxy-lignoceryl-CoA ↓ thiolase	Hydroxy-methyl-palmitoyl-CoA ↓ SCPX	Varanoyl-CoA ↓ SCPX
C22-CoA + Acetyl-CoA	Myristoyl-CoA + Propionyl-CoA	Choloyl-CoA + Propionyl-CoA

Fig. 38-1 Activation and subsequent β-oxidation of very long chain fatty acids, branched-chain fatty acids, and bile acid intermediates by the L- and D-specific pathways in peroxisomes. CoA, coenzyme A.

MFP = multifunctional protein
BC = branched chain
SCP = sterol carrier protein
Long chain acyl CoA-ligase and lignoceroyl-CoA ligase

Peroxisomal function is therefore influenced by metabolic state, nutrition, and pharmaceutical agents.

Reflecting this genetic and metabolic control, peroxisomes vary in tissues throughout the body and during development. In the nervous system of the rat, the peroxisomes are smaller, approximately 140 nm, and fewer than in the liver. They predominate in the first 2 weeks of life in the glia and neurons of the cerebrum, cerebellum, locus coeruleus, and spinal cord, but are fewer in the neurons of adult animals [Nagase et al., 2004]. They are rare in oligodendrocytes in neonatal or adult animals, but become prominent during myelin formation, and may lie adjacent to the outer lamellae that form the myelin sheath [Arnold and Holtzman, 1978]. The biochemical activities follow a similar pattern wherein the activities of catalase and peroxisomal acyl-CoA oxidase and oxidation of lignoceric acid in brain reach a peak at postnatal days 10–16 and then decline. This decline suggests that peroxisomes play a vital role during brain development and myelinogenesis, which may account for the severe brain abnormalities noted in the neonatal and infantile forms of these disorders, including neuronal migration defects.

Metabolic Function of Peroxisomes

Peroxisomes were named for the presence of hydrogen peroxide and catalase, which decomposes the hydrogen peroxide. The seminal observation by Lazarow and de Duve in 1976 that rat liver peroxisomes oxidized palmityl-CoA, followed in 1978 by the demonstration of enzymes of β-oxidation and production of acetyl-CoA by Lazarow and Fujiki [1985], led to the recognition of the importance of this organelle in biologic processes. It is now known that more than 40 enzymatic functions are found in the peroxisome. Some peroxisomal activities, such as oxidation of fatty acids and cholesterol synthesis, can occur in other cellular compartments as well. Certain reactions, however, occur exclusively in the peroxisome. These reactions include oxidation of very long chain fatty acids and pipecolic acid and certain steps in the synthesis of plasmalogens and bile acids. These reactions are abnormal in many peroxisomal disorders. The composition of enzymes within the peroxisome varies among species and within tissues in a species, as well as with maturation, metabolic state, and environmental factors. The following discussion focuses on those metabolic pathways that are unique and are used as markers in diagnosis.

Peroxisomal Fatty Acid Oxidation

Peroxisomal β-oxidation enzymes are distinct from their mitochondrial counterparts. The biochemical steps are similar, involving several distinct enzymes including an oxidase, multifunctional enzyme (displaying enoyl-CoA hydratase and 3-hydroxy acyl-CoA dehydrogenase activity), and 3-oxo acyl-CoA thiolase. It recently has become clear that several distinct oxidases, multifunctional proteins, and enzymes catalyzing the thiolytic cleavage exist. The two pathways, L- and D-specific, are depicted in Figure 38-1.

LONG-CHAIN ACYL-COENZYME A LIGASE AND LIGNOCEROYL-COENZYME A LIGASE

Initially it was thought that a single acyl-CoA ligase that activated long-chain (C10–C18) fatty acids was involved in oxidation of fatty acids and that it was common to mitochondria,

microsomes, and peroxisomes [Miyazawa et al., 1985]. This enzyme is localized to the cytoplasmic side of the peroxisomal membrane, unlike other peroxisomal enzymes, which are in the matrix [Mannaerts et al., 1982]. Subsequently, a series of investigations led to the recognition of a closely related but separate enzyme, which is a ligase for very long chain fatty acids and is referred to as lignoceryl-CoA ligase or synthetase [Singh et al., 1988]. This enzyme is active toward lignoceric acid (C24:0) and hexacosanoic acid (C26:0). Unlike long-chain ligase, very long chain fatty acid ligase is absent in mitochondria. Singh et al. [1984] demonstrated that lignoceric acid is oxidized exclusively in the peroxisome. It is unclear if the very long chain fatty acid ligase plays any role in the pathogenesis of peroxisomal disorders.

ACYL-COENZYME A OXIDASES

The straight-chain acyl-CoA oxidase is synthesized in the mature form containing the carboxyl-terminal PTS1 [Miyazawa et al., 1987]. The oxidase is most active toward saturated and unsaturated fatty acids with 12- to 18-carbon chain lengths. The oxidase for bile acid intermediates and branched-chain fatty acids is a separate enzyme in humans [Casteels et al., 1990; Ferdinandusse et al., 2003; Scheperse et al., 1990].

BIFUNCTIONAL OR MULTIFUNCTIONAL ENZYMES

In both peroxisomal β-oxidation systems, the hydration step (enoyl-CoA hydratase) and the dehydrogenation step (3-hydroxyacyl-CoA dehydrogenase) are catalyzed by multifunctional enzymes (MFEs). The originally identified "bifunctional enzyme," known as either MFE1 or L-bifunctional protein (L-BP), is L-specific. Human deficiency of the D-specific enzyme, referred to as either MFE2 or D-bifunctional protein (D-BP), causes a failure in the oxidation of very long chain fatty acids and branched-chain fatty acids. MFE2 was found to be identical to 17-hydroxysteroid dehydrogenase type 4 and has a domain at its carboxyl terminus that resembles sterol carrier protein 2 (SCP2), an important intracellular sterol and lipid-binding and transport protein [van Grunsven et al., 1999].

THIOLASES

3-Ketoacyl-CoA thiolase is the enzyme for the L-specific pathway and was characterized and cloned first [Bout et al., 1988; Hashimoto, 1982]. Unlike other peroxisomal enzymes but similar to mitochondrial enzymes, it is synthesized as a precursor and converted to the mature form by cleavage of a leader sequence. The peroxisomal targeting sequence for thiolase is located at the amino-terminal end [Swinkels et al., 1991] and was the first protein in which the PTS2 signal was characterized. The thiolytic cleavage in the D-specific pathways is catalyzed by sterol carrier protein X (SCPX). This 58-kDa protein has an amino-terminal thiolase domain that is a phylogenetic equivalent of the mitochondrial and peroxisomal thiolases [Igual et al., 1992].

Oxidation of Unsaturated Fatty Acids

Degradation of monounsaturated and polyunsaturated fatty acids has been demonstrated to occur in peroxisomes, in addition to chain shortening of long-chain dicarboxylic acids [Ferdinandusse et al., 2001; Hiltunen et al., 1986; Kolvraa and Gregersen, 1983; Schulz and Kunau, 1987]. An example of a polyunsaturated fatty acid that requires peroxisomal oxidation is docosahexaenoic acid, which has an important role in retina and brain development, and is known to be deficient in certain peroxisomal disorders [Moser et al., 1999; Watkins et al., 2001].

Branched-Chain Fatty Acid Oxidation and Phytanic Acid α-Oxidation

Branched-chain fatty acids are channeled into the D-specific pathway. The relevant enzymes include branched-chain acyl-CoA oxidase, MFE2, and sterol carrier protein, which functions as thiolase (see Figure 38-1). Phytanic acid has a β-methyl group that blocks β-oxidation and therefore must be α-oxidized first. After activation to its CoA derivative, phytanic acid is α-hydroxylated by phytanoyl CoA α-hydroxylase, the enzyme defective in classic Refsum's disease [Jansen et al., 1997; Mihalik et al., 1997]. The α-hydroxy phytanoyl CoA is then degraded by a lyase to pristanic acid and formate [Croes et al., 1997]. The pristanic acid then can enter β-oxidation through the branched-chain pathway.

Bile Acid Synthesis

Cholesterol is converted in the liver to cholic acid and chenodeoxycholic acid by a series of enzymatic steps localized to several subcellular compartments. Pedersen and Gustafsson [1980] first demonstrated that the peroxisomal fraction of rat liver catalyzes the conversion of an intermediate product of this pathway, tri- or tetrahydroxy-5-β-cholestanoic acid (trihydroxycholestanoic acid), to cholic acid. Subsequently, Kase et al. [1986] reported that the conversion of trihydroxycholestanoic acid to cholic acid, and of dihydrocholestanoic acid to chenodeoxycholic acid also took place in peroxisomes and was deficient in patients with Zellweger's syndrome. Shortening of the cholesterol side chain by β-oxidation resulting in the formation of bile acids is analogous to fatty acid oxidation and uses the enzymes of the D-specific peroxisomal β-oxidation pathway. The oxidase for trihydroxycholestanoic acid–CoA is separate from that of fatty acids and in humans also is believed to function as a branched-chain fatty acid oxidase (see Figure 38-1). A cytochrome P-450 catalyzing the hydroxylation of the C26/27 carbon of cholesterol in bile acid synthesis and formation of taurine conjugates of bile acid also has been localized to peroxisomes [Gutierrez et al., 1988; Kase and Bjorkheim, 1989]. In peroxisomal disorders, an increase in plasma and urine bile acid intermediates can be used as a diagnostic criterion.

Plasmalogen Synthesis

Plasmalogens are ether phospholipids and constitute 5–20 percent of phospholipids in mammalian cell membranes [Snyder, 1972]. They are abundant in myelin, in which they constitute one-third of the myelin phospholipids [Norton and Autilio, 1966]. Although the role of ether phospholipids is not fully elucidated, they appear to have important roles as antioxidants in membrane dynamics, storage of polyunsaturated fatty acids, and signal transduction [Brites et al., 2004].

Plasmalogen synthesis is initiated by the acylation of dihydroxyacetone phosphate by dihydroxyacetone phosphate acyltransferase. Experimental studies in cultured skin fibroblasts demonstrate that ATP is required to overcome the latency of dihydroxyacetone phosphate acyltransferase, a finding that is compatible with an ATP-linked translocation of the substrate across the peroxisomal membrane [Wolvetang et al., 1990]. The second enzyme, alkyl-dihydroxyacetone phosphate synthase, replaces the acyl group with a long-chain alcohol [Hajra and Bishop, 1982]. Both enzymes involved in these initial steps of introducing the ether bond into ether phospholipids are located on the inner surface of peroxisome membranes. The third step is the reduction of the alkyl-dihydroxyacetone phosphate to 1-alkyl glycerol-3-phosphate by the enzyme acyl/alkyl-dihydroxyacetone phosphate reductase, which is present in both peroxisomes and microsomes [Datta et al., 1990]. All subsequent steps of synthesis occur in the microsomes. A method developed by Roscher et al. [1985] determines the ratio of the activities in peroxisomal and microsomal components, and has proved to be of value in the study of peroxisomal disorders, many of which feature a marked reduction in plasmalogen synthesis.

Prostaglandin Degradation

Peroxisomes are involved in the chain shortening of prostaglandins F_{2a} [Diczfalusy and Alexson, 1988] and E_2 [Schepers et al., 1986]. Tiffany et al. [1991] demonstrated that basal and interleukin-1-stimulated synthesis of prostaglandin E_2 increased in a group of patients with X-linked adrenoleukodystrophy.

Amino Acid Metabolism

D-AMINO ACID OXIDASE

D-Amino acid oxidase is a flavoprotein with stereospecific activity toward D-amino acids and greatest activity toward D-proline. The kidney has the highest level of activity, although the enzyme is widely distributed in vertebral tissues. The role of D-amino acids as neurotransmitters has recently attracted attention [Errico et al., 2009].

ALANINE-GLYOXALATE AMINOTRANSFERASE

Alanine-glyoxalate aminotransferase is a pyridoxal phosphate-dependent enzyme that catalyzes the transamination of glyoxalate to glycine, with alanine serving as the amino group donor. The subcellular localization of alanine-glyoxalate aminotransferase is species-dependent; it is present in peroxisomes in humans, rabbits, guinea pigs, and macaques, whereas it is mitochondrial in cats and dogs. It is present in both organelles in the rat, mouse, and hamster. The complementary DNA (cDNA) sequence of alanine-glyoxalate aminotransferase has been determined, and the subcellular localization appears to be determined by the targeting signal at the amino terminus [Danpure, 1995; Noguchi and Takada, 1979; Noguchi et al., 1978]. Of great interest is the observation that the mitochondrial targeting signal active in the rat enzyme is not expressed in humans. In some patients with hyperoxaluria type 1, this is altered, resulting in targeting of the alanine-glyoxalate aminotransferase to mitochondria instead of to the peroxisomes [Purdue et al., 1990]. In hyperoxaluria, the defective alanine-glyoxalate aminotransferase results in the conversion of glyoxalate to oxalic acid, which causes oxaluria and nephrocalcinosis.

PIPECOLIC ACID OXIDASE

L-Pipecolic acid is a component of an alternate lysine degradation pathway and is oxidized by L-pipecolic acid oxidase to α-aminoadipic acid. This enzyme contains flavin, and its subcellular localization is species-dependent. The major site of oxidation is peroxisomal in humans and monkeys, and mitochondrial in rabbits [Mihalik and Rhead, 1989]. The enzyme has been identified in human liver and has been reported to be deficient in Zellweger's syndrome [Mihalik et al., 1989; Wanders et al., 1988a]. The human enzyme most closely resembles the bacterial monomeric sarcosine oxidases [Dodt et al., 2000]. Isolated increases in pipecolic acid have been reported in normal adults and may be a benign trait [Vallat et al., 1996]. Pipecolic acid elevation has also been seen in pyridoxine-responsive seizures, but this is due not to defects in the oxidase, but rather to the antiquitin (*ALDH7A1*) gene, which affects other aspects of the pathway [Bennett et al., 2009].

Classification of Peroxisomal Disorders

Peroxisomal disorders may be divided into two categories:
1. disorders of peroxisome assembly or biogenesis
2. single-enzyme defects [Raymond, 2001].

In the first, the peroxisome fails to form, and abnormalities of multiple peroxisomal functions are present. It is understood that these disorders are defects in protein importation using the PTS1 and PTS2 targeting sequences or membrane incorporation. This group of biogenesis disorders can be further divided by their clinical and biochemical features into the Zellweger spectrum disorders and rhizomelic chondrodysplasia punctata. The second major group consists of a growing number of disorders in which a genetically determined abnormality of a single peroxisomal enzyme is present and peroxisomal structure is intact.

All of these disorders are, in actuality, single-gene and ultimately single-protein deficiencies, but the downstream consequences of the first group affect more than one peroxisomal pathway, resulting in multiple diagnostic abnormalities. With the emergence of DNA-based diagnosis, the utility of this division may require reassessment. An overview of diagnostic evaluation of peroxisomal disorders is provided in Figure 38-2.

Conditions Resulting from Defective Peroxisome Biogenesis

Conditions resulting from defective peroxisome biogenesis are listed in Box 38-1; Zellweger's syndrome and rhizomelic chondrodysplasia punctata are the respective prototypes. Clinical and biochemical variation between these two types of assembly defects still makes it useful to discuss them separately, although it is important to recognize that these disorders were described on a clinical basis before details of the cell and molecular biology of peroxisomal disorders was known, and hence they were assigned names based on the clinical features, pathologic findings, or biochemical defects that identified them.

Molecular Etiology of Disorders of Peroxisome Assembly

Cell complementation studies were instrumental in the early understanding of the genetics of peroxisomal assembly disorders. Identification of complementation groups provided

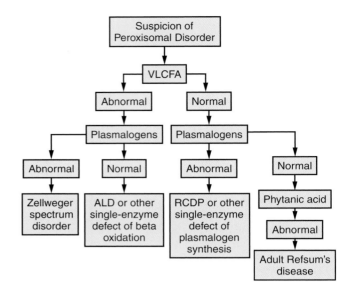

Fig. 38-2 Diagnostic evaluation of peroxisomal disorders. Confirmatory genetic or biochemical testing may be required. ALD, adrenoleukodystrophy; RCDP, rhizomelic chondrodysplasia punctata; VLCFA, very long chain fatty acid.

cell lines that are homogeneous with respect to their gene defect. In conjunction with the use of other molecular biology tools, including the study of yeast and other cell types and the emergence of computerized genomic databases, a new understanding of the molecular underpinnings of the peroxisome assembly disorders has been attained [Lazarow, 1995]. These disorders result from defects in the *PEX* genes. A complex interaction of peroxins is necessary for the biogenesis of peroxisomes, and a defect in any of these proteins impairs the process. The final common pathway is peroxisomal dysfunction, with the respective clinical syndromes.

From the study of complementation groups, it was determined that peroxisomal disorders comprise up to 16 complementation groups [Moser et al., 1995]. A majority of the identified groups included persons with Zellweger's syndrome and milder variations of that condition. One complementation group, however, contained all of the patients with rhizomelic chondrodysplasia punctata, and no overlap between this clinical group and the others was identified. It has subsequently been determined that Zellweger spectrum disorders are secondary to PTS1-mediated pathways including *PEX5*, and that rhizomelic chondrodysplasia punctata is secondary to mutations in *PEX7*, the receptor for PTS2 proteins.

The most common causes of Zellweger spectrum disorders are mutations in either *PEX1* or *PEX6*, although to date, 13 *PEX* genes have been identified as potential causes of these disorders (Table 38-1). *PEX1* and *PEX6* encode AAA ATPases. Their exact role in matrix protein importation is not certain, but it is evident that they interact. Overexpression of *PEX6* or *PEX1* can correct mild deficiencies of the other [Germain-Lee et al., 1997; Reuber et al., 1997]. *PEX1* defects account for more than 65 percent of cases of such defects [Steinberg et al., 2003; Weller et al., 2003]. A degree of phenotype correlation with the causative mutation has been noted. A single base-pair deletion results in a severe phenotype, and G843D allows a milder phenotype [Collins and Gould, 1999]. Because it is known that *PEX1* and *PEX6* interact, the mutation G843D affects this interaction [Weller et al., 2003].

Table 38-1 Disorders of Peroxisome Biogenesis

Gene	Complementation Group	Chromosome Localization	Protein Name	Protein Family or Domain	Percentage of Patients with ZSD Phenotype*
PEX1	1	7q21–22	Peroxisome biogenesis factor 1	AAA ATPase	68
PXR1 (PEX5)	2	12p13.3	Peroxisomal targeting signal 1 receptor	C-terminus TPR domains N-terminal WxxxF/Y repeats	1.5
PEX12	3	17q21.1	Peroxisome assembly protein 12	C-terminal zinc binding RING	4.1
PEX6	4	6p21.1	Peroxisome assembly factor-2	AAA ATPase	10.7
PEX10	7	1p36.32	PAP 10	C-terminal zinc binding RING	4.6
PEX26	8	22q11.2	PEX26 protein	PMP, N-terminal cytosolic, C-terminal peroxisomal	6.6
PEX16	9	11p12–p11.2	PMP PEX16	Orphan	0.5
				C-terminal zinc binding RING	1.0
PXMP3 (PEX2)	10	8q21.1	PAF-1		
PEX3	12	6q23	PAP PEX3	Orphan	1.5
PEX13	13	2p15	PMP PEX13	C-terminal SRC homology domain	1.0
PXF (PEX19)	14	1q22	Peroxisomal farnesylated protein	Farnesylated at C-terminus	0.5
PEX14	–	1p36.2	PMP PEX14	SH3-binding motif PxxP	
PEX7	11	6q21–q22.2		WD40 repeats containing protein	

* Percentage of patients is adapted from the experience of the Kennedy Krieger Institute and Johns Hopkins Hospital DNA Diagnostic Laboratory [Steinberg et al., 2003]. All PEX7 patients are rhizomelic chondrodysplasia punctata; other *PEX* genes express Zellweger spectrum disorder (ZSD). PMP, peroxisome membrane protein.

Zellweger Spectrum Disorders

Zellweger's syndrome (cerebrohepatorenal syndrome) was first described by Bowen and associates [Bowen et al., 1964; Opitz, 1985]. Subsequently, the disorders neonatal adrenoleukodystrophy and infantile Refsum's disease were described as separate entities. Although classic Zellweger's syndrome is the most severe form with a characteristic phenotype, clinical overlap exists between it and the other forms. All of the Zellweger spectrum disorders share morphologic and biochemical abnormalities, and genetic understanding of the underlying mutations has been obtained in many cases. In view of this overlap, it appears prudent at this time to retain a portion of this clinical nomenclature and refer to the group as Zellweger spectrum disorders.

Clinical and Pathologic Features

ZELLWEGER'S SYNDROME

Zellweger's syndrome is a multiple congenital anomaly syndrome characterized by craniofacial abnormalities, eye abnormalities, neuronal migration defects, hepatomegaly, chondrodysplasia punctata, and near-complete absence of peroxisomes. The craniofacial features include a high forehead, hypoplastic supraorbital ridges, epicanthal folds, midface hypoplasia, and a large fontanel (Figure 38-3). The head circumference usually is normal. Reported ocular abnormalities include cataracts, glaucoma, corneal clouding, Brushfield spots, optic nerve hypoplasia, and pigmentary retinal abnormalities. Severe weakness and hypotonia manifest in the newborn period, often accompanied by seizures and apnea [Heymans, 1984; Wilson et al., 1986]. Most affected infants have oromotor dysfunction and require tube feeding. Little psychomotor development ensues, and the average life span is limited, with most affected children surviving for 12–24 months. The facial appearance, Brushfield spots, and profound hypotonia may lead to a consideration of Down syndrome, although the chromosomal determination will eliminate that as a consideration.

Striking abnormalities of neuronal migration unique to Zellweger's syndrome are evident in the cerebral hemispheres as areas of pachygyria or polymicrogyria localized to the opercular region. In the cerebellum, the Purkinje cells form scattered heterotopias throughout the cortex and in the granule cell layer. Laminar discontinuities involving the olivary nucleus are noted, which also are unique to Zellweger's syndrome [Evrard et al., 1978; Volpe and Adams, 1972]. Studies of *PEX* gene knockout mice have demonstrated similar neuropathologic changes [Baes et al., 1997; Faust, 2003; Faust et al., 2001; Gressens et al., 2000; Janssen et al., 2000, 2003].

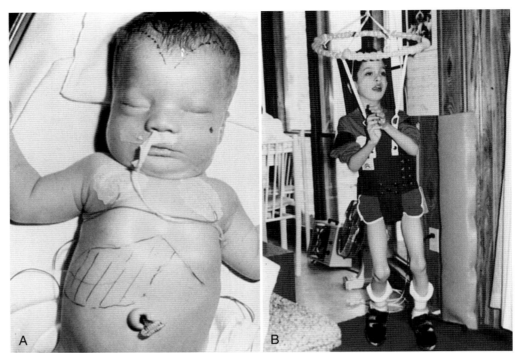

Fig. 38-3 Cerebrohepatorenal syndrome of Zellweger. A, Note the prominent forehead, large fontanel, hypertelorism, epicanthal folds, hypotonia, and hepatomegaly. **B,** Milder form of generalized peroxisomal disorder: 10-year-old boy with ataxia, significant mental retardation, visual loss secondary to retinitis pigmentosa, absence of speech, and sensorineural hearing loss. Liver biopsy showed micronodular cirrhosis and very few, abnormally small peroxisomes.

N-methyl-D-aspartate (NMDA)-mediated abnormalities may contribute to the clinical findings seen in the most severely affected persons [Gressens et al., 2000].

Multiple other abnormalities have been reported. The eyes demonstrate loss of retinal ganglion cells and gliosis of the optic nerve [Cohen et al., 1983]. Retinal pigmentary degenerative changes are associated with absent electroretinograms [Hittner et al., 1981]. Hepatomegaly (present in 78 percent of patients) with periportal fibrosis may result in significant cholestasis (in 59 percent) and jaundice, micronodular cirrhosis (in 37 percent), and hypoprothrombinemia [Heymans, 1984]. Excessive iron deposition has been noted, which diminishes with age [Gilchrist et al., 1976]. Renal cortical cysts of varied sizes are present in 97 percent of patients studied pathologically but may be missed by ultrasound analyses [Bernstein et al., 1974; Heymans, 1984]. The adrenal gland demonstrates changes similar to those in X-linked adrenoleukodystrophy, with cytoplasmic lamellar inclusions consisting of cholesterol esterified with very long chain fatty acids [Goldfischer et al., 1983]. Skeletal abnormalities include clubfoot, thumb rotation, and stippled chondral calcification of the patella and acetabulum in 50 percent of patients [Heymans, 1984].

NEONATAL ADRENOLEUKODYSTROPHY AND INFANTILE REFSUM'S DISEASE

The neonatal form of adrenoleukodystrophy was described by Ulrich et al. [1978] in a male infant with neonatal seizures and severe developmental delay. Postmortem examination at 18 months revealed adrenal atrophy and cytoplasmic inclusions typically seen in X-linked adrenoleukodystrophy; therefore, the disease was considered to be a connatal form of adrenoleukodystrophy. The multiple peroxisomal defects were first recognized in 1982 by Mobley and co-workers and substantiated later by others [Kelley et al., 1986; Partin and McAdams, 1983; Wanders et al., 1987]. Hyperpipecolicacidemia

was described in 1968 by Gatfield and associates in a male infant with neurodegenerative disease and an enlarged liver, who died at 27 months of age. A marked excess of pipecolic acid was noted in the tissues and body fluids. In 1975, Danks and colleagues demonstrated excess pipecolic acid in Zellweger's syndrome, and in 1988, Wanders and associates described a generalized peroxisomal dysfunction in that disorder, including the original case of Gatfield and associates [Wanders et al., 1988c]. The term infantile phytanic acid storage disease, a possible variant of Refsum's disease, was used by Scotto et al. [1982] to describe the disorder in three unrelated males aged 3–6 years with hepatomegaly, dysmorphism, mental retardation, sensorineural hearing loss, and retinitis pigmentosa. The investigators noted that the liver biopsy specimen contained inclusions similar to plant chloroplasts that included phytol, which led to the measurement and recognition of increased phytanic acid levels, as in classic Refsum's disease. The generalized peroxisomal dysfunction was documented by Poulos et al. [1984, 1986], and later by Poll-The et al. [1986a, b] and Wanders et al. [1986b].

We now have a clear understanding that alteration in *PEX* genes may result in clinical phenotypes that are less severe than in Zellweger's syndrome. Even in the milder forms, patients generally have mental retardation, retinal degeneration, and motor handicaps. Dysmorphism is less severe than in Zellweger's syndrome; renal cysts may be absent, and no radiographic stippling of the cartilages is seen. Although neonatal adrenoleukodystrophy and infantile Refsum's disease have in the past been split into distinct clinical presentations, this division can no longer be supported in light of more recent information on the genetic mechanism. This was already apparent from the clear clinical overlap between Zellweger's syndrome and neonatal adrenoleukodystrophy and infantile Refsum's disease. In addition, attempts to differentiate between these milder phenotypes either genetically or biochemically do not reliably predict the clinical course.

Patients with milder forms may present in the neonatal period with mild to moderate dysmorphism, hypotonia, poor feeding, and hepatomegaly with micronodular cirrhosis. Motor and cognitive development usually is delayed. Even with hypotonia, patients may be able to walk, although gait often is ataxic. Retinal pigmentary degeneration may not become evident until the age of 4–6 months and often results in visual loss in the first years of life. Electroretinograms show profound abnormalities in nearly all affected persons and do not correlate well with vision in this population. Sensorineural hearing loss is associated with limited language development [Aubourg et al., 1986; Boltshauser et al., 1982; Budden et al., 1986; Poll-The et al., 1987; Scotto et al., 1982; Torvik et al., 1988; Wanders et al., 1990a; Weleber et al., 1984]. Adrenal dysfunction may develop with age [Govaerts et al., 1989; Poll-The et al., 1987]. Liver dysfunction often is present and detectable by persistent elevation of liver enzymes. A bleeding diathesis that responds to vitamin K also may develop, and in several children, esophageal varices were observed, consistent with portal hypertension. Several investigators have reported postmortem studies in patients aged 8 months to 12 years [Challa et al., 1983; Chow et al., 1992; Powers and Moser, 1998; Torvik et al., 1988]. The liver demonstrated micronodular cirrhosis, and the adrenal glands were hypoplastic. Lipid-laden macrophages were present in the liver, lymph nodes, and certain areas of the cerebral white matter. The only cerebral malformation was a variable hypoplasia of the cerebellar granular layer and a migrational defect of the Purkinje cells. Retinal abnormalities include a loss of ganglion cells, gliosis of the nerve fiber layer, and bileaflet inclusions in the pigment epithelium and macrophages [Cohen et al., 1983].

Optic atrophy seen in patients with neonatal adrenoleukodystrophy/infantile Refsum's disease has been confused with Leber's optic atrophy [Ek et al., 1986], and the association of retinal pigmentary degeneration and sensorineural hearing loss has led to misdiagnosis as Usher's syndrome [Kelley et al., 1986; Noetzel et al., 1983].

Life span is variable, and patients have survived to adulthood [Kelley et al., 1986; Poll-The et al., 1987]. Several older patients have now been described. All identified patients have been visually impaired, with sensorineural hearing loss.

A progressive leukodystrophy, with variable age at onset, has been reported in a number of patients. This disorder results in loss of previously acquired skills, and, in most cases, progresses to a vegetative state and death. Unlike in X-linked adrenoleukodystrophy, the rate of progression has been highly variable.

Clinical recognition of these disorders may present some uncertainty because of nonspecific abnormalities and phenotypic variability. Disorders of peroxisome biogenesis commonly manifest in the neonatal period, and patients come to attention because of hypotonia, seizures, or liver disease. Evaluation appropriately focuses on a search for cytogenetic abnormalities, acute treatable metabolic disorders, and structural liver disease. Later in childhood, patients often are mistakenly diagnosed as having cerebral palsy, X-linked adrenoleukodystrophy, mitochondrial disease, or lysosomal disorders. The possibility of a disorder of peroxisome biogenesis should be considered in children with any of the following features:

1. psychomotor retardation
2. dysmorphism
3. hypotonia
4. hepatomegaly
5. seizures
6. retinal pigmentary changes/absent electroretinogram
7. sensorineural hearing loss
8. renal cysts
9. aberrant calcific stippling
10. adrenal insufficiency.

After analyzing 40 cases, Theil et al. [1992] subdivided the clinical characteristics into major and minor features. They suggest that the combined presence of three major features (present in more than 75 percent of patients) and one or more minor features (present in 50–75 percent) warrants biochemical investigation for peroxisomal disease. Other investigators have pointed out that, in view of the lack of specificity and ease of testing, strict screening criteria are not warranted, and the possibility of neonatal adrenoleukodystrophy and infantile Refsum's disease should be considered in more children with previously undiagnosed developmental delay [Moser and Raymond, 1998].

All of the disorders in this group are inherited in an autosomal-recessive fashion, so it is important for genetic counseling that an accurate diagnosis be arrived at expeditiously. Carrier detection is possible only by DNA analysis if the molecular defect has been identified in the index case [Shimozawa et al., 1992]. Carrier detection is not possible by biochemical determination in blood or fibroblasts.

Laboratory Diagnosis

The diagnostic abnormalities present in patients with Zellweger spectrum disorders are listed in Table 38-2. A major diagnostic biochemical abnormality is the increased amount of very long chain fatty acids, which are fatty acids with carbon chains of more than 22. They also are elevated in single-enzyme defects

Table 38-2 Diagnostic Biochemical Plasma Profile of Peroxisomal Disorders

	Very Long Chain Fatty Acid	Red Blood Cell Plasmalogens	Pipecolic Acid*	Phytanic Acid*
Zellweger spectrum disorder	↑↑	↓↓	↓	↑
Rhizomelic chondrodysplasia punctata	N1	↓↓	N1	↑
Adrenoleukodystrophy	↑	N1	N1	N1
L-bifunctional enzyme deficiency	↑↑	N1	N1	↑
Adult Refsum's disease	N1	N1	N1	↑↑

N1, normal.
* May be age dependant.

of peroxisomal β-oxidation, so their presence is nonspecific, and other studies are required for this diagnosis. Very long chain fatty acid accumulation here is due to the reduction of peroxisomal β-oxidation, which is greater in Zellweger's syndrome than in milder forms. A virtual absence of peroxisomal acyl-CoA oxidase and bifunctional enzyme has been demonstrated in the liver of patients with Zellweger's syndrome [Suzuki et al., 1986; Tager et al., 1985]. It should be noted, however, that very long chain fatty acids are not elevated in rhizomelic chondrodysplasia punctata and other peroxisomal disorders (e.g., acatalasemia) that do not involve lipid oxidation, and normal levels do not exclude all peroxisomal disorders.

Because the first two steps of plasmalogen synthesis are peroxisomal functions, a reduction of plasmalogen levels is noted in patients with peroxisome biogenesis defects. Deficient levels of dihydroxyacetone phosphate acyltransferase have been used for diagnostic purposes in skin fibroblasts, amniocytes, chorionic villus samples, red blood cells, leukocytes, and platelets [Besley and Broadhead, 1987; Datta et al., 1984; Schutgens et al., 1985; Wanders et al., 1985, 1986a]. Webber et al. [1987] have demonstrated that the K_m values and other properties of the residual enzyme are normal, suggesting that the enzyme is not defective but is abnormally labile in the cytosol because of failure of transport into the peroxisome. Plasmalogens are reduced to 5 percent of control values in Zellweger's syndrome [Heymans et al., 1984; Wanders et al., 1986a].

An age-related increase in the levels of phytanic acid occurs in all of the peroxisome biogenesis disorders, including rhizomelic chondrodysplasia punctata, although not to the extent seen in classic adult Refsum's disease. The accumulation of phytanic acid was demonstrated first in infantile Refsum's disease [Scotto et al., 1982] and later in Zellweger's syndrome [Poulos et al., 1984]. Poulos et al. [1988] demonstrated that pristanic acid is elevated in disorders of peroxisome biogenesis. This elevation was later confirmed to be due to an impaired capacity to oxidize pristanic acid [Singh et al., 1990]. These findings are unlike those in classic Refsum's disease, in which the defect involves the conversion of phytanic acid to pristanic acid. Thus, oxidation of pristanic acid is a peroxisomal function that is disrupted in disorders of peroxisome biogenesis [Watkins et al., 1990].

Normally, bile acid intermediates, such as trihydroxycholestanoic acid and dihydroxycholestanoic acid, are absent or present in low concentrations. In Zellweger spectrum disorders, however, they constitute 30–50 percent of total plasma bile acids [Clayton et al., 1987; Eyssen et al., 1985; Gustafsson et al., 1983; Hanson et al., 1979; Mathis et al., 1980; Monnens et al., 1980; Poulos and Whiting, 1985]. Bile acid intermediates also may be abnormal in single-enzyme defects, such as peroxisomal bifunctional enzyme deficiency.

The impaired activity of L-pipecolic acid oxidase results in increased accumulation of pipecolic acid in plasma and increased excretion of pipecolic acid in urine of patients with Zellweger spectrum disorders [Kelley and Moser, 1984; Mihalik et al., 1989; Wanders et al., 1988a]. Pipecolic acid levels in blood and urine are age-dependent, but an excess can be demonstrated in all patients, irrespective of age [Dancis and Hutzler, 1986]. Medium- and long-chain dicarboxylic acids accumulate and are excreted in urine, suggestive of a partial block in the degradation of long-chain dicarboxylic acids [Bjorkheim et al., 1984; Rocchiccioli et al., 1986].

In Zellweger's syndrome, the number of catalase-containing particles in liver or kidney biopsy specimens is reduced [Goldfischer et al., 1973; Small et al., 1988], although today biopsy rarely is needed for diagnosis. A reduction in the number of peroxisomes also occurs in neonatal adrenoleukodystrophy and infantile Refsum's disease but, as expected, is less severe than in Zellweger's syndrome. The catalase is cytosolic rather than particulate in catalase-containing particles. Although, in the past, peroxisomes were considered absent, Santos et al. [1988] demonstrated membranous structures called peroxisomal ghosts that contain peroxisomal membrane proteins. This finding has been substantiated by other investigators, who demonstrated the presence of major membrane proteins in skin fibroblasts from patients with Zellweger's syndrome, some of which were quite abundant [Gaertner et al., 1991; Suzuki et al., 1989]. These ghosts lack the matrix enzyme catalase and some or all of the matrix proteins. Schram et al. [1986] have reported that peroxisomal β-oxidation enzymes, which normally are located in the peroxisome matrix, are formed at a normal rate but are rapidly degraded in the cytosol. The mitochondrial abnormalities observed are considered secondary [Trijbels et al., 1983].

Prenatal Diagnosis

Cultured amniocytes or chorionic villus cells can be used to diagnose all of the disorders of peroxisome biogenesis. A variety of biochemical strategies have been used and focus on the type and degree of biochemical abnormality. Two independent techniques, the measurement of very long chain fatty acid β-oxidation [Moser et al., 1984a; Solish et al., 1985] and plasmalogen synthesis [Roscher et al., 1985; Schutgens et al., 1985], have demonstrated accurate diagnosis when performed by laboratories experienced in these methodologies. Molecular genetic techniques may be used in families in which the mutation has been identified and pre-implantation genetic diagnosis has been performed [Al-Sayed et al., 2007].

Therapy

Because many of the abnormalities are present in the affected fetus, potential for therapy is limited at present and likely to remain so. Treatment is primarily supportive, targeting, as appropriate, liver dysfunction with vitamin K for prothrombin deficiency, tube feeding, and antiepileptic medication. In the milder phenotypes, rehabilitative approaches, including communication training and physical and occupational therapy, are helpful.

Attempts to normalize some of the biochemical abnormalities include oral ether lipid therapy [Holmes et al., 1987; Poulos et al., 1990; Wilson et al., 1986] and dietary restriction of very long chain fatty acids [Van Duyn et al., 1984] and phytanic acid [Greenberg et al., 1987; Steinberg, 1989]. These approaches may normalize plasma levels of very long chain fatty acids, phytanic acid, and red blood cell plasmalogens. The clinical effectiveness of these interventions, however, has yet to be demonstrated because of the phenotypic variability of these disorders. Ursodeoxycholic acid can reduce levels of bile acid intermediates and has the potential to prevent liver damage [Colombo et al., 1990]. Dietary therapy with docosahexaenoic acid replaces low levels in plasma and red blood cells of patients with Zellweger's syndrome, neonatal adrenoleukodystrophy, and infantile Refsum's disease [Martinez et al., 1993,

1994]; however, it is ineffective in improving clinical function [Mahmood et al., 2010]. Peroxisome proliferators, such as clofibrate, do not induce the formation of catalase-containing peroxisomes or improve clinical status [Lazarow et al., 1985].

Rhizomelic Chondrodysplasia Punctata

Rhizomelic chondrodysplasia punctata is characterized by severe shortening of limbs, mental retardation, and early death [Spranger et al., 1971]. A striking reduction in plasmalogen synthesis exceeding that seen in Zellweger's syndrome led to the recognition of a peroxisomal defect in this disorder [Heymans et al., 1985, 1986]. Subsequent studies have revealed the following triad of biochemical defects:

1. marked reduction of plasmalogen levels resulting from impaired plasmalogen synthesis [Heymans et al., 1984]
2. impaired oxidation of phytanic acid with increased plasma levels [Hoefler et al., 1988]
3. presence of 3-oxoacyl-CoA thiolase in the precursor form. The levels of very long chain fatty acids are normal, suggesting that the immature thiolase is catalytically active. Despite the presence of catalase in the particulate fraction, peroxisomal structure may not always be normal. Heymans et al. [1986] described two patients in whom peroxisomes were absent in some hepatocytes, but large or irregularly shaped in others.

The clinical features (Figure 38-4A) include disproportionate shortening of the proximal portions of the extremities, short stature, microcephaly, dysmorphic facial appearance, cataracts, ichthyosis, and severe mental retardation. Radiologic highlights include shortening of the proximal limbs, metaphyseal cupping, and disturbed ossification with epiphyseal and extra-epiphyseal calcification (see Figure 38-4B). Lateral views of the spine reveal coronal clefts of the vertebral bodies (see Figure 38-4C). Epiphyseal stippling involves mainly the knee, hip, elbow, and shoulder, and is uncommon in the vertebral column. The clinical features resemble those seen in warfarin embryopathy and should be differentiated from those of the milder autosomal-dominant form (Conradi–Hunermann type) and the X-linked forms of chondrodysplasia punctata, in which no biochemical abnormalities of peroxisomal function are detectable [Schutgens et al., 1988].

Rhizomelic chondrodysplasia punctata in a 9-month-old female with the classic triad of biochemical abnormalities, but with less severe disability, has been recognized. Her mentation and limb length were normal, despite radiographic evidence of chondrodysplasia punctata [Poll-The et al., 1991]. Other mildly affected patients have been identified, and many persons with an adult Refsum phenotype have alterations in *PEX7* [Braverman et al., 2002; van den Brink et al., 2003].

The immature form of thiolase appears to be enzymatically active in patients with rhizomelic chondrodysplasia punctata because the levels of very long chain fatty acids are not increased and very long chain fatty acid oxidation is normal. Alternatively, small amounts of mature enzyme undetected by the immunoblot technique may be present. Balfe et al. [1990] reported that, in rhizomelic chondrodysplasia punctata and in some cases of Zellweger's syndrome, the immature thiolase is present in a subcellular particle with a lower density than in normal peroxisomes or mitochondria, and speculated that this density difference may be related to peroxisome ghosts described by Santos et al. [1988].

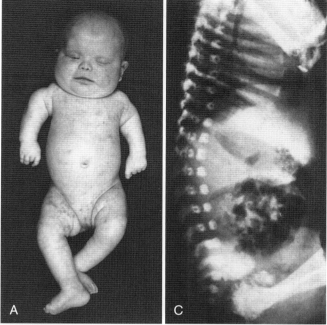
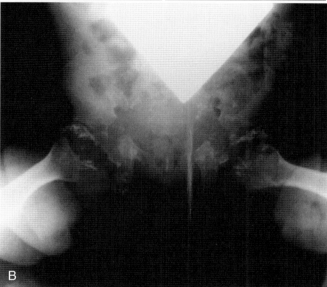

Fig. 38-4 Rhizomelic chondrodysplasia punctata A, Newborn with midface hypoplasia, hypertelorism, severe shortening of proximal portions of limbs, and ichthyosis. **B,** Radiographic evidence of shortened proximal limbs, metaphyseal cupping, and stippling of the chondral epiphyses. **C,** Vertebrae show coronal clefts, which fused later. (**A** and **B,** *Courtesy of Dr. B McGillivary, Vancouver, British Columbia.* **C,** *Courtesy of Dr. J Dorst, Johns Hopkins Hospital, Baltimore, Maryland.*)

The diagnosis is confirmed by the impaired plasmalogen synthesis and elevated phytanic acid with reduced phytanic acid oxidation. Prenatal diagnosis using cultured amniocytes or chorionic villus samples is available. Duff et al. [1990] have reported on the prenatal diagnosis of rhizomelic chondrodysplasia punctata by ultrasound analysis. As suggested by the presence of the biochemical triad with normal intelligence and normal limb length reported by Poll-The et al. [1991], the phenotype of rhizomelic chondrodysplasia punctata is more varied than was previously recognized and cautions against the previous assumptions of these diagnostic criteria for prenatal diagnosis.

Rhizomelic chondrodysplasia punctata is inherited in an autosomal-recessive manner. The disease results from a defect in *PEX7*, which encodes the receptor for PTS2. Several mutations have been noted in the *PEX7* gene in patients with rhizomelic chondrodysplasia punctata; however, the L292ter found in more than half of affected genes probably indicates a Northern European founder effect [Braverman et al., 2000, 2002].

Treatment is very limited and consists of palliative orthopedic care and cataract removal. Although dietary restriction of phytanic acid has been proposed, no evidence indicating that it affects outcome is available. The recent development of a mouse model offers the potential to understand the pathogenesis and attempt therapies in this serious disorder [Braverman et al., 2010].

Defects of Single Peroxisomal Enzymes

Defects of Single Peroxisomal β-Oxidation Enzymes

Adrenoleukodystrophy

The first clinical cases of what is known as X-linked adrenoleukodystrophy were described in 1923 by Siemerling and Creutzfeldt. The X-linked mode of inheritance was suggested by Fanconi et al. [1963]. A key observation of characteristic lamellar lipid-soluble cytoplasmic inclusions in the adrenal cortical cells and brain macrophages of patients with childhood adrenoleukodystrophy was made by Powers et al. [1980]. Similar inclusions were observed in men with Addison's disease and spastic paraparesis by Budka et al. [1976], and by Griffin et al. [1977], and the related condition was named adrenomyeloneuropathy. Similar histopathologic changes observed in a symptomatic child and an adult within a kindred strengthened the assertion that, despite the phenotypic variation, the same disease process was present. Igarashi et al. [1976] defined the biochemical defect by demonstrating that the inclusions in the adrenal cortex and cerebral white matter consisted of cholesterol esters with a striking excess of saturated unbranched fatty acids of 24- to 30-carbon chain length, of which C26:0 and C25:0 were the most abundant. This excess of very long chain fatty acids in cultured skin fibroblasts, plasma, or red blood cells is useful for diagnostic purposes [Kawamura et al., 1978; Moser et al., 1981; Tanaka et al., 1986, 1990; Tsuji et al., 1981].

BIOCHEMICAL AND MOLECULAR BASIS

The peroxisomal β-oxidation pathway consists of four enzymatic steps (as outlined in Figure 38-1). Before the substrates can enter this pathway, the acyl residues require activation by transfer of a coenzyme A. For very long chain fatty acids entering the L-specific β-oxidation pathway, lignoceryl-CoA ligase (also referred to as lignoceryl-CoA synthetase) is the activating enzyme. Deficiency of this enzyme initially was implicated as the basis of the very long chain fatty acid accumulation in X-linked adrenoleukodystrophy. Singh and co-workers [1984] demonstrated that the capacity to oxidize the C24:0 and C26:0 fatty acids was reduced in patients with X-linked adrenoleukodystrophy. Studies by Wanders et al. [1988c],

indicated that the defect involves the capacity to form the CoA derivative of very long chain fatty acid, because the capacity to oxidize lignoceryl-CoA is intact. It is known that the genetic basis for X-linked adrenoleukodystrophy is mutations of the *ABCD1* gene, which encodes a PMP, an ATP-binding cassette protein [Mosser et al., 1993], and the gene for this protein is located on the X chromosome in the Xq28 region. It remains unclear how mutations in this nonenzyme membrane protein affect the function of lignoceryl-CoA ligase [Wanders et al., 2010]. The following other peroxisomal proteins with homology to ABCD1 have been described:
1. ALDR, adrenoleukodystrophy-related protein
2. PMP70, PMP of 70 kDa [Kamijo et al., 1990]
3. PMP70R, PMP70-related protein.

All of these proteins are located within the peroxisomal membrane and contain an ATP-binding cassette motif. It has been hypothesized that they are involved in the transport of other proteins or possibly substrates for peroxisomal pathways across the peroxisome membrane. Experimental data indicate that these proteins form homodimers and heterodimers [Valle and Gartner, 1993]. Multiple mutations in *ABCD1* have been identified in patients with X-linked adrenoleukodystrophy, and no phenotype correlation has been identified [Kemp et al., 2001; Kok et al., 1995]. Several mouse models of X-linked adrenoleukodystrophy are now available [Lu et al., 1997].

CLINICAL AND PATHOLOGIC FEATURES OF X-LINKED ADRENOLEUKODYSTROPHY AND ADRENOMYELONEUROPATHY

Table 38-3 summarizes the different phenotypes of patients with X-linked adrenoleukodystrophy. These patients all demonstrate accumulation of very long chain fatty acid, and molecular studies have confirmed *ABCD1* gene mutations. Various phenotypes have been recognized as occurring within the same pedigree, so neither the genetic mutation nor the biochemical abnormality predicts the clinical presentation.

Childhood Cerebral Form of Adrenoleukodystrophy

The childhood cerebral variant is the most common and fulminant form of X-linked adrenoleukodystrophy. Affected boys are normal until 4–8 years of age, when they manifest behavior

Table 38-3 Phenotypes among X-Linked Adrenoleukodystrophy Hemizygotes

Type	Frequency (%)
Childhood cerebral	33–39
Adolescent cerebral	4–7
Adult cerebral	2–3
AMN	26–32
Addison's only	13–17
Asymptomatic	7–18

AMN, adrenomyeloneuropathy.
(Adapted from the North American data of the Kennedy Krieger Institute [Bezman and Moser, 1998].)

problems and failure in school as a result of rapid regression of auditory discrimination, spatial orientation, speech, and writing. Seizures occur in 30 percent of patients and in rare instances may be the initial sign. The magnetic resonance imaging (MRI) scan reveals parieto-occipital white matter lesions (in 85 percent of patients) or frontal lesions (in 15 percent) at this stage, with contrast accumulation at the leading edge of the lesion [Duda and Huttenlocher, 1976; Eiben and DiChiro, 1977; Kumar et al., 1987] (Figure 38-5). Rapid clinical deterioration leads to spastic quadriparesis, swallowing difficulty, and visual loss, culminating in a vegetative state usually within 2 years of the initial signs and symptoms. Although males come to medical attention because of the neurologic deficits, impaired cortisol response can be identified by adrenocorticotropic hormone stimulation in 85 percent of this group [Moser et al., 1991b].

Adolescent Cerebral Form of Adrenoleukodystrophy

Patients with the adolescent cerebral form of adrenoleukodystrophy manifest signs and symptoms of cerebral involvement, as described previously, between 10 and 21 years of age.

Adult Cerebral Form of Adrenoleukodystrophy

In the adult cerebral form of adrenoleukodystrophy, dementia, psychiatric disturbances, seizures, and spastic paraparesis develop after age 21 [Bresnan and Richardson, 1979; Esiri et al., 1984; James et al., 1984; Kitchin et al., 1987; Sereni et al., 1987; Turpin et al., 1985]. Patients may be misdiagnosed as having multiple sclerosis, brain tumor, or schizophrenia, and demonstrate rapid deterioration similar to that in the childhood cerebral form. Therefore, patients with these clinical presentations and adrenal insufficiency or leukodystrophy should be evaluated for a positive family history; in addition, measurement of plasma very long chain fatty acids is warranted.

Adrenomyeloneuropathy

The neurologic manifestations of adrenomyeloneuropathy, an adult form of adrenoleukodystrophy, consist of an insidious onset and slow progression of spastic paraparesis, impaired vibratory sense in the lower extremity, and bladder or bowel dysfunction. Onset is typically in the third decade of life. The primary pathology involves the spinal cord with loss of myelinated axons in the corticospinal tracts, nucleus gracilis, and dorsal spinocerebellar tracts [Budka et al., 1983; Probst et al., 1980; Schaumburg et al., 1977]. Sural and peroneal nerves reveal a loss of large and small myelinated fibers.

The development of cerebral demyelination has been seen in approximately 15–20 percent of men with adrenomyeloneuropathy [van Geel et al., 2001]. This pathologic change needs to be differentiated from long tract findings on MRI [Loes et al., 2003]. Cerebral disease is similar in time course to the childhood form of the disease and leads to dementia, spasticity, blindness, and death. Approximately half of patients with adrenomyeloneuropathy appear to have some degree of cerebral involvement, with mild to moderate abnormalities noted on MRI in 46 percent [Kumar et al., 1995] (see Figure 38-5). These abnormalities consist most frequently of parietal-occipital white matter and optic radiation involvement.

Adrenal insufficiency, or Addison's disease, precedes the onset of neurologic symptoms in 42 percent of patients; in some, this may occur 3–35 years earlier. Adrenal insufficiency was evident in 67 percent of patients in our series. Serum testosterone levels were abnormally low in 22 percent of our patients, and early-onset sexual dysfunction occurred in one-third.

Adrenoleukodystrophy with Addison's Disease Only

The diagnosis of adrenoleukodystrophy with Addison's disease only includes the patients who have isolated Addison's disease in the absence of neurologic signs and symptoms, and is more common than was previously recognized. A study conducted in an endocrine clinic found that 5 of 8 male Addisonian patients had the biochemical defect of adrenoleukodystrophy [Sadeghi-Nejad and Senior, 1990]. Recognition of these patients is vital for genetic counseling and to monitor for the development of adrenomyeloneuropathy or cerebral symptoms later on. Onset of adrenal dysfunction does not correlate with neurologic involvement.

Asymptomatic Patients with the Biochemical Defect of Adrenoleukodystrophy

In asymptomatic patients with the biochemical defect of adrenoleukodystrophy, diagnosis may be accomplished by measurement of plasma very long chain fatty acids during screening tests of relatives of symptomatic patients. These persons may be of any age. The elevation of very long chain fatty acid levels in these males is comparable with that in severely affected family members. At present, it is uncertain why the abnormal increase of very long chain fatty acids is not associated with disease in some patients. A 62-year-old man in this category whose brother died at the age of 48 years with the adult cerebral form of adrenoleukodystrophy has been identified. The unaffected brother had no evidence of adrenal insufficiency but, when re-examined by the same neurologist 4 years later, demonstrated signs of corticospinal tract involvement compatible with mild adrenomyeloneuropathy. Several asymptomatic men demonstrate an impaired cortisol response to adrenocorticotropic hormone stimulation, suggesting that they have adrenal involvement and are presumed to be at risk for developing adrenomyeloneuropathy.

Symptomatic Heterozygotes

Between 10 and 20 percent of the women who are carriers for the adrenoleukodystrophy gene manifest myelopathy resembling that in adrenomyeloneuropathy between the third and fifth decades of life [Dooley and Wright, 1985; Heffungs et al., 1980; Morariu et al., 1982; Moser et al., 1980; Naidu et al., 1986; Noetzel et al., 1987; O'Neill et al., 1982, 1984; Penman, 1960; Pilz and Schiener, 1973]. Long tract signs and diminished vibration sense in the legs are present in two-thirds of the patients, although only 25 percent complain of symptoms. Approximately 14 percent have severe spinal involvement requiring assistance with ambulation, and 5 percent have dementia [Naidu and Moser, 1990]. In contrast with males, adrenal insufficiency rarely occurs in these women [El-Deiry et al., 1997].

Elevation of very long chain fatty acids in plasma or skin fibroblasts allowed identification of 85 percent of obligate heterozygotes in one series [Moser et al., 1983]. The remaining cases can be identified by molecular analysis for the gene defect.

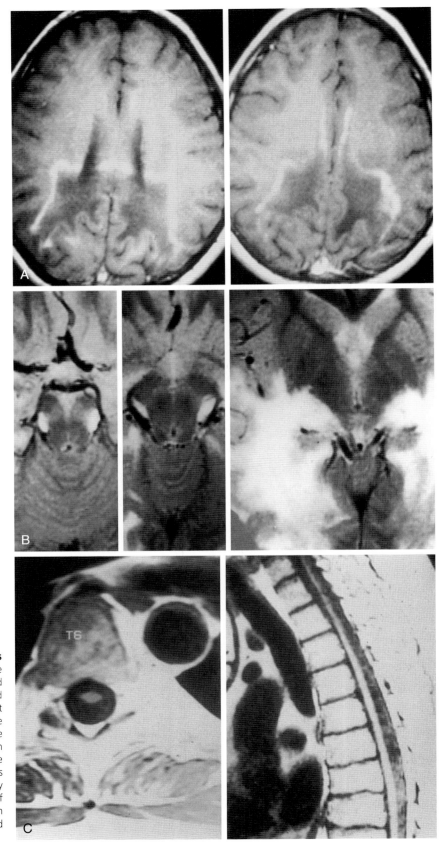

Fig. 38-5 Magnetic resonance imaging (MRI) studies in adrenoleukodystrophy. A, Typical alteration of the blood–brain barrier at the edge of the demyelinated lesion in childhood adrenoleukodystrophy demonstrated on gadolinium-enhanced MRI. **B,** The discrete but continuous auditory pathway involvement from the lateral lemniscus in the pons to the medial geniculate bodies at the midbrain level to the temporal cortex can be seen. MRI permits precise correlation between the location of the lesion and cognitive deficits; the findings may explain the early auditory comprehension deficiency seen in childhood adrenoleukodystrophy. **C,** MRI study of the spine in X-linked adrenoleukodystrophy. Views in axial (left) and lateral (right) planes demonstrate cord atrophy, particularly in the thoracic regions.

Mutation analysis helps identify heterozygotes once the mutation in the index case is known [Boehm et al., 1999]. Migeon et al. [1981] studied fibroblast clones from heterozygotes and identified two types of cells; one had a normal fatty acid pattern, and the pattern in the other cell type was similar to that in affected males, reflecting X-inactivation status. To determine if differential X-inactivation accounts for the clinical variability in heterozygotes, an indirect immunofluorescence analysis of ALDP, the protein defective in X-linked adrenoleukodystrophy, has been applied to skin fibroblasts. Previous studies have reported that 70 percent of males with X-linked adrenoleukodystrophy lack immunoreactivity for ALD protein (ALDP). As a result of differential X-inactivation, heterozygotes from these informative families have a mixed population of normal and ALDP-deficient cells. Despite considerable variation, a positive correlation is noted between immunonegative cells and clinical severity. No correlation is seen between immunoreactivity and either very long chain fatty acid levels or age alone. When age is considered, however, the correlation between severity and ALDP immunoreactivity is strengthened. Thus, differences in patterns of X-inactivation appear, in part, to contribute to the variable severity of the disease seen in the X-linked adrenoleukodystrophy heterozygotes [Naidu et al., 1997].

PATHOGENESIS OF ADRENOLEUKODYSTROPHY

The main biochemical defect is the striking excess of very long chain fatty acids, which accumulate in the cholesterol ester fraction, primarily in the adrenal gland and cerebral white matter. Theda et al. [1987] noted that, in areas of brain where myelin was intact, there was a 20-fold excess of C26:0 in the phosphatidylcholine fraction, whereas the cholesterol ester fraction had a normal fatty acid composition. The enrichment with C26:0 in the cholesterol ester fraction reported by earlier investigators [Brown et al., 1983; Igarashi et al., 1976; Menkes and Corbo, 1977; Molzer et al., 1981; Ramsey et al., 1979; Reinecke et al., 1985; Taketomi et al., 1987] was present only in zones undergoing active demyelination and, to a lesser extent, where myelin had been replaced by glial tissue. They concluded that increased very long chain fatty acids in phosphatidylcholine could be the primary event and that the excess in the cholesterol ester fraction is due to myelin breakdown.

The accumulation of very long chain fatty acids in X-linked adrenoleukodystrophy is not as severe as in disorders of peroxisome biogenesis or single-peroxisomal β-oxidation enzyme defects. Red cell membrane microviscosity is increased in X-linked adrenoleukodystrophy [Knazek et al., 1983], which may impair functional capacity. This finding also is suggested by studies in human adrenal gland cultures, where the addition of C26:0 fatty acid to the culture medium resulted in an impaired cortisol response to adrenocorticotropic hormone [Whitcomb et al., 1988]. Cholesterol esterified with very long chain fatty acids is a poor substrate for cholesterol ester hydrolase, which may limit steroid production [Ogino and Suzuki, 1981].

The pathogenesis of the nervous system lesion has been more difficult to discern. It has been presumed that elevation of very long chain fatty acids results in the axonopathy seen in patients with adrenomyeloneuropathy and in women who are carriers. It is not clear, however, why rapid, inflammatory demyelination affecting the cerebral white matter tracts develops in certain persons. The levels of very long chain fatty acids in plasma or skin fibroblasts or the capacity to metabolize very long chain fatty acids in cultured fibroblasts [Boles et al., 1991] do not differ in males with the childhood form from those in men with adrenomyeloneuropathy or other forms. No correlation exists between severity of the neurologic disease and levels of very long chain fatty acids. Antoku et al. [1991], however, reported that patients with childhood cerebral adrenoleukodystrophy had higher levels of very long chain fatty acids in mononuclear cells than did patients with adrenomyeloneuropathy, even though levels in plasma and erythrocytes demonstrated no difference. The inability to distinguish the various forms prospectively hampers genetic counseling and choice of therapeutic modalities. These observations have led to the conclusion that very long chain fatty acid excess alone is not sufficient to explain cerebral demyelination and that other factors must play a role in the phenotypic variability.

The presence of the perivascular lymphocytic infiltration in the white matter of the cerebral forms provides evidence of immunologic involvement as one additional factor [Powers and Moser, 1998]. This is not seen in the adrenal gland or other leukodystrophies. Typing of the lymphocytic cells in brain from four patients with the cerebral form of adrenoleukodystrophy examined postmortem revealed 59 percent T cells, 34 percent T4 cells, 16 percent T8 cells, 24 percent B cells, and 11 percent monocytes [Griffin et al., 1985]. This pattern is similar to that found during a cellular immune response in the central nervous system. Bernheimer et al. [1983] reported increased levels of IgG and IgA in brain from patients with adrenoleukodystrophy, similar to that in patients with multiple sclerosis. Boutin et al. [1989] suggest that interleukin-2 plays an important role. McGuinness et al. [1995] demonstrated an elevation in tumor necrosis factor-α (TNFα) in the leading edge of areas of active demyelination. More recently, there is evidence that very long chain fatty acids are toxic to the microglia and their involvement in the disease cascade is being determined [Eichler et al., 2008]. The collective evidence implies that an immunologic mechanism contributes to the rapid progression of white matter lesions, possibly in response to the altered lipid composition in brain of patients with adrenoleukodystrophy. Segregation analyses suggest the existence of a modifier gene that potentially affects this immune response [Smith et al., 1991]. Further studies in this area may identify factors that contribute to the pathogenesis of the nervous system lesions.

THERAPIES FOR ADRENOLEUKODYSTROPHY

The two forms of therapy under intensive investigation are dietary restriction and bone marrow transplantation. Based on the observations of Kishimoto et al. [1980] that the very long chain fatty acids accumulating in the brain of patients with adrenoleukodystrophy were partly of dietary origin, a diet that restricted very long chain fatty acid intake was developed [Brown et al., 1982; Van Duyn et al., 1984]. This diet had no effect on the levels of plasma very long chain fatty acids or on the clinical course. Rizzo et al. [1986] reported that cultured skin fibroblasts synthesized saturated very long chain fatty acids, including C26:0, and that the rate of this synthesis was reduced by the addition of monounsaturated fatty acids, such as oleic acid. As saturated and monounsaturated fatty acids are elongated to very long chain fatty acids by the same microsomal elongation system, presumably the addition of oleic acid reduces synthesis of saturated very long chain fatty acids by competing for the same enzyme system [Bourre et al., 1976].

These findings led to clinical trials with oral glyceryl trioleate in combination with dietary restriction of very long chain fatty acids. This dual therapy achieved a 50 percent reduction of the levels of saturated very long chain fatty acids in plasma, as well as a statistically significant improvement in peripheral nerve function in patients with adrenomyeloneuropathy [Moser et al., 1991a; Rizzo et al., 1987]. Subsequently, erucic acid (C22:1) was demonstrated to be more effective in reducing synthesis of saturated very long chain fatty acids; therefore, glyceryl trioleate was combined with glyceryl trierucate. A dramatic normalization of the level of C26:0 in plasma occurred within a month [Moser et al., 1995; Rizzo et al., 1989], and the microviscosity of the red cell membranes returned to normal [Knazek et al., 1983].

Unfortunately, this regimen does not alter the course of the childhood cerebral form of adrenoleukodystrophy [Uziel et al., 1990]. In open, uncontrolled studies, the effects on the clinical course of the adult form have been uncertain but generally unimpressive [Aubourg et al., 1993; Kaplan et al., 1995]. Further studies are planned in presymptomatic males: controlled studies, in men with adrenomyeloneuropathy. Symptomatic heterozygotes have been managed with glyceryl trioleate/glyceryl trierucate and dietary restriction therapy without significant improvement, as in their male counterparts. Prophylactic treatment is not recommended for asymptomatic heterozygotes.

The results of bone marrow transplantation in mildly affected patients are encouraging [Aubourg et al., 1990; Lockman et al., 1993; Loes et al., 1994; Peters et al., 2004]. In patients with more advanced disease, transplantation has not resulted in halting the course and may be associated with worsening of the neurologic status immediately after the procedure; therefore, this procedure is not advised [Moser et al., 1984b; Weinberg et al., 1988]. In patients with advanced disease, neither dietary therapy nor bone marrow transplantation is effective. Immunosuppression with cyclophosphamide did not arrest the rapid progression of the illness [Naidu et al., 1988a; Stumpf et al., 1981]. Recently, gene therapy with a lentivirus vector has been successfully used in three boys with early cerebral disease. This advancement in the field potentially offers additional avenues of treatment for many individuals who could not previously undergo transplantation [Cartier et al., 2009].

Males at risk for developing the childhood form of X-linked adrenoleukodystrophy (younger than 10 years of age) require appropriate monitoring. MRI should be performed on a yearly basis. Because MRI abnormalities become evident at least 12 months before onset of neurologic symptoms, periodic neurologic examination is not sufficient for monitoring these patients. Timely assessments are especially important because the best outcomes with bone marrow transplantation are in patients identified at an early stage of cerebral disease. Appropriate adrenal monitoring also is indicated in identified patients.

NEWBORN SCREENING FOR XALD

A biochemical assay using tandem mass spectroscopy and the standard newborn blood spot has been developed recently and has been found to be highly sensitive and specific. If this is subsequently incorporated into newborn screening programs, it will most likely change the proportion of males coming to attention in the presymptomatic phase, and will also improve their care and management [Hubbard et al., 2009].

Contiguous Deletion of the XALD Gene

Corzo and co-workers identified three males in the newborn period who demonstrated abnormalities suggestive of a defect of L-bifunctional enzyme [Corzo et al., 2002]. Very long chain fatty acids were elevated; other findings included hypotonia and liver disease. All three patients died in the first year of life. Further investigation demonstrated large deletions of *ABCD1*, including the promoter region, with extension of these 5' deletions into contiguous genes, including the DNA marker *DXS1356E*. The investigators proposed the name "contiguous *ABCD1 DXS1357E* deletion syndrome" (CADDS) for this phenotype. The specific role of the additional genetic areas is uncertain at present. Two of the mothers were determined to be carriers for these deletions, indicating the importance of correct diagnosis of single-enzyme defects of peroxisomal β-oxidation.

Acyl-CoA Oxidase Deficiency

Two siblings and an unrelated female patient have been reported to have acyl-CoA oxidase deficiency [Kyllerman et al., 1990; Poll-The et al., 1988a]. A large deletion of the gene encoding this enzyme was reported in the siblings [Fournier et al., 1994]. Dysmorphism, hypotonia, feeding difficulties, and intractable neonatal seizures were the presenting features. Little motor or cognitive development occurred in the first 2 years of life. Ocular involvement with extinguished electroretinography and white matter involvement with abnormal contrast enhancement were present. Adrenal insufficiency was not evident, but elevated serum adrenocorticotropic hormone and low cortisol levels were present in one patient. No organomegaly was present. Although the clinical characteristics resembled those in the milder forms of peroxisome biogenesis disorders, the following two features distinguished it from the Zellweger spectrum disorders:

1. Peroxisomes in the liver were abundant and appeared larger than normal.
2. Except for increased levels of very long chain fatty acids in the range of values consistent with Zellweger's syndrome, all other peroxisomal function studies, such as levels of phytanic acid, pipecolic acid, bile acid intermediates, and plasmalogen levels, were normal.

Immunoblot studies revealed absence of acyl-CoA oxidase in the liver, and other peroxisomal β-oxidation enzymes were normal [Poll-The et al., 1988a]. Cultured skin fibroblasts had a reduced capacity to oxidize lignoceric acid and peroxisomal palmitoyl-CoA oxidase. The first prenatal diagnosis of isolated acyl-CoA oxidase deficiency was made by Wanders et al. [1990b]. In amniotic fluid, measurements of very long chain fatty acids were significantly elevated, but levels of bile acid intermediates were normal. In amniocytes, very long chain fatty acids were markedly increased, but plasmalogen biosynthesis was normal. Immunoblot analysis of amniocytes and the aborted fetal liver tissues demonstrated that all components of acyl-CoA oxidase were absent, whereas the bifunctional protein and mature form of thiolase were normal.

Bifunctional Enzyme Deficiency

Watkins et al. [1988] described a patient without dysmorphism or organomegaly who had significant hypotonia and neonatal seizures. Mental retardation was severe, and death occurred at 5½ months. Neuropathologic abnormalities included polymicrogyria and focal cortical heterotopias, similar to those in peroxisome biogenesis disorders [Kaufmann et al., 1996; Naidu et al., 1988b]. The liver had normal-appearing peroxisomes. Biochemical studies revealed elevation of very long chain fatty acids and bile acid intermediates; all other peroxisomal functions were normal. Postmortem immunoblot studies of liver demonstrated the absence of the bifunctional protein; other peroxisomal β-oxidation enzymes were present. The mRNA for the bifunctional protein was normal, indicating defective translation of the mRNA or abnormal post-translational processing, such as defective peroxisomal import mechanisms.

Although bifunctional enzyme deficiency bears some clinical resemblance to the acyl-CoA deficiency with elevation of very long chain fatty acids, a significant difference is the additional accumulation of bile acid intermediates (trihydroxycholestanoic acid) as well [Watkins et al., 1995]. The reason for trihydroxycholestanoic acid accumulation is evident in Figure 38-1, which demonstrates that the initial oxidation step for bile acid intermediates and very long chain fatty acids occurs by separate enzymes, whereas the subsequent step at the level of the bifunctional enzyme is common to both systems. Another patient with similar clinical features was found to have a functionally inactive bifunctional protein, although immunologic studies revealed normal amounts of the enzyme [Wanders et al., 1990c]. This patient is presumed to have a different mutation from the one described previously.

3-Oxoacyl-CoA Thiolase Deficiency

The entity 3-oxoacyl-CoA thiolase deficiency was first described by Goldfischer and co-workers in 1986 and called pseudo-Zellweger syndrome because of the presence of normal peroxisomes in the liver despite a clinical resemblance to Zellweger's syndrome. Biochemically, the levels of very long chain fatty acids and bile acid intermediates were increased, but phytanic acid level was normal. A re-examination of material from one of these cases demonstrated that the infant, in fact, had a defect in bifunctional enzyme. The clinical existence of a thiolase deficiency is therefore not proved [Ferdinandusse et al., 2002].

Trihydroxycholestanoic Acid-CoA Oxidase Deficiency

Christensen et al. [1990] described an unusual female patient who demonstrated normal development until 18 months of age, when she deteriorated, with clinical manifestations including ataxia, dysarthria, and dry skin. By 5 years of age, she was severely incapacitated, with hearing loss and mental retardation. At this stage she had normal findings on computed tomography (CT) scan, absence of retinal degeneration, and normal liver function and nerve conduction velocities. Because the phytanic acid level was elevated, she was placed on a diet low in phytanate, after which she demonstrated significant improvement in gait, hearing, and speech. The most prominent biochemical abnormality, however, was an elevation in bile acid intermediates with normal very long chain fatty acid concentration, presumed to be secondary to a defect in trihydroxycholestanoic acid-CoA oxidase. Because phytanic acid oxidase levels were normal in cultured fibroblasts, the elevation in phytanic acid is believed to result from inhibition of phytanate oxidation by the accumulating bile acid intermediates.

Peroxisomal α-Methylacyl-CoA Racemase Defect

Several patients with adult-onset neurologic findings, including spasticity, sensory motor neuropathy, seizures, and retinitis pigmentosa, have been described. Very long chain fatty acid levels were normal, but elevations in C27 bile acid intermediates and pristanic acid were found. Phytanic acid was mildly elevated. Because pristanic acid β-oxidation was reduced, the activity of α-methylacyl-CoA racemase (AMACR) was examined and found to be deficient. AMACR is involved in the interconversion of (R)- and (S)-stereoisomers of α-methyl branched-chain fatty acyl-CoA esters, including pristanoyl-CoA, and the interconversion of the CoA esters of dihydroxycholestanoic acid and trihydroxycholestanoic acid. Its physiologic function is to produce the (S)-stereoisomers because only these serve as substrate for branched-chain acyl-CoA oxidase [Ferdinandusse et al., 2000].

Single-Enzyme Defects of Plasmalogen Synthesis

Patients with defects in acyl-dihydroxyacetone phosphate transferase [Wanders et al., 1992] or alkyl-dihydroxyacetone phosphate synthase [Wanders et al., 1994] have a marked deficiency of plasmalogens. They differ from patients with defects of PEX7 because they metabolize phytanic acid and process thiolase normally. In most instances, however, the clinical picture resembles that in rhizomelic chondrodysplasia punctata. This similarity has led to the consideration that all of the clinical abnormalities in rhizomelic chondrodysplasia punctata are attributable to a deficiency of plasmalogens. Isolated dihydroxyacetone phosphate-AT deficiency also may manifest with a milder phenotype of rhizomelic chondrodysplasia punctata [Clayton et al., 1994].

Acatalasemia

Acatalasemia demonstrates clinical heterogeneity, with presentations ranging from absence of symptoms (in the Swiss variant) to oral ulcers, presumed to be secondary to peroxide-generating bacteria, in a severe Japanese variant. The Japanese patients have greatly reduced catalase activity; however, the electrophoretic mobility of the residual enzyme is normal. By contrast, the symptom-free patients with the Swiss variant have a large amount of catalase, but it demonstrates greater than normal heat lability. Studies by Crawford et al. [1988] report that the Japanese variant involves a regulatory mutation in which the gene is not transcribed, whereas in the Swiss variant, a structural mutation renders the enzyme unstable. The human catalase gene has been localized to 11p13 and cloned [Junien et al., 1980; Quan et al., 1986].

Hyperoxaluria Type I

Primary hyperoxaluria type I does not involve the nervous system, but does highlight an important pathogenic mechanism in peroxisomal disorders. It is inherited as an autosomal-recessive trait. Clinical onset is in childhood or adolescence. Patients present with urolithiasis and renal failure. Increased urinary excretion of oxalate (more than 50 mg/1.73 m^2 of body surface per day), glycolate (more than 70 mg/1.73 ^{2} per day), and occasionally glyoxylate is diagnostic. In 1986, Danpure and Jennings demonstrated that the enzyme alanine-glyoxalate aminotransferase, which converts glyoxylate to glycine, is deficient in patients with this disorder [Danpure and Jennings, 1986]. Latta and Brodhel [1990] noted that this disorder accounted for 2–2.7 percent of children with end-stage renal disease. In human liver, this enzyme is peroxisomal [Danpure and Jennings, 1986], and the activity varies in affected patients, correlating with the severity of the disease [Danpure and Jennings, 1988]. A milder pyridoxine-responsive form of the disease has a less severe reduction of the enzyme [Wanders et al., 1988b]. Liver biopsy establishes the enzyme defect, but peroxisomes are present and intact in the liver [Iancu and Danpure, 1969]. The functions of other peroxisomal enzymes are normal. Danpure et al. [1989a] and Cooper et al. [1988] noted that in one-third of the patients with diminished but not absent alanine-glyoxalate aminotransferase, the enzyme is misdirected to the mitochondria, instead of its normal localization in humans to the peroxisome. The alanine-glyoxalate aminotransferase cDNA has been sequenced from eight patients with hyperoxaluria type I in whom the alanine-glyoxalate aminotransferase was localized to the mitochondria, and three new mutations were identified. One of these encoded a glycine to arginine substitution at residue 170 and was unique to these patients, but the two other mutations also were present in 5–10 percent of the control population [Purdue et al., 1990]. Nishiyama et al. [1991] have reported a point mutation encoding a serine to proline mutation at residue 205 in a patient in whom alanine-glyoxalate aminotransferase activity was nearly absent and who thus differed from the other group.

Diagnosis is established by the demonstration of deficient alanine-glyoxalate aminotransferase activity in a liver biopsy specimen [Danpure and Jennings, 1986; Danpure et al., 1987]. Prenatal diagnosis has been achieved by second-trimester fetal liver biopsy [Danpure et al., 1989b] and, in the future, could be achieved by DNA analysis of amniocytes or chorionic villus sampling. The estimated incidence of this disorder is 1 in 5 million to 15 million children; family studies demonstrate an increased incidence of parental consanguinity [Latta and Brodhel, 1990].

An exciting therapeutic advance has been a combination of liver and kidney transplantation with extremely favorable results [McDonald et al., 1989; Morgan and Watts, 1989; Ruder et al., 1990; Watts et al., 1987]. Some of the mildly affected patients respond to pyridoxine [Wanders et al., 1988b; Watts et al., 1979]. MacCollin et al. [1991] have described a patient with normal intelligence, ataxia, peripheral neuropathy, and calcium oxalate stones. Peroxisomes were absent. A marked increase in very long chain fatty acid and pipecolic acid was documented, with catalase present in the cytosolic fraction. This patient's case is the only recorded case of hyperoxaluria in association with abnormal peroxisome biogenesis and multiple peroxisomal enzyme involvement.

Peroxisomal Glutaryl-CoA Oxidase Deficiency

The first patient with peroxisomal glutaryl-CoA oxidase deficiency was identified at 11 months, when the child was presented for failure to thrive and vomiting (in particular, post-prandial vomiting), by Bennett et al. [1991]. Urinary glutaric acid level was 500 mmol per mole of creatinine, whereas the normal level is less than 2 mmol. The glutaricaciduria was responsive to riboflavin 200 mg given twice daily. At the age of 5 years 8 months, the patient was judged to be developmentally normal, although this outcome may have been attributable to the vitamin therapy. Detailed metabolic investigations ruled out glutaricaciduria types I and II. The activity of peroxisomal glutaryl-CoA oxidase was reduced to less than 10 percent of control values. Of interest, loading studies demonstrated that the glutaric acid was derived from lysine, presumably through the same pathway in which pipecolic acid is an intermediate. This case represents a peroxisomal cause of glutaricaciduria distinct from the well-known mitochondrial disorders resulting in glutaricaciduria types I and II.

Classic Adult Refsum's Disease

Classic adult Refsum's disease is a rare disorder of autosomal-recessive inheritance; originally described by Refsum [1946], it is characterized by retinitis pigmentosa, peripheral polyneuropathy, cerebellar ataxia, and increased cerebrospinal fluid protein. Biochemical identification is by the increased plasma levels of phytanic acid with normal pristanic acid. In this condition, the capacity for hydroxylation of phytanoyl-CoA has been lost. Low phytanic acid oxidation also is seen in human cells lacking PEX7, the receptor for PTS2, suggesting that the enzyme defective in Refsum's disease is targeted to peroxisomes by a PTS2.

The enzyme deficiency of phytanoyl-CoA hydroxylase A and the gene defect in this disease have been identified conclusively [Jansen et al., 1997; Mihalik et al., 1997] and are the primary cause of adult Refsum's disease. The gene PAHX is localized to chromosome 10, and patients with Refsum's disease are homozygous for inactivating mutations in PAHX. It must be emphasized, however, that a substantial number of adult patients with the same phenotypic features have now been identified as having mutations in PEX7 [Jansen et al., 1997], and mutational analysis is required for definitive diagnosis. Therapy consists of restriction of dietary phytanic acid and symptomatic treatment.

Mulibrey Nanism

Mulibrey nanism is a rare disorder of autosomal-recessive inheritance that manifests with prenatal and postnatal growth failure, hepatomegaly, pericardial constriction, and characteristic facial features. Mulibrey stands for "muscle-liver-brain-eye," and features of this disorder include yellow dots on the fundi, muscular weakness, enlarged cerebral ventricles, increased incidence of Wilms' tumor, and cutaneous nevus flammeus [Kallijarvi et al., 2002; Lapunzina et al., 1995]. Patients have normal intelligence. It is more common in the Finnish population. It is due to defects in TRIM37 located on 17q22–q23. This gene encodes RING-B-box-coiled-coil protein, which is localized to the peroxisome. Patients with TRIM37 mutations do have normal peroxisome morphology, and other PTS1-containing matrix proteins are not affected. No abnormality is seen in very long chain fatty acid concentration or other biochemical measures. TRIM37 apparently lacks a PTS1 signal, but uptake of this protein was lacking in cell lines defective for *PEX1* and *PEX5*. The exact role in peroxisomal function is not known at present [Avela et al., 2000; Kallijarvi et al., 2002]. The demonstration of this disorder as involving the peroxisome highlights an important point in going forward in the identification of peroxisomal disorders. Current screening strategies have focused on known biochemical features, and expansion of our understanding will require newer diagnostic modalities.

Current and Future Outlook

With expanding clinical phenotypes, peroxisomal disorders are now included as standard considerations in the differential diagnosis for a variety of neurologic findings in infants, children, and adults. As new peroxisomal functions are being identified, they have provided insight into mechanisms involving biogenesis of the organelle and control of protein import. Their vital role encompassing neuronal migration in fetal brain development through membrane integrity in the axons in adults is being appreciated. All of the disorders can be recognized by noninvasive biochemical and genetic tests, providing valuable information for genetic counseling. These disorders may be severely debilitating or fatal, but therapeutic options are becoming available.

The complete list of references for this chapter is available online at **www.expertconsult.com**.
See inside cover for registration details.

Neurotransmitter-Related Disorders

Matthew T. Sweney and Kathryn J. Swoboda

The term neurotransmitter disorders constitutes a broad and increasingly complex spectrum of neurologic conditions associated with defects in the production, transport, release, and reuptake of a variety of chemical compounds involved in neurotransmission. This chapter provides an overview of such disorders, with a primary emphasis on those associated with a dopamine or serotonin deficiency state.

Neurologic symptoms associated with dopamine deficiency are broad, and range from extremely mild and subtle alterations in mood or gait to a classic exercise-induced dystonic gait abnormality and an infantile-onset parkinsonism syndrome. In recessive inborn errors of dopamine metabolism associated with tetrahydrobiopterin (BH_4) deficiencies, neurologic symptoms are often more severe and accompanied by hyperphenylalaninemia, which can be detected on newborn screening. Associated serotonin deficiency is present in most of these disorders. Even when these disorders are ascertained by newborn screening, repletion of neurotransmitter precursors may not be sufficient, resulting in global developmental impairment, fluctuating tone abnormalities, eye movement abnormalities, encephalopathy, ataxia, and seizures.

Diseases related to dysfunction of other neurotransmitter systems (i.e., gamma-aminobutyric acid [GABA], glutamate, and glycine, among others) are more difficult to characterize in humans, likely due to their breadth of function and inadequate methods of detection. None the less, developments in neurophysiologic research indicate that manifestations of these disorders are equally as diverse as in monoaminergic systems, including seizures, ataxia, hypotonia, oculomotor dyspraxia, and developmental delay. In addition, there are new, seemingly specific neurotransmitter systems (e.g., orexins and their role in narcolepsy) that are the target of much investigation. As yet, these systems are covered elsewhere, or outside the scope of the present topic.

Screening for this group of disorders occurs primarily by recognition of key neurologic symptoms. For example, symptoms such as exercise-induced dystonia and childhood-onset parkinsonism have a greater likelihood of an associated dopamine deficiency state. However, the wide spectrum of phenotypes associated with dopamine deficiency states and overlap with other disorders with shared features can make accurate identification and diagnosis of these disorders challenging. The routine availability of increasingly more sophisticated diagnostic tools, including cerebrospinal fluid neurotransmitter metabolite studies, cerebrospinal fluid and urine pterin studies, neuroimaging studies, phenylalanine loading studies, enzymatic assays in blood cells or skin fibroblasts, and molecular studies, have greatly increased our ability to diagnose and treat patients with monoaminergic neurotransmitter abnormalities accurately. Amino acid neurotransmitter disorders, such as GABA transaminase deficiency and succinic semialdehyde dehydrogenase deficiency, are currently detectable via cerebrospinal fluid studies as well, however much remains to be elucidated about these diseases.

For ease of classification, these disorders can be divided into five groups:
1. monoaminergic neurotransmitter deficiency states with hyperphenylalaninemia
2. monoaminergic neurotransmitter deficiency states without hyperphenylalaninemia
3. amino acid neurotransmitter dysmetabolism
4. secondary neurotransmitter deficiency states
5. undefined neurotransmitter deficiency states (Table 39-1).

Monoaminergic Neurotransmitter Deficiency States with Hyperphenylalaninemia

Overview

The neurotransmitter deficiency in infants in this group arises as a result of defects in BH_4 metabolism (Figure 39-1). Patients are usually identified by elevated phenylalanine levels on newborn screening, as BH_4 is required for phenylalanine hydroxylation in the liver. The accompanying neurotransmitter deficiency results from the lack of BH_4, an obligatory co-factor required for the synthesis of catecholamines and serotonin. Although most academic biochemical genetics clinics that monitor children with phenylketonuria systematically perform the additional studies required to diagnose this group of disorders, children occasionally are not identified until they have progressive neurologic symptoms or clear evidence of developmental delay despite a phenylalanine-restricted diet. In the past, these patients were referred to as atypical phenylketonurics. In some cases, such afflicted infants are overlooked because screening is performed before an adequate interval of protein intake, resulting in a false-negative result on newborn testing.

Approximately 1–3 percent of patients with hyperphenylalaninemia have an associated BH_4 deficiency state. It is critical to identify such children so that BH_4 and neurotransmitter

Table 39-1 Primary Monoaminergic Neurotransmitter Deficiency Disorders

Disorder	Phenotypic Features	Locus	Inheritance
ELEVATED PLASMA PHENYLALANINE			
6-Pyruvoyltetrahydrobiopterin synthase deficiency*	Encephalopathy, dystonia, spasticity, axial hypotonia, autonomic symptoms, oculogyric crises, seizures	11q22.3–23.3	AR
Dihydropteridine reductase deficiency*		4p15.31	AR
GTP cyclohydrolase deficiency*		14q22.1–22.2	AR
Primapterinuria	Benign hyperphenylalaninemia	10q22	AR
NORMAL PLASMA PHENYLALANINE			
GTP cyclohydrolase deficiency*	Exercise-induced dystonia, gait disorder, writer's cramp, restless leg syndrome, tremor	14q22.1–22.2	AD
Aromatic L-amino acid decarboxylase deficiency*	Dystonia, spasticity, torticollis, axial hypotonia, limb rigidity, autonomic symptoms, psychomotor retardation, oculogyric crises	7p11	AR
Sepiapterin reductase deficiency*	Parkinsonian symptoms, psychomotor retardation, behavioral disturbances	2p14p12	AR
Tyrosine hydroxylase deficiency*	Gait disturbance, infantile parkinsonism, dystonia, speech delay	11p15.5	AR
Tryptophan hydroxylase deficiency*	Ataxia, speech delay, hypotonia, psychomotor retardation	11p15.3	AR
Dopamine β-hydroxylase deficiency*	Orthostatic hypotension, lethargy, ptosis	9q34	
Monoamine oxidase A deficiency	Mild mental retardation, tendency to violent or aggressive behavior	Xp11.23	XR

* Disorder associated with a dopamine deficiency state.
AD, autosomal-dominant; AR, autosomal-recessive; GTP, guanosine triphosphate; XR, X-linked recessive.

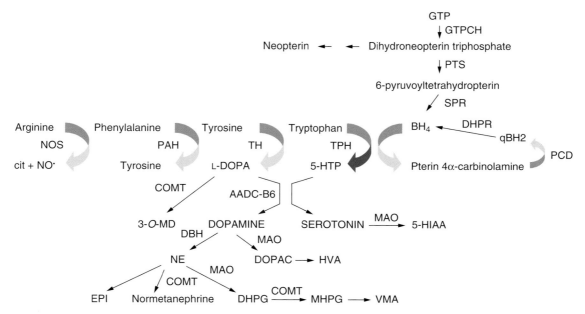

Fig. 39-1 Synthesis and catabolism of catecholamine and indoleamine neurotransmitters. AADC, aromatic L-amino acid decarboxylase; B$_6$, pyridoxine; COMT, catechol O-methyltransferase; DBH, dopamine β-hydroxylase; DHPG, dihydrophenyl glycine; DHPR, dihydropteridine reductase; DOPAC, dihydroxyphenylacetic acid; EPI, epinephrine; 5-HIAA, 5-hydroxyindoleacetic acid; 5-HTP, 5-hydroxytryptophan; GTPCH, guanosine triphosphate cyclohydrolase; HVA, homovanillic acid; MAO, monoamine oxidase; MHPG, methoxy 4 hydroxyphenylglycol; NE, neoepinephrine; NOS, nitric oxide synthase; PAH, phenylalanine hydroxylase; PCD, pterin-4α-carbinolamine dehydratase; PTS, 6-pyruvoyltetrahydropterin synthase; qBH2, quinonoid dihydropterin; SPR, sepiapterin reductase; TH, tyrosine hydroxylase; TPH, tryptophan hydroxylase; VMA, vanillylmandelic acid.

precursors can be supplemented as early as possible. The two most commonly identified disorders in children presenting with hyperphenylalaninemia in the newborn period are 6-pyruvoyltetrahydropterin synthase deficiency, accounting for 60 percent of mutations in atypical phenylketonurics, and dihydropteridine reductase deficiency, affecting 30 percent of cases [Longo, 2009]. 6-Pyruvoyltetrahydropterin synthase deficiency results in inadequate BH_4 synthesis; dihydropteridine reductase deficiency results in decreased regeneration of BH_4 from dihydrobiopterin (see Figure 39-1). Both are autosomal-recessive disorders in which hyperphenylalaninemia results from a deficiency of BH_4. Because of the involvement of BH_4 in catecholamine and serotonin synthesis, such infants also have a manifest deficiency of neurotransmitter metabolites in addition to hyperphenylalaninemia. Other conditions in this category include autosomal-recessive guanosine triphosphate cyclohydrolase (GTPCH) deficiency and primapterinuria (Table 39-2).

Role of BH_4 in the Central Nervous System

Because BH_4 is required for the hydroxylation of aromatic amino acids, its importance in the central nervous system (CNS) becomes immediately apparent. Tyrosine and tryptophan are required for the synthesis of catecholamines and serotonin. A BH_4-dependent process can be strongly suspected when plasma phenylalanine levels return to normal after BH_4 supplementation. A dose of 5–10 mg/kg of BH_4 is the usual recommended dose for correction of peripheral hyperphenylalaninemia, and 10–20 mg/kg per day has been recently advocated in classic phenylketonuria. Because BH_4 crosses the blood–brain barrier poorly, lifelong supplementation with the neurotransmitter precursors L-DOPA and 5-hydroxytryptophan, along with carbidopa to prevent peripheral decarboxylation, is necessary in most of the disorders mentioned earlier. A much higher dose of BH_4, approximately 20 mg/kg, can return BH_4 levels in the cerebrospinal fluid to normal, but it remains prohibitively expensive, and no studies exist as to the possible additional benefit of such a regimen. Dosing can be monitored by assessing clinical response and periodically

measuring cerebrospinal fluid levels of neurotransmitter metabolites [Hyland, 2007]. Verifying normalization of serum prolactin levels has been advocated, but sensitivity is limited, as is detection of overadministration of precursors [Concolino et al., 2008]. The greater requirement of tyrosine hydroxylase for BH_4 in comparison with tryptophan hydroxylase may explain the more severe impairment in the catecholaminergic system compared with the serotonergic system.

Nitric oxide synthase is yet another enzyme with an absolute requirement for BH_4 for the oxidation of arginine to nitric oxide. The inability to replete normal levels of BH_4 in the CNS with oral administration in its currently used doses may be one reason that many children with BH_4-deficient disorders develop lifelong cognitive and developmental impairments despite other treatments. Nitric oxide also plays a critical role in CNS injury and neuroprotective mechanisms, and reduced efficiency of this enzyme may result in an imbalance of neuronal injury and vascular dysregulation and repair.

6-Pyruvoyltetrahydropterin Synthase Deficiency

6-Pyruvoyltetrahydropterin synthase catalyzes the elimination of inorganic triphosphate from dihydroneopterin triphosphate to form 6-pyruvoyltetrahydropterin. Patients have elevated neopterin to biopterin ratios in urine and plasma. Reduced 6-pyruvoyltetrahydropterin synthase activity can be documented in red blood cells. In the classic form of the disorder, patients have reduced catecholamine and serotonin metabolites and an increased neopterin to biopterin level in cerebrospinal fluid. Patients are usually detected by newborn screening, as with phenylketonurics. They exhibit progressive signs of neurologic involvement in the first few months of life, including extrapyramidal signs, axial and truncal hypotonia, hypokinesia, feeding difficulties, choreoathetotic or dystonic limb movements, and autonomic symptoms. Many of these patients, despite early diagnosis and supplementation with BH_4 and neurotransmitter precursors, continue to manifest delay in

Table 39-2 Metabolite Patterns Observed in Urine, Plasma, and Cerebrospinal Fluid in the Inherited Disorders Affecting Dopamine and Serotonin Metabolism

	Phe	BH_4	BH_2	Neop	Sep	Prim	HVA	5-HIAA	3OMD
GTPCH (Recessive)	↑ (P)	↓ (U, CSF)	N	↓ (U, CSF)	N	N	↓ (CSF)	↓ (CSF)	N
GTPCH (Dominant)	N	↓ (CSF)	N	↓ (CSF)	N	N	↓ (CSF)	± ↓ (CSF)	N
6PTPS	↑ (P)	↓ (U, CSF)	N	(U, CSF)	N	N	↓ (CSF)	(CSF)	N
6PTPS (Mild)	(P)	(U)	N	(U)	N	N	N	N	N
SR	N	(CSF)	(CSF)	N	↑ (CSF)	N	(CSF)	(CSF)	N
PCD	↑ (P)	↓ (U)	N	N	N	N	(U)	N	N
DHPR	(P)	↓ (U) ± ↓ (CSF)	↑ (U, CSF)	N	N	N	↓ (CSF)	↓ (CSF)	N
TH	N	N	N	N	N	N	↓ (CSF)	N	N
AADC	N	N	N	N	N	N	↓ (CSF)	↓ (CSF)	↑ (P, CSF, U)

AADC, aromatic L-amino acid decarboxylase; BH2, 7,8-dihydrobiopterin; DHPR, dihydropteridine reductase; 5-HIAA, 5-hydroxyindoleacetic acid; GTPCH, guanosine triphosphate cyclohydrolase; HVA, homovanillic acid; N, normal; Neop, neopterin; P, plasma; PCD, pterin α-carbinolamine dehydratase; Phe, phenylalanine; Prim, primapterin; Sep, sepiapterin; 6PTPS, 6-pyruvoyltetrahydropterin synthase; SR, sepiapterin reductase; TH, tyrosine hydroxylase; 3OMD, 3-O-methyldopa; U, urine; ↓, decreased; ↑, elevated.

(From Hyland K. Inherited disorders affecting dopamine and serotonin: Critical neurotransmitters derived from aromatic amino acids. J Nutr 2007;137:1568–72S.)

development [Dudesek et al., 2001]. A "peripheral" form of the disorder is associated with nearly one-third of known mutations with the human *PTS* gene [Thony and Blau, 2006], and is characterized by normal central neurotransmitter levels and less significant or transient hyperphenylalaninemia [Niederwieser et al., 1987]. Patients with the peripheral form have an excellent prognosis for normal neurologic development, provided the hyperphenylalaninemia is corrected by diet or BH_4 administration.

Dihydropteridine Reductase Deficiency

Dihydropteridine reductase deficiency manifests in a variety of phenotypes, all with hyperphenylalaninemia. The clinical presentation is similar to that of central 6-pyruvoyltetrahydropterin synthase deficiency. Without folinic acid to restore methyltetrahydrofolate status in the CNS, these patients can have progressive calcification of the basal ganglia and subcortical regions, despite treatment with BH_4 and neurotransmitter precursors [Woody et al., 1989]. A juvenile variant has been reported in which siblings were developmentally normal until 6 years of age, at which time they developed progressive encephalopathy, epilepsy, and pyramidal, cerebellar, and extrapyramidal features on clinical examination [Larnaout et al., 1998]. Diagnosis can be confirmed by the pattern of urine pterins and documentation of abnormal dihydropteridine reductase activity in skin fibroblasts [Milstien et al., 1980]. Results of phenylalanine loading tests are abnormal, and phenylalanine status improves or returns to normal with BH_4 supplementation. Cerebrospinal fluid neurotransmitter and pterin analysis reveals reduced concentrations of homovanillic acid and 5-hydroxyindoleacetic acid, decreased or normal BH_4 levels, and elevated dihydrobiopterin levels.

Autosomal-Recessive Guanosine Triphosphate Cyclohydrolase Deficiency

Although most mutations in GTPCH to date have been documented in association with autosomal-dominant dopa-responsive dystonia, or Segawa's disease, these patients do not have hyperphenylalaninemia on routine plasma screening studies. Patients with the autosomal-recessive form of GTPCH deficiency, however, present in a fashion similar to patients with dihydropteridine reductase deficiency and 6-pyruvoyltetrahydropterin synthase deficiency. Such patients have severe global developmental impairment, marked hypotonia of the trunk and axial muscles, eye movement abnormalities, limb hypertonia, and convulsions; autonomic symptoms include temperature dysregulation, excessive diaphoresis, and blood pressure lability caused by the associated catecholamine deficiency. They typically have absent GTPCH activity in blood cells, liver, and skin fibroblasts. By contrast, patients with autosomal-dominant dopa-responsive dystonia have preservation of some GTPCH activity in liver because of their heterozygous status, enough to maintain normal phenylalanine levels under usual circumstances. Cerebrospinal fluid neurotransmitter metabolite analysis reveals low concentrations of homovanillic acid and 5-hydroxyindoleacetic acid, and low neopterin and biopterin levels.

Pterin-4α-Carbinolamine Dehydratase Deficiency (Primapterinuria)

Pterin-4α-carbinolamine dehydratase deficiency, or primapterinuria, is a cause of mild hyperphenylalaninemia [Blau et al., 1988; Adler et al., 1992]. These infants are usually identified on newborn screening but generally have a benign course with normal development. Phenylalanine hydroxylase catalyzes the conversion of phenylalanine to tyrosine, during which BH_4 is converted to the unstable carbinolamine 4α-hydroxytetrahydrobiopterin [Citron et al., 1993]. Carbinolamine dehydratase catalyzes the dehydration of carbinolamine to quinonoid dihydropterin (qBH2). The decreased rate of dehydration is responsible for the production of 7-biopterin in some mildly hyperphenylalaninemic individuals [Thony et al., 1998]. Urine studies reveal an excess of 7-substituted pterins, reduced biopterin levels, and an increased neopterin to biopterin ratio.

Monoaminergic Neurotransmitter Deficiency States without Hyperphenylalaninemia

Overview

Neurotransmitter deficiency disorders not associated with hyperphenylalaninemia span an increasingly complex spectrum of clinical phenotypes, ranging from ataxia and mental retardation to spastic diplegia to exercise-induced dystonia. The lack of ascertainment by way of newborn screening and increasingly broad phenotypic spectrum make these disorders as a group much more challenging to recognize. Other than autosomal-dominant dopa-responsive dystonia, the remaining disorders in this category are all inherited in an autosomal-recessive fashion with the exception of monoamine oxidase A deficiency, a rare X-linked recessive disorder. In general, heterozygous carriers for mutations in this group do not have a discernible phenotype, with rare exceptions in tyrosine hydroxylase deficiency and combined monoamine oxidase A and B deficiency.

Segawa's Disease or Autosomal-Dominant Dopa-Responsive Dystonia

The best-described and most widely identified entity among this group of disorders is autosomal-dominant dopa-responsive dystonia caused by GTPCH deficiency, or Segawa's disease [Segawa et al., 1976]. Identification and treatment of this disorder can be extremely rewarding because patients often benefit greatly from directed treatment of the associated dopamine deficiency state [Harwood et al., 1994]. Patients with a classic presentation of exercise-induced dystonia are not difficult to recognize. This diagnosis should also be considered in patients with spastic diplegia, especially when significant fluctuation in gait or worsening gait at the end of the day is noted, and in patients with more atypical presentations, including writer's cramp, asymmetric limb dystonia, tremor, or restless leg-type symptoms. In patients with a classic presentation, many clinicians can make the diagnosis on a presumptive basis, after observing remission of symptoms with a trial of L-DOPA/carbidopa.

As of 2009 there are more than 85 known mutations of the *GCH-1* gene, and in a large review of dopa-responsive dystonia, it was found that 60 percent are point mutations [Clot et al., 2009]. Although inheritance is autosomal-dominant, penetrance is incomplete, and variable expressivity among family members with the same mutation is well documented [Steinberger et al., 1998]. For instance, one might see spastic diplegia, writer's cramp, restless leg syndrome, and more typical exercise-induced dystonia phenotypes among different members of the same family. The female to male ratio in sporadic cases is 4:1, and investigators have confirmed increased penetrance of *GTPCH-I* gene mutations in females [Ichinose et al., 1994; Furukawa et al., 1998]. Of note, a review of 47 patients with *GCH-1* mutations or deletions found 40 patients manifested dystonic symptoms in the first decade of life [Clot et al., 2009].

Not surprisingly, mood and sleep disorders appear to be unusually prevalent in families with the disorder. Recent study of the neurologic and psychiatric phenotype of affected individuals within three extended families showed a higher frequency of major depressive disorder and obsessive-compulsive disorder, as well as disrupted sleep in 55 percent of patients [Van Hove et al., 2006]. These data help to support the idea that the disease carries an increased burden of attentional difficulties, anxiety, dysphoria, depression, and sleep disorders.

Cerebrospinal fluid neurotransmitter metabolite and pterin studies are helpful in confirming the diagnosis in these patients and can help characterize the degree of associated dopamine and serotonin deficiency. Phenylalanine loading is also valuable in confirming a suspected diagnosis but is not specific to the disorder, as phenylketonuria heterozygotes also manifest delayed phenylalanine clearance. GTPCH activity can be measured directly in skin fibroblasts. Urine pterin analysis serves as the first step in evaluation, with urine biopterin levels being low in autosomal-dominant GTPCH deficiency. Cerebrospinal fluid analysis should be performed before institution of a treatment trial of L-DOPA/carbidopa because treatment results in increased levels of homovanillic acid and 3-*O*-methyldopa. The typical pattern in cerebrospinal fluid in dopa-responsive dystonia resulting from GTPCH deficiency is a low homovanillic acid level, normal or low 5-hydroxyindoleacetic acid level, and reduced BH_4 level. Patients who are heterozygous for a GTPCH mutation, despite their normal blood phenylalanine levels on routine screening, have abnormal phenylalanine metabolism if they are stressed by administration of an oral phenylalanine load. If cytokine-stimulated fibroblast enzyme analysis of biopterin metabolism is not feasible or patients decline a cerebrospinal fluid examination and have an otherwise typical presentation, an oral phenylalanine loading test may be helpful in supporting the diagnosis. Phenylalanine is administered orally to the fasting patient at a dose of 100 mg/kg. Serum phenylalanine and tyrosine levels are obtained at baseline and 1, 2, and 4 hours after loading. An elevated phenylalanine to tyrosine ratio and delayed clearance of phenylalanine are typical in patients with GTPCH deficiency because BH_4 levels are typically reduced. Gene sequencing is available for confirmation of diagnosis, but has not yet supplanted biochemical studies as the diagnostic standard.

Treatment with L-DOPA/carbidopa leads to significant benefit or resolution of motor symptoms in the majority of patients with Segawa's disease within a few weeks. However, compound heterozygotes or patients with long-standing or more severe motor manifestations, such as parkinsonism or long-standing spastic paraparesis, may require more careful titration of dosing, with gradual adjustment during a period of several months. Mood manifestations, such as depression and anxiety, often respond to L-DOPA treatment to some degree, but some patients have additional benefit from directed treatment of their associated serotonin deficiency, either with the serotonin precursor 5-hydroxytryptophan or with a serotonin reuptake inhibitor. Anecdotal evidence suggests that anticholinergic agents may also help ameliorate postural dystonia and tremor [Segawa et al., 1976].

Aromatic L-Amino Acid Decarboxylase or Dopa-Decarboxylase Deficiency

Aromatic L-amino acid decarboxylase is a pyridoxine-dependent enzyme that decarboxylates L-DOPA and 5-hydroxytryptophan to make dopamine and serotonin, respectively. Patients with this disorder typically present in the first few months of life with dystonia or intermittent limb spasticity, axial and truncal hypotonia, oculogyric crises, autonomic symptoms, and ptosis [Hyland et al., 1992]. Neonatal symptoms, including poor suck and feeding difficulties, ptosis, lethargy, and hypothermia, are common. Neurologic signs and symptoms are clearly evident within the first few months of life in all patients described to date. These patients demonstrate multisystemic involvement with a wide array of neurologic difficulties, including problems with sleep, attention, emotional regulation, and cognitive function that extend well beyond their motor difficulties. As they get older, gross motor delays with fluctuating tone, ataxia, and expressive speech impairment are prominent features, even in the patients with the best outcomes.

The phenomenology of the movement disorder is remarkably similar among the cases and, not surprisingly, shares a number of features in common with children with BH_4 deficiency disorders, such as 6-pyruvoyltetrahydropterin synthase deficiency and dihydropteridine reductase deficiency, and the autosomal-recessive form of GTPCH deficiency. Intermittent oculogyric crises and limb dystonia, generalized athetosis, and an overall paucity of voluntary movement become evident between 1 and 6 months of age. Tongue thrusting, ocular convergence spasm (Figure 39-2), myoclonic jerks, and episodes of sudden loss of head control or episodes resembling flexor spasms are common and frequently lead to a clinical diagnosis of epilepsy. Oculogyric crises, orofacial dystonia, torticollis, limb tremor with attempted voluntary movement, and blepharospasm are often the most compelling evidence supporting a defect in dopaminergic transmission. Breath-holding or apneic spells, paroxysmal sweating, nasal congestion, sudden respiratory or cardiorespiratory arrest, unresponsiveness associated with hypoglycemia, intermittent hypothermia, and feeding and gastrointestinal issues are manifestations of the often profound autonomic dysfunction these patients demonstrate [Swoboda et al., 2003]. First- and second-degree relatives of affected individuals have been shown to have a high incidence of psychiatric disorders, including depression, psychosis, suicide, or suicide attempts [Manegold et al., 2009].

Cerebrospinal fluid neurotransmitter metabolites demonstrate a characteristic pattern: low homovanillic acid and 5-hydroxyindoleacetic acid levels; markedly elevated 3-*O*-methyldopa, 5-hydroxytryptophan, and L-DOPA; and

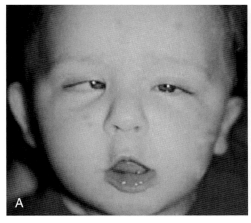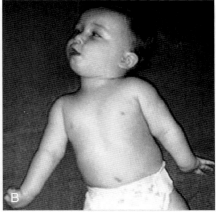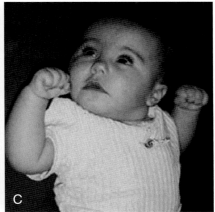

Fig. 39-2 Episodic neurologic manifestations in aromatic L-amino acid decarboxylase deficiency. A, Ocular convergence spasm, ptosis, and orofacial dystonia. **B,** Torticollis and limb dystonia. **C,** Torticollis and limb rigidity.

normal biopterin and neopterin levels. Plasma L-DOPA is markedly elevated. Urine catecholamines may be reduced or elevated, specifically with vanillactic acid, despite normal preliminary organic acid results [Manegold et al., 2009; Abeling et al., 1998, 2000].

Although some children benefit in terms of the underlying movement disorder, treatment is complex, and these patients are vulnerable to an array of medication-related side effects. Instead of replacement of neurotransmitter precursors, as in the BH_4 deficiency-related disorders, the use of neurotransmitter receptor agonists or strategies to hinder reuptake or metabolism of endogenously produced neurotransmitters is necessary. Reported benefit has been noted in a subset of patients with monoamine oxidase inhibitors, dopamine receptor agonists, anticholinergic agents, pyridoxine, and, in rare cases associated with a defect in the gene encoding aromatic L-amino acid decarboxylase at the dopa-binding site, L-DOPA [Swoboda et al., 1999]. Dopamine receptor antagonists, such as clozapine, have been proposed as a new therapeutic option, given their increase in aromatic L-amino acid decarboxylase activity in a mouse model [Allen et al., 2009].

However, in spite of a variety of treatment interventions directed at ameliorating the effects of the associated neurotransmitter deficiency state, overall clinical outcomes in aromatic L-amino acid decarboxylase deficiency remain poor. All patients have had some degree of cognitive impairment, and there is increasing evidence of a gender-dependent discrepancy in severity, with females demonstrating the most severe phenotypes [Pons et al., 2004].

Sepiapterin Reductase Deficiency

Sepiapterin reductase catalyzes the (NADP) reduction of carbonyl derivatives, including pteridines, and plays an important role in BH_4 biosynthesis. Somewhat surprisingly, the first identified cases had normal plasma phenylalanine and urine pterin levels [Bonafe et al., 2001b]. Blau and colleagues have hypothesized that peripheral tissues can use alternative carbonyl, aldose, and dihydrofolate reductases to perform the last two steps in BH_4 biosynthesis. Therefore, BH_4 levels in the liver are likely to be normal, probably explaining the absence of hyperphenylalaninemia in these patients. In addition, it is likely

that low dihydrofolate reductase activity in the brain allows accumulation of dihydrobiopterin that inhibits tyrosine and tryptophan hydroxylases and uncouples neuronal nitric oxide synthase, leading to neurotransmitter deficiency and neuronal cell death. Thus, identification of low cerebrospinal fluid neurotransmitter levels and the presence of elevated cerebrospinal fluid dihydrobiopterin is crucial for making the diagnosis in these patients.

Few patients have been described to date [Neville et al., 2005; Blau et al., 2001; Bonafe et al., 2001a]. Dystonic posturing, oculogyric crises, spasticity, tremor, ataxia, and psychiatric disturbances have been reported. The largest and most recent study reviewed clinical phenotypes in seven children, showing uniform early motor delay and diurnal variation in motor symptoms, with a high frequency of oculogyric crises, dystonia, and hypotonia [Neville et al., 2005]. All had cognitive delay to some extent, and some had parkinsonian symptoms and bulbar involvement. Also, in all cases, significant motor improvement resulted from low-dose L-DOPA/carbidopa therapy (range 1–6 mg/kg/day), although cognitive outcomes were not changed by therapy. In addition to L-DOPA/carbidopa therapy, there has been anecdotal improvement with the use of selegiline, a monoamine oxidase B inhibitor that prolongs the half-life of dopamine at the synapse. Cerebrospinal fluid neurotransmitter metabolite and pterin analysis reveals low levels of homovanillic acid and 5-hydroxyindoleacetic acid and high levels of biopterin, dihydrobiopterin, and sepiapterin. Diagnosis can be confirmed by documenting low sepiapterin reductase activity in skin fibroblast cultures.

Tyrosine Hydroxylase Deficiency or Autosomal-Recessive Dopa-Responsive Dystonia

Tyrosine hydroxylase deficiency, sometimes referred to as autosomal-recessive Segawa's disease, displays a diverse phenotype ranging from exercise-induced dystonia to progressive gait disturbance and tremor in childhood to severe infantile parkinsonism [Bodeau-Pean et al., 1999; De Lonlay et al., 2000; de Rijk-Van Andel et al., 2000]. A wide range of symptoms can be associated with tyrosine hydroxylase deficiency, with mild, moderate, and severe phenotypes. In a large review of dopa-responsive dystonia, tyrosine hydroxylase deficiency accounted for less than 5 percent of all cases [Clot et al., 2009].

In the mildest cases, walking or running may be clumsy, but little else may be noticed, at least initially. Abnormal posturing may be evident when the child is stressed or later in the day. These symptoms may progress slowly as the child gets older. Sometimes, one side of the body may seem weaker, or the child may begin to toe-walk because of hamstring or heel-cord tightness. Sometimes these children are diagnosed with cerebral palsy; other times, they are simply considered clumsy or uncoordinated. Some children demonstrate attentional difficulties or mild articulation disorders. Essentially, all children with mild symptoms are readily treated with medication.

In moderately affected cases, children demonstrate an abnormal gait. Children may demonstrate dystonic posturing while walking or with attempts to walk on their heels or toes. Some children are ataxic or have significant spasticity. Speech delay may be present. Many of these children are diagnosed with cerebral palsy. Some demonstrate involuntary eye movement problems, characterized either by brief upward eye-rolling movements when they are fatigued or stressed, or by frank oculogyric crises. The majority of these children have an excellent response to treatment, but full benefit may take many months.

In the most severe cases, children are severely disabled and affected from early infancy. This is referred to as the infantile Parkinson's disease variant. Infants may demonstrate muscle tightness and rigidity, arching, tremor and poor muscle control, and involuntary eye movements. They may have ptosis. They usually have speech delay and often demonstrate difficulties in feeding, chewing, or swallowing. Constipation is common. Whereas most children tend toward increased muscle tone and even rigidity, there are children who have generalized low muscle tone, with poor head control and inability to sit unsupported. They often demonstrate torticollis. They may have difficulty directing their hands to a toy, generating a flinging hand motion. Occasionally, children suffer from intermittent color changes, unexplained low body temperature or fevers, low blood glucose level, and difficulty regulating blood pressure. These symptoms are more likely to occur during another illness the child may be experiencing. Children in the more severely affected group of patients are more difficult to treat, and several medications may be needed to modulate symptoms. They are unusually vulnerable to side effects of dopaminergic agonists or precursors, which can result in excessive movement and irritability. Response may be slow, with some continued benefit during months to years, but it may not result in the complete resolution of all symptoms. Some children have had persistent mental retardation, encephalopathy, and motor disability in spite of directed treatment of their underlying dopamine deficiency state.

Low tyrosine hydroxylase activity results in significant cerebrospinal fluid catecholamine deficiency, as demonstrated by low homovanillic acid concentrations; cerebrospinal fluid concentrations of 5-hydroxyindoleacetic acid, neopterin, and biopterin are normal. It is more difficult to distinguish these children from those with secondary neurotransmitter deficiency states because phenylalanine loading studies are normal, and enzymatic assays for confirmation of a suspected diagnosis are not presently available. Confirmation by molecular testing is extremely helpful, particularly in providing adequate counseling for parents about recurrence risks with future pregnancies. Children have a paucity of autonomic features, suggesting a compensatory peripheral mechanism, except in children with the severe infantile parkinsonism variant. In four patients whom the author has observed, including one patient with the severe infantile parkinsonism variant, peripheral plasma catecholamine levels have been normal, although reduced urine homovanillic acid levels have been noted. Caution should be taken to monitor blood glucose concentration in the setting of prolonged fasting, such as before a magnetic resonance imaging (MRI) study.

Patients variably respond to L-DOPA/carbidopa, and some have complete reversal of symptoms. The exception to this is the patient with the severe infantile parkinsonism form. These patients sometimes tolerate L-DOPA poorly, with excessive dyskinesia, irritability, and reflux, or have incomplete or inadequate response with regard to their motor manifestations of the disorder [Brautigam et al., 1999; Dionisi-Vici et al., 2000]. When diagnosis occurs late in such patients, motor development must be recapitulated, and continued slow improvement during months is to be expected. Typical features in infants affected by the severe infantile parkinsonism variant include rigidity, tremor, bradykinesia, oculogyric crises, and severe psychomotor delay.

Treatment with L-DOPA/carbidopa alone may lead to severe dyskinesias with marked on-off effects in such patients. Addition of dopamine agonists such as selegiline or anticholinergic agents like trihexyphenidyl can provide significant benefit and help promote the gradual on-going attainment of motor skills and ability to ambulate independently, but such achievements may occur over years, rather than months or weeks, in the most severely affected patients. Whereas more mildly affected patients may tolerate 1–3 mg/kg of L-DOPA per dose, 2–4 times per day, severely affected infants and younger children require L-DOPA quantities as low as 0.2 mg/kg/dose. Breaking standard formulations of L-DOPA/carbidopa into more than two doses per tablet is not advisable because the amount of carbidopa will then be insufficient to help enhance transport of L-DOPA across the blood–brain barrier and to minimize peripheral side effects, such as nausea, reflux, decreased appetite, and vomiting. Carbidopa should be maintained at a minimum of approximately 1 mg/kg/dose up to 25 mg per dose, no matter the L-DOPA requirement. Slow institution of small, compounded doses of L-DOPA/carbidopa, along with selegiline (monoamine oxidase B inhibitor) and an anticholinergic agent such as trihexyphenidyl, may be more beneficial than L-DOPA/carbidopa alone [Haussler et al., 2001]. Selegiline doses may also require compounding because low-dose formulations are not available for use in infants. Frequent side effects of excessive dosing include eating disorders, nightmares, and insomnia. Dosing should be started in the range of 0.1 mg/kg and increased as tolerated. Patients with a mild form of the disorder, such as an isolated gait disorder or exercise-induced dystonia, respond well to monotherapy with L-DOPA/carbidopa and rarely develop dyskinesia.

Although inheritance to date in most families seems to be recessive, at least one family has been described in which the father of the affected proband had mild exercise-induced dystonia responsive to therapy, raising the possibility that tyrosine hydroxylase deficiency could present in an autosomal-dominant fashion in some families with a milder phenotype [Furukawa et al., 2001].

Tryptophan Hydroxylase Deficiency

Tryptophan hydroxylase catalyzes the BH_4-dependent hydroxylation of tryptophan to 5-hydroxytryptophan, which is then decarboxylated to form serotonin. Tryptophan hydroxylase expression is limited to certain cells in the CNS and periphery, including raphe neurons, pinealocytes, mast cells, mononuclear leukocytes, beta cells of the islets of Langerhans, and enterochromaffin cells of the gut. Patients with presumed tryptophan hydroxylase deficiency have been described, although it is not yet certain that their symptoms result from tryptophan hydroxylase deficiency [Raemaekers et al., 2001]. Clinical features, consisting of ataxia, speech delay, mild psychomotor retardation, and hypotonia, are nonspecific. Cerebrospinal fluid neurotransmitter metabolite and pterin studies demonstrate the expected low 5-hydroxyindoleacetic acid with normal homovanillic acid, neopterin, and biopterin levels. Mutations in the gene encoding tryptophan hydroxylase have not yet been identified, although identification of isoforms specific to nervous tissue will likely facilitate future research [Invernizzi, 2007].

Dopamine β-Hydroxylase Deficiency

Dopamine β-hydroxylase is the enzyme that converts dopamine to norepinephrine. Presenting symptoms of this disorder have been largely attributed to the importance of this enzyme in postganglionic sympathetic neurons [Robertson et al., 1986]. Patients with severe deficiency of this enzyme, however, cannot synthesize norepinephrine, epinephrine, and octopamine in CNS or peripheral autonomic neurons. Dopamine acts as a false neurotransmitter for noradrenergic neurons. Neonates with dopamine β-hydroxylase deficiency can have episodic hypothermia, hypoglycemia, and hypotension, leading to early death. Survivors do fairly well until late childhood, when overwhelming orthostatic hypotension profoundly limits their activities. The hypotension can be so severe as to lead to convulsive syncope with recurrent clonic seizures [Robertson et al., 1991].

Most patients have been identified as young adults. Observation of severe orthostatic hypotension in a patient whose plasma norepinephrine/dopamine ratio is much less than 1 supports the diagnosis. Orthostatic hypotension, particularly after exercise, and ptosis are constant features. General lethargy and lassitude improve dramatically and blood pressure becomes normal with treatment with D,L-threo-dihydroxyphenylserine, a synthetic amino acid that is converted to norepinephrine by aromatic L-amino acid decarboxylase. Whether these patients suffer from attention problems or other subtle cognitive deficits has not been adequately studied. Patients may undergo personality change, becoming more "aggressive" with treatment.

Monoamine Oxidase Deficiency

Monoamine oxidase is a mitochondrial enzyme involved in the catabolism of biogenic amines. Monoamine oxidase A, the primary type in fibroblasts, preferentially degrades serotonin and norepinephrine. Monoamine oxidase B, the primary type in platelets and in the brain, preferentially degrades phenylethylamine and benzylamine. These enzymes are critical in the neuronal metabolism of catecholamine and indoleamine neurotransmitters. The genes are closely linked on the X chromosome, near the Norrie's disease locus, and only affected boys

have been identified to date [Schuback et al., 1999]. Comparisons of the neurochemical characteristics of previously described patients with combined monoamine oxidase A and B deficiency and selective monoamine oxidase A deficiency have led to an improved understanding of the roles of monoamine oxidase A and monoamine oxidase B in the metabolic degradation of catecholamines and other biogenic amines, including serotonin and the trace amines.

Monoamine Oxidase A Deficiency

Brunner described a family with an X-linked nondysmorphic mild mental retardation and a tendency to aggressive or violent behavior, including arson, attempted rape, exhibitionism, and attempted suicide [Brunner et al., 1993b]. Urine studies revealed marked disturbance of monoamine metabolism. Normal platelet monoamine oxidase B activity suggested that the unusual behavior pattern in this family might be caused by isolated monoamine oxidase A deficiency, which was later confirmed by identification in all affected males of a point mutation leading to premature termination of the protein [Brunner et al., 1993a].

Measurement of 3-methoxy-4-hydroxyphenylglycol, a metabolite of norepinephrine, in plasma is the most sensitive index of monoamine oxidase A activity in humans and can be used to screen potential cases. Monoamine oxidase A enzyme activity can be measured directly from fibroblasts. The inability to identify additional patients, despite screening of at-risk males with mental retardation or a behavioral phenotype, makes it likely that this disorder is rare [Segawa et al., 1976], although report of a knockout mice strain involving monoamine oxidase A with enhanced aggression will likely provide new directions for research [Scott et al., 2008]. Interestingly, a high-activity monoamine oxidase A promoter allele has been found with increased frequency in women with panic disorder [Deckert et al., 1999]. A possible association of decreased enzyme activity in women with bipolar disorder has also been reported [Preisig et al., 2000].

Monoamine Oxidase B Deficiency

Isolated monoamine oxidase B deficiency has not yet been reported in a patient. Two brothers with a microdeletion, including the Norrie locus and monoamine oxidase B, however, had features consistent with Norrie's disease alone, with congenital blindness and progressive hearing loss caused by cochlear degeneration in adolescence. These patients had neither abnormal behavior nor mental retardation, leading the authors to conclude that monoamine oxidase A plays a more significant role than does monoamine oxidase B in the metabolism of biogenic amines, and monoamine oxidase B deficiency alone may have a primarily neurochemical phenotype: that of increased phenylethylamine in urine [Lenders et al., 1996].

Monoamine Oxidase A and B Deficiency

Conclusions about the phenotype of individuals with combined deficiency of monoamine oxidase A and monoamine oxidase B come primarily from a study of a single boy with a microdeletion at Xp14 involving the Norrie locus and documented severe deficiency of monoamine oxidase A and B activity [Collins et al., 1992]. He was severely mentally retarded and blind, and he had other neurologic features, including myoclonus and tendency for motor stereotypies. Because Norrie's disease is an X-linked recessive disorder, obligate carriers would not be expected to have symptoms. In this family, two obligate carriers had normal intelligence. The proband's mother had psychiatric symptoms characterized by "chronic hypomania and schizotypal features," however, and both carriers had low monoamine oxidase activity.

Disorders of Amino Acid Neurotransmitters

Amino acid neurotransmitters are the main inhibitory and excitatory messengers in the nervous system. Although the list of proposed neurotransmitters is long, relatively few have been found to play a role in human neurologic disease. Among these, disorders of GABA and glycine have undergone the most study, yet current understanding is far from complete. Glycine, a simple amino acid with ubiquitous function, has both excitatory and inhibitory properties. Glycine encephalopathy, formerly referred to as nonketotic hyperglycinemia, is a disorder of glycine degradation that typically manifests with neonatal encephalopathy, lethargy, hypotonia, myoclonus, and apnea. It will be touched on briefly, as more extensive review occurs elsewhere in this text. Disorders of GABA degradation will also be reviewed (Figure 39-3), with specific emphasis on succinic semialdehyde dehydrogenase deficiency, the most common and best characterized. Previously, it was thought that disordered GABA synthesis might be related to the clinical entity of pyridoxine-responsive epilepsy; however, recent elucidation of the epileptogenic mechanism has proven it to be due to lysine degradation [Mills et al., 2006] and so it will not be discussed in this chapter.

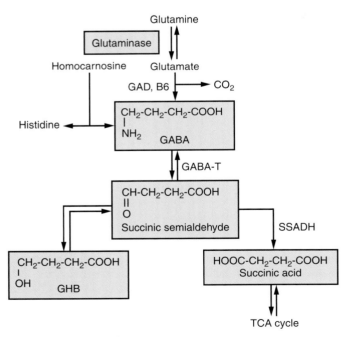

Fig. 39-3 The gamma-aminobutyric acid metabolism pathway. GABA-T, gamma-aminobutyric acid transaminase; GAD, glutamate decarboxylase; GHB, gamma-aminohydroxybutyrate; SSADH, succinic semialdehyde dehydrogenase; TCA, tricarboxylic acid. *(From Pearl PL, Gibson KM. Clinical aspects of the disorders of GABA metabolism in children. Curr Opin Neurol 2004;17:107–113.)*

Gamma-Aminobutyric Acid Transaminase Deficiency

GABA is the major inhibitory neurotransmitter of the brain, derived primarily from glutamate, the major excitatory neurotransmitter. The first step of the GABA degradation pathway involves GABA transaminase, which removes an amino group from GABA and adds it to alpha-ketoglutarate, thus replenishing glutamate and re-establishing the closed loop system known as the GABA shunt. GABA transaminase deficiency is a rare, autosomal-recessive disorder characterized by abnormal development, seizures, and high levels of GABA in serum and cerebrospinal fluid [Pearl and Gibson, 2004]. Publications to date have presented limited family and case studies, all of which have had poor outcomes. Definitive diagnosis can be made by measurement of GABA transaminase activity in liver, lymphocytes isolated from whole blood, or Epstein–Barr virus-transformed cultured lymphocytes [Gibson et al., 1985].

Succinic Semialdehyde Dehydrogenase Deficiency

Succinic semialdehyde dehydrogenase deficiency is an autosomal-recessive inborn error of metabolism associated with a defect in the metabolism of GABA [Gibson et al., 1998]. Phenotypic features range from nonspecific global developmental delay and hypotonia to ataxia, severe mental retardation, visual impairment, and seizures. The course of the disease is somewhat unique in regard to other neurotransmitter abnormalities in that it is not intermittent or episodic, making distinction from static encephalopathies challenging [Pearl et al., 2009]. Neuropsychiatric symptoms are prominent and include sleep disorders, inattention, hyperactivity, and anxiety [Pearl et al., 2009]. Generalized epilepsy affects nearly half of patients, with over half having abnormal electroencephalograms (EEGs) [Pearl et al., 2009]. MRI is commonly abnormal in patients with succinic semialdehyde dehydrogenase deficiency, with increased T2-weighted signal in the globus pallidi, subcortical white matter, cerebellar dentate nucleus, and brainstem [Pearl et al., 2009].

Urine organic acid screening to detect elevated 4-hydroxybutyric acid is the most easily available screening strategy, but GABA levels in cerebrospinal fluid and urine are also elevated. Improvement of seizures in a mouse model of the disorder was demonstrated with treatment with vigabatrin or a GABA B receptor antagonist [Hogema et al., 2001]. Unfortunately, this medicine has not been consistently helpful in humans and there is considerable risk involved with its administration. Investigations into other potential therapies, including taurine, the ketogenic diet, and GABA B receptor antagonists is currently under way in mouse models [Pearl et al., 2009].

Secondary Neurotransmitter Deficiency States

Menkes' disease is an X-linked recessive disorder in which affected males have progressive encephalopathy, spasticity, seizures, and sparse, brittle hair. The primary defect is reduced or absent function of the copper-transporting ATPase ATP7A. Multiple copper-dependent enzymes can be secondarily affected, including dopamine β-hydroxylase, leading to secondary autonomic involvement and norepinephrine deficiency.

Recently, plasma monoamine monitoring has been posed as a method of early detection in Menkes' disease [Kaler et al., 2008].

Hyperekplexia, or "startle disease," is a heterogeneous disorder caused by defects in the a_1 subunit of the glycine receptor [Shiang et al., 1993]. The disorder occurs in autosomal-dominant and autosomal-recessive forms, and is characterized predominantly by stimulus-sensitive myoclonus. Transient hypertonia and hypokinesia in infancy in some families with the disorder has led to the designation "stiff baby syndrome." Dubowitz et al. [1992] described an infant with classic startle disease, in whom the cerebrospinal fluid concentrations of GABA were substantially lower than normal during the first weeks of life. Infants with hyperekplexia have higher than expected rates of sudden infant death syndrome.

Later in life, patients develop involuntary myoclonus, markedly hyperactive brainstem reflexes, and a momentary generalized jerking on falling asleep. An exaggerated startle response persists throughout life; sudden, unexpected acoustic or tactile stimuli can precipitate a brief attack of intense rigidity with falling. Congenital dislocation of the hip and inguinal and abdominal hernias, presumably caused by increased intra-abdominal pressure, are more frequent in affected families. Dramatic improvement of symptoms occurs in most patients with clonazepam.

Neurodegenerative disorders associated with on-going cell loss are sometimes associated with reductions in neurotransmitter metabolites. Such abnormalities have been seen in patients with leukodystrophy and progressive encephalopathy phenotypes in which a primary defect in neurotransmitter or pterin metabolism could not be identified. Certain patients may still benefit from directed treatment of the underlying neurotransmitter deficiency. For example, in one young patient with an otherwise undefined leukodystrophy, supplementation with L-DOPA/carbidopa markedly ameliorated his lower limb spasticity. None the less, he continued to have progressive neurologic involvement with time.

Periods of hypoxia or ischemia can lead to secondary deficiencies of serotonin and dopamine, as demonstrated by low levels of homovanillic acid and 5-hydroxyindoleacetic acid in cerebrospinal fluid. In addition, BH_4 levels are low and neopterin levels can be elevated. This presents a confusing pattern that mimics the metabolite profile observed in 6-pyruvoyltetrahydropterin synthase deficiency. The absence of hyperphenylalaninemia and the presence of signal abnormalities in the basal ganglia, thalamus, and cortex consistent with hypoxic-ischemic encephalopathy allow differentiation.

Undefined Neurotransmitter Deficiency States

Increasingly, with more widespread testing of cerebrospinal fluid neurotransmitter metabolites, patients are being identified with documented neurotransmitter deficiency states that do not fit easily into any of the preceding diagnostic categories, and the nature of their underlying defects remains unknown. These include patients with a wide variety of movement disorder phenotypes, encephalopathy, or seizures.

Additional studies are needed to determine the precise defects affecting neurotransmitter levels and to ascertain whether they are primary or secondary. In addition to neurotransmitter deficiency, excess levels of neurotransmitter metabolites have also been seen in some cases. The etiology in these patients remains uncertain at this time, but it may imply an underlying receptor defect, with secondary upregulation.

A careful history of medications or herbal supplements is important because some agents, such as serotonin reuptake inhibitors, could theoretically increase serotonin metabolite levels. Overall, cerebrospinal fluid neurotransmitter metabolite and pterin assays provide powerful tools to help better characterize patients with otherwise undefined or poorly defined neurologic disorders.

Approach to Treatment in Patients with Neurotransmitter Deficiency States

Because patients with neurotransmitter deficiency disorders caused by tyrosine hydroxylase or BH_4 deficiency have been deficient for prolonged periods before treatment, they can be extremely sensitive to initiation of neurotransmitter precursors. Starting with extremely conservative dosages, increasing the dosage slowly during weeks or months, and ensuring that peripheral aromatic L-amino acid decarboxylase is fully blocked by providing ample carbidopa can make the transition to treatment much easier. The rate or degree to which children respond depends on a variety of factors, including age at diagnosis, specific disorder and mutation, presence or absence of associated hyperphenylalaninemia, and presence or absence of central BH_4 deficiency. In general, optimism about improvement is warranted.

Institution of neurotransmitter precursor treatment may lead to new problems, such as intermittent dyskinesia related to a peak dose effect, changes in appetite, gastroesophageal reflux, diarrhea, and constipation. These problems, greatest in the first few weeks of institution of treatment, tend to improve with time. With regard to replacement of L-DOPA, use of a slow-release form of the medication may theoretically be ideal. However, such formulations are dosed, not for use in children, but for use in adults with Parkinson's disease. In addition, dividing standard dosage forms marketed for adults makes adequate dosing in infants and young children a significant challenge. Thus, ideal dosage forms may need to be formulated in compounded preparations, rather than through commercially marketed dosage preparations. Support for parents and children during this often difficult period of transition from initiation of treatment to adjustment of medications is critical because these patients will likely require neurotransmitter precursor replacement throughout their lifetimes.

In a disorder such as aromatic L-amino acid decarboxylase deficiency, in which direct receptor agonists may be indicated, only adult formulations of these often-potent medications are available, making the use of compounding necessary. Giving more frequent and lower doses throughout the day may be necessary in some children.

Although patients with primary neurotransmitter deficiency states are more likely to respond optimally to treatment, patients with secondary neurotransmitter deficiency may have some symptomatic benefit from directed treatment of their underlying neurotransmitter deficiency state.

Neurologic Disorders Characterized by Excess Neurotransmitter Levels

Glycine Encephalopathy

Glycine encephalopathy, formerly referred to as nonketotic hyperglycinemia, is a heterogeneous disorder associated with insufficient activity of various components of the mitochondrial glycine cleavage system. The enzyme system for cleavage of glycine is composed of four protein components: P protein, a pyridoxal phosphate-dependent glycine decarboxylase; H protein, a lipoic acid-containing protein; T protein, a tetrahydrofolate-requiring enzyme; and L protein, a lipoamide dehydrogenase. Nonketotic hyperglycinemia may be caused by a defect in any one of these enzymes. It is an autosomal-recessive disorder with several reported phenotypes, including the classic severe neonatal form, an infantile variant, a mild-episodic childhood variant, a late-onset form, and a benign reversible form [Hamosh and Johnston, 2001].

Most patients described to date have the neonatal and most severe phenotype, likely because it is the most distinctive phenotype. These patients present shortly after birth with lethargy, encephalopathy, hypotonia, myoclonic jerks, and apnea. EEG generally reveals a burst-suppression pattern. Those who survive the neonatal period generally develop intractable seizures and profound mental retardation. Patients with the infantile form have seizures and variable cognitive impairment after a short period of apparently normal development. In the mild-episodic form, patients typically present some time after infancy with mild psychomotor retardation, and may manifest episodes of delirium, chorea, and vertical gaze palsy during febrile illness. In the late-onset form, children present with progressive spastic diplegia and optic atrophy. They generally do not have seizures, and intellectual function is preserved.

Diagnosis is best made by documenting an increased cerebrospinal fluid to plasma glycine ratio [Applegarth and Toone, 2001]. In the neonatal form of nonketotic hyperglycinemia, cerebrospinal fluid glycine level can be 30 times normal. Plasma glycine level is also typically high, but it can be in the normal range. A cerebrospinal fluid to plasma ratio above 0.08 is usually considered diagnostic, but mildly affected cases can have ratios of 0.04–0.1 [Applegarth and Toone, 2001]. (In rare cases, cerebrospinal fluid to plasma ratios are normal, and only elevations in plasma glycine occur [Jackson et al., 1999].) Confirmation of diagnosis requires enzyme analysis in liver or transformed lymphoblasts [Christodoulou et al., 1993]. Treatment with dextromethorphan and sodium benzoate has led to variable improvement in seizure control and behavioral problems in some patients [Boneh et al., 1996; Hamosh et al., 1998].

Leukoencephalopathy with Vanishing White Matter

Leukoencephalopathy with vanishing white matter (also known as childhood ataxia with central white matter hypomyelinization) is a heterogeneous autosomal-recessive leukodystrophy characterized by progressive ataxia, motor impairment, and encephalopathy, in which episodic deterioration is associated with infection or minor head trauma [van der Knaap et al., 1997]. A wide range of onset has been reported in the dozen patients described to date. Cerebrospinal fluid glycine is elevated and can be helpful in confirming the diagnosis [van der Knaap et al., 1999]. At least two genes have been noted to have mutations in patients with this disorder: *EIF2B5* and *EIF2B2*, the first translation initiation factors implicated in human disease [Leegwater et al., 2001]. This disorder is described in more detail in Chapter 71.

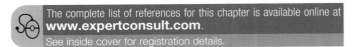

Phakomatoses and Allied Conditions

Elizabeth A. Thiele and Bruce R. Korf

The disorders referred to as phakomatoses are notable for their dysplastic nature and tendency to form tumors in various organs, particularly the nervous system. Bielschowsky observed these characteristic features in neurofibromatosis and tuberous sclerosis complex [Bielschowsky, 1914, 1919], and van der Hoeve called particular attention to these disorders and named the disease category the "phakomatoses" (Greek *phakos*, "mole" or "birthmark") [Van der Hoeve, 1923]. Von Hippel–Lindau disease and Sturge–Weber syndrome were thought to belong to this category of diseases [Van der Hoeve, 1923, 1932] and Louis-Bar identified a syndrome, ataxia-telangiectasia, that she believed also had the typical clinical characteristics of the phakomatoses [Louis-Bar, 1941]. Some of these conditions have been referred to as "neurocutaneous disorders" because of the frequent involvement of the skin in addition to the nervous system. Cutaneous features are not present in all phakomatoses, however (e.g., von Hippel–Lindau syndrome), and many include features outside the skin and nervous system, so the term can be misleading. Box 40-1 lists disorders associated with specific cutaneous findings; Table 40-1 summarizes the phakomatoses.

This chapter surveys the clinical features of the three major phakomatoses: neurofibromatosis, tuberous sclerosis complex, and von Hippel–Lindau syndrome. Also included in this chapter are a number of additional disorders that are commonly considered along with the phakomatoses, including vascular malformation syndromes, pigmentary disorders, and several other rare disorders. Ataxia-telangiectasia is considered in detail in Chapter 67 on the hereditary ataxias.

The Neurofibromatoses

It was only with the report of Young et al. [1970] that the distinction between a peripheral and a central form of neurofibromatosis came to be recognized. The classification was formalized by the National Institutes of Health (NIH) Consensus Development Conference in 1987 [Stumpf, 1988], with the peripheral form of neurofibromatosis referred to as NF1, and the central form, the hallmark of which is bilateral vestibular schwannomas, called NF2. The distinction between the disorders was subsequently verified when the two genes were found to be distinct, first by mapping and later by cloning. More recently, a third disorder, referred to as schwannomatosis, has been split out [MacCollin et al., 2005]. This disorder is characterized by the development of multiple schwannomas of cranial nerves except the vestibular nerve, and of spinal and peripheral nerves.

Neurofibromatosis Type 1

Neurofibromatosis type 1 (NF1) is transmitted as an autosomal-dominant trait and is notable for its great variability of expression. It can involve not only the peripheral and central nervous systems, but also many other systems, including the skin, bone, endocrine, gastrointestinal, and vascular systems. Although von Recklinghausen is credited with the initial clinical and pathologic account of this disease in 1882 [von Recklinghausen, 1882], he cited Tilesius for the first description of a patient with multiple fibrous skin tumors. Wishart [Wishart, 1822] and Smith [Smith, 1849] also provided clinical accounts of the disorder before the report of von Recklinghausen, although early reports failed to recognize the distinction between the disorders known as NF1 and NF2. Diagnostic criteria for NF1 are presented in Box 40-2.

Clinical Characteristics

In NF1, the usual presenting signs are cutaneous manifestations. These skin changes include café-au-lait macules, cutaneous neurofibromas, hypopigmented macules, patchy and diffuse areas of hyperpigmentation, juvenile xanthogranulomas, and angiomas. Café-au-lait macules usually are present at birth and range in size from a few millimeters to centimeters [Crowe et al., 1956] (Figure 40-1). They do not significantly increase in number after the first 2 years of life. Six or more café-au-lait macules measuring at least 5 mm across before puberty or 15 mm after puberty constitute one diagnostic criterion for NF1. Rare persons with variant forms of neurofibromatosis, such as spinal neurofibromatosis [Messiaen et al., 2003; Korf et al., 2005], may lack café-au-lait macules, and one rare NF1 gene mutation is associated with café-au-lait macules and no neurofibromas in affected individuals [Upadhyaya et al., 2007]. Individuals with mutation in the *SPRED1* gene may also present with multiple café-au-lait macules, skinfold freckles, and macrocephaly, but do not appear to develop neurofibromas or other tumor-related NF1 complications [Brems et al., 2007; Messiaen et al., 2009]. Nevertheless, in a majority of children who present with six or more café-au-lait macules and do not have an alternative diagnosis, signs of NF1 eventually develop [Korf, 1992]. Usually the second sign to appear is skinfold freckling [Crowe, 1964] (Figure 40-2). Freckles begin in the inguinal region in children at 3–4 years of age, and eventually appear in the axillae, at the base of the neck, and in the inframammary region in females. Areas of freckling also can

Box 40-1 Neurocutaneous Disorders: Specific Cutaneous Abnormalities and Associated Disorders

Hyperpigmented lesions

- Neurofibromatosis 1
- Epidermal nevus syndrome
- Neurocutaneous melanosis
- Incontinentia pigmenti

Hypopigmented lesions

- Tuberous sclerosis complex
- Hypomelanosis of Ito

Angiomatous lesions

- Sturge–Weber syndrome
- Maffucci's syndrome
- Klippel–Trenaunay–Weber syndrome

Hemihypertrophy

- Proteus syndrome
- Klippel–Trenaunay–Weber syndrome
- Neurofibromatosis type 1

Retinal involvement

- Tuberous sclerosis complex
- Von Hippel–Lindau disease

Hamartomas/tumors

- Neurofibromatosis type 1
- Neurofibromatosis type 2
- Schwannomatosis
- Tuberous sclerosis complex

Table 40-1 Phakomatoses and their Clinical Features

Syndrome	Common Non-neurologic Features	Common Neurologic Features
Neurofibromatosis type 1	Café-au-lait spots, malignant peripheral nerve sheath tumor, skeletal dysplasia	Neurofibromas, optic glioma, learning disabilities
Neurofibromatosis type 2	Posterior subcapsular cataract	Vestibular schwannomas, other cranial and peripheral nerve schwannomas, meningiomas, ependymomas
Schwannomatosis		Schwannomas
Tuberous sclerosis complex	Hypopigmented macules, collagenous plaques, angiofibroma, renal angiomyolipoma, pulmonary lymphangiomyomatosis, periungual fibromas	Cortical dysplasias, subependymal nodules, subependymal giant cell astrocytomas, seizures
Sturge–Weber syndrome	Port-wine stain	Leptomeningeal angiomatosis, seizures
von Hippel–Lindau disease	Ocular hemangioblastoma, renal cell carcinoma, pheochromocytoma, endolymphatic sac tumor	Hemangioblastomas
Maffucci's syndrome	Multiple endochondromas	
Epidermal nevus syndrome	Epidermal nevus, skeletal dysplasia	Seizures, developmental impairment
Parry–Romberg syndrome	Facial hemiatrophy	
Neurocutaneous melanosis	Multiple melanocytic nevi, melanoma	Leptomeningeal melanosis, seizures, hydrocephalus, Dandy–Walker malformation
Klippel–Trenaunay–Weber syndrome	Hemihypertrophy, angioma	Macrocephaly, hydrocephalus
Incontinentia pigmenti	Females only; hyperpigmented skin lesions, abnormalities of teeth, hair, and bone	Seizures, developmental impairment
Hypomelanosis of Ito	Hypopigmented skin lesions	Seizures
Wyburn–Mason syndrome	Retinal arteriovenous malformations	Cerebral arteriovenous malformations

Box 40-2 Diagnostic Criteria for Neurofibromatosis 1

- Six or more café-au-lait macules more than 5 mm in greatest diameter in prepubertal children, and more than 15 mm in greatest diameter in postpubertal children
- Two or more neurofibromas of any type or one plexiform neuroma
- Freckling in the axillary or inguinal regions
- Optic pathway glioma
- Two or more Lisch nodules (iris hamartomas)
- A distinctive osseous lesion, such as sphenoid dysplasia or thinning of long bone cortex, with or without pseudarthrosis
- Diagnosis of NF1 in a first-degree relative (parent, sibling, or offspring) according to foregoing criteria

(Modified from Stumpf D. Consensus development conference of neurofibromatosis. Arch Neurol 1988;45:575–578; Gutmann DH et al. The diagnostic evaluation and multidisciplinary management of neurofibromatosis 1 and neurofibromatosis 2. JAMA 1997;278: 51–57.)

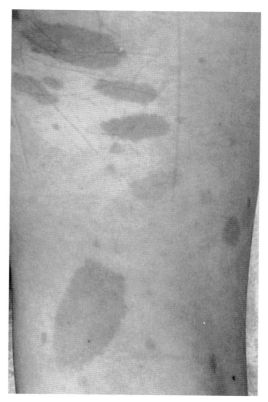

Fig. 40-1 **Multiple café-au-lait spots.**

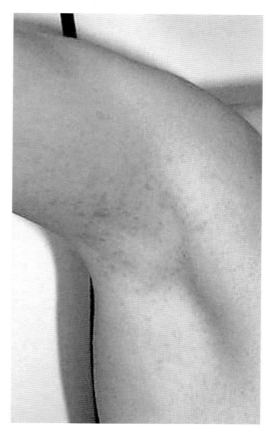

Fig. 40-2 **Axillary freckling.**

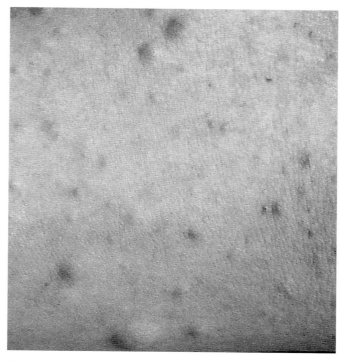

Fig. 40-3 **Multiple cutaneous neurofibromas.**

be found over the trunk and extremities. Diffuse, patchy areas of hyperpigmentation also may appear, sometimes overlying plexiform neuromas [Riccardi, 1980]. Areas of hypopigmentation or hypovascularity also may occur. Juvenile xanthogranulomas appear as firm yellowish papules in infants and young children, and eventually regress. Although an association with leukemia has been suggested [Zvulunov, 1996], this has not been verified.

Cutaneous neurofibromas are a prominent finding in NF1 and are located in the dermis or adjacent to it (Figure 40-3). They are discrete, soft or firm papules, ranging in size from a few millimeters to several centimeters, can be flat, sessile, or pedunculated, and can be readily impressed into the skin below. Neurofibromas can develop at any time and in any location, and may affect any component of the peripheral nervous system, from the dorsal root ganglion to the terminal nerve twigs. Plexiform neuromas represent tumors that involve a longitudinal section of nerve and can involve multiple branches of a major nerve [Korf, 1999]. Near the surface of the body they can cause thickening and hypertrophy of the skin and soft tissues (Figure 40-4). They may occur deeper in the body and be detected only by imaging [Tonsgard et al., 1998]. Tumors of the orbit or limbs can cause major physical deformity. Plexiform neurofibromas can be congenital lesions, often growing rapidly in the early months of life; they then may remain quiescent for long periods of time or grow unpredictably. The tumors are easily visualized by magnetic resonance imaging (MRI), and display a characteristic "target sign." Volumetric MRI may be helpful in following their growth [Dombi et al., 2007; Cai et al., 2009]. Neurofibromas originating at the dorsal roots may grow in a dumbbell shape and invade the spinal canal (Figure 40-5), sometimes causing spinal cord compression. The gastrointestinal tract can also be affected by growth of neurofibromas or ganglioneuromas. These tumors can cause intestinal obstruction or bleeding.

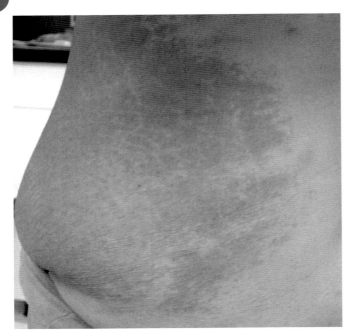

Fig. 40-4 Truncal plexiform neurofibroma with overlying hyperpigmentation.

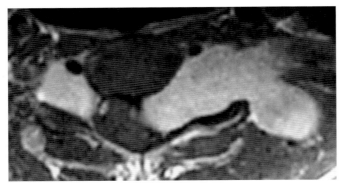

Fig. 40-5 Magnetic resonance imaging scan showing bilateral spinal tumors, with displacement of the cord by the larger tumor on the right side of the photo.

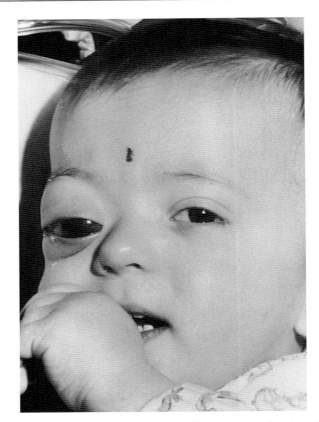

Fig. 40-6 Orbital plexiform neurofibroma associated with buphthalmos.

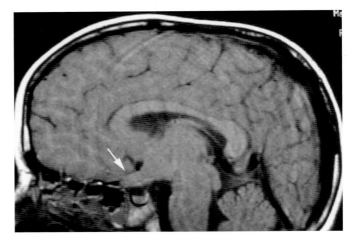

Fig. 40-7 Sagittal magnetic resonance imaging scan of brain showing a glioma of the optic chiasm (arrow).

Ophthalmologic features of NF1 include Lisch nodules, glaucoma, and optic glioma. Iris Lisch nodules are melanocytic hamartomas that are highly specific to NF1 [Lisch, 1937; Lewis and Riccardi, 1981]. Their appearance is age-dependent, usually beginning at the age of approximately 6 years. Lisch nodules occur in approximately 95 percent of adults with the disorder [Lubs et al., 1991] and are therefore helpful in diagnosis. Glaucoma usually occurs when a plexiform neurofibroma involves the upper eyelid (Figure 40-6) [Morales et al., 2009]. Orbital plexiform neurofibroma, arising from the trigeminal nerve, often is associated with sphenoid dysplasia, and can present with pulsating exophthalmos or enophthalmos [Jacquemin et al., 2002].

Optic pathway gliomas are found in approximately 15 percent of patients [Lewis et al., 1984]. Most are asymptomatic, but these tumors can manifest with symptoms of decreased visual acuity, visual field defects, or precocious puberty [Listernick et al., 2007]. The glioma can involve the optic nerves, chiasm, optic radiations, and hypothalamus (Figure 40-7); it rarely manifests as the diencephalic syndrome of infancy or precocious puberty. Optic gliomas are pilocytic astrocytomas, but often are slow-growing.

Aside from optic gliomas, astrocytomas of the cerebrum, brainstem, and cerebellum are the most common intracranial tumors encountered in NF1 [Albers and Gutmann, 2009]. Malignant peripheral nerve sheath tumor occurs in upwards of 8–13 percent of affected persons [Evans et al., 2002]. These manifest with pain or sudden growth, usually within a pre-existing plexiform neurofibroma [D'Agostino, Soule and Miller, 1963]. Various other neoplastic disorders occur more frequently in patients with NF1 than in the general population, including leukemia, especially juvenile myelomonocytic leukemia [Stiller, Chessells and Fitchett, 1994] and pheochromocytoma [Walther et al., 1999a].

Macrocephaly and short stature are common in NF1 and scoliosis has been reported to occur in 10–40 percent of patients [Crawford and Herrera-Soto, 2007]. Scoliosis usually does not develop before the age of 6 years and most commonly involves the thoracic spine. Bowing of the tibia, fibula, and other long bones can be present in early life, with occurrence of spontaneous fractures at the junction of the middle and distal thirds of the bone shaft, resulting in pseudarthrosis [Elefteriou et al., 2009; Stevenson et al., 1999]. Non-ossifying fibromas may occur and can present with pain or fracture [Howlett et al., 1998]. There is also evidence for decreased bone mineral density in children and adults with NF1, which may contribute to an increased risk of fracture [Stevenson et al., 2008; Kuorilehto et al., 2005].

Approximately 50 percent of patients have learning disabilities, with no specific pattern unique to those with NF1 [Hyman, Arthur Shores and North, 2006]. Both verbal and nonverbal disabilities occur, as well as attention-deficit disorder [Mautner et al., 2002] and hypotonia [Souza et al., 2009]. Fewer than 10 percent have mental retardation, and most of these patients have large deletions of the *NF1* gene [Kayes et al., 1994]. Seizures occur in approximately 6–10 percent of patients [Korf, Carrazana and Holmes, 1993]. The pathogenesis of the cognitive phenotype is not known. Abnormal cortical architecture and heterotopias have been reported in the brains of some patients with severe cognitive deficits [Rosman and Pearce, 1967]. It has been suggested that the areas of enhanced T2 signal intensity characteristically seen in the brains of children with NF1 (Figure 40-8) may be associated with learning disabilities [Hyman et al., 2007]. These lesions occur in the basal ganglia, brainstem, cerebellum, and internal capsule; tend to disappear with age [Hyman et al., 2003; Ferner et al., 1993]; and are characterized by increased myelin water content and gliosis [DiPaolo et al., 1995].

Vascular anomalies in NF1 include regions of intimal proliferation and fibromuscular changes in small arteries [Friedman et al., 2002]. Renal artery stenosis can lead to hypertension in children [Fossali et al., 2000], and involvement of other vessels can cause vascular insufficiency or hemorrhage as a result of arterial wall dissection [Hinsch et al., 2008]. Stenosis of the internal carotid artery can lead to moyamoya disease and stroke [Cairns and North, 2008], although lesions often are asymptomatic. The stenotic changes can arise spontaneously in children with NF1, but frequently develop after radiation therapy for brain tumors in young children [Kestle, Hoffman and Mock, 1993].

Pathology

Neurofibromas consist of a mixture of cell types, including Schwann cells, fibroblasts, perineurial cells, and mast cells [Pineda, 1965]. They are polyclonal [Fialkow et al., 1971], but genetic studies have confirmed that the "tumor cell" is the Schwann cell [Sherman et al., 2000; Zhu et al., 2002], or in the case of dermal neurofibromas, stem cells referred to as skin-derived precursors [Le et al., 2009]. The other cell types present in the lesion apparently proliferate as a secondary phenomenon, perhaps in response to stimulation by cytokines [Yang et al., 2003]. Mast cells are present in large numbers and have been suspected of being a source of cytokines [Yang et al., 2008]. In plexiform neurofibromas, the pathologic process extends across multiple nerve fascicles instead of occurring at a focal site in a nerve, and may extend across branches of a larger nerve. Malignant peripheral nerve sheath tumor manifests as a malignant tumor of Schwann cell origin, although sometimes rhabdoid elements are present in such tumors [Buck, Mahboubi and Raney, 1977]. Most, if not all, of these neoplasms arise from pre-existing tumors, usually plexiform neurofibromas. The pathology of other NF1-associated lesions is less well understood than that of the neurofibroma.

Genetics

NF1, inherited as an autosomal-dominant trait, has an estimated prevalence of 1 in 3000; about half of cases are new mutations [Crowe, Schull and Neel, 1956; Huson, Harper and Compston, 1988]. The *NF1* gene is located at 17q11.2 and encodes a 3818-amino-acid protein referred to as neurofibromin [Cawthon et al., 1990a, b; Viskochil et al., 1990; Wallace et al., 1990]. Neurofibromin is expressed in multiple cell types but is highly expressed in Schwann cells, oligodendrocytes, and neurons [Daston et al., 1992]. The protein includes a functional GTPase-activating protein (GAP) domain that regulates conversion of Ras-guanosine triphosphate to Ras-guanosine diphosphate [Ballester et al., 1990; Xu et al., 1990a, b]. Ras is a membrane-bound intracellular signaling molecule that is activated by complexing with guanosine triphosphate (GTP) on ligand binding to membrane receptor tyrosine kinases. GAP proteins regulate this process by stimulating a GTPase activity that is intrinsic to Ras [Bernards, 2003]. Neurofibromin functions as a tumor suppressor gene with respect to neurofibroma formation [Sherman et al., 2000; Cichowski and Jacks, 2001; Zhu et al., 2002]. The germline mutation of one NF1 allele constitutes the first "hit"; the second hit is a somatic mutation [Upadhyaya et al., 2004] in a Schwann cell that causes that cell to proliferate and attract other cells, such as mast cells, fibroblasts, and perineurial cells, which also proliferate. These cells, being heterozygous for the *NF1* mutation, may be hypersensitive to cytokine stimulation [Vogel et al., 1995]. Transformation to malignancy requires additional genetic changes, such as mutation of p53 [Legius et al., 1994]. Biallelic *NF1* gene mutation also occurs in melanocytes within café-au-lait macules

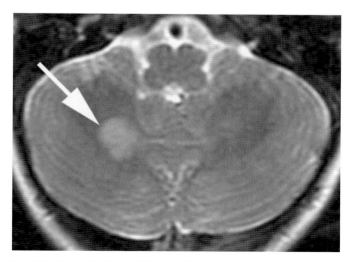

Fig. 40-8 Area of enhanced T2 signal intensity in cerebellum (arrow).

[Maertens et al., 2007] and in dysplastic bone tissue [Stevenson et al., 2006]. It is unclear whether other dysplastic lesions also occur as a result of a tumor suppressor mechanism, or whether haploinsufficiency of neurofibromin expression itself causes these lesions. Mice rendered heterozygous for an *NF1* mutation do display cognitive deficits [Costa et al., 2002], suggesting that haploinsufficiency might account for some of the NF1 phenotype.

NF1 exhibits a wide range of variability of expression and complete penetrance. Mutations are widely scattered across the gene and include a wide variety of mutational mechanisms [Messiaen et al., 2000]. Most of the mutations lead to decreased level of expression of neurofibromin or complete lack of expression. Few genotype–phenotype correlations have been established. Large deletions that include the *NF1* gene and multiple contiguous genes over a 1.5-Mb region tend to lead to a particularly severe form of NF1, with mental retardation, early onset of large numbers of neurofibromas, facial dysmorphism, and increased risk of cancer [De Raedt et al., 2003; Kayes et al., 1994; Wu et al., 1995]. Another variant form of neurofibromatosis, familial spinal neurofibromatosis, may represent an additional genotype–phenotype correlation. Persons with this disorder have multiple spinal neurofibromas and subcutaneous tumors but lack skinfold freckling and dermal tumors, and tend to have missense mutations or splicing mutations [Korf, Henson and Stemmer-Rachamimov, 2005]. Individuals with a three-base deletion in exon 17 have only café-au-lait spots and do not develop neurofibromas [Upadhyaya et al., 2007]. Approximately 50 percent of cases of NF1 occur sporadically, as a result of a new mutation of the *NF1* gene. Because of the high penetrance of the disorder, unaffected parents of a sporadically affected child have a low risk of recurrence, barring the rare instance of germline mosaicism [Lazaro et al., 1995]. Somatic mosaicism for NF1 may manifest with segmental distribution of features [Tinschert et al., 2000; Vandenbroucke et al., 2004]. Genetic testing for diagnosis of NF1 is available on a clinical basis. It is used to confirm a diagnosis in patients who fulfill only a single diagnostic criterion, to characterize patients with unusual clinical presentations, and to enable prenatal testing. The discovery of mutation in the *SPRED1* gene accounting for patients with multiple café-au-lait spots but lacking other features of NF1 [Brems et al., 2007] (now referred to as "Legius syndrome"), provides additional rationale for genetic testing in young children with multiple café-au-lait spots. The majority of mutations are found in the *NF1* gene, making it cost-effective to begin with *NF1* testing, followed by *SPRED1* testing if no *NF1* mutation is found [Messiaen et al., 2009].

Management

Treatment of patients with neurofibromatosis is symptomatic. Affected persons should be followed on a regular basis by a physician who is familiar with the disorder to recognize treatable complications early and to provide anticipatory guidance and counseling. Genetic counseling should be provided. Controversy surrounds the use of imaging, especially MRI, in screening patients with NF1. Most of the lesions that will be identified are not amenable to treatment, so such testing may create needless anxiety, and in children the procedure carries the risks associated with sedation. The value of the "baseline" examination is questionable because most of the lesions of NF1 are slow-growing and will be followed both clinically and by imaging once they come to attention [Listernick et al., 1994]. Current consensus guidelines do not recommend routine imaging [Gutmann et al., 1997], although care should be individualized for specific clinical needs.

Neurofibromas of the peripheral nerves need not be removed unless they are subject to repeated irritation and trauma or develop malignant change. Some plexiform neuromas can be removed for cosmetic reasons, although complete resection is difficult and regrowth is common [Needle et al., 1997]. Malignant tumors are managed with appropriate neurosurgical measures, radiation therapy, and chemotherapy. Optic gliomas tend to behave in an indolent manner and therefore are followed clinically without treatment in asymptomatic children [Listernick et al., 2007]. Symptomatic tumors most often are treated with chemotherapy [Packer et al., 1997]; radiation therapy may be associated with second malignant tumors [Sharif et al., 2006] or moyamoya disease [Desai et al., 2006; Kestle, Hoffman and Mock, 1993]. Malignant peripheral nerve sheath tumors tend to be highly malignant, so early diagnosis is essential [Evans et al., 2002]. Patients with unexplained pain or growth of a neurofibroma should be evaluated, with consideration of biopsy. Positron emission tomography (PET) scanning may be helpful in distinguishing a malignant peripheral nerve sheath tumor from plexiform neurofibroma [Ferner et al., 2000; Karabatsou et al., 2009; Warbey et al., 2009].

Clinical trials of drugs to treat specific complications are ongoing. These include the use of statins to treat learning disabilities [Krab et al., 2008] and several experimental treatments for neurofibromas [Babovic-Vuksanovic et al., 2007; Gupta et al., 2003; Packer and Rosser, 2002; Packer et al., 2002].

Neurofibromatosis Type 2

Clinical Characteristics and Pathology

Diagnostic criteria for NF2 are presented in Box 40-3 [Gutmann et al., 1997; Stumpf, 1988; Baser et al., 2002]. The defining feature of NF2 is the occurrence of bilateral vestibular schwannomas. Age at onset is highly variable, ranging from early childhood to the seventh decade and beyond [Evans 1999; Mautner et al., 1993]. In view of this variability in age at onset of vestibular tumors, NF2 also should be considered in patients with early onset of associated tumors or those with combinations of associated tumors.

Vestibular schwannomas commonly manifest with tinnitus and/or hearing loss, and may cause problems with balance [Evans, 1999]. Audiology and auditory brainstem-evoked response testing can be helpful, but definitive diagnosis is based on MRI findings (Figure 40-9). Early tumors may be confined to the internal auditory canal and require careful search with thin MRI slices to be detected. Schwannomas can occur along any other cranial nerve, the fifth being most common after the eighth. Schwannomas also may occur along spinal nerves, with the potential for causing radiculopathy or cord compression, or along peripheral nerves. In some patients, a polyneuropathy develops as a result of Schwann cell proliferation around peripheral nerves [Gijtenbeek et al., 2001; Hagel et al., 2002]. Dermal schwannomas appear as plaquelike lesions, often with associated hair growth. Café-au-lait macules are not a reliable indicator of NF2, unlike in NF1 [Mautner et al., 1997]. Other major central nervous system tumors associated with NF2 are meningiomas and ependymomas. Multiple meningiomas may

---

Box 40-3 Diagnostic Criteria for Neurofibromatosis 2

Confirmed NF2*

- Bilateral vestibular schwannomas
  or
- A first-degree relative with NF2
  and either
- Unilateral vestibular schwannoma before age 30 years
  or any two of
- Meningioma, schwannoma, ependymoma, juvenile lens opacity

Presumptive NF2

- Unilateral vestibular schwannoma before age 30 years and at least one of: meningioma, schwannoma, ependymoma, juvenile lens opacity
  or
- Two or more meningiomas and unilateral vestibular schwannoma before age 30 years or at least one of: meningioma, schwannoma, ependymoma, juvenile lens opacity

Manchester Criteria†

- Bilateral vestibular schwannomas
  or
- A first-degree relative with NF2
  and either
- Unilateral vestibular schwannoma or any two of: meningioma, schwannoma, ependymoma, neurofibroma, posterior subcapsular lenticular opacity
  or
- Unilateral vestibular schwannoma and any two of: meningioma, schwannoma, ependymoma, neurofibroma, posterior subcapsularlenticular opacity
  or
- Two or more meningiomas and unilateral vestibular schwannoma or any two of: meningioma, schwannoma, ependymoma, neurofibroma, posterior subcapsular lenticular opacity

(Based on

* Gutmann DH et al. The diagnostic evaluation and multidisciplinary management of neurofibromatosis 1 and neurofibromatosis 2. JAMA 1997;278: 51–57.
† Baser ME et al. Evaluation of clinical diagnostic criteria for neurofibromatosis 2. Neurology 2002;59(11):1759–1765.)

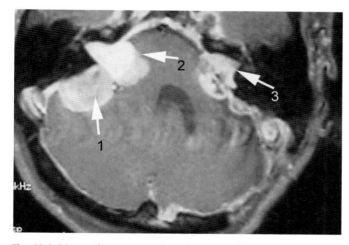

Fig. 40-9 Magnetic resonance imaging scan of brain from a person with NF2 showing a meningioma (arrow 1) and two vestibular schwannomas (arrows 2 and 3). The tumor indicated by arrow 3 has been partially resected.

not be surgically resectable and can be responsible for significant morbidity. Virtually the entire NF2 phenotype is characterized by proliferative lesions; the one exception is the occurrence of posterior subcapsular cataracts or cortical wedge opacities [Pearson-Webb et al., 1986].

Genetics

NF2 is transmitted as an autosomal-dominant trait with complete penetrance and variable expression. Prevalence is estimated at approximately 1 in 60,000, and birth incidence at 1 in 30,000 [Evans, 2009; Evans et al., 2010]. Approximately half of cases occur sporadically as a result of new mutation. The *NF2* gene was mapped to chromosome 22 [Rouleau et al., 1987], and the responsible gene was identified by two groups in 1993 [Rouleau et al.,

1993; Trofatter et al., 1993]. The protein is variously referred to as schwannomin or merlin (the latter an acronym for moesin, ezrin, and radixin-like protein]. Merlin is a cytoskeletal protein that appears to play a role in the control of cell growth in tissues [Xiao, Chernoff and Testa, 2003]. Schwannomas are clonal tumors, and the *NF2* gene acts as a tumor suppressor in formation of these tumors, as well as other NF2-associated tumors [Seizinger et al., 1987]. Genetic testing for NF2 is available for diagnostic purposes. Some genotype–phenotype correlations have been identified; specifically, missense or splicing mutations tend to predict milder disease than do mutations that lead to protein truncation [Parry et al., 1996; Ruttledge et al., 1996]. Somatic mosaicism for *NF2* mutation may produce localized disease or ameliorate disease severity [Baser et al., 2000a].

Management

Patients benefit from multidisciplinary care at a center with experience in dealing with the varied manifestations of the disorder [Evans et al., 1993]. Management of tumors associated with NF2 is primarily surgical [Evans et al., 2005]. Timing of surgery and the decision to treat one or both vestibular tumors depends on tumor size, degree of hearing loss, and involvement of other cranial nerves or compression of the brainstem. Stereotactic radiosurgery is also used for the treatment of vestibular schwannomas [Battista, 2009], though there may be an increased risk of malignancy in residual tumor [Baser et al., 2000b]. Recent trials with the vascular endothelial growth factor (VEGF) inhibitor bevacizumab have shown promising results in reduction in size of vestibular schwannomas [Plotkin et al., 2009; Mautner et al., 2010].

Schwannomatosis

Schwannomatosis is a more recently recognized entity [MacCollin et al., 1996; Evans et al., 1997], characterized only by the occurrence of schwannomas on cranial and spinal nerves

Box 40-4 Diagnostic Criteria for Schwannomatosis

- Patient does not fulfill diagnostic criteria for NF2, and has no vestibular schwannoma on high-resolution MRI and no *NF2* mutation

Definite Diagnosis

- Age over 30 years AND two or more nonintradermal schwannomas, at least one with histologic confirmation

or

- One pathologically confirmed schwannoma plus a first-degree relative who meets the above criteria

Possible Diagnosis

- Age under 30 years AND two or more nonintradermal schwannomas, at least one with histologic confirmation

or

- Age over 45 years AND two or more nonintradermal schwannomas, at least one with histologic confirmation

or

- Radiographic evidence of a schwannoma and first-degree relative meeting the criteria for definite schwannomatosis

Segmental

- Meets criteria for either definite or possible schwannomatosis but limited to one limb, or five or fewer contiguous segments of the spine

(From MacCollin M et al. Diagnostic criteria for schwannomatosis. Neurology 2005;64(11):1838–1845; Baser ME et al. Increasing the specificity of diagnostic criteria for schwannomatosis. Neurology 2006;66(5):730–732.)

other than the vestibular nerve. It often manifests with pain or nerve compression. Diagnostic criteria are provided in Box 40-4. Schwannomatosis is most commonly sporadic, but familial cases have been observed, in which case inheritance is autosomal-dominant with incomplete penetrance. The gene responsible for the disorder is designated *INI1* (also designated *SMARCB1*; Hulsebos et al., 2007; Boyd et al., 2008], and encodes a protein component of a chromatin remodeling complex. It is located on chromosome 22 near the *NF2* locus but is distinct from that locus. Symptomatic tumors are treated surgically. Many patients require management for chronic pain.

Tuberous Sclerosis Complex

Tuberous sclerosis complex is a disorder of autosomal-dominant inheritance that affects multiple organ systems, resulting in manifold clinical expressions. Tuberous sclerosis complex is currently recognized as one of the most common single-gene disorders seen in children and adults, with an estimated incidence of 1 in 5800 live births [Osborne et al., 1991] The first description of tuberous sclerosis complex was by von Recklinghausen, who described a newborn who had died of respiratory distress and was found at postmortem examination to have multiple cardiac tumors and a "great number of cerebral scleroses [von Recklinghausen, 1862]." Bourneville usually is credited with the first detailed description of the cerebral manifestations of the disease, describing "sclérose tubéreuse," indicating the superficial resemblance of the lesions of a potato [Bourneville

and Brissard, 1880]. He attached no significance to the facial skin rash of his first patient, calling it acne rosacea, but he and Brissard believed that the renal tumors and cerebral scleroses were associated findings [Bourneville and Brissard, 1900]. Facial angiofibromas, previously referred to as adenoma sebaceum, were independently described in several reports, but Vogt emphasized the association of adenoma sebaceum and the cerebral scleroses described by Bourneville [Vogt, 1908]. He also described a "classic" triad of clinical features comprising mental retardation, intractable epilepsy, and adenoma sebaceum, which is now known to be present in less than one-third of patients with tuberous sclerosis complex.

Clinical Characteristics

Diagnostic criteria are provided in Box 40-5. The clinical presentation of tuberous sclerosis complex depends on the age of the patient, the organs involved, and the severity of involvement. Of importance, both the brain and the skin

Box 40-5 Diagnostic Criteria for Tuberous Sclerosis Complex

Major Features

- Facial angiofibromas or forehead plaque
- Nontraumatic ungual or periungual fibroma
- Hypopigmented macules (more than 3)
- Shagreen patch (connective tissue nevus)
- Cortical tuber
- Subependymal nodule
- Subependymal giant cell astrocytoma
- Multiple retinal nodular hamartomas
- Cardiac rhabdomyoma, single or multiple
- Lymphangiomyomatosis
- Renal angiomyolipoma

Minor Features

- Dental pits (more than 14), randomly distributed
- Hamartomatous rectal polyps
- Bone cysts
- Cerebral white matter radial migration lines
- Gingival fibromas
- Nonrenal hamartomas
- Retinal achromic patch
- "Confetti" skin lesions
- Multiple renal cysts

Diagnostic Certainty Criteria

Definite TSC

- 2 major features or
- 1 major feature + 2 minor features

Probable TSC

- 1 major feature + 1 minor feature

Possible TSC

- 1 major feature or
- 2 or more minor features

(From Roach ES et al. Tuberous sclerosis complex consensus conference: Revised clinical diagnostic criteria. J Child Neurol 1998;13(12):624–8.)

have more than one major criterion for diagnosis; therefore, a diagnosis of definite tuberous sclerosis complex can be based on skin findings alone, or on neuroimaging findings alone.

Epilepsy is the most common presenting symptom in tuberous sclerosis complex and also is the most common medical disorder. In up to 80–90 percent of persons with tuberous sclerosis complex, seizures will develop during their lifetime, with the onset most frequently in childhood [Gomez, 1999; Thiele, 2004; Chu-Shore et al., 2009]. A majority of children with tuberous sclerosis complex have the onset of seizures during the first year of life, and approximately one-third develop infantile spasms. Almost all seizure types can be seen in persons with tuberous sclerosis complex, including tonic, clonic, tonic-clonic, atonic, myoclonic, atypical absence, partial, and complex partial. Only "pure" absence seizures are not observed.

Infantile spasms will develop in approximately one-third of children with tuberous sclerosis complex, although some reports suggest an incidence as high as 75 percent [Riikonen and Simell, 1990; Fukushima et al., 1998; Hamano et al., 2003; Husain et al., 2000]. Tuberous sclerosis complex is thought to be the most common single cause of infantile spasms, and in some series, 25 percent of symptomatic infantile spasms are secondary to tuberous sclerosis complex. Partial complex seizures precede infantile spasms in approximately one-third of patients with tuberous sclerosis complex in whom infantile spasms develop [Curatolo et al., 2001, 2002]. A strong association between the presence of infantile spasms in tuberous sclerosis complex and subsequent developmental impairment has been noted, although children with tuberous sclerosis complex and infantile spasms can have a normal cognitive outcome [Goh et al., 2005; Yamamoto et al., 1987; Muzykewicz et al., 2009].

The electroencephalogram (EEG) in infantile spasms associated with tuberous sclerosis complex often demonstrates hypsarrhythmia or modified hypsarrhythmia. It is important to realize, however, that the EEG, although usually abnormal, frequently does not have the features of hypsarrhythmia; in some series, up to 70 percent of children with tuberous sclerosis complex and infantile spasms did not have the characteristics of hypsarrhythmia [Curatolo et al., 2001]. Several reports have characterized the EEG patterns of persons with tuberous sclerosis complex and have found a high incidence of abnormalities, including diffuse slowing and epileptiform features [Ganji and Hellman, 1985; Westmoreland, 1999; Muzykewicz et al., 2009].

Tuberous sclerosis complex is associated with a wide range of cognitive and behavioral manifestations. Approximately one-half of persons with tuberous sclerosis complex have normal intelligence, whereas the other half have some degree of cognitive impairment, ranging from mild learning disabilities to severe mental retardation. A bimodal distribution of cognitive abilities is evident, with affected persons falling into a severely cognitively impaired group or a group with normal intelligence [Gillberg et al., 1994; Winterkorn et al., 2007]. Risk factors for cognitive impairment include a history of infantile spasms, intractable epilepsy, and a mutation in the *TSC2* gene. Persons with tuberous sclerosis complex, particularly those with cognitive impairment, also are at high risk for developmental disorders. Autistic spectrum disorders affect up to 50 percent of persons with tuberous sclerosis complex [Wiznitzer, 2004; Curatolo et al., 2004; Smalley, 1998], and attention-deficit

hyperactivity and related disorders also are common, affecting approximately 50 percent of the patients [de Vries and Watson, 2008]. During adolescence and adulthood, anxiety disorders, depression, or mood disorders develop in a majority of patients with tuberous sclerosis complex [Muzykewicz et al., 2007; Raznahan et al., 2006; Pulsifer et al., 2007].

Cutaneous manifestations are found in up to 96 percent of patients with tuberous sclerosis complex [Gomez et al., 1987; Webb et al., 1996]. Angiofibroma, the skin manifestation initially described in the disorder as adenoma sebaceum, typically appears between the ages of 1 and 4 years and can progress through childhood and adolescence [Gomez et al., 1987; Webb et al., 1996; Pampiglione and Moynahan, 1976]. These lesions typically are pink or red papules that appear in patches or in a butterfly distribution on or about the nose, cheeks, and chin (Figure 40-10).

Hypopigmented, oval, or leaf-shaped macules, ranging from a few millimeters to several centimeters in length and scattered over the trunk and limbs, are commonly seen [Fitzpatrick, 1991]. The lesions often are apparent at birth and can appear more prominent during the first several years of life as the child's body size and surface area increase. In fair-skinned persons, visualization of these hypopigmented spots is facilitated by using a Wood's light, an ultraviolet light that accentuates the hypopigmented spots [Fitzpatrick et al., 1968; Roth and Epstein, 1971]. At least three types of hypopigmented macules occur: polygonal (similar to a thumbprint) is the most frequent shape (0.5–2 cm); an ash leaf-shaped hypopigmented macule is characteristic but is not the most common shape (1–12 cm); and the third common type is a confetti-shaped arrangement of multiple, tiny white macules (1–3 mm) [Fitzpatrick, 1991] (Figure 40-11). Histologic assessment of the hypopigmented spots usually demonstrates a normal number of melanocytes, and on electron microscopy a reduction in the number,

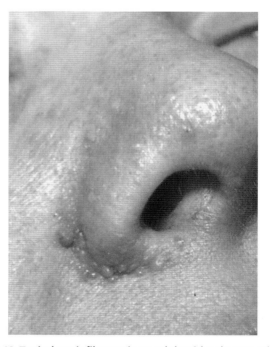

Fig. 40-10 Typical angiofibroma in an adult with tuberous sclerosis complex. *(Courtesy of Dr. TN Darling, Uniformed Services University of Health Sciences, Bethesda, MD.)*

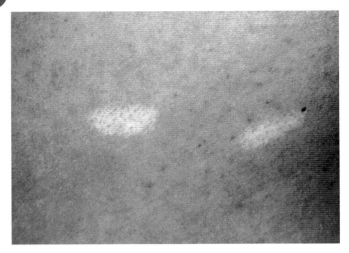

Fig. 40-11 Hypopigmented macule in a child with tuberous sclerosis complex. *(Courtesy of Dr. TN Darling, Uniformed Services University of Health Sciences, Bethesda, MD.)*

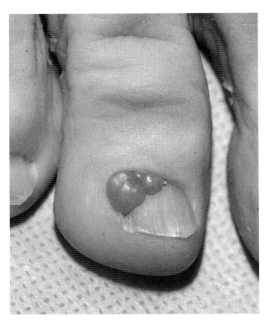

Fig. 40-13 Periungual fibroma on finger of a patient with tuberous sclerosis complex. *(Courtesy of Dr. TN Darling, Uniformed Services University of Health Sciences, Bethesda, MD.)*

diameter, and melanization of melanosomes in the melanocytes from the white macule is seen [Jozwiak and Schwartz, 2003]. If hypopigmented macules occur on the scalp, the affected person will have poliosis, or a patch of gray or white hair [McWilliam and Stephenson, 1978].

Another skin manifestation currently considered a major criterion for clinical diagnosis of tuberous sclerosis complex is the shagreen patch, a connective tissue hamartoma that is distributed asymmetrically on the dorsal body surfaces, particularly on the lumbosacral skin (Figure 40-12). In a majority of the cases, the shagreen patch is characterized by multiple and small areas of connective tissue hamartoma, ranging in size from a few millimeters to 1 cm. Present from birth, the shagreen patch is more easily identified as the child grows and body surface area increases. Subungual or periungual fibromas (Koenen's tumors) are present in at least 20 percent of patients and usually first appear during adolescence, although they can be seen earlier. These typically involve the toes more often than the fingers [Barroeta and Grinspan Bozza, 1962] (Figure 40-13). Oral fibromas or papillomas occur in about 10 percent of patients and usually are found on the anterior aspect of the gingiva [Papanyothou and Verzirtzi, 1975]. Dental enamel pits have

been found in all adult patients with tuberous sclerosis complex, compared with 7 percent of controls [Hoff et al., 1975; Mlynarczyk, 1991; Weits-Binnerts et al., 1982].

The kidneys are frequently affected in persons with tuberous sclerosis complex, and after neurologic manifestations, renal involvement is the most common cause of morbidity and mortality [Franz, 2004]. The two main types of renal lesions are angiomyolipoma and renal cysts. Angiomyolipoma are present in up to 80 percent of patients with tuberous sclerosis complex and can develop in either childhood or adulthood [Rakowski et al., 2006]. Persons with tuberous sclerosis complex can have multiple small angiomyolipomas on the surface of the kidneys, throughout the kidney, or one or more larger lesions. The larger lesions are considered to be at greater risk of becoming symptomatic, particularly when they reach 4–6 cm in size. They can produce nonspecific complaints such as flank pain, but they also carry a risk of potentially life-threatening hemorrhage from rupture of dysplastic, aneurysmal blood vessels in the angiomyolipoma. Renal cysts are seen in fewer than 20 percent of persons with tuberous sclerosis complex and are rarely, if ever, symptomatic. Polycystic kidney disease occurs in 3–5 percent of patients with tuberous sclerosis complex and, when present, usually reflects a contiguous gene syndrome, because the polycystic kidney disease gene is adjacent to the *TSC2*-tuberin gene on chromosome 16 [Brook-Carter et al., 1994].

The cardiac manifestation, rhabdomyoma, is seen in 50–60 percent of persons with tuberous sclerosis complex [Jozwiak et al., 1994]. Typically, rhabdomyomas, which can frequently be detected prenatally, are maximal at birth and early childhood, and undergo spontaneous regression during the first few years of life. If symptomatic, they result in outflow tract obstruction or valve dysfunction. If the lesions involve the cardiac conduction system, they can predispose the patient to dysrhythmias not only in infancy and childhood, but also throughout life.

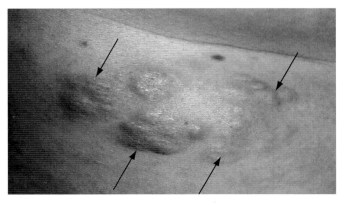

Fig. 40-12 Shagreen patch (arrows) over the lumbosacral region of an adolescent with tuberous sclerosis complex. *(Courtesy of Dr. TN Darling, Uniformed Services University of Health Sciences, Bethesda, MD.)*

Pulmonary involvement in tuberous sclerosis complex includes lymphangioleiomyomatosis, multifocal micronodular pneumocyte hyperplasia, and pulmonary cysts. While multifocal micronodular pneumocyte hyperplasia is seen fairly commonly in both men and women with tuberous sclerosis complex, lymphangioleiomyomatosis is thought to occur almost exclusively in women. Although lymphangioleiomyomatosis was once thought to be quite rare, affecting less than 1 percent of women, recent studies have found such abnormalities in up to 40 percent of women with tuberous sclerosis complex, many of whom are asymptomatic [Moss et al., 2001].

Retinal hamartomas are relatively common, affecting at least 50 percent of patients, although typically they are not clinically significant [Rowley et al., 2001]. A nodular (mulberry) tumor can be seen on or about the optic nerve head, and round or oval gray–yellow glial patches can be central or peripheral. The large retinal tumors can be cystic [Walsh and Hoyt, 1969; Messinger and Clarke, 1937]. Papilledema is not present, except in those patients with an intracranial mass lesion that obstructs the normal circulation of the cerebrospinal fluid, resulting in increased intracranial pressure [Kapp et al., 1967].

Hamartomas also can be found in other organ systems, including stomach, intestine, colon, pancreas, and liver. Hepatic angiomyolipoma and cysts have been reported in up to 24 percent of persons with tuberous sclerosis complex and are thought to be asymptomatic and nonprogressive [Fricke et al., 2004]. Sclerotic and hypertrophic lesions of bone often can be seen, although these typically are not symptomatic.

Clinical Laboratory Testing

As a result of the multi-organ involvement in tuberous sclerosis complex, a variety of clinical testing is recommended both at time of diagnosis and subsequently, to monitor for involvement and allow appropriate intervention (Table 40-2).

Table 40-2 Diagnostic and Follow-Up Management in Tuberous Sclerosis Complex

Evaluation	Initial Testing	Follow-up Testing
Neuroimaging	At diagnosis	Every 1–3 years until age 20
Neuropsychologic testing	At diagnosis	At school entry and as indicated
Electroencephalogram	If seizures occur	As indicated
Opthalmologic examination	At diagnosis	As indicated
Echocardiogram, electrocardiogram	At diagnosis	As indicated
Renal ultrasound examination	At diagnosis	Every 1–3 years, more frequently as indicated
Chest computed tomography	At onset of adulthood (women only)	As indicated

(From Roach ES et al. Tuberous sclerosis consensus conference: Recommendations for diagnostic evaluation. National Tuberous Sclerosis Association. J Child Neurol 1999;14(6):401–407.)

Neuroimaging studies, particularly MRI and also computed tomography (CT), are important in confirming the diagnosis of tuberous sclerosis complex, demonstrating cortical tubers, subependymal nodules (Figure 40-14), and subependymal giant cell tumors (Figure 40-15). Brain MRI is the preferred

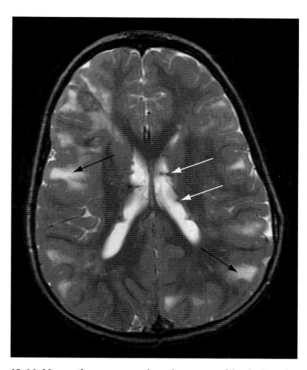

Fig. 40-14 Magnetic resonance imaging scan of brain in tuberous sclerosis complex, showing cortical tubers (black arrows) and subependymal nodules (white arrows).

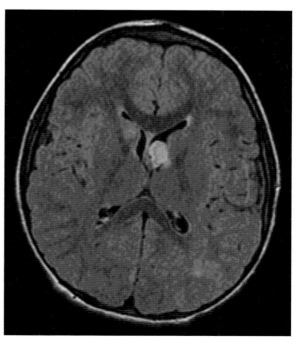

Fig. 40-15 Computed tomography scan of brain in tuberous sclerosis complex, showing subependymal giant cell tumor.

imaging modality, because it allows better delineation of cortical tubers and other cortical abnormalities, such as radial migration lines. The imaging characteristics of tubers change with the age of the patient, which is thought to be related to myelination. In neonates, tubers appear hyperintense on T1 sequences and hypointense on T2. With increasing age, tubers appear isointense on T1 and hyperintense on T2. In addition to T1- and T2-weighted MRI sequences, fluid-attenuated inversion recovery (FLAIR) sequences appear most useful for identifying tubers and other cortical and subcortical abnormalities. Both CT and MRI can identify subependymal nodules; calcification of the nodules is readily apparent on CT scan. In view of the risk of development of subependymal nodules into subependymal giant cell tumors, which occurs in 5–10 percent of persons with tuberous sclerosis complex, follow-up neuroimaging is recommended annually if possible until the age of 20 years [Goh et al., 2004; Roach et al., 1999]. For unclear reasons, subependymal giant cell tumors lose the propensity to grow after early adulthood.

Pathology

Tuberous sclerosis complex is a multisystem disorder of cellular migration, proliferation, and differentiation, resulting in the development of hamartias and hamartomas. The major pathologic features in the brain include cortical tubers, subependymal nodules, and subependymal giant cell tumors. Cortical tubers are found in the cortex and subcortical white matter, typically located at the gray–white junction. They vary widely in size and distribution among patients with tuberous sclerosis complex and may extend centrally in a linear or wedge-shaped zone spanning the full thickness from the ventricular wall to the cortical surface. Histologically, tubers consist of dysplastic, hypomyelinated aggregates of abnormal glial and neural elements, with glia-derived cells and astrocytes predominating. A distinguishing feature of cortical tubers is the giant cell – an enlarged, bizarre-appearing neuron – or large cells with both neuronal and glial characteristics. As noted previously, many children with tuberous sclerosis complex may experience learning difficulties, as a result of mental retardation or autistic spectrum disorders. Risk factors include early seizure onset, infantile spasms, and an intractable seizure disorder. Correlation between the severity of cognitive deficits and epilepsy with tuber burden is thought probable, although the data are limited. Distinct from cortical tubers, subependymal nodules do have growth potential and are located around the wall of the lateral ventricle, consisting of astrocytes arising from the subependymal zone and protruding into the ventricles. Subependymal nodules most commonly occur at the caudothalamic groove in the vicinity of the foramen of Monro, and it is thought that they arise from remnants of the germinal matrix in that region.

Genetics

Tuberous sclerosis complex is transmitted as an autosomal-dominant trait with variable penetrance and an estimated incidence of 1 in 5800 live births worldwide [Gomez, 1999]. Wide phenotypic variability of clinical manifestations and severity has been noted, even within families having the same mutation [Lyczkowski et al., 2007]. Currently, no known effect of paternal or maternal age or of birth order on disease phenotype has been recognized. Approximately two-thirds of cases are sporadic and the result of apparent spontaneous mutations. Both somatic and germline mosaicism have been described in many patients [Kwiatkowska et al., 1999; Verhoef et al., 1999].

Two genes, *TSC1* and *TSC2*, have been identified for tuberous sclerosis complex. A disease causing mutation in one of these two genes can be identified in approximately 85 percent of persons with Definite tuberous sclerosis complex according to current criteria [Kwiatkowski et al., 2003]. *TSC1* located at 9q34; it was cloned in 1997, and the protein product, hamartin, was identified and characterized [Sampson et al., 1989; Smith et al., 1990; Connor and Sampson, 1991; Haines et al., 1991; Hornigold et al., 1997; van Slegtenhorst et al., 1997]. The *TSC2* gene is located on 16p13 [Kandt et al., 1992; Consortium, 1993] and encodes a protein referred to as tuberin.

Tuberin and hamartin interact with one another and function as tumor suppressor molecules. Loss of heterozygosity has been identified in hamartomas from persons with *TSC1* and *TSC2* mutations, particularly in kidney and lung tissue, but less commonly in cortical tubers or subependymal giant cell astrocytomas [Henske et al., 1996]. Tuberin has GTPase-activating properties, similar to the NF1 protein product. Hamartin and tuberin are components of the mammalian target of rapamycin (mTOR) pathway, which is involved in many functions, including regulation of cell size [Gao and Pan, 2001; Potter et al., 2001; Tapon et al., 2001; Crino et al., 2006; Huang and Manning, 2008]. In vivo, it appears that tuberin can be phosphorylated by Akt, at least in part regulating its activity. In normal cells, the tuberin/hamartin complex acts as an inhibitor of mTOR activity. On growth factor stimulation or other stimuli, however, tuberin is phosphorylated by Akt, which leads to the inactivation of inhibitory activity of TSC1/TSC2 and resultant cell growth. In cells containing mutations affecting the function of hamartin or tuberin, mTOR and S6 kinase activities are significantly increased, and cell growth is no longer regulated by the PI3-kinase-TSC1/TSC2 signaling pathway, which is thought to lead to the development of hamartoma.

Management

Tuberous sclerosis complex affects most organ systems, and management and treatment recommendations vary according to organ manifestations (see Table 40-2). Affected persons, both children and adults, should be managed with regular follow-up evaluations by a physician who is familiar with tuberous sclerosis complex, to recognize treatable manifestations early and to provide anticipatory guidance and counseling.

With regard to neurologic manifestations, management focuses on treatment of epilepsy and behavioral disorders and on identification of learning disabilities. Treatment of epilepsy in tuberous sclerosis complex is similar to that for partial epilepsies resulting from other causes, and includes antiepileptic medications, the vagus nerve stimulator, and the ketogenic diet [Thiele, 2004]. Vigabatrin is particularly effective in treating infantile spasms in patients with tuberous sclerosis complex [Curatolo et al., 2008]. Epilepsy surgery has a very important role in the management of patients who have pharmacoresistant epilepsy [Weiner et al., 2004; Jansen et al., 2007].

Rapamycin, an mTOR antagonist, has been shown to reduce the size of subependymal giant cell tumors and renal angiomyolipoma in tuberous sclerosis complex, and may also reduce the progression of pulmonary lymphangioleiomyomatosis

[Bissler et al., 2008; Franz et al., 2006]. In animal models of tuberous sclerosis complex, rapamycin has also been shown to prevent epilepsy if given prenatally, and to improve cognitive deficits [Zeng et al., 2008; Ehninger et al., 2008]. On-going multicenter trials are evaluating the role of rapamycin and other mTOR antagonists in the management of tuberous sclerosis complex.

Von Hippel–Lindau Disease

Von Hippel–Lindau disease is inherited as an autosomal-dominant trait and is characterized by retinal, cerebellar, and spinal hemangioblastomas, cystic tumors of the pancreas, kidney, and epididymis, renal cell carcinoma, endolymphatic sac tumors, and, in some families, pheochromocytoma. The basic pathologic lesion is a capillary hemangioblastoma. The retinal lesions, originally described by Panas and Remy, were not recognized as hemangioblastomas [Panas and Remy, 1879]. Fuchs posited that the retinal lesions were arteriovenous malformations [Fuchs, 1882], and Collins believed that the retinal lesions were hemangioblastomas [Collins, 1894]. Von Hippel believed that the retinal lesions were hemangioblastomas but labeled them as angiomatosis retinae [von Hippel, 1911]. The postmortem examination in one patient with retinal lesions reported by von Hippel revealed cerebellar tumor, hypernephroma, and cystic lesions of the pancreas, kidney, and epididymis. Lindau recognized the similarity of the tissue type of the retinal lesions and some cerebellar tumors, and also observed that the same type of tumor occasionally was found in the medulla and spinal cord [Lindau, 1926].

Clinical Characteristics

Retinal hemangioblastoma is one of the earliest manifestations of the disease, and although it has been reported in early childhood [Ridley et al., 1986; Webster et al., 1999], it usually is first observed during the third decade of life (Figure 40-16A). The early retinal lesion has the appearance of an aneurysmal dilatation of a peripheral retinal vessel; typically, tortuous vessels later manifest, with an arteriovenous pair leading to small, elevated retinal lesions [Macmichael, 1970]. These lesions commonly are located in the retinal periphery and can easily be overlooked unless careful ophthalmoscopy is performed. Fluorescein angiography is helpful in demonstrating the lesion [Atuk et al., 1979; Augsburger et al., 1981; Greenwald and Weiss, 1984]. An accumulation of fluid beneath the retina can occur, and retinal detachment with progressive visual loss commonly is observed as the first manifestation of retinal abnormality [Goldberg and Duke, 1968; Kupersmith and Berenstein, 1981; Hardwig and Robertson, 1984; Webster et al., 1999]. Wong et al. studied 335 Von Hippel–Lindau patients with hemangioblastomas in at least one eye and found unilateral tumors in 42.1 percent and bilateral tumors in 57.9 percent [Wong et al., 2008a]. Vascular proliferation leading to visual loss has been reported in rare patients [Wong et al., 2008b].

Although they usually affect the cerebellum [Slater et al., 2003], central nervous system hemangioblastomas sometimes are found in the medulla [Pavesi et al., 2010] and spinal cord [Kanno et al., 2009], and rarely occur in the cerebral hemispheres. The tumor usually is found in patients after the third decade of life, but has been reported to occur rarely

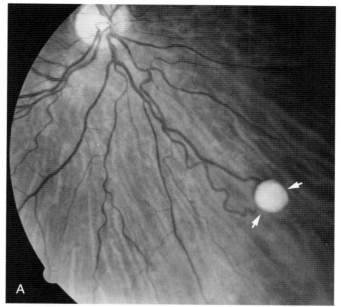

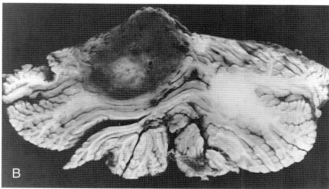

Fig. 40-16 Von Hippel–Lindau disease. A, Typical round, elevated, whitish-red retinal lesion. These retinal angiomatous hamartomas can be located centrally near the optic disc or peripherally. **B,** Cerebellar hemangioblastoma. Note the typical paramedial and superficial location of the tumor. (**A,** *Courtesy of Dr. Creig Hoyt, University of California Medical Center, San Francisco, CA.*)

in children; initial symptoms and signs are those of a space-occupying lesion of the posterior fossa. Symptoms and signs tend to be associated with tumors that display a cystic component [Slater et al., 2003]. Hemangioblastomas of the medulla or spinal cord are associated with syringomyelia in approximately 80 percent of patients [Salazar and Lamiell, 1980]. The tumor rarely is found in the supratentorial region, and can occur in the pituitary gland, third ventricle, or cerebral hemispheres (i.e., frontal, temporal, parietal, and parieto-occipital lobes].

A variety of renal lesions has been found in von Hippel–Lindau disease, including benign cysts, hemangiomas, adenomas, and malignant hypernephromas. Cystic lesions vary in size, ranging from a few millimeters to several centimeters across, and, although they can occur unilaterally, these lesions are more often bilateral and multiple [Melmon and Rosen, 1964]. The cystic lesions can be so extensive that they mimic polycystic kidney disease. A prominent cause of morbidity and mortality is renal cell carcinoma, occurring with a frequency next to that of the retinal and cerebellar hemangioblastoma [Neumann et al., 1998].

Cystic lesions can also occur in the pancreas, adrenal gland, and epididymis. Other organs less commonly affected with cystic changes include the liver, spleen, and lung. Endolymphatic sac tumors associated with von Hippel–Lindau disease can cause hearing loss [Manski et al., 1997]. Pheochromocytomas occur more often in patients with von Hippel–Lindau disease than in the general population and tend to cluster in certain families. Walther et al. diagnosed pheochromocytoma in 64 of 246 patients with von Hippel–Lindau and found an association with missense mutations in the *VHL* gene [Walther et al., 1999b].

The retinal hemangioblastoma diagnosis usually is established by careful ophthalmoscopy with fluorescein retinal angiography, revealing the vascular characteristics of the lesions. Cranial MRI scans demonstrate the cerebellar hemangioblastoma or those tumors affecting the medulla and spinal cord. Intra-abdominal cystic lesions can be visualized by CT, MRI, or ultrasonography. Other laboratory studies that can assist in diagnosis include erythrocyte count and hematocrit determination, which can be elevated in patients with cerebellar hemangioblastoma or renal carcinoma because of the increased erythropoietin activity of the cyst fluid. The absence of polycythemia, however, does not exclude the diagnosis of the tumor. Patients with central nervous system tumors commonly have increased protein concentration of the cerebrospinal fluid. A 24-hour urine assay for catecholamines and metanephrines should be performed to screen for the presence of pheochromocytoma. Genetic testing of the von Hippel–Lindau gene is clinically available.

Pathology

The tumors usually are well circumscribed, can be solid or cystic, and usually are found in the paramedial aspect of the cerebellar cortex (see Figure 40-16B). Characteristic microscopic features include large numbers of thin-walled, closely packed blood vessels lined by plump endothelial cells; the cells are separated by large, pale cells and incorporated in the elaborate network of reticulin fibers.

Genetics

Von Hippel–Lindau disease is inherited as an autosomal-dominant trait. It is estimated to affect about 1 in 36,000 persons [Maher et al., 1991]. Penetrance is found to be nearly complete on careful evaluation. The gene is located on 3p25–26 [Latif et al., 1993], and encodes a protein that regulates a cellular system that senses and responds to hypoxia [Kaelin, 2005]. The *VHL* gene functions as a tumor suppressor; hence, homozygous mutation occurs in tumors, leading to loss of function and constitutive activation of the hypoxia-sensing pathway. Genetic testing is available and has revealed that specific mutations tend to be found in families with von Hippel–Lindau disease associated with pheochromocytoma [Nordstrom-O'Brien et al., 2010]. Von Hippel–Lindau disease has been subdivided into type 1, in which all of the manifestations may be present except for pheochromocytoma, and type 2, which includes the full set of features. Type 2 is further divided into 2A (pheochromocytoma and other manifestations, but not renal cell carcinoma), 2B (all features), and 2C (isolated pheochromocytoma). [Nordstrom-O'Brien et al., 2010] categorized mutations in 945 Von Hippel–Lindau families. A wide variety of mutations were found in type 1 families, whereas 83 percent of type 2 families had missense mutations. Nonsense and frameshift mutations were more frequent in type 1 families.

Management

Affected individuals should be provided a program of surveillance to insure early recognition of treatable complications. Recommendations of the VHL Family Alliance are provided in Table 40-3. Poulsen et al. reviewed records for 59 Danish Von Hippel–Lindau patients, noting that semi-annual MRIs were not sufficient to prevent neurological complications, and instead recommended annual evaluations [Poulsen et al., 2010]. They also noted CNS hemangioblastomas in 18 percent of children younger than 15 years and in one 8-year-old. Retinal hemangioblastomas should be carefully followed by serial ophthalmologic evaluations when the lesions are small. If, however, visual loss or retinal detachment occurs, the lesions can be treated by either laser photocoagulation or cryocoagulation [Webster et al., 1999]. Central nervous systems lesions are usually treated surgically [Pavesi et al., 2008] or with stereotactic radiation therapy [Kano et al., 2008; Karabagli et al., 2010]. Medications that inhibit angiogenesis are being explored as possible nonsurgical therapies [Sardi et al., 2009].

Table 40-3 Recommendations for Surveillance of Individuals with von Hippel–Lindau disease

Surveillance	Infancy	Age 2–10 years	Age 11–19 years	Age >20 years
Ophthalmologic examination	Initial eye exam	Annual	Every 6 months	Annual
24-hour urine collection for catecholamines and metanephrines		Annual	Annual	Annual
Ultrasound examination of abdomen		Annual from 8 years of age	Annual	Annual, and abdominal CT every other year
MRI of brain and spine with gadolinium		As clinically indicated	Every 1–2 years or as clinically indicated	Every 2 years and before and after pregnancy
Audiology assessment		Every 2–3 years or as clinically indicated	Every 1–2 years or as clinically indicated	Every 2 years or as clinically indicated

(Modified from VHL Family Alliance, www.vhl.org/handbook/vhlhb4.php#Suggested.)

Sturge–Weber Syndrome (Encephalofacial Angiomatosis)

Sturge–Weber syndrome is characterized by presence of a facial angioma (port-wine stain, or nevus flammeus) and an ipsilateral leptomeningeal angioma; it has an incidence currently estimated at 1 case in 20,000–50,000 persons [Comi, 2007]. Schirmer initially described a patient with a facial vascular nevus who had associated buphthalmos, but he did not mention the central nervous system lesion [Schirmer, 1860]. Sturge initially described this syndrome by providing the clinical findings of a 6-year-old girl with a facial nevus who also had angiomas of the lips, gingiva, palate, floor of the mouth, uvula, and pharynx [Sturge, 1879]. The child had buphthalmos and was hemiparetic, and Sturge suggested that she had a similar vascular nevus of the underlying brain. Not until 1897, however, did Kalischer perform the first neuropathologic study of a patient with similar findings, demonstrating that Sturge's initial contention of cerebral involvement by vascular nevus was correct [Kalischer, 1897]. Associated intracranial calcification was later described by Weber [Weber, 1929].

Clinical Characteristics

Sturge–Weber syndrome, which occurs sporadically, is characterized by angiomas involving the leptomeninges and ipsilateral skin of the face, typically in the ophthalmic (V1) and maxillary (V2) distributions of the trigeminal nerve. It can extend to other facial areas, including the lips, gingiva, palate, tongue, pharynx, and larynx. The neck, trunk, and extremities also can be involved, either ipsilaterally or contralaterally to the facial angioma. The angioma also can involve the nasopharynx, mucous membrane, and ocular choroidal membrane, resulting in glaucoma in approximately 25 percent of patients (Figure 40-17). Additional ocular findings include iridic heterochromia, strabismus, optic atrophy, and dilated retinal veins. In the brain, the associated ipsilateral leptomeningeal angioma most commonly involves the parietal and occipital regions, but also may involve the temporal region and, on occasion, can affect both hemispheres. Dimitri reported that these patients had intracranial calcifications observed on the skull radiographs and described the typical serpentine "tram-track sign" of calcific intracranial densities [Dimitri, 1923].

Neurologic manifestations vary and depend on location and extent of the leptomeningeal angioma. Seizures occur in 75–90 percent of patients with Sturge–Weber syndrome and may be refractory to treatment [Bebin and Gomez, 1988; Takeoka and Riviello, 2010]. It is hypothesized that the seizure activity results from cortical irritability caused by the leptomeningeal angioma, resulting in regional hypoxia, ischemia, and gliosis, although associated cortical dysgenesis also may be involved. Seizure manifestations are primarily partial motor (40 percent), although some patients can have primary or secondary generalized tonic-clonic (20 percent) and both partial and generalized seizures (40 percent) [Chao, 1959; Bebin and Gomez, 1988]. Other types of seizure activity occur less frequently. Unfortunately, refractory epilepsy develops in a significant number of patients with Sturge–Weber syndrome, ranging in series from 11 to 83 percent [Takeoka, 2010]. Surgical procedures, including focal cortical resection, hemispherectomy, and corpus callosotomy, should be considered if seizure activity proves medically intractable.

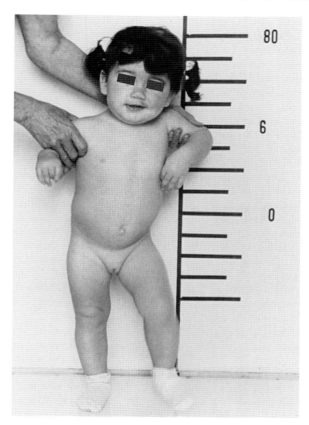

Fig. 40-17 A 20-month-old girl with Sturge–Weber syndrome. Note the facial angioma affecting primarily the upper face. In addition, she had a contralateral hemiparesis and hemiatrophy.

Persons with Sturge–Weber syndrome also are at risk for hemiparesis contralateral to the leptomeningeal angioma, which is seen in approximately 33 percent of the patients. The hemiparesis can result from ischemia with venous occlusion and thrombosis due in part to venous congestion resulting from failure of cortical vein development [Hebold, 1913; Chao, 1959; Alexander, 1972; Chamberlain et al., 1989]. Transient weakness also may result from seizure activity, and may become more severe and less transient with recurrent seizure activity. Leptomeningeal venous angiomas can arise in the absence of any facial angioma; although secondary cerebral signs and symptoms similar to those of Sturge–Weber syndrome can occur, these patients are more appropriately considered to have leptomeningeal angiomatosis.

Persons with Sturge–Weber syndrome also are at risk for developmental delay and mental retardation, which occur in 50–60 percent of the patients and are more likely in those with bilateral leptomeningeal involvement [Bebin and Gomez, 1988] and in those with a history of seizures [Sujansky and Conradi, 1995; Comi, 2007]. Headaches also are common, occurring in up to 60 percent of affected persons, and are thought to be secondary to the vascular abnormalities, giving symptoms consistent with migraine [Maria et al., 1999]. EEG studies document decreased amplitude and frequency of electrocerebral activity over the affected hemisphere. Diffuse, multiple, and independent spike foci commonly are present [Aminoff, 1992; Sassower et al., 1994].

Hemianopsia in young patients also is difficult to determine but is believed to occur in about one-quarter to one-half of patients. About one-third of patients have glaucoma, and approximately half of these have buphthalmos ipsilateral to the facial angioma. Glaucoma can be unilateral or bilateral, regardless of whether the facial angioma is bilateral.

Intracranial calcification is evident on radiographs in 90 percent of adult patients. Calcifications uncommonly are present at birth but are manifest in virtually all patients by the end of the second decade of life [Nellhaus et al., 1967]. The intracranial calcifications typically assume a linear, parallel configuration ("tram-track sign") or a convolutional pattern most commonly seen in the parietal or parieto-occipital regions [Thomas-Sohl et al., 2004] (Figure 40-18). Cranial CT and MRI scans are complementary in evaluating the cerebral changes of Sturge–Weber syndrome, in that the MRI demonstrates thickened cortex, decreased convolutions, and abnormal white matter, whereas cranial CT scans demonstrate more definitively the characteristic calcification. Cranial MRI scans (T2-weighted images) reveal smaller, nonspecific foci of hypointense signal [Chamberlain et al., 1989; Thomas-Sohl et al., 2004]. Gadolinium enhancement may reveal pial angioma, thereby allowing early diagnosis of Sturge–Weber syndrome before calcification [Sugama et al., 1997].

Cerebral angiography discloses decreased cerebral venous drainage with dilatation of the deep cerebral veins. Various other vascular abnormalities have been demonstrated in approximately one-third of patients and include thrombotic lesions, dural venous sinus abnormalities, and arteriovenous malformations [Bentson et al., 1957]. PET provides a sensitive measure of the extent of cerebral metabolic impairment. Serial PET scans in children with Sturge–Weber syndrome can be useful and, when used with other neuroimaging studies, document the progression of the disease [Chugani et al., 1989].

Pathology

Sturge–Weber syndrome is thought to be caused by the presence of residual embryonal blood vessels and their secondary effects on surrounding tissues. During development, a vascular plexus develops around the cephalic portion of the neural tube, under the ectoderm that subsequently becomes facial skin. This plexus forms during the sixth week of gestation and regresses at approximately the ninth week. It is thought that failure of this regression results in residual vascular tissue, subsequently forming the angiomata of the leptomeninges, face, and ipsilateral eye. Neuropathologic studies have demonstrated thickened, hypervascularized leptomeninges that involve the occipital, parietal, or temporoparietal region primarily (Figure 40-19). These meningeal vessels generally are small and tortuous, and rarely enter the underlying brain substance. Calcific deposits are present in the walls of some small cerebral vessels but more commonly are found in the outer pyramidal and molecular cortical layers. Biochemical assays have demonstrated increased calcium content of the gray and white matter, with normal iron content. The pathophysiology of the deposition of intracerebral calcium is not well understood [Weber, 1929; Tingey, 1956; Wachswulth and Lowenthal, 1979; Thomas-Sohl et al., 2004].

Management

Treatment for the neurologic manifestations of Sturge–Weber syndrome includes management of seizure activity and headaches. Approximately 50 percent of children with seizures achieve control with administration of appropriate antiepileptic drugs. Those patients with seizure disorders refractory to medical treatment should be carefully considered for epilepsy surgery with resection of the affected lobe(s) or hemispherectomy. Rochkind and colleagues reported that seizure control after surgery was better in those patients who received antiepileptic drugs [Rochkind et al., 1990]. Aspirin therapy may reduce the incidence of strokelike episodes, and is typically used in individuals with either recurrent vascular events or progressive neurologic deficits [Roach et al., 1985; Comi, 2007]. Treatment options for the facial angioma include laser therapy using various pulsed-dye lasers, as well as pulsed-light sources, and other laser therapies. The current recommendation

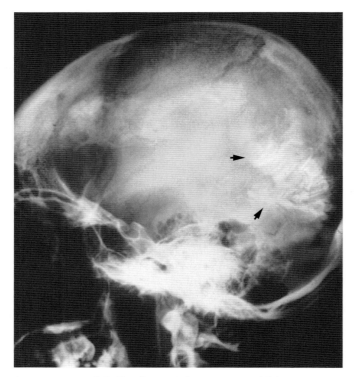

Fig. 40-18 Lateral skull radiograph from a young child with Sturge–Weber syndrome, demonstrating parallel linear calcifications (the "tram-track sign").

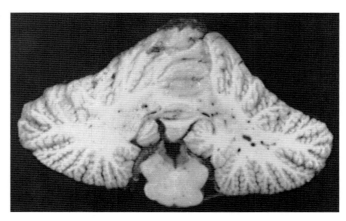

Fig. 40-19 Section of the cerebellum and brainstem in Sturge–Weber Syndrome. There is notable cerebeller atrophy. *(Courtesy of Dr. Nathan Malamud, University of California Medical Center, San Francisco, CA.)*

is to begin treatment as early as possible; infants have received treatment during the first week of life. Treatment of glaucoma, if present, consists of control of intraocular pressure, to prevent optic nerve injury, by medical or surgical intervention. The management of patients with Sturge–Weber syndrome requires the skill of an attentive physician, psychologist, and social worker.

Maffucci's Syndrome

Maffucci's syndrome is a rare congenital disease characterized by multiple enchondromas with secondary hemangiomas, phlebolithiasis, and malformations of bone. Occasionally, associated skin changes, including patches of vitiligo, café-au-lait spots, and other hyperpigmented patches and nevi, are seen. The reported cases are sporadic, and no gender predilection exists. A related disorder, Ollier's disease, is characterized by multiple endochondromas without hemangiomas. The initial report of this syndrome by Maffucci described a 40-year-old woman who had multiple enchondromas, some of which had undergone sarcomatous changes [Maffucci, 1881]. Her four children had no stigmata of the disease. Maffucci syndrome's generally is a sporadic occurrence. Hopyan et al. have identified mutations in the gene encoding the parathyroid hormone/parathyroid hormone-related protein type 1 receptor (PTHR1) in persons with endochondromatosis, suggesting the possibility that the disorder is inherited as autosomal-dominant, with most cases due to new mutation [Hopyan et al., 2002]. Couvineau et al. identified germline *PTHR1* mutations in 1 of 61 patients with Ollier's disease, but in none of 23 patients with Maffucci's syndrome [Couvineau et al., 2008].

The enchondromas affect the small bones of the hands and feet, or any bone preformed in cartilage; they are apparent during the first few years of life. Initially, a small, firm nodule 1–2 cm in diameter usually is found on digital bone; the nodule is readily palpable. Additional, similar nodules appear shortly thereafter. They are unilateral in about 40 percent of patients and, if bilateral, are strikingly asymmetric [Bean, 1955, 1958]. During childhood, the enchondromas increase in size, ultimately resulting in malformations of the limbs and trunk (Figure 40-20). Patients generally are of small stature and have a distinctive appearance resulting from their deformities. About 20–30 percent of affected individuals have enchondromas that undergo sarcomatous changes [Albregts and Rapini, 1995; Ranger et al., 2009; Ramina et al., 1997]. Neurologic symptoms may result from

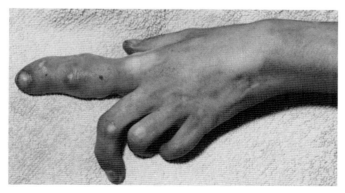

Fig. 40-20 Multiple enchondromas of the digits, typically observed in Maffucci's syndrome.

skull-base chondrosarcomas or from rare gliomas. Cutaneous hemangiomas become apparent during the first decade of life and are not necessarily found in the areas of enchondromas. They can be superficial or deep, and they may affect the lips, tongue, palate, or cheeks. Visceral hemangiomas involving the esophagus, ileum, and anal mucosa have been reported. Patients have cavernous hemangiomas and lymphangiomas. Associated angiofibromas, hemangiomas, hemangioendotheliomas, teratomas, thecomas, and pancreatic adenocarcinomas have been reported [McDermott et al., 2001].

No single treatment plan exists, because each patient must be individually managed. Some bone deformities can be corrected, to a variable degree, by orthopedic procedures. Patients with neurologic signs and symptoms secondary to an intracranial osteoenchondroma can benefit from surgical excision. Primary brain tumors are treated by appropriate neurosurgical measures, which can be followed by radiation therapy, chemotherapy, or both. The partial or complete removal of hemangiomas or lymphangiomas can be accomplished by reconstructive surgical procedures or by dermatologic methods, including laser techniques. Finally, the physician must provide realistic supportive care to the patient and family, recognizing the notable limitations of any palliative surgical procedure.

Epidermal Nevus Syndrome

Epidermal nevus syndrome is a heterogeneous group of disorders characterized by patchy cutaneous hamartomatous lesions, central nervous system abnormalities, and various other manifestations (Table 40-4). Most of these disorders occur sporadically and are highly variable in their presentation [Vidaurri-de la Cruz et al., 2004; Happle, 1991]. Nevi can take various forms, including verrucous, sebaceous, and lentiginous, and may evolve over the years. They tend to follow the lines of Blaschko and manifest early in life. Central nervous system manifestations include unilateral lissencephaly, a paucity of white matter, excessive and heterotopic gray matter, apparent schizencephaly, unilateral colpocephaly, and hemimegalencephaly [Hager et al., 1991; Zhang et al., 2003]. Associated neurologic abnormalities include mental retardation and convulsive disorders, occurring in approximately 60 percent of patients; ocular abnormalities in up to 50 percent of patients; and corticospinal tract dysfunction in a smaller number of patients [Holden and Dekaban, 1972; Kurokawa et al., 1981]. Cortical resection has been helpful in some instances [Maher et al., 2003], but no other definitive treatment exists.

The patchy manifestations of these disorders have suggested the possibility that they result from somatic mosaicism; this has been demonstrated in some instances of Proteus syndrome, where mosaicism for *PTEN* has been found [Hobert and Eng, 2009; Orloff and Eng, 2008].

Parry–Romberg Syndrome (Facial Hemiatrophy)

Parry–Romberg syndrome, which typically has onset between 5 and 15 years of age, is characterized by a progressive ipsilateral loss of facial soft tissue, cartilage, and bone. This tissue loss usually involves the tissues between the nose and nasolabial fold or above the maxilla, but progresses to affect most of the ipsilateral face during the ensuing years. The tongue, the

Table 40-4 **Classification of Epidermal Nevus Syndrome**

Disorder	Features	Genetics
Sebaceous nevus syndrome	Congenital sebaceous nevus, neurologic dysfunction, skeletal, ocular anomalies	Sporadic
Nevus comedonicus syndrome	Congenital hyperkeratotic papules of follicular origin on face, neck, chest, abdomen, arms; ipsilateral eye and skeletal defects; seizures, mental retardation	Sporadic
Becker nevus syndrome	Hyperpigmented plaque associated with hair growth; smooth muscle hyperplasia, rib defects, breast hypoplasia	Sporadic (more common in males)
Phakomatosis pigmentokeratotica	Sebaceous and speckled lentiginous nevus; ipsilateral weakness, hypohydrosis; seizures, mental retardation	Sporadic
Proteus syndrome	Epidermal nevi; asymmetric overgrowth of soft tissues and bone	Sporadic; some with mosaic *PTEN* mutations
Congenital hemidysplasia with ichthyosiform nevus and limb defects (CHILD)	Ichthiosiform nevus; skeletal aplasia or hypoplasia; abnormalities in brain, lung, heart, kidneys	X-linked dominant; mutations in 3β-hydroxysteroid dehydrogenase gene

For additional information, see Happle R. How many epidermal nevus syndromes exist? A clinicogenetic classification. J Am Acad Dermatol 1991;25:550–556; Vidaurri-de la Cruz H. Epidermal nevus syndromes: Clinical findings in 35 patients. Pediatr Dermatol 2004;21(4): 432–439.

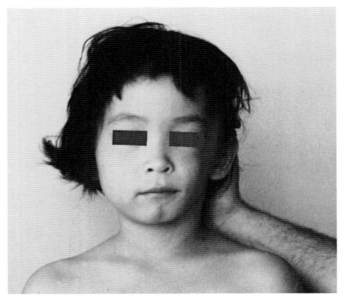

Fig. 40-21 Hemifacial atrophy as manifested in Parry–Romberg syndrome.

gums, and the soft palate may also become involved. The eyelashes, eyebrows, and hair on the involved side can be affected, and ipsilateral blanching of the hair or alopecia can occur (Figure 40-21). Progression of this atrophic process generally lasts between 2 and 10 years, and is believed to cease by the end of the second or beginning of the third decade of life [Wartenberg, 1945; Wolf and Verity, 1974; Rischbieth, 1976; Stone, 2003].

In addition to atrophy of the facial tissues, various other neurologic deficits have been reported, including recurrent headaches, trigeminal neuralgia, ipsilateral Horner's syndrome, contralateral partial seizures, and hemiparesis [Stone, 2003]. Moreover, an unusual association of the syndrome with multiple benign tumors has been described. Scleroderma and lipodystrophy must be clinically differentiated from this disease. Cranial CT can be normal or document cerebral atrophy; contralateral intracerebral calcification has been described [Asher and Berg, 1982]. No typical or consistent neuropathologic findings have been reported. No specific treatment for the syndrome exists; however, various reconstructive surgical procedures, often using grafts of autogenous fat after disease stabilizes, can result in reasonably good cosmetic results [Hintringer et al., 1991; Mayro et al., 1991].

Neurocutaneous Melanosis

Neurocutaneous melanosis is a rare, nonfamilial, embryonic, neuroectodermal dysplasia characterized by abnormally pigmented cutaneous areas (e.g., giant hairy pigmented nevi, multiple hyperpigmented cutaneous nevi, large congenital melanocytic nevi) and leptomeningeal melanosis [DiRocco et al., 2004]. Virchow [Virchow, 1859] first reported the topographic distribution of melanotic cells in the arachnoid, but Rokitansky provided the initial clinical description of this condition with his report of a 14-year-old, mentally retarded, hydrocephalic girl who had a giant pigmented nevus over her back and multiple hyperpigmented skin lesions [Rokitansky, 1861]. At postmortem examination, a brown–black pigmentation of the pia overlying the cerebral cortex was noted. Van Bogaert named this condition neurocutaneous melanosis [Van Bogaert, 1948].

Diagnosis is usually made in infants and children younger than 2 years of age; however, the condition is present at birth. No gender predilection exists. All patients have areas of abnormal skin hyperpigmentation, the most common pattern of which is multiple giant hairy pigmented nevi. Giant hairy nevi usually have a "bathing suit" or cape-shaped distribution. In one series of 289 patients with large congenital melanocytic nevi, 33 had manifest central nervous system melanosis, wherein the nevi were present in the posterior axial location on the head, neck, back, and/or buttocks. "Satellite" nevi were present in 31 of the 33 patients [DeDavid et al., 1996]. Lovett et al. [Lovett et al., 2009] reviewed a series of 26 patients with large congenital melanocytic nevi who underwent MRI, and found six with neurocutaneous melanosis. The presence of multiple satellite lesions and midline location for pigmented lesions were predictive of neurological involvement.

Melanoblasts, normally present in the pia mater, are manifested by small brown–black pigmented flecks in the leptomeninges, which are most frequently distributed over the ventral aspect of the lower medulla. These cells are the presumed source of melanoma originating in the central nervous system. The leptomeninges are thickened and infiltrated by melanin-containing cells that are diffuse or arranged in sheets. Localized areas of intracerebral brown–black pigmentation are relatively common and most often are found in the cerebellar cortex.

The clinical presentation of neurocutaneous melanosis depends on the location and extent of involvement of this leptomeningeal lesion. Hydrocephalus is commonly encountered because of cerebrospinal fluid pathway obstruction in the basilar cisterns, the arachnoid villi over the cerebral hemispheric convexities, or both, and intraspinal melanotic arachnoid cyst, lipoma, and intraspinal lipoma have been described as obstructed [Kasantikul et al., 1989; van Heuzen et al., 1989]. Association with Dandy–Walker malformation has been reported [Schreml et al., 2008]. Behavioral abnormalities and recurring seizures can occur, as well as cranial nerve dysfunction and signs of spinal cord and root involvement [Pavlidou et al., 2008]. Findings on cerebrospinal fluid examination can be normal; however, the protein level usually is elevated, and glucose concentration is decreased. Cytologic examination usually reveals abnormal melanin-containing cells [Fox, 1972]. In one study of MRI scans of seven patients with neurocutaneous melanosis, five had regions of T1 shortening in the cerebellum, three of whom also had T2 shortening. Five patients had regions of T1 shortening in the anterior temporal lobes. Other areas of involvement included the pia mater over the cerebellum, pons, medulla, and left parietal lobe. Only two lesions demonstrated enhancement, edema, or necrosis, and both lesions were found to be malignant melanomas at biopsy [Barkovich et al., 1994].

Attempts to treat hydrocephalus by a shunting procedure are palliative. There is a risk of melanoma. The prognosis for neurocutaneous melanosis generally is poor, regardless of the variety of treatment methods used, which include radiation therapy, chemotherapy, or both, and patients rarely live beyond the age of 20 years, though one report suggests a role for aggressive chemotherapy in associated melanoma [Subbiah and Wolff, 2010].

Klippel–Trénaunay–Weber Syndrome

Klippel–Trénaunay–Weber syndrome initially was believed to be characterized only by cutaneous and/or subcutaneous hemangiomas, varicosities, and hypertrophy of the soft tissues and bone of a limb. Additional associated anomalies later recognized included macrocephaly; hydrocephalus; lymphangiomas; hemangiomas of the trunk, intestine, and bladder; and abnormalities of the digits [Klippel and Trénaunay, 1900; Lian and Alhomme, 1945; Meine et al., 1997; Parkes Weber, 1907]. Klippel–Trénaunay–Weber syndrome usually occurs sporadically but has been found to be associated, at least in some patients, with translocations that disrupt the AGGF1 gene, which encodes a protein involved in angiogenesis [Tian et al., 2004]. Hu et al. [2008] also demonstrated association of single nucleotide polymorphisms in this gene with Klippel-Trénaunay-Weber syndrome.

Jacob et al. [1998] reviewed findings in 252 patients, and found port-wine capillary malformations in 98 percent, venous malformations in 72 percent, and limb hypertrophy in 67 percent. Typical skin lesions usually are present at birth but may not be recognized until several years later. They can be single or multiple, and affect the face, trunk, and limbs. The vascular lesions are variable and include capillary hemangiomas, nevus flammeus, telangiectasias, varicosities, phlebectasias, and arteriovenous fistulae; lymphangiectasis also can be present. Vascular lesions usually are found in areas of limb hypertrophy. Rarely, patients with large vascular lesions have a bleeding diathesis; thrombophlebitis can occur, as well as thromboembolic phenomena. Varicosities of various sizes commonly are present and, although usually found in the lower limbs, also can be found on the scalp, chest, and torso [Inceman and Tangun, 1969].

Limb hypertrophy usually is apparent at birth. Prenatal diagnosis has been made by ultrasonography [Hatjis et al., 1981]. Lymphedema can be present. An inordinately progressive growth of the affected body part eventually occurs, leading to the development of various other abnormalities. Abnormal growth of one leg, for example, can result in a pelvic tilt and scoliosis, but the patient's overall height is not significantly changed [Lindenauer, 1965]. The legs are affected more commonly than the arms.

Additional abnormalities include megalocornea, glaucoma, iridic heterochromia, syndactyly, polydactyly, macrodactyly, and clinodactyly. Hemangiomas of the tongue, pharynx, larynx, and bladder have been described, and labial and scrotal lesions are common. Macrocephaly often is present, and seizures and mental retardation have been reported. Less frequently, associated abnormalities include congenital heart malformations and imperforate anus [Banhayan, 1971; Lindenauer, 1965; Hall, 1971].

Any treatment plan for these patients must be individualized and requires a multidisciplinary team. Nonsurgical management involves compression of the involved limb. MRI or CT venography [Mavili et al., 2009; Bastarrika et al., 2007] can be performed if any vascular surgical procedure is contemplated. Some vascular lesions can be treated with cryotherapy, laser therapy, or sclerotherapy, whereas others can be surgically removed [Redondo et al., 2009; Gloviczki and Driscoll, 2007]. An osteotomy or epiphyseal stapling procedure can occasionally benefit patients with limb hypertrophy, but limb amputations may be required in others.

Incontinentia Pigmenti (Bloch–Sulzberger Syndrome)

Incontinentia pigmenti is transmitted as an X-linked dominant trait, predominantly affecting females [Lenz, 1961]. Most hemizygous males apparently die in utero; rare affected males usually are mosaics or have a 47,XXY karyotype [Kenwrick et al., 2001]. The gene has been identified and is referred to as NEMO; it encodes a protein that participates in the nuclear factor kappa B (NF-κB) signaling pathway [Smahi et al., 2000]. The syndrome is characterized by various hyperpigmented skin lesions that can be apparent at birth and by commonly associated abnormalities involving the central nervous system, eyes, hair, teeth, and bone.

Garrod [1906] likely provided the first description of this syndrome with his report of the case of a 2-year-old, mentally retarded, spastic diplegic girl who had a whorled pattern of brown skin pigmentation on her trunk and limbs. Bardach [1925], however, is most often credited with the first clinical description of the syndrome in twin sisters; Bloch [1926], Sulzberger [1938], and Sieman [1929] each later defined the syndrome more clearly. Bloch introduced the term incontinentia pigmenti, which is still used.

The skin manifestations have been described as having three stages: The first stage typically is characterized by vesiculobullous lesions present at birth or during the first several weeks of life. These lesions appear in groups or in a linear distribution over the trunk and limbs, following the lines of Blaschko. A preponderance of eosinophils is found in the vesicular fluid, and the peripheral blood also can exhibit an eosinophilia. The lesions rupture, resulting in oozing and crusting, and can persist for months. The second stage is characterized by evolution into verrucous lesions beginning after the sixth week of life. The third stage typically is characterized by hyperpigmented brown or gray–brown macular lesions that follow the lines of Blaschko. These pigmented skin lesions usually become more prominent during the first few years of life and then gradually fade. The decrease of abnormal pigmentation may continue throughout adolescence, and in some patients the pigmentation can completely disappear [Carney, 1976].

One-third to one-half of patients have symptoms and signs of neurologic abnormalities manifested by developmental retardation, corticospinal tract dysfunction, and seizures [Carney, 1976]. Microcephaly and hydrocephaly may occur. Approximately one-third of patients have ocular abnormalities, including optic atrophy, papillitis, abnormal retinal pigmentation, nystagmus, strabismus, and cataracts. Visual loss occurs in about 8 percent of patients. The most common ocular abnormalities are retinal detachment and a fibrovascular retrolental membrane [Heathcote et al., 1991].

There are often associated ectodermal and skeletal anomalies [Carney, 1976]. Skin changes include atrophic scarring and alopecia, and nails can be flat and thin, commonly with transverse ridges. Skeletal abnormalities include spina bifida, hemivertebrae, accessory ribs, and syndactyly. Delayed dentition, pegged teeth, and abnormal crown formation are also seen.

Skin biopsy specimens obtained early in the course of the disease demonstrate a perivascular inflammatory infiltrate composed principally of eosinophils. The verrucous stage is characterized by hyperkeratosis and epidermal hyperplasia, and the third stage is notable for hyperpigmentation, with numerous melanophages found within the dermis. Electron microscopic examination of these lesions documents defects of the basement membrane, with melanocytic dendritic processes containing melanosomes and melanin granules extending into the dermis.

Few neuropathologic studies are available. Some reports have described micropolygyria, cortical atrophy, and small areas of leukomalacia; however, these findings can be nonspecific and unrelated to the disease process [Hauw et al., 1977]. MRI studies suggest that the underlying cerebral pathology may be microvascular infarcts associated with the occlusion of small vessels [Hennel et al., 2003; Lee et al., 1995].

Treatment remains symptomatic and supportive. Recent case reports indicate some success in treating early skin lesions with corticosteroids [Kaya et al., 2009] or topical tacrolimus [Jessup et al., 2009].

Incontinentia Pigmenti Achromians (Hypomelanosis of Ito)

Incontinentia pigmenti achromians initially was described by Ito [Ito, 1951] and has been known as systemic achromic nevus and hypomelanosis of Ito. Typical skin changes occur as hypopigmented lesions on any part of the head, trunk, or limbs, either unilaterally or bilaterally. The configuration of the hypopigmented lesions may manifest as linear streaks or whorls of hypopigmentation that follow the lines of Blaschko. The skin lesions are congenital. Multiple associated anomalies are common and can involve the central nervous system or the peripheral nervous system, eyes, and bone [Takematsu et al., 1983; Hamada et al., 1967, 1979]. Common central nervous system abnormalities include mental retardation, language disabilities, seizures, and motor system dysfunction. Ocular abnormalities include strabismus, epicanthic folds, myopia, optic nerve hypoplasia, and hypopigmentation of the fundus; rarely, corneal asymmetry, pannus, and atrophic irides with irregular pupillary margins have been reported. Cataracts and retinal detachments also have been reported. Visual loss has not been reported in patients with incontinentia pigmenti achromians [Takematsu et al., 1983; Weaver et al., 1991].

Characteristic histologic features of skin biopsy specimens include dyskeratosis, increased dermal mastocytes, and pilosebaceous abnormalities. Electron microscopy reveals few melanosomes, sparsely dendritic melanocytes, and a reduction in the number of melanosomes in keratinocytes [Schwartz et al., 1977].

In one study [Ruggieri et al., 1996], MRI was performed in 13 affected patients, and anomalies of the white matter were observed in 7. Abnormal signals in white matter were located primarily in the parietal, periventricular, and subcortical regions of both hemispheres, and asymmetry of the cerebral and cerebellar hemispheres was observed in each of two patients. A correlation between the white matter changes and neurologic symptoms and signs was noted.

Hypomelanosis of Ito occurs sporadically and in many cases has been found to be associated with mosaicism for chromosomal abnormalities. The abnormal cells may be confined to the skin lesions and therefore are detected only by cytogenetic analysis of cultured fibroblasts obtained by skin biopsy. No single chromosome abnormality accounts for all cases; rather, it appears that the streaky hypopigmentation associated with the disorder, or sometimes patches of hyperpigmentation following Blaschko's lines, are the cutaneous manifestation of mosaicism for various genes or chromosomal regions [Ritter et al., 1990; Taibjee et al., 2004; Zajac et al., 1997; Flannery, 1990].

Wyburn–Mason Syndrome (Retinocephalic Angiomatosis)

One of the first descriptions of a retinal vascular malformation was by Magnus [1874], who viewed it as a medical curiosity. Yates and Paine [1930] reported an extensive retinal and ipsilateral cerebral arteriovenous malformation in a patient who died from cerebral hemorrhage, but the association of a unilateral arteriovenous malformation of the retina, brain, and parts of the face and head initially was described in a postmortem examination report by Brock and Dyke [1932]. Bonnet et al. [1937] emphasized the importance of a coexisting tortuous angioma of the fundus in patients with intracranial arteriovenous malformations. In 1943, Wyburn–Mason described the clinical syndrome in detail [1943]. Although known as Bonnet–Dechaum–Blanc syndrome in Europe and as Wyburn–Mason syndrome in the United Kingdom and the United States, the condition is more appropriately called a retinocephalic vascular malformation. The syndrome is thought to result from an embryonic abnormality in the development of the optic nerve pathway and related vessels from its origin in the mesencephalon all the way to the projection to the retina.

Wyburn–Mason [1943] reviewed reports of 27 patients with retinal angiomas and found signs of intracranial arteriovenous malformations in 22 patients. He later surveyed reports of 20 other patients with midbrain arteriovenous malformations and found 14 of those with associated retinal arteriovenous malformations. He then suggested that the syndrome was more common than had been suspected and that patients with vascular malformations of the retina or brain were likely to have other organs similarly affected. Because many of his patients had not been studied with cerebral angiography and only two patients had neuropathologic confirmation of the lesion, his suggestions were criticized, and the syndrome has been considered rare [Bech and Jensen, 1958]. Schmidt et al. [2008] reviewed the 121 patients with retinal arteriovenous malformations in the literature, and found that 27 had typical retinocephalic angiomatosis, 25 lacked the facial skin lesions, 57 had apparent isolated retinal arteriovenous malformations, and 12 had retinal arteriovenous communications and neurologic signs, but no neuroradiologic evidence of cerebral arteriovenous malformations. The retinal lesions are unilateral and readily observed by ophthalmoscopy. The vascular malformation affects one or all retinal vessels, which are notably dilated and tortuous. Ocular enlargement, conjunctival hyperemia,

and proptosis usually occur; a cranial bruit is commonly present. Visual function of the involved eye is rarely normal, and the visual loss varies according to the severity of the vascular malformation. The retrobulbar soft tissue and optic nerve commonly are affected by the malformed vessels [Hoyt and Cameron, 1968; Reck et al., 2005].

The intracranial vascular malformation usually is deep within the brain substance and can involve the mesencephalon, diencephalon, and basal ganglia, extending to the visual pathways and chiasm. Variable involvement of the cranial nerves occurs, including the third, sixth, seventh, and eighth nerves; nystagmus and Parinaud's syndrome have been reported. Corticospinal tract dysfunction can be unilateral or bilateral, and some patients are ataxic [Hoyt and Cameron, 1968; Theron et al., 1974]. Approximately one-half of patients have vascular malformations that affect the palate, oral mucosa, maxilla, and mandible. Cutaneous lesions also can occur, manifesting as angiomas or punctate erythematous lesions.

The diagnosis of this syndrome is initially considered when the retinal vascular lesion is observed. Cranial CT and MRI scans clearly demonstrate arteriovenous malformation, but only cerebral angiography reliably delineates the extent of the lesion [Fujita et al., 1989; Hopen et al., 1983]. No beneficial treatment method is currently available for this syndrome. The surgical removal of part or all of the extensive vascular malformation cannot be performed with any practical success, and the use of rigorous radiologic interventional techniques has been unsuccessful.

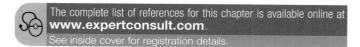

Degenerative Disorders Primarily of Gray Matter

Rose-Mary N. Boustany and Mohamad K. El-Bitar

This chapter groups together the seemingly disparate entities of Rett's syndrome (RTT), Menkes' disease, Alpers' disease, and various forms of Batten's disease. The first assumption is that they are neurodegenerative diseases that progress after a relatively normal period of early development. That is true for most, with the exception of Menkes' disease, in which affected children are abnormal from birth. The second assumption is that cerebral and cerebellar cortex and deep gray structures are affected, with neuronal loss occurring in most and defective cellular function occurring in all. The third and most tenuous assumption is that the white matter or myelin is spared or only secondarily affected because of Wallerian degeneration. As more is learned about the cellular pathobiology of these disorders, it has become apparent that myelin and white matter are affected in a primary way and not as a result of neuronal loss or malfunction. Great strides have been made in defining the underlying genetics and molecular defects of these diseases. The next frontier is to understand the functions of the identified proteins and to devise intelligent, effective, and targeted therapies for these devastating disorders.

Rett's Syndrome

Rett's syndrome is an X-linked disease that primarily affects females. It is the second leading cause of mental retardation in females, with an incidence of 1 case per 10,000–22,000 females [Hagberg et al., 1985; Kozinetz et al., 1993]. All ethnicities are equally affected. The hallmarks of this syndrome are a period of normal development followed by regression of speech and development of stereotypical hand gestures. The genes that cause this syndrome are *MECP2*, which maps to the Xq28 locus, *CDKL5* (cyclin-dependent kinase-like 5) gene (previously known as *STK9*) located in Xp22 [Scala et al., 2005; Kalscheue et al., 2003; Evans et al., 2005], *Netrin G1* gene, located on chromosome 1 [Borg et al., 2005], and *FOXG1* gene, located in 14q12 [Ariani et al., 2008]. The MECP2 protein is thought to be necessary for the maintenance of neurons during the later stages of development and after neuronal maturation is complete. The structure and function of the MECP2 protein continue to be the focus of intense scrutiny. Although this syndrome has many severe manifestations, approximately 50 percent of affected individuals live into the third decade of life. Despite the advances in knowledge about the cause and defects of Rett's syndrome during the past decade, treatment remains primarily supportive.

History

Rett's syndrome was first reported in 1966 by Dr. Andreas Rett [Rett, 1966]. This initial case report was followed in 1978 with a publication about Japanese female patients with a particular pattern of symptoms, including mental retardation and stereotypical hand-wringing [Ishikawa et al., 1978]. It was not until 1983, when Hagberg et al. [1983] published a case report of 35 female patients, that Rett's syndrome gained international attention. Intense investigation of Rett's syndrome over the past 20 years led to identification of the genetic defect in 1999 [Amir et al., 1999], 2005 [Borg et al., 2005; Scala et al., 2005; Kalscheue et al., 2003; Evans et al., 2005], and 2008 [Ariani et al., 2008].

Clinical Description

The diagnosis of Rett's syndrome is based on a set of clinical observations accompanied by changes in various laboratory test results. The clinical criteria for classic Rett's syndrome were established in the 1980s [Hagberg et al., 1985; Trevathan and Moser, 1988], and include loss of speech, seizures, mental retardation, and classic motor (specifically hand) movements. Criteria for atypical Rett's syndrome were reported in 1993 [Hagberg and Gillberg, 1993]. More than 75 percent of patients have classic Rett's syndrome, whereas 25 percent have atypical Rett's syndrome variants [Hagberg, 2002].

In classic Rett's syndrome (Table 41-1), the newborn initially appears developmentally normal. This period is followed by deceleration of head growth, loss of purposeful hand movements, development of stereotypic hand movements, and gait dyspraxia. These five criteria must be met for the diagnosis of classic Rett's syndrome [Hagberg, 1995]. The chronology of these symptoms is critical for the diagnosis. Normal development is typical for the first 3–6 months of life. Deceleration in the rate of head growth occurs between 3 months and 4 years. Patients lose the ability to use their hands in a purposeful manner between 9 months and 2.5 years. Stereotypic hand movements appear between 1 and 3 years of age, and a dyspraxic gait manifests between 2 and 4 years of age if the patient is ambulatory.

Clinical manifestations of classic Rett's syndrome are grouped into four stages: early onset (3–6 months of age), regression (1–4 years of age), stabilization, and late motor impairment (after the age of 3 years) [Jellinger, 2003]. The early-onset stage is characterized by developmental delay,

Table 41-1 Obligatory Criteria for the Diagnosis of Rett's Syndrome

Manifestation	Age	Comments
Period of normal neonatal development	0–6 mo	Prenatal or perinatal period into the first 6 months of life, sometimes longer
Stagnation of rate of head circumference growth	3 mo–4 yr	Normal at birth, then decelerates
Loss of purposeful hand skills	9 mo–2.5 yr	Communicative dysfunction, social withdrawal, mental deficiency, loss of speech or babbling
Classic stereotypic hand movements	1–3 yr	Hand-washing or hand-wringing and variants, including clapping and tapping, are common
Gait or posture dyspraxia Absence of organomegaly, optic atrophy, retinal changes, or delayed intrauterine growth	2–4 yr	Truncal "ataxia"

(Data from Hagberg B. Clinical manifestations and stages of Rett syndrome. Ment Retard Dev Disabil 2002;8:61–65, and from Percy AK. Clinical trials and treatment prospects. Ment Retard Dev Disabil 2002;8:106–111.)

deceleration of head growth [Neul and Zoghbi, 2004; Schultz et al., 1993], onset of autistic-like behavior, and classic hand-wringing [Jellinger, 2003]. Weight and height percentiles for age also decrease; the median values fall below the fifth percentile by age 7 years [Percy, 2002]. Although Rett's syndrome can manifest earlier, clear signs of a central nervous system abnormality are usually not evident until 6 months of age [Akbarian, 2003]. The second stage of the syndrome is characterized by cognitive decline and regression [Hagberg, 2002]. Loss of speech and purposeful hand movements, emergence of stereotypic movements, seizures, breathing irregularities, other signs of autonomic instability, inattentive behavior, and hypotonia appear [Hagberg, 2002; Jellinger, 2003; Kerr et al., 2001]. The third stage consists of stabilization of symptoms; this stage differentiates Rett's syndrome clinically from other pediatric neurodegenerative disorders. Sometimes there is a return of communication skills, with preservation of remaining ambulatory skills. This stage is also known as the pseudostationary stage because slow neuromotor regression continues [Hagberg, 1995]. In patients older than 3 years, bradykinesia and rigidity set in [Fitzgerald et al., 1990]. Stabilization can last years to decades. Late motor impairment begins when ambulation ceases; this signals the end of the stabilization or pseudostationary stage. This final stage of Rett's syndrome is characterized by nonambulation and severe disability. The length of late motor impairment is variable and can last decades.

Common clinical manifestations of classic Rett's syndrome include stereotypic hand movements, intense staring, breathing irregularities, bruxism, sleep disturbances and night laughter, scoliosis, lower limb spasticity and dystonia, seizures, swallowing dysfunction, constipation, gastroesophageal reflux, and small, bluish or red feet. The stereotypic hand movements occur while the individual is awake. These gestures are individualized, but they typically include continuous and repetitive twisting, wringing, knitting, and clapping motions. The intense eye communication may be compensatory for the loss of speech. This eye pointing has been observed in many individuals with Rett's syndrome. The breathing irregularities are of two types: hyperventilation and breath-holding. Typically, they occur only while the individual is awake, but can also occur during sleep [d'Orsi et al., 2009a].

Periods of apnea can last 30–40 seconds, and they disrupt stretches of hyperventilation. Most individuals with Rett's

syndrome experience sleep disturbances. It has also been reported that up to 90 percent of young children interrupt sleep with night laughter.

Although it is not pathognomonic, many individuals with Rett's syndrome have early growth retardation of their feet. The nails and skin demonstrate trophic changes, and the skin is cool to touch and discolored with a blue–red color. Autonomic dysregulation may produce some of these changes. The scoliosis in Rett's syndrome is a double-curve deformation that develops during the first decade of life. Most commonly, the double curve has a longer upper curve and a shorter lower curve. The incidence of scoliosis increases with age, occurring in 8 percent of preschool patients and 80 percent of patients older than 16 years. Abnormalities of the lower extremities in Rett's syndrome include asymmetric distal dystonia, mild spasticity, and feet that tend to orient in a flexed and supinated position.

Seizures are reported in 30–80 percent of individuals with Rett's syndrome. The electroencephalogram (EEG) is always abnormal after the age of 2 years. Early-onset seizures were reported in patients with *CDKL5* [Artuso et al., 2010] and *Netrin G1* gene mutations [Borg et al., 2005]. Prevalence of drug-resistant epilepsy in RTT patients with *MeCP2* mutations was 16 percent. No significant relationship was found between clinical severity of drug-resistant epilepsy and quantitative or qualitative EEG scores. In addition, no significant relationship was found between the drug-resistant epilepsy and the RTT genotype category, or a specific *MECP2* genotype [Buoni et al., 2008]. Myoclonic status had been misdiagnosed as a movement disorder of gait impairment [Pelc and Dan, 2009; d'Orsi et al., 2009b]. Infrequent clinical manifestations of classic Rett's syndrome include bloating, violent screaming, abnormal nociception, pain insensitivity [Devarakonda et al., 2009], hyperkalemic distal renal tubular acidosis [Assadi et al., 2006], and cardiac arrhythmias [Acampa and Guideri, 2006]. Bloating or air swallowing is generally mild, but 5–10 percent of individuals with Rett's syndrome demonstrate severe bloating. Massive gastric dilatation, with total necrosis and perforation due to bloating, has been reported [Baldassarrea et al., 2006]. The gastrointestinal disturbances are attributed to changes within the autonomic nervous system. Screaming typically is encountered in teenage patients. The screaming may be associated with ill-defined pain, but no known pathology can be found. Occasionally, patients have abnormally prolonged responses or insensitivity to pain. Children and adults with Rett's syndrome are at substantially increased risk of fracture. The lower limbs, especially the femur, are particularly susceptible and patients with the *R270X* and *R168X* mutations genotype are especially vulnerable. The presence of epilepsy also increased fracture risk [Downs et al., 2008]. Although a decreased life span is characteristic for this syndrome, many patients survive into adulthood [Sekul and Percy, 1992], with 50 percent remaining alive in their 30s [Akbarian, 2003].

The atypical Rett's syndrome variants include a forme fruste variant, early seizure type variant, late childhood regression variant, preserved speech variant, and congenital Rett's syndrome. Diagnosis of atypical Rett's syndrome is complex. The criteria for variants of classic Rett's syndrome, as outlined by Hagberg and Skjeldal [1994], are especially helpful (Box 41-1). Forme fruste is the most common atypical variant, accounting for about 80 percent of nonclassic Rett's syndrome. There is a wide variability of function in forme fruste; it is a milder variant. It is seldom diagnosed before 8–10 years of age, and it is usually suspected in older individuals who are just beginning to develop symptoms of Rett's syndrome. The early-onset seizure variant is linked to mutations in *CDKL5* and *Netrin G1* gene and manifests with early epilepsy onset between the first week and 5 months, hand stereotypies, severely impaired psychomotor development, and severe hypotonia [Artuso et al., 2010; Borg et al., 2005]. The late childhood regression form is characterized by a normal head circumference and by a more gradual and later onset (late childhood) of regression of language and motor skills. The preserved speech variant was first described in 1992 [Zappella, 1992]. It is characterized by the preservation of speech, but preserved head size and obesity are also common features [Zappella, 1992; Zappella et al., 2001]. There is some debate about whether the preserved speech variant is part of the autistic spectrum disorders, as well as the Rett's syndrome spectrum [Percy et al., 1990]. Congenital Rett's syndrome is rare. It differs from classic Rett's syndrome because of the absence of the 3- to 6-month period of normal development [Hagberg and Skjeldal, 1994]. It is linked to mutations in *FOXG1* gene [Ariani et al., 2008].

Clinical Diagnostic Tests

Routine Laboratory Tests

Levels of lactate, pyruvate, and glutamate are increased in cerebrospinal fluid [Budden et al., 1990; Lappalainen et al., 1997a]. Cerebrospinal fluid testing yields decreased levels of β-phenylalanine, substance P, and gangliosides [Lekman et al., 1991; Matsuishi et al., 1997; Satoi et al., 2000]. There are increased levels of biogenic amines and creatine in the urine [Lekman et al., 1990]. Plasma levels of levels of β-endorphin and prolactin are decreased [Fanchetti et al., 1986]. The increased levels of lactate and pyruvate in the cerebrospinal fluid may result from hyperventilation [Budden et al., 1990], whereas the decreased levels of cerebrospinal fluid β-phenylalanine are caused by dysregulation of the dopaminergic pathways in patients with Rett's syndrome [Satoi et al., 2000]. The levels of IgA and IgG antibodies to gluten and gliadin proteins found in grains and to casein found in milk are significantly increased in girls with Rett's syndrome [Reichelt and Skjeldal, 2006].

Box 41-1 Defining Variants of Rett's Syndrome

Inclusion Criteria

1. A girl of at least 10 years of age with mental retardation of unexplained origin
2. And three of the six primary criteria defined below
3. And six of the eleven supportive manifestations defined below

Primary Criteria

1. Partial or subtotal loss of acquired fine finger skill in late infancy or early childhood
2. Loss of acquired single words, phrases, or nuanced babble
3. Stereotypic Rett's syndrome hand movements, with hands together or apart
4. Early deviant communicative ability
5. Deceleration in head growth of two standard deviations below the mean (even if head growth or circumference is still within normal limits)
6. Rett's syndrome profile
   - Stage I – early-onset stagnation
   - Stage II – period of regression
   - Stage III – recovery of some contact and communicative abilities after stage II. Slow neuromotor regression that lasts through school age and adolescence
   - Stage IV – late motor deterioration. Slow neuromotor regression that lasts through school age and adolescence

Supportive Manifestations

1. Breathing irregularities (e.g., hyperventilation, breath-holding)
2. Bloating or air swallowing
3. Teeth grinding
4. Gait dyspraxia
5. Neurogenic scoliosis or high kyphosis (in ambulant girls)
7. Development of abnormal lower limb neurology
8. Small, blue or cold, impaired feet; autonomic or trophic dysfunction
9. Abnormal electroencephalogram, consistent with Rett's syndrome
10. Unprompted laughing or screaming spells
11. Impaired or delayed nociception
12. Intensive eye communication (i.e., eye pointing)

Neurophysiologic Tests

The EEG is abnormal in Rett's syndrome. Initial abnormalities are noticed in the rapid eye movement stage of sleep [Kudo et al., 2003]. During the stabilization stage of Rett's syndrome, a slow spike-wave pattern resembling that in Lennox–Gastaut syndrome is observed [Glaze, 1987]. After 3 years of age, there is a decrease in alpha activity with a subsequent increase in theta activity [Bashina et al., 1994]. Evoked potential studies indicate intact visual and auditory peripheral pathways and dysfunction of central cortical pathways involved in processing and integration of sensory information in young girls with Rett's syndrome. Somatosensory-evoked potentials can be characterized by "giant" responses, suggesting cortical hyperexcitability [Glaze, 2005]. There is a prolongation of somatosensory-evoked responses in older patients, suggesting involvement of the upper spinal cord and spinothalamic tracts [Bader et al., 1989]. Results of nerve conduction studies are consistent with an axonopathy and denervation indicative of lower motor dysfunction [Jellinger et al., 1990]. Impairment of the autonomic nervous system in Rett's syndrome is suggested by an increased incidence of long QT intervals during electrocardiographic recordings and diminished heart rate variability [Glaze, 2005].

Neuroimaging Studies

Initial cranial computed tomographic (CT) scans and magnetic resonance imaging (MRI) are normal. As the patient ages and neurologic symptoms develop, generalized atrophy of the cerebral hemispheres and decreased volume of the caudate nucleus become apparent [Reiss et al., 1993]. Imaging of the basal ganglia reveals decreased volume of the caudate head [Dunn et al., 2002]. Commonly, there is a decrease in gray and white matter volumes, specifically within the frontal and temporal regions, and of the midbrain and cerebellum [Subramaniam et al., 1997]. Hypoperfusion of the prefrontal and temporoparietal regions is also reported [Lappalainen et al., 1997b]. Although imaging studies can help in making the diagnosis, there is no correlation between spectroscopic changes and clinical status [Gokcay et al., 2002]. One study reported an association between the level of hypoperfusion and early-onset Rett's syndrome [Lappalainen et al., 1997b]. In more recent MR spectroscopy studies of RTT patients with *MeCP2* mutations, NAA/Cr ratios decreased and myoinositol/Cr ratios increased with age. The mean glutamate and glutamine/Cr ratio was increased. The mean NAA/Cr ratio decreased in RTT patients with seizures and with increasing clinical severity score. Compared to patients with *T158X*, *R255X*, and *R294X* mutations, and C-terminal deletions, patients with the *R168X* mutation tended to have the greatest severity score and the lowest NAA/Cr ratio. Decreasing NAA/Cr and increasing myoinositol/Cr with age are suggestive of progressive axonal damage and astrocytosis in RTT, respectively, whereas increased glutamate and glutamine/Cr ratio may be secondary to increasing glutamate/glutamine cycling at the synaptic level [Horska et al., 2009].

Pathology

Brain

Gross findings include generalized atrophy of the frontal and temporal regions, the cerebellum, and especially the vermis. The corpus callosum decreases in size by as much as 30 percent [Oldfors et al., 1990; Reiss et al., 1993]. The brain is the only organ that is decreased in size compared with height [Armstrong et al., 1999]. Cerebellar volume is reported to remain relatively normal. The average weight of a brain from a patient with Rett's syndrome is about 950 g, equivalent to the weight of a brain from a developmentally normal 1-year-old child [Armstrong, 2000]. More importantly, the brain weight does not continue to decrease with age, because Rett's syndrome is not a progressive neurodevelopmental disorder in the classic sense.

There are many microscopic findings in brain tissue from Rett's syndrome patients. Neuronal size is decreased, but cell

density in the cerebral cortex, thalamus, basal ganglia, amygdala, and hippocampus is increased [Bauman et al., 1995]. The previous findings contrast with a report of an overall decrease in the number of neurons in the frontal cortex, the temporal cortex, and the cholinergic nucleus basalis of Meynert [Belichenko et al., 1994; Kitt and Wilcox, 1995]. Decreases in dendritic branching and dendritic number are found in the frontal, motor, and subicular areas [Armstrong, 1997; Armstrong et al., 1995; Cornford, 1994]. In addition to decreases in dendritic number and branches, shortening of the apical and basilar dendritic branches within these same regions of the brain has been reported [Armstrong et al., 1998]. Afferent neurons have decreased synaptic contacts. The striatum and internal pallidum exhibit hypochromia, whereas hypomyelination is observed in the substantia nigra pars compacta [Jellinger et al., 1988]. The neocortex has decreased expression of microtubule-associated protein 2, and disruption of the cytoskeleton within the neocortex is apparent [Kaufmann et al., 1995]. The caudate nucleus and putamen exhibit reduced levels of dopamine transporter protein [Wong et al., 1998]. Degenerative changes of the substantia nigra, caudate nucleus, and putamen have been demonstrated in neuropathological and neurochemical studies of RTT brains. Stereotypies and other movement disorders present in RTT could be interpreted as signs of dysfunction of the nigrostriatal-dopaminergic pathway [Kitt and Wilcox, 1995; Wenk, 1995].

There are conflicting results regarding the expression of nerve growth factor in Rett's syndrome patients. One study documented no reduction in the cortical levels of nerve growth factor [Wenk and Hauss-Wgrzyniak, 1999], and others demonstrated large decreases in the expression of nerve growth factor and the neurotrophic tyrosine kinase type receptor, which binds to nerve growth factor with high affinity [Lipani et al., 2000]. Adults with Rett's syndrome also have axonal degeneration, loss of motor neurons, loss of spinal ganglion cells, and decreased glutamate and gamma-aminobutyric acid type B (GABA B) receptor density [Oldfors et al., 1988; Blue et al., 1999]. Blue et al. [1999] reported age-specific alterations in amino acid neurotransmitter receptors within the basal ganglia of adults.

Electron microscopy of neurons depicts distinct abnormalities [Papadimitriou et al., 1988]. These changes include abnormal neurites that are filled with lysosomes and laminate bodies. Axonal swellings, large mitochondria, and membranous multilamellar bodies are seen. Although electron microscopy reveals intraneuronal inclusion bodies that contain lipofuscin-like material, there are no other characteristics of a lipid storage disorder.

Muscle

Type I and type II fiber atrophy is sometimes seen on muscle biopsy [Wakia et al., 1990]. Decreased cytochrome c oxidase and succinate cytochrome c reductase activities in muscle biopsies have also been reported [Coker and Melnyk, 1991]. The myocardium has no gross abnormalities. The atrioventricular node has an abnormal or immature rearrangement of muscle fibers within the conduction system [Armstrong, 1997]. Electron microscopy of muscle biopsy specimens reveals dumbbell-shaped mitochondria with foamy vacuoles [Ruch et al., 1989].

Genetics

Rett's syndrome is an X-linked dominant disorder that has been mapped to the Xq28 locus [Ellison et al., 1992; Sirianni et al., 1998]. Although most cases of Rett's syndrome are sporadic, genetic mapping was possible because familial inheritance does occur, and there is concordance in monozygotic twins [Jellinger, 2003]. Mutations within the methyl-CpG binding protein 2 gene (*MECP2*) cause 70–80 percent of reported cases of Rett's syndrome in females [Auranen et al., 2001; Van den Veyver and Zoghbi, 2002]. This gene was identified in 1999 [Amir et al., 1999]. Most mutations in males lead to fetal demise. Although DNA mitochondrial mutations are found in some cases of Rett's syndrome, there is no indication that mitochondrial DNA plays a part in the development of this syndrome [Nielson et al., 1993; Colantuoni et al., 2001]. Mutations within *MECP2* have also been linked to childhood-onset schizophrenia, Angelman's syndrome, and mild mental retardation [Watson et al., 2001].

The MECP2 protein has three known functional domains: an amino-terminal methyl-CpG binding domain [Lewis et al., 1992], a transcriptional repressor domain, and a carboxyl-terminal domain [Chandler et al., 1999]. The MECP2 protein binds to methylated CpG dinucleotides by the methyl-CpG binding domain [Nan et al., 1993]. The transcriptional repressor domain interacts with various co-repressor complexes and disrupts transcription [Nan et al., 1996, 1997]. The nuclear localization signal (NLS), consisting of amino acid residues 265–271, is contained within the transcriptional repressor domain. The biochemical function of the carboxyl-terminal region is unknown [Kriaucionis and Bird, 2003]. Seventy percent of the mutations within *MECP2* are in eight hotspots affecting translation of the following amino acids: R106, R133, T158, R168, R255, R270, R294, and R306. Seven of these eight mutation hotspots affect arginine, which contains a CpG in its codon. These mutations may result from unrepaired deamination of 5-methylcytosine. This mechanism is thought to cause one-third of all point mutations that lead to human genetic disease [Cooper and Youssoufian, 1988]. Eighty percent of females with classic Rett's syndrome have nonsense or frameshift mutations within the *MECP2* gene [Van den Veyver and Zoghbi, 2002].

Genotype–Phenotype Correlation

Genotype–phenotype correlation has been attempted, but it is complicated by *MECP2* gene X-chromosome inactivation. This inactivity allows a mother with a mutation of *MECP2* to have a normal phenotype because of skewing of X-chromosome inactivation. If this mother has a daughter with the mutation of *MECP2* but balanced X-chromosome inactivation, the daughter will have Rett's syndrome [Amir et al., 2000]. Despite the problems with X-chromosome inactivation, many studies of genotype–phenotype correlations exist. It is reported that truncated mutations of *MECP2* are more severe than missense mutations [Chae et al., 2002; Cheadle et al., 2000; Monros et al., 2001]. The location of the truncation generally does not affect the phenotype [Bienvenu et al., 2000; Giunti et al., 2001; Huppke et al., 2000; Satoi et al., 2000; Amir et al., 2000] reported that truncation mutations led to increased levels of homovanillic acid in cerebrospinal fluid and to increased respiratory problems. The same study reported an increased incidence of scoliosis in cases of missense mutations.

Huppke et al. [2002] examined mutations from 123 patients with Rett's syndrome. They determined that mutations affecting the NLS caused the most severe phenotype. They also reported that deletions within the carboxyl terminus caused the least severe clinical presentation. Truncations result in more severe disease than missense mutations, except when the truncation affects the carboxyl terminus. Single-amino acid mutations cause less severe phenotypes, presumably because they lead to mild impairment of protein function [Laccone et al., 2002].

Rett's Syndrome Variants

Most of the mutations within *MECP2* cause classic Rett's syndrome. Twenty-nine cases of the preserved speech variant of Rett's syndrome have mutations within the *MECP2* gene [Conforti et al., 2003; Hoffbuhr et al., 2001; Huppke et al., 2000; Neul and Zoghbi, 2004; Nielsen et al., 2001; Obata et al., 2000; Weaving et al., 2003; Yamashita et al., 2001; Zappella et al., 2001]. These mutations were evenly distributed among the three known functional domains of the *MECP2* gene: the methyl-CpG binding domain, the transcriptional repressor domain, and the carboxyl-terminal domain. Mutations resulting in less severe phenotypes (i.e., mutations within the carboxyl terminus or a truncation after the NLS motif) were common in patients with the preserved speech variant of Rett's syndrome. Patients with the preserved speech variant who had mutations normally associated with severe disease had skewed X-chromosome inactivation (92:8 in one case), explaining the less severe phenotypes [Hoffbuhr et al., 2001; Zappella et al., 2001].

MECP2 *Mutations in Males*

Three outcomes occur in males: Rett's syndrome, severe encephalopathy with neonatal fatality, and mild neuropsychiatric phenotypes [Geerdink et al., 2002; Villard et al., 2000; Wan et al., 1999; Zeev et al., 2002]. The classic form of Rett's syndrome can occur in males [Jan et al., 1999]. Although similar mutations are seen in males and females with this disease, there is a report of a unique mutation within *MECP2* that causes Rett's syndrome in males [Ravn et al., 2003]. Male siblings of female Rett's syndrome patients with identical *MECP2* mutations develop a severe encephalopathy and die by 1–2 years of age. These mutations typically affect the methyl-CpG binding domain or the NLS portion of the MECP2 protein.

Rett's syndrome is produced as a result of somatic mosaicism, meaning there is a mixed population of cells with the wild type of *MECP2* and mutated *MECP2* [Armstrong et al., 2001; Clayton-Smith et al., 2000; Topcu et al., 2002]. Males with Rett's syndrome have a unique genetic composition. Klinefelter's syndrome (46,XXY) allows phenotypic males to replicate the somatic mosaicism achieved by females and avoid neonatal fatality [Leonard et al., 2003; Schwartzman et al., 2001]. There are case reports of Rett's syndrome occurring in a phenotypic male, in whom the *SRY* region of the Y chromosome that produces "maleness" is translocated on to an X chromosome, so that a phenotypic male is genotypically a female (46,XX) [Maiwald et al., 2002]. Mutations in the *MECP2* gene also occur in males with mental retardation and no other symptoms of Rett's syndrome. These mutations generally affect the carboxyl terminus of the methyl-CpG binding domain region of the MECP2 protein [Couvert et al., 2001; Kleefstra et al., 2002; Yntema et al., 2002a]. Whether these mutations contribute to the phenotypes observed, or are normal polymorphisms, is being explored [Laccone et al., 2002; Yntema et al., 2002b].

Cell Biology

Because Rett's syndrome is caused primarily by mutations within the *MECP2* gene, it is necessary to understand the function and interactions of the MECP2 protein. The *MECP2* gene encodes a protein with three known functional domains: the methyl-CpG binding domain, the transcriptional repressor domain, and the carboxyl terminus. Human MECP2 has 48 amino acids (about 80 kDa) [Akbarian, 2003]. The methyl-CpG binding domain contains 85 amino acids [Nan et al., 1993] and binds to single- and double-methylated CpG dinucleotides [Bird and Wolfe, 1999; Lewis et al., 1992]. There is a correlation between the capability of the methyl-CpG binding domain to bind to pericentromeric heterochromatic regions of DNA and the ability of the protein to repress methylated promoters [Kudo et al., 2003]. Residues R111, R133C, and R134C within the methyl-CpG binding domain are thought to come into contact with methylated cystines. Mutations affecting R111 cause the MECP2 protein to lose its binding ability to heterochromatic DNA and its capability to repress transcription. Mutations resulting in R133C or R134C affect neither of the aforementioned protein properties. The MECP2 protein associates with chromatin remodeling complexes and aids in the regulation of the structure and function of chromatin.

The transcriptional repressor domain is 100 base pairs (bp) long, and it interacts with various co-repressor complexes [Nan et al., 1997]. One of these complexes is the Sin3A co-repressor complex. This complex contains histone deacetylases 1 and 2, which remove acetyl groups from histones and create a compressed form of chromatin that then inhibits or represses gene expression [Nan et al., 1998]. The action of the transcriptional repressor domain is partially reversed by trichostatin A, a histone deacetylase inhibitor. This finding suggests that repression by means of the transcriptional repressor domain is caused by histone deacetylation. *MECP2* recruits these histone deacetylases and other chromatin remodeling complexes to methylated CpG dinucleotides. This leads to chromatin condensation that interferes with the binding of transcription complexes [Akbarian, 2003]. The transcriptional repressor domain has also been seen to bind to *TFIIB* (also designated *GTF2B*), *SKI* (a proto-oncogene), *DNMT1* (which codes for a DNA methyltransferase), and *SUV39H1* (which codes for a histone methyltransferase), although the importance of these interactions is unknown [Fuks et al., 2003; Kaludov and Wolffe, 2000; Kimura and Shiota, 2003]. Repression can be mediated in other ways, because the MECP2 protein binds to general transcription factors and interferes with the binding of transcription complexes. The transcriptional repressor domain is able to repress transcription when bound as far as 2000 bp from the transcription initiation site. The carboxyl terminus is thought to be involved in the binding of MECP2 to naked and nucleosomal DNA. Specifically, the carboxyl-terminal region of the MECP2 protein binds to DNA that is coiled around histone octamers [Chandler et al., 1999].

The MECP2 protein is mostly located within the nucleus of cells, and a small portion is seen within the perikarya [Kaufmann et al., 1995]. Although MECP2 binds throughout chromosomes, binding is most dense around pericentromeric heterochromatic regions of DNA. Forty percent of methyl-CpGs (i.e., binding sites for the methyl-CpG binding domain) are found within pericentromeric heterochromatic DNA. The immunoreactivity of MECP2 is increased around centromeric and perinucleolar heterochromatin. MECP2 does not associate with ribosomal DNA, despite its many methylations. MECP2 distribution is regulated by unknown factors and does not simply distribute to where methylated CpGs are found. The MECP2 protein is thought to play a role in the maintenance of neuronal nuclei in the later stages of development and within the mature brain [Akbarian, 2003]. It is hypothesized that MECP2 makes chromatin more stable and less accessible to transcription factors by anchoring chromatin fibers into the nuclear matrix.

There are reduced levels of dopamine, serotonin, and their metabolites, homovanillic acid and 5-hydroxy-indoleacetic acid, in Rett's syndrome [Lekman et al., 1990]. Some researchers have noticed a decreased density of postsynaptic D_2 receptors in older patients with Rett's syndrome [Dunn, 2001], whereas others describe increased specific binding at D_2 receptors. The latter finding implies that the decreased levels of dopamine are causing increased levels or density of postsynaptic receptors [Chiron et al., 1993; Dunn et al., 2002]. The D_1 receptor density is unchanged [Wenk, 1995]. Jellinger et al. [1990] proposed that the different densities of postsynaptic receptors within the dopaminergic pathways might be age-specific. Increased choline concentrations and decreased choline acetyltransferase levels are thought to result from problems within the cholinergic system in the forebrain [Gokcay et al., 2002]. The frontal cortex and striatum have decreased levels of ferritin [Sofic et al., 1987]. Decreased levels of binding protein for the benzodiazepine receptor in the frontotemporal, parietal, and occipital regions of the brain also have been reported [Yamashita et al., 1998]. Significantly increased oxidative stress markers (intraerythrocyte non-protein-bound iron, plasma non-protein-bound iron, free F2-isoprostanes, esterified F2-isoprostanes, total F2-isoprostanes, and protein carbonyl concentrations) were evident in Rett's syndrome subjects and associated with reduced arterial oxygen levels compared to controls. Biochemical evidence of oxidative stress was related to clinical phenotype severity and lower peripheral and arterial oxygen levels. Pulmonary $\dot{V}/\dot{Q}$ mismatch was found in the majority of the Rett's syndrome population. These data identify hypoxia-induced oxidative stress as a key factor in the pathogenesis of classic Rett's syndrome [De Felice et al., 2009].

Animal Models

In a model of MECP2-null mice, males and females were affected. Homozygous female mice and heterozygous male mice were developmentally normal for the first several weeks of life, but they died soon after neurologic symptoms appeared [Chen et al., 2001; Guy et al., 2001]. This model replicates the genetic component of Rett's syndrome, but it was difficult to study because of the rapid deterioration and early death of the animals after symptoms appeared. Shahbazian et al. [2002] developed a mouse model that has a truncation mutation within the *MECP2* gene with a less severe phenotype than the MECP2-null mice. The truncated protein mimics a commonly observed human mutation, and it is partially functional, containing the methyl-CpG binding domain and transcriptional repressor domain. This group observed that the mice appeared developmentally normal up to 6 weeks after birth. After this period of normal development, the mice developed neurologic symptoms, including tremors, motor impairment, hypoactivity, seizures, kyphosis, and the classic forearm movements associated with human Rett's syndrome [Shahbazian et al., 2002b]. Random X-inactivation causes a variety of phenotypes due to a single genotype in females, which makes analysis of the mouse model difficult [Young and Zoghbi, 2004]. One solution is to use male mice, because they are not subject to random X-inactivation.

Luikenhuis et al. [2004] overexpressed MECP2 in postmitotic neurons of homozygous MECP2-null mice. These mice did not display any neurologic symptoms, and they were developmentally equivalent to the control population. In normal mice, *MECP2*-encoded RNA is not expressed until about 10 days after conception, and it reaches adult levels by 16 days after conception. It has been postulated that the defect in Rett's syndrome involves neuronal maintenance and maturation, and therefore affects developmental stability. Ballas et al. found that the loss of *MeCP2* occurs not only in neurons but also in glial cells of Rett brains, and that mutant astrocytes from a Rett mouse model, and their conditioned medium, failed to support normal dendritic morphology of either wild-type or mutant hippocampal neurons [Ballas et al., 2009]. This suggests that astrocytes in the Rett brain carrying *MeCP2* mutations have a non-cell autonomous effect on neuronal properties, probably as a result of aberrant secretion of soluble factor(s).

Pathogenesis

The timeline of MECP2 expression suggests that it is needed in the later phase of cortical development in neonates and after maturation in adults. MECP2 is expressed in normal fetal brains until 20 weeks' gestation, after which it disappears from the cerebellum. It disappears from the brainstem after the perinatal period. MECP2 does not reappear in the brain until after adolescence. Lack of MECP2 during any of these developmental periods may lead to synaptic and neuronal dysfunction of the catecholaminergic neurons in patients with Rett's syndrome [Itoh and Takashima, 2002]. Mice with MECP2 overexpressed in postmitotic neurons are rescued from the Rett's syndrome phenotype. A decrease in MECP2 in postmitotic neurons during the later stages of development is sufficient to cause Rett's syndrome [Chen et al., 2001], but MECP2 deficiency in neuronal precursors is probably not a major contributor to the pathogenesis in Rett's syndrome.

MECP2 causes transcriptional repression, and loss of function of this protein may cause an imbalance between transcription and gene silencing, leading to dysregulated gene expression and pathologic changes. Some groups have found no evidence for MECP2 transcriptional repression in neurons or glia. Gene expression studies found an increase in glial transcription, in contrast to the predicted decrease. Levels of presynaptic proteins, however, were decreased. MECP2 may be causing perturbations within the presynaptic signal transduction pathway [Colantuoni et al., 2001]. The critics

of this theory point out that these studies were performed on postmortem brains, suggesting that relevant time points in gene expression may have been missed. Additional evidence argues against MECP2 deficiency unsilencing transcription and causing Rett's syndrome. Affymetrix GeneChip analysis of MECP2-deficient human fibroblasts did not demonstrate any large-scale dysregulation of gene expression. There were only small differences in gene expression in presymptomatic, early symptomatic, and late symptomatic MECP2-deficient mouse brains [Tudor et al., 2002].

If MECP2 does not act as a transcriptional repressor, it may play a maintenance role during development. MECP2-encoded mRNA is undetectable in the mouse forebrain during midgestation [Coy et al., 1999]. Immunohistochemical studies in nonhuman primates and mice demonstrate MECP2 expression in neuronal nuclei correlates with neuronal maturity, and levels of expression are highest in the adult cerebral cortex [Akbarian et al., 2001]. In human cerebral cortex, MECP2 is seen only in Cajal–Retzius cells, the earliest maturing neurons [Marin-Padilla, 1998], at 14 weeks' gestation. At 26 weeks' gestation, MECP2-immunoreactive neurons are seen in the deeper, more differentiated cortical layers. MECP2 neuronal immunoreactivity increases with age. Only about 10 percent of cells are immunoreactive during the third trimester of pregnancy, but approximately 80 percent of neurons demonstrate immunoreactivity for MECP2 at 10 years of age [Shahbazian et al., 2002a]. These findings are also seen in rodents and nonhuman primates. The observation that MECP2 expression is decreased in immature neurons and elevated in mature neurons suggests a role for MECP2 in neuronal maintenance. MECP2 expression studies show high levels of the protein in mature neurons but not in glia or astrocytes.

MECP2 may also play a role in cell division. Removing pericentromeric heterochromatin or disrupting heterochromatin silencing by inhibition of histone deacetylases in *Drosophila* and yeast reduced chromosome transmission during cell division [Henikoff, 2001]. Because MECP2 associates with pericentromeric heterochromatin, it may influence cell division.

Treatment

Rett's syndrome has no cure. The treatments available have been empirically derived and are designed to combat specific symptoms. Antiepileptic agents include carbamazepine, valproic acid, and lamotrigine. The use of L-DOPA and dopamine agonists to increase motor ability in Rett's syndrome patients is controversial [Zappella, 1990]. A study of the treatment of Rett's syndrome with folate and betaine did not find any objective evidence of improvement [Glaze et al., 2009]. Zinc sulfate, lithium, and antidepressants have been demonstrated to increase central brain-derived neurotropic factor (BDNF) levels or signaling in human as well as animal studies. Thus, it is proposed that these agents could have therapeutic potential for RTT subjects [Tsai, 2006]. The breathing irregularities associated with Rett's syndrome can be treated with naltrexone, an opiate antagonist. Naltrexone (1–3 mg/kg/day) can reduce disorganized breathing and increases oxygen saturation levels [Percy, 2002]. Use of high-fat, high-calorie diets is recommended in the late stages of the disease, and it has been suggested that individuals with Rett's syndrome require a higher protein intake [Motil et al., 1999]. Feeding by means of a gastrostomy tube is sometimes indicated

[Jellinger, 2003]. Constipation in Rett's syndrome has been managed with high-fiber foods, enemas, mineral oils, milk of magnesia, and polyethylene glycol or MiraLax, with varying degrees of success. Orthopedists and physical therapists routinely see individuals with Rett's syndrome. The goals are to improve balance, enhance flexibility, and strengthen atrophying muscles. Bracing for scoliosis is necessary when a 25° curvature exists, and surgery is advised when the curvature exceeds 40°. Speech and occupational therapy are occasionally used to improve communication.

Small-scale clinical trials using L-carnitine and the ketogenic diet have been completed. L-Carnitine has been reported to improve the respiratory features of Rett's syndrome [Ellaway et al., 2001], and the ketogenic diet may reduce seizure frequency during the first 3 months, but no long-term clinical trials have been reported. A comprehensive, life-span approach to the management of scoliosis in Rett's syndrome is recommended that takes into account factors such as physical activity, posture, and nutritional and bone health needs. Surgery should be considered when the Cobb angle is approximately 40–50° and must be supported by specialist management of anesthesia, pain control, seizures, and early mobilization. Evidence- and consensus-based guidelines were successfully created and have the potential to improve care of a complex comorbidity in a rare condition and stimulate research to improve the current limited [Downs et al., 2009].

Menkes' Disease

Menkes' disease is an X-linked disorder caused by mutations in the *ATP7A* gene. The protein it encodes is necessary for absorption of copper from the intestinal epithelium and for transport of copper across the blood–brain barrier. The reported incidence is 1 case per 100,000 to 300,000 persons. Menkes' disease has three variants: classic disease, mild disease, and occipital horn syndrome. In classic disease, a 2- to 3-month period of normal development is followed by severe neurologic regression characterized by seizures, hypotonia, visual impairment, and failure to thrive. Death ensues by 4 years of age. Kinky, coarse, and lightly pigmented hair is pathognomonic for this disease, although many other phenotypic features may be observed. Connective tissue disorders are common in all three variants because of dysfunction of the cupric enzyme lysyl oxidase. Two biochemical markers, decreased serum copper and ceruloplasmin, in conjunction with clinical manifestations, aid in the diagnosis. The only available treatment is replacement therapy using copper histidine. Early intervention is essential for the therapy to be neuroprotective.

History

The story of the discovery of Menkes' disease begins in the 1930s, when veterinary physicians in Australia noticed the importance of copper for the normal development of sheep [Bennetts and Chapman, 1937]. They observed that mothers that grazed in copper-deficient pastures had offspring with cerebral demyelination, ataxia, and porencephaly. They concluded that copper deficiency in sheep was associated with ataxia and a demyelinating disease. The disease was described in 1962 by John Menkes [Menkes et al., 1962]. He described five males of English–Irish heritage who had "peculiar" hair, failure

to thrive, and a neurodegenerative disorder. The syndrome was initially called Menkes' kinky hair syndrome in reference to the unique appearance of the hair of these patients. The basis for Menkes' disease was not known until the association was made with the illness in sheep [Danks et al., 1972, 1973]. The distinctive hair found in the copper-deficient sheep and in patients provided the necessary link. Serum testing revealed that patients who had this distinctive hair also had decreased serum copper and ceruloplasmin levels. Danks et al. [1972, 1973] then concluded that Menkes' disease was a human example of a neurodevelopmental disorder caused by copper deficiency. In 1993, three groups used positional cloning to discover the *ATP7A* gene [Chelly et al., 1993; Mercer et al., 1993].

Clinical Description

Menkes' disease typically occurs in males. Its occipital horn syndrome variant is also known as X-linked cutis laxa [Danks, 1995]. In classic Menkes' disease, there is a period of normal development that typically lasts for 2–3 months [Kaler, 1994]. Developmental regression follows, with seizures, hypotonia, and failure to thrive [Kaler, 1998]. Patients exhibit severe mental retardation with symptoms of neurodegeneration [Mercer, 1998]. Most individuals with classic Menkes' disease die between the ages of 7 months and 4 years [Bankier, 1995]. Occipital horn syndrome is characterized by a less severe genetic mutation that results in a connective tissue disorder.

The characteristic findings in classic Menkes' disease are related to the patient's hair. Commonly described as steel-woolish, the hair on the scalp and eyebrows is short, sparse, coarse, and twisted. The amount of hair is decreased, and it is generally shorter on the sides of the head. The color is often light, with white, silver, and gray being common. Light microscopy of hair reveals three characteristic findings [Kaler, 1998; Moore and Howell, 1985]:

1. Pili torti is a 180° twisting of the hair shaft that is pathognomonic for Menkes' disease.
2. Trichoclasis is a transverse fracture of the hair shaft.
3. Trichoptilosis is longitudinal splitting of the hair shaft.

Hypopigmentation is common but not the rule, and is caused by a deficiency of catechol oxidase. Patients typically have large jowls, sagging cheeks, large ears, and a high-arched palate. The skin appears loose at the nape of the neck, in the axillae, and on the trunk. Delayed tooth eruption and pectus excavatum are common, and the incidence of umbilical hernias is increased. Nephrocalcinosis and chronic renal failure have also been reported [Balestracci et al., 2009].

Classic Menkes' disease has several distinctive neurologic findings. These patients exhibit truncal hypotonia with poor head control, hyperactive deep tendon reflexes, impaired visual fixation or tracking, and cortical adducted thumbs. There is increased appendicular tone, and asymmetric growth failure that appears shortly after neurodegeneration begins. EEGs are moderately or severely abnormal, and hypsarrhythmia occurs frequently [Venta-Sobero et al., 2004]. Ophthalmologic findings common in Menkes' disease include myopia, strabismus, and problems with visual fixation and tracking.

Connective tissue disorders are common in the three variants. Pelvic ultrasound and cystograms reveal diverticula of the urinary bladder [Daly and Rabinovitch, 1981; Harke et al., 1977].

Associated vascular disorders include lumbar and iliac artery aneurysms [Adaletli et al., 2005]. Skull and skeletal radiographs are notable for Wormian bones in the skull, metaphyseal spurring of the long bones, and anterior flaring or multiple fractures of the ribs [Adams et al., 1974; Capesius et al., 1977; Koslowski and McCrossin, 1979; Stanley et al., 1976]. Congenital skull fracture, related to global osteopenia, subdural hematoma, intrauterine growth delay, and lethal outcome, is reported in neonatal Menkes' disease [Veit-Sauca et al., 2009]. MRI demonstrates white matter changes and impaired myelination, cerebral blood vessel tortuosity, ventriculomegaly, and diffuse cerebral atrophy [Faerber et al., 1989; Johnsen et al., 1991]. White matter lesions localized in the deep periventricular white matter in the absence of diffuse cortical atrophy [Lee et al., 2007], and transient temporal lobe lesions related to vasogenic and cytotoxic edema [Ito et al., 2008] were reported.

Patients with occipital horn syndrome have hyperelastic skin and may develop other connective tissue disorders, including aortic aneurysms, hernias, bladder diverticula, and skeletal abnormalities, which most likely result from lysyl oxidase deficiency. The characteristic occipital horns are symmetric exostoses protruding from the occipital bone and pointing down. These may be present around 1–2 years of age, but are usually detected only around 5–10 years of age and continue to grow up to early adulthood [Tümer and Moller, 2009]. These individuals also have mild mental retardation and autonomic dysfunction that manifests as syncope, hypothermia, and diarrhea [Byers et al., 1980]. The severity of mild Menkes' disease falls between that in the classic form and the much milder occipital horn syndrome [Procopis et al., 1981]. It is important for patients with milder variations of Menkes' disease to have frequent vision examinations because ophthalmologic problems can greatly impair functioning of affected individuals.

Clinical and Biochemical Diagnoses

The clinical diagnosis of Menkes' disease is supported by specific laboratory findings [Poulsen et al., 2002]. Early diagnosis of affected newborns is necessary for the institution of appropriate therapy and survival. A high index of suspicion based on clinical grounds is essential because supportive laboratory findings may be problematic in the first few months of life.

Initially, few or no neurologic manifestations occur [Gunn et al., 1984]. Kinky hair with light hair pigmentation is most suggestive of Menkes' disease. The pili torti pathognomonic for Menkes' disease are usually seen only in older patients. The diagnosis should be considered for a neonate born after premature labor and delivery with large cephalohematomas, unexplained hypothermia or hypoglycemia, jaundice requiring phototherapy, pectus excavatum, and inguinal or umbilical hernias [Kaler, 1998].

The classic biochemical markers of Menkes' disease are low serum levels of copper and ceruloplasmin. Decreased intestinal copper absorption leads to low levels of copper in the plasma, liver, and brain. In contrast, copper stores are increased in the duodenum, kidney, spleen, pancreas, and skeletal muscle [Heydorn et al., 1975; Horn, 1984; Williams and Atkins, 1981].

Early laboratory diagnosis of neonates is complicated by the fact that copper and ceruloplasmin concentrations are normally low in healthy newborns, and these values can overlap with those typically found for older patients with Menkes' disease [Lockitch et al., 1986, 1988]. Copper egress assay in cultured fibroblasts is the definitive diagnostic study at this age, but the test is lengthy and requires several weeks of cell culture. Rapid diagnosis of Menkes' disease can be achieved by measurement of plasma catecholamines or polymerase chain reaction (PCR) detection of known deletions or point mutations in the *ATP7A* gene. The copper deficiency in Menkes' disease affects the function of many enzymes requiring copper. Dopamine mono-oxygenase is one of the cuproenzymes that is dysfunctional in Menkes' disease, resulting in abnormal plasma catechol concentrations in newborns and fetuses [Kaler et al., 1993a, 1993b, 1993c]. The plasma catecholamine profile is considered to be the most rapid and reliable way to diagnose Menkes' disease during the neonatal period. Patients with Menkes' disease have high plasma dopamine and low norepinephrine levels. Considered alone, neither dopamine nor norepinephrine levels have perfect sensitivity, whereas the ratio of dopamine to norepinephrine is high in all affected patients. Analogously, levels of the dopamine metabolite, dihydroxyphenylacetic acid, and the norepinephrine metabolite, dihydroxyphenylglycol, were imperfectly sensitive, whereas the dihydroxyphenylacetic acid to dihydroxyphenylglycol ratio is high in all patients. Plasma dihydroxyphenylalanine and the ratio of epinephrine to norepinephrine levels are high in affected neonates [Goldstein et al., 2009]. Increased urine ratios of homovanillic acid/vanillylmandelic acid (HVA/VMA) have been proposed as a screening tool for Menkes' disease also [Matsuo et al., 2005]. PCR methods are helpful in the diagnosis of partial deletions and point mutations when they are already identified for a specific family. The DNA-based technologies used for screening *ATP7A* for point mutations are chemical cleavage mismatch detection [Das et al., 1994], single-strand conformational polymorphism analysis [Tumer et al., 1997], and dideoxy fingerprinting [Moller et al., 2000]. PCR-based methods for screening *ATP7A* for large partial deletions include multiplex PCR, genomic PCR, and reverse transcriptase PCR [Poulsen et al., 2002]. These PCR methods are useful in neonatal and prenatal diagnosis, and they are helpful for carrier screening.

Prenatal diagnosis and identification of carrier status are important for families that are at risk for Menkes' disease. Assays looking for increased levels of copper in cultured fibroblasts also can be used for prenatal diagnosis and for testing of potential carriers [Goka et al., 1976; Poulsen et al., 2002; Tümer et al., 2003], but random X-inactivation renders carrier testing using this technique uninformative when negative. The only definitive tests that can exclude this disease are DNA-based assays.

An important component of all variants of Menkes' disease is connective tissue involvement. Deoxypyridinoline is a cross-linking residue of type I collagen and is a good marker for lysyl oxidase activity, the cuproenzyme deficiency that is responsible for the connective tissue disorders observed in these patients. Deoxypyridinoline has been proposed as a marker for the presence of connective tissue disorders associated with Menkes' disease [Kodama et al., 2003].

Genetics

Menkes' disease is an X-linked disease, and one-third of cases are thought to represent new mutations [Haldane, 1935]. The gene responsible for Menkes' disease, *ATP7A*, was discovered in 1993 [Chelly et al., 1993; Mercer et al., 1993; Vulpe et al., 1993]. The gene encodes the copper transporting ATPase known as ATP7A [Mercer, 1998]. ATP7A is part of a highly conserved family of cation-transporting ATPase proteins [Odermatt et al., 1993; Pederson and Carafoli, 1987]. This protein family includes the protein WD that is defective in Wilson's disease. The *ATP7A* gene (formerly known as *MNK*) is located at Xq13.2–q13.3 [Tümer et al., 2003]. It has 23 exons and is about 140 kb long [Dierick et al., 1995]. *ATP7A* is 8.5 kDa. About 357 different mutations have been identified and are distributed as follows: nonsense mutations 18 percent, splice-site mutations 16 percent, missense mutations 17 percent, partial insertions 4 percent, minus mutations 5 percent, partial deletions 17 percent, chromosomal mutations 1 percent, and small indels 22 percent [Møller et al., 2009].

Occipital horn syndrome results from point mutations (75 percent), chromosomal rearrangements (about 1 percent), and large or partial deletions (about 15 percent) in the *ATP7A* gene [Liu et al., 1999; Tümer et al., 1999]. Severe classic Menkes' disease RNA contains low levels of active ATP7A mRNA, whereas mild variants of Menkes' disease have higher levels of active ATP7A mRNA. Occipital horn syndrome has 20–35 percent residual ATP7A mRNA in cultured cells, whereas classic Menkes' disease has lower levels of mRNA in the cells [Kaler, 1994, 1998]. Decreased mRNA levels result from premature stop codons, missense mutations, frame shifts, and other deletions or mutations that affect RNA splicing [Das et al., 1995]. Patients with the identical deletion or mutation may have different clinical outcomes [Tümer et al., 2003]. This finding suggests that other modifying genes or proteins must play a role in the pathogenesis of this disease. Alternatively, other pathways for copper transport may exist at the cellular level.

Alternate splice products of *ATP7A* exist. One of the splice variants lacks exon 10, but the product is in-frame. This exon encodes transmembrane domains 3 and 4. This protein may act as a copper transporter, but it may not be able to function as a copper-transporting ATPase. It is also possible that alternate exons exist within intronic sequences.

Biochemistry

The genetic mutation of the *ATP7A* gene leads to problems with copper transport within the body. Normally, ATP7A allows efflux of copper from gut epithelium into the portal circulation, transport of copper across the blood–brain barrier, and transfer of copper that is reabsorbed by the kidney back into circulation. ATP7A protein deficiency results in an inability of the body to absorb copper from the gastrointestinal tract in amounts required to satisfy nutritional needs, as well as in impaired use and handling of the copper that is absorbed from the intestine. Copper is mobilized from the cytoplasm of cells so that it can be incorporated into secretory pathways [Tümer et al., 2003]. The mutation of a copper-transporting ATPase causes impaired cellular copper efflux, leading to increased intracellular copper concentrations. Patients with Menkes' disease have high concentrations of copper in gut epithelial cells, and they absorb little copper from their diet. Copper accumulates in kidney tubules. At high levels, copper causes lipid peroxidation, protein cleavage, enzyme inhibition, and DNA damage. Normally, basal intracellular stores are maintained at low levels [Rae et al., 1999; Voskoboinik and Camakaris, 2002]. The disease is caused by a decreased amount of the ATP7A protein, or it can result from alterations to the protein that impair its ability to transport copper.

ATP7A has 6–8 transmembrane domains, and it transports Cu^{2+} ions using energy from adenosine triphosphate (ATP)

hydrolysis [Vulpe et al., 1993]. The protein has several known motifs or domains within it, such as the ATP binding domain. The phosphorylation motif (DKTG) contains an aspartic acid that becomes phosphorylated during the protein's cycle (present in all P-type ATPases). The cation transduction motif (CPC) features a conserved proline, which plays a role in the conformation changes that occur with cation transport [Silver et al., 1989]. There are six metal binding sites (MBSs) in the amino-terminal region of ATP7A. The consensus sequence of the MBS is GMxCxxC. Although human ATP7A has six different forms of MBS, microbial cells show that only one or two are necessary for a functional protein [Odermatt et al., 1993; Solioz et al., 1994]. Human ATP7A does not need an MBS, demonstrated by the fact that mutations in all six MBSs do not stop ATP7A from functioning [Forbes et al., 1999; Payne and Gitlin, 1998; Tsivkovskii et al., 2002]. The MBS may act as a sensor for intracellular copper levels, and it may play a regulatory role when concentrations are low [Goodyer et al., 1999; Strausak et al., 1999; Voskoboinik and Camakaris, 2002]. ATP7A also features a magnesium-binding motif (TGE), the "hinge" domain of the protein, and a phosphorylation motif (DKTG).

ATP7A-encoded mRNA is found is most cell types, but it is missing in liver. ATP7B, the protein mutated in Wilson's disease (Table 41-2), transports copper in the liver [Vulpe et al., 1993; Paynter et al., 1994]. ATP7A and ATP7B are members

Table 41-2 Comparison of Menkes' Disease and Wilson's Disease

Characteristic	Menkes' Disease	Wilson's Disease
Inheritance pattern	X-linked recessive	Autosomal-recessive
Location	Xq13.3	13q14.3
Incidence	1:300,000	1:100,000
Clinical manifestations	Onset at birth Cerebral degeneration Global delay Kinky hair Pili torti Abnormal facies Hypopigmentation Arterial rupture or thrombosis Bone changes or cutis laxa	Dysarthria Kayser–Fleischer rings
Laboratory test findings	↓Serum Cu ↓Serum ceruloplasmin ↑Intestinal or kidney Cu ↓ Liver Cu	↓ Serum Cu ↓ Serum ceruloplasmin ↑ Urinary Cu ↑ Liver Cu
Prognosis	Lethal in classic cases Death <3 yr	Can be treated effectively with chelating agents
Gene product	1500-amino acid copper-binding ATPase	1411-amino acid copper-binding ATPase
Location, expression	All tissues except liver	Liver, kidney, and placenta
Mutation	Partial deletions in 15 percent; most others are point mutations	Point mutations and small rearrangements

of the P-type ATPases group IB family, as are bacterial heavy metal transporters [Tsivkovskii et al., 2002; Voskoboinik et al., 2001]. *ATP7A* has been localized to the *trans*-Golgi compartment under basal conditions [Petris et al., 1996]. This is consistent with the ability of ATP7A to supply cuproenzymes (i.e., lysyl oxidase) that are in secretory pathways. There is continuous recycling of ATP7A between the plasma membrane and the *trans*-Golgi compartment [Petris and Mercer, 1999]. ATP7A traffics to the plasma membrane with increased extracellular copper concentrations and is endocytosed back to the *trans*-Golgi compartment after extracellular levels decrease to normal. Copper-dependent vesicular trafficking moves ATP7A from the plasma membrane to the *trans*-Golgi network and back. Lower organisms have two copper ATPases, but this is unnecessary in humans because ATP7A traffics between the two areas where such ATPases are needed [Yuan et al., 1997]. Cu(I) may be the type of copper used by ATP7A as its substrate. It is unknown whether Cu(I) becomes Cu(II) before or after it is released in the Golgi lumen.

Menkes' disease is caused by mutations that result in a substitution of highly conserved amino acids or those in highly conserved motifs. Any mutation that affects the structure and function of the *ATP7A* gene will lead to disease [Guy et al., 2001]. Mutations that induce Menkes' disease include those that abolish the Mg^{2+} binding domain [Seidel et al., 2001] and those that change the cation transduction motif. Classic Menkes' disease is usually caused by a premature truncation, typically occurring before the first transmembrane domain and resulting in loss of all catalytic activity. Occipital horn syndrome and mild Menkes' disease usually result from missense or splice mutations. It is unknown how much catalytic activity is needed to result in a milder phenotype (i.e., ATP7A still able to absorb sufficient amounts of intestinal copper and enable its delivery to the requisite enzymes) [Tümer et al., 1997]. A case study of a patient with occipital horn syndrome showed that the splice mutation allowed 2–5 percent of ATP7A transcripts to be produced. This amount of protein was sufficient to allow partial absorption of copper from the gut epithelium and partial transport across the blood–brain barrier [Møller et al., 2000]. There was, however, too little protein for lysyl oxidase to function correctly. Between 2 and 5 percent of ATP7A activity is the proposed amount of protein necessary to decrease the severity of the Menkes' disease phenotype.

Most of the clinical manifestations of Menkes' disease can be explained by understanding which cuproenzymes are affected. Intracellular copper is necessary for oxidative reactions. Most clinical symptoms are caused by dysfunction of dopamine mono-oxygenase, peptidylglycine mono-oxygenase, cytochrome c oxidase, lysyl oxidase, and Cu/Zn superoxide dismutase (SOD), tyrosinase, and sulfhydryl oxidase.

Dopamine mono-oxygenase, also known as dopamine β-hydroxylase, is part of the catecholamine biosynthetic pathway. In Menkes' disease, there is complete or partial deficiency of dopamine β-hydroxylase. This deficiency causes abnormal plasma and cerebrospinal fluid patterns. The degree of deficiency can be evaluated by looking at norepinephrine concentrations or the ratio of dihydroxyphenylalanine to dihydroxyphenylglycol. Cases of Menkes' disease with deficient dopamine β-hydroxylase exist that have normal plasma and cerebrospinal fluid concentrations of norepinephrine. It is unknown why compensatory mechanisms are active in some patients but not in others. In the mouse model of Menkes' disease, normal concentrations of norepinephrine are observed in certain areas of the brain [Prohaska and Bailey, 1994]. The dopamine β-hydroxylase deficiency causes temperature instability, hypoglycemia, eyelid ptosis, and loss of sympathetic adrenergic function [Biaggioni et al., 1990; Robertson et al., 1986].

Peptidylglycine mono-oxygenase is a cuproenzyme necessary for the removal of the carboxyl-terminal glycine residue from neuroendocrine precursors, including gastrin, cholecystokinin, vasoactive intestinal peptide, corticotropin-releasing factor, calcitonin, vasopressin, and thyrotropin-releasing hormone [Eipper et al., 1983, 1992]. When this enzyme is deficient, these neuroendocrine factors have 100- to 1000-fold decreased bioactivity. Affected animal models of Menkes' disease have decreased peptidylglycine mono-oxygenase activity within their brains [Prohaska and Bailey, 1995]. The decreased activity of these neuroendocrine factors contributes to the phenotype of Menkes' disease.

Cytochrome c oxidase is a copper-dependent enzyme that is deficient in Menkes' disease. The decreased cytochrome c oxidase activity causes a subacute necrotizing encephalomyelitis without the severe lactic acidemia that is generally associated with complex IV defects [DiMauro et al., 1990; Robinson, 1989; Robinson et al., 1987]. Peripheral hypotonia and muscle weakness in patients with Menkes' disease is partially caused by decreased activity of this enzyme.

The normal function of lysyl oxidase (protein lysine 6-oxidase) is to deaminate lysine and hydroxylysine during the first step of collagen cross-link formation [Siegel, 1979]. ATP7A may be needed to transport copper into the *trans*-Golgi for use by lysyl oxidase. Deficiency of lysyl oxidase decreases the strength of connective tissue in certain tissues or organs and leads to a host of connective tissue disorders that usually are associated with Menkes' disease, including vascular tortuosity [Royce and Steinmann, 1990], bladder diverticula [Daly and Rabinovitch, 1981; Harke et al., 1977], and gastric polyps. ATP7A deficiency affects lysyl oxidase more profoundly than any of the other cuproenzymes [Gacheru et al., 1993]. It is possible that other cuproenzymes can acquire copper from cytoplasmic carriers without using ATP7A (an intermediate carrier), and this may explain why some mutations of ATP7A lead to the less severe occipital horn syndrome.

Cu/Zn SOD is also deficient in this disease [Rohmer et al., 1977]. Lowered levels of Cu/Zn SOD can increase susceptibility to damage by oxygen free radicals. It is not known whether decreased Cu/Zn SOD causes any developmental regression, because animal models without Cu/Zn SOD have normal development [Reaume et al., 1996] Postmortem studies of patients with Menkes' disease have found increased levels of manganese SOD, which may be a compensatory change for the decreased levels of Cu/Zn SOD [Shibata et al., 1995]. It is unknown whether the decrease in this enzyme contributes to the phenotype observed in Menkes' disease. Tyrosinase and sulfhydryl oxidase act on pigment formation and cross-linking of keratin, respectively; hence the manifestations of hypopigmentation, abnormal hair, and dry skin [Horn and Tümer 2002].

Pathology

Kidney

Copper accumulation within the kidneys leads to problems with renal reabsorption. Animal models of Menkes' disease demonstrate an accumulation of copper within the proximal tubules of the kidney [Kodama and Murata, 1999]. Beta$_2$-microglobulin is absorbed by the renal proximal tubules. Urinary β_2-microglobulin levels rise with increasing age of Menkes' disease patients, regardless of whether they undergo treatment [Ozawa et al., 2003].

Brain

Microscopy of tissues from animal models of Menkes' disease reveals an increased number of apoptotic cells within the neocortex and the hippocampus [Rossi et al., 2001]. Postmortem cerebral cortex and cerebellum analysis showed downregulation of genes involved in myelination, energy metabolism, and translation, with the cerebellum being more sensitive to copper deficiency [Liu et al., 2005]. Brain CT scans demonstrate atrophy that is generalized or diffuse. Brain MRI reveals infarcts that result from tortuous arteries [Venta-Sobero et al., 2004]. MRI also demonstrates white matter disturbances, ventriculomegaly, and diffuse atrophy [Faerber et al., 1989].

Connective Tissue

Urinary diverticula can be seen on pelvic ultrasound and cystography. Bone abnormalities are common and include Wormian bones in the skull, metaphyseal spurring of the long bones, and anterior flaring and multiple fractures of the ribs [Adams et al., 1974; Stanley et al., 1976].

Pathogenesis

Defective copper trafficking explains most changes seen in Menkes' disease. The body's nutritional needs for copper are crucial in the first 12 months of life. Brain growth and motor development are most rapid during this phase. Neurodevelopment and motor development are processes that require copper [Berg, 1994]. Expression of BCL2, an anti-apoptotic protein, is decreased in children with Menkes' disease. Decreased levels of copper lead to mitochondrial damage that causes decreased levels of BCL2 [Rossi et al., 2001]. These decreased levels of BCL2 may explain the increased number of apoptotic cells seen in the brain of the animal model, as well as the mechanism behind neurodegeneration in Menkes' disease.

Phenotypic differences in animal models and in humans appear to depend on the amount of functional *ATP7A*-encoded mRNA. During different stages of development, the various organs and tissues have different copper requirements. If the requirement is not met, the organ or tissue undergoes developmental failure.

Animal Models

Complete deficiency of the Menkes' protein in mice causes lethality before birth, whereas humans can survive for a limited time without ATP7A [Mercer, 1998]. The murine homolog of ATP7A is Atp7a [Levinson et al., 1994; Mercer et al., 1994]. Just as in humans, there are a variety of observed phenotypes, with most of them reflecting their human counterparts. The severity of the murine phenotypes depends on the amount of *ATP7A*-encoded mRNA. Four murine genotypes are used to study Menkes' disease:

1. Jax brindled, akin to classic Menkes' disease, does not respond to copper treatment.

2. Macular brindled corresponds to classic Menkes' disease. Mice are hypopigmented because of catechol oxidase deficiency. They have severe neurologic deficits and die about 15 days after birth if untreated. However, if copper is given before the seventh day of life, the mice are able to survive [Fujii et al., 1990; Mercer, 1998].

3. Viable brindled corresponds to mild Menkes' disease. These mice are similar to the other brindled mutants, but they have increased viability.

4. Blotchy corresponds to occipital horn syndrome. These mice display less severe phenotypes than the other mutants. Their defects are mostly limited to connective tissue abnormalities. Assays reveal that full-length Atp7a-encoded mRNA is present [Levinson et al., 1994; Mercer et al., 1994].

Treatment

Treatment of Menkes' disease is limited to supportive therapy and supplementation with parenteral copper histidine. Unlike nutritional copper deficiency, Menkes' disease cannot be cured by copper replacement. Copper histidine is more effective in patients with milder phenotypes. A small subset of patients can achieve normal neurodevelopment. Early detection and intervention are critical for the copper histidine treatment to have an effect. Daily copper injections may improve the outcome in Menkes' disease if started within days after birth [Kaler et al., 2008]. Many individuals with Menkes' disease fare poorly, with little or no developmental improvement despite early intervention. Older patients with neurologic signs of Menkes' disease demonstrate little improvement with copper histidine replacement. Therapy may, however, reduce irritability and allow for calmer sleeping patterns and minor improvements in personal and social development [Kaler, 1998]. These minor responses to therapy may help lessen the burden placed on caretakers. Copper histidine therapy helps the neurologic signs and symptoms of Menkes' disease, but it has no effect on connective tissue disorders associated with this disease.

Early copper histidine replacement therapy is most effective in patients with milder phenotypes who have some residual copper transport activity. These milder variants result from mutations that do not affect the regions of ATP7A necessary for catalytic activity and allow for residual levels of copper transport. The beneficial response to copper histidine therapy can be predicted by PCR-based analysis of mutations.

Future Directions

Improved therapeutic strategies are critical for better outcomes. Biochemical approaches to bypass the block in copper absorption from the intestine and allow requisite copper absorption are needed. Affected individuals must be identified early to initiate treatment before manifestations of neurologic signs and symptoms occur. This is the period when treatment has the most potential. ATP7A is necessary for the transport of copper through the blood–brain barrier. To prevent neurologic developmental regression, other ways of delivering copper stores to the brain must be identified. The symptoms of Menkes' disease result from the dysfunction of multiple cuproenzymes, and copper must be made available to these enzymes to reduce the non-neurologic symptoms experienced by these patients [Kaler, 1998]. Although advances have been made in early detection of affected individuals, there has been little progress in finding ways to deliver copper to the necessary cuproenzymes or through the blood–brain barrier. Because classic Menkes' disease is the result of the partial or complete absence of the traditional copper transport pathway, identification of alternate routes may allow the delivery essential for normal development.

Alpers' Disease

Alpers' disease is a fatal, progressive disease that affects the gray matter of the brain [Simonati et al., 2003]. This disease was initially described formally in 1931 [Alpers, 1931]. Alpers' disease is known by other names: diffuse progressive degeneration of the gray matter, poliodystrophia cerebri progressiva, degeneration of the cerebral gray matter of Alpers' [Ford et al., 1951], diffuse cerebral degeneration of infancy [Blackwood et al., 1963], progressive poliodystrophy [Dreifuss and Netsky, 1964], spongy glioneuronal dystrophy [Klein and Dichgans, 1969], spongy degeneration of the gray matter [Janota, 1974], Alpers–Huttenlocher syndrome [Huttenlocher et al., 1976], and progressive neuronal degeneration of childhood with liver disease [Harding et al., 1986]. Characteristic manifestations include neurologic deterioration, intractable seizures, and liver failure [Harding, 1990]. There is no known treatment. The clinical manifestations of Alpers' disease are caused by myriad genetic defects with various forms of inheritance. Most of the genetic mutations that lead to Alpers' disease are still unknown.

History

While visiting a colleague's laboratory in Hamburg, American neuropathologist Bernard Alpers conducted a detailed study of a 4-month-old girl who died after a month of intractable seizures. The patient had a normal birth and normal development until age 4 months. There was necrosis of the deep gray matter nuclei and diffuse loss of ganglion cells in the third layer of the cortex. Alpers believed that the degeneration had a toxic cause. Many similar case reports have been made since then. Huttenlocher et al. [1976] were first to report that the neuronal degeneration was associated with liver failure. The pattern of inheritance has been postulated to be autosomal-recessive [Sandbank and Lerman, 1972]. A mitochondrial defect leading to Alpers' disease has also been hypothesized [Naviaux et al., 1999]. The disease most likely has several causes, accounting for subtypes such as hepatocerebral or myopathic Alpers' disease.

Clinical Description

Alpers' disease is a clinical diagnosis that is documented on MRI but confirmed on postmortem examination. The disease is a diagnosis of exclusion, but specific clinical findings suggest its presence. Characteristic manifestations are liver failure, refractory seizures, and psychomotor retardation [Wefring and Lamvik, 1967]. Patients with Alpers' disease are developmentally normal initially. Onset can occur between 1 month and 25 years of age [Harding et al., 1995]. Onset is more common during a patient's infancy and adolescence, with most cases showing initial symptoms in infancy, usually before the age of 5. Death occurs between 3 months and 12 years of age, with most patients dying before the age of 3 years. The

course of Alpers' disease is variable, alternating between periods of development, degeneration, and mild recovery or stasis. Rare cases of Alpers' disease have been reported in individuals as old as 25 years. Because of the variable age of onset, Alpers' disease has been categorized as having juvenile, infantile, and prenatal forms [Frydman et al., 1993; Harding et al., 1995; Montine et al., 1995; Simonati et al., 2003; Worle et al., 1998]. Prenatal Alpers' disease has been described in one family, and it is characterized by microcephaly, intrauterine growth retardation, retrognathia, joint limitations, and chest deformity. The infantile form manifests with early onset, a slowly progressive course, and late-occurring severe signs and symptoms. The juvenile form of Alpers' disease is identical to the infantile form, but it is notable for a peripheral ataxia resulting from central and peripheral sensory axonopathy.

In addition to the classic triad of symptoms (i.e., psychomotor retardation, intractable seizures, and liver failure), patients with Alpers' disease may have other manifestations. Hypotonia may occur initially [Egger et al., 1987]. Ataxia, febrile illness, and cortical blindness are less common [Naviaux and Nguyen, 2004]. A progressive ataxia that involves the sensory pathways has been described. This occurrence is similar to other sensory neuropathies caused by mitochondrial disorders [Fadic et al., 1997].

Liver failure is a complication that manifests late in the course of the disease [Smith et al., 1996], and it is usually the cause of death. Most cases of liver failure in these patients were attributed to hepatotoxicity caused by antiepileptic drugs, specifically valproic acid. However, some cases of liver failure and identical hepatic histology have occurred in patients who did not receive antiepileptic drugs. Valproic acid may cause hepatotoxicity in some cases of Alpers' disease, but it cannot explain all cases. Orthotopic liver transplantation has not been helpful in cases with liver failure. Liver transplantation in patients with Alpers' disease has been associated with neurologic deterioration [Delarue et al., 2000; Kayihan et al., 2000]. Complications of neuronal degeneration can lead to death from respiratory failure or primary hypoventilation.

Clinical Diagnostic Tests

Initial laboratory test results can be normal. Liver function test results can be elevated initially, although this finding is rare [Egger et al., 1987]. Values are elevated in the later stages of the disease because of liver cirrhosis. There are no specific in vivo serum or cerebrospinal fluid markers for Alpers' disease, and the diagnosis must rely on neuropathologic evaluation. Lactate levels may be raised in the blood, and the protein and lactate levels may be elevated in the cerebrospinal fluid [Worle et al., 1998]. Positive cerebrospinal fluid oligoclonal bands, and very high immunoglobulin (Ig) G synthesis rate and IgG index were also reported [Bao et al., 2008]. Elevated cerebrospinal fluid neopterin, interleukin (IL)-6, IL-8, interferon (IFN)-c, reduced cerebrospinal fluid 5-methyltetrahydrofolate (5-MTHF), and increased serum, as well as cerebrospinal fluid folate receptor blocking autoantibodies, are present [Hasselmann et al., 2009].

Cranial CT scans demonstrate progressive atrophy and low densities in the occipital and temporal lobes. There is involvement of the cortex and the white matter [Kendall et al., 1987; Flemming et al., 2002]. Generalized atrophy is common throughout the brain in the later stages of the disease. Multiple findings are apparent on conventional MRI scans. These include diminished white matter and cortical thinning of the frontal, posterotemporal, and occipital lobes [Barkovich et al., 1993]. Lesions of the thalamus also have been reported. Occipital lobe atrophy is widespread. Proton MR spectroscopy reveals increased cerebrospinal fluid levels of lactate [Charles et al., 1994] and a reduced *N*-acetylaspartate to creatine ratio. The increase in lactate marks the switch from oxidative to anaerobic metabolism. *N*-acetylaspartate is an indicator of neuronal viability [Neumann-Haefelin et al., 2000].

EEG findings correlate with the lesions seen on MRI that are most apparent in the occipital lobes. The EEG of Alpers' disease is described as slow (<1 Hz) with high-amplitude activity (0.2–1.0 mV). Lower-amplitude polyspikes are also recognized on the EEG. This pattern is seen in 75 percent of patients, but it may be present only transiently in periodic bursts [Martinez-Mena et al., 1998]. These bursts increase in number and duration as the disease progresses. Unilateral occipital rhythmic high-amplitude delta with superimposed (poly)spikes (RHADS) was described in convulsive status epilepticus in Alpers' patients [Wolf et al., 2009]. Mild axonal sensory neuropathy was reported, as was central-peripheral sensory axonopathy in a juvenile case of the syndrome [Simonati et al., 2003]. There can be a loss of visual-evoked potentials [Martinez-Mena et al., 1998]. The triad of requisite clinical symptoms and MRI and EEG findings suggests the diagnosis of Alpers' disease.

Pathology

Alpers originally described the neuronal pathology as cortical lesions with reactive gliosis, demyelination, nerve cell loss, spongy degeneration, and accumulation of neutral lipids. The occipital cortices are usually involved, and involvement can be symmetric or asymmetric. Patchy cerebral cortical destruction usually is worst within the striate cortex. Striate cortex involvement is a hallmark of Alpers' disease [Harding, 1990; Harding et al., 1986]. Because of the destruction of the visual cortices, patients often have cortical blindness [Charles et al., 1994; Dietrich et al., 2001; Parsons et al., 2000]. Multiple case studies have described the cortical destruction as neuronal loss, spongiosis, astrocytosis, and gliosis. Milder changes are seen in the parietal cortices [Montine et al., 1995]. Necroses in the hippocampi, lateral geniculate nuclei, amygdala, substantia nigra, and dorsal columns may be evident. In patients with severe liver failure in the late stages of Alpers' disease, Alzheimer's disease type II astrocytes are seen. The white matter is only minimally affected.

Premortem liver biopsies reveal lobular disarray, microvesicular steatosis, and inflammation with acute and chronic hepatocyte necrosis [Narkewicz et al., 1991]. Common hepatic findings at autopsy are fibrosis, regenerative nodules, hepatocyte dropout, bile duct proliferation, fatty changes, and bile stasis. Pancreatitis is infrequently observed in these patients. Muscle biopsies may contain ragged red fibers and cytochrome c oxidase-negative fibers when Alpers' disease is caused by a mitochondrial defect. A subset of patients with Alpers' disease lacks any detectable energy metabolism defect and has normal hepatic histology [Frydman et al., 1993].

Biochemistry

The clinical manifestations of Alpers' disease have several causes. Abnormalities within the citric acid cycle of leukocytes, cultured fibroblasts, and hepatocytes due to a defect in pyruvate metabolism or mitochondria have been suggested [Gabreels et al., 1984; Prick et al., 1981]. These defects result in deficiencies of cytochrome c oxidase, pyruvate cocarboxylase, and mitochondrial electron transport chain complex I. Mitochondrial DNA (mtDNA) polymerase gamma activity is less than 5 percent of normal in muscle and liver cells [Naviaux and Nguyen, 2004]. Immunoreactive subunits of the mtDNA polymerase are still present in patients. The deletion that causes the reduced amount of mtDNA polymerase is small because detectable levels of protein are still present. Southern blot analysis of two infants with Alpers' disease revealed decreased mtDNA in muscle, liver, brain, and fibroblasts. The loss of mtDNA may be tissue-specific [Tesarova et al., 2004].

Genetics

The mode of transmission of Alpers' disease is understood, and it is consistent between families. Case studies and biochemical evidence support autosomal-recessive inheritance and maternal or mitochondrial inheritance patterns. Cases with autosomal-recessive inheritance patterns have no mitochondrial deficiencies [Harding, 1990]. Simonati et al. [2003] observed that, although the disease affects both genders, there appears to be a mild male predominance. The same group also observed that children with juvenile Alpers' disease do not have depletion or significant mutations in mtDNA.

Two mutations within the polymerase gamma gene (*POLG*) are associated with Alpers' disease: G2899T and G1681A. G2899T causes a premature stop codon (Glu873Stop). Some Alpers' disease patients are heterozygous for the *POLG* mutation Glu873Stop. It has been theorized that this stop codon is incomplete and allows a small number of ribosomes to be read. The number of ribosomes that are able to bypass the premature stop codon may be regulated in an age- and tissue-dependent manner, allowing Alpers' disease to manifest at different ages and in different tissue types. In *Drosophila melanogaster*, proteins are regulated in a tissue-specific manner by changing the ratio of short to long forms of the protein [Robinson and Cooley, 1997]. The premature stop codon in *POLG* may change the ratio and cause tissue-dependent regulation.

The G1681A causes an Ala167Thr substitution. This corresponds to the linker region of the POLG protein. *POLG* is located on chromosome 15q24–26 [Zullo et al., 1997]. No other polymerase can be substituted for decreased POLG activity. POLG is the only polymerase of the 15 known DNA polymerases that has a mitochondrial import signal. Mutations within *POLG* are found in other mitochondrial diseases: progressive external ophthalmoplegia (autosomal-recessive and dominant forms) [Van Goethem et al., 2002, 2003], ophthalmoparesis, sensory ataxia, neuropathy, dysarthria, and male infertility. Children homozygous for the G2899T mutation are affected with Alpers' disease, whereas control groups consisting of patients with neuromuscular diseases or patients with other mitochondrial diseases do not have this mutation. Many patients with Alpers' disease are heterozygous for G1681A, but the mutation is not specific. Heterozygous G1681A mutations are also seen in ophthalmoparesis, both types of progressive external ophthalmoplegia, and in the asymptomatic parents of children with Alpers' disease.

Pathogenesis

Alpers' disease was originally believed to be a complication of concomitant hypoxia and epilepsy. Comparisons with status epilepticus cases are not valid because the cortical lesions in the two diseases differ significantly. Others have proposed that the underlying defect is metabolic. Alpers' disease most likely can be caused by multiple metabolic defects. The cerebral destruction of the striate cortex in Alpers' disease may result from a novel form of hepatocerebral toxicity, which is different from that seen in Wilsonian hepatocerebral degeneration. The possibility of a viral infection has been raised after brain tissue from a patient who died from Alpers' disease was injected into hamsters, and caused a spongiform encephalopathy [Rasmussen et al., 2000].

Management

There is no known treatment for Alpers' disease. It is important to recognize this disease early and avoid the use of valproic acid, because this increases the incidence of hepatotoxicity in these patients. Plasma alanine aminotransferase (AAT) can be used as an index of liver cell damage. Vigabatrin, which suppresses AAT activity, is better avoided in Alpers' patients [Williams et al., 1998]. Although some patients may respond to antiepileptic medications early in their disease course, the seizures become refractory to treatment. Treatment with oral leucovorin (5-formyl-tetrahydrofolate) in a patient with increased serum as well as cerebrospinal fluid folate receptor-blocking autoantibodies was initiated at 0.25 mg/kg b.i.d., and later increased to 4 mg/kg twice daily; this resulted in improvement of seizure frequency and communicative abilities [Hasselmann et al., 2009]. Ketogenic diet is reported to cause clinical and EEG improvement [Joshi et al., 2009].

Neuronal Ceroid-Lipofuscinosis: Batten's Disease

The neuronal ceroid-lipofuscinoses, or Batten's disease, comprise a group of inherited neurodegenerative diseases of childhood caused by defects in different genes and proteins. Their unifying clinical hallmarks are seizures, blindness, cognitive and motor decline, and early death. Eight genes and their protein products have been identified to account for 8 of the 10 or more described clinical entities: CLN1/protein palmitoyl thioesterase (PPT1), CLN2/tripeptidyl peptidase (TTP1), CLN3/battenin, CLN5, CLN6, CLN7/MFSD8 (major facilitator superfamily), CLN8/EPMR, and CLN10/CTSD (cathepsin D) [Siintola et al., 2007]. The clinical types are classic infantile (INCL/CLN1); classic late infantile (LINCL/CLN2); variant late infantile Finnish (CLN5); variant late infantile, also known as Costa Rican or Portuguese but not limited to these populations (CLN6); classic juvenile (JNCL/CLN3); Scottish juvenile (CLN1); epilepsy with mental retardation (EPMR/CLN8); Turkish variant infantile, previously classified as CLN7 (with defects in the *CLN8* gene); a second type of Turkish variant,

infantile due to CLN7/MFSD8 defects; CLN9 variant (CLN9; gene to be identified); and a number of adult-onset variants that are dominantly or recessively inherited (CLN4, gene to be identified) [Boustany, 1996; Goebel et al., 1999; Mole, 2004] (Table 41-3). Naturally occurring mouse models with defects in either Ctsf (cathepsin F) [Tang, 2006], Clcn-3 [Yoshikawa et al., 2002], or Clcn-7 [Kasper et al., 2005] result in an NCL-like phenotype, but mutations within these genes have not yet been reported in humans.

Most of the variants manifest neuronal and photoreceptor programmed cell death. Massive neuronal loss is documented as cerebral and cerebellar cortical atrophy on CT scans and by MRI, and photoreceptor loss as attenuated a and b waves is demonstrated on electroretinograms (ERGs). Autofluorescent material accumulates in these cells. Ultrastructural features characteristic for the clinical types consist of granular osmiophilic deposits (GRODs) in INCL, curvilinear bodies in LINCL, curvilinear and fingerprint-like inclusions in JNCL, and combinations of these features in the others. These inclusions have been observed in neurons, liver, muscle, conjunctival, and other cell types from affected patients.

A plethora of novel information has emerged over the past decade regarding the genetics, molecular and cell biology, and biochemistry of this group of disorders. [Gao et al., 2002; Persaud-Sawin et al., 2004; Puranam et al., 1997; Ranta et al., 1999; Schulz et al., 2004; Sleat et al., 1997]. Three of the proteins identified, protein palmitoyl thioesterase, tripeptidyl peptidase, and cathepsin D, are soluble lysosomal proteins, although INCL, LINCL, and congenital NCL are not typical lysosomal storage diseases. Two other proteins, CLN6 and CLN8, are resident proteins in the endoplasmic reticulum, and CLN3 is a protein that traffics between Golgi, early recycling endosomes, and lipid rafts in the plasma membrane. CLN3, CLN6, and CLN8 are hydrophobic membrane proteins. CLN5 is characterized as a lysosomal membrane glycoprotein. There are many naturally occurring animal models. Two of these, the nclf mouse and the New Zealand Southhampshire sheep, are models for CLN6. The mnd mouse is a model for CLN8. Transgenic models for INCL, LINCL, and CLN6-deficient variant LINCL and CLN10 also are available.

Diagnosis is primarily made on clinical grounds, documented by appropriate neuroradiologic and electrophysiologic studies, and confirmed by the appropriate enzymatic (PPT1 or TTP1 activity in CLN1 and CLN2 deficiencies, respectively) or DNA-based laboratory tests. Ultrastructural examination of skin fibroblasts continues to be a valuable diagnostic tool, particularly for identification of novel clinical variants not accounted for by the known genetic defects. Abnormal ultrastructural findings in the setting of a convincing clinical picture is what led to pursuit of the cause, genetics, and biochemistry of the CLN8-, CLN6-, CLN9-, and CLN10-deficient human variants.

Treatment options are beginning to expand beyond anticonvulsants and supportive nutritional and physical measures. Targeted therapies have been used in patients with known biochemical and cell biologic processes, such as cysteamine in INCL; flupirtine in INCL, LINCL, variant forms of LINCL, JNCL, and CLN6- and CLN9-deficient variants [Batten and Mayou, 1915; Dhar et al., 2002; Mayou, 1904]; and mycophenolate mofetil in JNCL. Gene- and protein-based delivery systems are being developed for the classic late infantile and infantile types with defects in soluble proteins, and they are

Table 41-3 Batten's Disease Variants

Gene	Eponym for Clinical Presentation	Age of Onset	Affected Ethnicities	Main Clinical Features	EM-Detected Protein	Diagnostic Tests	MRI and CT125 Findings	Protein Type, Location
CLN1* PPT1	CLN1 disease, infantile	9–18 mo	Primarily Finnish, described in others	Seizures, cognitive and motor decline, blindness, microcephaly	GRODs, saposins A and D	PPT1 enzymatic assay, gene-based test, skin biopsy, isoelectric EEG by age 3 yr	Signal loss in the thalami, T2-weighted high signal intensity for periventricular rims, cerebral atrophy	Soluble lysosomal protein, lysosome
	CLN1 disease, late infantile	2–4 yr	Italian, American, Finnish	Seizures, cognitive and motor decline, blindness, microcephaly	GRODs	PPT1 enzymatic assay, gene-based test, skin biopsy	Diffuse cerebral and cerebellar atrophy	Soluble lysosomal protein, lysosome
	CLN1 disease, juvenile	6 yr	English	Behavioral problems, seizures, cognitive and motor decline, blindness	N/a	PPT1 enzymatic assay, gene-based test, skin biopsy	Cerebral, cerebellar, and thalamic atrophy	Soluble lysosomal protein, lysosome
	CLN1 disease, adult	22 yr		Mood disorders, hallucinations, visual loss	GRODs	PPT1 enzymatic assay, gene-based test, skin biopsy	Diffuse cerebral and cerebellar atrophy	Soluble lysosomal protein, lysosome
CLN2† TPP1	CLN2 disease, late infantile	2.5–3.5 yr	Pan-ethnic	Seizures, ataxia, cognitive and motor decline, retinitis pigmentosa	Curvilinear inclusions, subunit C or 9 of ATP synthase	TTP1 enzymatic assay, gene-based test, giant occipital EEG spike, ERG	Increased T2 periventricular signal; signal loss in thalami; caudate, cerebral, and cerebellar atrophy	Soluble lysosomal protein, lysosome and PM
CLN3	CLN3 disease, juvenile	4–8 yr	Northern European, described in many others	Retinitis pigmentosa, seizures, echolalia, psychosis, dystonia, tremor, bradycardia	Fingerprint or curvilinear inclusions, subunit C or 9 of ATP synthase	Gene-based test, ERG	Cerebellar and cerebral atrophy, caudate and putamen atrophy, decreased thalamic density	Membrane protein, PM, Golgi, early endosomes, lipid rafts
CLN4‡	CLN4 disease, adult ANCL, Kufs' disease, dominant forms known as Parry's disease	30 yr		Early dementia, psychosis; type A myoclonic seizures; type B extrapyramidal signs and facial dyskinesias	Fingerprint inclusions, pigmentation, subunit C of ATP synthase	Clinical, pathologic examinations; exclude other dementias	Normal or mild cerebral cortical atrophy	Unknown
CLN5	CLN5 disease, late infantile	5–7 yr	Finnish	Clumsiness, visual failure, cognitive and motor decline, seizures	Curvilinear or fingerprint inclusions, subunit C of ATP synthase, saposins A and D fingerprint profiles, often condensed, and occasionally associated with lipid droplets	Gene-based test	Severe early cerebellar atrophy, cerebral atrophy	Soluble lysosomal glycoprotein, lysosome, ER

Continued

Table 41-3 Batten's Disease Variants—cont'd

Gene	Eponym for Clinical Presentation	Age of Onset	Affected Ethnicities	Main Clinical Features	EM-Detected Protein	Diagnostic Tests	MRI and CT125 Findings	Protein Type, Location
	CLN5 disease, juvenile	4–9 yr	Colombian, French Canadian, Irish, UK, Dutch, mixed Caucasian	Clumsiness, visual failure, cognitive and motor decline, seizures	Fingerprint, curvilinear, and granular patterns	Gene-based test	Diffuse cerebral and cerebellar atrophy	Soluble lysosomal glycoprotein, lysosome, ER
	CLN5 disease, adult	17 yr	Mixed Caucasian	Motor difficulty, cognitive regression, and visual loss		Gene-based test	N/a	Soluble lysosomal glycoprotein, lysosome, ER
CLN6	CLN6 disease, late infantile or early juvenile	4–6 yr	Costa Rican, Portuguese, Czech, Indian, Pakistani	Loss of speech, seizures, retinitis, cognitive and motor decline	Fingerprint, curvilinear, or rectilinear inclusions; lipid drops; subunit C of ATP synthase	Gene-based test	Increased T2 periventricular signal, cerebellar and cerebral atrophy, decreased T2 signal for thalamus and putamen	Membrane protein, ER, PM
CLN7‡ MFSD8	CLN7 disease, late infantile	5–7 yr	Turkish, Italian, Dutch, Czech, Greek, Albanian		Fingerprint or curvilinear inclusions		Similar to findings for CLN2, CLN6	Unknown
CLN8	CLN8 disease, EPMR	5–10 yr	Finnish	Seizures increased with puberty and decreased with age; clumsiness, dysarthria, decreased cognition, agitation, decreased visual acuity	Curvilinear inclusions, fine GRODs, lipid drops, subunit C of ATP synthase, saposin D	Gene-based test, EEG	Cerebral cortical atrophy	Membrane protein, ER, ER–Golgi intermediate compartment
CLN8	CLN8 disease, late infantile, vLINCL Turkish (previously classified as CLN7)	2–7 yr	Turkish, German, Pakistani, Israeli, Italian	Loss of speech, seizures, retinitis, cognitive and motor decline	Curvilinear or fingerprint inclusions, subunit C of ATP synthase	Clinical, exclude CLN2, CLN5, CLN6 forms	Cerebral cortical atrophy	Membrane protein, ER, ER–Golgi intermediate compartment
CLN9‡	CLN9 disease, juvenile, vJNCL	4–8 yr	Serbian, German	Myoclonus, seizures, cognitive and motor decline	Fingerprint or curvilinear inclusions, GRODs, subunit C of ATP synthase	EM, increased cell growth, decreased cell adhesion, GeneChip analysis	Cerebellar and cerebral cortical atrophy	Unknown

* Rare cases of adolescent and adult forms of CLN1 deficiency have been described. The *CLN1* gene is also designated *PPT1*.
† Patients with CLN2 deficiency of later onset survive into the fourth and fifth decades.
‡ *CLN4*, *CLN7*, and *CLN9* genes are unidentified.

ANCL, adult neuronal ceroid-lipofuscinosis; ATP, adenosine triphosphate; CLN, ceroid-lipofuscinosis, neuronal; CT, computed tomography; EEG, electroencephalogram; EM, electron microscopy; EPMR, epilepsy with mental retardation; ER, endoplasmic reticulum; ERG, electroretinography; GRODs, granular osmiophilic deposits; INCL, infantile neuronal ceroid-lipofuscinosis; JNCL, juvenile neuronal ceroid-lipofuscinosis; LINCL, late infantile neuronal ceroid-lipofuscinosis; MFSD, major facilitator superfamily; MRI, magnetic resonance imaging; PM, plasma membrane; PPT1, palmitoyl protein thioesterase-1; TPP1, tripeptidyl peptidase-1; v, variant.

being tested in transgenic mouse models. Stem cell replacement is being explored in animal models as potential therapy for these terminal diseases, as well as in terminal CLN2 and CLN1 human cases.

A clinical rating scale, the Unified Batten Disease Rating Scale (UBDRS), was developed to assess motor, behavioral, and functional capability in JNCL [Marshall et al., 2005]. This scale should be of assistance in evaluating novel treatment strategies mentioned.

History and Terminology

The first clinical description of neuronal ceroid-lipofuscinosis was that of the juvenile form by Stengel [1826]. This was soon followed by clinical and pathologic descriptions by Batten, Mayou, Spielmeyer, Vogt, and Sjögren [Batten and Mayou, 1915; Mayou, 1904; Spielmeyer, 1923; Vogt, 1909]. The *CLN3* gene responsible for the juvenile form (JNCL) was discovered in 1995 [Lerner et al., 1995]. The late infantile form (LINCL) was described by Jansky and Bielchowski in 1908 and 1913 [Jansky, 1908]. These two variants were previously referred to as Batten's disease, a term that now refers to all variants. The adult form, or Kufs' disease, an early-onset dementia with seizures and absence of visual findings, was described in 1925 [Dom et al., 1979]. The adult form (ANCL) has been described in sporadic cases and familial cases, with some families suggesting a dominant pattern of inheritance. Chromosomal location of the *CLN4* gene or genes responsible for the adult disease remains unknown.

The term neuronal ceroid-lipofuscinosis was introduced by Zeman and Dyken in 1969 as a descriptive term referring to the autofluorescent, waxy, dusky lipid accumulating in neuronal endosomes, reminiscent of lipofuscin, the aging pigment [Zeman et al., 1970]. The infantile form (INCL) was described by Hagberg and then by Haltia and Santavuori in 1973 [Hagberg et al., 1968; Haltia et al., 1973a, 1973b; Santavuori et al., 1973]. The *CLN1* gene was identified in 1995, followed by the *CLN2* gene responsible for LINCL [Sleat et al., 1997]. Other types have been described since then, including variant late infantile forms and early juvenile forms due to defects in the *CLN5*, *CLN6*, and *CLN8* genes [Gao et al., 2002; Ranta et al., 2001; Savukoski et al., 1998; Wheeler et al., 2002]. A CLN9 form is also described that is clinically similar to the juvenile form [Lin et al., 2001; Schulz et al., 2004]. The *CLN9* gene remains to be characterized.

The terminology is confusing because it was established before many variants or clinical forms were defined and before any of the genes were identified. The terms INCL, LINCL, JNCL, and ANCL were initially chosen to separate the forms according to age of onset. This holds true for the main classic variants described. Since discovery of the various genes, many atypical cases have been described with variable ages of onset. It has, therefore, been decided to refer to these diseases by a unified nomenclature, illustrated by the following example: CLN1 disease infantile; CLN1 disease late infantile; and so on, as referred to in Table 41-3 [Mole et al., 2010].

The decision to name the genes *CLN*, as opposed to neuronal ceroid-lipofuscinosis or *NCL* genes, is most unfortunate, because it causes confusion with yeast cyclin genes, especially in scientific and medical literature searches. The decision to refer to all forms as Batten's disease, although historically incorrect, is a simple and practical one, because of the length and wordiness of neuronal ceroid-lipofuscinoses. The term Batten's disease has been universally adopted and accepted by family groups, private foundations, and U.S. government agencies.

Major Neuronal Ceroid-Lipofuscinosis Clinical Types or Syndromes

The clinical features, laboratory tests, pathology, biochemistry, and genetics are summarized for each of the major types (see Table 41-3).

Infantile Neuronal Ceroid-Lipofuscinosis

INCL (i.e., Haltia–Santavuori variant, CLN1-defective, PPT1-deficient form) is caused by a deficiency in palmitoyl protein thioesterase. The function of this lysosomal thioesterase is to remove fatty acids attached in thioester linkages to cysteine residues in proteins [Schriner et al., 1996]. The first description of this disease was in 1968 by Hagberg et al. [1968]. A comprehensive clinical and pathologic characterization of this autosomal-recessive disorder was provided later from Finland [Haltia et al., 1973b; Santavuori et al., 1973].

CLINICAL DESCRIPTION

The Finnish cases represent the most severe form of the disease. Development is normal until 10–18 months of age. Deceleration of head growth can start as early as 5 months of age. Developmental arrest, hypotonia, and ataxia ensue. All children become microcephalic. Visual impairment is apparent at 1 year of age, and children are blind by the age of 2 years. Optic atrophy, thinned retinal vessels, and a discolored, brownish macula are seen funduscopically. Frequent myoclonic jerks begin after year 1, and many affected children develop generalized seizures. Hand-knitting movements reminiscent of Rett's syndrome are observed early but disappear by age 2 years. By the third year of life, patients are bedridden, hypotonic, irritable, and spastic. At age 5 years, severe flexion contractures, acne, hirsutism, and rarely, precocious puberty are observed. Children with INCL have an increased risk of hypothermia and bradycardia late in the course, especially during anesthesia due to impaired thermoregulation. These children should be carefully monitored and warming interventions applied during operative procedures [Miao et al., 2009]. Most children die between the ages of 7 and 13 years. There are rare cases in which the age of onset may be as late as 4 years. A distinct adolescent phenotype reminiscent of the classic juvenile variant has been described in some patients of Scottish descent [Mitchison et al., 1998].

CLINICAL DIAGNOSTIC TESTS

The single best diagnostic test is measurement of PPT1 enzyme activity in leukocytes [Das et al., 1998]. Enzyme activity can be measured from a dried blood spot on filter paper or from cultured fibroblasts. In the proper clinical setting, an enzyme activity less than 5 percent of normal is diagnostic for INCL. Salivary PPT1 measurement also is reported as a reliable method of diagnosis [Kohan et al., 2005]. DNA diagnostics are also widely available. Before the availability of the enzyme assay or DNA diagnostics for this disease, the diagnosis was based on the clinical presentation and electron microscopic examination of skin or other available tissue. The characteristic finding is membrane-bound GRODs, which typically are seen in endothelial, periepithelial, and autonomic nerve cells of the submucosal myenteric nerve plexus, but they also have been reported in other cell types. The EEG may initially be normal but then reveals lack of sleep spindles and absence of the attenuation in amplitude seen with eye opening by the ages of 16–24 months. There is gradual loss of amplitude, and the EEG becomes isoelectric by age 3 years. The ERGs, visual-evoked responses, and somatosensory-evoked responses are also abnormal but tedious to demonstrate in young children, and they are not needed for the diagnosis. The ERG is abnormal, with cone function affected before rod function. CT and MRI findings are present early and include signal loss in the thalami and cerebral atrophy with high-signal-intensity, thinned periventricular rims. Postmortem T2-weighted MRI scans reveal a remarkable hypointensity of the gray matter with respect to the white matter. Prenatal diagnosis has been performed on chorionic villus samples as early as 11 weeks, and it can be achieved by examining amniocytes at a later stage (16–18 weeks). Initially, electron microscopic or ultrastructural studies were performed to look for GRODs, but the PPT1 enzyme assay and a DNA analysis can be performed instead. Prenatal diagnosis using allele specific primer extension (ASPE) is also reported [Zhong et al., 2005]. There remains a role for electron microscopy when enzymatic diagnosis is not available, when enzyme activities and DNA analysis are not clear-cut, or when identification of the existing mutation is absent. Ideally, all three diagnostic methods should be used because of the importance of the decision, based on these results, to be taken by the family, treating obstetrician, and geneticist. The diagnosis of a normal or carrier fetus should be confirmed at birth by analysis of cord blood.

PATHOLOGY

At the time of death, brain weight is drastically reduced to 250–400 g. Serial pathologic studies in Finland revealed progressive cortical neuronal loss beginning at 1 year of age, with a subtotal loss of neurons by 4 years. Giant Betz cells and neurons of the hippocampal CA1 and CA4 sectors are relatively preserved. Reactive astrocytes become more prominent with time. GRODs are apparent in neurons and macrophages as early as 8 weeks' gestation. Ultimately, cerebellar Purkinje cells and granule cells are destroyed and are replaced by a rim of Bergman glia. The white matter appears gliotic. The brainstem and basal ganglia are also involved. The spinal cord is relatively preserved with anterior horn cells that demonstrate storage only. Storage granules can be seen in many different tissues of the body, but tissue destruction is reserved for the brain and retina [Goebel and Wisniewski, 2004; Wisniewski et al., 2004b].

BIOCHEMISTRY, CELL BIOLOGY, AND PATHOPHYSIOLOGY

There is loss of function of PPT1, which removes long-chain fatty acids attached in thioester linkage to the cysteine residues of proteins. Proteins containing the fatty acylated cysteine residues are usually found at the inner plasma membrane leaflet. Normally, reversible acylation and deacylation of these may have impact on protein–protein and protein–lipid membrane interactions. S-acylated proteins are degraded in lysosomes, and this function also may be impaired in INCL. INCL, like other neuronal ceroid-lipofuscinosis disorders, differs from other storage diseases in that the material that accumulates in the cell has no demonstrable link to the actual defect and may be a secondary occurrence. PPT1 is located in the lysosome and taken up in a mannose-6 phosphate-dependent manner, but it is also activated at neutral and basic pH, and likely functions in the lysosome and elsewhere in the cell. PPT1 co-localizes with synaptophysin to presynaptic vesicles in neurons. Sphingolipid activator proteins A and D accumulate in storage cytosomes, probably as a secondary phenomenon [Tyynela et al., 1993]. There are reported abnormalities in brain sphingomyelin and other phospholipids, levels of which are decreased in the INCL brain. There are reports of increased rates of apoptosis in lymphocytes, cultured lymphoblasts, and fibroblasts from patients, as well as neurons rendered deficient in PPT1 [Cho et al., 2001].

Increased apoptosis is a common finding in a number of neurodegenerative disorders, such as Alzheimer's disease, Parkinson's disease, amyotrophic lateral sclerosis, and other forms of Batten's disease. Recognizing the defect in deacylation of S-acylated proteins and the increased apoptosis rate of PPT1-deficient cells and neurons has led to some targeted therapies (see "Management and Treatment").

GENETICS

All cases of INCL in Finland are caused by an identical common missense mutation (R122W, arginine to tryptophan) that leads to an unstable protein that is degraded in the endoplasmic reticulum [Mole et al., 1999]. At 1 in 70, the carrier frequency is high in Finland, and the incidence of the disease is 1 case per 20,000 individuals. The incidence in the United States has never been accurately computed, but it probably accounts for about 20 percent of all diagnosed cases of Batten's disease. A juvenile-onset variant of this disorder was first described in a person from Scotland; it has a threonine to proline substitution at position 75 [Mitchison et al., 1998]. This mutation and another with a premature stop codon at arginine 151 account for most alleles from patients in the United States, all of whom have Irish or Scottish ancestry. The former is found in juvenile cases and the latter in infantile cases. At least 40 mutations in the CLN1 gene have been described.

MANAGEMENT AND TREATMENT

Supportive therapies are still the mainstay. Muscle relaxants, including baclofen and benzodiazepine derivatives, are given to combat irritability, sleep problems, athetosis, spasticity, and rigidity. Lamotrigine, valproic acid, and many of the benzodiazepine derivatives are used to manage the seizures and the previously described symptoms. Pain is a common feature that is helped by these medications. Physical therapy plays a role early in the course and delays the onset of painful contractures.

In a mouse model for PPT1 deficiency, virally mediated CLN1 gene delivery has cleared storage and improved the clinical condition of these neurologically impaired mice. This therapy is being developed for use in humans. Enzyme replacement is a theoretical possibility, although protein delivery to the central nervous system is not trivial. Under development are methods to chemically open the blood–brain barrier or chemically camouflage proteins to enable them to cross it selectively. Bone marrow replacement has failed, but stem cell therapies are being explored. Gene therapy using intravitreal injection of AAV2-PPT1 increased enzyme levels in the eye and correlated with improvements in the histological abnormalities and mixed rod/cone and pure cone functions in murine models. In addition, PPT1 activity was detected in the brain following intravitreal injection [Griffey et al., 2005]. A clinical trial is using phosphocysteamine, a safe oral drug that deacylates proteins and is anti-apoptotic, is on-going. Clinical efficacy is unknown, but the drug clears storage material and decreases apoptosis in vitro [Zhang et al., 2001]. Flupirtine is an oral anti-apoptotic drug with analgesic, antispasmodic, and weak antiepileptic properties that protects PPT1-deficient cells from apoptosis. It is approved for use as an analgesic and antispasmodic in Europe, but it has not been approved by the U.S. Food and Drug Administration (FDA). Its clinical efficacy in INCL remains unknown.

Late Infantile Neuronal Ceroid-Lipofuscinosis or Late Infantile Batten's Disease

LINCL (i.e., Jansky–Bielchowski, CLN2-defective, TPP1-deficient form) results from a deficiency of lysosomal tripeptidyl peptidase. The defect was discovered by comparing mannose-6-phosphate-modified lysosomal proteins from a normal and an LINCL-affected brain [Sleat et al., 1997]. It was first described by Jansky in 1908 and then by Bielchowski in 1913. It is the most pan-ethnic of neuronal ceroid-lipofuscinosis disorders, having been described in European, Middle Eastern, Chinese, Pakistani, and Indian patients. It is the second most common form of Batten's disease in the United States, although the total number of cases at any time is less than 500, making it an orphan disease according to the FDA. It is thought that a large number of cases originate from Europe.

CLINICAL DESCRIPTION

LINCL manifests with a generalized seizure disorder and ataxia due to unrecognized, frequent absence seizures occurring between the ages of 2.5 and 3.5 years. Within 6 months, vision, motor, and cognitive skills deteriorate rapidly. Affected children are blind by age 4 years because of tapetoretinal degeneration. Most children are nonambulatory and mute by age 5 years, and they require gavage feeding. In addition to prolonged, generalized tonic-clonic seizures, all have frequent myoclonic jerks, which are most prominent in the face but are also observed in the trunk and extremities. An early hypotonia gives way to severe spasticity with flexion contractures. Autoregulation of vascular tone is lost, resulting in mottled, cold hands and feet. Hypothalamic involvement leads to temperature instability vacillating between hyperthermia and hypothermia. Hyperthermia often leads to unnecessary fever evaluations. Copious secretions and shallow breathing resulting from poor chest wall excursions often cause pneumonias. Sepsis and uncontrollable seizures are frequently the cause of death at the end of the first decade or in the early teens [Boustany, 1996; Zhong et al., 2000]. Some atypical cases have a later onset and protracted course [Wisniewski et al., 2004c].

CLINICAL DIAGNOSTIC TESTS

The most definitive test is measurement of TPP1 enzyme activity when the clinical history and course fit the description. Typically, enzyme activity less than 5 percent of normal is diagnostic for LINCL. This test can be performed on leukocytes, cultured fibroblasts, or amniocytes, and on dried blood from a filter paper. Salivary PPT1 measurement is also reported as a reliable method of diagnosis [Kohan et al., 2005]. DNA-based diagnosis is also available, but it is more tedious, particularly if the specific family mutation or mutations are not known. In this instance, the diagnostic laboratory excludes the most commonly reported mutations first. Before availability of enzyme or DNA diagnosis, ultrastructural study of a skin biopsy provided objective proof for the disease. The appearance of curvilinear bodies enclosed within unilamellar endosomes in multiple cell types (i.e., endothelial cell, pericyte, Schwann cell, and others) is the most characteristic feature. Rarely, few fingerprint profiles may be seen. Electron microscopy continues to be a valuable diagnostic tool when other forms of diagnosis are not available and in evaluating atypical cases. It has sometimes led to identification of novel neuronal ceroid-lipofuscinosis variant. The ERG reveals reduced amplitudes early in the course of this illness, even before changes of thinned vessels and pale discs become apparent. The process is extinguished within a few months of presentation. Characteristic giant occipital polyspike-spike discharges are seen on the EEG in response to a single flash of light or to low-frequency, repetitive stimulation. These discharges represent the early phase of an exaggerated visual-evoked response. Wave amplitudes of visual-evoked and somatosensory-evoked responses are also high. These tests are seldom used diagnostically. Neuroimaging studies often help to confirm the diagnosis. An initial CT or MRI scan may be normal, but usually within 6 months of onset and before the age of 4 years, cerebral and cerebellar atrophy is prominent. Within 2 years of onset, there is a 40 percent loss of volume of the cerebellum and a fivefold increase in lateral ventricle to hemisphere volume ratio. Caudate and thalamic volumes are markedly reduced compared with age-matched controls, and there is relative preservation of brainstem volume early in the course [Boustany and Filipek, 1993]. Prenatal diagnosis may be possible using ASPE [Zhong et al., 2005].

PATHOLOGY

Brain weight at the time of death is markedly diminished to between 250 and 700 g. The calvarium is thickened and the sulci are prominent, particularly in the occipital regions. Cerebellar folia are prominent, the ventricles are widened, and laminar necrosis is observed. There is massive neuronal loss, with some neurons preserved in layer III. Those cells demonstrate meganeurites. Purkinje and granule cells are almost completely absent from the cerebellum. The putamen and subthalamic nuclei, as well as nuclei in the brainstem, manifest neuronal loss. There is pallor of the white matter. A reactive astrocytosis is seen with activation of microglia, but monocyte-derived macrophages seen in chronic and acute inflammation are conspicuously absent. This absence suggests that the initial event in LINCL is neuronal destruction and loss, with a secondary, reactive gliosis.

The small number of remaining neurons has distended cell bodies and granular cytoplasm. This material is positive for periodic acid–Schiff (PAS), Luxol fast blue, and Sudan black B in light microscopy sections. White matter appears relatively intact, strongly speaking against a primary inflammatory component in LINCL. Condensed chromatin identified by electron microscopy, upregulation of BCL2 protein, and positive terminal deoxynucleotidyl transferase dUTP nick end labeling

(TUNEL) stains all provide evidence for the occurrence of apoptosis, a feature common to multiple neurodegenerative diseases [Puranam et al., 1995, 1997]. There is strong reactivity with an antibody to subunit C of mitochondrial ATP synthase [Johnson et al., 1995]. The reason for this is still unknown, but it may represent a form of apoptosis observed in neurodegenerative illnesses called mitopsis.

Ultrastructurally, neurons and many other cells contain curvilinear inclusions enclosed within a single membrane. Frequently, these inclusions are admixed with fingerprint profiles. This is more commonly observed in cells outside the central nervous system, such as smooth muscle cells, eccrine sweat glands, endothelial cells, and pericytes. Before the availability of enzymatic diagnosis, prenatal diagnosis was determined by analyzing the ultrastructure of amniocytes obtained at 16–17 weeks' gestation [Wisniewski et al., 2004a].

BIOCHEMISTRY

LINCL is caused by defects in a pepstatin-insensitive lysosomal tripeptidyl peptidase that normally removes tripeptides from the amino terminus of proteins. The defect was discovered by comparing mannose-6-phosphorylated glycoproteins from a normal and an LINCL-affected brain. TPP1 is a 46-kDa protein with strong similarity to bacterial proteases. Subunit C or 9 of mitochondrial ATP synthase accumulates. It is unknown how or whether this relates to the TPP1 deficiency. Other neuronal ceroid-lipofuscinosis disorders with normal TPP1 activity (i.e., CLN3, CLN4, CLN6, and CLN8 forms) also accumulate subunit C. It is most likely a secondary process and may be related to the increase in apoptotic activity observed in CLN2, CLN3-, CLN6-, and CLN8-deficient cells. TPP1 deficiency and measurement of its activity constitute the cornerstone of diagnostic tools available to the clinician for objective diagnosis of LINCL. This test can also be performed on dried blood filter paper spots.

GENETICS

LINCL is an autosomal-recessive disorder that appears to be pan-ethnic, with cases diagnosed from many countries on all continents except Africa. There is a notable lack of African and Jewish cases. It is the second most common form of Batten's disease in the United States, accounting for one-third of diagnosed cases. More than 53 mutations have been described. In the United States, two common mutations account for 65 percent of diagnosed cases. One is a nonsense mutation, Arg208X, and the other affects a splice junction site, IVS5-1G>C. The few cases with a milder course and later onset carry one of these two mutations on one allele and an Arg447His on the other. A mouse model for this disease has been developed [Sleat et al., 2004].

MANAGEMENT AND TREATMENT

Treatment is primarily supportive. Areas requiring attention include seizures that become uncontrollable with antiepileptic drug monotherapy. Single or combined use of valproic acid, clonazepam, and clorazepate is helpful, particularly in the early stages. There is also a role for phenobarbital, zonisamide, and levetiracetam. Gavage feeding becomes a necessity by age 5–7 years, when frequent pneumonias imply difficulty in swallowing and aspiration. Attention should be given to development of contractures. Bone marrow transplantation has been

tried and has failed [Lake et al., 1997]. Gene and enzyme replacement strategies are being developed and soon may be tried in a developed mouse model. Gene replacement achieved by a number of strategically placed burr holes in three patients with advanced disease is being evaluated. Stem cell therapy also is being developed as a treatment option. It has been proposed that oral use of an anti-apoptotic drug such as flupirtine may slow the progression of this disease. The safety of this drug and its analgesic, antispasmodic, and weak antiepileptic effects make it particularly attractive [Dhar et al., 2002]. Its efficacy in LINCL remains unproven.

Variant Late Infantile Forms

Several variant late infantile types (i.e., vLINCL; Finnish type: CLN5-deficient form; Costa Rican/Portuguese/Lake Cavanaugh variant: CLN6-deficient form; northern epilepsy or epilepsy with mental retardation [EPMR] and Turkish vLINCL or tLINCL: CLN8-deficient form) have been described, with an age of onset between 5 and 8 years and a clinical profile reminiscent of the late infantile type but with a more protracted course.

Three genes have been described. The gene for the variant Finnish type, CLN5, was the first to be identified. This rare variant is mostly restricted to a region in Finland and has been found in 16 families, with one Swedish and one Dutch case also reported. Northern epilepsy and its gene, CLN8, were identified in cases from the northeast part of Finland. A subset of Turkish cases with variant LINCL are also caused by mutations in the CLN8 gene. The variant LINCL type referred to as Costa Rican/Portuguese or CLN6-deficient has been identified in patients of Venezuelan, Pakistani, and Indian descent, as well as in a case from the United States. It had been previously described as an early juvenile form, and it is also referred to as the Lake Cavanaugh variant [Gao et al., 2002; Savukoski et al., 1998; Wheeler et al., 2002].

CLINICAL DESCRIPTION

For the Finnish variant LINCL (i.e., CLN5-deficient form), the initial symptoms are motor clumsiness at age 4.5 years, followed by cognitive decline at age 6 years and by generalized and myoclonic epilepsy at age 8 years. Blindness due to macular degeneration is evident by age 8 years. Children lose the ability to ambulate by age 10 years, and most die between the ages of 14 and 34 years.

For northern epilepsy or EPMR (i.e., CLN8-deficient form) [Ranta et al., 1999], the first stage of disease occurs from age 5 to puberty, and is characterized by frequent but short generalized tonic-clonic convulsions and complex partial seizures, as well as by cognitive decline to a low average level. After puberty, the second stage is notable for slowness of movement and a slowing of the rate of cognitive decline. In the final stage of the illness, seizures diminish in frequency, but mental dullness and cognitive decline lead to moderate mental retardation by the end of the third decade. This stage is also notable for clumsiness, ataxia, and impaired vision. Age at death varies from 17 years to late middle age.

For Turkish vLINCL (i.e., tLINCL or CLN8-deficient form), the clinical phenotype is substantially more severe than that of EPMR. Patients present between the ages of 2 and 5 with severe seizures. Intellectual decline, blindness, and behavioral problems follow and are prominent by age 8 or 9 years. By 10 years of age, most of the children are wheelchair-bound.

For the Costa Rican/Portuguese vLINCL/Lake Cavanaugh variant (i.e., CLN6-deficient form) [Teixeira et al., 2003], the initial presenting symptoms at the age of 4 years are ataxia and speech difficulties after a period of normal development. Visual failure due to retinitis pigmentosa, myoclonic jerks, and seizures are accompanied by ataxia and intellectual decline. Death occurs in the early to middle teens.

CLINICAL DIAGNOSTIC TESTS

Presenting symptoms suggesting classic LINCL or JNCL with atypical features, normal TPP1 enzyme activities, absence of vacuolated lymphocytes, and a normal CLN3 gene screen strongly suggest one of the variant LINCL types. Electron microscopic results of a skin biopsy, the patient's ethnic background, and subtle characteristic clinical features for one of these subtypes may tip the scale in favor of one of the LINCL variants over the others. Fingerprint and rectilinear structures favor the Finnish variant. A combination of curvilinear and fingerprint bodies favors the Costa Rican/Portuguese variant. Electron microscopic findings for the Finnish CLN8 variant include loose curvilinear-like structures, and electron microscopic assessment of the Turkish variant demonstrates dense fingerprint profiles in addition to dark amorphous material. The definitive confirmatory test is DNA-based proof of defects in one of the relevant genes: *CLN5*, *CLN6*, or *CLN8*. MRI scans of Costa Rican/Portuguese/Venezuelan CLN6-deficient patients and those with Finnish vLINCL demonstrate severe cerebral and cerebellar cortical atrophy, low densities in the thalami and basal ganglia, and hyperintensities of the white matter. MRI scans of patients with tLINCL demonstrate cerebellar and cerebral atrophy, and tissue loss in the brainstem. The EEGs for all of these variants record large-amplitude occipital spikes in response to low-frequency photic stimulation.

PATHOLOGY

In cases of Finnish variant LINCL (i.e., CLN5-deficient form), the brain weighs about 500 g at postmortem examination. Most notable is the severe cerebellar atrophy. Findings are otherwise quite similar to those for classic LINCL. There is strong immunoreactivity to subunit C or 9 of mitochondrial ATP synthase and weak immunoreactivity to the saposins. Electron microscopic findings are notable for the presence of rectilinear profiles and curvilinear and fingerprint bodies [Goebel and Wisniewski, 2004; Goebel et al., 1999; Topcu et al., 2004; Wisniewski et al., 2004b].

For the Costa Rican/Portuguese vLINCL/Lake Cavanaugh variant (i.e., CLN6-deficient form), the brain weighs between 600 and 900 g at postmortem examination. Neuronal loss is pervasive and particularly prominent in neocortex layer V. Although granule cells in the cerebellum are completely eliminated, some Purkinje cells remain. There is strong immunoreactivity with subunit C of mitochondrial ATP synthase in neuronal tissues. It is, however, absent from peripheral organs. At the electron microscopic level, there are primarily fingerprint bodies and, to a lesser extent, rectilinear profiles in the brain. Rectilinear, fingerprint, and curvilinear components are found in organs.

For northern epilepsy or EPMR (i.e., CLN8-deficient form), the brain weight at postmortem examination has been in excess

of 100 g but less than 1600 g. The brain may appear entirely normal, or mild atrophy can be observed. Most storage material is seen in layer III of the cortex. Neuronal loss is most prominent in cortex layer V. Deep gray structures and cerebellar Purkinje cells demonstrate little storage. There is strong reactivity with antibodies to β-amyloid, subunit C, and saposin D. Ultrastructure of the storage bodies demonstrates curvilinear bodies and granular material.

For Turkish vLINCL or tLINCL (i.e., CLN8-deficient form), no pathology reports are available in the literature. The ultrastructure of skin fibroblasts reveals the presence of curvilinear, rectilinear, and fingerprint profiles [Topcu et al., 2004].

GENETICS

For the Finnish vLINCL (i.e., CLN5-deficient form), the major mutation accounting for 94 percent of Finnish cases is a 2-bp deletion in exon 4 (c.1175delAT). There is a minor Finnish mutation, D279N, and two other mutations, W75X and c669insC, reported in rare Dutch and Swedish cases.

For the Costa Rican/Portuguese vLINCL/Lake Cavanaugh variant (i.e., CLN6-deficient form), more than 19 mutations are recognized. The most prevalent are the nonsense mutation (c.214G>T) reported in 20 Costa Rican families and the 3-bp deletion (I154del) in 6 Portuguese families [Teixeira et al., 2003]. Other mutations have been described in those of Venezuelan, Indian, Pakistani, Greek, U.S., Trinidadian, or East Indian ancestry. The nclf mouse is a naturally occurring model for CLN6-deficient vLINCL [Mole, 2004].

For northern epilepsy or EPMR (i.e., CLN8-deficient form) and variant Turkish tLINCL, one mutation, R24G, accounts for all patients with northern epilepsy. The four other mutations result in the more severe phenotype of tLINCL. Two missense mutations (R204C and W263C) occur in exon 3, and two others, L16M and T170M, occur in exon 2 and are also missense mutations. R204C occurs in the conserved TLC lipid-sensing domain and predicts a potential role for CLN8 in the sphingolipid synthetic pathways. The mnd mouse is a naturally occurring mouse model for CLN8-deficient forms of neuronal ceroid-lipofuscinosis [Ranta et al., 2004].

BIOCHEMISTRY AND CELL BIOLOGY

CLN6 and CLN8 are transmembrane proteins that reside in the endoplasmic reticulum. The CLN5 protein has been reported as being a transmembrane protein in some papers and a secreted lysosomal glycoprotein in others [Holmberg et al., 2004; Savukoski et al., 1998]. CLN5 has been reported to co-immunoprecipitate with CLN2 protein and with CLN3 protein [Vesa et al., 2002]. This interaction implies that these are dynamic proteins that most likely exist in many subcellular locations and that they may functionally interact, forming a complex whereby one protein may substitute for the other. This finding can have great implications for therapy, because some of these proteins, such as CLN2, are soluble and amenable to protein or gene replacement therapy, whereas transmembrane proteins, such as CLN3, are not.

MANAGEMENT AND THERAPY

Treatment for these variants is almost identical to that outlined for the classic LINCL and JNCL types. The relatively mild northern epilepsy variant responds very well to monotherapy with clonazepam. Patients have been reported to remain seizure-free for a number of years on this drug. Seizure frequency in this variant tends to wane with age.

MFSD8/CLN7

Siintola et al. identified the novel gene, major facilitator superfamily (MFS) domain containing 8 (MFSD8), for Turkish vLINCL in 2007. The gene was identified after homozygosity mapping of 10 families, for which known human *NCL* loci and homologous genes (*CLCN3* and *CLCN7*) causing NCL-like phenotypes in animal models were excluded by haplotype analysis [Siintola et al., 2007]. *CLN7/MFSD8* mutations are now reported from India, the Netherlands, Italy, Czech Republic, Albania, and Greece [Kousi et al., 2009].

CLINICAL DESCRIPTION

The age of presentation varies between 3 and 8 years. Patients present with delayed speech development, stereotypic hand movements, and sleep disorders. Later, myoclonic, clonic, and nocturnal seizures develop. These respond to medical therapy, then become refractory. In some patients, the presenting feature is epilepsy. Status epilepticus has been also reported. Progressive neurological decline and psychological symptoms of agitation and aggressiveness occur in late childhood. Axial akinesia, hypertonia, palilalia, and blindness ensue. Patients become disabled, cannot walk without support, and become wheelchair-bound at the end stages. Death usually occurs in late childhood but some patients survive till the second and third decade. Patients with missense mutation in exon 5 (c.362a>g /p.Tyr121Cys) were reported to have unaffected vision [Siintola et al., 2007; Stogmann et al., 2009].

CLINICAL DIAGNOSTIC TESTS

Brain MRI reflects cerebellar and cerebral atrophy and increased signal intensity in white matter, with evidence of delayed white matter maturation [Siintola et al., 2007]. EEG documents slow background activity, multifocal epileptic discharges [Siintola et al., 2007], and occipital epileptiform activity [Aiello et al., 2009]. Eye ground examination reveals retinopathy and optic atrophy [Siintola et al., 2007].

PATHOLOGY

Peripheral blood lymphocytes show vacuoles. Skin biopsy reveals vacuoles with fingerprint profiles. Rectal biopsy contains neuronal curvilinear bodies [Siintola et al., 2007]. Electron microscopy performed in skin fibroblasts details fingerprint profiles, curvilinear bodies, and granular osmiophilic deposits [Aiello et al., 2009].

BIOCHEMISTRY

MFSD8 is predicted to encode 518 amino acids of an approximately 58-kDa protein with 12 predicted transmembrane domains. In an in vitro translation assay, hemagglutinin-tagged MFSD8 proteins were detected as approximately 60-kDa bands on denaturing polyacrylamide gel electrophoresis, in agreement with the calculated molecular weight of the protein. *MFSD8* appears to be evolutionarily conserved, since a basic local alignment search tool (BLAST) search for regions of local sequence similarity returned several homologs for *MFSD8* in different species. In each vertebrate species, *MFSD8* has a single ortholog.

The two identified missense mutations (p.Gly310Asp and p.Gly429Asp) change the highly conserved glycines that reside in the predicted eight and tenth transmembrane domains, respectively, to aspartic acids. Two of the mutations (c.697ArG and c.1102GrC) may change highly conserved amino acids (p.Arg233Gly and p.Asp368His, respectively), and may result in changes in the protein structure and/or function. Alternatively, they may affect splicing of the transcript, because they change sequences at the exon–intron junctions in the 3' ends of exons 7 and 11, and thus may lead to production of abnormal mRNAs and/or proteins [Siintola et al., 2007].

GENETICS

Analysis of genome-wide single nucleotide polymorphism (SNP) data in families with vLINCL revealed three regions on chromosomes 4, 8, and 15, with heterozygosity log of odds (HLOD) scores >2. Ninety known putative genes were identified. After excluding TRAM1L1 and TRPC3 by sequencing, six homozygous mutations in *MFSD* were identified. Homozygous nonsense mutation c.894TrG, in exon 10, creates a premature stop codon (p.Tyr298X) predicted to truncate the protein by 221 aa. Homozygous missense mutations c.929GrA (p.Gly310Asp) in exon 10 and c.1286GrA (p.Gly429Asp) in exon 12, respectively, affect amino acids that are conserved across vertebrates. Homozygous nucleotide changes at the exon–intron junctions may either change an amino acid or affect the splicing of the transcript. An arginine to glycine transition at the second-to-last nucleotide of exon 7 (c.697Arg; p.Arg233Gly) and a transversion of G to C at the last nucleotide of exon 11 (c.1102GrC; p.Asp368His) are two examples. Both Arg233 and Asp368 are conserved in vertebrates. Intronic mutation (c.754_2TrA) was identified in intron 8 [Siintola et al., 2007]. Other mutations reported are a missense mutation in exon 5 (c.362a>g/p.Y121C) [Stogmann et al., 2009], nonsense mutations (p.Arg35Stop, p.Glu381Stop, p.Arg482Stop), missense mutations (p.Met1Thr, p.Gly52Arg, p.Thr294Lys, p.Pro447Leu), splice site mutations (c.863+3_4insT, c.863+1G>C), 17-bp deletion predicting a frameshift and premature protein truncation (c.627_643del17/p.Met209IlefsX3) [Aiello et al., 2009], missense mutation in exon 12 (c.1398C>T) [Aldahmesh et al., 2009], and other mutations in Indian and European families [Kousi et al., 2009].

MANAGEMENT AND TREATMENT

Supportive therapies are the mainstay. Levetiracetam and valproic acid are used to manage seizures early in the disease. Physical therapy plays a role early on and may delay the onset of severe disabilities.

Juvenile Neuronal Ceroid-Lipofuscinosis or Juvenile Batten's Disease

Although cases of JNCL (i.e., JNCL, Spielmeyer–Vogt–Batten–Mayou, CLN3-defective or deficient form) from all over the world have been described, there is a preponderance of cases with Northern European ancestry (i.e., Finland, Iceland, Norway, Sweden, Denmark, Germany, and Holland). There is a notable absence of African or Jewish cases. Japanese, Portuguese, Polish, British, Turkish, Moroccan, and Lebanese cases and cases from other countries have been described. It is the most prevalent type of neuronal ceroid-lipofuscinosis in the United States [Boustany, 1996]. JNCL was the first Batten variant to be recognized, and the gene responsible for it, *CLN3*, was the first to be cloned [Lerner et al., 1995]. Description of the first juvenile cases is credited to a Danish physician, Otto Christian Stengel [Stengel, 1826]. The genetic nature of the illness was established in the Norwegian family he described, who had four affected siblings. Because they were raised in different geographic areas by different family members, an environmental cause for the illness was eliminated.

CLINICAL DESCRIPTION

Early development is normal. The first sign of trouble is decreased central vision caused by retinitis pigmentosa. This sets in between 4 and 6 years of age. These children are followed by ophthalmologists as normal children with retinitis pigmentosa. They ultimately are enrolled in schools for the visually impaired. Patients become completely blind between the ages of 10 and 14 years, but sometimes even later. Retinal findings include macular retinal pigment epithelium atrophy, pigment stippling, epiretinal membrane, bull's eye maculopathy, retinitis with the appearance of peripheral bone spicules, and variable disk pallor [Hainsworth et al., 2009]. Complete blindness is accompanied by a disturbed sleep–wake cycle and insomnia. Retrospectively, a subset of affected children may manifest difficult behavior between the ages of 7 and 9 years. By age 10 years, cognitive decline sets in. The diagnosis is first suspected by teachers, who may be familiar with this condition in the pediatric visually impaired population. Seizures make their appearance as early as age 12 years, but they often do not occur until 14 years of age. Early-onset seizures that are difficult to control often foretell a more rapidly declining course. Speech becomes echolalic. Perseveration of speech and actions becomes routine. A cogwheel rigidity of the limbs sets in. Patients walk with a stooped, shuffling gait reminiscent of patients with Parkinson's disease. An intention tremor of variable severity is often observed.

Patients generally plateau in their middle teens. A large number become depressed and agitated, and a small number become aggressive and psychotic. These adolescents often have a positive family history for unipolar or bipolar illness. Treatment is often necessary. It can aggravate extrapyramidal signs and symptoms. Hallucinations are common. They can, however, be of a pleasant and repetitive nature. A number of patients have imaginary friends with names and include them in their daily routine. Growth and physical maturity are not affected, which can make sexual development a problem, particularly for teenage girls. Contraception is often sought by parents for affected teenage daughters. Late-stage symptoms include drooling, difficulty swallowing, and weight loss. These problems are obviated by the use of feeding tubes. Temperature instability, with episodes of extreme hypothermia down to 92°F, alternating with hyperthermia, points to hypothalamic involvement. Seizures increase in number and are difficult to control. Some patients develop a cardiomyopathy or sick sinus syndrome with bradycardia. Most patients succumb in their early to mid-20s to seizures and cardiopulmonary arrest. A small number can survive into the fourth decade of life.

CLINICAL DIAGNOSTIC TESTS

When clinical suspicion is strong, DNA-based *CLN3* gene tests can confirm the diagnosis (see "Genetics"). The EEG is abnormal from age 9 years onward. Large-amplitude spike and slow-wave complexes are observed. CT and MRI scans may initially be normal and can remain so until age 12 years. Ultimately, cerebral atrophy with gaping sulci and large ventricles is the norm. Cerebellar atrophy is often present. Morphometric MRI measurements indicate loss of hemispheric, caudate, thalamic, and lenticular volumes [Boustany and Filipek, 1993]. There is a low signal in the white matter seen in T2-weighted images. Positron emission tomography (PET) has demonstrated decreased glucose use that starts in the calcarine area and progresses to involve all gray matter structures. The latter two techniques are not done routinely on patients, but when carried out, they can help to understand disease progression better. The ERG is often abnormal, even before the patients complain of decreased vision. Visual-evoked potentials reveal reduced-amplitude potentials, and somatosensory-evoked potentials are enhanced, but these are not particularly useful tests. The ultrastructure of the skin biopsy sample is often helpful, particularly if the common 1-kb deletion is absent from one or both alleles. Schwann cells, endothelial cells, pericytes, neurons, macrophages, and eccrine sweat glands all contain inclusions. Fingerprint-like inclusions enclosed by a unit membrane are typical. Curvilinear inclusions are frequently seen, sometimes within the same cell. Vacuolated lymphocytes are a hallmark of JNCL, but these have to be processed swiftly and correctly, otherwise the number of false-positive results becomes high. Unfortunately, very few diagnostic laboratories can accurately evaluate vacuolated lymphocytes. Skin fibroblast electron microscopy is a more robust test that has proved extremely helpful over the years.

PATHOLOGY

Brain weight at the time of death is 450–1100 g. There is thinning of the cortical mantle. There is moderate neuronal loss with gliosis and accumulation of autofluorescent material. This material is Sudan black B- and PAS-positive. Meganeurites are seen in the basolateral amygdaloid complex and in cortical layer V. Purkinje cell and granule cell dropout is observed in the cerebellum. Electron microscopy reveals apoptotic neurons with dark, shrunken, and fragmented chromatin in the cerebral cortex. A number of neurons are TUNEL stain-positive, confirming the existence of apoptotic neurons. Surviving neurons demonstrate immunoreactivity with antibodies to BCL2, a neuroprotective protein, and to subunit C or 9 of mitochondrial ATP synthase. Lipopigment accumulates in anterior horn cells of the spinal cord and the receptor cells of the organ of Corti. In neuronal cells, fingerprint profiles predominate, whereas in non-neuronal cells, curvilinear inclusions are common.

BIOCHEMISTRY, CELL BIOLOGY, AND PATHOPHYSIOLOGY

An initial observation was that ceramide, the pro-apoptotic lipid second messenger, was elevated in JNCL brains [Puranam et al., 1999]. This elevation correlated with the identification of apoptosis in JNCL brains and anti-apoptotic amino acid stretches within the CLN3 protein [Persaud-Sawin et al., 2002]. In addition to ceramide, galactosyl-ceramide, glucosylceramide, ceramide trihexoside, and sphingomyelin levels are elevated, pointing to sphingolipid overproduction [Persaud-Sawin et al., 2004]. The CLN3 protein is upregulated in a number of human and mouse cancer cell lines and in solid colon cancer specimens [Rylova et al., 2002]. The CLN3 protein localizes to the Golgi, early recycling endosomes, and lipid rafts in plasma membranes. The VYFAE motif within the CLN3 protein is embedded in a larger galactosylceramide lipid raft binding domain. In CLN3-deficient cells, mutant CLN3 incorrectly localizes to late endosomes and lysosomes, and mutant CLN3 protein and galactosylceramide, an important component of lipid rafts, remain stuck in the Golgi, never reaching the plasma membrane and lipid rafts. Reversal of this after restoring CLN3 to the deficient cells suggests that CLN3 normally functions as a galactosylceramide transporter from the Golgi to lipid rafts by recycling endosomes. This may explain the increase in apoptosis that is often initiated from lipid rafts and the increased production of sphingolipids in an attempt to rectify the galactosylceramide deficiency in lipid rafts [Rusyn et al., 2008].

GENETICS

JNCL is the most common form of Batten's diseases in the United States. This autosomal-recessive disease has a prevalence of 7 per 100,000 live births in Iceland and 0.71 per 100,000 live births in Germany. The prevalence decreases as the distance from Scandinavian countries increases, and the prevalence in the United States therefore is much lower. JNCL is classified as an orphan disease, according to FDA guidelines.

The gene has 15 exons, which translates into a protein that is 438 amino acids long. The hydrophobic protein has 5–7 potential transmembrane domains. This protein is highly conserved among species, indicating a significant role for cell maintenance. Thirty-six mutations have been described. The same 1.02-kb deletion accounts for 85 percent of cases in the United States. DNA-based carrier testing is available, provided the family mutation is known. Prenatal diagnosis has been performed using ultrastructure and DNA-based tests as early as 11 weeks' gestation. It is best to confirm diagnosis again at birth using cord blood.

MANAGEMENT AND TREATMENT

JNCL is the most challenging of the clinical types to manage. Although initially seizure control is easily achieved with one drug, as the disease advances, some patients progress to having over 100 seizures per day despite use of a multitude of antiepileptic medications. The seizures are of mixed type, including generalized, myoclonic, and partial complex seizures. The emotional and psychiatric aspects of this disorder present a therapeutic dilemma. Many patients require antipsychotic drugs and mood stabilizers, which lower seizure threshold and aggravate parkinsonian symptoms. Insomnia is a problem that should be addressed with the use of benzodiazepines and other drugs. Weight loss becomes an issue in the final few years. It requires gastrostomy tubes for adequate provision of calories, liquids, and anticonvulsants. Anecdotal reports of the use of the anti-apoptotic medication flupirtine suggests improved seizure control and sleep patterns. Of those patients that develop bradycardia, only a handful have needed pacemakers placed. Nonconventional therapies based on findings in a small number of patients positive for GAD-65 and anti α-fetoprotein antibodies [Castaneda and Pearce, 2008] includes a trial of modulators of the immune system by a variety of ways, including oral prednisone and mycophenolate mofetil (Cellcept). The latter has been FDA-approved for human clinical trials [personal communication to R-MB, NCL

Resource, UK]. Eight patients with JNCL positive for GAD65 antibodies were treated with oral prednisolone 0.75 mg/kg/day, maximum dose of 40 mg, for 10 days each month. Two had a significant increase in verbal IQ, alertness, and ability to move on days 3–4 of treatment. This effect lasted just a few days beyond therapy, only to reappear during the next month with treatment [Aberg et al., 2008].

Death ensues, on average, in the early to middle 20s, with some patients dying as young as age 13 and others surviving to age 40 years. The average survival has increased with the advent of vigorous treatment of infections, use of feeding tubes, and better antiepileptic drugs. Unfortunately, because CLN3 is a membrane protein, there is little enthusiasm for protein or gene replacement strategies. Stem cell approaches have not been explored but may some day have a role in therapy. Bone marrow transplantation is not effective. There are multiple mouse models for this disease. The hope for lessening the burden of JNCL continues to rely on achievement of a better understanding of the pathobiology and biochemistry of this disorder.

CLN9-Deficient Juvenile-like Variant

Two German brothers and two American sisters of Serbian descent had been clinically diagnosed with the JNCL variant before identification of the *CLN3* gene [Lin et al., 2001; Schulz et al., 2004]. When DNA from these cases was examined, it was determined that they had no defects in the *CLN3* gene, and they had normal levels of CLN3 mRNA. Analysis of cDNA from CLN3-, CLN1-, CLN2-, and CLN6-deficient variants, together with cDNA from these unknown cases, using Affymetrix GeneChips, revealed a distinctive gene profile that grouped them together as a separate variant (Figure 41-1). Results of enzyme assays and molecular tests for all other known neuronal ceroid-lipofuscinosis variants were normal.

CLINICAL DESCRIPTION

The clinical course for CLN9-deficient juvenile-like variant is almost identical to that of JNCL, with decreased vision occurring at age 4 years, cognitive decline at age 6 years, and ataxia and rigidity by age 9 years. These patients develop dysarthria and scanning speech, and are mute by age 12 years. One of the German brothers developed hallucinations and behavior problems. All four patients developed intractable seizures in their early to middle teens, which eventually diminished. Retinitis with pigmentary changes was documented in one of the two brothers. One of the brothers died of pneumonia at age 15 years, and the other died at age 19 years after suffering from

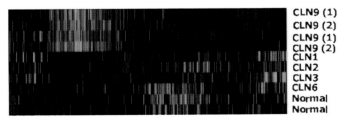

Fig. 41-1 Partial dendrogram depicting gene expression pattern for CLN1-, CLN2-, CLN3-, CLN6-, CLN9-deficient and normal fibroblast RNA. Upregulated genes are red, downregulated genes are green, and no change from control is black. Notice the similarity of gene expression in the CLN9(1) and CLN9(2) patients. CLN, ceroid-lipofuscinosis, neuronal.

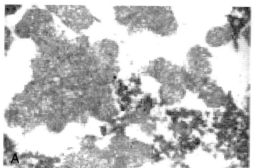
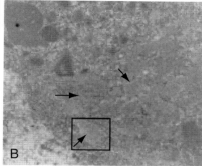
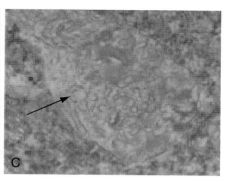

Fig. 41-2 Electron micrographs of CLN9-deficient frontal cortex. A, Notice the secondary lysosomes with curvilinear bodies (magnification × 18,400). **B,** Granular osmiophilic deposits (GRODs) are denoted by arrows, and curvilinear bodies are denoted by a framed arrow (magnification × 45,400). **C,** Enlarged inset from B (magnification × 96,000).

swallowing difficulties and many seizures. The two sisters remain alive. One is in her early 20s and has been bedridden since she was 14 years old. She has well-controlled seizures and requires a feeding tube. The younger sister is now 12 years old and is following a similar course.

CLINICAL DIAGNOSTIC TESTS

The ERG documented diminished wave amplitudes in one of the brothers with JNCL variant. The EEGs in all four patients demonstrated slowing and frequent polyspike discharges.

Electron micrographs of lymphocytes indicate numerous membrane-bound inclusions containing a mixture of electron-dense storage material and fingerprint patterns. CT and MRI scans showed progressive cerebral and cerebellar cortical atrophy. Abnormal signal intensity was observed in the periventricular white matter. A diagnostic brain biopsy from one of the sisters depicts neurons that contain granular osmiophilic inclusions and curvilinear bodies.

PATHOLOGY

The brain weight of the older brother at the time of death was 1140 g. Neurons were ballooned with fine, granular material. Large neurons remaining in the cerebral cortex and the deep gray structures were ballooned. The substantia nigra and nuclear thalami had moderate to severe astrogliosis, as did the spinal cord. The storage material was stained gray with Sudan black, and it had a yellow autofluorescence. The ultrastructure of neurons reveals GRODs and curvilinear bodies (Figure 41-2). Neurons also demonstrated immunoreactivity to subunit C or 9 of mitochondrial ATP synthase.

GENETICS

Chromosomal location of the underlying *CLN9* gene remains unknown, but candidate genes include those encoding for proteins that impact the ceramide synthetic and catabolic pathways. The small number of affected cases has precluded traditional linkage analysis studies.

BIOCHEMISTRY AND CELL BIOLOGY

Although the gene remains unidentified, the biochemistry and cell biology of this variant are well understood. CLN9-deficient cells have a distinctive morphology and phenotype. Cells are small and rounded rather than elongated, and they have prominent nucleoli, as seen by filipin staining. They have rapid growth rates because of increased DNA synthesis, but they have an increased sensitivity to apoptosis. They have an adhesion defect, and a number of the genes involved in cell adhesion and apoptosis are dysregulated, as determined by gene profiling [Schulz et al., 2004]. Gene expression of cyclins A2, B1, C, E2, G1, and T2 were increased. Cyclin D1, encoded by a proto-oncogene involved in malignant transformation of breast tissue, was significantly downregulated, as was member 1A of the tumor necrosis factor superfamily.

Expression of subunits of cytochrome c oxidases and glutathione *S*-transferase was also increased. Ceramide, sphingomyelin, lactosylceramide, ceramide trihexoside, and globoside levels were decreased by 60–100 percent. The key regulating enzyme in the ceramide de novo synthetic pathway, serine palmitoyl transferase, was three- to fourfold upregulated, suggesting a block further downstream. The low levels of glycosphingolipids can explain the defect in cell adhesion observed in CLN9-deficient fibroblasts.

MANAGEMENT AND TREATMENT

Treatment is similar to that outlined for the JNCL variant. Flupirtine used empirically in the two sisters has led to stabilization of the course and better control of seizures. After the entire sphingolipid pathway and its perturbations are better defined for this variant, it will become possible to use drugs to correct defects in the pathway. CLN9 protein may be a regulator of dihydroceramide synthase. 4-hydroxyphenyl retinamide (4-HPR), an activator of the enzyme, could be developed as a treatment for CLN9-deficient patients [Schulz et al., 2006].

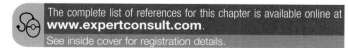

Channelopathies

Kelly Knupp, Julie A. Parsons, and Amy R. Brooks-Kayal

Introduction

Channelopathies are a group of genetically and phenotypically heterogeneous neurological disorders that result from genetically determined defects in ion-channel function. Channelopathies are considered phenotypically heterogeneous because mutations in the same gene can cause different diseases; they are considered genetically heterogeneous because mutations in different genes can result in the same disease phenotype. Mutations of ion channels can alter the activation, ion selectivity, or inactivation of the mutated channel. Neurological manifestations of channelopathies fall into several clinical phenotypes: epilepsy, pain, migraine, ataxia, movement disorders, and muscle disorders (myotonia and weakness).

Ion channels are transmembrane glycoprotein pores that control the excitability of neurons and muscle cells by mediating the flow of charged ions in and out of cells. Channels are typically composed of different protein subunits, each encoded by a different gene. There are two major classes of ion channels: voltage-gated and ligand-gated. Voltage-gated ion channels are activated and inactivated by changes in membrane voltage and are identified according to the principal ion conducted through the channel (e.g., sodium, potassium, calcium, or chloride). Activation and opening of voltage-gated channels have different effects (depolarization, repolarization, or hyperpolarization of the cell membrane), depending on what ion they gate and its charge, the electrochemical gradient for that ion (which determines which direction the ion flows when the channel is opened), and where the channels are located on the cell. Sodium channel opening results in the generation of the action potential (i.e., depolarization). Opening of potassium channels repolarizes cell membranes after action potential firing and maintains the resting membrane potential. Calcium channels are important for the generation of muscle contraction, neurotransmitter release, and intracellular signaling via second messengers. Opening of voltage-gated chloride channels results in the hyperpolarization of cells.

Ligand-gated channels are heterogeneous complexes composed of multiple protein subunits that are activated by the binding of their respective agonists. Several ligand-gated channels are present in the peripheral and central nervous systems. Gamma-aminobutyric acid $(GABA)_A$ receptors mediate most of the fast synaptic inhibition in the brain outside of the fetal and early neonatal periods. They are anion-selective and gate primarily chloride, which flows into the cell, causing hyperpolarization upon $GABA_A$ receptor activation. Glutamate is the primary excitatory neurotransmitter in the central nervous system and binds to three types of ligand-gated, cation-selective receptor channels: N-methyl-D-aspartate (NMDA), α-amino-3-hydroxy-5-methylisoxazole-4-propionic acid (AMPA), and kainate. Glutamate receptors gate either sodium only (most AMPA and all kainate receptors), or sodium and calcium (NMDA receptors and some subtypes of AMPA receptors). Nicotinic acetylcholine receptors are nonselective cation channels permeable to Na^+ and K^+, and in some subtypes Ca^{2+}; they are located on certain neurons and on the postsynaptic side of the neuromuscular junction. Opening of nicotinic receptors causes depolarization of the plasma membrane and activation of voltage-gated ion channels that can effect the release of neurotransmitters and activate intracellular signaling cascades.

Epilepsy Syndromes

As basic science advances and the etiology of several epilepsy syndromes is discovered, ion channelopathies have been identified involving sodium, potassium, and calcium channels. Ligand-gated channels such as GABA receptors and nicotinic receptors also have been implicated. Identifying these syndromes will likely lead to unique treatments for this group of patients.

Dravet's Syndrome (Severe Myoclonic Epilepsy of Infancy, Severe Myoclonic Epilepsy of Infancy – Borderline)

Clinical Features

Dravet's syndrome was described first by Charlotte Dravet in 1978 and then in the publication *Advances in Epileptology* in 1982 [Dravet et al., 1982]. Dravet described a group of children using the name "severe myoclonic epilepsy of infancy" (SMEI). Over time, it became recognized that some children have an incomplete form of the disease, leading to the terminology of "severe myoclonic epilepsy of infancy – borderline."

These children classically begin to have seizures in the first year of life, typically in the setting of fever and usually characterized by prolonged seizures with hemiconvulsions. The laterality of seizures can alternate with each individual seizure and often evolve into status epilepticus. In the second year of life, other seizure types may begin to emerge, including absence, myoclonic, and generalized tonic–clonic seizures, as well as partial seizures typically occurring without fever. Tonic seizures are rare and, if they do occur, tend to be brief and nocturnal. Myoclonus can be either generalized, focal, or both. Photo-induced seizures occur in some of these children and self-induced seizures have been reported. Throughout childhood, fever continues to be a common provoker of seizures and these seizures are often very difficult to control.

An interesting feature of Dravet's syndrome is the presence of "obtundation status." This involves episodes of nonconvulsive status with intermixed myoclonus, at times building up to rhythmic bilateral jerking resembling a generalized clonic seizure. The duration can be hours to days, with slowed responsiveness or waxing and waning alertness. The electroencephalogram (EEG) will often demonstrate diffuse delta activity with intermixed focal and diffuse spikes. Myoclonus may not correlate with spike discharges, except with larger more generalized rhythmic myoclonic jerks. Hospitalization may be required for effective treatment. Some children may have several characteristics of localization-related epilepsy and occasionally have undergone surgical treatment of seizures before the syndrome has been identified.

Development is universally normal in the first year of life. As seizure types become more varied and more frequent, there is often developmental regression or cessation of developmental progress. Severe mental retardation is present in many children with Dravet's syndrome, but the degree of cognitive impairment is associated with seizure control in many patients [Wolff et al., 2006]. Behavioral issues seem to become more of a concern after age 2. Hyperactivity and autistic traits can be present and very prominent. As children enter into adolescence, hyperkinetic behavior tends to improve and is replaced with overall slowed behavior. Ataxia may also become prominent.

Not all children with Dravet's syndrome present with what are now considered the classical features, as described above. Some children may not have all of the varied seizure types and have little developmental regression. Myoclonic seizures need not be present for a diagnosis to be made. These seemingly less affected children continue to be exquisitely sensitive to seizure exacerbation due to elevated body temperature, as well as to anticonvulsants that are sodium channel blockers (e.g., carbamazepine, phenytoin, fosphenytoin, oxcarbazepine, lamotrigine, and zonisamide). In some cases these features may suggest the diagnosis. Recently, this syndrome was recognized in a large percentage of children (11 of 14) presenting with seizures and encephalopathy after receiving vaccines (vaccine encephalopathy) [Berkovic et al., 2006]. Logically, it would seem that, for many children, their first fever likely occurs with the first or second set of immunizations. A child was reported to have "hemiconvulsion-hemiplegia syndrome" after a prolonged episode of hemiconvulsion, and subsequently was identified to have the genetic mutation associated with Dravet's syndrome [Sakakibara et al., 2009].

Since gene testing has become available for this syndrome, it appears that the phenotype is broader than initially appreciated. The diagnosis of severe myoclonic epilepsy of infancy no longer seems to be an appropriate label; therefore the eponym "Dravet's syndrome" is now the preferred name, encompassing both groups of children. As more children are found to have a similar gene mutation, the true phenotype of this syndrome will likely evolve.

Genetics/Pathophysiology

Mutations in a sodium channel, SCN1A, were initially identified in 7 of 7 children with severe myoclonic infantile epilepsy [Claes et al., 2001]. Approximately 80 percent of children with a clinical diagnosis of Dravet's syndrome have a mutation in this gene. This channel was initially implicated in generalized epilepsy with febrile seizures plus (GEFS+; see below). The sensitivity to body temperature in both of these syndromes led investigators to evaluate for mutations in the SMEI population. The majority of the children with Dravet's syndrome have a de novo mutation, although some of the families have a higher than expected history of febrile seizures. The phenotype of patients can be predicted by mutation in most cases, as the majority of patients have a truncation mutation or a mutation that affects the function of the channel pore. Patients with less severe phenotypes often have point mutations that do not result in as severe an effect on the function of the sodium channel, although the correlation of specific SCN1A mutation to phenotype is not a tight one.

Recent discoveries related to the cell type-specific localization of SCN1A added to our understanding of how loss of function of a sodium channel, logically a cause of hypoexcitablity of individual neurons, could lead to network hyperexcitabilty and, consequently, seizures. This seeming contradiction can be explained by the finding that the loss of SCN1A function leads to selective loss of sodium channel function in inhibitory interneurons [Yu et al., 2006], causing inhibitory dysfunction and secondary hyperexcitability.

Clinical Laboratory Tests

EEG findings are typically normal in the first year of life, but evolve to demonstrate generalized and multifocal abnormalities. A photoconvulsive response can be seen, and diffuse background slowing can become more prominent as children age. No characteristic pattern is diagnostic of Dravet's syndrome, as is seen in Lennox–Gastaut or Doose's syndrome; in fact, there can be some overlap between these syndromes and Dravet's syndrome, making accurate diagnosis challenging. EEG findings can fluctuate, and a small percentage of patients may continue to have normal EEGs; over time, a decrease in epileptiform abnormalities has been reported in older patients.

Magnetic resonance imaging (MRI) in patients with Dravet's syndrome is usually without any focal abnormalities. In one study that evaluated 58 children with Dravet's syndrome, 60 percent had SCN1a mutations and 22 percent had abnormal MRI findings, the majority with cortical atrophy and others with cerebellar atrophy, white matter hyperintensity, mesial temporal sclerosis, and focal cortical dysplasia. Abnormal findings were more likely in patients without a genetic mutation [Striano et al., 2007]. Other studies have suggested that mild, diffuse atrophy and ventriculomegaly may develop over time.

Genetic testing is appropriate in patients suspected to have Dravet's syndrome. Early diagnosis may avoid extensive and expensive metabolic testing and inadvertent exacerbation of seizures by certain medications, as well as providing prognostic information for the family. However, as the phenotype expands, using genotype to provide an accurate prognosis may become more problematic.

Treatment

Seizure control is the primary treatment goal in this disorder. Medications that are known to block the sodium channel often will exacerbate seizures and should be avoided [Guerrini et al., 1998]. Prior to clinical diagnosis, a worsening of seizures while being treated with one of these medications should raise suspicion of Dravet's syndrome. Topiramate, valproic acid, benzodiazepines, and levetiracetam have been helpful. Non-pharmacologic treatments, such as vagal nerve stimulation or the ketogenic diet [Caraballo and Fejeman, 2006], have been useful in some patients. Combination therapy with stiripentol, clobazam, and either depakote or topiramate has been reported to be more effective than other combinations of medication. In an initial report by Chiron et al., 15 of 21 patients responded to stiripentol [Chiron et al., 2000]. Acetazolamide has not been shown to be beneficial. A recent report with the calcium channel blocker, verapamil, has suggested that this may be helpful, but more research is required [Iannetti et al., 2009].

Avoidance of hot temperatures, both environmental and elevated body temperature, has been used by many families to reduce seizures. Antipyretics, such as acetaminophen, have been helpful, although there is a recent report of four children with transient liver abnormalities that may be associated with use of this medication [Nicolai et al., 2008]. Helmets may be indicated in some patients. Due to the severity of the cognitive impairment, appropriate support must be initiated for the family [Nolan et al., 2008]. Medications for behavioral issues may also be necessary (see Chapter 49).

Generalized Epilepsy with Febrile Seizures Plus (GEFS+)

Clinical Features

This is a familial epilepsy syndrome characterized by febrile seizures in childhood in several generations of family members, often with continuation of febrile seizures into adulthood. Some seizures related to fever may be prolonged. Some family members may also have generalized epilepsies, such as absence epilepsy, myoclonic astatic epilepsy, or, rarely, Dravet's syndrome. Seizure types include generalized tonic clonic, myoclonic, absence, and atonic seizures. There is variable penetrance of seizures in these familial cohorts. Phenotype also varies among family members. Many family members may have resolution of seizures by age 12. The majority of these patients have normal development and intelligence. There has also been a report of temporal lobe epilepsy with mesial temporal sclerosis associated with the SCN1A mutation [Mantegazza et al., 2005].

Genetics/Pathophysiology

SCN1B was a mutation first reported in a large family with this syndrome [Wallace et al., 1998]. Mutations in other sodium channels – SCN1A [Escayg et al., 2000a] and SCN2A [Sugawara et al., 2001] – have been found subsequently. The majority of these mutations have been point mutations. In patients with SCN1A mutations, a difference in phenotype from GEFS+ and Dravet's syndrome can often be predicted, given the location of the mutation (distance from the pore), as well as alteration in transcription of the gene. Nonsense and truncation mutations are more likely to be associated with Dravet's syndrome. Sodium channel mutations do not account for all of the mutations in GEFS+; there also have been reports of mutations identified in GABA$_A$ receptor subunit genes, GABRG2 and GABRD (gamma 2 and delta subunits) [Harkin et al., 2002]. GABA$_A$ receptors are ligand-gated chloride channels that provide the majority of inhibition in brain beyond the neonatal period, and mutations resulting in GABA$_A$ receptor

dysfunction result in increased central nervous system excitability that has been associated with a number of genetic epilepsies.

Treatment

There has been little published discussion of the treatment of these syndromes. For patients with sodium channel mutations, avoidance of sodium channel blockers is wise. Treatment when necessary with broad-spectrum anticonvulsants is thought to be useful. Avoidance of temperature changes and routine use of fever control measures may be of some benefit.

Benign Familial Neonatal Seizures

Clinical Features

Benign familial neonatal seizures are an autosomal-dominant epilepsy presenting with seizures in the first or second week of life, most commonly starting on day of life 2 or 3, resolving within weeks to months. Most seizures have stopped at 4–5 months of life. Seizures are usually multifocal clonic seizures or focal seizures. The feature suggesting this entity is the presence of similar seizures in parents and first-degree relatives, occurring at the same age. Development is characteristically normal during this time period, as well as after seizures stop. Fifteen percent of children will develop epilepsy later in life, usually in childhood or as a young adult. There are some children who progress to medically refractory epilepsy with encephalopathy [Steinlein et al., 2007].

Genetics/Pathophysiology

Mutations in potassium channels KCNQ2 [Singh et al., 1998; Biervert et al., 1998] and KCNQ3 [Charlier et al., 1998] (found on chromosomes 20 and 8 respectively) have been reported in families with benign neonatal seizures. These mutations also have been reported in some families with benign rolandic epilepsy [Hahn and Neubauer, 2009]. Recently, mutations in these genes also have been reported in a small percentage of patients with idiopathic generalized epilepsy, suggesting it may play some role in the etiology of these epilepsies. Mutations can cause alteration in function or complete loss of function of the potassium channel. Approximately 50 percent of mutations lead to shortening of expressed protein [Heron et al., 2007]. The age specificity of the seizures in this disorder is thought to emanate from brain developmental changes during the neonatal period. GABA, which acts as an inhibitory neurotransmitter later in life, can be excitatory in the early neonatal period due to developmental changes in the chloride gradient that result in opening of GABA$_A$ receptor chloride channels, producing membrane depolarization in early development rather than membrane hyperpolarization, as it does in mature neurons. In contrast, opening of potassium channels is hyperpolarizing throughout development, and due to the paucity of GABAergic inhibition, potassium channel-mediated inhibition is uniquely critical in the newborn. This may explain why impairment or absence of potassium channel inhibition results in seizures specifically at this time and why only a small fraction of patients with KCNQ2/3 mutations have seizures later in life.

Clinical Laboratory Tests

EEG generally demonstrates normal interictal features, although at the time of seizure there is an electrographic correlate. MRI is expected to be normal. Other causes of seizures, such as neonatal infection and metabolic abnormalities, should be excluded.

Developmental Delay, Epilepsy and Neonatal Diabetes (DEND)

This is a rare syndrome, presenting with neonatal diabetes, developmental delay, seizures and mild dysmorphic features, which has been associated with a mutation in the *KCNJ11* gene that encodes for a subunit of the adenosine triphosphate (ATP)-sensitive potassium channel. This channel is found on pancreatic islet cells, as well as neurons, and neonates with this disorder usually present with diabetes and subsequently develop seizures and global developmental delay [Gloyn et al., 2004]. Dysmorphic features, including downturned mouth, bilateral ptosis, prominent metopic suture, and contractures, have also been described [Gloyn et al., 2004]. There have been reports of infantile spasms in some of these children [Bahi-Buisson et al., 2007], as well as others with tonic-clonic and myoclonic seizures. Seizures have been very refractory to traditional antiepileptic medications. In contrast, patients are very responsive to treatment with sulfonylurea medications such as glibenclamide, leading to improvement in diabetes as well as developmental outcomes and seizures.

Other "Idiopathic" Epilepsies

Autosomal-Dominant Nocturnal Frontal Lobe Epilepsy

Autosomal-dominant nocturnal frontal lobe epilepsy is a familial epilepsy characterized by frontal lobe seizures that typically occur at night and usually present as arousal from sleep with bizarre hypermotor behaviors, such as spinning, thrashing and rocking. Seizures can occur several times per night. Nicotinic receptor mutations have been found in many of these familial cohorts [Steinlein et al., 1995], although there are several families for which no gene mutation has been identified. These ligand-gated receptors allow sodium and potassium to cross the cell membrane. Many patients are responsive to carbamazepine and phenytoin.

Benign Familial Infantile–Neonatal Seizures

Benign familial infantile–neonatal seizures is an epilepsy syndrome that has been described as being similar to benign neonatal seizures but occurs at a slightly older age. Mutations have been found in a sodium channel, *SCN2A1*, in some cohorts [Herlenius et al., 2007].

Childhood Absence Epilepsy

Childhood absence epilepsy has been linked to mutations in GABA receptors (*GABRA1* and *GABRG2*) [Baulac et al., 2001; Wallace et al., 2001] and chloride channels (*CLCN2*). Mutations have also been described in a calcium channel, *CACNA1H*, but this mutation may represent an ethnic variant present in Chinese Han patients, as these findings were not present in a large European cohort [Chen et al., 2003]. The families with *CLCN2* also had members with generalized tonic-clonic seizures on awakening and juvenile myoclonic epilepsy [Baykan et al., 2004].

Juvenile Myoclonic Epilepsy

Juvenile myoclonic epilepsy is a seizure disorder that usually presents in adolescents with myoclonic seizures that are more likely to occur in the early morning after awakening, as well as generalized tonic-clonic seizures that also tend to occur in the morning hours. Several gene mutations have been found in these patients, although the majority of patients have yet to have an underlying etiology determined. It appears that, similar to childhood absence epilepsy, this is likely a polygenic disorder. Channels that have been identified include GABA receptors (*GABRA1* and *GABRD*) [Cossette et al., 2002], calcium channels (*CACNB4*) [Escayg et al., 2000b], and chloride channels (*CLCN2*) [Baykan et al., 2004]. In addition, a gene that is not a direct channel gene but enhances calcium influx into the cell and can stimulate programmed cell death (*EFHC1*) [Suzuki et al., 2004] has also been identified as being involved in this epilepsy syndrome.

Familial Pain Syndromes

Several pain syndromes have been associated with sodium channel mutations. This is not surprising, as sodium channels are located on spinal sensory neurons in the dorsal root ganglion.

Clinical Features

INHERITED ERYTHROMELALGIA, PRIMARY ERYTHERMALGIA

Inherited erythromelalgia (IEM), or primary erythermalgia, is a pain syndrome characterized by episodes of redness and swelling of the hands and feet, associated with burning pain. These episodes can be triggered by mild warmth or exercise. Many patients prefer to avoid or are unable to wear socks and shoes due to heat inducing an episode. Some patients also report involvement of the ears, nose, and other parts of their face, as well as the upper legs. Erythema can become constant, and edema may be associated [Drenth and Waxman, 2007]. Families have reported symptoms starting in the first year of life. Age of onset can vary from childhood to adulthood, and can be familial or sporadic [Drenth et al., 2008; Han et al., 2009]. About 15 percent of cases are familial, and in these cases onset is often in the first decade of life.

PAROXYSMAL EXTREME PAIN DISORDER

Paroxysmal extreme pain disorder (PEPD), formerly called familial rectal pain, is characterized by severe pain, which most commonly occurs in the perirectal region but can also involve genitals, limbs, and face, especially the periorbital region. Pain is associated with flushing. Stimulation of the region by bowel movements, contact in the perianal region, eating, or sudden changes in temperature can induce pain episodes. Areas of pain and redness can spread to other parts of the body, including orbits and face. Cardiac abnormalities, occurring at the time of the episode, have been reported in some of these cases. In addition, harlequin skin changes and pupillary abnormalities have been seen. Tonic episodes that are nonepileptic in nature can occur with the pain episodes and are secondary to the intense severity of the pain. Episodes can last seconds to minutes, and rarely 1–2 hours. Onset is usually sudden and very commonly the paroxyms are provoked. Limb attacks can be associated with weakness lasting up to 24 hours after the pain has resolved. Constipation is a common problem due to the episodes being induced by passing stool. Symptoms have been reported as early as at the time of delivery and have been suspected to occur in utero [Fertleman et al., 2007].

CONGENITAL INDIFFERENCE TO PAIN

Congenital indifference to pain is a syndrome characterized by insensitivity to pain and loss of smell. The sensory examination is normal, differentiating this syndrome from a peripheral neuropathy. Patients are aware of a stimulus but do not experience pain in relation to the stimulus. These patients can experience fractures, burns, and other significant injury without pain. Due to this inability to appreciate pain, fractures and foot injuries may be present for several days without notice. Patients may have frequent injury to the fingertips that goes unnoticed due to lack of awareness of injury. Individuals can differentiate between hot and cold, but lack the ability to determine whether an object is hot enough to cause injury. There are no signs of peripheral neuropathy on clinical examination or neurophysiological testing. There are also no abnormalities of the autonomic nervous system.

Genetics/Pathophysiology

Mutations in *SCN9A*, a sodium channel, have been associated with IEM and PEPD. Mutations are thought to lead to hyperexcitability of the sodium channel. Mutations in IEM allow the channel to be activated by smaller than normal depolarizations and the channel remains open longer, once activated. Familial cohorts with IEM have demonstrated mutations in this channel [Drenth et al., 2005], although a study looking at a more heterogeneous population with IEM only found 1 of 15 patients with a mutation [Drenth et al., 2005], suggesting that other factors might also be involved in this disease. Mutations in PEPD lead to prolonged action potentials and repetitive neuronal firing when stimulated [Jarecki et al., 2008]. Mutations in this same channel that lead to *loss* of function are associated with congenital indifference to pain [Goldberg et al., 2007; Nilsen et al., 2009]. It remains unclear why different mutations lead to different phenotypes and different pain syndromes.

Treatment

Treatment for IEM, including use of sodium channel blockers, has not been very effective, although there have been reports of some relief with lidocaine, mexiletine [Choi et al., 2009], and carbamazepine [Fischer et al., 2009]. Response to medications may vary with different mutations. Carbamazepine has been helpful in treating PEPD, but topiramate and gabapentin have not.

Congenital indifference to pain does not have a specific treatment, but patients need to be observed carefully for occult injuries, including fracture, joint injuries, and burns, as well as mouth and hand injuries. Establishing a daily routine to monitor for injuries is important.

Migraine and Ataxia Syndromes

Familial Hemiplegic Migraines

Clinical Features

Familial hemiplegic migraine often presents in the first or second decade of life with severe headache, often unilateral, and is associated with unilateral weakness that can last up to 24 hours,

or rarely several days. Coma has been reported in a small number of patients. Some patients can have a less impressive clinical presentation with unilateral paresthesias and hemianopsia. Rarely, seizures can occur during hemiplegia. In some patients, ataxia and dysarthria can be seen between attacks, or for a short duration while recovering from an attack. Family members also have been reported with benign paroxysmal torticollis of infancy [Giffin et al., 2002], although this is rare and it is unclear whether this is or is not related to the gene mutation.

Headaches can at times have features of basilar migraine, including vertigo, visual symptoms, tinnitus, dysarthria, and ataxia. Some patients have been reported to have progressive ataxia later in life [Terwindt et al., 1998]. In addition, cognitive impairment has been noted in affected patients [Marchioni et al., 1995].

At times, hemiplegic migraines have been reported after minor head trauma and can be associated with the occurrence of delayed cerebral edema. There may initially be a lucid period that is followed by the development of focal or diffuse cerebral edema, observed with neuroimaging, along with symptoms of encephalopathy, coma, and occasionally seizures. Rarely, this syndrome can result in death.

Genetics/Pathophysiology

Many patients with familial hemiplegic migraine have a calcium channel mutation (*CACNA1A*) [Stam et al., 2008]; if this is present, patients seem to be more likely to have ataxia and coma, and to be more prone to delayed cerebral edema after minor head injury [Terwindt et al., 1998; Kors et al., 2001; Stam et al., 2009]. Mutations in *CACNA1A* also have been reported in patients with alternating hemiplegia of childhood, which phenotypically has some overlap with hemiplegic migraine [de Vries et al., 2008], as well as in patients with episodic ataxia type 2 (see below) and spinocerebellar ataxia type 6. Mutations in *SCN1A* and in *ATP1A2* also have been found in some patients with this clinical syndrome [De Fusco et al., 2003; Dichgans et al., 2005a]. Interestingly, febrile seizures also have been reported in patients with mutations in either *SCN1A* or *ATP1A2* [de Vries et al., 2009; De Fusco et al., 2003].

Clinical Laboratory Tests

MRI findings are not pathognomonic, but cerebellar atrophy [Terwindt et al., 1998], particularly in the superior cerebellar vermis, has occasionally been reported. MR spectroscopy of this region demonstrated metabolic abnormalities consistent with neuron loss [Dichgans et al., 2005b]. EEG during events can demonstrate slowing in the affected hemisphere, and mild asymmetries with minimal unilateral slowing have been noted on EEGs performed between episodes [Marchioni et al., 1995].

Treatment

Most commonly, patients are treated with acetazolamide, calcium channel blockers, such as verapamil, or a trial of other standard migraine prophylactic drugs (tricyclic antidepressants, beta blockers). Limited correlation exists between drug response and hemiplegic migraine type.

Episodic Ataxia

Clinical Features

This disorder is characterized by intermittent periods of ataxia, (also see Chapter 67). There are two commonly described disorders: episodic ataxia type 1 and type 2. They differ slightly from one another in clinical presentation, allowing clinical separation.

Type 1 has frequent, brief episodes of ataxia, involving ataxic gait and slurred speech, that can be precipitated by strong emotional outbursts, sudden movements, and exercise. Episodes can last several seconds to minutes in duration and typically occur several times a day. In addition, there usually is evidence of muscle hyperexcitability manifested by the presence of myokymia clinically and electrographically. Some family members have reported seizures and isolated myotonia.

Episodic ataxia type 2 involves primarily truncal ataxia, with more prolonged periods of ataxia lasting hours to days. Eye movement abnormalities are sometimes present. Episodes can be induced by stress or exercise. Myokymia is not often present. Some patients can have slowly progressive cerebellar features that are often very subtle. Cerebellar atrophy also has been reported. Migraine symptoms can be present in both types of episodic ataxia but are more common in type 2; they may have many features consistent with basilar migraine, including vertigo, nausea, and occipital pain.

Genetics/Pathophysiology

Both disorders are inherited in an autosomal-dominant fashion, although penetrance is not always complete. Ion channel abnormalities also have been found in both disorders. Type 1 has been associated with point mutations in *KCNA1*, located on chromosome 12 [Browne et al., 1994]. This is a potassium channel that has no intervening introns. Episodic ataxia type 2 has been linked to mutations in *CACNA1A* (a calcium channel). Mutations that interfere with splicing or lead to a premature stop have been linked to the episodic ataxia type 2 phenotype [van den Maagdenberg et al., 2002]. This appears to lead to loss of function of the calcium channel. Familial hemiplegic migraine (see above) and spinocerebellar ataxia type 6 (see below) also have been reported to have mutations in this gene.

Clinical Laboratory Tests

Electromyography (EMG) is helpful with episodic ataxia type 1 in identifying and/or confirming myokymia. MRI also maybe useful, especially in episodic ataxia type 2, and should be performed to rule out other underlying etiologies of ataxia.

Treatment

Acetazolamide and carbamazepine have both been reported to lead to reduction and severity of events.

Spinocerebellar Ataxia

Clinical Features

Several progressive ataxias have been described and reported as due to a variety of etiologies (see Chapter 67). Channelopathies are responsible for one subtype, now called spinocerebellar ataxia type 6. This presents as a slowly progressive cerebellar degeneration with ataxia, dysmetria, and other cerebellar signs as a prominent clinical feature. Spasticity and cranial neuropathies are not prominent. There can be some overlap with episodic ataxia type 2, with episodes of truncal ataxia lasting for several hours to days and often precipitated by stress or exertion. There also may be some features associated with basilar migraine or familial hemiplegic migraine.

Genetics/Pathophysiology

Spinocerebellar ataxia type 6 has been reported to be associated with triplet repeats in the *CACNA1A* gene [Zhuchenko et al., 1997]. Unlike the gene changes associated with other triplet repeat disorders, this one seems relatively stable and is a smaller expansion than that typically seen in association with an abnormal phenotype. It is unclear if symptoms are related to channel dysfunction or the cytotoxic effects of the repeat, as is seen in other diseases. The overlap between these phenotypes suggests that there is a pathological role in the abnormal function of the calcium channel. Mutations in this gene also have been reported in cohorts with familial hemiplegic migraine – which usually have point mutations. Cohorts with episodic ataxia type 2 also have been reported to have mutations in this gene that often lead to splicing errors or premature stops.

Clinical Laboratory Tests

MRI is helpful, as many symptomatic episodic ataxia patients will have cerebellar atrophy.

Treatment

Supportive treatment is recommended. Patients with episodes of headaches may be helped by the treatments outlined for the episodic ataxias and familial migraine syndromes.

Muscle Channelopathies

Contraction in skeletal muscle occurs by generating and propagating action potentials. The release of intracellular calcium stores triggers mechanical contraction. This process is dependent on proper functioning of ion channels. Mutations in muscle ion channel genes have been identified, which cause a variety of diseases collectively called muscle channelopathies. Voltage-gated ion channels share similar structural features. The ion-conducting pores are selective for a specific ion. Mutations in muscle channel genes cause changes in channel function that alter membrane excitability and cause neuromuscular symptoms. Understanding the pathophysiological mechanisms involved in these diseases is an on-going focus of many studies. Clinical symptoms and their underlying neurophysiology are being linked with abnormal muscle membrane function. The overall incidence of muscle channelopathies is estimated at 1 in 100,000 [Meola et al., 2009].

Skeletal muscle disorders associated with ion channelopathies produce symptoms of myotonia, weakness, or both [Hudson et al., 1995]. Table 42-1 summarizes the various disorders (see also Chapter 96).

Myotonia Congenita

Myotonia congenita is a chloride channel disorder. Both dominant and recessive forms of this channelopathy exist. Thomsen's disease is autosomal-dominant, while Becker's disease is autosomal-recessive. Both have myotonia as the primary symptom.

Table 42-1 **Muscle Channelopathies**

Disorder	Clinical Features	Inheritance	Chromosome	Gene
Chloride channelopathies				
Myotonia congenita				
Thomsen's disease	Myotonia	AD	7q35	CLCN1
Becker's type myotonia disease	Myotonia and weakness	AR	7q35	CLCN1
Sodium channelopathies				
Paramyotonia congenita	Paramyotonia	AD	17q13.1–13.3	SCN4A
HyperKPP	Periodic paralysis with myotonia and paramyotonia	AD	17q13.1–13.3	SCN4A
HypoKPP	Periodic paralysis	AD	17q13.1–13.3	SCN4A
Potassium-aggravated myotonia				
Myotonia fluctuans	Myotonia	AD	17q13.1–13.3	SCN4A
Myotonia permanens	Myotonia	AD	17q13.1–13.3	SCN4A
Acetazolamide-responsive myotonia	Myotonia	AD	17q13.1–13.3	SCN4A
Calcium channelopathies				
HypoKPP	Periodic paralysis	AD	1q31–32	CACNA1S
Anderson–Tawil syndrome	Periodic paralysis, cardiac arrhythmia, skeletal abnormalities	AD	17q23	$K^{ir}2.1$
Malignant hyperthermia	Anesthetic-induced delayed relaxation	AD	19q13.1	RYR1

AD, autosomal-dominant; AR, autosomal-recessive; CACNA1S, skeletal muscle voltage-gated calcium channel gene; CLCN1, skeletal muscle voltage-gated chloride channel gene; HyperKPP, hyperkalemic periodic paralysis; HypoKPP, hypokalemic periodic paralysis; $K^{ir}2.1$, potassium channel gene; RYR1, ryanodine receptor gene; SCN4A, skeletal muscle voltage-gated sodium channel gene.

Clinical Features

Symptoms of painless generalized myotonia develop in the first or second decade of life in myotonia congenita. Characteristics of this disorder include a "warm-up phenomenon" in which repeated muscle movements relieve the myotonia and stiffness that occur with sudden physical exercise after a period of rest. A similar response is seen in individuals with myotonic dystrophy. In contrast, some sodium channel myotonias demonstrate increasing stiffness with repetitive movement, which is a paramyotonic response.

In both dominant and recessive forms of myotonia congenita, prominent muscle hypertrophy occurs and is most notable in the legs. Grip and eyelid closure myotonia is noted. Lid lag may be present. Strength, muscle stretch reflexes, and cerebellar and sensory testing are normal. The warm-up phenomenon can be demonstrated during the examination by having the patient sit or recline for 10 minutes, then attempt to stand, run, or walk suddenly.

Patients with Becker's or autosomal-recessive myotonia congenita may have transient muscle weakness on initiation of movement after a period of rest or quiescence. Muscle strength normalizes after several muscle contractions. Both forms of myotonia congenita are more severe in men than women [Platt and Griggs, 2009].

Genetics

The point mutation for the skeletal muscle chloride channel is located on chromosome 7q35 [Koch et al., 1992]. Both recessive and dominant forms are due to mutations in the voltage-gated chloride channel gene (CLCN1).

Pathophysiology

In normal skeletal muscle, a nerve stimulus causes depolarization of the sarcolemma, propagating an action potential that results in muscle contraction, followed by relaxation. Increased excitability of the muscle fibers in myotonia results in a single nerve stimulus causing repetitive action potentials. Skeletal muscle has a high chloride conductance, which accounts for up to 85 percent of resting membrane conductance [Bryant and Morales-Aguilera, 1971]. In myotonia congenita, reduced sarcolemmal chloride conductance causes enhanced excitability of the muscle cells, resulting in myotonic discharges [Lipicky et al., 1971].

Clinical Laboratory Tests

Myotonia congenita is usually diagnosed clinically. The presence of repetitive discharges on EMG, both on insertion as well as with voluntary contraction, can be used for conformation. Muscle biopsy is unnecessary.

In patients suspected of having myotonia congenita, other myotonic disorders should be considered, including myotonic dystrophy, paramyotonia congenita, and periodic paralyses.

Treatment

Medications used to treat myotonia are acetazolamide, mexiletine, procainamide, quinine, phenytoin, carbamazepine, and dantrolene. Exercise may temporarily relieve the muscle stiffness.

Sodium Channel Disorders

Paramyotonia Congenita (Eulenberg's Disease)

Paramyotonia congenita is a syndrome consisting of episodic paralysis and myotonia that is triggered by cold and exercise. As opposed to the warm-up phenomenon seen in patients with myotonia congenita, paradoxical myotonia that quickly worsens with exercise can be demonstrated. Facial muscles (particularly eyelids), pharyngeal muscles, and hand muscles are particularly involved. The legs are more mildly affected

[Miller et al., 2004]. Myotonia may be present for a brief time, but weakness may persist for hours. Muscle hypertrophy is present in about 30 percent of patients [Matthews et al., 2008]. Paramyotonia congenita is present from infancy and symptoms manifest within the first decade of life.

GENETICS

Paramyotonia congenita is caused by a mutation of the *SCN4A* gene, with exons 22 and 24 being active areas of interest [Matthews et al., 2008].

PATHOPHYSIOLOGY

Episodes of weakness experienced by individuals with paramyotonia congenita are caused by intermittent loss of fiber excitability. This is due to persistent depolarization of the membrane resting potential, as sodium channels do not inactivate completely, resulting in a persistent influx of sodium current [Cannon, 2006].

CLINICAL LABORATORY TESTS

Muscle biopsy is rarely necessary, but shows an absence of type 2B fibers. Clinical electrophysiology may be useful as the compound muscle action potential (CMAP) will show a gradual and prolonged decrement after exercise. With repeated exercise testing and muscle cooling, the decrement is exacerbated [Fournier et al., 2006].

TREATMENT

Counseling regarding decreased exposure to cold and strenuous exercise as precipitants for myotonia is recommended. If symptoms are mild, no further treatment may be necessary. In patients with more severe disease, the medications previously listed for myotonia may be used.

Hyperkalemic Periodic Paralysis

Hyperkalemic periodic paralysis shares features with paramyotonia congenita. The disorder can occur at any age, but may appear in infancy. The frequency of attacks increases during adolescence, and decreases after the fourth decade [Miller et al., 2004]. Mild myotonia of the eyelids and finger extensors may be noted on examination between attacks. Myotonia may be cold-induced but is not exacerbated by exercise [Subramony et al., 1986], which distinguishes it from paramyotonia congenita. Moderate exercise may trigger attacks of flaccid muscle weakness, which may be brief or last for several hours. Attacks also may be precipitated or made worse by eating foods containing high potassium, exposure to cold, rest after moderate exercise, glucocorticoids, or emotional stress [Lehmann-Horn et al., 2004]. Permanent weakness may develop in older individuals [Bradley et al., 1990]. Before confirming a diagnosis of hyperkalemic periodic paralysis, other causes of potassium elevation should be excluded. Adrenal insufficiency, rhabdomyolysis, hypoaldosteronism, or medications such as angiotensin-converting enzyme inhibitors should be ruled out.

Genetics

Between 60 and 70 percent of patients have a mutation in the *SCN4A* gene on chromosome 17, which encodes skeletal muscle voltage-gated sodium channels [Fontaine et al., 1990]. Genetic testing should focus on the common sites of mutations (T704M and M1592V) in the *SCN4A* gene. It has also been confirmed that hyperkalemic periodic paralysis and paramyotonia congenita are allelic disorders [Ptacek et al., 1991]. These are inherited in autosomal-dominant fashion.

Pathophysiology

Abnormal inactivation of voltage-gated sodium channels causes membrane depolarization. The abnormal sodium channel gating creates a gain of function, resulting in increased sodium current that depolarizes affected muscle and leads to weakness [Venance et al., 2006].

Clinical Laboratory Tests

Serum potassium elevation by 1.5–3 mmol/L during an attack and electrocardiogram changes (peaked T waves) confirm the diagnosis. Myotonia is detectable on EMG in approximately 50 percent of patients [Lehmann-Horn et al., 2004] and supports the diagnosis. Muscle biopsy in patients with periodic paralysis may exhibit vacuoles and tubular aggregates.

Treatment

Carbohydrate-rich meals, ongoing mild exercise, avoidance of potassium-rich foods, and exposure to cold may prevent or mitigate attacks. For frequent attacks, use of acetazolamide or thiazide diuretics may be beneficial. Glucose and insulin therapy may be required to treat an acute attack.

Potassium-Aggravated Myotonias

There are several other myotonic disorders, all associated with allelic point mutations in the gene encoding SCN4A. All are characterized by stiffness following ingestion of potassium or strenuous exercise. All share the absence of sensitivity to cold. Myotonia fluctuans is a mild form of myotonia precipitated by rest and resolved with continued exercise. The onset of myotonia is delayed for 10 or more minutes after exercise. Pain sometimes accompanies the myotonia, but muscle weakness is not a feature [Heine et al., 1993]. Acetazolamide-responsive myotonia (atypical myotonia congenita) is a painful myotonia precipitated by exercise and is insensitive to cold [Ptacek et al., 1994a]. Myotonia permanens is a very severe disorder, with EMG showing continuous myotonic activity. As a result, generalized muscle hypertrophy is noted, as well as serum creatine kinase elevation.

Calcium Channel Disorders

Hypokalemic periodic paralysis, the most frequent cause of periodic paralysis, is an autosomal-dominant disorder. Two different forms exist: a myopathic form and a paralytic form. The pure paralytic form is the most common and is present in 60 percent of cases. The onset of symptoms is between 5 and 16 years of age. Attacks are often precipitated by carbohydrate-rich meals or by exercise followed by a period of rest. As a consequence, many patients have attacks early in the morning. Exposure to cold may also be an inciting event.

Most attacks last between 4 and 6 hours, but may be longer. Some patients will experience proximal weakness; some have a more diffuse paralysis. Extraocular and respiratory muscles are not involved. Recurrent attacks typically wane over 30 years. The myopathic form is seen in approximately 25 percent of cases. Progressive fixed weakness develops in the legs. This weakness may occur in the absence of paralytic symptoms.

A positive family history and the characteristics of paralysis render a clinical diagnosis. During an attack, potassium concentrations may be as low as 1.5 mmol/L, but may also be only slightly below normal values. Electrocardiogram changes of bradycardia, prolonged PR and QT intervals, and flattened T waves are present. Secondary causes of hypokalemia, such as renal or gastrointestinal potassium wasting, or use of medications such as thiazide, should be excluded prior to diagnosing this condition.

Genetics

Mutations in the *CACNA1S* gene account for about 70 percent of cases of hypokalemic periodic paralysis [Ptacek et al., 1994b]. *CACNA1S* codes for the dihydropyridine receptor. The gene maps to chromosome 1q31–32. About 12 percent of patients have a mutation in the *SCN4A* gene [Jurkat-Rott et al., 2000]. There may be further gene heterogeneity to account for other patients who do not test positive for either of these mutations.

Pathophysiology

In hypokalemic periodic paralysis, the mechanism for depolarization-induced attacks of weakness is not well characterized. A loss of function leading to reduced current density and slower activation is a result of calcium channel mutations. There are also sodium channel mutations that enhance inactivation, producing a net loss of function defect as well [Venance et al., 2006].

Clinical Laboratory Tests

Vacuolar myopathy, centralization of nuclei, and fiber type disproportion are noted on histopathology in biopsies from patients with the myopathic form of hypokalemic periodic paralysis. EMG does not show evidence of myotonia.

Treatment

In patients with normal renal function, oral potassium chloride is the treatment of choice. A low-sodium diet and chronic potassium supplementation may help to prevent attacks. Acetazolamide may also be beneficial [Links et al., 1988].

Andersen–Tawil Syndrome

Andersen–Tawil syndrome is characterized by periodic paralysis, cardiac ventricular ectopy, and skeletal abnormalities [Tawil et al., 1994]. It was first described in 1971 [Andersen et al., 1971]. Clinical symptoms of intermittent weakness begin in the first or second decade. Episodes can be triggered by prolonged rest or rest following exertion. Proximal weakness may develop and be permanent. Potassium may be elevated, normal, or reduced during attacks, and levels do not correlate well with the frequency or severity of weakness. ECG abnormalities include prolonged QT interval, prominent U waves, premature ventricular contractions, ventricular bigeminy, and polymorphic ventricular tachycardia. Patients with ventricular ectopy may be asymptomatic, or may present with palpitations, syncope, or cardiac arrest [Tristani-Firouzi et al., 2002]. The physical phenotype includes small mandible, hypertelorism, low-set ears, clinodactyly, syndactyly, and a broad nasal bridge [Donaldson et al., 2004]. The disorder is autosomal-dominant and maps to chromosome 17q23, which includes the *KCNJ2* gene that encodes the *kir2.1* potassium channel receptor.

Malignant Hyperthermia

Malignant hyperthermia is an autosomal-dominant inherited disorder that is characterized by a rapid rise in body temperature, muscular rigidity, and necrosis triggered by administration of certain anesthetic agents (e.g., halothane) with or without concurrent administration of a depolarizing muscle relaxant, such as succinylcholine. Increased sarcoplasmic reticulum calcium concentration results in constant muscle contraction and hyperthermia. Untreated, the disorder can be fatal.

Central core and multiminicore myopathy is associated with an increased risk of malignant hyperthermia. Because of the risk of malignant hyperthermia in patients with underlying muscle disease, precautions should be taken before any surgical procedures performed on these patients.

Genetics

Normal contraction of skeletal muscle depends on interaction between the ryanodine receptor and the dihydropyridine receptor. The ryanodine receptor encodes the skeletal muscle sarcoplasmic reticulum calcium release gene. The receptor maps to chromosome 19. The dihydropyridine receptor encodes the voltage-dependent calcium channel. Mutations in the *RYR1* gene account for 50–70 percent of cases of malignant hyperthermia [McCarthy et al., 2000]. Mutations also have been identified in the *CACNA2D1* and *CACNA1S* calcium channel genes [Jurkat-Rott et al., 2002].

Pathophysiology

Hypersensitive channels caused by mutations in the *RYR1* gene allow efflux of calcium from the sarcoplasmic reticulum into the muscle cell. Sustained muscle contraction and rigidity result, which also causes an elevation in body temperature. This excessive muscle contraction results in depletion of ATP and increased glycogenolysis, which produces lactic acidosis and a metabolic acidosis. Oxygen consumption is escalated and results in hypoxemia and hypercapnia with excess carbon dioxide production. Patients may develop rhabdomyolysis, hyperkalemia, and complications, including renal failure or cardiac dysrhythmia and arrest [Platt and Griggs, 2009].

Clinical Laboratory Tests

Confirmation of malignant hyperthermia is sought by contracture testing. This procedure relies on the in vitro response of freshly biopsied muscle to various concentrations of caffeine and halothane, which raise the intracellular calcium content. Test sensitivity is almost 100 percent and specificity 87–90 percent [Allen et al., 1998].

Treatment

Recognition of the syndrome of malignant hyperthermia is of utmost importance in rapid treatment. Anesthesia should be immediately discontinued. Acidosis should be corrected, and treatment of elevated body temperature using cooling blankets or cooled intravenous fluids should be initiated. If rhabdomyolysis and myoglobinuria are present, then volume loading and diuretics may be needed. Dantrolene is the specific pharmacologic therapy used, as it inhibits calcium release from the sarcoplasmic reticulum. Failure to recognize and treat malignant hyperthermia as an emergency can cause increased mortality.

The complete list of references for this chapter is available online at **www.expertconsult.com**. See inside cover for registration details.

Global Developmental Delay and Mental Retardation/ Intellectual Disability

Elliott H. Sherr and Michael I. Shevell

Definitions

Global developmental delay and mental retardation are related, complementary, nonsynonymous terms featuring both common and distinctive characteristics. In a manner analogous to cerebral palsy, each is a symptom complex highlighting a clinically recognizable entity that is etiologically heterogeneous, and which mandates a particular evaluation, management, and intervention approach. Both can be conceptualized as neurodevelopmental disabilities that can be defined as early-onset, chronic disorders that share the essential feature of a predominant disturbance in the acquisition of cognitive, motor, language, or social skills, which has a significant and continuing impact on the developmental progress of an individual [APA, 1994]. Diagnosis of these disorders occurs against a backdrop of a wide variation in "normality" of what can be highly individualized developmental trajectories that may not be smooth [Darrah et al., 2003]. Clear boundary lines may not be evident, mandating diagnosis over time rather than at a single point of clinical contact.

The consensus definition put forward in 2002 by the American Association on Mental Retardation (AAMR) defines mental retardation as "a disability characterized by a significant limitation both in intellectual functioning and in adaptive behavior as expressed in conceptual, social, practical, and adaptive skills." This disability originates before the age of 18 [AAMR, 2002] and manifests with severe problems in the individual's capacity to perform (i.e., impairment), ability to perform (i.e., activity limitations), and opportunity to function (i.e., participation restrictions) [WHO, 2001]. Correct and consistent application of this definition requires an awareness of five inherent contextual assumptions:

1. Limitations in current functioning are to be considered within the context of an individual's typical community environments.
2. Valid assessments must consider, reflect, and be sensitive to linguistic and cultural diversity.
3. Limitations coexist with strengths.
4. By describing limitations, a profile of needed supports can be conceptualized.
5. With appropriate sustained support, the life function of an individual with mental retardation can often be improved.

The present definition of mental retardation extends far beyond the traditional concept of a general subaverage level of intellectual function, as captured in a single numerical measurement such as an intelligence quotient (IQ). The recent emerging emphasis on functional behaviors and contextual factors is altering both the construct of disability and appropriate relevant terminology whereby the term "intellectual disability" is replacing "mental retardation." The terms are essentially synonymous and both are used concurrently at present; however, it can be foreseen that "intellectual disability" will suplant "mental retardation" in the near future.

For the young child, the term global developmental delay has emerged to describe a disturbance across a variety of developmental domains [Batshaw and Shapiro, 1997; Fenichel, 2001; Kinsbourne and Graf, 2001; Majnemer and Shevell, 1995; Shevell et al., 2000; Simeonsson and Simeonsson, 2001]. Such a child has limitations or delay in the acquisition of developmental and functional skills that are both observable and measurable within the context of the natural progression of infants and young children [Shevell, 2008]. The latest consensus definition used by the American Academy of Neurology (AAN) practice parameter statement defines global developmental delay operationally as a significant delay in two or more developmental domains (e.g., gross/fine motor, cognitive, speech/language, personal/social, activities of daily living) [Shevell et al., 2003]. Typically, if there is delay in two domains, this implies delay across all domains.

Global developmental delay and intellectual disability are frequently diagnosed on the basis of experienced clinical judgment in advance of or as a substitute for detailed standardized assessments. Potential errors in measurements create a zone of uncertainty or range of confidence captured in the concept of the standard error of measurement (SEM) [Reschly, 1987]. This contributes to a conceptual hesitation regarding the application of strict numerical cutoffs. Accuracy is increased by repeated application of a particular measure over a longitudinal time interval [Batshaw, 1993]. The precise relationship between the diagnoses of mental retardation and global developmental delay must still be determined [Petersen et al., 1998; Yatchmink, 1996]; however, limitations and delay in the widespread acquisition of developmental skills, especially language, may be a harbinger of later intellectual disability.

Epidemiology

Much information has been ascertained regarding the prevalence and causes of mental retardation; however, interpretation of these data necessitates an understanding of the assumptions inherent in these analyses. The operational parameters for mental retardation usually include an intelligence quotient (IQ) value that is 2 standard deviations below the mean (IQ below 70), identification before the age of 18, and difficulties in adaptive functioning. Although definitions are arbitrary, they allow for agreement on standardization of measurement. Assuming a normal distribution of IQ scores, approximately 2.25 percent of individuals will have an IQ below 70. Many of these individuals (given the high correlation between scores on IQ tests and standardized adaptive functioning tests) will also have adaptive difficulties, meeting the definition of mental retardation. Early population-based studies seem to have confirmed this point. Hagberg and Kyllerman [1983] documented a rate of mental retardation of 2 percent; 1.5 percent had mild mental retardation (IQ of 50–70), and 0.5 percent had moderate or severe mental retardation (IQ of less than 50). The population studied and the instruments used can influence the rate of mild mental retardation, but they seem to have little effect on the rate of severe mental retardation. The prevalence rates for mild mental retardation in 15 subsequent studies varied from 5 to 80 cases per 1000 people, with an average prevalence of 35 per 1000. In contrast, in 37 studies the prevalence of severe mental retardation varied only between 2.5 and 7 per 1000, with an average of 3.6 per 1000 [Leonard and Wen, 2002].

Because the highest percentage of children with mental retardation are in the mild range, any change between measured populations in mental retardation definitions or in the type or severity of deleterious environmental exposures (e.g., poor education, nutrition, environmental toxins, such as lead) can have a significant effect on the overall numbers of children with mild mental retardation. One of the more comprehensive investigations of mental retardation, the Metropolitan Atlanta Developmental Disabilities Study, identified a smaller than average rate for mild mental retardation (IQ of 50–70) of 8.4 per 1000, whereas that for severe mental retardation, at 3.6 per 1000, was consistent with the meta-analysis average [Boyle et al., 1996; Yeargin-Allsopp et al., 1997]. This study also documented two additional observations about the prevalence of mental retardation: race disparity and gender imbalance. The Atlanta study found that mental retardation was overrepresented by 50 percent among blacks relative to the white population [Yeargin-Allsopp et al., 1995], and that the male to female ratio was 1.4:1.0. A California study reported a similar rate of racial disparity for all categories of mental retardation and found that there was a substantial increased risk associated with low birth weight and maternal age [Croen et al., 2001]. Additional maternal influences observed in this study that increase the risk for mental retardation include poor nutritional status, tobacco smoking, and alcohol consumption. Paternal smoking also increases the risk of having affected children. In almost every study, gender disparity is a consistent finding, with males accounting for 20–40 percent more of the cases than females. A significant component of this difference may be related to X chromosome disorders, but studies have shown that maternal smoking or low birth weight has a more direct effect on IQ in male infants, suggesting that this disparity has many causes [Leonard and Wen, 2002].

Although there is considerable variation in the numbers of individuals diagnosed with mental retardation, there is less disagreement about the known causes of mental retardation and the high percentage of cases with unknown causes. For classification purposes, mental retardation cases are often grouped by prenatal, perinatal, and postnatal causes. The prenatal group includes known genetic syndromes and chromosomal disorders, central nervous system malformations, and toxic or infectious causes. Perinatal conditions include birth asphyxia, stroke, and infection. Postnatal conditions include infection, toxins (e.g., lead), and injury, such as nonaccidental trauma. Using this classification, the Metropolitan Atlanta Study found that 87 percent of children with mild mental retardation and 57 percent of moderately to severely affected children did not have identified causes. A similar breakdown – 77 percent for mild and 65 percent for severe cases – was found in the California study. Among the causes identified, chromosomal defects were the most common, accounting for 25 percent of all causes of mental retardation among more than 4.5 million live births in California; Down syndrome was the single most common known chromosomal cause. Other causes of retardation, including infection, central nervous system anomalies, and metabolic or endocrine causes, accounted for up to 8 percent of the total. In this analysis, low birth weight and other environmental exposures were not counted as biomedical causes, although they were associated with increased risk, as previously mentioned. Better focus on how these environmental influences affect ultimate IQ is essential for prevention and early intervention.

Many individuals with severe or mild mental retardation are unable to become productive members of society and require institutionalized or group-home care. The economic costs to society are substantial. In a Dutch study, mental retardation was the disease category with the largest health-care costs, almost equal to the economic impact of stroke, heart disease, and cancer combined [Meerding et al., 1998]. An analysis by the U.S. Centers for Disease Control and Prevention (CDC) estimates lifetime costs of more than $1 million dollars per person with mental retardation, which is more than that for cerebral palsy, hearing loss, or vision impairment [CDC, 2004].

History and Ethics

The first to draw a clear distinction between mental retardation and mental illness was the English philosopher John Locke, who wrote in his essay *Concerning Human Understanding* (1690), "Herein seems to lie the difference between idiots and madmen, that madmen put wrong ideas together and reason from them, but idiots make very few or no propositions and reason scarce at all." The development of intelligence testing by Alfred Binet and Theodore Simon in 1905 ushered in an era of a more rigorous, scientific approach to defining mental retardation that became the basis for formulating an approach to its comprehensive management [Sherr and Ferriero, 2003].

Early 20th-century definitions of mental retardation focused on its incurability with permanent predetermined limitations and consistent prevention of participation in society (e.g., "mental deficiency is a state of incomplete mental development of such a kind and degree that the individual is incapable of adapting himself to the normal environment of his fellows in such a way to maintain existence independently of supervision, control or external support"; [Tredgold, 1937]). In the middle of the 20th century, adaptive behavior limitations were added as criteria for diagnosing mental retardation [Heber, 1961]. This addition was meant to implement a reduction in rigid reliance on IQ scores and to better reflect the social characteristics of the disability that is attached to mental retardation. Adaptive behavior deficiency was conceptualized as problems in maturation, learning, or social adjustment that were based on difficulties in adjusting to ordinary demands. By 1973, the AAMR definition of mental retardation required concurrent manifested deficits in general intellectual function and adaptive behavior [Grossman, 1973]. A 1992 AAMR definition specified the adaptive skill areas affected and emphasized limitations in current functioning across the individual's life span [Luckasson et al., 1992]. As captured in the most recent effort of consensus definition, adaptive deficits lead to both activity limitations and participation restrictions that necessitate contextually driven systems of support to enable the individual's fullest actualization of inherent potential and broadest societal integration [AAMR, 2002].

Evolution of the concept of mental retardation has been marked by an on-going debate regarding the nature of intelligence and its measurement. Despite the changing nuances of its definition, the primary criterion for diagnosing mental retardation over time has always been a deficit in intellectual ability [Gottfredson, 1997]. Factor analysis of data obtained from administering cognitive tests to large groups of individuals permitted the objectification of a unifactorial latent trait (i.e., general intelligence) to account for the variance between cognitive scores [Spearman, 1927]. Within this framework, intelligence was conceptualized as general mental capability that includes the ability to reason, solve problems, think abstractly, plan, and learn from experience [Carroll, 1997]. In essence, it is a reflection of a person's ability to comprehend his or her surroundings. In contradistinction to the established unifactorial position of intelligence, several theoretical models of intelligence as a multidimensional construct have been put forward, with each intelligence component featuring distinctive developmental trajectories, problem-solving, and information-processing capacities [Gardner, 1993]. Validation by standardized and quantifiable measures of these intriguing and intuitively appealing constructs of intelligence remains elusive.

Historical controversy exists regarding the mechanisms by which intelligence can be measured and the social, cultural, and ethnic contexts of its measurement [Gould, 1981]. Establishing cutoff points for the labeling of "subaverage intellectual functioning" has also been problematic [MacMillan et al., 1995], especially with the single application of a particular measure and with scores that fall near the cutoff point within the range of the test SEM. IQ scores have also unfortunately been used at various historical points to further biologically determinist agendas and potentially to demonize minority groups [Gould, 1981].

A survey of the past century reveals a remarkable trajectory in the treatment of those affected by mental retardation or global developmental delay in Western society. With the prominence of eugenics (i.e., science of the improvement of the human race by better breeding) in the first part of the 20th century, those with mental retardation were targeted for involuntary eugenic sterilization in many jurisdictions [Kevles, 1985; Parent and Shevell, 1998; Proctor, 1988]. The global emphasis after World War II on individual civil rights resulted in national and international mandates that provided for legislative and judicial protection for the intellectually disabled from active discrimination (e.g., Americans with Disabilities Act of 1990 is but one national example). Early educational, rehabilitation, and school programs financed by public funds for those at risk of developmental disability or affected by mental handicap (e.g., Early Intervention Amendments to the Education of the Handicapped Act, Education for All Handicapped Children Act) have been implemented. These mandates for protection against discrimination and service provision exist with broad community and political support, providing a level of class protection not previously encountered. Legal standards have been upheld consistently by judicial authorities.

The medical care of individuals with global developmental delay and intellectual disability has been included in the thrust of broad medical principles. A common morality has emerged, framed by a generally accepted understanding of socially approved norms of human conduct [Shevell, 2009a]. Within this framework, ethical behavior is driven by mutually recognized duties and obligations. Within the medical sphere of human interactions, these duties and obligations focus on issues of autonomy, beneficence, non-maleficence, and justice [Bernat, 2002].

The absence of the capacity for competence (defined as "the ability to understand the context of the decision, the choices available, the likely outcomes of the varying choices, and to rationally process this information to make a decision"), together with minority age (typically less than 18 years), renders the pediatric patient with global developmental delay or intellectual disability doubly vulnerable with respect to ethical issues [Bernat, 2002]. The cornerstone of ethical modern medical practice is the respect for individual autonomy reflected in the primacy accorded to informed consent in all aspects of medical decision-making [Faden et al., 1986]. For those unable ever to provide informed consent, a "best interest" model for decision-making must be implemented that mandates careful selection of responsible proxy decision-makers and consideration of the risks and benefits for intervention from the unique perspective of the affected individual [Shevell, 1998]. Consensus exists that cognitive disability alone should never be the only reason to withhold or withdraw care. Developmentally appropriate models of assent that respect the cognitive capacity of the intellectually disabled offer an alternative to enhance our ethical efforts and are increasingly a feature of clinical practice. A determined effort must be made not to use the challenges faced in ethical practice with this population to abandon efforts through research to improve all aspects of care and outcome [Shevell, 2002].

Justice concerns itself with the fair distribution within society of what ultimately are limited resources in a broader socioeconomic context [Outka, 1974]. An appropriate standard would be objectively applied, equally valuing individual worth. Within the health-care sector, access frequently requires effective advocacy, which may favor better publicly organized and financially enabled disease advocacy groups.

Diagnosis

Definitions and Testing

Accurate diagnosis of global developmental delay or intellectual disability is an essential precondition to proper management and service provision. Accurate diagnosis serves many functions, including understanding the specific associated medical and psychiatric complications, eligibility for service and support provision and its specific attributes, family counseling, and legal recognition of disability [Shevell, 2009b].

The diagnosis of intellectual disability, as presently defined, requires demonstration of significant limitations in intellectual functioning and adaptive behavior [AAMR, 2002]. Intelligence, conceptualized as general mental capabilities, is represented "objectively" by an IQ score obtained through proper application of an appropriate assessment measure [Hernstein and Murray, 1994]. Adaptive behavior refers to skills (i.e., conceptual, social, and practical) that a person learns in order to function within the context of the expectations and challenges of everyday life. Limitations in these skills affect the ability to respond to changes and demands encountered, affecting performance in daily life and participation in available opportunities. Multiple standardized, age-appropriate measures have been normed and validated on normal populations to assess adaptive behavior skills [Spreat, 1999]. For intellectual function and adaptive behavior, a significant limitation thought sufficient to trigger possible inclusion under the rubric of intellectual disability is performance at least 2 standard deviations below the mean for an appropriate test [AAMR, 2002]. Some of the standardized measures for the evaluation of intellectual, neurodevelopmental, and behavioral testing are summarized in Table 43-1, and a qualitative description of IQ and index scores on Wechsler tests that categorize intelligence levels is provided in Table 43-2.

Table 43-1 Measures for Evaluation of Intellectual, Neurodevelopmental, and Behavioral Progress

Test Name, Age Range Of Subjects, And Test Publication Data	Test Description	Administration and Scoring Information
DEVELOPMENTAL TESTS		
Bayley Scales of Infant Development, Second Edition (Bayley II)		

16 days to 3 years 6 months 15 days Nancy Bayley, The Psychological Corporation, 1993, www.psychcorp.com (Bayley III, 2005)	Standardized assessment of cognitive, motor, and behavioral development for children aged 1–42 months
	Mental Scale has 178 items, Psychomotor Scale has 111 items, and Behavior Rating Scale has 30 items
	Mental Scale yields a normalized standard score called the Mental Development Index, evaluating a variety of abilities, including sensory/perceptual acuities, learning, and problem-solving; verbal communication; abstract thinking; and mathematical concept formation
	Motor Scale assesses skills of degree of body control, large muscle coordination, finer manipulatory skills of the hands and fingers, dynamic movement, dynamic praxis, postural imitation, and stereognosis
	Behavior Rating Scale assesses the child's relevant test-taking behaviors and measures the following factors: attention/arousal, orientation/engagement, emotional regulation, and motor quality
		Yields: Mental Development Index (MDI) and Psychomotor Development Index (PDI); and five behavior factors: Attention/Arousal, Orientation/Engagement, Emotional Regulation, Motor Quality, and Total Behavior Rating
		MDI and PDI means = 100, SD = 15
		Behavior ratings as percentile ranks:
		  Non-optimal: 1–10th
		  Questionable: 11–25th
		  Within normal limits: 26–99th
		Administration time: younger, about 30 minutes; older, about 60 minutes

Bayley Infant Neurodevelopmental Screener (BINS)		
3 months to 24 months Glen P Aylward, The Psychological Corporation, 1995, www.psychcorp.com	Screening test to identify infants who are developmentally delayed or have neurologic impairments Four domains: Neurological Functions/Intactness (N), Receptive Functions (R), Expressive Functions (E), and Cognitive Processes (C) The infant is administered 11 or 13 items and scored as optimal or non-optimal performance Total scores can range from 0 to 11 or 13, with a higher score indicating better functioning This screen can be used to prompt a more comprehensive evaluation	Yields: A Total Score summing performance across the four domains Chart shows age-appropriate cut-off values for high, moderate, or low risk for developmental delay or neurologic impairments Administration time: 10 minutes
Denver Developmental Screening Test II (Denver II)		
Birth to 6 years WK Frankenburg and JB Dodds et al., Denver Developmental Materials, 1992, www.denverii.com	Surveillance and monitoring instrument to determine if a child's development is within the normal range. Acquired skills are checked off on a chart, and results demonstrate in a graphic manner the child's pattern of developmental skills compared with age-mates It is not intended as a diagnostic tool and may be more appropriate as a developmental chart or inventory rather than as a screener Four domains: Personal-Social, Language, Fine Motor-Adaptive, and Gross Motor; 125 items	If a child fails items that are successfully completed by 90 percent of younger children, delay may be suspected, and further evaluation may be needed

Continued

Table 43-1 Measures for Evaluation of Intellectual, Neurodevelopmental, and Behavioral Progress—cont'd

Test Name, Age Range Of Subjects, And Test Publication Data	Test Description	Administration and Scoring Information
INTELLIGENCE OR COGNITIVE TESTS		
Wechsler Intelligence Scale for Children, Fourth Edition (WISC-IV)		
6 years 0 months 0 days to 16 years 11 months 30 days David Wechsler, The Psychological Corporation, 2003 (Spanish version, 2005), www.psychcorp.com	This test of intellectual or cognitive ability for school-age children is part of a series that includes the WPPSI-III (see below) for preschool and primary ages and the WAIS-III for adolescents and adults It is the most commonly used intelligence test for school-age children Ten core subtests and five optional subtests	Yields: Verbal Comprehension Index (VCI), Perceptual Reasoning Index (PRI), Working Memory Index (WMI), Processing Speed Index (PSI), and Full Scale Intelligence Quotient (FSIQ) Subtest means = 10, SD = 3 Index and IQ means = 100, SD = 15 Administration time: 65–80 minutes for core subtests
Wechsler Preschool and Primary Scale of Intelligence, Third Edition (WPPSI-III)		

2 years 6 months 0 days to 7 years 3 months 30 days
  Preschool level: 2 years 6 months 0 days to 3 years 11 months 30 days
  Primary level: 4 years 0 months 0 days to 7 years 3 months 30 days
 	
David Wechsler, The Psychological Corporation, 2002, www.psychcorp.com
	Test of young children's intellectual ability
	  Preschool: four core subtests and one optional subtest
	  Primary: seven core subtests and seven optional subtests
		Yields:
		  Preschool: Verbal IQ (VIQ), Performance IQ (PIQ), and Full Scale IQ (FSIQ); and optional General Language Composite (GLC)
		  Primary: Verbal IQ (VIQ), Performance IQ (PIQ), Processing Speed Quotient (PSQ), and Full Scale IQ (FSIQ); and optional General Language Composite (GLC)
		Subtest means = 10, SD = 3
		IQ, PSQ, GLC means = 100, SD = 15
		Administration times:
		  Preschool: 35–40 minutes for all
		  Primary: 40–50 minutes for core subtests

Stanford-Binet Intelligence Scales, Fifth Edition (SB5)		
2 years 0 months to 85 years+ Gale H Roid, Riverside Publishing, 2003, www.riversidepublishing.com	Assessment of intelligence and cognitive abilities Two domains: Verbal (V) and Nonverbal (NV) Each has five factors of cognitive ability: Fluid Reasoning (FR), Knowledge (KN), Quantitative Reasoning (QR), Visual-Spatial Processing (VS), and Working Memory (WM) Use of Change-Sensitive Score (CSS) makes it possible to compare changes in an individual's scores over time if retested	Yields: ten subtest scores and four types of composite scores – five factor indices, two domain scales (Verbal IQ and Nonverbal IQ), Abbreviated Battery IQ, and the Full Scale IQ of all 10 subtests Change-Sensitive Scores (CSS) are criterion-referenced (rather than norm-referenced) and therefore reference absolute levels of ability from the 2-year-old level to the adult level Subtest score means = 10, SD = 3 Index and IQ means = 100, SD = 15 Change-Sensitive Scores range = 376-592, from 2-year-old level to adult (most fall in the range of 420–530); 500 is an average score for an individual 10 years 0 months old Administration time: 50–60 minutes for all ten subtests
Differential Ability Scales (DAS)		

2 years 6 months to 17 years 11 months
  Preschool level: 2 years 6 months to 5 years 11 months
  School-age level: 6 years 0 months to 17 years 11 months
 	
Colin D. Elliott, The Psychological Corporation, 1990 (DAS-II, 2006), www.psychcorp.com
	Test of cognitive ability and of basic academic skills; includes nine cognitive and three achievement subtests
	For language-impaired and non-English-speaking children, the examiner can obtain Special Nonverbal Composite
		Yields: Cognitive:
		  General Conceptual Ability (GCA) score and cluster scores of Verbal Ability and Nonverbal Ability for Preschool level Verbal Ability, Nonverbal Reasoning Ability, and Spatial Ability for school-age level
		Academic Achievement: Basic Number Skills, Spelling, and Word Reading scores
		Subtest T-score means = 50, SD = 10
		General Conceptual Ability (GCA), Cluster, and Academic Achievement means = 100, SD = 15
		Administration time:
		  Full cognitive battery, 45–60 minutes
		  Academic achievement tests, 15–25 minutes

Table 43-1 Measures for Evaluation of Intellectual, Neurodevelopmental, and Behavioral Progress—cont'd

Test Name, Age Range Of Subjects, And Test Publication Data	Test Description	Administration and Scoring Information
Leiter International Performance Scale, Revised (Leiter-R)		
2 years 0 months to 20 years 11 months Gale H Roid and Lucy J Miller, Stoelting Company, 1997, www.stoelting.com	Totally nonverbal test of intelligence and cognitive abilities Two domains: Visualization and Reasoning (VR) for measuring IQ, and Attention and Memory (AM) There are 10 subtests in each domain Includes four social-emotional rating scales (by Examiner, Parent, Self-Rating, and Teacher) Nonverbal tasks, especially suited for children and adolescents who are nonverbal, do not speak English, or use English as Second Language (ESL); speech-hearing-motor impaired; attention-deficit hyperactivity disorder (ADHD), autistic; delayed; disadvantaged; or traumatic brain injury (TBI)	Yields: 20 subtests Five composite scores: Fluid Reasoning, Fundamental Visualization, Spatial Visualization, Attention, and Memory; and Brief IQ (based on four VR subtests) and Full Scale IQ scores Growth-scale scores for subtests and IQ in a metric that can track growth over time if retested Subtest score means = 10, SD = 3 Composite and IQ score means = 100, SD = 15 Administration time: VR, about 40 minutes; AM, about 35 minutes
Comprehensive Test of Nonverbal Intelligence (CTONI)		
6 years to 90 years Donald D Hammill, Nils A Pearson, and J Lee Wiederholt, The Psychological Corporation, 1997, www.psychcorp.com	Test measures nonverbal reasoning abilities and estimates intelligence of individuals who experience undue difficulty in language (e.g., bilingual, language other than English, deaf) or fine motor skills. It can be administered orally in English or in pantomime. No oral responses, reading, writing, or object manipulation are required; responses are made by pointing to alternative choices Analogical Reasoning, Categorical Classifications, and Sequential Reasoning in two different contexts: pictures of familiar objects and geometric designs; and solving problems Six subtests: Pictorial Analogies, Pictorial Categories, Pictorial Sequences, Geometric Analogies, Geometric Categories, Geometric Sequences	Yields: three composite scores – Nonverbal Intelligence Quotient, Pictorial Nonverbal Intelligence Quotient, and Geometric Intelligence Quotient – and an overall score Subtest means = 10, SD = 3 Composite and overall means = 100, SD = 15 Administration time: 1 hour
NEUROPSYCHOLOGICAL TESTS		
NEPSY (NE for neuro and PSY for psychology)		

3 years 0 months to 12 years 11 months
    Younger: 3 years 0 months to 4 years 11 months
    Older: 5 years 0 months to 12 years 11 months
Marit Korkman, Ursula Kirk, and Sally Kemp, The Psychological Corporation, 1997, www.psychcorp.com (NEPSY-II, 2007)
	Test of neuropsychological development in preschool and early school-age children
	Subtests can be used in various combinations, according to the needs of the child
	Five domains: Attention and Executive Functions, Language, Sensorimotor Functions, Visuospatial Processing, and Memory and Learning
	    Younger: 11 core (and 1 extended) subtests
	    Older: 14 core (and 5 extended) subtests
		Yields: subtest and five domain scores
		Subtest Scaled Score means = 10, SD = 3
		Core Domain Score means = 100, SD = 15
		Percentile ranks:
		    ≤2% well below expected level
		    3–10% below expected level
		    11–25% borderline
		    26–75% at expected level (most children in each age group)
		    >75% above expected level
		Administration times:
		    Core: younger, 45 minutes; older, 65 minutes
		    Full: younger, 1 hour; older, 2 hours

Delis–Kaplan Executive Function System (D-KEFS)		
8 years to 89 years Dean C Delis, Edith Kaplan, and Joel H Kramer, The Psychological Corporation, 2001, www.psychcorp.com	Test of executive function in older school-age children and adults evaluates component processes of tasks thought to be especially sensitive to frontal lobe dysfunction, such as flexibility of thinking, inhibition, problem-solving, planning, impulse control, concept formation, abstract thinking, and creativity in verbal and spatial modalities Nine stand-alone tests	Yields: nine test scores Scaled score means = 10, SD = 3 Administration time: 90 minutes for all nine tests

Continued

Table 43-1 Measures for Evaluation of Intellectual, Neurodevelopmental, and Behavioral Progress—cont'd

Test Name, Age Range Of Subjects, And Test Publication Data	Test Description	Administration and Scoring Information
INDIRECT FUNCTIONAL RATINGS BY PARENT OR CAREGIVER		
Vineland Adaptive Behavior Scales, Second Edition (Vineland-II)		
0 to 89 years (parents/caregivers) 3 to 21 years 11 months (teachers) Sara S Sparrow, Domenic V Cicchetti, and David A Balla, American Guidance Service (AGS), 2004, www.agsnet.com	A measure of personal and social skills as reported by the parent or caregiver Four domains: Communication, Daily Living Skills, Socialization, and Motor Skills, with 11 subdomains The Survey Interview, Expanded Interview, and Parent/Caregiver Rating Forms contain an optional maladaptive behavior domain for pinpointing undesirable behaviors that may interfere with adaptive functioning	Yields: 11 subdomain scores, 4 domain scores, and an overall Adaptive Behavior Composite Subdomain score means = 10, SD = 3 Domain and Adaptive Behavior Composite score means = 100, SD = 15 Administration Time: Survey Interview and Parent/Caregiver Rating Forms, 20–60 minutes
Infant Development Inventory		
Birth to 18 months Harold Ireton, Behavior Science Systems, 1994, www.childdevelopmentreview.com	A measure of skills as reported by parent/caregiver Five areas: Social, Self-Help, Gross Motor, Fine Motor, and Language The child's level of development in each area is determined by asking the parent, "What's your baby doing?" and by observing the infant. The questionnaire can be completed by the parent or done as an interview The child's level of development in each area is compared with the child's actual age	Yields: a profile of development in the five areas compared with age norms of children from birth to 21 months Administration time: 10 minutes
Child Development Inventory		
15 months to 6 years Harold Ireton and Edward J. Thwing, Behavior Science Systems, 2005, www.childdevelopmentreview.com	A measure of skills as reported by the parent or caregiver Nine scales: Social, Self-Help, Gross Motor, Fine Motor, Expressive Language, Language Comprehension, Letters, Numbers, and an overall General Development On an inventory of the child's observed developmental skills, parents answer "yes" (present or already acquired) or "no" (not yet) There are 270 statements about the child's behavior and 30 problem items describing various symptoms and behavior problems	Yields: profile of development in the eight behavior domains and of the overall level of development compared with age norms of children between the ages of 1 year and 6.5 years The age level assigned to each behavior item was defined as the age at which at least 75% of parents answered "yes" to that statement Administration time: 30–50 minutes

(Courtesy of Rita J Jeremy, Ph.D., Developmental Psychologist, Department of Pediatrics, University of California, San Francisco, CA.)

Table 43-2 Qualitative Description of IQ and Index Scores on Wechsler Tests

Score	Classification	Percentage Included in Theoretical Normal Curve
130 and above	Very superior	2.2
120–129	Superior	6.7
110–119	High average	16.1
90–109	Average	50.0
80–89	Low average	16.1
70–79	Borderline	6.7
69 and below	Extremely low	2.2

Widely used measures for intelligence testing for children (5 to 16 years old) include the Wechsler Intelligence Scale for Children III (WISC-III) [Wechsler, 1991], the Cognitive Assessment System (CAS) [Naglieri and Das, 1997], and the Kaufman Assessment Battery for Children (K-ABC) [Kaufman and Kaufman, 1983]. For adults, the Wechsler Adult Intelligence Scale III (WAIS-III) is widely used [Wechsler, 1997]. The Stanford–Binet IV has applicability for children and adults [Thorndike et al., 1986]. The Wechsler Preschool and Primary Scale of Intelligence – Revised (WPPSI-R) [Wechsler, 1967] has been standardized for children as young as 3 years and has recognized limitations in interpretability [Sattler, 1982]. The standard for a systematic measurement of adaptive behavior from birth to adulthood has been the Vineland Adaptive Behavior Scale (VABS) [Sparrow et al., 1984], although acceptable alternatives exist, including the AAMR Adaptive Behavior Scale (ABS) [Lembert et al., 1993; Nihira et al., 1983], the Scales of Independent Behavior – Revised (SIB-R) [Bruininks et al., 1996], the Comprehensive Test of Adaptive Behavior – Revised (CTAB-R) [Adams, 1999], and the Adaptive Behavior Assessment System (ABAS) [Harrison and Oakland, 2000].

For an accurate diagnosis of global developmental delay, careful attention must be paid to its underlying concept and operational definition [Shevell, 1998, 2002, 2003, 2006]. A significant delay (i.e., greater than 2 standard deviations below the mean) needs to be demonstrated in two or more developmental domains exclusive of the qualitative impairment in language and social interaction that has been used to define an autistic spectrum disorder. Practically, delay in the child with global developmental delay is typically evident across all developmental domains. The practitioner should be aware of the general psychometric properties of testing instruments, their intended domains of evaluation and potential sources of error, and inherent standard error of measurement.

Standardized tests for assessment of infant, toddler, or pre-school child development exist and include the Bayley Scales of Infant Development (2nd edition) [Bayley, 1993], the Battelle Developmental Inventory [Newborg et al., 1984], and the Denver Developmental Screening Test (2nd edition) [Frankenburg et al., 1992]. Frequently, rather than using a broad developmental instrument, domain-specific measures are individually applied and an overall assessment arrived at. Examples of domain-specific developmental measures include the following groups:

1. Motor profile: Alberta Infant Motor Scale (AIMS) [Piper and Darrah, 1994], the Peabody Developmental Motor Scales (PDMS) [Folio and Dubose, 1974], the Bruininks–Oseretsky Test of Motor Proficiency (BOTMP) [Bruininks, 1978].
2. Language skills: Peabody Picture Vocabulary Test – Revised (PPVT-R) [Dunn and Dunn, 1997], Expressive One Word Picture Vocabulary Test – Revised (EOWPVT-R) [Gardner, 1990], the Clinical Linguistic and Auditory Milestone Scales (CLAMS) [Capute and Accardo, 1991], the Clinical Evaluation of Language Function (CELF, 4th edition) [Semel et al., 2003], and the Slossen Intelligence Test (SIT) [Slossen, 1983].
3. Behavior and activities of daily living: Vineland Adaptive Behavior Scale (VABS) [Sparrow et al., 1984], Pediatric Evaluation of Disability Inventory (PEDI) [Haley et al., 1992], and the Pediatric Functional Independent Measure (WeeFIM) [Msall et al., 1994].
4. Increasingly being utilized in both clinical and research settings in this population are measures of participation and quality of life. These include the Children's Assessment of Participation and Enjoyment [King et al., 2004], Assessment of Life Habits [Fougeyrollas and Noreau, 2002], the Peds QL [Varni et al., 2006], and the KIDSCREEN [Erhart et al., 2009].

Often, diagnosis may be initially formulated or, less frequently, entirely based on clinical judgment [AAMR, 2002]. To be valid, such clinical judgment must be based on extensive direct experience with individuals with global developmental delay or intellectual disability. Typically, clinical judgment may be necessary because of various social, cultural, and linguistic contexts or because of unavailability, inappropriateness, or delay in the administration of standardized assessment procedures. Validation of clinical judgment is increased by direct observation, reliance on reliable third-party informants, input from an interdisciplinary team skilled in multidimensional standardized assessments, and repeated observations of an individual over time.

Advances in Diagnostic Testing

How does the clinician approach the diagnostic evaluation of a child with global developmental delay or intellectual disability? The AAN practice parameter and evidence report for global developmental delay [Shevell et al., 2003; Michelson et al., 2011] provide a framework for such an evaluation (Figure 43-1). The recommendations incorporate a combination of broad screening tools and disease-specific testing based on a heightened pretest probability, given identifying clinical features. Correctly applied, each has a reasonable pretest probability (>1 percent)

of diagnosis. The current algorithm begins with a complete clinical assessment. For those patients in whom a specific diagnosis is considered, targeted testing is recommended, whether this be an MRI for an asymmetric physical examination or methylation testing for Angelman's syndrome. For the remaining patients a step-wise approach is recommended that begins with array comparative genomic hybridization (CGH), followed by chromosomal karyotype if that is negative. This recommendation is an outgrowth of many recent studies showing the enhanced utility of array CGH to detect clinically relevant chromosomal changes, and is also recommended by a consortium of clinical genetics laboratories and clinicians [Miller et al., 2010; Michelson et al., 2011]. Fragile X is recommended to evaluate mildly affected children of both genders and MeCP2 the gene that causes Rett syndrome testing is considered important in severely affected females. If these tests are unrevealing, the algorithm recommends conducting head magnetic resonance imaging (MRI; with single proton spectroscopy, where that is available). If this approach is not diagnostic, comprehensive metabolic testing is then recommended (see Figure 43-1). This then diverges based on an a priori consideration of a specific diagnosis. As all these diagnostic tools advance (a discussion of some recent advances are expanded upon below), these algorithms will continue to change to reflect these technical improvements. Regardless, clinical judgment will still be tantamount.

Genomic Microarray

Genomic microarray technology is an evolving platform that arrays a representation of the human chromosome on a glass slide and hybridizes fluorescently labeled control and patient DNA to detect copy number changes in the genome [Bejjani et al., 2005]. The first-generation chips had approximately 3000 elements spaced approximately every 1.0 Mb [Pinkel et al., 1998]. Newer-generation chips have been developed that completely cover the genome (i.e., tiling arrays) using more than 100,000-oligonucleotide spots [Ishkanian et al., 2004]. All of these platforms aim to identify interstitial copy number changes or copy number variants. Initially, this approach has been used very successfully to identify chromosomal regions (and genes) involved in cancer progression. Studies done thus far suggest that this approach will likely find many additional regions that are implicated in neurodevelopmental disabilities, even in the setting of prior normal high-resolution karyotyping [Harada et al., 2004; Shaw-Smith et al., 2004; Engels et al., 2007; Shevell et al., 2008]. Many studies in autism, mental retardation, and cohorts with multiple congenital anomalies (who also have neurodevelopmental disabilities) show that a few loci occur repetitively and at a much higher frequency in affected individuals than in controls [Berkel et al., 2010; Koolen et al., 2006; Sharp et al., 2008]. This type of large-scale analysis can provide clinicians with the necessary information to advise families about the significance of these genetic findings.

However, one challenge that arises from this whole-genome analysis is distinguishing normal variation from disease-causing changes, particularly in cases in which the genetic variation has never been reported previously in the literature, or has been reported but its incidence in cases and controls is not well documented. The first step is to establish whether a documented copy number change is de novo or familial; this is essential with respect to determining the possible pathogenicity of such changes [Speicher and Carter, 2005],

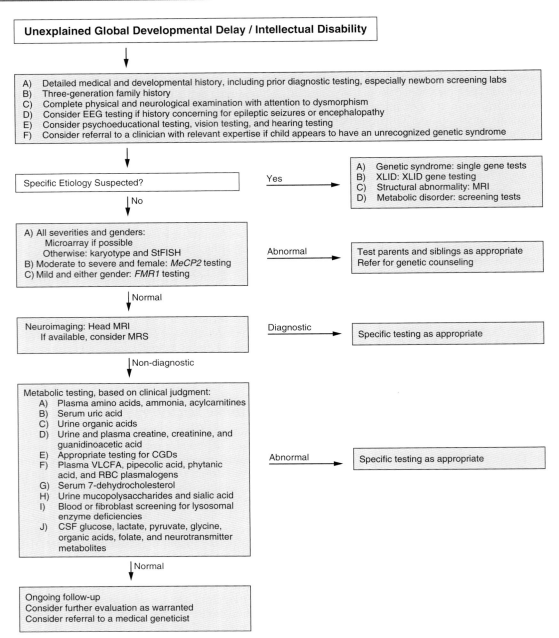

Fig. 43-1 Algorithm for the evaluation of the child with unexplained global developmental delay or intellectual disability. A detailed history, a complete physical examination, psychoeducational testing, and screening tests for visual and hearing deficits are recommended for all children with GDD/ID. EEG is recommended when there is concern about seizures or an epileptic encephalopathy. In children with features suggesting a specific etiology, genetic testing, neuroimaging, and metabolic testing may be useful for confirmation. For children without features suggesting a specific etiology, testing can be done in a stepwise or parallel manner for genetic abnormalities, structural brain abnormalities, and metabolic abnormalities. Although an extensive list of metabolic tests is provided in this algorithm, there is insufficient evidence to make specific recommendations as to which testing sequence would have the greatest diagnostic yield. The algorithm is explained in greater detail in the Clinical Context section of this guideline. CGD = congenital disorder of glycosylation, CSF = cerebrospinal fluid, EEG = electroencephalogram, RBC = red blood cell, MRI = magnetic resonance imaging, MRS = magnetic resonance spectroscopy, VLCFA = very long chain fatty acids, XLID = X-linked intellectual disability. This algorithm is based on data contained in an evidence-based review on this topic [Michelson et al, 2011]. *(Report of the Quality Standards Subcommittee of the American Academy of Neurology and the Practice Committee of the Child Neurology Society. Neurology 2011, in press.)*

although there is an increasing number of reported cases now in which inherited loci have been shown to correlate with disease presentation [Girirajan et al., 2010; Kumar et al., 2008; Shinawi et al., 2009; Weiss et al., 2008]. As we continue to make strides in genetics that move away from simple mendelian disorders, this concept of "partial penetrance" will grow in clinical relevance. The establishment of comprehensive, computerized, publicly available genotype–phenotype databases will aid in the process of establishing pathogenicity of these less common

copy number changes in the future [Speicher and Higgins, 2007].

Advances in Imaging

High-quality MRI has significantly advanced the ability to detect many brain malformations. Certain studies suggest that MRI is useful for detecting abnormalities in up to 50 percent of children with developmental delay. In some cases, such as bifrontal poly-microgyria, lissencephaly, and bilateral periventricular nodular heterotopia, certain genes are known to cause these inherited syndromes [Gaitanis and Walsh, 2004]. For most cases, the genetic or other cause of the malformation has yet to be determined. Proton MR spectroscopy measures the resonance of molecules in the brain. Given the unique resonance frequencies of many molecules, their abundance can be noninvasively measured. This approach has been useful for detecting changes in cerebral lactate in mitochondrial disorders, and for observing the absence of creatine in the three disorders of creatine deficiency [Stromberger et al., 2003], another cause of potentially treatable nonsyndromic mental retardation [Schulze, 2003]. This technique also has been useful for the detection of abnormalities in succinic semialdehyde dehydrogenase deficiency [Ethofer et al., 2004], and for those changes that precede the changes on conventional T2-weighted MRI for X-linked adrenoleukodystrophy patients [Eichler et al., 2002].

Another mode of MRI that holds promise for refinement of diagnostics is diffusion tensor imaging (DTI). Predicated on the assumption that water molecules most likely diffuse along the trajectory of axons within the white matter, DTI can measure this water diffusion and, by employing certain algorithms, can approximate the position and direction of the major white matter tracts in the cerebrum. This approach should refine the imaging results for mental retardation or autism in which no changes can be identified by conventional MRI [Barnea-Goraly et al., 2004].

Proteomics in Disease Analysis

Practical and theoretical concerns limit exclusive reliance on genetic information to understand the causes of mental retardation (even including only those that are genetically based). Proteomics potentially offers a rapid means to screen individuals for many specific diseases within a general category, particularly when the proteins are expressed in the blood or other tissue that is readily available for analysis. For example, the true prevalence of mitochondrial dysfunction as a cause of mental retardation is unknown, but some studies suggest that mitochondrial abnormalities can be detected in a high percentage of patients with developmental delay, seizures, and hypotonia [Fillano et al., 2002; Marin-Garcia et al., 1999]. Mitochondrial genetics are too complex to be approached directly, because most patients are thought to have autosomal-recessive mitochondrial disease, and hundreds of genes are necessary for proper mitochondrial function. In cases of maternal inheritance, this problem can be addressed by full sequencing of the mitochondrial genome in muscle samples of affected individuals. Given that the mitochondrial genome contains only 16,500 base pairs (bp), this is a feasible goal in the short term. Investigators have begun to undertake whole mitochondrial proteomics approaches (i.e., combining immunocapture with mass spectrometry peptide fingerprinting) to determine the quantitative values for the specific polypeptides in these multiprotein complexes [Lib et al., 2003]. Missing subunits can be readily identified, and the post-translational modifications (e.g., phosphorylation) can be monitored [Schulenberg et al., 2004].

Etiology

General Considerations

The known specific causes of mental retardation are too numerous to be listed here. The term mental retardation returns more than 1200 entries in the Online Mendelian Inheritance in Man site alone, and this catalogs only identifiable genetic causes. Mental retardation usually is classified by prenatal, perinatal, postnatal, and undetermined causes (Table 43-3). In most studies, the largest category of known primary causes is genetic or chromosomal [Leonard and Wen, 2002]. Many of the environmental causes, such as low birth weight and prematurity, are measured as risk factors and do not rise to the level of actual biomedical causes. Just as the prevalence varies, the percentage of mental retardation resulting from each group of causes varies by location and by definitions. In a California epidemiologic study of mental retardation, 75 percent of the known cases of mental retardation were due to chromosomal aberrations, whereas fewer than 3 percent were caused by any endocrine or metabolic abnormality [Croen et al., 2001]. In a Taiwanese study, 82 percent of all the chromosomal causes of mental retardation were a result of Down syndrome, but these data were collected before the clinical use of subtelomeric fluorescent in situ hybridization (FISH) probes [Hou et al., 1998]. In some regions of the world, cretinism from severe iodine deficiency occurs in up to 2–10 percent of the population of isolated communities [Delange et al., 2001]. Mild mental impairment from iodine deficiency occurs five times more frequently than cretinism, making iodine deficiency the most common preventable cause of mental retardation. Treatment during the first trimester has a significant effect on the frequency of cretinism [Cao et al., 1994]. In regions of mainland China with iodine deficiency, children score on average 10 IQ points less than cohorts in iodine-rich regions. This link between iodine deficiency and mental retardation also has a strong genetic component, because specific alleles for the deiodinase type II gene and the ApoE4 allele confer a significantly greater risk of mental retardation when the pregnant mother is iodine-deficient [Guo et al., 2004; Wang et al., 2000]. Despite the tremendous wealth of information about the causes of mental retardation, the cause remains unknown in most individuals. Genetic and epidemiologic approaches likely will continue to make progress toward unraveling and treating these currently unelucidated causes.

Genetic Causes

Some of the most significant advances in our understanding of the genetic causes of mental retardation have come from work addressing X-linked mental retardation, including mental retardation due to the fragile X syndrome or other genes.

Fragile X Syndrome

The fragile X syndrome, caused by inactivation of the *FMR1* gene, has an estimated prevalence of 1 in 3000 males and is one of the most common causes of mental retardation [Crawford et al., 2001]. Expansion of the trinucleotide sequence CGG to more than 200 copies results in CpG methylation and inactivation of the *FMR1* gene. Patients have narrow and elongated faces, large protruding ears, macro-orchidism, and joint hyperlaxity. Up to 20 percent have epilepsy, and most have complex partial seizures [Willemsen et al., 2004]. Carrier females and males with somatic mutations have various levels of intellectual impairment; studies demonstrate that the amount of the residual FMR protein detected in hair roots correlates well with IQ [Willemsen et al., 2003]. Research on the FMR protein has shown that it participates in the transport of mRNA and the regulation of protein translation

Table 43-3 **Categories and Causes of Mental Retardation**

Categories	Causes

Prenatal	Genetic
	    Chromosomal (e.g., trisomy 21, Prader–Willi syndrome, Williams' syndrome, translocations)
	    Syndromic single gene (e.g., fragile X, Rubinstein–Taybi, Coffin–Lowry syndromes)
	    Nonsyndromic single gene (e.g., oligophrenin [*OPHN1*], *FMR2* mutation)
	    Metabolic (e.g., phenylketonuria, galactosemia, Smith–Lemli–Opitz syndrome)
	Acquired
	    Fetal alcohol syndrome
	    Other maternal substance abuse
	    Nutritional (e.g., maternal phenylketonuria, iodine deficiency)
	    Infection (e.g., rubella, toxoplasmosis, cytomegalovirus, human immunodeficiency virus)
	    Stroke
	Unknown causes (most likely genetic but can be acquired)
	    Clinical syndromes without genetic diagnoses (e.g., Schinzel–Giedion, Marinesco–Sjögren, Marden–Walker syndromes)
	    Multiple congenital anomaly and mental retardation

Perinatal	Birth asphyxia Infection (herpes simplex virus encephalitis or group B streptococcus meningitis) Stroke (embolic or hemorrhagic) Very low birth weight, extreme prematurity Metabolic (e.g. hypoglycemia, hyperbilirubinemia)
Postnatal-environmental	Toxins (e.g., lead) Infection (e.g., *Haemophilus influenzae* b meningitis, arbovirus encephalitis) Stroke Trauma (consider nonaccidental source) Poor nutrition Poverty
Undetermined	Familial Nonfamilial

in neuronal dendrites [Zalfa et al., 2003]. This function perhaps explains the paucity of dendrites seen in autopsy series of these patients [Greenough et al., 2001]. Although previous studies suggested that premutation male carriers (55–200 repeats) were asymptomatic, later work from Hagerman and colleagues [1988] documented a progressive neurologic disorder, the fragile X-associated tremor/ataxia syndrome (FXTAS). After the age of 50, male patients present with intention tremor and cerebellar ataxia, and they may have cognitive decline [Jacquemont et al., 2004]. This syndrome, which is unique to these premutation males, may result from an increase in expanded repeat *FMR1* mRNA that is consistent with a toxic "gain of function" mechanism [Hagerman and Hagerman, 2004]. Because the level of FMR protein correlates with disease severity, a number of investigators have tried to identify demethylating or hyperacetylating drugs as a means to activate *FMR1* transcription [Chiurazzi et al., 1998, 1999]. Although these methods do not offer treatment for patients, this approach is generating new agents that can be tested for their ability to activate *FMR1* without associated toxicity.

Other X-Linked Mental Retardation Conditions

The increased prevalence of mental retardation in males and the relative ease of detecting the familial transmission of X-chromosome mutations have facilitated the effort to uncover the genes on the X chromosome that cause mental retardation. Many excellent reviews have detailed the syndromic and nonsyndromic forms of X-linked mental retardation [Chelly and Mandel, 2001; Gecz, 2004]. Since 1996, more than 15 genes have been identified as causes of nonsyndromic mental retardation without other associated organ involvement or significant dysmorphology (Table 43-4).

An initial assumption had been that these genes would work directly at the level of the synapse. In certain cases, in vitro and animal model data confirm this idea. For example, the protein neuroligin on the postsynaptic membrane, and its binding partner neurexin on the presynaptic side, have been shown to promote synapse formation in vitro [Dean et al., 2003; Scheiffele et al., 2000]. Some reports have shown that two X-linked neuroligin genes (*NLGN3* and *NLGN4*) are implicated in mental retardation and autism [Jamain et al., 2003; Laumonnier et al., 2004]. Similarly, multiple genes that participate in signaling through the small G protein RHO are mutated in many cases of X-linked mental retardation: *GDI1*, *PAK3*, *OPHN1*, and *ARHGEF6* [Ramakers, 2002]. In a mouse gene deletion of oligophrenin (*OPHN1*), there were clear deficits in the formation of spines along dendrites, the critical subcellular structure on which central nervous system excitatory synapses form [Govek et al., 2004]. However, involvement in synapse formation does not preclude possibly important roles more generally in organ and body development. For example, further analysis showed that mutations in oligophrenin are also found in patients with epilepsy, profound cerebellar hypoplasia, and cerebral cortical atrophy [Bergmann et al., 2003; Philip et al., 2003]. The genes *ARX* and *MECP2* can cause syndromic mental retardation (as in patients with X-linked lissencephaly with ambiguous genitalia [XLAG] and Rett's syndrome) and nonsyndromic mental retardation, depending on the severity of the mutation [Gomot et al., 2003; Sherr, 2003]. These observations demonstrate the complexity of understanding how genetic alteration causes mental retardation, what form it takes, and how genotype may correlate with phenotype.

Table 43-4 Genes Implicated in X-linked Mental Retardation

Gene	Function	Locus	Study
GENES PRIMARILY IMPLICATED IN NONSYNDROMIC MENTAL RETARDATION			
PAK3	P21 (CDKN1A)-activated kinase 3	Xq23	Allen et al., 1998
GDI1	Guanosine triphosphate (GTP) dissociation inhibitor 1	Xq28	D'Adamo et al., 1998
IL1RAPL1	Interleukin 1 receptor accessory protein-like 1	Xp21.3	Jin et al., 2000
ARHGEF6	Rac/Cdc42 guanine nucleotide exchange factor 6	Xq26.3	Kutsche et al., 2000
SLC6A8	Creatine transporter 8	Xq28	van der Knaap et al., 2000
FACL4	Long-chain fatty acid-coenzyme A ligase 4	Xq23	Meloni et al., 2002
AGTR2	Angiotensin II receptor, type 2	Xq23	Vervoort et al., 2002
FTSJ1	S-adenosylmethionine-binding protein	Xp11.23	Freude et al., 2004
DLG3	Synapse-associated protein 102 (anchoring protein)	Xq13.1	Tarpey et al., 2004
NLGN3	Neuroligin 3 (postsynaptic receptor)	Xq13.1	Jamain et al., 2003
NLGN4	Neuroligin 4 (binds neurexin)	Xp22.32	Laumonnier et al., 2004
PQBP1	Polyglutamine binding protein 1	Xp11.23	Kalscheuer et al., 2003
RPS6KA3	Serine/threonine kinase	Xp22.12	Chechlacz and Gleeson, 2003
ZNF41	Zinc-finger protein involved in chromatin activation	Xp11.3	Shoichet et al., 2003
GENES IMPLICATED IN SYNDROMIC AND NONSYNDROMIC MENTAL RETARDATION			
OPHN	Rho-GTPase activating protein (cerebellar hypoplasia)	Xq12	Billuart et al., 1998
ARX	Aristaless-related homeobox (X-linked lissencephaly with ambiguous genitalia [XLAG])	Xp22.11	Sherr, 2003
MECP2	Methyl-CpG binding protein 2 (Rett's syndrome)	Xq28	Gomot et al., 2003

Nonsyndromic Autosomal Mental Retardation

The inheritance pattern of X-linked diseases accelerates the discovery of genes. However, because nonsyndromic mental retardation is not clinically unique, it is difficult to link families together by common features to find causative genes. In the only autosomal-recessive mental retardation gene identified, a single 4-bp deletion was found in the synapse-localized serine protease neurotrypsin [Molinari et al., 2002]. Although this same 4-bp deletion was identified in another proband with mental retardation, no confirmatory mutations were identified. Investigators have used an inclusive approach, sequencing candidate genes in many dozens of mental retardation families that link to the X chromosome. Looking for additional autosomal-recessive mental retardation genes by this approach will increase the complexity more than 20-fold.

Other Etiologic Considerations

Several questions arise when considering the causes of mental retardation that guide the clinician in evaluating patients and help the researcher focus on the underlying pathophysiology. What is the prevalence of any genetic cause for mental retardation and how many genes can cause mental retardation? Will cases of mild mental retardation be caused by less severe mutations in these same, already discovered, genes or in a completely different subset? How many cases of mental retardation will be found to be caused by genetic factors alone, environmental factors alone, or the interplay between the two, as has been demonstrated for iodine deficiency?

Evaluation of the Patient

History

The assessment of a child with suspected global developmental delay or intellectual disability begins with a detailed history, and much time and effort should be directed to this evaluation [Shevell, 1998, 2002, 2006, 2009c]. Fundamental to this process is obtaining a careful family history, searching for other affected family members with similar or other potentially relevant neurologic impairments. The possible presence of early postnatal deaths should be questioned. Parental or intrafamilial consanguinity needs to be ascertained, along with the ethnic heritage of the parents. Clues to consanguinity (which may not be willingly acknowledged by parents) include origin from the same village or sharing of the same last name within the family tree. The mother's prior gestational history and her pregnancy with the affected child must be carefully probed, seeking evidence for adverse events or toxin exposures and clues to intrauterine difficulties. Timing and mode of delivery should be determined, and the reason for any forceps application or cesarean section must be identified. Birth weight, Apgar scores, head circumference measurement at birth, and duration of postnatal hospital stay are important objective markers of newborn health status. Difficulties in the newborn nursery, especially pertaining to possible clues for a neonatal encephalopathy (e.g., seizures, feeding difficulties prompting gavage), must be searched for and carefully documented. Box 43-1 lists commonly accepted risk factors for later developmental disability that can be apparent on maternal, gestational, or neonatal history-taking.

Box 43-1 Factors that Increase the Risk of Neonatal Mortality and Mental Retardation

Maternal Factors

- Complications of pregnancy
- Perinatal factors
- Neonatal factors
- Age younger than 16 or older than 40 years (over 35 years for a primigravida)
- Cervical abnormalities (e.g., incompetence, tumor)
- Consanguinity
- Contracted pelvis
- Women statistically at higher risk: unmarried, short, thin, malnourished, uneducated, nonwhite, low-income
- Other diseases and disorders
  - Bacteriuria
  - Diabetes mellitus
  - Drug addiction
  - Malnutrition
  - Nephritis
  - Phlebitis
  - Proteinuria
  - Renal hypertension
  - Thyroid disease
- History of abortion, stillbirth, neonatal death, live or stillborn infants weighing less than 1500 g, abruptio placentae, circumvallate placenta
- Hemorrhagic shock

- Polyhydramnios
- Vaginal bleeding in the second or third trimester
- Cesarean section after trial of labor

Conditions at Birth

- Cyanosis
- Need for resuscitation
- Poor Apgar score
- Presence of respiratory distress
- Gestational age of less than 30 weeks
- Hypoxic-ischemic encephalopathy
- Intrauterine hypoxia associated with prolapsed umbilical cord, abruptio placentae, or toxemia of pregnancy
- Midforceps delivery or breech presentation
- Abnormal sucking, feeding, or crying
- Anomalies
- Asymmetry of face and extremities
- Hyperbilirubinemia
- Hypotonia
- Injuries
- Need for an incubator or oxygen
- Poor weight gain or malnutrition
- Seizures
- Vomiting and fever

(Data from Denhoff E. Cerebral palsy, the preschool years. Springfield, IL: Charles C Thomas, 1967; from Pearson PH. The physician's role in diagnosis and management of the mentally retarded. Pediatr Clin North Am 1968;15:835.)

The domain of first concern is the age at which this concern became manifested to the parents; it should be documented. The timing of developmental milestones across developmental domains should be determined for the affected child. Observant parents can usually and reliably recall motor skills in the first year of life, such as when their child rolled over, sat, crawled, cruised, and took the first steps. Parental recall of meaningful speech and language milestones is often not as certain [Majnemer and Rosenblatt, 1994]. The possibility of any loss or regression of previously acquired developmental skills should be specifically questioned, as this would mandate a different and more urgent approach to etiologic evaluation and follow-up. Current skill level in the various developmental domains and the degree of independence in activities of daily living must be ascertained. For the school-age child, important points include scholastic history, with special reference to actual school and classroom placement, and identification of the provision of any supplemental educational resources.

Coexisting medical problems, with particular reference to possible seizure disorders or feeding difficulties, should be questioned. Sleeping and problematic behaviors (e.g., aggressive, inappropriate, or self-injurious) may be particular concerns of the parents and are often under-appreciated by health professionals. The past medical history, including possible chronic medical conditions, prior hospital admissions, or surgical procedures, should be documented. Past and current medications prescribed, their indications, and their effects (beneficial or deleterious) must be assessed. The current social situation of the child and family must be carefully probed with reference to items such as socioeconomic status, parental educational attainment, marital status and home living arrangements, child custody, and existing support services. The examiner must determine whether the patient has access to appropriate rehabilitation services (e.g., occupational therapy, physiotherapy, speech therapy, special education, psychology), and whether previous relevant evaluations or laboratory investigations have been conducted.

By the end of the history-taking, the clinician should have clear ideas regarding evidence of a static or progressive encephalopathy; an approximate idea of the developmental and functional level of the affected child; the possible timing of an underlying cause; the possibility of an underlying etiologic cause; the social or rehabilitation status of the affected child; and the possibility of associated and relevant medical or behavioral conditions.

Physical Examination

Ideally, the physical examination begins with careful observation of the child as the history is being taken. The delayed child often presents a challenge to the clinician with respect to the formal examination because of inherent features, such as short attention span and limitations in understanding and cooperation. The availability of a play area with appropriate toys, including paper, crayons, dolls, and representational toys, that is amenable to observation by the examiner may allow for a nonintrusive and noninvasive assessment of developmental skills, dexterity, inquisitiveness, behavior, and interaction with the surroundings and others. Much of the neurodevelopmental examination can take place during extended history-taking by observation alone. In the older child, language skills, both spontaneous and responsive, expressive and receptive, should be established, together with an understanding of simple cognitive concepts (i.e., size, shape, analogies, action, commonalities, numbers).

The general physical examination should specifically ascertain possible dysmorphology, hepatosplenomegaly, and cutaneous markers of the phakomatoses. The spine should be carefully inspected, including the sacral region, to look for dermal sinuses, hair tufts, or other subtle signs of spinal dysraphism. Height and weight should be plotted. Genetic catalogs are indispensable for an accurate recognition of specific syndromes.

Current and previous occipitofrontal circumference should be obtained and plotted, with particular attention directed at microcephalic or macrocephalic measurements or changing percentile values over time. In cases of microcephaly or macrocephaly, the parental occipitofrontal circumferences also should be obtained and plotted. The head shape and status of the anterior and posterior fontanels in the infant, together with the sutures, should be observed. Determination of the presence of any focal or asymmetric neurologic findings is the primary objective of the formal neurologic examination. Careful evaluation of vision, in addition to aiding in a definitive diagnostic process, is indicated to minimize the contribution of potentially correctable visual impairment to the burden of disability. Similarly, this approach applies to evaluating for possible gross auditory impairments in the office setting.

Within the clinical office setting, several test instruments exist for use as objective screening assessments of development during the first years of life (i.e., Denver Developmental Screening Test [Frankenburg and Dodds, 1967], the Denver II [Frankenburg et al., 1992], and the CAT/CLAMS [Capute and Accardo, 1991], which focuses on language- and non-language-based reasoning abilities). These may be supplemented or complemented by the use of parent-based questionnaires (e.g., Child Developmental Inventory [Ireton, 1992], and Ages and Stages Questionnaire [Bricker, 1999]) that provide an aspect of objective developmental screening. Observed signs and symptoms and their association with various diagnostic entities that can result in global developmental delay or intellectual disability are summarized in Boxes 43-2 to 43-10. Definitive diagnosis of these associated entities often requires specific laboratory testing.

Box 43-2 Eye Abnormalities

Cataracts

- Cerebrotendinous xanthomatosis
- Cockayne's syndrome
- Cretinism
- Down syndrome
- Galactosemia
- Lowe's syndrome
- Marinesco–Sjögren syndrome
- Myotonic dystrophy
- Pseudohypoparathyroidism
- Rubella (gestational)
- Trichothiodystrophy

Cherry-red spot in macular area

- GM$_1$ gangliosidosis (generalized)
- Neuraminidase deficiency
- Niemann–Pick disease type A
- Tay–Sachs disease

Chorioretinitis

- Clouding of cornea
- Congenital lues
- Cytomegalic inclusion body disease
- Hunter's syndrome
- Hurler's syndrome
- Lowe's syndrome
- Prenatal rubella (gestational)

Corneal ulcers

- Familial dysautonomia

Dislocated lenses

- Homocystinuria

- Sulfite oxidase deficiency

Glaucoma

- Lowe's syndrome
- Rubinstein–Taybi syndrome
- Sturge–Weber syndrome

Nystagmus

- Hyperpipecolatemia
- Hypervalinemia
- Joubert's syndrome

Photophobia

- Cockayne's syndrome
- Hartnup's disease
- Homocystinuria

Retinitis pigmentosa

- Ataxia-telangiectasia
- Cockayne's syndrome
- Hallervorden–Spatz syndrome
- Hyperpipecolatemia
- Kearns–Sayre syndrome
- Laurence–Moon–Biedl syndrome
- Mitochondrial encephalomyopathies
- Neuronal ceroid-lipofuscinosis
- Scleral telangiectasia

Vertical supranuclear gaze palsy

- Niemann–Pick disease type C
- Tauopathy dementia (progressive supranuclear palsy)

Box 43-3 **Seizures**

Generalized tonic-clonic seizures

- Argininosuccinic aciduria
- Neuronal ceroid-lipofuscinosis
- Citrullinemia
- Glycogen synthetase deficiency
- Hyper-beta-alaninemia
- Hyperammonemia
- Hyperlysinemia
- Hyperornithinemia-hyperammonemia and homocitrullinuria hyperprolinemia I
- Hypoglycemia, particularly associated with glycogen storage diseases I, III, IV, and VII, and idiopathic hypoglycemia of infancy
- Joseph's disease
- Ketotic hypoglycemia
- Kinky hair disease (Menkes' disease)
- Lactic acidosis
- Lysine intolerance with periodic ammonia intoxication
- Maple syrup urine disease
- Methionine malabsorption syndrome
- Mitochondrial encephalomyopathies (e.g., *MERRF* [now *MT-TK*], *MELAS* defects)

- Nonketotic hyperglycinemia
- Phenylketonuria
- Severe myoclonic epilepsy of infancy (*SCN1A* defect)
- Tay–Sachs disease
- X-linked infantile spasm syndrome (*ARX* [also called *ISSX*] mutation)

Seizures in the neonatal period

- Argininosuccinic aciduria
- Hyperammonemia I and II
- Hyperprolinemia I
- Hypoglycorrhachia (*GLUT1* [now designated *SCL2A1*] deficiency syndrome)
- Hypoxic-ischemic encephalopathy
- Isovaleric acidemia
- Joseph's disease
- Lactic acidosis
- Maple syrup urine disease
- Mitochondrial encephalomyopathy
- Methylmalonic acidemia
- Propionic acidemia

Box 43-4 **Skin Abnormalities**

Café au lait spots

- Ataxia-telangiectasia
- Bloom's syndrome
- Neurofibromatosis
- Tuberous sclerosis

Depigmented nevi

- Tuberous sclerosis

Eczema

- Phenylketonuria

Linear nevus

- Linear sebaceous nevus of Jadassohn

Malar flush

- Homocystinuria

Photosensitivity

- Hartnup's disease
- Tryptophanuria

Rash

- Biotinidase deficiency
- Holocarboxylase synthetase deficiency

Synophrys

- Cornelia de Lange syndrome
- Cretinism

Box 43-5 **Hearing Abnormalities**

Conduction deafness

- Hunter's syndrome
- Hurler's syndrome

Hyperacusis

- GM$_1$ gangliosidosis (generalized)
- Krabbe's disease
- Subacute sclerosing panencephalitis
- Sulfite oxidase deficiency
- Tay–Sachs disease

Sensorineural deafness

- CHARGE syndrome (i.e., coloboma, heart defects, atresia choanae, retardation of growth and development, genitourinary problems, and ear anomalies) [Menenzes and Coker, 1990]
- Kearns–Sayre syndrome
- MELAS syndrome (i.e., mitochondrial myopathy, encephalopathy, lactacidosis, and stroke)
- MERRF syndrome (i.e., myoclonus epilepsy associated with ragged red fibers)
- Refsum's disease

Laboratory Testing

Laboratory testing is directed at establishing the possible cause of the individual's delay or intellectual disability [Schaefer and Bodensteiner, 1992]. This testing may be confirmatory, directed

Box 43-6 Vomiting

- Hyperammonemia (all types)
- Hyperglycinemia
- Hyperlysinemia
- Hypervalinemia
- Increased intracranial pressure
- Lactic acidosis
- Maple syrup urine disease
- MELAS syndrome (i.e., mitochondrial myopathy, encephalopathy, lactacidosis, and stroke)

Box 43-7 Hair Abnormalities

Fine hair

- Homocystinuria
- Hypothyroidism

Friable and tufted hair (trichorrhexis nodosa)

- Argininosuccinic aciduria
- Kinky hair disease (Menkes' disease)

Loss of scalp hair

- Familial lactic acidosis with necrotizing encephalopathy

Premature gray hair

- Ataxia-telangiectasia
- Progressive cerebral hemisphere atrophy

White hair (patches)

- Methionine malabsorption syndrome
- Tuberous sclerosis

Box 43-8 Hepatosplenomegaly

- Argininosuccinic aciduria
- Gaucher's disease
- Glycogen storage disease types I and III
- GM1 gangliosidosis (generalized)
- Hydroxykynureninuria
- Hyperpipecolatemia
- Mucopolysaccharidoses
- Neuronal ceroid-lipofuscinosis
- Niemann–Pick disease

Box 43-9 Metabolic Acidosis

- Ketotic hypoglycemia
- Lactic acidosis
- Maple syrup urine disease
- Methionine malabsorption syndrome
- Methylmalonic acidemia
- Mitochondrial encephalomyopathy
- 5-Oxoprolinuria (pyroglutamic aciduria)
- Propionic acidemia

at a suggested cause from the history and/or physical examination, or it may be undertaken on a screening basis, directed at finding a previously unsuspected cause. Some data exist on the diagnostic yield of various laboratory investigations of community-derived samples of children with global developmental delay or mental retardation, with older series restricted to more severe variants of institutionalized individuals [Hagberg and Kyllerman, 1983; Hunter et al., 1980; McLaren and Bryson, 1987], and more recent series derived from ambulatory community settings [Srour et al., 2006]. Controversy exists regarding the extent to which diagnostic investigations should be undertaken for a developmentally delayed or cognitively disabled child. However, consensus does exist that an all-inclusive "shotgun" approach is not warranted or feasible from medical, personal, or economic viewpoints [Shevell et al., 2003]. Laboratory testing is undertaken in the spirit that, although yield may be lower than in other clinical situations, the potential value of a definitive etiologic diagnosis from individual and familial perspectives may be substantial. Technologic advances, especially in the domains of genetic testing and neuroimaging, have resulted in improved diagnostic yield and precision. This is reflected in improved etiologic yield in community samples studied retrospectively and prospectively [Majnemer and Shevell, 1995; Shevell et al., 2000; Srour et al., 2006]. Aiding the formulation of a rational approach to laboratory investigations in this clinical population is the AAN practice parameter evidence report (see Figure 43-1) [Shevell et al., 2003; Michelson et al., 2011], the American College of Medical Genetics consensus [Curry et al., 1997], and the AAP technical document [Moeschler and Shevell, 2006] on this topic.

Routine metabolic testing for an extensive list of potential inborn errors of metabolism cannot presently be justified [Carson and Neill, 1962; Henderson et al., 1981; Reinecke et al., 1983]. However, diagnostic vigilance needs to be maintained for these disorders, given the implication for treatment, prognosis, and recurrent risk [Papavasiliou et al., 2000]. Clinical situations suggesting a possible inborn error of metabolism that should prompt careful and detailed metabolic testing include family history, parental consanguinity, documented developmental regression, suggestive dysmorphology, involvement of nonectodermal organ systems, and possible white matter involvement observed on imaging or peripheral electrophysiologic studies.

For the globally or intellectually delayed child without an apparent cause after history and physical examination, current recommendations would include beginning with microarray testing, followed, if clinically indicated, by a karyotype and high-resolution MRI [Miller et al., 2010; Michelson et al., 2011]. As mentioned above, if specific causes are considered, they should be tested for early on in the diagnostic evaluation. For instance, if the affected child is a male and his maternal uncles are similarly affected, there is good evidence to suggest that sequencing X chromosome mental retardation genes would be a high-yield diagnostic approach [Michelson et al., 2011].

Neuroimaging has greatly enhanced the clinical practice of neurology and improved etiologic yields. Although largely of little additional value in early reported studies [Lingham et al., 1982; Moeschler et al., 1981], later studies have indeed emphasized the added value of neuroimaging in detecting cerebral dysgenesis, acquired injury of various causes, or disturbances in white matter maturation [Bouhadiba et al., 2000; VanBogaert et al., 1992]. The superiority of MRI over

Box 43-10 Other Abnormalities

Anterior horn cell disease (includes electrodiagnostic evidence of normal nerve conduction time in the presence of muscular denervation potentials)

- Neuroaxonal dystrophy
- Beta-methyl-crotonyl CoA decarboxylase deficiency

Ataxia (partial representative list)

- Argininosuccinic aciduria
- Ataxia-telangiectasia
- Cockayne's syndrome
- Guanosine triphosphate (GTP) cyclohydrolase deficiency (dopa-responsive dystonia)
- Hartnup's disease
- Hyperammonemia from any cause
- Joubert's syndrome
- Kearns–Sayre syndrome
- l-2-α-hydroxyglutaric aciduria
- Marinesco–Sjögren syndrome
- Metachromatic leukodystrophy
- Mitochondrial disorders
- Neuronal ceroid-lipofuscinosis
- 5-Oxoprolinuria (pyroglutamic aciduria)
- Partington's syndrome (*ARX* defect)
- Pyruvate decarboxylase deficiency
- Tryptophanuria

Broad thumbs and toes

- Rubinstein–Taybi syndrome [Rubinstein and Taybi, 1963]

Choreoathetosis

- Dentatorubral pallidoluysian atrophy
- Glutaricaciduria type I
- Huntington's chorea
- Joseph's disease
- Lesch–Nyhan disease
- Pantothenate kinase-associated neurodegeneration (PKAN)
- Phenylketonuria

Dystonia

- Alexander's disease
- Canavan's disease
- Enlarged head
- GM2 gangliosidosis (generalized)
- GTP cyclohydrolase deficiency (dopa-responsive dystonia)
- Histiocytosis X
- Hydrocephalus

- Mitochondrial disorders
- Mucopolysaccharidoses
- Pelizaeus–Merzbacher disease
- PKAN
- Sandhoff's disease
- Spongy degeneration
- Subdural effusion
- Subdural hematoma
- Tay–Sachs disease
- Wilson's disease

Fat pad distribution, abnormal

- Congenital disorders of glycosylation
- Cornelia de Lange syndrome
- Micromelia

Odors

- Isovaleric acidemia
- Maple syrup urine disease
- Methionine malabsorption syndrome
- Phenylketonuria

Peripheral neuropathy (includes electrodiagnostic evidence of decreased conduction time)

- Cockayne's syndrome
- Krabbe's syndrome
- Metachromatic leukodystrophy
- Niemann–Pick disease

Short stature

- Bird-headed dwarf (Seckel type)
- Cockayne's syndrome
- Cornelia de Lange syndrome
- Cretinism
- Leprechaunism [Dekaban, 1965]
- Mucolipidoses
- Mucopolysaccharidoses
- Prader–Willi syndrome
- Rubinstein–Taybi syndrome

Tremor

- Citrullinemia
- Hartnup's disease
- Hyperpipecolatemia
- Hypersarcosinemia

computed tomography (CT) has made it the imaging modality of choice contingent on local availability and individual sedation restrictions.

Similar to metabolic studies, electrophysiologic studies, such as electroencephalography, should be undertaken only in the situation of a suspected coexisting paroxysmal disorder or evidence of language regression or behavioral abnormalities suggestive of an epilepsy syndrome, such as Landau–Kleffner

or electrical status epilepticus during slow-wave sleep [Sheth, 1998]. Visual- and auditory-evoked potentials are of use in assessing the integrity of the visual and auditory systems in the young, uncooperative child.

The presence of certain clinical features predicts the success or failure of the etiologic search. Documented neonatal difficulties, microcephaly, focal neurologic findings, and positive family history all suggest an enhanced possibility of success. Coexisting autistic features have been found to be a negative predictor of detecting an underlying cause [Shevell et al., 2000; Srour et al., 2006].

Consultation and Follow-up

Concerns about the developmental and functional patterns highlighted at the time of specialty evaluation should prompt referrals to other health professionals with different but complementary expertise, permitting a multidisciplinary, comprehensive evaluation of the affected child [Shevell, 2002, 2006, 2009c]. These professionals, in addition to documenting various deficits objectively in a standardized way, usually assume responsibility for implementing goal-directed therapeutic interventions, and serve as conduits to appropriate community-based, long-term rehabilitation and educational resources. These health professionals represent occupational therapy (e.g., fine motor, activities of daily living, feeding), physical therapy (i.e., gross motor), speech and language pathology (i.e., language), and psychology (e.g., cognition, social, behavioral). Specific care needs, such as tube feeding, respite care, or financial difficulties, may prompt nursing or social service intervention. Vision and hearing screening is important because of the high frequency of potentially correctable primary sensory impairments in this population, and results should prompt ophthalmologic and audiologic evaluations [Kwok et al., 1996; Menacker, 1993; Warburg, 1994]. Concerns regarding a possible genetic cause or specific behavioral issues may require the expertise and intervention of genetic or psychiatric services.

A key part of the evaluation of the delayed or intellectually disabled individual is a second visit. This second visit is needed to review the results of laboratory investigations, integrate the reports of the various health professionals consulted, characterize the type and level of developmental disability, ascertain the provision of rehabilitation or relevant educational services, counsel the family appropriately, and by ascertaining developmental progress, exclude the possibility of a progressive encephalopathy or neurodegenerative process. Frequently, the opportunity exists to reconsider and refine the diagnostic evaluation over a longer interval because the child neurologist frequently participates directly in the on-going care of the child with developmental delay or intellectual disability who has coexisting and often challenging conditions requiring continuing medical management.

Medical Management of Coexisting Conditions

With a greater drive to incorporate intellectually disabled individuals into the community comes a better awareness of the unique and challenging profile of their psychiatric and medical issues, and of how best to optimize their treatment to improve quality of life and outcome for both the individual and family.

Psychiatric Disorders in the Mentally Retarded

The prevalence of coexistent Axis I psychiatric conditions and challenging, disruptive, or injurious (towards self or others) behaviors is higher among patients with intellectual disability than among people in the general population [Marco, 2009].

These conditions are generally under-recognized and under-treated. Under-recognition is the byproduct of several factors:
1. Conceptual differentiation of intellectual disability and mental illness is relatively recent.
2. The clinical phenomenology of mental disorders is altered by declining intellectual and verbal capabilities.
3. Comprehensive and thorough evaluation of affective and behavioral domains is time-consuming and often beyond the scope of expertise of the individual practitioner [Marco, 2009].

Diagnosis of challenging behavior and mental illness in those with developmental delays or intellectual disabilities requires modification in recognition that both takes into account developmental and cognitive abilities, and focuses on behavioral domains and standards for inferential diagnosis in the absence of objective markers. Multiple screening tools have been developed to assist in recognition. These include the Developmental Behavioral Checklist for Pediatrics (DBC-P) [Clarke et al., 2003], the Children's Depression Inventory [Meins, 1993], and the Psychiatric Assessment Schedule for Adults with Developmental Disability Checklist (PAS-ADD checklist) [Mohr et al., 2005], amongst other instruments.

In one population-based study, 40 percent of mental retardation patients had a Diagnostic and Statistical Manual of Mental Disorders (DSM-IV) diagnosis, one-fourth of this group had more than one diagnosis, and these disorders caused severe impairment in everyday functioning for more than one-half of patients. Of these mental retardation patients, 22 percent had anxiety disorders, 5 percent had mood disorders, and 25 percent had disruptive disorders. The most common diagnoses were specific phobias (17.5 percent), attention-deficit hyperactivity disorder (14.8 percent), and oppositional defiant disorder (13.9 percent). However, of all the children with a DSM-IV diagnosis, only 27 percent were receiving specific help for any of these problems [Dekker and Koot, 2003]. For those whose diagnoses caused severe impairment, only 41 percent received professional help. As is the case for the diagnosis of mental illness in children generally, eliciting a careful history from the parents or caretakers is essential to the accurate diagnosis and to the evaluation of treatment efficacy. Based on reasonable clinical inference, some modifications in specific diagnostic criteria are occasionally necessary.

Treatment of Psychiatric Disorders

Several studies support medical therapies for the treatment of psychiatric conditions in the intellectually disabled population. The newer neuroleptics (especially risperidone) have been effective for behavioral disorders, particularly aggression and impulsivity, in patients with mental retardation or autism, or both [Snyder et al., 2002]. However, side effects can include intolerable weight gain, particularly at higher doses [Cohen et al., 2001]. Other atypical antipsychotic agents, such as quetiapine and aripiprazole, have less effect on weight and may be effective for aggressive and aberrant behavior [Sajatovic, 2003; Stigler et al., 2004]. Clonidine has been effective for hyperactivity, hypersensitivity, and the less aggressive impulsive behaviors [Agarwal et al., 2001]. Methylphenidate is now available in varied long-acting formulations and has been effective for many patients with mental retardation [Aman et al., 2003; Pearson et al., 2004a, 2004b]; it is the most common class of medications used for fragile X syndrome males, in whom up to

67 percent showed a positive response in a controlled study [Hagerman et al., 1988]. Anxiety and compulsive and perseverative behaviors and mood symptoms can be managed with selective serotonin reuptake inhibitors (SSRIs). In particular, SSRIs have been shown to be helpful for the treatment of social anxiety and withdrawal [Santosh and Baird, 1999]. Chapter 49 reviews the psychopharmacologic agents that can be used for the treatment of some of these disorders.

Treatment of Epilepsy

Approximately 15–20 percent of intellectually disabled individuals also have epilepsy, a rate 10 times higher than the general population [Kelly et al., 2004; Mayville and Matson, 2004]. Many of these patients have intractable epilepsy. When treating seizures in these individuals, the same guidelines apply as for patients without intellectual disability: minimize side effects (i.e., sedation, altered mentation, behavioral changes) while eliminating or substantially reducing the number of seizures. Since many individuals with intellectual limitations will be unable to express their response to the medication verbally, the physician must be alert to other means of assessing side effects and seizure reduction. In the case of young children living at home, their parents or other primary caretakers can provide reasonable estimates of these parameters. In the case of multiple caretakers or of patients residing in assisted living environments, special care must be taken to ensure the accuracy and reliability of reporting between different observers. Clarification of which seizure types to record and maintaining a seizure diary before alteration of the medication regimen can help achieve this goal. In some instances, use of standardized instruments, such as the Glasgow epilepsy outcome measure, may be helpful [Espie et al., 2001]. Drug treatment should be guided primarily by the type of epilepsy. Patients with Lennox–Gastaut syndrome have responded well to lamotrigine, infantile spasms to vigabatrin, and nonsyndromic generalized seizures to valproic acid. In general, avoidance of barbiturates and benzodiazepines is preferable because of the propensity for sedation and impairment of cognition [Coulter, 1997]. Polypharmacy, with its cumulative and synergistic potential for side effects, should also be avoided whenever possible [Marco, 2009]. Intractable epilepsies may respond to the ketogenic diet, placement of a vagal nerve stimulator, or, especially if lesional in origin, surgical resection. Callosotomy is still rarely utilized for intractable atonic seizures.

Sleep Disorders

The most common sleep problem in the general population and among the developmentally impaired is insufficient sleep [Didde and Sigafoos, 2001]. Preadolescents sleep 9–10 hours per night, with sleep latencies of 20 minutes or more. Seizures during sleep are a frequent cause of sleep disruption. For generalized seizure disorders, one study determined that 34 percent of seizures occurred upon arousal to the waking state, 45 percent occurred only in sleep, and 21 percent occurred both diurnally and nocturnally [Marco, 2009]. Specific sleep epilepsy disorders, such as electrical status epilepticus of sleep, Landau–Kleffner syndrome, and nocturnal frontal lobe epilepsy, should be considered [Lancioni et al., 1999]. Many patients with intellectual disability also have hypotonia or extensive central nervous system abnormalities, or both, and central and obstructive sleep apnea is a common complication.

Obstruction can occur at the pharyngeal level because of corticobulbar and bulbar weakness, or because of the inability of the muscles of respiration to overcome the normal change in airway resistance produced by progression from waking to non-rapid eye movement sleep to rapid eye movement sleep. This problem is exacerbated by the loss of muscle tone seen in rapid eye movement sleep. Since the circadian clock within the suprachiasmatic nucleus is chronobiologic and requires light input from the retina to entrain a rhythm, patients who are blind or who have had profound brain injury may suffer from disorganized sleep architecture.

In patients with a sleep problem, obtaining an accurate sleep history that includes sleep hygiene, nighttime awakenings, and daytime behavior is essential. If this approach is not informative, a formal sleep study with polysomnography may be indicated [Harvey and Kennedy, 2002]. Melatonin has been particularly useful for this population and has been effective for patients with global developmental delay and sleep disturbance in general [Coppola et al., 2004].

Vision and Hearing Impairment

Individuals with global developmental delay and intellectual disability are at an elevated risk for sensory impairment involving either hearing, vision, or both [MMWR, 1997]. These impairments may be congenital or acquired in origin, but often remains undiagnosed and untreated. This is indeed unfortunate, as early identification and treatment of these sensory impairments can improve overall outcome for these individuals [Yoshinaga-Itano, 2003]. Vigilant and early hearing and vision screening in this population should be a standard of clinical practice.

Feeding and Nutritional Disorders

Difficulties with nutritional intake, gut motility, and growth (i.e., failure to thrive) are common in individuals with global developmental delay and intellectual disability [Canadian Pediatric Society, 1994]. Oral motor incoordination and apraxia are frequent consequences of the underlying primary neurologic dysfunction. Altered esophageal sphincter tone, combined with oral motor incoordination, predisposes to gastro-esophageal reflux and frequent aspirations. Furthermore, the gastro-esophageal reflux may lead to pain and irritability that provoke additional management challenges. Swallowing studies employing video fluoroscopy are an indispensable tool for assessing upper gastrointestinal function. Both medical and behavioral interventions are available to improve feeding competency and comfort, but at times, the placement of a percutaneous feeding tube may be necessary if recurrent pain, aspiration, and malnutrition that limits functional status persists [Marco, 2009]. Enteric feeding may substantially improve quality of life for the affected individual and appreciably diminish the burdens of care upon the family [Sanders et al., 1990].

Pharmacologic Treatment of Cognitive Impairment

Pharmacologic treatment of cognitive impairment is a prominent goal of clinicians and researchers. There are tantalizing studies in animal models and some preliminary data from studies of patients. Unfortunately, there is not yet solid evidence supporting a role for pharmacologic enhancement of cognition in the mental retardation population as a whole. The animal model for the Rubinstein–Taybi syndrome exemplifies the potential of this approach [Bourtchouladze et al., 2003]. Rubinstein–Taybi syndrome, which manifests with mental retardation and characteristic physical findings (i.e., broad thumbs and toes, short stature, and craniofacial anomalies), occurs in approximately 1 in 125,000 births and is caused by mutations in the cAMP-responsive element binding protein (CREB)-binding protein (CBP). Many patients with Rubinstein–Taybi syndrome are heterozygous for de novo CBP truncation mutations or deletions involving the gene, implying that the phenotype is expressed in an autosomal-dominant fashion. Analogously, CBP heterozygous knockout (+/−) mice share features with Rubinstein–Taybi syndrome patients, whereas the CBP homozygous knockout (−/−) pattern in mice is embryonically lethal. In one study, treatment with inhibitors of phosphodiesterase-4 resulted in an improvement in cognitive performance for the CBP +/− mice [Bourtchouladze et al., 2003]. A similar improvement in cognition was demonstrated in the mouse model of neurofibromatosis type 1. Neurofibromatosis type 1 results from an autosomal-dominant heterozygous mutation in neurofibromin [Costa and Silva, 2002]. Additional experimental data suggest that overactivation of the small GTP protein RAS by the mutant neurofibromin is the cause of cognitive dysfunction. Inhibition of RAS through pharmacologic manipulation (i.e., farnesyl transferase inhibitors) or by genetic modification increases cognitive performance in neurofibromatosis type 1 mice and improves physiologic correlates for learning [Costa et al., 2002], such as long-term potentiation.

Successful changes in cognitive function in patients have been much more limited, and most reports are uncontrolled and anecdotal. One open-label study with these methodologic limitations suggested that donepezil (a cholinesterase inhibitor) improved language performance in patients with Down syndrome [Heller et al., 2003].

Outcome and Prognosis

The vast majority of developmentally delayed or intellectually disabled children presently remain at home with the best caregivers possible – a loving, supportive, and nurturing family. This represents a dramatic historical shift from the previous standard of segregated institutionalization that persisted until the latter half of the twentieth century. However, the child's family should not be taken for granted, nor should the burden placed on the family be underestimated. Supportive counseling is often necessary to help family members accept the diagnosis, plan realistically for the future, and deal with any feelings of anger, guilt, loneliness, or even shame that are often regrettably but understandably experienced. The emotional states experienced by parents of a delayed child resemble those experienced during bereavement [Batshaw, 1993; Kübler-Ross, 1969]. Parental stress is often elevated over the long term and parents will frequently experience fatigue, isolation, and financial hardship [Majnemer and Limperopoulos, 2009]. Support to lessen the family burden, especially in the context of severe delay or intellectual disability, such as short-term respite care, frequently needs to be sought and made available to ensure family health and well-being. Access to available governmental supplemental financial resources should be facilitated. Siblings of the delayed child are often overlooked and are prone to more frequent peer and behavior problems [Bagenholm and Gillberg, 1991].

Longitudinal studies suggest continued intellectual development in those with mild or moderate delay [Eyman and Widaman, 1987; Hogg et al., 1988], and the absence of such improvement in those with severe or profound intellectual disability. Functional attainment for the child with severe neurodevelopmental disability by age 6 typically represents the functional attainment with respect to ambulation, feeding, toileting, and self-hygiene for the life span [Strauss et al., 1997]. Greater developmental progress has occurred in those provided home or foster care rather than institutional or residential care [Eyman and Widaman, 1987]. In the United States, federal law mandates with public funds the provision of early educational and rehabilitation services to the preschool child with a developmental disability and appropriate educational services to the school-age child, regardless of the severity of the mental impairment. The long-term benefits of early intervention remain speculative in the absence of definitive longitudinal studies, but a beneficial trend for sustained intervention in a programmatic approach with targeted screening and intervention at key points in the life span is suggested [Majnemer, 1998].

Pragmatically, the focus should be on short-term achievable goals that assist in improving functional capacity, especially with respect to obtaining independence in activities of daily living. Life skills and vocational training are viable and important objectives for those with mild or moderate intellectual disability, and appear to be integral to achieving a sense of self-worth and self-esteem. Clinical judgment suggests that continued progress implies the potential for even further future progress and remains a good prognostic sign, in contradistinction to a long-term plateau in developmental skills.

Studies have consistently demonstrated that early childhood developmental delays are correlated with later academic difficulties during the school years [Shapiro et al., 1990]. Persisting functional and developmental disabilities have also been demonstrated in longitudinal prospective studies, as well as suggesting a prognostic validity to the diagnostic label of global developmental delay [Shevell et al., 2005]. The degree of initial delay predicted functional attainment (i.e., what a child does do) to a greater extent than developmental attainment (what a child can do). The capacity of a family potentially to advocate on behalf of their child, as reflected in a higher socioeconomic status, resulted in better functional attainment, suggesting potential modifiability that should enable broader rehabilitation services provision across the spectrum of individuals and families with developmental disabilities.

The transition to adult life can be challenging for the intellectually disabled individual and involved family members. Transition concerns issues related to living situations (independent or assisted), limited access to entitlements, opportunities for participation, sexuality, and employment (sheltered or supported) [Batshaw, 1993], and the locus of medical care provision (i.e., pediatric to adult). Deterioration in ability or adaptive function has not been manifested in cohorts followed through this transitional phase [Eyman and Widaman, 1987]. Severe childhood intellectual disability can predict later adult dependence and disability, but investigators are only now evaluating the transition to adulthood of populations raised in an era after segregation to residential institutions [Clarke and

Clarke, 1988]. Family involvement in transition planning and an individual's educational attainment and ability to acquire basic living skills have been key factors in the successful adjustment to adult life [Reiter and Palnizky, 1996]. Individuals with mild to moderate intellectual disability have had higher unemployment rates than the general population and a tendency for placement in segregated (i.e., sheltered) environments [Kraemer and Blacher, 2001]. Periodic, on-going support often has been found to be a necessary precondition for continued employment. Since employment has been linked to a better quality of life and self-esteem, it should be sought for the individual patient or collectively for the class of individuals affected [Kraemer et al., 2003]. Since psychiatric and behavioral disorders occur with increased frequency in intellectually disabled individuals, this may be an added factor to precluding social inclusion and also a challenge to sufficient psychiatric service provision [O'Brien, 2000].

The life expectancy of a child with mild to moderate intellectual disability who is in good general health without evidence of cardiorespiratory disease or severe epilepsy can be considered similar to that of the general pediatric population. Significant mobility limitations (e.g., quadriplegia with inability to roll or sit independently), lack of functional hand use, and feeding dependency (especially the placement of a gastrostomy tube) have been associated with limitations in life expectancy. Other important variables include the nature of associated disabilities and the severity of coexisting medical conditions, together with the availability and accessibility of quality medical care. However, a temporal trend is evident, with life expectancy improving overall for those with intellectual disability, even for the most severely affected individuals [Eyman et al., 1990; Piloplys et al., 1998; Strauss et al., 1997; Strauss et al, 2008].

Acknowledgments

The authors wish to thank Rita J Jeremy, Ph.D., Developmental Psychologist, Department of Pediatrics, University of California, San Francisco for her assistance in preparation of the tables containing information on measures for evaluation of intellectual, neurodevelopmental, and behavioral progress, and Alba Rinaldi for her secretarial assistance. MS was supported by the MCH Foundation during the writing of this manuscript.

 The complete list of references for this chapter is available online at **www.expertconsult.com**.
See inside cover for registration details.

Cognitive and Motor Regression

David J. Michelson and Stanford K. Shu

Introduction

Diseases in which there is a gradual loss of cognitive function can be described as progressive encephalopathies (PE). A number of toxic, infectious, inflammatory, and neoplastic disorders of the central nervous system (CNS) can have subacute to chronic presentations, and must be considered in the differential diagnosis of patients initially presenting with PE, but this chapter is primarily focused on the diagnostic challenge posed by patients with genetic disorders that present with progressive neurological dysfunction.

One challenge posed by these disorders relates to their being individually rare and thus generally unfamiliar to clinicians. A second challenge relates to phenotypic variability, as many of the inborn errors of metabolism (IEMs) that had been known by one or more "classic" phenotypes are now known to vary greatly in presentation, based on the degree of the enzymatic defect. For example, neonatal encephalopathy and multi-organ failure may result from the complete deficiency of an enzyme, whose partial deficit may cause only nonspecific psychiatric symptoms in adulthood.

Pathophysiology

Most genetic causes of PE can be classified as an IEM or neurodegenerative disorder (ND). The IEMs are themselves frequently divided into three groups, based on pathophysiology. In the first group are those disorders in which symptoms of acute or chronic intoxication are caused by the intracellular and extracellular (and thus measurable in blood, urine, and cerebrospinal fluid) accumulation of the compounds proximal to the defective enzyme. This includes errors of amino acid catabolism (e.g., phenylketonuria and maple syrup urine disease), organic acid catabolism (e.g., methylmalonic aciduria and propionic acidemia), urea synthesis (e.g., ornithine transcarbamylase deficiency and argininemia), sugar catabolism (e.g., galactosemia and hereditary fructose intolerance), metal transport (e.g., Wilson's disease and Menkes' disease), and porphyrin metabolism. Because the placenta acts to maintain homeostasis, these disorders are unlikely to cause embryonic toxicity. Most patients develop symptoms in infancy and childhood, following a symptom-free period whose length depends in part on the degree of enzyme deficiency. Other circumstances, such as fever, illness, and diet changes, can also influence the timing and severity of symptoms.

The second group of IEMs are those in which symptoms are due, at least in part, to the inability of the brain and other organs to produce or utilize sufficient energy for normal function. Energy deficiency can result from defective function of the mitochondria, including defects of pyruvate transport and modification, the Krebs cycle enzymes, fatty acid oxidation enzymes, and the respiratory chain enzymes that allow for aerobic metabolism. Energy deficiency can also result from defects in cytoplasmic enzymes, such as those responsible for glycogen synthesis, glycolysis and gluconeogenesis, insulin secretion and responsiveness, creatine synthesis and transport, and the pentose phosphate pathway. It is not uncommon for children with IEMs causing energy defects to present with congenital dysmorphism or cerebral dysgenesis.

The third group of IEMs are typically thought of as storage disorders, in which incompletely catabolized complex molecules accumulate within neuronal and extraneuronal tissues and cause progressive neurologic symptoms and somatic changes. This would include the mucopolysaccharidoses, the oligosaccharidoses, and the lysosomal storage disorders. Some authors expand this third group to include disorders of complex molecule synthesis and catabolism that do not result in measurable storage, including the peroxisomal disorders, congenital disorders of glycosylation, and disorders of cholesterol biosynthesis.

Genetic disorders causing PE, which are not known to have a specific metabolic basis but which result in the progressive loss of neurons, usually demonstrated as progressive atrophy on neuroimaging, are classified as neurodegenerative. While the diagnosis of a ND previously relied solely on clinical features and expert pattern recognition, the past decades have seen elucidation of the genetic basis for most and the pathophysiologic basis for many. Those NDs in which the pathophysiology remains unclear are often subdivided into those affecting the brain homogenously (diffuse encephalopathies) and those tending to affect the cerebral cortex (poliodystrophies), cerebral white matter (leukodystrophies), basal ganglia (corencephalopathies), cerebellum, or to preferentially affect the brainstem.

Epidemiology

Although the causes of PE are individually rare, the combined incidence of PE has been estimated to be as high as 1 in 2000 live births [Surtees, 2002]. Much of what has been published regarding these disorders has been retrospective and focused on individual conditions, providing little basis for a discussion of their collective epidemiology. A few studies have been notable exceptions.

An early paper examining the experience with PE at two large academic centers in the United States found that, of 1218 admissions to their child neurology services over the course of 10 years, 341 patients were diagnosed with 1 of more than 50 disorders causing neurological dysfunction [Dyken and Krawiecki, 1983]. Table 44-1 shows the results of their analysis of the relative frequency of the various diagnoses. Although 72 percent of the cases studied had a genetic or metabolic disorder causing PE, the study also included a significant number of children with pure lower motor neuron syndromes and acquired injuries due to infection, immunologic disorders, refractory epilepsy, chronic environmental insults, nutritional deficiencies, and iatrogenic factors. A study from the Children's Hospital of Lahore, Pakistan [Sultan et al., 2006], found that, of the 1273 children admitted to the neurology service from 2004 to 2005, 66 were diagnosed with PE and most received a specific diagnosis. The most common diagnoses, in descending order of frequency, were metachromatic leukodystrophy (14 cases), adrenoleukodystrophy (11), subacute sclerosing panencephalitis (8), Wilson's disease (6), Friedreich's ataxia (5), liposis (4), Gaucher's disease (3), Alexander's disease (2), and pantothenate kinase-associated neurodegeneration (PKAN) (2). More than half of the patients underwent funduscopic examination, electroencephalography, and cerebrospinal fluid examination as part of their diagnostic work-up.

Following the initial description in 1996 of 10 cases of new variant Creutzfeldt–Jakob disease (nvCJD) affecting young adults in the United Kingdom [Will et al., 1996], several countries instituted prospective surveillance programs to collect data on patients with PE to better identify additional cases of nvCJD. Although these studies have relied on reports from pediatricians and have been unable to describe absolute incidence or prevalence figures, they have reported relative

Table 44-1 Diagnosis in 340 Cases of Developmental Regression

Diagnosis	Number of Cases
POLIODYSTROPHIES*	**129**
Lysosomal storage disorders	39
Hypoxic poliodystrophy	29
Idiopathic poliodystrophy	24
West's syndrome	17
Lennox–Gastaut syndrome	9
Metabolic poliodystrophy	4
Toxoplasmosis	3
Post-vaccine poliodystrophy	3
Lowe's syndrome	1
LEUKODYSTROPHIES†	**71**
SSPE	26
ADEM and MS	17
Adrenoleukodystrophy	8
Metachromatic leukodystrophy	5
Pelizaeus–Merzbacher disease	4
Krabbe's disease	4
Phenylketonuria	2
Cockayne's syndrome	2

Table 44-1 Diagnosis in 340 Cases of Developmental Regression—cont'd

Diagnosis	Number of Cases
Canavan's disease	1
Alexander's disease	1
Maple syrup urine disease	1
CORENCEPHALOPATHIES‡	**26**
Idiopathic corencephalopathy	8
Huntington's disease	5
Mitochondrial disorders	4
Dystonia musculorum deformans	2
Hallervorden–Spatz syndrome	2
Ataxia-telangiectasia	1
Congenital indifference to pain	1
Infantile neuroaxonal dystrophy	1
Riley–Day syndrome	1
Wilson's disease	1
DIFFUSE ENCEPHALOPATHIES	**63**
Tuberous sclerosis	19
Idiopathic encephalopathy	17
Hyperammonemic disorders	6
Mitochondrial disorders	4
Neurofibromatosis	4
Achondroplasia	2
Organic acidurias	2
Letterer–Siwe disease	2
Sturge–Weber syndrome	2
Zellweger's syndrome	2
Homocystinuria	1
Incontinentia pigmenti	1
Sjögren–Larsson syndrome	1
SPINOCEREBELLOPATHIES§	**51**
Spinal muscular atrophy	19
Hereditary spastic paraplegia	12
Acute cerebellar ataxia	8
Infantile polymyoclonus	4
Charcot–Marie–Tooth disease	2
Friedreich's ataxia	2
Marinesco–Sjögren syndrome	1
OPCA	1
Spinocerebellar degeneration	1
Refsum's disease	1

* Poliodystrophies = predominant cortical involvement.
† Leukodystrophies = predominant cerebral white-matter involvement.
‡ Corencephalopathies = predominant basal ganglia involvement.
§ Spinocerebellopathies = predominant spinal cord and cerebellar involvement.
ADEM, acute disseminated encephalomyelitis; MS, multiple sclerosis; OPCA, olivopontocerebellar atrophy; SSPE, subacute sclerosing panencephalitis.
(From Dyken P, Krawiecki N. Neurodegenerative diseases of infancy and childhood. Ann Neurol 1983;13:351–364.)

prevalences within their areas. The first report from the surveillance done in the UK [Devereux et al., 2004] collected and analyzed pediatric cases of progressive intellectual and neurological deterioration (PIND) over a 5-year span. The cases included children who had:

1. progressive deterioration over more than 3 months
2. the loss of already attained intellectual or developmental abilities
3. the development of abnormal neurological signs.

The study excluded children with intellectual and neurological deterioration after a nonprogressive insult, such as encephalitis, trauma, or global hypoxic-ischemic injury, but did include children with seizure disorders who otherwise met the case definition and children carrying diagnoses that could be expected to lead to progressive deterioration in the future. Of the 798 cases collected, 577 had a confirmed diagnosis, 6 had definite or probable nvCJD, and 211 had no clear etiologic diagnosis at the time of publication but did not have clinical features suggestive of nvCJD. There were nearly 100 different confirmed diagnoses, but more than one-quarter of the cases were explained by the five most common: mucopolysaccharidosis type III (Sanfilippo's syndrome), adrenoleukodystrophy, late infantile neuronal ceroid-lipofuscinosis, mitochondrial diseases, and Rett's syndrome. Higher rates of prevalence and of consanguinity were reported in families of South Asian origin. A follow-up of the UK study [Verity et al., 2010a] reported a confirmed etiologic diagnosis in 1047 of the 2493 cases of PIND that had been collected by 2008, with nearly one-quarter of cases again explained by the five most common diagnoses: neuronal ceroid-lipofuscinoses, mitochondrial diseases, mucopolysaccharidoses, gangliosidoses, and peroxisomal disorders. The most recent update of the study [Verity et al., 2010b] reported that, after 12 years, 147 different etiologies were found to explain 1114 of the 2636 cases of PIND collected. In total, only 6 children with confirmed or probable nvCJD had been identified. The 30 most common diagnoses identified in the study are presented in Table 44-2.

A survey-based study conducted in Australia [Nunn et al., 2002] identified 230 cases of childhood PE in a 2-year period, with 134 patients having Rett's syndrome, 20 having a lysosomal storage disorder, 16 having a leukodystrophy, and 15 having a mitochondrial disease. A study done in Oslo, Norway, gathered cases of pediatric PE over an 18-year period from the area's one children's hospital and from the national diagnostic laboratory for metabolic diseases [Strømme et al., 2007]. The authors excluded patients with diseases in which cognitive impairment was either atypical (e.g., spinocerebellar ataxia

Table 44-2 Common Diagnoses in 1114 Cases of Progressive Encephalopathy

Diagnosis	Number of Cases
LEUKOENCEPHALOPATHIES	**183**
Metachromatic leukodystrophy	59
Krabbe's disease	33
Pelizaeus–Merzbacher disease	17
Canavan's disease	13
Vanishing white matter disease	11

Table 44-2 Common Diagnoses in 1114 Cases of Progressive Encephalopathy—cont'd

Diagnosis	Number of Cases
Aicardi–Goutières syndrome	10
Alexander's disease	10
Other	31
NEURONAL CEROID-LIPOFUSCINOSES	**141**
NCL late infantile	73
NCL juvenile	44
NCL infantile	22
Other	2
MITOCHONDRIAL	**122**
Leigh's syndrome	17
NARP (including NARP/MILS)	17
Other	88
MUCOPOLYSACCHARIDOSES	**102**
Mucopolysaccharidosis IIIA (Sanfilippo's syndrome)	69
Mucopolysaccharidosis IIA (Hunter's disease)	15
Other	18
GANGLIOSIDOSES	**100**
GM$_2$ gangliosidosis type 1 (Tay–Sachs disease)	41
GM$_2$ gangliosidosis type 2 (Sandhoff's disease)	33
GM$_1$ gangliosidosis	23
Other	3
PEROXISOMAL	**69**
Adrenoleukodystrophy	56
Other	13
OTHER METABOLIC	**95**
Niemann–Pick disease type C	38
PKAN/NBIA	21
Menkes' disease	16
Glutaric aciduria type 1	10
Molybdenum co-factor deficiency	10
NONMETABOLIC	**135**
Rett's syndrome	60
Huntington's disease	22
Cockayne's disease	15
Neuroaxonal dystrophy	12
Ataxia telangiectasia	9
Subacute sclerosing panencephalitis	9
Rasmussen's syndrome	8

MILS, maternally inherited Leigh's syndrome; NARP, neuropathy, ataxia, and retinitis pigmentosa; NBIA, neurodegeneration with brain iron accumulation; NCL, neuronal ceroid-lipofuscinosis; PE, progressive encephalopathy; PKAN, pantothenate kinase-associated neurodegeneration (previously Hallervorden–Spatz disease).
(From Verity et al., The epidemiology of progressive intellectual and neurological deterioration in childhood. Arch Dis Child 2010b.)

and spinal muscular atrophy) or typically seen only late in the course (multiple sclerosis). Also, unlike the studies already discussed, this study excluded disorders, such as regressive autism and Rett's syndrome, in which intellectual deterioration may be seen early in the course but typically stabilizes. They reported a total of 84 cases of PE, of which they classified two-thirds as metabolic, one-third as neurodegenerative, and 2, both due to HIV/AIDS, as infectious. The metabolic and neurodegenerative cases were further subcategorized as shown in Table 44-3.

There were 28 children with disorders of subcellular organelles (23 lysosomal, 3 mitochondrial, and 2 peroxisomal) and 27 with disorders of intermediary metabolism (11 organic acidurias, 6 fatty acid oxidation disorders, 4 urea cycle disorders, 4 galactosemia, and 2 unspecified). The neurodegenerative cases included 10 children with a specific diagnosis (1 ataxia telangiectasia, 2 Cockayne's syndrome, 1 megalencephalic leukoencephalopathy with subcortical cysts, 3 microphthalmia and brain atrophy, 1 pontocerebellar hypoplasia and infantile spinal muscular atrophy, and 2 Schinzel–Gideon syndrome) and 17 in which only the portion of the CNS most affected could be specified (8 cerebellum, 3 cerebral cortex, 3 cerebral white matter, 1 basal ganglia, 1 cerebellum and basal ganglia, and 1 cerebellum and brainstem). Analysis of the study data found that there was a 7-fold increase in risk of PE in children of Pakistani origin, due largely to the predominantly autosomal-recessive inheritance pattern for causes of PE and the much higher incidence of reported consanguinity in that community [Strømme et al., 2010]. It was estimated that 30 percent of all cases of PE, and at least 50 percent of the cases in children of Pakistani origin, would have been prevented if the practice of consanguinous marrage were avoided.

The same authors [Strømme et al., 2008] used local population data to calculate an overall incidence rate for PE of 6.43 per 100,000 person years (95 percent CI 5.15–7.97), with the age-specific rates being highest for infants <1 year old (79.9 per 100,000 person years) and lowest for children over 5 years (0.65 per 100,000 person years). They also found that the age at diagnosis averaged 0.5 years for patients with metabolic diseases and 4.5 years for patients with neurodegenerative diseases, and that children with neonatal onset and metabolic etiology had the highest risk of mortality.

Diagnostic Evaluation

Every child with a suspected developmental disorder should be subjected to a thorough clinical evaluation that includes a detailed medical and developmental history, family history, review of systems, and physical examination. The two features that most suggest a PE are:

1. the gradual loss of previously acquired milestones or intellectual abilities
2. the development of neurological signs and symptoms following a period of normal growth and development.

These features are most readily observed when disorders have a later onset and more rapid deterioration, as is often seen in the cerebral forms of adrenoleukodystrophy [Moser et al., 2007]. PE may be difficult to recognize when disorders have a very early onset, develop very slowly, or prevent even initial development from being normal. A variety of metabolic and genetic conditions have been diagnosed in children initially thought to have cerebral palsy due to static encephalopathy [Gupta and Appleton, 2001], and those that have been reported in the literature are listed in Table 44-4. This experience suggests that

Table 44-3 Diagnoses in 84 Cases of Progressive Encephalopathy in Oslo, Norway

Diagnosis	Number of Cases
METABOLIC	**55**
Subcellular organelles	28
Lysosomal	23
Mitochondrial	3
Peroxisomal	2
Intermediate metabolism	27
Organic aciduria	11
Fatty acid oxidation defect	6
Urea cycle disorder	4
Galactosemia	4
Unspecified	2
NEURODEGENERATIVE	**27**
Specified	10
Unspecified	17
INFECTIOUS	**2**

(From Strømme P et al. Incidence rates of progressive childhood encephalopathy in Oslo, Norway: A population based study. BMC Pediatr 2007;7:25.)

Table 44-4 Progressive Encephalopathy Reported to Present as Cerebral Palsy

Finding	Etiologic Diagnoses
Hypotonia	Duchenne muscular dystrophy Infantile neuroaxonal dystrophy Mitochondrial encephalopathy
Dystonia	3-methylcrotonyl CoA carboxylase deficiency 3-methylglutaconic aciduria Dopa-responsive dystonia Glutaric aciduria type I Juvenile dystonic lipidosis Juvenile neuronal ceroid-lipofuscinosis Leigh's disease Lesch–Nyhan syndrome Pelizaeus–Merzbacher disease Rett's syndrome
Spasticity	Adrenoleukodystrophy Adrenomyeloneuropathy Arginase deficiency Hereditary progressive spastic paraplegia Holocarboxylase synthetase deficiency Metachromatic leukodystrophy
Ataxia	Angelman's syndrome Ataxia telangiectasia GM_1 gangliosidosis NARP Niemann–Pick disease type C Congenital disorder of glycosylation Posterior fossa tumor X-linked spinocerebellar ataxia

NARP, neuropathy, ataxia, and retinitis pigmentosa.

children with a diagnosis of cerebral palsy should undergo further evaluation for neurodegenerative disorders when any of the following conditions is identified: no definite history of a preceding injury, a family history of neurologic symptoms, a history of parental consanguinity, or inadequately explained oculomotor abnormalities, involuntary movements, ataxia, muscle atrophy, or sensory loss. Children with recurrent, unexplained episodes of altered mental status, vomiting, or abnormal movements should be strongly suspected of having an IEM, such as a mitochondrial disease, aminoacidopathy, organic aciduria, or urea cycle enzyme defect.

Conversely, children who do not have a progressive neurological disease can undergo clinical deterioration resulting from medication side effects, intercurrent medical or psychiatric illnesses, or the evolution of existing hydrocephalus, spasticity, dystonia, or seizures. Some epileptic and neurodevelopmental disorders are associated with loss of acquired skills or cognitive function, but the deterioration is not relentlessly progressive and there is often no discernible destructive process occurring in the CNS. This situation is seen in children with epileptic encephalopathies, such as Dravet's syndrome, West's syndrome, and Lennox–Gastaut syndrome, in which neurodevelopment plateaus or regresses at the onset of seizures but may progress again in the future. The regression in language and social skills seen in cases of idiopathic autism is also distinguishable in this way from PE due to metabolic and neurodegenerative disorders.

The critical elements of the clinical evaluation are no different from those discussed in the evaluation of children with nonprogressive neurodevelopmental disorders, which is discussed in detail in Chapter 43. To establish the progressive nature of the child's symptoms or clinical findings, however, it can be particularly helpful to review any records of the child's appearance and abilities to which the caregivers can provide access, including photographs, videotapes, and examples of the child's writing and drawing. Repeated examinations over months or even years may be necessary to uncover subtle regression in some children.

Primary motor and sensory functions are readily assessed by the screening neurologic examination, even in uncooperative children, but higher cortical functions are far more difficult to evaluate. The collective observations of clinicians, parents, and teachers who suspect subtle cognitive decline should be supplemented by those of a child psychologist who is trained to administer age-specific tests and to give an appropriate assessment of the impact of potential confounders, such as primary sensory and motor deficits, inattentiveness, shyness, behavior problems, and cultural and language differences [Sparrow and Davis, 2000]. Children with PE generally have sufficiently impaired social and occupational functioning from loss of higher cortical function to be described as suffering dementia, although the term is rarely applied.

Disturbances of higher cortical function are well characterized and localized in adult patients with acquired and degenerative disorders, including amnesia (i.e., disturbed ability to form new memories or to recall previously learned information), aphasia (i.e., difficulty with the expression or comprehension of language), apraxia (i.e., difficulty carrying out learned motor tasks not caused by weakness or incoordination), agnosia (i.e., difficulty recognizing or identifying objects or sounds not caused by sensory loss), and disturbed executive functioning (i.e., poor planning, organizing, sequencing, and

abstracting). The definitions and localizations of the most commonly encountered cognitive disturbances are listed in Table 44-5.

Laboratory Testing

When PE is suspected, a timely evaluation that results in a specific diagnosis can be of great value. Although specific treatments are available for only a minority of diseases, an etiological diagnosis is helpful in relieving caregivers of anxiety and uncertainty; empowering caregivers to become involved in support and research networks; limiting further diagnostic testing, which may be costly or invasive; and improving understanding of:

1. treatment and prognosis
2. anticipation and management of associated medical and behavioral comorbidities
3. counseling regarding recurrence risk
4. ability to prevent recurrence through screening for carriers and prenatal testing.

In all cases, the diagnostic tests employed should be tailored to the presentation of the child should generally proceed from least to most invasive. Consideration should be given to the early identification or exclusion of all potentially treatable causes of the patient's symptoms.

One approach to the laboratory evaluation of children with nonspecific PE is outlined in Table 44-6, which lists screening tests that might be applicable to all such children, as well as basic studies for infectious, toxic, endocrinologic, genetic, neoplastic, metabolic, autoimmune, and nutritional disorders that may be suspected on the basis of the history or the results of the initial screening tests. The results of these tests will often suggest the need for:

1. further neuroimaging with magnetic resonance angiography, venography, or spectroscopy
2. further electrophysiologic testing with electroretinography or electromyography
3. further metabolic screening via loading tests or tissue biopsies for microscopy or enzyme analysis.

Another approach to the evaluation of a patient who may have a rare disease with which the clinician is unfamiliar is to use an interactive database to generate a broad differential diagnosis [Segal, 2007]. Simulconsult (www.simulconsult.com) is a web-based program of this kind that is freely available to clinicians and students. As each piece of clinical information about a patient is entered, including the age of onset of symptoms and pertinent negatives, the program re-orders the diagnoses on its suggested differential and updates the suggestions it makes for what additional pieces of clinical and laboratory data would most help in distinguishing between them. Currently, the program has information on more than 2300 predominantly metabolic and genetic neurological disorders, including more than 120 that are suggested when the finding of "regression (loss or deterioration of milestones)" is entered. A broad differential can help clinicians to avoid cognitive pitfalls that commonly contribute to diagnostic error and delay [Norman and Eva, 2010], including the biases of availability and representativeness (favoring familiar diagnoses over less well-known diagnoses or disease variants) and those of framing and premature closure (favoring findings that confirm rather than question a pre-existing diagnosis).

Table 44-5 Cortical Localization of Cognitive Impairments

Cognitive Impairment	Clinical Features	Cortical Localization
APHASIA		
Sensory (Wernicke)	Altered discrimination of sounds (phonetic errors) and substitution of sounds and syllables (phonemic errors), or words and phrases (verbal paraphasias)	Dominant posterosuperior temporal gyrus
Motor (Broca)	Disturbed speech production with loss of fluency and syntax	Dominant inferior frontal gyrus
Conduction	Poor repetition, despite normal fluency and comprehension	Dominant arcuate fasciculus
Alexia with agraphia	Isolated deficits in reading and writing language	Dominant supramarginal and angular gyri
Dysprosody (sensory, motor, and conduction)	Impaired discrimination, production, or repetition of the intonation, melody, or phrasing of language	Nondominant perisylvian cortex, with homology with the corresponding aphasia in the dominant hemisphere
AGNOSIA		
Visual	Impaired recognition of colors (achromatopsia), object classes (visual object agnosia), or specific objects (prosopagnosia)	Bilateral occipitotemporal visual association cortex
Tactile	Decreased perception of object shape (astereognosis), weight, and texture	Contralateral parietal cortex
Auditory	Inability to recognize verbal (word deafness) or nonverbal (amusia) sounds	Bilateral temporoparietal cortex
Spatial	Inattention toward one side of the world or self that is partial (extinction) or complete (neglect)	Nondominant parietal cortex
APRAXIA		
Ideational	Inability to perform or recognize learned motor skills, resulting from loss of mechanical knowledge	Dominant inferior parietal cortex
Ideomotor	Inability to copy gestures or use tools without errors in positioning, orientation, movement, and timing	Contralateral motor cortex
Limb-kinetic	Loss of finger dexterity	Contralateral and dominant premotor and supplementary motor cortex
Gerstmann's syndrome	Impairments in writing (dysgraphia), performing arithmetic calculations (dyscalculia), distinguishing right from left, and identifying fingers (finger agnosia)	Dominant angular gyrus of the parietal lobe

The individual disorders causing PE in childhood are too numerous to discuss in detail in this chapter, but they are presented in the tables that follow, grouped by age of presentation, the presence or absence of associated somatic signs, and the neurological presentation itself. Treatable disorders are highlighted in boldface and the reader is directed to the appropriate chapter of this textbook for further details regarding clinical presentation, diagnostic testing, and disease management.

We begin with Table 44-7, which classifies the common metabolic disorders presenting in neonates based on clinical features, degree of acidosis and ketosis, and the results of tests for ammonia, lactate, glucose, calcium, and cell counts. For infants from 1–12 months old, disorders causing PE have been grouped into those associated with somatic abnormalities (Table 44-8), those with specific or suggestive neurological signs (Table 44-9), and those that typically cause slowly progressive developmental delays without more specific findings (Table 44-10). For children between the ages of 1 and 5 years, the disorders causing PE have been grouped into three different categories: those with somatic signs (Table 44-11), those with paraparesis (Table 44-12), and those with ataxia and incoordination (Table 44-13). The disorders causing PE in later childhood, between the ages of 5 and 15 years, have been divided into those that present with seizures and ataxia (Table 44-14), extrapyramidal signs, such as dystonia or choreoathetosis (Table 44-15), severe and diffuse CNS signs, including seizures and visual loss (Table 44-16), polymyoclonus (Table 44-17), cerebellar ataxia (Table 44-18), polyneuropathy (Table 44-19), and psychiatric symptoms (Table 44-20). Finally, disorders that may present with PE in late adolescence and adulthood are listed in Table 44-21.

Up-to-date information about the sensitivity and availability of tests for specific genetic disorders is available through the Gene Tests website (www.genetests.org), maintained by the University of Washington at Seattle through funding from the National Institutes of Health. Some genetic tests can be performed on a research basis through direct communication and cooperation between the clinician and research laboratory.

Management

The specific cause of childhood PE can be difficult to uncover, with about half of the cases in large epidemiologic surveys having no etiologic diagnosis. Still, as a small number of disorders can be at least ameliorated by medical therapies, there is a sense of both hope and urgency to the diagnostic work-up. Caregivers can be expected to have a great number of questions

Table 44-6 Screening Diagnostic Tests for Nonspecific Progressive Encephalopathy

Type of Screening	Tests
General evaluation	Neuroimaging (MRI with and without contrast preferable to CT) Electroencephalogram (capturing wake and non-REM sleep) Comprehensive metabolic panel Complete blood count Ophthalmologic examination (by specialist if possible) Audiologic testing
ADDITIONAL SCREENING	
Autoimmune disorder	Serum sedimentation rate (Westergren), antinuclear antibody titer, complement levels
Autonomic disorder	Histamine skin test, sweat testing
Endocrinopathy	Serum T_4, TSH, ACTH, and cortisol
Genetic disorder	Genomic microarray (preferable to karyotype) *MECP2* mutation screening
Infection	CSF cell count, glucose, protein CSF bacterial, fungal, and viral cultures CSF HIV and HSV by polymerase chain reaction CSF fungal antigens CSF test for prion proteins CSF for viral antibodies (measles, mumps)
Intoxication	Serum lead and thin-layer chromatography Urine screen for drugs of abuse
Metabolic disorder	Serum amino acids, lactate, pyruvate, ammonia Serum carnitine (free and total) and acylcarnitines Serum cholesterol and lipid panel, very long-chain fatty acids Lymphocyte vacuolization, lysosomal enzyme analysis Urine organic acids, metabolic screen, porphyrins CSF lactate, amino acids, and neurotransmitter metabolites
Neoplastic disorder	CSF for cytologic analysis CSF and serum for paraneoplastic antibodies
Nutritional disorder	Serum niacin, thiamin, pyridoxine, cobalamine, vitamin E Serum homocysteine, methylmalonic acid

ACTH, adrenocorticotropic hormone; CSF, cerebrospinal fluid; CT, computed tomography; HIV, human immunodeficiency virus, HSV, herpes simplex virus, MRI, magnetic resonance imaging; REM, rapid eye movement; TSH, thyroid stimulating hormone.

Table 44-7 Classification of Inborn Errors Presenting in the Neonatal Period (0–3 Months)

Clinical Type	Acidosis Ketosis	Other Signs	Possible Diagnosis*	Elective Methods of Investigation
Neurologic deterioration (intoxication type) Abnormal movements Hypertonia	Acidosis 0 DNPH +++ Acetest 0/±	NH_3 N or ↑± Lactate N Blood count N Glucose N Calcium N	**Maple syrup urine disease (special odor)**	Amino acid (plasma, urine)
Neurologic deterioration (intoxication type) Dehydration	Acidosis ++ Acetest ++ DNPH 0/±	NH_3 ↑+/++ Lactate N or ↑± Leukopenia Thrombocytopenia Glucose N or ↑+ Calcium N or ↓+	**Organic acidurias (MMA, PA, IVA, MCD) Ketolysis defects**	Organic acid (urine) Carnitine (plasma) Carnitine esters (urine, plasma)
Neurologic deterioration (energy deficiency type) With liver or cardiac symptoms	Acidosis ++/± Acetest 0 DNPH 0	NH_3 ↑±/++ Lactate ↑±/++ Blood count N Glucose ↓+/++ Calcium N or ↓+	**Fatty acid oxidation and ketogenesis defects (GA II, CPT II, CAT, VLCAD, MCKAT, HMG CoA lyase)**	As above, plus: Loading test Fasting test Fatty acid oxidation studies (lymphocytes or fibroblasts)
Neurologic deterioration (energy deficiency type) Polypnea Hypotonia	Acidosis +++/+ Acetest ++/0 Lactate +++/+	NH_3 N or ↑± RBCs ↓ or N Glucose N or ↓± Calcium N	Congenital lactic acidoses (PC, **PDH**, Krebs cycle, respiratory chain) **MCD**	Plasma redox states ratios (L:P, 3OHB:AA) Organic acid (urine) Polarographic studies Enzyme assays (muscle, lymphocytes, fibroblasts)

Continued

Table 44-7 Classification of Inborn Errors Presenting in the Neonatal Period (0–3 Months)—cont'd

Clinical Type	Acidosis Ketosis	Other Signs	Possible Diagnosis*	Elective Methods of Investigation
Neurologic deterioration (intoxication type) Moderate hepatocellular disturbances Hypotonia Seizures Coma	Acidosis 0 (alkalosis) Acetest 0 DNPH 0	NH$_3$ ↑+/+++ Lactate N or ↑+ Blood count N Glucose N Calcium N	**Urea cycle defects** **Triple H syndrome** **Fatty acid oxidation defects** (GA II, CPT II, VLCAD, LCHAD, CAT) **PA, MMA, IVA**	Amino acids (plasma, urine) Organic acids (urine) Orotic acid (urine) Liver or intestine enzyme studies (CPS, OTC)
Neurologic deterioration Seizures Myoclonic jerks Severe hypotonia	Acidosis 0 Acetest 0 DNPH 0	NH$_3$ N Lactate N or ↑+ Blood count N Glucose N	NKH SO ± XO **Pyridoxine dependency** **3-Phosphoglycerate dehydrogenase** Peroxisomal disorders Trifunctional enzyme Respiratory chain **Neurotransmitter disorders** CDG syndrome Cholesterol biosynthesis disorders	Amino acids (plasma, CSF) Organic acids (urine) VLCFA, phytanic acid (plasma) Acylcarnitine profile (plasma) Lactate (plasma) Neurotransmitters (plasma, urine, CSF) Isoelectric focusing of transferrin (plasma) Cholesterol (plasma)
Hepatomegaly Hypoglycemia	Acidosis ++/+ Acetest +	NH$_3$ N Lactate ↑+/++ Blood count N Glucose ↓++	**Glycogenosis type I** (Acetest −) **Glycogenosis type III** (Acetest ++) **Fatty acid oxidation** **Fructose diphosphatase**	Fasting test Loading test Enzyme studies (liver, lymphocytes, fibroblasts) Organic acids (urine) Acylcarnitine profile (plasma) Insulin (plasma)
Hepatomegaly Jaundice Liver failure Hepatocellular necrosis	Acidosis +/0 Acetest +/0	NH$_3$ N or ↑+ Lactate ↑+/++ Glucose N or ↓++	**Galactosemia** **Hereditary fructose intolerance** **Tyrosinosis type I** Neonatal hemochromatosis Respiratory chain disorders	Enzyme studies Iron-ferritin (salivary glands) Organic acid (urine) Polyols Succinyl acetone
Hepatomegaly Cholestatic jaundice ± Failure to thrive ± Chronic diarrhea	Acidosis 0 Ketosis 0	NH$_3$ N Lactate N Glucose N	α$_1$-antitrypsin **Inborn errors of bile acid metabolism** CDG syndrome **Cerebrotendinous xanthomatosis** Cholesterol metabolism Citrin Peroxisomal disorders Niemann–Pick type C **LCHAD** Mevalonate kinase	Bile acids (plasma, urine) Protein electrophoresis Organic acid (urine) Acylcarnitine profile VLCFA, phytanic acid, pipecolic acid (serum) Isoelectric focusing of transferrin (serum) Fibroblast studies
Hepatosplenomegaly storage signs (coarse facies, ascites, hydrops fetalis, macroglossia, bone changes, cherry-red spot, vacuolated lymphocytes) ± Failure to thrive ± Chronic diarrhea	Acidosis 0 Acetest 0 Ketosis 0 DNPH 0	NH$_3$ N Lactate N or ↑ Blood count N Glucose N Hepatic signs ±	CDG syndrome **Congenital erythropoietic porphyria** Galactosialidosis GM$_1$ gangliosidosis ISSD (sialidosis type II) I-cell disease Mevalonic aciduria Niemann–Pick disease type IA MPS VII Transaldolase	Enzyme studies (lymphocytes, fibroblasts) Glycosaminoglycans (urine) Oligosaccharides (urine) Polyols (HPLC) Porphyrins (urine) Sialic acid (urine)

* Disorders shown in bold type are treatable.
N, normal; ±, slight; ++, marked; +++, significant; ↑, increased; ↓, decreased; 0, absent or negative.
CAT, carnitine acylcarnitine translocase deficiency; CDG, congenital disorder of glycosylation; CPS, carbamyl phosphate synthetase deficiency; CPTII, carnitine palmitoyltransferase II; CSF, cerebrospinal fluid; DNPH, 4-dinitrophenylhydrazine; GA II, glutaric aciduria II; HMG-CoA lyase, 3-hydroxy-e-methylglutaryl-coenzyme A; HPLC, high-performance liquid chromatography; ISSD, infantile sialic acid storage disease; IVA, isovaleric acidemia; LCAD, long-chain acyl CoA dehydrogenase; LCHAD, 3-hydroxy long-chain acyl CoA dehydrogenase; MCD, multiple carboxylase deficiency; MCKAT, medium-chain ketoacyl-CoA thiolase deficiency; MMA, methylmalonic acidemia; MPS VII, mucopolysaccharidosis type VII; MSUD, maple syrup urine disease; NKH, nonketotic hyperglycemia; OTC, ornithine transcarbamylase deficiency; PA, propionic acidemia; PC, pyruvate carboxylase; PDH, pyruvate dehydrogenase; RBCs, red blood cells; SO, sulfite oxidase; VLCAD, very long-chain acyl-CoA dehydrogenase deficiency; VLCFA, very long chain fatty acids; XO, xanthine oxidase.
(Adapted from Scriver et al., The Metabolic and Molecular Basis of Inherited Disease, online edition, www.ommbid.com.)

Table 44-8 Progressive Encephalopathy in Infancy (1–12 Months) with Obvious Somatic Symptoms

Main Sign	Other Signs	Onset	Diagnosis*	Evaluation	Chapter
Visceral changes	Hepatosplenomegaly Coarse facies Joint stiffness	0–3 mo	GM$_1$ gangliosidosis	Oligosaccharides (urine) Mucopolysaccharides (urine) Acid β-galactosidase (leukocytes) *GLB 1* genetic studies	36
			Mucolipidosis II (I-cell disease)	Oligosaccharides (urine) Neuraminidase (fibroblasts) *GNPTAB* genetic studies	36
			Sialidosis type II	Sialic acid (urine, fibroblasts) UDP-GlcNAc 2-epimerase activity (fibroblasts) *GNE* genetic studies	36
	Cherry-red spot Vacuolated lymphocytes	6–12 mo	Niemann–Pick disease type A	Acid sphingomyelinase (lymphoblasts or cultured skin fibroblasts) Bone marrow (sea-blue histiocytes) *SMDP1* genetic studies	36
			Niemann–Pick disease type C (lactosyl ceramidosis)	Intracellular cholesterol esterification (cultured fibroblasts) Filipin staining Bone marrow (sea-blue histiocytes) *NPC1* and *NPC2* genetic studies	36
	Bone changes Hepatosplenomegaly Opisthotonos Spasticity Vegetative state	1–6 mo	Gaucher's disease	β-glucocerebrosidase (leukocytes) Bone marrow *GBA* genetic studies	36
	Hepatomegaly Digestive signs Retinitis pigmentosa	0–6 mo	Peroxisomal disorders	Very long chain fatty acids, phytanic acid, pristanic acid, pipecolic acid, phytanoyl-CoA hydroxylase *PHYH* and *PEX7* genetic studies	38
			Congenital disorders of glycosylation	Isoelectric focusing of transferrin Genetic studies	35
Hair and skin abnormalities	Steely, brittle hair	3–6 mo	Menkes' disease (X-linked)	Ceruloplasmin (serum) 24-hour copper collection (urine) *ATP7A* genetic studies	41
			Trichothiodystrophy family of disorders	Sulfur in hair sample	41
	Trichorrhexis nodosa		**Argininosuccinic aciduria**	Ammonia Amino acids *ASL* genetic studies	33
	Ichthyosis Brittle hair Spastic paraplegia	1–6 mo	Congenital disorder of glycosylation	Isoelectric focusing of transferrin Genetic studies	35
			Serine deficiency syndrome	Amino acids (serum)	32
			Sjögren–Larsson syndrome	Fatty aldehyde dehydrogenase Skin fibroblasts *FALDH* genetic studies	32
	Alopecia Cutaneous rashes Ketoacidosis Hyperlactacidemia	3–12 mo	**Biotinidase deficiency**	Biotinidase activity (serum) *BTD* genetic studies	32
			Respiratory chain disorders	Lactate, pyruvate, ammonia Amino acids (serum) Organic acids (urine) Muscle biopsy Genetic studies	37
	Peculiar fat pads on buttocks Thick, sticky hair Episodic multi-organ failure (liver, cardiac tamponade)	1–3 mo	Congenital disorder of glycosylation	Isoelectric focusing of transferrin Genetic studies	34
	Cyanosis (generalized) Methemoglobinemia Hypertonicity	0–6 mo	Methemoglobinemia due to cytochrome b5 reductase deficiency	Methemoglobin NADH-cytochrome b5 reductase deficiency *DIA 1* genetic studies	37

Continued

Table 44-8 **Progressive Encephalopathy in Infancy (1–12 Months) with Obvious Somatic Symptoms—cont'd**

Main Sign	Other Signs	Onset	Diagnosis*	Evaluation	Chapter
	Kernicterus Athetosis	1–3 mo	**Crigler–Najjar syndrome**	Bilirubin UDPGT 1A1 enzyme activity *UGT 1A1* genetic studies	85
	Acrocyanosis Petechiae Chronic diarrhea Attacks of lactic acidosis	1–3 mo	Ethylmalonic aciduria	Lactate, pyruvate Organic acids (urine) Acylcarnitine profile *ETHE1* genetic studies	68
Megaloblastic anemia	Failure to thrive Pigmentary retinopathy	1–3 mo	**Inborn errors of folate metabolism**	Folate (serum, CSF) Lactate, pyruvate, ammonia Organic acids (urine) Amino acids (serum) Homocysteine (urine) Genetic studies	32
			Inborn errors of cobalamin metabolism	Lactate, pyruvate, ammonia Organic acids (urine) Amino acids (serum) Homocysteine (urine) Genetic studies	32
			Hereditary orotic aciduria	Ammonia Amino acids (serum) UMPS enzyme analysis *OTC* genetic studies	32
Cardiac abnormalities	Cardiomyopathy	0–6 mo	D2-hydroxyglutaric acidemia	Lactate, pyruvate Organic acids (urine) *L2HGDH* genetic studies	32
	Heart failure		Respiratory chain disorders	Head MRI Lactate, pyruvate Ammonia Organic acids, ketones (urine) Amino acids (serum) Muscle biopsy	37
	Heartbeat disorders		Congenital defects of glycosylation	Isoelectric focusing of transferrin Genetic studies	35
Ocular symptoms	Cherry-red spot Hydrops fetalis	0–3 mo	GM$_1$ gangliosidosis	Oligosaccharides and mucopolysaccharides (urine) Acid β-galactosidase (leukocytes) *GLB 1* genetic studies	36
			Galactosialidosis	β-Galactosidase (serum) Neuraminidase (serum)	36
			Sialidosis type I	Sialic acid (urine) UDP-GlcNAc 2-epimerase enzyme activity *GNE* genetic studies	36
	Myoclonic jerks Macrocephaly	3–12 mo	GM$_2$ gangliosidosis (Tay–Sachs disease)	Hexosaminidase A (serum) *HEXA* genetic studies	36
			Sandhoff's disease	Hexosaminidase A and B *HEXB* genetic studies (serum)	36
	Optic atrophy Macrocephaly	1–6 mo	Canavan's disease	*N*-acetyl aspartate (urine) Aspartoacylase activity (fibroblasts) *APSA* genetic studies	71
	Nystagmus Dystonia Stridor	3–12 mo	Pelizaeus–Merzbacher disease (X-linked)	Head MRI *PLP1* genetic studies	71
	Retinitis pigmentosa	0–3 mo	Disorder of glycosylation Lysosomal storage disease Mitochondrial disorders Peroxisomal disorders	See Chapter	35 36 37 38

Table 44-8 Progressive Encephalopathy in Infancy (1–12 Months) with Obvious Somatic Symptoms—cont'd

Main Sign	Other Signs	Onset	Diagnosis*	Evaluation	Chapter
	Abnormal eye movements		Dopamine β-hydroxylase deficiency	CSF neurotransmitter	39
	Strabismus		Congenital disorders of glycosylation	Isoelectric focusing of transferrin Genetic studies	35
	Supranuclear paralysis		Gaucher's disease	β-glucocerebrosidase (leukocytes) Bone marrow *GBA* genetic studies	36
			Niemann–Pick disease type C	Intracellular cholesterol esterification (cultured fibroblasts) Filipin staining Bone marrow (sea-blue histiocytes) *NPC1* and *NPC2* genetic studies	36

* Disorders shown in bold type are treatable.
CSF, cerebrospinal fluid; MRI, magnetic resonance imaging; NADH, nicotinamide adenine dinucleotide; UDP, uridine diphosphate; UMPS, uridine monophosphate synthetase.
(Adapted from Scriver et al., The Metabolic and Molecular Basis of Inherited Disease, online edition.)

Table 44-9 Progressive Encephalopathy in Infancy (1–12 Months) with Specific or Suggestive Neurologic Signs

Main Sign	Other Signs	Onset	Diagnosis*	Evaluation	Chapter
Extrapyramidal signs	Major parkinsonism	0–3 mo	Inborn errors of biopterin metabolism	Newborn screening Phenylalanine CNS neurotransmitter studies *PAH* genetic studies	39
			Aromatic amino acid decarboxylase deficiency	CSF neurotransmitters	39
			Tyrosine hydroxylase deficiency	CSF neurotransmitters	39
	Choreoathetoid movements Self-mutilation Aggressiveness	3–6 mo	Lesch–Nyhan syndrome (X-linked)	Urate/creatinine (urine) Hypoxanthine-guanine phosphoribosyltransferase (HPRT) (blood) *HPRT1* genetic studies	68
	Bilateral athetosis Hypertonicity	0–6 mo	Cytochrome b5 reductase deficiency	Methemoglobin NADH-cytochrome b5 reductase deficiency *DIA* 1 genetic studies	37
	Cyanosis	0–12 mo	Methemoglobinemia	CBC, reticulocyte count, lactate dehydrogenase, bilirubin, haptoglobin Comprehensive metabolic panel, hemoglobin electrophoresis, NADH-dependent methemoglobin reductase (platelets, granulocytes, and fibroblasts) Cytochrome b5 reductase (red blood cells)	68
	Dystonia Laryngeal stridor	3–12 mo	Pelizaeus–Merzbacher disease (X-linked)	Head MRI *PLP* 1 genetic studies	71
	Kernicterus	1–3 mo	**Crigler–Najjar syndrome**	Bilirubin (serum) UGT1A1 enzyme activity (liver) *UGT1A1* genetic studies	85
	Acute onset Pseudoencephalitis Choreoathetosis Dystonia	9–12 mo	**Glutaric aciduria type I**	Lactate, pyruvate Organic acid (urine) *GCDH* genetic studies	32
	Low creatinine	0–12 mo	**Cerebral creatine deficiency (GAMT deficiency)**	Guanidinoacetate (GAA), creatine, and creatinine (urine and plasma) *GAMT, GATM,* or *SLC6A8* genetic studies GAMT enzyme, AGAT enzyme, or creatine uptake (fibroblasts)	32

Continued

Table 44-9 **Progressive Encephalopathy in Infancy (1–12 Months) with Specific or Suggestive Neurologic Signs—cont'd**

Main Sign	Other Signs	Onset	Diagnosis*	Evaluation	Chapter
	Spastic paraplegia Ataxia Epilepsy		**Cerebral folate deficiency**	Folate (serum, CSF) Lactate, pyruvate, ammonia Organic acids (urine) Amino acids (serum) Homocysteine (urine) Genetic testing	39
	Leigh's syndrome		**Pyruvate dehydrogenase deficiency**	Lactate, pyruvate, ammonia (serum) Amino acids (serum and urine) Pyruvate dehydrogenase (leukocytes) Genetic studies	32
Painful pyramidal hypertonia	Opisthotonus	0–12 mo	Krabbe's disease	Galactocerebrosidase (leukocytes) *GALC* genetic studies	71
			Gaucher's disease type III	β-glucosylceramidase (leukocytes) *GBA* genetic studies	36
			Niemann–Pick disease type C	Intracellular cholesterol esterification (cultured fibroblasts) Filipin staining Bone marrow (sea-blue histiocytes) *NPC1* and *NPC2* genetic studies	36
Early infantile spasms	Spasticity	0–12 mo	Glycine encephalopathy (nonketotic hyperglycinemia)	Glycine (CSF and serum) *AMT*, *GLDC* genetic studies Glycine cleavage enzyme (liver)	32
			Sulfite oxidase deficiency	Lactate, pyruvate, ammonia Organic acids (urine) Amino acids (serum/urine) Urothion and thiosulfate (urine) *SUOX*, *MOCS2*, and *GEPH* genetic studies	32
			Maple syrup urine disease	Lactate, pyruvate, ammonia Organic acids (urine) Amino acids (serum)	32
			Menkes' kinky hair disease	Ceruloplasmin (serum) 24-hour copper collection (urine) *ATP7A* genetic studies	41
			Multiple carboxylase deficiency	Ammonia, amino acids (serum) Organic acids (urine) Biotinidase, carnitine, and acylcarnitine (serum) *BTD* genetic studies	31
			Organic acidurias	Lactate, pyruvate, ammonia Organic acids (urine) Amino acids (serum)	31
Macrocephaly	Cherry-red spot Myoclonic jerks Startle response to sound Megaloencephaly Tonic spasms Opisthotonos	6–12 mo	Tay–Sachs disease	Hexosaminidase A *HEX A* genetic studies	36
			Sandhoff's disease	Hexoasaminidase A and B	36
		3–6 mo	Canavan's disease	*N*-acetyl aspartate (urine) Aspartocylase activity (fibroblasts) *APSA* genetic studies	71
			Alexander's disease	Head MRI Rosenthal fibers (brain biopsy) *GFAP* genetic studies	71
Ocular symptoms	Optic atrophy Incessant crying Irritability Peripheral neuropathy (abnormal nerve conduction velocity)	3–6 mo	Krabbe's disease (infantile)	Galactocerebrosidase (leukocytes) *GALC* genetic studies	71

Table 44-9 **Progressive Encephalopathy in Infancy (1–12 Months) with Specific or Suggestive Neurologic Signs—cont'd**

Main Sign	Other Signs	Onset	Diagnosis*	Evaluation	Chapter
	Dystonia Choreoathetosis	9–12 mo	**Glutaric aciduria type I**	Lactate, pyruvate Organic acid (urine) *GCDH* genetic studies	32
			L-2-hydroxyglutaric aciduria	Lactate, pyruvate Organic acids (urine) *D2HGDH* genetic studies	31
	Developmental delay Progressive irritability Limb hypertonia Cardiomyopathy	1–3 mo	Respiratory chain disorders (complex I)	Lactate, pyruvate, ammonia Organic acids (urine) Amino acids (serum) Muscle biopsy Genetic studies	37
Recurrent attacks of neurologic crisis	Mental regression Failure to thrive Hyperventilation attacks Various neurologic signs (optic atrophy, ataxia, peripheral neuropathy, intention tremor)	3–12 mo	Leigh's syndrome/ NARP	Lactate, pyruvate, ammonia Organic acids (urine) Amino acids (serum) Muscle biopsy Genetic studies	37
	Strokelike episodes	1–12 mo	**Urea cycle defects**	Ammonia, amino acids, acylcarnitine profile, glucose (serum) organic acids (urine)	33
			Maple syrup urine disease	Lactate, pyruvate, ammonia Organic acids (urine) Amino acids (serum)	32
			Organic acidemias	Lactate, pyruvate, ammonia Organic acids (urine) Amino acids (serum)	32
			Glutaric acidemia I	Lactate, pyruvate, ammonia Organic acids (urine) Amino acids (serum)	32
	Thromboembolic accidents	1–12 mo	Congenital defects of glycosylation	Isoelectric focusing of transferrin Genetic studies	35
			Classic homocystinuria	Homocysteine (serum and urine) Cystathionine β-synthase (CBS) enzyme activity *MTHFR* genetic studies	32

* Disorders shown in bold type are treatable.
AGAT, arginine glycine amidinotransferase; CBC, complete blood count; CNS, central nervous system; CSF, cerebrospinal fluid; GAMT, guanidinoacetate N-methyl transferase; MRI, magnetic resonance imaging; NADH, nicotinamide adenine dinucleotide; NARP, neuropathy, ataxia, and retinitis pigmentosa.
(Adapted from Scriver et al., *The Metabolic and Molecular Basis of Inherited Disease,* online edition.)

Table 44-10 **Progressive Encephalopathy in Infancy (1–12 Months) without Suggestive Neurologic Signs**

Main Sign	Other Signs	Onset	Diagnosis*	Evaluation	Chapter
Clear developmental arrest	Infantile spasms Hypsarrhythmia Autistic features	3–12 mo	**Classic untreated phenylketonuria**	Newborn screening, amino acids (serum), pterins (urine), dihydropteridine reductase (plasma) *PAH* genetic studies	32
			Inborn errors of biopterin metabolism	Newborn screening Phenylalanine CSF neurotransmitter studies *PAH* genetic studies	39
			Peroxisomal disorders	Very long chain fatty acids, phytanic acid, pristanic acid, pipecolic acid, phytanoyl-CoA hydroxylase *PHYH* and *PEX7* genetic studies	38
			Rett's syndrome	*MECP2* genetic studies	31

Continued

Table 44-10 Progressive Encephalopathy in Infancy (1–12 Months) without Suggestive Neurologic Signs—cont'd

Main Sign	Other Signs	Onset	Diagnosis*	Evaluation	Chapter
Lack of clear developmental arrest, resembling a static encephalopathy	Frequent autistic features Poor feeding Failure to thrive Hypotonia Seizures	0–24 mo	**Hyperammonemia (late-onset subacute form)**	Lactate, pyruvate, ammonia Amino acids (serum) Organic acids (urine)	32
			4-Hydroxybutyric aciduria	Lactate, pyruvate, ammonia Amino acids (serum) Organic acids (urine)	32
			L-2-Hydroxyglutaric aciduria	Lactate, pyruvate, ammonia Amino acids (serum) Organic acids (urine)	32
			D-2-Hydroxyglutaric aciduria	Lactate, pyruvate, ammonia Amino acids (serum) Organic acids (urine)	32
			Mevalonic aciduria	Mevalonate kinase (lymphoblasts)	32
	With diverse neurologic findings simulating cerebral palsy	0–24 mo	Adenylosuccinase deficiency	Succinyladenosine/succinyl-5-amino-4-imidazolecarboxamide riboside (CSF)	32
			Dihydropyrimidine dehydrogenase	Uracil, thymine, and 5-hydroxymethyluracil (urine) *DPYD* genetic studies	32
			3-methylglutaconic aciduria	Lactate, pyruvate, ammonia, amino acids (serum), organic acid (urine) *OPA3* genetic studies	32
			Fumarase deficiency	Organic acids (urine) Fumarate hydratase (fibroblasts) *FH* genetic studies	32
			Other organic acidurias	Lactate, pyruvate, ammonia Organic acids (urine) Amino acids (serum)	32
			Cerebral creatine deficiency	Guanidinoacetate (GAA), creatine, and creatinine (urine and plasma) *GAMT*, *GATM*, or *SLC6A8* genetic studies GAMT enzyme, AGAT enzyme, or creatine uptake (fibroblasts)	32
			3-phosphoglycerate dehydrogenase deficiency	Serine and glycine (CSF) Amino acids (serum) *PHGDH* genetic studies	32
			3-phosphoserine phosphatase deficiency	Serine and glycine (CSF) Amino acids (serum) *PSPH* genetic studies	32
			Homocystinuria (iridodonesis, lens dislocation)	Homocysteine (serum and urine) Cystathionine β-synthase (CBS) enzyme activity *MTHFR* genetic studies	32
			Sialuria disease (ocular nystagmus)	Sialic acid (urine) Sialic acid (lysosome) UDP-GlcNAc 2-epimerase activity *GNE* genetic studies	36
			Neurotransmitter disorders	CNS neurotransmitter studies	39
			Angelman's syndrome	15q11.2–13 genetic studies	31
			Blood–brain barrier glucose carrier deficiency	Glucose (CSF/blood) *Glut1-DS* genetic studies	34

* Disorders shown in bold type are treatable.

AGAT, arginine glycine amidinotransferase; CNS, central nervous system; CSF, cerebrospinal fluid; GAMT, guanidinoacetate N-methyl transferase; UPD, bifunctional UDP-N-acetylglucosamine 2-epimerase/N-acetylmannosamine kinase.

(Adapted from Scriver et al., The Metabolic and Molecular Basis of Inherited Disease, online edition.)

Table 44-11 Progressive Encephalopathy in Early Childhood (1–5 Years) with Somatic Signs

Main Sign	Other Signs	Onset	Diagnosis*	Evaluation	Chapter
Coarse facies	Skeletal changes Hepatosplenomegaly Hirsutism Corneal opacities Joint stiffness	2–3 yrs	**Hurler's syndrome** (mucopolysaccharidosis type I)	α-L-iduronidase (leukocytes, fibroblasts, plasma) Glycosaminoglycans (urine) *IDUA* genetic studies	36
		1–2 yrs	Hunter's syndrome (X-linked) (mucopolysaccharidosis II)	Iduronate 2-sulfatase (I2S) (leukocytes, fibroblasts, plasma) Glycosaminoglycans (urine) *IDS* genetic studies	36
		3–5 yrs	Sanfilippo's syndrome (mucopolysaccharidosis type III)	Glycosaminoglycans (urine) Heparan *N*-sulfatase (fibroblasts) *N*-acetyl-α-D-glucosaminidase (fibroblasts) Acetyl-CoA: α-glucosaminide acetyltransferase (fibroblasts) *N*-acetylglucosamine-6-sulfate sulfatase (fibroblasts)	36
		2–4 yrs	Pseudo-Hurler's polydystrophy (mucolipidosis III)	Oligosaccharides (urine) Glycosaminoglycans (urine) UDP-*N*-acetylglucosamine: lysosomal hydrolase *N*-acetylglucosamine-1- phosphotransferase (GNPTA) (fibroblasts) *GNPTAB* genetics studies	36
	Subtle bone changes Hepatosplenomegaly Vacuolated lymphocytes ± lens/corneal opacities	2–6 yrs	α-Mannosidosis (gingival hyperplasia)	α-mannosidase (leukocytes) *MAN2B1* genetic studies	36
		1–2 yrs	Fucosidosis (angiokeratoma)	Oligosaccharides (urine) α-fucosidase (fibroblasts) *FUCA1* genetic studies	36
		1–5 yrs	Aspartylglucosaminuria (macroglossia, leukopenia, joint laxity)	Oligosaccharides (urine) Aspartylglucosaminidase (blood, fibroblasts) *AGA* genetic studies	36
		1–2 yrs	Multiple sulfatase deficiency (Austin's disease) (ichthyosis)	Arylsulfatase A, B, and C (serum) Oligosaccharides (urine) *SUMF 1* genetic studies	36
Hepatosplenomegaly	Vertical supranuclear ophthalmoplegia Progressive dementia Myoclonic jerks	2–6 yrs	Niemann–Pick disease type C (late infantile form)	Intracellular cholesterol esterification (cultured fibroblasts) Filipin staining Bone marrow (sea-blue histiocytes) *NPC1* and *NPC2* genetic testing	36
Splenomegaly + hepatomegaly	Osseous lesions Various neurologic signs (ataxia, supranuclear ophthalmoplegia, myoclonus)	1–6 yrs	Gaucher's disease type III (subacute neuronopathy)	β-glucosylceramidase (leukocytes) *GBA* genetic studies	36
Major visual impairment or ocular signs	Blindness Corneal clouding in first year Cytoplasmic membranous bodies in cells (conjunctiva, fibroblasts, liver, spleen)	1–2 yrs	Mucolipidosis type IV	Gastrin (skin) Lysosomal inclusions (skin, conjunctiva) *MCOLN1* genetic studies	36
	Retinitis pigmentosa Deafness	1–5 yrs	Peroxisomal disorders	Very long chain fatty acids, phytanic acid, pristanic acid, pipecolic acid, phytanoyl-CoA hydroxylase *PHYH* and *PEX7* genetic studies	38

Continued

Table 44-11 Progressive Encephalopathy in Early Childhood (1–5 Years) with Somatic Signs—cont'd

Main Sign	Other Signs	Onset	Diagnosis*	Evaluation	Chapter
			Usher syndrome type II	Clinical features Genetic studies	34
	Cataracts Joint laxity Severe hypotonia Low plasma citrulline, ornithine, and proline Preprandial hyperammonemia	1–5 yrs	Pyrroline-5-carboxylate synthetase deficiency	Ammonia Amino acids (serum)	32

* Disorders shown in bold type are treatable.
(Adapted from Scriver et al., The Metabolic and Molecular Basis of Inherited Disease, online edition.)

Table 44-12 Progressive Encephalopathy in Early Childhood (1–5 Years) with Paraparesis

Main Sign	Other Signs	Onset	Diagnosis*	Evaluation	Chapter
Flaccid paraparesis ± pyramidal signs	Abnormal nerve conduction velocity High protein content in CSF fluid Dysarthria Dementia Blindness	12–18 mo	Metachromatic leukodystrophy	Arylsulfatase A (leukocytes) *ARSA* genetic studies	71
Flaccid paraparesis	Normal nerve conduction velocity No change in CSF protein Optic atrophy Early mental regression Denervation atrophy on EMG	6–24 mo	Neuroaxonal dystrophy (Seitelberger's disease)	EMG with NCS Axonal spheroids (sural nerve biopsy) *PLA2G6* genetic studies	71
			Schindler's disease	α-N-acetylgalactosaminidase (fibroblasts) *NAGA* genetic studies	36
Progressive spastic diplegia	Ataxia resembling subacute degeneration of the cord	6–24 mo	**Methylmalonic aciduria and homocystinuria (Cbl C)**	Lactate, pyruvate, ammonia (serum) Organic acids (urine) Amino acids (serum) Homocysteine (serum and urine) Cobalamin levels Genetic studies	32
			Homocystinuria (Cbl E, F, G)	Lactate, pyruvate, ammonia (serum) Organic acids (urine) Amino acids (serum) Homocysteine (serum and urine) Cobalamin levels Genetic studies	32
	Scissoring or "tiptoe" gait Irritability Hyperactivity Ataxia Seizures Psychosis Hyperargininemia High orotic acid excretion	2 mo–5 yrs	**Arginase deficiency**	Ammonia (serum) Amino acids (serum) *ARG1* genetic studies	33
	Bilateral optic atrophy Ataxia Spasticity Cognitive deficits		3-Methylglutaconic aciduria, type III (Costeff's syndrome)	Lactate, pyruvate Organic acids (urine) *OPA3* genetic studies	32

* Disorders shown in bold type are treatable.
CSF, cerebrospinal fluid; EMG, electromyography; NCS, nerve conduction studies.
(Adapted from Scriver et al., The Metabolic and Molecular Basis of Inherited Disease, online edition.)

Table 44-13 Progressive Encephalopathy in Middle to Late Childhood (1–5 Years) with Ataxia and Incoordination

Main Sign	Other Signs	Onset	Diagnosis*	Evaluation	Chapter
Normal organic acid excretion	Ataxia with choreoathetosis Oculocephalic asynergia Conjunctival telangiectasias Lymphoid tissue node atrophy Sinopulmonary infections Low IgA level	18 mo–3 yrs	Ataxia-telangiectasia	α-fetoprotein (serum) *ATM* genetic studies	68
	Ataxia Difficulty in walking Mental deterioration (speech)	6 mo–4 yrs	GM$_1$ gangliosidosis (Landing's disease)	Acid β-galactosidase in leukocytes *GLB 1* genetic studies	36
	Spastic quadriparesis Pseudobulbar signs Normal vision, CSF, and nerve conduction velocity		**Biotin-responsive basal ganglia disease**	Head MRI Biotin trial *SLC19A3* genetic studies	32
	Ataxia Spinocerebellar degeneration Psychotic behavior Spasticity Seizures	2–4 yrs	GM$_2$ gangliosidosis (Tay–Sachs disease, Sandhoff's disease) (late infantile form)	Hexosaminidase A (leukocytes) *HEX A* genetic studies	36
	Ataxia Pyramidal signs (hemiplegia, paraplegia) Vision loss Peripheral neuropathy Normal CSF and nerve conduction velocity in 50% Acute onset common	6 mo–3 yrs	Krabbe's disease (late infantile form)	Galactocerebrosidase (leukocytes) *GALC* genetic studies	71
	Ataxia Muscular atrophy in lower extremities Disequilibrium Dyskinesia Walking tiptoe with support Contractures of the knees Strokelike episodes Abnormal nerve conduction velocity (peripheral neuropathy)	3 mo–6 yrs	Congenital defects of glycosylation	Isoelectric focusing of transferrin Genetic studies	35
	Seizures and myoclonic jerks Uncoordinated movements Postictal coma Transient hemiplegia Hepatic symptoms (jaundice, high transaminases) Hyperlactatemia	3 mo–3 yrs	POLG-related disorder (Alpers–Huttenlocher syndrome, progressive external ophthalmoplegia)	*POLG* genetic studies	37
	Extrapyramidal disorder Dyskinesia Epilepsy Neurologic regression Failure to thrive Low plasma creatinine		Cerebral creatine deficiency (GAMT deficiency)	Guanidinoacetate (GAA), creatine, and creatinine (urine and plasma) *GAMT, GATM,* or *SLC6A8* genetic studies GAMT enzyme, AGAT enzyme, or creatine uptake (fibroblasts)	32
	Leukoencephalopathy Ataxia-spasticity Optic atrophy Vanishing white matter	1–5 yrs	Disease of vanishing white matter with hyperglycorrhachia	Head MRI Eukaryotic translation initiation factor 2B (lymphoblast) *EIF2B* genetic studies	71
	Ataxia-dysarthria retardation Optic atrophy, nystagmus Mental retardation Leukoencephalopathy	3 mo–5 yrs	Leukoencephalopathy with disturbance of polyol metabolism	Ribose 5-phosphate isomerase (plasma/CSF) Magnetic resonance spectroscopy *RPIA* genetic studies	71

Continued

Table 44-13 **Progressive Encephalopathy in Middle to Late Childhood (1–5 Years) with Ataxia and Incoordination—cont'd**

Main Sign	Other Signs	Onset	Diagnosis*	Evaluation	Chapter
Abnormal organic acid excretion	Progressive ataxia Intention tremor Slight extrapyramidal signs Cerebellar atrophy Spongiform encephalopathy L-2-hydroxyglutaric aciduria	2–3 yrs	L-2-hydroxyglutaric aciduria (L-2-hydroxyglutaric)	L-2 hydroxyglutaric acid (CSF/plasma) Lactate, pyruvate (serum) Organic acids (urine) *L2HGDH* genetic studies	32
		1–3 yrs	**Inborn errors of cobalamin metabolism**	Lactate, pyruvate, ammonia Organic acids (urine) Amino acids (serum) Homocysteine (urine) Genetic studies	32
	Ataxia Peripheral neuropathy Recurrent attacks of lethargy Hyperlactatemia	1–5 yrs	**Pyruvate dehydrogenase deficiency**	Lactate, pyruvate, ammonia (serum) Organic acids (urine) Amino acids (serum) *PDHA-1* genetic studies	32
	Ataxia Intention tremor Muscular weakness	1–5 yrs	Respiratory chain disorders	Lactate, pyruvate, ammonia (serum) Organic acids (urine) Amino acids (serum) Muscle biopsy	37
			MERRF syndrome	Lactate, pyruvate (serum) Organic acids (urine) Muscle biopsy *MT-TK, MT-TF, MT-TP* genetic studies	37
	Retinitis pigmentosa Dysarthria Myoclonic epilepsy Associated or not with multi-organ failure	2 mo–5 yrs	3-methylglutaconic aciduria	3-methylglutaconate (3-MGC) and 3-methylglutaric acid (3-MGA) (urine) *OPA3* genetic studies	32
	Ataxia Peripheral neuropathy Abnormal nerve conduction velocity Retinitis pigmentosa Progressive cardiomyopathy Recurrent attacks of hypoketotic hypoglycemia and of myoglobinuria	6 mo–4 yrs	Long-chain acyl-CoA-dehydrogenase deficiency	Lactate, pyruvate, acylcarnitine profile, acylglycine profile, total and free carnitine (serum) Organic acids (urine) *ACADL* genetic studies	37
	Ataxia Subacute degeneration of the cord Megaloblastic anemia	Infancy to childhood	**Methylmalonic aciduria and homocystinuria**	Lactate, pyruvate, ammonia (serum) Organic acids (urine) Amino acids (serum) Homocysteine (serum and urine) Cobalamin levels Genetic studies	32
			Homocystinuria	Lactate, pyruvate, ammonia (serum) Organic acids (urine) Amino acids (serum) Homocysteine (serum and urine) Cobalamin levels Genetic studies	32
Acute attacks resembling encephalitis and increasingly severe choreoathetosis	Macrocephaly Temporal lobe atrophy and bilateral basal ganglia damage	1–3 yrs	**Glutaric aciduria type I (glutaric, methylglutaconic)**	Lactate, pyruvate (serum) Organic acid (urine) *GCDH* genetic studies	32

Table 44-13 Progressive Encephalopathy in Middle to Late Childhood (1–5 Years) with Ataxia and Incoordination—cont'd

Main Sign	Other Signs	Onset	Diagnosis*	Evaluation	Chapter
	Dystonia Athetosis Chronic diarrhea	Birth to adulthood	**Methylmalonic acidemia (methylmalonic)**	Lactate, pyruvate, ammonia, amino acids (serum) Organic acid (urine) Homocysteine (serum and urine) Vitamin B$_{12}$ (serum) Skin biopsy Genetic studies	32
			Propionic acidemia (methylcitrate, tiglylglycine)	Lactate, pyruvate, ammonia, amino acids (serum) Organic acid (urine) Amino acids (serum) *PCA* and *PCB* genetic studies	32
		Infancy to childhood	**Homocystinuria (CblE, CblF, CblG)**	Lactate, pyruvate, ammonia (serum) Organic acids (urine) Amino acids (serum) Homocysteine (serum and urine) Cobalamin levels Genetic studies	32

* Disorders shown in bold type are treatable.
AGAT, arginine glycine amidinotransferase; CSF, cerebrospinal fluid; GAMT, guanidinoacetate N-methyltransferase; MERRF, myoclonic epilepsy with ragged red fibers; MRI, magnetic resonance imaging.
(Adapted from Scriver et al., The Metabolic and Molecular Basis of Inherited Disease, online edition.)

Table 44-14 Progressive Encephalopathy in Middle to Late Childhood (5–15 Years) with Seizures and Ataxia

Main Sign	Other Signs	Onset	Diagnosis*	Evaluation	Chapter
Seizures, ataxia, and frequent falling	Rapidly advancing psychomotor degeneration Hypotonia Ataxia Myclonic jerks Early-flattening EEG Blindness	1–2 yrs	Santavuori–Hagberg disease (infantile ceroid-lipofuscinosis)	Electron microscopy (skin, lymphocytes, conjunctiva) Palmitoyl-protein thioesterase 1 (PPT1) (leukocytes) Tripeptidyl-peptidase 1 (TPP-1) (leukocytes) Cathepsin D (CTSD) (leukocytes) Genetic studies	36
	Akinetic myoclonic absence Polymyoclonus Cerebellar ataxia Retinitis pigmentosa Typical EEG on slow-rate photic stimulation Vacuolated lymphocytes	2–4 yrs	Jansky–Bielschowsky disease (late infantile ceroid-lipofuscinosis)	Electron microscopy (skin, lymphocytes, conjunctiva) Palmitoyl-protein thioesterase 1 (PPT1) (leukocytes) Tripeptidyl-peptidase 1 (TPP-1) (leukocytes) Cathepsin D (CTSD) (leukocytes) Genetic studies	36
	Rapid regression Myoclonic seizures Muscular hypotonia Spasticity Corneal blindness Optic atrophy Severe osteoporosis	6–24 mo	Schindler's disease	α-N-acetylgalactosaminidase (fibroblasts) *NAGA* genetic studies	36

Continued

Table 44-14 Progressive Encephalopathy in Middle to Late Childhood (5–15 Years) with Seizures and Ataxia—cont'd

Main Sign	Other Signs	Onset	Diagnosis*	Evaluation	Chapter
	Myoclonic epilepsy, volitional and intentional myoclonias Muscular weakness Cerebellar ataxia Hyperlactacidemia Optic atrophy Deafness	4–15 yrs	MERRF syndrome (respiratory chain disorders)	Lactate, pyruvate (serum) Organic acids (urine) Muscle biopsy *MT-TK, MT-TF, MT-TP* genetic studies	37
	With splenomegaly and hepatomegaly	2–6 yrs	Niemann–Pick disease type C and related disorders (late infantile form)	Intracellular cholesterol esterification (cultured fibroblasts) Filipin staining Bone marrow (sea-blue histiocytes) *NPC1* and *NPC2* genetic studies	36
	With supranuclear ophthalmoplegia	0–12 mo	Gaucher's disease type III (subacute neuronopathy)	β-glucosylceramidase (leukocytes) *GBA* genetic studies	36
	Seizures and myoclonic jerks Uncoordinated movements Postictal coma Transient hemiplegia Hepatic symptoms (jaundice, high transaminases) Hyperlactatemia	1–2 yrs	POLG-related disorder (Alpers–Huttenlocher, progressive external ophthalmoplegia syndrome)	*POLG* genetic studies	37
	Autistic behavior Loss of speech Regression of high-level achievements Stereotyped movements of fingers Acquired microcephaly Secondary epilepsy	1–2 yrs	Rett's syndrome	*MECP2* genetic studies	31

* Disorders shown in bold type are treatable.
EEG, electroencephalography; MERRF, myoclonic epilepsy with ragged red fibers.
(Adapted from Scriver et al., The Metabolic and Molecular Basis of Inherited Disease, online edition.)

Table 44-15 Progressive Encephalopathy in Middle to Late Childhood (5–15 Years) with Predominant Extrapyramidal Signs

Main signs	Onset	Diagnosis*	Evaluation	Chapter
Torsion Dystonia No mental retardation	6–10 yrs	**Dystonia musculorum deformans (idiopathic distortion dystonia)**	*TOR1A* genetic studies	68
Dystonia of lower extremities Gait difficulties No or minimal axial dystonia Normal intellect Diurnal fluctuation of dystonia Dopa-responsive	5–10 yrs	**Segawa's disease (GTP cyclohydrolase deficiency)**	Pterins (CSF) GTP cyclohydrolase (GTPCH1) (fibroblasts) *GCH1* genetic studies	68

Table 44-15 Progressive Encephalopathy in Middle to Late Childhood (5–15 Years) with Predominant Extrapyramidal Signs—cont'd

Main signs	Onset	Diagnosis*	Evaluation	Chapter
Lens dislocation Moderate mental retardation Marfanoid morphology	5–15 yrs	**Classic homocystinuria**	Lactate, pyruvate, ammonia (serum) Organic acids (urine) Amino acids (serum) Homocysteine (serum and urine) Cystathionine β-synthase (CBS) enzyme activity *MTHFR* genetic studies	32
Progressive disorder of locomotion Dystonic posture Choreoathetosis Severe mental regression Retinitis pigmentosa Acanthocytosis	5–15 yrs	Pantothenate kinase deficiency (Hallervorden–Spatz syndrome)	Head MRI Acanthocytes (peripheral smear) Lipoprotein (plasma) *PANK2* genetic studies	68
Generalized parkinsonian rigidity or gross postural and intention tremor Scholastic failure Psychiatric abnormalities Hepatic signs Kayser–Fleischer ring	10–15 yrs	**Wilson's disease**	Ceruloplasmin and copper (serum) 24-hour copper assay (urine) Copper (liver) *ATP7B* genetic studies	68
Rigidity Fine tremor abolished by movements Dementia Seizures Dominant inheritance	10–15 yrs or later	Huntington's chorea	*HTT (HD)* genetic studies	68
Parkinsonism (no tremor) Rigidity Moderate hypokinesia Brisk tendon jerks Difficulties in reading and writing Alacrima Dysphagia due to achalasia Hypoglycemia due to selective cortisol deficiency	10–15 yrs	**Familial glucocorticoid deficiency**	Comprehensive metabolic panel, morning cortisol, renin, aldosterone, dihydroxyepiandrosterone sulfate (serum) ACTH stimulation test Very long chain fatty acids to rule out adrenoleukodystrophy 17-hydroxyprogesterone levels rule out congenital adrenal hyperplasia Pituitary hormone evaluation	68
Subacute encephalopathy Dysarthria, dysphagia External ophthalmoplegia Cogwheel rigidity Dystonia Central necrosis of basal ganglia	5–10 yrs	**Biotinidase deficiency (biotin-responsive basal ganglia disease) (multiple carboxylase deficiency)**	Biotinidase (serum) Lactate, pyruvate (serum) Organic acids (urine) *BTD* genetic studies	32

* Disorders shown in bold type are treatable.
ACTH, adrenocorticotropic hormone; CSF, cerebrospinal fluid; GTP, guanosine triphosphate; MRI, magnetic resonance imaging.
(Adapted from Scriver et al., The Metabolic and Molecular Basis of Inherited Disease, online edition.)

Table 44-16 Severe, Diffuse, Progressive Encephalopathy in Middle to Late Childhood (5–15 Years)

Main Signs	Other Signs	Diagnosis*	Evaluation	Chapter
Visceral signs	Hepatosplenomegaly	Niemann–Pick disease type C	Intracellular cholesterol esterification (cultured fibroblasts) Filipin staining Bone marrow (sea-blue histiocytes) NPC1 and NPC2 genetic studies	36
	Splenomegaly	Gaucher's disease type III	β-glucosylceramidase (leukocytes) GBA genetic studies	36
No visceral signs	Abnormal nerve conduction velocity High CSF protein	Metachromatic leukodystrophy (juvenile form)	Arylsulfatase A (leukocytes) ARSA genetic studies	71
	High CSF protein Adrenal dysfunction	Adrenal leukodystrophy	Very long chain fatty acids (serum) ACTH levels (serum) ACTH stimulation test ABCD1 genetic studies	71
	Ophthalmoplegia Peripheral neuropathy Various signs	Leigh's syndrome/NARP	Lactate, pyruvate, ammonia (serum) Organic acids (urine) Amino acids (serum) Muscle biopsy Genetic studies	37
	Paraplegia	Krabbe's disease (infantile form)	Galactocerebrosidase (leukocytes) GALC genetic studies	71
	Tremor Ataxia	GM_1 and GM_2 gangliosidoses (juvenile form)	Acid β-galactosidase in leukocytes GLB 1 genetic studies Hexosaminidase A (leukocytes) HEX A genetic studies	36
Multi-organ failure	Lactic acidemia	**Respiratory chain disorders**	Lactate, pyruvate, ammonia (serum) Organic acids (urine) Amino acids (serum) Muscle biopsy	37
	Peripheral neuropathy	Peroxisomal biogenesis defects	Very long chain fatty acids, phytanic acid, pristanic acid, pipecolic acid, phytanoyl-CoA hydroxylase PHYH and PEX7 genetic studies	38

* Disorders shown in bold type are treatable.
ACTH, adrenocorticotropic hormone; CSF, cerebrospinal fluid; NARP, neuropathy, ataxia, and retinitis pigmentosa.
(Adapted from Scriver et al., The Metabolic and Molecular Basis of Inherited Disease, online edition.)

Table 44-17 Progressive Encephalopathy in Middle to Late Childhood (5–15 Years) with Polymyoclonus

Main Sign	Other Signs	Onset	Diagnosis	Evaluation	Chapter
Generalized epilepsy	Polymyoclonus Dementia Neurologic deterioration Ataxia	14–20 yrs	Lafora's disease	Skin biopsy (Lafora bodies) EPM2A and EPM2B genetic studies	56
Intellectual deterioration	Loss of sight Retinitis Polymyoclonus Ataxia Extrapyramidal signs Vacuolated lymphocytes	5–12 yrs	Neuronal ceroid-lipofuscinosis	Electron microscopy (skin, lymphocytes, conjunctiva) Palmitoyl-protein thioesterase 1 (PPT1) (leukocytes) Tripeptidyl-peptidase 1 (TPP-1) (leukocytes) Cathepsin D (CTSD) (leukocytes) Genetic studies	36
Predominant seizures	Myoclonic epilepsy Dementia Splenomegaly Osseous signs	7–10 yrs	Gaucher's disease type III	β-glucosylceramidase (leukocytes) GBA genetic studies	36

Table 44-17 Progressive Encephalopathy in Middle to Late Childhood (5–15 Years) with Polymyoclonus—cont'd

Main Sign	Other Signs	Onset	Diagnosis	Evaluation	Chapter
Cerebellar ataxia	Myoclonic jerks Cherry-red spot	4–10 yrs	Late-onset GM$_2$ gangliosidosis (Sandhoff's disease, Tay–Sachs disease)	Hexosaminidase A and B (leukocytes) *HEXA* genetic studies *HEXB* genetic studies	36
Hepatomegaly	Splenomegaly Ophthalmoplegia	5–10 yrs	Niemann–Pick disease type C	Intracellular cholesterol esterification (cultured fibroblasts) Filipin staining Bone marrow (sea-blue histiocytes) *NPC1* and *NPC2* genetic testing	36
Myoclonic epilepsy	Ataxia Lactic acidosis	All ages	Respiratory chain disorders (MERRF, etc.)	Lactate, pyruvate, ammonia (serum) Organic acids (urine) Amino acids (serum) Muscle biopsy	37

MERRF, myoclonic epilepsy with ragged red fibers.
(Adapted from Scriver et al., The Metabolic and Molecular Basis of Inherited Disease, online edition.)

Table 44-18 Progressive Encephalopathy in Middle to Late Childhood (5–15 Years) with Predominant Cerebellar Ataxia

Main Sign	Other Signs	Diagnosis*	Evaluation	Chapter
Little to no mental deterioration	Dysarthria Pes cavus Cardiomyopathy Spinocerebellar degeneration	Friedreich's ataxia	Cardiac echocardiogram *FXN* (previously *FRDA*) genetic studies	68
	Variable	Spinocerebellar ataxias	Genetic studies	68
	Chronic diarrhea Low cholesterol Acanthocytosis	**Abetalipoproteinemia (Bassen–Kornzweig)**	Stool fat studies Peripheral smear (acanthocytes) β-lipoprotein (serum) *MTTP* genetic studies	68
	Retinitis pigmentosa Peripheral neuropathy	Peroxisomal disorders	Very long chain fatty acids, phytanic acid, pristanic acid, pipecolic acid, phytanoyl-CoA hydroxylase *PHYH* and *PEX7* genetic studies	38
		Congenital disorders of glycosylation	Isoelectric focusing of transferrin Genetic studies	35
		Refsum's disease	Phytanic acid, pristanic acid (plasma) Pipecolic acid (plasma) Erythrocyte plasmalogen concentration Di- and trihydroxycholestanoic acid (serum) Phytanoyl-CoA hydroxylase (fibroblasts) *PHYH, PEX7,* and/or *AMACR* genetic studies	38
	Oculocephalic asynergia Conjunctival telangiectasias	Ataxia-telangiectasia	α-fetoprotein (serum) *ATM* genetic studies	68
Significant mental deterioration and dementia		Lafora's disease	Skin biopsy (Lafora bodies) *EPM2A* and *EPM2B* genetic studies	56
		Cerebrotendinous xanthomatosis	Cholestanol, cholesterol (plasma) Bile alcohols (plasma and urine) Cholestanol and apolipoprotein B (CSF) Sterol 27-hydroxylase (fibroblasts) *CYP27A1* genetic studies	71

Continued

Table 44-18 Progressive Encephalopathy in Middle to Late Childhood (5–15 Years) with Predominant Cerebellar Ataxia—cont'd

Main Sign	Other Signs	Diagnosis*	Evaluation	Chapter
		GM$_1$, GM$_2$ gangliosidoses	Acid β-galactosidase in leukocytes *GLB 1* genetic studies Hexosaminidase A (leukocytes) *HEXA* genetic studies	36
		Gaucher's disease	β-glucocerebrosidase (leukocytes) Bone marrow *GBA* genetic studies β-glucosylceramidase (leukocytes) *GBA* genetic studies	36
		Niemann–Pick disease type C	Intracellular cholesterol esterification (cultured fibroblasts) Filipin staining Bone marrow (sea-blue histiocytes) *NPC1* and *NPC2* genetic studies	36
		Krabbe's disease (juvenile form)	Galactocerebrosidase (leukocytes) *GALC* genetic studies	71
		Metachromatic leukodystrophy	Arylsulfatase A (leukocytes) *ARSA* genetic studies	71
		Respiratory chain disorders	Lactate, pyruvate, ammonia (serum) Organic acids (urine) Amino acids (serum) Muscle biopsy	37

* Disorders shown in bold type are treatable.
CSF, cerebrospinal fluid.
(Adapted from Scriver et al., The Metabolic and Molecular Basis of Inherited Disease, online edition.)

Table 44-19 Progressive Encephalopathy in Middle to Late Childhood (5–15 Yrs) with Predominant Polyneuropathy

Other Signs	Diagnosis*	Evaluation	Chapter
Acute attacks	**Porphyrias**	Porphobilinogen, uroporphyrins I and III, coproporphyrins I and III, pre-coproporphyrin (urine)	103
	Tyrosinemia type I	α-fetoprotein, PT, PTT, AST, ALT, GGT (serum) Lactate, pyruvate, ammonia, amino acids (serum) Organic acids (urine) Fumarylacetoacetic acid hydrolase (FAH) (fibroblasts) *FAH* genetic studies	32
Progressive with demyelination	β-mannosidase	Glycosaminoglycans and oligosaccharides (urine) β-mannosidase (leukocytes) *MANBA* genetic studies	36
	Charcot–Marie–Tooth disease	Electromyography with nerve conduction studies Genetic studies based on family history	89
	Krabbe's disease	Galactocerebrosidase (leukocytes) *GALC* genetic studies	71
	Metachromatic leukodystrophy	Arylsulfatase A (leukocytes) *ARSA* genetic studies	71
	Mitochondrial neurogastrointestinal encephalomyopathy (MNGIE)	Deoxyuridine, thymidine (plasma) Thymidine phosphorylase (leukocytes) *TYMP* genetic studies	37

Table 44-19 Progressive Encephalopathy in Middle to Late Childhood (5–15 Yrs) with Predominant Polyneuropathy—cont'd

Other Signs	Diagnosis*	Evaluation	Chapter
	Peroxisomal biogenesis defects	Very long chain fatty acids, phytanic acid, pristanic acid, pipecolic acid, phytanoyl-CoA hydroxylase (serum) *PHYH* and *PEX7* genetic studies	38
	Refsum's disease	Phytanic acid, pristanic acid, pipecolic acid, very long chain fatty acids, di- and trihydroxycholestanoic acid (serum) Plasmalogen (erythrocytes) Phytanoyl-CoA hydroxylase (fibroblasts) *PHYH, PEX7*, and/or *AMACR* genetic studies	38
Progressive – predominantly axonal	**Abetalipoproteinemia**	Stool fat studies Peripheral smear (acanthocytes) β-lipoprotein (serum) *MTTP* genetic studies	89
	α-Methyl acyl-CoA racemase (AMACR)	Pristanic acid AMACR enzyme analysis (fibroblasts) *AMACR* genetic studies	38
	Cerebrotendinous xanthomatosis	Cholestanol, cholesterol (plasma) Bile alcohols (plasma and urine) Cholestanol and apolipoprotein B (CSF) Sterol 27-hydroxylase (fibroblasts) *CYP27A1* genetic studies	71
	Congenital disorders of glycosylation	Isoelectric focusing of transferrin Genetic studies	35
	Leigh's disease	Lactate, pyruvate, ammonia (serum) Organic acids (urine) Amino acids (serum) Muscle biopsy Genetic studies	37
	Respiratory chain disorders	Lactate, pyruvate, ammonia (serum) Organic acids (urine) Amino acids (serum) Muscle biopsy	37
	Ornithine aminotransferase	Amino acids, ammonia (serum) Ornithine amino transferase (fibroblasts) *OAT* genetic studies	38
	△1-Pyrroline-5-carboxylate synthase deficiency	Amino acids, ammonia (serum)	32
	Pyruvate decarboxylase deficiency (pyruvate dehydrogenase complex deficiency)	Lactate, pyruvate, ammonia, amino acids (serum) Organic acids (urine) Enzyme analysis (leukocytes or fibroblasts) *PDHA1* genetic studies	32
	Long-chain acyl CoA-dehydrogenase deficiency (3-hydroxy-acyl CoA dehydrogenase deficiency [3-hydroxydicarboxylic and 3-hydroxy-acylcarnitine esters])	Lactate, pyruvate (serum) Organic acids (urine) Acylcarnitine profile *ACADL* genetic studies	37
	Peroxisomal biogenesis defects	Very long chain fatty acids, phytanic acid, pristanic acid, pipecolic acid, phytanoyl-CoA hydroxylase (serum) *PHYH* and *PEX7* genetic studies	38
	Serine deficiency	Amino acids (serum) Serine and glycine (CSF)	32
	Trifunctional enzyme deficiency	Lactate, pyruvate (serum) Organic acids (urine) Acylcarnitine profile *HADHA* and *HADHB* genetic studies	94

* Disorders shown in bold type are treatable.

ALT, alanine aminotransferase; AST, aspartate aminotransferase; CSF, cerebrospinal fluid; GGT, gamma-glutamyl transferase; PT, prothrombin time; PTT, partial thromboplastin time.

(Adapted from Scriver et al., The Metabolic and Molecular Basis of Inherited Disease, online edition.)

Table 44-20 **Progressive Encephalopathy in Middle to Late Childhood (5–15 Years) with Predominantly Psychiatric Symptoms**

Diagnosis*	Evaluation	Chapter
X-linked adrenoleukodystrophy	Very long chain fatty acids (serum) ACTH levels (serum) ACTH stimulation test *ABCD1* genetic studies	71
Cerebrotendinous xanthomatosis	Cholestanol, cholesterol (plasma) Bile alcohols (plasma and urine) Cholestanol and apolipoprotein B (CSF) Sterol 27-hydroxylase (fibroblasts) *CYP27A1* genetic studies	71
Cobalamin defects (Cbl C)	Lactate, pyruvate, ammonia Organic acids (urine) Amino acids (serum) Homocysteine (urine) Genetic testing	32
Classic homocystinuria	Lactate, pyruvate, ammonia (serum) Organic acids (urine) Amino acids (serum) Homocysteine (serum and urine) Cobalamin levels Genetic studies	32
Huntington's chorea (juvenile form)	*HTT* (*HD*) genetic studies	68
Krabbe's disease	Galactocerebrosidase (leukocytes) *GALC* genetic studies	71
Methylene tetrahydrofolate reductase deficiency	Homocysteine (urine) *MTHFR* genetic studies	103
Metachromatic leukodystrophy	Arylsulfatase A (leukocytes) *ARSA* genetic studies	71
Niemann–Pick disease type C	Intracellular cholesterol esterification (cultured fibroblasts) Filipin staining Bone marrow (sea-blue histiocytes) *NPC1* and *NPC2* genetic studies	36
Neuronal ceroid-lipofuscinosis	Electron microscopy (skin, lymphocytes, conjunctiva) Palmitoyl-protein thioesterase 1 (PPT1) (leukocytes) Tripeptidyl-peptidase 1 (TPP-1) (leukocytes) Cathepsin D (CTSD) (leukocytes) Genetic studies	36
Pantothenate kinase deficiency (Hallervorden–Spatz)	Head MRI Acanthocytes (peripheral smear) Lipoprotein (plasma) *PANK2* genetic studies	68
Pyruvate carboxylate deficiency (Leigh's disease)	Lactate, pyruvate, ammonia (serum) Organic acids (urine) Amino acids (serum) Muscle biopsy Genetic studies	37
Sanfilippo's syndrome	Heparan *N*-sulfatase (fibroblasts) *N*-acetyl-alpha-D-glucosaminidase (fibroblasts) Acetyl-CoA: alpha-glucosaminide acetyltransferase (fibroblasts) *N*-acetylglucosamine-G-sulfate sulfatase (fibroblasts) Glycosaminoglycans (urine) Genetic studies	36
Urea cycle defects	Lactate, pyruvate, ammonia, amino acids (serum) Organic acids (urine) Genetic studies	33
Wilson's disease	Ceruloplasmin and copper (serum) *ATP7B* genetic studies	68

* Disorders shown in bold type are treatable.
ACTH, adrenocorticotropic hormone; CSF, cerebrospinal fluid; MRI, magnetic resonance imaging.
(Adapted from Scriver et al., The Metabolic and Molecular Basis of Inherited Disease, online edition.)

Table 44-21 **Progressive Encephalopathy in Adulthood (15–70 Years)**

Predominant Signs	Diagnoses*	Evaluation	Chapter
Ataxia	**Cerebrotendinous xanthomatosis**	Cholestanol, cholesterol (plasma) Bile alcohols (plasma and urine) Cholestanol and apolipoprotein B (CSF) Sterol 27-hydroxylase (fibroblasts) *CYP27A1* genetic studies	71
	Galactosialidosis	Neuraminidase, β-galactosidase, cathepsin A (fibroblasts) *CTSA* genetic studies	36
	Hexosaminidase deficiencies	Hexosaminidase A and B *HEXA* and *HEXB* genetic studies	36
	Metachromatic leukodystrophy	Arylsulfatase A (leukocytes) *ARSA* genetic studies	71
	3-methylglutaconic aciduria	Organic acids (urine) *OPA3* genetic studies	32
	Niemann–Pick disease type C	Intracellular cholesterol esterification (cultured fibroblasts) Filipin staining Bone marrow (sea-blue histiocytes) *NPC1* and *NPC2* genetic studies	36
Peripheral sensory polyneuropathy	α-Methyl acyl-CoA racemase	Pristanic acid *AMACR* enzyme analysis (fibroblasts) *AMACR* genetic studies	38
	Congenital disorders of glycosylation	Isoelectric focusing of transferrin Genetic studies	35
	Long-chain acyl CoA-dehydrogenase deficiency (3-hydroxy-acyl CoA dehydrogenase deficiency [3-hydroxydicarboxylic and 3-hydroxy-acylcarnitine esters])	Lactate, pyruvate (serum) Organic acids (urine) Acylcarnitine profile *ACADL* genetic studies	37
	Peroxisomal biogenesis defects	Very long chain fatty acids, phytanic acid, pristanic acid, pipecolic acid, phytanoyl-CoA hydroxylase (serum) *PHYH* and *PEX7* genetic studies	38
	Trifunctional enzyme deficiency	Lactate, pyruvate (serum) Organic acids (urine) Acylcarnitine profile *HADHA* and *HADHB* genetic studies	94
Psychosis	**Cerebrotendinous xanthomatosis**	Cholestanol, cholesterol (plasma) Bile alcohols (plasma and urine) Cholestanol and apolipoprotein B (CSF) Sterol 27-hydroxylase (fibroblasts) *CYP27A1* genetic studies	71
	Cobalamin defects (Cbl C)	Lactate, pyruvate, ammonia Organic acids (urine) Amino acids, total and free carnitine, vitamin B_{12} (serum) Homocysteine (urine) Genetic testing	32
	Hexosaminidase deficiencies	Hexosaminidase A and B *HEXA* and *HEXB* genetic studies	36
	Classic homocystinuria	Lactate, pyruvate, ammonia (serum) Organic acids (urine) Amino acids (serum) Homocysteine (serum and urine) Cobalamin levels Genetic studies	32
	Huntington's chorea	*HTT* (*HD*) genetic studies	68
	Lafora's disease	Skin biopsy (Lafora bodies) *EPM2A* and *EPM2B* genetic studies	56

Continued

Predominant Signs	Diagnoses*	Evaluation	Chapter
	Metachromatic leukodystrophy	Arylsulfatase A (leukocytes) *ARSA* genetic studies	71
	Neuronal ceroid-lipofuscinosis (Kufs' disease)	Electron microscopy (skin, lymphocytes, conjunctiva) Palmitoyl-protein thioesterase 1 (PPT1) (leukocytes) Tripeptidyl-peptidase 1 (TPP-1) (leukocytes) Cathepsin D (CTSD) (leukocytes) Genetic studies	36
	Niemann–Pick disease type C	Intracellular cholesterol esterification (cultured fibroblasts) Filipin staining Bone marrow (sea-blue histiocytes) *NPC1* and *NPC2* genetic studies	36
	Ornithine transcarbamylase deficiency	Lactate, pyruvate, ammonia, amino acids (serum) Organic acids (urine) *OTC* genetic studies	33
	Wilson's disease	Ceruloplasmin and copper (serum) 24-hour copper assay (urine) Copper (liver) *ATP7B* genetic studies	68
Extrapyramidal signs	GM₁ gangliosidosis	Acid β-galactosidase in leukocytes *GLB 1* genetic studies	36
	Hexosaminidase deficiencies	Hexosaminidase A and B *HEXA* and *HEXB* genetic studies	36
	Huntington's chorea	*HTT* (*HD*) genetic studies	68
	Neuronal ceroid-lipofuscinosis (Kufs' disease)	Electron microscopy (skin, lymphocytes, conjunctiva) Palmitoyl-protein thioesterase 1 (PPT1) (leukocytes) Tripeptidyl-peptidase 1 (TPP-1) (leukocytes) Cathepsin D (CTSD) (leukocytes) Genetic studies	36
	Niemann–Pick disease type C	Intracellular cholesterol esterification (cultured fibroblasts) Filipin staining Bone marrow (sea-blue histiocytes) *NPC1* and *NPC2* genetic testing	36
	Wilson's disease	Ceruloplasmin and copper (serum) *ATP7B* genetic studies	68
Hemiparesis or paraparesis with little cognitive deterioration	Adrenomyeloneuropathy	Very long chain fatty acids (serum) ACTH levels (serum) ACTH stimulation test *ABCD1* genetic studies	71
	Krabbe's disease (late-onset form)	Galactocerebrosidase (leukocytes) *GALC* genetic studies	71
	Peroxisomal disorders	Very long chain fatty acids, phytanic acid, pristanic acid, pipecolic acid, phytanoyl-CoA hydroxylase (serum) *PHYH* and *PEX7* genetic studies	38
Myoclonic epilepsy	Galactosialidosis	Neuraminidase, β-galactosidase, cathepsin A (fibroblasts) *CTSA* genetic studies	36
	Lafora's disease	Skin biopsy (Lafora bodies) *EPM2A* and *EPM2B* genetic studies	56
	Mucolipidosis I (sialidosis type I)	Oligosaccharides (urine) Neuraminidase, β-galactosidase (fibroblasts) *NEU1* genetic studies	36
	Neuronal ceroid-lipofuscinosis (Kufs' disease)	Electron microscopy (skin, lymphocytes, conjunctiva) Palmitoyl-protein thioesterase 1 (PPT1) (leukocytes) Tripeptidyl-peptidase 1 (TPP-1) (leukocytes) Cathepsin D (CTSD) (leukocytes) Genetic studies	36

* Disorders shown in bold type are treatable.
ACTH, adrenocorticotropic hormone; CSF, cerebrospinal fluid; MRI, magnetic resonance imaging.
(Adapted from Scriver et al., The Metabolic and Molecular Basis of Inherited Disease, online edition.)

and concerns that will require a large amount of time, patience, and sensitivity on the part of the clinician. Even when disease-specific treatments are not available, the clinician can be of great assistance in maintaining the child's quality of life. Efforts should be made early in the course to direct the child to other sources of supportive care, including rehabilitation specialists, nutritionists, special education instructors, and speech, occupational, and physical therapists. When possible, the child's caregivers should be referred to a social worker who can help them obtain financial support, nursing care, and social support networks.

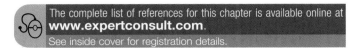

The complete list of references for this chapter is available online at **www.expertconsult.com**.
See inside cover for registration details.

Developmental Language Disorders

Ruth Nass and Doris A. Trauner

Introduction

Developmental language disorder (DLD; also known as Specific Language Impairment – SLI) is a condition in which a child with normal intelligence and hearing fails to develop language in an age-appropriate fashion. DLD is a clinical diagnosis, based on the presence of a normal nonverbal IQ, evidence of expressive and/or receptive language at least 1.5 standard deviations below the mean for age, and absence of other specific conditions such as autism, mental retardation, metabolic or genetic disorders, or severe environmental deprivation. The prevalence of DLD varies widely in different reports with a range of 1–11 percent [Bishop, 2002a; Shriberg et al., 1999]. Box 45-1 lists normal language milestones as a baseline for assessing a child's developing language competence.

Pathophysiology

The underlying neural dysfunction that causes DLD is not known. Studies over the past 30 years have suggested that DLD is the result of a deficit in processing rapid auditory information. Evidence for this hypothesis comes from research showing that children with DLD have difficulty discriminating both nonspeech and speech sounds that are presented rapidly or very briefly in time [Tallal et al., 1993; Tallal and Benasich, 2002]. Some investigators argue for a speech-specific processing deficit [Mody et al., 1997], while others believe that the deficit is more general and that processing of all auditory information is slowed in DLD, whether the information presented is linguistic or nonlinguistic (e.g., environmental sounds) [Cummings and Ceponiene, 2010]. Studies using event-related brain potentials (ERPs) have demonstrated clear differences between DLD and control children, with language-impaired individuals having delayed N400 responses to incongruous picture–word combinations [McArthur et al., 2009].

MRI studies have shown relatively subtle differences between the brains of DLD and controls. Some children and adults with DLD (as well as relatives of DLD probands) do not have the typical planum temporale asymmetry pattern [Jackson and Plante, 1996; Gauger et al., 1997]. The absence of the typical planum asymmetry may be the result of aberrant neurogenesis, which leads to reduced cell development in the perisylvian regions or atypical patterns of cell death. Atypical right-biased asymmetries have also been reported in the prefrontal region [Jernigan et al., 1991]. An extra sulcus in the inferior frontal gyrus was associated with a history of DLD [Clark and Plante, 1998] in a group of 41 neurologically normal adults. DLD children may have decreased white-matter volumes in a left-hemispheric network comprising the motor cortex, the dorsal premotor cortex, the ventral premotor cortex, and the planum polare in the superior temporal gyrus [Jancke et al., 2007]. Rare reports document right hemisphere abnormalities in the DLD child that are suggestive of a right hemisphere contribution to language acquisition [Plante et al., 2001]. Trauner et al. [2000], in a series of 35 children with DLD, found evidence of structural abnormalities in one-third of the children. These included ventricular enlargement (n = 5), central volume loss (3), and white-matter abnormalities (4). The findings were consistent with bilateral white-matter disruption, and suggested that connectivity between different brain regions important for language development might be disrupted in DLD.

Other structural differences in brain development have been observed in some individuals with specified DLD types. Perisylvian abnormalities of varying degrees and associated with language disorders of varying severity have been reported, particularly in verbal dyspraxia and the phonological syntactic syndromes (see below for nosology). Complete opercular agenesis has been reported in association with suprabulbar palsy (Worster–Drought syndrome). Polymicrogyria has also been reported in the perisylvian region in children with DLD. Patients with the most extensive disease have the greatest language impairments, while those with posterior parietal polymicrogyria have milder symptoms [Guerreiro et al., 2002; Nevo et al., 2001]. One form of DLD, semantic pragmatic syndrome, has been reported in patients with agenesis of the corpus callosum and with hydrocephalus, which supports a possible localization in the subcortex and its connections or a disconnection effect. Consistent with this, callosal size may be decreased in some children with DLD [Preis et al., 2000]. In the KE family (see below) the caudate nucleus and inferior frontal gyrus are reduced in size bilaterally, while the left frontal opercular region (pars triangularis and anterior insular cortex) and the putamen bilaterally have a greater volume of gray matter [Watkins et al., 2002a]. An insufficient dosage of a critical forkhead transcription factor during embryogenesis may lead to malformations of regions of the brain necessary for speech and language development [Lai et al., 2001].

Metabolic imaging suggests abnormalities in the left temporal region and may vary by DLD subtype. Some children with DLD may be right hemisphere language-dominant [Bernat and

Box 45-1 **Normal Language Milestones**

Receptive

- Some words understood by 9 months
- Follows one-step commands by 12 months without being cued by a gesture

Expressive

- Cooing – 2 months
- Babbling – 6 months
- Variable babble – 8 months
- One word other than dada and mama – 12 months
- 10–50 words used meaningfully – 16–20 months
- 2-word phrases – 20–24 months
- Points to at least one body part and to named objects and people on command – 20 months
- Vocabulary >200 words – 2 years
- 2-word combinations – 2 years
- Follows 2-part commands – 2 years
- Sentences of 3–4 words – 3 years
- Compound and complex sentences – 4 years
- Passive voice – 6 years

Altman, 2003]. Whitehouse and Bishop [2008] compared language organization in four groups of adults – those with persisting SLI, those with a history of SLI, those on the autistic spectrum (ASD) with language impairment, and matched controls – using functional transcranial Doppler ultrasonography (fTCD), which assesses blood flow through the middle cerebral arteries. The participants were asked to generate words starting with a given letter silently and then later were required to verbalize these words. All of the participants in the SLI-history group and the majority of participants in the ASD (81.8 percent) and typical (90.9 percent) groups had greater activation in the left compared to the right middle cerebral arteries, while the majority of participants in the persistent SLI group had bilateral (27 percent) or right hemisphere (55 percent) language function. The investigators suggest that atypical language dominance may be a marker of persisting SLI. All 17 of the DLD children studied by Im et al. [2007] had grossly normal magnetic resonance imaging (MRI); however, 87.5 percent had decreased metabolic activity on positron emission tomography (PET) studies, most frequently in the thalamus, but also in both frontal, temporal, and right parietal areas, and significantly increased metabolism in both occipital areas as compared to a control group. Children with SLI showed significantly lower cerebral blood flow (CBF) values in the right parietal region and in subcortical regions compared to an attention-deficit hyperactivity disorder (ADHD) group. In addition, the DLD group had symmetric CBF distributions in the left and right temporal regions, whereas the ADHD group showed the usual asymmetry with left-sided hemispheric predominance in the temporal regions. The findings provide further evidence of anomalous neurodevelopment with deviant hemispheric lateralization as an important factor in the etiology of SLI. They also point to the role of subcortical structures in language impairment in childhood [Ors et al., 2005].

Although DLD is often referred to as "specific" language impairment, individuals with this disorder often have other accompanying problems, including abnormalities in gross and fine motor function [Trauner et al., 2000; Visscher et al., 2007]. These findings are indicative of more global neurological dysfunction and may reflect the fact that language disorders do not occur in isolation, but are merely the most prominent symptom of a more widespread neural network malfunction. Stuttering is a disorder involving the rhythm and fluency of speech production, as opposed to language. The stutterer knows what s/he wishes to say but cannot get the words out without significant dysfluency and hesitation. The neurobiological basis of stuttering has been the subject of a number of recent studies [Brown et al., 2005; Watkins et al., 2008]. During speech production, regardless of fluency or auditory feedback, stutterers showed overactivity relative to controls in the anterior insula, cerebellum, and midbrain bilaterally, and underactivity in the ventral premotor, rolandic opercular and sensorimotor cortex bilaterally, and Heschl's gyrus on the left. These results are consistent with a recent meta-analysis of functional imaging studies in developmental stuttering. Overactivity occurred in the midbrain, at the level of the substantia nigra, and extended to the pedunculopontine nucleus, red nucleus, and subthalamic nucleus. This overactivity is consistent with suggestions in previous studies of abnormal function of the basal ganglia or excessive dopamine in stutterers. Underactivity of the cortical motor and premotor areas was associated with articulation and speech production. Analysis of the diffusion data revealed that the integrity of the white matter underlying the underactive areas in ventral premotor cortex was reduced in people who stutter. The white matter tracts in this area, via connections with posterior superior temporal and inferior parietal cortex, provide a substrate for the integration of articulatory planning and sensory feedback, and via connections with primary motor cortex, a substrate for execution of articulatory movements. These data would lead to the conclusion that stuttering is a disorder related primarily to disruption in the cortical and subcortical neural systems supporting the selection, initiation, and execution of motor sequences necessary for fluent speech production [Watkins et al., 2002b]. A recent meta-analysis of these studies identified three "neural signatures" of stuttering: people who stutter show more activity than fluent-speaking controls in the cerebellar vermis and in the right anterior insular cortex, with an "absence" of activity in the auditory cortices in the superior temporal lobe [Brown et al., 2005]. These abnormal levels of activity were observed during speech production, regardless of the presence or absence of stuttered speech during scan acquisition. Surprisingly, the meta-analysis did not reveal abnormal levels of activity in the basal ganglia circuitry, despite early imaging work on small samples showing abnormal metabolism.

In summary, multiple avenues of research indicate that DLD is associated with impaired processing of auditory information, with electrophysiological abnormalities found during linguistic (and some nonlinguistic) tasks, suggesting that there are disrupted neural networks in DLD. Further, brain structure is aberrant in individuals with DLD, but there is no single pattern observed across all studies.

Factors Associated with DLD

As with many neurodevelopmental disorders, there is a higher incidence of DLD in males. One recent study showed a ratio of 1.66:1 males to females in a group of children with communication disorders [McLeod and McKinnon, 2007]. The cause for

Box 45-2 Disorders Known to be Associated with Language Delay/Impairment

Genetic Disorders

- Fragile X syndrome
- Klinefelter's syndrome
- Prader–Willi syndrome
- Angelman's syndrome
- Williams' syndrome
- Homocystinuria
- Tuberous sclerosis
- Isodicentric chromosome 15
- Mitochondrial encephalopathies
- Fatty acid oxidation defects
- Amino acidopathies (e.g., Hartnup's disease, phenylketonuria)

Epileptic Syndromes

- Infantile spasms
- Lennox–Gastaut syndrome
- Landau–Kleffner syndrome
- Rolandic epilepsy

Congenital and Developmental Disorders

- Congenital rubella syndrome
- Neuronal migration defects

the gender differences is not known. A number of biological and environmental risk factors for DLD have been identified. Box 45-2 lists a number of disorders associated with language impairment. Low birth weight and prematurity, as well as prenatal exposure to drugs (e.g., cocaine) and to cigarettes, adversely affect language development [Lewis et al., 2007]. Although frequent episodes of otitis media have been suggested as causing language impairment, there is little evidence from controlled studies to indicate a causal relationship. Intermittent hearing loss may interfere with language development in at-risk children, but is not likely to cause long-term language issues in otherwise normally developing children. Other environmental factors that may potentially adversely affect language development have been studied. For example, early and excessive TV exposure has been associated with language delay. Children who started watching television before 12 months of age and watched television for more than 2 hours per day were approximately six times more likely to have language delays than children without such early TV exposure [Chonchaiya et al., 2008]. Such associations, however, do not indicate causation.

Language impairment is seen in association with specific neurological and genetic disorders [Nass and Frank, 2010]. For example, perisylvian polymicrogyria (or congenital bilateral perisylvian syndrome) is a disorder of defective neuronal migration that has a spectrum of neurological impairments that include severe epilepsy and cognitive impairment. In some children with this condition, language impairment is the most prominent feature [Brandao-Almeida et al., 2008]. Language impairment has been described in children with neurofibromatosis type 1, although those individuals often have other cognitive deficits and learning disabilities as well. Language impairment is also prominent in a number of chromosomal disorders, including Down, Klinefelter's, and fragile X syndromes.

Epileptic encephalopathies, particularly Landau–Kleffner syndrome (LKS), may present with language impairment as an isolated or primary symptom [Kleffner and Landau, 2009]. Children with LKS typically have greater receptive than expressive language dysfunction, although they may become completely aphasic and mute in the course of the disease process. Rolandic epilepsy, often considered to be "benign", may be complicated by DLD and learning disabilities [Lillywhite et al., 2009].

Genetics

Heritability rates for DLDs run as high as 0.5 [Byrne et al., 2009], but they are very variable and are affected by the criteria used to diagnose DLD. The median incidence rate for language difficulties in the families of children with language impairment runs as high as 35 percent, compared with a median incidence rate of 11 percent in control families [Stromswold, 1998]. Increased monozygotic versus dizygotic twin concordance rates indicate that heredity, not just shared environment, is responsible for familial clustering [Bartlett et al., 2002; Stromswold, 2001]. Heritability is substantially higher if DLD is identified based on referral to speech and language pathology services [Bishop and Hayiou-Thomas, 2008] than if it is identified by language test scores. Childhood language disorders that are demonstrated in population screening are likely to have different phenotypes and different etiologies than clinically referred cases. It is also possible, however, that familial cases are more likely to come to the attention of specialists since the parents are more attuned to the problem and recognize it earlier in subsequent children.

Studies using genome-wide scanning have implicated a number of gene loci, but the same loci have not been found in a reproducible fashion [SLI Consortium, 2002; Grigorenko, 2009]. One exceptional family stands out. In the three-generation KE family, half the members are affected with a severe speech and language disorder that is transmitted as an autosomal-dominant monogenic trait involving the *FOXP2* forkhead-domain gene [Watkins et al., 2002b]. Notably, however, a recent screening of 270 4-year-olds with DLD was negative for the *FOXP2* mutation [Meaburn et al., 2002]. It is unlikely that there will prove to be specific genes whose function would be restricted to forming the genetic basis for speaking and language acquisition. It is much more likely that there are many genes that contribute to a variety of functions, and that these genes form networks that are recruited in the process of forming language-related representations during language acquisition [Grigorenko, 2009]. The definition of the phenotype forming the basis for specific genetic studies is crucial. To date, in addition to the KE family phenotype, nonword repetition has proven the most useful phenotype in molecular genetic research [SLI Consortium, 2004; Vernes et al., 2008]. The issue of pleiotropy, or the impact of the same genes on multiple phenotypes, has also been discussed in the literature on DLD, given the substantive overlap in regions of linkage for a variety of developmental disorders, such as speech and sound disorders (SSD) and developmental dyslexia [Miscimarra et al., 2007; Stein et al., 2004], and SLI and autism [Tager-Flusberg and Joseph, 2003]. Once again, whether these are true examples of pleiotropy or outcomes of the imprecision of phenotype definitions is yet to be determined [Grigorenko, 2009].

Diagnosis

DLD is a clinical diagnosis based on a delay in language development for expected age, in the absence of mental retardation, hearing impairment, environmental deprivation, or psychiatric disorders. In children for whom formal language assessments are conducted, a score of 1.5 or more standard deviations from the normative mean on a standardized test of language is considered diagnostic for DLD.

Box 45-3 lists warning signs that suggest a DLD during the first 3 years. Language delay can be diagnosed very early, whether the delay is primarily expressive only or mixed receptive and expressive. Before the age of 2 years, however, delay may not always equal disorder. Research on late-talking toddlers reveals a lack of homogeneity within the population of children with a vocabulary delay at 2 years of age. In a recent study, only about 40 percent of children retained the diagnosis of DLD at ages 3 and 4 years [Dale et al., 2003]. This is particularly true if the early language delay was primarily expressive. Children with receptive language impairments are more likely to have a persistent DLD. The pattern of receptive language development is highly predictable during the elementary school years. In a study of 184 children age-assessed at three time points – 7 years, 8 years, and 11 years of age – receptive language disorder was associated with declining rates of language growth over time [Law et al., 2008]. Thus, concern for poor language prognosis should be heightened when receptive language deficits are identified.

Although expressive language delays have more variable outcomes by school age, many children with early language delay who appear to "catch up" go on to have language-based learning disabilities (e.g., dyslexia). It is therefore important to recommend periodic reassessment of a child's language and academic functioning after an early language delay has been diagnosed.

Another basis sometimes suggested as a means of screening for DLD is the presence of a large discrepancy between nonverbal intelligence and language capabilities [Klee et al., 2000; Aram et al., 1992]. However, this means of identification of DLD may have variable results, depending on the tests used. Various discrepancy criteria have been used to identify children with developmental language disorders [Bishop, 2004]. In one study of young children clinically designated as having a developmental language disorder, the diagnosis was suspected only 40–60 percent of the time, using variations of the Stanford–Binet IQ test/Test of Language Development discrepancy score. A nonverbal IQ/specific language test performance discrepancy criterion of 1 standard deviation (e.g., Wechsler Performance IQ versus the Peabody Picture Vocabulary Test, Token Test, Rapid Automatized Naming, or Sentence Repetition) identified 34 percent of very low birth weight 7-year-olds and 45 percent of controls as having a developmental language disorder. A 2 standard deviation discrepancy yielded 14 percent and 19 percent frequency in the two groups, respectively [Aram et al., 1992]. Evaluating a group of adolescents, Miller and Gilbert [2008] had similar problems using discrepancy scores to diagnose SLI. They too found that nonverbal IQ scores are dependent on the test being used and the group being tested. The discrepancies were greater in those with SLI than in those with normal language. Thus, using the difference between a language measure and a particular nonverbal IQ measure may result in diagnosis with one test and not another, and potentially different diagnoses (DLD or not) in the same child. Both under- and over-diagnosis occur using seemingly standardized criteria over a broad age range. Thus, this method of assessing for DLD is not the recommended approach.

Speech articulation disorders may be found in isolation or in association with language disorders. Early articulation errors are common and usually mild. However, if there are other features, e.g., excessive drooling or inability to chew food properly, or if a child is not able to be understood virtually 100 percent of the time by age 4 years, this should raise concern about a more serious condition, such as oromotor apraxia. A thorough oral motor examination by the physician will identify apraxia in the severe cases. Milder forms may require a more extensive oral motor assessment by a speech pathologist or pediatric occupational therapist.

Box 45-3 Warning Signs of a Developmental Language Disorder

Limitations in Expressive Language

- Has feeding problems related to sucking, swallowing, and chewing
- Fails to vocalize to social stimuli and fails to vocalize two syllables at 8 months
- Produces few or no creative utterances of three words or more by age 3

Limitations in Vocabulary

- Has small repertoire of words understood or used, and acquires new words slowly or with difficulty

Limitations in Comprehending Language

- Relies too much on contextual cues to understand language

Limitations in Social Interaction

- Rarely interacts socially, except to have needs met

Limitations in Play

- Has not developed symbolic, imaginative play by age 3
- Does not play interactively with peers

Limitations in Learning Speech

- Expressive speech contains numerous articulation errors or is unintelligible to unfamiliar listeners

Limitations in Using Strategies for Language Learning

- Uses unusual or inappropriate strategies for age level, e.g., overuses imitation (echolalia), does not imitate verbalizations of others (dyspraxia), does not use questions for learning ("why" questions)

Limitations in Attention for Language Activities

- Shows little interest in book reading, talking, or communicating with peers

(Modified with permission from Nelson NW. Childhood Language Disorders in Context: Infancy through Adolescence. New York: Macmillan, 1993; Hall N. Developmental language disorders. Semin Pediatr Neurol 1997;4:77–85.)

Nosology of Developmental Language Disorders

The proper nosology of the DLDs is debated. The DSM-IV-TR [APA, 2000] subtypes of communication disorders (expressive language disorder, mixed receptive–expressive language disorder, phonological disorder, stuttering, and communication disorder, Not Otherwise Specified (NOS)) are rather nonspecific. The subtypes discussed here are more specific and focus on psycholinguistic features. The subtypes are named for the linguistic areas that are most problematic [Rapin, 1996; Table 45-1 and glossary of terms, Box 45-4) Depending on subtype, DLDs vary in their characteristic features, etiology, prognosis, and treatment response.

Articulation and Expressive Fluency Disorders

Pure Articulation Disorders

Articulatory skills improve with age and, as with language development, the normal range is considerable. Most children (70 percent) speak intelligibly by age 2 years. Unintelligible speech is the exception at age 3 years (15 percent). However, almost 50 percent of children at age 4 years still have articulation difficulties. A common problem is defective use of *th* or *r* sounds. At kindergarten entry, one-third of children still have minor to mild articulation defects, but speech is unintelligible in less than 5 percent.

Stuttering and Cluttering

Stuttering is a disorder in the rhythm of speech. The speaker knows what to say, but is unable to say it because of an involuntary, repetitive prolongation or cessation of a sound. Some

Box 45-4 Glossary of Terms used in Describing Linguistic Functions

Functors	The small words of the language, like prepositions, conjunctions, etc. These are also called closed-class words because they are limited in number
Lexicon	The words in a language; the dictionary of word meanings
Mean length of utterance (MLU)	The number of morphemes per utterance
Morpheme	The smallest meaningful unit in a language, occurring either in a word or as a word. A compound word, like "compounding," is made up of three morphemes: com-pound-ing. Prefixes, suffixes and inflected endings like -ed, -s, and -ly are also morphemes
Phoneme	A distinct sound unit in a language. In English, there are 46: 9 vowels and 37 consonants
Phonology	The rules a speaker follows when combining speech sounds
Pragmatics	The communicative intent of speech rather than its content, e.g. asking a question at the right time and in the right way
Prosody	The melody of language: the tone of voice used to ask questions, for example, or show emotion
Semantics	The meaning of words; their definition
Syntax	The grammar of a language; the acceptable relationship between words in a sentence

Table 45-1 Subtypes of Developmental Language Disorders

	Receptive Expressive Verbal Auditory Agnosia	Phonological Syntactic	Expressive Verbal Dyspraxia	Phonological Programming	Higher-Order Semantic Pragmatic	Lexical Syntactic
COMPREHENSION – RECEPTIVE						
Phonology	↓↓	↓				
Syntax	↓↓	↓				↓
Semantics	↓↓	?			↓↓	↓
PRODUCTION – EXPRESSIVE						
Semantics (lexical)	↓↓				↓↓	↓
Syntax	↓↓	↓↓	?	?		↓
Phonology	↓↓	↓↓	↓↓	↓		
Repetition	↓↓	↓	↓		↑	↓
Fluency	↓↓	↓	N1 or ↓	N1 or ↓	N1 or ↑	↓
Pragmatics	N1 or ↓	N1 or ↓			↓↓	↓

NI = normal; ↓ = impaired; ↓↓ = very impaired; ↑ = atypically enhanced; ? = unknown
(Modified from Nass R, Ross G. Disorders of higher cortical function in the preschooler. In: David R, ed. Child and Adolescent Neurology. St. Louis, MO: Mosby, 1997; Rapin I. Preschool Children with Inadequate Communication. London: Mackeith, 1996.)

degree of dysfluency is common as language skills evolve during the preschool years, particularly as the mean length of utterance (MLU) reaches 6–8 words between ages 3 and 4 years. However, stuttering, in contrast to developmental dysfluency, is probably a linguistic disorder (errors occur at grammatically important points in the sentence), as well as a motor planning problem [Logan, 2002]. Stuttering is often a genetic trait. Although the cause of developmental stuttering is unknown, the main theories are anomalous dominance and abnormalities of interhemispheric connections [Foundas et al., 2001]. Stuttering occurs more frequently in children with other DLDs and with mental retardation [Gordon, 2002]. Cluttering, by contrast, as seen in fragile X syndrome, is characterized by incomplete sentences and short outbursts of two- to three-word phrases, along with echolalia, palilalia (compulsive repetition reiterated with increasing rapidity and decreasing volume), perseveration, poor articulation, and stuttering.

Stuttering may provide a clue to the genetics of language disorders. For example, the typically observed onset of stuttering is between the ages of 3 and 6 years, and reports indicate natural, unassisted recovery rates of 75 percent [Yairi and Ambrose, 1999]. Thus, the prevalence of stuttering as a lifetime disorder is much lower than its incidence (0.5–1 percent vs. 4–5 percent, respectively; Bloodstein, 1995; Felsenfeld, 2002]. Yet childhood stuttering is a significant risk factor for other DLDs that develop later in life, even if stuttering disappears. It is possible that this "continuity" of developmental transformation is due to the presence of particular dimensions of the complex phenotypes common to all DLDs [Grigorenko, 2009].

Phonological Programming Disorder

Children with the phonological programming disorder have fluent speech, and their MLU approaches normal. Despite initially poor intelligibility, serviceable speech is expected. Language comprehension is relatively preserved. Most such children show delayed rather than deviant phonology, and improve 1–7 years after their preschool diagnosis. It is debatable whether this disorder is a severe articulation problem or a mild form of verbal dyspraxia [Shriberg and Kwiatkowski, 1994]. The fact that patients with the phonological programming disorder have more difficulty learning manual signs than do controls supports an association with dyspraxia [Bradford and Dodd, 1994; Bishop, 2002a]. A pre-remediation paired associate learning task may help select the best remediation method for each child because some are better with symbols and some with signs [Pearce et al., 1987]. An adult aphasia equivalent does not exist.

Verbal Dyspraxia

The speech of children with verbal dyspraxia [Nevo et al., 2001], also called dilapidated speech [Ferry et al., 1975], is extremely dysfluent. These children are unable to convert an abstract phonological representation into a set of motor commands to the articulators [Bishop, 1992], or, put in other terms they have a deficit in phonology–motor conversion [Thoonen et al., 1997]. Utterances are short and laboriously produced. Phonology is impaired and includes inconsistent omissions, substitutions, and distortions of speech sounds. Consonant substitutions can be divided into substitutions by place of articulation, manner of articulation, and voicing. Children with dysarthria make voicing errors that distort, while children with dyspraxia make place substitution errors [Maassen, 2004].

In conversation, they make phrasal errors [Maassen, 2004]. Syntactic skills are difficult to assess in the face of dysfluency. Language comprehension is relatively preserved, but many children do have noticeable receptive language problems. Many require speech and language therapy for prolonged periods. Children with verbal dyspraxia who do not develop intelligible speech by age 6 years are unlikely to acquire it later. The frequency with which nonverbal praxis deficits – buccal-lingual dyspraxia (e.g., positioning muscles of articulation) and generalized dyspraxia or clumsiness – coexist with verbal dyspraxia is unknown. The presence of a more diffuse disorder of praxis has significant therapeutic implications because children with verbal dyspraxia may depend on signing and writing skills for communication [Shriberg et al., 1997]. Developmental coordination disorder (DCD) is commonly comorbid with speech/language learning disabilities [Visscher et al., 2007]. Young children who are in early intervention programs for speech/language delays may have significant coordination difficulties that will become more evident at kindergarten age, when motor deficits begin to impact self-care and academic tasks [Gaines and Missiuna, 2007]. The use of nonspeech oral motor treatments (NSOMTs) in the management of apraxia is controversial. At this time there is no evidence to support their use [Powell, 2008]. Although often accompanied by other neurological symptoms, verbal dyspraxia most resembles the adult aphasia called aphemia.

Disorders of Receptive and Expressive Language

Phonological Syntactic Syndrome

Phonological syntactic syndrome (also called mixed receptive expressive disorder, expressive disorder, and nonspecific formulation-repetition deficit) is probably the most common DLD [Korkman and Hakkinen-Rihu, 1994]. The high frequency of this subtype is consistent with the view that impaired inflectional morphology is a hallmark of DLD [Rice and Wexler, 1996]. The phonological disturbances consist of omissions, substitutions, and distortions of consonants and consonant clusters in all word positions. The production of unpredictable and unrecognizable sounds makes speech impossible to understand. The syntactic impairment consists of a lack of functors and an absence of appropriate inflected endings. Plurals, third person singulars, past tense, auxiliary verb *be*, *the* and *a*, infinitives – to, and case markings on pronouns are particularly vulnerable. Grammatical forms are atypical, not just delayed. Whereas a typically developing young child may say "baby cry" or "a baby crying," children with the phonological syntactic syndrome produce deviant constructions, such as "the baby is cry." Telegraphic speech is common. The presence or absence of difficulties in other language areas is variable. Overall, comprehension is relatively, although not wholly, spared. Semantic skills tend to be intact. Repetition, pragmatics, and prosody may be normal. Autistic children with this DLD subtype produce a significant amount of jargon.

Neurological dysfunction is especially frequent in this DLD subtype. Feeding problems due to sucking, swallowing, and chewing difficulties are common, and drooling is often persistent. The neurological examination may reveal signs of pseudobulbar palsy, oromotor apraxia, hypertonia, and incoordination. This DLD most resembles Broca's aphasia in adults.

Verbal Auditory Agnosia

Despite intact hearing, meaningful language is not understood by children with verbal auditory agnosia (VAA) (also called generalized low performance and global dysfunction). VAA may occur on a developmental basis, and as an acquired disorder, the Landau–Kleffner syndrome [Billard et al., 2009]. VAA is common in low-functioning children with autism. VAA best supports the theory that DLDs result from difficulty with processing basic sensory information entering the nervous system in rapid succession [Tallal and Benasich, 2002].

The outcome from the developmental form of VAA is generally poor. The outcome from the acquired disorder is somewhat better with approximately one-third of patients having a good outcome. VAA is seen in adults with acquired bitemporal lesions.

Higher-Order Language Disorders

Semantic Pragmatic Syndrome

Children with the semantic pragmatic syndrome (also called repetition strength and comprehension deficit, language without cognition, and cocktail party syndrome in children with hydrocephalus usually with accompanying meningomyeloceles) are fluent speakers, even verbose. Vocabulary is often large and somewhat formal. Parents are often encouraged by the child's sizeable vocabulary, only to find later that the verbosity did not indicate superior cognitive skills. Many children have trouble with meaningful conversation and informative exchange of ideas. They talk to talk. Pragmatic skills are lacking. Children with semantic pragmatic syndrome often show deficits in prosody; their speech has a monotonous, mechanical, or sing-song quality. They cannot convey the additional pragmatic intentions that prosody affords, such as speaking with the proper emotion or indicating by tone of voice that they are asking a question. Comprehension may be impaired. Phonological and syntactic skills are generally intact [Rapin and Allen, 1998]. Semantic pragmatic syndrome is often seen in higher-functioning autistic children [Bishop, 2002a].

Repetition strength in the setting of fluent speech with impaired comprehension characterizes the adult aphasia syndrome of transcortical sensory aphasia. Difficulties with prosody and pragmatics suggest right hemisphere dysfunction.

Lexical Syntactic Syndrome

The lexical syntactic syndrome is relatively common, occurring in approximately 15 percent of children with DLD. Speech is generally dysfluent, even to the point of stuttering, because of word-finding difficulties and poor syntactic skills, with many hesitancies and false starts. Both literal and semantic paraphasias are common. Lexical deficits may not be specific to this DLD subtype. Most children with DLD have delays in word acquisition and less lexical diversity than their age-matched counterparts. Verbs appear to be the most difficult lexical category for them to learn. Some have questioned whether their difficulties with verbs cause collateral damage, i.e., contribute to syntactic problems [Leonard and Deevy, 2004]. Syntax is immature but not deviant. Phonology is spared, and therefore speech is intelligible. Repetition is generally better than spontaneous speech. In conversation, idiom use is better than spontaneous speech. During narratives fourth-graders with DLD evidence higher disruption rates at phrase boundaries than do their age-matched peers, reflecting the lexical and syntactic deficits in children with DLD [Guo et al., 2008]. Pragmatics may be impaired, particularly when this syndrome occurs in autistic children. Comprehension is generally acceptable, although complex questions and other linguistic forms taxing higher-level receptive syntactic skills are often deficient.

No clear counterpart for the lexical syntactic syndrome exists among the acquired aphasias of adulthood, despite overlap with anomic aphasia, conduction aphasia, and transcortical aphasia.

Outcome of Developmental Language Disorders

The occurrence of a DLD, even when it appears to resolve, may affect later social-emotional adjustment, educational achievement, and vocational choices. Short- and long-term behavioral, social-emotional, and psychiatric problems are associated with early language problems [Irwin et al., 2002; Jerome et al., 2002]. Language delays were not associated with behavior problems among toddlers, except that toddlers aged 18–30 months with language delays appeared to show elevated social withdrawal relative to typically developing toddlers [Rescorla et al., 2007]. Using data from Child Behavior Checklists completed by teachers and parents, Coster et al. [1999] found that behavior problems were common in DLD children in elementary school, occurring in 32 percent of their sample, and those problems tended to be internalizing rather than externalizing.

Emotional and behavioral problems often surface as DLD children enter school. In school-age children with speech and language problems, the frequency of ADHD ranges from 30 to 49 percent, and the frequency of behavioral and emotional problems ranges from 10–22 percent to 50 percent [Beitchman et al., 1996; Cantwell and Baker, 1987]. The incidence of dyslexia and other learning disabilities in children earlier diagnosed with DLD is up to 50 percent in some studies [Eisenmajer et al., 2005]. Children with early language impairment had higher rates of anxiety disorder (particularly social phobia) and antisocial personality disorder in young adulthood compared with nonimpaired children. The majority of participants with anxiety disorders had a diagnosis of social phobia. Trends were found toward associations between language impairment and overall and antisocial personality disorder rates [Beitchman et al., 2001]. In some, but not all, studies the biggest differentiating factor between those with and those without a psychiatric diagnosis was the degree of language deficit [Cantwell and Baker, 1987; Beitchman et al., 2001]. In preschool children with DLD, nonverbal intelligence is the best single predictor of overall long-term outcome, and severity of language problems is the best predictor of later language skills. Preschool language skills are the best single predictor of later reading ability and disability [Aram and Nation, 1980]. Even children with good receptive skills who speak late may be at risk for continuing subtle language difficulties and later reading and language-based academic difficulties [Rescorla et al., 1997]. Thus, both screening and follow-up studies of children with DLD are important. Persisting, although often subtle, language or communication problems in adolescence and beyond have been reported in as many as 90 percent of individuals with earlier diagnosed DLD [Conti-Ramsden et al., 2001; Rescorla,

2002, Young et al., 2002]. Follow-up of 112 individuals with DLD into adult life demonstrated lower levels of functioning in the areas of communication, educational attainment, and occupational status compared with their typical peers [Johnson et al., 2009]. Interestingly, the adults with DLD did not perceive their quality of life to be worse than that of their peers. Such studies, however, do indicate the need for continued surveillance of individuals with DLD and adequate guidance in terms of academic and career choices.

Evaluation of the Child with Suspected DLD

The differential diagnosis of a child with language impairment is listed in Box 45-5. The work-up of the child with a DLD (Box 45-6) must include an assessment of hearing and an

---

Box 45-5 Differential Diagnosis of Language Delay/Disorder

- Hearing loss
- Mental retardation
- Severe oral motor dysfunction
- Autistic spectrum disorders
- Developmental language impairment
- Selective mutism
- Other psychiatric disorders
- Landau–Kleffner syndrome/epileptic encephalopathies

Box 45-6 Evaluation of a Child with Suspected Language Disorder

- Complete neurodevelopmental and family history and neurological examination (including social interaction and communicative behaviors)
- Hearing test
- Office developmental screen (e.g., Denver Developmental Test [Frankenburg et al., 1992], McArthur Communicative Development Inventory [Fenson et al., 1993]; Children's Communication Checklist [Norbury et al., 2004]; Peabody Picture Vocabulary Test [Dunn and Dunn, 2001]; Preschool language scale [Zimmerman et al., 2011]; Early Language Milestones [Coplan et al., 2006]) may be helpful
- Psychometric testing to establish general cognitive function (a nonverbal intelligence test such as the Leiter International Performance Scale – Revised or the Test of Non-Verbal Intelligence-P:4 or I:3 [TONI-P:4, Brown et al., 2010] is most appropriate in a language-impaired child)
- Depending on history and examination, other tests to consider:
  - Sleep EEG
  - Overnight video EEG monitoring
  - MRI of brain
  - Karyotype, fragile X chromosome or DNA study, fluorescent in situ hydridization (FISH) probes
  - Metabolic screen (e.g., urine organic acids, blood amino acids)

---

assessment of overall level of cognitive functioning. A number of metabolic disorders can present with isolated language disorders, so in some circumstances a metabolic screen is appropriate [Vodopiutz et al., 2007]. Mitochondrial disorders, as well as organic acidemias, may have language impairment as their primary feature, particularly in the first few years of life. Mucopolysaccharidosis type III (Sanfilippo Syndrome), as well as juvenile Tay–Sachs disease, may present early with what appears to be an isolated language delay. Those children will eventually develop progressive neurologic deterioration, but initially such conditions should be considered in the differential diagnosis of a child with unexplained language delay. Similarly, some other syndromes present with predominantly language issues in association with their distinctive dysmorphic features [Nass and Frank, 2010]. Children with congenital cleft palate and those with velocardiofacial syndrome may have specific language impairments not explained solely by the facial deformity [Goorhuis-Brouwer et al., 2003; Priester and Goorhuis-Brouwer, 2008].

There is no indication for an EEG or imaging studies in a child with DLD unless there is a history of a language regression, abnormal findings on the neurological examination, or an indication that the child might have seizures.

Treatment

Whether intensive early therapy changes the long-term outcome to an appreciable degree remains to be determined [Tyler, 2002; Forrest, 2002; Warren and Yoder, 2004]. Treatment of language-disordered preschool children varies according to the kind of language impairment, as well as its degree of severity. Children with a moderate to severe language impairment, who suffer associated social, cognitive, and behavioral difficulties, are best treated in a therapeutic nursery or special education preschool for language-impaired children. Mildly impaired children can often do well in a regular nursery program combined with individual speech-language therapy. Play materials are used by the speech-language therapist with the preschool child in a directive way. Every activity becomes a language activity, in that the child's actions are given words by the therapist. Play activities are also a helpful way to engage children with severe expressive difficulties. Pleasurable activities involving the mouth, such as blowing bubbles, or initiating mouth movements and sounds, as well as nonvocal imitative games, such as hand clapping, have been found to foster language acquisition. Formal language work typically begins at the phonologic level, involving repetition of sounds and sound sequences to encourage fluency. Treatment of receptive disorders often necessitates the use of visual modalities, such as signs and gesture. Less severe disorders of comprehension are addressed through practiced structuring of conversations with the child. Developmental language-disordered children with severe comprehension deficits rarely progress in treatment as well as children with primary expressive disorders.

Another focus for language remediation is driven by different theoretical frameworks [Dunn, 1997]. One approach involves identifying specific linguistic deficits (e.g., problems with morphology) and targeting them for remediation. Another approach involves identifying specific DLD subtypes and addressing them in remediation [Law, 2004]. This approach means, for example, that a child's level of comprehension is taken into account in selecting a strategy for improving language production. A third approach aims to detect a core cognitive processing deficit to be targeted for intervention. A fourth approach emphasizes the neuropsychological profile. In contrast to the other approaches, which are deficit-centered, the neuropsychological approach defines and uses children's strengths to remediate their weaknesses; it also takes into account the child's temperament and neurodevelopmental status to determine their learning styles and develop optimal methods for remediating targeted deficits. To date, no formal study has compared the efficacy of these approaches.

In the classroom, some accommodations may be necessary in order for the child with DLD to succeed. Children with DLD may have associated ADHD and/or learning disabilities, and may require additional help from a resource specialist or tutor. They may require additional time for giving reports and for taking tests. Whenever possible, presentation of oral information should be accompanied by visual aids. In support of previous research, children with DLD have problems with inferencing, linking directly observed or stated information to likely outcomes. They also have limited working memory capacity, and they are more likely to make errors related to inattention. In a recent study, narrative abilities of 6-year-old children were linked to their verbal working memory [Dodwell et al., 2008]. The information the DLD group heard was harder to access than information they had been able to generate themselves based on a series of pictures. Such findings suggest that children with DLD are likely to be at a disadvantage in classroom situations, particularly for information presented aurally and if the information is complex. The use of pictorial aids may help them encode the information. They may also benefit from having information broken into manageable (shorter) units.

When necessary, medications for treatment of ADHD should be considered. Since there is a high incidence of secondary emotional problems and self-esteem issues associated with DLD, referral for psychological counseling should be considered as soon as these problems become apparent. Families should be informed about their child's condition and be encouraged to provide a positive and supportive environment. A multidisciplinary approach, including physician, speech-language pathologist, teacher, psychologist, and parents, provides the most effective means of helping children with DLD.

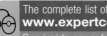

The complete list of references for this chapter is available online at **www.expertconsult.com**.
See inside cover for registration details.

Dyslexia

Sally E. Shaywitz and Bennett A. Shaywitz

Developmental dyslexia (or specific reading disability) is defined as an unexpected difficulty in accuracy or fluency of reading for an individual's chronological age, intelligence, level of education, or professional status. Dyslexia is, at its core, a problem with phonological processing: that is, getting to the elemental sounds of spoken language, affecting both spoken and written language. As a consequence, individuals who are dyslexic require accommodations for their lack of reading and/or oral fluency. As dyslexic children progress in school, given good instruction, reading accuracy often improves; however, lack of fluency persists and remains a lifelong problem. Dyslexia is the most common and most comprehensively studied of the learning disabilities, affecting 80 percent of all individuals identified as learning-disabled. Historically, dyslexia in adults was first observed in the latter half of the 19th century, and developmental dyslexia in children was first reported in 1896 [Morgan, 1896]. Although the diagnosis and implications of dyslexia were often uncertain in the past, advances in our knowledge of the epidemiologic, neurobiologic, and cognitive influences on the disorder allow it to be approached within the framework of a traditional medical model. This chapter reviews these advances and their implications for the approach to children and adults with dyslexia.

Definition

Perhaps the most consistent and enduring core of the definition is the concept of dyslexia as an unexpected difficulty in reading. "Unexpected" refers to the presence of a reading difficulty in a child (or adult) who appears to have all of the factors (intelligence, motivation, exposure to reasonable reading instruction) present to be a good reader but who continues to struggle [Shaywitz, 1998]. Recent evidence provides empiric support for defining dyslexia as an unexpected difficulty in reading. Using data from the Connecticut Longitudinal Study, we [Ferrer et al., 2010] demonstrated that, in typical readers, reading and IQ development are dynamically linked over time. Not only do reading and IQ track together over time, they also influence one another. Such mutual interrelationships are not perceptible in dyslexic readers, suggesting that reading and cognition develop more independently in these individuals (Figure 46-1). These findings provide the first empirical demonstration of a coupling between cognition and reading in typical readers, confirming the general public perception that if you are a good reader, you are likely to be very intelligent and, conversely, if you struggle to read, you may be less intelligent. These new data demonstrating a developmental uncoupling between cognition and reading in dyslexic readers

indicate that dyslexia is a special case that violates the assumption that reading and IQ are always linked, and confirm that, in dyslexia, one can be highly intelligent and still struggle to read.

Our findings of an uncoupling between IQ and reading in dyslexia, and the influence of this uncoupling on the developmental trajectory of reading, provide evidence to support the conceptual basis of dyslexia as an unexpected difficulty in reading in children who otherwise have the intelligence to learn to read but struggle to read fluently. Based on dynamic models, the uncoupling of reading and cognition observed demonstrates that, in the special case of dyslexia, a child or adult can be both bright and accomplished along with a much lower level of reading than expected for a person of that level of intelligence, education, or professional status. It also demonstrates that, in dyslexia, the reading difficulty is unexpected for an *individual's* level of intelligence or education; that is, the difficulty is defined as a disparity existing *within* the individual. The implication is that, for individuals who are dyslexic, the appropriate comparison is between a person's ability and his/her reading. Thus, in dyslexia, a highly intelligent person may read at a level above average but below that expected, based on his/her intelligence, education, or accomplishments. These new findings provide an explanation for the "unexpected" nature of developmental dyslexia and also supply the long-sought empirical evidence for the seeming paradox involving cognition and reading in individuals with developmental dyslexia.

More challenging has been the question of how to operationalize the unexpected nature of dyslexia. Thus, using differing methods and criteria, definitions have attempted to capture the "unexpected" nature of dyslexia by requiring a discrepancy of a certain degree between a child's measured IQ and his reading achievement. For example, schools have typically relied on criteria based on an absolute discrepancy, most commonly one or one-and-one-half standard deviations between standard scores on IQ and reading tests. We want to emphasize that the difficulty has been not with the concept of a disparity, but rather with the real-life practical effect of implementing this model in a primary school setting. For example, children who were clearly struggling as early as kindergarten or first grade had to wait, often until third grade or later, until their failure in reading was of such a magnitude that they met discrepancy requirements. Attempts to clarify the criteria by meta-analyses comparing discrepant to simply low-achieving poor readers (defined on the basis of a reading score below a certain cut point, e.g., below a standard score of 90) find overlap between the two groups on reading-related constructs but differences on IQ-related measures [Stuebing et al., 2002].

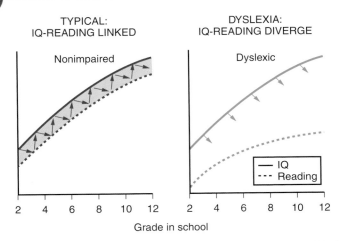

Fig. 46-1 Uncoupling of reading and IQ over time: empirical evidence for a definition of dyslexia. Left, In typical readers, reading and IQ development are dynamically linked over time. Right, In contrast, dyslexic readers, shows that reading and IQ development are dissociated and one does not influence the other. *(Data adapted from Ferrer E et al. Uncoupling of reading and IQ over time: empirical evidence for a definition of dyslexia. Psychological Science; 2010.)*

In addition, studies examining growth curve models for low-achieving and discrepant readers indicate comparable reading plateaus (level of reading achievement) reached by the two groups but with the IQ-discrepant readers showing the lowest achievement level at any IQ level during the school years [Francis et al., 1996]. Not only do poor readers identified by either discrepancy or low-achievement criteria resemble one another on measures of reading and growth rates of reading, but each group also differs along multiple dimensions from groups of typically achieving boys and girls [Lyon et al., 2001].

These findings have strong educational implications. It is not valid to deny the education services available for disabled or at-risk readers either to low-achieving, nondiscrepant children, or to those children who are not low-achieving but who, at the same time, are reading below a level expected for their ability. The observed similarity of the discrepant and low-achieving groups in reading-related constructs argues for identification approaches that include both low-achieving children and those struggling readers who are discrepant but who do not satisfy an arbitrary cut point for designation as low-achieving. Seventy-five percent of children identified by discrepancy criteria also meet low-achievement criteria in reading; the remaining 25 percent who meet only discrepancy criteria may fail to be identified and yet still be struggling to read [Shaywitz et al., 1992].

Difficulties in identifying younger children based solely on a discrepancy score bring into focus the fact that dyslexia, as most other disorders in medicine, is a clinical diagnosis. Accordingly, while it may not yet be possible to demonstrate a quantitative disparity between ability and achievement in the lowest grades, it is still possible to demonstrate the fundamental concept of an unexpected difficulty in reading. Here, a history of core symptoms (weaknesses and strengths, see below), observation of oral reading demonstrating inaccurate and lack of fluent reading, and cognitive and psychological processing test scores indicating reading and, particularly in younger children, phonological processing difficulties (as well

as strengths discussed below) should provide the necessary evidence to diagnose dyslexia. Dyslexia is neither diagnosed nor accurately represented by a single score on a test, but by consideration of a broader clinical picture conforming to the known characteristics of the disorder.

Epidemiology

Epidemiologic data indicate that, like hypertension and obesity, dyslexia fits a dimensional model. Within the population, reading ability and reading disability occur along a continuum, with reading disability representing the lower tail of a normal distribution of reading ability [Shaywitz et al., 1992]. Dyslexia is perhaps the most common neurobehavioral disorder affecting children, with prevalence rates ranging from 5 to 17.5 percent [Interagency Committee on Learning Disabilities, 1987; Shaywitz, 2003]. Longitudinal studies, prospective [Francis et al., 1996; Shaywitz et al., 1999] and retrospective [Bruck, 1992; Felton et al., 1990], indicate that dyslexia is a persistent, chronic condition; it does not represent a transient developmental lag (Figure 46-2). Over time, poor readers and good readers tend to maintain their relative positions along the spectrum of reading ability [Francis et al., 1996; Shaywitz et al., 1995].

Etiology

Dyslexia is both familial and heritable [Pennington and Gilger, 1996]. Family history is one of the most important risk factors, with 23–65 percent of children who have a parent with dyslexia reported to have the disorder [Scarborough, 1990]. A rate among siblings of affected persons of approximately 40 percent and among parents of 27–49 percent [Pennington and Gilger, 1996] provides opportunities for early identification of affected

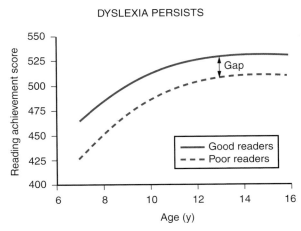

Fig. 46-2 Trajectory of reading skills over time in nonimpaired and dyslexic readers. Numbers on the ordinate are Rasch scores (W scores) from the Woodcock–Johnson reading test [Woodcock and Johnson, 1989], and numbers on the abscissa are ages in years. Dyslexic and nonimpaired readers improve their reading scores as they get older, but the gap between the dyslexic and nonimpaired readers remains. Dyslexia is a deficit, not a developmental lag. *(Adapted from Shaywitz S. Overcoming dyslexia: A new and complete science-based program for reading problems at any level. New York: Alfred A. Knopf, 2003. Copyright 2003 by S. Shaywitz. Adapted with permission.)*

siblings and often for delayed but helpful identification of affected adults. Given that dyslexia is familial and heritable, initial hopes that dyslexia would be explained by one or just a few genes have been disappointing. Thus, along with a great many common diseases, genome-wide association studies (GWAS) in dyslexia have so far identified genetic variants that account for only a very small percentage of the risk – less than 1 percent [Meaburn et al., 2008]. Current evidence suggests "that common diseases involve thousands of genes and proteins interacting on complex pathways" [Duncan, 2009], and that, similar to experience with other complex disorders (heart disease, diabetes), it is unlikely that a single gene or even a few genes will identify people with dyslexia. Rather, dyslexia is best explained by *multiple* genes, each contributing a *small* amount of the variance. Thus, current evidence suggests that the etiology of dyslexia is best conceptualized within a multifactorial model, with multiple genetic and environmental risk and protective factors leading to dyslexia.

Cognitive Influences

Among investigators in the field, there is a strong consensus supporting the phonologic theory. This theory recognizes that speech is natural and inherent, but that reading is acquired and must be taught. To read, the beginning reader must connect the letters and letter strings (i.e., the orthography) to something that already has inherent meaning – the sounds of spoken language. In the process, a child has to develop the insight that spoken words can be pulled apart into the elemental particles of speech (i.e., phonemes) and that the letters in a written word represent these sounds [Shaywitz, 2003]; such awareness is largely deficient in dyslexic children and adults [Liberman and Shankweiler, 1991; Shankweiler et al., 1979; Shaywitz, 2003]. Results from large and well-studied populations with reading disability confirm that, in young school-age children [Stanovich and Siegel, 1994] and in adolescents [Shaywitz et al., 1999], a deficit in phonology represents the most robust and specific correlate of reading disability [Morris et al., 1998; Ramus et al., 2003]. Such findings form the basis for the most successful and evidence-based interventions designed to improve reading [Report, 2000].

Implications of the Phonologic Model of Dyslexia

Reading comprises two main processes: decoding and comprehension [Gough and Tunmer, 1986]. In dyslexia, a deficit at the level of the phonologic module impairs the ability to segment the spoken word into its underlying phonologic elements. As a result, the reader experiences difficulty, initially in spoken language and then in written language. The phonologic deficit is domain-specific; that is, it is independent of other, nonphonologic abilities. In particular, the higher-order cognitive and linguistic functions involved in comprehension, such as general intelligence and reasoning, vocabulary [Share and Stanovich, 1995], and syntax [Shankweiler et al., 1995], are generally intact. This pattern – a deficit in phonologic analysis contrasted with intact higher-order cognitive abilities – offers an explanation for the paradox of otherwise intelligent, often gifted people who experience great difficulty in reading [Ferrer et al., 2010; Shaywitz, 1996, 2003].

Neurobiologic Studies

Neural Systems for Reading

Our understanding of the neural systems for reading emerged more than a century ago, with descriptions of adults who (usually due to a stroke) suddenly lost their ability to read, a condition termed acquired alexia. These postmortem studies, pioneered by Dejerine as early as 1891, suggested that a portion of the left posterior brain region (which includes the angular gyrus and supramarginal gyrus in the inferior parietal lobule and the posterior aspect of the superior temporal gyrus) is critical for reading [Dejerine, 1891]. Another left posterior brain region, one more ventral in the occipito-temporal area, was also described by Dejerine [Dejerine, 1892] as critical in reading. Within the last two decades, the development of functional brain imaging, particularly functional magnetic resonance imaging (fMRI), has provided the most consistent and replicable data on the location of the neural systems for reading and how they differ in dyslexic readers. fMRI is noninvasive and safe, and can be used repeatedly, properties which make it ideal for studying people, especially children. The signal used to construct MRI images derives from the determination of the blood oxygen level-dependent (BOLD) response; the increase in BOLD signal in regions that are activated by a stimulus or task results from the combined effects of increases in the tissue blood flow, volume and oxygenation, and in cognitive tasks the changes are typically in the order of 1–5 percent. Details of fMRI are reviewed in Anderson and Gore [1997], Frackowiak et al. [2004], and Jezzard et al. [2001]. To date, fMRI in dyslexic individuals can be carried out reliably only at a group level. The technology for determining brain activation at an individual subject level remains a work in progress.

Reflecting the language basis for reading and dyslexia, three neural systems critical in reading and dyslexia are localized in the left hemisphere (Figure 46-3): two left hemisphere

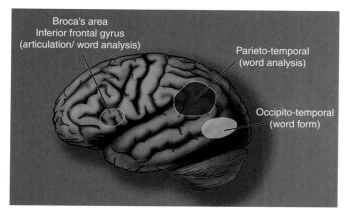

Broca's area
Inferior frontal gyrus
(articulation/ word analysis)

Parieto-temporal
(word analysis)

Occipito-temporal
(word form)

© Sally Shaywitz, *Overcoming Dyslexia*, 2003

Fig. 46-3 Neural systems for reading. Three neural systems for reading are illustrated for the surface of the left hemisphere: an anterior system in the region of the inferior frontal gyrus (Broca's area), which is believed to serve articulation and word analysis, and two posterior systems, one in the occipito-temporal region, which is believed to serve word analysis, and a second in the occipito-temporal region (the word-form area), which is believed to serve for the rapid, automatic, fluent identification of words. *(Adapted from Shaywitz S. Overcoming dyslexia: A new and complete science-based program for reading problems at any level. New York: Alfred A. Knopf, 2003. Copyright 2003 by S. Shaywitz. Adapted with permission.)*

posterior systems, one around the occipito-temporal region and another in the left occipito-temporal region, and an anterior system around the inferior frontal gyrus (Broca's area) [Brambati et al., 2006; Helenius et al., 1999; Kronbichler et al., 2006; Nakamura et al., 2006; Paulesu et al., 2001; Shaywitz et al., 2002; Shaywitz et al., 2003; Shaywitz et al., 1998].

Many brain imaging studies in children and adults with developmental dyslexia (see below) have documented the importance of the left occipito-temporal system in reading, and its properties involving word analysis, operating on individual units of words (e.g., phonemes). In our figure we refer to the occipito-temporal system, which encompasses portions of the supramarginal gyrus in the inferior parietal lobule, portions of the posterior aspect of the superior temporal gyrus, and in some studies, may even encompass portions of the angular gyrus in the parietal lobe. The second posterior reading system is localized in the left occipito-temporal area, which Cohen and Dehaene have termed the visual word-form area (VWFA) [Cohen et al., 2000; Dehaene et al., 2005; Vinckier et al., 2007]. Just how the VWFA functions to integrate phonology (sounds) and orthography (print) is as yet unknown, though some have suggested that visual familiarity, phonological processing, and semantic processing all make significant but different contributions to activation of the word-form region [Cohen et al., 2004; Henry et al., 2005; Johnson and Rayner, 2007; Xue et al., 2006]. Still another reading-related neural circuit involves an anterior system in the left inferior frontal gyrus (Broca's area), a system that has long been associated with articulation and also serves an important function in word analysis [Fiez and Peterson, 1998; Frackowiak et al., 2004].

The Reading Systems in Dyslexia in Children and Adults

Converging evidence from many laboratories around the world has demonstrated what has been termed "a neural signature for dyslexia": that is, inefficient functioning of left posterior reading systems during reading real words and pseudowords, and often what has been considered as compensatory overactivation in other parts of the reading system. This evidence from functional brain imaging has, for the first time, made visible what previously was a hidden disability (Figure 46-4).

For example, in a study from our own research group, we [Shaywitz et al., 2002] used fMRI to study 144 dyslexic and nonimpaired boys and girls as they read pseudowords and real words. Our results indicated significantly greater activation in typical readers than in dyslexic readers during phonologic analysis in the posterior reading systems. Our data converge with reports from many investigators using functional brain imaging in dyslexia that show a failure of left hemisphere posterior brain systems to function properly during reading (reviewed in Richlan et al. [2009]; Shaywitz and Shaywitz [2005]). Recent studies report similar findings in German [Kronbichler et al., 2006] and Italian [Brambati et al., 2006] dyslexic readers.

Development of Reading Systems in Dyslexia

While converging evidence points to three important neural systems for reading, few studies have examined age-related changes in these systems in typical readers or in dyslexic

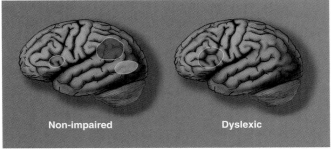

© Sally Shaywitz, *Overcoming Dyslexia*, 2003

Fig. 46-4 Neural signature for dyslexia. A neural signature for dyslexia is illustrated in this schematic view of left hemisphere brain systems in (left) nonimpaired and (right) dyslexic readers. In typical readers, the three systems provided in Figure 46-3 are shown. In dyslexic readers, the anterior system is slightly overactivated compared with systems of typical readers; in contrast, the two posterior systems are underactivated. This pattern of underactivation in left posterior reading systems is referred to as the neural signature for dyslexia. *(Adapted from Shaywitz S. Overcoming dyslexia: A new and complete science-based program for reading problems at any level. New York: Alfred A. Knopf, 2003. Copyright 2003 by S. Shaywitz. Adapted with permission.)*

children. We [Shaywitz et al., 2007] used fMRI to study age-related changes in reading in a cross-sectional study of 232 dyslexic and nonimpaired boys and girls as they read pseudowords. Findings indicated that the neural systems for reading that develop with age in typical readers differ from those that develop in dyslexic readers. Specifically, a system for reading that develops with age in dyslexic readers involves a more posterior and medial system, in contrast to a more anterior and lateral system within the left occipito-temporal area in typical readers. Interestingly, this difference in activation patterns between the two groups of readers has parallels to reported brain activation differences observed during reading of two Japanese writing systems: Kana and Kanji. Left anterior lateral occipito-temporal activation, similar to that seen in typical readers, occurred during reading Kana [Nakamura et al., 2005]. Kana script employs symbols that are linked to the sound or phonologic element (comparable to English and other alphabetic scripts). In Kana and in alphabetic scripts, children initially learn to read words by learning how letters and sounds are linked and then, over time, these linkages are integrated and permanently instantiated as a word form.

In contrast, posterior medial occipito-temporal activation, comparable to that observed in dyslexic readers, was noted during reading of Kanji script [Nakamura et al., 2005]. Consideration of the mechanisms used for reading Kanji compared to Kana provides insights into potentially different mechanisms that develop with age in dyslexic contrasted to typical readers. Kanji script uses ideographs where each character must be memorized, suggesting that the left posterior medial occipito-temporal system functions as a memory-based system. It is reasonable to suppose that, as dyslexic children mature, this posterior medial system supports memorization rather than the progressive sound–symbol linkages observed in typical readers. There is also evidence that, as they mature, dyslexic readers are not able to make good use of sound–symbol linkages and, instead, come to rely on memorized words. For example, phonologic deficits continue to characterize struggling readers even as they enter adolescence and adult life [Bruck, 1992; Shaywitz et al., 1999], and persistently poor adult readers read words by memorization so that they are able to read familiar words but have difficulty reading unfamiliar words [Shaywitz et al., 2003].

Thus, these results support and now extend previous findings to indicate that the system responsible for the integration of letters and sounds, the left anterior lateral occipito-temporal system, is the neural circuit that develops with age in typical readers. And conversely, dyslexic readers, who struggle to read new or unfamiliar words, come to rely on an alternate system, the left posterior medial occipito-temporal system, that functions via memory networks.

Furthermore, functional brain imaging has provided, for the first time, evidence demonstrating that dyslexic readers require the accommodation of extra time on high-stakes standardized tests. Thus, although dyslexic readers exhibit an inefficiency of functioning in the left occipito-temporal word-form area, they appear to develop ancillary systems involving areas around the inferior frontal gyrus in both hemispheres, as well as the right hemisphere homolog of the left occipito-temporal word-form area [Shaywitz et al., 2002]. While these ancillary systems allow the dyslexic reader to read accurately, dyslexic readers continue to read nonfluently. Inefficient functioning in this system for skilled reading has very important practical implications for the dyslexic reader – it provides the neurobiological evidence for the biologic necessity for the accommodation of additional time on high-stakes tests (Figure 46-5).

Implications of Brain Imaging Studies

The brain imaging studies reviewed above provide neurobiological evidence that illuminates and clarifies current understanding of the nature of dyslexia and its treatment. For example, brain imaging has taken dyslexia from what had previously been considered a hidden disability to one that is visible; the findings

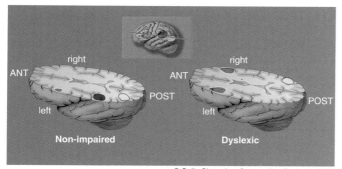

© Sally Shaywitz, *Overcoming Dyslexia*, 2003

Fig. 46-5 Compensatory neural systems and the neural basis for the requirement for extended time for dyslexic students on high-stakes testing. The image is a cutaway view of the brain showing the left and right hemispheres. Typical readers activate three left hemisphere neural systems for reading: an anterior system and two posterior systems. Dyslexic readers have inefficient functioning in the left hemisphere posterior neural systems for reading, but compensate by developing anterior systems in the left and right hemispheres and the posterior homolog of the visual word-form area in the right hemisphere. *(Adapted from Shaywitz S. Overcoming dyslexia: A new and complete science-based program for reading problems at any level. New York: Alfred A. Knopf, 2003. Copyright 2003 by S. Shaywitz. Adapted with permission.)*

of inefficient functioning in posterior reading systems are often referred to as a "neural signature for dyslexia." These findings should eliminate any thoughts of whether dyslexia is real or a "valid" diagnosis; even more so, these cutting-edge converging data from imaging laboratories worldwide should encourage the use of the word dyslexia, for it has meaning and relevance at levels reaching to the basic neural architecture in reading and its inefficient functioning in struggling readers. These findings, too, are universal, having been demonstrated in readers of English and other alphabetic scripts with very similar findings in readers of logographic languages as well.

Diagnosis

At all ages, dyslexia is a clinical diagnosis. The clinician seeks to determine, through history, observation, and psychometric assessment, if there are unexpected difficulties in reading (i.e., difficulties in reading that are unexpected for the person's age, intelligence, or level of education or professional status) and associated linguistic problems at the level of phonologic processing. There is no one single test score that is pathognomonic of dyslexia. As with any other medical diagnosis, the diagnosis of dyslexia should reflect a thoughtful synthesis of all the clinical data available. Dyslexia is distinguished from other disorders that may prominently feature reading difficulties by the unique, circumscribed nature of the phonologic deficit, one not intruding into other linguistic or cognitive domains.

Reflecting the core phonological deficit, a range of downstream effects is observed in spoken, as well as in written, language. In the young child, problems with spoken language include late speaking, mispronunciations, and confusing words that sound alike, such as saying "recession" when the individual meant to say "reception." In bright young adults, problems with spoken language often take the form of difficulties with word retrieval, such as needing time to summon an oral response, or difficulties in not appearing glib, in making subtle mispronunciations, or in avoiding using words that the individual knows but is fearful of mispronouncing when speaking. As a consequence, a dyslexic individual's spoken vocabulary is often considerably smaller than his/her listening vocabulary. These spoken language difficulties are a problem especially during high-stakes oral examinations, where the dyslexic young adult's difficulty in oral fluency is intrepreted by the examiner as not knowing the material, when, in fact, he knows the material very well.

In the preschool child, a history of language delay or of not attending to the sounds of words (e.g., trouble learning nursery rhymes or playing rhyming games with words, confusing words that sound alike, mispronouncing words) and trouble learning to recognize the letters of the alphabet, along with a positive family history, represent important risk factors for dyslexia. In the school-aged child, presenting complaints most commonly center on school performance – "she's not doing well in school" – and often parents (and teachers) do not appreciate that the reason is a reading difficulty. A typical picture is that of a child who may have had a delay in speaking, does not learn letters by kindergarten, has not begun to learn to read by first grade, and has difficulty consistently sounding out words. The child progressively falls behind, with teachers and parents puzzled about why such an intelligent child may have difficulty learning to read. The reading difficulty is unexpected with respect to the child's ability, age, or grade. Even after acquiring decoding skills, the child typically remains a slow reader. Bright dyslexic children may laboriously learn how to read words accurately, but they do not become fluent readers because they do not recognize words rapidly and automatically. Dysgraphia and spelling difficulties are often present and accompanied by laborious note-taking. Self-esteem is frequently affected, particularly if the disorder has gone undetected for a long period (Box 46-1) [Shaywitz, 2003].

In an accomplished adolescent or young adult, dyslexia is often reflected by slowness in reading or choppy reading aloud that is unexpected in relation to the level of education or professional status, such as graduation from a competitive college or completion of medical school and a residency. In bright adolescents and young adults, a history of phonologically based reading difficulties, requirements for extra time on tests, and current slow and effortful reading (i.e., signs of a lack of automaticity in reading) are the sine qua non of a diagnosis of dyslexia. In summary, at all ages, a history of difficulties getting to the basic sounds of spoken language, of laborious and slow reading and writing, of poor spelling, and of requiring additional time in reading and in taking tests provides indisputable evidence of a deficiency in phonologic processing, which serves as the basis for and the signature of a reading disability.

Dyslexia is conceptualized as fitting what is referred to as a "sea of strengths" model, with strengths in higher cognitive functions surrounding the weakness in phonological awareness and fluent reading [Shaywitz, 2003]. Thus, the same individual who struggles to retrieve words and reads slowly with effort may have significant strengths in conceptual abilities, problem-solving, verbal reasoning, the ability to grasp the big picture, and what has been referred to as creative

or out-of-the-box thinking. Indeed, it is just these higher-level strengths that make it imperative for individuals who have dyslexia to receive the accommodations (e.g., extra time) they require in order to demonstrate their abilities.

Assessment of Pre-reading and Reading

Even before the time at which a child is expected to read, a child's readiness to read or at-risk status for specific reading disability may be assessed by measurement of the skills, especially phonologic, related to reading success. After a predictable developmental pathway, children's phonologic abilities can be evaluated beginning at about age 4 years. Such tests mainly are centered on a child's ability to focus on phonemes, the basic particles of spoken language. Initial tests typically ask what word rhymes with another or what spoken word begins (or ends) with the same sound as another. At more advanced levels, tests ask children to pronounce a spoken word after a sound is removed, such as "can you say steak without the t sound?" (sake) or "can you count the number of sounds you hear in man?" (three sounds). In general, as a child develops, he or she gains the ability to notice and to manipulate smaller and smaller parts of spoken words. Tests of phonologic capabilities and reading readiness are becoming increasingly available; one such test is the Comprehensive Test of Phonological Processing in Reading (CTOPP, PRO-ED), which is nationally standardized for age 5 through adult years. In addition to phonology, knowledge of letter names and sounds is the strongest predictor of a child's readiness to read. An appropriate battery of tests for the early recognition of reading problems includes tests of phonology, letter names and sounds, vocabulary, print conventions, and listening comprehension. Tests of reading are

---

Box 46-1 Clues to Dyslexia Beginning in Second Grade and Beyond

Problems in Speaking

- Mispronunciation of long or complicated words
- Speech that is not fluent (pausing or hesitating often); lots of "ums"
- Use of imprecise language
- Inability to find the exact word
- Struggle to retrieve words: "It was on the tip of my tongue."
- Need for time to summon an oral response, inability to come up with a verbal response quickly when questioned
- Lack of glibness, especially if put on the spot
- Spoken vocabulary smaller than listening vocabulary; hesitation to say aloud words that might be mispronounced
- Oral presentations often underestimate knowledge of the individual

Problems in Reading

- Very slow progress in acquiring reading skills
- Lack of a strategy to read new words
- Trouble reading unknown (new or unfamiliar) words that must be sounded out
- The inability to read small "function" words such as that, an, in
- Fear of reading out loud
- Oral reading that is choppy and labored

- Disproportionately poor performance on multiple-choice tests
- Inability to finish tests on time
- Disastrous spelling
- Reading that is very slow and tiring
- Messy handwriting but with excellent facility at word processing
- Extreme difficulty learning a foreign language
- Reading whose accuracy improves over time, though it continues to lack fluency and is laborious
- Lowered self-esteem, with pain that is not always visible to others
- Avoidance of reading – gains knowledge from sources other than reading, e.g., audiobooks, discussions, film
- Lack of fluency in reading increases attentional demands – vulnerable to noise, reading tiring
- Comprehension – often higher than word-reading accuracy or fluency
- Sacrifice of social life for studying
- Anxiety around test-taking or reading/speaking aloud
- Noted success, with accommodations, in a range of professions, including writing, science, medicine, architecture, law, journalism
- A history of reading, spelling, and foreign language problems in family members

(From © Shaywitz S. Overcoming Dyslexia. New York: Alfred A Knopf, 2003:123–124.)

also useful because they allow comparison of a child's reading skills with his peers at a time when he should be beginning to read [Shaywitz, 2003]. The importance of such early assessments is that they can identify at-risk children early on, so that these boys and girls can be provided with the effective, evidence-based reading interventions now available.

In the school-age child, one important element of the evaluation is how accurately the child can decode words (i.e., read single words in isolation). This element is measured with standardized tests of single real word and pseudoword reading such as the Woodcock–Johnson III (Riverside) and the Woodcock Reading Mastery Test – Revised – Normative Update (Pearson Psychocorp). Pseudoword reading, measuring the ability to decode nonsense or made-up words, is a particularly useful test. Because the words are made up, and the child has not seen them before and therefore could not have memorized the words, each nonsense word must be sounded out. Tests of nonsense word reading are referred to as word attack. Silent reading comprehension may be assessed by the Woodcock test. Reading fluency, the ability to read accurately, rapidly, and with good intonation, is a critical but often overlooked component of reading. The ability to read words fluently is an indication that these words are read automatically, without the need to apply attentional resources. Fluency is generally assessed by asking the child to read aloud, either passages or single words. For example, the Gray Oral Reading Test – Fourth Edition (GORT-4, Pearson–PsychCorp) consists of 13 increasingly difficult passages, each followed by five comprehension questions; scores for accuracy, rate, fluency, and comprehension are awarded. Such tests of oral reading are particularly helpful in identifying a child who is dyslexic; by its very nature, oral reading forces a child to pronounce each word. Listening to a struggling reader attempt to pronounce each word leaves no doubt about the child's reading difficulty. In addition to the reading aloud of passages, single-word reading efficiency may be assessed using the Test of Word Reading Efficiency (TOWRE, PRO-ED), a test of speeded oral reading of individual words. Children who struggle with reading often have trouble spelling. In reading, the written word is decoded into its constituent sounds; in spelling, sounds in a spoken word are encoded into letters. The Wide Range Achievement Test, Revised (WRAT-R, PAR) and the Test of Written Spelling-4 (PRO-ED) are among the tests that measure spelling.

For informal screening by primary care physicians in an office setting, it is recommended that the physician listen to the child read aloud from his own grade-level reader. Keeping a set of graded readers available in the office serves the purpose and does not require children to bring their own schoolbooks. Oral reading is a very sensitive measure of reading accuracy and reading fluency. A set of read-aloud paragraphs appropriate for children in the primary grades can be found in Appendix 46-1.

The most consistent and telling sign of a reading disability in an accomplished young adult is slow and laborious reading and writing. Failure to recognize or to measure the lack of automaticity in reading may be the most common error in the diagnosis of dyslexia in older children and in accomplished young adults. Simple word identification tasks cannot detect a dyslexic accomplished enough to be in honors high-school classes or to graduate from college and attend law, medical, or any other graduate-degree school. Such an individual may have compensated to some degree in reading accuracy, but will remain a dysfluent reader. Accordingly, tests relying on the accuracy of word identification alone are inappropriate to use to diagnose dyslexia in accomplished young adults; tests of word identification reveal little or nothing of their struggles to read. It is important to recognize that, because they assess reading accuracy but not automaticity (speed), the kinds of reading tests commonly used for school-age children may provide misleading data on bright adolescents and young adults. The most critical tests are those that are timed; they are the most sensitive to a phonologic deficit in a bright adult. However, there are very few standardized tests for young adult readers that are administered under timed and untimed conditions; the Nelson–Denny Reading Test (Riverside Publishing) represents an exception. Any scores obtained on testing must be considered relative to peers with the same degree of education or professional training.

Appendix 46-1

Three reading samples are provided [Hiebert, 2003]. They can be photocopied and given to young patients as reading tests for informal screening of dyslexia during an office visit. The superscript numbers indicate word counts.

Reading Sample for Children Beginning Second Grade
Office Jobs
There are many kinds of offices. However, most people who work in offices spend their time inside. One kind of office is a[25] bank. People keep their money in banks. Another kind of office is a doctor's office. People go to doctors' offices when they are sick.

People[50] who work in offices often work in teams. In banks, teams keep the money safe. In doctors' offices, teams make sure that sick people get[75] the help they need. In offices, everyone on a team works together to get the job done.[92]

Reading Sample for Children in Second Grade
Jobs That Help You
There are many people who do jobs that help you. You see and talk to some of these people, such as[25] your teacher or doctor. Teachers help you learn. Doctors help you stay well.

You don't see all the people who do jobs that help you.[50] You are not likely to see the people who built your school or the writers of the books you read. You are not likely to[75] see the people who make the pens you use to write or the paper on which you write. Around the world, many people are doing jobs that help you.[104]

Reading Sample for Children in Third Grade
Selling Things
Many companies don't sell their bikes to people. They sell their bikes to stores. Then these stores sell the bikes to people.

Store[25] owners need to have money to pay a company for the bikes. Store owners also need a place to sell the bikes. They need sales[50] people to help people choose a bike. Store owners need to pay their sales people, too.

Store owners also need to set the price of[75] a bike. This price should be more than the store owner paid for it. However, the bike should cost the same as or less than[100] bikes in other stores. After all, many people compare different stores' prices.[112]

(From Hiebert E. QuickReads. Parsippany, NJ: Modern Curriculum Press, 2003. © 2003 by Pearson Education, Inc. Used by permission.)

Physical and Neurologic Examination and Laboratory Tests

A general physical examination has a very limited role in the evaluation of individuals with dyslexia. Primary sensory impairments should be ruled out, particularly in young children. The examination should be governed by any nondyslexic symptoms that indicate specific areas of concern. Results of the routine neurologic examination are usually normal for children who are dyslexic. Laboratory measures, such as imaging studies, electroencephalograms, or chromosome studies, are ordered only if there are specific clinical indications not relating to dyslexia. As mentioned earlier, functional imaging is currently restricted to research studies of *groups* of typical compared to dyslexic readers, and is not sensitive enough to be used for clinical diagnosis of individual children or adults.

Outcome: Phonologic Deficit in Adolescence and Adult Life

Lack of fluency and deficits in phonologic coding continue to characterize dyslexic readers, even in adolescence; performance on phonologic processing measures contributes most to discriminating between dyslexic and typical adolescent readers and typical and superior adolescent readers as well [Shaywitz et al., 1999]. Dyslexia does not spontaneously remit, nor do these children demonstrate a lag mechanism for "catching up" in the development of reading skills. However, many dyslexic readers can become quite proficient in reading a finite domain of words that recur in their area of special interest, usually words that are important for their careers. For example, an individual who is dyslexic in childhood may in adult life become interested in molecular biology and learn to decode words that form a minivocabulary important in molecular biology. Such an individual, although able to decode words in this domain, still exhibits evidence of his early reading problems when reading unfamiliar words, which then are read accurately but not fluently and automatically [Ben-Dror et al., 1991; Bruck, 1994; Lefly and Pennington, 1991; Shaywitz et al., 1999]. Because they are able to read words accurately (albeit very slowly), dyslexic adolescents and young adults may mistakenly be assumed to have "outgrown" their dyslexia. Data from studies of children with dyslexia who have been followed prospectively support the notion that, in adolescents, the rate of reading and the facility with spelling may be most useful clinically in differentiating average from poor readers in students in secondary school, college, and even graduate school. These older dyslexic students may be similar to their unimpaired peers on untimed measures of word recognition but continue to suffer from the phonologic deficit that makes reading less automatic, more effortful, and slow.

Treatment

The management of dyslexia demands a life-span perspective. Early on, the focus is on remediation of the reading problem. As a child matures and enters the more time-demanding setting of secondary school, the emphasis shifts to incorporate the important role of providing accommodations. Effective intervention programs provide children with systematic instruction in each of the critical components of reading

and practice that is aligned with that instruction. The goal is for children to develop the skills that will allow them to read and understand the meaning of familiar and unfamiliar words they may encounter and to read these words fluently.

As in other areas of medicine, knowledge is being accrued to inform the practice of evidence-based education. Based on a prior consensus report from the National Research Council [Snow et al., 1998] and on the results of its own analysis, the National Reading Panel [Report, 2000] reported that five critical elements were necessary to teach reading effectively: phonemic awareness (i.e., ability to focus on and manipulate phonemes – speech sounds – in spoken syllables and words); phonics (i.e., understanding how letters are linked to sounds to form letter–sound correspondences and spelling patterns); fluency (i.e., ability to read accurately, rapidly, and with good intonation); vocabulary; and comprehension strategies. The National Reading Panel emphasized that these elements must be taught systematically and explicitly, rather than in a more casual, fragmented, or implicit manner. Such systematic phonics instruction is more effective than "whole-word" instruction, which teaches little or no phonics or teaches phonics haphazardly or using a "by-the-way" approach.

Fluency is of critical importance because it allows for the automatic, attention-free recognition of words, permitting these attentional resources to be directed to comprehension. Although it is generally recognized that fluency is an important component of skilled reading, it is often neglected in the classroom. The most effective method to build reading fluency is a procedure referred to as guided repeated oral reading with feedback and guidance. Typically, the teacher models reading a passage aloud, and the student rereads the passage repeatedly to the teacher, another adult, or a peer, receiving feedback until he or she is able to read the passage correctly. The evidence indicates that guided repeated oral reading has a clear and positive impact on word recognition, fluency, and comprehension at a variety of grade levels, and applies to all students – good readers and those experiencing reading difficulties. The evidence is less secure for programs for struggling readers that encourage large amounts of independent reading (i.e., silent reading without any feedback to the student). Even though independent silent reading is intuitively appealing, the evidence is insufficient to support the notion that reading fluency improves in struggling readers. No doubt there is a correlation between being a good reader and reading large amounts; however, there is a paucity of evidence indicating that there is a causal relationship such that poor readers who read more will become more fluent.

In contrast to teaching phonemic awareness, phonics, and fluency, interventions for reading comprehension are not as well established. In large measure, this reflects the nature of the very complex processes influencing reading comprehension. The limited evidence indicates that the most effective methods to teach reading comprehension involve teaching vocabulary and strategies that encourage an active interaction between reader and text.

Large-scale studies have focused on younger children, and there are few or no data available on the effect of these training programs on older children. The data on younger children are extremely encouraging, indicating that using evidence-based methods can remediate and even prevent reading difficulties in primary school-aged children [Foorman et al., 2003; Shaywitz, 2003; Torgesen et al., 1999].

Attentional Mechanisms in Reading and Dyslexia

For almost two decades, the central dogma in reading research has been that the generation of the phonological code from print is modular: that is, automatic, not attention-demanding, and not requiring any other cognitive process. Recent findings now present a competing view, suggesting that attentional mechanisms play a critical role in reading and that disruption of these attentional mechanisms plays a causal role in reading difficulties. These data, reviewed by us previously [Shaywitz and Shaywitz, 2008], provide one of the most exciting new developments on the horizon: the potential use of pharmacologic agents that influence not only attention, but reading as well. Randomized clinical trials of such agents are currently in progress and may lead to a role for pharmacotherapy in reading as an adjunct to the reading interventions discussed above.

Accommodations

An essential component of the management of dyslexia in students in secondary school, college, and graduate school incorporates the provision of accommodations. High-school and college students with a history of childhood dyslexia often present a paradoxical picture; they are similar to their unimpaired peers on measures of word recognition and comprehension, but they continue to suffer from the phonologic deficit that makes reading less automatic, more effortful, and slow. Neurobiologic data provide strong evidence for the necessity of extra time for readers with dyslexia (see Figure 46-5). Functional MRI data demonstrate that, in the word-form area, the region supporting rapid reading functions inefficiently. Readers compensate by developing anterior systems bilaterally and the right homolog of the left word-form area. Such compensation allows for accurate reading, but it does not support fluent or rapid reading [Shaywitz et al., 2002]. For these readers with dyslexia, the provision of extra time is an essential accommodation; it allows them the time to decode each word and to apply their unimpaired higher-order cognitive and linguistic skills to the surrounding context to get at the meaning of words that they cannot entirely or rapidly decode. While readers who are dyslexic improve greatly with additional time, providing additional time to nondyslexic readers results in very minimal to lack of improvement in scores. Although providing extra time for reading is by far the most common accommodation for people with dyslexia, other helpful accommodations include allowing the use of laptop computers with spelling checkers, and access to recorded books. (Recordings read by actual people are available from Learning Ally formerly Recording for the Blind and Dyslexic, 800-221-4792 or audible.com, while digitized materials are read by artificial voice on Kindle or Kurzweil readers.) Other helpful accommodations include providing access to syllabi and lecture notes, tutors to "talk through" and review the content of reading material, alternatives to multiple-choice tests (e.g., reports or projects), waivers of high-stakes oral exams and a separate, quiet room for taking tests [Shaywitz, 2003]. With such accommodations, many students with dyslexia are successfully completing studies in a range of disciplines, including medicine.

Dyslexia and the Sea of Strengths

Dyslexia is conceptualized as a "sea of strengths" in higher cognitive functions surrounding the weakness in phonological awareness and fluent reading [Shaywitz, 2003]. Thus, the same individual who struggles to retrieve words and reads slowly with effort may have great strengths in conceptual abilities, problem-solving, verbal reasoning, the ability to grasp the big picture, and what has been referred to as creative or out-of-the-box thinking. Indeed, it is just these higher-level strengths that make it imperative for individuals who have dyslexia to receive the accommodations (e.g., extra time) they require in order to demonstrate their abilities. It is important to appreciate that phonologic difficulties in dyslexia are independent of intelligence. Many highly intelligent boys and girls have reading problems that are often overlooked and even ascribed to "lack of motivation." In counseling their patients who are dyslexic, physicians should bear in mind that many outstanding writers, lawyers, physicians, and scientists, including Nobel laureates, such as Niels Bohr in physics (1925) and Baruj Benacerraf (1984) and Carol Greider (2009) in physiology or medicine, are dyslexic. More information regarding the relationship between dyslexia and creativity may be found on the website of the Yale Center for Dyslexia and Creativity, www.dyslexia.Yale.edu.

People with dyslexia and their families frequently consult their physicians about unconventional approaches to the remediation of reading difficulties; there are very few credible data to support the claims made for these treatments, such as optometric training, medication for vestibular dysfunction, chiropractic manipulation, and dietary supplementation. Physicians should be aware that there is no one program that remediates reading difficulties; a number of programs following the guidelines provided earlier have proved to be highly effective in teaching struggling children to read.

Conclusions and Implications

Within the last two decades, overwhelming evidence from many laboratories has converged to indicate the cognitive basis for dyslexia. Dyslexia represents a disorder within the language system and, more specifically, within a particular subcomponent of that system: phonologic processing. Advances in imaging technology and the development of tasks that sharply isolate the subcomponent processes of reading allow the localization of phonologic processing in brain and provide, for the first time, the potential for elucidating a biologic signature for reading and reading disability. Results from laboratories using functional brain imaging indicate an inefficient functioning of left hemisphere posterior brain systems in childhood and adult dyslexic readers while performing reading tasks, with an additional suggestion for an associated increased reliance on ancillary systems, such as those in the frontal lobes and right hemisphere posterior circuits. The discovery of neural systems serving reading has significant implications. At the most fundamental level, it has made a heretofore hidden disability visible.

Acknowledgments

The work described in this chapter was supported by grants from the National Institute of Child Health and Human Development (P50 HD25802, RO1 HD046171, R01 HD057655), by the Yale Center for Dyslexia and Creativity, and by Eli Lilly Ltd.

 The complete list of references for this chapter is available online at **www.expertconsult.com**. See inside cover for registration details.

Attention-Deficit Hyperactivity Disorder

David E. Mandelbaum

Attention-deficit hyperactivity disorder (ADHD) has been described as the most common neurobehavioral disorder in childhood [Cantwell, 1996]. Prevailing opinion characterizes ADHD as a disorder of executive function attributable to abnormal dopamine transmission in the frontal lobes and frontostriatal circuitry. In large part, this concept is based on the clinical efficacy of medications affecting catecholamine transmission in these regions.

The first reference to behavior now associated with ADHD was by George Still in 1902, who referred to a deficit of "moral control." Within the context of this broad concept, he made the following observation: "A notable feature in many of these cases of moral deficit without general impairment of intellect is a quite abnormal incapacity for sustained attention" [Still, 1902]. Strauss and Lehtinen [1947] used the term "minimal brain damage syndrome" to describe children with cognitive and behavioral deficits. In 1962, Clements and Peters coined the term "minimal brain dysfunction" to describe functional abnormalities in children in whom brain damage could not be demonstrated. Although widely accepted, this concept came under immediate challenge, as it included too heterogeneous a group of children [MacKeith, 1963]. The subsequent emphasis on attention and its neurologic substrate, the frontal lobe and frontostriatal circuitry, represents a refinement of the definition of the condition.

Diagnosis of Attention-Deficit Hyperactivity Disorder

ADHD is a clinical diagnosis based on criteria in the fourth edition of the Diagnostic and Statistical Manual of Mental Disorders (DSM-IV) (Box 47-1). Criteria are divided into two lists of symptoms, one for inattention and another for hyperactive-impulsive behavior. Based on the number of items identified, there are three classifications: ADHD/I (primarily in-attentive type), ADHD/HI (primarily hyperactive-impulsive type), and ADHD/C (combined type). The revised diagnostic criteria of DSM-IV, with the inclusion of the three subtypes, increased the number of females, preschoolers, and adults with ADHD [Lahey et al., 1994]. Increased numbers in these groups resulted in an increase in the prevalence of ADHD from 3–5 percent with the DSM-III-R to about 12 percent; ADHD/I alone has been estimated to have a prevalence between 5.4 and 9 percent [Baumgaertel et al., 1995; Wolraich et al., 1996].

It has been proposed that the core deficit in ADHD is impairment of behavioral inhibition, which leads to the other symptoms of ADHD. This model of impaired behavioral inhibition is limited to ADHD/HI and ADHD/C (i.e., those with hyperactive or impulsive symptoms) and excludes children with ADHD/I (i.e., those with inattention only) [Barkley, 1997]. The observation that overflow movements were the most discriminating finding between hyperactive boys (without learning disabilities) and normal control subjects seems to support the concept of impaired behavioral inhibition [Denckla and Rudel, 1978]. If this formulation is widely accepted, future classifications may call for separate diagnostic entities, such as attention-deficit disorder and behavioral-inhibition disorder. Some investigators have proposed that all three ADHD subtypes can be explained as disorders of attention or executive function (other than response inhibition), with symptoms of hyperactivity and impulsivity resulting from these impairments [Brown, 2000; Chhabildas et al., 2001; Weiss and Weiss, 2002]. Others also distinguish ADHD/HI and ADHD/C from ADHD/I, but they posit that the symptoms of hyperactivity and impulsivity can result from poor inhibitory control or differences in motivational style characterized by delay aversion [Sonuga-Barke, 2002].

A review of the literature regarding the hypothesis that ADHD represents a primary deficit in executive control defined executive function as comprising "at least four factors: (1) response inhibition and execution, (2) working memory and updating, (3) set-shifting and task-switching and (4) interference control" [Willcutt et al., 2005]. There were significant differences between children with and without ADHD on tasks assessing executive function. Six of eight studies assessing working memory found impaired working memory in children with ADHD. The most consistent effects were observed in measures of response inhibition, vigilance, and planning; children with combined and inattentive types of ADHD differed from controls and did not differ from each other, whereas children with hyperactive-impulsive ADHD had minimal executive function impairment, suggesting that executive function weaknesses are primarily associated with inattention, rather than hyperactivity-impulsivity symptoms. The observation that fewer than half of the children with ADHD had significant impairment of any specific task of executive function, and that the correlation, while significant, tended to be small in magnitude, led the authors to conclude that their findings "do not support the hypothesis that executive functions deficits are the single necessary and sufficient cause of ADHD

Box 47-1 Diagnostic Criteria for Attention-Deficit/Hyperactivity Disorder

A. Either (1) or (2):

(1) Six (or more) of the following symptoms of **inattention** have persisted for at least 6 months to a degree that is maladaptive and inconsistent with developmental level:

Inattention

- often fails to give close attention to details or makes careless mistakes in schoolwork, work, or other activities
- often has difficulty sustaining attention in tasks or play activities
- often does not seem to listen when spoken to directly
- often does not follow through on instructions and fails to finish schoolwork, chores, or duties in the workplace (not due to oppositional behavior or failure to understand instructions)
- often has difficulty organizing tasks and activities
- often avoids, dislikes, or is reluctant to engage in tasks that require sustained mental effort (such as schoolwork or homework)
- often loses things necessary for tasks or activities (e.g., toys, school assignments, pencils, books, or tools)
- is often easily distracted by extraneous stimuli
- is often forgetful in daily activities

(2) Six (or more) of the following symptoms of **hyperactivity-impulsivity** have persisted for at least 6 months to a degree that is maladaptive and inconsistent with developmental level:

Hyperactivity

- often fidgets with hands or feet or squirms in seat
- often leaves seat in classroom or in other situations in which remaining seated is expected
- often runs about or climbs excessively in situations in which it is inappropriate (in adolescents or adults, may be limited to subjective feelings of restlessness)

- often has difficulty playing or engaging in leisure activities quietly
- is often "on the go" or often acts as if "driven by a motor"
- often talks excessively

Impulsivity

- often blurts out answers before questions have been completed
- often has difficulty awaiting turn
- often interrupts or intrudes on others (e.g., butts into conversations or games)

B. Some hyperactive-impulsive or inattentive symptoms that caused impairment were present before age 7 years

C. Some impairment from the symptoms is present in two or more settings (e.g., at school [or work] and at home)

D. There must be clear evidence of clinically significant impairment in social, academic, or occupational functioning

E. The symptoms do not occur exclusively during the course of a pervasive developmental disorder, schizophrenia, or other psychotic disorder and are not better accounted for by another mental disorder (e.g., mood disorder, anxiety disorder, dissociative disorder, or a personality disorder)

Code based on type:

314.01 Attention-Deficit/Hyperactivity Disorder, Combined Type: If both Criteria A1 and A2 are met for the past 6 months

314.00 Attention-Deficit/Hyperactivity Disorder, Predominantly Inattentive Type: if Criterion A1 is met but Criterion A2 is not met for the past 6 months

314.01 Attention-Deficit/Hyperactivity Disorder, Predominantly Hyperactive-Impulsive Type: if Criterion A2 is met but Criterion A1 is not met for the past 6 months

Coding note: For individuals (especially adolescents and adults) who currently have symptoms that no longer meet full criteria, "In Partial Remission" should be specified.

---

in all individuals with the disorder. Instead executive function difficulties appear to be one of several important weaknesses that comprise the overall neuropsychological etiology of ADHD" [Willcutt et al., 2005].

Inhibitory deficits and delay aversion in ADHD can be dissociated by specific types of tasks; either deficit alone is only moderately associated with ADHD, whereas these two deficits combined correctly classify nearly 90 percent of children with ADHD. Thus a formulation was proposed in which executive functions (EF) are divided into cognitive aspects, associated with dorsolateral prefrontal cortex ("cool" EF), in contrast to the affective aspects, associated with orbital and medial prefrontal cortex ("hot" EF). Inattention symptoms were attributed to deficits in "cool" EF, whereas hyperactivity-impulsivity symptoms reflected "hot" EF deficits. The authors noted that "the neuroanatomical substrates of cortical-striato-thalamo-cortical circuitry are now revealed to include spirals of one directional information from 'hot' ventral-medial/orbital/ventral striatal regions to dorsolateral/superior medial/anterior striatal 'cool' regions to even 'cooler' premotor and motor circuits" [Castellanos et al., 2006].

The use of the word "often" in the list of symptoms, coupled with qualification "to a degree that is maladaptive and

inconsistent with developmental level," lends an element of subjectivity to this diagnostic schema. Symptom rating scales for parents and teachers have been developed to assist in the ascertainment of diagnostic criteria [Conners, 1997]. The use of broader rating scales, such as the Child Behavior Checklist, provides information regarding the presence of other disorders, such as conduct disorder, oppositional defiant disorder (ODD), and anxiety disorder [Achenbach, 1991; Vaughn et al., 2000], which may warrant diagnoses other than ADHD [Jensen et al., 1997]. The Yale Children's Inventory was developed to ascertain the presence of attentional deficits and learning disabilities [Shaywitz et al., 1986]. A comprehensive review of evaluation issues in ADHD concluded that no single test can be used to make the diagnosis and that it is up to the clinician "to choose a battery of measures that satisfies what is, to some degree, an individually determined level of diagnostic certainty" [Nass, 2005]. The American Academy of Pediatrics has endorsed the Vanderbilt ADHD rating scales for parents and teachers [Wolraich et al., 2003a, b] and has provided a complete "tool kit," including a cover letter to teachers and scoring information, on the internet (http://www.nichq.org/about/index.html).

Developmental variability in the presentation of ADHD, and the inconsistency of behavior of children with ADHD in different settings and at different times in the same setting, add to the diagnostic confusion. In preschool children, in particular, the prevalence of ADHD-type symptoms [Blackman, 1999; Palfrey et al., 1985] and the transient nature of such symptoms in many cases [Barkley, 1998] make this a difficult diagnosis. Efforts have been made to provide a more objective basis for the diagnosis of ADHD, such as computerized continuous performance tests [Conners, 1985] or tests of variables of attention [Greenberg, 1993]. However, the correlation of these measures of attention with the behavioral disorder is not sufficient for their use as replacements for the behavioral criteria of DSM-IV [Barkley, 1991].

The motor examination may help distinguish between children with a learning disorder and those with ADHD; it is best to evaluate a child between the age of 5 years and the onset of puberty, a period of rapid change in motor development, when quantitative examination of the motor system, such as the Physical and Neurological Examination for Soft Signs (PANESS) [Denckla, 1985], may demonstrate evidence of motor disinhibition [Denckla, 2003].

Controversies in the Diagnosis of Attention-Deficit–Hyperactivity Disorder

The DSM-IV clinical criteria for diagnosing ADHD (see Box 47-1) indicate a number of qualifications that are too often ignored, resulting in an incorrect diagnosis [American Psychiatric Association, 1994]. The text explicitly states that the findings need to be present "to a degree that is maladaptive and inconsistent with developmental level." Behavior that may not be typical but is not maladaptive does not warrant a diagnosis of ADHD. Similarly, unreasonable expectations of a child at a young age may result in a false diagnosis. The diagnostic criteria are followed by a number of statements regarding the context of the symptoms. Item C states, "Some impairment from the symptoms is present in two or more settings (e.g., at school [or work] and at home)." This provision allows for the possibility that a child in an inadequate school environment, perhaps with excessive class size, hostile peers, or inexperienced teachers, may present with findings that are unique to that setting rather than represent a disorder of attention. Similarly, a chaotic home environment may explain the child's presentation. The importance of verifying the presence of symptoms in two or more settings is underscored by a study that found an increase in the incidence of ADHD diagnoses in: states with school accountability laws; students with older or nonwhite teachers; children from a single-parent family, from the lowest income quintile, with a US-born father, or born to a young (<18 years) or older (>38 years) mother [Schneider and Eisenberg, 2006]. Item D reiterates that "there must be clear evidence of clinically significant impairment in social, academic, or occupational function."

Perhaps most important is item E, which states, "The symptoms do not occur exclusively during the course of a pervasive developmental disorder, schizophrenia, or other psychotic disorder and are not better accounted for by another mental disorder (e.g., mood disorder, anxiety disorder, dissociative disorder, or a personality disorder)." If a child has symptoms that meet the diagnostic criteria for ADHD in the context of these other disorders, treatment should be directed at these other conditions before concluding that the child has a disorder of attention. Not addressed in item E of the DSM-IV criteria are studies that have demonstrated that children with specific neurologic disorders can present with symptoms that meet criteria for ADHD but are attributable to the neurologic disorder rather than a primary disorder of attention. A study by Walters et al. [2000] demonstrated symptoms of impaired attention and hyperactivity in children diagnosed with restless leg syndrome; treatment of the sleep disturbance resolved the so-called ADHD symptoms. Disordered breathing during sleep has also been found to manifest with symptoms consistent with ADHD [Gottlieb et al., 2003]. There are reports of children with focal epileptic discharges having symptoms suggestive of ADHD that resolved when the spike activity was suppressed with antiepileptic drugs [Holtmann et al., 2003; Laporte et al., 2002]. Many symptoms of ADHD are prevalent in individuals with neurogenetic syndromes as part of the behavioral phenotype [Pelc and Dan, 2008]. Future versions of the DSM should add neurological disorders (e.g., sleep disorders, epilepsy, neurogenetic syndromes) to the list of conditions in item E that must be excluded before ADHD is diagnosed. Refining the diagnosis of ADHD will facilitate ascertainment of the physiological and genetic underpinnings of ADHD and its treatment.

The question of conditions coexisting with ADHD is quite complex. Should a diagnosis of ADHD be reserved for individuals with an isolated disorder of attention, hyperactivity, or impulsivity, with an alternative classification used to describe children who meet DSM-IV criteria for ADHD in the context of other neurodevelopmental problems? Denckla [2003] used the term pseudo-ADHD to describe children with comorbidities or confounding factors. In a paper describing a father and son both with orbitofrontal epilepsy and associated attention difficulties and hyperactivity, the term attention-deficit hyperactivity syndrome was used to make a distinction from the specific disorder of ADHD [Powell et al., 1997], analogous to the distinction between Parkinson disease and parkinsonism. It has been proposed that ADHD be divided into subgroups based on the patterns of comorbidity [Biederman et al., 1991].

The presumption that a response to psychostimulant medication indicates that the underlying problem is ADHD can lead to an erroneous diagnosis. Psychostimulant medications can ameliorate depression [Janowsky, 2003], chronic fatigue syndrome [Turkington et al., 2004], and daytime somnolence caused by sleep disorders [Happe, 2003; Ivanenko et al., 2003], and enhance normal individuals' cognitive functioning and behavior [Rapoport et al., 1978]. A positive response to psychostimulants has no diagnostic significance.

Neurobiology of Attention-Deficit Hyperactivity Disorder

Advances in structural and functional imaging, clinical neurophysiologic techniques, and molecular genetics have been applied to the evaluation of children with ADHD and have provided important insights into this condition. However, inconsistency in the inclusion and exclusion criteria among studies, particularly related to comorbidity, limits comparisons between studies and their conclusions.

Structural Imaging

Cortical Structures

Reports of reductions in volume of prefrontal regions, more so in the right than left hemisphere, have been described in children with ADHD [Castellanos et al., 1996; Filipek et al., 1997]. A later study further localized involvement to prefrontal and premotor areas [Mostofsky et al., 2002]. In this study of 12 males with ADHD, children with conduct, mood, and anxiety disorders were excluded, but 3 children with coexistent ODD were included. A study involving other brain regions reported reductions in total cerebral volume with a negative correlation between gray-matter volumes and symptom severity [Castellanos et al., 2002]. However, the impact of coexisting conditions on anatomic findings was not considered or described (i.e., it was unclear if there was an association between severity of symptoms and coexisting conditions). Serial examinations found that most volume differences between ADHD and control subjects remained stable; however, the size of the caudate nucleus, which initially was smaller in the ADHD group, became comparable with that in the control group during adolescence. This finding reflected a greater rate of reduction in caudate size in the normal than in the ADHD group. Normalization of the caudate nucleus in adolescents with ADHD may relate to the observation that ratings for hyperactivity and impulsivity are decreased in that age group compared with those in younger children [Hart et al., 1995]. A study using serial magnetic resonance imaging (MRI) scans to measure cortical thickness over time found that typically developing children without ADHD reached peak cortical thickness in the frontal cortex between the ages of 7 and 8 years. In contrast, children with ADHD reached this developmental milestone between the ages of 10 and 11 years. Both groups of children underwent cortical thinning from this peak point of thickness throughout adolescence [Shaw et al., 2007]. A subsequent study compared repeated neuroimaging studies of children with ADHD not taking psychostimulants to an age-matched group of children with ADHD who were taking psychostimulant medication during the inter-scan interval. Comparison was also made to a group of children without ADHD. The decision whether or not to treat with psychostimulants was left up to the treating physician and the family, thus was not randomly assigned. A comparison of the groups taking stimulants and not taking stimulants showed no significant differences in gender, IQ, or clinical characteristics. The neuroanatomic analysis revealed that there was more rapid cortical thinning in the group *not* taking psychostimulants (0.15 mm/yr) compared to the group taking psychostimulants (0.03 mm/yr). Thus, whereas at baseline there were no significant group differences in cortical thickness, at the end of the study the non-treatment group had a significantly thinner cortex than the treatment group. The authors hypothesize that the "psychostimulant induced increases in age appropriate levels of cognition and action, and perhaps underlying localized fronto-parietal neural activity, might foster cortical development within the normal range" [Shaw et al., 2009].

Subcortical Structures

Findings in the basal ganglia have been inconsistent, with reports of volume reductions in the right caudate nucleus and globus pallidus [Castellanos et al., 1996] or in the left caudate [Filipek et al., 1997]. The study by Castellanos et al. [1996] included children with "mild–moderate" conduct disorder (CD), ODD, anxiety disorder, and reading disorders. However, re-analysis of the data by excluding the children who had CD or ODD found a more robust correlation between volume reductions in the right prefrontal, caudate, and globus pallidus and ADHD. In the study by Filipek et al. [1997], children with co-existent conditions were excluded. In addition to the anatomic differences between children with ADHD and control subjects, this study revealed differences in structural abnormalities between children with ADHD who were considered responders to psychostimulants and those who were not. A study of monozygotic twins discordant for ADHD [Castellanos et al., 2003] revealed reduced caudate volume in the affected twin. In another report on twins discordant for ADHD [Sharp et al., 2003], fathers of twins discordant for ADHD had lower ADHD scores than fathers of ADHD singletons. The rate of breech presentation was greater in affected twins than affected singletons. The data suggested that the discordant twins represented non-genetic instances of ADHD, possibly caused by injury in utero, and that the caudate abnormalities in these individuals might not be pertinent to ADHD that is genetic in nature. No abnormalities have been reported in the putamen, and there have been few studies of the globus pallidus in children with ADHD [Durston et al., 2003]. A study utilizing large deformation diffeomorphic mapping (LDDMM) found that boys with ADHD had significant shape differences and decreases in overall volume of the basal ganglia compared to controls, whereas girls with ADHD did not have volume or shape differences. Children with comorbidities, including other neuropsychiatric disorders, conduct disorders, mood disorder, generalized anxiety disorder, obsessive-compulsive disorder, learning disabilities, or speech and language disorders, were excluded from this analysis [Qiu et al., 2009].

Cerebellum

Reductions in total cerebellar volume [Castellanos et al., 1996, 2002] and in the volume of the cerebellar vermis alone in ADHD compared with control subjects have been described [Castellanos et al., 2001; Mostofsky et al., 1998]. These differences could have been caused by different methods for serially measuring volume, making comparisons between studies difficult. These studies included children who had a high percentage of coexistent conditions, such as ODD, CD, and learning, mood, and anxiety disorders, but the decreased volume of the cerebellar vermis in the ADHD group remained when children with disruptive behavioral disorders were removed from the analysis. However, the subgroup with ADHD and coexisting mood or anxiety disorders had the smallest vermian volumes.

Functional Imaging

The clinical benefit from medications affecting catecholamine levels has led to a focus on frontostriatal circuitry and dopamine pathways in ADHD. Functional magnetic resonance imaging (fMRI) studies have demonstrated abnormal activation of frontostriatal regions in children with ADHD. In normal children, maturation is associated with increased activation of the ventral frontostriatal regions and improved inhibitory control [Durston et al., 2002]. A comparison of ADHD with normal control subjects demonstrated greater frontal activation and lower striatal activation during response inhibition in 10 children with ADHD (8 ADHD/C, 2 ADHD/I; children with high comorbidity scores were excluded). Administration of methylphenidate also resulted in improved performance in a test of response inhibition, associated with increased frontal activation in ADHD children and control subjects, and increased striatal activation in the children with ADHD [Vaidya et al., 1998].

Single-photon emission computed tomography (SPECT) has been used to investigate children with ADHD. One study compared 8 adolescents with "pure" ADHD against 11 with ADHD and coexistent conditions during a test of variables of attention (TOVA) [Lorberboym et al., 2004]. Children with coexistent conditions (e.g., ODD, CD, mood disorders, learning disorder alone or in combination) had decreased temporal lobe perfusion in response to the TOVA compared with the pure ADHD children, who had some but not statistically significant decreases in frontal lobe perfusion. Regional differences in perfusion between the two groups may explain the better rate of response to stimulants in the pure ADHD group and suggests that different treatments for the two groups may be warranted.

Untreated adults with ADHD (with no psychiatric comorbidity) have increased striatal dopamine transporter (DAT) levels compared with normal control subjects (as measured by binding to technetium-99m TRODAT-1, the first ^{99m}Tc-labeled ligand identified by SPECT that specifically binds DAT), which decreased after 4 weeks of methylphenidate treatment [Krause et al., 2000]. This finding, along with increased striatal activity on positron emission tomographic (PET) scanning in adolescents with ADHD compared with normal control subjects [Ernst et al., 1999], suggests a role for excess dopaminergic activity in the striatum or nucleus accumbens in persons with ADHD [Solanto, 2002].

Proton MR spectroscopy has also been used to study children with ADHD [Sparkes et al., 2004]. N-acetyl-aspartate (NAA), glutamate/glutamine/γ-aminobutyric acid (Glx), choline, and creatine (Cre) levels in the right prefrontal cortex and left striatum during a test of response inhibition were compared between ADHD children and a control group. A negative correlation between the NAA/Cre ratio and reaction time in the ADHD group was found, compared with a positive correlation in the control group. Children with ADHD with NAA/Cre levels more comparable with those in controls also had much longer reaction times. These findings were thought to reflect preferential use of the prefrontal cortex by children with ADHD during tasks of response inhibition. Of the 8 children with ADHD in this study, 5 had ODD, and 1 had a generalized anxiety disorder; the interpretation of these results, as they apply to ADHD compared with other disorders, is unclear.

Clinical Neurophysiology

Event-related potential (ERP) studies in ADHD children suggest a lack of frontal lobe inhibitory processes, particularly in pathways involving the anterior cingulate cortex. In one study using a Go/NoGo task designed to assess inhibition, no significant performance differences were found between children with ADHD and normal control subjects [Smith et al., 2003]. However, children with ADHD had larger ERPs

than the control group to a warning stimulus that provided no information helpful for task performance, suggesting a lack of inhibition to an irrelevant stimulus in the ADHD group. A second study found shorter-latency and higher-amplitude ERPs that were thought to reflect an inhibitory process in the ADHD group [Falkenstein et al., 1999]. These findings suggested that children with ADHD need to trigger inhibition processes earlier and more strongly to achieve the same behavioral performance as control subjects. Individuals in this study likely did not represent a pure ADHD group because they had higher scores in oppositional, delinquent, and aggressive behaviors and social problems. A third study found that the children with ADHD and without coexisting conditions had significantly longer reaction times to target stimuli and made significantly more omission errors than the control group, but did not differ in the number of commission errors [Fallgatter et al., 2004]. The ERP data indicated diminished activation of the anterior cingulate cortex in the Go/NoGo trials in the ADHD group, suggesting deficits in prefrontal response control. This deficit in prefrontal response control was distinguished from deficits in response inhibition. Because the latter study excluded ADHD children with comorbidity, it more strongly suggests that abnormalities in activation of the anterior cingulate cortex may be specific to ADHD.

Genetic Studies

Concise reviews of advances in the genetics of ADHD, including findings that may account for the ADHD subtypes, comorbidities and responses to specific medications, are provided in a commentary and editorial in journal issues devoted to this topic. As summarized by DV Pauls: "there is overwhelming evidence that ADHD is inherited and that genetic factors play a significant role in its manifestation" [Pauls, 2005; Faraone, 2006]. Evidence of dopaminergic involvement has led to molecular genetic studies of dopamine transporter and receptor genes [Kent, 2004]. Pursuit of the DAT gene (SLC6A3, formerly designated DAT1) was in part caused by the fact that psychostimulant medications inhibit activity of DAT. An association between ADHD and the 480-base pair alleles at a variable number tandem repeat (VNTR) in SLC6A3 has been reported [Cook et al., 1995]. A subsequent study confirmed these findings and demonstrated a significant relation between SLC6A3 high-risk alleles and the number of hyperactive-impulsive symptoms, but not inattentive symptoms [Waldman et al., 1998]. The study involved 117 probands, all but one of whom met criteria for ADHD; the remaining child had ODD. Most children with ADHD frequently had symptoms of or were diagnosed with ODD, CD, and depression or dysthymia. Two subsequent studies, one with a similar rate of coexisting conditions [Palmer et al., 1999] and one with a much lower rate [Swanson et al., 2000], failed to replicate the association between SLC6A3 and ADHD.

The dopamine D4 receptor gene (DRD4) has also been associated with ADHD. A 48-base pair VNTR in the third exon of DRD4, also referred to as the DRD4 7-repeat allele, was suggested based on a review of previous studies [Faraone et al., 2001]. Children with ADHD who had the 7-repeat allele had a greater degree of impulsivity (i.e., faster and less accurate responses), were significantly more active (based on Actigraph measures), and had greater total ADHD symptoms scores than those without the allele. However, no differences were seen using measures of attention or response inhibition. The ADHD children with the 7-repeat allele also had higher rates of ODD and CD.

A third dopamine receptor gene, *DRD5*, has been linked to ADHD. One study that examined a number of candidate genes, including *DRD3*, *DRD4*, *DRD5*, and genes for four enzymes involved in dopamine metabolism, found no significant association between the children with ADHD and genetic polymorphisms [Payton et al., 2001]. However, the 138 ADHD children in this study frequently had coexisting conditions, including ODD (57.5 percent), CD (11.6 percent), and tic (12.3 percent), anxiety (2.7 percent), and depressive (1.4 percent) disorders. Another study also included children with coexistent conditions (Tourette's syndrome or tics in 34 percent, CD or ODD in 25 percent, anxiety or depression in 8 percent), and linkage to *DRD5* only reached significance when restricted to the children who had a response to methylphenidate [Tahir et al., 2000]. Information was not provided about whether the methylphenidate responders had fewer coexisting conditions. Linkage of the *DRD4* gene to methylphenidate responders was also observed. However, this study found an inverse relationship between DRD4 and DSM scores and comorbidity ratings.

Studies of DNA from ADHD probands, parents, and healthy controls found a significant association of ADHD with two *NET1* single-nucleotide polymorphisms and two *DRD1* single-nucleotide polymorphisms. There was no association with polymorphisms in ten other genes previously reported as candidate genes. There were no significant differences in anatomic brain MRI measurements between the children with *NET1* or *DRD1* gene types; nor was there a relationship between the genetic findings and cognitive or behavioral measures. This study represented the first replication of a previously described association between ADHD and polymorphisms in *NET1* and *DRD1* genes [Bobb et al., 2005].

In a study of a group of children from families of European descent with an ADHD proband, the ADHD probands were assessed by a child psychiatrist; parental ADHD was assessed through the use of an ADHD self-report scale. The ADHD cohort consisted of 335 parent–child trios of European descent and a set of 2026 ethnically matched, disease-free children as a control group. There was no significant difference in copy number variants (CNV: deletions, duplications, or size) between the patient and control groups. A search for CNVs spanning more than ten consecutive single-nucleotide polymorphisms (SNPs) for deletions, or more than twenty SNPs for duplications present in at least one parent, along with one or more related probands, but not in the controls, yielded 158 deletions and 64 duplications from 154 probands. These CNVs encompassed or overlapped 229 distinct genes, with the largest family of genes affected being the olfactory receptor superfamily. Twenty-two of these genes had previously been implicated in various neurological and neuropsychiatric disorders, including Tourette's syndrome (2 genes), autism (4 genes), and schizophrenia (15 genes). An additional 8 genes had been recently identified as having structural variants in autism and schizophrenia. Reviewing the gene set for genes associated with nervous system development, function, and behavior, the authors found genes associated with learning, cognition, and hindbrain development. Two genes, the *PTPRD* and *GRM5* genes, were thought to be particularly interesting putative candidate genes for ADHD; one, involving the protein tyrosine phosphatase gene, was detected in four unrelated ADHD probands. Two of the four

ADHD probands with the *PTPRD* deletion reported symptoms consistent with restless leg syndrome. All three children in a family found to have the *GRM5* variant met the criteria for ADHD; the *GRM5* gene, a glutamatergic receptor gene, has been postulated to play a role in ADHD. Thus the CNVs found in this ADHD were significantly enriched for genes reported as candidate genes in other neuropsychiatric disorders and in neurodevelopmental pathways [Elia et al., 2009].

Other Potential Causes of Attention-Deficit Hyperactivity Disorder

Data reported from the National Longitudinal Survey of Youth [NLSY, 1979] associated hours of television watched per day at ages 1 and 3 years with parental reports of attentional problems at age 7 [Christakis et al., 2004]. The children did not necessarily have clinically diagnosed ADHD; rather, they were scored as having attentional problems by the parents. Although the interaction between environmental influences and genetic endowment is well accepted, such preliminary data suggest the need for further investigation because of issues of cause and effect, limitations in adjusting for confounders, potential for biased reporting, and selective recall.

Coexisting Conditions

Many children who present with symptoms suggestive of ADHD have neurologic or psychiatric conditions that are the cause of those symptoms (e.g., depression, sleep disorders, epilepsy). There are other instances in which multiple conditions coexist. The implications for management are significant. Just as correction of a sleep disorder may resolve the symptoms of inattention, hyperactivity, or impulsivity, addressing a child's previously undiagnosed learning disability may resolve these symptoms. Alternatively, a child may have both problems, and remediation of the learning disability may still leave him or her with inattention, hyperactivity, or impulsivity that must be independently addressed. It has been proposed that ADHD be divided into subgroups based on the patterns of comorbidity [Biederman et al., 1991]. ADHD and CD have been posited to be distinct disorders [Schachar and Tannock, 1995]. From a practical standpoint, most studies of children with ADHD and coexisting CD treated with psychostimulants demonstrated a reduction in physical and nonphysical aggression and had improvement of ADHD symptoms [Spencer et al., 1996]. Antidepressants also reduced symptoms of aggression and ADHD in these children. Anxiety disorder has been shown to be transmitted independently from ADHD in families [Perrin and Last, 1996], suggesting that these two conditions are distinct disorders. Most studies of children with ADHD and coexisting anxiety or depression found a reduced response in ADHD symptoms when treated with psychostimulants compared with children only with ADHD [Spencer et al., 1996].

Inasmuch as ADHD and mood instability include impulsivity and behavioral problems in their definitions, both involve impairment in executive function, and there are findings of overlapping neuroanatomical abnormalities and treatments, it has been proposed that mood instability be considered a core feature of ADHD, rather than a comorbidity [Skirrow et al., 2009].

A review of the overlapping symptoms associated with ADHD and sleep disorders noted that many children with primary sleep disorders have symptoms highly suggestive of ADHD. Conversely, many children with ADHD are reported to have sleep disturbances, which may be primary, attributable to the side effects of medication, or a result of comorbid conditions, such as ODD, depression, and/or anxiety disorders. A comorbid sleep disorder may significantly increase the daytime impairment in a child with ADHD. It was recommended that all children presenting with ADHD symptoms be clinically assessed for the presence of sleep problems [Owens, 2005].

Reading disability and ADHD are two distinct disorders that may occur together [Shaywitz et al., 1995]. There is evidence of genetic linkage for ADHD and reading disability to the same region on the short arm of chromosome 6. This connection may represent a pleiotropic effect (i.e., the same gene increasing susceptibility to more than one disorder) [Willcutt et al., 2002]. A survey of audiologists and pediatricians found that, although auditory processing disorder and ADHD/I have symptoms in common, there were features that allowed them to be distinguished from each other [Chermak et al., 2002].

A meta-analysis of the literature reporting on tests of overall cognitive ability in ADHD analyzed data from 137 studies in which full-scale IQ scores for children with ADHD were compared to a healthy control group. The ADHD groups had significantly lower full-scale IQ scores relative to the control groups, with an average decrement of 9 points in the full-scale IQ; the verbal and performance IQs were lower in the ADHD group. There was no difference in ADHD subtypes, although the number of children with ADHD/I was small. The authors concluded that these findings "may indicate that the disorder is characterized by mild global cognitive inefficiencies or by multiple specific deficits affecting several cognitive abilities." They raised the possibility that the decrement could also be attributable to test-taking differences between the groups. In support of this latter possibility, the authors found that the effect size of the full-scale IQ was largest when ability was based on the complete test, as opposed to estimates from subtests; the larger effect on the complete test could possibly be due to longer testing times in studies using a full intellectual assessment battery, with decreasing performance over time caused by deficient sustained attention in the ADHD group. The authors expressed surprise at the finding that for only a few of the measures was the effect size for executive functioning tasks significantly larger than effect sizes for the full-scale IQ. Only the academic achievement tests and CPT (continuous performance tests) measures displayed substantially larger effects than the full-scale IQ; the WCST (Wisconsin card sorting task)-variables, SST (stop signal task)-probability of inhibition, and MFFT (matching familiar figures test)-time tests had smaller effect sizes than full-scale IQ. In a comparison of the mean effect size of tests of executive versus nonexecutive functions, there was greater impairment in the tests of executive function. The authors allowed for the possibility that impairment of executive function accounted for differences in overall ability, inasmuch as measures of overall ability are heavily influenced by executive function. Academic measures of spelling and arithmetic were significantly more sensitive to ADHD than overall cognitive abilities measured by full-scale IQ; the authors commented that achievement measures "may be useful not only for screening co-morbid learning disabilities but also for characterizing behavioral and motivation deficits resulting from executive dysfunction" [Frazier et al., 2004].

Diagnostic Evaluation

ADHD is a clinical diagnosis; there are no diagnostic, laboratory, or cognitive tests [Nichols and Waschbusch, 2004]. A child presenting with symptoms suggestive of ADHD should undergo hearing and vision screening, potentially treatable problems that may be mistaken for ADHD. If the child's difficulties are predominantly in the school setting, an evaluation for learning disabilities should be pursued, with educational remediation if problems are identified. Social stressors may also be a significant factor [Biederman et al., 2002], which may justify intervention by social services agencies. In general, routine diagnostic testing is not needed in the evaluation of a child for ADHD [American Academy of Pediatrics, 2000]. However, specific testing may be indicated in some circumstances.

Laboratory Studies

Features in the history or on examination may lead to specific tests for disorders manifesting as or coexisting with ADHD, such as hypothyroidism [Rovet, 2002], hyperthyroidism [Suresh et al., 1999], or phenylketonuria [Antshel and Waisbren, 2003]. Reports of an association between lead exposure and ADHD have been inconsistent [Eppright et al., 1997; Tuthill, 1996]. Depending on the results of such laboratory studies, therapy targeting the specific condition may be initiated. An uncontrolled study reported improvement in the parents', but not the teachers', Connors Rating Scales scores in children with ADHD treated with iron supplementation, even though they were not iron-deficient [Sever et al., 1997]. Better studies are needed before concluding that routine testing of or supplementation with iron or screening for iron deficiency is advisable.

Electroencephalography

Studies reporting an increased frequency of epileptiform discharges in children with ADHD [Duane et al., 2003; Holtmann et al., 2003; Richer et al., 2002] and reports of ADHD-type symptoms resolving when spike activity was suppressed with antiepileptic drugs [Holtmann et al., 2003; Laporte et al., 2002] have led to proposed guidelines for obtaining an electroencephalogram (EEG). These include a history of clinical events suggesting a seizure (even if only nocturnal or febrile), perinatal stress, head trauma, fluctuating behavioral manifestations, or a family history of epilepsy [Duane, 1996].

Sleep Studies

A sleep history should be obtained. If the results suggest a diagnosis of a sleep disorder or if there is a strong family history of sleep disorders, a sleep study should be considered [Gottlieb et al., 2003; Owens, 2005; Thunstrom, 2002; Walters et al., 2000].

Imaging Studies

There are few clinical indications for performing neuroimaging in children with ADHD. ADHD has been reported in association with head trauma [Gerring et al., 2000; Wassenberg et al., 2004], prematurity [Foulder-Hughes and Cooke, 2003], perinatal injury [Toft, 1999], and neurofibromatosis [Rosser and Packer, 2003]. However, if the child is clinically stable, the presence of ADHD symptoms does not call for imaging studies beyond those indicated for the primary condition.

Treatment

Pharmacologic Therapy

In the 1930s, Charles Bradley administered benzedrine (an amphetamine) to children with a history of neurologic and behavioral problems in whom he had done a lumbar puncture in an attempt to stimulate secretion of cerebrospinal fluid by the choroid plexus and diminish headaches after lumbar puncture. Although benzedrine did not affect the incidence of headaches, the childrens teachers reported major improvement in learning and behavior in a number of children that lasted the entire time they were treated [Gross, 1995]. A subsequent open trial of benzedrine in children with neurologic and behavioral problems who had normal intelligence resulted in improved learning, a greater interest in and a higher quality of their schoolwork, behavioral and social improvements, and increased voluntary control [Bradley, 1937]. However, the use of medication in children was viewed unfavorably in the medical and educational community, and it was not until the 1960s, when methylphenidate was found to be effective in the treatment of attention disorders, that stimulant use was accepted by physicians and parents [Clements and Peters, 1962]. Between 1990 and 1998, there was a 3.7-fold increase in the diagnosis of ADHD, and prescription of stimulants for children 5–18 years old increased from 11.5 to 42 per 1000 [Robison et al., 2002].

Recently, and controversially, the American Heart Association recommended that all children placed on stimulant medications for ADHD should have a screening electrocardiogram (EKG) [Vetter et al., 2008]. The American Academy of Pediatrics concluded that this is neither necessary nor recommended and, instead, recommended cardiovascular screening based on personal, past, and family histories and the cardiovascular examination [Perrin et al., 2008]. Cases of children and adolescents who had a sudden unexplained death were reviewed and a determination was made as to whether toxicology studies revealed evidence of stimulant use at the time of death. Comparison was made to a group of children and adolescents who died as passengers in motor vehicle accidents, in whom toxicology screens were performed. The study excluded children with cardiac conditions, including a history of prolonged QT interval in the deceased or any first-degree relative, history of sudden death among first-degree relatives, conduction disorders in the deceased, and evidence of cardiac disease or any abnormal anatomic findings on autopsy, including cardiomegaly, cardiac hypertrophy, and cardiomyopathy. Ten of 564 sudden unexplained death cases (1.8 percent) had evidence of stimulant use at the time of death, compared to 2 out of 564 motor vehicle accident cases (0.4 percent). The odds ratio of 7.4 was significant at p = 0.02 level of significance. The authors cautioned about potential bias in such a study, but concluded that the finding represents "a significant association or 'signal' between sudden unexplained death and the use of stimulant medication, specifically methylphenidate" [Gould et al., 2009]. An accompanying editorial pointed out that sudden unexplained death is a rare event and "that it is not possible to quantify the risk beyond estimating that it is very small," adding that the findings "underscore the fact that stimulants are not innocuous, their therapeutic use requires careful diagnostic assessment, diligent safety screening and ongoing monitoring," and that "when making treatment decisions, clinicians need to apply the current, still incomplete, evidence to the care of individual patients by carefully considering the type and severity of symptoms, availability of different treatments, expected benefits and potential risks" [Vitiello and Towbin, 2009]. Given the exclusion criteria in this published review, it would appear that routine EKGs would not have had an impact on the rate of sudden unexplained death.

Table 47-1, derived from a review of pharmacotherapy in ADHD [Biederman et al., 2004], summarizes information regarding drug class, dose range, dosing schedule, indications, common adverse effects, and comments by the investigators.

Stimulant Medications

Stimulant drugs, sympathomimetic agents structurally similar to endogenous catecholamines, act centrally and peripherally by enhancing dopaminergic and noradrenergic transmission. Stimulants have been demonstrated to improve cognitive ability, school performance, and behavior [Barkley and Jackson, 1977; Famularo and Fenton, 1987; Rapport et al., 1988]. A study of children with ADHD with a high degree of comorbidity (ODD, 10 percent; CD, 30 percent; anxiety disorder, 17 percent; dyslexia, 32 percent) found differential effects of methylphenidate on various attentional functions at different doses [Konrad et al., 2004]. Specifically, alertness and focused and sustained attention improved in a linear fashion with increasing dose; inhibition and set-shifting were enhanced at a low dose but worsened at a moderate dose; and divided attention did not change at all. The different dose–response relationships for various cognitive and behavioral functions were explained by differential effects of these agents in different brain regions [Solanto, 2002]. The positive effects of methylphenidate on cognitive functions were caused by facilitation of dopaminergic activity in some brain regions, whereas improvement in hyperactivity and impulsivity was mediated by reduction in dopaminergic stimulation in other brain regions. This study did not uncover any differences in the response to methylphenidate between children with ADHD/C versus ADHD/I, nor was there any effect of comorbidity. Such data suggest that a single measure of response to stimulant treatment may be insufficient because different doses may be necessary to improve particular functions.

The response to methylphenidate in a group of 28 preschoolers (3–5 years old), as measured using behavioral ratings by teachers and parents, documented improvement, with 82 percent rated as having normal behavior after treatment, higher than the rate generally achieved in older children [Short et al., 2004]. With the exception of decreased appetite, there were no adverse side effects. The investigators speculate that the higher normalization rate for preschoolers than elementary school children may be a function of fewer demands placed on the preschooler (e.g., shorter school day, no homework).

The most commonly reported side effects of stimulants include appetite suppression and sleep disturbance. Absorption of stimulant medications is not notably affected when taken with or after meals, which may ameliorate appetite suppression [Green, 2001]. Insomnia can be a side effect from the medication but may also be caused by a rebound effect as the medication effect subsides. This distinction is important because, in the latter situation, a late afternoon or evening dose of stimulant medication may ease falling asleep

Table 47-1 Major Drug Classes Used in the Pharmacotherapy of Attention-Deficit Hyperactivity Disorder*

Drug	Total Daily Dose	Daily Dosage Schedule	Main Indications	Common Adverse Effects/Comments
STIMULANTS				
Dextroamphetamine	0.3–1 mg/kg	2 or 3 times	ADHD	Insomnia, decreased appetite Depression, psychosis (rare, with very high doses) Increased heart rate and blood pressure (mild) Possible growth reduction with long-term use Withdrawal effects and rebound phenomena
Mixed salts of L- and D-amphetamine	0.5–1.5 mg/kg	1 or 2 times	ADHD	Regular form has 6-hour duration of action Extended release form has 10–12-hour duration of action
Lisdexamfetamine	30–70 mg (total)	Daily	ADHD	Less abuse potential than dextroamphetamine
Methylphenidate	1–2 mg/kg	1–3 times	ADHD	Regular forms have 3–4-hour duration of action Extended release forms have 8–12-hour duration of action
Methylphenidate patch	10–30 mg/9 hours (total)	Daily	ADHD	
Dexmethylphenidate	0.5–1 mg/kg	2 or 3 times	ADHD	
Magnesium pemoline	1.0–2.5 mg/kg	1 or 2 times	ADHD	Associated with rare, serious hepatotoxicity and requires monitoring of liver function tests
Modafinil	200–400 mg (total)	Daily	Narcolepsy	Fewer peripheral sympathomimetic effects than amphetamines
NSRIs				
Atomoxetine	0.5–1.4 mg/kg	1 or 2 times	ADHD ± comorbidity Enuresis (?) Tic disorder (?) Depression/anxiety disorders (?)	Mechanism of action: noradrenergic-specific reuptake inhibitor Mild or moderate appetite depression Gastrointestinal symptoms Mild initial weight loss Mild increase in blood pressure, pulse No ECG conduction or repolarization delays Not abusable
TRICYCLIC ANTIDEPRESSANTS				
Tertiary amines Imipramine Amitriptyline Clomipramine	 2.0–5.0† mg/kg 2.0–5.0† mg/kg 2.0–5.0† mg/kg	 1 or 2 times 1 or 2 times 1 or 2 times	ADHD Enuresis Tic disorder Anxiety disorders (?) OCD (clomipramine)	Mixed mechanism of action (noradrenergic/serotonergic) Secondary amines more noradrenergic Clomipramine primarily serotonergic Narrow therapeutic index Overdoses can be fatal Anticholinergic effects: dry mouth, constipation, blurred vision Weight loss Mild increase in diastolic blood pressure and ECG conduction parameters with daily doses >3.5 mg/kg

Table 47-1 Major Drug Classes Used in the Pharmacotherapy of Attention-Deficit Hyperactivity Disorder—cont'd

Drug	Total Daily Dose	Daily Dosage Schedule	Main Indications	Common Adverse Effects/Comments
Secondary amines				
Desipramine	2.0–5.0[†] mg/kg	1 or 2 times		
Nortriptyline	1.0–3.0[†] mg/kg	1 or 2 times		
MAOIs			Atypical depression Treatment-refractory depression	Difficult medicines to use in juveniles
Phenelzine	0.5–1.0 mg/kg	2 or 3 times		Reserved for refractory cases
Tranylcypromine	0.5–1.0 mg/kg	2 or 3 times		Severe dietary restrictions (i.e., high-tyramine foods)
Selegiline	0.5–1.0 mg/kg	2 or 3 times		Drug–drug interactions
				Hypertensive crisis with dietetic transgression or with certain drugs
				Weight gain
				Drowsiness
				Changes in blood pressure
				Insomnia
				Liver toxicity (remote)
OTHER ANTIDEPRESSANTS				
SSRIs			MD, dysthymia	Serotonergic mechanism of action
Fluoxetine	0.3–0.9 mg/kg	1 time, in ar	OCD	Large margin of safety
Paroxetine	0.3–0.9 mg/kg	1 time, in ar	Anxiety disorders	No cardiovascular effects
Citalopram	0.3–0.9 mg/kg	1 time, in ar	Eating disorders	Irritability
Sertraline	1.5–3.0 mg/kg	1 time, in ar	PTSD (?)	Insomnia
Fluvoxamine	1.5–4.5 mg/kg	1 time, in ar		Gastrointestinal symptoms
				Headaches
				Sexual dysfunction
				Withdrawal symptoms more common with short-acting drugs
				Potential drug–drug interactions (cytochrome P-450)
Bupropion (SR)	3–6 mg/kg	2 times	ADHD	Mixed mechanism of action (dopaminergic/noradrenergic)
			MD	Irritability
			Smoking cessation	Insomnia
			Anti-craving effects (?)	Drug-induced seizures at doses >6 mg/kg
Venlafaxine (XR)	1–3 mg/kg	1 time	Bipolar depression (?)	Contraindicated in bulimics
			MD	Mixed mechanism of action (serotonergic/noradrenergic)
			Anxiety disorders	Similar to SSRIs
			ADHD (?)	Irritability
			OCD (?)	Insomnia
				Gastrointestinal symptoms
				Headaches
				Potential withdrawal symptoms
				Blood pressure symptoms

Table 47-1 Major Drug Classes Used in the Pharmacotherapy of Attention-Deficit Hyperactivity Disorder—cont'd

Drug	Total Daily Dose	Daily Dosage Schedule	Main Indications	Common Adverse Effects/Comments
Nefazodone	4–8 mg/kg	1 time	MD Anxiety disorders OCD (?) Bipolar depression (?)	Mixed mechanism of action (serotonergic/noradrenergic) Dizziness Nausea Potential interactions with nonsedating antihistamines, cisapride (cytochrome P-450) Rare, serious hepatotoxicity Less manicogenic (?)
Mirtazapine	0.2–0.9 mg/kg	1 time, in the afternoon	MD Anxiety disorders Stimulant-induced insomnia (?) Bipolar depression (?)	Mixed mechanism of action (serotonergic/noradrenergic) Sedation Weight gain Dizziness Less manicogenic (?)
NORADRENERGIC MODULATORS				
α2-Agonists Clonidine	0.003–0.010 mg/kg	2 or 3 times	Tourette disorder ADHD Aggression/self-abuse Severe agitation Withdrawal symptoms	Sedation (frequent) Hypotension (rare) Dry mouth Confusion (with high dose) Depression Rebound hypertension Localized irritation with transdermal preparation
Guanfacine (see text for information on long acting form of Guanfacine)	0.015–0.05 mg/kg	1 or 2 times		Same as clonidine Less sedation, hypotension
β-Blockers Propranolol	1–7 mg/kg	2 times	Aggression/self-abuse Severe agitation Akathisia	Risk for bradycardia and hypotension (dose-dependent) and rebound hypertension Bronchospasm (contraindicated in asthmatics) Rebound hypertension on abrupt withdrawal

* Doses are general guidelines and must be individualized with appropriate monitoring. Weight-corrected doses are less appropriate for obese children and adult doses should not be exceeded in older or larger children. When high doses are used, serum levels may be obtained to avoid toxicity.
† Dose adjusted according to serum levels (therapeutic window for nortriptyline).
ADHD, attention-deficit hyperactivity disorder; DR, delayed release; ECG, electrocardiographic; IR, immediate release; MAOIs, monoamine oxidase inhibitors; MD, mood disorder; MR, mental retardation; NSRIs, norepinephrine-specific reuptake inhibitors; OCD, obsessive-compulsive disorder; OROS, oral osmotic; PTSD, post-traumatic stress disorder; SR, sustained release; SSRIs, selective serotonin reuptake inhibitors; XR, extended release.
(Adapted from Biederman J et al. Evidence-based pharmacotherapy for attention-deficit hyperactivity disorder. Int J Neuropsychopharmacol 2004;7:77.)

[Chatoor et al., 1983]. Uncommonly, there have been reports of mood disturbances and lethargy after stimulant use [Wilens and Biederman, 1992]. Stimulants may also affect heart rate and blood pressure, but in healthy children, this change is unlikely to have clinical significance [Brown et al., 1984; Short et al., 2004]. There have been reports of psychostimulants inducing or exacerbating tic disorders, but subsequent studies have not found this to be a universal problem [Spencer et al., 1999]. Although this possibility should be discussed with children and their families, the presence of tics in a child with ADHD or a family history of tics is not an absolute contraindication to the use of psychostimulants. Concerns are often expressed regarding an increased risk of substance abuse in children treated with psychostimulants [Biederman et al., 1995b], but there is no supporting evidence. One study found that pharmacologic treatment for ADHD actually decreased the risk of subsequent substance abuse [Biederman et al., 1999]. There also have been reports of a decrease in the height of children taking stimulant medications [Safer et al., 1972], but other studies indicated no effect [Gross, 1976]. The reported decrease in height may reflect a transient maturational delay associated with ADHD, rather than a growth-stunting effect of medication [Spencer et al., 1998]. A longitudinal study [MTA Cooperative Group, 2004] revealed that children treated with medication had a reduced height gain compared with those who were not treated. Growth suppression was still evident during the second year of treatment in the group treated continuously, indicating that this was a persistent effect. The observation that there was less growth suppression in the children who were not treated continuously suggests that interrupting treatment with stimulant medication may limit growth suppression, supporting the concept of drug holidays to address this side effect. However, there have been reports of behavioral deterioration when stimulant medications are abruptly discontinued [Biederman et al., 2004].

The most commonly used drugs in the stimulant class include methylphenidate, dextroamphetamine, and mixed salts of L-and D-amphetamine. Although in the same class, these drugs have slightly different mechanisms of action, and patients may respond differently to each of them [Greenhill et al., 1998]. A review of double-blind, controlled trials of stimulant medications, published from 2005 through 2008, discussed the properties of the various formulations, including immediate, extended-release, and transdermal forms of methylphenidate, dexmethylphenidate, immediate- and extended-release forms of mixed amphetamine salts, and lisdexamfetamine, indicated which preparations can be opened and sprinkled into food and which medications were available as liquid or chewable tablets [Chavez et al., 2009]. The authors emphasized that a lack of response to one stimulant does not predict a response to other stimulants and a trial with a different agent is warranted if the initial treatment fails. ADHD subtype was not felt to dictate treatment choice. Results of studies comparing short- and long-acting preparations have been inconsistent [Fitzpatrick et al., 1992; Pelham et al., 1987, 1990]. Greydanus et al. [2009], in their review of the various classes of medication for treatment of ADHD, conclude: "despite intense pharmacologic advertisements, there are no short-acting or long-acting psychostimulants that are proven to be superior to the others."

Methylphenidate

Methylphenidate has fewer side effects than amphetamine [Efron et al., 1997]. In the standard formulation, methylphenidate reaches peak concentrations between 1 and 3 hours after oral intake. It is rapidly and extensively metabolized by nonmicrosomal hydrolytic esterases in the liver and other tissues, with an average half-life of 3 hours. In children, the starting dose is 0.3 mg/kg in the morning, rounded to the nearest 5-mg tablet [Drugdex Drug Evaluations, 2009]. It can be useful to have teachers complete a behavior checklist before and after initiation of treatment (preferably without being aware of exactly when the medication is started) to assess efficacy. If, after 1–2 weeks, there is inadequate benefit, the dose can be increased to 0.6 mg/kg. With an average half-life of 3 hours, a morning dose does not persist through the afternoon. Increasing the morning dose may increase the duration of the effect. Alternatively, a second dose 3–4 hours after the initial dose may be necessary. A dose in the middle to late afternoon to facilitate completion of homework may also be warranted. Alternatives to multiple daily doses are the long-acting formulations of methylphenidate. These formulations reach peak concentration 6–8 hours after oral intake, obviating the need for a midday dose. When using the longer-acting formulations, the entire daily dose is given in the morning. If there is no significant improvement in symptoms at a total daily dose of 1–2 mg/kg, alternate medication should be considered.

The regular formulation of methylphenidate is available in 5-, 10-, and 20-mg tablets (Ritalin). There are multiple extended-release formulations that use different mechanisms to achieve their sustained-release effect; they are available in 10- and 20-mg tablets (Metadate ER); 10-, 20-, and 30-mg capsules (Metadate CD); 20-, 30-, and 40-mg capsules (Ritalin LA); and 18-, 27-, 36-, and 54-mg tablets (Concerta).

Methylphenidate can also be administered by the transdermal route, in the form of a methylphenidate patch (Daytrana Transdermal System). The side effect profile is the same as for other forms of methylphenidate; however, the patch allows for a steadier rate of administration over a longer period. The patch is available in 12.5-, 18.75-, 25-, and 37.5-cm^2 sizes. The recommendations include applying the patch 2 hours before the desired effect and removing the patch 9 hours after application (or earlier if a shorter duration of effect is desired). For children 6–12 years of age, the recommended dose titration begins with the 12.5 cm^2 patch, which delivers 10 mg over 9 hours, at a rate of 1.1 mg/hour and increasing, in steps to the 37.5 cm^2 patch, which delivers 30 mg over 9 hours, at a rate of 3.3 mg/hour. A double-blind, placebo-controlled, randomized trial performed for FDA approval of this formulation found no evidence of improved efficacy when the dose was increased from 20 mg to 30 mg over 9 hours [Drugdex Drug Evaluations, 2009].

Dexmethylphenidate

Dexmethylphenidate is the D-threo-enantiomer of methylphenidate. A PET study found specific binding of the D-enantiomer to dopamine transporters in the basal ganglia, whereas the L-enantiomer had widespread, nonspecific binding [Ding et al., 1995]. Studies comparing dexmethylphenidate and methylphenidate have concluded both to be effective in ADHD, but dexmethylphenidate has a longer duration [Keating and

Figgitt, 2002]. The time to peak concentrations after oral intake is similar to that of methylphenidate (i.e., between 1 and 3 hours) and, like methylphenidate, it is rapidly and extensively metabolized by nonmicrosomal hydrolytic esterases in liver and other tissues, with an average half-life of about 2 hours. In children, the starting dose of dexmethylphenidate is one-half of the methylphenidate dose (0.15 mg/ kg in the morning, rounded to the nearest 2.5-mg tablet) [Drugdex Drug Evaluations, 2009]. If, after 1–2 weeks, there is inadequate benefit, the dose can be increased in 2.5-mg increments, to a maximum of 20 mg/day. The report of longer clinical efficacy than methylphenidate (despite the similar half-life) may eliminate the need for a midday dose, depending on the clinical response. There is no evidence that giving the D-isomer (dexmethylphenidate) at one-half of the dose of the D,L-enantiomer (methylphenidate) confers any clinical advantage. Dexmethylphenidate is available in 2.5-, 5-, and 10-mg tablets (Focalin).

Lisdexamfetamine

Lisdexamfetamine, a prodrug of dextroamphetamine, is rapidly absorbed in the gastrointestinal tract and converted to dextroamphetamine; thus its efficacy in ADHD is similar to that of dextroamphetamine. The T_{max} of lisdexamfetamine is 1 hour, but the T_{max} of dextroamphetamine, the active agent, is 3.5 hours after a single dose of lisdexamfetamine. The longer T_{max} of dextroamphetamine, when given in the form of lisdexamfetamine, allows for once-a-day dosing and is thought to decrease the abuse potential of this formulation. The recommended starting dose is 30 mg/day, with upward titration by 10–20 mg increments to a maximum dose of 70 mg/day. Lisdexamfetamine comes in 20, 30, 40, 50, 60, and 70 mg capsules [Drugdex Drug Evaluations, 2009].

Dextroamphetamine

Dextroamphetamine has a time to peak concentration of 60–160 minutes and is metabolized in the liver. The average half-life of dextroamphetamine is 10–12 hours, but this varies considerably with urinary pH; at a urine pH of less than 6.6, more than two-thirds of unmetabolized drug is excreted in the urine, whereas at a urine pH greater than 6.7, it is less than one-half. The initial dose of dextroamphetamine is 0.15–0.3 mg/kg (rounded to the nearest 5 mg) [Drugdex Drug Evaluations, 2009]. This dose can be gradually increased to desired effect up to a peak dose of approximately 1 mg/kg/day. Dextroamphetamine's longer half-life compared with methylphenidate may obviate the need for a midday dose. An extended-release preparation of dextroamphetamine eliminates the need for midday dosing. The regular formulation of dextroamphetamine is available in 5-mg tablets (Dexedrine); the extended-release formulation is available in 5-, 10-, and 15-mg capsules (Dexedrine Spansules).

Adderall is a combination of four amphetamine salts (D-amphetamine saccharate, D-amphetamine sulfate, D,L-amphetamine sulfate, and D,L-amphetamine aspartate), with a 3:1 ratio of D-isomer to L-isomer. The time to peak concentration and half-life are similar to those for dextroamphetamine. The initial dose of Adderall is 2.5 or 5 mg, with weekly increments based on the response to a maximum dose of 1.5 mg/kg/day, up to about 40 mg. The half-life of Adderall is such that a midday dose may or may not be necessary.

Adderall is available in 5-, 7.5-, 10-, 12.5-, 15-, 20-, and 30-mg tablets. Adderall XR capsules, with one-half of the contents in a delayed-release formulation, eliminate the need for midday dosing; the entire daily dose is given in the morning. Adderall XR is available in 5-, 10-, 15-, 20-, 25-, and 30-mg capsules.

Noradrenergic Potentiation

Atomoxetine

Atomoxetine (Strattera) is a norepinephrine-specific reuptake inhibitor that is effective in the treatment of children with ADHD. In a study comparing atomoxetine to methylphenidate and placebo, the response rate to atomoxetine and methylphenidate was essentially identical, and both were better than placebo. Appetite suppression was somewhat lower in atomoxetine compared with methylphenidate (22 percent versus 32 percent), and there was significantly less insomnia on atomoxetine (7 percent versus 27 percent) [Spencer et al., 2002]. Atomoxetine is metabolized by the cytochrome P-450 (CYP) 2D6 pathway. Peak plasma concentrations of atomoxetine occur 1–2 hours after oral administration. In extensive metabolizers (most patients), atomoxetine half-life is 4–5 hours. Substantial decreases in clearance and prolongation of the half-life are seen in poor metabolizers. The starting dose is 0.5 mg/kg/day, with gradual increase to a target dose of 1.2 mg/kg/day. In poor metabolizers (about 7 percent of the population), the half-life is substantially longer, and the dose requirement may be much lower. Depending on the response, midday dosing may be required for extensive metabolizers. Food does not affect absorption [Drugdex Drug Evaluations, 2009]. Because atomoxetine is not a controlled substance in the United States, prescriptions with multiple refills can be provided, and renewals can be done over the phone, in contrast to the procedures for stimulant medications. Atomoxetine is available in 10-, 18-, 25-, 40-, and 60-mg capsules. In December 2004 the Food and Drug Administration (FDA) asked the manufacturer to add a bolded warning about severe liver injury to the labeling, indicating that the medication should be discontinued in patients who develop jaundice or laboratory evidence of liver injury. In September 2005 the FDA directed the manufacturer to revise the labeling further to include a boxed warning regarding an increased risk of suicidal thinking in children and adolescents being treated with this drug.

Other agents

Modafinil, a central nervous stimulant, the mechanism of action of which is uncertain, lacks the peripheral sympathomimetic effects seen with amphetamines. Modafinil has been approved for the treatment of excessive daytime sleepiness associated with narcolepsy, obstructive sleep apnea, and shift-work sleep disorder. Studies of its efficacy in ADHD have found it to be more effective than placebo in ameliorating ADHD symptoms and comparable to methylphenidate in efficacy. The doses studied were 340 and 425 mg/day in children weighing less than or more than 30 kg, respectively [Swanson et al., 2006]. Modafinil is available in 100- and 200-mg oral tablets [Drugdex Drug Evaluations, 2009].

Armodafinil, the longer lived, R-enantiomer of modafinil, is available as 50-, 150-, and 250-mg tablets; it has the same mechanism of action and the same clinical indications as

Modafinil. No studies have been done on the efficacy of armodafinil in ADHD; presumably it would have efficacy similar to that of modafinil [Drugdex Drug Evaluations, 2009].

Nonstimulant Medications

It is estimated that at least 30 percent of children diagnosed with ADHD do not respond to or tolerate stimulant medications [Spencer et al., 1996]. Most studies have reported a reduced rate of response to psychostimulants in children with ADHD and anxiety or depression [Spencer et al., 1996]. The failure to respond to psychostimulants suggests the possibility of an incorrect diagnosis. However, genetic studies have suggested that children with ADHD respond differently to methylphenidate, depending on whether they were homozygous or heterozygous for the 10-repeat allele at dopamine transporter gene *SLC6A3* [Loo et al., 2003; Rhode et al., 2003; Winsberg and Comings, 1999].

Tricyclic Antidepressants

Other agents found to be effective in the treatment of ADHD include tricyclic antidepressants (TCAs). In one study, comorbidity with conduct disorder, depression, or anxiety, or a family history of ADHD did not result in a differential response to desipramine [Biederman et al., 1989]. In studies comparing TCAs with stimulants, TCAs appear to improve behavioral symptoms more consistently than cognitive function [Rapport et al., 1993].

Desipramine

Desipramine, a tricyclic antidepressant, is metabolized in the liver by the CYP-2D6 pathway, with an average half-life of 17.1 hours. For the 7 percent of the population with decreased activity of this enzyme, the half-life may be as long as 77 hours [Drugdex Drug Evaluations, 2009]. The effective dose of desipramine is lower and onset of action sooner for ADHD than for depression [Green, 2007]. The starting dose of desipramine is 1 mg/kg/day, with gradual increments to a maximum of 5 mg/kg/day. This medication may be given once daily or in divided doses, depending on the response. For slow metabolizers, the dose requirement is much lower, and once-daily dosing should be sufficient.

There have been case reports of sudden death in children treated with desipramine [Riddle et al., 1991]. Although a subsequent epidemiologic study did not find greater risk of sudden death with desipramine [Biederman et al., 1995b], it has been suggested that a baseline EKG be obtained before initiating treatment and that serial EKGs be obtained after significant dose increments and periodically during treatment [Biederman et al., 2004].

Alpha-Adrenergic Agonists

The α-adrenergic agents clonidine and guanfacine have been widely used for treatment of ADHD, despite few clinical studies. The success of these agents for Tourette's syndrome and other tic disorders [Leckman et al., 1991] has made them especially useful in children with ADHD and tic disorders, particularly if a trial of stimulant medication resulted in exacerbation of tics. Reports of three deaths of children taking a combination of methylphenidate and clonidine prompted reviews that found no evidence of an adverse methylphenidate–clonidine interaction [Fenichel, 1995; Popper, 1995].

Nevertheless, if there is a plan to prescribe this combination, a review of this literature and discussion of risks and benefits with the parents are advisable. Guanfacine appears to have an advantage over clonidine because it has a longer half-life and is less sedating [Hunt et al., 1995]. Guanfacine reaches a peak concentration after oral intake in 1–4 hours and is metabolized in the liver, with an average half-life of 17 hours [Drugdex Drug Evaluations, 2009]. The starting dose is 0.015 mg/kg/day (to the nearest 0.5 mg), with a gradual increase to a maximum of 0.05 mg/kg or 4 mg/day, based on the clinical response [Biederman et al., 2004]. The half-life of guanfacine should allow for once-daily dosing, although in clinical studies it was administered in 2–4 divided doses [Chappell et al., 1995; Hunt et al., 1995]. Guanfacine is available in 1 and 2 mg tablets. An extended release form of guanfacine is also available in 1-, 2-, 3-, and 4-mg tablets, which must be swallowed whole. The recommended starting dose is 1 mg/day with therapeutic benefit demonstrated at doses from 0.05 mg/kg/day up to 0.12 mg/kg/day to a maximum of 4 mg/day [Drugdex Drug Evaluations, 2009]. Other agents reported to be effective in ADHD are reviewed in Table 47-1.

Future directions include studies of AMPA (ampakine) receptor modulators, nicotinic acetylcholine receptor antagonists, dopamine agonists (which are effective in the treatment of restless leg syndrome), atypical antipsychotics (e.g., aripiprazole and risperidone), selective noradrenaline reuptake inhibitors and gamma-aminobutyric acid (GABA) B receptor antagonists [Greydanus et al., 2009].

Nonpharmacologic Therapies

Children with ADHD need a school environment with minimal distractions, and with seating that is somewhat isolated and close to the front of the classroom in front of the teacher [Shaywitz and Shaywitz, 1984]. The setting should be fairly structured, with organizational techniques such as checklists and homework assignment pads, and an uncluttered desk at home devoted exclusively to schoolwork.

A multicenter clinical trial of various treatment strategies for ADHD [MTA Cooperative Group, 1999] concluded that stimulants were more effective than behavioral therapies for ADHD symptoms. The combination of stimulants and behavioral therapy resulted in improved social skills but did not significantly improve ADHD symptoms over stimulants alone. A review of treatment modalities of children diagnosed with ADHD in the period from 1995 to 1999 found that among children diagnosed with ADHD, 24 percent also had mental illness. The most frequent treatments were stimulant medication alone (42 percent), stimulant medication combined with psychotherapy or mental health counseling (32 percent), and psychotherapy or mental health counseling alone (10.8 percent). Fifteen percent of children received no treatment other than office visits for initial and follow-up medical care. The percentage of children receiving psychotherapy or mental health counseling alone or in combination with stimulant medication increased with age, and males were more likely than females to receive treatment [Robison et al., 2004].

Biofeedback Programs

Various forms of computer training programs have been studied in treating children with ADHD. Such working memory training programs improved working memory capacity in children with ADHD and adults without ADHD. Improvement generalized to nonpracticed tasks involving prefrontal cortex. In children with ADHD, the improvement in working memory was associated with a decrease in head movements [Klingberg et al., 2002]. Children with ADHD trained to modify their slow cortical potentials also have an increase in contingent negative variation during a continuous performance task compared with those who did not receive training. Associated with this electrophysiologic phenomenon were fewer impulsivity errors on the continuous performance task, suggesting that the contingent negative variation increase represented a neurophysiologic correlate of improved self-regulatory capabilities [Heinrich et al., 2004].

The use of an EEG biofeedback program has been compared with the effectiveness of methylphenidate [Fuchs et al., 2003]. Children were trained to increase the power of the sensory motor rhythm (12 to 15 hertz) and low beta activity (15 to 18 hertz). Assignment to the biofeedback versus methylphenidate group was based on parental preference. Two-thirds of parents chose the biofeedback training program, raising issues of selection bias, and there was no placebo arm in this study. After 3 months, both groups had significant improvements in all four subscales on the TOVA, as well as on a behavior rating scale. Changes in the EEG as a result of biofeedback were not monitored in this study. A previous study using biofeedback reported greater improvement on the TOVA in participants with significant EEG changes than in those without changes (although there were improvements in both groups) [Lubar et al., 1995]. There was no correlation between behavioral changes reported by the parents and changes in the EEG. This study did not include a control group. A study of EEG biofeedback that used a control group (i.e., association between EEG patterns and feedback to the participants was random) found no benefit from EEG biofeedback [Heywood and Beale, 2003]. The investigators noted that, had the data analysis excluded the dropouts and failed to control for behavioral trends unrelated to the EEG biofeedback training, it would have led to the erroneous conclusion that the treatment was effective.

A study assessing the gait of a group of 16 children with ADHD under "usual" and "dual task" conditions found that dual tasking caused a significant decrease in stride time variability in the ADHD group, which was unexpected and the opposite of the anticipated result. After methylphenidate was taken, dual tasking no longer significantly affected stride time variability in the ADHD group. Methylphenidate and dual tasking had similar effects on gait variability, but opposite effects on gait speed, with methylphenidate increasing gait speed and dual tasking slowing it down. It was hypothesized that children with ADHD walk more rhythmically in the dual-tasking condition, opposite to the effect observed in healthy adults, due to a higher attentional level (vigilance) created by presenting the children with a cognitive challenge. Alternatively, the additional cognitive load may have created an "automatic pilot" of gait [Leitner et al., 2007]. This might explain the reported effects of biofeedback and other interventions involving cognitive activity.

Complementary and Alternative Medications

A survey of parents of children referred for evaluation of ADHD reported that 54 percent of the parents used complementary and alternative medicine (e.g., acupuncture, nutritional supplements) for the child's ADHD symptoms in the prior year [Chan et al., 2003]. Only 11 percent of the parents discussed using such interventions with their child's physician. A review of the literature on the role of nutritional factors in ADHD, including food additives, sugars, food allergies or sensitivities, and essential fatty acids, identified methodological problems with negative studies without similar discussion of problems with positive studies, possibly revealing bias of the authors [Schnoll et al., 2003]. Nevertheless, the summary statement is reasonably cautious: "There is increasing evidence that there is a subset of children with behavioral problems who are sensitive to one or more food components that may precipitate or contribute to their hyperactive behavior. Research indicates that it is futile to try to identify a specific food or substance that will precipitate negative behavior in all hyperactive children."

A placebo-controlled, double-blind study of dietary supplementation with omega-3 and omega-6 fatty acids in children with developmental coordination disorder, defined in the DSM-IV as a specific impairment of motor function independent of general ability [American Psychiatric Association, 1994], found a statistically significant improvement in reading, spelling, and ADHD-related symptoms after 3 months in the treatment group, compared to placebo. There was no improvement in the score on a movement assessment battery. Of the 102 children with data at 3 months, there were 32 children who had baseline scores on a parent rating scale exceeding 2 standard deviations above the general population average for DSM-IV criteria for ADHD; of these, 16 were in the treatment group and 16 were in the placebo group. After 3 months, 7 of the 16 children in the treatment group were no longer in the clinical range for ADHD symptoms, while only 1 of 16 in the placebo group was no longer in the clinical range for ADHD [Richardson and Montgomery, 2005]. In contrast, a review of the biology of essential fatty acids (EFAs) in brain function and studies of EFAs in children with ADHD found that uncontrolled, open-label studies reported that EFA supplementation improved ADHD symptoms; however, randomized controlled trials did not show treatment effects; in some cases, there were better results for the placebo group. The authors concluded that the available evidence "does not support the use of EFA supplements as a treatment for children with ADHD" [Raz and Gabis, 2009]. It should be emphasized that the latter review was of studies that recruited children with a diagnosis of ADHD, in contrast to the former study that recruited children with a diagnosis of developmental coordination disorder.

Outcome

ADHD persists into adulthood. The symptoms of ADHD may be less obvious after the individual is older [Hart et al., 1995]. The incidence of ADHD in adults depends on diagnostic criteria and whether historical data are obtained from the patients or their parents [Weiss and Weiss, 2002]. The finding that adolescents and young adults with ADHD had more car accidents with bodily injuries indicates that this is a serious problem, even in older children and adults [Barkley et al., 1993].

Conclusions

There is still much research required for achieving a fuller understanding of ADHD, not least of which is agreeing on a precise definition, including appropriate exclusion criteria, so that treatment studies can be compared, and anatomic and genetic studies can be done on phenotypically homogeneous groups. Available evidence suggests that there may be value in distinguishing ADHD/I from ADHD/HI and ADHD/C and in separating cases with comorbidity, because these groups have different characteristics and different responses to treatment. Also, the controversy over the safety of psychostimulants has to balance the evident, but very small, risk of serious adverse effects against the well-documented benefit, including evidence suggesting anatomical, as well as functional, normalization. A crucial role for the physician assessing a child for the possibility of ADHD is recognizing features in the presentation that suggest alternative diagnoses.

The complete list of references for this chapter is available online at **www.expertconsult.com**.
See inside cover for registration details.

Autistic Spectrum Disorders

Deborah G. Hirtz, Ann Wagner, and Pauline A. Filipek

The autistic spectrum disorders (ASD) represent a wide continuum of associated cognitive and neurobehavioral deficits, including deficits in socialization and communication, with restricted and repetitive patterns of behaviors [American Psychiatric Association, 1994, 2000]. The terms autism and autistic spectrum disorders are used interchangeably throughout this chapter and refer to the broader umbrella of pervasive developmental disorders (PDD), as defined by the Fourth Edition of the *Diagnostic and Statistical Manual of Mental Disorders* [American Psychiatric Association, DSM-IV, 1994; DSM-IV-TR, 2000].

Historical Perspective of the DSM

Although Kanner [1943] first described a syndrome of "autistic disturbances" in 11 children who shared "unique" and previously unreported patterns of behavior, including social remoteness, obsessiveness, stereotypy, and echolalia, the first set of formal diagnostic criteria for this disorder was not formulated until the 1970s [Ritvo and Freeman, 1978; Rutter and Hersov, 1977]. In the DSM-III [American Psychiatric Association, 1980], the term "autism" was included for the first time, and was clearly differentiated from childhood schizophrenia and other psychoses under a new diagnostic umbrella of pervasive developmental disorders; the possible PDD diagnoses included the terms infantile autism (onset before age 30 months) and childhood-onset pervasive developmental disorder (onset after age 30 months), with each further subclassified as full syndrome present or residual state. The DSM-IIIR [American Psychiatric Association, 1987] broadened the spectrum of PDD and narrowed the specific diagnoses to two: autistic disorder and PDD – not otherwise specified (PDD-NOS). The DSM-IV [1994] and DSM-IV-TR [2000] included five possible diagnoses under the PDD umbrella: autistic disorder, Asperger's disorder, childhood disintegrative disorder, Rett's syndrome, and PDD-NOS/atypical autism. With an anticipated publication date of 2013, DSM-V [in press] will most likely eliminate the term PDD and instead will use autistic spectrum disorders as the umbrella term, with autistic disorder and atypical autism as the two possible diagnostic categories (Box 48-1).

Clinical Features of ASD

All individuals on the autistic spectrum demonstrate deficits in three core domains: reciprocal social interactions, verbal and nonverbal communication, and restricted and repetitive behaviors or interests [American Psychiatric Association, 1994, 2000]. There is marked variability in the severity of symptoms across patients, and cognitive function can range from profound mental retardation through the superior range on conventional IQ tests. Symptoms and signs are discussed in detail in the DSM-IV, in the monograph edited by Rapin [1996], in the Wing Autistic Disorders Interview Checklist – Revised [Wing, 1996], and in numerous additional publications [Allen, 1988; Allen and Rapin, 1992; Barbaro and Dissanayake, 2009; Filipek et al., 1999; Greenspan et al., 2008; Rapin and Tuchman, 2008; Zwaigenbaum et al., 2009] (Box 48-2).

Qualitative Impairment in Social Interactions

The criteria in this domain refer to a *qualitative* impairment in reciprocal social interactions, not to the absolute lack of social behaviors. Behaviors range from total lack of awareness of another person to the presence of eye contact that is not used to modulate social interactions. The qualitative nature of this and the communication domains were first included in the DSM-IV [1994].

As infants, some autistic children do not lift up their arms or change posture in anticipation of being held. They may or may not cuddle, or even stiffen when held, and often do not look or smile when making a social approach. The characteristic give-and-take in lap play that is seen in typically developing infants and toddlers is often missing. Typically developing infants and toddlers often take great delight in using their newfound "pointer" finger to request or to show; those with ASD usually do not point to request or show/share. Older children often do not point things out or use eye contact to share the pleasure of seeing something with another person, which is called joint attention or social referencing.

Some children do make eye contact, often only in brief glances, but the eye contact is usually not used to get someone's attention. Others may make inappropriate eye contact by turning someone else's head to gaze into their eyes. Autistic children may appear to ignore a familiar or unfamiliar person because of a lack of social interest. Some children do make social approaches, although their conversational turn-taking or modulation of eye contact is often grossly impaired. At the opposite extreme of social interactions, some children may make indiscriminate approaches to strangers (e.g., climb into the examiner's lap before the parent has entered the room, be unaware of psychologic barriers, or be described as a child that continuously and inappropriately "gets in your face").

Some children with autism indicate little or no interest in other children or adults and prefer to play alone, away from others. Others play with adults nearby or sit on the outskirts of other children's play and engage in parallel play or simply watch the other children. Some children involve other children in designated, often repetitive play, but often only as

Box 48-1 DSM IV and Proposed DSM V Categories

DSM-IV and DSM-IV-TR [APA, 1994, 2000]

- Pervasive developmental disorders (PDD)
  - Autistic disorder
  - Asperger's disorder
  - Childhood disintegrative disorder
  - Rett's syndrome
  - PDD – not otherwise specified (NOS), atypical autism

Proposed DSM-V [APA, in press]

- Autism spectrum disorders

"assistants," without heeding any suggestions from the other children. Some prefer to serve in the passive role in other children's play, such as the infant in a game of house, and follow others' directions. Other children may seek out one specific child with whom there is a limited solitary interest that dominates the entire relationship.

Autistic children may also have no age-appropriate friends, and older children often are teased or bullied. A child may "want friends" but usually does not understand the concept of the reciprocity and sharing of interests and ideas inherent in friendship. They may refer to all classmates as friends; one telling example is the child who said, "Oh, I have many, many, 29 friends, but none of them likes me." Verbal children may have one friend, but the relationship may be limited or may focus only on a similar circumscribed interest, such as a particular computer game. Often, children gravitate to either older peers, in which case they play the role of followers, or to much younger peers, in which case they become the leaders.

Qualitative Impairment in (Verbal and Nonverbal) Communication

The communication deficits seen in the autistic spectrum are far more complex than presumed by simple speech delay, and they are similar to the deficits seen in children with developmental language disorders or specific language impairments [Allen and Rapin, 1992]. Expressive language function across the autistic spectrum ranges from complete mutism to verbal fluency, although fluency is often accompanied by many semantic (i.e., word meaning) and verbal pragmatic (i.e., use of language to communicate) errors. Some mute autistic children do not respond to their names, and often, they are initially presumed to be severely hearing-impaired.

In early infancy, some children with ASD do not babble or use any other communicative vocalizations, and they are described as quiet babies. Some children have absolutely no spoken language when speech should be developing, and they fail to compensate with facial expressions or gestures. A typically developing infant or toddler may pull his or her mother over to a desired object and then will clearly point to the object they request. In contrast, a characteristic behavior of many autistic children is to use another person's hand mechanically to point to the desired object, an action called hand-over-hand "pointing." Other "independent" children make no demands or requests of the parents but learn to climb at a young age and acquire the desired object for themselves.

A common feature of verbally fluent children is their inability to initiate or sustain a conversation, which requires two or more parties communicating in a give-and-take fashion on a mutually agreed topic. Although they may be able to respond relatively well to, ask questions of, or talk "at" another person, the reciprocity inherent in a conversation is often difficult for individuals with ASD.

Box 48-2 DSM-IV/DSM-IV-TR Diagnostic Criteria for 299.00 Autistic Disorder

A. A total of six (or more) items from 1, 2, and 3, with two from 1 and at least one each from 2 and 3:

1. Qualitative impairment in social interaction, manifested by at least two of the following:
   a. Marked impairment in the use of multiple nonverbal behaviors, such as eye-to-eye gaze, facial expression, body postures, and gestures, to regulate social interaction
   b. Failure to develop peer relationships appropriate to developmental level
   c. Lack of spontaneous seeking to share enjoyment, interests, or achievements with other people (e.g., by lack of showing, bringing, or pointing out objects of interest)
   d. Lack of social or emotional reciprocity
2. Qualitative impairment in communication, as manifested by at least one of the following:
   a. Delay in or total lack of the development of spoken language (not accompanied by an attempt to compensate through alternative modes of communication, such as gesture or mime)
   b. In individuals with adequate speech, marked impairment in the ability to initiate or sustain a conversation with others

   c. Stereotyped and repetitive use of language or idiosyncratic language
   d. Lack of varied, spontaneous make-believe or social imitative play appropriate to developmental level
3. Restrictive, repetitive, and stereotypic patterns of behavior, interests, and activities, as manifested by at least one of the following:
   a. Encompassing preoccupation with one or more stereotyped and restricted patterns of interest that is abnormal in intensity or focus
   b. Apparently inflexible adherence to specific nonfunctional routines or rituals
   c. Stereotyped and repetitive motor mannerisms (e.g., hand or finger flapping, twisting or complex entire-body movements)
   d. Persistent preoccupation with parts of objects

B. Delays or abnormal functioning occurs in at least one of the following areas, with onset before age 3 years: (1) social interaction, (2) language as used in social communication, or (3) symbolic or imaginative play.

C. The disturbance is not better accounted for by Rett's disorder or childhood disintegrative disorder.

(From American Psychiatric Association. Diagnostic and statistical manual of mental disorders, 4th edn. Washington, DC: American Psychiatric Association, 1994.)

A hallmark of autistic speech is immediate or delayed echolalia. Immediate echolalia refers to immediate noncommunicative repetition of words or phrases – the child is simply repeating exactly what was heard without synthesizing the intrinsic language. This ability is a crucial aspect of normal language development in infants under the age of 2 years, but it becomes pathologic when still present as the sole and predominant expressive language after the age of about 18–24 months.

Delayed echolalia or scripts refers to the use of highly ritualized phrases that have been memorized, such as from videos, television, commercials, or overheard conversations. The origin of this stereotypic language does not necessarily have to be clearly identifiable. Many older autistic children incorporate the scripts in an appropriate conversational context, which can give much of their speech a rehearsed and often more fluent quality relative to the rest of their spoken language. Children also demonstrate difficulties with pronouns or other words that change in meaning with context and they often reverse pronouns or refer to themselves in the third person or by name. Others may use literal idiosyncratic phrases or neologisms. Verbal autistic children may speak in detailed and grammatically correct phrases, which are none the less repetitive, concrete, and pedantic. If a child's answers to questions seem to "miss the point," further history and conversation with the child should be elicited because this is also a hallmark of autistic language deficits.

Some autistic children do not appropriately use miniature objects, animals, or dolls in pretend play. Others use the miniatures in a repetitive, mechanical fashion without evidence of representational play. Some highly verbal children may invent a fantasy world that becomes the sole focus of repetitive play. A classic example of the lack of appropriate play is the fluent autistic preschooler who "plays" by repeatedly reciting a soliloquy of the old witch scene verbatim from *Beauty and the Beast* while manipulating dollhouse characters in sequence precisely according to the script. When given the same miniature figures and dollhouse but instructed to play something other than Beauty and the Beast, this child is incapable of synthesizing any other play scenario.

Restricted, Repetitive, and Stereotypic Patterns of Behaviors, Interests, and Activities

Some verbal autistic children ask the same question repeatedly, regardless of what reply is given, or they engage in highly repetitive, perseverative play. Others are preoccupied with special interests that are highly unusual. For example, many children are fascinated with dinosaurs, but autistic children may amass exhaustive facts about every conceivable type of dinosaur and about which museums house which particular fossils; these children often repeatedly "share" their knowledge with others, regardless of the others' interest or suggestions to the contrary.

Many autistic children are so preoccupied with "sameness" in their home and school environments or routines that little can be changed without prompting a tantrum or other emotional disturbance. For example, some insist that all home furnishings remain in the same position, that all clothing to be a particular color, or that only one specific set of favored sheets be used on the bed. Others may eat only from a specific plate when sitting in a specific chair in a specific room, which may

not necessarily be the kitchen or dining room. Some children may insist on being naked while in the home but insist on wearing shoes to the dinner table. This inflexibility may also pertain to familiar routines, such as taking only a certain route to school, entering the grocery store only by one specific door, or never stopping or turning around after the car starts moving. Many parents may not be aware that they are following certain rituals to avoid the emotional upheaval, or they may be aware but are too embarrassed to volunteer such information. Within this context, some children have distinct behavioral repertoires that they use to sustain sameness, even when not imposed externally. By adulthood, many of these rituals may evolve to more classic obsessive-compulsive symptoms.

Some children have obvious stereotypical movements, such as florid hand-clapping or arm-flapping whenever excited or upset, which is pathologic if it occurs after the age of about 18–24 months. Running aimlessly, rocking, spinning, bruxism (teeth grinding), toe-walking, or other odd postures are commonly seen in autistic children. Others may repetitively tap the back of the hand in a less obtrusive manner, or touch or smell items. In higher-functioning youngsters, the stereotypic movements may become "miniaturized" as they get older into more socially acceptable behaviors, such as pill rolling [Bauman, 1992; Rapin, 1996].

Many children demonstrate the classic behavior of lining up toys, videotapes, or other favored objects, but others may simply collect things for no apparent purpose. Many are preoccupied with repetitive actions, such as opening and closing doors, drawers, to flipping the tops of trash cans, or turning light switches repetitively off and on. Others repetitively flick string, elastic bands, measuring tapes, or electric cords. Younger autistic children love spinning objects or themselves. Others are often particularly fascinated with water, and they especially enjoy transferring water repetitively from one vessel into another.

Asperger's Disorder

The validity of Asperger's disorder as an entity separate from high-functioning (verbal) children with ASD remains controversial [Ariella Ritvo et al., 2008; Frith, 2004; Howlin, 2003; Macintosh and Dissanayake, 2004; Sanders, 2009; Schopler, 1996; Witwer and Lecavalier, 2008; Woodbury-Smith and Volkmar, 2009], and Asperger's disorder will most likely not be included as a separate entity under the ASD umbrella in DSM-V [in press]. Clinically, the diagnosis of Asperger's disorder is often inappropriately given as an alternative, more acceptable, "A-word" to high-functioning autistic children [Bishop, 1989]. The similarity and overlap of signs and symptoms of Asperger's disorder with nonverbal learning disabilities (NLD) additionally expand the spectrum of these developmental disorders [Harnadek and Rourke, 1994; Klin et al., 1995; Rourke, 1989]; a recent report, however, demonstrates a lack of difficulty with spatial- or problem-solving tasks – a main principle in the NLD model – in a small cohort of children with Asperger's disorder [Ryburn et al., 2009].

In sharp contrast to autistic disorder, DSM-IV-TR Asperger's criteria state that "there are no clinically significant delays in early language (e.g., single words are used by age 2, communicative phrases by age 3)" [2000, p. 81]. Normal or near-normal cognitive function is also the rule, including self-help skills, "adaptive behavior (other than in social interaction), and curiosity about the environment in childhood" [1994, p. 77]. Although absence of language *delay* is required for diagnosis, the DSM-IV definition of single words by age 2 and communicative phrases by age 3 is none the less considerably outside the recognized norm for language development [Coplan and Gleason, 1993; Rossetti, 1990; Sanders, 2009; Zimmerman et al., 2002]. Asperger's criteria for the qualitative impairments in social interaction and restrictive and repetitive patterns of behaviors and activities are identical to those for autistic disorder (for a recent review, see Woodbury-Smith and Volkmar [2009]).

High verbal skills are the rule in Asperger's disorder, which typically leads to later clinical recognition than with autistic disorder [Volkmar and Cohen, 1991; Woodbury-Smith and Volkmar, 2009]. Despite the DSM-IV definition [1994, 2000], language in Asperger's disorder is clearly not typical or normal. For example, there usually is pedantic and poorly intoned speech, poor nonverbal pragmatic or communication skills, and intense preoccupation with circumscribed topics, such as the weather or railway timetables [Ghaziuddin and Gerstein, 1996; Klin et al., 1995; Wing, 1981]. Individuals with Asperger's use fewer personal pronouns, temporal expressions, and referential expressions [Colle et al., 2008]. They often exhibit deficits in the semantics and verbal pragmatics of language, resulting in concrete and literal speech; their answers often miss the point. They also demonstrate deficits in general receptive language [Koning and Magill-Evans, 2001; Noterdaeme et al., 2009; Saalasti et al., 2008] and in prosodic comprehension [Jarvinen-Pasley et al., 2008]. Szatmari et al. [1995] further define this disorder by the complete lack of delayed echolalia, pronoun reversal, or neologisms in language production.

Socially, individuals with Asperger's disorder are usually unable to form true friendships. Because of their naive, inappropriate, one-sided social interactions and lack of empathy, they may be ridiculed by their peers. Often, they cease their attempts to develop friendships because of the cruel ridicule and then remain extremely socially isolated. Fine and gross motor deficits have been described, including clumsy and uncoordinated movements and odd postures [Jansiewicz et al., 2006; Klin et al., 1995; Nishitani et al., 2004; Rinehart et al., 2006; Wing, 1981]. However, frank motor apraxia is an inconsistent finding [Dziuk et al., 2007; Mostofsky et al., 2006].

Autistic Regression and Childhood Disintegrative Disorder

Approximately 22–35 percent of autistic children initially appear to develop normally until at least 12 months of age, followed by loss of language and/or social skills [Baird et al., 2008; Meilleur and Fombonne, 2009; Rogers, 2004; Tuchman and Rapin, 1997; Wiggins et al., 2009]. Loss of language skills has been found to be specific for ASD [Kurita, 1996; Pickles et al., 2009]. Parents usually report that infants were socially responsive, smiled, waved bye-bye, and said some words, but they then suddenly or gradually stopped speaking and seemed to withdraw. In an on-going surveillance program, Wiggins et al. [2009] found that, not surprisingly, children with a known ASD diagnosis had a higher rate of parentally reported regression than those identified with ASD through the retrospective record review (26 percent vs. 17 percent, respectively). Regression occurred at a median age of

24 months; boys were more likely to demonstrate regression than girls, and at earlier ages. Children who experienced regression were diagnosed with ASD much earlier (mean age 4.2 years) than those without regression (mean age 6.2 years) [Shattuck et al., 2009].

One difficulty hindering a better understanding of autistic regression involves the disentangling of age at onset from age at recognition [Chawarska et al., 2007; Volkmar et al., 1985]. Many children thought by parents to be normal in the first 18 months may indeed show signs or symptoms on retrospective evaluation of home movies and videotapes by as early as 12 months of age [Baranek, 1999; Goldberg et al., 2003; Maestro et al., 2005; Osterling and Dawson, 1994, 1999; Ozonoff et al., 2005; Werner and Dawson, 2005]. Goldberg et al. [2008] found significant concordance between parental report and retrospective analysis of home videotapes of regression only in the language domains.

As recently reviewed by Tuchman [2006, 2009], there is considerable controversy surrounding the relation between autistic regression and epilepsy, with regression associated with an epileptiform electroencephalogram (EEG) approximately 20 percent of the time. Studies report both higher [Hrdlicka, 2008; Kobayashi and Murata, 1998] and lower rates [Baird et al., 2008; Tuchman et al., 1991] of epilepsy in regression. The behavioral phenotypes of autistic regression, Landau–Kleffner syndrome (LKS), and continuous spike-wave during slow-wave sleep (CSWS) overlap considerably, and may represent distinct syndromes based on age of regression, degree and type of regression, and frequency of epilepsy and EEG abnormalities [Tuchman, 2009]. Children with LKS and isolated language regression are more likely to have epileptiform EEGs and seizures than those with an autistic regression [McVicar et al., 2005].

Mitochondrial disorders have recently been reported to be associated with autism, and with regression in particular [Poling et al., 2006]. In a cohort of 25 patients with ASD and definite or probable mitochondrial disease by the Modified Walker and Mitochondrial Disease Criteria [Bernier et al., 2002; Wolf and Smeitink, 2002], Weissman found that 56 percent experienced regression of previously acquired skills; 64 percent of the regressions were multiple, and 43 percent had the regression(s) after 3 years of age [Weissman et al., 2008]. Shoffner et al. [2009] found that 61 percent of children with ASD and mitochondial disease experienced a regression, 71 percent associated with and 29 percent without fever.

By DSM-IV definition, childhood disintegrative disorder (CDD) refers to the rare phenomenon of normal early development until at least age 24 months, followed by the loss of language, social, play, or motor skills which culminate most often in symptoms of autism. Previously called Heller's syndrome, dementia infantalis, or disintegrative psychosis, CDD usually occurs between 36 and 48 months of age but may occur up to age 10 years [American Psychiatric Association, 1994, 2000]. There is, therefore, much overlap between CDD and autistic regression, which has led to significant controversy [Hendry, 2000; Malhotra and Gupta, 2002]. The category of CDD will most likely be retained in DSM-V [in press] under the umbrella of ASD; however, the diagnostic criteria may be changed to reflect the increased understanding of the phenomenon of regression in autism. The lower age limit of CDD will most likely be increased to age 3 years, with autistic regression occurring prior to age 3 years remaining under autism.

CDD is considered rare, with recent epidemiological data suggesting a prevalence estimate of 2 per 100,000 [Fombonne, 2002b, 2009]. It is usually associated with more severe autistic symptoms than is early-onset autism, including profound loss of cognitive skills resulting in mental retardation. There is a 4:1 male predominance and a mean age of onset of 29 ± 16 months; more than 95 percent demonstrate symptoms of speech loss, social disturbances, stereotyped behaviors, resistance to change, anxiety, and deterioration of self-help skills [Kurita et al., 2004a, b; Mouridsen, 2003; Volkmar and Rutter, 1995]. The risk of epilepsy may be as high as 70 percent [Mouridsen et al., 1999]. Children with CDD after age 3 years are more likely to have seizures than those who regress before age 24 months [Klein et al., 2000; Shinnar et al., 2001; Wilson et al., 2003]. Treatment experience in CDD has been generally limited to anticonvulsant therapy for seizures, although Mordekar et al. [2009] recently reported amelioration of behavior, language, and motor regression after corticosteroid treatment in two children with CDD, seizures, and/or epileptiform EEG patterns.

Pervasive Developmental Disorder – Not Otherwise Specified and Atypical Autism

The diagnosis of atypical autism or PDD-NOS is used when clinically significant autistic symptoms are present involving reciprocal social interactions, verbal or nonverbal communication, or stereotyped behavior, interests, and activities, but criteria are not met for a specific diagnostic category under the umbrella of autistic spectrum or pervasive developmental disorders (e.g., a child who does not meet the required 6 of 12 criteria for the diagnosis of autistic disorder) [American Psychiatric Association, 1994, 2000]. Children whose symptoms are atypical or not as severe are coded under this diagnosis. It should be noted that the DSM-IV definition of PDD-NOS required that a child meet *only 1 of the 12 criteria* in any of the three core domains; in DSM-IV-TR, the definition was changed to require impairment in the development of reciprocal social interaction and either impairment in verbal and nonverbal communication skills or the presence of stereotyped behavior, interests, and activities. It is expected that this diagnostic category will be eliminated in the DSM-V [in press, Box 48-3].

Epidemiology

The reported prevalence of autism has dramatically increased, and it is now recognized as one of the most common developmental disorders. Most studies come from industrialized countries, but there is increasing awareness of autism and other developmental disabilities in less developed communities around the world. For many years after autism was first described in the 1940s, prevalence was considered to be 2–4 cases per 10,000 children [Wing and Potter, 2002]. Fombonne [2003a] reviewed a total of 32 epidemiological studies published from 1966 through 2001. For the 16 studies published from 1966 to1991, the median prevalence was 4.4 per 10,000; for the 16 studies published from 1992 to 2001, the median was 12.7 per 10,000.

The Centers for Disease Control and Prevention (CDC) examined children in metropolitan Atlanta, Georgia, who were 3–10 years old in 1996, and found a prevalence of children who were diagnosed with ASD of 3.4 per 1000 (CI = 3.0–3.7) [Yeargin-Allsopp et al., 2003]. A 2002 CDC survey of 400,000 children aged 8 years (born in 1994) found a prevalence of 6.6 per 1000 with a wide variation across the 14 states in the study [ADDM, 2007]. Most recently, the CDC reported a prevalence rate of 9.0 per 1000 in 2006 in 307,790 8-year-old children across 11 states [ADDM, 2009]. All of these CDC studies relied on abstraction of health and education records.

Higher numbers have been more recently reported in other studies that relied on active screening and diagnosis of populations of children. The prevalence of ASDs in 55,000 British 8- and 9-year-old children was 11 per 1000 [Baird et al., 2006b], and in a separate study of children ages 5–9 years, cases were documented at a rate of 1 per 100, but the authors thought that not all cases were likely to have been found [Baron-Cohen et al., 2009]. Based on the most recent parent-reported U.S. diagnostic survey, the prevalence for ASD was as high as 11 per 1000 [Kogan et al., 2009]. Definitions used, screening methods, diagnostic criteria, and completeness of sampling varied in these studies; all have methodologic issues affecting prevalence results [Bresnahan et al., 2009; Charman et al., 2009; Hertz-Picciotto and Delwiche, 2009; King and Bearman, 2009; Nassar et al., 2009].

A number of factors contribute to this apparent increase. Diagnostic criteria have evolved and broadened; the concept of autism is now defined as autistic disorder plus the broader autistic spectrum disorders, including Asperger's syndrome and PDD-NOS; there is now co-diagnosis with known medical disorders such as fragile X syndrome, Tourette's syndrome (TS) and Down syndrome; and the growing public awareness among parents and teachers has led, in developing countries, to earlier and more accurate diagnoses. The increased availability of services [Nassar et al., 2009] and the ability to diagnose children at younger ages [Parner et al., 2008] may influence the frequency of diagnosis. Children earlier diagnosed as mentally retarded may have met current criteria for autism [King and Bearman, 2009; Nassar et al., 2009; Prior, 2003]. Bishop et al. [2008] found that up to 60 percent of adults previously diagnosed with developmental language disorder would meet more recent criteria for PDD. Case ascertainment methodology is also a factor, because using multiple sources and broad population screening increases the number of cases found. There are little data on prevalence in older populations.

Clearly, a substantial proportion of the increase seen in autism is due to factors such as a combination of better, more population-based studies and changes in the diagnostic criteria and age at diagnosis. However, the increase cannot be solely attributed to known factors and there may, in fact, be a true increase in incidence. It is important for etiologic reasons and for public health and educational planning to ascertain whether the rise in cases is genuine, if it is continuing, and to what degree. The CDC is monitoring the prevalence of autism over time in a number of U.S. sites using consistently applied ascertainment and diagnostic protocols [Croen et al., 2002a; Fombonne, 2003a].

The proportion of children with ASDs who had IQs less than or equal to 70 ranged from about 30–50 percent in the CDC's Autism and Developmental Disabilities Monitoring Network. A higher proportion of females had cognitive

Box 48-3 Proposed Revision to 299.00 in DSM-V: Autism Spectrum Disorder

Must meet criteria 1, 2, and 3:

1. Clinically significant, persistent deficits in social communication and interactions, as manifest by all of the following:
   a. Marked deficits in nonverbal and verbal communication used for social interaction
   b. Lack of social reciprocity
   c. Failure to develop and maintain peer relationships appropriate to developmental level
2. Restricted, repetitive patterns of behavior, interests, and activities, as manifested by at least TWO of the following:
   a. Stereotyped motor or verbal behaviors, or unusual sensory behaviors
   b. Excessive adherence to routines and ritualized patterns of behavior
   c. Restricted, fixated interests
3. Symptoms must be present in early childhood (but may not become fully manifest until social demands exceed limited capacities)

Rationale

- New name for category, autism spectrum disorder, which includes autistic disorder (autism), Asperger's disorder, childhood disintegrative disorder, and pervasive developmental disorder not otherwise specified
  - Differentiation of autism spectrum disorder from typical development and other "nonspectrum" disorders is done reliably and with validity, while distinctions among disorders have been found to be inconsistent over time, variable across sites, and often associated with severity, language level, or intelligence, rather than features of the disorder
  - Since autism is defined by a common set of behaviors, it is best represented as a single diagnostic category that is adapted to the individual's clinical presentation by inclusion of clinical specifiers (e.g., severity, verbal abilities, and others) and associated features (e.g., known genetic disorders, epilepsy, intellectual disability, and others.) A single-spectrum disorder is a better reflection of the state of knowledge about pathology and clinical presentation; previously, the criteria were equivalent to trying to "cleave meatloaf at the joints"
- Three domains become two:
  1. Social/communication deficits
  2. Fixated interests and repetitive behaviors
     - Deficits in communication and social behaviors are inseparable and more accurately considered as a single set of symptoms with contextual and environmental specificities
     - Delays in language are not unique nor universal in autism spectrum disorder and are more accurately considered as

a factor that influences the clinical symptoms of autism spectrum disorder, rather than defining the autism spectrum disorder diagnosis

- Requiring both criteria to be completely fulfilled improves specificity of diagnosis without impairing sensitivity
- Providing examples for subdomains for a range of chronological ages and language levels increases sensitivity across severity levels from mild to more severe, while maintaining specificity with just two domains
- Decision based on literature review, expert consultations, and workgroup discussions; confirmed by the results of secondary analyses of data from Collaborative Programs of Excellence in Autism (CPEA) and Studies to Advance Autism Research and Treatment (STAART), University of Michigan, Simons Simplex Collection databases

- Several social/communication criteria were merged and streamlined to clarify diagnostic requirements
  - In DSM-IV, multiple criteria assess the same symptom and therefore carry excessive weight in making diagnosis
  - Merging social and communication domains requires a new approach to criteria
  - Secondary data analyses were conducted on social/communication symptoms to determine the most sensitive and specific clusters of symptoms and criteria descriptions for a range of ages and language levels
- Requiring two symptom manifestations for repetitive behavior and fixated interests improves specificity of the criterion without significant decrements in sensitivity. The necessity for multiple sources of information, including skilled clinical observation and reports from parents/caregivers/teachers, is highlighted by the need to meet a higher proportion of criteria
- The presence, via clinical observation and caregiver report, of a history of fixated interests, routines, or rituals and repetitive behaviors considerably increases the stability of autism spectrum diagnoses over time and the differentiation between autism spectrum disorder and other disorders
- Reorganization of subdomains increases clarity and continues to provide adequate sensitivity while improving specificity through provision of examples from different age ranges and language levels
- Unusual sensory behaviors are explicitly included within a subdomain of stereotyped motor and verbal behaviors, expanding the specification of different behaviors that can be coded within this domain, with examples particularly relevant for younger children
- Autism spectrum disorder is a neurodevelopmental disorder and must be present from infancy or early childhood, but may not be detected until later because of minimal social demands and support from parents or caregivers in early years

(American Psychiatric Association. Proposed Revisions to 299.00 Autistic Disorder in DSM-V, 2010. Retrieved 28 February 2010, from http://www.dsm5.org/Proposed Revisions/Pages/proposedrevision.aspx?rid=94#.)

impairment compared to males. The mean male to female ratio is 4:1 or greater for the milder forms, but as severity of cognitive impairment increases, the male to female ratio decreases to 1.3:1 [Yeargin-Allsopp et al., 2003]. The rate of PDD-NOS is approximately 1.5 times that of autistic disorder; the rate of Asperger's disorder is one-fourth that of autistic disorder. Children with autistic disorder and a

measurable IQ of less than 50 are more likely than those who are high-functioning to be female and to have minor physical anomalies, neuroimaging abnormalities, microcephaly, and epilepsy [Nicolson et al., 1999]. Those with specific, known inherited conditions, such as tuberous sclerosis or phenylketonuria, are likely to be more severely cognitively impaired [Rutter et al., 1994].

Risk Factors

Sibling Studies

The risk of ASDs in a sibling has been reported to be 3–8 percent when there is one affected child [Chakrabarti and Fombonne, 2001; Micali et al., 2004]. However, a recent report from Japan by Sumi et al. [2006] found gender differences in the risk for subsequent siblings: general sibling risk was 10 percent, 7.7 percent if the proband was male, and 20.0 percent if the proband was female. The risk is 25 percent if there are already two siblings with ASD [Folstein and Rosen-Sheidley, 2001].

Infant siblings of children with autism have garnered recent research attention as a high-risk group with the hope of identifying the earliest warning signs of ASD [Barbaro and Dissanayake, 2009; Brian et al., 2008; Cassel et al., 2007; Elder et al., 2008; Elsabbagh and Johnson, 2007; Elsabbagh et al., 2009a, b; Goldberg et al., 2005; Ibanez et al., 2008; Iverson and Wozniak, 2007; Landa and Garrett-Mayer, 2006; Landa et al., 2007; Loh et al., 2007; Merin et al., 2007; Mitchell et al., 2006; Sigman et al., 2004; Toth et al., 2007; Zwaigenbaum et al., 2005, 2007; see Rogers [2009] for a recent review]. Age at entry into the studies varies considerably, and one might anticipate that parents of those infants enrolled at later ages might have already recognized warning signs that prompted their participation in the study. This may contribute to the fact that the rate of an eventual diagnosis of ASD also varies highly across the studies, reported as 10 percent for infants enrolled by 5 months of age [Iverson and Wozniak, 2007], 14 percent for those enrolled between 12 and 23 months of age [Yoder et al., 2009], 23 percent for those enrolled between 6 and 12 months of age [Brian et al., 2008], and 62 percent for those enrolled by 18 months of age [Landa and Garrett-Mayer, 2006]. As a result, the true sibling recurrence rate cannot be currently ascertained through the available studies.

Developmental differences in infant siblings who are later diagnosed with an ASD (Sib-ASD) appear to emerge by around 12 months of age, with the developmental gap widening at a decreasing rate over the second year of life [Brian et al., 2008; Rogers, 2009; Stone et al., 2007; Yoder et al., 2009]; to date, studies have not reported significant differences at 6 months of age. Delays in fine and gross motor development have been noted by some [Landa and Garrett-Mayer, 2006] but not all studies [Iverson and Wozniak, 2007; Ozonoff et al., 2008; Toth et al., 2007]. Although stereotypic behaviors are "expected" in infants during the course of motor development [Thelen, 1979], specific atypical and repetitive behaviors (specifically spinning, rotating, rolling, and, most commonly, unusual visual regard of toys) occurred more frequently at 12 months of age [Ozonoff et al., 2008], and Loh et al. [2007] found that arm-waving at 12 and covering of the ears at 18 months of age occurred significantly more often in Sib-ASD.

Delays in verbal and nonverbal communication have been noted in Sib-ASD, beginning only at 12 months of age by almost every research group [Gamliel et al., 2007; Goldberg et al., 2005; Landa and Garrett-Mayer, 2006; Landa et al., 2007; Toth et al., 2007; Yirmiya et al., 2006; Yoder et al., 2009; Zwaigenbaum et al., 2005]. However, no consistent specific deficits have emerged to date across the studies as characteristic of Sib-ASD. Response to name has been explored by several researchers, as well [Brian et al., 2008; Nadig et al., 2007; Yirmiya et al., 2006; Zwaigenbaum et al., 2005], and Sib-ASD responded typically at 6 months, but not at 12 months of age.

Studies of response to joint attention in Sib-ASD have found fewer responses in the second year of life [Cassel et al., 2007; Presmanes et al., 2007; Sullivan et al., 2007], particularly in those situations requiring both head turn and verbal prompt [Presmanes et al., 2007]. Yoder et al. [2009] found that the response to joint attention at 12 months was predictive of degree of social impairment and eventual ASD diagnosis at 3 years of age. Zwaigenbaum et al. [2005] were able to differentiate Sib-ASD infants on imitation of body, oral, and object acts, which was not found in high-risk infants who did not develop ASD [Toth et al., 2007].

Neonatal Intensive Care and Prematurity

Matsuishi et al. [1999] first reported a significantly increased rate of ASD in children born between 1983 and 1987, with a mean gestational age of 35.4 ± 4.6 weeks, requiring neonatal intensive care, and who were followed up between 5 and 8 years of age using DSM-III-R criteria [APA, 1987]; a history of meconium aspiration was significantly more common in those children with ASD than in the comparison groups of children with cerebral palsy and those with typical development. Badawi et al. [2006] also have reported an increased rate of ASD at 5 percent in term neonatal intensive care unit (NICU) survivors of newborn encephalopathy, defined as either seizures alone or any two of the following lasting for longer than 24 hours: abnormal consciousness, difficulty maintaining respiration (of presumed central origin), difficulty feeding (of presumed central origin), and abnormal tone and reflexes [Badawi et al., 1998].

Several recent publications have documented a much higher rate of positive screening for ASD in infants with extreme prematurity using the Modified Checklist for Autism in Toddlers (M-CHAT) [Robins and Dumont-Mathieu, 2006; Robins et al., 2001] and other screening instruments. Limperopoulos et al. [2008] found a 25 percent rate of positive screening for ASD at 18–24 months of age in 91 infants who were less than 1500 g and 31 weeks' gestation at birth. Kuban et al. [2009] noted a 22 percent rate of positive M-CHAT screens in 988 NICU survivors at 24 months of age who were less than 28 weeks' gestation at birth and who were followed in the multicenter ELGAN study. Major motor, cognitive, visual, and hearing impairments appeared to account for more than half of the positive M-CHAT screens in this cohort. Even after the toddlers with those impairments were eliminated, 10 percent of children – nearly double the expected rate – screened positive.

In a large Swedish population-based study, Buchmayer et al. [2009] reported that the increased risk of autistic disorders related to preterm birth was mediated primarily by prenatal and neonatal complications that occur more commonly among preterm infants, predominantly pre-eclampsia, but also intracranial hemorrhage, cerebral edema, low Apgar scores, and seizures. Limperopoulos [2009] suggests that the incidence of ASD among survivors of preterm birth is inversely related to gestational age. If so, as survival rates continue to improve in extremely premature infants, the resulting morbidity of ASD may also continue to increase. As noted by Fombonne [2006], it is important that all practitioners have a heightened awareness of these risk factors to screen toddlers and preschoolers with suboptimal perinatal histories systematically.

Other Risk Factors

Risk of ASD is higher with increasing age of mothers, and independently, with increasing age of fathers [Durkin et al., 2008]. In a large population of children born between 1989 and 1994, mothers older than 35 years were three times more likely to have an autistic child than women younger than 20 years [Croen et al., 2002a]. One California study found that, when adjusted for age of the other parent and other covariates, risk of autism increases by up to 40 percent for each 10-year increase in maternal age and by 20–25 percent for each 10-year increase in paternal age [Grether et al., 2009a]. In another study also from California, maternal age was linearly correlated with risk but increased paternal age was a risk factor only in mothers over 30 years old [Shelton et al., 2010]. Some studies found that socioeconomic level does not affect risk [Bhasin and Schendel, 2007; Larsson et al., 2005], but in another study, women with a postgraduate education were twice as likely to have an autistic child as women with less than a high-school education [Croen et al., 2002b]. Risk was also increased in multiple births (RR = 1.7; 95 percent CI = 1.4–2.0) and in black children (RR = 1.6, 95 percent CI = 1.5–1.8) [Croen et al., 2002a].

Advanced parental age and some of the other risk factors for autism that have been suggested may act through increasing risk for de novo mutations. There may also be mutagens in the environment, such as mercury, cadmium, nickel, trichloroethylene, and vinyl chloride. Factors associated with vitamin D deficiency may cause mutations as vitamin D contributes to repair of DNA damage [Kinney et al., 2010]. The number of fetal ultrasounds does not seem to be associated with increased risk [Grether et al., 2009b], and perinatal risk factors associated with fetal distress (other than breech presentation) did not contribute significantly to risk [Bilder et al., 2009].

Pathophysiology and Etiology

Animal Models

No single animal model exists for autism, but several animal models that exhibit some of the major features of autism have provided an opportunity to understand the neural substrates of functional impairments. In the macaque monkey, social behavior is mediated by the amygdala, temporal cortex, orbitofrontal cortex, and superior temporal gyrus [Lord et al., 2000]. In another monkey model (rhesus), bilateral removal of the medial temporal lobes leads to abnormal social behavior during maturation that resolves in adults [Bachevalier, 1994; Machado and Bachevalier, 2003]. Symptoms include abnormal social interaction, absence of facial and body expression, and stereotypic behaviors. Social anxiety and fear have been studied in primates [Amaral, 2002] and in rats [Wolterink et al., 2001], and are related to amygdaloid circuitry.

A behavioral syndrome in Lewis rats with analogies to autism is the result of Borna disease virus infection in neonates [Pletnikov et al., 2003; Weissenbock et al., 2000]. Neonatal infection produces specific behavioral abnormalities, with disturbances in sensorineural development, lower startle responsiveness, and abnormal social play. Proprioceptive systems were abnormal that involved use of hind-limbs and balance. Pathologically, Borna disease virus induces regional neuronal loss in the cerebellum. This model provides some insights into mechanisms of pre- and perinatal infection causing damage to the developing brain, but it does not indicate that Borna disease virus is an etiologic agent in autism.

Other animal models have been developed by knocking out different candidate genes [Lijam et al., 1997], by oxytocin and vasopressin administration [Insel et al., 1999], and by exposing embryos to teratogens such as valproic acid [Ingram et al., 2000]. Behavioral studies have focused on social interaction and memory deficits. Because the neurexin 1-alpha gene has been linked to ASD phenotypes, a knockout mouse model has been developed with analogies to at least one core domain of ASD [Etherton et al., 2009].

Neuropathology

Abnormalities in major cortical and subcortical brain structures have been found through postmortem and magnetic resonance imaging (MRI) studies of autistic subjects. Comprehensive examination of nine autistic postmortem brains was carried out by Kemper and Bauman [1994]. They described three major findings: curtailment of normal development in forebrain neurons, which were smaller and more densely distributed than normal; an apparent congenital decrease in the number of Purkinje cells; and age-related changes in cell size and the number of neurons in the diagonal band of Broca, the cerebellar nuclei, and the inferior olive.

These neuropathologic findings may account for many clinical features of autism. Perinatally acquired lesions in limbic system structures could lead to disruption in memory processes involved in the ability to learn new information. In contrast, striatal and cortical areas involved in habitual memory were spared, potentially relating to the need for sameness, narrow interests, and capacity for rote memory. Disruption of cerebellar function may lead to a number of motor and sensory system deficiencies, including mental imagery, anticipatory planning, and timing and integration of sensory and motor information [Kemper and Bauman, 1998]. Support of brain-tissue banking is critical to continued research into the neuropathologic underpinnings of autism [Pickett, 2001].

Another approach to determining the neuropathologic underpinnings of autism has been suggested by Rodier [2002]. She found that children exposed to thalidomide in the first trimester developed autism at an increased rate, supporting the idea that the brain abnormality originates at the time of closure of the neural tube [Rodier et al., 1996]. This finding was corroborated by postmortem examination of a brain from a subject with autism not exposed to thalidomide, but whose mother was an alcoholic, showing near-complete absence of the facial nucleus and superior olive and narrowing of the brainstem between the trapezoid body and inferior olive. This deficit was reproduced in an *HOXA1*-knockout mouse model and by exposing rat embryos to valproic acid on the day of neural tube closure [Ingram et al., 2000]. The investigators concluded that central nervous system injuries occurring during or just after neural tube closure can lead to selective loss of neurons derived from the basal plate of the rhombencephalon, and this finding may indicate that the initiating injury in some individuals with autism takes place around the time of neural tube closure.

Additional supporting evidence for this theory comes from a Nova Scotia cohort of 61 autistic children [Rodier et al., 1997]. Forty-two percent of these children with autism had posterior rotation of the external ears, compared with 18 percent of controls. They postulated that this could have been associated with a disruption of otic disc formation in the fourth week of embryonic life and that ear anomalies found in some children with autism could possibly be a marker for initiating events in utero.

An important additional neuropathologic finding described by Casanova et al. [2008, 2002] is the finding of abnormalities in the structure of minicolumns in the brain of autistic individuals. Minicolumns consist of 80–100 neurons, and they are believed to be the smallest unit of functional organization in the cortex. In autistic individuals, the minicolumns were described as more numerous but smaller than those of controls and with less space in between. This structural difference may cause the firing of too many processing units at once and prohibit the units from coherently responding to signals. Over-arousal or under-arousal could easily result. This abnormality could also be responsible for the increased incidence of seizures in individuals with autism.

Neuroimaging

Both structural and functional imaging have contributed to the understanding of autism. Quantitative volume analysis using MRI has provided information that the outer layers of white matter are enlarged in autistic subjects compared with controls. Herbert et al. [2005, 2004] compared 13 subjects with high-functioning autism, 14 subjects with developmental language disorder, and 14 controls. The inner zones of white matter were not different in autistic subjects from those in controls, but the outer zone of white matter was larger than controls in autistic individuals and subjects with developmental language disorder. In the autistic group, frontal lobe enlargement was proportionally greater than other areas, but not in the developmental language disorder sample. These areas myelinate relatively late, beginning in the second half of the first year and continuing into the second year of life and later, which is consistent with the timing of increased head circumference seen in autistic subjects. By the time autistic children are 2–4 years old, 90 percent have above-average brain volume, and 37 percent have developmental macrocephaly, defined as brain volume exceeding 2 standard deviations above the normal mean for age [Courchesne et al., 2001]. This finding suggests an on-going postnatal process that primarily affects interhemispheric and cortical connections.

In other studies, children with ASDs were found to have significantly increased cerebral volumes compared with normal and with developmentally delayed children, and white-matter enlargement was seen [Sparks et al., 2002]. There was greater enlargement of the frontal cortex [Carper et al., 2002] compared with other lobes, and reduced amygdala volume [Aylward et al., 1999]. Juranek et al. [2006] also found a positive correlation between amygdalar volume, particularly the right side, and anxiety levels as measured by the Child Behavior Checklist in a cohort of 42 children with ASD, which supports evidence for a neurobiologic relationship between symptoms of anxiety and depression with amygdalar structure and function.

Courchesne et al. [2003] have found specific neuroanatomic abnormalities, increased cerebellar and cerebral white matter, and cerebral cortical gray matter in 2- to 3-year-old children compared with controls, but not in older children or adolescents with autism. Frontal lobes were most affected with greatest involvement in the dorsolateral and medial prefrontal cortex. A widely debated finding in the MRI literature is reduction in size of one or another subregion of the cerebellar vermis [Courchesne et al., 1994a, b, 1988; Hashimoto et al., 1995]. Other investigations have failed to replicate these findings [Filipek, 1995; Hardan et al., 2001; Piven and Arndt, 1995].

Increasing evidence from functional MRI studies (fMRI) points to changes in activation and synchronization of cortical networks. Functional connectivity is lowered, leading to deficits in language, social cognition, motor planning, and perception [Levy et al., 2009]. Autistic children have profound deficits in face-recognition tasks [Klin et al., 1999]. Technologies involving the use of eye-tracking devices and fMRI have yielded important information regarding the pathways for face recognition in autism. The fusiform face area (on the lateral aspect of the fusiform gyrus) is hypoactive as seen by fMRI, and the degree of hypoactivation strongly correlates with the degree of disability [Critchley et al., 2000; Kanwisher et al., 1997; Pierce et al., 2001; Schultz et al., 2000]. Hubl et al. [2003] saw lower blood oxygen-level dependent signals in ten autistic subjects during face processing than in controls, and they observed higher activation in the medial occipital gyrus, an area related to processing objects. Schultz et al. [2000] also found lower activation in autistic subjects in the right fusiform gyrus, but they identified higher activity in the right inferior temporal gyrus. Mechanisms that underlie learning of novel movement patterns are different in children with autism compared to controls, and may lead to impaired skill development [Gidley Larson and Mostofsky, 2008].

Serotonin

Elevated blood levels of serotonin (5-hydroxytryptamine – 5HT) in autistic subjects, first reported in 1961 [Schain and Freedman, 1961], are caused by an elevation within circulating platelets, an increase in the serotonin transporter concentration, and a decrease in $5HT_2$ receptor binding [Cook and Leventhal, 1996]. Elevated concentrations of a low-molecular-weight peptide that increases the uptake of 5HT into platelets [Pedersen et al., 1999] was demonstrated in autistic subjects. Elevation of platelet serotonin levels has been well studied and generally replicated.

It has been hypothesized that, if siblings of children with autism have higher platelet 5HT levels, it may indicate a higher familial risk [Piven et al., 1991b]. A familial pattern of hyper-serotonemia was confirmed by Leboyer et al. [1999] in a sample of 62 autistic subjects and 122 first-degree relatives. Levels of whole-blood 5HT did not change with age in subjects with autism but did change in controls. There does not seem to be a correlation between 5HT levels and specific defined phenotypes [Kuperman et al., 1987]. However, Leboyer et al. [1999] suggested that the level of 5HT in blood could be considered an intermediate or surrogate phenotype that could be correlated with DNA polymorphisms in the 5HT transporter gene.

Serotonergic disturbances, including defects in 5HT transporter expression and decreases in plasma tryptophan, may play a role in the pathophysiology of autism [Croonenberghs et al., 2000; Marazziti et al., 2000]. 5HT has an important role in central nervous system development, affecting social behavior, sleep, aggression, anxiety, and affective regulation, and it plays a role in the modulation of synaptogenesis [Chugani, 2002]. It may have a role in the development of neuropathologic abnormalities in the hippocampus, amygdala, and cerebellum [Bauman and Kemper, 1994] and in thalamocortical connections. Depletion of 5HT in critical developmental periods may also cause a decrease in growth of dendritic spines [Yan et al., 1997]. Using positron emission tomography (PET) scans, Chugani et al. [1997] found alterations of 5HT synthesis in the frontal and thalamic pathways that are important for language production and sensory integration.

About one-half of the patients with Smith–Lemli–Opitz syndrome, a malformation syndrome with mental retardation that is caused by an inborn error in cholesterol biosynthesis [Opitz et al., 2002], exhibit autistic behavior. A mouse model of the Smith–Lemli–Opitz syndrome was created by eliminating *DHCR7*, which encodes 7-dehydrocholesterol reductase, the terminal enzyme required for cholesterol biosynthesis [Waage-Baudet et al., 2003]. These knockout mice have a 300 percent increase in 5HT immunoreactivity in hindbrains compared with control mice, and 5HT-immunoreactive cells are present in unusual locations and represent an increase in the total number of 5HT neurons and fibers. These observations provide a basis for the autistic phenotype seen in Smith–Lemli–Opitz syndrome, and they support the focus of therapeutic interventions aimed at modulation of the serotonergic system.

Vaccines

There has been public concern about a potential relation between autism and vaccines, undermining the confidence of some parents in accepting the recommended vaccinations. Symptoms of autism generally are noticed first in the second year of life, although they may be recognized only in retrospect, and this is when the measles-mumps-rubella vaccine is given. Targets of concern have been the measles-mumps-rubella vaccine itself and thimerosal, the mercury-containing preservative that was used in childhood vaccines until its removal between 1999 and 2002.

Multiple studies concluded that there was no increase in risk of autistic disorder with exposure to the measles-mumps-rubella vaccine [Chen et al., 2004; Dales et al., 2001; Fombonne and Chakrabarti, 2001; Kaye et al., 2001; Madsen and Vestergaard, 2004; Taylor et al., 1999]; see monograph by Offit [2008]. Additional data derived from passive surveillance systems also consistently failed to detect an association [Patja et al., 2000; Peltola et al., 1998; Plesner et al., 2000]. There has been no evidence that the incidence of regressive autism has increased after administration of the measles-mumps-rubella vaccine. The measles-mumps-rubella vaccine has been given at a constant rate since 1979 in the United States, 1982 in Finland, and 1998 in the United Kingdom and Denmark, but rates of autism have steadily risen [Klein and Diehl, 2004]. The Immunization Safety Review Committee of the Institute of Medicine of the National Academies (IOM) [Stratton et al., 2001] concluded that there was consistent evidence of no causal association between administration of the measles-mumps-rubella vaccine and autism.

However, the IOM report did not think there was sufficient evidence to accept or reject a causal association between exposure to thimerosal and autism [McCormick, 2003]. Exposure to thimerosal is a concern because mercury is a known neurotoxin, and there are claims of abnormal levels of mercury in autistic children who respond to chelation therapy. There are no studies involving low doses, and the pharmacokinetics of ethyl mercury in human infants is unknown. Almost all studies available regarding mercury toxicity are related to exposure to methyl rather than ethyl mercury, and the clinical picture of mercury poisoning from any dose, duration, or age of exposure is different from that of autism [Nelson and Bauman, 2003]. Analysis of data from California, Sweden, and Denmark [Stehr-Green et al., 2003] found that, although thimerosal exposure from vaccines was eliminated in Sweden and Denmark by the early 1990s, the incidence of autism was accelerated. This finding was confirmed by a retrospective cohort study [Verstraeten et al., 2003].

A claim has been made that persistent measles virus found in the gastrointestinal tract of ten children with autism and bowel symptoms was causally related to their autism [Wakefield et al., 1998]. Wakefield's hypothesis was that measles-mumps-rubella vaccine is a risk factor for children with regressive autism. However, there was no clear clinical description of the subjects, there were no controls, and the history and timing of regression was determined years later retrospectively. Most of the other authors have since rescinded the conclusions of this study [Murch et al., 2004], the paper has been officially retracted by the *Lancet* [Dyer, 2010; Godlee et al., 2011]. Taylor et al. [1999] found 6.6 percent of children with autism had regression and bowel symptoms, but the onset of symptoms was not associated with the measles-mumps-rubella vaccine. Another prospective report [Fombonne and Chakrabarti, 2001] did not find any association in a large, prospective sample. Further strong evidence against the association of autism with persistent measles virus in the gastrointestinal tract or measles-mumps-rubella exposure came from a case control study by Hornig et al. [2008]. Gastrointestinal tissue samples from children with autism, 90 percent of whom showed behavioral regression, and from controls, was examined for presence of measles virus RNA in a blinded study, with results consistent over three laboratory sites [Hornig et al., 2008]. There were no differences between case and control groups in the presence of measles virus RNA, and gastrointestinal symptom and autism onset were unrelated to timing of the measles-mumps-rubella vaccine.

Diagnostic Evaluation and Screening

ASDs can be reliably diagnosed in children as young as 2 years [Lord, 1995; Moore and Goodson, 2003], and early intervention is beneficial [Lord, 1995; National Research Council, 2001]. However, the average age of diagnosis is reported as 3–6 years [Howlin and Moore, 1997; Mandell et al., 2002], and it has remained fairly stable over the past decade. There is evidence that age of diagnosis varies as a function of ethnicity and socioeconomic status [Mandell et al., 2002]. Parents often report concerns about their child's social and communication skills, and they seek medical assistance long before a formal diagnosis is obtained.

The American Academy of Pediatrics and the CDC launched an awareness campaign to sensitize pediatricians and parents to the early symptoms of autism, to encourage caregivers to listen to parents' concerns, and to encourage parents to be assertive in making sure that their concerns are addressed. The campaign includes evaluating strategies for screening and developing resources and tools for physicians. The CDC website offers downloadable educational information and screening instruments: http://www.cdc.gov/ncbddd/autism/hcp-screening.html.

The American Academy of Pediatrics Council of Children with Disabilities recently published a set of guidelines [Johnson and Myers, 2007; Myers and Johnson, 2007] on the identification and management, respectively, of children with ASD. Risk factors that should call attention to the possibility of ASD include having a sibling with ASD, or when there is parental, other caregiver, or pediatrician concern.

Screening and Diagnostic Instruments

Symptoms of ASDs vary with characteristics of the child, including age, IQ, and temperament. Although all children with ASDs share core features, there is great heterogeneity within this population. Some characteristics, such as repetitive behavior, are more common at certain ages and levels of cognitive functioning. This heterogeneity poses challenges to recognition during typical medical appointments.

The Child Neurology Society and American Academy of Neurology published a "Practice Parameter for the Screening and Diagnosis of Autism" [Filipek et al., 1999, 2000a]. A two-level approach is recommended. Level 1 involves developmental screening as part of routine well-child care, followed by an ASD-specific screen for children identified with developmental delay. Level 2 involves formal diagnostic procedures to determine whether the child has ASD. This level of diagnostic evaluation is conducted by an experienced clinician, and it uses information gleaned from the medical history, neurologic evaluation, and developmental testing to determine the child's developmental profile.

Instruments for Autistic Spectrum Disorders Screening

"Red flags" for language development can be easily recognized and should engender prompt referral (Box 48-4). Screening instruments for ASDs are in various stages of development. Presented here are those that have reported good psychometric properties (although they all need further development and psychometric evaluation) and that are available for use by clinicians. These instruments are most sensitive when they follow general developmental screening and are applied when a child has already been identified with delayed or atypical development. Some of these instruments are also being validated for use in the general population as a first-step screening, which would be desirable in many settings. However, administration of ASD-specific screening tools after screening for and identification of atypical development is the method with the most sensitivity (i.e., probability of correctly identifying a child with ASD) and specificity (i.e., proportion of non-ASD cases correctly identified).

Box 48-4 Red Flags for Language Development

Prompt referral should be made for any of the following:
- No vocalizations by 6 months
- No polysyllabic babbling or gestures by 12 months
- No spontaneous (not echoed) single words by 16 months
- No spontaneous phrases by 24 months
- No spontaneous sentences by 36 months
- Any loss of babbling, single words, or phrases, including response to name

---

The Checklist for Autism in Toddlers (CHAT) [Baird et al., 2000, 2001] was developed in Great Britain, and it is most useful in screening children 18–24 months old. It was designed for use in the general population and to be administered in the home by a medical caregiver. The CHAT is intended to be cost-effective and sensitive to early signs of ASD. Parents respond to nine items asking about their child's social orienting behaviors, such as pretend play, joint attention, and pointing. The clinician completes five items after observing the child. Unfortunately, when administered in the general population, the sensitivity has been disappointing, with high rates of false-negative results. The developers recommend a screen-rescreen procedure (at 18 and again at 19 months), which increases specificity to within acceptable limits [Charman et al., 2002, 2007].

Scambler et al. [2001] conducted a small study in which they demonstrated better sensitivity (65 percent) and specificity (100 percent) when using the CHAT to distinguish children with autism from among a group already identified with developmental problems. They improved on this further by developing their own criteria (i.e., Denver Criteria) for defining risk status. The CHAT worked best with children whose developmental level was within the 18- to 24-month range, despite them being older in chronologic age. The sample size was small, and the Denver Criteria were developed ad hoc. Although the CHAT looks promising for this type of use, more validation is needed. Development of this tool is on-going, and there are attempts at modifications to improve sensitivity and specificity within the general population.

The Modified Checklist for Autism in Toddlers (M-CHAT) [Robins and Dumont-Mathieu, 2006; Robins et al., 2001] relies only on parent report. There is a 23-item questionnaire completed by a parent. If results of the checklist indicate possible risk for autism, there is a follow-up parent interview. The use of this follow-up interview increases the sensitivity and specificity of the instrument, especially when used in a general pediatric population that has not already been screened for developmental disorders [Kleinman et al., 2008].

The Screening Tool for Autism in Two-Year-Olds (STAT) [Stone et al., 2000, 2008] is composed of interactive items administered by a clinician to children 24–35 months old. It is designed to identify children with autism disorders (not the full range of ASDs) from a population of children identified with developmental delays. The STAT quantifies behaviors in four domains: play, requesting, directing attention, and motor imitation. The instrument requires training in administration and scoring, and it takes about 20 minutes to complete. Strong psychometric properties are reported, although they are derived from small samples, and there is need for further development (e.g., evaluation of usefulness with the full range of ASDs) [Stone et al., 2004]. Preliminary results also suggest that the tool is useful in identifying autism in at-risk toddlers down to 14 months of age [Stone et al., 2008]. The investigators suggest that the qualitative information obtained during the screening can be used to inform intervention goals for individual children. In some settings, this may outweigh the inconvenience of the need for training and the relatively longer administration time.

The screening instruments previously described are designed for early diagnosis. Unfortunately, not all children are diagnosed early, and a neurology practice is likely to encounter older children referred for possible autism. The Social Communication

Questionnaire [Berument et al., 1999; Rutter et al., 2003a] was developed to identify older, higher-functioning individuals with ASD. It is a 40-item, parent-completed questionnaire for children 4 years old and older. In a large sample of children referred for possible ASD diagnoses, the instrument performed well when differentiating ASDs from other diagnoses. It also demonstrated good sensitivity and specificity in identifying ASD in school-age children with special learning needs [Charman et al., 2007].

Instruments for ASD Diagnosis

The Childhood Autism Rating Scale (CARS) is a clinician-rated diagnostic instrument for use with children older than 2 years [Chlebowski et al., 2010]. It should be administered by a clinician who is experienced with ASDs. The clinician should view a training videotape before using this rating scale. It takes 30–45 minutes to administer. The CARS is widely recognized and used in clinical settings. Psychometric properties are good to excellent, although in some of these reports, the sample population is not well described. Because the CARS was developed before publication of the DSM-IV [American Psychiatric Association, 1994] and ICD-10 [World Health Organization, 1992], it is less helpful in distinguishing between subgroups within the broader category of ASDs.

The Autism Diagnostic Interview – Revised (ADI-R) [Lord et al., 1994; Rutter et al., 2003b], a structured parent interview, and the Autism Diagnostic Observation Schedule (ADOS) [Lord et al., 1994; Luyster et al., 2009] are considered the gold standards for the diagnosis of autism. These instruments differentiate between autism disorder and PDD-NOS with definitive thresholds. They were developed for use in research, but both have become commercially available for clinical use. The procedures are time-consuming and costly, and they require extensive training. As a result, they are most likely to be used in research or specialty clinics for ASDs and are not widely used in general clinical practice.

The ADI-R is a comprehensive interview with a parent or caregiver that probes for autistic symptoms in the spheres of social relatedness, communication, and ritualistic or perseverative behaviors. It asks about current behavior and about behavior in early childhood, when the classic symptoms of autism are most likely to be observed. The interview takes at least 1.5 hours to complete.

The ADOS is a semistructured, observational assessment that includes investigator-directed activities to evaluate communication, reciprocal social interaction, play, stereotypic behavior, restricted interests, and other abnormal behaviors. The procedure takes about 30–45 minutes to complete. Five modules are available, including a new research module for toddlers under 30 months of age. Each of the other four modules corresponds to a developmental level, so the instrument can be used with individuals of all ages and all levels of functional impairment. The ADOS is an observation of current behavior, and it must be combined with a clinical interview to obtain historical information. An algorithm can be used to convert ADOS scores into a severity metric, which facilitates comparison of scores across modules, making it useful to track changes in functioning over time [Gotham et al., 2008].

The reliability of a diagnosis is always increased when multiple sources of information are obtained and synthesized. When more than one standardized instrument is used, there is always a possibility of obtaining conflicting results, with the same individual meeting a threshold cutoff on one instrument but not another. For this reason, diagnoses should be undertaken by clinicians with extensive training and experience in the diagnosis of ASD.

The Neurologic Evaluation in Autism

Neurologic Examination

Most investigators report that a small proportion of autistic children have frank macrocephaly or megalencephaly. The distribution of head size is clearly shifted upward, with the mean approximately at the 75th percentile [Bailey et al., 1993; Bolton et al., 1994; Courchesne, 2004; Davidovitch et al., 1996; Lainhart, 2003; Lainhart et al., 2006; Woodhouse et al., 1996]. Some investigators have observed that a large head circumference correlates with higher IQ and tends to be a familial trait [Filipek et al., 1992; Miles et al., 2000]. The large head circumference is not usually present at birth, but it may appear in early to middle childhood with increased rates of growth [Lainhart, 1997; Mason-Brothers et al., 1990; Mraz et al., 2009]. Head circumference is generally normal by adolescence and adulthood [Aylward et al., 2002], as is postmortem brain weight by adulthood [Bauman and Kemper, 1997]. Microcephaly is more common in autistic subjects than in controls, and it is associated with abnormal physical morphology, medical disorders, lower IQ, and seizures [Fombonne et al., 1999; Miles et al., 2000].

Abnormalities in the neurologic examination may include hypotonia, which was observed in about 25 percent of 176 autistic children and in 33 percent of 110 nonautistic, developmentally delayed children. Spasticity was found in less than 5 percent of either group (exclusionary criteria for this sample included the presence of lateralizing gross motor findings) [Rapin, 1996]. Motor apraxia was identified in almost 30 percent of autistic children with normal cognitive function; in 75 percent of retarded, autistic children; and in 56 percent of a nonautistic, retarded control group [Dziuk et al., 2007; Mari et al., 2003; Ming et al., 2007; Mostofsky et al., 2006; Rapin, 1996; Smith and Bryson, 2007; Vernazza-Martin et al., 2005; Williams et al., 2004]. Characteristic motor abnormalities include motor stereotypies, which occurred in more than 40 percent of autistic children but in only 13 percent of the nonautistic control group [Rapin, 1996]. Hand or finger mannerisms, body rocking, and unusual posturing are reported in 37–95 percent of individuals, and they often manifest during the preschool years [Lord, 1995; Rapin, 1996; Rogers et al., 2003]. There may be considerable overlap in the repertoire of stereotypic movements that autistic children and normal or mentally retarded children display, but they are more prevalent in children with autism especially, most particularly those who are low-functioning [Singer, 2009].

Clinical Testing

Evaluation of Hearing

Many children diagnosed with autism are first described by parents as acting "as if deaf." However, most children with autism have normal hearing function. Rosenhall et al. [1999] performed audiologic evaluations on 199 children and adolescents with autism and found that pronounced to profound bilateral hearing loss or deafness was present in 3.5 percent of all cases, a prevalence greater than that for the general population but similar to the rate for individuals with mental retardation. However, the rate of hearing loss in this study was equivalent across all levels of cognitive functioning. In contrast, hyperacusis was commonly found; it affected almost 20 percent of the autistic sample. Tharpe et al. [2006] found that, as might be expected, behavioral responses of children with autism were elevated and less reliable, relative to those of typically developing children. In addition, approximately half of the children with autism demonstrated abnormal behavioral responses to tones (but not to speech sounds), despite having normal to near-normal hearing sensitivity as determined by other audiometric measures. Audiologic evaluation or brainstem auditory-evoked potential testing should be performed in all children with autism so that, if indicated, appropriate referrals can be made for aural habilitation [American Speech-Language-Hearing Association, 1991; Filipek et al., 1999, 2000a; Johnson and Myers, 2007; Myers and Johnson, 2007].

Lead Level

Children with developmental delay who spend an extended period in the oral-motor stage of play (when everything "goes into their mouths") are at increased risk for lead toxicity, especially in certain environments [Filipek, 2005]. The prevalence of pica in this group can result in high rates of substantial and often recurrent exposure to lead and other metals [Shannon and Graef, 1997]. All children with developmental delay or who are at risk for autism should have a periodic lead screen until the pica disappears [Centers for Disease Control and Prevention, 1997; Shannon and Graef, 1997].

Electroencephalography

There is currently insufficient evidence to recommend for or against the use of routine screening EEGs in autistic patients. A recent review found that epileptiform EEG abnormalities were present in 10.3–72.4 percent of patients and subclinical abnormalities in 6.1–31 percent [Kagan-Kushnir et al., 2005]. The authors concluded that further research is needed about the significance of the EEG abnormalities in the absence of clinical epilepsy (see section on epilepsy p. 14).

Metabolic Testing

The reported co-occurrence of autistic-like symptoms in individuals with inborn errors of metabolism has led to consideration of screening tests as part of the assessment of patients with severe developmental impairment [Steffenburg, 1991]. Although the percentage of children with autism who prove to have an identifiable metabolic disorder has traditionally been considered to be less than 5 percent [Dykens and Volkmar, 1997; Rutter, 1997; Rutter et al., 1994], the recent recognition of the potential association between autism and mitochondrial disorders is bringing this figure into question. Most biochemical analyses are useful only as research tools in the on-going effort to understand the biology of autism, but metabolic testing clearly is indicated by a history of lethargy, cyclic vomiting, early seizures, dysmorphic or coarse features, mental retardation, questionable newborn screening, or birth outside of the United States [Filipek, 2005]. Although

on-going research studies may produce evidence to the contrary, at present, selective metabolic testing should continue to be initiated only in the presence of suggestive clinical and physical findings [Curry et al., 1997; Filipek et al., 1999, 2000b].

Neuroimaging Studies

Routine neuroimaging to evaluate a child with autism and macrocephaly is not warranted unless there is evidence of lateralizing signs on neurologic examination. A review of neuroimaging reports for children with autism found a very low prevalence of focal lesions or other abnormalities, none of which turned out consistently to be more than coincidental findings. PET and single-photon emission computed tomography (SPECT) are used only as research tools and are not indicated in the diagnostic evaluation of autism [Filipek, 2005; Filipek et al., 1999, 2000a].

Tests of Unproven Value

Unsupported claims have led a number of parents to subject their children to various tests in the hope of finding a treatable cause of autism. There is inadequate evidence to support routine clinical testing of individuals with autism for trace elements in the hair [Shearer et al., 1982; Wecker et al., 1985], celiac antibodies [Pavone et al., 1997], allergies (particularly food allergies caused by gluten, casein, and *Candida* and other molds) [Lucarelli et al., 1995], immunologic or neurochemical abnormalities [Cook et al., 1993; Singh et al., 1997; Yuwiler et al., 1992], micronutrients such as vitamin levels [Findling et al., 1997; LaPerchia, 1987; Tolbert et al., 1993], intestinal permeability [D'Eufemia et al., 1996], stool analysis, urinary peptides, thyroid function [Hashimoto et al., 1991], or erythrocyte glutathione peroxidase [Michelson, 1998].

Coexistent Medical Conditions

Feeding Disturbances and Gastrointestinal Problems

Feeding habits and food preferences of children with autism typically are unconventional. Bowers [2002] performed an audit of referrals of autistic children to a dietetic service over a 3-month period and found that, despite selective food preferences in 46 percent, the majority of children had intakes that met or exceeded dietary reference values.

Although there have been reports of gastrointestinal complaints in children with autism dating back more than 30 years [Goodwin et al., 1971; Walker-Smith and Andrews, 1972], the gastrointestinal tract only recently has become a significant focus of study [Filipek, 2005]. In one survey of 500 parents of autistic children, almost 50 percent reported loose stools or frequent diarrhea [Lightdale et al., 2001b]. Other studies found that 19–24 percent of children with autism reported gastrointestinal symptoms, with constipation identified in 9 percent [Fombonne and Chakrabarti, 2001], and diarrhea in 17 percent [Molloy and Manning-Courtney, 2003].

In contrast, others have found that the frequency of gastrointestinal symptoms in ASD is not as common as the literature from gastroenterology clinics might suggest [Black et al., 2002; DeFelice et al., 2003; Kuddo and Nelson, 2003; Mouridsen et al., 2009; Peltola et al., 1998; Taylor et al., 2002]. The recent consensus panel [Buie et al., 2010] reviewed the available literature and concluded that evidence-based recommendations for diagnostic evaluation and management of gastrointestinal problems in children with ASD were not yet available, but that individuals with ASD should receive the same standard of care in the diagnostic work-up and treatment of gastrointestinal concerns, as should occur for patients without ASD. Providers should be aware that problem behavior in patients with ASD may be the primary or sole symptom of underlying medical conditions, including gastrointestinal disorders.

In addition, the consensus panel found that available research data do not support the use of a casein-free diet, a gluten-free diet, or combined gluten-free/casein-free (GFCF) diet as a primary treatment for individuals with ASD. To date, only one small randomized, double-blind crossover study has been published. Similar results were found in both the GFCF diet and non-diet-treated groups [Elder, 2008].

Sleep Disturbances

Sleep disturbances, and particularly abnormalities in sleep-wake cycles, have been a recognized feature of autism for over 25 years (see Didde and Sigafoos [2001]; Ivanenko and Johnson [2008]; Richdale [1999]; and Stores and Wiggs [1998] for reviews). The majority of children with autism have sleep problems, often severe, and usually involving extreme sleep latencies, lengthy nighttime awakenings, shortened night sleep and early morning awakenings [Glickman, 2009; Honomichl et al., 2002; Johnson et al., 2009; Johnson and Malow, 2008; Patzold et al., 1998; Richdale and Schreck, 2009; Schreck and Mulick, 2000; Souders et al., 2009]. Children with autism also have more unusual and obligatory bedtime routines: e.g., requiring that parents hold them, lie down with them, or sit beside their bed; that all family members go to bed at the same time; or that curtains or bedclothes be positioned in a certain way. If these routines are not performed exactly, the result is usually a tantrum or other angry outburst. As might be expected, only the autistic children *always* followed their bedtime routine [Patzold et al., 1998], and the presence of sleep problems was significantly associated with parental stress [Richdale et al., 2000]. Schreck et al. [2004] recently suggested that both the quantity and quality of sleep per night predicted overall autism scores, as measured by the Gilliam Autism Rating Scale (GARS) [Gilliam, 1995], social skills deficits, and stereotypic behaviors. It is unclear whether sleep disorders in children with autism cause daytime maladaptive behaviors, simply allow them to continue, or actually worsen pre-existing problems [Wiggs and Stores, 1996].

Hering et al. [1999] compared the results of parental questionnaires with electronic movement activity recordings (actigraphy) in three groups of children: group 1 consisted of autistic children whose parents reported sleep difficulties; group 2, autistic children whose parents did not report sleep difficulties; and group 3, typically developing children. The initial questionnaires showed that 50 percent of children in group 1 had sleep disorders versus only 20 percent in group 2 and none in group 3. When sleep was quantified using actigraphy, there were no differences in patterns of sleep between groups 1 and 2, except for more early morning awakening in group 1. These findings support the need for objective study methodologies in these samples. Diomedi et al. [1999] compared

polysomnograph parameters in adult autistic individuals, who demonstrated a significant reduction of rapid-eye-movement (REM) sleep, increased interspersed wakefulness, and increased number of awakenings with reduction of sleep efficiency, relative to normal controls (see Harvey and Kennedy [2002] for a comprehensive review of polysomnography in autism and other developmental disabilities).

Epilepsy

Epilepsy occurs frequently in children with autism; approximately one-third will develop epilepsy by adulthood, and all seizure types occur [Volkmar and Nelson, 1990]. There is a bimodal distribution of age of onset, with peaks occurring at younger than 5 years and during adolescence [Spence and Schneider, 2009; Tuchman and Rapin, 2002], and with the rate of epilepsy increased among those with mental retardation or underlying medical conditions. The presence of cerebral palsy or focal motor findings also increases risk. Tuchman et al. [1991] found a prevalence of epilepsy of 14 percent among 314 autistic children, but many were younger than adolescent age; in autistic children with normal or near-normal cognitive function, the risk of epilepsy was less than 10 percent by age 10 years. The rate was 27 percent in the presence of severe mental retardation and 67 percent for those with severe mental retardation and a motor deficit. In a subgroup of 160 children with ASD, normal intelligence, no associated cause, and no family history, the cumulative probability of epilepsy was 6 percent, similar to a rate of 8 percent for children with developmental language disorders. The risk of epilepsy in children with Asperger's disorder and PDD-NOS was less than 10 percent.

Spence and Schneider [2009] recently reviewed the role of epilepsy and epileptiform EEGs in ASD. They found that the rate of epilepsy, even in idiopathic cases of autism with normal IQ, was indeed significantly higher (13–17 percent) [Canitano, 2007; Canitano et al., 2005; Hara, 2007] than the risk in the general population (1–2 percent). Reports have also focused on the presence of subclinical epileptiform abnormalities [Akshoomoff et al., 2007; Baird et al., 2006a; Canitano, 2007; Chez et al., 2006; Gabis et al., 2005; Giannotti et al., 2008; Giovanardi Rossi et al., 2000; Hara, 2007; Hrdlicka et al., 2004; Hughes and Melyn, 2005; Kim et al., 2006; Rossi et al., 1995; Spence and Schneider, 2009]. Kim et al. [2006] found epileptiform abnormalities in the absence of electrographic and clinical seizures in 19 of 32 children referred for prolonged video EEG monitoring for possible seizure activity. Chez et al. [2006] noted epileptiform EEG abnormalities during sleep in 61 percent of almost 900 children with ASD without a history of epilepsy. Other studies, however, report much lower rates [Canitano, 2007; Gabis et al., 2005; Hara, 2007; Parmeggiani et al., 2007], which may be due to differences in sample characteristics and the use of routine EEGs versus prolonged video monitoring. The high rates of isolated epileptiform abnormalities represent a possible objective physiologic finding in ASD, and the treatment of these discharges in the absence of documented seizures is controversial, pending future well-designed longitudinal studies [Spence and Schneider, 2009].

Autism may follow infantile spasms [Riikonen and Amnell, 1981]. Chugani et al. [1996] found that, among children with infantile spasms, those with bitemporal glucose hypometabolism were likely to manifest autism with severe language impairment and mental retardation. In a recent large population-based study, infantile spasms predicted high risk for ASD, but this was, to a large extent, explained by the association of ASD with the symptomatic origin of the seizures [Saemundsen et al., 2008].

Seizures in children with autism should be treated as they would be in children without autism, with even more attention than usual paid to the possible behavioral and cognitive side effects of antiepileptic drugs. Occasionally, it may be difficult to distinguish repetitive and stereotypic behaviors from symptoms of temporal lobe seizures, and inattention from absence seizures may be construed as abnormal, autistic behavior. It is often necessary to use sedation to obtain EEGs for children with autism.

Congenital Blindness

The comorbidity of autism and congenital blindness has received relatively meager attention in the autism research literature. Autistic symptomatology has been anecdotally associated with congenital blindness (CB) for decades; in some studies up to 30 percent of children with CB were also described as being autistic (see reviews by Cass [1998]; Hobson and Bishop [2003]; Hobson et al. [1999]. Rogers and Newhart-Larson [1989] reported a diagnosis of autism in all five boys studied with Leber's congenital amaurosis. Ek et al. [1998] found that 56 percent of premature babies with retinopathy of prematurity (ROP) had both autistic disorder and mental retardation, and, of those, one-third had coexistent cerebral palsy; in comparison, only 14 percent of those with hereditary retinal disease had autistic disorder. Janson [1993] postulated that, in blind children with ROP, a behavior pattern of unresponsivity and stereotypic object manipulation emerges between 12 and 30 months to distinguish autistic and non-autistic children with CB. Msall et al. [2004] followed children with ROP at ages 5 and 8 years, and found that 23 percent had epilepsy, 39 percent cerebral palsy, and 44 percent learning disabilities. Of the children with no or minimal light perception or totally detached retinas bilaterally, 9 percent were autistic, as compared with only 1 percent of those with more favorable visual status.

Cass et al. [1994] reported that, of an entire sample of over 600 congenitally blind children of differing etiologies, only 17 percent demonstrated no evidence of additional disabilities and were developing normally at age 16 months when first studied. Subsequently, 31 percent had a regression in their development occurring between 16 and 27 months of age; children who regressed tended to have disorders of central nervous system/optic nerve/retina, while children who did not regress had a purely optical cause for their blindness (e.g., congenital cataracts or glaucoma). The more "central" pathophysiology of the blindness in the regression cohort was subsequently confirmed by neuroimaging studies; the children with developmental regression had more central nervous system lesions than those who did not regress [Waugh et al., 1998].

Brown et al. [1997] reported that almost half of their sample with CB met criteria for autism, and that, even in CB without autism, there were significantly more "autistic features" than seen in matched sighted children. Brown et al. [1997] and Hobson et al. [1999] compared congenitally blind (of various etiologies) and sighted autistic children and noted remarkably similar clinical features. The authors' clinical impressions were that blind autistic children were less severely impaired than sighted autistic children; none was abnormal in listening response, but most were markedly abnormal in body and object use. Mukaddes et al. [2007] examined 257 blind children for autism, and identified 30 (12 percent) who met criteria for DSM-IV Autistic Disorder. Differentiating factors between those CB children with and without autism included severity of blindness, cerebral palsy, and intellectual level, with greater neurological impairments and more severe blindness in those with CB and autism.

Known Genetic and Other Conditions associated with Autism

Known single-gene defects and diagnosed medical conditions account for about 10 percent of cases of autism [Chakrabarti and Fombonne, 2001; Fombonne, 2002a], and there may be subtle but qualitative differences in the symptoms of ASD in specific syndromes. Bolton et al. [1991] and Rutter et al. [1993] found that 8.1 percent of 151 individuals with autism had specific associated medical conditions, including fragile X syndrome, bilateral deafness, cerebral palsy, multiple congenital abnormalities, and identified chromosomal anomalies. About 3.8 percent had other medical concerns that were less likely to be associated with etiologic factors. The possibility of finding any associated medical condition rises with increasing degrees of mental retardation – approaching 50 percent among persons at the severe and profound levels of cognitive dysfunction [Scott, 1994]. In a survey of multiple studies, the fraction of patients with autism who have an associated medical condition of potential etiologic significance was 0–17 percent, with a mean of 6 percent [Fombonne, 2003a, b]. Defined mutations, genetic syndromes, and metabolic diseases account for up to 20 percent of autistic patients [Benvenuto et al., 2009a, b].

These studies investigated the prevalence of medical disorders in populations of individuals with autism. It is important to differentiate that perspective from the prevalence of an autistic phenotype *in a population of individuals with the given disorder*. Tuberous sclerosis complex (TSC) and fragile X syndrome (FraX) are prime examples to illustrate this concept. In a population of *individuals with autism*, only a few will have a diagnosis of TSC or FraX; however, in a population of *individuals with TSC or FraX*, over 50 percent will have a diagnosis of autism. It is therefore important to recognize the autistic phenotype in associated genetic-metabolic and syndromic conditions to optimize intervention plans for these children and adults [Moss and Howlin, 2009].

Fragile X Syndrome

Fragile X syndrome is second only to Down syndrome in terms of a known chromosomal cause of mental retardation. Between 21 and 50 percent of boys with fragile X syndrome are on the autistic spectrum [Moss and Howlin, 2009], and 0–6 percent of autism populations have fragile X syndrome (median of six studies 0.75 percent) [Fombonne et al., 1997b]. A milder presentation of autistic symptoms is more common, and symptoms tend most frequently towards social anxiety, extreme shyness, and gaze avoidance [Roberts et al., 2007].

Summarizing data across 40 studies, Fisch [1992] found virtually identical pooled proportions of fragile X syndrome in autistic males and in mentally retarded males. These studies suggested that autism and fragile X syndrome may occur together, but the prevalence of these cases is much lower than originally thought, and that fragile X syndrome is not a major etiologic factor in autism.

Tuberous Sclerosis Complex

TSC has been strongly associated with autism and identified more frequently in individuals with mental retardation and most commonly in those with epilepsy [Gutierrez et al., 1998; Kandt, 2003]. Rates of ASD in TSC most consistently range between 24 and 60 percent [Moss and Howlin, 2009]. The incidence of autistic individuals with TSC complex has been estimated to be between 0.4 and 4 percent in epidemiologic studies [Chudley et al., 1998; Fombonne et al., 1997b; Smalley, 1998]. This rate increases to 8–14 percent for autistic individuals with epilepsy [Gillberg, 1991].

PET studies of children with TSC and autism have revealed changes in the deep cerebellar nuclei and caudate nuclei that were not seen in nonautistic TSC subjects [Asano et al., 2001], but the presence of cortical tubers in the temporal lobes did not increase the risk for autism.

15q Syndrome

A chromosomal abnormality that occurs in 1–4 percent of autistic individuals involves the proximal long arm of chromosome 15q11–q13 [Browne et al., 1997; Schroer et al., 1998], which is the most frequent of the currently identifiable chromosomal disorders associated with autism. The clinical phenotype is highly variable, ranging from profound psychomotor retardation to normal nonverbal cognitive scores [Filipek et al., 2000c]. The duplication is usually maternally inherited, and involves the area roughly corresponding to the Prader–Willi/Angelman critical region (PWACR) of approximately 4 million base pairs. The additional genetic material may be interstitial, producing a trisomy of 15q11–q13, which may or may not be inverted, or may be a separate marker chromosome, producing a tetrasomy of this region. Over 100 individuals with autism and this chromosomal anomaly have been reported in the literature to date (see Schanen [2006] for a recent review). In addition to *MECP2* deletions, Longo et al. [2004] also found 15q11–q13 duplications in 3 out of 63 (4.7 percent) patients with Rett's syndrome.

Chromosome 22q11 Deletion Syndrome/Velocardiofacial Syndrome

Shprintzen et al. [1981] first described velocardiofacial syndrome (VCFS), which is characterized by cleft palate, cardiac malformations (usually a ventricular septal defect), typical facies (tubular nose, narrow palpebral fissures, and retruded jaw), learning disabilities and/or mental retardation, microcephaly, short stature, central nervous system vascular malformations, and seizures [Coppola et al., 2001; Perez and Sullivan, 2002; Roubertie et al., 2001]. It is now known to be caused by a microdeletion in the *TBX1* gene on chromosome 22q11.2, and its prevalence is estimated at 1 in 4000 [Bassett and Chow, 1999]. Gothelf et al. [2001, 2004] reported that 16–25 percent will develop psychotic disorder by adolescence; the prevalence

of schizophrenia in VCFS is 25 times that of the general population, and up to 40 percent meet criteria for attention-deficit hyperactivity disorder (ADHD), and 33 percent for obsessive-compulsive disorder. Kozma [1998] was the first to report comorbid autism in VCFS, with associated severe mental retardation. Subsequent studies found that 20–30 percent of VCFS subjects met criteria for autistic disorder, and over 50 percent for an ASD; over 50 percent had mental retardation [Chudley et al., 1998; Fine et al., 2005; Kates et al., 2007; Niklasson et al., 2001, 2002; Roubertie et al., 2001; Vorstman et al., 2006].

Autism has also been associated with neurofibromatosis [Fombonne et al., 1997b; Gillberg and Forsell, 1984; Marui et al., 2004; Mouridsen et al., 1992; Williams and Hersh, 1998], Smith–Lemli–Opitz syndrome [Bukelis et al., 2007; Cohen et al., 2005; Martin et al., 2001; Sikora et al., 2006; Tierney et al., 2006], cerebral folate deficiency [Moretti et al., 2005, 2008; Ramaekers et al., 2007], and biotinidase deficiency [Zaffanello et al., 2003], as well as the classic example of phenylketonuria [Baieli et al., 2003; Chen and Hsiao, 1989; Miladi et al., 1992].

Mitochondrial Disorders

Coleman and Blass [1985] first reported an association of lactic acidosis with autism over 20 years ago, which was corroborated by Laszlo et al. [1994]. Lombard [1998] postulated a mitochondrial etiology for autism, based on, among other things, his unpublished anecdotal observations of carnitine deficiency. Functional neuroimaging methodologies have also related autism and deficient energy metabolism in the brain [Chugani et al., 1999; Levitt et al., 2003; Minshew et al., 1993].

Clark-Taylor and Clark-Taylor [2004] reported a child with autism who also had an abnormal acyl-carnitine profile with elevations of unsaturated fatty-acid metabolites C14:1 and C14:2 and ammonia, and alterations of tricarboxylic acid cycle energy production. Filipek et al. [2003] first reported evidence of mitochondrial dysfunction in two autistic children with inverted duplications of chromosome 15q11–q13. They also found that free and total carnitine and pyruvate were significantly reduced, while ammonia, lactate, and alanine levels were considerably elevated in 100 asymptomatic autistic children in a clinic population, suggestive of mild mitochondrial dysfunction [Filipek et al., 2004]. In a population-based study, Oliveria et al. [2005] found hyperlacticacidemia in 20 percent, with a definite mitochondrial respiratory chain disorder identified in 7.2 percent of 120 children with ASD.

Filiano et al. [2002] reported a group of 12 children presenting with hypotonia, intractable epilepsy, autism, and developmental delay (HEADD syndrome), who demonstrated reduced levels in specific mitochondrial respiratory activities encoded by mitochondrial DNA, with a majority also showing mitochondrial structural abnormalities. Several additional reports have appeared in the literature recently, describing specific mitochondrial DNA abnormalities associated with ASD [Graf et al., 2000; Kent et al., 2008; Pons et al., 2004; Smith et al., 2009]. Weissman et al. [2008], in a record review of 25 children with ASD and mitochondrial disorders, found clinical abnormalities uncommon in idiopathic autism, including constitutional symptoms, especially excessive fatigability, significant non-neurologic medical histories, marked delay in early gross motor milestones, and unusual patterns of regression.

Knowledge of mitochondrial function and dysfunction is presently expanding exponentially and concurrently with knowledge of the neurobiology and genetics of autism; further research will elucidate the validity and extent of mitochondrial dysfunction in individuals with autism [Lerman-Sagie et al., 2004; Zecavati and Spence, 2009].

Down Syndrome

Down syndrome is the most common chromosomal cause of mental retardation, occurring in approximately 1 in 1000 live births [Bell et al., 2003; Iliyasu et al., 2002]. Although once considered implausible, the comorbidity of autism and Down syndrome is not rare [Bregman and Volkmar, 1988; Ghaziuddin, 1997, 2000; Ghosh et al., 2008; Howlin et al., 1995; Lowenthal et al., 2007; Molloy et al., 2008, 2009; Wakabayashi, 1979; Wing and Gould, 1979]. In fact, Down's original phenotypic description [1887, pp. 6–7] describes the autistic phenotype. In epidemiological studies, the prevalence of Down syndrome in individuals with autism ranges from 0 to 16.7 percent (see Fombonne et al. [2003] for a review). Some studies that screened samples with Down syndrome for autism found relatively low rates of autism, ranging from 1.0 to 2.2 percent; other series have reported that as many as 39 percent of subjects with Down syndrome also meet criteria for autism [Capone et al., 2005; Ghaziuddin et al., 1992; Gillberg et al., 1986; Kent et al., 1999; Lowenthal et al., 2007; Lund, 1988; Starr et al., 2005; Turk and Graham, 1997] (see Moss and Howlin [2009] for a recent review).

Howlin et al. [1995] eloquently championed the importance of recognizing autism in children with Down syndrome. Although autism diagnoses are typically made in the preschool years, they noted later ages of autistic diagnoses in all cases reported in the literature (range from 7 years to adulthood). This singular diagnostic view creates unnecessary stress for families, and prevents them from using supports and interventions available to families with an autistic child. Reasons for the lack of recognition of autistic signs in Down syndrome are unclear. The stereotyped personality of individuals with Down syndrome is outgoing, affectionate, easy-going, placid, cheerful, highly social, and verbal. Yet, children with comorbid Down syndrome and autism are very different from other children with Down syndrome, demonstrating classic deficits in sociability, immediate and delayed echolalia, poor developmental progress in communication skills, motor stereotypies and ritualistic behaviors or interests, and adaptive behaviors. Even though autism may not be common in Down syndrome, it should be considered in the range of diagnostic possibilities for all individuals with this syndrome.

Williams–Beuren Syndrome

Williams–Beuren syndrome (WBS) is a rare disorder first described over 40 years ago [Beuren et al., 1962; Williams et al., 1961], and caused by a microdeletion on chromosome 7q11.23 that includes the gene for elastin [OMIMTM, 2000]. The association between WBS and autism has not been widely studied, and there are only few cases of comorbidity formally reported in the literature [Feinstein and Singh, 2007; Gillberg and Rasmussen, 1994; Herguner and Mukaddes, 2006; Klein-Tasman et al., 2009; Reiss et al., 1985]. WBS and autism have traditionally been thought to show opposing patterns of cognitive strength and weakness.

By definition, individuals with autism often have poor verbal and nonverbal communication skills. In contrast, despite significant early language delay, many individuals with WBS have been described as showing relative sparing of expressive language and linguistic functioning, including high-level syntax and semantics [Bellugi et al., 2001], story-telling and narrative enrichment strategies involving affective prosody and a sense of drama [Reilly et al., 1990], and a reliance on stereotypic, adult phrases [Udwin and Yule, 1990]. Recently however, investigators have more specifically characterized the atypical language development in WMS for example, referential language precedes referential pointing, the opposite of what is seen in normal development. Noted that referential language precedes referential pointing in WBS, the opposite of what is seen in typical language development. Toddlers with WBS also do not spontaneously use the pointing gesture in free-play situations. Laing et al. [2002] reported that, despite superficially "good social skills," children with WBS were deficient at both initiating and responding to triadic interactions (e.g., child–interlocutor–object), which are essential for joint attention and referential uses of language. Laws and Bishop [2004] demonstrated that children with WBS indeed have difficulties with social relationships and a semantic-pragmatic language disorder (described by some as "loquaciousness"), particularly with inappropriate initiation of conversation and the use of stereotyped conversation; they also have a restricted range of interests, specialized factual knowledge and usual vocabulary. The authors suggested that, "Far from representing the polar opposite of autism, as suggested by some researchers, WBS could seem to share many of the characteristics of autistic disorder" [2004, p. 45].

Prader–Willi and Angelman's syndromes

Described as "sister imprinting disorders" [Cassidy et al., 2000], Angelman's syndrome (AS) and Prader–Willi syndrome (PWS) are each the result of either a deletion or uniparental disomy (UPD) in the PW-AS critical region of chromosome 15 (see Clayton-Smith and Laan [2003] for a review). AS, coined the "happy puppet syndrome" [Bower and Jeavons, 1967], presents with severe motor and intellectual retardation, ataxia, hypotonia, epilepsy, absence of speech, and unusual "happy" facies, and has been associated with ASD in recent years [Bonati et al., 2007; Moss and Howlin, 2009; Pelc et al., 2008; Peters et al., 2004; Pickler and Elias, 2009; Steffenburg et al., 1996; Trillingsgaard and Stergaard, 2004; Veltman et al., 2005; Zafeiriou et al., 2007]. Thompson and Bolton [2003] reported one case of Angelman's syndrome and paternal UPD, and discussed the milder AS symptomatology associated with UPD, including a lack of autistic features.

Genomic imprinting is a form of epigenetic modification in which allele silencing is specific to the parent of origin. This occurs in Angelman's syndrome, caused by molecular abnormalities that include deletion of a maternally derived copy of the 15q11–q13 chromosomal region. Children with Angelman's syndrome have many overlapping features of autism [Peters et al., 2004]. Two types of imprinting defects may cause Angelman's syndrome: inherited deletions of the imprinting center, which are primarily genetic but also have secondary epigenetic effects, and imprinting defects that have no identifiable DNA sequence abnormality [Jiang et al., 2004].

PWS is characterized by obesity, muscular hypotonia, mental retardation, short stature, hypogonadotropic hypogonadism, and small hands and feet. It appears that PWS results from UPD or deletion of the paternal copies of the imprinted small nuclear ribonucleoprotein polypeptide N (*SNRPN*) and *necdin* genes, and possibly others as well. Several recent reports note an association between PWS and ASD [Descheemaeker et al., 2002, 2006; Dimitropoulos and Schultz, 2007; Feinstein and Singh, 2007; Greaves et al., 2006; Milner et al., 2005; Veltman et al., 2005]. Veltman et al. [2004] found that maternal UPD cases of PWS would be more likely to exhibit ASD than would cases with deletions in the PWACR. Therefore, the extent of the associations of AS and PWS with autism remains unclear to date, particularly the differential effects of UPD, as compared with deletions of the responsible genes.

Genetic Studies

Although Bettelheim [1967] espoused the theory that autism was caused by parental behavior (the "refrigerator mother"), it has become clear that autism is a complex genetic disorder. Twin studies provide strong evidence that autism is genetic, involving multiple genes and variable expression. The concordance rate for autistic disorder in monozygotic twins has been reported as 36–90 percent [Bailey et al., 1995; Folstein and Rutter, 1977; Ritvo et al., 1989; Steffenburg et al., 1989], compared with 0–23 percent in dizygotic twins [Bailey et al., 1995]. However, when twin pairs are evaluated for a broader autistic phenotype that includes communication and social disorders and stereotypic behaviors, the concordance rate is 92 percent for monozygotic twins and 10 percent for dizygotic twin pairs.

In families of children with autism, characteristics known as the broader autism phenotype are more common than in controls [Fombonne et al., 1997a; Pickles et al., 2000]. These characteristics include difficulty with communication and language, including delayed onset [Folstein et al., 1999], social reticence or phobias, and preference for routine and difficulty with change [Pickles et al., 2000; Piven et al., 1991a] or obsessive-compulsive traits [Hollander et al., 2003]. These traits are not usually associated with difficulties in function [Folstein and Rosen-Sheidley, 2001]. Milder impairments in social and communicative skills also occur in siblings and relatives of probands more often than in controls [Bailey et al., 1998; Szatmari et al., 2000]. Relatives are more likely to have traits within the broader autism phenotype if a proband is higher- rather than lower-functioning [Nicolson and Szatmari, 2003], and if there are multiple probands with autism [Spence, 2004].

It was formerly felt that there were multiple genes that, in various combinations, confer small to moderate effects on the autism phenotype. Using entire-genome screens in families with more than one affected member, autism or autistic traits has been linked to various shared genetic markers that are regions of interest inherited by affected persons more frequently than would be expected by chance. Multiple collaborative groups have facilitated the identification of regions of interest. One consortium recently identified a common genetic variant associated with autism on chromosome 5p14.4 [de Vries, 2009]. Many of these identified markers have not been verified in other populations, and it has been difficult to find robust common variants [Levy et al., 2009]. Using new whole-genome DNA microarray technologies, or high-density screening platforms, progress has been made in identifying structural

abnormalities, from microscopic to submicroscopic: e.g., copy number variations (CNVs), microdeletions, and rearrangements. Environmental factors may act to influence the risk for de novo mutations. There may be many ASD cases attributable to multiple interacting genes interacting with environmental factors, but the more recent thinking is that there are also multiple rare variants or CNVs, most commonly deletions, that have a primary effect on producing the autism phenotype. These may be inherited or may arise de novo. CNVs may account for up to 10 percent of nonfamilial cases of ASD, and about 2 percent of familial cases [Sebat et al., 2007]. Deletion variations are seen more frequently in sporadic than in familial cases of ASD. Chromosome microarray testing (CMA) has been reported to have the highest detection rate for patients with ASD, even though many of the copy number variants seen do not have known significance [Shen et al., 2010].

ASD candidate genes have been identified using whole-genome approaches. Candidate genes are selected for study, often through known genetic disorders or animal models, because they are known to affect developmental processes that may be involved in the pathogenesis of autism. Candidate genes that interfere with synaptic maturation or function have emerged as a plausible reason for the aberrant structural and functional connectivity seen in ASDs [Levy et al., 2009].

Studies of serotonin transporter genes have yielded conflicting results [Betancur et al., 2002; Kim et al., 2002; Klauck et al., 1997; Maestrini et al., 1999; Persico et al., 2000; Tordjman et al., 2001; Yirmiya et al., 2001]. Glutamate transporter genes were found to be upregulated in postmortem studies [Purcell et al., 2001], and the glutamate receptor-6 gene (*GRIK2*, formerly designated *GLUR6*) was expressed in brain regions involving learning and memory [Jamain et al., 2002]. Another candidate gene involves oxytocin. Oxytocin levels affect social behavior, and two genome-wide screens have found linkage to a locus containing the oxytocin receptor gene [Auranen et al., 2002; Shao et al., 2002].

Many of the genes identified to date involve cell adhesion pathways [Betancur et al., 2009], including Shank 3, a synaptic protein that regulates synaptic scaffolding organization, along with neuroligins [Durand et al., 2006]. Neuroligins are important in excitatory synapses and synaptogenesis; defects may affect cognitive development and communication. De novo structural chromosome variations are seen in cases both with and without intellectual disability [Geschwind, 2009]. A region of interest on chromosome 7q has been identified that is associated with developmental language disorders; because a core feature of autism is a communication disorder, it is possible that autism and severe language impairment could share a gene in this region [Ashley-Koch et al., 1999; Badner and Gershon, 2002; Folstein and Rosen-Sheidley, 2001; IMGSAC, 1998, 2001]. The 7q region also contains a gene called *RELN* that codes for a protein thought to help neurons migrate to their proper location.

Epigenetics

Exogenous factors can modify the control of gene expression. Epigenetics refers to the stable and heritable or potentially heritable changes in gene expression that do not involve a change in DNA sequence [Jiang et al., 2004]. Epigenetic mechanisms involve a signal or stimulus that changes gene expression and may help to explain the onset of symptoms in autism after a period of apparently normal development; it may also play a role in how the environment affects phenotypic expression. Chromosomes originating from one parent may have an abnormal epigenotype that leads to modulation of DNA methylation, which causes gene silencing [Bjornsson et al., 2004a, b].

Genetic Counseling

If one child in a family has ASD, the risk for subsequent siblings is elevated [Chakrabarti and Fombonne, 2001; Micali et al., 2004], and is higher if the child with autism is a girl [Sumi et al., 2006]. Rates of mental retardation without autism are not increased in families with ASDs, suggesting that the mental retardation is part of the autistic disorder, not a separate condition. There is no prenatal test to identify autism, but it is important to look for physical or dysmorphic features in the identified autistic child that may suggest a diagnosable genetic condition such as fragile X syndrome [Miles and Hillman, 2000] or tuberous sclerosis complex.

Cytogenetic methods of karyotyping and molecular analyses for fragile X, and the implications of a cytogenetic or molecular diagnosis for other family members, justify their routine inclusion in the diagnostic evaluation of a child with autism [Abdul-Rahman and Hudgins, 2006; Battaglia and Carey, 2006; Challman et al., 2003; Curry et al., 1997; Filipek, 2005; Herman et al., 2007; Marshall et al., 2008]. Current data do not support extensive clinical genetic testing of all children with ASD [Johnson and Myers, 2007]. However, fluorescent in situ hybridization (FISH) studies targeted for specific deletions or duplications – such as is seen in the 15q syndrome, for example – may prove useful in individual cases. Subtelomeric FISH screening in ASD has failed to identify any abnormalities in a total of 225 subjects [Battaglia and Bonaglia, 2006; Keller et al., 2003; Wassink et al., 2007].

Even if the karyotyping appears normal, a microarray comparative genomic hybridization test (aCGH) is advised. aCGH studies identify CNVs, microdeletions, and microduplications that otherwise would go undetected [Christian et al., 2008; Miller et al., 2010]. As such techniques become more available, they should be extended to children without dysmorphic features, as microdeletions and microduplications are common among those with no dysmorphic features as well [Lintas and Persico, 2009]. When there are implications of a cytogenetic or molecular diagnosis for other family members, especially when another pregnancy may be a possibility, their inclusion in the diagnostic evaluation of a child with autism is recommended [American College of Medical Genetics: Policy Statement, 1994]. Prenatal genetic testing is not recommended, because almost all of the recognizable genetic or genomic abnormalities responsible for ASD are not detectable, with the exception of very rare major chromosomal rearrangements.

Even if no genetic condition is revealed, genetic counseling should include a discussion of the risks of recurrence of ASDs in a subsequent child and the lack of ability to diagnose this prenatally [Folstein and Rosen-Sheidley, 2001; Sumi et al., 2006]. The goal of counseling is to provide as much information as possible but to leave decision-making and interpretation of the genetic information to the families.

Additional studies are needed to understand the role of genetics and environmental influences in autism. Questions can be answered only with increasingly large and varied populations and by advances in phenotypic characterization. It is important to encourage families, particularly those with multiple affected members, to participate in clinical research.

Pharmacologic Therapy

The goal of pharmacologic treatment for children with autism is to improve symptoms and specific behaviors. Target symptoms include anxiety, repetitive motor behaviors, obsessive-compulsive symptoms, impulsivity, depression, mood swings, agitation, hyperactivity, aggression, and self-injurious behavior. Although no medications directly impact cognitive impairment, controlling these symptoms should allow the child to maximize benefit from educational and behavioral treatments that are more directed toward the core impairments. Almost all of these medications are prescribed off-label. There are a relatively small number of randomized, prospective, double-blind, placebo-controlled trials and very little long-term follow-up.

Dosing should start with low amounts and be slowly escalated with careful attention to possible side effects, the most common of which is activation, defined as overactivity, agitation, or emotional lability. Weight gain and metabolic changes are common side effects of neuroleptics [Correll et al., 2009], and the long-term consequences are of particular concern in children, as they may require treatment for an extended time. Target symptoms should be clearly defined, and new drugs should be tried for a sufficient length of time to determine their usefulness. One caution to keep in mind is that sedation in response to pharmacotherapy may be mistaken for a positive response [Volkmar and Pauls, 2003]. It is important to work with teachers and families to monitor a therapy's effectiveness and side effects. Drug treatment should be one facet of a comprehensive, multidisciplinary treatment approach that includes structured special educational techniques, language or communication interventions, behavior modification, and parent training.

Neuroleptic Agents

Neuroleptics that block dopamine receptors, such as haloperidol, thioridazine, and trifluoperazine, were used until the development of drugs that were more effective in blocking serotonin receptors. Haloperidol decreased motor stereotypies, hyperactivity, withdrawal, and negativism in children with autism [Anderson et al., 1989]. Common side effects are sedation and weight gain [Campbell et al., 1997].

The newer atypical neuroleptics include risperidone, clozapine, olanzapine, and quetiapine. They modulate dopamine (D_2) and serotonin $(5HT_2)$ receptors [Buitelaar and Willemsen-Swinkels, 2000]. Risperidone and aripiprazole have been approved by the Federal Drug Administration (FDA) for the treatment of irritabilty (including aggression, self-injurious behavior, temper tantrums, and mood swings) in school-age children and adolescents with autistic disorder. However, these agents have been associated with weight gain, prolactin increases, and sedation in some patients.

In an 8-week multisite, double-blind, randomized trial of risperidone in 101 children with ASD [McCracken et al., 2002], a relatively low dose of 0.5–3.5 mg/d improved irritability, hyperactivity, and stereotypies. Treatment effects were maintained over 16 weeks of treatment, and discontinuation of the medication resulted in return of behavioral symptoms [Aman et al., 2005]. Side effects included weight gain that averaged 6 pounds over 8 weeks, and mild to moderate fatigue in about half of the children. There was a very low incidence of acute extrapyramidal symptoms. These results have been replicated in children [Hellings et al., 2006; Shea et al., 2004] and adults [Hellings et al., 2006]. Luby et al. [2006] conducted a small trial of risperidone with 24 younger children (ages 2.5–6) with ASD. There was a modest but statistically significant improvement on a global autism rating scale compared to the placebo group after 6 months. Significantly greater weight gain and elevated prolactin levels were observed in the treatment group. A double-blind, placebo-controlled trial with 31 autistic adults [McDougle et al., 1998] similarly found decreased irritability, repetitive behavior, and overall behavioral symptoms in the group treated with risperidone.

An 8-week double-blind, randomized, placebo-controlled trial with aripiprazole in 218 children and adolescents with autistic disorder compared three doses of the drug (5, 10, or 15 mg/d) to placebo [Marcus et al., 2009]. All doses demonstrated improvement in irritability, although only the 5 mg/day group reached statistical significance, possibly due to a high placebo response (35 percent). Improvement was reported within 2 weeks, at a point at which all participants were taking the lowest dose. About 10 percent of the participants withdrew from the study because of adverse effects; the most common side effect leading to discontinuation was sedation. Extrapyramidal symptoms were reported in 23.1 percent of the treatment group, compared to 11.8 percent in the placebo group, and more subjects in the treatment groups received medication to treat these symptoms. Aripiprazole was associated with a higher incidence of weight gain than placebo, although no participants discontinued treatment for this reason.

Other atypical neuroleptics studied with similar results include olanzapine and ziprasidone, although they were assessed only in open trials [Malone et al., 2001] or with very small number of participants [Hollander et al., 2006b].

Concern about side effects has led to some comparisons studies. Miral et al. [2008] compared haloperidol and risperidone in 30 children and adolescents with autistic disorder. Both agents were effective in reducing tantrums, aggression, and self-injury. Risperidone was slightly superior to haloperidol in improving disruptive behavior. There was a significant worsening of extrapyramidal symptoms reported in the group treated with haloperidol. Similar levels of weight gain occurred in each group, and there was a greater increase in prolactin in individuals taking risperidone. Remington et al. [2001] compared haloperidol to the serotonin reuptake inhibitor, clomipramine, in 36 children and adults (ages 10–36 years) with ASD. Haloperidol was superior to clomipramine in reducing irritability and hyperactivity. Neither medication was superior to placebo in reducing stereotypies or inappropriate speech. There was a higher dropout rate in the clomipramine group due to side effects, particularly behavioral activation.

Opiate Antagonists

Several published trials used naltrexone, a long-acting opiate antagonist that can be taken orally. The hypothesis for benefit is that autism is associated with hypersecretion of brain opioids, including beta-endorphins, and that many symptoms of autism are similar to those induced by opiate administration, such as decreased socialization, repetitive stereotypic movements, and motor hyperactivity [Feldman et al., 1999]. Naltrexone in doses of 1.0 mg/kg daily in 23 autistic children decreased restlessness and hyperactivity [Campbell et al., 1993] in a parallel study design. Side effects were mild gastrointestinal symptoms, appetite decrease, and drowsiness. In a randomized, double-blind, crossover design, naltrexone was associated with modest improvement of behavior in 11 of 24 children, but no improvement in learning occurred [Kolmen et al., 1995]. In a separate, similarly designed study that looked specifically at communication skills, no benefit was seen [Feldman et al., 1999]. Studies by Willemsen-Swinkels and colleagues [Willemsen-Swinkels et al., 1995a, b, 1996, 1999] also failed to prove any benefit, and in some children, stereotypic behaviors were increased.

Serotonin Reuptake Inhibitors

Symptoms causing major disruption in autism, such as anxiety and repetitive and ritualized behaviors, can impair learning. Because of the efficacy of serotonin reuptake inhibitors (SRI; e.g., clomipramine, fluoxetine, sertraline, fluvoxamine, and paroxetine) on anxiety and obsessive-compulsive symptoms, and the finding of serotonin system abnormalities in individuals with autism [Chandana et al., 2005], there has been considerable interest in treating disruptive behaviors in autism with these agents. Results of open-label and observational studies have been mixed but encouraging for the reduction of ritualistic behavior, anxiety, and aggression, as well as behavioral rigidity, obsessive-compulsive disorder symptoms, and stereotypies [e.g., Brasic et al., 1994; Cook and Leventhal, 1996; Cook et al., 1992; DeLong et al., 2002; Fatemi et al., 1998; Hollander et al., 2000; Martin et al., 2003; Owley et al., 2005; Sanchez et al., 1995, 1996; Steingard et al., 1997]. However, results of recent double-blind, placebo-controlled, randomized trials have been mixed, and suggest that efficacy of SRIs may be moderated by age, with better responsivity in adults than in children. Additionally, the evidence for possible developmentally sensitive altered regulation of serotonin synthesis in autistic children provides a rationale for giving serotonergic drugs to very young autistic children in order to improve synaptic plasticity during periods of brain development. Controlled clinical trials enrolling very young children are difficult to undertake, but at least one is in process.

A randomized, double-blind, placebo-controlled trial enrolling adults with autism found improvement in one-half of the fluvoxamine-treated patients compared with placebo, with reduction of repetitive thoughts and behavior, maladaptive behavior, language, social relatedness, and aggression [McDougle et al., 1996]. There were few side effects at a mean dose of 270 mg/day. A crossover trial of six adults using the selective SRI fluoxetine demonstrated significant improvement in obsessive behaviors and anxiety, and PET scans demonstrated fluoxetine-elevated metabolic rates in the right frontal lobes [Buchsbaum et al., 2001].

Results of trials in children, however, have been less encouraging. Low-dose liquid fluoxetine (mean dose of 10 mg/day) was superior to placebo on a measure of repetitive behaviors, but not on a measure of clinician-rated global improvement, in 39 children and adolescents with autism in a randomized, crossover trial [Hollander et al., 2005]. Agitation resulted in a dose reduction in 16 percent of the subjects in the fluoxetine group, compared with 5 percent in the placebo group, but this difference was not statistically significant.

A large double-blind, randomized, placebo-controlled trial of citalopram in children and adolescents with ASD has failed to find the predicted effects on repetitive behaviors. A multisite study with 149 children with ASD (ages 5–17 years) and high levels of repetitive behavior evaluated the efficacy of citalopram in reducing those behaviors [King et al., 2009]. In 12 weeks of treatment with a flexible dose schedule, citalopram did not separate from placebo in the primary outcome measures of repetitive behavior and global improvement. The mean citalopram dose was 16.5 (SD = 6.5) mg/d. Citalopram levels and high parent-reported compliance to treatment suggest that this was an adequate trial and the doses were similar to those previously reported to be effective in open trials. Adverse events were significantly more likely to occur in the citalopram-treated group. The most frequently reported side effects were activation, stereotypy, diarrhea, insomnia, and dry skin or pruritus. Two subjects treated with citalopram had seizures. Of note, there was a high placebo response rate (34 percent), which underscores the need for placebo-controlled clinical trials.

In summary, SRIs, selective SRIs, and other medications affecting serotonin and dopamine levels can reduce specific symptoms of autism, such as ritualized behaviors, stereotypies, rigid behaviors, aggression, and anxiety in adults. Large multi-site clinical trials with children found that SRIs did not reduce repetitive behavior, or other disruptive behaviors, in children with ASD. While SRIs appear to be generally safe, children may be particularly sensitive to the behavioral activation of these drugs [Buitelaar and Willemsen-Swinkels, 2000]. Seizures have emerged under SRI treatment in clinical trials in a few instances, although this is a seizure-prone population and it is not clear whether the medications were causal. Additionally, there has been concern about reports of an association of fluoxetine and possibly other selective SRIs with suicidal ideation in depressed children, and the FDA has recommended that children on these medications should be very carefully monitored.

Stimulants and Drugs to Treat Hyperactivity

Hyperactivity is an important target symptom that can be potentially improved with psychostimulant medication [Handen et al., 2000; Quintana et al., 1995]. The Research Units on Pediatric Psychopharmacology (RUPP) Autism Network [Posey et al., 2007; Research Units on Pediatric Psychopharmacology Autism Network, 2005a] conducted a randomized, double-blind, placebo-controlled trial of methylphenidate in children with ASDs and high levels of hyperactivity and/or impulsiveness. Doses at the 0.25 and 0.5 mg/kg level were effective in reducing hyperactivity and impulsivity, but less effective in reducing inattention, at 4 weeks and after 8 weeks' continuation. The response rate was about 35 percent compared to typical response rates of around 70 percent in non-PDD children with ADHD. About 18 percent of subjects withdrew due to side effects, primarily irritability. Other common side effects included decreased

appetite and trouble falling asleep. Some children responded best to lower doses of methylphenidate. Observational data was available on a subset of 33 study participants, suggesting that the benefits of methylphenidate extended to some aspects of social interactions, self-regulation, and affect [Jahromi et al., 2009].

Atomoxetine is a nonstimulant medication for ADHD that inhibits the presynaptic norepinephrine transporter. In a placebo-controlled, double-blind crossover study with 16 children with ASD and ADHD symptoms, atomoxetine was more effective than placebo in reducing hyperactivity. The response rate was similar to that reported for methylphenidate in children with ASD, and the mean highest dose was 44.2 (SD = 21.9) mg/d. Side effects, including gastrointestinal symptoms, fatigue, and racing heart were common but transient [Arnold et al., 2006]. Only one participant terminated the study due to intolerance of side effects.

Two small placebo-controlled trials found that clonidine, an adrenergic receptor agonist, had some effect in decreasing irritability and hyperactivity [Fankhauser et al., 1992; Jaselskis et al., 1992] in children and adults with autistic disorder.

There is little evidence for any beneficial effect on hyperactivity using the selective SRIs. Naltrexone, however, has improved hyperactivity [Campbell et al., 1993; Kolmen et al., 1995; Willemsen-Swinkels et al., 1995a, b, 1996, 1999] in small randomized, controlled trials. In clinical trials testing the efficacy for atypical antipsychotics for severe behavior disturbance, hyperactivity was decreased with risperidone [Hellings et al., 2006; McCracken et al., 2002; Research Units on Pediatric Psychopharmacology Autism Network, 2005b; Shea et al., 2004].

Antiepileptic Drugs

Several antiepileptic drugs have been used for behavioral manifestations of autism, particularly for treating intense rapid mood shifts. In open-label studies, levetiracetam [Rugino and Samsock, 2002] and divalproex sodium [Hollander et al., 2001] appeared to be well tolerated and to improve repetitive behavior, impulsivity, and mood stability. A retrospective study of topiramate in children and adolescents with ASDs suggested that the drug reduced misconduct, hyperactivity, and inattention in 8 of 15 patients. Two randomized, placebo-controlled trials, however, have had mixed results. Lamotrigine was not better than placebo on several parent-report and clinician ratings of disruptive behavior and autism symptoms in a double-blind, randomized, controlled trial of 28 children [Belsito et al., 2001]. Children in both groups showed improvement. In a small placebo-controlled, double-blind trial of levetiracetam in 8- to 17-year-olds (n = 20), there was no difference from placebo on measures of behavioral disturbance, repetitive behavior, and autism symptoms [Wasserman et al., 2006]. In a randomized, double-blind, controlled trial with 13 individuals (mean age = 9 years), divalproex sodium was better than placebo in decreasing repetitive behavior [Hollander et al., 2006a]. Patients with the most robust response had repetitive behaviors of the compulsive type, as opposed to stereotypies. This small trial hypothesized a specific target (repetitive behavior), as opposed to global improvement, and the participants demonstrated high levels of that behavior at baseline. The results need replication in a larger trial.

It has been hypothesized that the mechanism of benefit from these medications might be their effect on subclinical seizures, which have been reported to occur in this population. However, there is no evidence and no controlled trials investigating whether treatment with anticonvulsants in children with autism who have epileptiform discharges but no clinical seizures might improve behavioral outcomes in children with autism [Spence and Schneider, 2009].

Cholinesterase Inhibitors

Acetylcholine (ACh) plays a significant role in attention and memory performance. Acetylcholinesterase inhibitors (AChE) slow the breakdown of ACh. This is the presumed mechanism by which cholinesterase inhibitors, such as donepezil, slow decline in memory, attention, and learning in Alzheimer's disease. Animal studies have suggested that administration of these agents early in development may also enhance learning in a prospective way. Because postmortem studies have found abnormalities of the cholinergic system and its nicotinic receptors in the brains of individuals with autism [Lee et al., 2002; Perry et al., 2001], there is growing interest in the potential benefit of these drugs in ameliorating neurodevelopmental disorders [Yoo et al., 2007].

Preliminary data provides some support for pursuing larger trials. A retrospective examination of effects of donepezil in eight children with autism suggested improvements in irritability and hyperactivity, but memory and attention were not measured [Hardan and Handen, 2002]. A randomized, controlled 6-week trial was conducted with 43 children with ASDs, examining the effects of donepezil (2.5 mg/d) [Chez et al., 2003]. The investigators concluded that the drug improved language and reduced overall autistic features. However, the statistical analyses pooled blinded and nonblinded data, leaving the results susceptible to confounders such as placebo effects. A prospective, open-label study with 13 children and adolescents with autism treated for 12 weeks with galantamine found reductions in irritability and social withdrawal [Nicolson et al., 2006]. The efficacy of cholinesterase inhibitors is yet to be demonstrated in rigorously designed and replicated trials.

In summary, a number of medications, particularly atypical neuroleptics, psychostimulants, and SRIs, can help decrease specific symptoms associated with autism, such as behavioral outbursts, stereotypic or compulsive behaviors, aggression, anxiety, inattention, and oppositional behavior (Table 48-1; also see chapter 49). Reduction in these behaviors can improve quality of life and promote better opportunities for learning. However, there must be careful attention to matching the medication with the targeted behavior, and to possible developmental differences in treatment response. Side effects are common, and must be monitored closely and weighed carefully against the benefits of the drugs. Unfortunately, there is currently no pharmacologic treatment that has been demonstrated to address effectively the deficits in language, cognition, and social understanding that are core features of autism.

Complementary and Alternative Medicine

A significant number of families seek complementary or alternative medicine treatments, few of which have been studied in well-designed trials [Levy and Hyman, 2008]. One survey [Levy and Hyman, 2003] found that 32 percent of 284 children at a Pennsylvania regional autism center were using complementary and alternative medicine. The investigators suggested that it is important to respect the parents' belief if the complementary medicine is not toxic, but if the treatment is potentially harmful, negotiating a safer replacement practice should be attempted. Examples of the more commonly used treatments include nutritional supplements, melatonin, hormones, glutein- and caseine-free diet, immunoglobulins, secretin, and chelation therapy.

A review [Nye and Brice, 2005] of vitamin B_6 and magnesium concluded that the few studies available were inconclusive and samples sizes were too small for an adequate test of efficacy. A double-blind, placebo-controlled study of pyridoxine and magnesium in 10 patients found no benefit but no significant side effects [Findling et al., 1997].

Dimethylglycine, a nutritional supplement closely related to the inhibitory transmitter glycine, has been proposed [Rimland, 1990] as helpful for autistic children and adults, but it was ineffective in two double-blind, placebo-controlled trials [Bolman and Richmond, 1999; Kern et al., 2001].

Plasma fatty acid levels have been found to be decreased in children with autism when compared with typical controls [Sliwinski et al., 2006; Vancassel et al., 2001], leading to interest in supplementation with omega-3 fatty acids. One small, randomized, double-blind, placebo-controlled pilot study with 13 children reported a nonsignificant trend toward improvement in hyperactivity after 6 weeks of treatment [Amminger et al., 2007]. Mild gastrointestinal side effects were noted.

Melatonin therapy has been used to treat the sleep disturbances in ASD, based on low plasma levels or urinary excretion of melatonin [Kulman et al., 2000; Mulder et al., 2010]. Melke et al. [2008] reported mutations and polymorphisms in the acetylserotonin methyltransferase (*ASMT*) gene, which encodes the last enzyme of melatonin synthesis, which result in dramatic decreases in *ASMT* transcripts in blood cell lines. Anecdotal and open-label studies of melatonin therapy have suggested significant improvements in sleep architecture in children with ASD [Andersen et al., 2008; Giannotti et al., 2006; Levy and Hyman, 2008]. Three recent double-blind, placebo-controlled crossover studies were performed in a total of 70 children with ASD using regular (5 mg in Garstang and Wallis [2006]; 3 mg in Wirojanan et al. [2009]) or 5 mg controlled-release melatonin [Wasdell et al., 2008]. Up to 94 percent of children derived significant benefits in sleep without evidence of significant side effects. Larger long-term, double-blind, placebo-controlled crossover studies will be needed to document the efficacy of melatonin across the behavioral subtypes of ASD.

Another popular treatment for ASDs is a gluten-free, casein-free diet. A small randomized, double-blind crossover study was conducted with 15 children with autism on a 12-week GFCF diet [Elder, 2008]. There were no statistically significant differences in autistic symptomatology or urinary peptide levels when participants were on the GFCF diet. The study did, however, demonstrate the feasibility of such a study and the need for an adequately powered trial.

Immunoglobulin has been administered intravenously in open trials [DelGiudice-Asch et al., 1999; Plioplys, 1998] and not found to be useful. A double-blind, placebo-controlled trial of oral human immunoglobulin was conducted with 125 children and adolescents who had autism and persistent

Table 48-1 Clinical Trials for Pharmacologic Treatment in ASD*

Drug	Dose	Age[†]	Efficacy	Side Effects	Reference
NEUROLEPTIC AGENTS					
Risperidone	0.25–2.5 mg/d <20 kg 0.5–2.5 mg/d 20–45 kg 0.5–3.5 mg/d >45 kg Mean = 2.4 mg/d	5–17	Decreased tantrums, aggression, self-injury, hyperactivity	Weight gain; increased appetite; transient sedation	McCracken et al., 2002
Risperidone	1.2–2.9 mg/d child Mean = 2.0 mg/d 2.4–5.3 mg/d adult Mean = 3.6 mg/d	8–56	Decreased irritability, hyperactivity	Increased appetite; weight gain; sedation	Hellings et al., 2006
Risperidone	0.01–0.06 mg/kg/d Mean = 1.17 mg/d	5–12	Decreased irritability, hyperactivity, noncompliance, conduct problems	Weight gain; transient somnolence; mildly increased heart rate and blood pressure	Shea et al., 2004
Risperidone	0.5–1.5 mg/d Mean = 1.14 mg/d	2.5–6	Minimal improvement in global autism severity scores	Weight gain; increased prolactin levels	Luby et al., 2006
Risperidone	1.0–10.0 mg/d	18–43	Reduced repetitive behavior, aggression, self-injury, property destruction	Transient sedation	McDougle et al., 1998
Aripiprazole	5 mg/d, 10 mg/d, or 15 mg/d	6–17	Reduced irritability, hyperactivity, stereotypy at all doses	Sedation, EPS, weight gain	Marcus et al., 2009
Aripiprazole	2–15 mg/d	6–10	Reduced irritability, hyperactivity, stereotypy, inappropriate speech; global improvement	Decreased prolactin level, weight gain, EPS	Owen et al., 2009
OPIATE ANTAGONISTS					
Naltrexone	1.0 mg/kg/d	3–8	No improvement over placebo in behavior and learning	None greater than placebo	Kolmen et al., 1997
Naltrexone	1.0 mg/kg/d	3–8	No improvement in communication skills	Not reported	Feldman et al., 1999
Naltrexone	40 mg/d	3–7	Decreased hyperactivity, improved attention	Not reported	Willemsen-Swinkels et al., 1995b
Naltrexone	20 mg/d	3–7	Decreased hyperactivity and improved attention by teacher, but not parent, report	No side effects	Willemsen-Swinkels et al., 1996
SEROTONIN REUPTAKE INHIBITORS					
Fluvoxamine	Mean dose= 276.7 mg/d	18–53	Reduced repetitive thoughts and behavior, and aggression; improved social communication	Transient nausea and sedation	McDougle et al., 1996
Fluoxetine	4.8-20 mg/d Mean=10.6 mg/d; 0.38 mg/kg/d	5–17	Modest reduction in repetitive behaviors, but no improvement in global functioning	Agitation requiring dose reduction	Hollander et al., 2005
Citalopram	2.5-20 mg/d Mean=16.5 mg/d	5–17	No improvement in repetitive behavior or global functioning	Increased energy, inattention, impulsivity, hyperactivity, stereotypy, diarrhea, insomnia, dry skin	King et al., 2009
Fluoxetine	Not reported	5–17	No improvement in repetitive behavior	Not reported	Neuropharm, unpublished
STIMULANTS					
Methylphenidate	0.125, 0.250, or 0.500 mg/kg t.i.d.	5–14	Reduced inattention, distractibility, hyperactivity, and impulsivity	Irritability, decreased appetite, difficulty falling asleep, emotional outbursts	RUPP, 2005a, b

Table 48-1 Clinical Trials for Pharmacologic Treatment in ASD—cont'd

Drug	Dose	Age[†]	Efficacy	Side Effects	Reference
Atomoxetine	20–100 mg/d Mean = 44.2 mg/d	5–15	Reduced hyperactivity, impulsivity, social withdrawal	Transient nausea and fatigue	Arnold et al., 2006
ANTIEPILEPTIC DRUGS					
Lamotrigine	Mean = 5.0 mg/kg/d	3–11	No improvement greater than placebo in disruptive behavior and autism symptoms	None greater than placebo	Belsito et al., 2001
Levetiracetam	20–30 mg/kg/d Mean = 862.5 mg/d	5–17	No improvement over placebo in disruptive behavior	None greater than placebo	Wasserman et al., 2006
Divalproex sodium	500–1500 mg/d Mean = 822.92 mg/d	5–40	Reduction in compulsive-type repetitive behavior	None greater than placebo	Hollander et al., 2006a, b

* Includes only double-blind, randomized, placebo-controlled trials.
† Age in years.
EPS, Extrapyramidal symptoms.

gastrointestinal symptoms [Handen et al., 2009]. There was no significant benefit on gastrointestinal symptoms, measures of autistic symptomatology, or behavior disturbances.

Reported dramatic improvement after the administration of secretin as part of endoscopy in three autistic children [Horvath et al., 1998] led to widespread use by parents. Subsequent blinded, randomized trials did not substantiate its efficacy [Carey et al., 2002; Chez et al., 2000; Coniglio et al., 2001; Corbett et al., 2001; Dunn-Geier et al., 2000; Esch and Carr, 2004; Kaminska et al., 2002; Kern et al., 2002, 2004; Levy et al., 2003; Lightdale et al., 2001a; Molloy et al., 2002; Owley et al., 1999; Ratliff-Schaub et al., 2005; Sponheim et al., 2002; Sturmey, 2005; Unis et al., 2002; Williams et al., 2005]. These trials included single- and repeated-dose protocols.

Proponents of chelation therapy suggest that mercury and other heavy metals may be poorly eliminated by children with autism and that it interferes with neurodevelopment via modulation of immune function and other biochemical systems. Despite the lack of scientific evidence of a link between exposure to mercury or other heavy metals and autism, chelation is widely used. One trial [Adams et al., 2009a, b] administered dimercaptosuccinic acid (DMSA) to 69 children with ASD. Those who had a high urinary excretion of toxic metals (n = 49) were then randomized to either DMSA or placebo for an additional six administrations. Some participants in both groups demonstrated improvement of measures of autism symptoms and disruptive behavior, but there were no significant differences between the two groups, and no comparative group that did not receive any treatment. There were no serious adverse effects reported, although a significant increase in excretion of potassium and chromium was noted. No placebo-controlled studies have examined the safety or efficacy of chelation for treating autism, and deaths resulting from hypocalcemia have been reported from the inappropriate use of a chelator, edetate disodium (EDTA) [Brown et al., 2006], including one boy with autism.

It is challenging to perform clinical trials enrolling children with autism, but without well-designed, blinded studies, safe and effective therapies cannot be determined. Problems include standardization of diagnoses, heterogeneity of target problem behaviors, and lack of cooperation of subjects. Many outcome measures are available, including global measures (Clinical Global Impression of Severity) and others targeted to specific symptoms. Whenever feasible, parents should be encouraged to participate in clinical trials to make progress in validating new pharmacologic and behavioral therapies. Information about on-going trials and their locations can be found at www.clinicaltrials.gov.

Educational and Behavioral Interventions

The core deficits associated with autism affect all aspects of the individual's life, necessitating a comprehensive approach to intervention [Lord and Bailey, 2002; Wetherby et al., 1997]. A primary source of intervention for most children with ASDs is through the educational system. The Individual with Disabilities Education Act (IDEA) ensures a "free and appropriate" public education to "children" between the ages of 3 and 21 who have been diagnosed with learning disabilities. This act specifically covers autistic disorder, but whether the full range of ASDs is covered depends on the particular state's definition of disabilities. The quality and extent of services that are provided vary from one community to another, even within a particular school district.

Numerous comprehensive early intervention programs for young children with ASDs have been developed and described [Dawson and Osterling, 1997; National Research Council, 2001; Rogers and Vismara, 2008; Seida et al., 2009]. The National Research Council [2001] provides descriptions of ten model programs considered representative of well-described, comprehensive treatment programs with at least some empiric support. Given the great heterogeneity in the population with ASDs, intervention programs must be tailored to the needs of the individual.

The National Research Council [2001] report describes the common elements of successful early intervention programs and makes several recommendations:

- Intervention should begin as soon as an ASD diagnosis *is suspected.*
- Intervention should include active engagement in instructional programming for at least 25 hours per week, with full-year programming.

- Intervention should include repeated, planned teaching opportunities that are one-to-one designs or delivered in a very small group, with individualized goals.
- Intervention should include family support and parent training.
- Intervention programs should have low student to teacher ratios, such as 2:1.
- Program evaluation and assessment of the child's progress should be on-going.
- Priority of intervention should focus on six specific areas:
  1. Functional spontaneous communication
  2. Social instruction delivered throughout the day in various settings
  3. Play skills
  4. Cognitive development
  5. Proactive approaches to problem behaviors
  6. Functional academics.

Methods based on applied behavior analysis for teaching skills and facilitating more appropriate and adaptive behaviors have been extensively tested for their effectiveness in children and adults with autism and other developmental disabilities [Dunlap and Fox, 1999; Lovaas, 1987; McEachin et al., 1993; Sheinkopf and Siegel, 1998; Smith et al., 2000]. In the most rigorously designed studies of intensive early intervention programs based on applied behavior analysis (ABA), effectiveness is demonstrated at the group level, but response is variable. At the group level, baseline IQ and language skills predict better response to treatment. However, prediction at the individual level is not yet established [Rogers and Vismara, 2008].

ABA and comprehensive programs based on applied behavioral analysis are established on principles of behavior modification. By carefully analyzing the causes and consequences of a particular behavior, identifying an opposite, competing behavior (i.e., desired behavior), and consistently altering the consequences so that the desired behavior is rewarded, the instructor can teach new skills or transform inappropriate behaviors into more acceptable ones. This relatively simple principle has been developed into techniques that have been highly effective for teaching new skills, increasing the frequency of appropriate or adaptive behaviors, and decreasing the frequency of inappropriate or maladaptive behaviors.

Behavioral techniques can be used to work on very specific social behaviors, such as making appropriate greetings and appropriate modes of expressing affection, sharing, and playing interactively. Behaviors that have the potential to generalize to other settings should be taught. For instance, teaching a child to make eye contact with a speech therapist is of limited use unless the child also makes eye contact when conversing with parents, peers, and others. One way to increase generalization is to help parents reinforce and apply the behavioral techniques at home and in the community. For this reason, good behavioral programs always contain a parent-training component. When parents are taught how to apply behavioral techniques, with on-going coaching, they can be effective in smoothing out interactions between the individual with an ASD and other family members.

Parents are most likely to learn ABA techniques when enrolling their children in a comprehensive treatment program. An alternative to enrollment in a comprehensive school-based program is home-based ABA. In this type of program, parents hire an expert to train the parent and paraprofessionals, who administer the treatment in shifts. As these comprehensive treatment programs have evolved, there have been trends toward teaching parents to implement the programs, toward using the behavior-management techniques in settings that are more naturalistic and during typical activities, and toward developing goals based on the child's unique developmental profile [Ingersoll et al., 2001]. There is also a trend, at least when applied to programs for children and adults with developmental disabilities, away from emphasizing the consequences of a behavior and toward an emphasis on understanding the triggers of a behavior, proactively providing cues or rehearsal of the appropriate behavior, making changes in the environment to avoid or minimize those triggers, and teaching more adaptive or appropriate responses when the triggers cannot be avoided.

Some comprehensive treatment programs derive strategies from a developmental theoretical framework. For instance, the Denver Model [Rogers et al., 2000] emphasizes the need to establish interpersonal relationships as a foundation to achieving other developmental milestones. Although most of these programs have not been extensively evaluated using rigorous scientific trials, there are theoretical reasons and some preliminary scientific evidence that they can be useful for many children with ASDs [National Research Council, 2001; Rogers, 1998]. An adaptation of the Denver Model for toddlers (18–30 months old), called the Early Start Denver Model (ESDM), was compared to usual community care in a randomized, controlled trial [Dawson et al., 2010]. The ESDM intervention is a parent-delivered treatment applied in the home for 20 hours per week. Intervention began at a mean of 23 months of age. Techniques taught to parents incorporate the developmental techniques from the Denver Model and applied behavior analysis. In this study, children in the ESDM model showed significantly greater improvements in IQ, language, and adaptive skills than the community-treated children with ASD. The gains were greater after 2 years than after 1 year, suggesting benefits from on-going intervention.

Many well-established programs combine elements of behavioral and developmental orientations [Marcus et al., 2000; McGee et al., 2000]. Some have specifically evaluated the effectiveness of the parent-training components of their programs. Parent-training models that are promising based on evidence provided by their developers include the Learning Experiences Alternative Program for Preschoolers and Their Parents [Strain and Cordisco, 2000], the Denver Model [Rogers et al., 2000], the Individualized Support Program at the University of South Florida [Dunlap and Fox, 1999], the Pivotal Response Training Model [Koegel et al., 1999], and the Douglas Developmental Center Program [Harris et al., 2000]. Whatever the theoretical underpinning, well-established and effective programs always include an emphasis on parent–child relationships and overall family support [Dawson and Osterling, 1997]. There is evidence that parents can learn to use these methods and that doing so helps them feel better in general, and more satisfied and confident in their parenting role [Koegel et al., 1996; Ozonoff and Cathcart, 1998; Schreibman, 1997, 2005; Sofronoff and Farbotko, 2002]. One study [Aman et al., 2009] demonstrated that adding a parent training program to medication management for severe behavior disturbances in ASD was more beneficial than medication intervention alone, and allowed for maintenance on a lower dose of the medication.

There is much less evidence when considering intervention programs or treatment options for older children, adolescents, and adults with ASDs. Core deficits in social understanding and social relationships are concerns throughout the life span, and social skills training (SST) is often a component of a treatment plan. Group-based SST programs show promise, but have not been rigorously evaluated [Williams White et al., 2007]. The inclusion of nonautistic peers to assist with SST may be important, but again, rigorous studies are needed [Chan et al., 2009]. A small randomized, controlled trial tested the efficacy of the Program for the Education and Enrichment of Relational Skills (PEERS) for adolescents with ASD [Laugeson et al., 2009]. This group-based intervention integrates parents into the program to help with generalization of skills into the home and community. Results of this study demonstrated benefits in social skills and increased frequency of peer socialization.

The PEERS program described above was originally developed for children with ADHD, and adapted for use with teens with ASD. Similarly, cognitive behavior therapy (CBT) for children with anxiety disorder has been adapted to treat anxiety in high-functioning ASD. A randomized, controlled trial of CBT for anxiety in 7–11-year-old children with ASD demonstrated benefit in reducing anxiety symptoms [Wood et al., 2009]. These studies suggest that adapting evidence-based interventions for specific symptom domains and comorbid symptoms in ASD is a reasonable strategy, but there remains a great need for rigorously designed research to demonstrate efficacy.

Although the needs of individuals with ASDs change over time, there is need for lifelong support. In particular, transitions (e.g., to high school, to higher education or vocational training, or to independent or assisted living) are critical periods during which supports already in place may be lost because of changes in eligibility or funding sources.

Resources for Families

An enormous amount of information is available to families on the Internet; they often need specific counseling regarding evaluation of treatments that are espoused without adequate scientific study. The American Academy of Pediatrics has a useful website (http://www.aap.org/healthtopics/autism.cfm). The National Institutes of Health website (www.nih.gov) can be searched for current research, as can those of specific institutes, including the National Institute of Neurological Disorders and Stroke (www.ninds.nih.gov), National Institute of Child Health and Human Development (www.nichd.nih.gov), and the National Institute of Mental Health (www.nimh.nih.gov). The CDC's National Center for Birth Defects and Developmental Disabilities has a website (http://www.cdc.gov/ncbddd/autism/index.html) devoted to providing evidence-based information on ASD and its treatment, including links to resources. The National Dissemination Center for Children with Disabilities (www.nichcy.org) has information on special education laws and on educational practices.

Another effort, the First Signs program, is developing methods to inform physicians about the importance of early identification of autism, and it provides resources, including screening tools and referral guidelines. The First Signs website (http://www.firstsigns.org) includes recommendations and information about obtaining autism screening instruments. Educational tools for families can be found on the Exploring Autism website (http://www.exploringautism.com). An organization for autism research has a useful parent's guide to understanding research on autism (www.researchautism.org). For practitioners, the AAN/CNS practice parameter for evaluation of children with autism and the detailed background paper can be found on the For OC Kids website: (http://www.childneurologysociety.org/resources/practiceparameters).

Disclaimer

The views expressed in this chapter are those of the authors and do not necessarily reflect the official position of the National Institute of Mental Health, the National Institute of Neurological Diseases and Stroke, the National Institutes of Health, or any other part of the U.S. Department of Health and Human Services.

The complete list of references for this chapter is available online at **www.expertconsult.com**.
See inside cover for registration details.

Neuropsychopharmacology

Rebecca Rendleman and John T. Walkup

Introduction

Historically, very few safe and effective medications were available to treat pediatric neuropsychiatric disorders. Children received either no treatment, or treatment that emphasized psychological or behavioral interventions. With a growing evidence base of tolerable and effective psychotropic medications, psychopharmacology has become standard practice for many neuropsychiatric disorders, resulting in increased use of medications in children [Zito, 2007; Zito et al., 2003] and broadening of the practitioner base for prescribing [Olfson et al., 2002].

The database for the safety and efficacy of psychotropic medications in children has increased dramatically in the past decade, although much remains to be done. There is support for the short-term efficacy of many commonly prescribed psychotropics, but there is limited data on their long-term efficacy and safety, the comparative efficacy of psychological and pharmacologic treatments, and the best practices for combining psychological and pharmacologic interventions. For example, there are excellent efficacy and safety data for the short-term treatment of attention-deficit hyperactivity disorder (ADHD) with stimulants [Greenhill et al., 2006; Jensen et al., 2001], of anxiety disorders with selective serotonin reuptake inhibitors [Birmaher et al., 2003; RUPP, 2001; Rynn et al., 2001; Walkup et al., 2008], of obsessive-compulsive disorder (OCD) with clomipramine and selective serotonin reuptake inhibitors [DeVeaugh-Geiss et al., 1992; Geller et al., 2001, 2004; March et al., 1998; POTS, 2004; Riddle et al., 2001], of depression with selective serotonin reuptake inhibitors [Emslie et al., 1997, 2002, 2009; TADS, 2004], and of schizophrenia [Findling et al., 2008b; Haas et al., 2009b; Kryzhanovskaya et al., 2009; Kumra et al., 1996, 2008], bipolar disorder [Delbello et al., 2002, 2006, 2008; Findling et al., 2005, 2009a; Haas et al., 2009a; Tohen et al., 2007], and irritability and behavioral dysregulation in different pediatric disorders with atypical antipsychotics [Aman et al., 2002; Hollander et al., 2006; McCracken et al., 2002; Owen et al., 2009]. In contrast, there remain very little data from placebo-controlled efficacy studies on the short-term benefit of mood stabilizers (e.g., lithium, anticonvulsants) for neuropsychiatric disorders [Wagner et al., 2006, 2009]. There is little information on the long-term usefulness of any psychotropic medication and also increasing concern about the long-term effects of psychotropic drugs on growth and development [MTA, 2004; Nilsson et al., 2004; Swanson et al., 2006; Weintrob et al., 2002]. Although medication combinations are commonly used in children [Martin et al., 2003], studies of medication combinations are uncommon [Abikoff et al., 2005; Delbello et al., 2002].

The expansion of the evidence base in pediatric neuropharmacology has been due, in large part, to the National Institute of Mental Health (NIMH)'s support of partnership between government, academic institutions, and drug companies [Satcher, 2001], and to legislation supporting medications studies in children. In 1997, the passage of the Food and Drug Administration (FDA) Modernization Act mandated the study of medication in children and offered 6-month patent extensions to pharmaceutical companies who studied their products in pediatric populations. As a result, a number of efficacy and safety studies of newer medications targeting a variety of disorders in children and adolescents emerged and contributed to a growing evidence base of medications that have FDA pediatric labeling. The list of psychotropic medications that have FDA approval for use in the treatment of psychiatric conditions in children has grown (Table 49-1). However, a number of studies supporting the safety and efficacy of psychotropic medication (e.g., stimulants for ADHD in children with tics [TSSG, 2002]; selective serotonin reuptake inhibitors for childhood anxiety [Ipser et al., 2009]) are not reflected in current labeling, leaving clinicians in an awkward position as to whether to prescribe medications with evidence for efficacy but without an FDA indication or appropriate labeling. Additionally, older medications that have gone off patent have no labeling, have FDA labeling but have not been subject to the rigorous study, or have out-of-date labeling. As a result, many psychotropic medications prescribed for children are prescribed off-label. Off-label use of medications increased in the past two decades for a variety of indications, including stimulants for children younger than 5 years, selective serotonin reuptake inhibitors for OCD and anxiety, and atypical antipsychotics for aggression. Increased off-label use resulted from downward extension of a current indication to a younger age group (e.g., stimulants in children younger than 5 years, antidepressants in teens and children) and the availability of newer medications with a reduced potential for serious side effects. Sometimes, off-label use has been extremely helpful (e.g., selective serotonin reuptake inhibitors for anxiety disorders), but some off-label prescribing may not be helpful. For example, based on its low side-effect profile, a few positive case reports and open trials, and an aggressive marketing campaign, gabapentin was prescribed for the treatment of bipolar affective disorder; however, subsequent controlled trials have not supported its efficacy [Frye et al., 2000; Pande et al., 2000].

There has also been an increased interest in the perceived safety of commonly prescribed psychotropic agents in children. Although short-term efficacy studies have often demonstrated safety, post-marketing studies have raised some concerns: for example, data suggesting growth suppression with stimulants [MTA, 2004; Swanson et al., 2006] and antidepressants [Nilsson et al., 2004; Weintrob et al., 2002]; increased risk of

Table 49-1 Labeled and Off-label Use of Neuropsychopharmacologic Agents in Children and Adolescents

Drug	Labeled Use in Children and Adolescents	Off-label Use/Clinical Practice in Children and Adolescents
Stimulants		
Amphetamine, mixed salts	ADHD ($\geq$3 yrs - IR, $\geq$6 yr - ER, Narcolepsy ($\geq$6 yrs, IR only)	
Dextroamphetamine	ADHD ($\geq$6 yrs), Narcolepsy ($\geq$6 yrs)	
Methylphenidate	ADHD ($\geq$6 yrs), Narcolepsy ($\geq$6 yrs)	
Pemoline	None (withdrawn 2005)	ADHD
Atomoxetine	ADHD ($\geq$6 yrs)	
Clonidine	ADHD (6–17 yrs - ER)	Aggression, Tic disorders
Guanfacine	ADHD (6–17 yrs - ER)	Aggression, Tic disorders
Benzodiazepines		As a group - agitation, catatonia
Clonazepam	None	
Lorazepam	Anxiety ($\geq$12 yrs), Insomnia ($\geq$12 yrs)	
Tricyclic Antidepressants		As a group – depression, anxiety disorders, ADHD and pain syndromes
Amitriptyline	Depression ($\geq$12 yrs)	
Clomipramine	OCD (>10 yrs)	
Desipramine	None	
Imipramine	Enuresis	
Nortriptyline	Depression	
Buproprion	None	Depression, ADHD
Serotonin Norepinephrine Re-uptake Inhibitors		
Desvenlavaxine	None	Depression, anxiety disorders
Duloxetine	None	Depression, Chronic pain
Venlafaxine	None	Depression, Anxiety disorders, ADHD
Mirtazapine	None	Depression, Anxiety disorders
Serotonin Re-uptake Inhibitors		As a group - depression, anxiety disorders
Citalopram	None	
Escitalopram	Depression ($\geq$12 yrs)	
Fluoxetine	OCD ($\geq$7 yrs), Depression ($\geq$8 yrs)	
Fluvoxamine	OCD ($\geq$8 yrs)	
Paroxetine	None	
Sertraline	OCD ($\geq$6 yrs)	
Lithium	Bipolar Disorder ($\geq$12 yrs)	Aggression
Anticonvulsants		As a group - bipolar disorder, aggression, mood instability
Carbamazepine	Seizure disorders	
Gabapentin	Seizure disorders	
Lamotrigine	Seizure disorders	
Topiramate	Seizure disorders	
Valproate	Seizure disorders	
Typical Neuroleptics		As a group – psychotic disorders
Chlorpromazine	Severe behavioral disturbances	
Haloperidol	Psychosis, tics, severe behavioral disturbance	
Piimozide	Tics	
Atypical Neuroleptics		As a group – psychotic disorders, Tourette's syndrome, aggression
Aripiprazole	Irritability in Autistic Disorder (6-17 yrs) Bipolar I Disorder ($\geq$10 yrs), Schizophrenia ($\geq$13 yrs)	
Clozapine	None	
Olanzapine	Bipolar I Disorder ($\geq$13 yrs), Schizophrenia ($\geq$13 yrs)	
Quetiapine	Bipolar I Disorder ($\geq$10 yrs), Schizophrenia ($\geq$13 yrs)	
Risperidone	Irritability in Autistic Disorder (6-17 yrs), Bipolar I Disorder ($\geq$10 yrs), Schizophrenia ($\geq$13 yrs)	
Ziprasidone	None	

IR = immediate release, ER = extended release
ADHD, Attention Deficit Hyperactivity Disorder, OCD, Obsessive –Compulsive Disorder

suicidal ideation in youth [Hammad et al., 2006] and young adults [Stone et al., 2009] with antidepressants; and weight gain and metabolic syndrome with antipsychotics [Fraguas et al., 2010; Correll, 2008]. These adverse events and public concern about the use of medications, particularly in children, have reinforced the importance of on-going research to elucidate the efficacy and safety of psychotropic medications.

The decision about whether to use pharmacologic interventions mandates careful consideration of the benefits and the risks of treatment and of the ability to monitor treatment safely [AACAP, 2009]. To justify the use of medications, the child must first have a disorder or target symptoms with the potential for pharmacologic responsiveness. Second, the child's level of impairment must cross a threshold of severity such that failure to treat with medication, given all the potential risks, would cause more harm. Third, the child's symptoms must be unresponsive or insufficiently responsive to nonpharmacologic interventions, or these interventions are not readily available in the community. Finally, the clinician must have the time available to monitor patients adequately – not only for common, and also for rare and important adverse events (e.g., suicidal ideation or behavior). Safe prescribing of medications for children also requires detailed documentation of the decision-making process and an active monitoring plan for outcome and adverse events.

The likelihood of a child with a neuropsychiatric disorder or symptoms presenting to a pediatric neurology practice is high. To treat these children effectively, the pediatric neurologist must have the ability to collect and integrate information from multiple sources (i.e., child, family, school, and other agencies) and to make a diagnostic formulation and treatment plan that addresses the neuropsychiatric symptoms and psychosocial factors that affect the delivery of care and the assessment of outcome. Given the rapidly changing nature and increasing complexity of modern clinical care, pediatric neurologists need to define their comfort level in assessing and treating neuropsychiatric disorders and to determine how this may influence the scope of their practice. For neurologists who treat neuropsychiatric disorders, it is critical to keep abreast of this evolving field, especially new safety data and data on the efficacy of nonpharmacological treatment, e.g., behavioral treatment for tics [Piacentini et al., 2010], that influence the standard of care. This may require a team of colleagues, including psychologists and psychiatrists, who can be involved in the assessment and treatment of these children with complex neuropsychiatric needs.

This chapter provides an overview of the major classes of medications used in pediatric neuropsychopharmacology, including stimulant medications, antidepressants, mood stabilizers, anxiolytics, α_2-agonists, and antipsychotics. In-depth discussions regarding comprehensive psychiatric assessments and multimodal treatments can be found in the basic textbooks in child psychiatry. The American Academy of Child and Adolescent Psychiatry (AACAP) and the American Psychiatric Association (APA) have developed and published practice guidelines that summarize current thinking about the assessment and treatment of pediatric neuropsychiatric disorders.

Stimulants

This section briefly describes the use of stimulants and non-stimulants in the treatment of ADHD (Table 49-2; also see Chapter 47).

Clinical Applications

Stimulants have been in clinical use since 1937, when it was observed that a group of children in residential treatment showed marked improvement in their behavior with benzedrine (D- and L-amphetamine) [Bradley, 1937]. Since then, the criteria for ADHD have been refined, and other stimulant medications have been evaluated and consistently found efficacious in numerous placebo-controlled studies [Jensen et al., 2001]. Approximately 70–80 percent of school-age patients with ADHD have a positive response to stimulant medication. Although behavioral treatment may be considered, in head-to-head studies medication alone is more beneficial than behavioral therapy alone in children 5 years of age and older. The combination of medication and behavioral therapy is specifically helpful for oppositional behavior and children with ADHD and anxiety [Jensen et al., 2001].

Based on clear evidence of efficacy, the stimulant medications have been used to address attention, hyperactivity, and impulsivity in those with pervasive developmental disorders and in younger children. For many years, stimulant medications were viewed as poorly effective or contraindicated for hyperactivity in children with autism and pervasive developmental disorders. However, in the first large, randomized, controlled trial in this population, methylphenidate demonstrated efficacy. The response rate was less robust than in typically developing children, and rates of adverse events were higher, with nearly 1 in 5 youngsters having to stop treatment [RUPP, 2005]. A single test dose of stimulant may be useful to identify children for whom a longer stimulant trial is contraindicated [Di Martino et al., 2004]. Children who experience a significant worsening of ADHD (e.g., hyperactivity and irritability) or other symptoms (i.e., tics or stereotypies) with a single dose may be excluded from further stimulant treatment [Di Martino et al., 2004].

Preschoolers with ADHD represent another specialized population for whom the use of stimulants may be considered. The Preschoolers with ADHD Treatment Study (PATS), a large randomized, placebo-controlled trial of methylphenidate in children of ages 3–5 years, demonstrated that methylphenidate at doses greater than 2.5 mg three times a day were effective in reducing ADHD in youngsters unresponsive to psychosocial intervention. Again, response rates were less robust than that observed in school-age children, and adverse effects were more common [Greenhill et al., 2006]. Furthermore, methylphenidate may reduce growth rates, even in short-term treatment, and requires careful monitoring of weight and height [Swanson et al., 2006].

Despite substantial data supporting the efficacy of stimulants, their use in children remains controversial. The lay public and media have expressed concerns about the potential for overdiagnosis of ADHD and overuse of stimulant medications in children. However, despite the dramatic increases in stimulant use in the past 10 years [Zito et al., 2003], there is little evidence to support this claim. According to the U.S. Surgeon General, most children with psychiatric disorders are not assessed or treated [Satcher, 2001], and the ratio of stimulant use to prevalence of ADHD is less than 1:1, suggesting that undertreatment is a more prevalent and important issue [Jensen et al., 1999]. Stimulant medications have also come under public scrutiny because of concerns about safety. Concerns about worsening tics, growth suppression, enhancing risk for addiction and, more recently,

Table 49-2 Stimulant and Nonstimulant Medications for Attention-Deficit-Hyperactivity Disorder: Preparations, Pharmacology, and Dosing

Drug	Preparation	Pharmacology	Dosing
Methylphenidate, immediate release	Ritalin (5-, 10-, and 20-mg tablets) Methylin (5-, 10-, and 20-mg tablets; 2.5-, 5-, and 10 mg chewable tablets; 5 mg/5ml or 10 mg/5ml oral solution	Time to peak plasma conc = 1-2 hr Half-life = 2.3 hr	Age ≥6 yr: 5 mg qam or twice a day; increase dose by 5 to 10 mg weekly; maximum daily dose 60 mg Optimum dose between 0.3 and 0.7 mg/kg/dose, given twice a day or three times a day (total dose = 0.6 to 2.1 mg/kg/daily)
Methylphenidate, sustained release	Ritalin SR (20-mg tablets)	Time to peak plasma conc = 4-5 hrs Duration of action = 8 hr	Once daily dosing of Ritalin SR corresponds to the titrated 8 hour dose of immediate-release methylphenidate (eg Ritalin SR 20 mg daily = Ritalin 10 mg po twice a day)
Methylphenidate, extended release	Methylin ER (10-, 20-mg tablets)	Time to peak plasma conc = 4.7 hrs Duration of action = 8 hrs	Once daily dosing of Methylin ER corresponds to titrated 8 hour dose of immediate-release methylphenidate
	Metadate ER (10- and 20-mg tablets)	Time to peak plasma conc = 4.5 hrs Duration of action = 8 hrs	Once daily dosing of Metadate ER corresponds to titrated 8 hour dose of immediate-release methylphenidate
	Metadate CD (10-, 20-, 30-, 40-, 50- and 60-mg capsules)	Bimodal release of methylphenidate Time to peak plasma conc 1st peak = 1.5 hr Time to peak plasma conc 2nd peak = 4.5 hr	Once-daily dosing of Metadate CD corresponds to titrated 8 hour dose of immediate release methylphenidate; may be opened and sprinkled on food
	Ritalin LA (10-, 20-, 30-, and 40-mg capsules)	Bimodal release of methylphenidate Time to peak plasma conc 1st peak = 1-3 hrs Time to peak plasma conc 2nd peak = 5-7 hrs	Once-daily dosing of Ritalin LA corresponds to titrated 8 hour dose of immediate release methylphenidate; may be opened and sprinkled on food
	Concerta (18-, 27-, 36-, 45- and 54-mg trilayer core tablets)	Bimodal release of methylphenidate Time to peak plasma conc 1st peak = 1-2 hr Time to peak plasma conc 2nd peak = 6-8 hr	Initiate 18 mg daily, increase gradually until clinical response achieved or maximum daily dose of 54 mg in children and 72 mg in adolescents.
Dexmethylphenidate, immediate release (d-enantiomer of methylphenidate)	Focalin (2.5-, 5- and 10-mg tablets)	Time to peak plasma conc = 1–1.5 hr Half life = 2.2 hr	Initial dose of 2.5 mg once- or twice-daily, increase gradually until clinical response achieved or maximum dose of 10 mg twice a day.
Dexmethylphenidate, Extended release	Focalin XR (5-, 10-, 15-, and 20-mg capsules)	Bimodal release of methylphenidate Time to peak plasma conc 1st peak = 1.5 hr Time to peak plasma conc 2nd peak = 6.5 hr	Initial dose of 5 mg once daily, increase gradually until clinical response achieved or maximum daily dose of 30 mg, may be opened and sprinkled on food.
Dextroamphetamine, immediate release	Dexedrine (5-mg tablets)	Time to peak plasma conc = 2-3 hr Half life = 10 hours	Ages 3-5 yr: 2.5 mg/day; increased 2.5 mg once or twice weekly Age ≥6 yr: initial dose of 5 mg/day; increase by 5 mg once or twice weekly; maximum of 40 mg/day Optimum dose: 0.15 to 0.5 mg/kg/dose given twice a day or three times a day (total dose = 0.3 to 1.5 mg/kg/day)
Dextroamphetamine, sustained release	Dexedrine Spansules (5-, 10-, and 15-mg spansules)	Time to peak plasma conc = ~8 hr Half life = 12 hr	Once daily dosing, dosing strategy same as immediate release form
Lisdexamfetamine (prodrug of dextroamphetamine)	Vyvanse (20-, 30-, 40-, 50-, 60- and 70-mg tablets)	Time to peak plasma conc of active metabolite = 3.5 hr	Ages ≥6 yr: initial dose of 30 mg daily; increase by 10 or 20 mg weekly; maximum dose of 70 mg/day.
Amphetamine, mixed salts	Adderall (5-, 7.5-, 10-, 12.5-, 15-, 20-, and 30-mg tablets)	Time to peak plasma conc = 3 hr Half life = 7-8 hr	Once or twice daily dosing Age 3-5 yr: 2.5 mg/day; increase by 2.5 mg once or twice weekly Age ≥6 yr: initial dose of 5 mg/day; increase by 5 mg once or twice weekly; maximum of 40 mg/day Optimum Dose: 0.15 to 0.5 mg/kg/dose given twice a day or three times a day (total dose = 0.3 to 1.5 mg/kg/day)
Amphetamine, mixed salts, extended release	Adderall XR (5-, 10-, 15-, 20-, 25-, and 30-mg tablets)	Time to peak plasma conc = 7 hr	Once daily dosing Age ≥6: initial dose 5-10 mg daily, increase by

Continued

Table 49-2 Stimulant and Nonstimulant Medications for Attention-Deficit-Hyperactivity Disorder: Preparations, Pharmacology, and Dosing—cont'd

Drug	Preparation	Pharmacology	Dosing
			5-10 mg once or twice weekly for a maximum daily dose of 30 mg/day; may be opened and sprinkled on food
Pemoline	Cylert (18.75-, 37.5-, and 75-mg tablets – not available in the US)	Time to peak plasma conc = 2-4 hr Half Life = 12 hr	Age ≥6: initial dose of 37.5 mg/day; increase by 18.75 mg/week until clinical response or maximum dose of 112.5 mg/day.
Atomoxetine	Strattera (10-, 18-, 25-, 40-, and 60-mg tablets)	Time to peak plasma conc Half life = 5.2 hr	Children and adolescents <70 kg: initial dose of 0.5 mg/kg/day using once or twice daily dosing; increase weekly as tolerated to a target dose of 1.2 mg/kg/day. If suboptimal response by 3-4 weeks, may increased to 1.4 mg/kg/day or 100 mg whichever is less. Children, adolescent and adults >70 kg: initial dose of 40 mg/day; increase weekly as tolerated to 80 mg; if less than optimal response by 3-4 weeks, may increase to 100 mg if tolerated.
Clonidine	Catapres (0.1-, 0.2-, and 0.3-mg tablets) Catapres TTS (0.1-, 0.2-, and 0.3-mg patch) Kapvay (0.1- and 0.2-mg extended release tablets)	Time to peak plasma conc = 3-5 hrs Half life = 12-16 hrs	Age ≥6: initial dose 0.05 mg at bedtime, increase slowly over 2-3 weeks to 0.15 to 0.3 mg/day in divided doses. Clonidine patch is applied once/week and may be substituted once stable oral dose has been achieved. Extended release: initial dose 0.1 mg daily, increase weekly by 0.1 mg given twice a day to maximum of 0.4 mg/day
Guanfacine	Tenex (1- and 2-mg tablets)	Time to peak plasma conc = 1-4 hrs Half life = 16 hrs	Immediate release: initial dose 0.5 mg at bedtime, increase to total dose of 3 mg/day.
	Intuniv (1-, 2-, 3-, and 4-mg extended release tablets)	Time to peak plasma conc = 5 hrs Half life = 18 hrs	Extended release: initial dose 1 mg, increase weekly to max dose of 4 mg/day

sudden death, although not substantiated by the evidence, remain important issues for families considering stimulant medications in their child. Some studies actually suggest that children with ADHD who are treated with stimulant early in life have a lower risk of substance abuse than children with ADHD who are not treated [Wilens et al., 2003], but such evidence may not be as reassuring to parents as one would hope. Prudent practice therefore necessitates an evaluation that leads to confidence in the diagnosis, fully informed consent, and use of appropriate doses with close monitoring, combined with effective and available psychosocial treatments. Detailed discussion, in the assessment and treatment phases, with the family and teachers, backed up by full documentation in the medical record, is essential. During the dose adjustment phase, children often are monitored for side effects, including blood pressure, pulse, height, and weight. After a maintenance dose is achieved, visit intervals can vary from 1–4 months.

Pharmacology

Stimulants are sympathomimetic drugs that directly stimulate α- and β-adrenergic receptors. They also stimulate the release of dopamine from presynaptic nerve terminals and inhibit dopamine reuptake. The exact mechanism for efficacy on attention and hyperactivity in ADHD is unknown. Stimulant medications are available in immediate-release and sustained-release preparations (see Table 49-2).

Clinical Management

ASSESSMENT

A neuropsychiatric assessment of inattention, impulsivity, and hyperactivity involves gathering information from multiple sources, including the child, parents, teacher, therapist, or other individuals involved with the child (e.g., day-care providers and coaches). Information can be gathered through clinical interview; patient, parent, and teacher rating scales; neuropsychological testing; and medical evaluation, including laboratory screening [AACAP, 1997]. The diagnostic criteria for ADHD are detailed in the Diagnostic and Statistical Manual of Mental Disorders, Fourth Edition, Text Revision (DSM-IV-TR [APA, 2000]). A thorough neuropsychiatric assessment is necessary because inattention, impulsivity, and hyperactivity can be complications of medical conditions, and they are commonly caused by other neuropsychiatric disorders. Children with ADHD often have co-occurring neuropsychiatric disorders, which can make it difficult to determine accurately whether ADHD symptoms are attributable to ADHD or to the co-occurring conditions. Medical and developmental problems in the differential include vision or hearing deficits, seizures, chronic medical illnesses, sleep deprivation, and poor nutrition [Pliszka, 2007]. Children who have unidentified intellectual deficits, learning disabilities, speech and language problems, or substance abuse may appear to exhibit ADHD symptoms. Neuropsychiatric conditions, such as anxiety disorders, depressive disorders, and bipolar disorder, have disturbances in attention, impulse control, and activity level that can be especially difficult to distinguish from ADHD.

Identification of co-occurring conditions and risk factors for adverse effects is essential because some medications may be contraindicated, or medication management may require dosing modification or closer monitoring. For example, a patient with co-occurring ADHD and anxiety or depression may prompt the clinician to initiate treatment with an antidepressant first rather than a stimulant, depending on which of the two conditions is more impairing. A child with a pervasive developmental disorder may have limited response to stimulants or may have an adverse behavioral reaction that can be severe. Similarly, despite evidence that stimulants are unlikely to cause tic worsening relative to placebo [Kurlan, 2003], a patient with a personal or family history of tic disorders may develop tics de novo or experience a worsening of existing tics during an initial stimulant trial.

A medical evaluation to "clear" a child before initiating most psychotropic medications, including stimulants, is prudent. The evaluation should include a recent medical history and a physical examination completed by the primary care provider. Any significant change in health during treatment requires repeat evaluation. Choice of laboratory screening procedures and imaging studies is guided by the medical history and findings on physical or neurologic examination. These may include lead level, thyroid function tests, genetic screening, metabolic studies, magnetic resonance imaging, sleep studies, and electroencephalography (EEG). Other assessments may be indicated, including occupational therapy, physical therapy, speech and language evaluation, and neuropsychology [AACAP, 1997]. For stimulant medications, baseline height, weight, family or personal history of a tic disorder, and family or personal history of cardiac disease, including nonvasovagal syncope and sudden death, are also important. Although baseline electrocardiograph (EKG) screening for all children has been advocated by some, at present the American Academy of Pediatrics and the American Heart Association do not recommend EKG screening of all patients, but rather that the need for an EKG be considered by the treating clinician based on physical exam and history [Vetter et al., 2008].

Completing a baseline sexual history is often overlooked by physicians when treating adolescents because of the clinician's lack of training or discomfort with the topic. Monitoring for sexual side effects after medication initiation is essential because psychotropic medications can have a significant impact on sexual functioning and may affect the patient's physical and mental health. Sexual side effects can be the cause of otherwise unexplained medication nonadherence. Some psychotropic medication can interact with oral contraceptives, rendering contraceptives ineffective, and psychotropic medications may have teratogenic effects.

INITIATING MEDICATION AND DOSE TITRATION

Pharmacotherapy is only one component in the treatment of children and adolescents with ADHD. Patients and families should be informed of the benefits and limitations of medications and the importance of nonpharmacological interventions in maximizing the benefits of treatment, including appropriate school placement, behavior management training for parents, and consistency and structure at home and at school. Practitioners may not have the full range of skills necessary for the management of all aspects of ADHD, and the prescribing physician may wish to develop a treatment team to meet the often-complex needs of children with ADHD.

The starting dose of methylphenidate is 5 mg, given twice daily and dispensed after breakfast and lunch to minimize appetite-suppressant effects. The dose is increased at weekly intervals by increments of 5–10 mg until the therapeutic effect is achieved or side effects are encountered. The manufacturer recommends a maximum daily dose of 60 mg [Ritalin, 2004]; however, some clinicians exceed this figure if higher doses are necessary to control symptoms and the patient is not experiencing adverse effects. Detailed informed consent and adequate monitoring and documentation are essential for safe prescribing. Severity of symptoms, after-school activities, or homework demands may warrant a late-afternoon dose. An alternative method is to calculate the dose by weight [Dulcan, 1990]. The target dose falls between 0.3 and 0.7 mg/kg, administered 2–3 times each day (total dose of 0.6–2.1 mg/kg/day).

With d-amphetamine and mixed salts preparations, the starting dose for children between the ages of 3 and 5 years is 2.5 mg/day, with incremental increases of 2.5 mg weekly until a therapeutic response is achieved. For children 6 years or older, the starting dose is 5 mg given once or twice each day, with weekly increases of 5 mg until a therapeutic response is achieved. The manufacturer does not recommend exceeding 40 mg/day [Adderall, 2004; Green, 2007]. As with methylphenidate, some clinicians use higher doses if clinically indicated. Dosing by weight, the optimum dose may fall between 0.15 and 0.5 mg/kg, administered twice or three times daily, with a maximum daily dose of 0.3–1.5 mg/kg/day [Dulcan, 1990].

Sustained-release preparations have been around for a long time but the options were limited until the mid 1990s. Earlier sustained-release preparations of methylphenidate and d-amphetamine were viewed clinically as less reliable than their immediate-release counterparts [Birmaher et al., 1989; Fitzpatrick et al., 1992; Pelham et al., 1987], and head-to-head comparisons of their efficacy compared to their immediate-release counterparts were lacking. Over the past decade, new and novel delivery systems have developed, which has significantly increased the range of available sustained-release preparations. In clinical practice, many patients experience comparable or greater benefit from sustained-release preparations because of the convenience of once-daily dosing, avoiding dosing at school, increasing compliance, and reducing rebound effects.

MONITORING STIMULANTS

On-going monitoring of medication efficacy involves assessment of the patient's level of functioning in school, family, community, and peer groups. Data are collected from behavioral observations during office visits, and parent and teacher reports and rating scales. Patients require monitoring of possible side effects that can occur with short-term and long-term stimulant use. Heart rate, blood pressure, weight, height, appetite, sleep, and emergence of or changes in tic severity should be assessed routinely.

Some clinicians consider the use of "drug holidays" on weekends or during the summer to limit children's exposure to stimulants and minimize possible long-term adverse effects, such as low weight and growth suppression. However, the practice of drug holidays is controversial because it may result in the rapid return of symptoms and accompanying impairment [Martins et al., 2004; Spencer et al., 2006]. To identify patients who may do well with drug holidays, clinicians can review symptoms and impairment from times of the day when children are not benefiting from stimulants, such as early morning or later in the evening. If patients do well during these times, it may be reasonable to consider more extended time off stimulants. Drug holidays should be planned for times when there are no important school or social activities and they should be reserved for patients whose families can provide adequate structure, behavior management, and supervision during these periods.

Although hyperactive symptoms tend to improve as children mature, inattention and impulsivity often persist. Long-term stimulant treatment may be necessary, as up to 80 percent of ADHD children continue to have symptoms into adolescence and 65 percent into adulthood [Barkley, 1996; Weiss and Hechtmann, 1993].

Adverse Effects

Although most children tolerate stimulant medications well, some do not. The most common side effects of stimulants are insomnia and nervousness [Ritalin, 2004]. Some children with ADHD experience sleep disturbance before exposure to stimulants. The child's pre-existing sleep history should be obtained, including other factors that may contribute to sleep disturbance (e.g., poor sleep hygiene, caffeine use, oppositional behavior, separation anxiety). Ironically, some children experience difficulty falling asleep related to hyperactivity, and they may actually benefit from a small dose of stimulant to help them stay in bed and fall asleep. In group comparisons, dosing three times daily with short-acting stimulants versus dosing two times daily was not found to increase sleep disturbance [Kent et al., 1995; Stein et al., 1996]; however, new-onset sleep delay after starting stimulants may be associated with a stimulant dose that is too high overall or with dosing stimulants too late in the day. Difficulty with falling asleep because of stimulants can be addressed with a combination of dose adjustment, improved sleep hygiene (i.e., straightforward ritual for falling asleep, and removal of distractions, such as televisions, video games, homework, and night lights, from the room), cooler room temperatures, room-darkening shades, avoidance of late-afternoon or evening doses of stimulants, switching to a different stimulant, or addition of a sedating medication with ADHD treatment effects, such as clonidine [Brown and Gammon, 1992; Prince et al., 1996] or guanfacine.

Short-term reductions in expected weight gain and height have been reported in many studies [MTA, 2004; Swanson et al., 2006], although this has not been universally reported [Spencer et al., 2006; Zeiner, 1995]. Overall, the risk of growth suppression appears mild in school-age children but is moderate in preschool-age children. The Preschool ADHD Treatment Study (PATS) reported an annual reduction in growth rate of 20 percent for height and 50 percent for weight in preschoolers treated with methylphenidate compared to those that were not on stimulants [Swanson et al., 2006]. Because the impact on weight is likely mediated by stimulant-induced appetite suppression, administering stimulant doses immediately after meals [Swanson et al., 1983], allowing the child to eat later in the evening after the appetite suppressant effect of the stimulant has abated, or allowing drug holidays on weekends or evenings may mitigate these effects.

The possibility of growth suppression with long-term use of stimulants remains a controversial topic. Longitudinal studies of children with ADHD treated with stimulants followed into adulthood have not revealed any reduction in height or weight compared to adults who were never exposed to stimulants [Hechtman et al., 1984; Klein and Mannuzza, 1988]. The apparent lack of impact on adult height was thought to result from the discontinuation of stimulants in adolescence. An alternative theory proposes that this pattern of growth is inherent in children with ADHD and not related to stimulant treatment. The dysregulation of several neurotransmitter systems associated with ADHD may alter neuroendocrine function, including those involving growth [Spencer et al., 1998]. It is not clear whether growth suppression identified in the NIMH Multimodal Treatment Study of ADHD (MTA) or PATS studies will continue and have a long-term impact, resolve with stimulant discontinuation, or resolve on its own [Spencer et al., 1998].

Historically, stimulant treatment has been associated with the emergence of tics [Borcherding et al., 1990] or the exacerbation of pre-existing tics [Law and Schachar, 1999]. Children at risk appeared to be those with a personal history or family history of tic disorders. However, the effect on tics is not absolute. In placebo-controlled trials, low to moderate doses of methylphenidate improve attention and behavior in children with chronic tic disorders without significantly worsening tics [Castellanos et al., 1997; Gadow et al., 1995, 1999]. In the Treatment of ADHD in Children with Tics (TACT) study, tic increases categorized as an adverse event occurred in nearly equal numbers of subjects on placebo (22 percent), clonidine (26 percent), and methylphenidate (20 percent). These data suggest that 20–26 percent of youngsters with tics will experience tic worsening shortly after initiation of any medication treatment, including placebo, lending support to the hypothesis that tic increases observed after starting stimulants reflect the natural waxing and waning of tic severity.

Although the product information for the stimulants warns of possible decreases in seizure threshold, no increase in seizure frequency was observed in children treated with stimulants who had co-occurring ADHD and seizure disorder [Feldman et al., 1989; Wroblewski et al., 1992]. There is no increased risk of addiction from appropriate treatment with stimulants for ADHD. Adolescents with ADHD treated with stimulants were less likely to abuse stimulants [Faraone and Wilens, 2003; Hechtman, 1985].

Concerns that stimulants may increase the risk of sudden unexplained death in children followed the publication of case reports and small case series in the early 1990s [Nissen, 2006]. A recently published case-control study comparing 564 cases of sudden death in children of 7–19 years with matched controls who died as passengers in motor vehicle traffic accidents over an 11-year period in the U.S. revealed an association between unexplained sudden death and use of stimulants [Gould et al., 2009]. This finding has enhanced concern that sudden death may be a rare side effect of stimulant use in children. However, the study design does not permit the establishment of causality. The possibility that having ADHD itself confers additional risks for sudden death must be considered, as should the co-occurring increased incidence of risk-taking behavior and substance abuse [Vitiello and Towbin, 2009]. Strategies for managing the cardiac risk of stimulants have been published [Vetter et al., 2008].

Despite the impact on a broad range of ADHD symptoms, including irritability, stimulant medications can be associated with undesirable changes in mood and behavior [Gadow et al., 1992]. Some of these changes occur when the stimulant is reaching peak serum concentrations, or they may occur when serum concentrations are waning – so-called rebound effects. Effects associated with peak concentrations include dysphoria, anxiety, agitation, or the "zombie" effect (i.e., over-focused and passive). Rebound effects include overactivity, talkativeness, excitability, irritability, and insomnia [Rapoport et al., 1978; Zahn et al., 1980]. It is often difficult to determine whether such rebound symptoms are the re-emergence of ADHD symptoms once the patient is off stimulants or true withdrawal or rebound symptoms. These adverse behavioral effects can be managed in a variety of ways, including dose reduction or medication discontinuation, and by improving late-afternoon coverage by adding a low dose of immediate-release stimulant or by switching to a long-acting stimulant [Pliszka, 2007]. Youngsters who experience these side effects on one of the stimulants do not necessarily have the same behavioral effects on another stimulant, and switching to another stimulant or alternative medication can be useful. Clinicians should be comfortable using all stimulant preparations to optimize treatment effects and minimize side effects.

Pemoline (Cylert©), a long acting stimulant with a novel structures has been associated with rare cases of acute hepatic failure [Shevell, 1997]. In 2005, the FDA withdrew labeling of pemoline for use in the treatment of ADHD, and subsequently the pharmaceutical companies voluntarily agreed to stop sales and manufacture of pemoline [Hogan, 2000].

Drug Interactions

If stimulant medications are administered concomitantly or within 2 weeks of receiving monoamine oxidase inhibitors, there is a risk of precipitating a hypertensive crisis. Methylphenidate may inhibit the metabolism of coumarin anticoagulants, some anticonvulsants (e.g., phenobarbital, phenytoin, carbamazepine, primidone), and tricyclic antidepressants (e.g., imipramine, desipramine, clomipramine). Foods and beverages with caffeine may increase both efficacy and adverse effects. Amphetamines inhibit adrenergic blockers. Gastrointestinal acidifying agents, including citrus juices, lower absorption of amphetamines. Urinary acidifying agents increase urinary excretion of methylphenidate. Both types of acidifying agents can lower blood levels and efficacy of amphetamines.

The safety of combining stimulants, especially methylphenidate, with clonidine has been controversial. Clonidine has been helpful in managing sleep disturbance related to ADHD or stimulant treatment [Wilens et al., 1994]. The combination appears to help children with ADHD and co-occurring oppositional and conduct disorder [Hunt et al., 1990]. The combination also appears useful in the treatment of ADHD in children with tic disorders [TSSG, 2002; Wilens et al., 2003]. Concerns about the interaction developed after the report of four deaths of children who apparently received clonidine and methylphenidate, as well as other medications in some cases [Fenichel, 1995]. Although the cases did not have a clear pattern of causality [Sallee et al., 2000a; Wilens et al., 1999], clinicians are more cautious about prescribing this combination. When combining clonidine and stimulants, careful screening is recommended for a personal and family history of cardiac abnormalities, arrhythmias, and nonvasovagal syncope, and a baseline and follow-up EKG may be warranted.

Nonstimulant Medications

Atomoxetine

Clinical Applications

Atomoxetine is a nonstimulant medication that is approved by the FDA for the treatment of ADHD in adults and in children 6 years old and up. It is a selective norepinephrine reuptake inhibitor that is structurally more similar to fluoxetine than to stimulant medications.

Atomoxetine potentially offers several advantages over stimulant medications: longer duration of action, lower misuse or abuse potential, lower risk of rebound effects, lower risk of precipitating tics or psychosis, and ease of prescribing because duplicate or paper prescriptions are not required and multiple refills are possible. Effectiveness of atomoxetine in children has been supported by placebo-controlled trials [Kelsey et al., 2004; Spencer et al., 2002]. Atomoxetine doses of 1.2 and 1.8 mg/kg/day administered in divided doses were superior to placebo and atomoxetine in a dose of 0.5 mg/kg/day; there was no clear superiority of 1.8 versus 1.2 mg/kg/day. Early clinical trials used twice-daily dosing, but once-daily dosing also appears effective [Michelson et al., 2004]. Longer-term treatment (9 months) with atomoxetine appears to be safe and well tolerated [Michelson et al., 2004]. Children maintained therapeutic effect and demonstrated superior psychosocial functioning compared to children who received placebo [Kratochvil et al., 2002]. When compared with methylphenidate treatment, atomoxetine was associated with comparable therapeutic effects [Michelson et al., 2003]. Efficacy of atomoxetine in adults with ADHD was demonstrated at doses of 60–120 mg/day [Strattera, 2010].

Pharmacology

Atomoxetine is well absorbed through the gastrointestinal tract and is metabolized by the liver, predominantly by cytochrome P-450 2D6 (CYP2D6). A small percentage of the population (approximately 7 percent of whites and 2 percent of African Americans) has reduced activity of the cytochrome P-450 isoenzyme system. These individuals are considered to be "poor metabolizers" of medications whose predominant method of metabolism is this isoenzyme. Poor metabolizers can be expected to achieve higher than expected plasma concentrations on a given dose and a prolonged half-life compared with those with normal CYP2D6 activity. The half-life of atomoxetine in poor metabolizers is 21.6 hours, compared with 5.2 hours in normal metabolizers. Atomoxetine is 98 percent bound to plasma proteins, primarily serum albumin [Strattera, 2010].

Clinical Management

Children should undergo standard psychiatric and medical assessment for ADHD (see "Clinical Management of Stimulant Medication"). No laboratory screening is required, although obtaining baseline and follow-up liver function studies should be considered in view of reports of severe acute liver dysfunction [Lim et al., 2006]. Baseline values for weight, heart rate, and blood pressure should be obtained. Concomitant use of medications with cardiovascular effects and medications that inhibit cytochrome P-450 may necessitate dosage adjustment. Although the determination of cytochrome P-450 metabolizer status is available, it appears to be unnecessary because regular dosing parameters provide the opportunity for assessment of outcome and adverse events that may be experienced by poor metabolizers.

In children, the usual starting dose of atomoxetine is 0.5 mg/kg/day, given in the morning or divided into morning and late-afternoon doses. Starting with a split dosing regimen may decrease gastrointestinal side effects and irritability. Decreasing side effects on initiation will ultimately lead to better compliance. The dose can be consolidated after a target dose is achieved. The dose may be increased every 3 days to a target dose of 1.2 mg/kg/day. For adults or for children and adolescents weighing more than 70 kg, atomoxetine may be initiated at 40 mg/day. The dose may be increased gradually every 3 days to a maximum dose of 80 mg. If there is an inadequate response after a 2- to 4-week trial, the dose may be increased to 100 mg/day. Patients taking atomoxetine concomitantly with potent inhibitors of CYP2D6 should be maintained at the initial dose for at least 4 weeks before a dosage increase is considered. Dosage reduction is required in patients with hepatic impairment [Strattera, 2010].

In clinical practice, combination therapy may be used during initiation and titration of atomoxetine, especially in children with severe ADHD symptoms. The effectiveness and tolerability of combining atomoxetine with methylphenidate in children who have not responded to monotherapy have been reported in a few patients [Brown, 2004]. Discontinuation of atomoxetine does not require dose tapering. Abrupt discontinuation of atomoxetine has not been associated with an acute discontinuation syndrome [Wernicke et al., 2003].

Adverse Effects

The most common side effects of atomoxetine in children and adolescents are upset stomach, decreased appetite, nausea, vomiting, dizziness, tiredness, and mood swings. Atomoxetine was associated with increases in heart rate of 6 beats per minute, and increases in systolic and diastolic blood pressure of 1.5 mmHg compared with placebo. In an analysis of short-term and long-term treatment with atomoxetine, increased systolic blood pressure was observed in adults, and increased diastolic blood pressure occurred in children and adolescents. Heart rate increased in both groups, and no prolongation of the QTc interval was observed [Strattera, 2010]. Seizures and prolonged QTc intervals were reported after an overdose with atomoxetine [Sawant and Daviss, 2004]. During post-marketing experience, several cases of significant liver injury in children treated with atomoxetine have been reported [Lim et al., 2006; Stojanovski et al., 2007]. Lilly Research Laboratories subsequently reviewed all hepatobiliary events during clinical trials and through post-marketing voluntary adverse events reporting, and identified three cases of probable severe, reversible liver injury related to atomoxetine use [Bangs et al., 2008]. Strattera labeling now warns that severe liver injury is possible and states that atomoxetine should be discontinued and not restarted when laboratory tests show liver injury or when there is clinical evidence of jaundice. Use in patients with liver disease probably should be avoided.

Drug Interactions

Inhibitors of CYP2D6 may increase serum concentrations of atomoxetine. Atomoxetine does not have significant effects on the cytochrome P-450 system. Combination with monoamine oxidase inhibitors may precipitate a hypertensive crisis. Atomoxetine has potential interactions with cardiovascular agents and adrenergic agonists. Albuterol's tendency to increase heart rate and blood pressure may be potentiated by atomoxetine. No increase in the cardiovascular effects of methylphenidate was observed when atomoxetine was added, and no interactions between atomoxetine and other protein-bound medications have been observed [Strattera, 2010].

Alpha$_2$-Agonists

Clinical Applications

Two $\alpha2$ agonists, clonidine (Catapres®, Kapvay®) and guanfacine (Tenex®, Intuniv®) are prescribed in the treatment of ADHD, Tourette's syndrome, aggressive or self-injurious behavior, and the physiological symptoms of anxiety. In 2009, extended release guanfacine (Intuniv®) was the first $\alpha2$-agonist to be approved by the FDA for treatment of ADHD in children and adolescents. More recently extended release clonidine (Kapvay®) has also been found effective and given FDA approval for treatment of ADHD in children and adolescents. In clinical practice, clonidine and guanfacine are second-line treatments for ADHD.

Clonidine is available in immediate-release and extended-release (ER) formulations. Immediate-release clonidine has been shown to improve behavior of children with ADHD; however, the degree of its effect in a meta-analysis was less than that of stimulants, and it was associated with many side effects [Connor et al., 1999]. The largest randomized controlled study to compare clonidine, methylphenidate, and the combination directly confirmed this earlier analysis [Palumbo et al., 2008]. Greatest improvement is seen with hyperactivity and impulsivity [Hunt, 1987; Hunt et al., 1982] and with frustration tolerance [Hunt, 1987] than with distractibility [Palumbo et al., 2008]. Children have been maintained on immediate-release clonidine for up to 5 years with continued benefit [Hunt et al., 1990, 1991]. Recently, clonidine ER was found effective in 2 randomized controlled trials (RCTs) in patient age 6-17 years (Kapvay, 2010, Kollins et al., 2011). One RCT used clonidine ER monotherapy and one RCT used clonidine ER as adjunctive therapy to a stimulant. To date, only the RCT with adjunctive therapy has been published in a peer reviewed journal (Kollins et al., 2011).

The combination of clonidine and methylphenidate has been helpful in adolescents with co-occurring ADHD and oppositional or conduct disorder [Hunt et al., 1990]. This combination allowed the dose of methylphenidate to be reduced by 40 percent [Hunt et al., 1990]. In children with co-occurring ADHD and tic disorders, those treated with clonidine experienced improvements in both conditions [Steingard et al., 1993]. A randomized controlled trial of clonidine, alone and in combination with methylphenidate, in children with ADHD and tics (TACT Trial) showed that clonidine was equally effective as methylphenidate but that the combination was most effective for treating ADHD symptoms [TSSG, 2002]. Clonidine has been used to treat sleep disturbances in children with ADHD [Wilens et al., 1994], and it appears to be helpful in managing severe aggression [Kemph et al., 1993]. Studies of clonidine in youngsters with Tourette's syndrome show mixed results [Leckman et al., 1982], but significant improvements in tics and behavior have been reported [Cohen et al., 1980; Comings et al., 1990; Leckman et al., 1991].

Guanfacine is available in immediate-release and extended-release (ER) formulations through different manufacturing companies. Limited data exist on immediate-release guanfacine in children. One open trial demonstrated its effectiveness in ADHD [Hunt et al., 1995]. Findings for patients with ADHD and Tourette's syndrome have been mixed [Chappell et al., 1995; Horrigan and Barnhill, 1995]. Results of more recent studies have been more promising [Scahill et al., 2001]. More data are available on the extended-release formulation (Intuniv®). Randomized, double-blind, placebo-controlled studies have demonstrated efficacy of guanfacine ER for treatment of symptoms of ADHD in short-term treatment [Biederman et al., 2008; Sallee et al., 2009b]. Continued efficacy is seen in longer-term treatment of up to 24 months [Sallee et al., 2009a]. Review of data suggests that guanfacine ER may be most effective in younger children and children with ADHD, combined type [Biederman et al., 2008].

Pharmacology

Clonidine and guanfacine immediate release are well absorbed from the gastrointestinal tract. Clonidine reaches peak plasma levels 3–5 hours after oral administration and has a half-life of 12–16 hours. Clonidine ER reaches peak plasma levels about 5 hours later than clonidine immediate release and has a similar half-life (Kapvay, 2010). Guanfacine reaches peak plasma levels between 1 and 4 hours and has a half-life of about 16 hours. Guanfacine ER reaches peak plasma levels at about 5 hours and has a slightly longer half-life of 18 hours [Intuniv, 2011]. Clonidine is also available in a transdermal patch.

Clonidine and guanfacine exert agonist effects on presynaptic α_2-adrenergic receptors in the sympathetic nuclei of the brain, resulting in decreased release of norepinephrine from presynaptic nerve terminals. In the central nervous system (CNS), α_2-adrenergic agonists are thought to regulate noradrenergic activity in the locus ceruleus [Arnsten et al., 1988].

Clinical Management

Before the initiation of clonidine or guanfacine, baseline EKG, heart rate, and blood pressure should be obtained. A history of syncope or cardiovascular disease is a relative contraindication. Heart rate and blood pressure should be monitored regularly during therapy for hypotension and bradycardia.

Clonidine is initiated at a 0.05-mg dose taken at bedtime, gradually titrating the dose over several weeks to 0.15–0.3 mg/day in divided doses. Clonidine is also available in a transdermal patch, which may have the advantage of increased medication compliance and more stable blood levels. After a therapeutic dose of oral clonidine is achieved, the equivalent patch can be substituted [Catapres, 2010]. Clonidine ER is initiated at 0.1 mg at bedtime and increased weekly by 0.1 mg to a maximum dose of 0.4 mg divided twice daily (Kapvay, 2010).

Guanfacine immediate release offers the advantage over clonidine of a longer half-life and therefore less frequent dosing, and it may cause less sedation than clonidine [Hunt et al., 1995]. It is initiated at 0.5 mg at bedtime and is titrated up to a maximum of 3 mg/day. Guanfacine ER has the greatest ease of administration and allows once-daily dosing. It is initiated at 1 mg daily and increased weekly to a maximum daily dose of 4 mg/day [Intuniv, 2011].

Adverse Effects

The most common side effects of clonidine and guanfacine include sedation, dizziness, fatigue, dry mouth and eyes, nausea, hypotension, and constipation [Catapres, 2010; Intuniv, 2011]. Syncope has been reported in 1 percent of children on guanfacine ER [Intuniv, 2011]. Clonidine in patch form may be associated with contact dermatitis, which may be reduced by changing its location on the body. Because of the risk of rebound hypertension with abrupt discontinuation, these medications should be prescribed only to patients with reliable medication compliance. Likewise, the dose should be tapered gradually when discontinuing the medication [Catapres, 2010; Intuniv, 2011].

Case reports of sudden death in children treated with clonidine has raised concerns about the cardiovascular safety of clonidine by itself or in combination with methylphenidate [Fenichel, 1995]. The most commonly reported cardiovascular side effect is bradycardia in patients taking clonidine either alone or in combination with methylphenidate [Chandran, 1994; Connor et al., 2000; Daviss et al., 2008], although this has not been universally reported [Kofoed et al., 1999; Leckman et al., 1991; Wilens et al., 2003]. One study reported prolongation of the PR interval that was not clinically significant [Connor et al., 2000], and one study reported bradycardia accompanied by a variety of EKG changes, which was confounded by concomitant treatment with other medications with potential for cardiovascular side effects [Chandran, 1994]. Some studies have suggested that the risk for bradycardia is higher when clonidine is given concomitantly with methylphenidate [Connor et al., 2000], but others have shown no additional risk [Daviss et al., 2008; Leckman et al., 1991]. To date, studies of guanfacine ER have not reported any EKG abnormalities considered to be serious adverse events, although a few subjects have been noted with clinically asymptomatic bradycardia [Biederman et al., 2008; Sallee et al., 2009a]. Practitioners should monitor bradycardia in patients taking clonidine.

Drug Interactions

Clonidine may potentiate the CNS-depressant effects of alcohol and sedating medications. The manufacturer advises caution in combining clonidine with medications that affect cardiac conduction and sinus node function because of potential additive effects, such as bradycardia and atrioventricular block [Catapres, 2010].

Antidepressants

Tricyclic Antidepressants

Clinical Applications

Tricyclic antidepressants are approved for the treatment of depression in adults and adolescents (Table 49-3). Placebo-controlled studies have demonstrated the efficacy of tricyclic antidepressants in the treatment of depression in adults, but studies enrolling children and adolescents have yielded inconsistent results. Some open studies show no significant response to tricyclic antidepressants [Kashani et al., 1984; Kramer and Feiguine, 1981]. Others suggest efficacy of desipramine, imipramine, and nortriptyline [Boulos et al., 1991; Geller et al., 1986; Ryan et al., 1986]. Placebo-controlled studies, however, do not support efficacy [Geller et al., 1989, 1990; Puig-Antich et al., 1987]. The lack of efficacy in placebo-controlled trials may be related to methodological problems, such as a small number of subjects, types of subjects enrolled (with depression that is either too mild or too severe), and the high placebo response rates in many studies. The use of tricyclic antidepressants for the treatment of depression in children and adolescents has declined because of their equivocal efficacy and safety in this population and the availability of antidepressants with a more favorable side-effect profile (i.e., selective serotonin reuptake inhibitors). Clomipramine has been approved for use in children 10 years of age or older for OCD, following publication of several randomized, controlled trials [DeVeaugh-Geiss et al., 1992; Leonard et al., 1989]. However, clomipramine is used less commonly for OCD than selective serotonin reuptake inhibitors and is considered second-line treatment in clinical practice, in part because of a less favorable side-effect profile.

Although amitriptyline is still commonly used in neurologic settings for adults, its side-effect profile in doses effective for the treatment of anxiety and depression is often prohibitive –

Table 49-3 **Representative Tricyclic Antidepressants Used in the Clinical Neuropsychopharmacology**

Drug	Preparations	Pharmacokinetics	Dosing
Imipramine	Tofranil (imipramine hydrochloride) (10-, 25-, and 50- mg tablets) Tofranil-PM (imipramine pamoate) (75-, 100-, 125-, and 150-mg capsules)	Time to peak plasma conc = 1-2 hr Half life = 8-16 hr.	Initiate at 25 mg/day and increase by 25 mg/day every 4-6 weeks while monitoring serum conc and electrocardiograms Therapeutic serum conc = combined serum conc of imipramine and desipramine, 125 to 250 ng/ml.
Nortriptyline hydrochloride	Pamelor (10-, 25-, 50-, and 75- mg capsules) Pamelor (10 mg/5 ml soln)	Time to peak plasma conc = 7-8.5 hr Half-life = 16-90 hr	Initiate at 10 mg/day and increase by 10 mg/day every 4-6 days while monitoring serum conc and electrocardiogram Therapeutic serum conc = 60-100 ng/ml
Clomipramine hydrochloride	Anafranil (10-, 25-, 50-, and 75- mg capsules)	Time to peak plasma conc = 2-6 hr Half-life = 19-37 hr Time to steady state = 2-3 wk	Initiate at 25 mg/day and increase gradually while monitoring serum conc and electrocardiogram to a maximum dose of 3 mg/kg or 200 mg/day whichever is lower

particularly sedation and weight gain. Nortriptyline, the primary metabolite of amitriptyline, is often better tolerated at treatment doses and has the benefit of an established target blood level for antidepressant efficacy that is unique among the tricyclic antidepressants. Because clinical trials do not support the efficacy of any tricyclic antidepressant for anxiety or depression in children or adolescents, they should not be considered first-line treatments. However, tricyclic antidepressants may be considered an alternative for children with anxiety and depression who cannot tolerate the selective serotonin reuptake inhibitors.

Tricyclic antidepressants have been prescribed as third-line treatments for patients with ADHD who have failed adequate trials of stimulants, who could not tolerate the adverse effects of stimulants, and who had co-occurring conditions such as depression, anxiety, tic disorders [Wilens et al., 1993], or enuresis. Studies have demonstrated significant improvement in ADHD symptoms with imipramine, nortriptyline [Saul, 1985; Wilens et al., 1993], and desipramine [Biederman et al., 1986, 1989; Gastfriend et al., 1984]. However, tricyclic antidepressants appear to be less effective than methylphenidate [Rapoport et al., 1974], and are associated with a large dropout rate over time due to loss of efficacy or side effects [Quinn and Rapoport, 1975].

Studies of imipramine in the treatment of separation anxiety disorder and school refusal have yielded inconsistent findings [Bernstein et al., 2000; Gittelman-Klein and Klein, 1971; Klein et al., 1992]. The largest double-blind, placebo-controlled study of adolescents with school refusal and comorbid depression and anxiety found greatest improvement in school attendance in youngsters who received a combination of imipramine and cognitive behavioral therapy when compared to youngsters receiving cognitive behavioral therapy alone [Bernstein et al., 2000]. Case reports describe the usefulness of tricyclic antidepressants in the treatment of panic disorder [Ballenger et al., 1989; Black and Robbins, 1990], but no placebo-controlled trials have been carried out.

Imipramine appears to be effective in treating enuresis as an initial agent.[Fritz et al., 2004], and in children who have failed nonpharmacological interventions and desmopressin [Gepertz and Neveus, 2004]. Efficacy appears to be correlated with serum concentration [Fritz, 1994].

Clomipramine is approved for the treatment of OCD in adults and children older than 10 years. In short-term clinical trials, clomipramine has demonstrated superiority over placebo [DeVeaugh-Geiss et al., 1992; Leonard et al., 1989] in reducing

symptoms of OCD and preventing relapse [Leonard et al., 1991]. Improvement in clomipramine-treated subjects was sustained during 1-year open treatment [DeVeaugh-Geiss et al., 1992].

Pharmacology

Tricyclic antidepressants are divided into two groups, based on the number of methyl groups bonded to the nitrogen atom of the side chain. Tertiary amines (i.e., imipramine, amitriptyline, clomipramine, trimipramine, and doxepin), which have two methyl groups, are metabolized into secondary amines. Several secondary amines, which have one methyl group, are marketed as independent entities, including desipramine (metabolite of imipramine), nortriptyline (metabolite of amitriptyline), and protriptyline (metabolite of trimipramine).

Tricyclic antidepressants differ from each other in their ability to block the reuptake of norepinephrine and serotonin (5HT), and act as competitive antagonists at muscarinic, histaminic (H_1), and adrenergic (α_1, α_2) receptors. Their therapeutic mechanism of action is thought to result from their effect on norepinephrine and serotonin systems in the brain. Clomipramine distinguishes itself from other tricyclic antidepressants in its relatively potent inhibition of serotonin reuptake in addition to its noradrenergic activity. Tricyclic antidepressant activity at central and peripheral muscarinic, histaminic, and adrenergic receptors is not thought to be involved in the clinical response, but rather is associated with side effects.

Tricyclic antidepressants are well absorbed in the gastrointestinal tract. They are metabolized in the liver by the cytochrome P-450 system. Although multiple isoenzymes are involved in their metabolism (i.e., CYP1A2, CYP2D6, CYP3A4, and CYP2C), the CYP2D6 isoenzyme is of particular importance. About 7 percent of the population are poor metabolizers, with reduced activity of CYP2D6. This results in increased plasma concentrations of tricyclic antidepressants and other medications metabolized by CYP2D6 compared with most of the population.

Co-administration of the tricyclic antidepressants with medications that inhibit cytochrome P-450 (e.g., some selective serotonin reuptake inhibitors) can result in clinically significant interactions. These drug interactions may result in discernible changes in efficacy or exacerbation of common tricyclic antidepressant side effects. Specifically, such interactions may result in elevated blood levels of tricyclic antidepressants, leading to a silent but potentially significant impact on cardiac conduction (i.e., prolonged QTc interval). EKG monitoring is required for patients taking such drug combinations.

Clinical Management

ASSESSMENT

As with ADHD, assessment for anxiety disorders and depression requires the gathering of information from multiple sources, including the child, parents, school, therapist, and others involved with the child. Information can be gathered through clinical interview, other informants, self-reports, and medical evaluation, including laboratory screening. Diagnostic criteria for anxiety disorders and depressive disorders are detailed in the DSM-IV TR [APA, 2000].

The diagnostic evaluation of children with depression and anxiety should also determine whether other coexisting conditions are present. Risk factors for adverse effects with tricyclic antidepressants should be identified: family and personal history of bipolar disorder; nonvasovagal syncope, history of cardiac disease (especially arrhythmias, conduction abnormalities, and sudden death); use of concomitant medications; hepatic disease; pregnancy; and narrow-angle glaucoma.

A medical evaluation is required before initiating tricyclic antidepressants. A physical examination should have been completed within the past 1 year. A baseline EKG, orthostatic blood pressure and heart rate, complete blood cell count (CBC), electrolyte determination, renal and hepatic function tests, thyroid function tests, and urinalysis should be performed [Green, 2007]. Other laboratory screening measures may be indicated, based on findings in the history or physical examination.

INITIATION AND TITRATION OF TRICYCLIC ANTIDEPRESSANTS

Dosing strategies, as well as the utility of serum blood levels of tricyclic antidepressants, are not as well established in children and adolescents as for adults, but the literature does provide some guidance. Imipramine may be initiated at 25 mg and increased by 25 mg every 4–6 days. Because there is large variability in plasma drug concentration with a given dose of tricyclic antidepressants among individuals, monitoring of serum concentration has been recommended [Biederman et al., 1989; Geller et al., 1986]. A combined serum concentration of imipramine and its primary metabolite, desipramine, in the range of 125–250 ng/mL is considered therapeutic for the treatment of depression. Higher serum concentrations within this range have correlated with higher response rates compared with placebo in the treatment of pediatric depression [Puig-Antich et al., 1987]. Serum concentrations greater than 250 ng/mL have not improved response rates and were associated with increased side effects [Preskorn et al., 1989]. Low doses of imipramine are recommended for treatment of enuresis, not to exceed 15 mg in children and 75 mg in adolescents [Fritz et al., 2004].

Nortriptyline is not FDA-approved for any indication in children and adolescents, but the limited studies to date have not reported serious adverse effects [Geller et al., 1989, 1992]. Although studies of nortriptyline in depressed adults reveal correlation between response and serum blood level with a therapeutic window of 50–150 ng/mL, correlations between therapeutic efficacy and serum nortriptyline levels have not been consistently established in pediatric populations [Geller et al., 1989, 1992]. A useful algorithm has been published for nortriptyline dosing, based on steady state plasma levels determined 24 hours after a single test dose of 25 mg in 5–9-year-olds and 50 mg in 10–17-year-olds for treatment of depression [Geller et al., 1985]. As the half-life is significantly shorter in children and adolescents, twice-daily dosing is recommended and there may be value in monitoring serum concentrations [Geller et al., 1986]. The therapeutic range for nortriptyline is postulated to be 60–100 ng/mL [Geller and Carr, 1988; Geller et al., 1987]. EKGs should be obtained at baseline and after steady-state plasma levels are achieved [Geller et al., 1987].

Clomipramine may be initiated at 25 mg/day and increased gradually over the course of 2 weeks to a maximum dose of 100 mg/day or 3 mg/kg/day, whichever is less. After 2 weeks, the dose may be gradually increased to 200 mg/day or 3 mg/kg/day, whichever is less. To allow tolerance to side effects and to avoid toxicity, slow titration is recommended after the first 2 weeks, because steady-state plasma concentrations may not be reached for 2–3 weeks.

Because of the risk of adverse cardiac effects, serial EKGs are recommended with the use of all tricyclic antidepressants. They should be obtained at baseline, at the middle point in titration, and at the final dose [Elliot and Popper, 1990/1991]. The following parameters have been suggested as safety parameters for cardiovascular monitoring:
1. PR interval: no greater than 210 milliseconds
2. QRS interval: widening no greater than 30 percent above baseline
3. QTc interval: less than 450 milliseconds
4. Heart rate: maximum of 130 beats per minute
5. Systolic blood pressure: maximum of 130 mmHg
6. Diastolic blood pressure: maximum of 85 mmHg.

Adverse Effects

Side effects of tricyclic antidepressants include sedation, weight gain, orthostatic hypotension, and anticholinergic side effects (i.e., dry mouth, constipation, blurred vision, and urinary retention). Serious anticholinergic effects may occur, including paralytic ileus, exacerbation of narrow-angle glaucoma, and the anticholinergic syndrome ("mad as a hatter, dry as a bone, blind as a bat, hotter than a hare").

Eight sudden deaths have been reported in children and adolescents taking tricyclic antidepressant medications [Popper and Zimnitzky, 1995; Riddle et al., 1993; Varley and McClellan, 1997]. Six were taking desipramine and two were taking imipramine. Although the role of the tricyclic antidepressants in these tragic deaths is unclear, it has been speculated that the cause of death was cardiac in nature, most likely due to malignant arrhythmias. After the reports, child psychiatrists have become more cautious about prescribing tricyclics in general, carefully screening patients at risk for adverse effects and monitoring cardiac status with serial EKGs [Elliot and Popper, 1990/1991]. It is not clear whether the vulnerability to such medication effects can be determined from routine monitoring of cardiac function. Those who experience increased QTc above that which is considered safe while on tricyclic antidepressants should be monitored closely, and the dose should be adjusted downward until resolution of QTc prolongation.

Behavioral side effects include early and acute increases in anxiety or depression. Tricyclic antidepressants may also induce manic episodes or rapid cycling in patients with a history of bipolar disorder. A family history of bipolar disorder may be a risk factor for this effect, but such a history is not a contra-indication for the use of antidepressants. A discontinuation syndrome (i.e. nausea, headache, and malaise), hypomania, or mania may result from abrupt cessation of antidepressants [Haddad, 2001] and may be associated with manic reactions [Narayan and Haddad, 2010]. The FDA mandated a black box warning regarding increases in suicidal ideation for all antidepressants (see "Selective Serotonin Reuptake Inhibitors").

Drug Interactions

Tricyclic antidepressants have multiple drug interactions. The product information for each of the tricyclic antidepressants provides details of specific drug interactions. A combination of tricyclic antidepressants and monoamine oxidase inhibitors can precipitate a hypertensive crisis requiring immediate medical treatment. Early signs and symptoms include headache, stiff neck, palpitations, sweating, nausea, and vomiting.

Medications that inhibit CYP2D6 activity, such as fluoxetine, paroxetine, and haloperidol (refer to prescribing information for other inhibitors), result in increased serum concentrations of tricyclic antidepressants and increased risk for tricyclic antidepressant side effects. Decreased serum concentrations may be caused by cigarette smoking, lithium, ascorbic acid, ammonium chloride, barbiturates, and primidone. Oral contraceptives may induce hepatic enzymes and decrease tricyclic antidepressant serum concentrations. Tricyclic antidepressants may block the activity of antihypertensives (e.g., guanethidine, propranolol, clonidine). Tricyclic antidepressants may increase the sedative effects of other drugs, such as over-the-counter cold medications, alcohol, opioids, anxiolytics, and hypnotics.

Selective Serotonin Reuptake Inhibitors

Clinical Applications

The selective serotonin reuptake inhibitors, including citalopram, escitalopram, fluvoxamine, fluoxetine, paroxetine, and sertraline, have FDA approval for a number of mood, anxiety, and eating disorders in adults (Table 49-4). In children and adolescents, fluoxetine, fluvoxamine, and sertraline have FDA approval for OCD; fluoxetine also has FDA approval for major depression. Escitalopram has FDA approval for major depression in adolescents (12 years and older). These indications are based on large-scale, randomized, controlled trials for OCD [Geller et al., 2001; March et al., 1998; Riddle et al., 2001] and major depression [Emslie et al., 1997, 2002, 2009; TADS, 2004]. Other large, randomized, controlled trials of the agents have been completed, but not all have been published. Published trials demonstrating efficacy include citalopram for depression [Wagner et al., 2004b]; fluoxetine [Birmaher et al., 2003], fluvoxamine [RUPP, 2001], and sertraline [Walkup et al., 2008] for separation, social, and generalized anxiety; sertraline for depression [Wagner et al., 2003] and generalized anxiety [Rynn et al., 2001]; paroxetine [Wagner et al., 2004a] and venlafaxine [March et al., 2007] for social phobia, and fluoxetine for stereotypies in children with autistic spectrum disorder [Hollander et al., 2001].

Table 49-4 Selective Serotonin Re-uptake Inhibitors

Drug	Preparations	Pharmacokinetics	Dosing
Citalopram	Celexa (10-, 20- and 40- mg tablets; 10 mg/5 ml oral soln)	Time to peak plasma conc = 4 hr Half life = 35 hr Time to steady state = 1 wk Linear kinetics with dosage ↑	Initiate at 10-20 mg/day; titrate to maximum of 40 mg/day.
Escitalopram	Lexapro (5-, 10- and 20 mg tablets; 5 mg/5 ml oral soln)	Time to peak plasma conc = 5 hr Half life = 27-32 hr Time to steady state = 1 wk Linear kinetics with dosage ↑	Initiate at 10 mg, titrate to maximum dose of 20-30 mg/day.
Fluoxetine	Prozac (10- and 20- scored tablets: 10-, 20- and 40- mg pulvules and capsules; 20 mg/5 ml oral soln)	Time to peak plasma conc = 6-8 hr Half life (chronic administration) = 7 days (fluoxetine), = 16 days (norfluoxetine) Time to steady state = 4-6 wks Nonlinear kinetics with dosage ↑	Initiate at 10 to 20 mg, increase weekly as clinically indicated, maximum daily dose of 20-60 mg/day.
Fluvoxamine	Luvox (25-, 50- and 100-mg tablets) Luvox CR (100- and 150-mg extended release capsule)	Time to peak plasma conc = 3 hr Half life = 15 hr Time to steady state = 10-14 days Linear kinetics at low dose Nonlinear kinetics at high dose	Initiate at 25 or 50 mg/day, increase by 25-50 mg weekly, maximum 200 mg/day in children and 300 mg/day in adolescents
Paroxetine	Paxil (10- and 20- mg scored tablets, 30- and 4-mg tablets, 10 mg/5 ml oral suspension)	Time to peak plasma conc = 5 hr Half life - 21 hr Time to steady state = 10 days Nonlinear kinetics with dosage ↑	Initiate at 5 mg daily, increase weekly by 5-10 mg, maximum of 50-60 mg/day.
Sertraline	Zoloft (25-, 50- and 100-mg scored tablets; 20 mg/ml oral concentrate)	Time to peak plasma conc = 4-8 hr Half life = 26 hr Time to steady state = 1 wk Linear kinetics	Initiate at 25 mg (ages 6-12 yr) or 50 mg (ages 13-17 yr); increase weekly by 25 to 50 mg as needed, maximum dose of 200 mg/day.

The use of the selective serotonin reuptake inhibitors for depression and anxiety disorder increased significantly in the 1990s, with upwards of 1–2 percent of teens being prescribed these medications for any indication [Olfson et al., 2002]. Despite the marked increase in use, the prevalence of disorders in children and adolescents that are potentially responsive to the selective serotonin reuptake inhibitors (e.g., depression and anxiety disorders) is much greater (minimum prevalence of 3–5 percent) than the number of children who are taking these medications (1–2 percent), suggesting overall under-utilization of these evidenced-based treatments.

In 2004, the FDA issued a black box warning for increased risk of suicidal ideation and behavior in children and adolescents using all antidepressants. This warning was based on the analysis of data from 24 short-term, placebo-controlled trials of nine antidepressant drugs, involving a total of over 4400 children and adolescents being treated for major depressive disorder, OCD, and other psychiatric disorders. Results of this analysis showed an increased risk of suicidal thoughts and behavior in the treatment groups compared to placebo (approximately 4 percent versus 2 percent). Since this time, prescriptions of antidepressants in pediatric populations have fallen off and recent reports suggest that rates of youth suicide increased after many years of decline [Gibbons et al., 2007]. There is no evidence that the prevalence of mood disorders in children has diminished over this same time period, or that patients who are identified as being depressed are being offered alternative treatments to medication. This is especially ironic, as the current evidence base suggests the limited value of non-pharmacological approaches to the treatment of depression [TADS, 2004].

Pharmacology

PHARMACODYNAMICS

The pharmacodynamic profiles of the selective serotonin reuptake inhibitors are very similar. Their beneficial effects are thought to be associated with their ability to block neuronal reuptake of serotonin, and the low side-effect profile is associated with their low affinity for other receptors. Although some individuals may do better on one selective serotonin reuptake inhibitor than another, comparative treatment trials suggest similarity in efficacy across all agents in this class. The selective serotonin reuptake inhibitors may demonstrate benefit in as little as 1 week, with substantial benefit occurring in 8–12 weeks. Improvement may continue at a more gradual rate for up to 6–12 months. Despite the similarity in pharmacodynamics, the selective serotonin reuptake inhibitors are very different in chemical structure and pharmacokinetics in ways that may impact their use. Very little is known about the pharmacodynamics or pharmacokinetics of the selective serotonin reuptake inhibitors in children and adolescents. The following information pertains to adults, unless stated otherwise.

PHARMACOKINETICS

Citalopram

Peak blood levels of citalopram (Celexa®) occur at about 4 hours, with a half-life of about 35 hours. Single- and multiple-dose pharmacokinetics of citalopram are linear throughout the standard dose range (10-40 mg/day). Steady-state plasma concentrations are reached in approximately 1 week. Citalopram is metabolized in the liver to a number of mostly inactive metabolites. Citalopram appears to have limited ability to inhibit cytochrome P-450 isoenzymes; inhibition of these isoenzymes is primarily responsible for the demethylation of citalopram. CYP3A4 and CYP2C19 do not appear to affect citalopram blood levels or half-life significantly. The (S)-enantiomer of citalopram is mostly responsible for the serotonin reuptake [Dietz and Robinson, 2005].

Escitalopram

Escitalopram (Lexapro®) is the (S)-enantiomer of a 50:50 racemic mixture of (R)- and (S)-enantiomers of citalopram. The (S)-enantiomer in escitalopram is approximately 100 times more potent at serotonin reuptake inhibition than the (R)-enantiomer. Evidence suggests that adolescents metabolize escitalopram more quickly than adults but once-daily dosing is adequate [Lexapro, 2009]. Steady state is achieved in about 1 week. The pharmacokinetic profiles of escitalopram for single and multiple doses are linear in the range of doses used clinically (10–30 mg/day). Escitalopram is metabolized primarily in the liver by CYP3A4, CYP2C19, and other enzymes. The primary metabolites are found in lesser concentrations in the plasma than escitalopram and are not thought to be clinically active. In a similar way to citalopram, it is not anticipated that escitalopram will inhibit cytochrome P-450 or be inhibited by medication that inhibits the cytochrome P-450 system [Lexapro, 2009].

Fluoxetine

Fluoxetine (Prozac®) reaches peak plasma levels approximately 6–8 hours after oral administration and is almost completely protein-bound. Fluoxetine is extensively metabolized in the liver to norfluoxetine (active metabolite) through a variety of isoenzymes of the cytochrome P-450 system. The kinetic profiles are generally nonlinear, with chronic plasma levels not directly linked to dose. With chronic administration, the half-life of fluoxetine and norfluoxetine increases to 7 days and up to 16 days, respectively. Steady-state concentrations are therefore delayed for up to 4–6 weeks. In pediatric populations, the steady-state concentrations of fluoxetine in children were 2 times higher than in adolescents at the same dose, mostly attributable to weight, although the overall levels were still within the range seen in studies of adult populations [Prozac, 2009]. The long duration of activity can have potential benefits (e.g., on-going medication exposure with occasional missed doses, and single-dose weekly administration for the sustained-release fluoxetine) and some risks – side effects may emerge as the plasma level increases 4–6 weeks after initiation of treatment, and newly prescribed medications may interact with fluoxetine or norfluoxetine for up to 4 weeks after fluoxetine discontinuation. The prolonged half-life may be problematic for patients who do not tolerate the medication, develop manic reactions, or have other problematic behavioral side effects [Reinblatt et al., 2009; Reinblatt and Riddle, 2006], when the need to discontinue and clear the medication from the body is critical.

Fluvoxamine

Fluvoxamine (Luvox®) reaches peak plasma levels in up to 8 hours after oral administration and up to 12 hours with the extended-release preparation. Pharmacokinetic profiles are nearly linear in the lower range of treatment doses, with a loss of linearity with higher doses. The half-life of fluvoxamine increases slightly from 15 hours to between 17 and 22 hours after single and multiple doses, respectively. Steady-state plasma levels are usually achieved within 10–14 days. Fluvoxamine undergoes extensive metabolism in the liver to a number of clinically inactive metabolites, but the specific cytochrome P-450 isoenzymes involved are unknown. Fluvoxamine does inhibit CYP1A2 and, to a lesser extent, CYP3A4 and CYP2D6, resulting in potentially significant drug interactions, including tertiary amine tricyclic antidepressants (e.g., imipramine, clomipramine), some benzodiazepines, propranolol, warfarin, and theophylline [van Harten, 1995]. Pharmacokinetic studies suggest that children, especially young girls, metabolize fluvoxamine more slowly and that they therefore may require lower treatment doses and have steady-state plasma levels that are 2–3 times that seen in adolescents [Labellarte et al., 2004].

Paroxetine

Paroxetine (Paxil®) reaches peak plasma concentrations at approximately 5 hours, and the average terminal half-life is about 21 hours after chronic administration of 30 mg/day. Steady-state paroxetine plasma levels are reached after about 10 days. Pharmacokinetics were nonlinear for multiple dosing and approximately eight times what would be expected based on single-dose kinetics. A nonlinear kinetic profile results from the saturation of CYP2D6, which is primarily responsible for paroxetine metabolism. Paroxetine undergoes extensive first-pass metabolism to a number of metabolites, none of which appears to have any significant clinical activity. Paroxetine appears to be a strong inhibitor of cytochrome P-450, which suggests the potential for clinically meaningful drug–drug interactions. Pediatric data suggest that children metabolize paroxetine more quickly than adults but that once-daily dosing is likely adequate [Findling et al., 1999].

Sertraline

Sertraline (Zoloft®) reaches peak plasma concentrations at approximately 4–8 hours after a 2-week period of oral administration, with an average terminal half-life of about 26 hours. Steady-state sertraline plasma levels are reached after about 1 week. Pharmacokinetic profiles were linear for single doses in the treatment range of 50–200 mg/day. Sertraline undergoes extensive first-pass metabolism by multiple cytochrome P-450 isoenzymes to N-desmethylsertraline, which is substantially less clinically active than sertraline. Sertraline does not appear to be a strong inducer or inhibitor of cytochrome P-450; coupled with the fact that sertraline is metabolized by multiple isoenzymes, this suggests that few clinically meaningful drug–drug interactions should occur. Pediatric data suggest that, although children metabolize sertraline more quickly than adults, they may require lower doses because of their lower body weight to avoid excessive plasma levels [Zoloft, 2009].

Clinical Management

ASSESSMENT

The assessment of mood and anxiety disorders before initiation of a selective serotonin reuptake inhibitor is similar to that described earlier for the tricyclic antidepressants. Assessment requires gathering information from multiple sources, including the child, parents, school, therapist, or others involved with the child. Information can be gathered through clinical interview, other informants, self-reports, and medical evaluation, including laboratory screening. Diagnostic criteria for anxiety disorders and depressive disorders are detailed in the DSM-IV TR [APA, 2000].

The diagnostic evaluation should pay particular attention to conditions that may coexist with depression, such as anxiety disorders and ADHD. Risk factors for adverse effects of selective serotonin reuptake inhibitors should be identified, and should include a family and personal history of bipolar disorder, history of suicidal ideation or behavior, sensitivity to other selective serotonin reuptake inhibitors, concurrent medications that could inhibit or could be inhibited by the selective serotonin reuptake inhibitor, pregnancy, and hepatic or renal disease.

No medical evaluation is required before initiating selective serotonin reuptake inhibitor treatment, but it may be prudent to clear a child medically by means of a medical history and physical examination, including baseline height and weight and targeted laboratory examination, as indicated by the history or physical examination findings.

INITIATION AND TITRATION OF DOSE

For all of the selective serotonin reuptake inhibitors, treatment usually is initiated with a low dose that is adjusted upward slowly at weekly intervals. Because the time–response pattern for the selective serotonin reuptake inhibitors occurs over a minimum of weeks, aggressive titration often leads to early side effects and may result in early discontinuation of the medication and the need to start again with another medication. Starting low and slowly titrating may allow the patient time to develop some tolerance to some of the side effects. However, going too slowly may put the patient at risk for being undertreated. Dosing of selective serotonin reuptake inhibitors is usually recommended in the morning because of activating side effects, and in the evening for individuals who feel sedated on the medication.

Citalopram

Citalopram comes in 20- and 40-mg scored tablets. Treatment doses range from 10-40 mg/day in adults. In industry-sponsored clinical trials of citalopram in children, patients were started on 20 mg/day, with the option of going up to 40 mg/day at week 6. Citalopram 20-mg tablets are scored, allowing beginning doses of 10 mg/day.

Escitalopram

Escitalopram comes in 5-, 10-, and 20-mg tablets. The 10- and 20-mg tablets are scored. The one positive double-blind, placebo-controlled study in adolescents used standard adult dosing of 10–20 mg/day [Emslie et al., 2009].

Fluoxetine

Fluoxetine comes in 10-, 20-, and 40-mg pulvules; 10-mg scored tablets; and Prozac Weekly, which contains approximately 90 mg of fluoxetine in a time-released preparation. Fluoxetine is also available in a liquid (20 mg/5 mL). In most clinical trials of fluoxetine in children and adolescents, dosing began at 10 mg/day for 1–2 weeks, with a subsequent increase to 20 mg. The dose is often held at this level up to 4–6 weeks before going to 30 or 40 mg/day [TADS, 2004]. Doses as high as 60 mg/day have been used in clinical trials, but maximum doses are used only if this dose is reached after a patient has demonstrated partial benefit after 10–12 weeks of treatment [TADS, 2004].

Fluvoxamine

Fluvoxamine comes in 25-, 50-, and 100-mg scored tablets. In clinical trials of fluvoxamine in children, dosing began at 25 or 50 mg/day and increased by 50 mg on a weekly basis to a maximum dose of up to 200 mg/day. Average therapeutic doses at the end of treatment were between 150 and 200 mg/day [Riddle et al., 2001]. In clinical trials, the method of titration often leads to the highest safe dose rather than least effective dose. With slower dosage adjustment, it may be possible to establish benefit at lower doses. This is particularly true for prepubertal children (especially girls), who may metabolize fluvoxamine more slowly and have higher blood levels than teens and adults [Labellarte et al., 2004].

Paroxetine

Paroxetine comes in 10-, 20-, 30-, and 40-mg tablets. The 10- and 20-mg tablets are scored. Paroxetine is also available in a suspension of 10 mg/5 mL. In adults, initial treatment can begin with 20 mg, given once daily in the morning or evening. Doses are increased by 10 mg/day every 7–10 days to a maximum dose of 50 mg. In clinical trials, final doses for adults ranged from 20 to 50 mg/day. For children, dosing can start as low as 5 mg/day.

Sertraline

Sertraline comes in 25-, 50-, and 100-mg scored pills or tablets and in a concentrate of 20 mg/mL. Generally, 50 mg/day given as a single dose appears to be as effective as other doses for most conditions. Dosing can begin at 25 or 50 mg/day. For those who do not respond or only partially respond, higher doses may be necessary. Clinical trials enrolling adults and children using sertraline have usually used doses up to 200 mg/day as tolerated. One clinical trial of sertraline in children demonstrated efficacy on a fixed dose of 50 mg/day [Rynn et al., 2001]; however, higher doses up to 140 mg/day are well tolerated [Walkup et al., 2008].

Adverse Effects

COMMON EFFECTS

The product information for each medication should be consulted for a comprehensive review of adverse events and warnings. Given the similar pharmacodynamic properties of the selective serotonin reuptake inhibitors, it is not surprising that their adverse-event profiles are also similar. In placebo-controlled trials of the selective serotonin reuptake inhibitors, a few adverse effects occurred significantly more often on active medication than on placebo. These include nausea or other gastrointestinal symptoms, insomnia, and anxiety or agitation. Other adverse effects that occur more often on active medication but are less common overall include apathy or somnolence, tremor, sweating, sexual dysfunction, and allergic reactions, including rash. The most common causes of medication discontinuation, other than lack of efficacy, are the behavioral or psychiatric side effects, such as anxiety or agitation.

Although clinicians usually think of adverse effects as physical changes for selective serotonin reuptake inhibitors, the behavioral and psychiatric adverse effects and their impact on growth and development are a greater concern and require review with the patient and parent before starting treatment. (For review, see Walkup and Labellarte [2001].) Perhaps the most important of these effects is activation, which occurs in about 10–20 percent of patients [March et al., 1998; Reinblatt et al., 2009; RUPP, 2001]. This activation syndrome (distinct from the mood improvement effects of the antidepressants) can result in a number of complaints, including anxiety, mental restlessness, increased activity level or akathisia, increased impulsivity, and disinhibition. This activation is very similar to but milder than what some children experience when they take diphenhydramine. Activation effects usually appear very early in treatment or after a dose change. Patients do not appear to develop tolerance to these symptoms, but they resolve with dose reduction or discontinuation, consistent with the pharmacokinetics of the medication.

Much less common but also serious are manic and hypomanic reactions. In clinical trials, manic reactions are much less common (1–2 percent) than activation, occur later in treatment after a period of improvement, do not always go away with dose reduction or discontinuation, and may require medical intervention to control. Core symptoms of mania include euphoria, grandiosity, decreased need for sleep, and increased goal-directed activities. It is critical to differentiate activation effects from manic reactions, as activation effects likely have little prognostic significance beyond potential sensitivity to other selective serotonin reuptake inhibitors, whereas manic reactions may have prognostic significance for the later development of mania.

Children with anxiety and mood disorders who benefit from selective serotonin reuptake inhibitor treatment do not always have uniform outcomes. For most, symptom relief is associated with return to normal and appropriate function. However, some children, especially those with behavioral problems or those at risk for other behavioral problems (i.e., poor parental discipline and monitoring), may present with increasing behavior problems after successful treatment of anxiety and depression. For example, a child with severe oppositional behavior may have a reduction of such behavior during a depressive episode due to psychomotor slowing or social withdrawal, but may actually have more behavioral difficulties with normalization of mood or decreased anxiety. Parents of youngsters at risk for or with a history of behavior problems need to be more active about structure and limit setting to manage the behavioral difficulties that can complicate recovery.

Children with anxiety and mood disorders also experience an evolution of symptoms over time. Children first presenting with separation anxiety at age 8 years may evolve into a generalized anxiety disorder or have periods of recurrent depression in their middle to late teens. As this can occur during the course of treatment, parents may be confused about whether medication treatment actually causes these changes in the progression of symptoms. Educating the patient and family regarding the progression of symptoms and the course of illness and treatment is helpful so that changes in the clinical course are, to some degree, anticipated and can be dealt with more easily.

The selective serotonin reuptake inhibitors have also been reported to induce an apathy syndrome. Although it may manifest early in treatment, those with anxiety and depression may not be sensitive to this subtle medication effect until after a period of recovery. Awareness of the potential for apathy improves the likelihood that it will be recognized. Even though patients who have experienced apathy can readily differentiate it from depression or sedation, careful interviewing may be required to make these differentiations. Apathy responds to dose reduction; however, dose reductions required to eliminate apathy may lead to loss of symptom control. Patients who report loss of response, not feeling like themselves, or feeling better but numb, or who appear to have lost interest without significant depressive symptoms should be interviewed closely to assess for apathy [Hoehn-Saric et al., 1990; Reinblatt and Riddle, 2006].

Sexual side effects are not commonly documented in clinical trials with children and adolescents, but in clinical practice, it is not uncommon for physicians to find that teens begin to complain spontaneously about sexual side effects when they explore their sexual responsiveness when alone or with another person. Awareness of sexual side effects can make it more likely that these effects are identified and managed, and that that they will not lead to poor adherence, discontinuation, and loss of treatment response. Dose reduction, changing to antidepressants with a lower risk for sexual side effects, or the addition of medication that may improve sexual function (i.e., bupropion or stimulants) have all been reported to be effective [Woodrum and Brown, 1998].

Although epistaxis is common in children and adolescents, some children experience increased rate or severity of epistaxis and increased bruising. Such changes appear to be an effect of the selective serotonin reuptake inhibitors on platelet functions, not on coagulation factors [Lake et al., 2000] and may be reflected in prolonged bleeding times.

Selective serotonin reuptake inhibitors, specifically fluoxetine, have been associated with change in the rate of linear growth. This was first reported in a small case series [Weintrob et al., 2002] and in a review of the large fluoxetine database [Nilsson et al., 2004]. It appears that the deceleration of growth stopped with medication discontinuation and recurred in one case when the medication was restarted [Weintrob et al., 2002]. It is not clear whether this is an effect of all the selective serotonin reuptake inhibitors or specific to fluoxetine. It is possible that this effect may be mediated by selective serotonin reuptake inhibitor-induced sleep disruption and resulting impact on growth hormone, and is not mediated by reduction in appetite, as can occur with the stimulants. It does not appear to affect all children uniformly. Because the follow-up period in these reports is relatively short, it is unclear whether children can catch up while on medication or whether medication discontinuation is required for children to obtain their optimal height. The assessment of changes in growth can be complicated by the potential effects of psychiatric disorders on growth [Pine et al., 1996].

In general cardiac side effects from SSRIs are rare. However, citalopram can cause prolongation of the QT interval and the FDA recently issued a safety alert indicating that doses over 40 mg were no longer recommended as this potentiated risk for torsades de pointes.

Although there are no data to suggest that selective serotonin reuptake inhibitor treatment leads to drug-seeking behavior (i.e., is addictive), some individuals do appear to have a discontinuation syndrome with abrupt discontinuation [Ditto, 2003]. There are three complications to abrupt discontinuation. The first complication is a withdrawal reaction that includes flu-like symptoms, such as malaise and gastrointestinal symptoms, but it may also include unusual symptoms, such as sensory or psychological disturbances. Some patients with abrupt discontinuation also experience an abrupt return of symptoms, including suicidal risk. Ironically, case reports suggest that abrupt discontinuation of antidepressants can be associated with hypomanic reactions [Narayan and Haddad, 2010]. Antidepressants with shorter half-lives appear to be more commonly associated with discontinuation syndromes than selective serotonin reuptake inhibitors with longer half-lives.

ANTIDEPRESSANTS AND RISK FOR SUICIDAL BEHAVIOR

Antidepressants have long carried warnings in their product labeling regarding the increased risk for suicidal ideation and behavior (i.e., suicidality) early in the course of treatment. The mechanism of this effect has never been clear, but it is commonly attributed to the positive energizing effects of antidepressants outpacing the improvement in mood and suicidality. For example, a patient with depression, psychomotor retardation, and suicidality, when treated with antidepressants, may experience increased energy and be capable of acting on suicidal impulses. After approximately 10 years of market exposure, concerns about the development of suicidality on antidepressants, especially the selective serotonin reuptake inhibitors, prompted a complete review by the British Medical and Healthcare Product Regulatory Agency and the U.S. FDA, and ultimately led to stronger warnings within the product information. In the United States, this means that all antidepressants must carry a black box warning regarding the risk for suicidality while on antidepressants early in the course of treatment and the need for close monitoring.

The data on which these new warnings are based include more than 24 randomized, controlled clinical trials (>4000 subjects) of the newer nontricyclic antidepressants [Hammad et al., 2006], completed for the purpose of extended exclusivity under the FDA Modernization Act [FDA, 1998]. Although a number of methodological limitations plague the analysis of these studies, it appears that there is a small but significant increased risk for more suicidality adverse events on active medication (about 4 events per 100 patients) versus placebo (about 2 events per 100 patients). There does not appear to be a groupwise risk for emergence or worsening of suicidal behavior for the medications, but the data do support an association with activation syndrome. Although the risk appears to be small (number needed to harm is about 50), the fact that, in these same studies, there is marginal antidepressant efficacy suggests that more caution is required when considering the use of these medications [Hammad et al., 2006]. In contrast to the industry-sponsored studies completed for exclusivity, National Institutes of Health (NIH)-funded studies of the treatment of depression and anxiety in children suggest significant benefit for the selective serotonin reuptake inhibitors [Birmaher et al., 2003; Emslie et al., 1997, 2009; RUPP, 2001; TADS, 2004; Walkup et al., 2008]. The big difference between industry-sponsored and NIH-sponsored clinical trials is the large placebo response rate in industry-sponsored trials, with resulting smaller effect sizes than those observed in NIH-funded trials. The increased risk for suicidality previously observed was principally seen in depressed patients, and its use for other indications, such as anxiety disorders, may not share this increased risk [Bridge et al., 2007]. This may be an important consideration for child neurologists because they are more likely to use selective serotonin reuptake inhibitors for such purposes.

The risk for suicide is higher overall among teenagers and less so in younger children.

Drug Interactions

The product information for each of the selective serotonin reuptake inhibitors provides detailed information regarding specific drug interactions. Because the number of individual interactions is too high to describe here, general principles are discussed. Adverse drug–drug interactions occur most commonly with highly protein-bound medications and with medications that significantly inhibit or induce cytochrome P-450 isoenzymes. Drug–drug interactions can result in loss (e.g., anticonvulsant combinations) or increase in benefit (e.g., cyclosporine and ketoconazole), increase in noticeable side effects (e.g., sedation), and an increase in side effects that can only be identified with careful monitoring (e.g., QTc prolongation). As a class, the selective serotonin reuptake inhibitors have more and more frequent drug–drug interactions because most of the selective serotonin reuptake inhibitors inhibit cytochrome P-450 isoenzymes. Most result in increased benefit of the co-administered agent or increase in noticeable side effects. The caution with using the selective serotonin reuptake inhibitors lies when they are combined with medications that have clinical effects, such as QTc prolongation, that require active monitoring to identify. Ironically, medications used in neuropsychiatry, such as the antipsychotics (e.g., pimozide) and tricyclic antidepressants (e.g., desipramine), have a potential for producing cardiac conduction effects. Careful monitoring is indicated when using selective serotonin reuptake inhibitors in combination with medication that may affect the QTc interval.

Serotonin-Norepinephrine Reuptake Inhibitors

Clinical Applications

The serotonin-norepinephrine reuptake inhibitors, which include duloxetine, venlafaxine, and desvenlafaxine, have FDA approval for treatment of depression and anxiety disorders in adults. Duloxetine also has FDA approval for treatment of fibromyalgia and diabetic neuropathic pain in adults. Venlafaxine has also shown promise in the treatment of ADHD in adults [Findling et al., 1996], and in co-occurring major depressive disorder and ADHD in adults [Hornig-Rohan and Amsterdam, 2002]. The use of serotonin-norepinephrine reuptake inhibitors in children and adolescents is off-label. At present, the only published randomized controlled studies of serotonin-norepinephrine reuptake inhibitors in pediatric populations include a positive trial of venlafaxine ER for social phobia [March et al., 2007], and equivocal trials for generalized anxiety disorder [Rynn et al., 2007] and depression [Emslie et al., 2007]. Two small open-label studies of venlafaxine in children and adolescents with ADHD suggest potential benefit for impulsivity and hyperactivity [Findling et al., 2007; Olvera et al., 1996] but were complicated by a high dropout rate due to adverse effects, including behavioral activation [Olvera et al., 1996]. A few case reports have been published on the successful use of duloxetine in youngsters with chronic pain and comorbid major depressive disorder [Meighen, 2007]; essentially, no data are available on use of desvenlafaxine. This review will limit its discussion to venlafaxine use in children and adolescents, given the limited data for duloxetine and desvenlafaxine.

Pharmacology

VENLAFAXINE

Venlafaxine is available in immediate-release tablets (Effexor®) and extended-release capsules (Effexor XR®). In adults, venlafaxine at doses of less than 150 mg/day selectively inhibit serotonin reuptake, and at higher doses, inhibit both serotonin and norepinephrine reuptake. Venlafaxine does not have significant activity at muscarinic, histaminic, or α-adrenergic receptors. It is well absorbed through the gastrointestinal tract, metabolized by the liver, and excreted in the urine. The serum half-lives of venlafaxine and its active metabolite, O-desmethylvenlafaxine, are about 5 and 11 hours, respectively (Table 49-5) [Effexor, 2009]. The pharmacodynamic behavior of venlafaxine ER is not well understood in children and adolescents, although some preliminary work suggests that there is no clear relationship between dose and plasma serotonin and norepinephrine [Emslie et al., 2007; Findling et al., 2007]. Various dosing strategies have been employed in clinical trials with higher dosing strategies used in youngsters with mood and anxiety symptoms and lower dosing strategies in youngsters with ADHD. In studies of depression, children under 40 kg were begun at 37.5 mg daily and increased weekly up to 112.5 mg; children of 40–49 kg also began at 37.5 mg and increased weekly up to 150 mg, and children over 50 kg were titrated up to a maximum daily dose of 225 mg daily [Emslie et al., 2007], although most individuals did not require the upper limits of these dosing strategies. Dosing strategies for venlafaxine in studies of ADHD used lower doses, ranging from 0.5 mg to 2.0 mg/kg daily in divided doses.

Adverse Effects

In adults, common adverse events associated with venlafaxine include asthenia, sweating, nausea, constipation, anorexia, vomiting, somnolence, dry mouth, dizziness, nervousness, anxiety, tremor, blurred vision, and sexual dysfunction. In addition, venlafaxine has been associated with increases in diastolic blood pressure that appear dose-dependent, especially with doses above 300 mg daily [Effexor, 2009]. In children and adolescents, treatment-emergent side effects include asthenia, anorexia, nausea, weight loss, abdominal pain, dizziness, somnolence, and nervousness [Emslie et al., 2007; March et al., 2007; Rynn et al., 2007]. Small increases in diastolic blood pressure have been reported in randomized clinical trials but were not considered clinically significant. Venlafaxine appears to have one of the highest rates of treatment-emergent suicide-related behaviors (relative risk of 8.84 percent) compared to other antidepressant medication in children and adolescents [Hammad et al., 2006], and has been associated with other treatment-emergent behavioral abnormalities, including hostility, overactivity, and agitation.

Drug Interactions

Venlafaxine or venlafaxine ER is contraindicated to be used in conjunction with a monoamine oxidase inhibitor and requires a 14-day washout period. Additionally, venlafaxine should only be used cautiously in conjunction with triptans due to the increased risk of serotonin syndrome. Although venlafaxine is metabolized by the CYP2D6 isoenzyme, the combined serum concentration of venlafaxine and its active metabolite does not appear to be altered by poor metabolizers [Effexor, 2009].

Table 49-5 Other Antidepressants

Drug	Preparation	Pharmacodynamic actions	Pharmacokinetic properties	Dosing
Buproprion	Wellbutrin (75 mg- and 100-mg tablets Wellbutrin SR (100-, 150- and 200-mg tablets Wellbutrin XL (150- and 300-mg tablets)	Weak inhibitor of neuronal uptake of NE and dopamine	Time to peak plasma conc (IR) = 2 hr Time to peak plasma conc (SR) = 3 hr Time to peak plasma conc (XL) = 5 hr Half life = 21 hr (chronic administration) Time to steady state = 8 days	Immediate release: initiate at 50 mg/day, increase by 50 mg weekly, Optimum dose: 100-250 mg/day or 3-6 mg/kg/day divided three times a day. Maximum dose 450 mg/day given three times a day with maximum of 150 mg per dose. Sustained release: Maximum dose 400 mg/day given twice a day with maximum of 200 mg per dose Extended release: maximum 450 mg/day given once daily
Venlafaxine	Effexor (25-, 37.5-, 50-, 75- and 100-mg tablets) Effexor XR (37.5-, 75- and 150-mg extended release capsules)	At low doses, inhibits 5HT re-uptake At high doses, inhibits 5HT and NE re-uptake	Time to peak plasma conc (IR) = 2 hr venlafaxine, 3 hr ODV* Time to peak plasma conc (ER) = 5.5 hr venlafaxine, 9 hr ODV Half Life = 5 hr venlafaxine, 11 hr ODV Time to steady state = 3 days	Initiate at 25 to 37.5 mg daily, increase weekly up to 112.5 mg/day (<40kg) or 150 mg/day (40 – 49 kg) or 200 mg/day (>50 kg).
Mirtazapine	Remeron (15- and 30-mg scored tablets) Remeron SofTab (15-, 30- and 45-mg orally disintegrating tablets	Antagonism of 5HT2 and 5HT3 receptors, H1 histaminic receptors, and presynaptic α2 adrenergic receptors	Time to peak plasma conc = 2 hr Half Life = 20-40 hr (females > males) Time to steady state = 5 days	Initiate at 7.5 mg/day at bedtime and rapidly adjust upward to 30-45 mg/day to avoid low dose side effects.

*O-desmethylvenlafaxine – active metabolite of venlafaxine; IR, immediate release, SR, sustained release; ER, extended release

Other Antidepressants

Bupropion

CLINICAL APPLICATIONS

Bupropion (Wellbutrin®, Zyban®) is FDA-approved for the treatment of depression, nicotine dependence, and smoking cessation in adults 2009 [Wellbutrin, 2009]. Off-label uses of bupropion include monotherapy in the treatment of depression in children and adolescents, augmentation of selective serotonin reuptake inhibitor therapy in the treatment of depression [Lam et al., 2004], management of selective serotonin reuptake inhibitor-induced sexual side effects [Masand et al., 2001], and as a second-line agent in the treatment of ADHD. Bupropion may improve symptoms of ADHD in prepubertal children [Casat et al., 1989; Simeon et al., 1986]. Effect sizes of bupropion and placebo differences were smaller than for standard stimulant medications [Casat et al., 1989]. However, bupropion appeared to have comparable efficacy compared with methylphenidate in a double-blind, crossover-design study [Barrickman et al., 1995]. Adolescents with depression [Glod et al., 2003] and adolescents with ADHD and co-occurring depression [Daviss et al., 2001] demonstrated improvement with bupropion.

PHARMACOLOGY

Bupropion is available in immediate-release tablets (Wellbutrin®, Zyban®) and extended-release tablets (Wellbutrin SR®, Wellbutrin XL®). The mechanism of action in ameliorating depression is unknown. In animals, bupropion selectively inhibits noradrenergic neurons in the locus ceruleus and inhibits the reuptake of dopamine, but it does not have significant activity at α-adrenergic, cholinergic, or histaminic receptors. Bupropion is well absorbed through the gastrointestinal tract, with a peak serum concentration attained in 2–3 hours and a half-life of 14–21 hours. Steady-state concentrations are achieved in 8 days. Steady-state plasma levels achieved with the extended-release form were about 85 percent of the immediate-release preparation. Bupropion is 80 percent bound to serum albumin. It is metabolized by the liver (primarily by CYP2B6) and excreted in urine and feces. Although bupropion has been found to induce its own metabolism in animals, this has not been specifically studied in humans (see Table 49-5) [Wellbutrin, 2009].

CLINICAL MANAGEMENT

In addition to the standard assessment for ADHD or depression, possible risk factors for adverse effects with bupropion should be identified. Bupropion has been associated with seizures in approximately 0.4 percent of patients treated at doses up to 450 mg/day. The risk of seizures appears to be strongly associated with peak serum concentrations and dose. The incidence of seizures appears to increase significantly above daily doses of 450 mg and with rapid dose titration [Wellbutrin, 2009]. The risk of seizures with bupropion increases with conditions that lower the seizure threshold, such as preexisting seizure disorder, metabolically unstable anorectic or bulimic patients, or those with head trauma, CNS tumors, concomitant use of medications that lower seizure threshold, excessive use of alcohol, and abrupt withdrawal of alcohol or sedatives. Patients with hepatic cirrhosis may have impaired metabolism of bupropion, resulting in elevated bupropion levels and increased risk of seizures, even at modest doses. No specific laboratory tests are recommended by the manufacturer before initiation. To minimize the risk of seizures, the manufacturer recommends that clinicians titrate bupropion slowly and divide the dose three times per day (immediate release), with each single dose no greater than 150 mg to avoid large peak serum concentrations. The dose should not exceed 450 mg/day for immediate-release preparations and 400 mg/day for extended-release preparations [Wellbutrin, 2009].

Bupropion has not been FDA-approved for use in children or adolescents. Conservative dosing strategies begin at 50 mg/day and are increased by 50 mg/day at weekly intervals [Simeon et al., 1986]. Optimal doses in studies have ranged from 100 mg to 250 mg/day in prepubertal children [Clay et al., 1988; Simeon et al., 1986] or 3–6 mg/kg/day [Conners et al., 1996]. No incidence of seizure was reported in these studies. If symptoms fail to respond to therapeutic doses of bupropion over this period, the medication should be tapered slowly to avoid adverse effects.

ADVERSE EFFECTS

Common adverse effects include agitation, dry mouth, insomnia, headache, nausea, vomiting, constipation, and tremor [Wellbutrin, 2009]. Neuropsychiatric side effects have been observed in some patients, including psychotic symptoms and confusion. In general, antidepressants carry a risk of inducing manic symptoms in patients with bipolar affective disorder. The risk of inducing mania with bupropion is thought to be less than with tricyclic antidepressants and selective serotonin reuptake inhibitors [Sachs et al., 1994] . Bupropion has been reported to exacerbate tics in children with co-occurring ADHD and Tourette's syndrome [Spencer et al., 1993].

DRUG INTERACTIONS

Because bupropion is metabolized by CYP2B6, plasma concentrations may increase if it is given concomitantly with inhibitors of this enzyme (e.g., orphenadrine, cyclophosphamide). Bupropion inhibits CYP2D6 and potentially increases the plasma concentrations of other medications metabolized by this isoenzyme (e.g., tricyclic antidepressants and some selective serotonin reuptake inhibitors). The combination of bupropion with monoamine oxidase inhibitors may precipitate a hypertensive crisis. Both Wellbutrin® and Zyban® contain bupropion, and this combination is contraindicated because of an increased risk of seizure. Concurrent use of L-DOPA and bupropion has been associated with an increased rate of adverse effects [Wellbutrin, 2009].

Mirtazapine

CLINICAL APPLICATIONS

Mirtazapine (Remeron®) is available in 15-, 30-, and 45-mg tablets and orally disintegrating tablets. It is FDA-approved for the treatment of major depressive disorder in adults. In short-term studies, it appears to be more effective than placebo and comparable to amitriptyline in improving depressive symptoms [Bremner, 1995; Claghorn and Lesem, 1995]. Use of mirtazapine is off-label for any indication in children and adolescents. Two unpublished randomized, placebo-controlled studies of mirtazapine in children and adolescents failed to show superiority of mirtazapine to placebo for depression. One open-label study of mirtazapine showed improvement in children and adolescents with social phobia, although tolerability was limited due to weight gain and high discontinuation rate for adverse events [Mrakotsky et al., 2008].

PHARMACOLOGY

Mirtazapine increases synaptic levels of norepinephrine and serotonin through antagonism of α_2-adrenergic receptors in the CNS. It is an antagonist at $5HT_2$ and $5HT_3$ receptors, increasing relative $5HT_1$ activity. Mirtazapine has antagonist activity at H_1 histaminic, α_1-adrenergic, and muscarinic receptors. Mirtazapine is well absorbed from the gastrointestinal tract. It reaches peak concentration in 2 hours, and its elimination half-life is in the range of 20–40 hours. Mirtazapine is metabolized by the liver and excreted in the urine. The isoenzymes CYP2D6, CYP1A2, and CYP3A4 are involved in its metabolism (see Table 49-5) [Remeron, 2007].

CLINICAL MANAGEMENT

In clinical practice, the sedating and appetite-stimulating effects of mirtazapine may be useful for patients who suffer from insomnia, agitation, decreased appetite, or anxiety as part of their depressive syndrome. Patients may be started at 7.5 mg (orally disintegrating tablets cannot be split) to 15 mg at bedtime. The dose may be increased up to a maximum of 45 mg daily at intervals of 1–2 weeks [Remeron, 2007]. More rapid dose escalation and uses of higher doses may actually be associated with fewer side effects, especially sedation and increased appetite [Preskorn, 2000].

ADVERSE EFFECTS

Common side effects of mirtazapine include sedation, dizziness, nausea, increased appetite, weight gain, and increased serum levels of cholesterol. Effects on sedation and appetite decrease at higher doses of mirtazapine [Preskorn, 2000]. Less common side effects include liver enzyme elevations (i.e., aspartate transaminase) greater than three times the upper limit of the normal range and induction of mania or hypomania. Mirtazapine has been associated with rare cases of neutropenia or agranulocytosis in premarketing clinical trials [Remeron, 2007].

DRUG INTERACTIONS

Mirtazapine may have additive effects if combined with alcohol or other CNS depressants. Mirtazapine is not a potent inhibitor of CYP2D6, CYP1A2, or CYP3A4. Combination of mirtazapine and monoamine oxidase inhibitors may induce a hypertensive crisis [Remeron, 2007].

Anxiolytics

Anxiety disorders are one of the most prevalent categories of childhood and adolescent psychopathology. Approximately 8.9 percent of prepubertal children [Costello, 1989] in a general pediatric sample and approximately 8.7 percent of an adolescent sample [Kashani and Orvaschel, 1988] met criteria for at least one anxiety disorder. Anxiety disorders in children tend to have a chronic course with low remission rates [Keller et al., 1992]. Co-occurring conditions, such as other anxiety disorders [Kendall et al., 2010, Straus and Last, 1993], depression

[Bernstein and Borchardt, 1991; Kashani and Orvaschel, 1988], and ADHD [Anderson et al., 1987; Last et al., 1987] are common.

Treatment of anxiety disorders in children and adolescents is multimodal, including psychoeducational and cognitive behavioral therapy, family therapy, school interventions, and pharmacotherapy [Connolly and Bernstein, 2007]. Choices include tricyclic antidepressants, selective serotonin reuptake inhibitors, benzodiazepines, and α₂-agonists and β-blockers. Selective serotonin reuptake inhibitors are the pharmacologic treatment of choice. Tricyclic antidepressants may be a reasonable choice for patients with co-occurring depression [Bernstein et al., 1996], ADHD [Pliszka, 2003], or enuresis [Fritz et al., 2004], or who cannot tolerate selective serotonin reuptake inhibitors. The role of benzodiazepines is limited to the short-term management of anxiety symptoms. In cases of severe anxiety, they may be added to tricyclic antidepressants or selective serotonin reuptake inhibitors for acute management of anxiety symptoms until the therapeutic effects of the antidepressants emerge. In clinical practice, the use of benzodiazepines is limited by concerns about possible abuse or dependence, drug diversion, and adverse cognitive effects.

Benzodiazepines
Clinical Applications

Benzodiazepines are classified as sedative-hypnotic medications. They act as sedatives or anxiolytics at low doses and sleep-inducing hypnotics at high doses. Although rapidly effective in relieving symptoms, they carry a risk of tolerance, dependence, and withdrawal with long-term use. These effects may be avoided by using only moderate doses for short-term therapy (1–2 weeks) [Sadock and Sadock, 2007]. Benzodiazepines differ from each other with regard to relative potency and half-life. In contrast to long-half-life benzodiazepines, short-half-life benzodiazepines are associated with less daytime sedation, more frequent dosing, earlier and more severe withdrawal syndromes, rebound insomnia, and anterograde amnesia. Long-half-life benzodiazepines require less frequent dosing and have a less severe withdrawal syndrome, but high plasma concentrations of the drug may accumulate and cause signs of toxicity over time [Sadock and Sadock, 2007].

Case reports and small open trials indicate that clonazepam and alprazolam may be helpful in treating anxiety disorders in children and adolescents [Biederman, 1987; Kutcher and MacKenzie, 1988; Simeon and Ferguson, 1987]. However, placebo-controlled studies have not supported their use [Graae et al., 1994; Simeon et al., 1992].

With the availability of more effective anxiolytics (e.g., selective serotonin reuptake inhibitors, tricyclic antidepressants), benzodiazepines are not considered first-line treatment for anxiety disorders in children and adolescents. However, benzodiazepines can be useful for the short-term management of specific anxiety-provoking situations, such as medical procedures, or as short-term adjunctive treatment with selective serotonin reuptake inhibitors in the initial treatment of severe anxiety disorders. Chronic administration of benzodiazepines for anxiety should be undertaken only after patients have failed more effective treatments for anxiety, including other medications and behaviorally oriented psychotherapy.

Additionally, benzodiazepines, most notably lorazepam, have been found effective for the treatment of catatonia. Higher doses than are typical for treatment of anxiety are often required (Caroff et al., 2004).

Pharmacology

Benzodiazepines are well absorbed from the gastrointestinal tract. They are extensively metabolized in the liver and excreted in urine. Benzodiazepine plasma concentrations are sensitive to medications that inhibit or induce cytochrome P-450 isoenzymes

Table 49-6 Benzodiazapines: Pharmakokinetic Properties, Dosing and Drug Interactions

Drug	Preparations	Dose Equiv.	Half-Life	Dosing	Drug Interactions
Alprazolam	Xanax (0.25-, 0.5-, 1-, and 2- mg tablets) Xanax XR (0.5-, 1-, 2- and 3-mg tablets)	0.25	6-27 hr	Initial dose (IR) of 0.25 mg/day if < 40 kg, or 0.5 mg if > 40 kg Maximum dose of 0.04 mg/kg/day in divided doses twice a day or four times a day	CNS depressants (additive effects) Inhibitors of cytochrome P-450 34A (↑ plasma concentrations) Fluvoxamine and fluoxetine (↑ plasma conc) Oral contraceptives (↑ plasma conc)
Clonazepam	Klonopin (0.5- 1.0- and 2-mg tablets) Klonopin wafer (0.125-, 0.5-, 1- and 2-mg oral disintegrating tablet)	0.5	>20 hr	Initial dose of 0.25- 0.5 mg/day, increase by 0.25-0.5 mg every 3-4 days or more quickly agitation or catatonia Maximum dose = 2 mg/day for anxiety, higher for agitation, catatonia.	CNS depressants (additive effects) Inhibitors of cytochrome P-450 34A (↑ plasma concentrations) Fluoxetine – no interaction Inducers of cytochrome P-450 (eg carbamazapine, phenytoin - ↓ plasma conc)
Diazepam	Valium (2-, 5-, and 10-mg tablets) Diazapam injectable (5mg/ml)	5	>20 hr (increases with age)	Initial dose of 1 to 2.5 mg three times a day or four times a day, increase gradually as needed and tolerated	CNS depression (additive effects) Inhibitors of cytochrome P-450 34A (↑ plasma concentrations)
Lorazepam	Ativan (0.5-, 1-, and 2-mg tablets) Ativan Injectable (2 mg/ml, 4 mg/ml)	1	6-20 hr	Usual daily dose of 1 to 6 mg/day, higher doses may be required for catatonia	CNS depression (additive effects) Inhibitors of cytochrome P-450 34A (↑ plasma concentrations)

IR, immediate release

(see "Drug Interactions"). Benzodiazepines activate gamma-aminobutyric acid (GABA) benzodiazepine binding sites, which open chloride channels, resulting in a reduced rate of neuronal firing and muscle activity (Table 49-6) [Sadock, 2007].

Clinical Management

In considering benzodiazepine therapy for a patient, the clinician should inquire about any possible history of substance abuse, as combined use of benzodiazepines and other CNS depressants can be lethal [Moody, 2004], and benzodiazepines can also be abused or diverted [Longo and Johnson, 2000]. Family history of substance abuse may identify patients who are at risk for drug abuse or dependence, and household members with substance use histories may indicate a risk for drug diversion. Concomitant use of medications and co-occurring medical conditions that may affect the metabolism of benzodiazepines should be identified. The patient and family should be informed about the risks of tolerance, dependence, and withdrawal effects, as well as possible effects on cognitive and motor functioning. During treatment, the clinician must ensure that medications are not overused, abused, or diverted, and should monitor for possible adverse cognitive or behavioral side effects. After the treatment trial is complete, the medication should be tapered slowly because of the potential for withdrawal and rebound anxiety [Coffey, 1993; Kutcher et al., 1992].

Adverse Effects

The most frequent adverse effects in children and adolescents are sedation, drowsiness, and decreased mental acuity [Biederman, 1991]. Benzodiazepines may cause paradoxical behavioral disinhibition, which manifests as increased agitation, aggression, and hyperactivity. This has been described with clonazepam in children [Graae et al., 1994] and adolescents [Reiter and Kutcher, 1991]. Anterograde amnesia also has been associated with benzodiazepines, particularly high-potency benzodiazepines [Uzun et al., 2010].

Benzodiazepine therapy carries a risk of tolerance, dependence, and withdrawal effects. Abrupt discontinuation or rapid dose reduction has been associated with seizures, delirium, and withdrawal symptoms [Uzun et al., 2010].

Drug Interactions

Additive CNS depression may occur when benzodiazepines are administered concomitantly with other CNS depressants, such as alcohol. Disulfiram may decrease the clearance of diazepam and chlordiazepoxide. Because benzodiazepines are metabolized by cytochrome P-450 isoenzymes, inhibitors and inducers of these isoenzymes can significantly alter the plasma concentration of benzodiazepines. Clonazepam and phenytoin decrease each other's plasma concentrations. Valproate may increase plasma concentrations of lorazepam [Depakote, 2009].

Buspirone

Clinical Applications

Buspirone (BuSpar®) is approved for use in the treatment of anxiety disorders and for short-term relief of symptoms of anxiety [Buspar, 2010]. It is typically used in the treatment of generalized anxiety disorder. Buspirone does not appear to be effective as monotherapy in other anxiety disorders, such as post-traumatic stress disorder, panic disorder [Sheehan et al., 1988], or social phobia [van Vliet et al., 1997]. Although

randomized, controlled trials do not support the use of buspirone to augment selective serotonin reuptake inhibitors in partial responders, some patients with depression [Dimitriou and Dimitriou, 1998] and OCD [Jenike et al., 1991] may benefit.

Open trials of buspirone in adolescents with generalized anxiety disorder [Kutcher et al., 1992] and children and adolescents with varied anxiety disorders [Simeon, 1991] demonstrate benefit. Additionally, buspirone appeared to improve anxiety and irritability in children with pervasive developmental disorders [Buitelaar et al., 1998] and may improve anxiety and aggression symptoms in some hospitalized children [Pfeffer et al., 1997]. However, two large unpublished, industry-sponsored, randomized, controlled trials in children and adolescents with generalized anxiety disorder did not demonstrate benefit [Buspar, 2010]. Buspirone offers several potential benefits over benzodiazepines, including lack of euphoric effects, performance impairment, abuse potential, and withdrawal symptoms with discontinuation. Although buspirone appears to be as effective as benzodiazepines in decreasing psychic symptoms of anxiety, it appears to be less effective for somatic symptoms of anxiety, and the onset of therapeutic effect may be delayed 2–4 weeks [Kutcher et al., 1992].

Pharmacology

Buspirone differs from benzodiazepines in that it has no activity at the GABA-benzodiazepine receptor complex. Buspirone acts as a partial agonist or mixed agonist/antagonist at $5HT_{1A}$ receptors, as an agonist at postsynaptic dopamine receptors, and as an antagonist at presynaptic autoreceptor and postsynaptic sites in the CNS. Buspirone is rapidly absorbed from the gastrointestinal tract. Only 4 percent of the dose reaches systemic circulation because of extensive first-pass metabolism. Buspirone is metabolized in the liver, primarily by the CYP3A4 isoenzyme. Its primary metabolite, 1-pyrimidinylpiperazine (1-PP), has clinical activity. The elimination half-life is about 2–4 hours in all age groups and is prolonged by renal or hepatic impairment. Unlike adolescents or adults, prepubertal children show the highest concentration of the active metabolite, 1-PP, after oral administration of buspirone at doses of 15–60 mg/day, which may account for higher incidence of side effects in this group [Salazar et al., 2001]. The onset of clinical response may appear within the first 2 weeks of therapy, but optimal therapeutic effect is usually delayed [Kutcher et al., 1992].

Clinical Management

Laboratory screening is not required before prescribing buspirone. The typical starting dose is 5 mg taken 2–3 times daily, with gradual increases to 15 mg taken three times daily. Younger children may be started at 2.5–5 mg/day and gradually increased to a total dose of 20–30 mg/day, administered in divided doses 2–3 times daily [Scahill and Martin, 2002].

Adverse Effects

The most common adverse effects of buspirone are dizziness, headache, drowsiness, and lightheadedness [Buspar, 2007]. Side effects in adults appear to be dose-related and to decrease over time [Feighner and Cohn, 1989]. CNS depression is less common than in benzodiazepines. Behavioral activation, including agitation, aggression and euphoric mania, has been described in prepubertal children [Pfeffer et al., 1997].

Drug Interactions

Combination of buspirone and monoamine oxidase inhibitors may result in a hypertensive crisis, requiring emergency medical attention. Because of reports of liver transaminase elevations with the concomitant use of buspirone and trazodone, the manufacturer recommends monitoring liver function when prescribing this combination. Because buspirone is highly protein-bound, it may displace other medications that are protein-bound and increase their free plasma level. Inducers of CYP3A4 may decrease plasma levels of buspirone. Alternatively, inhibitors of CYP3A4 (e.g., fluvoxamine, erythromycin, grapefruit juice) may increase the serum concentration of buspirone. Increased serum concentrations of haloperidol have been reported when combined with buspirone [Buspar, 2010].

Mood Stabilizers

The term mood stabilizers refers to medications used to treat severe, fluctuating moods, including depression and mania in bipolar disorder. Mood stabilizers have antimanic and antidepressant properties and treat specific mood states without negatively impacting other mood states (i.e., worsening depression when mania is treated, or vice versa).

The diagnosis of bipolar disorder in children is controversial for a number of reasons. Historically, it was thought not to exist in children; the presentation of bipolar disorder in children does not always resemble the presentation in adults; there is the perception of overdiagnosis; and with limited evidence of efficacy, use of medications for bipolar disorder in prepubertal children is rising. Although juvenile bipolar disorder has sometimes been overdiagnosed [Carlson, 1990], it is often under-recognized, or misdiagnosed as schizophrenia or disruptive behavior disorders [Carlson et al., 1994]. The phenotype of juvenile bipolar disorder has not been well defined and different investigators have utilized varying criteria [DelBello and Grcevich, 2004; Leibenluft et al., 2006]. Efforts to operationalize the diagnosis of juvenile bipolar disorder better are on-going [Leibenluft et al., 2003]. Bipolar children can, but are not likely to, exhibit classic symptoms of adult bipolar disorder. Rather, children with bipolar disorder are more likely to exhibit atypical manic or mixed-mood symptoms [Swann et al., 2005]. Adding to the complexity of making the diagnosis is the broad differential diagnosis and co-occurrence of other neuropsychiatric disorders [McClellan et al., 2007].

Evidence supporting the use of mood stabilizers to treat the acute episodes of mood disturbances and for prophylactic use during the maintenance phase of bipolar disorder [APA, 2002] will be reviewed. Mood stabilizers used in clinical practice can be grouped into four categories:

- lithium, which is approved for use in the acute treatment of mania and for mania prophylaxis in adults
- anticonvulsants approved for use in adults with bipolar disorder (e.g., valproic acid, lamotrigine, carbamazepine)
- antipsychotics approved for use in adults, children, and adolescents with bipolar disorder (e.g., risperidone, olanzapine, quetiapine)
- anticonvulsants prescribed off-label in all age groups (e.g., gabapentin, oxcarbazepine).

Each mood stabilizer is not equally effective for all phases of the disorder or as prophylaxis. In adults, lithium, valproate, carbamazepine, risperidone, olanzapine, ziprasidone, aripiprazole, and quetiapine are currently approved for treating acute mania. Lamotrigine, seroquel, and olanzapine are labeled for use during the depressive phase of bipolar disorder [Calabrese et al., 1999; Evins, 2003]. Lithium, lamotrigine, quetiapine, olanzapine, and aripiprazole are FDA-approved for use during the maintenance phase of treatment as prophylaxis against recurrent episodes.

Combining medications in the treatment of bipolar affective disorder in adults is common. Typical treatment consists of long-term maintenance with a mood stabilizer as prophylaxis. An antipsychotic or an additional mood stabilizer may be added to stabilize the acute symptoms of a manic episode [Drug treatments for bipolar disorder, 2005; Narayan and Haddad, 2010]. During a depressive episode, an antidepressant, lamotrigine, or atypical antipsychotic may be added while cautiously monitoring for the possible emergence of antidepressant-induced manic or rapid-cycling symptoms [Drug treatments for bipolar disorder, 2005; Narayan and Haddad, 2010].

The pediatric literature is less well developed than that for adults and is complicated by diagnostic variability between studies. However there is an emerging evidence base for the treatment of bipolar I disorder. In the past several years, risperidone, olanzapine, quetiapine, and aripiprazole were FDA-approved for treatment of bipolar I disorder in youngsters 10 years and older (with the exception of olanzapine, which is 13 years and older). Additionally, lithium is FDA-approved for use in youngsters of 12 years and older for bipolar disorder, although the evidence base for this labeling is not robust and results from a downward extension of the adult literature. As with childhood depression, children with bipolar affective disorder are thought to be less responsive to medication compared with adults [McClellan et al., 2007]. Combination of mood stabilizers [Findling et al., 2003], or a mood stabilizer with an antipsychotic [Kafantaris, 1995], is sometimes required to stabilize acute manic symptoms. Studies looking at efficacy of combination therapies in children and adolescents are lacking.

Given the complexity of making an accurate diagnosis, the treatment-resistant nature of pediatric bipolar illness, and the complicated regimens of medication sometimes required, the average pediatric neurologist may wish to request a consultation from a child psychiatrist if faced with a patient with possible bipolar disorder.

Lithium

Clinical Applications

Lithium is FDA-approved for use in the treatment of bipolar affective disorder. It is effective in managing acute manic and depressive episodes, preventing or diminishing the intensity of subsequent episodes in maintenance treatment, and decreasing mood instability between episodes [Goodwin and Jamison, 2007]. Data in children and adolescents with bipolar disorder are limited and offer mixed results. Several earlier studies showed good response rates [DeLong and Aldershof, 1987; Strober et al., 1990; Varanka et al., 1988], although this was not universally demonstrated [Carlson et al., 1992]. These studies were largely uncontrolled and naturalistic, varied in diagnostic criteria, and included mixed diagnostic groups (e.g., bipolar I, bipolar II, bipolar not otherwise specified (NOS)), making interpretation of results difficult. A more recent large open-label study has provided additional support for the use of lithium in adolescents with bipolar disorder [Kafantaris et al., 2003], although the need for larger randomized, controlled studies of children and adolescents in both the acute and maintenance phases is recognized and protocols are currently in development [Findling et al., 2008a]. Lithium also has been used with positive results in the treatment of severe aggression in adults [Sheard, 1975] and children [Campbell et al., 1984; DeLong and Aldershof, 1987; Malone et al., 2000].

Pharmacology

Lithium is an alkali metal, similar to sodium and potassium, and it is available in salt form as lithium carbonate or lithium citrate. Lithium has effects at the cellular level (i.e., cell membrane ion channels and cyclic adenosine monophosphate second-messenger cellular processes) and in neurotransmitter systems. However, the specific mechanism of action is unclear [Lenox and Wang, 2003].

Lithium is available in immediate-release and sustained-release preparations. Ninety percent of immediate-release lithium is absorbed by the gastrointestinal tract; 60–90 percent of extended-release lithium is absorbed. Immediate-release lithium reaches peak serum levels in 1–1.5 hours (4–12 hours for the extended-release form), and it is almost completely excreted in urine, with the remainder excreted in the feces and breast milk. Lithium has a half-life of about 20 hours and reaches steady-state levels after 1 week of administration [FDA, 2010].

Clinical Management

Before starting lithium therapy, the patient should be screened for conditions that may contraindicate or complicate lithium therapy, such as pregnancy, renal disease, or diabetes mellitus. A medical evaluation should be completed, including an EKG, laboratory screen for electrolytes, kidney and thyroid function tests, CBC, urinalysis, and urine pregnancy screen.

Lithium is started at dosages ranging from 300 to 600 mg/day. Formulas [Weller et al., 1986] and nomograms [Alessi et al., 1999; Geller and Fetner, 1989] have been developed to guide lithium dosing in pediatric populations. Trough lithium levels (10–12 hours after last dose) are drawn when steady state is achieved, at least 5 days after initiating lithium or changing the dose. The recommended therapeutic serum levels range from 0.6 to 1.2 mEq/L in adults, although therapeutic level has not been firmly established in children. Lithium levels between 0.8 and 1.0 mEq/L may offer the best prophylaxis against mania, whereas lower levels may be adequate for prophylaxis against depression [Severus et al., 2005, 2009]. Lithium levels above the therapeutic range increase the risk of toxicity. Early therapeutic effects may be detected at 10–14 days after achieving a therapeutic level; however, there is often a significant lag of 4–6 weeks [Kowatch et al., 2000]. Between 4 and 6 weeks of lithium at therapeutic serum concentrations constitutes an adequate trial. Because several days are required to achieve therapeutic plasma concentrations, antipsychotic medications may be necessary to stabilize severe mania acutely, especially if psychotic symptoms are present.

After mood symptoms are stabilized, lithium levels should be routinely checked every 3–6 months. Other indications to obtain a lithium level include symptoms of toxicity, worsening side effects, and breakthrough mood symptoms. Urinalysis, renal evaluation [Jefferson, 2010], and thyroid function tests should be repeated every 3–6 months to monitor for the emergence of subclinical renal and thyroid dysfunction (Table 49-7).

Stabilization of manic symptoms may be prolonged up to several years [Biederman et al., 1998]. Lithium should be continued for at least 18 months after manic symptoms have been stabilized [APA, 2002] because discontinuation of lithium therapy, especially abrupt discontinuation, is associated with increased relapse rates [Strober et al., 1990].

Adverse Effects

Side effects of lithium are polydipsia, polyuria or enuresis, gastric distress (i.e., nausea, vomiting, and diarrhea), weight gain, tremor, fatigue, leukocytosis, acne, and mild cognitive impairment [Alessi et al., 1999; Silva et al., 1992]. Serious renal side effects are rare and include nephrotic syndrome, features of distal renal tubular acidosis, nonspecific interstitial fibrosis, and renal failure [Alessi et al., 1999; Gelenberg and Schoonover, 1991]. Lithium therapy can induce alterations in thyroid function tests and produce hypothyroidism [Alessi et al., 1999]. Lithium can have rare cardiac side effects, including first-degree atrioventricular block, irregular sinus rhythm, and increased premature ventricular contractions [Gelenberg and Schoonover, 1991]. Reversible conduction abnormalities in children have been demonstrated on their EKGs [Campbell et al., 1972]. Studies examining the long-term effects of lithium treatment of children are lacking. Intrauterine exposure to lithium during the first trimester has been associated with teratogenic effects, most commonly Ebstein's anomaly of the tricuspid valve [Giles and Bannigan, 2006]. Lithium has been associated with pseudotumor cerebri in children [Kelly et al., 2009].

Drug Interactions

Lithium levels are affected by medications or conditions that can alter the body's fluid and electrolyte status. Dehydration and extremely low salt intake can result in elevated lithium levels. Likewise, an extremely high salt intake can result in lowered lithium levels. Many medications, such as diuretics, nonsteroidal anti-inflammatory drugs, and tetracycline, can cause an increase in lithium levels by influencing renal clearance [Finley et al., 1995].

Lithium is commonly used in combination with other psychotropic medications in the treatment of bipolar disorder. However, a number of case reports have described neurotoxicity occurring rarely when combined with other mood-stabilizing medications, including antipsychotic medications [Finley et al., 1995].

Valproic Acid

Clinical Applications

Valproic acid is approved for the treatment of seizures, migraine prophylaxis, and the manic phase of bipolar affective disorder in adults [Depakote, 2009]. The initial support for use of valproic acid in child psychiatric practice came from the adult literature. The evidence for its use in the treatment of juvenile bipolar disorder, however, is limited. Although some support for the use of valproic acid was derived from earlier case series and open trials [Henry et al., 2003; Kowatch et al., 2000; Wagner et al., 2002], a large, double-blind, randomized, placebo-controlled trial did not demonstrate superiority of divalproex extended release over placebo in the acute phase management of bipolar disorder [Wagner et al., 2009]. Divalproex sodium has also been shown in small studies to benefit children and adolescents with explosive temper and mood lability [Donovan et al., 2000] and for treatment of core symptoms of autism and associated symptoms of affective instability, aggression, and impulsivity [Hollander et al., 2001].

Table 49-7 Mood Stabilizers: Baseline Assessment, Monitoring, and Adverse Effects

Drug	Preparations	Baseline Assessments	Monitoring	Adverse Effects
Lithium immediate release Lithium, sustained release	Lithium carbonate (150-, 300-, and 600-mg capsules) Lithium carbonate (300-mg tablets) Lithium citrate syrup (8mEq/ml) Lithobid (300-mg tablets) Eskalith CR (450-mg tablets)	Laboratory screening: thyroid function tests, electrolytes, renal function tests, complete blood count, urinalysis, pregnancy test, Electrocardiogram	Lithium level (target of 0.8-1 ng/mL) during dose titration, every 3-6 months or with signs of toxicity or breakthrough symptoms. Urinalysis, thyroid-stimulating hormone, and renal function tests every 3-6 months or earlier with signs of toxicity.	Sedation, nausea, tremor, acne, weight gain, polydipsia, polyuria, enuresis, renal dysfunction, leukocytosis, hypothyroidism, and electrocardiographic changes.
Valproic acid Divalproex Sodium	Depakene (250-mg capsule) Depakene syrup (250 mg/5mL) Depakote (125-, 250-, and 500-mg delayed release tablets) Depakote (250- and 500-mg tablets) Depakote sprinkles (125-mg capsules with coated particles)	Laboratory screening: liver function tests, pancreatic enzymes, complete blood count, pregnancy test	Valproic acid level (target of 80-100 ng/mL) during dose titration, every 3-6 months, or with signs of toxicity or breakthrough symptoms Liver function tests, complete blood count, and pancreatic enzymes every 3-6 months or with signs of toxicity.	Sedation, nausea, weight gain, thrombocytopenia, elevated liver function tests, liver failure, pancreatitis, polycystic ovary syndrome.
Carbamazepine	Tegretol (200-mg scored tablets; 100-mg chewable tablets, 100 mg/5mL susp) Tegretol XR (extended release) (100-, 200-, and 300-mg tablets) Carbatrol (extended release) (100-, 200-, and 300-mg capsules)	Laboratory screening: liver function tests, complete blood count, electrolytes, pregnancy test	Carbamazepine level (target of 4-12 mg/mL) during dose titration, every 3-6 months, or with signs of toxicity or breakthrough symptoms. Liver function tests, complete blood count, and electrolytes every 3-6 months or with signs and symptoms of toxicity Monitor for rash	Nausea, vomiting, anorexia, ataxia, sedation, tremor, aplastic anemia, agranulocytosis, elevated liver function tests, hepatitis, cholestasis, life threatening skin conditions.
Oxcarbazepine	Trileptil (150-, 300-, and 600-mg tablets, 300mg/5mL suspension)	None	No routine laboratory monitoring but consider following serum sodium in patients at increased risk of hyponatremia Monitor for rash	Diplopia, dizziness, somnolence, fatigue, nausea, benign and rarely life threatening rashes, and hyponatremia
Lamotrogine	Lamictal (25-, 50-, 150-, and 200-mg tablets; 2-, 5-, and 25-mg chewable dispersible tablets) Lamictal ODT (25-, 50-, 100- and 200-mg oral disintegrating tablets)	None	Monitor for rash	Dizziness, ataxia, somnolence, headache, diplopia, blurred vision, nausea, vomiting, rash Serious rashes requiring hospitalization and discontinuation include Steven's Johnson syndrome (0.8% of pediatric population), toxic epidermal necrolysis
Topirimate	Topomax (25-, 50-, 100-, and 200-mg tablets; 15- and 25-mg sprinkle capsules)	None	No routine laboratory monitoring unless clinically indicated (i.e., electrolytes for symptoms of metabolic acidosis)	Fatigue, ataxia, confusion, impaired concentration and memory, sedation, agitation, anorexia with weight loss, kidney stones, diplopia and metabolic acidosis
Gabapentin	Neurontin (100-, 300-, and 400-mg capsules; 600- and 800-mg film coated tablets; 250 mg/5mL solution)	None	No routine monitoring	Dizziness, ataxia, sedation, fatigue, nystagmus, dyspepsia, peripheral edema, diplopia and amblyopia, hyperactivity and aggression.

Pharmacology

The mechanism of action of valproic acid is unidentified, although it is known to increase brain concentrations of the inhibitory neurotransmitter GABA. Valproic acid is available in several preparations: valproate (Depakene® capsules); valproate syrup (Depakene® syrup); divalproex (Depakote®); divalproex capsules with coated particles (Depakote Sprinkle®); divalproex sodium, delayed-release tablets (Depakote®); and divalproex sodium in extended-release tablets (Depakote ER®).

Valproate rapidly converts to valproic acid in the stomach. Divalproex dissociates into valproic acid in the gastrointestinal tract. Valproic acid is rapidly and almost entirely absorbed from the gastrointestinal tract. Peak plasma concentrations are achieved 1–4 hours, 3–5 hours, and 7–14 hours after oral administration of valproate, divalproex, and extended-release tablets, respectively. Food intake can retard the time to peak plasma concentrations, although this has little clinical consequence once steady-state concentrations have been achieved. Valproic acid binds plasma proteins; therefore, the presence of other protein-binding drugs can increase the unbound or free fraction of valproic acid. Conversely, the addition of valproate with another protein-bound drug can increase the unbound or free fraction of the other drug. Renal and hepatic insufficiency can reduce protein binding, which can increase unbound valproate. Additionally, plasma protein binding of valproic acid is dependent on drug concentration. Concentrations of free valproic acid increase at serum levels above 100 mg/mL. Peak and trough concentrations with delayed-release tablets and capsules containing coated particles may differ from the equivalent dose of valproic acid. Valproic acid is metabolized in the liver and excreted predominantly in the urine [Depakote, 2009]. No therapeutic serum concentrations for the treatment of behavioral or psychiatric disorders have been determined.

Clinical Management

In addition to the routine psychiatric or neurologic history, patients should be asked about risk factors affecting treatment with valproate, including pregnancy, disorders of metabolism, hepatic or renal disease, concomitant medications, and coagulation disorders. Laboratory screening should include liver function tests and a CBC, and a pregnancy test in females [Danielyan and Kowatch, 2005]. Parents should be educated about potential signs of hepatic or pancreatic toxicity and polycystic ovary disease.

Recommended initial dosing of valproic acid is 10–15 mg/kg/day, given in divided doses two or three times per day. Dosage may be increased by 5–10 mg/kg/day at weekly intervals [Depakote, 2009]. The manufacturer's maximum recommended dosage is 60 mg/kg/day. However, starting at lower doses and using slower upward adjustments of dose may be required for tolerability. Although therapeutic levels for treating mania have not been established, achieving a plasma concentration of 85–110 mg/L [Kowatch et al., 2000] is needed to consider a trial adequate for determining outcome in an individual patient. Divalproex extended release allows for once-daily dosing.

In adult psychiatry, an oral loading dose of valproate is sometimes used to achieve a therapeutic plasma concentration and to gain rapid control over mania. The tolerability of an oral loading dose of divalproex sodium was examined in children and adolescents [Good et al., 2001]. A loading dose of 15 mg/kg/day resulted in therapeutic plasma levels by day 5 of treatment and it was well tolerated. Dosage adjustment was required for overweight children, in order to avoid supratherapeutic drug levels [Good et al., 2001]. Total valproic acid levels should be checked when steady state is reached, after any dosage change, after conversion to a different preparation of valproate, for signs of toxicity, or for a change in clinical status.

Maintenance involves monitoring of the therapeutic response and side effects and requires laboratory screening. Liver enzymes, CBC, and serum valproic acid levels should be periodically monitored, although the exact frequency of testing has not been determined. Initially, monitoring may be done every 3–6 months for the first year and semiannually thereafter (see Table 49-7).

Adverse Effects

Adverse effects include sedation, nausea, vomiting, gastrointestinal upset, increased appetite, weight gain, and hair loss. Rare side effects include thrombocytopenia, platelet dysfunction, prolonged bleeding time, elevation in liver transaminase levels, and lactate dehydrogenase, and can occur without clinical symptoms. Children younger than 2 years appear to have an increased risk of hepatotoxicity, and extreme caution should be used in this population. This heightened risk may result from an undiagnosed metabolic or mitochondrial disorder. In particular, children with urea cycle defects, such as ornithine transcarbamylase deficiency, should not receive this medication. Carnitine supplementation should be considered when prescribing this medication, as this may facilitate the processing of valproate in the mitochondrial β-oxidation pathway. Valproate has also been associated with rare cases of hyperammonemic encephalopathy [Barrueto and Hack, 2001; Elgudin et al., 2003], which occurs more commonly with polypharmacy and with associated liver dysfunction [Verrotti et al., 1999]. One case reported in the child psychiatry literature manifested as increased aggression and confusion, an EEG with symmetric 5- to 6-Hz waves, elevated serum ammonia levels, and normal levels of serum liver transaminases [Yehya et al., 2004]; the situation resolved with valproic acid discontinuation. Elevated ammonia levels have also been observed in the absence of encephalopathy, but the clinical relevance of such laboratory abnormalities is unclear. Other reports suggest that oral carnitine can be useful in reducing ammonia levels [Bohan et al., 2001]. Rare cases of pancreatitis have been reported [Depakote, 2009]. Cases of polycystic ovary disease have been reported in some women treated with valproate for seizure disorder [Isojarvi et al., 1993]. It is unclear whether this is related to the medication or is an endocrine abnormality related to the epilepsy [Davis et al., 2000]. Intrauterine exposure to valproic acid during the first trimester is associated with neural tube defects [Depakote, 2009].

Drug Interactions

As it is metabolized by the cytochrome-P450 system, valproic acid has many interactions with medications that are also metabolized by this system. Medications that may increase valproic acid concentrations include erythromycin, selective serotonin reuptake inhibitors, guanfacine, and aspirin. Medications that may decrease concentrations of valproate include carbamazepine. Additionally, valproic acid may result in increases in concentration of other anticonvulsants (phenytoin, phenobarbital, primidone, carbamazepine, and lamotrigine), tricyclic antidepressants, diazepam, and warfarin. Great caution should be utilized when valproic acid is used in combination with lamotrigine due to enhanced risk of Stevens–Johnson syndrome. When valproic acid is combined with antipsychotics, CNS depressant effects and extrapyramidal side effects may increase. Valproic acid may increase lithium-associated tremor [Danielyan and Kowatch, 2005].

Carbamazepine

Clinical Applications

Limited data are available on the efficacy of carbamazepine for the treatment of bipolar disorder children and adolescents. Justification for its use in clinical practice has rested on the adult literature, which is difficult to interpret. Carbamazepine was superior to placebo and comparable to lithium [Lerer et al., 1987; Small et al., 1991] in improving manic symptoms. However, it was not as effective as valproate, and patients on carbamazepine required adjunctive medication to achieve stabilization [Vasudev et al., 2000]. Similarly, in children, carbamazepine was as effective as lithium but less so than valproic acid [Kowatch et al., 2000]. Carbamazepine may be helpful in the depressive phase of bipolar disorder [Dilsaver et al., 1996].

Through the induction of hepatic enzymes carbamazepine can have multiple drug interactions that complicate combined pharmacotherapy in the management of bipolar disorder. Clinicians and patients may prefer carbamazepine to the other mood stabilizers because of its reduced tendency to cause weight gain.

Pharmacology

Carbamazepine is structurally related to tricyclic antidepressants. It reduces activity at sodium and calcium channels, resulting in reduced synaptic transmission. It is available in immediate-release forms (e.g., Tegretol® tablets, chewable tablets, suspension) and extended-release capsules (i.e., Tegretol XR®). It is slowly absorbed from the gastrointestinal tract. The plasma half-life gradually decreases over 3–5 weeks from 25–65 hours to approximately 12–17 hours due to autoinduction. Steady-state concentrations are achieved in 2–4 days. Between 75 and 90 percent of the drug is bound to plasma proteins. It is metabolized in the liver and excreted in the urine [Tegretol, 2009].

Clinical Management

Patients should be evaluated for medical conditions that may contraindicate use of carbamazepine, including liver disease, hematologic disorders, immune disorders, cardiac disease, and pregnancy. Laboratory screening should include a urine pregnancy screen, liver function tests, and a CBC. Because laboratory screening can fail to predict impending hepatic and hematologic complications, parents should be aware of signs and symptoms indicating serious adverse effects, such as rash, symptoms of aplastic anemia or agranulocytosis, and hepatitis or cholestasis. Sexually active patients should be informed of its teratogenic effects and the possible decrease in effectiveness of oral contraceptives [Tegretol, 2009].

Dosage is initiated at 100–300 mg/day, increasing as tolerated while monitoring blood levels. Therapeutic blood levels in the treatment of mania have not been established. Recommended levels are the same as those for seizure disorder, 4–12 mg/mL [Rosenberg et al., 1994]. Blood levels should be checked 5 days after initiating or changing doses, and again in 4 weeks because of an anticipated reduction in plasma levels due to autoinduction. Although it is recommended that liver function tests, bilirubin levels, and CBCs be routinely checked every 3 months, the utility of such testing in predicting serious hepatic or hematologic complications is questionable (see Table 49-7). Hyponatremia resulting from carbamazepine use is rare in children, and if it is clinically suspected, sodium levels should be obtained.

Adverse Effects

The most common adverse effects are nausea, vomiting, sedation, and ataxia [Tegretol, 2009]. Carbamazepine can cause benign elevations in liver transaminases; hepatitis, indicated by elevated liver transaminase levels greater than three times normal; and cholestasis, indicated by elevations in bilirubin and alkaline phosphatase. Carbamazepine therapy has been associated with leukopenia in 1–2 percent of patients, and agranulocytosis or aplastic anemia in 1 of 250,000 patients. Although blood dyscrasias are not always predicted by leukopenia, CBCs are recommended at 3- to 6-month intervals. Other adverse effects observed with carbamazepine include cognitive or behavioral disturbance [Carpenter and Vining, 1993], CNS toxicity, altered cardiac conduction, and life-threatening dermatologic conditions (i.e., exfoliative dermatitis, toxic epidermal necrolysis, and Stevens–Johnson syndrome). Intrauterine exposure has been associated with neural tube defects and other fetal malformations [Rosa, 1991]. Case reports of manic reactions to carbamazepine may be related to its antidepressant structure [Myers and Carrera, 1989].

Drug Interactions

Carbamazepine is an inducer of CYP3A4, leading to decreased plasma concentrations of medications metabolized by this isoenzyme. Several medications that are commonly combined with carbamazepine in psychiatric practice may be affected, including anticonvulsants (e.g., lamotrigine, clonazepam, valproic acid), antidepressants (e.g., bupropion, clomipramine, desipramine, imipramine, nefazodone), and antipsychotics (e.g., clozapine, fluphenazine, haloperidol, olanzapine, ziprasidone). Carbamazepine levels can be increased by fluoxetine, lamotrigine, valproate, cimetidine, and erythromycin. Coadministration of carbamazepine with nefazodone results in inadequate levels of nefazodone and its active metabolite, and is therefore contraindicated. Combination with lithium or antipsychotics may increase the risk of adverse neurologic effects (e.g., drowsiness, dizziness, ataxia) [Tegretol, 2009].

Other Mood Stabilizers

Although lithium and valproate are first-line pharmacologic treatments for bipolar disorder in adults [APA, 2002], many children and adolescents do not respond adequately to these medications and cannot tolerate the side effects or the requirement of laboratory monitoring. In clinical practice, newer anticonvulsants are beginning to be used for the treatment of bipolar disorder. These medications include oxcarbazepine, lamotrigine, gabapentin, and topiramate. Many of these newer anticonvulsants have a more favorable adverse effect profile and do not require blood tests. Support for their use in clinical practice, however, has been primarily based on case reports and open trials. Use of these medications is more appropriate for patients with bipolar disorder who are unresponsive to traditional therapies or cannot tolerate traditional agents.

Lamotrigine

CLINICAL MANAGEMENT

Lamotrigine (Lamictal®) is approved for use in the treatment of epilepsy and for prophylaxis of mania during maintenance therapy for type 1 bipolar disorder [Lamictal, 2009]. In adults, lamotrigine appears to be helpful in the treatment of patients with bipolar depression [Calabrese et al., 1999; Evins, 2003], some patients with rapid-cycling bipolar disorder [Bowden et al., 1999; Calabrese et al., 2000; Frye et al., 2000], and as a prophylactic agent to prevent or attenuate recurrences of bipolar episodes [Bowden et al., 2003; Calabrese et al., 2000, 2003; McElroy et al., 2004]. Data on lamotrigine in pediatric bipolar disorder are limited to case series and open-label trials but suggest that, in adolescents, lamotrigine may be effective for the treatment of bipolar depression [Chang et al., 2006; Kusumakar and Yatham, 1997] and for the maintenance treatment of bipolar disorder [Pavuluri et al., 2009].

PHARMACOLOGY

Lamotrigine (Lamictal®) is a member of the phenyltriazine class of antiepileptic drugs and is chemically unrelated to other antiepileptic drugs. The mechanism of action of lamotrigine is unknown in both epilepsy and bipolar disorder. Lamotrigine may exert its effect on sodium channels and modulate release of excitatory amino acids, such as glutamate and aspartate [Lamictal, 2009]. Lamotrigine is available in scored tablets (Lamictal®), chewable dispersible tablets (which can be chewed or dissolved in juice), and orally disintegrating tablets (Lamictal ODT®). Lamotrigine is rapidly absorbed through the gastrointestinal tract, metabolized in the liver, and excreted in urine. Pharmacokinetic studies reveals that lamotrigine clearance is influenced by total body weight and by co-administration of other antiepileptic drug therapy. Specifically, children tend to have a higher lamotrigine clearance than adults, especially those under 30 kg, and may require a higher weight-corrected dose. As with adults, the clearance of lamotrigine is affected by concurrent antiepileptic drug treatment [Lamictal, 2009].

CLINICAL MANAGEMENT

Because supporting data are limited in pediatric populations, the use of lamotrigine in children and adolescents for the treatment of bipolar disorder should be reserved for those who have failed alternative treatments and demonstrate persistent disabling symptoms.

Before initiating treatment, a urine pregnancy test should be obtained. The patient and family should be educated about the risk of serious rash or hypersensitivity reaction (i.e., Stevens–Johnson syndrome), and instructed on how to recognize the signs and symptoms requiring immediate medical attention and the need for a slow titration [Joe et al., 2009] and slow retitration after discontinuation to avoid the rash.

Dosing for treatment of pediatric bipolar disorder is not established, but existing published reports in adolescent populations used gradual titration of lamotrigine over 6–8 weeks, starting at 12.5–25 mg with weekly or biweekly increments of 12.5–25 mg up, reaching doses between 100 and 200 mg daily based on clinical response [Chang et al., 2006; Pavuluri et al., 2009]. A painstaking approach to dose adjustment decreases the risk for rash, including Stevens–Johnson syndrome [Joe et al., 2009]. Doses were adjusted for adolescents on valproate with initial dosing of 12.5 mg, with weekly increments of 12.5 mg for a maximum daily dose between 50 and 100 mg daily. There are published dosing recommendations for pediatric patients who are being treated for epilepsy with and without concomitant antiepileptic drug treatment [Lamictal, 2009]. For children between the ages of 2 and 12 years who are not on other antiepileptic medications, 0.3 mg/kg/day of lamotrigine is administered in one or two divided doses (rounded down to the nearest 5 mg) for the first 2 weeks. During the third and fourth week, 0.6 mg/kg/day is administered in two divided doses (rounded down to the nearest 5 mg). The dose may be titrated up in increments of 0.6 mg/kg/day (rounded down to the nearest tab) every 2 weeks. The usual maintenance dose of seizures ranges from 4.5 to 7.5 mg/kg/day. For pediatric patients older than 12 years, 25 mg of lamotrigine is administered daily during the first 2 weeks of treatment. The dose is increased to 50 mg/day for the third and fourth week and given in two divided doses. The dose may be increased by increments of 50 mg/day every 1–2 weeks (see Table 49-7). Maintenance dosage ranges from 225 to 375 mg daily, given in two divided doses. Dosing must be adjusted upward for children taking concomitant carbamazepine, phenytoin, phenobarbital, or primidone, which increases lamotrigine clearance, and dosing must be reduced for children taking concomitant valproate, which decreases lamotrigine clearance; physicians are referred to the product prescribing information for detailed recommendations regarding dosing with valproate and other antiepileptic medications [Lamictal, 2009].

ADVERSE EFFECTS

Common adverse effects observed in clinical studies include dizziness, ataxia, somnolence, headache, diplopia, blurred vision, nausea, vomiting, and rash [Lamictal, 2009]. Lamotrigine has been associated with serious rashes requiring hospitalization and discontinuation of treatment. The manufacturer reports the incidence of Stevens–Johnson syndrome as 0.8 percent in the pediatric population, which is higher than that observed in adult populations. Rare cases of toxic epidermal necrolysis and rash-related death have been reported. Potential risk factors for serious rash are concomitant use of valproate, rapid dose escalation, and higher than recommended starting doses. Most rashes emerge during the first 6–8 weeks of treatment [Lamictal, 2009]. Rashes have been reported in 10 percent of patients in clinical trials. As it is difficult to distinguish a benign rash from the early stages of a more serious rash, the manufacturer recommends discontinuation of treatment at the first sign of a rash, unless it is clearly not medication-related. Rare but potentially life-threatening hypersensitivity reactions have occurred with lamotrigine. Symptoms such as fever and lymphadenopathy, with or without a rash, should prompt immediate evaluation and possible discontinuation of treatment.

Lamotrigine accumulates in melanin-rich tissues, such as skin and the eye. Clinical trials did not detect ophthalmologic adverse effects; however, no long-term data are available. Lamotrigine inhibits dihydrofolate reductase; administration of lamotrigine to rats reduced serum folate levels. Low folate levels have been associated with teratogenic effects [Lamictal, 2009].

DRUG INTERACTIONS

Any drug interaction that might lead to higher blood levels or longer duration of action may increase the risk for rash. Valproate, for example, decreases clearance of lamotrigine and may increase the risk of potentially life-threatening rashes [Lamictal, 2009]. In contrast, carbamazepine, phenytoin, phenobarbital, and primidone increase clearance of lamotrigine and may require dosing adjustments.

Oxcarbazepine

CLINICAL APPLICATIONS

Oxcarbazepine is a 10-keto analog of carbamazepine and is currently approved for both monotherapy and adjunctive therapy for partial seizures in children and adolescents. Data in adults suggest that oxcarbazepine is efficacious for treatment of acute mania [Hirschfeld and Kasper, 2004]. Data are limited for treatment of pediatric bipolar disorder, but oxcarbazepine was not superior to placebo in the one published randomized, placebo-controlled trial in children and adolescents with bipolar I disorder [Wagner et al., 2006].

PHARMACOLOGY

The mechanism of action of oxcarbazepine (Trileptal®) in the treatment of seizures and bipolar disorder is unknown. Oxcarbazepine is well absorbed after oral administration and is rapidly reduced in the liver to the active 10-monohydroxy metabolite (MHD), which is responsible for its pharmacologic activity. The MHD is conjugated with glucuronic acid and almost entirely excreted in the urine. The half-life of the oxcarbazepine is 2 hours and the half-life of the MHD is 9 hours. Dose adjustments are not required with mild to moderate hepatic insufficiency, but are required with renal disease [Trileptil, 2009].

DRUG INTERACTIONS

Oxcarbazepine has little activity on most of the cytochrome P-450 enzymes, with the exception of CYP2C19 and CYPCA4/5. Due to its activity on the CYPCA4/5 isoenzyme, it can reduce plasma concentrations of oral contraceptives and cyclosporine. Additionally, plasma levels of oxcarbazepine and its active metabolite are lowered in the presence of inducers of the P450 enzyme system, including carbamazepine, phenytoin, and phenobarbital. Unlike carbamazepine, oxcarbazepine does not induce its own metabolism and is not highly protein-bound: therefore, its co-administration with other medications is less complex [Trileptil, 2009].

CLINICAL MANAGEMENT

As efficacy has not been established, dosing requirements for treatment of pediatric bipolar disorder are unknown. Dosing for pediatric epilepsy is weight-based. It is recommended that oxcarbazepine should be started at 8–10 mg/kg daily in divided doses, not to exceed a total dose of 600 mg. The dose may be increased over a period of 2 weeks to a target dose (900 mg if <30 kg, 1200 mg if <40 kg, and 1800 mg if >40 kg) [Trileptil, 2009]. Although rapid dose escalation is possible, there is suggestion that slower titration of oxcarbazepine improves tolerability [Wagner et al., 2006].

ADVERSE EFFECTS

Common adverse effects reported in the pediatric literature included diplopia, dizziness, somnolence, fatigue, nausea and rash. Although not common, hyponatremia and serious rashes, including Stevens–Johnson syndrome, have been reported [Trileptil, 2009].

Gabapentin

CLINICAL APPLICATIONS

Gabapentin (Neurontin®) is approved as a treatment for postherpetic neuralgia in adults and as an adjunctive therapy for treatment of partial seizures in children and adults [Neurontin, 2009]. Case reports and open studies of gabapentin as adjuvant therapy in adult bipolar patients were promising; however, double-blind trials have not confirmed efficacy in mania as monotherapy [Frye et al., 2000] or adjunctive treatment [Pande et al., 2000], or in treatment of resistant rapid-cycling bipolar disorder [Evins, 2003; Yatham et al., 2002]. Data are very sparse on mood or behavioral symptoms in pediatric populations. One small case series suggested that gabapentin may reduce irritability in children with severe neurologic impairment [Hauer et al., 2007], but there are no safety or efficacy data in pediatric bipolar disorder.

PHARMACOLOGY

Gabapentin (Neurontin®) is available in capsules, tablets, and solution. Plasma half-life is 5–7 hours. It is not metabolized by the liver and is excreted unchanged in the urine. It is not protein-bound and has no clinically significant drug interactions [Neurontin, 2009].

CLINICAL MANAGEMENT

Pediatric dosing for partial seizures is established, and for adolescents typically ranges from 900 mg to 1800 mg daily [Neurontin, 2009]. Clinical trial data do not indicate any routine monitoring of laboratory screens. No therapeutic plasma concentrations have been established (see Table 49-7).

ADVERSE EFFECTS

Gabapentin is generally well tolerated. Common side effects include dizziness, ataxia, sedation, fatigue, and nystagmus. Less common side effects include dyspepsia, peripheral edema, diplopia, and amblyopia [Neurontin, 2009]. Behavioral side effects are possible and include aggression and hyperactivity [Lee et al., 1996; Tallian et al., 1996].

Topiramate

CLINICAL APPLICATIONS

Topiramate (Topamax®) is approved for migraine prophylaxis in adults, monotherapy of partial and primary generalized tonic-clonic seizures for ages 12 years and up, adjunctive therapy for partial seizures and primary generalized tonic-clonic seizures for ages 2 years and up, and for seizures associated with

Lennox–Gastaut syndrome for ages 2 years and up [Topomax, 2009]. In adults, despite early promise that topiramate may be effective as adjunctive therapy in treatment-resistant bipolar disorder [Ghaemi et al., 2001; Vieta et al., 2002] and for management of acute mania or rapid-cycling bipolar disorder [Chengappa et al., 1999; McElroy et al., 2000], placebo-controlled trials did not demonstrate superiority over placebo in the acute management of mania [Kushner et al., 2006]. Data are quite limited in pediatric populations. Retrospective chart reviews of outpatient and inpatient children and adolescents with bipolar disorder treated with topiramate as an adjuvant mood stabilizer indicated response rates of 73 percent for mania [Barzman et al., 2005; DelBello et al., 2002], but the only double-blind, placebo-controlled trial was terminated prematurely when the adult trials failed to show efficacy [Delbello et al., 2005]. Potential advantages of topiramate over other mood stabilizers are its weight-neutral and appetite-suppressive effects [Chengappa et al., 1999; McElroy et al., 2000]. Topiramate augmentation of olanzapine for the treatment of pediatric bipolar disorder helped to limit weight gain compared to youngsters treated with olanzapine alone, although did not confer any benefit on mood stabilization [Wozniak et al., 2009].

PHARMACOLOGY

Topiramate (Topomax®) is available in tablets or sprinkle capsules, which are bioequivalent. Its absorption is rapid, reaching peak plasma concentrations at 2 hours. Antacids can decrease absorption of topiramate. Plasma elimination half-life is 21 hours, and steady state is reached in about 4 days. About 70 percent of topiramate is excreted unchanged in the urine. The remainder is metabolized in the liver [Topomax, 2009].

CLINICAL MANAGEMENT

Topiramate should be initiated at 25–50 mg daily (1–3 mg/kg/day), with small weekly increases of 1–3 mg/kg/day to minimize adverse effects. The recommended total daily dose in the treatment of seizures is 5–9 mg/kg/day or 400 mg in divided doses [Topomax, 2009]. No guidelines are available for dosing in pediatric bipolar disorder. Lower doses, 50–100 mg daily, of topiramate given adjunctively with olanzapine were effective in limiting weight gain [Wozniak et al., 2009]. Monitoring the plasma concentration is unnecessary, unless topiramate is used concomitantly with phenytoin or carbamazepine (see Table 49-7).

ADVERSE EFFECTS AND DRUG INTERACTIONS

Adverse effects include fatigue, ataxia, confusion, impaired concentration and memory, sedation, agitation, anorexia with weight loss, kidney stones, and diplopia. Topiramate may decrease systemic levels of bicarbonate, leading to a metabolic acidosis. Consequently, slow titration, clinical observation, and laboratory monitoring are advised. Carbamazepine, valproic acid, and phenytoin can lower the plasma concentration of topiramate. Topiramate may increase the concentration of phenytoin and decrease that of valproic acid [Topomax, 2009].

Dopamine Receptor Antagonists: Typical Antipsychotics

Dopamine receptor antagonist is a term used to refer to a medication that is a high-affinity antagonist of dopamine receptors. Other terms used to refer to these drugs include typical antipsychotics, neuroleptics, and major tranquilizers. The first antipsychotic, chlorpromazine, was initially used in the early 1950s in France to manage preoperative anxiety and postoperative shock. When it was found to have a calming effect on patients with schizophrenia and mania, it gained widespread use in psychiatry. Unfortunately, these patients developed neurologic side effects, including extrapyramidal symptoms, associated with short- and long-term use of chlorpromazine.

Other antipsychotic agents were developed that were effective in treating a variety of psychiatric conditions, but they could not escape the risk of producing extrapyramidal symptoms. Uncovering their pharmacodynamic properties led to more sophisticated drug development. The antipsychotic effects of these medications are thought to be mediated through the inhibition of dopamine binding at dopamine D_2 receptors, resulting in the reduction of dopaminergic neurotransmission in the CNS. The neurologic side effects appear to be mediated by dopamine antagonism in the nigrostriatal pathway. Other side effects associated with antipsychotics result from activity at adrenergic, cholinergic, and histaminic receptors.

Dopamine receptor antagonists are distinguished from serotonin–dopamine antagonists, also called novel or atypical antipsychotics or second-generation antipsychotics. In contrast to typical antipsychotics, the serotonin–dopamine antagonists have a higher ratio of serotonin type 2 to dopamine D_2 receptor blockade. Additionally, they have reduced risk of short- and long-term neurologic side effects and are superior in treating negative symptoms of schizophrenia and acute mania. Unfortunately, as patients and clinicians gained experience with serotonin–dopamine antagonists, other adverse effects, such as weight gain, hyperglycemia, and hyperlipidemia, were recognized [McEvoy et al., 2005].

Serotonin–dopamine antagonists have become first-line medications in the treatment of schizophrenia in adults, largely due to their lessened risk of extrapyramidal side effects and tardive dyskinesia [Lehman et al., 2004], and for similar reasons are appealing to the clinical practice of child psychiatry. However, recent published data from head-to-head comparisons of first- and second-generation antipsychotics in the treatment of schizophrenia in adult and pediatric populations have revealed no significant difference in efficacy and reinforce the continued role of these earlier medications [Lewis et al., 2006; Sikich et al., 2008]. Additionally, typical antipsychotics continue to be used in certain neuropsychiatric diagnoses such as Tourette's syndrome, and when excessive weight gain and metabolic abnormalities result from atypical antipsychotics.

Common Characteristics of Typical Antipsychotics

The common characteristic among typical antipsychotics is their ability to antagonize dopamine receptors in the CNS. Activity in the mesocortical region is presumed to result in their therapeutic effects, and their neurologic side-effect profile is attributed to activity in the nigrostriatal region. Dopamine receptor blockade in the tuberoinfundibular tract may result in endocrine effects from elevated prolactin levels [Sadock and Sadock, 2007].

Typical antipsychotics can be classified by their chemical structure. In clinical practice, classification according to dopamine receptor binding potency is more practical. High-potency antipsychotics (e.g., haloperidol, fluphenazine, pimozide) are more likely to cause extrapyramidal symptoms, whereas low-potency antipsychotics (e.g., chlorpromazine, thioridazine) are more likely to cause side effects mediated by cholinergic (e.g., dry mouth, constipation), α_1-adrenergic (e.g., vasodilatation and orthostatic hypotension), and histaminic receptor activity (e.g., sedation, weight gain) (Table 49-8) [Sadock and Sadock, 2007].

Side effects of dopamine receptor antagonists include orthostatic hypotension, peripheral anticholinergic effects (i.e., dry mouth, blurred vision, constipation, urinary retention, and mydriasis), central anticholinergic effects (i.e., agitation, delirium, hallucinations, seizures, and coma), hyperprolactinemia, leukopenia, agranulocytosis, jaundice, photosensitivity, decreased seizure threshold, and weight gain. Thioridazine has been associated with irreversible retinal pigmentation. Chlorpromazine has been associated with skin pigmentation and deposits in the lens and cornea, which usually do not affect vision [Sadock and Sadock, 2007].

Rarely, cardiotoxicity and sudden death have been associated with some typical antipsychotics, especially low-potency antipsychotics. Thioridazine can cause prolongation of the QT interval, arrhythmias, and torsades de pointes (i.e., a form of ventricular tachycardia). Chlorpromazine can cause prolongation of the QT and PR intervals. Both have been associated with sudden death. Pimozide, especially when combined with CYP3A4 inhibitors, has been associated with cardiotoxicity [Sadock and Sadock, 2007].

Neurological side effects of dopamine receptor antagonists include parkinsonism, dystonias, akathesia, and dyskinesias (collectively called extrapyramidal symptoms), and are more commonly observed with the high-potency antipsychotics (Table 49-9). Children and adolescents appear to be more sensitive than adults to these side effects [Correll, 2008]. Symptoms of parkinsonism include cogwheel rigidity, shuffling gait, bradykinesia, masklike facies, stooped posture, coarse tremor, perioral tremor (i.e., rabbit syndrome), and akinesia (i.e., lack of initiative). Symptoms may be managed by reducing the dose of the antipsychotic or by adding anticholinergic medications, such as benztropine, or antihistamines, such as diphenhydramine.

Acute dystonic reactions, which are sustained muscular contractions, tend to occur early in the course of treatment, usually within hours to days. They may be painful and frightening to patients and families who are not forewarned of this possible side effect. Dystonias may involve the eyes (i.e., oculogyric crisis), neck (i.e., torticollis or retrocollis), tongue, jaw, or entire body (i.e., opisthotonos). Use of 1–2 mg of intramuscular benztropine or 25–50 mg of oral or intramuscular diphenhydramine can relieve acute dystonias within several minutes. Continued maintenance dosing with benztropine may prevent subsequent dystonias. Although it is possible to prevent parkinsonism and acute dystonias with prophylactic benztropine or diphenhydramine, the potential negative effects of the increased anticholinergic burden, including confusion, and enhanced peripheral effects, such as constipation and urinary retention, must be carefully considered.

Akathisia is a persistent, uncomfortable restlessness. Patients may constantly rock or pace around the room and secondarily feel anxious and dysphoric. Extreme cases have described patients developing suicidal ideation and behavior [Van Putten and Marder, 1987]. This symptom can be challenging to diagnose, as it can mimic psychomotor agitation and mislead clinicians into increasing the antipsychotic dose. In children, akathisia can be accompanied by insomnia and can be mistaken for ADHD. Dosage reduction or propranolol sometimes brings relief [Correll, 2008].

Dyskinesia associated with dopamine receptor antagonists refers to a potentially irreversible syndrome of involuntary

Table 49-8 Representative Antagonists: Comparison of Potency, Side-Effect Profile, and Dosing

Drug	Preparations	Potency	Sedative Effect	Anti-cholinergic Effect	Extra-pyramidal Effect	Dosing
Chlorpromazine	Thorazine (10-, 25- 50-, 100-, and 200-mg tablets; 10mg/ 5mL syrup; 30 mg/ml and 100 mg/ml concentrate; 25- and 100- mg suppositories) Thorazine Spansules (30-, 75- and 150mg sustained release capsules)	Low	High	High	Low	Age ≤12 yr: 0.25 mg/kg every 4 to 6 hr as needed Age >12 yr: 10 mg three times a day to 25 mg four times a day: titrate with increases of 25 to 50 mg one or twice a week
Haloperidol	Haldol (0.5-, 1-, 2-, 5-, 10- and 20-mg tablets)	High	Low	Low	High	Initial dose of 0.5 mg/day; increased gradually by 0.5 mg every 5-7 days until therapeutic effect is achieved or increase is prohibited by side effects.
Pimozide	Orap 1- and 2-mg tablets)	High	Low	Low	High	Initial dose of 0.05 mg/kg; increase gradually by 0.5 mg once or twice per week until therapeutic effect is achieved or maximum tolerability; maximum dose of 10 mg/ day or 0.2 mg/kg/day.

Table 49-9 **Extrapyramidal Symptoms Associated with Antipsychotic Medications**

Neurologic Side Effects	Time Course	Symptoms	Intervention
Parkinsonism	Within 5–90 days of initiation	Cogwheeling ridigity, shuffling gait, bradykinesia, masklike facies, stooped posture, coarse tremor, perioral tremor (rabbit syndrome), akinesia (lack of initiative) ataraxia (indifference to the environment)	Anticholinergic Medications: benzotropine (Cogentin) or diphenhydramine (Benadryl)
Acute dystonia	Within hours to days of initiation	Slow, sustained muscular contractions involving any part of the body, which may be painful: eyes (oculogyric crisis), neck (torticollis or retrocollis), tongue, jaw, whole body (opisthotonos)	Intramucular anticholinergic medications
Akathisia	Any time during treatment	Motor restlessness and muscular discomfort	Decrease dose of neuroleptic add anticholingergic medication or propronolol
Withdrawal Dyskinesia	During taper or discontinuation of neuroleptic Duing crossover from high potency antipsychotic to lower potency neuroleptic	Involuntary choreoathetoid movements in muscles of the head (perioral movements, lip smacking, grimacing, tongue protrusion, lateral jaw movements), trunk (trunk twisting and pelvic thrusting) and extremities.	Monitor severity of movements with objective ratings; Taper antipsychotic more slowly Consider Branched-chain amino acid if significant functional impairment
Tardive dyskinesia	Any time during treatment, risk increases with duration of treatment	Same as for withdrawal dyskinesia	Monitor severity of movements with objective ratings Decrease or discontinue antipsychotic Switch to different antipsychotic Consider use of clozapine
Neuroleptic malignant syndrome	Any time during treatment	Muscle rigidity, fever, autonomic instability, delirium, elevated creatine phosphokinase, leukocytosis, rhabdomyolysis, myoglobinuria, renal failure	Emergency medical treatment and immediate discontinuation of antipsychotic

choreoathetoid movements, which have a delayed onset of action compared to other neurological side effects. These movements commonly involve orofacial muscles but can involve any muscle group, including muscles of the extremities, trunk, and diaphragm. Two types of dyskinesias are described – withdrawal dyskinesias and tardive dyskinesia. Withdrawal dyskinesia occurs in the context of lowering or discontinuing dopamine receptor antagonists. It can also be observed when cross-tapering from a high-potency antipsychotic to a lower-potency antipsychotic [Correll, 2008]. Children and adolescents are vulnerable to the development of withdrawal dyskinesias, with rates as high as 30 percent [Campbell et al., 1997; Kumra et al., 1998]. With early identification and management, withdrawal dyskinesias are frequently reversible but can persist for months following medication discontinuation. Branched-chain amino acid may be effective in ameliorating withdrawal dyskinesias that result in significant functional impairment in children and adolescents [Kafantaris et al., 2005]. In contrast to withdrawal dyskinesias, tardive dyskinesia may occur any time during treatment, is not specifically associated with drug discontinuation, and has greater potential to become irreversible. The presence of pre-existing involuntary movements should be assessed at baseline with objective rating scales, such as the Abnormal Involuntary Movement Scale (AIMS). Serial assessments should be completed after 3 months and annually during antipsychotic therapy [Correll, 2008]. An increase in involuntary movements should prompt a discussion with the patient and family about treatment options. There are no consistently useful treatments for tardive dyskinesia, although symptom reduction may occur with lowering or discontinuing the medication when clinically feasible, or with a switch to an antipsychotic of a different class. Symptoms of

tardive dyskinesia can be ameliorated by increasing the dose of antipsychotic (masking the symptoms), but continued exposure may make tardive dyskinesia symptoms worse over time.

Neuroleptic malignant syndrome is a rare and potentially fatal adverse effect, which may occur any time during treatment with antipsychotics, but may be more likely to occur in the first 2 weeks [Addonizio et al., 1987]. The frequency of occurrence has been 0.02–2.44 percent with typical antipsychotics [Khan and Farver, 2000]. It is characterized by symptoms in four major areas: autonomic instability, extrapyramidal symptoms, hyperpyrexia, and altered mental status. Specific symptoms include muscle rigidity, fever, sweating, increased blood pressure and heart rate, confusion, agitation, and renal insufficiency. Laboratory findings include leukocytosis; elevated levels of serum creatine phosphokinase, liver transaminases, and myoglobin; and myoglobinuria. In a review of 49 cases of neuroleptic malignant syndrome, the mortality rate among children was 27 percent, and the mortality rate among adolescents was 13 percent [Latz and McCracken, 1992]. Treatment involves immediate hospitalization for supportive treatment and discontinuation of the antipsychotic drug.

Haloperidol

Clinical Applications

Haloperidol (Haldol®) is approved for the treatment of psychotic disorders and Tourette's syndrome in children, adolescents, and adults. In addition, it is approved for use in treating children with severe behavioral disorders, including ADHD, that have not responded to non-pharmacologic interventions or non-antipsychotic medications [Haldol, 2001]. In clinical practice, haloperidol is sometimes administered intramuscularly to stabilize acutely agitated and aggressive patients who pose an immediate threat to themselves or others, when alternative measures have failed. Haloperidol appears to be effective in children with schizophrenia [Green et al., 1992; Spencer et al., 1992]. It appears to be effective in improving behavior in children with autism [Anderson et al., 1984; Joshi et al., 1988] and in reducing tics in Tourette's syndrome [Shapiro et al., 1989].

Pharmacology

Haloperidol is a high-potency dopamine receptor antagonist. It is available in oral tablets, an oral concentrate, parenteral preparations (intramuscular or intravenous), and depot intramuscular injections (Haldol decanoate®). Oral haloperidol is well absorbed from the gastrointestinal tract and undergoes first-pass metabolism in the liver. Peak plasma concentrations are reached within 2–6 hours. Peak plasma haloperidol concentration occurs 10–20 minutes after intramuscular injection. Peak pharmacologic action occurs within 30–45 minutes in agitated patients. In psychotic patients, improvement may be seen within 30–60 minutes, and the effects increase over the next 2 hours. Haldol decanoate® is released slowly, with peak concentrations occurring 6–7 days after injection. Steady-state concentrations are achieved in approximately 3 months with monthly injections. Haloperidol is metabolized by the liver and excreted in urine and feces [Haldol, 2001].

Clinical Effects

For children between the ages of 3 and 12 years, haloperidol may be initiated at 0.5 mg/day. The dose may be increased by increments of 0.5 mg at 5- to 7-day intervals to a clinically therapeutic dose. Dosing recommendations for psychotic disorders is 0.05–0.15mg/kg/day. For nonpsychotic behavior disorders and Tourette's syndrome, the therapeutic range is 0.05–0.075 mg/kg/day [Haldol, 2001].

Adverse Effects

Adverse effects of haloperidol are characteristic of high-potency typical antipsychotics (see "Common Characteristics of Typical Antipsychotics"). Rates of acute dystonic reaction with haloperidol have been observed to be 16.7 percent and 25 percent in children treated for schizophrenia [Green et al., 1992; Spencer et al., 1992]. The rate of withdrawal dyskinesia observed in a long-term study in autistic children was 33.9 percent. Higher cumulative dose, female gender, and perinatal complications appeared to increase risk [Campbell et al., 1997]. In addition, dose-related anxiety, dysphoria, and other affective changes have been reported in children with Tourette's syndrome treated with haloperidol [Bruun, 1988].

Drug Interactions

Medications that inhibit the cytochrome P-450 isoenzyme system can increase serum concentrations of haloperidol and therefore increase risks for adverse effects.

Pimozide

Clinical Applications

Pimozide (Orap®) is labeled for use in the treatment of Tourette's syndrome in patients who have failed to respond to standard treatment and experience severe impairment from tics. Pimozide has been shown to be effective in decreasing tics in pediatric and adult populations [Sallee et al., 1997; Shapiro and Shapiro, 1984; Shapiro et al., 1983]. However, the atypical antipsychotic risperidone appears to be more efficacious in decreasing tics when directly compared with pimozide [Bruggeman et al., 2001; Gilbert et al., 2004] and has a more favorable side-effect profile.

Pharmacology

Pimozide is a high-potency dopamine receptor antagonist. It is metabolized by the liver, primarily by CYP3A4 and to a lesser extent by CYP1A2, and excreted in urine. Mean serum half-life is about 55 hours [Scahill et al., 2006].

Clinical Management

Before beginning pimozide, the patient should undergo a thorough psychiatric and medical evaluation. Pimozide is contraindicated in patients with congenital long QT syndrome, with a history of arrhythmias, or with conditions that cause hypokalemia [Scahill et al., 2006]. Additionally, pimozide has the potential for many adverse drug interactions and a careful review of medications is indicated. Baseline measurements include laboratory screening (CBC, electrolytes, tests of renal and liver function, fasting glucose and lipids, height, weight, and baseline assessment of the extrapyramidal system [Correll, 2008].

Because pimozide can prolong the QT interval, EKGs should be obtained at baseline and during dose titration. The QTc interval should not exceed 0.47 seconds or increase more than 25 percent above baseline [Scahill et al., 2006]. A pediatric cardiologist should be consulted if the EKG is equivocal. As hypokalemia can adversely affect cardiac conduction, serial electrolytes are indicated.

Pimozide may be initiated at 0.05 mg/kg and gradually increased by 0.5 mg once or twice weekly. Doses greater than 0.2 mg/kg/day or 10 mg/day are not recommended [Scahill et al., 2006]. Efficacy (i.e., severity and frequency of tics) and safety (i.e., serial EKGs and serum electrolytes) of pimozide should be actively monitored over time.

Adverse Effects

Adverse effects of pimozide are those typical of high-potency antipsychotics (see "Common Characteristics of Typical Antipsychotics"). Pimozide has been associated with QT prolongation, serious cardiac arrhythmias, and sudden death. Use of pimozide with potent inhibitors of the CYP3A4 enzyme (macrolide antibiotics, protease inhibitors, azole antifungal agents and commonly used antidepressants, citalopram, escitalopram, and sertraline) is contraindicated by the FDA because of the risk of cardiotoxicity with these combinations [Scahill et al., 2006].

Atypical Antipsychotics

Common Characteristics

Serotonin–dopamine antagonists (also called atypical or second-generation antipsychotics) differ from typical antipsychotics in that they have a higher ratio of serotonin type 2 to dopamine type 2 receptor blockade. Risperidone, olanzapine, quetiapine, ziprasidone, and clozapine are serotonin–dopamine antagonists. Aripiprazole is commonly grouped with the second-generation antipsychotics but has an unique mechanism of action as a partial dopamine agonist. Each atypical antipsychotic possesses different affinities at dopamine, serotonin, adrenergic, cholinergic, and histaminic receptors, which result in different side-effect profiles and clinical effects (Table 49-10). Atypical antipsychotics offer advantages over typical antipsychotics in their ability to improve both the negative and positive symptoms of schizophrenia, their effectiveness as a treatment of acute mania and their lower risk of producing extrapyramidal symptoms. However, they may pose other health risks, including weight gain, insulin resistance, and hyperlipidemia [Sadock and Sadock, 2007].

Experience with serotonin–dopamine antagonists in children and adolescents is growing. In recent years, the FDA has approved individual serotonin–dopamine antagonists for use in the acute management of mania, schizophrenia, and irritability associated with autistic disorders in children and adolescents (see Table 49-1). Child prescribers welcomed the more favorable neurological adverse effects profile offered by these newer medications, and clinical experience has generally confirmed that children and adolescents had a lower risk of developing extrapyramidal symptoms. None the less, direct comparisons of serotonin–dopamine antagonists and dopamine receptor antagonists using rigorous methodology in children and adolescents have been limited [Kumra et al., 1996; Sikich et al., 2008]. Interestingly, in both of these studies, the extrapyramidal symptoms reported by patients on serotonin–dopamine antagonists did not differ substantially from that reported by patients on dopamine receptor antagonists, although the severity of extrapyramidal symptoms was greater on first- as compared to second-generation antipsychotics. With the exception of clozapine, dyskinesias have been reported with all of the serotonin–dopamine antagonists, although the available evidence does appear to support lower rates than that seen with the dopamine receptor antagonists [Correll and Kane, 2007].

Weight gain has emerged as one of the most common and troubling side effects for children and adolescents on the serotonin–dopamine antagonists. Olanzapine consistently confers the greatest risk of weight gain in pediatric patients [Correll, 2008]. In the Treatment of Early Onset Schizophrenia study, the olanzapine treatment arm was terminated early by the NIMH Data and Safety Monitoring Board when olanzapine showed greater increases in weight compared to risperidone or molindone in the absence of greater effectiveness [Sikich et al., 2008]. Olanzapine consistently confers the greatest risk of weight gain but significant weight gain occurs with quetiapine, risperidone, and aripiprazole [Fraguas et al., 2010]. Experience with ziprasidone has been limited and it remains to be seen whether it confers the same weight-sparing properties in children as it is reported to do in adults. Clinicians need to be sensitive to weight-gain effects because weight gain is likely to affect a child or adolescent's self-esteem and may lead to noncompliance with medications and relapse. Childhood obesity correlates with obesity in adulthood and confers additional long-term cardiometabolic risk [Dietz and Robinson, 2005]. Recommendations to increase exercise and to make healthier food choices may be effective with motivated patients and families.

Studies in adults have indicated that atypical antipsychotic medications are associated with metabolic disturbances, such as increased insulin resistance [Haupt and Newcomer, 2001], metabolic syndrome [McEvoy et al., 2005], and dyslipidemia [Lindenmayer et al., 2003]. Although data in pediatric populations are more limited, emerging evidence reveals that serotonin–dopamine antagonists can cause significant metabolic changes, even with short-term treatment, although metabolic syndrome and diabetes are uncommon [Correll et al., 2009]. Additionally, metabolic changes vary across the atypical antipsychotics. In one large prospective, naturalistic study, olanzapine and quetiapine showed significant increase in all lipid levels, while risperidone showed marked increase in triglycerides only. Aripiprazole appears to have minimal effect on metabolic parameters [Correll et al., 2009]. Managing antipsychotic weight gain with diet and exercise is recommended [Correll, 2008], but approaches with medications are also being explored [Maayan and Correll, 2010].

As with typical antipsychotics, elevated prolactin levels can develop with the serotonin–dopamine antagonists. The significance of asymptomatic elevations is not known. Risperidone and olanzapine show the greatest risk, while quetiapine and clozapine show the least risk [Correll, 2008]. Aripiprazole has been associated with low prolactin levels [Correll, 2008].

Cardiac effects have been noted with the serotonin–dopamine antagonists. Quetiapine and clozapine can cause dizziness and orthostatic hypotension, thought to be mediated by adrenergic blockade. QT prolongation has been observed with ziprasidone [Correll, 2008]. Clozapine has been linked to myocarditis in adults but this appears rare in children [Wehmeier et al., 2004].

Given the possible adverse effects of antipsychotics and our limited knowledge of their long-term safety, careful monitoring of pediatric patients is necessary. A comprehensive psychiatric evaluation should include an assessment for the risk of adverse effects. Personal and family medical history should pay attention to obesity, hypertension, diabetes, dyslipidemia, coronary artery disease, and sudden cardiac death. Sexual or reproductive dysfunction should be noted and lifestyle behaviors should be reviewed, including diet, exercise, smoking, substance abuse, and sleep hygiene. Recommended baseline measurements include laboratory screening (e.g., CBC, electrolytes, liver and renal function tests, thyroid function test, and fasting glucose and lipid levels), height, weight, and baseline assessment of extrapyramidal symptoms using clinician ratings (e.g., AIMS). A baseline EKG is recommended before initiating ziprasidone or clozapine [Correll, 2008].

Risperidone

Clinical Applications

Risperidone (Risperdal®) is labeled for use in the treatment of schizophrenia and the manic phase of bipolar disorder, either alone or in conjunction with lithium or valproate in adults. In pediatric populations, risperidone is labeled for use in the treatment of schizophrenia ($\geq$13 years), the acute manic phase of bipolar disorder ($\geq$10 years), and irritability associated with autism (5–16 years). The FDA labeling for risperidone in children and adolescents is based on a series of large, randomized controlled trials of the treatment of schizophrenia [Sikich et al., 2004, 2008], bipolar disorder [Haas et al., 2009a], and irritability and behavior problems in autistic children [McCracken et al., 2002]. Risperidone has also been found to be effective in conduct disorder [Findling et al., 2000], aggression in children with subaverage IQ [Aman et al., 2002], tic disorders [Bruggeman et al., 2001; Dion et al., 2002; Gaffney et al., 2002; Scahill et al., 2003], and co-occurring tic disorders and OCD [Bruggeman et al., 2001; Gaffney et al., 2002].

Table 49-10 **Serotonin-dopamine Antagonists: Comparison of Receptor Activity and Dosing**

Drug	Preparations	Dopamine Receptor Activity	Serotonin Receptor Activity	Anticholinergic Receptor Activity	Adrenergic Receptor Activity	Histaminic Receptor Activity	Dosing
Risperidone	Risperidal (0.25-, 0.5-, 1-, 2-, 3-, and 4-mg tablets) Risperidal M-Tab (0.5, 1-, 2-, 3-, and 4-mg tablets) Risperidal Oral Soln (1mg/ml)	D_2	$5HT_{2A}$		α_1, α_2	H_1	Mania or Schz*: initiate 0.5 mg/day, increase daily by 0.5 to 1 mg, effective range 0.5 to 6 mg/day. DBDs**: initiate at 0.25 to 0.5 mg/day, increase by 0.25 to 0.5 mg weekly; effective range 0.5 to 3mg/day
Olanzapine	Zyprexa (2.5-, 5-, 7.5- 10-, 15-, and 20-mg tablets Zyprexa Zydis (5-, 10-, 15-, and 20-mg tablets)	D_1-D_4	$5HT_{2A},$ $5HT_{T6,}$ $5HT_{2C}$	M_1-M_5	α_1	H_1	Mania or Schz*: Initiate 2.5 mg to 5 mg/day, Maximum dose of 20 mg/day.
Quetiapine	Seroquel (25-, 50-, 100-, 200-, 300-mg, and 400-mg tablets) Seroquel XR (50-, 150-, 200-, 300-, and 400-mg tablets)	D_1, D_2	$5HT_{1A,}$ $5HT_2$		α_1, α_2	H_1	Mania or Schz*: initiate 25 mg twice a day, increase by 50 to 100 mg increments in divided doses to target of 400 mg/day. effective range 400-600 mg.
Ziprasidone	Geodon (20-, 40-, 60-, and 80-mg tablets)	D_2, D_3, D_4	$5HT_{1D,}$ $5HT_{1A}$ $5HT_{2A,}$ $5HT_{2C}$		α_1	H_1	Initiate 20 mg daily and titrate to maximum of 160 mg/day in divided doses.
Aripiprazole	Abilify (2-, 5-, 10-, 15-, 20- and 30-mg tablets) Abilify Discmelt (10- and 15-mg tablets) Abilify Oral Soln (1mg/ml).	D_3, D_4 Partial D_2 agonist	$5HT_{1A,}$ $5HT_{2A}$		α_1	H_1	Mania or Schz*: initiate at 2-5mg/day, effective range 10-30 mg. Autistic Disorder: Initiate at 2 mg/day, target dose of 5-10mg/day. Maximum dose of 30 mg/day.
Clozapine	Clozaril (25- and 100-mg scored tablets)	D_1-D_5	$5HT_{2A,}$ $5HT_{2C,}$ $5HT_3$	M_1, M_3, M_5	α_1	H_1	Schz*: initiate at 12.5 - 25 mg/day, and increase 25-50 mg daily as tolerated to 300 mg/day in divided doses for adults. Slower titration in pediatric patients, effective range 350 - 550 mg/day divided twice a day or three times a day.

* Schz = Schizophrenia
** DBDs = Disruptive Behavior Disorders including irritability associated with autism.

Pharmacology

Risperidone is a serotonin–dopamine antagonist with activity at serotonin $5HT_{2A}$, dopamine D_2, α_1- and α_2-adrenergic, and histaminic H_1 receptors. It is available in tablets, solution, orally disintegrating tablets, and depot injectable preparations. It is well absorbed in the gastrointestinal tract and undergoes extensive first-pass metabolism in the liver by CYP2D6 to its active metabolite, 9-hydroxyrisperidone. The mean half-life of both forms is about 20 hours [Risperdal, 2010].

Clinical Management

Risperidone is an effective medication in a variety of disorders, but given the risk of adverse effects and limited knowledge of long-term effects, the clinician must consider alternative interventions, both nonpharmacological and pharmacological. A thorough risk–benefit analysis should be part of the informed consent discussion with the parent or guardian. Baseline assessment is as outlined in the "Common Characteristics of Atypical Antipsychotics" section. In the treatment of mania or schizophrenia, risperidone can be initiated at 0.25–0.5 mg/day, and increased daily by 0.5–1 mg to reach a target dose of 2.5 mg daily. Little additional benefit is observed at higher doses in randomized controlled trials. In the treatment of other conditions, such as disruptive behaviors or tics, lower doses and slower titration are recommended.

Adverse Effects

Risperidone can cause sedation, dizziness, orthostatic hypotension, increased appetite, weight gain, and extrapyramidal symptoms [Risperdal, 2010]. Risperidone is the most potent inducer of prolactin when compared to both typical and atypical antipsychotics. Some experts suggest that baseline and follow prolactin levels are advisable [Singh et al., 2010], although others suggest checking prolactin levels if a child or adolescent develops symptoms suggestive of hyperprolactinemia, such as amenorrhea, oligomenorrhea, sexual dysfunction, or galactorrhea [Correll, 2008]. Gastrointestinal symptoms, elevated transaminases, and fatty infiltrates in the liver have been described [Kumra et al., 1997]. Risperidone or its metabolite can prolong the QT interval in some patients, which can lead to cardiac arrhythmia if combined with medications having similar effects [Risperdal, 2010].

Drug Interactions

Risperidone may potentiate sedative and hypotensive effects of other medications. Clozapine may reduce clearance of risperidone. Certain selective serotonin reuptake inhibitors (fluoxetine and paroxetine) increase risperidone levels and may enhance risk of extrapyramidal symptoms. Co-administration with lithium and valproic acid does not result in any significant drug interactions, although co-administration with carbamazepine, a cytochrome P-450 enzyme inducer, lowers risperidone levels [Risperdal, 2010].

Olanzapine

Clinical Applications

In adults, olanzapine (Zyprexa®) is labeled for use as a treatment for schizophrenia, acute manic or mixed episodes of bipolar disorder, and prophylaxis in bipolar disorder. Additionally, it is labeled for use as an adjunct with lithium or valproate in the treatment of bipolar disorder. In pediatric populations, olanzapine is labeled for the short-term treatment of schizophrenia and bipolar manic or mixed episodes in adolescents of 13 years of age or older. The FDA labeling for olanzapine in children and adolescents is based on a series of large, randomized, controlled trials of the treatment of schizophrenia [Kryzhanovskaya et al., 2009] and of bipolar disorder [Tohen et al., 2007]. Additionally, olanzapine has been found useful in the treatment of autism [Malone et al., 2001; Potenza et al., 1999] and Tourette's syndrome [Stamenkovic et al., 2000].

Pharmacology

Olanzapine is a serotonin–dopamine antagonist with high activity at serotonin $5HT_{2A}$, $5HT_{2C}$, and $5HT_6$; dopamine D_{1-4}; α_1-adrenergic; and histaminic H_1 receptors. It has moderate activity at muscarinic M_{1-5} and serotonin $5HT_3$ receptors [Zyprexa, 2010]. Olanzapine is available in a tablet, oral disintegrating tablet (Zyprexa-Zydis®), and injectable form. It is well absorbed from the gastrointestinal tract. Approximately

40 percent of the dose is metabolized by first-pass metabolism. It reaches peak concentration in about 6 hours; its mean half-life is 30 hours [Zyprexa, 2010].

Clinical Management

Patients should undergo careful psychiatric assessment, with attention to conditions or risk factors that may complicate or contraindicate treatment with olanzapine. Specifically, obesity, insulin resistance, diabetes, dyslipidemias, cardiovascular disease, hepatic disease, and medications that could enhance weight gain or hepatic dysfunction should be reviewed. Baseline assessments are similar to those for all serotonin–dopamine antagonists and were previously reviewed under "Common Characteristics of Atypical Antipsychotics". Dosing is started at 2.5–5 mg/day and may be increased by increments of 2.5–5 mg weekly, not to exceed 20 mg/day. A more rapid titration may be required in the presence of severe agitation and psychosis of mania or schizophrenia. Weight, fasting glucose and lipid levels, liver transaminases, and AIMS should be monitored during on-going therapy [Correll, 2008].

Adverse Effects

Adolescents are prone to all of the same side effects of olanzapine as adults, but appear to be at increased risk for weight gain, sedation, elevations in total cholesterol, low-density lipoprotein (LDL) cholesterol, triglycerides, prolactin, and hepatic transaminase levels [Zyprexa, 2010]. Compared to the other atypical antipsychotics, olanzapine has consistently had the highest risk for weight gain [Consensus development conference on antipsychotic drugs and obesity and diabetes, 2004; Weiner et al., 2004]. A careful risk–benefit analysis should be considered and reviewed with parents before selecting this medication. Additionally, olanzapine has one of the highest risks for anticholinergic side effects of the serotonin–dopamine antagonists, and symptoms of constipation, urinary hesitancy or retention, and confusion should be followed. As with other antipsychotics, patients may experience extrapyramidal symptoms, tardive dyskinesia, and neuroleptic malignant syndrome [Zyprexa, 2010]. Patients with diabetes mellitus or those at risk for the disorder require very careful monitoring over the course of treatment for worsening symptoms.

Drug Interactions

Fluvoxamine, a potent CYP1A2 inhibitor, can increase serum concentrations of olanzapine [Zyprexa, 2010].

Quetiapine

Clinical Applications

In adults, quetiapine (Seroquel®) is labeled for use in the treatment of schizophrenia and the acute treatment of the manic phase of bipolar disorder, either alone or as an adjunct to lithium or valproate [Seroquel, 2010]. In pediatric populations, quetiapine is approved for the acute treatment of schizophrenia in adolescents of 13 years or older, and of mania associated with bipolar disorder in children and adolescents of 10 years or older. The studies that formed the basis for the FDA labeling of quetiapine in children and adolescents are as yet unpublished in peer-reviewed journals, but are described in the product information for Seroquel under the heading Clinical Studies [Seroquel, 2010]. Specifically, efficacy in the treatment of schizophrenia was established in a 6-week randomized, double-blind, fixed-dose (400 or 800 mg), placebo-controlled trial involving 222 patients. Both doses were superior to placebo on the primary efficacy measure, which was change from baseline on the Positive and Negative Syndrome Scale (PANSS). Efficacy in the treatment of mania was established in a 3-week randomized, double-blind, fixed-dose (400 or 600 mg), placebo-controlled, multicenter trial involving 277 patients. Both doses were superior to placebo in the primary efficacy measure, which was change from baseline of the Young Mania Rating Scale. Additionally, quetiapine has been found effective as an adjunct to divalproex in the treatment of adolescent mania [Delbello et al., 2002], and equally effective as divalproex as a monotherapy of adolescent mania [DelBello et al., 2006]. Two case reports describe usefulness of quetiapine in Tourette's syndrome [Mukaddes and Abali, 2003; Parraga et al., 2001]. In one small study of patients with autism and intellectual disability, quetiapine was ineffective [Martin et al., 1999].

Pharmacology

Quetiapine is a serotonin–dopamine antagonist similar to clozapine in its neurochemical profile. It has activity at serotonin $5HT_{1A}$ and $5HT_{T2}$; dopamine D_1 and D_2, α_1- and α_2-adrenergic; and histaminic H_1 receptors. Quetiapine is rapidly absorbed through the gastrointestinal tract, reaching peak plasma levels in 1–2 hours, and is extensively metabolized in the liver. The steady-state half-life is about 6 hours [Seroquel, 2010].

Clinical Management

For acute management of schizophrenia or mania, quetiapine may be initiation at 50 mg daily and increased by 50–100 mg daily, to reach a target dose of 400 mg. Additional increases may be required with a maximum daily dose of 800 mg daily. The drug is usually given in divided doses two or three times daily [Seroquel, 2010].

Adverse Effects

Adverse effects of quetiapine include dizziness, postural hypotension, dry mouth, and dyspepsia. Quetiapine was thought to have less risk of weight gain but recent data looking at quetiapine use in usual clinical practice point to a significant risk of weight gain in children and adolescents [Correll et al., 2009]. Quetiapine poses minimal risk of prolactin elevation [Correll, 2008]. Development of cataracts in dogs has been observed during animal testing. Lens changes have been observed in patients with long-term use of quetiapine. The manufacturer recommends a baseline ophthalmologic examination and serial examinations every 6 months during treatment [Seroquel, 2010].

Drug Interactions

Phenytoin and thioridazine increase clearance of quetiapine. Inhibitors of CYP3A4, such as ketoconazole, erythromycin, and protease inhibitors, decrease clearance of quetiapine, substantially increasing serum concentrations [Seroquel, 2010].

Ziprasidone

Clinical Applications

Ziprasidone (Geodon®) is labeled for use in the treatment of schizophrenia and manic or mixed episodes associated with bipolar disorder in adults. In clinical practice, its main advantage over other atypical antipsychotics in adults is its weight-neutral effects [Nasrallah, 2003;]. In pediatric populations, use of ziprasidone is off-label. It has been found effective in one large 4-week randomized, double-blind, placebo-controlled trial for the treatment of mania in children and adolescents 10 years of age or older at doses of 80–160 mg daily. These data have been presented at national meetings and the abstract has been published [Delbello et al., 2008]. Ziprasidone has also been used as a treatment in early-onset schizophrenia and schizoaffective disorder with a mean dose of around 120 mg [Ambler et al., 2006], and in tics associated with Tourette's syndrome [Sallee et al., 2000b]. Clinicians may be hesitant to use it because of its effects on the QT interval and the lack of data on safety and efficacy in the pediatric populations. In a study of 12 patients with autistic spectrum disorder, 6 were responders, and 2 patients with co-occurring bipolar disorder were rated much worse [McDougle et al., 2002].

Pharmacology

Ziprasidone (Geodon®) is an atypical antipsychotic with antagonistic activity at serotonin $5HT_{1D}$, $5HT_{2A}$, $5HT_{2C}$; dopamine D_2, D_3, and D_4; α_1-adrenergic; and histaminic H_1 receptors. It is an agonist at $5HT_{1A}$ receptors and inhibits uptake of serotonin and norepinephrine. Ziprasidone is well absorbed orally and reaches peak plasma level at 6–8 hours. Absorption is increased when ziprasidone is taken with food. Although highly protein-bound in plasma, drug interactions with other protein-bound medications are minimal. Ziprasidone is extensively metabolized in the liver. About one-third of ziprasidone's metabolic clearance is mediated by the CYP3A4 isoenzyme [Geodon, 2009].

Clinical Management

Before ziprasidone is initiated, a careful history must be obtained to identify possible contraindications, including concomitant use of drugs known to prolong the QT interval, family history and history of congenitally long QT syndromes, history of cardiovascular disease or cardiac arrhythmia, and conditions that place the patient at risk for electrolyte disturbances. Baseline examinations include serum electrolytes, renal and hepatic screens, fasting glucose and lipid panel, and CBC. Baseline EKG and follow-up after reaching final dosage are recommended, although the manufacturer does not give specific guidelines.

Ziprasidone is available in oral (ziprasidone hydrochloride) and injectable (ziprasidone mesylate) forms. Initial adult dosage of ziprasidone hydrochloride is 20 mg taken twice daily, which may be increased after a minimum of 2 days. Maximum dosage recommended by the manufacturer is 80 mg taken twice daily [Geodon, 2009]. Dosages in older children and adolescents required to treat psychotic disorders and mania are similar to adult dosing. The mean dosage used by Sallee and colleagues [Sallee et al., 2000b], in a study of ziprasidone in 28 children and adolescents with tic disorders, was 28 mg/day. Ziprasidone was initiated at 5 mg/day and adjusted upward to a maximum dose of 40 mg/day. Within this dosage range, ziprasidone was well tolerated with no cardiac adverse effects. In adults with schizophrenia, intramuscular ziprasidone can be used to control acute agitation in patients; 10–20 mg is given as a single dose. Use in patients who are already receiving oral ziprasidone should be avoided because the safety of concomitant oral and intramuscular ziprasidone has not been established [Geodon, 2009]. There is some evidence from case series that ziprasidone may be effective in the treatment of agitation in inpatient children and adolescents [Deshmukh et al., 2010].

Adverse Effects

The most common side effects reported in pediatric populations are sedation, insomnia, activation, weight gain, and extrapyramidal symptoms. In the study of early-onset schizophrenia and schizoaffective disorder, half of the patients developed significant activation, including some cases of frank hypomania or mania which led to discontinuation [Ambler et al., 2006]. Other side effects of ziprasidone include rash, orthostatic hypotension, seizures, and hyperprolactinemia. Ziprasidone has been associated with prolongation of the QT interval, which may increase the risk of fatal arrhythmias, such as torsades de pointes, or sudden death [Geodon, 2009].

Drug Interactions

Use of ziprasidone is contraindicated in patients who are taking medications that are known to prolong the QTc interval. Psychiatric medications in this category include thioridazine, chlorpromazine, droperidol, pimozide, and tricyclic antidepressants. Ziprasidone may potentially interact with medication that induces or inhibits CYP3A4 isoenzyme. It potentially has additive hypotensive effects when combined with hypotensive agents, and potential additive sedative effects when combined with CNS agents [Geodon, 2009].

Aripiprazole

Clinical Applications

Aripiprazole (Abilify®) is labeled for use in the treatment of schizophrenia and bipolar disorder in adults. It has been shown to be superior to placebo in managing positive and negative symptoms of schizophrenia [Marder et al., 2003]. Experience with aripiprazole in pediatric populations is growing, and aripiprazole has FDA approval for the acute treatment of schizophrenia in adolescents of 13 years or older, of manic or mixed episodes of acute mania in children and adolescents of 10 years or older, and for irritability associated with autistic disorder in children and adolescents of 6 years or older. The studies that formed the basis for FDA labeling were large, multicenter, randomized, double-blind, placebo-controlled trials in schizophrenia [Findling et al., 2008b], in acute mania [Findling et al., 2009b], and in irritability in autism [Marcus et al., 2009]. In addition, aripiprazole has been found to be useful in the treatment of conduct disorder [Findling et al., 2009a].

Pharmacology

Aripiprazole differs from other atypical antipsychotics in its pharmacodynamic properties. It has high affinity for dopamine D_2 and D_3, and serotonin $5HT_{1A}$ and $5HT_{2A}$, and moderate affinity for dopamine D_4, serotonin $5HT_2$ and $5HT_3$, α_1-adrenergic, and histamine H_1 receptors. It has novel properties compared to other serotonin–dopamine antagonists and serves as a partial agonist at dopamine D_2 and serotonin $5HT_{1A}$ receptors. It has no activity at cholinergic muscarinic receptors.

Aripiprazole is well absorbed, with peak plasma concentrations attained in 3–5 hours. It is highly bound to plasma proteins, and is metabolized by the liver. The isoenzymes CYP3A4 and CYP2D6 are involved in its metabolism [Abilify, 2010].

Clinical Management

Initial evaluations should incorporate an assessment of risk factors, including a history of cardiovascular disease, seizure disorder, pregnancy, and use of medications that potentially interact with aripiprazole. In the treatment of schizophrenia or mania, the recommended initial dose is 2 mg daily. The dose should be increased to 5 mg on day 3, and finally to the target dose of 10 mg. If the patient does not respond at this dose, subsequent increases can be made, but not higher than 30 mg daily. In the treatment of irritability associated with autistic disorder, the initial recommended dose is 2 mg, followed by slow upward titration to a target dose of 10–15 mg daily [Abilify, 2010].

Adverse Effects

Common side effects include somnolence, nausea, vomiting, esophageal dysmotility, dizziness, hypersalivation, tremor, and extrapyramidal symptoms [Abilify, 2010]. In a study of children and adolescents with conduct disorder, an initial dose of 0.2 mg/kg resulted in tolerability issues – namely, vomiting and sedation. A reduction in initial dose to 0.1 mg/kg and more gradual titration resolved these issues [Findling et al., 2009a].

Drug Interactions

Because aripiprazole is metabolized by CYP3A4 and CYP2D6, serum concentrations may be affected by medications that induce or inhibit these isoenzymes. Quinidine, fluoxetine, and paroxetine are potent inhibitors of CYP2D6 and can increase aripiprazole levels, necessitating dose reduction. Carbamazepine, an inducer of CYP3A4, can decrease Abilify levels. Aripiprazole does not appear to have any significant effect on the metabolism of drugs through the CP2D6, CYP2C9, or CYP3A4 enzymes [Abilify, 2010].

Clozapine

Clinical Applications

Clozapine (Clozaril®) is labeled in adults for the management of schizophrenia in patients who failed standard drug treatment, and for the reduction of suicidal behavior in patients with schizophrenia and schizoaffective disorder [Clozaril, 2010]. It is off-label for use in pediatric populations. Clozapine has been found effective in the management of treatment-refractory childhood-onset schizophrenia in randomized, double-blind comparison trials [Kumra et al., 2008; Shaw et al., 2006], but its use is limited by increased risk of adverse events. Additionally clozapine has been found to be effective in treating tardive dyskinesia in adult patients with schizophrenia [Lieberman et al., 1991; Spivak et al., 1997], and is the only antipsychotic for which the risk of tardive dyskinesia is considered minimal.

Pharmacology

Clozapine is a dibenzodiazepine that demonstrates antagonistic activity at dopamine D_1, D_2, D_3, and D_4, serotonin $5HT_{2a}$, $5HT_{1D}$, $5HT_{1A}$, $\alpha1$-adrenergic, muscarinic, and histaminic H_1 receptors [Clozaril, 2010]. It has weak antagonism of dopamine D_2 receptor compared to other antipsychotics, with only 40–50 percent occupancy of striatal D_2 receptors, which is postulated to be the reason that clozapine does not cause extrapyramidal side effects. Clozapine is rapidly absorbed orally, with peak plasma levels at 2 hours. Clozapine's elimination half-life increases with chronic administration and reaches 12 hours at steady-state dosing in less than 1 week. Clozapine is highly protein-bound and thus has potential for significant drug interactions. N-demethylclozapine, clozapine's principle metabolite, is thought to have pharmacological activity and may contribute to some of clozapine's unique properties [Weiner et al., 2004].

Clinical Management

Before initiating clozapine, the physician must assess medical history, looking for seizures, cardiac disease, agranulocytosis, substance use history, and concurrent medications or treatments with potential for drug interaction. The patient should undergo a physical examination and a check of vital signs. Baseline work-up should include CBC (specifically white blood count [WBC] and absolute neutrophil count [ANC]), liver function tests, lipid profile, thyroid stimulating hormone, EKG, and EEG. Clozapine is typically started at 12.5 mg 1–2 times daily, and increased in 12.5–25 mg increments up to 150 mg/daily by week 1 and 300 mg by the end of week 2. The typical dose range is 350–550 mg/day, divided 2–3 times. The dose is titrated according to clinical response, with younger patients likely requiring less than adults. Careful monitoring of vital signs is needed to evaluate for tachycardia and orthostatic hypotension. The value of clozapine levels in pediatric populations has not been established [Gogtay and Rapoport, 2008].

Adverse Effects

Common side effects are sedation, dizziness, tachycardia, hypotension, nausea, constipation, sialorrhea (excessive salivation), and weight gain. Seizures are reported in 4 percent of patients, with increasing risk at higher doses. Other less common adverse events include myocarditis, cardiomyopathy, eosinophilia, hepatitis, cerebrovascular accidents, and severe anticholinergic toxicity [Clozaril, 2010]. Agranulocytosis (ANC <500 mm^3) is a serious and potentially fatal adverse effect of clozapine, which is estimated to occur at a rate of 1 percent in adults. The period of greatest risk appears to be in the first 6 months of treatment, after which the rate drops off, but never goes to zero. The FDA requires monitoring of the WBC and ANC throughout the course of treatment. At present, the guidelines require that the CBC and ANC be monitored every week for the first 6 months, every other week for the second 6 months, and then monthly thereafter with uninterrupted treatment. Patients who develop a WBC between 3000 mm^3 and 3500 mm^3, or ANC between 1500 mm^3 and 2000 mm^3, or experience successive drops in their WBC or ANC require twice-weekly monitoring. If the WBC falls below 3000 mm^3 or ANC falls below 1500 mm^3, clozapine must be stopped. Re-challenge is possible if the ANC does not drop below 1000 mm^3 or CBC below 2000 mm^3, although the risk of repeated episodes of neutropenia is high. Clinicians are referred to the manufacturing guidelines for complete detail of monitoring requirements [Clozaril, 2010].

Experience with clozapine in the treatment of treatment-refractory, childhood-onset schizophrenia has shown that neutropenia is more common in children than in adults and is estimated to occur at a rate of 10–13 percent [Gerbino-Rosen et al., 2005; Gogtay and Rapoport, 2008]. Lithium has been used successfully as a pretreatment to mitigate risk of neutropenia, and during treatment with clozapine to boost ANC, although caution is warranted in administrating the two medications. With longer-term use, seizures and lipid abnormalities have been reported. Enuresis is common early in the course of treatment but does appear to improve after the first 4–6 months. In contrast to adults where extrapyramidal symptoms are not reported, akathisia has been reported in children and may respond to the addition of a beta blocker [Gogtay and Rapoport, 2008].

Drug Interactions

Clozapine may potentiate CNS depression when combined with alcohol or CNS-active drugs, such as benzodiazepines. Episodes of cardiovascular collapse have been reported in this context and can result in death [Clozaril, 2010]. Caution should be exercised when administering clozapine concurrently with drugs that cause agranulocytosis. Additionally, co-administration of anticholinergic drugs with clozapine should be avoided. Clozapine is metabolized by cytochrome P-450, and drugs that inhibit this enzyme system can result in elevated clozapine levels. Increased levels of clozapine occur with concurrent use with risperidone, paroxetine, fluoxetine, and fluvoxamine. Poor metabolizers of the P450 system are particularly at risk for elevated clozapine levels. Drugs that induce the P450 enzyme system (carbamazepine and phenytoin) may hasten metabolism of clozapine and thus lower the blood level, requiring dosage adjustment [Sadock and Sadock, 2007].

Conclusion

Increasing evidence for short-term efficacy of many psychotropic medications in children has led to an increased use and hopefully increased benefit for children with psychiatric disorders. With more opportunities for benefit comes increased concern regarding short- and long-term efficacy and safety and strategies for monitoring. Studies are needed to complete the psychopharmacology evidence base for psychotropic medications commonly used in children and, importantly, the development of methods to assess the long-term safety and efficacy of psychotropic agents in children. In addition, studies are needed to evaluate effective and, especially, efficient strategies for monitoring children on medication that can be integrated into today's complex models of physician practice.

Despite these many challenges, children can and do benefit from medications when treatment is provided in the context of a thorough diagnostic assessment that integrates information from multiple sources; knowledge of the available data for adults and children in the literature; knowledge of standards of community care, especially when prescribing medications off-label; an analysis of the risks and benefit of treatment options; appropriate involvement of the parent or guardian in the informed consent process; and close monitoring for adverse effects during therapy.

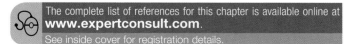

Pediatric Epilepsy: An Overview

Peter R. Camfield and Carol S. Camfield

After a first unprovoked seizure in childhood, the risk of a recurrence is about 50 percent, and after the second the risk is about 80 percent. By convention, epilepsy may be diagnosed only after a child has had two or more unprovoked seizures [Camfield et al., 1985a; Shinnar et al., 2000]. The term unprovoked implies that there has been no closely associated concurrent illness, fever, or acute brain injury. Recurrent seizures immediately after a head injury or associated with drug intoxication do not qualify for the diagnosis of epilepsy. Some specific provoking factors leading to reflex seizures are permitted, such as seizures provoked by patterns and flashes from video terminals for children with photosensitive epilepsy. Seizures are still viewed as unprovoked if they occur with stresses related to personal activity, such as sleep deprivation or severe emotional distress, unless these stresses are extreme.

Seizure Type and Epilepsy Syndrome

The definition of epilepsy allows for a tremendous variety of disorders. The seizure types, age of onset, cause, severity, comorbid conditions, response to medication, and clinical course vary widely. There are two main ways of grouping patients to bring an ordered approach to classification, treatment, and prognosis: seizure type and epilepsy syndrome. Both concepts continue to evolve. The International League against Epilepsy defined the seizure types listed in Box 50-1 [Commission on Classification and Terminology of the International League against Epilepsy, 1981]. There is a basic distinction between seizures with a generalized onset that seem to arise from everywhere in the cortex at once, and seizures with a partial or focal onset that begin in a defined area of cortex. A proposed update in the classification of epileptic seizures suggested that the distinction between simple partial and complex partial seizures is often difficult to assess and not needed [Engel, 2001].

A given seizure type may occur with many different associations. For example, a 2-year-old child with severe mental handicap may have generalized tonic-clonic seizures that are completely resistant to medication, or a normal teenager may have the same seizure type that is completely suppressed by medication. Factors beyond seizure type allow a more comprehensive diagnosis – an epilepsy syndrome diagnosis. Epileptic syndromes may have one or more seizure types, often with a characteristic interictal electroencephalogram (EEG). Each syndrome has a typical age of onset, a defined group of causes, sometimes a clear response to specific treatments, and sometimes a defined clinical course and prognosis. As with seizure types, syndromes have been classified as localization-related (focal) or generalized, and then subdivided into idiopathic (when microdysgenesis or a biochemical etiology is likely), symptomatic (when a diffuse or localized brain abnormality is known), and cryptogenic (when a diffuse or localized brain abnormality is suspected but unproven; Table 50-1). The term cryptogenic has been discouraged, as the detection of a structural lesion is dependent on the evolving quality of brain imaging and detection of a biochemical abnormality is dependent on the evolving understanding of genomic and proteomic abnormalities. In adults, localization-related epilepsy syndromes are most common, usually symptomatic, and caused by a localized, structural abnormality. Children have similar disorders, but there are many other important syndromes. The idiopathic partial and generalized syndromes all begin in childhood, and genetic influences are significant. The generalized symptomatic syndromes of childhood account for most intractable epilepsy in children [Arzimanogolou et al., 2004; Camfield and Camfield, 2003].

The International League Against Epilepsy (ILAE) classified febrile seizures as a special syndrome. Febrile seizures are the most common convulsive event in the human species. Because these seizures are provoked by fever, febrile seizures do not fit well with the usual definition of epilepsy, and few children with febrile seizures later develop unprovoked seizures. The disorder merits special consideration, as reviewed in Chapter 57.

The 1989 ILAE syndrome classification scheme is still in wide use, and most patients can be "forced" into one of the broad categories, but many children, especially those with symptomatic generalized epilepsy, do not meet the criteria for a more specific syndrome [Commission on Classification and Terminology of the International League Against Epilepsy, 1989]. There are many recently described epilepsy syndromes, but a newer, comprehensive syndrome classification system has been elusive. Advances in genetics have revealed that the same mutation may cause a variety of epilepsy syndromes, including partial and generalized epilepsies, even within the same family (see Chapter 52). This finding has been particularly well illustrated in large families with mutations in the gene coding for neuronal sodium channel – *SCN1A*.

Another evolving classification is "epilepic encephalopathy," defined as an epilepsy syndrome where the seizures and/or interictal EEG discharge have permanent deleterious effects on brain development. Examples would be West's syndrome with infantile spasms and hypsarrhythmia on EEG, Lennox–Gastaut syndrome with mixed generalized

Box 50-1 International Classification of Seizure Type

Partial Seizures

- Simple partial seizures
    - With motor signs
    - With somatosensory or special sensory hallucinations
    - With autonomic symptoms
    - With psychic symptoms
- Complex partial seizures
    - Simple partial followed by impairment of consciousness
    - With impaired consciousness at onset
- Partial seizures evolving to secondary generalized seizures
    - Simple partial seizures evolving to generalized
    - Complex partial seizures evolving to generalized
    - Simple partial seizures evolving to complex partial seizures

Generalized Seizures

- Absence seizures
    - Atypical absence seizures
- Myoclonic seizures
- Clonic seizures
- Tonic seizures
- Tonic-clonic seizures
- Atonic seizures

Unclassifiable Epileptic Seizures

(Adapted from the Commission on Classification and Terminology of the International League against Epilepsy. Proposal for revised clinical and electroencephalographic classification of epileptic seizures. Epilepsia 1981;22:489.)

Table 50-1 Proposal from the International Classification of Epilepsies and Epileptic Syndromes and Related Seizure Disorders of 1989 and the Listing of Epilepsy Syndromes Recognized in the Proposed 2001 ILAE Classification Scheme

1989 ILAE Classification*	2001 ILAE Proposal[†]
LOCALIZATION-RELATED (LOCAL, FOCAL, PARTIAL EPILEPSIES AND SYNDROMES	
Idiopathic (with Age-Related Onset)	
Benign childhood epilepsy with centrotemporal spikes	Benign childhood epilepsy with centrotemporal spikes
Childhood epilepsy with occipital paroxysms	Early-onset benign childhood occipital epilepsy (Panayiotopoulos type) *(new)* Late-onset childhood occipital epilepsy (Gastaut type) *(new)* Idiopathic photosensitive occipital lobe epilepsy *(new)*

Primary reading epilepsy	Primary reading epilepsy
	 Now called Reflex epilepsies, *which also includes:*
	   Other visual sensitive epilepsies
	   Primary reading epilepsy
	   Startle epilepsy

Symptomatic or Cryptogenic	
Chronic progressive epilepsia partialis continua	*(No longer listed; see Rasmussen's syndrome below)*
Syndromes characterized by seizures with specific modes of precipitation	*Now a Reflex epilepsy*

Temporal lobe epilepsies	Limbic epilepsies *(expanded)*
	   Mesial temporal lobe epilepsy with hippocampal sclerosis
	   Mesial temporal lobe epilepsy defined by specific etiologies
	   Other types defined by location and etiology
	 Neocortical epilepsies *(new)*
	   Rasmussen's syndrome *(new)*
	   Hemiconvulsion-hemiplegia syndrome
	   "Migrating partial seizures of infancy" *(new)*
	 Other types defined by location and etiology *(new)*
	   Familial temporal lobe epilepsies *(new)*
	   "Familial focal epilepsy with variable foci" *(new)*

Frontal lobe epilepsies	*(No longer listed, as location of onset of seizures is insufficient for classification of a syndrome)*
Parietal lobe epilepsies	*(No longer listed, as location of onset of seizures is insufficient for classification of a syndrome)*
Occipital lobe epilepsies	*(No longer listed, as location of onset of seizures is insufficient for classification of a syndrome)*

Table 50-1 Proposal from the International Classification of Epilepsies and Epileptic Syndromes and Related Seizure Disorders of 1989 and the Listing of Epilepsy Syndromes Recognized in the Proposed 2001 ILAE Classification Scheme—cont'd

1989 ILAE Classification*	2001 ILAE Proposal[†]
GENERALIZED EPILEPSIES AND SYNDROMES	
Idiopathic (with Age-Related Onset)	
Benign familial neonatal seizures	Benign familial neonatal seizures
Benign neonatal convulsions	Benign neonatal convulsions *(Diagnosis of epilepsy not now required)*
Benign myoclonic epilepsy in infancy	Benign myoclonic epilepsy in infancy Benign familial infantile seizures Benign infantile seizures (nonfamilial)
Childhood absence epilepsy	Childhood absence epilepsy Juvenile absence epilepsy *(new)*
Juvenile myoclonic epilepsy	Juvenile myoclonic epilepsy
Epilepsy with grand mal seizures on awakening	Epilepsy with generalized tonic-clonic seizures only *(renamed)*
Childhood absence epilepsy	Childhood absence epilepsy
Other generalized idiopathic epilepsies	Other undetermined epilepsies not defined above Juvenile absence epilepsy *(new)*
Juvenile myoclonic epilepsy	Juvenile myoclonic epilepsy Landau–Kleffner syndrome (LKS) *(new)* Epilepsy with continuous spike-and-waves during slow-wave sleep (other than LKS) *(new)* Progressive myoclonus epilepsies *(new)*
Epilepsies with seizures precipitated by specific modes of activation	*Now called Reflex epilepsies*
Cryptogenic or Symptomatic	
West's syndrome	West's syndrome
Lennox–Gastaut syndrome	Lennox–Gastaut syndrome
Epilepsy with myoclonic-astatic seizures	Epilepsy with myoclonic-astatic seizures
Epilepsy with myoclonic seizures	*(No longer listed)*
Epilepsy with myoclonic absences	Epilepsy with myoclonic absences
Early infantile epileptic encephalopathy with suppression burst	Ohtahara's syndrome *(renamed)*
Early myoclonic encephalopathy	Early myoclonic encephalopathy Myoclonic status in progressive encephalopathies *(new)*
Other symptomatic generalized epilepsies	
Specific syndromes	
Epileptic seizures complicating other disease states	
Epilepsies and syndromes undetermined whether focal or generalized with both generalized and focal seizures	
Neonatal seizures	*(No longer listed)*
Severe myoclonic epilepsy of infancy	Dravet's syndrome *(renamed)*
Epilepsy with continuous spike waves during slow-wave sleep	Epilepsy with continuous spike waves during slow-wave sleep (not LKS)
Acquired epileptic epilepsies (LKS)	Acquired epileptic epilepsies *(renamed)* (LKS) "Generalized epilepsies with febrile seizures plus" *(new)* Autosomal-dominant nocturnal frontal lobe epilepsy
Other undetermined epilepsies without unequivocal generalized or focal features	
Special syndromes	
Situation-related seizures	
Febrile convulsions	Febrile seizures *(renamed)*
Isolated seizures of isolated status epilepticus	*(No longer listed)*
Seizures occurring only with acute metabolic or toxic events	Drug or other chemically induced seizures *(expanded)* Alcohol withdrawal seizures Single seizures or isolated clusters of seizures Rarely repeated seizures (oligoepilepsy) Immediate and early post-traumatic seizures

* Modified from the 1989 International League Against Epilepsy (ILAE) Proposal.
[†] Modified from the 2001 ILAE Proposal. In this proposal there are no headings or subheadings, only a listing of epilepsy syndromes by specific syndrome name. Our format of presentation has indicated where syndromes are removed or renamed from the 1989 ILAE proposal or newly recognized in the 2001 proposal. Each syndrome was "forced" into the 1989 proposed schema.

seizures and nearly continuous slow spike wave EEG discharge, or Landau–Kleffner syndrome with relatively mild clinical seizures but very active bitemporal epileptic EEG discharge (see Chapter 56).

A new proposal for syndrome classification in 2001 is based on a five-axis system [Engel, 2001]. Axis 1 concerns ictal phenomenology (i.e., what the seizure looks like). Axis 2 is the specific seizure type. Axis 3 is the specific epilepsy syndrome, when it can be defined; axis 4 is the cause; and axis 5 describes the degree of impairment associated with epilepsy. This proposal comes with a more comprehensive list of epilepsy syndromes, although the system is less categorical than the 1989 classification [Commission on Classification and Terminology of the International League against Epilepsy, 1989]. The 2001 proposal has not been widely accepted, although it does serve well to alert the clinician to the many aspects of the epileptic diathesis in an individual patient. Table 50-1 highlights the differences between the two classification schemes by using each to characterize some accepted epileptic syndromes. A clinician interested in epilepsy should be conversant with the 1989 and 2001 classification schemes and must anticipate additional revisions.

Incidence

In developed countries, the overall incidence of childhood epilepsy from birth to 16 years is approximately 40 cases in 100,000 children per year [Camfield et al., 1996b; Hauser et al., 1993]. The incidence in the first year of life is about 120 in 100,000. Between 1 and 10 years of age, the incidence plateaus at 40–50 cases in 100,000 children, and then drops further in the teenage years to about 20 in 100,000. The details of incidence by year of life from the Nova Scotia childhood epilepsy study are illustrated in Figure 50-1. Hauser estimates that about 1 percent of all children will have at least one afebrile seizure by age 14 years, and that 0.4–0.8 percent will have epilepsy by age 11 years [Hauser and Hesdorffer, 1990]. In less developed countries, there is suggestive evidence for a higher incidence of childhood epilepsy, possibly related to higher incidence of trauma and central nervous system infections.

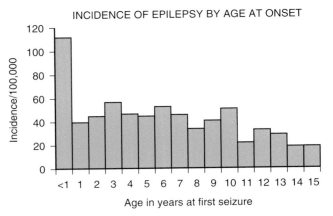

INCIDENCE OF EPILEPSY BY AGE AT ONSET

Fig. 50-1 Incidence of epilepsy by age of onset. *(From Camfield CS et al. Incidence of epilepsy in childhood and adolescents: A population based study in Nova Scotia from 1977–1985. Epilepsia 1996b;37:19.)*

Epilepsy types vary in incidence. Syndromes dominated by generalized tonic-clonic or partial seizures account for 75 percent of childhood epilepsy. Syndromes dominated by absence seizures account for approximately 15 percent, and the secondary generalized epilepsies account for 10 percent. The latter group includes most of the "catastrophic" epilepsy syndromes, such as West and Lennox–Gastaut syndromes [Camfield et al., 1996b]. Prevalence data for seizure type or epilepsy syndrome are not easily collated because of various definitions of active epilepsy. When active epilepsy was defined as receiving daily antiepileptic drugs or a seizure within the past 5 years, the prevalence of epilepsy in children was 4.3–9.3 in 1000 [Hauser and Hesdorffer, 1990]. Because some epileptic syndromes rarely remit, they contribute more to prevalence of epilepsy than its incidence. The relative prevalence of symptomatic generalized epilepsies is higher than their relative incidence. This finding means that physicians who focus on newly diagnosed children will encounter a predominance of benign epilepsy syndromes. Those primarily treating chronic cases will observe a higher proportion of more malignant seizure disorders. A population-based prevalence study from Finland found that the main seizure types for each patient were focal in 43 percent, with complex partial and partial with secondary generalization most common. For 44 percent, generalized seizures were dominant, with generalized tonic-clonic seizures most common. Overall, 45 percent had localization-related epilepsy syndromes, and 48 percent had generalized syndromes [Eriksson and Koivikko, 1997].

Differential Diagnosis

The diagnosis of epilepsy is based almost exclusively on a clinical history of two or more unprovoked seizures. Parents vary in their capacity to describe these frightening events, and physicians vary in their ability to ask good questions. Some children are misdiagnosed. A Dutch group of neurologists shared case descriptions of childhood seizure disorders and were able to agree about most diagnoses of epilepsy; however, in 207 cases of possible first seizures, there was disagreement in 35 percent [Van Donselaar et al., 1989] – even experts sometimes disagree. Studies of interobserver reliability have demonstrated important differences in observations when families and neurologists have reviewed the same video seizures, and neurologists often disagree with each other. Neurology residents and faculty often classify seizures differently based on written histories [Camfield and Camfield, 2003]. When the history is not clear-cut, it is better to wait for additional attacks before diagnosing epilepsy. A list of disorders in children that are frequently confused with epilepsy is found in Box 50-2. Reflex anoxic seizures associated with pallid or vasodepressor syncope or with cyanotic breath-holding are particularly likely to be misinterpreted [Stephenson, 1991] (see Chapter 64).

The EEG can be used to make the diagnosis of epilepsy only if a seizure is recorded – a rare event on routine EEG acquisition because most children with epilepsy have infrequent seizures. A small percentage of normal children have epileptiform activity on EEG but never have a seizure [Petersen and Eeg-Olofsson, 1968], and up to 40 percent of children with chronic epilepsy never demonstrate epileptiform discharges on interictal EEG [Camfield et al., 1995]. EEG findings may change significantly over time and reveal conflicting findings [Camfield et al.,

---

Box 50-2 Disorders that may Mimic Childhood Epilepsy

Confused with Generalized Tonic-Clonic Seizures

- Pallid syncope (reflex anoxic seizure)
- Vasodepressor syncope (reflex anoxic seizure)
- Cyanotic breath-holding attacks
- Collapsing attacks with cardiac dysrhythmias
- Cataplexy

Confused with Generalized Absence Seizures

- Behavioral staring attacks
- Complex partial seizures
- Tic disorder

Confused with Complex Partial Seizures

- Self-stimulatory behavior, especially in children with autistic spectrum disorders

- Sleep walking
- Night terrors
- Temper tantrums with amnesia for the rage event
- Benign paroxysmal vertigo
- Migraine-related disorders

Confused with Epileptic Myoclonus

- Physiologic hypnagogic myoclonus
- Benign infantile sleep myoclonus
- Startle disease

1995; Trojaborg, 1968]. An interictal EEG is often useful for syndrome clarification but must be interpreted in the clinical context.

Likewise, the diagnosis of epilepsy cannot be based on brain-imaging studies. The presence of an anomaly on magnetic resonance imaging (MRI) increases the possibility of epilepsy and, depending on the nature of the abnormality, increases the likelihood of a specific syndrome. For example, lesions typical of tuberous sclerosis in the first year of life increase the risk that a child will have West's syndrome.

Natural History of Childhood Epilepsy

Recurrence after a First Seizure

Many children are seen by a physician after a first unprovoked generalized tonic-clonic seizure, a few after a first complex partial seizure, but almost none after a single absence or myoclonic seizure. For children presenting after a single unprovoked seizure, there is an immediate question: Will it happen again? Berg and Shinnar's meta-analysis of the recurrence risk after a first seizure concluded that, overall, about 40 percent will have a second seizure [Berg and Shinnar, 1991; Shinnar et al., 1996]. There is much less information about the further recurrence risk after a second seizure, especially if medication is withheld. Current data suggest that the risk of a third seizure after a second is at least 80 percent [Camfield et al., 1985b; Shinnar et al., 2000; Hauser et al., 1998]. These observations validate the restriction of the diagnosis of epilepsy to those with two or more unprovoked seizures, because the concept of epilepsy implies a chronic, recurring disorder.

If a child has a single seizure, a small number of clinical features are helpful in predicting the risk of a second seizure. These include remote symptomatic cause, partial seizures, presence of intellectual or mental handicap, and possibly EEG spike discharge [Berg and Shinnar, 1991]. A normal child with a first generalized tonic-clonic seizure and a normal EEG has a recurrence risk of 20–30 percent, whereas a child with mental handicap, a partial seizure, and spike discharge on the EEG has a recurrence risk of 80–90 percent [Berg and Shinnar, 1991; Camfield et al., 1985b]. The value of MRI lesions in predicting recurrence after a first seizure has not been extensively evaluated [Arthur et al., 2008]. If a second seizure is to occur, it usually happens shortly after the first. At least 75 percent of recurrences happen within 6 months of the first, and most occur within a few weeks. Few recurrences are observed after 2 years.

Very few children presenting with a first seizure develop severe epilepsy. Of 407 children with a first seizure identified by Shinnar et al. [2000], only 13 percent went on to have more than 10 seizures over the next 10 years. However, 28 percent of those with two seizures had more than 10 subsequent seizures.

Starting Medication Treatment

There is little justification for beginning daily medication after a child's first unprovoked seizure because 60 percent of these children will never have another attack [Van Donselaar et al., 1989; Hirtz et al., 2003]. Population-based studies have found that medication prescription after the first seizure does not alter the recurrence rate, probably because of poor compliance in taking the medication [Camfield et al., 1985b; Hauser et al., 1982; Hirtz et al., 1984]. An open-label, randomized trial of medication versus no medication after a first seizure in 397 children and adults demonstrated a significant reduction in recurrences for those on medication over a 2-year treatment period [First Seizure Trial Group, 1993]. The risk of recurrence without treatment was 51 percent by 24 months, but there were still relapses in 25 percent of those randomized to medication (i.e., 2.8 times higher; 95 percent confidence interval [CI] = 1.9–4.2). When this cohort was followed for several more years, the eventual remission rate was the same for those treated or untreated after the first seizure [Musicco et al., 1997].

It has become common practice to prescribe medication after a second seizure. There is no evidence that the prescription of medication alters the long-term outlook of childhood epilepsy. There is convincing information that delaying antiepileptic drug treatment until the child has had up to 10 seizures does not alter the ease of seizure control or the long-term remission rate [Camfield et al., 1996a; Arts and Geerts, 2009]. In other words, if a child has few seizures, there is no evidence that each seizure facilitates the next. The main reasons to treat children with antiepileptic drugs are the avoidance of bodily injury from seizures and improvement in psychosocial function. Results from several studies indicate that injury is uncommon with most seizure types in children. Peters et al. [2001] described 79 children with benign rolandic epilepsy who together had more than 900 seizures over an 8.5-year period. There were no significant injuries. In a group of 59 children with generalized absence seizures followed over 15 years, Wirrell et al. [1997] observed that 16 had a serious physical injury as the result of a seizure. Kirsch et al. [2001] compared 31 cognitively normal children with epilepsy with best-friend controls and found no significant differences in injury number or severity. Hodgman et al. [1979] described 25 adolescents with generalized tonic-clonic epilepsy and observed that those with poorer seizure control were better able to communicate about seizures and had a better self-image. The "hidden handicap" for children with controlled seizures may have important effects on social adjustment. Epilepsy in children and adults has attracted social stigma in most cultures. Helping children deal with perceived and actual stigma may be an important part of treatment [Bandstra et al., 2008]. Once medication is started, most children still have more seizures. Only about 20 percent have "smooth-sailing epilepsy," meaning that they start medication, become immediately seizure-free, and later are able to discontinue medication successfully without ever having another seizure [Camfield et al., 1993]. Only 50 percent of children continue to receive the same medication 1 year after initiating treatment [Camfield et al., 1985b; Canadian Childhood Epilepsy Study Group, 1996; Verity et al., 1995]. The decision to start medication is often not the end of the seizure problem.

Long-Term Remission

For many children, epilepsy is transient, and with maturation, the problem seems to vanish. At the time of diagnosis, it is possible to predict that at least 50 percent of children will outgrow their disorder and be able to discontinue medication [Camfield et al., 1993]. The Dutch Study of Epilepsy in Childhood followed 453 newly diagnosed children and found that 64 percent were no longer receiving medication 5 years later [Arts et al., 2004; Arts and Geerts, 2009]. The longer the follow-up, the higher the proportion with remission of symptoms. In Rochester, Minnesota, 115 children with epilepsy beginning before age 10 years were followed through the Mayo Clinic record linkage system. Ten years later, 75 percent had been seizure-free for at least 5 years, and 51 percent no longer received medication [Hauser et al., 1993]. At the end of a remarkable 30-year follow-up study of children with epilepsy from a population-based sample in Turku, Finland, Sillanpaa [1993] found that 76 percent of survivors had been seizure-free for at least 3 years.

Across most studies, factors that predict which children will outgrow their epilepsy have included normal intelligence, normal neurologic examination findings, relatively small numbers of seizures at diagnosis (which makes complex partial seizures unlikely), age of the first seizure below about 12 years, and absence of a remote symptomatic cause (an identified brain problem that preceded the onset of epilepsy). In an 8-year follow-up study of a population-based study of 504 children with epilepsy from Nova Scotia, a predictive scoring system was developed; it is outlined in Table 50-2 [Sillanpaa et al., 1995]. Those with a good prognosis had an 80 percent chance of remission (i.e., seizure-free and no longer receiving medication). For those with one or more of these adverse factors, the chance of remission was less but still about 40 percent. The Dutch Study of Epilepsy in Childhood found comparable predictive variables and supplemented these with the clinical

Table 50-2 Scoring System for Remission of Childhood Epilepsy at the Time of Diagnosis

Variable	Score*
Age of first seizure (months)	
<12	99
12–144	142
>144	0
Intelligence	
Normal	111
Retardation	0
Previous neonatal seizures	
No	218
Yes	0
Number of seizures before starting medication	
1 or 2	72
3–20	123
>20	0

* Add the scores from this column. If the total score is greater than 495, the child is predicted to have remission of epilepsy.

(Adapted from Sillanpaa M et al. Predicting long term outcome of childhood epilepsy in Nova Scotia, Canada, and Turku: Validation of a simple scoring system. Arch Neurol 1995;52:589.)

course in the first 6 months of treatment. Rates of correct prediction were similar. Based on clinical features present at the time of diagnosis, it is possible to predict the long-term outcome with moderate accuracy. Surprisingly, most epilepsy syndromes do not have a definite outcome; however, a few specific syndromes allow an accurate prognosis [Camfield et al., 2003]. Epilepsy is always outgrown in cases of benign rolandic epilepsy, benign myoclonic epilepsy of infancy, and benign occipital epilepsy, early-onset type. Epilepsy is never outgrown by children with Rasmussen's syndrome, Lennox–Gastaut syndrome, or Dravet's syndrome. The Dutch and Nova Scotia studies were combined to allow study of 1055 newly diagnosed patients with at least 5 years of follow-up [Geelhoed et al., 2005]. Multivariate analysis that took into account clinical factors, syndrome diagnosis, and response to treatment in the first 6 months revealed that, at the time of diagnosis, a prognostic scoring scheme could correctly predict remission or no remission in about 70 percent. This means that, at the time of diagnosis, if parents ask "will the seizures be outgrown?", the physician will give the wrong answer in about one-third of cases.

Stopping Medication

About 60–70 percent of children with epilepsy who have become seizure-free for 1–2 years can successfully stop medication treatment [Berg and Shinnar, 1991; Dooley et al., 1996]. The rate of success is no greater if medication is continued for up to 5 years seizure-free [Hollowach-Thurston et al., 1982]. Factors that predict successful discontinuation of medication include generalized seizures, age of onset before 10–12 years, normal neurologic examination, and in some studies, resolution of interictal EEG spike discharges. Children with no adverse factors may have an 80–90 percent success rate. Each factor has an additive effect and those with all of the adverse factors may have only a 10–20 percent success rate.

If an initial discontinuation trial is unsuccessful, medication is usually restarted. About 50 percent of children again become seizure-free for sufficient time to try to discontinue medication a second time, with a 70 percent success rate [Camfield et al., 1993]. The remission rate for juvenile myoclonic epilepsy (JME) is low, although a recent population-based study suggested that eventually 40 percent will no longer require daily medication [Camfield et al., 2009]. Still, most experts suggest that medication for JME should be continued lifelong and that further attempts to discontinue medication after an initial failure are probably not warranted [Delgado-Escueta and Enrile-Bacsal, 1984].

A Scandinavian study randomized 207 children at the time of diagnosis of epilepsy to receive 1 or 3 years of treatment [Braathen and Melander, 1997]. If the child was seizure-free for the last 6 months of study, medication was discontinued. This practice meant that some of the children in the 1-year treatment group had been seizure-free for only 6 months before medication was stopped. The success rate for those in the short-treatment group was significantly less than for the 3-year group (53 percent vs. 71 percent). A Dutch study randomized 161 children with epilepsy that was controlled within 2 months of starting treatment to 6 months or 1 year of treatment. The 6-month group had a higher relapse rate when medication was stopped; however, by 2 years later, the rates of remission were identical [Peters et al., 1998]. None the less, for a substantial number of children, epilepsy was a short-lived disorder requiring only short-term medication use. Medication treatment for benign rolandic epilepsy often is not needed [Peters et al., 2001], and further studies will likely identify other children who do not require drug treatment.

Intractability

Defining intractable epilepsy is difficult, and many definitions have been suggested [Berg et al., 2006a]. For a study of 613 children with epilepsy from Connecticut, Berg and Shinnar [2001] defined intractability as a "failure, for lack of seizure control, of more than 2 first-line antiepileptic drugs with an average of more than one seizure per month for 18 months and no more than 3 consecutive months seizure free during that interval." There were 60 intractable cases in the first 24 months after diagnosis. The proportions of intractable patients in each major syndrome grouping were as follows: cryptogenic/symptomatic generalized, 34.6 percent; idiopathic generalized, 2.7 percent; other localization-related, 10.7 percent; and unclassified, 8.2 percent. Sillanpaa's [1993] follow-up study from Turku, Finland, defined intractability as one or more seizures per year in the past 10 years of follow-up. After 20 years of follow-up, 22 percent of the subjects met these criteria. Predictors of intractability included poor initial response to medication, remote symptomatic cause, and status epilepticus. The Dutch Study of Childhood Epilepsy (using Berg and Shinnar's definition of intractability), with 453 children followed for 5 years, found that 6 percent were intractable [Arts et al., 2004]. Camfield et al. [1993] defined intractability as "at least one seizure each three months for the last year of follow-up, with failure of at least 3 antiepileptic drugs." For those with partial and generalized tonic-clonic epilepsies, 8 percent of 511 children became intractable during an average of 8 years of follow-up. After 20 years of follow-up, 51 percent of 75 patients with childhood-onset symptomatic generalized epilepsy had intractable seizures. In this study, the major predictor was severe neurologic deficit at the time of diagnosis.

An important issue in the definition of intractability is the length of follow-up. In the clinical setting, many children with intractable epilepsy eventually become well controlled. In a series of 145 children with intractible seizures (i.e., less than one per month for at least 2 years) followed over 18 years, Huttenlocker and Hapke observed that 75 percent of normally intelligent children and 30 percent with mental handicap had complete or nearly complete seizure remission (i.e., less than one seizure per year) [Huttenlocker and Hapke, 1990]. In the Nova Scotia cohort, 39 patients with partial and generalized tonic-clonic epilepsies had intractable epilepsy after 7 years' follow-up. After 12.5 years of follow-up, 7 (18 percent) of 39 became seizure-free [Camfield et al., 1996a].

In contrast, when the history was reviewed retrospectively for adults undergoing a work-up for intractable epilepsy, it was common to find long periods of remission during childhood [Berg et al., 2006b]. Intractable epilepsy in childhood may spontaneously resolve and epilepsy in childhood may remit, only to re-emerge as intractable epilepsy in adulthood.

There is controversy about how the number of drug failures required before intractability can be declared. In a Scottish study of 470 newly treated adults, 47 percent became seizure-free with their first antiepileptic drug [Kwan and Brodie, 2000]. Only 11 percent gained control with subsequent medications. In children, the failure of a first drug is important but far less ominous [Camfield et al., 1997]. Of 417 eligible patients with partial and generalized tonic-clonic epilepsies with at least 4 years of follow-up, 83 percent were successfully treated with a single antiepileptic drug during the first year of treatment. Of these, 61 percent eventually had remission of epilepsy, and 4 percent had intractable seizures. Among the 17 percent who failed treatment with their first antiepileptic drug, 42 percent eventually had complete remission of epilepsy, although 29 percent developed intractable seizures. Children with absence epilepsies had nearly identical findings [Wirrell et al., 2001].

In summary, intractability for an individual child is difficult to predict before several years of antiepileptic drug treatment. Intractability appears to decrease with prolonged follow-up, although the burden of this wait-and-see approach may be substantial. Failure of a first antiepileptic drug is a risk factor for intractability but none the less many remit. As a general rule, consideration for epilepsy surgery should await failure of three appropriate drug treatments. Other factors influence this decision, including seizure severity, frequency, and duration of epilepsy.

Psychosocial Outcome for Children with Epilepsy

Children with epilepsy have high rates of behavior and cognitive problems that contribute to social dysfunction in childhood and in later adulthood, even if the epilepsy resolves. These issues are reviewed in more detail in Chapter 51. Austin et al. [2002] reported that, at the time of diagnosis, 40 percent of children were at significant risk of behavior problems, as judged by scores on the Child Behavior Checklist. Those with multiple recurrent seizures were at even higher risk.

The Isle of Wight study found that children with epilepsy had high rates of behavioral disorders [Rutter et al., 1970], which might have had their origins in social stigmatization, comorbid cognitive disorders, or medication effects. Oostrom et al. [2003] demonstrated greater cognitive and behavioral problems and the need for special educational assistance among 51 outpatient children with idiopathic or cryptogenic epilepsy compared with their classmate controls. Trostle [1988] reported that parents indicate a reluctance to have their normal children play with a child with epilepsy. Less than one-third of 20,000 U.S. high-school students indicated that they would date a person with epilepsy [Austin et al., 2002]. These behavioral, cognitive, and social stigma problems in childhood all point to grave concerns for the social adjustment and success of children with epilepsy after they reach adulthood.

Kokkonen et al. [1997] described the social outcome (by interview or questionnaire) of 81 young, "noninstitutionalized" adults from the catchment area of Oulu, Finland, compared with 211 randomly selected controls from the same birth cohort. At least 20 percent of this sample were unable to complete 9 years of education and presumably had severe learning disorders or mental retardation. They accounted for most of the poor social outcome, including a high rate of educational failure, failure to marry, and unemployment.

In Nova Scotia and Finland, children with "epilepsy only" were followed into young adulthood [Camfield et al., 1993; Jalava et al., 1997]. "Epilepsy only" meant having normal intelligence and no other neurologic handicaps. About 30 percent of each cohort had significant social adjustment problems, with decreased rates of stable relationships, marriage, social contacts, job satisfaction, and work achievement. Rates of unemployment or underemployment were high. Social outcome was not clearly related to epilepsy remission, and in the Nova Scotia study, variables related directly to epilepsy, such as age of onset, type of medication treatment, presence or absence of seizure remission, and frequency and severity of seizures, did not appear to predict social outcome in young adulthood [Camfield et al., 1993]. The strongest predictor of poor social outcome was the presence of a learning disorder, although predictive models were inaccurate; the main reasons for the unsatisfactory outcomes were unclear.

Wakamoto et al. [2000] studied 148 normally intelligent young adults (>20 years old) living in a rural district of Japan who had childhood-onset epilepsy. This population-based study found that 72 percent attended regular classes (versus 99 percent of those without epilepsy), 66 percent (versus 97 percent) entered high school, 67 percent (versus 95 percent) had employment, and 23 percent (versus 33 percent) married. There were 49 patients with mental handicap having a less satisfactory outcome: 14 percent attended regular class, 6 percent entered high school, 20 percent were employed, and 2 percent married.

Few studies have addressed the social outcome of children with specific epilepsy syndromes. Several studies have indicated a favorable outcome for adults with previous benign rolandic epilepsy (Loiseau et al., 1983; Peters et al., 2001). In the Nova Scotia study, 56 children with typical childhood absence epilepsy were followed to young adulthood [Wirrell et al., 1997] and compared with a similar cohort with mild juvenile rheumatoid arthritis. Those with absence had significantly greater problems with impulsive behavior, including a 34 percent risk of an unplanned pregnancy. Educational and work achievement, family and other social relationships, and alcohol abuse were more often unsatisfactory. Those with on-going seizures despite medication had greater problems; however, most of the poor social outcome was unrelated to epilepsy-specific factors. The findings in JME were similar – 24 normally intelligent patients followed for 20–30 years had an unemployment rate of 35 percent with many unplanned pregnancies and social isolation [Camfield and Camfield, 2009]. Therefore, childhood epilepsy may have a lifelong, serious effect on social function, an effect that is greater than some other chronic disorders of childhood. Intervention studies have not been undertaken; however, the role of learning disorders and inadequate education is clear. If the long-term social outcome is to be rectified, physicians must address these areas with an enthusiasm equal to the drug treatment of childhood epilepsy. Early referral to an epilepsy support group may be of benefit.

Mortality in Children with Epilepsy

Children with epilepsy have a 5.3 times higher risk of dying than the general population [Camfield, et al., 2002]. The causes that lead to this excess are direct complications of seizures (e.g., aspiration or cardiac arrhythmia), accidents caused by seizures (e.g., falling into a fire), comorbid conditions (e.g., decompensated hydrocephalus), and suicide or sudden unexpected death in epilepsy (SUDEP). Three large prospective studies have found that children with epilepsy but no neurological deficit have the same survival as the general population. [Callenbach et al., 2001; Berg et al., 2006; Camfield et al., 2002]. SUDEP is very rare (2 of 1777 newly diagnosed cases). The excessive mortality in childhood epilepsy is almost entirely accounted for by comorbid severe neurological problems, especially those that affect bulbar function. The clinician can reassure families of normal children with epilepsy that they do not face an increased risk of untimely death despite the frightening nature of seizures.

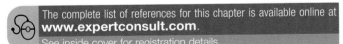

The complete list of references for this chapter is available online at **www.expertconsult.com**.
See inside cover for registration details.

Neurophysiology of Seizures and Epilepsy

Carl E. Stafstrom and Jong M. Rho

This chapter reviews the cellular basis for focal and generalized seizure activity and the factors that influence the enhanced susceptibility of the immature brain to seizures and epilepsy. Emphasis is placed on ion channels and synaptic transmission, and how their dysfunction can lead to the cellular hyperexcitability and hypersynchronous neuronal firing that characterize seizures. Finally, the mechanisms of actions of antiepileptic drugs (AEDs) are summarized.

A seizure is defined as abnormal neuronal firing leading to a clinical alteration of neurologic function (motor, sensory, autonomic, or psychological). Electrical activity underlying a seizure is the net product of biochemical processes at the cellular level occurring in the context of large neuronal networks and likely involves several key cortical and subcortical structures. The output of this activity is reflected on the surface electroencephalogram (EEG), which is the primary clinical tool for measuring normal and abnormal brain electrical activity. Epilepsy is the condition of recurrent spontaneous seizures arising from aberrant electrical activity within the brain. Epilepsy is not a singular disease, but rather is heterogeneous in terms of clinical expression, underlying causes, and pathophysiology (Table 51-1). An epilepsy syndrome refers to a group of signs and symptoms that usually occur together, such as seizure type, age of seizure onset, responsiveness to a particular AED, and characteristic EEG findings, genetics, and natural history. Epileptogenesis is the process by which neural circuits undergo structural or physiological changes, resulting in an enduring epileptic state.

At the cellular level, the two hallmark features of a seizure are neuronal hyperexcitability and neuronal hypersynchrony. Hyperexcitability refers to the reduced threshold for neuronal firing, while hypersynchrony is defined by neurons in a given area firing together. Therefore, a seizure reflects aberrant function at the level of both single neurons and the neuronal network.

Classification of Seizures

Seizures are broadly divided into two groups, depending on their site of origin and pattern of spread (Figure 51-1). Partial seizures arise from a localized region of the brain, and the associated clinical manifestations are related to the function ordinarily subserved by that area. Focal discharges can spread locally through synaptic and nonsynaptic mechanisms, distally to subcortical structures, and through commissural pathways

that may eventually involve the entire cortex; this evolution is believed to occur when focal seizures secondarily generalize. For example, a seizure arising from the left motor cortex may cause jerking movements of the right upper extremity. If epileptiform discharges subsequently spread to adjacent areas and eventually encompass the entire brain, it is described as a secondarily generalized tonic-clonic seizure.

Primary generalized seizures begin with abnormal electrical discharges in both hemispheres simultaneously and involve reciprocal thalamocortical connections (see Figure 51-1). The EEG signature of a primary generalized seizure is bilateral synchronous spike-wave discharges seen across all scalp electrodes. The manifestations of such widespread epileptiform activity can range from brief impairment of consciousness (e.g., an absence seizure) to rhythmic jerking movements of all extremities accompanied by loss of posture and consciousness.

Epilepsies or epilepsy syndromes have likewise been categorized into those in which seizures begin focally (partially) or throughout the brain (generalized), with further division into those that have a known etiology (symptomatic) and those that do not (idiopathic; many of these have a genetic basis) [Commission, 1989]. The classification of epilepsy syndromes is undergoing revision as new knowledge of epilepsy genetics and pathophysiology emerges [Engel, 2006].

Cellular Electrophysiology

Excitation/Inhibition Balance

Although there are differences in the mechanisms that underlie partial and generalized seizures, it is useful to view any seizure activity as a perturbation in the normal balance between inhibition and excitation. This imbalance can involve a localized region, multiple brain areas, or the entire brain, and often reflects a combination of increased excitation and decreased inhibition. However, the traditional concept of a seizure arising when the excitation/inhibition balance is altered is useful but oversimplified. It is now appreciated that factors once thought to be solely inhibitory (e.g., gamma-aminobutyric acid (GABA) synaptic transmission) can actually be excitatory in some circumstances (see Increased Seizure Susceptibility of the Immature Brain, below). Furthermore, synaptic inhibition is critical for certain normal brain rhythms and probably also plays a role in abnormal rhythmic activity, such as spike-wave discharges [Fritschy, 2008].

Table 51-1 **Examples of Pathophysiologic Defects Leading to Epilepsy**

Level of Brain Function	Condition	Pathophysiologic Mechanism
Neuronal network	Cerebral dysgenesis, post-traumatic scar, mesial temporal sclerosis (in TLE)	Altered neuronal circuits; formation of aberrant excitatory connections (i.e., sprouting)
Neuron structure	Down syndrome and other syndromes with mental retardation and seizures	Abnormal structure of dendrites and dendritic spines; altered current flow in neuron
Neurotransmitter synthesis	Pyridoxine (vitamin B_6) dependency	Decreased GABA synthesis; B_6, a co-factor for GAD
Neurotransmitter receptors, inhibitory	Angelman syndrome, juvenile myoclonic epilepsy	Abnormal GABA receptor subunits
Neurotransmitter receptors, excitatory	Nonketotic hyperglycinemia	Excess glycine leads to activation of NMDA receptors
Synapse development	Neonatal seizures	Many possible mechanisms, including the depolarizing action of GABA early in development
Ion channels (channelopathies)	Benign familial neonatal convulsions Dravet syndrome	Potassium channel mutations Sodium channel mutations

GABA, gamma-aminobutyric acid; GAD, glutamic acid decarboxylase; NMDA, N-methyl-D-aspartate; TLE, temporal lobe epilepsy.

Structural Correlates of Epilepsy: Hippocampus and Neocortex

Brain regions differ in their propensity to generate seizures, based on intrinsic membrane properties, synaptic organization, cell density, and pattern of cellular inteconnectivity. Even within the same brain region, cell types differ with regard to their excitability [Steriade, 2004]. The hippocampus and neocortex are particularly prone to seizure generation. The hippocampus, with its orderly laminar organization and trisynaptic excitatory circuitry, has been used extensively in electrophysiologic studies of seizure mechanisms [Schwartzkroin and Mueller, 1987].

Familiarity with hippocampal anatomy will facilitate understanding of the physiological concepts discussed below (Figure 51-2). The hippocampal formation consists of the dentate gyrus, hippocampus proper (i.e., Ammon's horn, with subregions CA1, CA2, and CA3), subiculum, and entorhinal cortex. These four regions are linked by prominent excitatory, largely unidirectional, feed-forward connections. The forward-projecting trisynaptic circuit begins with neurons in layer II of the entorhinal cortex that project axons to the dentate gyrus along the perforant pathway, where they synapse on granule cell and interneuron dendrites. Granule cells, the principal cell type of the dentate gyrus, send their axons, called mossy fibers, to synapse on cells in the hilus and in the CA3 field of Ammon's horn. Several classes of inhibitory interneurons within the dentate hilus modulate on-going excitatory neuronal activity [Lawrence and McBain, 2003]. CA3 pyramidal cells project to other CA3 pyramidal cells through local collaterals, to the CA1 field of Ammon's horn through Schaffer collaterals, and to the contralateral hippocampus. CA1 pyramidal cells send their axons into the subicular complex. Neurons of the subicular complex project to the entorhinal cortex and other cortical and subcortical targets.

Overview of Ion Channels

The key channels and receptors involved in normal and epileptic firing are summarized in Figure 51-3 and Table 51-2. Two major types of ion channels – voltage-gated and ligand-gated – are responsible for inhibitory and excitatory activity. Voltage-gated channels include sodium and calcium channels that function to depolarize the cell membrane toward the action potential threshold, while voltage-gated potassium channels largely dampen neural excitation. Voltage-gated channels are activated by membrane potential changes that alter the conformational state of the channel and allow selective passage of charged ions through a pore. Ligand-gated channels constitute the second type. In ligand-gated channels, a neurotransmitter (e.g., glutamate, GABA) is released from a presynaptic terminal (after presynaptic calcium influx) into the synaptic cleft and then binds with selective affinity to a membrane-bound receptor on the postsynaptic membrane. This binding activates a cascade of events, including a conformational shift to reveal an ion-permeant pore. Passage of ions across these channels results in depolarization (i.e., inward flux of cations) or hyperpolarization (i.e., inward flux of anions or outward flux of cations). Numerous ion channel mutations underlie epilepsy syndromes, giving rise to the concept of "epilepsy channelopathies" [Reid et al., 2009].

Voltage-Dependent Membrane Conductances

Depolarizing Conductances

A rapidly inactivating inward sodium conductance underlies the depolarizing (excitatory) phase of the action potential, and a non-inactivating, persistent sodium current can augment cell depolarization (e.g., produced by excitatory synaptic input) in the subthreshold voltage range; both are critical for regulation of neuronal firing and play a role in epilepsy [Stafstrom, 2007b; Ragsdale, 2008]. Many AEDs act in part through interactions with voltage-dependent sodium channels [Rogawski and Loscher, 2004]. Each sodium channel is composed of a complex of three polypeptide subunits: a major α subunit and two smaller β subunits that influence the kinetic properties of the α subunit. The shape of action potentials is determined by the types of α and β subunits present in an individual neuron [Catterall et al., 2005].

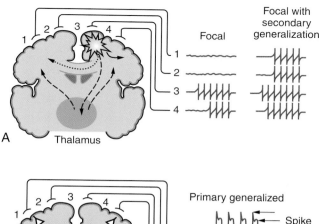

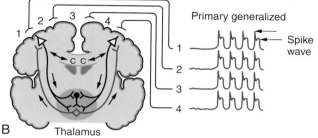

Fig. 51-1 Coronal brain sections depicting seizure types and potential routes of seizure spread. A, Focal area of hyperexcitability (star under electrode 3) and spread to adjacent neocortex (solid arrow under electrode 4) by the corpus callosum (dotted arrow) or other commissural pathways to the contralateral cerebral hemisphere or by subcortical pathways (e.g., thalamus, upward dashed arrows). Accompanying EEG patterns show brain electrical activity under electrodes 1–4. Focal epileptiform activity is maximal at electrode 3 and is seen at electrode 4 (left traces). If a seizure secondarily generalizes, activity may be seen synchronously at all electrodes after a delay (right traces). **B,** A primary generalized seizure begins simultaneously in both hemispheres. The characteristic bilateral synchronous spike-wave EEG pattern is generated by reciprocal interactions between the cortex and thalamus, with rapid spread by means of the corpus callosum (CC) contributing to the rapid bilateral synchrony. One type of thalamic neuron (black neuron) is a GABAergic inhibitory cell that displays intrinsic pacemaker activity. Cortical neurons (triangles) send impulses to thalamic relay neurons (blue diamond) and to inhibitory neurons, setting up oscillations of excitatory and inhibitory activity, which gives rise to the rhythmic spike-wave EEG pattern. *(From Stafstrom CE. An introduction to seizures and epilepsy: Cellular mechanisms underlying classification and treatment. In: Stafstrom CE, Rho JM, eds. Epilepsy and the ketogenic diet. Totowa, NJ: Humana Press, 2004;3–29. Reprinted with kind permission of Springer Science+Business Media.)*

Neurons also display voltage-gated inward calcium conductances. Calcium currents underlie burst discharges in hippocampal CA3 neurons. Activation of voltage-dependent calcium channels contributes to the depolarizing phase of the action potential, and can affect neurotransmitter release, gene expression, and neuronal firing patterns. Several distinct subtypes of calcium channels are distinguished on the basis of electrophysiologic properties, pharmacologic profile, molecular structure, and cellular localization [Catterall et al., 2003]. The molecular structure of voltage-gated calcium channels is similar to that of sodium channels. Voltage-dependent calcium channels are hetero-oligomeric complexes containing a principal pore-forming α-1 subunit and one or more smaller subunits (α_2, β, γ, δ) that are not obligatory for normal activity but modulate the kinetic properties of the channel.

Hyperpolarizing Conductances

Depolarizing sodium and calcium currents are counterbalanced by an array of voltage-dependent hyperpolarizing (inhibitory) currents, primarily mediated by potassium channels. Potassium channels represent the largest and most diverse family of voltage-gated ion channels, and they function to decrease neuronal excitation [Gutman et al., 2005]. The prototypic voltage-gated potassium channel is composed of four membrane-spanning α subunits and four regulatory β subunits that are assembled in an octameric complex to form an ion-selective pore. Potassium conductances include a leak conductance, which is a major determinant of the resting membrane potential; an inward rectifier (involving the flux of other ions), which is activated by hyperpolarization; a large set of delayed rectifiers, which are involved in the termination of action potentials and repolarization of the neuron's membrane potential; an A-current, which helps to determine interspike interval and affects the rate of cell firing; an M-current, which is activated by cholinergic muscarinic agonists and affects resting membrane potential and cell firing rate; and a set of calcium-activated potassium conductances, which are sensitive to intracellular calcium concentration and affect cell firing rate and interburst interval. (Rectification refers to differences in conductance depending on the direction of ion flow through the channel; rectification can also result from blocking of the pore by other ions.)

Modulation or facilitation of hyperpolarizing conductances can be viewed as potentially antiepileptic, and some newer AEDs act directly on voltage-gated potassium channels [Wickenden, 2002]. For example, topiramate induces a steady membrane hyperpolarization mediated by a potassium conductance, and levetiracetam blocks sustained repetitive firing by paradoxically decreasing voltage-gated potassium currents. Retigabine, an opener of Kv7 subtype potassium channels, has broad efficacy in animal seizure models and enhances activation of KCNQ2 and KCNQ3 potassium channels [Miceli et al., 2008]. This finding is particularly intriguing, given that mutations in genes encoding these proteins have been linked to a rare form of inherited epilepsy, benign familial neonatal seizures [Singh et al., 2003].

Synaptic Physiology

Inhibitory Synaptic Transmission

Synaptic inhibition is mediated by two basic circuit configurations. First, feedback or recurrent inhibition occurs when excitatory principal neurons synapse on to and excite inhibitory interneurons, which project back to the principal neurons and inhibit them (i.e., a negative-feedback loop). Second, feed-forward inhibition occurs when axons synapse directly on to inhibitory interneurons, which then inhibit downstream principal neurons.

GABA, the main inhibitory neurotransmitter in the mature mammalian central nervous system, is a neutral amino acid synthesized from glutamic acid by the rate-limiting enzyme glutamic acid decarboxylase. GABA released from axon terminals binds to at least two classes of receptors, GABA_A and GABA_B, which are found on almost all cortical neurons [Sieghart, 2006].

The GABA_A receptor is a macromolecular receptor complex consisting of an ion pore and binding sites for agonists and a

Fig. 51-2 Schematic of major pathways of excitatory synaptic transmission in the hippocampal formation. The hippocampal trisynaptic pathway begins with neurons in layer II of the entorhinal cortex that project axons to the dentate gyrus along the perforant path (1), where they synapse on granule cell dendrites. Dentate granule cells send their axons (called mossy fibers) to synapse on cells in the hilus and in the CA3 field of Ammon's horn (2). CA3 pyramidal cells project to the CA1 field of Ammon's horn by means of Schaffer collaterals (3). CA1 neurons send projections outward through the fornix to other brain regions and back to the subiculum. For simplicity, only the classic feed-forward projections of the trisynaptic pathway are shown. Omitted are the known backward projections and local circuit interactions.

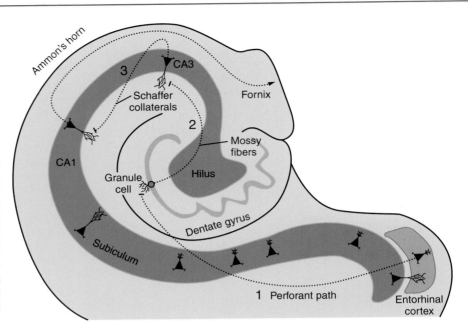

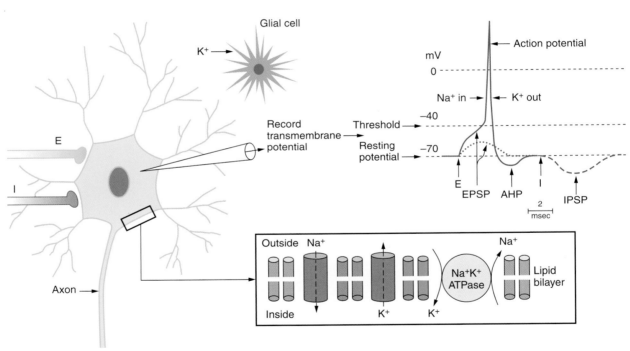

Fig. 51-3 Normal neuronal firing is illustrated by the schematic of a neuron with one excitatory (E) and one inhibitory (I) input. Right trace shows membrane potential (in millivolts [mV]), beginning at a typical resting potential (−70 mV). Activation of E leads to graded excitatory postsynaptic potentials (EPSPs), the larger of which reaches threshold (approximately −40 mV) for an action potential. The action potential is followed by an after-hyperpolarization (AHP), the magnitude and duration of which determine when the next action potential can occur. Activation of I causes an inhibitory postsynaptic potential (IPSP). The inset shows a magnified portion of the neuronal membrane as a lipid bilayer with interposed voltage-gated Na⁺ and K⁺ channels; the direction of ion fluxes during excitatory activation is indicated. After firing, the membrane-bound Na⁺-K⁺ pump and star-shaped astroglial cells restore ionic balance. *(From Stafstrom CE. An introduction to seizures and epilepsy: Cellular mechanisms underlying classification and treatment. In: Stafstrom CE, Rho JM, eds. Epilepsy and the ketogenic diet. Totowa, NJ: Humana Press, 2004;3–29. Reprinted with kind permission of Springer Science+Business Media.)*

variety of allosteric modulators, such as benzodiazepines and barbiturates, each differentially affecting the kinetic properties of the receptor. The GABA$_A$ receptor is a heteropentameric complex composed of combinations of several polypeptide subunits arranged in topographic fashion to form an ion channel. This channel is selectively permeable to chloride and bicarbonate ions. Seven types of subunits (α, β, γ, δ, ϵ, π, ρ) have been described, each with one or more subtypes [Wafford et al., 2004]. Although several thousand receptor isoforms are possible from differential expression and assembly

Table 51-2 Roles of Channels and Receptors in Normal and Epileptic Firing

Channel or Receptor	Role in Normal Neuronal Function	Possible Role in Epilepsy
Voltage-gated Na^+ channel	Subthreshold EPSP; action potential upstroke	Repetitive action potential firing
Voltage-gated K^+ channel	Action potential downstroke	Abnormal action potential repolarization
Ca^{2+}-dependent K^+ channel	AHP after action potential; sets refractory period	Limits repetitive firing
Voltage-gated Ca^{2+} channel	Transmitter release; carries depolarizing charge from dendrites to soma	Excess transmitter release; activates pathophysiologic intracellular processes
Non-NMDA receptor (i.e., AMPA)	Fast EPSP	Initiates PDS
NMDA receptor	Prolonged, slow EPSP	Maintains PDS; Ca^{2+} activates pathophysiologic intracellular processes
$GABA_A$ receptor	IPSP	Limits excitation
$GABA_B$ receptor	Prolonged IPSP	Limits excitation
Electrical synapses	Ultrafast excitatory transmission	Synchronization of neuronal firing
Na^+-K^+ pump	Restores ionic balance	Prevents K^+-induced depolarization

AHP, after-hyperpolarization; AMPA, α-amino-3-hydroxy-5-methyl-4-isoxazolepropionic acid; EPSP, excitatory postsynaptic potential; GABA, γ-aminobutyric acid; IPSP, inhibitory postsynaptic potential; NMDA, N-methyl-D-aspartate; PDS, paroxysmal depolarization shift.

of various subunits, only a limited number of functional combinations is likely to exist in the brain. Most functional $GABA_A$ receptors follow the general motif of containing either α and β or α, β, and γ subunits with variable stoichiometry. Because individual subunits may be differentially sensitive to pharmacologic agents, $GABA_A$ receptor subunits represent potentially useful molecular targets for new AEDs [Macdonald and Kang, 2009].

Activation of $GABA_A$ receptors on the somata of mature neurons generally results in the influx of chloride ions and consequent membrane hyperpolarization, inhibiting cell firing. In neurons of the immature brain, however, $GABA_A$ receptor activation causes depolarization of the postsynaptic membrane [Staley, 2006a]. This reversal of the conventional $GABA_A$ effect reflects a reversed chloride electrochemical gradient, a consequence of the evolving expression of cation chloride co-transporters during development (see Development of Neuro-transmitters, Receptors, and Transporters, below).

In addition to $GABA_A$ receptors, metabotropic $GABA_B$ receptors are located on postsynaptic membrane and presynaptic terminals [Bettler and Tiao, 2006]. $GABA_B$ receptors act through guanosine triphosphate (GTP)-binding proteins to control calcium or potassium conductances. Whereas $GABA_A$ receptors generate fast, high-conductance, inhibitory postsynaptic potentials close to the cell body, $GABA_B$ receptors on the postsynaptic membrane mediate slow, long-lasting, low-conductance inhibitory postsynaptic potentials, primarily in dendrites. Perhaps of greater functional significance, activation of $GABA_B$ receptors on axon terminals blocks neurotransmitter release. It is thought that $GABA_B$ receptors are associated with terminals that release GABA on to postsynaptic $GABA_A$ receptors. In such cases, activation of $GABA_B$ receptors reduces the amount of GABA released, resulting in disinhibition [Simeone et al., 2003]. Abnormalities of GABAergic function, including synthesis, synaptic release, receptor composition, trafficking or binding, and metabolism, can each lead to a hyperexcitable, epileptic state [Cossart et al., 2005; Macdonald and Kang, 2009].

Excitatory Synaptic Transmission

Glutamate, an excitatory amino acid, is the principal excitatory neurotransmitter of the mammalian central nervous system. Glutamatergic pathways are widespread throughout the brain, and excitatory amino acid activity is critical to normal brain development and activity-dependent synaptic plasticity [Simeone et al., 2004]. There are two broad classes of glutamate receptors – ionotropic and metabotropic. Ionotropic glutamate receptors are divided into N-methyl-D-aspartate (NMDA) and non-NMDA receptors, based on biophysical properties and pharmacologic profiles. Each subtype of glutamate receptor consists of a multimeric assembly of subunits that determine its distinct functional properties. An NMDA receptor consists of an NR1 subunit plus NR2A, NR2B, NR2C, NR2D, and/or NR3A.

The NMDA receptor contains a binding site for glutamate (or NMDA) and a recognition site for a variety of modulators (e.g., glycine, polyamines, MK-801, zinc). NMDA receptors also demonstrate voltage-dependent block by magnesium ions. When the membrane is depolarized and the magnesium block of the NMDA receptor is alleviated, activation of the NMDA receptor results in an influx of calcium and sodium ions. Calcium entry is central to the initiation of a number of second messenger pathways, such as stimulation of a variety of kinases that subsequently activate signal transduction cascades, leading to changes in transcriptional regulation. Activation of the NMDA receptor leads to generation of relatively slow and long-lasting excitatory postsynaptic potentials. These synaptic events contribute to epileptiform burst discharges, and NMDA receptor blockade results in the attenuation of bursting activity in many models of epileptiform activity [Kalia et al., 2008].

Non-NMDA ionotropic receptors are divided into α-amino-3-hydroxy-5-methyl-4-isoxazolepropionic acid (AMPA) and kainate receptors [Vincent and Mulle, 2009]. AMPA receptors are composed of combinations of GluR1, GluR2, GluR3, and/or GluR4 subunits, while kainate receptors are composed of combinations of GluR5, GluR6, GluR7, KA1, and/or KA2 subunits. AMPA receptors are responsible for the major part of the excitatory postsynaptic potential – fast-rising and brief in duration – generated by release of glutamate on to postsynaptic neurons. The depolarization generated by AMPA receptors is necessary for effective activation of NMDA receptors. Consequently, AMPA receptor antagonists block most excitatory synaptic activity. Non-NMDA receptors typically pass sodium current, but certain subunit combinations, such as a relative deficit of GluR2, GluR5, or GluR6, endow the receptor with increased calcium permeability, a finding that has implications for development, as well as for epilepsy (see Development of Neurotransmitters, Receptors, and Transporters below) [Rakhade and Jensen, 2009; Santos et al., 2009].

Metabotropic glutamate receptors represent a large, heterogeneous family of G-protein-coupled receptors that subsequently activate various transduction pathways – phosphoinositide hydrolysis and activation of adenylate cyclase and phospholipases C and D. Metabotropic receptors are important modulators of voltage-dependent potassium and calcium channels, nonselective cation currents, and ligand-gated receptors (i.e., GABA and glutamate receptors), and they can regulate glutamate release. Different metabotropic glutamate receptor subtypes are specific for different intracellular processes. Although ubiquitous within the central nervous system, subtypes of metabotropic receptors appear to be differentially localized. Metabotropic glutamate receptors have been implicated in a wide variety of normal neurologic processes (e.g., long-term potentiation) [Anwyl, 2009] and disease states (e.g., epilepsy) [Ure et al., 2006].

Abnormal Neuronal Firing

Specific pathophysiological mechanisms mediate each stage of seizure evolution, including transitions from a normal neuronal firing pattern to interictal epileptiform bursts, from interictal firing to seizure activity, and from the seizure to the postictal state [Stafstrom, 2004; Lado and Moshe, 2008]. Figure 51-4

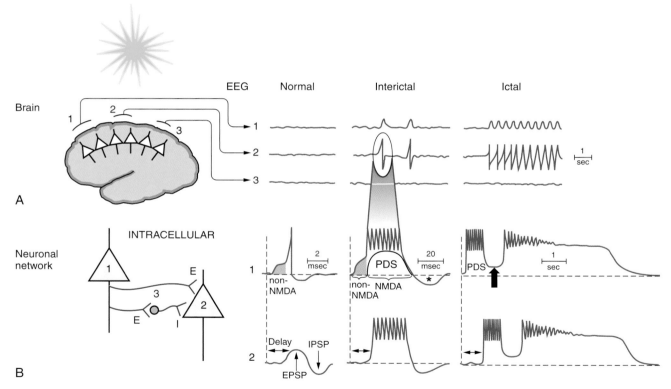

Fig. 51-4 **Abnormal neuronal firing at the levels of the brain (A) and a simplified neuronal network (B), consisting of two excitatory neurons (1 and 2) and an inhibitory interneuron (solid circle, 3).** EEG (top set of traces) and intracellular recordings (bottom set of traces) are shown for normal (left column), interictal (middle column), and ictal (right column) conditions. Numbered traces refer to like-numbered recording sites. Notice the time scale differences in different traces. **A,** Three EEG electrodes record activity from superficial neocortical neurons. In the normal case, activity is low-voltage and desynchronized (i.e., neurons are not firing together in synchrony). In the interictal condition, large spikes are seen focally at electrode 2 (and to a lesser extent at electrode 1, where they may be called sharp waves), representing synchronized firing of a large population of hyperexcitable neurons (expanded in time below). The ictal state is characterized by a long run of spikes. **B,** At the neuronal network level, the intracellular correlate of the interictal EEG spike is called the paroxysmal depolarization shift (PDS). The PDS is initiated by a non-NMDA-mediated, fast excitatory postsynaptic potential (EPSP) (shaded area), but it is maintained by a longer, larger, NMDA-mediated EPSP. The post-PDS hyperpolarization (asterisk) temporarily stabilizes the neuron. If this post-PDS hyperpolarization fails (right column, arrow), ictal discharge can occur. The lowest traces, recordings from neuron 2, show activity similar to that recorded in neuron 1, with some delay (double-headed arrow). Activation of inhibitory neuron 3 by firing of neuron 1 prevents neuron 2 from generating an action potential (i.e., the inhibitory postsynaptic potential [IPSP] counters the depolarization caused by the EPSP). If neuron 2 does reach firing threshold, additional neurons will be recruited, leading to an entire network firing in synchrony (i.e., a seizure). NMDA, *N*-methyl-D-aspartate. *(From Stafstrom CE. An introduction to seizures and epilepsy: Cellular mechanisms underlying classification and treatment. In: Stafstrom CE, Rho JM, eds. Epilepsy and the ketogenic diet. Totowa, NJ: Humana Press, 2004;3–29. Reprinted with kind permission of Springer Science+Business Media.)*

depicts EEG and intracellular changes that can be seen in normal, interictal, and ictal states. In the normal situation, action potentials are generated in neuron 1 when the membrane potential reaches threshold for firing. These discharges may influence the activity of an adjacent neuron (neuron 2) synaptically, resulting in an excitatory postsynaptic potential. An adjacent interneuron (neuron 3, which is inhibitory) may also be activated by a discharge from neuron 1 after a brief delay, giving rise to an inhibitory postsynaptic potential. The activity recorded in neuron 2 reflects the temporal and spatial summation of excitatory and inhibitory postsynaptic potentials.

If this integrative concept is extrapolated to thousands of synaptic contacts, it is easy to envision the "sculpting" or grading of individual cellular responses by degrees of inhibition. For discharges of a discrete group of hyperexcitable neurons to spread to adjacent areas, the epileptic firing must overcome the powerful inhibitory influences (inhibitory surround) that normally keep aberrant excitability in check. Therefore, even a single cell can influence the output of a network and contribute to hypersynchronous firing.

Paroxysmal Depolarization Shift

The intracellular correlate of the focal interictal epileptiform discharge on the EEG is known as the paroxysmal depolarization shift (PDS) [Gorji and Speckmann, 2009]. Initially, there is a rapid shift in the membrane potential in a depolarizing direction, followed by a burst of repetitive action potentials lasting several hundred milliseconds (Figure 51-5). The initial depolarization is mediated by AMPA receptors, whereas the sustained depolarization is a consequence of NMDA receptor activation. Afterward, the PDS terminates with a repolarization phase, primarily a consequence of inhibitory potassium and chloride conductances carried by voltage-gated potassium channels and GABA receptors. The prolonged period of hyperpolarization after the PDS is mediated by inhibitory conductances and constitutes a refractory period. PDS activity in several adjacent neurons would be expected to facilitate synchronous firing [LeDuigou et al., 2009].

Synchronizing Mechanisms

The hippocampal formation (see Figure 51-2) normally displays robust neuronal synchronization. Sharp waves, dentate spikes, theta activity, 40-Hz oscillations, and 200-Hz oscillations are all forms of neuronal synchronization that can be recorded in various regions of the hippocampal formation [Buzsaki and Draguhn, 2004]. Synchronization of neuronal activity appears to be intrinsic to the mechanism by which the hippocampus performs its normal functions. However, neuronal synchronization is also a hallmark of epilepsy and exaggerated synchrony among hippocampal neurons may directly generate seizures [Engel et al., 2009; Hughes, 2008]. Forms of synchronized activity that do not trigger seizures in a normal hippocampus may trigger epileptiform discharges in a hippocampus that has undergone selective neuronal loss, synaptic reorganization, or changes in receptor expression.

In the hippocampus, synchronizing mechanisms include inputs from subcortical nuclei and intrinsic interneuron-mediated synchronization. For example, high-amplitude theta activity is a salient feature of the normal hippocampus. The theta rhythm represents synchronized activity of hippocampal

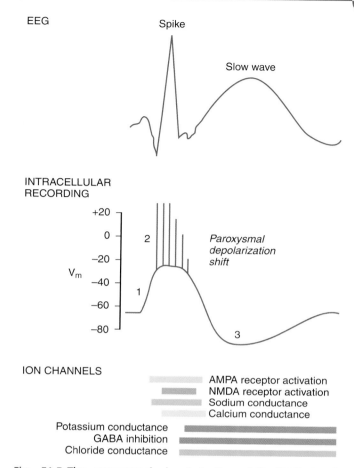

Fig. 51-5 The paroxysmal depolarization shift (PDS) is the intracellular correlate of an interictal spike on the surface EEG. The temporal correlations are illustrated for an interictal epileptiform discharge (top, spike and slow-wave complex), intracellular recording (middle), and sequence of ionic conductance changes. The PDS is initiated by excitatory conductances (top four bars) and terminated by inhibitory conductances (bottom four bars). The initial depolarization (phase 1), which is an excitatory postsynaptic potential (EPSP), is mediated by α-amino-3-hydroxy-5-methyl-4-isoxazolepropionic acid (AMPA) receptors and sustained by N-methyl-D-aspartate (NMDA) receptors, whereas the overriding action potentials (phase 2) are generated by voltage-gated sodium channels and calcium channels. Repolarization and after-hyperpolarization (phase 3) are mediated by inhibitory conductances (i.e., multiple voltage-gated potassium channels and chloride flux, such as through gamma-aminobutyric acid [GABA] receptors).

neurons and largely depends on input from the septum [Buzsaki and Draguhn, 2004]. Subcortical nuclei, such as the septum, have divergent inputs that target hippocampal interneurons. The divergent axon projections of interneurons and the powerful effect of the GABA$_A$ receptor-mediated conductances that they produce enable interneurons to entrain the activity of large populations of principal neurons. These characteristics make interneurons a very effective target for subcortical modulation of hippocampal principal cell activity.

Recurrent excitatory circuits are another substrate for neuronal synchronization. Recurrent excitatory collaterals are a normal feature of the hippocampal CA3 region. CA3 pyramidal cells form direct, monosynaptic connections with other CA3 pyramidal cells, contributing to the synchronized bursts that characterize this region [Traub et al., 2004a]. In the epileptic temporal lobe, synaptic reorganization and axonal sprouting may lead to aberrant recurrent excitation, providing a synchronizing mechanism in other parts of the hippocampal formation, including CA1, subiculum, entorhinal cortex, and dentate gyrus. In the dentate gyrus of the normal hippocampus, for example, granule cells form few or no monosynaptic contacts with neighboring granule cells. However, in the epileptic hippocampus, mossy fiber sprouting results in direct excitatory interactions among granule cells [Nadler, 2003] (Figure 51-6).

Mechanisms independent of chemical synaptic transmission may synchronize neuronal firing under some circumstances. Such nonsynaptic mechanisms include gap junctions, electrical field (i.e., ephaptic) effects, and changes in extracellular ion concentrations. Gap junctions allow electrical signals to pass directly between cells. Gap junctions are upregulated in epileptic brain tissue and blockade of gap junctions significantly affects the duration of seizure activity [Traub et al., 2004b]. Ephaptic effects, generated by current flow through the extracellular space, can enhance epileptogenic neuronal synchronization [Dudek et al., 1998]. Increases in extracellular potassium concentration have long been known to affect epileptic excitability and synchronization, and experiments have demonstrated clear epileptogenic effects of blocking potassium regulation (e.g., through inwardly rectifying potassium channels) [Traynelis and Dingledine, 1988; McBain et al., 1993].

Glial Mechanisms for Modulating Epileptogenicity

Glial contributions to epileptic mechanisms have been relatively neglected until recently [Wetherington et al., 2008]. Because the ionic balance between the intracellular and extracellular compartments is altered after neuronal activity (especially after repetitive discharges seen with seizures), there must exist mechanisms to restore ion homeostasis. Astrocytes are perhaps most closely associated with regulation of extracellular potassium levels (i.e., potassium buffering) because glial cell membranes are preferentially permeable to potassium. A variety of inwardly rectifying potassium channels mediate potassium uptake, and the association of glial endfeet with brain microvasculature provides a convenient "sink" for potassium release. Glial cell membrane potential changes are directly correlated with changes in extracellular potassium concentration, and blockade of potassium channels selective for glial cells results in neuronal hyperexcitability. Therefore, certain glial cells can modulate neuronal discharge by regulating extracellular potassium.

Another important role of glia is transporting synaptically released glutamate out of the extracellular space. Glia cell membranes are uniquely equipped for this role, possessing powerful glutamate transporters [Shigeri et al., 2004]. Rapid and efficient removal of extracellular glutamate characterizes normal, healthy brain tissue, and this is essential because residual glutamate would continue to excite surrounding neurons. Blockade of glutamate transporters (or knockout of the genes for these transport proteins) results in epilepsy or excitotoxicity [Meldrum et al., 1999].

Glial cells modulate excitability in other ways, as well. First, glia play a critical role in regulating extracellular pH by a proton exchanger and by bicarbonate transporter mechanisms. Even low levels of neuronal activity create significant pH transients. NMDA receptor function is very sensitive to pH. Second, glial cells are thought to release powerful neuroactive agents into the extracellular space. Glial glutamate release can excite neighboring neurons, and some investigations have suggested that other glia-related factors – such as the cytokine interleukin-1 – can have profound proconvulsant effects [Vezzani et al., 2008].

Physiology of Absence Epilepsy

The generalized spike-wave discharges accompanying absence seizures reflect a widespread, phase-locked oscillation between excitation (i.e., spike) and inhibition (i.e., slow wave) in mutually connected thalamocortical networks [McCormick and Contreras, 2001; Huguenard and McCormick, 2007].

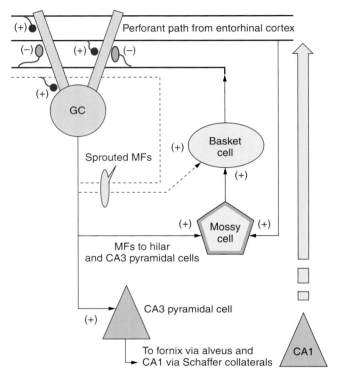

Fig. 51-6 Hippocampal circuitry and seizure-induced circuit reorganization. Granule cells (GC) receive their major input by the perforant path. The perforant path also stimulates hilar interneurons (e.g., mossy cells, basket cells) to provide feed-forward inhibition of the granule cells. Granule cell axons, the mossy fibers (MFs), make synaptic contact with CA3 pyramidal cells. Mossy fiber collaterals innervate the hilar interneurons, such as the mossy cell shown in the diagram. Mossy cells are excitatory to GABAergic basket cells that provide feedback inhibition to the granule cell. Sprouting of mossy fibers (in response to seizure-induced loss of CA3 pyramidal cells and hilar mossy cells) can result in enhanced excitation by forming autapses (i.e., an axon sprout synapsing with the dendrites of the same cell) and can augment synchronization by stimulating neighboring granule cells (not shown), contributing to epileptogenicity. It has been suggested that the sprouted mossy fibers may restore inhibition lost after seizure-induced death of hilar mossy cells by direct stimulation of deafferented (dormant) basket cells. *(From Sankar R et al. Paroxysmal disorders. In: Menkes JH et al., eds. Child Neurology, 7th ed. Philadelphia: Lippincott Williams & Wilkins, 2006;857–942.)*

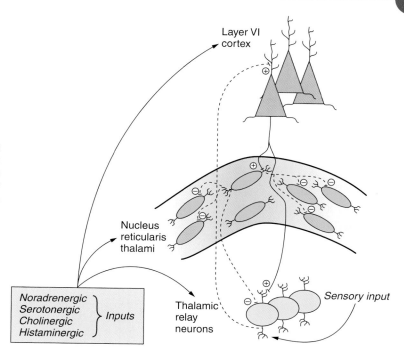

Fig. 51-7 Thalamocortical circuitry is thought to form the basis of normal oscillatory rhythms, which, when perturbed, can produce generalized spike-wave discharges seen with absence seizures. This circuitry involves excitatory projections from layer VI neocortical pyramidal neurons on to thalamic relay (TR) neurons and inhibitory neurons comprising the nucleus reticularis thalami (NRT). TR neurons send excitatory axons back to the neocortex. Activation of NRT neurons results in recurrent inhibition of adjacent neurons and TR neurons. The neurotransmitters at the excitatory (+) and inhibitory (−) synapses are thought to be glutamate and gamma-aminobutyric acid (GABA), respectively. Low-threshold (T-type) calcium channels and hyperpolarization-activated cation (HCN) channels in TR and NRT neurons help regulate intrinsic rhythmicity. Extrinsic modulatory influences on this circuitry include inputs from the forebrain and brainstem nuclei and the sensory inputs from other thalamic nuclei.

Pyramidal neurons from layer VI of the neocortex send excitatory projections to thalamic relay neurons and inhibitory GABAergic neurons comprising the nucleus reticularis thalami (Figure 51-7). Excitatory outputs of the thalamic relay neurons impinge on the apical dendrites of layer VI pyramidal neurons in the neocortex. This thalamocortical relay is a critical substrate for the generation of cortical rhythms and is influenced by sensory inputs (e.g., from the retina) and by several brainstem nuclei that constitute the origin of cholinergic, noradrenergic, serotonergic, and other projections. This reciprocal circuitry, which is responsible in large part for normal EEG oscillations during wake and sleep states, can become hyperactive and generate generalized spike-wave discharges or can be dampened to reduce spontaneous cortical rhythms. The anatomy implies that spike-wave discharges are interrupted at cortical or thalamic levels.

Although multiple ionic conductances are involved in rhythmic pacemaking activity, two channels are believed to play a key role in regulating thalamocortical activity. The first is a subtype of voltage-gated calcium channel known as the low-threshold (T-type) calcium channel. These channels are activated by small depolarizations of the plasma membrane. In many neurons, calcium influx through these channels triggers low-threshold spikes and activates a burst of action potentials [McCormick and Contreras, 2001; Perez-Reyes, 2003]. Such an excitatory burst is thought to underlie the spike portion of a generalized spike-wave oscillation. AEDs known to be clinically effective against absence seizures (e.g., ethosuximide, valproic acid) block T-type calcium currents.

The second important ion channel involved in the regulation of thalamocortical rhythmicity is the hyperpolarization-activated cation channel, responsible for the so-called h-current. These channels, densely expressed in the thalamus and hippocampus, are activated by hyperpolarization and produce a depolarizing current carried by an inward flux of sodium and potassium ions. This depolarization helps to bring the resting membrane potential toward threshold for activation of T-type calcium channels, which produces a calcium spike and a burst of action potentials. Hyperpolarization-activated cation channels are highly expressed in dendrites and are expressed to a lesser extent in the soma. They are also critically involved in developmental plasticity [Bender and Baram, 2008].

Unlike other voltage-gated conductances that can be labeled either inhibitory or excitatory, h-currents are both inhibitory and excitatory [Poolos, 2004; Dyhrfjeld-Johnsen et al., 2009]. Hyperpolarization-activated cation channels possess an inherent negative-feedback property; hyperpolarization activates certain cation channels, which then leads to depolarization that then deactivates these channels. The net effect of hyperpolarization-activated cation channel activation is a decrease in the input resistance of the membrane, which is the voltage change produced by a given synaptic current. H-currents tend to stabilize membrane potential around the resting potential, countering hyperpolarizing and depolarizing inputs. The relevance of hyperpolarization-activated cation channels in the pathogenesis of absence seizures was underscored by the demonstration that lamotrigine, an anti-absence agent, enhances dendritic h-currents in hippocampal pyramidal neurons and by the experimental finding that deletion of a specific hyperpolarization-activated cation isoform results in absence epilepsy [Ludwig et al., 2003].

With respect to antiepileptic action, it is uncertain whether known T-type calcium channel blockers, such as ethosuximide, in fact block absence seizures through interactions with this type of calcium channel [Huc et al., 2009]. Antagonists of GABA$_B$ receptors and dopaminergic agonists can also interrupt abnormal thalamocortical discharges in experimental absence epilepsy models [Snead, 1996]. GABA$_B$ receptors are involved in mediating long-lasting thalamic inhibitory postsynaptic potentials involved in the generation of normal thalamocortical rhythms, whereas brainstem monoaminergic projections disrupt these rhythms. Although it is appealing to think of absence seizures as a byproduct of dysfunction of the T-type calcium channel or h-channel, or both, the actual pathophysiologic mechanisms are probably much more complex [Hughes, 2009].

Increased Seizure Susceptibility of the Immature Brain

Seizure incidence is highest during the first decade and especially during the first year of life. Multiple physiologic factors (Table 51-3 and Figure 51-8) contribute to the increased susceptibility of the developing brain to seizures [Sanchez and Jensen, 2001; Velísková et al., 2004; Wong, 2005; Ben-Ari and Holmes, 2006; Silverstein and Jensen, 2007; Stafstrom, 2007a]. This information is mainly derived from experimental epilepsy models in rodents, in which a window of heightened excitability in the second postnatal week gives rise to a lowered seizure threshold. This period of hyperexcitability in the rodent is approximately analogous to the first year of life in the human infant [Avishai-Eliner et al., 2002].

Each seizure susceptibility factor alters the net brain excitatory–inhibitory balance in favor of enhanced excitation, and each involves a multiplicity of substrates and mediators, including ion channels, neurotransmitters and their receptors, structural changes in the maturing brain, and ionic gradients.

Seizure propensity in the very young involves a complex interplay between the timing of these cellular and molecular changes [Rakhade and Jensen, 2009]. Although there are disadvantages to the physiologic adaptations that make the immature brain especially vulnerable to hyperexcitability and seizure generation, such idiosyncrasies of early brain development also provide the opportunity to develop novel, age-specific therapies.

Development of Ionic Channels and Membrane Properties

The relative timing of ion channel development plays a major role in the enhanced excitability of the immature brain [Spitzer, 2006]. Sodium and calcium ion channels, which mediate neuronal excitation, develop relatively early. Action potentials persist longer in early development, and this prolonged excitation mediates a greater calcium current, particularly at the presynaptic terminal; these factors increase excitability by enhancing neurotransmitter release. However, the brain must achieve a critical balance; activity-driven calcium channel activation is necessary for normal developmental processes such as cellular differentiation, migration, and synaptogenesis, but excessive inward calcium current can cause seizures and neuronal damage. Mutations of the α-1 subunit of the sodium

Table 51-3 Factors Promoting Increased Seizure Susceptibility in the Developing Brain

Factor	Consequence	References
Input resistance and time constant: increased in immature neurons	Small inputs result in relatively large voltage changes	McCormick and Prince, 1987
Voltage-gated ion channels: earlier maturation of sodium and calcium channels, delayed development of potassium channels	Longer action potentials, shorter refractory periods, increased neuron firing	Spitzer, 2006
Synapse development: excitatory synapses appear before inhibitory synapses	Relative predominance of excitation over inhibition early in development	Swann et al., 1999
Synapse development: overexpression of excitatory synapses during critical period	Corresponds to window of heightened seizure susceptibility	Swann et al., 1999
Developmental changes in glutamate receptor subunits: NR2B/NR2A ratio favors prolonged depolarizing responses; NR2D relative overexpression reduces Mg^{2+} block	Favor relative hyperexcitability	Rakhade and Jensen, 2009
Late appearance of functional inhibitory synapses	Along with other factors favoring excitation, contributes to neuronal excitatory drive and lack of functional inhibition	Brooks-Kayal, 2005
Developmental changes in GABA$_A$ receptor function and Cl^- gradient	GABA is depolarizing early in life, enhancing excitability	Ben-Ari, 2002
Developmental changes in GABA$_A$ receptor subunits	Partially accounts for developmental differences in inhibitory effectiveness and benzodiazepine responsiveness	Brooks-Kayal, 2005
Developmental sensitivity to glutamate toxicity	Less glutamate-induced excitotoxicity early in development	Rakhade and Jensen, 2009
Immature GABA$_A$ binding pattern in substantia nigra	Proconvulsant effect	Velisek et al., 1995
Electrical synapses; more common early in development	Mechanism for enhanced synchrony of neuronal networks	Talhouka et al., 2007)
Immature homeostatic mechanisms: Na^+,K^+-ATPase, glial K^+ regulation, K^+-Cl^- cotransporters	Prolonged exposure to elevated extracellular K^+ leads to further neuronal depolarization	Haglund and Schwartzkroin, 1990

GABA, gamma-aminobutyric acid; NR, N-methyl-D-aspartate (NMDA) receptor.
(Adapted from Stafstrom CE et al. Consequences of epilepsy in the developing brain: Implications for surgical management. Semin Pediatr Neurol 2000;7:147.)

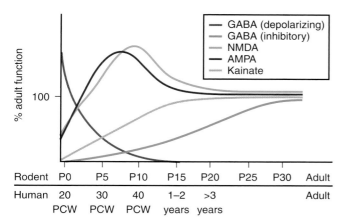

NEURONAL RECEPTOR EXPRESSION VS AGE

Fig. 51-8 Schematic depiction of changes in receptor expression in the developing brain. Relative changes in the expression of GABA receptors and glutamate receptor subtypes are shown relative to adult levels (100 percent). Human and rodent data are compared in the panel below the graph. Between about postnatal (P) day 4 in the rat (corresponding to postconceptual week [PCW] 28 in the human) until about P15 in the rodent (1–2 years of age in the human), there is a window of over-abundance of excitation. Excitatory glutamate receptor subtypes NMDA and AMPA (light blue and red lines) expression peaks during this time interval and GABA-induced depolarization (purple line) is high relative to GABA-induced inhibition (green line). These factors contribute to enhanced seizure predisposition in this age range. AMPA, α-amino-3-hydroxy-5-methyl-4-isoxazolepropionic acid; GABA, gamma-aminobutyric acid; NMDA, N-methy-D-aspartic acid. (*From Silverstein FS, Jensen FE. Neonatal seizures. Ann Neurol 2007;62:112–120. Wiley–Liss, Inc.)*

channel are responsible for a spectrum of developmental epilepsies, including generalized epilepsy with febrile seizures plus and Dravet syndrome (also known as severe myoclonic epilepsy of infancy) [Meisler and Kearney, 2005; Harkin et al., 2007; Stafstrom, 2009].

Through a large variety of potassium channels outward currents counter depolarizing influences and tend to stabilize membrane excitability. Potassium channels develop slightly later than sodium and calcium channels. During a window of development, the net balance of ion fluxes favors excitation [Rakhade and Jensen, 2009].

Intrinsic membrane properties, such as membrane resistance and time constant, contribute to the neuron's response to a synaptic input. During development, neurons have relatively higher membrane resistances and shorter time constants, and a depolarizing stimulus of a given amplitude and duration can have a greater effect in an immature neuron than in a mature one [McCormick and Prince, 1987]. Such electrical factors act in concert with ionic conductances to determine the magnitude of the membrane's response to a synaptic input.

Development of Neurotransmitters, Receptors, and Transporters

Excitatory synapses tend to form before inhibitory ones. Each glutamate receptor type, and each receptor subunit within the receptor type, possesses a distinct ontogenetic profile. For example, excitatory NMDA receptors are transiently over-expressed early in postnatal development, when they are needed for critical developmental processes [Simeone et al., 2004]. The early developmental stoichiometry of NMDA receptor subunits favors prolonged depolarizing responses. Early in development, NMDA receptor subunits NR2A, NR2B, and NR3A are elevated, favoring longer depolarizations, decreased sensitivity to blockade by magnesium ions, and enhanced calcium influx. All of these physiological adaptations favor depolarization, seizures, and excitotoxicity. Similarly, the developmental profile of AMPA receptors favors subunit stoichiometries (fewer combinations with GluR2 subunits) with enhanced calcium influx. Metabotropic glutamate receptors may also be expressed developmentally to favor seizure generation [Avallone et al., 2006].

Electrical synapses appear to be more prevalent in the developing brain than in the mature brain. Electrical synapses have been reported in several brain regions, including neonatal neocortex and hippocampus. Fast-acting electrical transmission can facilitate rapid synchrony of the neuronal network and precipitate seizures and excitotoxicity [Velazquez and Carlen, 2000; Talhouka et al., 2007].

GABA receptors also exhibit a developmental profile, with different expression of GABA$_A$ receptor subunits at different stages of development [Brooks-Kayal, 2005; Huang, 2009]. GABA's physiologic action also varies during development. Early in development, GABA exerts an excitatory action, rather than the inhibitory effect seen later. Emerging evidence suggests that GABA is depolarizing early in development because of the particular distribution of chloride ions (Figure 51-9) [Staley, 2006b]. In the developing brain (up to about the second week of life in rats, which corresponds roughly to a few months of age in humans), the intracellular chloride concentration is much higher than in mature neurons. This distribution is due to the presence of a membrane pump, called sodium, potassium, chloride co-transporter 1 (NKCC1), that actively influxes chloride ions, utilizing the energy stored in the transmembrane sodium gradient to import a potassium ion, along with one sodium ion and two chloride ions. NKCC1's activity results in an intracellular chloride concentration about 3–4 times greater than that found in mature neurons. Thus, when GABA$_A$ receptors are activated by GABA release from interneurons, the postsynaptic chloride-permeable channels open and chloride effluxes out of the neuron down its concentration gradient. Chloride efflux results in a loss of intracellular negativity and a depolarizing current; the membrane potential deviates toward the chloride equilibrium potential, which is several tens of millivolts less negative than resting potential (i.e., depolarizing). The resulting depolarizing current can lead to action potential generation. This membrane depolarization is sufficient to activate NMDA receptors and allow entry of calcium ions into the cell.

Even when GABA is depolarizing, another mechanism – shunting – can effectively produce inhibition by increasing membrane conductance. Shunting dissipates depolarizing synaptic currents without causing membrane potential change [Isaev et al., 2007]. That is, when chloride is passively distributed across the membrane, increasing chloride conductance will not generate transmembrane chloride currents. Therefore, the neonatal brain retains some inhibition, even in the face of depolarizing GABA action.

As development proceeds, the expression and activity of the NKCC1 transporter declines and another membrane pump is expressed, potassium chloride co-transporter 2 (KCC2) [Rivera et al., 1999]. KCC2 has the opposite action – it actively

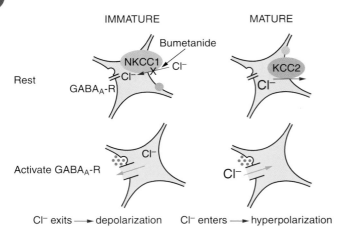

Fig. 51-9 The role of intracellular chloride concentration as a function of age on neuronal responses to GABA (orange dots). At early postnatal ages (left), intracellular chloride concentration is high due to the activity of a membrane transporter (NKCC1, green oval) that causes chloride influx; activation of GABA$_A$ receptors at this age (lower left) causes chloride efflux and depolarization. In the mature brain (right), NKCC1 expression is much reduced, whereas another chloride transporter (KCC2, pink oval) extrudes chloride, keeping the intracellular chloride concentration relatively low. Therefore, in the mature brain, activation of GABA$_A$ receptors (lower right) results in chloride influx and hyperpolarization of the neuron. Relative expression of the chloride transporters NKCC1 and KCC2 at the two ages is indicated by the sizes of the symbols, and relative intracellular chloride concentrations at the two ages is indicated by the sizes of the Cl$^-$ lettering. Bumetanide (upper left), a loop diuretic, blocks NKCC1 action and protects against neonatal seizures, probably by reducing the depolarizing action of GABA at immature ages. GABA$_A$-R, gamma-aminobutyric acid type A receptor; KCC2, potassium-chloride co-transporter 2; NKCC1, sodium-potassium-chloride co-transporter 1. *(Modified from Stafstrom CE. Neurobiological mechanisms of developmental epilepsy: translating experimental findings into clinical application. Semin Pediatr Neurol 2007;14:164–172. Reprinted with permission of Elsevier, Inc.)*

extrudes chloride to the outside of the neuron, leaving the intracellular compartment with a lower basal chloride concentration (see Figure 51-9). Binding of GABA to the GABA$_A$ receptor of a mature neuron that expresses KCC2 will cause channel opening and influx of chloride into the neuron, down its concentration gradient. Increased intracellular negativity will hyperpolarize the neuron, moving its membrane potential closer to the chloride reversal potential, which is more negative than resting potential. These actions will keep the neuron further from the threshold for action potential firing, comprising its inhibitory action.

The transition from GABAergic excitation to inhibition is an important physiological milestone. As glutamatergic synapses develop and begin to mediate their characteristic excitatory action, GABA switches to its mature inhibitory action (via change in expression of the chloride pumps described above; also see Figure 51-8). This time point also corresponds to other developmental milestones: namely, the appearance of GABA$_B$ inhibitory responses and disappearance of large oscillatory currents known as giant depolarizing potentials (GDPs) [Mohajerani and Cherubini, 2006]. GDPs are seen only at early ages, are dependent upon both NMDA and depolarizing GABA action, and function to facilitate the formation of synapses and neuronal circuits. The peak point of seizure susceptibility

resides during this transition, when GABA is still excitatory, excitation via glutamate receptors has not yet matured, and GABA$_B$ inhibition is not yet complete. This maximum susceptibility occurs around postnatal (P) day 10–14 in rats, corresponding to approximately term in humans, an observation of major relevance for neonatal seizures and their treatment.

Phenobarbital, which blocks GABA$_A$ receptors, is typically used to suppress seizures in the neonatal period, but its efficacy against neonatal seizures is imperfect [Painter et al., 1999]. GABA$_A$ receptor ontogeny is also associated with varying sensitivity to benzodiazepines, an observation relevant to seizure treatment. Therefore, novel approaches to the management of neonatal seizures are needed. In this regard, bumetanide, a diuretic similar to furosemide that blocks NKCC1 (see Figure 51-9), has been shown to suppress epileptic activity in brain slices and animal models [Dzhala et al., 2005], an effect that is enhanced with concomitant phenobarbital use [Dzhala et al., 2008].

Structural Maturation of the Brain and Seizure Susceptibility

In the developing brain, synaptic connections are formed and pruned as a function of neuronal activity. Neuronal activity also determines which connections remain stable and which are lost. Such changes are referred to as plasticity, a general phenomenon that likely influences the brain's capacity to learn and respond to the environment. The same properties that govern plasticity may also contribute to increased susceptibility for the epileptic network to synchronize in association with brain pathology or injury. For example, during the second week of life in the rat, the hippocampal CA3 region is characterized by an exuberance of excitatory connections between pyramidal cells that endow the region with heightened excitability and epileptiform activity [Swann, 2005]. These connections are later pruned, with stabilization of the excessive excitation seen during this developmental window.

Regulation of the Ionic Environment

The development of several ion transport mechanisms favors excitability early in life [Shigeri et al., 2004]. Expression of the chloride gradient depends on the development of the KCC2 transporter, which determines whether GABA mediates a depolarizing or hyperpolarizing effect. Expression of the sodium-potassium ion pump (Na$^+$,K$^+$-ATPase) also follows a developmental pattern [Haglund and Schwartzkroin, 1990]. Extracellular accumulation of potassium after neuronal activity (e.g., during a seizure) can further depolarize the neuronal membrane, exacerbating or prolonging ictal activity. The ability of glial cells to clear extracellular potassium improves with age.

Epileptogenesis in the Developing Brain

The discussion above emphasizes the mechanisms by which the immature brain is susceptible to seizures, or ictogenesis. The developing brain is also prone to the development of epilepsy, a process called epileptogenesis. While there is some overlap between mechanisms of ictogenesis and epileptogenesis, the latter term refers to the development of spontaneous recurrent seizures, either following a brain injury or due to a genetic predisposition. Intensive investigation is now focusing on ways in which the developing brain becomes epileptic, and importantly, on interventions to retard or prevent epileptogenesis.

Numerous factors likely play a role in epileptogenesis, and these are best considered according to a temporal sequence [Bender and Baram, 2007; Pitkanen and Lukasiuk, 2009; Rakhade and Jensen, 2009]. In the first hours to days following a precipitating brain injury or severe seizure, immediate early genes are activated that lead to transcription of proteins that alter subsequent excitability. In addition, after a seizure, many receptors and other proteins involved in excitability are phosphorylated, including potassium channels and $GABA_A$, AMPA, and NMDA receptors. Later, in the time frame of days to weeks, inflammation occurs, with elevations of cytokines and other inflammatory compounds, neurotrophic factors, ion channels, and neurotransmitter receptors. These changes presage chronic epileptogenic events that are expressed weeks to months later, including altered neurogenesis and gliosis. Therefore, the epileptogenic cascade progresses from changes at the gene level to changes at the structural level; hopefully, these multifactorial processes will provide biomarkers to identify which individuals are at most risk for the development of epilepsy and optimal ways to intervene in the process (Sankar and Rho, 2007).

Antiepileptic Drug Mechanisms

Procedures for Antiepileptic Drug Testing

Since the introduction of phenobarbital in 1912, dozens of AEDs have been approved for medical use by the U.S. Food and Drug Administration after extensive testing in a variety of animal seizure models and in human clinical trials. Until recently, the paradigms of drug discovery have been biased toward the development of drugs sharing properties exhibited by older agents, such as phenytoin and phenobarbital. Now, AED screening programs incorporate advances in molecular and cellular neurobiology, resulting in more rational screening programs, with new molecular targets being discovered beyond neuronal membrane-bound ion channels and enzymes involved in neurotransmitter metabolism and reuptake [Rogawski, 2006].

The two most commonly used models for the routine screening and identification of new AEDs are the maximal electroshock (MES) and subcutaneous pentylenetetrazol (PTZ) tests conducted with mice or rats [White et al., 2007]. MES tests the ability of a compound to eliminate the tonic extensor component of an electrically evoked seizure, whereas PTZ (a $GABA_A$ receptor antagonist) tests the ability of a drug to inhibit a generalized clonic seizure. MES seizures can be blocked by agents such as phenytoin and carbamazepine, which are effective in treating seizures with partial onset. In contrast, drugs effective in treating generalized absence seizures (e.g., ethosuximide) effectively inhibit PTZ-induced seizures. Valproic acid, a broad-spectrum agent, is effective in MES and PTZ tests, and is clinically effective against most seizure types. Alternative screeing tests are currently being used to assess AED effects on limbic seizures (e.g., 6-Hz test, kindling) and other seizure types [Barton et al., 2001; Bertram, 2007].

Despite the prevailing view that acute animal seizure models can predict efficacy against partial or generalized seizures in humans, there is a significant limitation of this strategy. These screening tests may fail to identify substances acting through novel mechanisms. Such is the case with levetiracetam, which is effective in the treatment of temporal lobe epilepsy but is inactive in the MES and PTZ models. A further confound is that potential AEDs are typically screened in adult animals, yet effects may be different at young ages.

Since 1993, many new AEDs have been approved for use in the United States – felbamate, gabapentin, lamotrigine, topiramate, tiagabine, oxcarbazepine, levetiracetam, zonisamide, pregabalin, lacosamide, rufinamide, and vigabatrin. Many of these agents were successful products of an extensive drug discovery campaign carried out in collaborative fashion by the National Institutes of Health, academic medical centers, and the pharmaceutical industry. Although the newer drugs appeared promising in early studies, particularly with regard to their side-effect profile, they have not yielded significantly higher clinical efficacy rates than older medications. The real impact of these newer drugs has been in diminished adverse effects and fewer drug interactions. Many children with epilepsy continue to experience intractable seizures and long-term cognitive impairment. Although AEDs are emphasized here, there is an urgent need to explore the mechanisms of action of alternative epilepsy treatments, such as dietary, surgical, and brain stimulation therapies.

Antiepileptic Drug Mechanisms of Action

Most AEDs exert their principal effects on the following molecular targets: $GABA_A$ receptors, glutamate receptors (both NMDA and non-NMDA), voltage-dependent sodium channels, and voltage-dependent calcium channels [Rogawski and Loscher, 2004]. Each AED is likely to have multiple mechanisms of action because there is no single action of an AED that can completely account for all of its clinical effects. Several AEDs block voltage-gated sodium channels, but the interactions with other molecular targets help to define a drug's clinical spectrum. Although this discussion focuses primarily on studies of hippocampal neurons and circuits, insights into antiepileptic mechanisms have emerged from studies of many neural tissues (e.g., spinal cord, peripheral nerve, neocortex) and experimental preparations [Rho and Sankar, 1999]. Putative molecular targets of clinically approved antiepileptic drugs are shown in Figure 51-10 and Figure 51-11, which depict key elements of central nervous system excitatory and inhibitory synapses, respectively.

For many years, the primary drugs of choice for the treatment of partial epilepsy have been phenytoin and carbamazepine. Both drugs cause voltage-, frequency-, and use-dependent block of sodium channels in a wide variety of neuronal preparations. Sustained, high-frequency, repetitive firing of neurons is limited by both agents at free plasma concentrations found in patients. Oxcarbazepine, a structural analog of carbamazepine that is reduced to a monohydroxy derivative, also blocks sustained repetitive firing and is effective only against partial seizures.

Although structurally unrelated to classic agents such as phenytoin and carbamazepine, lamotrigine blocks sodium channels in a voltage-, frequency-, and use-dependent manner. However, lamotrigine has a much broader spectrum of activity than phenytoin or carbamazepine, demonstrating efficacy against several forms of generalized seizures in addition to partial seizures. The mechanistic basis for this difference

CENTRAL EXCITATORY SYNAPSE

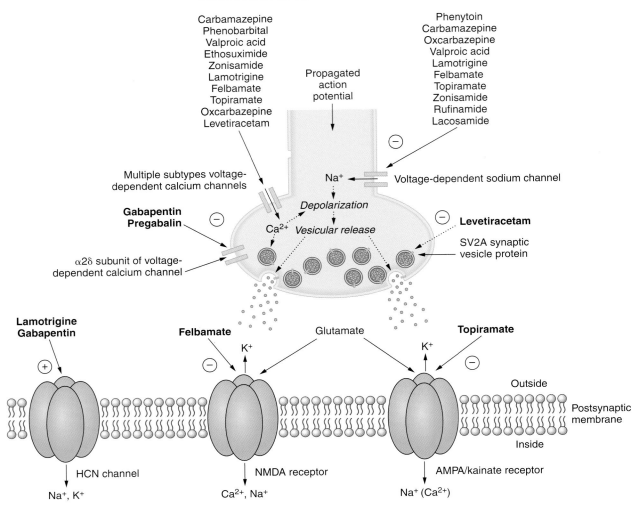

Fig. 51-10 Schematic diagram of an excitatory synapse in the central nervous system and the putative major sites of action of various antiepileptic drugs. Levetiracetam has been found to bind to a synaptic vesicle protein, SV2A, which is involved in exocytosis. AMPA, α-amino-3-hydroxy-5-methyl-4-isoxazolepropionic acid; HCN, hyperpolarization-activated cation; NMDA, N-methyl-D-aspartate. *(Adapted from Rho JM, Sankar R. The pharmacological basis of antiepileptic drug action. Epilepsia 1999;40:1471–1483. Reprinted with the permission of Blackwell Publishing Ltd.)*

may be related to the drug's enhancement of dendritic hyperpolarization-activated cation channels [Rogawski and Loscher, 2004].

The principal molecular targets of benzodiazepine and barbiturate antiepileptics are postsynaptic GABA$_A$ receptors. Binding of benzodiazepines or barbiturates to their respective recognition sites results in enhancement of GABA$_A$ receptor current. Two newer agents affecting the GABA system are vigabatrin, an irreversible inhibitor of the major GABA degradative enzyme, GABA transaminase, and tiagabine, a selective blocker of presynaptic GABA reuptake. Both vigabatrin and tiagabine elevate synaptic GABA levels.

Valproic acid is a broad-spectrum AED that induces a wide variety of biochemical and neurophysiologic changes in multiple neurotransmitter systems. Despite numerous studies, valproic acid's precise mechanisms of action remain a mystery. Investigation has focused on its multiple effects on the GABAergic system, resulting in elevated brain GABA levels. At therapeutic levels, valproic acid also diminishes sustained

repetitive firing of neocortical neurons, implicating actions on voltage-gated sodium channels as well.

Contrary to the prediction that gabapentin, a GABA analog, may act on GABAergic systems, gabapentin does not interact with GABA$_A$ or GABA$_B$ receptors, and does not affect GABA reuptake, synthesis, or metabolism. However, the existence of a specific binding site for gabapentin has been reported. Unlike other pharmacologic agents (e.g., flunarizine, dihydropyridines) that interact with the α$_1$ subunit of voltage-dependent calcium channels, gabapentin binds to the α$_2$δ subunit of the L-type calcium channel [Rogawski and Bazil, 2008]. Gabapentin (much like lamotrigine) enhances h-currents in hippocampal neurons, but the clinical significance of this remains unclear. Recent data confirms an interaction of gabapentin with GABA$_B$ receptor coupling to G-proteins and modulation of an inwardly rectifying potassium channel and N-type voltage-gated calcium channels. Whatever the relevant mechanisms of antiepileptic action, elevated brain GABA levels are found in patients taking gabapentin.

CENTRAL INHIBITORY SYNAPSE

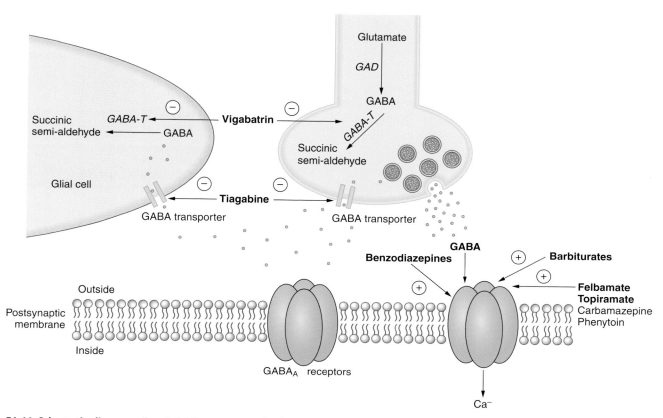

Fig. 51-11 Schematic diagram of an inhibitory synapse in the central nervous system, and the putative major sites of actions of various antiepileptic drugs. GABA, gamma-aminobutyric acid; GABA-T, GABA transaminase; GAD, glutamic acid decarboxylase. *(Adapted from Rho JM, Sankar R. The pharmacological basis of antiepileptic drug action. Epilepsia 1999;40:1471–1483. Reprinted with the permission of Blackwell Publishing Ltd.)*

Felbamate is the first pharmacologic agent to potentiate GABA_A receptor-mediated responses and inhibit NMDA receptor-mediated responses within the same drug concentration range [Rho and Sankar, 1999]. These dual actions may result in synergism with respect to seizure protection. Similarly, topiramate inhibits the AMPA or kainate subtype of glutamate receptor (specifically the GluR5 kainate receptor) and augments GABA_A receptor-mediated chloride currents [Rogawski and Loscher, 2004].

Zonisamide is a broad-spectrum agent that has a unique mechanistic profile [Rogawski and Loscher, 2004]. In cultured spinal cord neurons, zonisamide reduces sustained repetitive firing of action potentials, consistent with actions on voltage-gated sodium channels; in cultured neurons from rat cerebral cortex, zonisamide blocks low-threshold T-type calcium currents, which predicts efficacy against generalized spike-wave epilepsies.

Levetiracetam has challenged our conceptual understanding of relevant mechanisms of action. It failed the MES and PTZ tests in animals, but had a profound effect in retarding amygdala kindling in rats, and has proven clinical efficacy against partial and perhaps some generalized seizures. The strongest clue to identifying levetiracetam's principal molecular target is the demonstration of a specific high-affinity neuronal binding site [Kaminski et al., 2008]. Levetiracetam binds to a specific synaptic vesicle protein, SV2A, which is involved in neurotransmitter release. The exact mechanism by which

levetiracetam is dependent on SV2A for its antiepileptic action remains unknown [van Vliet et al., 2009].

The most recently approved AEDs in the United States are pregabalin, lacosamide, and rufinamide. Pregabalin, like gabapentin, seems to work by binding to the α2δ subunit of voltage-activated calcium channels, which reduces synaptic release of glutamate [Rogawski and Bazil, 2008]. Lacosamide reportedly possesses a novel mechanism of action – enhancing slow inactivation of sodium channels (older AEDs that block sodium channels do so by enhancing fast inactivation, which is mechanistically distinct) [Errington et al., 2008]. Whether this molecular mechanism will lead to enhanced seizure suppression is currently unkown, but it does represent an attempt to explore novel therapeutic approaches using physiologically relevant targets. Further preliminary evidence links lacosamide to modulation of collapsin-response mediator protein-2, which is involved in neuronal growth and plasticity; whether this action affects seizure suppression is unknown [Beydoun et al., 2009]. Rufinamide's mechanism of action is currently unknown, but preliminary results point to an effect on fast sodium channel inactivation [Arroyo, 2007].

Despite their diverse molecular actions, current AEDs fail to cure the disease; rather, they attempt to eliminate the major symptom – seizures – by dampening neuronal excitation, synchronization, and spread of seizure activity. There is little experimental evidence to support the idea that these drugs are truly antiepileptogenic. As epilepsy mechanisms are better understood, it may be possible to design more specific and rational interventions.

Summary

Epileptic seizures arise from a multiplicity of factors that regulate neuronal excitability and synchrony. Important mechanisms and substrates are believed to underlie seizure activity in the mature and the developing brain. There are unique differences in the ontogeny of ion channels and transporters that render the immature brain more susceptible to seizures than the adult brain. Although much has been learned about the molecular and cellular alterations that produce or accompany seizure activity, neurologists have yet to integrate these findings fully with the largely phenomenologic electroclinical observations and treatment responses in experimental animal models of epilepsy and in humans. In dissecting the basic neurophysiology of epilepsy, it is tempting to assign causality to any identifiable alteration that could theoretically enhance neuronal excitation. However, investigators frequently discover that it is not easy to identify the critical mediators and pathways in the processes of ictogenesis and epileptogenesis, and that, ultimately, seizures are a reflection of a complex array of perturbations occurring at multiple hierarchical levels of cell structure and function and as yet unpredictable consequences of neuronal network activity.

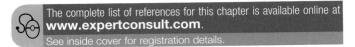

Genetics of Epilepsy

Maria Roberta Cilio and Susannah Cornes

Introduction

The concept of genetic epilepsy is that the condition is, as best as understood, the direct result of a known or presumed genetic defect in which seizures are the core symptom of the disorder [Berg et al., 2010]. The knowledge regarding the genetic contribution may derive from specific molecular genetic studies that have been well replicated and even become the basis of diagnostic tests. Alternatively, the central role of a genetic component may rely on evidence from appropriately designed family studies. This concept supersedes the term "idiopathic," defined in the 1989 classification for epilepsies [International League Against Epilepsy, 1989] as a form of epilepsy in which there is no underlying cause other than a possible hereditary predisposition and a presumed genetic etiology. Many of the traditional "idiopathic" epilepsies spontaneously remit during a predictable age range; as such, the term "idiopathic" has been used to imply "benign." This implication has now been discarded, and a genetic cause for epilepsy is no longer equated with a good prognosis.

The term "genetic" designates the fundamental nature of the disorder, while not excluding the possibility that environmental factors may contribute to the expression of the disease. Genetic epilepsies include epilepsies of varying prognoses, from the benign familial neonatal seizures to the more severe Dravet's syndrome. This field has seen a dramatic evolution of information in the past decade, both in defining new, rare cases of mendelian epilepsies, which provide insight into broader disease mechanisms, and in helping to define the substrates involved in the more complex inheritance patterns, which underlie most genetic epilepsy syndromes. Knowledge of the genetic epilepsies not only informs clinicians about the molecular biology of the disease, providing insights regarding normal brain function and mechanisms of epileptogenesis, but also has important consequences for clinical practice and genetic counseling [Andermann, 2009].

This chapter is intended to provide clinicians with updated information on the genetics of the epilepsies. It includes a comprehensive clinical review of the genetic epilepsies discovered so far and addresses newer concepts underlying genotype–phenotype correlation. A large section is devoted to the analysis of monogenic epilepsies with emphasis on epileptogenic channelopathies that have been intensively investigated in recent years. We review epilepsy syndromes in which one or more gene mutations or polymorphisms have been identified and syndromes in which a locus or loci has/have been mapped.

Epilepsy syndromes are organized by age at onset: neonatal (<44 weeks gestational age), infant (<2 years), child (2–12 years), and adolescent (12–18 years). Within each age group,

focal and generalized epilepsies are discussed, as relevant. This list of genetic epilepsies is constantly changing as new loci and genes are identified as the result of the effective collaborations between people working in clinical and laboratory settings. Indeed, some of the most exciting genetic discoveries in the field have been made possible by a careful definition of the phenotype by clinical epileptologists. On the other hand, epileptogenic gene mutations discovered by molecular biologists have also led to recognition of previously unidentified clinical forms of epilepsy.

Epilepsies of the Neonatal Period

Benign Familial Neonatal Seizures

Benign familial neonatal seizures (BFNS), is a rare autosomal-dominant epilepsy of the newborn characterized by recurrent, mainly focal seizures that begin in the first few days of life and remit after a few weeks or months. Seizures start with a tonic posture accompanied by other symptoms such as apnea and other autonomic features. The seizures often progress to focal or bilateral clonic jerks. Generalized seizures have also been reported. Seizures are usually brief, lasting for approximately 1–2 minutes, but may occur as many as 20–30 times a day. The postictal state is short-lived, and the neonates look normal in the interictal period [Ronen et al., 1993]. The interictal electroencephalogram (EEG) pattern either is normal or shows minimal focal or multifocal abnormalities. EEG patterns suggestive of poor prognosis, such as a burst-suppression or inactive EEG, have not been reported. The original description of the disease dates back to the work of Rett and Teubel, who described a four-generation family with nine individuals affected [Rett and Teubel, 1964]. In their original work, the authors emphasized the heritability of the disease and the absence of acquired origin. The term "benign" was added only few years later, to highlight the fact that most affected individuals experienced normal psychomotor development. Nevertheless, 5 percent of BFNS patients present with febrile seizures and 11 percent develop epilepsy later in life [Plouin and Anderson, 2005]. In rare infants, the outcome may be poor [Dedek et al., 2003; Borgatti et al., 2004; Steinlein et al., 2007], and a single family with myokymia later in life has been described [Dedek et al., 2001].

BFNS is the first epilepsy syndrome for which a gene could be localized [Singh et al., 1998; Charlier et al., 1998]. This disorder has been linked to mutations in the neuronal voltage-gated potassium channel subunits, *KCNQ2* and *KCNQ3* [Singh et al., 1998; Charlier et al., 1998], located on chromosome

20 (20q13.3) and on chromosome 8 (8q24), respectively. *KCNQ2* and *KCNQ3* subunits mediate the M-current, a neuronal-specific K$^+$ current, which plays a key role in controlling neuronal excitability [Biervert et al., 1998; Singh et al., 2003; Wang et al., 1998; Soldovieri et al., 2007]. The majority of cases, 56 percent, are associated with mutations in *KCNQ2*, with *KCNQ3* mutations accounting for only 6.6 percent [Deprez et al., 2009]. More than 60 mutations of *KCNQ2* have been reported so far, including missense, frameshift, nonsense, and splice-site mutations. Furthermore, submicroscopic deletions or duplications in *KCNQ2* have been shown to account for a significant proportion of unsolved BFNS cases, in which mutations are not detected by direct sequencing [Heron et al., 2007a], and have been found in about one-sixth of BFNS families.

The age dependency of BFNS has been explained by the peculiar spatial and temporal expression pattern of *KCNQ2* and *KCNQ3* subunits in human development [Kanaumi et al., 2008]. A high degree of expression of *KCNQ2* has been identified in the hippocampus, temporal cortex, cerebellar cortex, and medulla oblongata in fetal life. There is a decrease in expression of the gene after birth. The increased expression of *KCNQ3* during fetal life compared with infancy has also been confirmed.

Benign Familial Neonatal-Infantile Seizures

Benign familial neonatal-infantile seizures (BFNIS) is an autosomal-dominant benign epilepsy of the early infancy with a high degree of penetrance. Age of onset ranges from 2 days to 6 months in different family members, with a mean age of onset of 3 months. Seizures have a focal onset, often with eye deviation, apnea, cyanosis, and staring. Secondary generalization may follow. Similarly to BFNS, seizures may occur in clusters. The interictal EEG is normal or shows occasional central or posterior focal spikes [Heron et al., 2002; Herlenius et al., 2007]. Seizures abate by 1 year of life, with a low risk of recurrence.

Unlike the previously discussed "benign familial neonatal seizures," which are associated with potassium channel mutations, this syndrome has been linked to mutations in *SCN2A* [Heron et al., 2002], the alpha-2 subunit of the neuronal voltage-gated sodium channel [Berkovic et al., 2004a; Helbig et al., 2008]. Eight different mutations in ten families have been described so far [Heron et al., 2002; Berkovic et al., 2004b; Herlenius et al., 2007]. Mutations in *SCN2A* seem to be specific to this condition, with only very few cases being reported [Helbig et al., 2008]. The *SCN2A* mutations reported in association with BFNIS are all missense mutations. While the majority are predicted to be gain-of-function, more recently, Misra and colleagues reported three mutations that are a loss-of-function type [Misra et al., 2008]. An increase in the Na$^+$ current caused by modifications of voltage-dependent gating, or a reduction in the current caused by reduced channel expression or impaired gating kinetics, has the ultimate effect of increasing neuronal excitability, thus favoring seizure generation or propagation [Avanzini et al., 2007; Misra et al., 2008].

Neonatal Epileptic Encephalopathies

The International League Against Epilepsy (ILAE) defines two further neonatal epilepsy syndromes, early myoclonic encephalopathy and Ohtahara syndrome (early infantile epileptic encephalopathy). Both syndromes have been defined as epileptic encephalopathies with neonatal onset and a typical suppression-burst EEG pattern [Aicardi and Ohtahara, 2005]. They are associated with severe psychomotor retardation and grave prognosis [Djukic et al., 2006]. A distinguishing feature is the main seizure type, which is myoclonic in the case of early myoclonic encephalopathy, and tonic in the case of early infantile epileptic encephalopathy. Ohtahara syndrome has been linked to a gene encoding syntaxin binding protein 1 (*STXBP1*), which encodes a vesicle release protein and has been implicated in 35.7 percent of cases [Saitsu et al., 2008; Deprez et al., 2009]. *STXBP1* mutations have also been implicated in cases [Saitsu et al., 2008; Deprez et al., 2009] of mental retardation and nonsyndromic epilepsy [Hamdan et al., 2009]. Therefore, the role of *STXBP1* in epilepsy is interesting on a couple of levels. First, it extends the genetic epilepsies to include molecules involved in neurotransmission through vesicle release, in addition to the many known ion channel mutations. Second, it redefines a syndrome as "genetic," which might otherwise have been classified as "structural" or "metabolic." Thus far, only one other protein involved in synaptic vesicle transmission, Synaspin-1, has been linked to epilepsy and learning difficulties, as reported in one family [Garcia et al., 2004]. Testing for *STXBP1* may be useful in nonlesional cases of Ohtahara.

A second gene has recently been implicated in Ohtahara; an *ARX* protein truncation mutation has been found in one family [Fullston et al., 2010]. *ARX* is a homeobox gene located on the short arm of the X chromosome, and it has been implicated in a number of different syndromes including West's syndrome (see below), lissencephaly, and nonsyndromic X-linked mental retardation and epilepsy [Strømme et al., 2002]. Limited human and extensive mouse gene-expression studies show high levels of *ARX* expression in the fetal brain, particularly in the neuronal precursors of the germinal matrix and the ventricular zone. High levels of expression are also observed in the subventricular zone, the caudate nucleus, putamen, substantia nigra, corpus callosum, amygdala, and hippocampus [Bienvenu et al., 2002; Kitamura et al., 2002; Colombo et al., 2004; Poirier et al., 2004]. This expression during early development and predilection for neuronal tissue suggests that *ARX* has a pivotal function in neurodevelopment. Recently, homozygous mutations on *SLC25A22* have been described in case reports of consanguineous families with neonatal epileptic encephalopathies with suppression-burst [Molinari et al., 2005, 2009].

A final epileptic encephalopathy is characterized by early onset of a severe intractable seizure in girls with normal interictal EEG and severe hypotonia. The syndrome is associated with mutations in X-linked cyclin-dependent kinase-like 5 (*CDKL5*) [Bahi-Buisson et al., 2008a, b]. Mutations in the *CDKL5* gene have also been shown to cause infantile spasms and Rett's syndrome-like phenotype. Recent studies [Bahi-Buisson et al., 2008a, b] highlighted the key clinical features of this rare epileptic encephalopathy that should help establish a molecular diagnosis. In younger patients under 2 years of age, early-onset epilepsy is probably the most consistent sign in *CDKL5* mutations. In all cases, epilepsy starts within 3 months, often in the neonatal period, with very frequent seizures and an interictal EEG that is normal or indicates background slowing. At this age, neurologic examination reveals severe hypotonia and poor eye contact. Subsequently, a large proportion of patients develop epileptic encephalopathy characterized by the occurrence of infantile spasms with hypsarrhythmia, and then multifocal epilepsy. While brain magnetic resonance imaging

(MRI) might be normal at onset, it is usually found to be abnormal later in the course of the disease. Although it is non-specific, most patients exhibit cortical atrophy combined with hyperintensities in the temporal lobe white matter that could be related to abnormal myelination. The evolution of the disorder includes the appearance of hand stereotypies from the age of 18 months to 3 years, hand apraxia, sleep disturbances and deceleration of head growth [Bahi-Buisson et al., 2008a]. All girls with *CDKL5* mutations are severely delayed, with limited, if any, autonomy.

Epilepsies of Infantile Onset

Benign Familial Infantile Seizures

Benign familial infantile seizures (BFIS) syndrome was first described in 1992 by Vigevano and co-workers, who reported on cases with focal seizures in infancy, a family history of convulsions, benign outcome, and autosomal-dominant inheritance [Vigevano et al., 1992]. This syndrome is now included in the most recent classification and terminology proposed by ILAE [Engel, 2001]. Age of onset ranges from 4 to 8 months, with a peak around 6 months. Seizures typically occur in clusters of brief recurrent episodes of up to ten a day, never reaching true status epilepticus. Seizures are often characterized by head and eye deviation that may alternate in laterality for different attacks; even in the same patient, EEG recordings corroborate independent right and left seizure onset, confirming the alternating clinical pattern [Vigevano, 2005].

While the overall prognosis remains excellent in terms of remission from seizures, there is a risk of paroxysmal dyskinesias in later childhood [Lee et al., 1998; Demir et al., 2005]. BFIS is the least well characterized genetically, with multiple loci implicated but few candidate genes. Multiple authors have linked the syndrome to the pericentromeric region of chromosome 16 [Lee et al., 1998; Demir et al., 2005]. There has also been one report linking the syndrome to chromosome 19 [Guipponi et al., 1997], and one linking it to chromosome 1 in a family with hemiplegic migraine and a mutation in the *ATP1A2* gene, which encodes a sodium-potassium ATPase transporter [Vanmolkot et al., 2003]. In addition, mutations in *SCN2A* and *KCNQ2* have been described [Striano et al., 2006; Zhou et al., 2006], suggesting a possible overlap of clinical and genetic characteristics of the three benign epilepsy syndromes occurring in the neonatal or neonatal-infantile period.

Dravet's Syndrome

Dravet's syndrome, previously known as severe myoclonic epilepsy in infancy (SMEI), was described by Charlotte Dravet in 1978 [Dravet, 1978]. This entity is an epileptic encephalopathy, a condition in which the epileptiform abnormalities themselves are believed to contribute to the progressive disturbance in cerebral function [Engel, 2001]. Onset is at approximately 6 months of age in previously healthy children. Dravet's syndrome typically presents with prolonged hemiclonic or generalized febrile seizures, sometimes leading to status epilepticus. Myoclonic jerks, atypical absences, and complex partial seizures appear later in the course of the disease. Subsequently, children develop neurological deficits, such as ataxia and corticospinal tract dysfunction [Dravet et al., 1992], as well as psychomotor delay, behavioral disturbances, and significant learning problems [Wolff et al., 2006].

EEG findings may be normal at onset, and then show generalized, focal, and multifocal abnormalities, often associated with a strong photosensitivity. MRI is usually normal or, in a few cases, shows dilatation of the cisterna magna or slight diffuse atrophy [Dravet et al., 2005]. However, most recent neuroimaging techniques can identify hippocampal sclerosis in some patients during the course of the disease [Striano et al., 2007]. The onset during infancy and frequent association with prolonged febrile seizures help to distinguish the syndrome from epilepsy with myoclonic-astatic seizures, also known as Doose's syndrome.

Major advances have occurred in our understanding of Dravet's syndrome with elucidation of its association with *SCN1A* mutations. Since the report of Claes and colleagues in 2001 [Claes et al., 2001], the concept that *SCN1A* is the major gene responsible for Dravet's syndrome has been established [Fujiwara et al., 2003; Wallace et al., 2003; Fukuma et al., 2004]. The gene encodes the neuronal sodium channel NaV1.1 alpha subunit, which has four homologous regions, each encoding six transmembrane domains and a region controlling interactions with the permeable ion. Mutations have been found throughout the gene [Gambardella and Marini, 2009], and a website has been created to track the increasing number of mutations at http://www.scn1a.info. There are currently more than 300 known *SCN1A* mutations, with mutational rates in patients with Dravet's syndrome of 33–100 percent [Claes et al., 2003; Fukuma et al., 2004; Mulley et al., 2005; Sugawara et al., 2002; Nabbout et al., 2003; Wallace et al., 2003]. Mutations are commonly truncations, although missense mutations can occur [Claes et al., 2003; Kanai et al., 2004; Mulley et al., 2005]. Among *SCN1A* mutations, those associated with Dravet's syndrome are quite variable, including frameshift, nonsense, deletion, amplification, and duplication. However, simple missense mutations still account for 40 percent of cases [Mullen and Scheffer, 2009].

Mutations are usually de novo, although cases of germline mosaicism have been reported and should be taken into account for genetic counseling [Gambardella and Marini, 2009]. Patients for whom standard polymerase chain reaction (PCR) fails to detect an *SCN1A* mutation may undergo additional testing with multiplex ligation-dependent probe amplification, which detects microchromosomal copy number variations, such as deletions or duplications, in an additional 10–25 percent of PCR-negative cases [Madia et al., 2006; Mulley et al., 2006; Suls et al., 2006; Marini et al., 2009]. In terms of treatment for Dravet's syndrome, topiramate, stiripentol, valproate, clonazepam, and levetiracetam, as well as the ketogenic diet, have been effective. Lamotrigine and carbamazepine may induce seizure aggravation [Guerrini et al., 1998; Wakai et al., 1996].

The spectrum of *SCN1A*-related epilepsies has been extended in the past few years, and several subgroups related to Dravet's syndrome have now been reported, such as the syndrome of borderline SMEI (SMEB), characterized by a lack of myoclonic seizures and generalized spike-wave discharges, and the intractable childhood epilepsy with generalized tonic-clonic seizures (ICE-GTC), in which tonic-clonic seizures predominate [Osaka et al., 2007; Fujiwara, 2006; Rhodes et al., 2005]. *SCN1A* has also been implicated in cases of familial migraine [Cestele et al., 2008; Vahedi et al., 2009] and in a variety of other epilepsy syndromes. While no association has been found with simple febrile seizures [Petrovski et al., 2009] in the 5 percent of Dravet cases found to have familial mutations, family members often have other phenotypes, such as generalized epilepsy with febrile seizures plus (GEFS+) [Wallace et al., 2001b; Sijben et al., 2009]. In a recent comprehensive study, Harkin and colleagues have analyzed a cohort of 188 patients with various epileptic encephalopathies and found *SCN1A* mutations in 48 percent of patients, mainly novel; 96 percent were de novo [Harkin et al., 2007]. No patients with West's syndrome or progressive myoclonic epilepsy had an *SCN1A* mutation. However, mutations were not restricted to those with typical epileptic encephalopathies. Interestingly, a few patients with cryptogenic generalized or focal epilepsy, myoclonic-astatic epilepsy, and Lennox–Gastaut syndrome also carried mutations.

Because *SCN1A* is implicated in a variety of other epilepsy syndromes, some of which are more benign, there is new potential for confusion regarding prognosis for affected patients, and a new need for clinicians to understand the subtleties of genetic testing for *SCN1A* mutations. While many different *SCN1A* mutations have been identified in patients with Dravet's syndrome, most of which are unique to individuals, several recurrent mutations have also been found [Mulley et al., 2005]. Mutations are spread throughout the gene and, therefore, have different predicted functional effects on the protein [Kanai et al., 2004]. However, it is apparent that wherever and whatever the functional effects of these mutations are, they all lead to a similar seizure phenotype. Collating the available functional data on such mutations does result in an obvious explanation of the shared epilepsy phenotype; however, mathematical modeling has predicted an increased excitability via augmented action potential firing [Spampanato et al., 2004]. Mutations in *SCN1A* are collectively the most frequent genetic cause of epilepsy. Hence, further efforts to clarify the precise pathophysiology are likely to be important to the fundamental understanding of epileptogenesis.

Generalized Epilepsy with Febrile Seizures Plus

Generalized epilepsy with febrile seizures plus (GEFS+), mentioned above, was first described by Sheffer and Berkovic, and is associated with *SCN1A* mutations in roughly 10 percent of cases [Scheffer and Berkovic, 1997]. Mutations are generally missense, and the syndrome is characterized by an autosomal mode of inheritance, a broad spectrum of phenotypes, and a penetrance of 60 percent. Cases are mostly considered to have generalized epilepsy. The most common phenotype is characterized by the association of febrile seizures (FS), or febrile seizures extending beyond 6 years of age (febrile seizures plus, FS+), with afebrile generalized tonic-clonic seizures. This condition is a heritable syndrome, so clinical characteristics may be present in multiple family members. Less common phenotypes show the association of FS+ with absences, or myoclonic or atonic seizures, while the most severe phenotype includes myoclonic-astatic epilepsy. Partial seizures have also been reported, though rarely [Baulac et al., 1999].

West's Syndrome

The final syndrome to consider that has infantile onset and a genetic etiology, in a minority of cases, is West's syndrome. While the majority of cases of infantile spasms have no genetic

association, mutations in *ARX*, *Aristaless*-related homeobox gene, have been associated with cases of X-linked recessive infantile spasms or "ISSX" [Fullston et al., 2010]. Genetic testing may therefore be appropriate in cases in which multiple males are affected by infantile spasms and mental retardation; dystonia is also a feature [Poirier et al., 2008; Shinozaki et al., 2009]. A second, dominant form of ISSX has been associated with a balanced X-autosomal translocation that disrupts *CDKL5* (see Neonatal Epileptic Encephalopathies). A final syndrome of epilepsy and mental retardation limited to females has also been described [Deprez et al., 2009; Hynes et al., 2009; Depienne et al., 2009; Dibbens et al., 2008]. This syndrome is often associated with autistic, obsessive, or aggressive traits, and has been linked to various mutation of *PCDH19* (protocadherin 19). (For a broader review of infantile spasms, please refer to Chapter 56.)

Syndromes with Childhood Onset

Early- and Late-Onset Childhood Occipital Epilepsy

Early-onset benign childhood occipital epilepsy was first described by Panayiotopoulos in 1989 as an epilepsy syndrome characterized by the "ictal triad of nocturnal seizures, tonic deviation of the eyes and vomiting" [Panayiotopoulos, 1989]. The age of onset of Panayiotopoulos syndrome (PS) is typically between 3 and 5 years of age; it affects boys and girls equally and is characterized by a low seizure burden. However, seizures can be prolonged, are marked by autonomic features, and often involve alteration in consciousness. Seizures may march to involve clonic movement of the head and upper extremities or secondary convulsion. A minority of patients may develop seizures during the day. The syndrome is benign, with remission before age 12.

The EEG reveals normal background activity, but frequent surface-negative spike and slow-wave complexes over the occipital region, occurring singularly or repetitively with a frequency of 2–4 Hz. Discharges may be apparent bilaterally with a persistent voltage asymmetry or a shifting predominance, or they may be unilateral. The spike-wave complexes attenuate with eye-opening and fixation, and are induced in darkness or with eye closure. Generalized discharges may also be present, and were noted in 50 percent of the original series. Other focal discharges also occur. The occipital spike wave remains present despite treatment with antiepileptic medications, but tends to decrease with age [Capovilla et al., 2009].

The Gastaut type, also known as childhood epilepsy with occipital paroxysms (CEOP), was first described by Camfield in 1978 [Camfield et al., 1978] and elaborated by Gastaut in 1982 [Gastaut, 1982]. CEOP has a later onset, presenting between 3 and 16 years, and seizures are characterized by visual symptoms rather than gaze deviation. Visual symptoms may include amaurosis, phosphenes, illusions, or hallucinations, and may progress to involve automatisms or hemiclonic seizures. Events are followed by migraine and classically have a diurnal pattern. EEG abnormalities similarly involve occipital spike wave activated by eye closure. However, the prognosis is somewhat poorer in terms of chance for remission.

The Panayiotopoulos and Gastaut forms of CEOP are probably better viewed as a clinical spectrum. One-third of patients with CEOP appear to have a mixed syndrome, with features of both Panayiotopoulos and Gastaut forms [Taylor et al., 2008]. Similarly, while there is evidence for a genetic component to CEOP, with some reports of concordant monozygotic or dizygotic twins, the concordance does not appear to be higher in monozygotic twins, indicating that other epigenetic or environmental factors likely also play a role [Taylor et al., 2008]. Additionally, while a family history of epilepsy can be established in roughly 36 percent of patients with either form of childhood occipital epilepsy, affected family members have been found to have a variety of generalized or focal epilepsy syndromes rather than CEOP alone.

Benign Epilepsy with Centrotemporal Spikes

Benign epilepsy with centrotemporal spikes (BECTS) is the most common benign focal epilepsy of childhood, with an incidence of 10–20 per 100,000 in children under age 15. Onset occurs most commonly between 7 and 10 years, with a slight male predominance [Panayiotopoulos et al., 2008]. Seizures are focal and involve unilateral sensorimotor function of the face, speech arrest, and hypersalivation. Consciousness is generally maintained, although seizures may progress to become hemiconvulsive or generalized tonic-clonic.

The EEG reveals bilateral independent centrotemporal spikes reflecting a horizontal dipole with maximal negativity over the central region and maximal positivity over the frontal region. Epileptiform activity may be augmented in sleep and, rarely, other focal discharges or generalized spike wave has been reported. Three-quarters of rolandic seizures occur out of non-rapid eye movement (REM) sleep, often at sleep transitions.

Prognosis is excellent, with the majority of patients having fewer than ten seizures in total. Many will not require treatment with medications, and 10–20 percent will only have a single seizure. Remission occurs within 2–4 years of onset and prior to age 16 years. Rarely, and in the most severe 1 percent of cases, language and cognitive dysfunction can develop in association with significant activation of the EEG during sleep. Therefore, many view BECTS as being on a spectrum with other epilepsy syndromes, including Landau–Kleffner, atypical focal epilepsy of childhood, and epilepsy with continuous spike and wave during sleep (CSWS).

BECTS was classically believed to have a strong genetic component, probably based on the heritability of centrotemporal spikes, present in 11–48 percent of sibling pairs [Helbig et al., 2008], and early twin studies addressing overall heritability of the idiopathic epilepsy syndromes [Berkovic et al., 1998]. In addition, there have been case reports of mendelian inheritance patterns in families with variants of BECTS in which the disease is associated with dystonia [Guerrini et al., 1999] or with speech and language dysfunction [Hirsch et al., 2006; Roll et al., 2006; Scheffer et al., 1995b; Rudolf et al., 2009]. More recent twin studies, however, targeted to evaluate BECTS alone, have found relatively low concordance rates for the clinical syndrome, unlike the EEG trait of centrotemporal spikes, and suggest that nongenetic factors are important in the development of the phenotype [Vadlamudi et al., 2006]. While genetics is likely to play some role, given familial aggregation of the disease, the genetic risk appears to have been overestimated initially. Certainly, simple inheritance patterns only appear relevant in rare disease variants.

Childhood Absence Epilepsy

Childhood absence epilepsy (CAE) accounts for 5–15 percent of childhood epilepsy. It has a typical onset between 4 and 8 years of age, and there is a history of febrile seizures in 10–15 percent. Seizures are characterized by brief losses of awareness, lasting 10 seconds on average, and with a rapid return to baseline mental status within 2–3 seconds. Absences may be associated with a fixed blank stare, upward movement of the eyes, mild clonic, atonic, or tonic components, or quasi-purposeful movements. Tonic-clonic seizures occur in roughly 40 percent of patients but are infrequent, and absence status epilepticus occurs in as many as 10 percent. Myoclonic jerks are not typically seen.

Absences generally respond well to medical management, and remission is common. In the rare instance in which seizures persist into adulthood, they are often tonic-clonic in semiology, rather than absence. The EEG reveals a generalized 3-Hz spike wave that appears as an interictal trait, precipitated by hyperventilation, and in association with clinically apparent absence seizures.

CAE was previously categorized as an "idiopathic generalized epilepsy" (IGE) syndrome, along with juvenile myoclonic epilepsy (JME), juvenile absence epilepsy (JAE), and generalized epilepsy with tonic-clonic seizures. While the term "idiopathic" has now been abandoned, it may still be useful to think of these syndromes together in so far as their genetic underpinnings remain intertwined and without phenotypic specificity. Although rare families with mendelian inheritance patterns have been described for a subset of these syndromes [Cossette et al., 2002], polygenic inheritance, influenced by susceptibility genes, is widely accepted as accounting for the bulk of disease.

While the genetics for these previously categorized IGEs remains complex, a strong role for genetics has been established through twin studies, demonstrating concordance for monozygotic twins of approximately 70 percent [Lennox, 1951; Vadlamudi et al., 2004]. In families without twins, however, the risk to siblings is roughly 6 percent, and as a result, only about one-third of families will report a family history. Within families with multiple affected members, there is often phenotypic heterogeneity, although there is some evidence for segregation of absence versus myoclonic phenotypes [Winawer et al., 2005].

A number of genes have been implicated in CAE. Mutations in *GABRG2*, which encodes the γ-2 subunit of the neuronal gamma-aminobutyric acid (GABA)$_A$ receptor, have been implicated in the development of both CAE and febrile seizures [Wallace et al., 2001a; Kananura et al., 2002], as well as in GEFS+. Mutations in *GABRA1*, which encodes the alpha-1 subunit of the neuronal GABA$_A$ receptor, have been associated with CAE in one series [Maljevic et al., 2006], and with JME in another [Cossette et al., 2002]. There is also evidence that the GABA$_A$ receptor beta-3 subunit gene (*GABRB3*) may play a role in the development of CAE via reduced expression associated with mutation in its promoter [Urak et al., 2006]. In addition, malic enzyme 2, which plays a role in the synthesis of GABA, has been found to have a polymorphism associated with the adolescent-onset generalized epilepsies (JAE, JME, and generalized tonic-clonic seizures alone), conferring a sixfold increase in the odds of developing the disease [Greenberg et al., 2005].

Varied mutations in *CACNA1H*, the neuronal voltage-gated T-type calcium channel subunit, have also been implicated in

CAE [Chen et al., 2003]. This channel is thought to play a key role in generating the 3-Hz spike wave that is characteristic of absence seizures. However, *CACNA1H* appears to function as a broader susceptibility gene and has also been shown to play a role in other generalized epilepsies, such as JME, JAE, and myoclonic astatic epilepsy, as well as in febrile seizures and even temporal lobe epilepsy [Heron et al., 2007b]. Similarly, *CLCN2*, a voltage-gated chloride channel, has also been implicated broadly in CAE, JME, JAE, and epilepsy with tonic-clonic seizures [D'Agostino et al., 2004]. *SLC2A1*, which encodes the GLUT1 glucose transporter, has recently been implicated in early-onset absence epilepsy before age 4 years [Suls et al., 2009].

The complex polygenic inheritance patterns involved in CAE and other genetic generalized epilepsy syndromes reveal that a single epilepsy phenotype can be generated by combinations of varied mutations, and that, conversely, a given mutation can be associated with more than one phenotype. With on-going research, understanding how such varied genetic factors can contribute to the development of seizures should tell us a great deal about the pathophysiology of epileptogenesis.

Syndromes with Adolescent or Adult Onset

Juvenile Absence Epilepsy

Juvenile absence epilepsy (JAE) has an average age of onset of 12 years, representing a second peak in incidence after CAE with onset between 4 and 8 years. JAE is rarer than CAE, representing no more than 20 percent of absence epilepsy cases diagnosed. JAE is characterized by absence seizures, as described above for CAE, but there is a higher incidence of convulsive seizures, which occur in 80 percent, and myoclonus may occur in 15 percent, causing an area of overlap with JME.

The EEG reveals a generalized spike wave occurring ictally, interictally, and in response to hyperventilation. The spike wave is superimposed on a normal background and may be less regular or faster than is seen in CAE.

The course remains relatively benign, with few cases remitting but 80 percent responding well to first-line therapy. As noted above, there is evidence for polygenic inheritance, with many of the genes involved in CAE being also linked to JAE, and some evidence that there is more genetic overlap with CAE than with JME [Winawer and Shinnar, 2005].

Juvenile Myoclonic Epilepsy

Juvenile myoclonic epilepsy (JME) is believed to represent as much as 10 percent of all epilepsy cases. Onset occurs between ages 12 and 18 years. Seizures are often myoclonic, but generalized tonic-clonic occur in 95 percent. Events often begin just after awakening, and sleep deprivation and alcohol are commonly cited as triggers. Myoclonus most often involves the bilateral upper extremities, and as a result, it is common to elicit a history of difficulty eating breakfast, brushing teeth, or applying make-up in the morning. Generalized tonic-clonic seizures are often preceded by a period of increasing myoclonic jerks with preserved consciousness, allowing patients to predict their seizures on some occasions, despite the generalized onset. Absences are rare.

The EEG reveals generalized fast spike- and polyspike-wave activity that may have a frequency of 10–16 Hz during myoclonic jerks, or slow to 2–5 Hz with modest irregularity during more prolonged seizures. Generalized, fast-spike, and polyspike wave is also seen interictally superimposed on a normal background.

The prognosis for JME remains good, in so far as most cases are well controlled on medications, and as many as one-third may be able to cease medications during adulthood without relapse [Camfield and Camfield, 2009]. However, the disability associated with even rare convulsions should not be underestimated. In addition to the direct impact on morbidity and mortality, there are implications for driving privileges, and higher rates of unemployment have been reported [Camfield and Camfield, 2009].

As was discussed for CAE and JAE, JME has complex polygenic inheritance. There is a positive family history reported in 30–50 percent, and a number of common susceptibility genes have been identified to date. These genes include *GABRA1*, which encodes the alpha-1 subunit of the neuronal $GABA_A$ receptor and has been associated with CAE and JME [Maljevic et al., 2006; Cossette et al., 2002], and malic enzyme 2, which is associated with adolescent-onset generalized epilepsies and plays a role in synthesis of GABA. In addition, *CACNA1H* and *CLCN2*, which encode a voltage-gated T-type calcium channel and a voltage-gated chloride channel, respectively, have been broadly implicated in primary generalized epilepsies and even in temporal lobe epilepsy [Heron et al., 2007; D'Agostino et al., 2004].

There are additional genes implicated specifically in the development of the JME phenotype. Several authors have reported gene mutations in *EFHC1* associated with JME in a variety of affected families of differing origin [Suzuki et al., 2004; Annesi et al., 2007]. EFHC1 encodes a protein of unknown function with calcium-binding EF-hand motif, a helix-loop-helix structural domain found in a large family of calcium-binding proteins. There is evidence that the protein modulates apoptotic activity and R-type voltage-dependent calcium channel properties [Suzuki et al., 2004].

Epilepsy with Generalized Tonic-Clonic Seizures Alone

Previously known as epilepsy with generalized tonic-clonic seizures on awakening, this epilepsy syndrome was found to be associated with the adolescent onset of tonic-clonic seizures alone, without predilection for certain times of day or states [Reutens and Berkovic, 1995]. As a result, it is now referred to as epilepsy with generalized tonic-clonic seizures alone. The genetics of the syndrome are likely similar to those of CAE, JAE, and JME (see above), with complex polygenic inheritance of common susceptibility genes.

Autosomal-Dominant Nocturnal Frontal Lobe Epilepsy

Autosomal-dominant nocturnal frontal lobe epilepsy (ADNFLE) typically arises during the first (53 percent) or second (35 percent) decade of life, with a median age of onset of 8 years [Scheffer et al., 1995]. Clinically, the disease is characterized by nocturnal tonic or hypermotor activity, such as sitting up in bed, crawling into the bed, or being flung from bed with associated injury. Awareness is generally preserved, although there may be an inability to respond. Seizures occur in clusters and are most commonly reported soon after falling asleep or in the early hours of the morning. Clusters consist of a median of 6 attacks, but can range from 1 to 72, in extreme cases. Rarely, seizures are reported from naps or daytime wakefulness. Seizures are generally brief (median 60 seconds) and often accompanied by aura, which may awaken the subject from sleep prior to the first attack. The pattern and semiology of the seizures often lead to misdiagnosis with nocturnal parasomnia or other psychiatric or medical illness.

The EEG is notable for rare interictal epileptiform activity (16 percent) or slowing (22 percent), with the majority having no discernible interictal abnormalities (84 percent). The ictal EEG may show frontally predominant sharp- and slow-wave activity, or may fail to reveal a definite ictal pattern. Seizures most frequently arise from stage 2 sleep. Review of semiology often reveals prominent dystonic posturing.

Outcomes for ADNFLE are good, although the disease does not typically remit. Individuals demonstrate normal intellect and neurologic examination. The great majority requires antiepileptic medication, but less than one-third requires combination therapy. For example, in the description by Scheffer and coauthors [Scheffer et al., 1995], 32 percent of patients were well controlled on carbamazepine monotherapy, while 29 percent required more than one agent. There may be improvement in later life, with rare individuals successfully weaning medications after age 50 years.

The inheritance of ADNFLE is autosomal-dominant, as the name states, with a penetrance of 70–80 percent [Scheffer et al., 1995]. The phenotype has been associated with various mutations in genes encoding the alpha-4 (*CHRNA4*), beta-2 (*CHRNB2*), and alpha-2 (*CHRNA2*) subunits of the nicotinic acetylcholine receptor, as well as with a variant of the promoter for the corticotropin-releasing hormone (CRH). The acetylcholine receptor is a pentameric ion channel consisting of predominantly alpha-4 and beta-2 subunits. The second transmembrane domain of each subunit lines the ion channel pore and is the site for the majority of the mutations that have been described for *CHRNA4* [Steinlein et al., 1995; Weiland and Steinlein, 1996] and *CHRNB2* [Diaz-Otero et al., 2008; De Fusco et al., 2000; Phillips et al., 2001]. In fact, independent mutations in particular conserved amino acid residues in these domains have been demonstrated in families of differing ethnicity, suggesting that these sites play an important role in the development of the syndrome. Functionally, the mutations appear to alter the desensitization kinetics of the receptor, thereby contributing to hyperexcitability and seizure [Weiland et al., 1996]. In addition, in the case of *CHRNB2*, one of the mutations is associated with a more pronounced blockade of current by carbamazepine, suggesting a mechanism for treatment responsiveness.

Despite the evidence that the second transmembrane domain is important for the development of the disease, mutation of this region is not essential. One family has been described with ADNFLE and memory difficulties, associated with a mutation involving the third transmembrane region of *CHRNB2* [Bertrand et al., 2005], and another family has been described with a *CHRNA2* involving the first transmembrane domain of the receptor and affecting the receptor sensitivity to acetylcholine [Aridon et al., 2006]. Finally, despite an increasing number of nAChR mutations demonstrated in

families with ADNFLE, the majority of cases remain without a putative gene, despite screening for nAChR mutations. Recently, a variation in the promoter of the corticotropin-releasing hormone gene (*CRH*) has been linked to the disease in one family [Combi et al., 2005], and it is possible that several additional loci will be found to explain the remaining cases, potentially helping our understanding of the various intersecting mechanisms at play in the development of the phenotype.

Autosomal-Dominant Partial Epilepsy with Auditory Features

Autosomal-dominant partial epilepsy with auditory features (ADPEAF), also known as autosomal-dominant lateral temporal lobe epilepsy (ADLTE), is a heritable partial epilepsy first described by Ottman and co-workers in 1995 [Ottman et al., 1995], with onset ranging from the second to fourth decades; it is estimated to make up 19 percent of genetic partial epilepsies [Michelucci et al., 2009]. To date, at least 35 families from Europe, the United States, Australia, and Japan have been reported, adding up to over 200 cases [Michelucci et al., 2003]. Seizures are focal, with a frequency from several per month to as few as twice a year. Secondary generalization occurs once or twice a year in 79–90 percent of cases. Auditory auras occur in 27–64 percent of cases, depending on case series, and may consist of poorly formed sounds, such as buzzing or ringing (74 percent); well-formed sounds, such as specific songs or voices (11 percent); or sound distortions, such as volume changes or muffling (28 percent). A variety of other auras can occur, including visual (17 percent), psychic (16 percent), autonomic (12 percent), vertiginous (95), and other sensory (13 percent) [Winawer et al., 2000]. Aphasia may also occur and is reported in 17 percent of cases.

The interictal EEG is often normal, but may show temporal slowing or epileptiform transients arising from the temporal region. Ictal EEG reveals seizure activity arising from the temporal region. Prognosis is good, in so far as seizures can be rapidly controlled with antiepileptic medications; however, there is a tendency for them to recur when patients are weaned off medications.

Roughly half of cases are associated with an autosomal-dominant mutation in *LGI1*, or leucine-rich glioma inactivated 1 protein [Ottman et al., 2004; Michelucci et al., 2003; Kalachikov et al., 2002]. Over twenty distinct mutations have been described, resulting in truncations, deletions, or single amino acid substitutions. Rarely, mutations are associated with idiopathic generalized epilepsy syndromes in some family members as well [Ottman et al., 2004]. Penetrance for the mutations ranges from 54 to 71 percent. Families with ADPEAF, for which no mutation has been identified, are more likely to have autonomic features associated with their epilepsy (56 percent vs. 16 percent) in some series, possibly indicating a more mesial onset.

It is of note, that *LGI1* is one of few genes implicated in epilepsy that is not part of an ion channel, and its pathophysiologic role is under investigation. It has been shown to be downregulated in high-grade gliomas, although thus far there is no known connection between ADPEAF and increased risk for malignancy. In vitro studies show that the mutant form of LGI1 fails to be secreted [Michelucci et al., 2003], thereby inhibiting its ability to anchor to postsynaptic scaffolding proteins, where it plays a role in AMPA receptor-mediated synaptic transmission [Fukata et al., 2006]. Additional studies have found a role for the protein in presynaptic potassium channel assembly, with mutant forms of the protein resulting in changes in the inactivation kinetics of the channel [Schulte et al., 2006], and thereby potentially providing a mechanism for hyperexcitability.

Familial Partial Epilepsy with Variable Foci

Familial partial epilepsy with variable foci (FPEVF) is an autosomal-dominant focal epilepsy syndrome in which seizures may arise from different regions in various affected family members. The syndrome has been described in one Australian [Scheffer et al., 1998], one Dutch [Callenbach et al., 2003], one Spanish (Berkovic et al., 2004), and one large French–Canadian family [Xiong et al., 1999], with an age of onset ranging from the first to the third decade, median 7 years and mean 13 years. The syndrome is distinguished from the two other autosomal-dominant partial epilepsies (ADNFLE and ADPEAF) by the presence of daytime seizures, although nocturnal frontal lobe seizures often occur and may make identification of the syndrome more challenging. Seizures are most often preceded by autonomic, somatosensory, or sensory auras, may be followed by automatisms, and may be associated with hypermotoric, tonic, or tonic-clonic activity. Secondary generalization does occur. Auditory symptoms are not reported. While various family members may have different seizure symptoms, depending on the origin of their seizures, any given family member has one consistent seizure type throughout life.

With repeated EEGs, interictal abnormalities are found in roughly 50 percent of recordings and most often reveal epileptiform activity arising from the frontal or temporal regions. Ictal EEG shows focal onset to seizure activity. Imaging studies are generally normal. Prognosis is reasonable, in so far as patients maintain normal IQ and most achieve adequate control of their seizures; however, as many as half will require dual therapy with antiepileptic medications, and very few are able to be weaned off medications.

The syndrome has been linked to chromosome 22q in 3 of the 4 families [Callenbach et al., 2003; Xiong et al., 1999], with a penetrance of about 50 percent. In the remaining family, linkage was made to chromosome 2q [Sheffer et al., 1998], and some have suggested that this family may be clinically distinct due to a higher frequency of daytime seizures. A putative gene has not been identified for either linkage.

Other Mendelian Focal Epilepsies

While mesial temporal lobe epilepsy has classically been thought of as an acquired epilepsy syndrome, there is increasing appreciation for a genetic role in some variants. The genetic forms have been divided, based on whether there is associated hippocampal sclerosis or history of febrile seizures, and no putative genes have yet been identified, although linkage has been established in some cases.

In familial mesial temporal lobe epilepsy (FMTLE) without hippocampal sclerosis or febrile seizures, onset occurs in adolescence before age 18 years. Seizures are characterized by prominent psychic auras, such as déjà-vu, which often can be quite intense and frequent. Seizures with alteration in awareness, however, occur only infrequently, and secondary generalization is rare. EEG and MRI are normal and prognosis is good.

A linkage has been found to chromosome 4q in one family [Hedera et al., 2007]. No gene has been identified, and the area of interest has not been found to contain any homologs of previously identified genes involved in heritable epilepsies. The linkage study suggests autosomal-dominant inheritance with variable penetrance.

In FMTLE with hippocampal sclerosis, the mean age of onset is around 10 years and seizures are more likely to involve alteration in consciousness and postictal confusion, as is seen in nonfamilial MTLE. Preceding febrile seizures are reported in about 10 percent and MRI reveals varying degrees of hippocampal sclerosis. While most affected individuals have a benign course and may remit, refractoriness is seen in as many as one-third of affected family members. Currently, there is no genetic linkage or candidate gene [Gambardella et al., 2009].

FMTLE with febrile seizures has been described in two large families with different linkage. Onset is in the first or second decade without hippocampal sclerosis on MRI, and the course is usually benign. In the first family, digenic inheritance was suggested, with linkage to 18qter and 1q25–31 [Baulac et al., 2001]. In the second, linkage was found to 12q22–23.3 [Claes et al., 2004]. Of course, febrile seizures also occur in other inherited epilepsies, such as GEFS+, and are certainly not specific to these rare cases; rather, febrile seizures probably represent a broad marker for increased susceptibility to seizure.

It should also be noted that temporal lobe epilepsy can occur as part of other inherited syndromes, such as FPEVF, discussed above. Temporal lobe seizures are also a feature of familial occipitotemporal lobe epilepsy, described in one Belgian family. This inherited epilepsy has a variable age of onset (mean 21 years), with migraine with visual aura occurring independently of seizures in 50 percent of affected individuals. Seizures are typically partial without alteration of consciousness and frequently consist of visual phenomena. EEG and MRI are normal, and prognosis is good. The syndrome has linkage to 9q21–q22, with a dominant mode of inheritance and a penetrance of 75 percent [Deprez et al., 2007].

The final mendelian focal epilepsy described to date is partial epilepsy with pericentral spikes. This syndrome was described in one large Brazilian family of Portuguese ancestry. Onset occurs in the first or second decade of life, and seizures may be hemiclonic, hemitonic, generalized tonic-clonic, or focal, with or without alteration in consciousness. EEG shows evidence of spikes or sharp waves in the pericentral region. The prognosis is good, with seizures remitting spontaneously or with a single antiepileptic agent. Linkage has been found to chromosome 4p15 [Kinton et al., 2002].

Conclusion

Recent advances in our understanding of epilepsy syndromes have seen an end to the concept that genetic epilepsies are "idiopathic," or essentially benign. There is an increasing appreciation for the broad spectrum of genetic epilepsies, and the redefining of the term "genetic" merely to denote that the syndrome is best explained by a known or suspected genetic defect. In addition to many known ion channel mutations involved in the development of the genetic epilepsies, an increasing variety of other types of genes are now implicated, including vesicle release proteins, cyclin-dependent kinases, homeobox genes, and genes with, as of yet, unknown functions. The next steps include identifying additional genes, genotype–phenotype correlations, and functional activities of the abnormal proteins. This diversity of genetic substrates holds great promise for substantially expanding our understanding of epileptogenesis and our ability to treat those who continue to suffer seizures effectively in years to come.

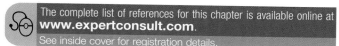

The complete list of references for this chapter is available online at **www.expertconsult.com**.
See inside cover for registration details.

Generalized Seizures

Gregory L. Holmes

As reviewed in Chapter 50, seizures are classified into two basic groups: partial and generalized [Commission on Classification and Terminology of the International League Against Epilepsy, 1981]. The International League Against Epilepsy (ILAE) Commission on Classification and Terminology has proposed a modification of the classification system of seizures and epilepsy [Berg et al., 2010]. Generalized seizures are those defined as occurring in bilaterally distributed networks whereas focal (partial) seizures involve networks limited to one hemisphere with either discretely localized or more widely distributed disturbances. While the proposed classification system has some advantages over the 1981 classification, it has not yet been widely used or endorsed by clinicians and in this chapter the older classification system will be used. Partial seizures involve only a portion of the brain at the onset but can spread, resulting in generalized tonic-clonic seizures. Primary generalized seizures are those in which the first clinical changes indicate initial synchronous involvement of both hemispheres without clinical, electroencephalographic (EEG), or other evidence of focal or partial onset. Impairment of consciousness is usual during generalized seizures, although some seizures, such as myoclonic, may be so brief that the level of consciousness cannot be assessed. The generalized seizures span a wide range of clinical presentations, ranging from the rather benign-appearing absence seizure to the dramatic and frightening generalized tonic-clonic seizure.

In most epidemiologic studies, primary generalized seizures are reported to be less common than partial seizures [Hauser and Kurland, 1975; Juul-Jensen and Foldspang, 1983]. For example, Hauser and Kurland [1975] and Juul-Jensen and Foldspang [1983] found that primary generalized seizures accounted respectively for 40.5 percent and 45.8 percent of the seizure types. Studies confined to children have been more variable. Todt [1984], in a study of children with seizures ranging in age from 3 to 16 years, found that 61.5 percent had primary generalized seizures, compared with only 26.6 percent of children between 2 months and 14 years of age in a series reported by Sofijanov [1982]. Of the primary generalized seizures, generalized tonic-clonic are the most common, followed by absence and myoclonic seizures [Hauser and Kurland, 1975].

These epidemiologic studies may be somewhat misleading. With improvement of diagnostic techniques in recent decades, especially with long-term video monitoring using EEG, it has become clear that the prevalence of primary generalized tonic-clonic epilepsy has been overestimated. In fact, most generalized tonic-clonic seizures begin as partial seizures and then generalize [Schmidt et al., 1983; Jobst et al., 2001].

This chapter discusses generalized tonic-clonic seizures and absence, clonic, tonic, and atonic seizures, along with the syndromes in which these are the predominant seizure type. Myoclonic seizures, which are generalized seizures, are reviewed in Chapter 56 and partial seizures in Chapter 54.

Generalized Tonic-Clonic Seizures

Clinical Features

Some children with generalized tonic-clonic seizures, or their parents, are aware of the impending seizure, hours or days before it occurs. The child may have a headache, insomnia, irritability, or a change in appetite. This prodrome is to be distinguished from an aura, which is a simple partial seizure that may occur before generalization of the seizure. Unlike the aura, the prodrome is not associated with any EEG epileptiform activity.

As indicated by the name, generalized tonic-clonic seizures have two distinct phases: tonic and clonic [Gastaut and Broughton, 1972]. Loss of consciousness usually occurs simultaneously with the onset of a generalized stiffening of flexor or extensor muscles – the tonic phase. The loss of consciousness usually is complete, and it is rare for patients to have any partial awareness of what happened during the seizure. During the tonic phase, prolonged extension of the back, neck, and all limbs often occurs. The eyes remain open, and a cry or yell is common. The tonic phase typically lasts 10–30 seconds and is followed by the clonic phase, which usually starts with a rapid tremor and then slows to massive jerks of the extremities and trunk. A decrescendo pattern to the frequency (although not necessarily the strength) of the jerks is seen as the seizure ceases. The clonic phase typically lasts 30–60 seconds.

Cyanosis is common and results from the arrest of ventilation during the tonic phase and insufficient short breaths during the following clonic phase. Pupillary dilatation, salivation, sweating, hyperthermia, and incontinence are common.

A postictal state always follows the clonic phase. The duration is quite variable. Some patients, even after a severe and prolonged seizure, respond within a minute or so, whereas other patients may be difficult to arouse for 20–30 minutes. Although the postictal phase initially consists of stupor, it may be followed by confusion or agitation.

In a number of syndromes, generalized seizures are a predominant feature. Epilepsy with so-called grand mal seizures on awakening is a syndrome in which the generalized tonic-clonic seizures occur only on awakening [Betting et al., 2006; Unterberger et al., 2001; Beghi et al., 2006]. In generalized epilepsy with febrile seizures plus, patients initially have febrile seizures; later, as the condition evolves, they experience afebrile generalized tonic-clonic or other types of generalized seizures [Abou-Khalil et al., 2001; Baulac et al., 2004; Scheffer and Berkovic, 1997; Wallace et al., 2001, 2002]. Generalized tonic-clonic or clonic-tonic-clonic seizures often can be a prominent component of juvenile myoclonic epilepsy, a condition discussed in Chapter 56. Children with Lennox–Gastaut syndrome may have generalized tonic-clonic seizures, although tonic seizures are the core seizure type in this syndrome.

Although their disorder currently is not classified as a syndrome, a distinct group of patients with photosensitive epilepsy have seizures provoked by flickering lights and have a photoconvulsive response to strobe light on EEG. The photoconvulsive response is characterized by spike-and-wave and multiple spike-and-wave complexes that are bilaterally synchronous, symmetric, and widespread (Figure 53-1). These should be contrasted with spikes that are time-linked with the photic stimulation and confined to the occipital region, which in children are normal. The photoconvulsive response may be self-limited and cease during stimulation or continue beyond the stimulation [Reilly and Peters, 1973]. The most effective frequency of the flash is 10–20 Hz.

The seizures evoked by photic stimulation usually are primary generalized in type: generalized tonic-clonic, absence, or myoclonic seizures. Although patients with partial seizures may have photoconvulsive responses during an EEG study, it is unusual for a partial seizure to be precipitated by photic stimulation [Jayakar and Chiappa, 1990]. Generalized epileptiform discharges during photic stimulation correlate with generalized seizures, whereas focal discharges are more commonly associated with partial seizures [Gilliam and Chiappa, 1995].

Photosensitive epilepsy can be classified into two major groups: (1) pure photosensitive epilepsy, in which clinical seizures occur only when the patient is exposed to the photic stimulus, and (2) photosensitive epilepsy, in which spontaneous seizures occur in addition to those induced by light stimulation [Binnie and Jeavons, 1992]. Precipitating stimuli that can produce a seizure include sunlight reflected from water, sunlight viewed through leaves of trees in a breeze or while driving along tree-lined streets, discotheque lighting, faulty fluorescent lamp ("nervous ballast"), television, and video games. Photosensitive epilepsy usually appears around puberty, with a mean age at onset of 14 years and a higher incidence in girls than in boys [Jeavons, 1982].

Differential Diagnosis

Difficulty is rarely encountered in correctly diagnosing generalized tonic-clonic seizures (formerly termed grand mal seizures). Generalized tonic-clonic seizures can be divided into those that are primarily generalized from onset and those that

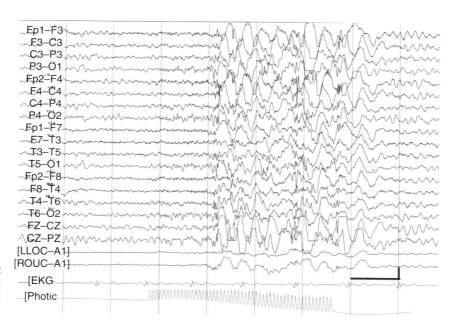

Fig. 53-1 Photoconvulsive response in a patient with primary generalized epilepsy. Note the burst of irregular spike-and-wave activity during the photic stimulation. (Calibration: 50 μV, 1 second)

Table 53-1 Comparison of Primary and Secondary Generalized Tonic-Clonic Seizures

	Primary GTC	Secondary GTC
Prodrome	Occasionally	Occasionally
Aura	Never	Frequently
Usual duration	1–3 min	1–3 min
Family history for seizures	Frequently	Occasionally
Acquired lesions	Rarely	Frequently
EEG		
Interictal	Normal or generalized spike-wave	Normal or focal or multifocal spikes
Photoconvulsive response	Frequently	Rarely
Hyperventilation	May activate spike-wave discharges	Usually does not activate epileptiform discharges

begin as partial seizures and then secondarily generalize [Schmidt et al., 1983; Jobst et al., 2001]. Differentiating features are listed in Table 53-1. On very rare occasions, generalized tonic-clonic seizures begin as another generalized seizure type such as absence [Niedermeyer, 1976] before evolving into tonic-clonic activity.

Breath-holding attacks, pseudoseizures (nonepileptic events), and syncope occasionally may resemble generalized tonic-clonic seizures. These are discussed in Chapters 64 and 65.

Electroencephalographic Findings

In patients with partial seizures with secondary generalization, the interictal EEG features are similar to those described for partial seizures. Patients with primary generalized tonic-clonic seizures typically have either normal interictal EEG activity or bursts of generalized spike-and-wave discharges. As with absence seizures, spike-and-wave or polyspike-and-wave activity can occur with photic stimulation and hyperventilation. Normal EEG activity, however, can be observed in patients with generalized tonic-clonic seizures.

The ictal EEG features begin suddenly and are widespread. The tonic phase usually begins as loss of background frequencies, with sudden generalized suppression of the background activity (flattening or attenuation of the EEG signal), followed by a gradual build-up of low-voltage fast spikes, usually starting at 20–40 Hz and then decreasing to 10 Hz, lasting up to 10 seconds, with a progressive increase in amplitude and decrease in frequency – the so-called "epileptic recruiting rhythm." This is followed by the clonic phase, with slow waves following the spikes. The spike-and-wave complexes gradually slow in frequency before stopping.

During the postictal phase, the EEG shows either suppression of background activity or diffuse slowing. The duration of the postictal changes is variable, with background abnormalities lasting minutes to even days following the seizure. Focal slowing during the postictal phase suggests that the seizure had a partial onset. The absence of any slowing during the postictal phase should raise the question of nonepileptic seizures.

Etiology

The etiology of seizures in children who have secondary generalized tonic-clonic seizures is the same as those described for partial seizures. Patients with primary generalized tonic-clonic seizures usually do not have structural lesions and often have a familial disorder, such as juvenile myoclonic epilepsy. The genetics of generalized tonic-clonic seizures are discussed in Chapter 52.

Initial Evaluation

The initial steps in the evaluation depend to a major degree on the patient's clinical status on first presentation to the physician. For example, the patient who arrives at the emergency department following a generalized seizure with fever and confusion is evaluated differently from the otherwise normal child who presents several hours after a generalized seizure. The former needs an urgent evaluation to look for an infectious etiology, such as meningitis or encephalitis, whereas the latter can be managed less hastily. This chapter deals with the evaluation and treatment indicated for patients with generalized seizures as their only presenting clinical sign.

In all children with their first seizure, a careful history should be obtained, with particular attention to whether the seizure was preceded by an aura or if the seizure had any focal features. An aura, focal onset to the seizures, or Todd's paralysis would suggest that the seizure had a partial onset. A review of potential precipitating factors, such as sleep deprivation or photic stimulation, may be useful in counseling the patient and the parents. A past medical history of birth asphyxia or trauma, head injury, prolonged febrile seizures, meningitis, or encephalitis may offer etiologic clues indicating that the seizures have a partial onset. A history of other neurologic symptoms should be sought. Headaches, especially those associated with vomiting or occurring at night, should raise the possibility of a structural lesion.

Although neuroimaging appears to have reduced the importance of the neurologic examination, abnormal findings, even if subtle, may provide clues to the location of seizure onset and etiology of the seizures. For example, asymmetries in facial expression or strength may indicate focal deficits, even in the presence of normal neuroimaging findings.

Diagnostic studies ordered depend on findings during the history and neurologic examination. Children with an unremarkable history other than for the seizures and with normal findings on neurologic examination typically require only an EEG and neuroimaging. An EEG should always be obtained because it may help differentiate partial from generalized seizures. Focal epileptiform activity or slowing would raise the possibility of a structural lesion.

Neuroimaging is recommended in all patients presenting with their first unexplained generalized tonic-clonic seizure, with the recognition that, in patients with normal neurologic examinations, the chance of finding a treatable lesion is quite low. Because generalized tonic-clonic may have a partial onset with subsequent rapid generalization, however, the seizure may be incorrectly diagnosed as primary generalized in type. In nonemergency settings, the imaging test of choice is a magnetic resonance imaging (MRI) scan. Computed tomography (CT) scans can be used in acute situations to determine whether a mass lesion and hemorrhage is present.

The need for further diagnostic testing, such as metabolic screening and cerebrospinal fluid examination, depends on the clinical presentation. In the absence of mental retardation, developmental regression, or abnormalities on neurologic examination, these studies usually are not indicated following the initial seizure.

Comorbidities Associated with Generalized Seizures

While a major goal in the treatment of epilepsy is stopping the seizures, it is not the only treatment goal. Patients with epilepsy are a risk for a number of comorbidities. Comorbidity refers to the co-occurrence of two supposedly separate conditions that occur together more than by chance (also see Chapter 62). Depression occurs more frequently in patients with epilepsy than in the normal population, so that epilepsy and depression are comorbidities. Comorbidities are not necessarily causal. For example, because epilepsy and depression are comorbidities does not mean that epilepsy caused the depression or depression caused the epilepsy. Rather, it is possible that both conditions have a common biological substrate or that another independent variable triggers one of the comorbidities. For example, epilepsy often leads to drug therapy, which could cause depression independently of the epilepsy.

Comorbidities associated with epilepsy include depression [Camfield and Camfield, 2009; Dunn et al., 1999], suicidality [Bridge et al., 2007; Tellez-Zenteno et al., 2007; Donner et al., 2001; McGregor and Wheless, 2006], attention-deficit hyperactivity disorder (ADHD) [Dunn and Kronenberger, 2005], conduct disorders [Dunn et al., 2009], anxiety [Caplan et al., 2005], cognitive impairment and learning disabilities [Fastenau et al., 2004; Aldenkamp et al., 2005], and migraine [Pellock, 2004].

Being aware of the comorbidities frequently associated with childhood epilepsy may influence the choice of antiepileptic drug (AED) used to treat the seizures. For example, lamotrigine and valproate may be helpful in treating both the primary generalized seizures and mood disturbance. Likewise, topiramate and valproate can treat both seizures and migraine. On the other hand, AEDs may exacerbate the comorbid condition. Topiramate can have adverse cognitive effects, while benzodiazepines and barbiturates can exacerbate ADHD and conduct disorders.

Medical Treatment

The medical treatment of generalized seizures that have a partial onset and secondarily generalize is, in general, the same as for the treatment of partial seizures. It is generally assumed that an AED that reduces the likelihood of partial seizures would also prevent partial seizures that secondarily generalize. However, it is possible that there may be a difference in the ability of an AED to prevent secondary generalization following the partial onset.

One of the issues is that, in many studies, partial seizures with secondary generalization are included along with primary generalized tonic-clonic seizures. In the United States, AEDs that have an indication for monotherapy or adjunctive therapy of generalized seizures include phenytoin and carbamazepine. However, while both drugs are effective in partial seizures, they can exacerbate primary generalized seizures [Perucca et al., 1998; Guerrini et al., 1998]. Studies examining efficacy and safety of AEDs in children with primary generalized epilepsy are very limited. Although a number of the newer AEDs are being used for the treatment of primary generalized tonic-clonic seizures, even in adults definitive evidence for their effectiveness is lacking [Faught, 2003; French et al., 2004]. In addition, data for adults and children often are combined when studies are reported. Antiepileptic drug studies done solely in children with primary generalized tonic-clonic seizures are limited. Although most of the newer antiepileptic drugs have been used in the treatment of generalized tonic-clonic seizures, their usefulness in children has not yet been established [Holmes, 2003; Jarrar and Buchhalter, 2003].

The major drugs typically used to treat primary generalized tonic-clonic seizures include valproate [Murphy and Delanty, 2000; Ramsay and DeToledo, 1997; Marson et al., 2007], lamotrigine [Mikati and Holmes, 1997; Trevathan et al., 2006; Marson et al., 2007], levetiracetam [Rosenfeld et al., 2009; Noachtar et al., 2008; Wheless, 2007], and topiramate [Biton et al., 1999; Marson et al., 2007]. Although phenobarbital is effective in the treatment of primary generalized tonic-clonic seizures, the adverse side effects profile has reduced its use as initial therapy for primary generalized tonic-clonic seizures [Taylor et al., 2001].

The four drugs most commonly used for primary generalized tonic-clonic seizures are reviewed briefly here. Additional information about AEDs is available in Chapter 59.

Valproate

Valproate (valproic acid and divalproex sodium) is widely used in children to treat primary generalized seizures, including generalized tonic-clonic seizures. In children with both absence and primary generalized tonic-clonic seizures, valproate is an excellent choice because it is efficacious in both conditions.

Valproate is approximately 90 percent protein-bound. Protein binding varies with drug plasma concentration, and the free fraction increases with increasing plasma concentration [Davis et al., 1994]. Therefore, with high blood levels of valproate, the free, or active, portion of valproate becomes greater, and toxicity may occur. In addition, drugs or endogenous substances, such as free fatty acids, can alter protein binding. The primary metabolism is by hepatic hydroxylation (mitochondrial beta oxidation) and conjugation with glucuronide. Eighty percent of an administered dose of valproic acid is metabolized through these two pathways and then excreted by the kidney [Levy et al., 2002]. The remainder of a dose is excreted in other oxidized metabolites. Drug interactions are common with valproate [Scheyer, 2002].

In children, the recommended starting dose is 10–15 mg/kg/day, with gradual increases by 5–10 mg/kg/day every week until therapeutic success is achieved or toxicity occurs. Although most patients do well with blood levels of 60–100 µg/mL, some patients tolerate blood levels up to 150 µg/mL.

Gastrointestinal toxicity includes anorexia, nausea, and indigestion. These symptoms may be reduced with the divalproex sodium preparations. Dose-related toxicities are action tremor (seen in 40 percent of adults, less frequently in children), elevated plasma transaminase (usually transient but a possible harbinger of serious hepatic disease), and hyperammonemia. Idiosyncratic toxicity includes hepatic necrosis (treatable with L-carnitine), thrombocytopenia, pancreatitis (in 0.5 percent, sometimes fatal), teratogenicity, and stupor and coma. The risk of hepatic fatality is greatest in children younger than 2 years and in patients taking valproic acid in combination with other AEDs [Dreifuss et al., 1987, 1989]. Toxic effects with long-term use are weight gain, hair loss, and platelet dysfunction. Routine monitoring of liver function tests, complete blood count, and valproate blood level determination is recommended.

Lamotrigine

Lamotrigine is a broad-spectrum AED that has a number of attractive features for childhood use. However, there is a risk of rash and the drug must be used with care. Lamotrigine has broad-spectrum efficacy, demonstrating efficacy in partial seizures, absences, tonic, atonic, and generalized tonic-clonic seizures [Besag et al., 1995; Eriksson et al., 1998; Duchowny et al., 2002]. It is indicated as adjunctive therapy for adults and in children with primary generalized seizures and generalized seizures in the Lennox–Gastaut syndrome in children over the age of 2 years. There are indications that the drug is useful in absence seizures.

Lamotrigine is rapidly and completely absorbed after oral administration. It undergoes hepatic metabolism and is excreted primarily as the 2-N-glucuronide metabolite. The elimination half-life of lamotrigine is highly dependent upon whether it is taken with other drugs. In children also taking carbamazepine, phenytoin, or phenobarbital, the elimination half-life is 7–15 hours. Co-administration with valproate (divalproex sodium, valproic acid) increases the elimination half-life of lamotrigine to 40–60 hours or more. The half-life of lamotrigine in children on no other medications is approximately 20 hours. Lamotrigine does not affect the plasma concentration of carbamazepine, phenobarbital, phenytoin, primidone, or valproate.

Lamotrigine is generally well tolerated in children [Duchowny et al., 2002]. The drug is not associated with behavioral or cognitive side effects. With high doses, particularly when used as adjunctive therapy, dizziness, diplopia, headache, ataxia, tremor, and nausea may occur.

Data from clinical trials with lamotrigine indicate that the risk of serious rash in pediatric patients is higher than in adults. The incidence of rash associated with hospitalization among adults treated with lamotrigine is 0.3 percent and the incidence among children is 1.0 percent [Messenheimer, 1998; Hirsch et al., 2006]. The incidence of cases reported as possible Stevens–Johnson syndrome is 0.1 percent for adult patients and 0.5 percent for pediatric patients. The risk of rash is higher in children who are taking valproate, presumably because it decreases the metabolism of lamotrigine. Most rashes occur during the first 6 weeks of therapy. The risk of rash is reduced by slow upward titration of dose.

In children between the ages of 2–12 years who are on enzyme-inducing drugs, such as phenytoin, phenobarbital, or carbamazepine, lamotrigine should be started at 0.6 mg/kg/day in two divided doses for the first 2 weeks, then 1.2 mg/kg/day for weeks 2–3. The dosage can then be increased by 1.2 mg/kg/day every 1–2 weeks. The typical maintenance dosage is 5–15 mg/kg/day. In children on valproate, the dosage should be 0.15 mg/kg/day for the first 2 weeks and then 0.3 mg/kg/day for the second 2 weeks. The dosage can be increased by 0.3 mg/kg/day every 2 weeks. The typical maintenance dose is 1–5 mg/kg/day.

A therapeutic range for lamotrigine plasma concentration has not been established. Preliminary data indicate that few patients have a good response with plasma concentrations below 5 μg per mL; patients with good responses usually have plasma concentrations of 5–15 μg per mL; patients with concentrations above 20 μg per mL often have side effects.

Levetiracetam

Levetiracetam is a broad-spectrum drug that is widely used in both children and adults for partial and generalized seizures [Carreno, 2007; Wheless, 2007]. It is rapidly and almost completely absorbed after oral administration. The absorption and elimination of levetiracetam are linear. Levetiracetam is not extensively metabolized in humans; the majority of the drug is excreted unchanged in the urine. The major metabolic pathway of levetiracetam is enzymatic hydrolysis of the acetamide group. Levetiracetam produces no inhibition of cytochrome P450 isoforms, epoxide hydrolase, or UDP-glucuronide enzymes. There are no reports of drug interactions between levetiracetam and AEDs or other drugs. The metabolites have no known pharmacological activity and are excreted in the urine. The elimination half-life is 4–8 hours in children. The pharmacodynamic effects of levetiracetam are longer than would be predicted by half-life and the drug can be given twice daily.

There are no reports of serious toxicity with levetiracetam. The drug is well tolerated in children [Wheless and Ng, 2002]. In children, headache, anorexia, somnolence, and mild

infection (otitis media, pharyngitis, and gastroenteritis) have been reported [Glauser et al., 2002]. These usually occur early in treatment and can be reduced by slow drug initiation and/or dose reduction. Levetiracetam has caused irritability and aggressiveness [Khurana et al., 2007]. Reversible treatment-emergent psychosis has been associated with levetiracetam therapy [Kossoff et al., 2001]. No hematological or hepatic disturbances have been reported and routine laboratory studies are not recommended.

The recommended starting dose is 10 mg/kg/day given twice daily. The dosage can be increased weekly or every 2 weeks by 10 mg/kg/day. The typical maintenace dosage is 30–40 mg/kg/day, although dosages above 60 mg/kg are usually well tolerated. Therapeutic blood levels of levetiracetam have not been established.

Topiramate

Topiramate has a broad spectrum of efficacy in children [Ormrod and McClellan, 2001], and has been found to be beneficial in the treatment of medically refractory primary generalized tonic-clonic seizures [Biton et al., 1999; French et al., 2004; Wheless, 2000].

Topiramate is rapidly absorbed and has very low protein binding [Bourgeois, 2000]. In the absence of enzyme-inducing drugs, 80 percent of a dose is excreted unchanged in the urine, with an elimination half-life of 20–30 hours. In the presence of enzyme-inducing drugs, 50–80 percent of a dose is excreted unchanged in the urine, with an elimination half-life of 12–15 hours in teenagers. The metabolic products of topiramate are formed in the liver and do not appear to be biologically active. Prepubescent children have a higher clearance and shorter elimination half-life than in adults [Bourgeois, 2000].

The recommended total dose of topiramate for pediatric patients (ages 2–16 years) is 5–9 mg/kg/day in two divided doses. Titration should begin at 25 mg (or less, based on a range of 1–3 mg/kg/day) nightly for the first week. The dose should then be increased at 1- or 2-week intervals by increments of 1–3 mg/kg/day (administered in two divided doses) to achieve optimal clinical response.

The most common side effects with topiramate are central nervous system-related: drowsiness, dizziness, decreased attention or impaired concentration, paresthesia, nervousness, confusion, and impaired memory. These side effects usually are mild to moderate, develop during the first weeks of therapy, and may decline over time. The central nervous system side effects appear to be fewer when topiramate is used for monotherapy than when it is used in polytherapy, and are less common in children than in adults. Weight loss [Ormrod and McClellan, 2001] and acidosis [Izzedine et al., 2004; Takeoka et al., 2001] can occur with topiramate therapy. Renal stones [Kuo et al., 2002; Lamb et al., 2004] and acute myopia [Coats, 2003] associated with secondary angle-closure glaucoma [Browne et al., 1974] have been reported. These side effects appear to be very rare in children.

Table 53-2 summarizes the AEDs used in the treatment of generalized tonic-clonic seizures and other generalized seizures in childhood. This listing is based on both efficacy and tolerability, and reflects the author's personal preferences. AED therapy should always be tailored to the needs of the particular patient.

Table 53-2 Antiepileptic Drugs of Choice in the Treatment of Seizures in Children

	GTC	Absence	Generalized Seizures Myoclonic	Tonic	Atonic
First choice	Valproate	Ethosuximide Lamotrigine Valproate	Valproate	Lamotrigine Valproate	Lamotrigine Valproate
Second choice	Lamotrigine Levetiracetam Topiramate	Levetiracetam Topiramate Zonisamide	Clonazepam Levetiracetam Rufinamide Zonisamide	Phenytoin Rufinamide Topiramate Felbamate (with caution)	Lamotrigine Rufinamide Topiramate Felbamate (with caution)

In addition to treating with AEDs, it is important to counsel the patient and parents about factors that could exacerbate seizures, such as sleep deprivation. Drugs that can lower seizure threshold, such as bupropion, should be avoided [Foley et al., 2006].

Absence Seizures

Clinical Features

Absence seizures, formerly termed petit mal seizures, are characterized by an abrupt cessation of activity, change in facial expression, and impairment of consciousness [Browne et al., 1974; Pearl and Holmes, 2008; Porter et al., 1973]. Absence seizures are not common, accounting for less than 10 percent of all seizure types [Hauser and Hersdorffer, 1990; Hauser and Kurland, 1975; Sofijanov, 1982]. Absence seizures may be the most common seizure type to go undetected. The prevalence of absence seizures is highest during the first 10 years of life and then drops dramatically to a very low level [Hauser and Kurland, 1975; Hertoft, 1963; Sato et al., 1976]. Absence seizures are more common in girls than in boys [Hertoft, 1963; Sato et al., 1976]. Typical absence seizures rarely start before the age of 2 years or after the teenage years [Sato et al., 1983; Sato, 1983]. In a study of 83 patients with absence seizures, Sato and co-workers [Sato et al., 1983] found the average age at onset was 3.8 years.

Absence seizures are classified as typical or atypical in type (Table 53-3). Typical absence seizures are short, rarely lasting over 30 seconds; as with other generalized seizures, they are never associated with an aura or postictal impairment. The sudden onset of impaired consciousness, usually associated with a blank facial appearance without other motor or behavioral phenomena, is characteristic. The degree of impairment

of consciousness is variable. Some children remember virtually everything that is said during the seizure, whereas for others, the entire duration of the seizure is "time lost."

Although the absence seizure is commonly thought to consist only of staring, in fact the behavioral changes associated with the seizure type usually are more complex. Most absence seizures are accompanied by motor, behavioral, or autonomic phenomena, and seizures characterized by only staring and altered consciousness are unusual. Penry et al. [1975] reviewed 374 absence seizures recorded on videotape from 48 patients and found simple absences, characterized by staring and cessation of activities, to constitute only 9.4 percent of the seizures. A majority of the patients had other clinical manifestations.

Automatisms, semipurposeful behaviors of which the patient is unaware and subsequently cannot recall, are very common with absence seizures [Holmes et al., 1987; Penry et al., 1975]. They either may be perseverative, reflecting continuation of preictal activities, or may arise de novo. Simple behaviors, such as rubbing the face or hands, licking the lips, chewing, grimacing, scratching, or fumbling with clothes, tend to be de novo automatisms. Complex activities, such as dealing cards, moving a chess piece, or handling a toy, are generally perseverative. Speech, if it occurs during the seizure, usually is perseverative and may be slow and slurred, but also may be totally normal [McKeever et al., 1983]. The longer the absence seizure lasts, the more likely automatisms are to occur [Penry et al., 1975].

Clonic or myoclonic components are common but may be quite subtle, most frequently consisting of blinking. Clonic activity also may be manifested by nystagmus, rapid jerking or trembling of the arms, or head nods. Alterations in muscle tone may lead to stiffening of the trunk or a fall. A study of 426 typical and 500 atypical absence seizures studied in

Table 53-3 Classification of Absence Seizures

Clinical Seizure Type	EEG – Interictal	EEG – Ictal
Typical absence a. Impairment of consciousness only b. With mild clonic components c. With tonic components d. With automatisms e. With autonomic components	Normal background; short bursts of regular and symmetrical 2.5–4-Hz spike wave; rare frontal or multifocal spikes, sharp waves; photoconvulsive response	Regular and symmetrical 2.5–4-Hz spike wave; often induced by hyperventilation or photic stimulation
Atypical absence	Abnormal background; short bursts of irregular, asymmetrical <2.5-Hz spike wave; multifocal spikes, sharp waves; photoconvulsive response rare	Bursts of irregular, asymmetrical <2.5-Hz spike wave; rarely induced by hyperventilation or photic stimulation

54 children using simultaneous EEG and video monitoring found myoclonic jerks in 13 percent of typical absences and 12 percent of atypical absences [Holmes et al., 1987]. Children with the syndrome of epilepsy with myoclonic absences have prominent myoclonus during the seizure.

Autonomic phenomena occasionally may be seen with absence seizures and include dilatation of the pupils, pallor, flushing, sweating, salivation, piloerection, and even urinary incontinence.

The frequency of absence seizures varies considerably from day to day and even from hour to hour. The number of absence seizures varies significantly with different environmental situations [Borkowski, et al., 1992; Pearl and Holmes, 2008]. Seizures are more likely to occur during periods of inactivity than when the child is busily engaged in a task. Fatigue also may dramatically increase seizure susceptibility.

A majority of children with typical absence seizures have normal findings on neurologic examination [Dalby, 1969; Sato, 1983]. When neurologic abnormalities are found, they usually are mild and nonprogressive. Most children with typical absence seizures have normal or mildly low intelligence [Dalby, 1969; Sato, 1983]. Compared with age-matched controls, children with absence seizures have lower general cognitive function with impaired visual-spatial skills and memory disturbances [Pavone et al., 2001]. Children with absence seizures have higher rates of behavioral problems and psychopathology than in the normal population [Ott et al., 2001].

Typical absence seizures may be associated with generalized tonic-clonic seizures in 40–60 percent of patients [Hertoft, 1963; Loiseau et al., 1983; Sato, 1983]. In most children, the generalized tonic-clonic seizures occur after onset of the absence seizures [Loiseau et al., 1983].

Although atypical absence seizures form a separate category of absences, overlap between the two seizure types is considerable, and they appear to represent a clinical continuum [Holmes et al., 1987]. Diminished postural tone, or tonic or myoclonic activity, is significantly more likely to be the initial clinical feature in atypical than in typical absences. Automatisms are less likely in atypical absences than in typical absences. Like typical absences, atypical absences have a distinct onset and ending, without auras or postictal symptoms. Although atypical absences usually are of longer duration than typical absences, a considerable amount of variability exists.

Atypical absences usually begin before the age of 5 years and often are associated with other seizure types and mental retardation. In children who have profound mental retardation, it may be difficult to detect subtle behavioral changes associated with the absence seizures. Many children with atypical absence seizures have Lennox–Gastaut syndrome.

Four syndromes are associated with typical absence seizures: childhood absence epilepsy (pyknolepsy), juvenile absence epilepsy, epilepsy with myoclonic absences, and juvenile myoclonic epilepsy.

Childhood Absence Epilepsy (Pyknolepsy)

Childhood absence epilepsy (pyknolepsy) describes typical absence seizures (i.e., both simple and complex) in children between the age of 3 years and puberty, who are otherwise normal. A strong genetic predisposition has been noted, and girls are more frequently affected. The absences are very frequent, occurring at least several times daily, and tend to occur in clusters. The EEG reveals a bilateral, synchronous, and symmetric 2.5- to 3-Hz spike-and-wave discharge with normal interictal background activity. The absences may remit during adolescence, but generalized tonic-clonic seizures occasionally may develop.

Juvenile Absence Epilepsy

Juvenile absence epilepsy begins around puberty and differs from pyknolepsy primarily in that the seizures are more sporadic. This syndrome may be confused with juvenile myoclonic epilepsy, because generalized tonic-clonic seizures and myoclonic seizures often are seen on awakening. Generalized tonic-clonic seizures are more common in children with this syndrome than in those with childhood absence epilepsy. Gender distribution is equal, and on EEG the spike-and-wave frequency often is slightly greater than 3 Hz.

Epilepsy with Myoclonic Absences

Epilepsy with myoclonic absences consists of typical absence seizures with a sudden onset and offset, in which the child has axial hypertonia with the trunk bent slightly forward and the arms and shoulders raised. In conjuction with the 3-Hz generalized spike and wave on the EEG, there are rhythmic jerks of the arms and shoulders [Genton and Bureau, 2006; Tassinari et al., 1992]. The condition should be differentiated from eyelid myoclonia with absences or Jeavons' syndrome, which is a generalized epileptic condition characterized by eyelid myoclonia with or without absences [Striano et al., 2009]. Epilepsy with myoclonic absences is often more difficult to treat than typical absence seizures.

Juvenile Myoclonic Epilepsy

Juvenile myoclonic epilepsy is a familial disorder that typically begins in the second decade of life and is characterized by mild myoclonic seizures, generalized tonic-clonic or clonic-tonic-clonic seizures (a variation of generalized tonic-clonic seizures in which an initial clonic phase precedes the usual pattern), and occasionally absence seizures. This syndrome is discussed in Chapter 56.

Differential Diagnosis

The primary diagnostic considerations in the child referred because of "staring attacks" include absence seizures, complex partial seizures, and daydreaming (Table 53-4). Complex partial seizures are more common than absence seizures and also are manifested by an alteration in consciousness with staring, automatisms, changes in tone, and autonomic symptoms. Complex partial seizures tend to be longer and less frequent, but clinically no absolute distinguishing factor may be present. The presence of an aura or postictal impairment is strongly suggestive of a complex partial seizure. In the child not on antiepileptic medications, 3 minutes of hyperventilation usually precipitates an absence seizure. It is unusual for complex partial seizures to be precipitated by hyperventilation. Abnormalities documented on the EEG constitute the best confirmation of either seizure type.

Daydreaming is associated with boredom, can be "broken" with stimulation, and is not associated with motor activity. Absence seizures, however, also can be terminated with

Table 53-4 Differential Diagnosis of Absence Seizures

Clinical and Laboratory Characteristics	Absence	Complex Partial	Daydreaming
Frequency/day	Multiple	Rarely >1–2	Situation-dependent
Duration	Frequently <10 sec; rarely >30 sec	Average duration >1 min; rarely <10 sec	Seconds to minutes
Aura	Never	Frequent	Never
Clonic component	Common; eyeblinking common	Rare	Never
Postictal impairment	Never	Frequent	Never
Seizures activated by			
Hyperventilation	Frequent	Rare	Never
Photic stimulation	Frequent	Rare	Never
EEG			
Interictal	Generalized spike wave	Focal spikes, sharp waves	Normal
Ictal	Generalized spike wave	Rhythmic spikes, sharp waves, or slow waves	Normal

stimulation and tend to increase during periods of relaxation and tiredness. Tics and pseudoseizures may need to be considered, as well. Normal findings on an EEG study that includes several trials of 3–5 minutes of hyperventilation, however, virtually rule out absence seizures. Repeated studies or prolonged monitoring occasionally may be necessary when diagnostic confusion persists.

Etiology

Both acquired and inherited factors are implicated in the etiology of absence seizures, reflecting the heterogeneity of the patient population. Genetic factors predominate in children with typical absence seizures, whereas acquired disorders are more common in children with atypical absences. The genetics of absence seizures are discussed in Chapter 52.

Initial Evaluation

The extent of the diagnostic evaluation required in patients with absence seizures is variable and depends somewhat on findings from the history and physical examination. All patients need a neurologic examination, with hyperventilation, and an EEG. Patients who have normal development, normal findings on neurologic examination, a history suggestive of typical absence seizures, and 2.5- to 4-Hz spike-wave discharges on an otherwise normal-appearing EEG require no further studies. Children with developmental delay, an abnormal neurologic examination, a history suggestive of atypical absences, or an EEG showing slow spike-and-wave (less than 2.5 Hz) discharges, background slowing, or focal epileptiform discharges should have neuroimaging, preferably MRI, and possibly more specific tests, such as metabolic studies and a lumbar puncture.

Electroencephalographic Findings

The EEG signature of a typical absence seizure is the sudden onset of 3-Hz generalized symmetric spike-and-wave or multiple spike-wave complexes (Figure 53-2). The voltage of the discharges often is maximal in the frontal-central regions. The frequency tends to be faster, about 4 Hz, at the onset and may slow to 2 Hz toward the end of a discharge lasting longer than 10 seconds.

Hyperventilation is a potent activator of typical absence seizures [Adams and Lueders, 1981; Dalby, 1969]. Failure to induce an absence seizure with several trials of hyperventilation of 3–5 minutes' duration in a child not receiving antiepileptic medication would make the diagnosis of typical absence seizures unlikely. Photic stimulation also may precipitate seizures, although the frequency of activation does not appear as high as with hyperventilation [Newmark and Penry, 1979].

When closely observed, children typically demonstrate behavioral changes with spike-and-wave discharges lasting longer than a few seconds. In studies of auditory reaction times, it has been found that responses are abnormal in 80 percent of the situations in which a stimulus is presented after onset of the spike-and-wave activity [Porter et al., 1973]. In a test of visual motor coordination in children with spike-and-wave activity on the EEG, discharges lasting longer than 3 seconds were associated with impaired function [Opp et al., 1992; Brown et al., 1974; Porter et al., 1973].

The interictal EEG in children with typical absence seizures typically shows a normal background. Brief bursts of generalized spike-and-wave activity, frontal spikes, or, less commonly, multifocal spikes can be seen. In absences, focal or multifocal spikes do not necessarily indicate a focal epileptiform process; rather, they may represent portions of generalized discharge that do not totally propagate uniformly to the cortex.

In atypical absences, the ictal EEG is more heterogeneous, showing 1.5- to 2.5-Hz slow spike-and-wave or multiple spike-and-wave discharges that may be irregular or asymmetric (Figure 53-3). Interictal EEG findings usually are abnormal, with background slowing and multifocal epileptiform features. The EEG features of typical and atypical absences are summarized in Table 53-3.

Pathophysiology

The observation that 3-Hz spike-and-wave discharges in absence seizures appear simultaneously and synchronously in all electrode locations led early investigators to speculate that the pathophysiologic mechanisms of absence seizures must involve "deep" structures with widespread connections between the two hemispheres.

A number of studies have demonstrated that the basic underlying mechanism in generalized absence epilepsies

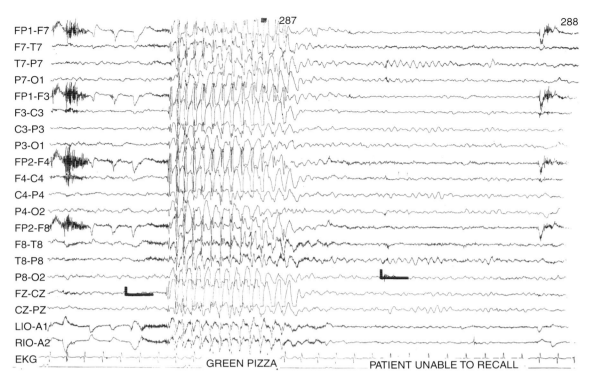

Fig. 53-2 EEG from a patient with typical absences. The technician said the phrase "green pizza" during the spike-and-wave discharge. After the absence seizure the patient did not recall the phrase (Calibration: 50 µV, 1 second).

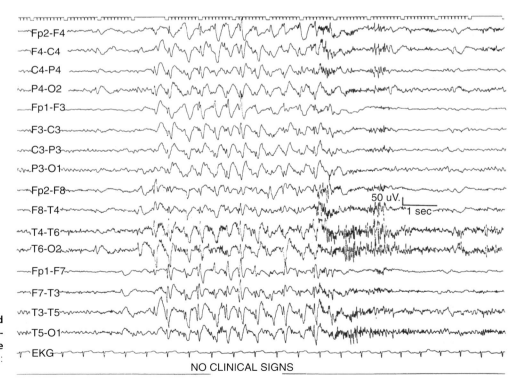

Fig. 53-3 Slow, irregular generalized spike-and-wave discharges in a patient with Lennox–Gastaut syndrome and atypical absences. (Calibration: 50 µV, 1 second).

involves thalamocortical circuitry and the generation of abnormal oscillatory rhythms in this neuronal network [Coulter and Zhang, 1994; Crunelli and Leresche, 2002; Hosford et al., 1995; Huguenard and Prince, 1994b; Steriade et al., 1993; Steriade and Conteras, 1998]. The neuronal circuits

that generate the oscillatory thalamocortical burst firing observed during absence seizures have now been identified. This circuit includes cortical pyramidal neurons, thalamic relay neurons, and the nucleus reticularis thalami (Figure 53-4) [Steriade and Llinas, 1988; Steriade et al., 1993]. The principal

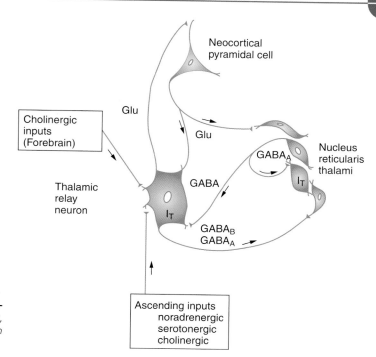

Fig. 53-4 **Principle neuronal populations and connections of thalamocortical circuits generating absence seizures.** T, T-current; Glu, Glutamatergic transmission. *(From Holmes GL. Basic mechanisms in epilepsy. Int Pediatr 1996;11:343.)*

synaptic connections of the thalamocortical circuit include glutamatergic fibers between neocortical pyramidal cells and the nucleus reticularis thalami, gamma-aminobutyric acid (GABA)-ergic fibers from nucleus reticularis thalami neurons that activate GABA$_A$ and GABA$_B$ receptors on thalamic relay neurons, and recurrent collateral GABAergic fibers from nucleus reticularis thalami neurons that activate GABA$_A$ receptors on adjacent nucleus reticularis thalami neurons. The nucleus reticularis thalami, therefore, is in a position to influence the flow of information between the thalamus and cerebral cortex [Snead, 1995]. The nucleus reticularis thalami cells undergo rhythmic burst firing during periods of sleep and continuous single-spike firing during wakefulness.

The cellular events that underlie the ability of nucleus reticularis thalami neurons to shift between an oscillatory and a firing mode include activation of the low-threshold, transient Ca^{2+} channels (T-channels) [Coulter et al., 1989, 1990; Crunelli and Leresche, 2002; Snead, 1995]. These channels appear to be important in the generation of absence seizures [Snead, 1995; Tsakiridou et al., 1995]. Mild depolarization of these neurons is sufficient to activate these T-channels and to allow the influx of extracellular Ca^{2+}. Further depolarization produced by Ca^{2+} inflow often exceeds the threshold for firing a burst of action potentials. After T-channels are activated, they become inactivated rather quickly – hence the name transient. T-channels require a lengthy, intense hyperpolarization to reverse their inactivation (a process termed deinactivation). The requisite hyperpolarization can be provided by GABA$_B$ receptors that are present on thalamic relay neurons. The interplay between GABA$_B$-mediated inhibition and the low-threshold T-type calcium channel therefore plays a critical role in generating the oscillating hyperpolarization/depolarization activity seen in the thalamus. In animal models of absences, GABA$_B$ agonists produce an increase in seizure frequency (by facilitating

deinactivation of T-channels), whereas GABA$_B$ antagonists reduce seizure frequency.

Recurrent collateral GABAergic fibers from the nucleus reticularis thalami neurons activate GABA$_A$ receptors on adjacent nucleus reticularis thalami neurons. Activating GABA$_A$ receptors in the nucleus reticularis thalami, therefore, results in reduction of GABAergic output to the thalamic relay neurons and serves to reduce hyperpolarization and delay deinactivation of the T-channels. In animal studies, injection of the GABA$_A$ agonists bilaterally into the nucleus reticularis thalami reduces absence seizure frequency. GABA$_A$ activation of thalamic relay neurons, however, would be expected to have the opposite effect, increasing hyperpolarization and deinactivation of the T-channel.

Abnormal oscillatory rhythms could be caused by abnormalities of the T-channel or enhanced GABA$_B$ function [Crunelli and Leresche, 2002; Snead, 1995]. In some animal models of absence seizures, T-channel activation in the nucleus reticularis thalami is significantly different than in control animals [Tsakiridou et al., 1995]. These aberrant T-channels may be one basis for absence seizures. In other animal models, an increase in GABA$_B$ receptors in thalamic and neocortical neuronal populations, compared with that in controls, has been described [Hosford et al., 1995]. Because an increase in GABA in the thalamic relay neurons would lead to enhanced hyperpolarization and consequently deinactivation of the T-channels, GABA$_B$ agonists produce an increase in seizure frequency, whereas GABA$_B$ antagonists reduce seizure frequency in rodent models of absence epilepsy [Hosford et al., 1992; Liu et al., 1992; Marescaux et al., 1992; Tsakiridou et al., 1995].

Supporting these animal findings are the clinical observations that three drugs efficacious in the treatment of absence seizures – valproic acid, ethosuximide, and trimethadione–suppress T-currents [Coulter et al., 1990]. In addition, some clinical evidence indicates that vigabatrin, which increases endogenous GABA levels and thereby increases the activation of GABA$_B$ receptors, worsens absence seizures in patients. Clonazepam, which activates GABA$_A$ levels in the nucleus reticularis thalami, can be an effective anti-absence drug [Huguenard and Prince, 1994a].

Treatment

AED therapy is recommended for children with absence seizures. Although not life-threatening, absence seizures may lead to poor school performance, ridicule, and accidents. Because even brief generalized spike-and-wave discharges can affect cognitive function, it is therefore reasonable to begin drug therapy in most patients once the diagnosis is secure.

In a randomized, controlled clinical trial of 453 children with childhood absence epilepsy who were randomly assigned to one of these three drugs, ethosuximide and valproic acid were more efficacious than lamotrigine whereas there were no significant differences among the three drugs with regard to discontinuation because of adverse events (Glauser et al., 2010). However, ethosuximide had less effect on attention than valproic acid. This study would suggest that when considering both efficacy and side effects ethosuximide is the drug of first choice for childhood absence epilepsy. A single agent should be chosen and, after appropriate laboratory studies, initiated at a low dose and gradually increased. AED levels may be helpful, but dose changes in either direction should follow clinical indications. On dosage modifications, drug levels should be obtained only after sufficient time has elapsed to reach steady-state serum concentrations.

In the United States, many physicians will begin therapy with ethosuximide, primarily because of the rare, but severe, hepatotoxicity and pancreatitis associated with valproic acid [Dreifuss et al., 1987, 1989; Penry and Dean, 1993]. Ethosuximide has proved over the past two decades to be a safe and effective AED used almost exclusively for absence seizures [Schneider, 1993; Perucca, 1990]. Valproic acid is equally effective and generally is considered the drug of choice in the patient who has both absence and generalized tonic-clonic seizures, because ethosuximide is not effective in the treatment of generalized tonic-clonic seizures. Lamotrigine appears to be a promising drug in the treatment of absence seizures [Frank et al., 1999; French et al., 2004; Holmes et al., 2008].

Benzodiazepines, such as clonazepam, may be effective, but they usually are reserved for refractory cases because of the relatively high incidence of drowsiness and behavioral side effects [Pearl and Holmes, 2008]. Topiramate [Cross, 2002; Wheless, 2000], levetiracetam [Cohen, 2003], and acetazolamide [Reiss and Oles, 1996] may be useful. Carbamazepine [Yang et al., 2003], vigabatrin [Yang et al., 2003], and tiagabine [Knake et al., 1999] should be avoided because they may exacerbate absence seizures.

In addition to obtaining an interim history, the clinician should always have the child perform a hyperventilation test at follow-up visits. Eliciting a seizure during hyperventilation strongly indicates that the epilepsy disorder is not totally controlled [Adams and Lueders, 1981].

The duration of therapy is variable, although a general rule is to discontinue therapy gradually after 2 seizure-free years have elapsed. Continued presence of spike-and-wave activity on the EEG indicates a high risk for relapse following discontinuation of the drug. Normal EEG findings while the child is on therapy, however, cannot be used as a firm indication that the child will remain seizure-free, because the anti-absence drugs can suppress spike-and-wave activity on the EEG.

Prognosis

Approximately two-thirds of children with childhood absence epilepsy can be expected to enter long-term remission [Wirrell, 2003]. Sato et al. [1976] identified favorable prognostic signs in absence seizures as a negative family history of epilepsy, normal EEG background activity, and normal intelligence. Nearly 90 percent of children with these characteristics stopped having absence seizures.

Juvenile absence epilepsy may occasionally persist into adulthood, however, and juvenile myoclonic epilepsy, as discussed later on, does not spontaneously remit [Wirrell et al., 1996]. As a rule, onset of generalized tonic-clonic seizures before absence seizures carries a poorer prognosis than that noted with the reverse order [Sato et al., 1976].

Clonic Seizures

Clinical Features

Clonic seizures are similar to generalized tonic-clonic seizures but are characterized by only rhythmic or semirhythmic contractions of a group of muscles. These jerks can involve any muscle group, although the arms, neck, and facial muscles are most commonly involved. The jerking often is asymmetric and irregular.

Differentiating a flurry of myoclonic seizures from a clonic seizure may be difficult. Clonic seizures, however, are associated with a more marked impairment of consciousness than is seen with a series of myoclonic seizures and typically include a postictal period, although this may be quite brief. Clonic seizures are more common in children than in adults and usually occur during the first few years of life.

Etiology and Prognosis

Clonic seizures are more likely to be symptomatic than are generalized tonic-clonic seizures. The prognosis is related to the etiology of the seizures.

Electroencephalographic Findings

The EEG may show fast activity, fast activity mixed with slow waves, or polyspike-and-wave discharges.

Tonic Seizures

Clinical Features

Tonic seizures are brief seizures (usually lasting less than 60 seconds), consisting of the sudden onset of increased tone in the extensor muscles [Egli et al., 1985; Holmes, 1988]. If standing, the patient typically falls to the ground. Electromyographic activity is dramatically increased in tonic seizures.

Impairment of consciousness during the seizure is characteristic, although when seizures are brief, this change may be difficult to detect. Tonic seizures frequently are seen in patients with Lennox–Gastaut syndrome, a disorder consisting of a mixed seizure disorder, mental retardation, and the EEG findings of a slow spike-and-wave pattern [Aicardi, 1988a, b;

Markand, 2003]. The seizures usually occur more frequently at night.

Tonic seizures frequently begin with a tonic contraction of the neck muscles, leading to fixation of the head in an erect position, widely opened eyes, and jaw clenching or mouth opening [Holmes, 1988]. Contraction of the respiratory and abdominal muscles often follows, sometimes leading to a high-pitched cry and brief periods of apnea. The tonic contractions may extend to the proximal musculature of the upper limbs, elevating the shoulders and abducting the arms. Asymmetric tonic seizures vary in severity, ranging from a slight rotation of the head to a tonic contraction of all of the musculature on one side of the body. Eyelid retraction, staring, mydriasis, and apnea also may occur [Aicardi, 1988b]. Occasionally, tonic seizures terminate with a brief clonic phase. Unlike in generalized tonic-clonic seizures, however, the clonic phase is abbreviated. Postictal impairment, with confusion, tiredness, and headache, is common. The degree of postictal impairment usually is related to the duration of the seizure.

Tonic seizures typically are activated by sleep and may occur repetitively throughout the night. They usually are more frequent during non-rapid eye movement (REM) sleep than during wakefulness and usually do not occur during REM sleep. Arousal from light sleep may occur after a tonic seizure. Because the child often does not wake up during the seizure, these seizures often go undetected.

Etiology and Prognosis

Tonic seizures usually occur in children with Lennox–Gastaut syndrome, which is discussed later.

Electroencephalographic Findings

The interictal EEG pattern in patients with tonic seizures usually is quite abnormal, consisting of slowing of the background, with multifocal spikes, sharp waves, and bursts of irregular spike-and-wave activity. The EEG ictal manifestations of tonic seizures usually consist of bilateral synchronous spikes of 10–25 Hz, of medium to high voltage, with a frontal accentuation. Simple flattening or desynchronization may also occur (Figure 53-5). Occasional multiple spike-and-wave or diffuse slow-wave activity may occur during a tonic seizure.

Atonic Seizures

Clinical Features

Atonic (astatic) seizures, or "drop attacks," are characterized by a sudden loss of muscle tone [Oguni et al., 1992, 1997]. They begin suddenly and without warning, and cause the patient, if standing, to fall quickly to the floor. Children with atonic seizures are more likely to fall backward than children with tonic seizures [Oguni et al., 1997]. Because muscle tone may be completely absent, the children have little means by which to protect themselves, and injuries often occur. The attack may be fragmentary and manifest as dropping of the head with slackening of the jaw or dropping of a limb.

At times, it may be difficult to distinguish epileptic from nonepileptic head drops. Children with head drops secondary to seizures often have a change in facial expression and subtle myoclonic extremity movements associated with the head drops. Head drops with a rapid head descent, followed by a slow recovery to the upright position, usually represent seizures [Brunquell et al., 1990].

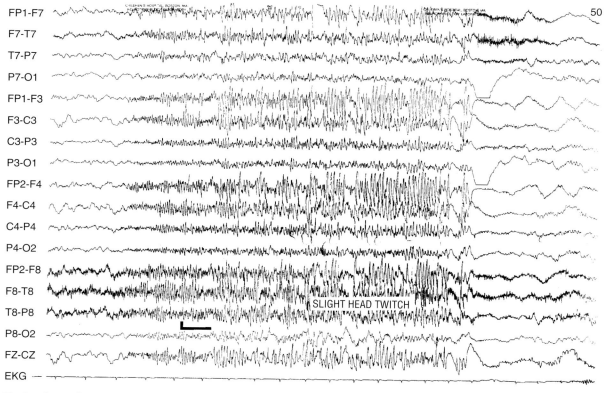

Fig. 53-5 Tonic seizure characterized by rapid discharge of rapid spikes. (Calibration: 50 μV, one second).

In atonic seizures, a loss of electromyographic activity is characteristic. Consciousness is impaired during the fall, although the patient may regain alertness immediately on hitting the floor. Atonic attacks are frequently associated with myoclonic jerks either before, during, or after the atonic seizure [Egli et al., 1985; Schneider et al., 1970]. This combination has been described as myoclonic-astatic seizures. Atonic seizures are rare [Egli et al., 1985; Ikeno et al., 1985]; a majority of children with drop attacks have myoclonic or tonic seizures [Ikeno et al., 1985].

Etiology and Prognosis

Atonic seizures usually occur in children with Lennox–Gastaut syndrome or Doose's syndrome. Doose's syndrome is discussed in Chapter 56.

Electroencephalographic Findings

Atonic seizures usually are associated with rhythmic spike-and-wave complexes varying from slow, 1- to 2-Hz, to more rapid, irregular spikes or multiple spike-and-wave activity.

Lennox–Gastaut Syndrome

Lennox–Gastaut syndrome is characterized by a mixed seizure disorder, of which tonic seizures are a major component, along with a slow spike-and-wave EEG pattern. The syndrome always begins in childhood and often is accompanied by mental retardation [Markand, 2003].

The child with Lennox–Gastaut syndrome typically has a mixture of seizure types. The most frequently occurring are tonic, tonic-clonic, myoclonic, atypical absences, and "head drops," which represent a form of atonic, tonic, or myoclonic seizures. Lennox–Gastaut syndrome is characterized by very frequent seizures, usually occurring multiple times per day. Tonic seizures, in particular, are a major problem in this syndrome [Aicardi, 1988b; Chevrie and Aicardi, 1972]. The tonic seizures usually are brief, lasting from a few seconds to a minute, with an average duration of about 10 seconds.

Myoclonic seizures, occurring either in isolation or as a component of an absence seizure, can occur in this disorder. In some patients, the myoclonus may be so prominent that some investigators have described a myoclonic variant of the Lennox–Gastaut syndrome [Aicardi, 1988b]. Atypical absence and generalized tonic-clonic seizures are seen in more than half of the patients with Lennox–Gastaut syndrome [Schneider et al., 1970]. Generalized tonic-clonic seizures usually cause the most concern to parents and often are the seizure type to precipitate hospitalization.

Mental retardation is present before the onset of seizures in 20–60 percent of patients [Aicardi, 1988b]. Some patients, with an idiopathic or cryptogenic etiology of their seizures, have normal intelligence quotient (IQ) scores or developmental histories before the onset of their seizures. The proportion of retarded patients increases with age because of the deterioration that frequently occurs in Lennox–Gastaut syndrome. Fluctuations in cognitive abilities may occur and are correlated to some degree with the intensity of EEG abnormalities. Behavioral problems also are common in Lennox–Gastaut syndrome, ranging from hyperactivity to frank psychotic and autistic behavior. Abnormalities on the neurologic examination have been reported in 30–88 percent of patients with Lennox–Gastaut syndrome [Kurokowa et al., 1980; Markand, 1977; Schneider et al., 1970].

Patients with Lennox–Gastaut syndrome typically have very frequent seizures [Markand, 1977; Papini et al., 1984]. It is not unusual for some children with this syndrome to have hundreds of seizures per day. Seizure frequency may vary during the course of a day, with the highest frequency during drowsiness and inactivity [Papini et al., 1984]. In addition, in many of the patients, a weekly or monthly periodicity in seizure frequency is observed that is unrelated to AED therapy [Aicardi, 1973]. Periods of prolonged repetitive seizures of a mixed type are interspersed with periods of relative freedom from attacks. During times when the child is seizure-free, marked improvements in alertness, motivation, and academic progress can be seen. Unfortunately, these periods usually are short-lived, leading to a great deal of frustration for the child, parent, school personnel, and medical professionals.

Electroencephalographic Findings

The hallmark of the EEG pattern in Lennox–Gastaut syndrome is the slow spike-and-wave discharge superimposed on an abnormal, slow background. The slow spike-and-wave or sharp-and-slow-wave complexes consist of generalized discharges occurring at a frequency of 1.5–2.5 Hz. The morphology, amplitude, and repetition rate may vary both between bursts and during paroxysmal bursts of spike-and-wave activity, and asymmetries of the discharge are frequent. The area of maximum voltage, although variable, usually is frontal or temporal in location. Often, sleep increases the number of epileptiform discharges, but these discharges may slow in frequency and become even more irregular than during the awake state (Figure 53-6). In REM sleep, the paroxysmal activity decreases markedly. Hyperventilation and photic stimulation rarely activate these discharges.

Etiology

The syndrome may arise de novo in a previously well child or may supervene in an already neurologically or medically handicapped patient. Lennox–Gastaut syndrome has been divided into primary and secondary cases. Primary refers to cases in which the etiology is idiopathic, whereas secondary refers to cases in which the disorder is symptomatic of a definable etiology. Markand [1977] was able to identify an underlying disorder in 64 percent of 83 patients, and Chevrie and Aicardi [1972] were able to do so in 66 percent of 80 patients. Other investigators, however, have reported a smaller incidence of identifiable causes in Lennox–Gastaut syndrome [Kurokowa et al., 1980; Schneider et al., 1970]. The causes of Lennox–Gastaut syndrome are listed in Box 53-1 and are similar to those seen in infantile spasms. In fact, in many patients with infantile spasms, (30–40 percent) the disorder will progress to Lennox–Gastaut syndrome [Kurokawa et al., 1980; Olmos-Garcia de Alba et al., 1984; Riikonen, 1996]. In some children with infantile spasms that evolve into Lennox–Gastaut syndrome the epileptic spasms continue to occur in series and become one of the seizure types (Donat and Wright, 1991).

Although a majority of patients with Lennox–Gastaut syndrome have a static disorder, degenerative disorders may occasionally manifest as this syndrome [Markand, 1977;

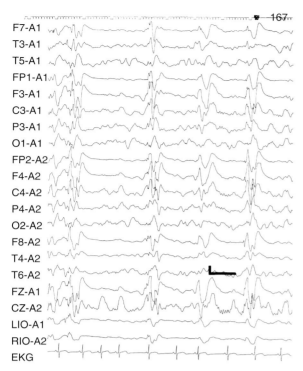

Fig. 53-6 Irregular spike and slow-wave complexes during sleep in a child with Lennox–Gastaut syndrome. (Calibration: 100 μV, one second).

Box 53-1 Common Disorders Associated with Lennox–Gastaut Syndrome

Prenatal

- Cerebral dysgenesis
- Tuberous sclerosis
- Congenital infection
- Stroke

Perinatal

- Hypoxia/ischemia
- Intracranial hemorrhage

Postnatal

- Meningitis/encephalitis
- Postinfectious
- Cerebral vascular disease
- Hypoxia/ischemia
- Status epilepticus
- Head injury
- Hypoglycemia
- Degenerative disorders

Pampiglione and Harden, 1977]. Genetic factors do not play a significant role in a majority of individuals with this disorder.

Treatment

Management of the child with Lennox–Gastaut syndrome is difficult. Because the degree of heterogeneity with this syndrome is considerable, the response to AED therapy is variable. Individualized treatment approaches are necessary.

Usually no single AED is effective in controlling all of the seizure types in Lennox–Gastaut syndrome. This frequently leads to polypharmacy. In addition, the sedating side effects of the AEDs may lead to an increase in seizure frequency. The other notable problem is tolerance. In patients who have an initial improvement, loss of efficacy often occurs after a few months of treatment. This decreased efficacy usually leads to an increase in dosage, often with accompanying side effects, or to additional polytherapy. Although polytherapy sometimes cannot be avoided, the physician must be aware of the potential for harm. Withdrawal of AEDs, particularly the barbiturates and benzodiazepines, may lead to improved alertness and an actual reduction in seizure frequency.

In the United States, valproate likely is the most commonly used drug in the treatment of Lennox–Gastaut syndrome. It is a broad-spectrum drug with effectiveness against all of the common seizure types in the syndrome. The lack of sedative side effects and the broad spectrum of action make the drug appealing. The drug has been associated with hepatotoxicity, however, particularly in children younger than 2 years of age. Phenytoin is considered by some investigators to be the drug of choice for tonic seizures. Intravenous phenytoin is used as a first-line drug for status epilepticus in Lennox–Gastaut syndrome (Richard et al., 1993) since benzodiazepines can precipitate tonic status epilepticus in Lennox–Gastaut syndrome [Tassinari et al., 1972].

Felbamate, released in the United States in 1993, was the first drug to be demonstrated to be effective in Lennox–Gastaut syndrome [Dodson, 1993a, b; The Felbamate Study Group in Lennox–Gastaut Syndrome, 1993]. After the drug was released, it was found to result in fatal aplastic anemia and hepatic failure. The overall risk of aplastic anemia for patients taking felbamate is estimated to be 1:5000, 100 times greater than the risk in the normal population, and the risk of fatal outcome is approximately 1:10,000 [Kaufman et al., 1997]. Felbamate-associated aplastic anemia has not been reported in children younger than 13 years [Brodie and Pellock, 1995; Pellock and Brodie, 1997]. Risk factors associated with aplastic anemia include a history of blood dyscrasia or of substantial toxicity to other AEDs, serologic or clinical evidence of an autoimmune disorder, and a history of treatment with felbamate for less than 1 year [Pellock, 1999].

Both lamotrigine [Donaldson et al., 1997; Motte et al., 1997] and topiramate [Guerreiro et al., 1997; Ormrod and McClellan, 2001; Sachdeo et al., 1999] have demonstrated efficacy in Lennox–Gastaut syndrome but rarely with total control of the seizures.

In a double-blind, placebo-controlled trial of lamotrigine in 169 patients with Lennox–Gastaut syndrome, either lamotrigine or placebo was added to the maintenance medications. After 16 weeks, 33 percent of children receiving lamotrigine and 16 percent of placebo recipients had more than a 50 percent reduction in seizure frequency [Motte et al., 1997]. In a double-blind, placebo-controlled, multicenter trial of topiramate for adjunctive therapy for Lennox–Gastaut syndrome, the frequency of drop attacks was reduced compared with that in the placebo group [Sachdeo et al., 1999].

The ketogenic diet (see Chapter 60), one of the oldest methods of treating childhood epilepsy, remains a reasonable therapy for children with seizures refractory to standard drug therapy [Vining et al., 1998; Wheless, 2004; Ferrie and Patel, 2009]. Although the diet was considered a therapy of last resort for many years, recent resurgence in interest has occurred, primarily owing to its success in several highly publicized cases. The diet consists of a high proportion of fats and small amounts of carbohydrate and protein, with a fat to carbohydrate and protein ratio of 4:1. Although it is clear that the child must remain in a state of ketosis for the diet to be effective, the basis of the therapeutic effectiveness of the ketogenic diet remains uncertain.

The resurgence in interest in the diet is appropriate because it does provide an attractive alternative in the treatment of childhood epilepsy. The literature supports the view that the ketogenic diet improves seizure control in a significant number of children with medically intractable epilepsy [Prasad et al., 1996; Rubenstein and Vining, 2004]. One-third to one-half of children appear to have an excellent response to the ketogenic diet in terms of a marked or complete cessation of seizures or reduction in seizure severity. In another one-third of the children, a partial reduction in seizure frequency or severity occurs; the remaining children have no appreciable benefit from the diet. Improvement in alertness and behavior often is seen when the child is placed on the diet. It is not clear whether this benefit is secondary to withdrawal of drugs, reduction in seizure frequency, or a direct result of the diet.

Aspects of the surgical evaluation of children with generalized epilepsies, including use of vagal nerve stimulators, are reviewed in Chapter 61.

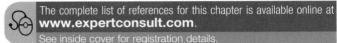

The complete list of references for this chapter is available online at **www.expertconsult.com**.
See inside cover for registration details.

Focal and Multifocal Seizures

Douglas R. Nordli, Jr.

Introduction

Focal or partial seizures originate in one region of the brain, where they may stay confined or spread to other areas. Multifocal seizures arise from multiple locations and constitute an important type of seizure in infancy and childhood. Both focal and multifocal types have been under-recognized in children, but modern epidemiologic studies show that focal epilepsies account for about 60 percent of all seizure disorders [Berg et al., 1999a,b; Sillanpaa et al., 1999]. The behavioral manifestations of focal seizures relate not only to the region of the brain involved during the ictal discharge, but also to the maturation of the nervous system and the integrity of the pathways necessary for clinical expression.

Focal seizures in the very young are subtler and less declarative than focal seizures seen later in life [Acharya et al., 1997; Hamer et al., 1999; Nordli et al., 1997]. This is particularly true in infants and children with diffuse encephalopathies, in whom brain immaturity, diffuse cerebral dysfunction, or both make manifestations of focal seizures difficult to recognize. Focal seizures also can be mistaken in older children when the presence of secondary convulsive movements prompts casual observers to label the event a "generalized tonic-clonic" seizure. With this misdiagnosis, critical elements of the seizures are overlooked. As described later, careful consideration of the unique features present in pediatric focal seizures can improve diagnostic accuracy.

In a majority of children with focal seizures, no focal structural lesion is present, and the seizures either are the expression of an idiopathic disorder (benign rolandic epilepsy) or are cryptogenic. This finding is in contrast to adults, in whom a focal seizure strongly implies the presence of a focal structural lesion (e.g., stroke, brain tumor). Instead, only 10 percent of children with focal seizures have brain tumors or strokes. In one large epidemiologic study, only 4 of 613 children with epilepsy had a brain tumor [Berg et al., 2000a].

The prognostic value of seizure classification by itself is limited, and a fuller understanding of the patient is achieved by making an epilepsy syndrome diagnosis. As pointed out in Chapter 50, two children with the same seizure type can have markedly different outcomes. Establishing an epilepsy syndrome diagnosis is the best way to determine on management options for different patients. An epilepsy syndrome diagnosis is preferred for assessing prognosis and treatment. Although it may not be possible to diagnose every child immediately on presentation, prospective population-based studies suggest that most children can ultimately be diagnosed with an epilepsy syndrome. Many factors contribute to the diagnosis of a syndrome, but in practice, three are most important:

1. age and development of the patient
2. type or types of observed seizures
3. interictal electroencephalogram (EEG) features.

Many well-known epilepsy syndromes are delineated by specific clinical triads comprising these factors. Accordingly, this chapter includes a discussion of epilepsy syndromes that frequently manifest with focal or multifocal seizures.

Children with multifocal seizures (three or more foci, involving both hemispheres) may have unfavorable forms of epilepsy (e.g., migrating partial seizures, Dravet's syndrome, symptomatic diffuse epileptogenic encephalopathies not otherwise specified). Although these epilepsies manifest with focal seizures, the children usually have evidence of concomitant diffuse cerebral dysfunction on clinical examination, developmental history, and interictal EEG studies. Correct diagnosis is particularly challenging in the group of children with focal seizures and evidence of widespread, diffuse, or multifocal cerebral dysfunction; too often, these patients end up in broad, poorly descriptive "wastebasket" categories, such as Lennox–Gastaut syndrome or generalized symptomatic epilepsy not otherwise specified. Lennox–Gastaut syndrome has particular diagnostic features and is not synonymous with diffuse symptomatic epilepsy, as discussed in Chapter 53. In summary, the importance of correctly recognizing focal seizures cannot be overstated.

Recognition of Focal Seizures in Children

Clinical features alone cannot always allow one to diagnose a focal seizure correctly. Rather, "focal seizure" is actually an electroclinical diagnosis. It usually is made following consideration of multiple factors related to the patient and the clinical event, but may require EEG confirmation, particularly in the very young. Still, a number of important clues can help point to the presence of focal seizures in children (Box 54-1). Experience using video EEG monitoring suggests that certain clinical features tend to have focal ictal EEG correlates [Nordli et al., 2001] (Figure 54-1).

Auras

Auras are special sensory or psychogenic phenomena that can be described only by the patient. They occur in a variety of forms and have important localizing value. Although the concurrent ictal EEG often does not reveal clear electrographic expression in most patients, auras are believed by most authorities to be the manifestation of discrete focal seizures. When a somatosensory aura is specific and an ictal EEG correlate is

Box 54-1 Seizure Semiology Indicating a Focal Seizure

- Aura
- Behavioral arrest (in most cases, although patients with absence also have behavioral arrest)
- Focal clonus
- Focal dystonic posture
- Focal limb automatisms

- Spasms (approximately one-quarter of patients with spasms have associated focal seizures)
- Tonic postures (particularly asymmetric tonic posture, although symmetric tonic postures also are seen in infants with focal seizures)
- Version (involving the head, eyes, or both)

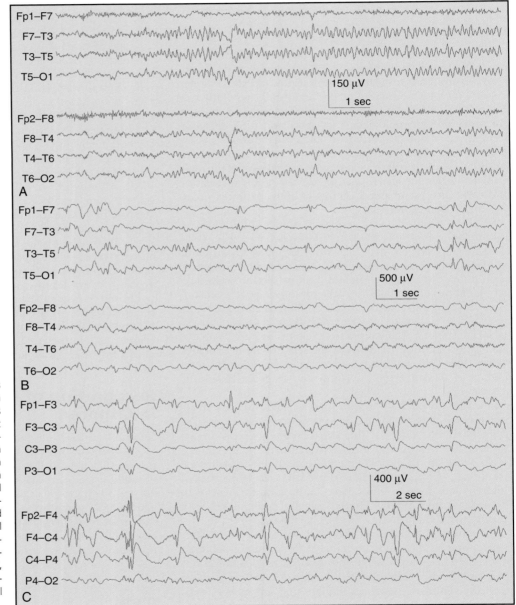

Fig. 54-1 Typical interictal findings on electroencephalogram (EEG) in children with focal seizures. A, This EEG from a child with benign rolandic epilepsy of childhood (BREC) shows focal stereotypic spikes appearing on a normal background. Notice that each spike closely resembles the others in morphology and location, as is typical of idiopathic localization-related epilepsies. **B,** By contrast, this EEG from a child with an epileptogenic focal structural lesion in the left temporal region demonstrates pleomorphic spikes and background slowing in the same region. **C,** EEGs from children with multifocal seizures often show multifocal interictal epileptiform discharges.

present, the ictal discharge is often low-voltage fast activity localized over the corresponding region of the sensory homunculus. Other auras arising from limbic structures often are "indescribable," or may have a fearful quality or include a feeling of epigastric discomfort. These discharges arise from subcortical structures, so the EEG may reveal little to no change, other than ipsilateral diffuse delta activity or a rhythmic theta-alpha pattern in the anterior to midtemporal region, particularly when the onset of activity is mesial temporal in location. Auras are a very reliable indicator of a focal seizure.

Automatisms

Limb automatisms are semipurposeful movements such as the rubbing, fumbling, or picking that may be seen in focal seizures. Oral automatisms, such as lip smacking, can occur with generalized absence seizures, but unilateral limb automatisms suggest a focal process. Well-developed distal limb automatisms are rarely seen in infants but become more common above age 6 years. When unilateral, automatisms are another helpful sign, indicating the presence of a focal seizure.

Behavioral Arrest

In some infants and young children, the most conspicuous feature of a focal seizure may be the sudden, abrupt cessation of on-going activity or a marked change in demeanor, as indicated by subtle but distinct changes in facial expression. Parents easily identify these features because they represent a clear paroxysmal alteration in the child's behavior. Parents are particularly well attuned to the nature of their child's habitual behavior, but these behavioral changes may be challenging for a person unacquainted with the child to identify on video tape. In the preverbal child, or in many children with special needs, it is impossible to ascertain alteration of consciousness reliably. Alteration of consciousness cannot be unambiguously inferred from behavior (e.g., daydreaming in school). To assess consciousness accurately, test items must be given and recall tested after the seizure. In children, this often is not possible, so the simple description of a behavioral arrest is more reliably used, rather than trying to infer if a seizure was truly "complex partial." Behavioral arrest seizures also have been described as hypomotor seizures. This description refers to a sudden reduction in the motor activity of the child. The electrographic ictal accompaniment often emanates from the temporal lobe or posterior quadrant and may be composed of monotonous rhythmic delta, rhythmic theta-alpha patterns with an electrographic "crescendo" appearance, or low-voltage fast discharges that subsequently evolve to other rhythms (Figure 54-2). In children above age 3 years, behavioral arrest may accompany both focal and generalized seizures (absence seizures), so in isolation it is not a reliable indicator of a focal seizure; however, since absence seizures rarely occur in children less than 2.5 years, it is likely to be the correlate of a focal seizure in this age group.

Dystonic Postures

A dystonic posture of a limb is a feature seen in focal seizures. It is infrequently seen in the very young but becomes more common in the school-age child. Dystonic postures of the hand are usually contralateral to the seizure focus. They may often be coupled with ipsilateral (to the seizure focus) limb automatisms. A unilateral dystonic posture suggests a focal seizure.

Focal Clonus

Hand or arm clonus (clonic seizure) is another reliable feature of focal epilepsy. This activity is easily recognized as ictal by the repetitive nature of the jerking, and the inability to suppress the motion by passive restraint. It usually is accompanied by runs of rhythmic spike discharges in the contralateral rolandic region, and is a reliable indicator of a focal seizure.

Spasms

Spasms can be recognized by their tendency to recur in clusters, many times in an almost periodic fashion, with a fairly constant interval between some of the individual spasms. Spasms have a quick or myoclonic component at the start, followed by a brief sustained posture (tonic phase), followed in turn by a relaxation. Spasms that are asymmetric, that occur in a child with hemiparesis or other focal pathology, or that are associated with marked interhemispheric asymmetries on EEG are most likely focal seizures. In about 25 percent of patients with spasms, clear electrographic focal seizures can be detected before, during, or after the cluster. The EEG accompaniment of spasms often contains diffuse electrodecrements, even if they are preceded by clear focal seizures [Kubota et al., 1999].

Tonic Postures

Tonic postures, both symmetric and asymmetric, are seen with focal seizures. It is surprising to observe how often symmetric tonic postures can occur as a manifestation of a focal seizure in infants, and also how unreliable asymmetries of tonic postures can be in localizing ictal onsets. It is possible that these tonic postures are generated in deeper brainstem or subcortical structures and are not direct manifestations of the ictal discharges. This finding would explain why some asymmetric tonic postures can be reversed by passive turning of the head during a seizure, in a fashion similar to the tonic neck reflex elicited in the newborn. As the child matures, symmetric tonic postures are seen less frequently as a manifestation of a focal epilepsy. Instead, tonic postures become more asymmetric and show more lateralizing features.

Version

Pronounced and sustained lateral version of the eyes (versive seizure) is rarely encountered as an ictal manifestation in infants or young children. When present, version is another indicator of a focal seizure. In contrast with older children and adults, in whom the electrographic discharge often is best developed in the contralateral frontotemporal region, the ictal discharge in infants is more often in the ipsilateral occipital lobe.

Seizure Classification: International League Against Epilepsy

The International League against Epilepsy (ILAE) Commission on Classification proposed a classification of seizures in 1981. This scheme was widely used for almost three decades. Recently, a new ILAE commission on classification proposed a substantial revision [Berg et al., 2010] (Box 54-2). Now, the term "focal" replaces the previous term "partial," and the obligatory separation of partial seizures into simple, complex, and secondary generalized has been discarded. Focal seizures still may be described further, if desired. One such way is to identify the degree of impairment. These and other descriptive terms are outlined in a previously published glossary [Blume et al., 2001] (Box 54-3). Examples of descriptors listed in the 2010 report include "without impairment of consciousness or awareness," "with impairment of consciousness or awareness," and "evolving to bilateral convulsive seizure." The reader

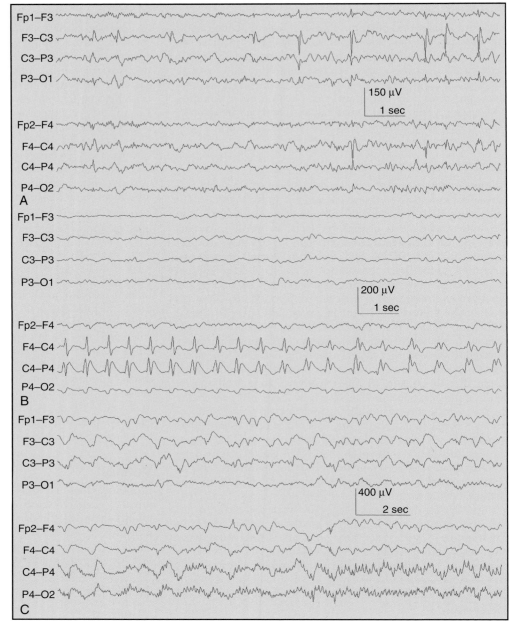

Fig. 54-2 Common infantile ictal patterns on electroencephalogram (EEG) in focal seizures. A, EEG during a behavioral arrest seizure shows an ictal discharge in the left temporal region. Notice the rhythmic build-up of fast activity. Ictal discharges usually have an evolution in frequency, amplitude, and spatial distribution (like a crescendo in music). **B,** During a clonic seizure involving the left arm, the EEG demonstrates an ictal correlate consisting of repetitive spikes in the right central region. Notice that the ictal discharge remains very localized. **C,** EEG obtained during a versive seizure with eyes deviating to the right, or the same side as for the ictal discharge, shows a fast ictal pattern superimposed on some rhythmic slowing in the right posterior head region.

Box 54-2 International Classification of Seizures

- Generalized Seizures
  - Tonic-clonic (in any combination)
  - Absence
  - Typical
  - Atypical
  - Absence with special features
  - Myoclonic absence
  - Eyelid myoclonia
  - Myoclonic
    - Myoclonic atonic
    - Myoclonic tonic
    - Clonic
    - Tonic
    - Atonic
- Focal Seizures
- Unknown
- Epileptic Spasms

Box 54-3 Further Descriptions of Focal Seizures

- Without impairment of consciousness or awareness
- With observable motor or autonomic components: roughly corresponds to the concept of "simple partial seizure." "Focal motor" and "autonomic" are terms that may adequately convey this concept, depending on the seizure manifestations
- Involving subjective sensory or psychic phenomena only: corresponds to the concept of an "aura," a term endorsed in the 2001 Glossary

- With impairment of consciousness or awareness: roughly corresponds to the concept of "complex partial seizure." "Dyscognitive" is a term that has been proposed for this concept [Blume et al., 2001]
- Evolving to a bilateral, convulsive seizure (involving tonic, clonic, or tonic and clonic components): this expression replaces the term "secondarily generalized seizure"

will note that these terms roughly equate to the older terms of simple, complex, and secondary generalized seizures. The important distinction is that these terms are no longer required but may be used by those who wish to maintain continuity with the 1981 classification. This adjustment appears minor, but is very useful because it is often not possible to determine alteration of consciousness reliably in the very young or in those with difficulties with communication. Lüders and colleagues have a logical and simple system that has been used internationally in major epilepsy centers (Lüders et al., 1999). Others have proposed a much-simplified semiologic classification system for use in the very young [Nordli et al., 1997]. Neither of these schemes has been endorsed by the ILAE [Nordli et al., 1997]. While seizures may sometimes be broadly classified using the most prominent and early feature of the seizure, the various combinations of features, patterns, and time course of the seizure cannot be adequately summarized in a single word or phrase. Nothing can replace a thorough and meticulous description of the seizure. Indeed, the historic narrative of the seizure, as described or observed by parents, is the single most helpful piece of information allowing proper diagnosis of the seizure disorder and should be recorded, as accurately as possible, with few or no editorial comments.

Epilepsy Syndromes with Focal Seizures

The ILAE classification of epilepsy syndromes is reviewed in Chapter 50. A recent modification of the ILAE classification eliminated the "focal" and "generalized" headings, along with the previous terms "idiopathic" and "symptomatic" (Box 54-4) [Borg et al., 2010]. One way to organize the recognized syndromes is by the specificity of the diagnostic criteria, further organized by age.

Neonatal Period

Benign Familial Neonatal Epilepsy

Of the three recognized epilepsy syndromes in neonates, only one has prominent focal seizures: *benign familial neonatal epilepsy* (BFNE). The other two syndromes, early myoclonic encephalopathy (EME) and Ohtahara's syndrome, may have accompanying focal seizures, but the predominant seizures are myoclonic, tonic, or epileptic spasms. BFNE was first described in 1964 by Rett and Teubel [Rett and Teubel, 1964]. Before the advent of newborn video-EEG recordings, it was thought that the seizures in this syndrome might be generalized, but subsequent recordings showed that the predominant seizures are focal clonic or adversive, even though

the accompanying EEG may show diffuse flattening at the onset. Ronen et al., reported the incidence as 14.4 per 100,000 live births [Ronen et al., 1999]. The clinical features have been thoroughly reviewed by Plouin [Plouin, 2008]. Most seizures (80 percent) start on the second or third day of life in term, otherwise healthy, newborns. Clinically, they usually begin with a diffuse tonic component, followed by a variety of motor and autonomic phenomena. Motor manifestations may include prominent oculofacial features, limb clonus, or both. Interictal EEG backgrounds are usually normal or may show a *théta pointu alternant* pattern, which consists of short bursts of rhythmic theta activity with sharply contoured components. Ictal EEGs have shown initial flattening, which may be focal or diffuse, followed by subsequent ictal rhythms. Family history, by definition, is positive and the inheritance is autosomal-dominant. Mutations in the genes encoding KCNQ2 and KCNQ3 account for the majority of cases. There are no official guidelines for treatment of BFNE and it is uncertain whether treatment is beneficial in the long run. There are clear regional preferences but phenobarbital, sodium valproate, and phenytoin have all been used. The long-term outcome is favorable, although 11 percent of patients may have epilepsy later in life [Plouin, 2008].

Infancy

There are at least four well-recognized syndromes occurring in infancy that may present with focal or multifocal seizures. Some proposed syndromes have features that overlap very closely with others. If one takes a broad view and lumps some of these variants together, then there are two syndromes with favourable outcomes, and two that are usually quite severe. Benign infantile epilepsy and benign familial infantile epilepsy share many clinical features but differ with regard to the family history. Epilepsy of infancy with migrating focal seizures and Dravet's syndrome are severe epilepsies with very different clinical features.

Benign Nonfamilial Infantile Seizures

Fukuyama in 1963 and later Watanabe were among the first to describe infants with the onset of epilepsy in the first 2 years of life with no known cause and excellent outcome [Fukuyama, 1963; Watanabe and Okumura, 2000]. Fukuyama originally described these seizures as generalized convulsions, but this was before the advent of modern video-EEG recordings and it is likely that these were actually focal seizures with secondary spread. Watanabe and colleagues described a case series in 1987 and noted clear focal features, describing these seizures as "complex partial" [Watanabe and Okumura, 2000]. Whether

Box 54-4 Electroclinical Syndromes Categorized by Age at Onset

Neonatal Period

- Benign familial neonatal epilepsy (BFNE)
- Early myoclonic encephalopathy (EME)
- Ohtahara's syndrome

Infancy

- Epilepsy of infancy with migrating focal seizures
- West's syndrome
- Myoclonic epilepsy in infancy (MEI)
- Benign infantile epilepsy
- Benign familial infantile epilepsy
- Dravet's syndrome
- Myoclonic encephalopathy in nonprogressive disorders

Childhood

- Febrile seizures plus (FS+) (can start in infancy)
- Panayiotopoulos' syndrome
- Epilepsy with myoclonic atonic (previously astatic) seizures
- Benign epilepsy with centrotemporal spikes (BECTS)
- Autosomal-dominant nocturnal frontal lobe epilepsy (ADNFLE)
- Late-onset childhood occipital epilepsy (Gastaut type)
- Epilepsy with myoclonic absences
- Lennox–Gastaut syndrome
- Epileptic encephalopathy with continuous spike-and-wave during sleep (CSWS)
- Landau–Kleffner syndrome (LKS)
- Childhood absence epilepsy (CAE)

Adolescence to Adulthood

- Juvenile absence epilepsy (JAE)
- Juvenile myoclonic epilepsy (JME)
- Epilepsy with generalized tonic-clonic seizures alone
- Progressive myoclonus epilepsies (PME)
- Autosomal-dominant epilepsy with auditory features (ADEAF)
- Other familial temporal lobe epilepsies

Less Specific Age Relationship

- Familial focal epilepsy with variable foci (childhood to adult)
- Reflex epilepsies

Distinctive Constellations

- Mesial temporal lobe epilepsy with hippocampal sclerosis (MTLE with HS)
- Rasmussen's syndrome
- Gelastic seizures with hypothalamic hamartoma
- Hemiconvulsion-hemiplegia-epilepsy

Epilepsies not Fitting Any of these Diagnostic Categories

These can be distinguished first on the basis of the presence or absence of a known structural or metabolic condition (presumed cause), and then on the basis of the primary mode of seizure onset (generalized vs. focal)

Epilepsies Attributed to and Organized by Structural-Metabolic Causes, Malformations of Cortical Development (Hemimegalencephaly, Heterotopias, etc.)

- Neurocutaneous syndromes (tuberous sclerosis complex, Sturge–Weber, etc.)
- Tumor
- Infection
- Trauma
- Angioma
- Perinatal insults
- Stroke
  Etc.

Epilepsies of Unknown Cause (Conditions with Epileptic Seizures Traditionally not Diagnosed as a Form of Epilepsy Per Se)

- Benign neonatal seizures (BNS)
- Febrile seizures (FS)

these are two separate conditions or one syndrome is a matter of some debate. In both cases, there is normal development before the onset of seizures. Imaging studies and metabolic tests are unremarkable. Onset is mostly within the first year of life in both cases. The interictal EEG is normal. In both cases, seizures may manifest with blank staring, and may be followed by secondary generalization in the Fukuyama type. Seizures may occur in clusters in both. The ictal focus is most often in the temporal region in the Watanabe form and in the centroparietal region in the Fukuyama type. Both demonstrate an excellent response to treatment and have normal development. Capovilla and colleagues have described another infantile epilepsy with excellent outcome. These infants have focal seizures and a characteristic interictal EEG finding of a "bell-shaped" discharge, which is maximal at the vertex [Capovilla and Vigevano, 2001]. Infants present between 8 and 30 months with relatively bland seizures characterized by motion arrest, some tonic stiffening, and oxygen desaturation. Seizures are infrequent and usually of short duration. The authors did not recommend treatment with antiepileptic drugs (AEDs) in most cases. A family history of epilepsy is present in half the cases and the outcome is very favorable.

Benign Familial Infantile Seizures

Vigevano and colleagues described cases with similar features but with a positive family history for infantile epilepsy [Vigevano et al., 1992]. In these patients there is a similar age of onset and normal development before the onset of seizures. Seizures usually start between 4 and 8 months of age, occur in clusters, have focal features including behavioral arrest, cyanosis, head/eye version, tonic stiffening of the limbs, and bilateral clonus. The interictal EEG is normal. The ictal EEG usually shows a fast rhythm beginning in the occipitoparietal region. Development is normal and the outcome is excellent. Treatment with antiepileptic medication is not mandatory. Since other family members may have experienced infantile seizures with a very favourable outcome, families may be very amenable to withholding treatment.

Epilepsy of Infancy with Migrating Focal Seizures

This condition was described by Coppola and others in 1995 [Coppola et al., 1995]. It is a severe and devastating epilepsy, with onset within the first 6 months of life in otherwise healthy infants.

Seizures are truly multifocal, with a variety of clinical manifestations that shift from side to side. They often involve head/eye version, eyelid twitching, limb jerks, and tonic stiffening of one or both limbs. Initially, seizures may begin with a simple behavioral arrest, subtle eye deviation, and some oral automatisms. The striking feature of this epilepsy is the nearly continuous nature of the seizures. At the start of the disorder, each individual seizure is brief; seizures tend to recur in groups, 5–30 seizures occurring during drowsiness several times per day. Seizures may cluster for days, and the severity increases over the course of days or months to the point where the seizures are more or less continuous. Developmental regression ensues in all affected infants, along with deceleration of head growth. Marsh and colleagues reported a series of infants with slightly better outcome, but even in this series of patients, mental retardation ranged from mild to severe [Marsh et al., 2005]. There is no known cause and treatment has been frustrating. In the original series, two patients benefited from a combination of clonazepam and stiripentol, while in another series two others benefited from treatment with potassium bromide [Okuda et al., 2000].

Dravet's Syndrome

Dravet's syndrome is another severe form of epilepsy affecting infants usually within the first year of life [Dravet et al., 2005]. Initial seizures are often hemiconvulsive and prolonged, and frequently are found in the setting of fever. Neurological examination and imaging studies are unremarkable. Subsequent seizure types may develop, including myoclonic jerks, and atypical absence and focal seizures. Athough development is usually normal prior to disease onset, children with Dravet's syndrome may experience a developmental regression that can result in severe global delays. It is not yet known whether modern treatments can prevent, delay, or reduce the severity of this regression. Despite the general trend not to rush to treatment with AEDs in most children with epilepsy, there is a strong suspicion that early and aggressive treatment is warranted in Dravet's syndrome once the diagnosis is secured [Arts and Geerts, 2009]. The diagnosis can be suspected in an infant with prolonged febrile seizures who later develops prolonged afebrile focal seizures, including hemiclonic convulsions [Millichap et al., 2009]. The majority of cases of Dravet's syndrome are associated with mutations in the *SCN1A* gene. In particular, truncating mutations or missense mutations involving the portion of the gene that encodes for the pore of the sodium channel are most common. Initially, EEGs may be normal, or show polyspikes in the posterior quadrant. In time, generalized spike-wave discharges develop, and children may have photoparoxysmal responses (Figure 54-3). Effective treatments include valproate, stiripentol, clobazam, topiramate, ketogenic diet, and bromides [Korff et al., 2007; Wheless 2009; Caraballo and Fejerman, 2006]. Other newer medications may be effective but have not yet been rigorously studied. Since drugs with sodium channel properties, like carbamazepine, phenytoin, and lamotrigine, may exacerbate Dravet's syndrome, newer medications that have pronounced sodium channel properties should probably be avoided [Guerrini et al., 1998]. Children with Dravet's syndrome may have gait disorders (walking with a stooped gait), fine motor skill difficulties, and dysarthria so comprehensive that multidisciplinary management of their disorder is warranted. Dravet's syndrome is also discussed in Chapter 55.

Myoclonic-astatic epilepsy, which was described by Doose, is sometimes confused with Dravet's syndrome. This is now called epilepsy with myoclonic-atonic seizures or myoclonic-atonic epilepsy (MAE). As in Dravet's syndrome, children can present with convulsive episodes early in life, but MAE usually begins *after* the first year of life, whereas almost all children with Dravet's syndrome start having seizures *in* the first year of life. The most conspicuous feature of MAE is the presence of myoclonic-atonic seizures, which begin with a sudden jerk and are followed by a drop attack. This sequence can be demonstrated on video-EEG, or with an ordinary EEG using polygraphic techniques. Absence seizures and sometimes tonic seizures may occur, but prolonged focal seizures are very unusual in MAE. Children with Dravet's syndrome often have myoclonus but it usually does not result in severe drop attacks. Children with MAE do not usually have mutations in the *SCN1A* gene. MAE is also discussed in Chapter 56.

Childhood

Panayiotopoulos' Syndrome

The ILAE recognized early-onset childhood epilepsy with occipital spikes (Panayiotopoulos type) and differentiated it from the later-onset occipital epilepsy, as described by Gastaut [Panayiotopoulos, 1999; Lada et al., 2003]. Panayiotopoulos' syndrome is about half as frequent as benign focal epilepsy with central-temporal spikes by some estimates, and carries an excellent prognosis. It is characterized by autonomic and behavioral disturbances, with vomiting, deviation of the eyes, and impairment of consciousness that can progress to convulsions. Seizures are long-lasting, often more than 3 minutes. The typical age at onset is 5 years. Occipital spikes may be present, but stereotypic spikes in other locations (cloned spikes) are reported, particularly as the child ages [Ohtsu et al., 2003] (Figure 54-4). Panayiotopoulos has indicated that diagnosis is important for several reasons, including the fact that prophylactic treatment may not be necessary.

Benign Focal Epilepsies of Childhood

Benign focal epilepsy with central-midtemporal spikes (also called central-temporal epilepsy or rolandic epilepsy) is most common in previously healthy children aged 4–13 years. It had previously been classified as an idiopathic localization-related epilepsy by the ILAE, but the widespread nature of the EEG features and the shifting laterality of the clinical expression could equally argue for a more diffuse or multifocal predisposition. Rolandic epilepsy has characteristic EEG and clinical features. In a comprehensive study performed in Connecticut, rolandic epilepsy represented 9.6–10.3 percent of all childhood epilepsies, determined at presentation and 2 years later [Berg et al., 2000]. In its pure form, it is not associated with structural lesions and severe neurocognitive deficits [Lundberg and Eeg-Olofsson, 2003]. When awake, children experience brief focal seizures, with twitching of one side of the face, anarthria, drooling, and paresthesias of the face, gums, tongue, or inner cheeks. These manifestations may be followed by hemiclonic movements or hemitonic posturing. These diurnal seizures are simple; consciousness is preserved. Postictal weakness (Todd's paralysis) of the involved face and limbs may occur. Most children have purely nocturnal seizures that

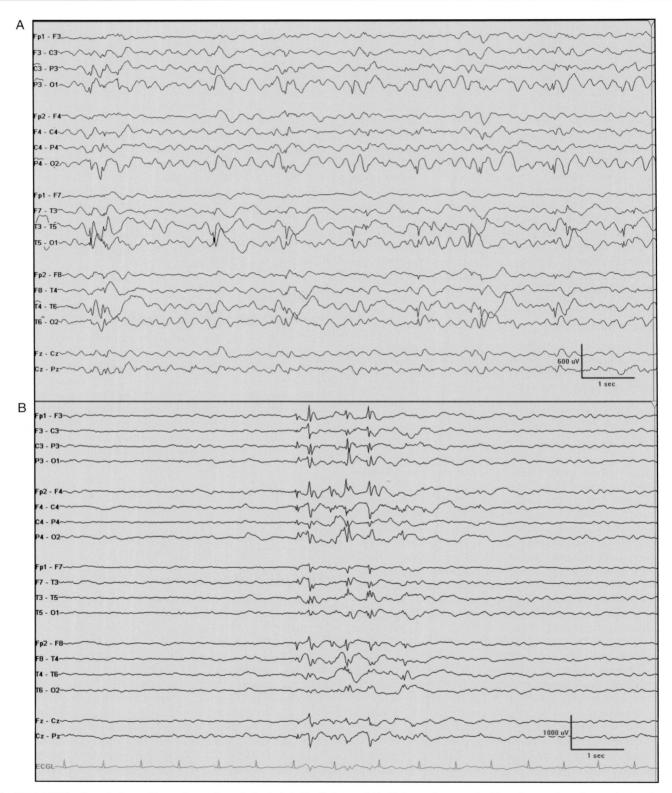

Fig. 54-3 EEG findings in Dravet's syndrome in an infant. A, In the first year of life EEGs may be normal, although posterior spikes and polyspikes are sometimes seen, as in this child at 10 months. **B,** Later, generalized spike and polyspike-wave discharges are noted. This is the same child 2 years later.

usually become secondarily generalized. In such cases, the focal onset of the seizure usually is not observed, but parents are alerted by the sounds of the secondarily generalized convulsion. The prognosis is good, and seizures remit by adolescence.

The EEG abnormality also resolves, although spikes may persist long after seizures have ceased.

Prior genetic studies indicate that the EEG trait itself is controlled by an autosomal-dominant gene with age-dependent

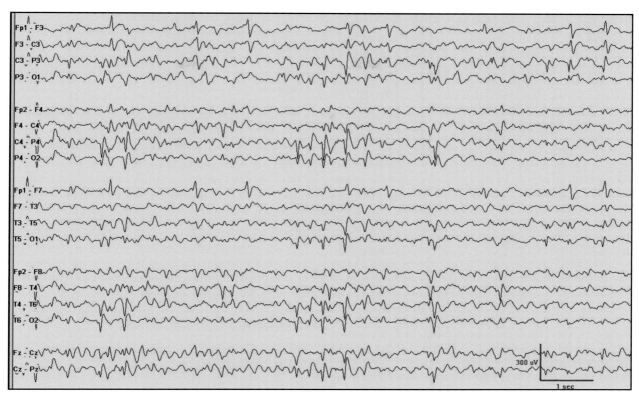

Fig. 54-4 **This EEG shows the highly stereotyped epileptiform discharges seen in a 3-year-old child with Panayiotopoulos' syndrome.** Occipital spikes are well known to occur in this syndrome, but spikes may be present in other locations as well.

penetrance [Bray and Wiser, 1965; Heijbel et al., 1975]. However, work done from recent multi-institutional twin studies suggests that the genetic contributions to the epilepsy per se appear to play a relatively minor role [Vadlamudi et al., 2006]. In the case of benign focal epilepsy with central-midtemporal spikes, more than half of siblings who have typical central-midtemporal spikes on EEG never have clinical attacks.

EEG findings are distinctive and diagnostic in benign focal epilepsy with central-midtemporal spikes. Focal di- or triphasic sharp waves of almost invariant morphology occur in the central and midtemporal regions (see Figure 54-1). Epileptiform discharges usually are of high voltage (greater than 100 mV), tend to occur in clusters, and activate dramatically during sleep, when they may seem almost continuous. In a single EEG, discharges may be unilateral, but with prolonged or repeated recordings, they are almost always bilateral. Lateralization may switch in serial tracings [Lerman, 1985]. Generalized spikes and spike-and-wave activity occasionally occur, although more often the spikes are maximal in either central region and are simply bisynchronous. "Benign" occipital spikes or multifocal spikes may coexist, especially in younger patients.

No correlation has been found between EEG findings and seizure occurrence or frequency. As a rule, EEG abnormalities are much more impressive than clinical seizure activity. Indeed, when central-midtemporal spikes are recorded in children without seizures, in whom EEGs are performed for other reasons, typical seizures eventually develop in only approximately half of the children. Furthermore, in symptomatic children, EEG abnormalities persist long after seizures cease. Thus, EEG does not provide assistance in making decisions about when or how long to treat. When treatment is elected because

of recurrent attacks that are interfering with the child's function or because of parental concern, carbamazepine and gabapentin are options. In some European countries, sulthiame (a drug not readily available in the United States) is used because of its reported beneficial effects of reducing spike frequency and clinical tolerance [Bast et al., 2003; Rating et al., 2000]. In addition, some authors are concerned that certain drugs (carbamazepine and lamotrigine, in particular) may aggravate this form of epilepsy [Cerminara et al., 2004; Parmeggiani et al., 2004], although such exacerbation appears to be rare [Corda et al., 2001].

Benign Focal Epilepsy with Occipital Spikes

Gastaut [1982] described another form of idiopathic localization-related epilepsy in children, in which visual symptoms, either amblyopia or hallucinations, are a common early feature of ictal events. The EEG shows stereotypic, high-voltage (200–300 mV) sharp-wave discharges over one or both occipital regions. Epileptiform activity is attenuated by eye opening and activated by sleep. Discharge morphology resembles that of central-midtemporal spikes. Background activity is normal. This electroclinical entity is more heterogeneous than benign focal epilepsy with central-midtemporal spikes. None the less, in a typical case, outcome usually is excellent, with complete resolution of clinical and EEG abnormalities in most children by 18 years of age. Like central-midtemporal spikes, occipital spikes do not correlate with clinical seizure activity or prognosis, and they often persist after seizures cease. Generalized spike-and-wave discharges and central-midtemporal spikes can coexist.

Acquired Epileptic Aphasia (Landau–Kleffner Syndrome)

Acquired epileptic aphasia, also known as Landau–Kleffner syndrome, is not a primary epileptic disorder, although epileptiform activity is one of the diagnostic criteria (see Chapter 55). Seizures occur in about 70 percent of cases but usually are infrequent. The syndrome is one of typically healthy children who acutely, or sometimes with a fluctuating course, lose previously acquired language skills. The aphasia begins with verbal auditory agnosia, and EEGs show abundant, high-voltage epileptiform activity that can be temporal, bitemporal, or generalized. Considerable slow-wave activity accompanies epileptiform discharges. In the early stages, EEG abnormalities may occur only during sleep, and throughout the illness, slow-wave sleep produces marked activation, sometimes with almost continuous generalized spike-and-wave activity. Review of original and subsequent cases of Landau–Kleffner syndrome does not support any single EEG feature or combination of features as being distinctive of this syndrome [Holmes et al., 1981; Landau and Kleffner, 1957]. AED treatment does not clearly alter the natural evolution of EEG abnormalities, clinical findings, or outcome, but corticosteroids may be of benefit [Lerman, 1991; Marescaux et al., 1990]. Subpial transections or focal resections are sometimes performed to treat acquired epileptic aphasia, but a surgical survey showed that they are rarely carried out and constitute less than 2 percent of all surgical procedures for epilepsy [Harvey et al., 2008].

Autosomal-Dominant Familial Nocturnal Frontal Lobe Epilepsy

Autosomal-dominant familial nocturnal frontal lobe epilepsy is characterized by clusters of brief hypermotor and tonic seizures with a nocturnal predominance. Onset typically is in childhood, and seizures may persist through life, with a wide variation in the severity of presentation. The ictal EEG shows bilateral anterior ictal discharges, but interictal findings usually are normal. Three different mutations in the gene encoding the alpha 4 subunit of a neuronal nicotinic acetylcholine receptor (*CHRNA4*) on chromosomal region 20q13.2 have been described, and other mutations in the gene encoding the beta 2 subunit of the neuronal nicotinic acetylcholine receptor (*CHRNB2*) on 1p21 were identified [Phillips et al., 1995, 2001]. Mutations in *CHRNA2* have also been noted, and currently, testing is clinically available for all three genes. The topic has been recently updated by Hirose and Kurahashi on GeneReviews. Carbamazepine is effective in 70 percent of individuals; some with mutations in *CHRNA4* respond better to zonisamide. At least one-third of patients may be refractory and require trials of multiple different AEDs. The susceptibility to seizures is lifelong, although the severity may lessen as patients reach middle age. The risk to each offspring of inheriting the mutant allele is 50 percent, but penetrance is estimated to be 70 percent and so the risk of inheriting the epilepsy is about 35 percent [Hirose and Kurahashi, 2010].

Adolescence–Adulthood

Autosomal-Dominant Epilepsy with Auditory Features

Mutations in *LGI1* cause autosomal-dominant partial epilepsy with auditory features, a form of familial temporal lobe epilepsy with auditory ictal manifestations. This disorder is characterized by simple partial seizures with auditory symptoms and secondary generalization. Sensory and psychic symptoms also may be present. Typical age at onset is in the first two decades [Ottman et al., 2004]. The most common auditory symptoms are simple, unformed sounds (e.g., buzzing, ringing).

Less Specific Age Relationship

Familial Focal Epilepsy with Variable Foci

Another epilepsy characterized by focal seizures but with a less specific age relationship is familial focal epilepsy with variable foci. Members of affected families have focal seizures with a variety of foci. The onset of seizures typically is in middle childhood, and attacks usually are easy to control. Seizure semiology varies among family members but is stereotypic for each affected person. In some reports, a pattern of nocturnal frontal lobe seizures suggested autosomal-dominant familial nocturnal frontal lobe epilepsy. Linkage to chromosome 22q has been found [Callenbach et al., 2003].

Distinctive Constellations

Mesial Temporal Lobe Epilepsy with Hippocampal Sclerosis

In mesial temporal lobe epilepsy with hippocampal sclerosis (MTLE with HS), seizures involving the limbic structures produce characteristic clinical and electrographic features. Patients may complain of a rising epigastric aura or an indescribable sensation. Propagation of the ictal discharges can cause alteration of consciousness. Observers can document alteration of consciousness by asking the child to carry out simple commands such as "point to the door," and to remember a peculiar test item such as "purple elephant." Amnesia can be ascertained by asking about this test item after the seizure is finished and the child's clinical condition has returned to baseline. Other characteristic clinical features that may evolve are ipsilateral picking automatisms and contralateral hand dystonic postures. Seizures may secondarily generalize; this sequence often begins with contralateral head and eye version, followed by contralateral clonus. This sequence represents a mature pattern, usually seen beyond the age of 6 years. In younger children, only fragments of this activity may be seen [Nordli et al., 2001].

Mesial temporal sclerosis (MTS) is a condition characterized by pathologic changes in the medial temporal region (Figure 54-5). It is a common cause of refractory temporal lobe seizures in adults that come to epilepsy surgery, but it is not commonly seen in population-based studies in children. Indeed, Berg et al. [2000a] found that only 3 children of 613 with epilepsy had evidence of hippocampal atrophy on their scans. One of these patients was later found to have a tumor. One possible explanation for this discrepancy is that mesial temporal sclerosis may be an acquired lesion. Indeed, pediatric operations for MTS are relatively rare worldwide [Harvey et al., 2008].

As mentioned, MTS frequently has been found in patients who have undergone temporal lobectomy for uncontrolled complex partial seizures [Corsellis and Meldrum, 1976]. Such sclerosis may also affect the amygdala and the parahippocampal gyrus. Patients who have undergone temporal lobectomy with subsequent pathologic documentation of MTS frequently

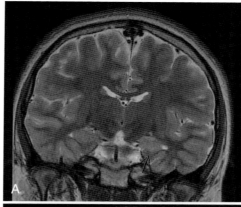
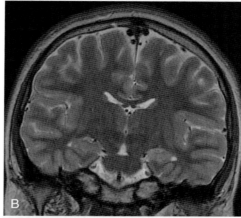
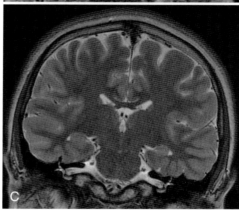

Fig. 54-5 Magnetic resonance image showing left mesial temporal sclerosis in an 8-year-old girl. A, The arrow shows increased T2 signal within the hippocampus. **B** and **C,** These images also demonstrate the reduced volume of the left hippocampus as compared with the right. The patient was seizure-free after resection of the left hippocampus.

experience prolonged febrile convulsions in infancy and early childhood. Ounsted et al. [1966] stressed that early-onset seizures and severe generalized tonic-clonic seizures, accompanied by a high frequency of temporal lobe attacks, were associated with an adverse prognosis. Meldrum [1978] stressed the metabolic process by which neuronal hippocampal changes could be produced by recurrent seizures. Prospective epidemiologic studies have failed to prove a clear connection between prolonged febrile convulsions and mesial temporal sclerosis, but experience at surgical centers suggests that many patients

with MTS have had prolonged febrile convulsions in early life. Magnetic resonance imaging (MRI) studies have shown acute and chronic changes in the hippocampi of children with prolonged febrile seizures [VanLandingham et al., 1998; Provenzale et al., 2008]. In these studies, increased T2 signal in the hippocampus was predictive of development of hippocampal atrophy. A large prospective study of children with febrile status epilepticus (FEBSTAT) is on-going in the US, which will hopefully address this important issue, but an association between prolonged febrile seizures and MTS appears likely from the published literature to date.

Brain MRI is very helpful in establishing the diagnosis of MTS [Woermann and Vollmar, 2009]. The afflicted hippocampus can be best visualized in coronal sequences obtained orthogonal to the long axis of the temporal lobe. Combinations of high-resolution images, inversion recovery sequences, and thin-cut images are used to compare the morphology, signal characteristics, and size of the hippocampus and adjacent structures. Characteristically, the interictal EEG shows focal pleomorphic interictal epileptiform discharges in the anterior to midtemporal region. Additional electrode placements, including anterior temporal and subtemporal leads, may assist in the detection and characterization of the interictal epileptiform discharges. The ictal EEG may reveal broad, relatively nonlocalizing, delta discharges at onset, but evolution to a rhythmic theta-alpha pattern within the first 10–20 seconds is a supportive feature. Patients with this lesion who have intractable epilepsy usually respond favorably to focal resection of the involved anterior temporal region. A randomized study of patients with temporal lobe epilepsy showed the superiority of surgical over medical management of MTS [Wiebe et al., 2001]. These results argue for early and aggressive surgical management of patients with intractable seizures resulting from MTS.

Epilepsia Partialis Continua and Rasmussen's Syndrome

Another important epilepsy constellation presenting with focal seizures is epilepsia partialis continua manifesting as Rasmussen's syndrome. Epilepsia partialis continua may be seen in a wide variety of clinical circumstances related to focal structural and metabolic lesions. In children, it may occur as a progressive entity with concurrent loss of motor skills [Rasmussen and McCann, 1968]. In a majority of patients, onset is before age 10 years. About two-thirds of children or their family members have an infectious or inflammatory illness before the onset of the epilepsia partialis continua. The first seizures are reported as generalized, and the intractable focal nature of the attack becomes apparent only over time. When fully established, the syndrome is characterized by unremitting seizure activity limited to part or one side of the body. Unlike those in more typical simple focal seizures of motor type, muscle movements usually are asynchronous in different muscle groups and seem to ebb and flow in waves, sometimes involving fewer muscles, sometimes more. The clinical course is marked by slow neurologic deterioration with development of hemiparesis, diminished mental capacity, and usually, hemianopia. Although progressive, the disease is only rarely fatal, and a permanent but stable neurologic deficit emerges.

Although childhood epilepsia partialis continua is considered the result of chronic encephalitis, the cause is unknown

[Andrews and McNamara, 1996]. Evidence of anti-glutamate receptor (anti-Glu R3) antibodies suggests that an autoimmune process may be involved, but this has not been substantiated. Focal motor seizures often are associated with myoclonus, which may appear early. Progressive motor deficits develop during the illness, as does loss of mental function. The seizures are extremely resistant to treatment, and the condition usually progresses to complete hemiplegia with progressive unilateral brain atrophy [Andermann, 1991].

EEG findings are variable, and their topography often is difficult to characterize precisely [Bancaud, 1985]. Most often, interictal EEGs show excessive dysrhythmic or rhythmic delta activity, which is usually bilateral but accentuated over a large area contralateral to the partial seizures. Epileptiform discharges are rarely well localized and often are sporadic, especially early in the illness. As the disease progresses, more abundant pleomorphic spike and sharp-wave discharges appear over an extensive area or in both hemispheres. With scalp recordings, it is usually difficult to recognize distinct ictal discharges, and correlation of EEG changes with muscle jerking is always poor to nonexistent.

The evaluation of patients with possible Rasmussen's syndrome is heavily dependent upon brain imaging, with important contributions from the clinical presentation and EEG. Progressive atrophy of one hemisphere, often heralded by a reduced size of the caudate along with a predominance of frontal atrophy, is strongly suggestive of this syndrome. Unilateral EEG findings of slowing, attenuation, and multiple populations of spikes predominantly within one hemisphere support the diagnosis. Patients with anti-GAD (glutamic acid decarboxylase) antibodies have been noted to have epilepsia partialis continua, but this can be easily excluded by a serum test searching for the presence of the antibodies. Children with Alpers' disease can present with epilepsia partialis continua and recurrent bouts of focal status epilepticus, but brain atrophy and EEG changes will be more widespread. Metabolic acidosis and strokelike episodes (MELAS) can also present with epilepsia partialis continua and may have increased T2 signal, particularly in the posterior regions. Serum lactate measurement will help to exclude this condition. Perhaps the most difficult diagnosis to exclude is cerebral vasculitis. The absence of substantial gadolinium enhancement and calcifications can help to argue against this diagnosis. A European consensus conference concluded that, if the patient has epilepsia partialis continua, the EEG features are unilateral, and the imaging findings show progressive atrophy, then Rasmussen's syndrome is highly likely and a brain biopsy is not needed [Bien et al., 2005]. In cases where the diagnosis is in doubt, the pathologic findings are microglial nodules and perivascular lymphocytes.

Immunomodulatory treatment with intravenous immunoglobulin or plasmapheresis has been tried and may ameliorate the clinical symptoms, including the epilepsy [Schmalbach and Lang, 2009]. The unanswered question is whether this approach can completely halt progression of the disease and avert the need for surgery. Even if successful, it is conceivable that medical treatment may only delay the inevitable definitive treatment: hemispherectomy. A complete disconnection of the involved hemisphere is necessary for good results. This can be achieved by a variety of surgical approaches, but a common modification of the standard anatomical hemispherectomy involves removing the temporal and inferior frontal lobes, thereby creating a window for the operating microscope.

The surgeon can then complete a disconnection of the corpus callosum, as well as the frontal and occipital lobes, without resecting those regions. This modification can reduce the need for ventriculoperitoneal shunting and other complications, but may have a higher failure rate because of the difficulty of completely disconnecting the inferior frontal lobe and insula. Even when successful, surgery may not be able to reverse the cognitive disabilities [Terra-Bustamante et al., 2009].

Epilepsies Attributed to and Organized by Structural Metabolic Causes

The recent ILAE revised terminology suggests this etiological group to replace the former symptomatic epilepsy designation [Berg et al., 2010]. Major causes of epilepsy in this group include cortical malformations, neurocutaneous syndromes, tumors, infections, trauma, vascular lesions, prenatal insults, and others. Epilepsy due to structural or metabolic causes may manifest at any age with focal seizures. The clinical presentation varies widely, depending on the age of the patient, degree of cerebral maturation, location of the epileptogenic focus, and integrity of the underlying nervous system.

Although partial seizures are more likely to be associated with focal hemispheric lesions than are generalized seizures, structural causes are rarely identified. In children, approximately 30–50 percent of these seizures have no determinable etiology, whereas others have vague putative causes, such as a difficult delivery at birth or early childhood head trauma that cannot be substantiated. Moreover, genetic factors evidently determine susceptibility to focal seizures. An important exception is infants, in whom the rate of brain abnormalities may be higher [Hsieh et al., 2010]. In the past, prenatal and perinatal complications were thought to cause pediatric seizure disorders, but more recent epidemiologic evidence suggests that cerebral malformations are the most commonly identified underlying cause. Berg et al. [2000a] found that 16 of 613 children with epilepsy had cortical malformations, whereas 13 had presumed intrauterine insults, 8 had a neurocutaneous syndrome, and 5 had intraventricular hemorrhage. Only 1 had an anoxic encephalopathy, and 3 had defined genetic or chromosomal abnormalities. Four patients had tumors, 3 had vascular lesions, and 3 had clear evidence of an infectious disorder (based on neuroimaging). Only 2 patients had neuroimaging findings indicating previous brain trauma.

Cortical Malformations

Cortical malformations are more commonly diagnosed today because of the widespread availability of MRI scanning and better appreciation of the subtle findings in some of these conditions. Of particular importance for focal seizures are focal and hemispheric malformations, including cortical dysplasia (Taylor types I and II), schizencephaly, isolated heterotopias, and hemimegalencephaly. Patients with lissencephaly may have focal seizures, but the widespread nature of the malformation places patients with this disorder in the generalized symptomatic epilepsy syndrome category. EEG clues to the presence of a cortical malformation may be the presence of periodic spikes or precocious fast rhythms early in life. This latter feature can be responsible for an incorrect EEG lateralization of the abnormal hemisphere in hemimegalencephaly. The electroencephalographer must be alert to the invariant peculiar quality of the precocious alpha rhythm over the involved hemisphere in this disorder, particularly during the first year of life.

Congenital and Perinatal Factors

Chromosomal pathologic conditions may result in malformations. Intrauterine infections, specifically cytomegalic inclusion disease, toxoplasmosis, and rubella, are well known for their ability to cause abnormal brain development. Syphilis, rare in many parts of the world, also may cause intrauterine brain infection, with severe neurologic residua. Maternal exposure to radiation during pregnancy or ingestion by the mother of teratogenic drugs also may lead to cerebral malformations. In addition to other manifestations, these disorders also may result in focal and multifocal seizures. An unusual seizure type, myoclonic spasms, sometimes results from intrauterine infections. Tuberous sclerosis may manifest during the first few months of life and may be accompanied by focal seizures or infantile myoclonic spasms. Other causes of seizures in the perinatal period are discussed in Chapter 16.

Brain Tumors

Tumors are an uncommon cause of seizures during childhood. Tumors occur less frequently in children than in adults, and are more commonly found in regions of the brain that are not predisposed to developing epileptogenic activity (e.g., thalamus, cerebellum, brainstem). None the less, focal seizures in children can be caused by tumors [Backus and Millichap, 1962]. In a study of 100 patients with seizures of focal origin, 4 had associated hemispheric gliomas and 2 had arteriovenous malformations. During the subsequent 10 years, temporal lobe tumors were discovered in 3 additional patients. A more recent study using a community-based approach and modern imaging techniques revealed brain tumors in only 4 of 613 children with epilepsy. One case each of ganglioglioma, astrocytoma grade II, dysembryoblastic neuroepithelial tumor, and oligodendroglioma was reported [Berg et al., 2000a].

Although MRI has facilitated the diagnosis of tumors, older studies clearly had a skewed perspective, owing to ascertainment bias. Tumors that are relatively less malignant and slow-growing are more often associated with seizures than are malignant tumors. Nevertheless, focal seizures accompanied by a history of headaches may be caused by tumor.

Postnatal Infectious Diseases

Seizures often are the first indication of bacterial meningitis in infants and children; moreover, seizures frequently are associated with established bacterial meningitis. The simultaneous presence of generalized seizures and fever generally suggests bacterial meningitis. Mechanisms of seizure production in bacterial meningitis include cortical vein and sagittal sinus thrombosis, primary involvement of the cortical tissue, cerebritis and subsequent abscess formation, and subdural effusions. Hydrocephalus and seizures may result from ependymitis, ventriculitis, or involvement of the meninges with subsequent impairment of spinal fluid absorption.

Focal or multifocal seizures may be associated with viral encephalitis. Many patients with viral encephalitis have only minor neurologic impairment, and their seizures may be transient. Conversely, severe encephalitis, resulting from herpes simplex virus or Epstein–Barr virus, both of which preferentially affect the temporal lobes, may result in severe sequelae with intractable seizures and permanent intellectual and memory dysfunction. Subacute sclerosing panencephalitis is associated with rubeola infection. This condition often is heralded by multifocal myoclonic seizures and focal and multifocal seizures. Diphtheria-pertussis-tetanus immunization may be followed by focal or generalized seizures. It generally is believed that these seizures are fever-induced and that pertussis encephalopathy is exceedingly rare. Parasitic infestation (see Chapter 82) may result in focal seizures. In particular, cysticercosis is accompanied by circumscribed cortical cysts and acute obstructive hydrocephalus. Echinococcosis is another parasitic infection that results in focal brain lesions. Tuberculosis with tuberculoma formation in the brain continues to be a problem in certain areas of the world.

Trauma

One of the most important consequences of traumatic brain injury is the development of convulsions, although the incidence depends on many factors, including injury severity. Epilepsy occurs more frequently after penetrating wounds [Raymont et al., 2010]. In closed head injuries, which constitute most of the wounds suffered by the general population, the incidence of traumatic epilepsy is relatively low. Cerebral damage during or near the time of birth may be manifested by early or late seizures. The effect of closed head injuries depends on the mechanical factors involved. In children, the most frequent traumatic causes of epilepsy are linear or depressed skull fractures. Except for some instances of early traumatic epilepsy after relatively trivial injury, the incidence of epilepsy after head trauma is generally proportional to the duration of post-traumatic amnesia.

Although epilepsy develops in nearly 50 percent of patients with penetrating head wounds and dural tears, seizures develop in only about 5 percent of patients after closed head injury [Jennett, 1975]. In a community-based study of 613 children with epilepsy in Connecticut, Berg and co-investigators found that only 2 children had neuroimaging findings consistent with trauma [Berg et al., 2000a].

Focal seizures may result from subdural hematomas in childhood; multifocal seizures can result from bilateral subdural hematomas. Bilateral subdural hematomas frequently are found in infants. Unless they are acute, an associated increase in the occipitofrontal circumference, along with increased tension of the anterior fontanel, is common. Nonaccidental trauma must be considered in the differential diagnosis in these cases, particularly with other associated features such as parenchymal brain lesions, retinal hemorrhages, or bone fractures.

Cerebrovascular Disease

Focal seizures in children rarely result from cerebrovascular disease [Chadehumbe et al., 2009]. Sturge–Weber syndrome (i.e., encephalofacial angiomatosis) usually manifests with a port-wine nevus in the distribution of one or more divisions of cranial nerve V. The associated angiomatosis is found over the ipsilateral cortex in the pia-arachnoid. The associated gyri are atrophied, and linear calcifications may be present, most often in the occipital lobes. Other features may include brain hypoplasia and focal seizures; hemiparesis may compromise the contralateral extremities [Thomas-Sohl et al., 2004]. Hemispherectomy often is indicated and likely should be undertaken early in life when seizures are intractable, and particularly when learning is impaired and a hemiplegia exists [Vining et al., 1997]. As a cautionary note, Kosoff and colleagues did not find a clear improvement in development in those children who underwent surgical treatment for their disease [Kossoff et al., 2002].

Management

Evaluation

Epilepsy syndromes can be identified by considering the age, functional developmental level of the child, clinical features of the seizures, and the interictal EEG findings. Those with favorable prognoses often occur against the backdrop of a normally developing child with either a normal interictal EEG or an EEG that shows highly stereotyped spikes. If the clinical features and EEG findings are not consistent with an epilepsy with a favorable prognosis, then MRI scanning is indicated. In the experience of Berg and colleagues, 177 of 613 children had symptomatic localization-related epilepsy, and findings on MRI were abnormal in 28.3 percent of these children [Berg et al., 2000a]. Any focal features on the neurologic examination or concerning interictal EEG characteristics (focal slowing, focal attenuation, focal polymorphic spikes) require follow-up imaging, and the location of the same findings can help to guide the MRI so that a specific target can be carefully examined (see Figure 54-1). Infants are a special category. While there are favorable forms of epilepsy in infancy, these are relatively uncommon. Indeed, recent imaging studies have suggested that all infants with recurrent seizures should have an MRI because of the low rate of generalized seizures and high rates of cortical malformations [Hsieh et al., 2010].

Berg et al. [2000a] studied 613 children with epilepsy. Neuroimaging was performed in a majority of these children (78.7 percent), but there was a very low rate of abnormalities in those with clear idiopathic localization-related epilepsy. Interictal EEG findings that suggest an idiopathic form of localization-related epilepsy include the presence of a normal background, lack of focal slowing, and stereotypic spikes in which each interictal epileptiform discharge closely resembles the other (see Figure 54-1). Guidelines for the evaluation of the first afebrile seizure have been published, and the recommendations concur that neuroimaging is not necessary in all cases [Hirtz et al., 2000].

Treatment

If the child is determined to have a favorable form of epilepsy presenting with focal seizures, then therapy should not be automatic, even if several seizures have occurred. It can be particularly useful to discuss precipitating factors with the parents and to give appropriate anticipatory guidance and counseling. A useful point to highlight is the importance of good sleep hygiene, keeping the same bedtime within an hour or so for weekdays and weekends. If therapy is warranted, carbamazepine, which is widely used in the United States, can be given, although many European practitioners avoid this drug because of concerns of aggravating the epilepsy. In Europe, valproate is still one of the most widely used medications [van de Vrie-Hoekstra et al., 2008]. A task force from the American Academy of Neurology and American Epilepsy Society recently reviewed the literature on AEDs for treatment of new-onset seizures and concluded that treatment could begin with any of the classic medications: carbamazepine, phenobarbital, phenytoin, or valproate. In addition, the task-force findings supported use of gabapentin, lamotrigine, oxcarbazepine, or topiramate as an alternative [French et al., 2004a]. A careful consideration of the side-effect profile of the various drugs in pediatrics is important before a specific AED is selected.

Four drugs, all released before 1978, have been most frequently used in pediatrics for focal seizures: carbamazepine, phenobarbital, phenytoin, and valproate. None is clearly superior to the others [Mattson et al., 1985], although randomized studies have found a disproportionately high incidence of side effects with phenobarbital [de Silva et al., 1996]. For this reason, chronic use of phenobarbital should be avoided, even in infants, unless special circumstances prevail. Most clinicians use carbamazepine as a first-line drug for management of epilepsies with focal seizures. Phenytoin was a favorite choice in the past, but cosmetic side effects and complicated kinetics make it less attractive than other agents. With valproate, a concern is the possibility of idiosyncratic, potentially fatal hepatotoxicity, particularly in children younger than 2 years of age who are receiving two or more antiepileptic agents [Dreifuss and Santilli, 1986].

At least ten new drugs have become widely available since 1993: felbamate, gabapentin, lacosamide, lamotrigine, levetiracetam, oxcarbazepine, rufinamide, topiramate, vigabatrin, and zonisamide. A comprehensive review of eight of these demonstrated that there was a general lack of well-designed randomized controlled trials in children and virtually no comparative efficacy trials [Hwang and Kim, 2008]. It might be tempting to rely on recommendations from experts but this information could be wrong and certainly is not a substitute for more definitive trials. A detailed understanding of the side effects and pharmacology of these medications are helpful. This has been recently reviewed by Sarco and Bourgeois, and medications are discussed in detail in Chapter 59 of this book [Sarco and Bourgeois, 2010].

In those epilepsies with multifocal seizures or focal seizures in combination with generalized seizures, drugs with a broad spectrum of action are usually preferred to those with action only against focal seizures. No published guidelines or practice parameters that apply to these patients are available. The literature on the subject is limited, so only anecdotal advice can be provided. These epilepsies appear to respond better to an agent with a wider spectrum of action, such as valproate. Newer agents offer the hope of better side-effect profiles with equivalent effectiveness (Table 54-1), but comparative data in children are not sufficient to permit a strong recommendation for their use as first-line treatment. The classic broad-spectrum agent is valproate, but newer agents with broad profiles include felbamate, lamotrigine, levetiracetam, topiramate, and zonisamide.

Refractory Focal Seizures

Evidence to guide the order of selection of AEDs for children with refractory focal seizures rationally is scarce. According to the most recently published practice parameters,

Table 54-1 Practical Guide to Antiepileptic Drugs

Drug*	Use	How Supplied	Dosing	Starting Dose (mg/kg/day)	Starting Dose Duration	Maintenance Dose (mg/kg/day)	Blood Level† (µg/mL)
Phenobarbital (1912)	Broad spectrum	Suspension: 20 mg/5 mL Tablets: 15, 30, 60, 100 mg	four times a day—two times a day	3-5	Immediate	3-8	15-45
Phenytoin (1938) [Dilantin]	Focal	Suspension: 125 mg/mL Chewable Infatabs: 50 mg Capsules: 30, 100 mg	four times a day—three times a day	4-7	Immediate	4-7	10-25
Primidone (1949) [Mysoline]	Broad spectrum	Suspension: 250 mg/5 mL Tablets: 50, 250 mg	three times a day	5	Average: 2-3 wk	15	PRM: 4-12 PB: 15-40
Ethosuximide (1958) [Zarontin]	Absence	Suspension: 250 mg/5 mL Capsules: 250 mg	two times a day	10	Average: 2-3 wk	15-40	40-120
Carbamazepine (1968) [Tegretol, Tegretol-XR, Carbatrol]	Focal	Suspension: 100 mg/5 mL Chewable tab: 100 mg Tablets: 200 mg; timed-release [Tegretol-XR]: 100, 200, 400 mg Sprinkles: 100, 200, 300 mg [Carbatrol]	two times a day‡—three times a day	5	Average: 2-4 wk	12-20	4-12
Valproate (1978) [Depakene, Depakote]	Broad spectrum	Suspension: 250 mg/5 mL [Depakene] Capsules: 250 mg [Depakene] Sprinkles: 125 mg Tablets: 125, 250, 500 mg	two times a day—three times a day	10	Average: 2-4 wk	30-60	50-120
Felbamate (1993) [Felbatol]	Broad spectrum	Suspension: 600 mg/5 mL Tablets: 400, 600 mg	three times a day—four times a day	15	Average: 2-4 wk	45	18-45
Gabapentin (1993) [Neurontin]	Focal	Suspension: 250 mg/5 mL Capsules: 100, 300, 400 mg Tablets: 600, 800 mg	three times a day—four times a day	15	Quick: 1 wk	30-45	5-15†
Lamotrigine (1994) [Lamictal]	Broad spectrum	Tablets: 25, 100, 150, 200 mg; chewable: 2, 5, 25 mg	two times a day	0.2 (with VPA); 0.5 (with CBZ/PHT)	Slow: 2-4 mo Slow: 6-8 wk	1-5 5-15	2-20†
Topiramate (1996) [Topamax]	Broad spectrum	Tablets: 25, 100, 200 mg Sprinkles: 15, 25 mg	two times a day	1-2	Average: 2-4 wk	5-10	2-25†
Tiagabine (1997) [Gabitril]	Focal	Tablets: 2, 4, 12, 16, 20 mg	two times a day—three times a day	0.05	Average: 2-4 wk	1-2	5-70†
Levetiracetam (1999) [Keppra]	Broad spectrum	Tablets: 250, 500, 750 mg Suspension: 100 mg/mL	two times a day—three times a day	10	Average: 2-4 wk	20-45	20-60†
Oxcarbazepine (2000) [Trileptal]	Focal	Suspension: 300 mg/5 mL Tablets: 150, 300, 600 mg	two times a day	8-10	Average: 2-4 wk	20-40	5-50†
Zonisamide (2000) [Zonegran]	Broad spectrum	Capsules: 100 mg	four times a day—two times a day	2-4	Average: 2-4 wk	4-12	10-40†
Diazepam rectal gel (1997) [Diastat]	Emergency	Pediatric: 2.5, 5 mg Universal: 10 mg Adult: 15, 20 mg	p.r.n.	0.2-0.5 mg/kg			0.2-1.5
Lacosamide (2009) [Vimpat]	Focal	50,100,150, 200 mg	two times a day	50 mg daily (adults only)	Average 2-4 wk	200-400 mg/day (adults only)	?
Rufinamide (2008) [Banzel]	Broad spectrum (LGS)	Tablets: 200, 400 mg	two times a day	10 mg/kg/day	Average 1-2 wk	45 mg/kg/day	?

* Year of availability is given in parentheses; trade names appear in brackets.
† Not well established.
‡ Twice-daily dosing with Tegretol-XR or Carbatrol.
CBZ, carbamazepine; LGS, Lennox-Gastaut syndrome; PB, phenobarbital; PHT, phenytoin; PRM, primidone; VPA, valproate.

gabapentin, lamotrigine, oxcarbazepine, and topiramate are useful adjunctive agents in the treatment of refractory pediatric focal seizures [French et al., 2004b]. Evidence was insufficient to make any recommendations concerning the use of levetiracetam, tiagabine, or zonisamide for the treatment of refractory focal seizures. Updated guidelines are probably in order.

Relevant comparative drug trials are lacking to assist the clinician in the selection of the best medications in most of the pediatric epilepsies. Considerations in management include the selection of the initial medication, the second or third choice for persistent seizures, and whether it is better to treat with combination therapy or monotherapy in refractory cases. Treatment strategies change over time, with the current trend being to use drugs in sequential monotherapy, although, in practice, some overlap between agents is almost always present. A recurrent theme that reverberates in the epilepsy community is rational polypharmacy versus sequential monotherapy. A pediatric consortium is needed to address the following issues:

1. For selected epilepsy syndromes, what is the best initial treatment?
2. What is the proper order for trial of medications if the first medication fails?
3. Do patients benefit from combination therapy or is sequential monotherapy superior?
4. For how long should a child be given a trial with medications if a focal lesion is present and seizures are intractable?

Long-Term Outcome and Multidisciplinary Issues

Pediatric epilepsy is more than just two afebrile seizures. Environmental and genetic factors that cause susceptibility to recurrent seizures also may increase the risk for other manifestations of central nervous system dysfunction, including psychopathology, attention difficulties, behavioral disorders, and socialization problems (see Chapter 62). Like the seizures themselves, these clinical features may be expressed only during special developmental windows and, if not promptly recognized and treated, can have long-lasting insidious effects. Sillanpaa et al. [1998] have found that children with epilepsy are at increased risk of failing to match the social, educational, and vocational achievement of their peers. A multidisciplinary team approach to epilepsy can address these concerns by effectively screening at-risk patients and referring affected children to health-care professionals with special expertise. This process moves in parallel with the medical evaluation of the seizures, but careful case management by experienced personnel also is required. Resources vary in different regions and facilities, but intermittent multidisciplinary meetings can facilitate optimal care. Specialized epilepsy centers often are staffed with such teams, and children with refractory epilepsies may benefit from these services. The ultimate goal of treatment is not just seizure control but also maximization of the long-term potential of the child with epilepsy.

Acknowledgments

I would like to recognize the contribution of the late Dr. Fritz Dreifuss to this chapter.

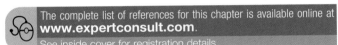

Epilepsy and Neurodevelopmental Disorders

Roberto Tuchman

Introduction

The association of epilepsy with neurodevelopmental disorders is now well established. Children with developmental epilepsies are at increased risk for cognitive [Hermann and Seidenberg, 2007], neurobehavioral [Hermann et al., 2008], and psychiatric disorders [Plioplys et al., 2007]. Specific factors associated with a higher risk of neuropsychological deficits in children with epilepsy include multiple seizures, use of antiepileptic drugs, etiology, and interictal epileptiform discharges (IEDs) on the initial electroencephalogram (EEG) [Fastenau et al., 2009]. In children with epilepsy, younger age at seizure onset, cognitive impairment, temporal or frontal lobe onset of seizures, and intractable epilepsy are associated with an increased likelihood of coexisting social, communication, and behavioral disorders [Hamiwka and Wirrell, 2009]. The multiple complex and confounding risk factors that account for the coexistence of epilepsy and neurodevelopmental disorders include etiology, associated disabilities, seizure type, frequency, duration, control, age of onset, and IEDs, as well as psychosocial factors and medication effects [Austin and Caplan, 2007].

The relationship between epilepsy and neurodevelopmental disorders also reflects common pathologies and mechanisms [Tuchman et al., 2009], and there is accumulating evidence to suggest that cognitive and behavioral impairments may precede the onset of seizures [Austin et al., 2001; Oostrom et al., 2003; Bhise et al., 2009; Fastenau et al., 2009]. On the other hand, there is evidence that recurrent seizures or IEDs can cause acute and long-lasting impairment of brain function and development [Holmes and Lenck-Santini, 2006; Galanopoulou and Moshe, 2009], and significant efforts are being made to determine how risk factors contribute to developmental outcomes in children with epilepsy [Austin and Fastenau, 2009]. The notion that epileptic activity, seizures, or IEDs can lead to cognitive and behavioral impairment above and beyond what might be expected from the underlying pathology is exemplified by the concept of epileptic encephalopathy [Berg et al., 2009]. This idea has important implications for treatment, especially in children with an epileptic encephalopathy, in whom early and successful treatment of seizures and interictal epileptiform activity may be crucial to positive neurodevelopmental outcomes [Freitag and Tuxhorn, 2005; Jonas et al., 2005; Lux et al., 2005; Arts and Geerts, 2009; Bombardieri et al., 2009].

Epilepsy is more frequent in children with intellectual disability [Goulden et al., 1991]; the behavioral, cognitive, and social aspects of epilepsy are multiple and diverse, and are discussed in Chapter 62. This present chapter focuses on the concept of epileptic encephalopathy and the association of epilepsy and IEDs with specific language impairments and autistic spectrum disorders (ASDs). In addition, the common mechanisms of disease and management of children with developmental epilepsies and neurodevelopmental disorders are addressed.

Epileptic Encephalopathies

The epileptic encephalopathies can occur at any age, but are more common and severe in the first decade of life as the brain is developing. Approximately 40 percent of epilepsies occurring during the first 3 years of life are associated with an epileptic encephalopathy [Guerrini, 2006]. Epileptic encephalopathy of childhood includes: early myoclonic encephalopathy (Ohtahara's or Aicardi's syndrome), severe myoclonic epilepsy of infancy (Dravet's syndrome), myoclonic-astatic epilepsy of early childhood (Doose's syndrome), infantile spasms (West's syndrome), Lennox–Gastaut syndrome, and Landau–Kleffner syndrome-continuous spike waves during slow-wave sleep [Engel, 2001].

The myoclonic epilepsies and infantile spasms are discussed in Chapter 56 and Lennox–Gastaut syndrome in Chapter 53. In this chapter, Dravet's syndrome, infantile spasms, Lennox–Gastaut syndrome, Landau–Kleffner syndrome, and continuous spike waves during slow-wave sleep will be discussed from a developmental perspective. Specifically, the impact of seizures and of IEDs on the developmental trajectories of children with these electroclinical syndromes will be emphasized.

Dravet's Syndrome

Dravet's syndrome is a genetically determined infantile epileptic encephalopathy, mainly caused by de novo mutations in the *SCN1A* gene [Scheffer et al., 2009]. Early development is normal, with seizures usually beginning in the first 10 months of life; these become frequent by 2–4 years of age, with focal and generalized myoclonus, atypical absences, and partial complex seizures, as well as seizures characterized by fluctuating alteration of consciousness with reduced postural tone and myoclonic jerks [Millichap et al., 2009]. Despite frequent seizures, the EEG is usually normal in the first 2 years of life and then usually progresses into spike and wave and multifocal discharges, although some children may have persistently normal interictal EEG studies [Korff et al., 2007]. Progressive decline or plateau in development occurs by 1–4 years of age, with intellectual disability and an autism phenotype commonly present, especially in those with more than five seizures per month [Scheffer et al., 2009].

Genes associated with Dravet's syndrome appear to have relevance to the neurodevelopmental disorders, such as ASDs. Specifically, a susceptibility locus for ASDs has been found on chromosome 2 in the vicinity of the epilepsy-involved genes *SCN1A* and *SCN2A* [Weiss et al., 2003], while *PCDH10* on chromosome 4 has been linked to ASDs in families with shared ancestry [Morrow et al., 2008]. Recently, a sporadic infantile epileptic encephalopathy that resembles Dravet's syndrome has been tied to mutations in *PCDH19* [Depienne et al., 2009]. These results hint strongly at possible shared molecular underpinnings between ASD and this epileptic encephalopathy.

Infantile Spasms

Infantile spasms constitute an age-specific seizure disorder, with a peak age of presentation between 4 and 8 months of age, a critical time of brain development [Zupanc, 2009]. There is a strong correlation between infantile spasms and intellectual disability [Trevathan et al., 1999], and the majority of children with infantile spasms develop intellectual disability and specific cognitive and behavioral deficits [Riikonen, 2001]. In addition, the association of infantile spasms and ASDs is well recognized [Riikonen and Amnell, 1981]; in children with infantile spasms the prevalence of ASDs is as high as 35 percent, depending on the severity of intellectual disability [Saemundsen et al., 2007], with a heightened risk of ASDs in the presence of identifiable structural lesions of the brain [Saemundsen et al., 2008]. Further, in children with infantile spasms, EEG epileptiform activity – particularly bilateral frontal EEG discharges and persistence of hypsarrhythmia – contributes to the development of the autism phenotype [Kayaalp et al., 2007].

One of the intriguing features of infantile spasms is that the severity and, to a certain extent, the frequency of seizures do not seem to correlate with the degree of cognitive impairment or the occurrence of regression [Riikonen, 1984; Bednarek et al., 1998]. It may be that the interictal EEG pattern of hypsarrhythmia associated with infantile spasms affects cortical and subcortical neuronal networks, resulting in abnormal synaptogenesis and poor developmental outcomes [Zupanc, 2009].

Lennox–Gastaut Syndrome

Lennox–Gastaut syndrome is an age-specific epileptic syndrome that peaks between 3 and 5 years; it is characterized by multiple seizure types that include tonic and atonic seizures, atypical absences, and myoclonic and generalized or focal seizures, in association with a characteristic EEG pattern of slow spike-and-wave complexes, often associated with multifocal epileptiform activity and runs of fast activity [Crumrine, 2002]. Approximately 20 percent of children with this epileptic syndrome have a history of infantile spasms [Markand, 2003]. Cognitive and behavioral abnormalities precede the clinical

seizures in approximately 20–60 percent of children with Lennox–Gastaut syndrome [Blume, 2001].

It has been suggested that the epileptic processes associated with this syndrome lead to patterns of abnormal activity and connectivity that compete with normal brain development, thus resulting in subsequent impairment or regression of cognition [Blume, 2004]. It is not known whether it is the underlying brain pathology, the burden of frequent seizures, the persistent epileptiform activity, or all of these factors that is responsible for the cognitive deficits in Lennox–Gastaut syndrome. The age specificity, typically frequent seizures, and unremitting epileptiform activity suggest that the epileptic activity occurring at a critical time in brain development contributes to a progressive disturbance in cerebral function.

Landau–Kleffner Syndrome-Continuous Spike Waves During Slow-Wave Sleep

Landau–Kleffner syndrome (LKS) is an acquired aphasia associated with an epileptiform EEG with spikes, sharp waves, or spike-and-wave discharges that are usually bilateral and occur predominantly over the temporal regions; in approximately 25 percent of children there are no clinical seizures [Landau and Kleffner, 1998]. Continuous spike-wave discharges during slow-wave sleep (CSWS), an epileptic encephalopathy associated with the EEG pattern of electrical status epilepticus during slow-wave sleep, with various seizure types, and with cognitive, motor, and behavioral disturbances, is, along with LKS, considered a sleep-related epileptic encephalopathy [Tassinari et al., 2009].

CSWS and LKS are epileptic encephalopathies with common clinical features, including seizures, regression, and epileptiform abnormalities that are activated by sleep [Nickels and Wirrell, 2008]. In CSWS there is a regression in global skills, while in LKS the primary clinical manifestation is a regression of language. The conceptual thinking is that there is a spectrum of disorders associated with activation of epileptiform activity during slow-wave sleep that includes LKS, CSWS, and "atypical" benign epilepsy with centrotemporal spikes (BECTS) [Fejerman, 2009; Scheltens-de Boer, 2009]. The implications are that the EEG abnormalities lead to regression in language, behavioral, and cognitive manifestations and that treatment requires reversal of the epileptiform pattern on the EEG. However, whether the frequency of the epileptiform discharges, as linked to the appearance or disappearance of electrical status epilepticus during slow-wave sleep, is responsible for the course of language, cognitive, and behavioral deterioration [Tassinari et al., 2000; Seri et al., 2009] remains an unanswered and controversial issue.

Seizures, Interictal Epileptiform Discharges, and Neurodevelopmental Disorders

In the epileptic encephalopathies, seizures and IEDs account for poor developmental outcomes, with intellectual disability, language, learning disorders, and ASDs occurring in a significant number of children with a history of an epileptic encephalopathy. From a different perspective, neurodevelopmental disorders are commonly associated with epilepsy and with IEDs. In general, this epileptic activity does not have a direct effect on modulation of the symptoms in children with neuro-developmental disorders.

IEDs, characterized by spikes or sharp waves that appear abruptly from the electrographic background, with or without an associated slow wave, are limited in duration and do not evolve in frequency and distribution over time, but can at times be responsible for disruption of cognitive and behavioral function [Fisch, 2003]. The concept that transitory changes in higher cortical functions can be secondary to EEG discharges not accompanied by seizures was proposed more than 60 years ago [Schwab, 1939]. The term transient cognitive impairment is used to describe individuals with epileptiform EEG discharges in association with a momentary disruption of adaptive cerebral function [Aarts et al., 1984; Binnie, 2003].

Studies by numerous investigators suggest that transient cognitive impairment is not a consequence of general impairment of attention, but is likely secondary to disruption of functions located in the region or regions of the brain where the epileptiform discharges arise [Kasteleijn-Nolst Trenite, 1995; Aldenkamp and Arends, 2004]. Specific functions, such as perception, reaction time, and scholastic performance, can be disrupted by brief epileptiform discharges in the absence of convulsive seizures [Shewmon and Erwin, 1988; Sengoku et al., 1990]. The spectrum of language and cognitive impairment secondary to an active epileptic focus, even in the absence of clinical seizures, is wide [Deonna and Roulet-Perez, 2005; Roulet-Perez and Deonna, 2006].

Specific Language Impairment

Specific language impairment is a developmental language disorder characterized by varying types and degree of dysfunction in expressive and receptive communication skills (see Chapter 45). Children with specific language impairments differ from children with acquired aphasia characteristic of the epileptic encephalopathies, such as LKS-CSWS, in that there is no regression of language skills. Nevertheless, the impairments of language in epilepsies such as BECTS raises interesting questions regarding the overlap and interactions of epilepsy, IEDs, and specific language impairments [Billard et al., 2009].

An increased association of seizures in children with specific language impairments has been found [Robinson, 1991; Echenne et al., 1992], with prevalence rates from 7–40 percent reflecting the cohort studied and the type and duration of the EEG recording [Parry-Fielder et al., 1997]. In one study that compared the rates of epilepsy in children with autistic spectrum versus developmental language disorders, the prevalence of epilepsy was 8 percent (14 of 168) in the nonautistic, language-impaired children. In addition, when the children were subtyped on the basis of language, the highest risk of epilepsy, regardless of whether the children had ASD or specific language impairment, was seen in those individuals with the most severe receptive language disorder [Tuchman et al., 1991; Klein et al., 2000]. A link between specific language impairment and IEDs during sleep has also been suggested [Parry-Fielder et al., 1997; Ballaban-Gil and Tuchman, 2000; Wheless et al., 2002]. However, the strength of this association has been questioned in a recent study in which 13 percent of children with specific language impairments had IEDs on a sleep EEG recording, which was not significantly different than the non-language-impaired control group [Parry-Fielder et al., 2009].

Autistic Spectrum Disorders

ASD is a broad classification that includes a heterogeneous group of individuals with behaviorally defined impairments in reciprocal social interaction, verbal and nonverbal communication, and restricted and repetitive behaviors (see Chapter 48). The prevalence of epilepsy in children with ASD is highly variable, depending on the study sample, with rates ranging from 5 to 46 percent [Spence and Schneider, 2009]. The major risk factor for epilepsy in children with ASD is moderate to severe intellectual disability [Amiet et al., 2008]. In children with ASD without severe intellectual disability, motor deficit, associated perinatal or medical disorder, or a positive family history of epilepsy, the prevalence of epilepsy is 6 percent, which is not significantly different than in nonautistic children with a specific language impairment [Tuchman et al., 1991]. The prevalence of ASD in individuals with epilepsy has not been investigated with the same intensity as that of epilepsy in ASD, although one study in a tertiary epilepsy clinic found that approximately 30 percent of children with epilepsy screened positive for ASD [Clarke et al., 2005].

The prevalence of IEDs in children with ASD and no clinical history of seizures may be as high as 60 percent [Chez et al., 2006], but varies depending on the cohort studied and the type of EEG performed, with most studies finding prevalence rates ranging from 6 to 31 percent [Kagan-Kushnir et al., 2005]. The higher prevalence of IEDs in children with specific language impairment and in those with ASD compared to the 1.5–4 percent rate of IEDs in the general population [Cavazzuti et al., 1980; Capdevila et al., 2008] has been a source of significant controversy. The significance of these findings remains unclear and is not unique, as IEDs have been reported in 6–30 percent of children with attention-deficit hyperactivity disorders [Hughes et al., 2000; Richer et al., 2002; Kaufmann et al., 2009], which is remarkably similar to the prevalence of IEDs in children with specific language impairment or ASDs without seizures. One suggestion is that the high prevalence of IEDs in all of these disorders is secondary to the neuropathological processes common to both epilepsy and neurodevelopmental disorders. However, the question of whether these IEDs may be a biomarker of prognostic or interventional significance in a subgroup of children with specific language impairment or with ASDs remains to be determined.

Regression

A key component of the concept of epileptic encephalopathy is that seizures or the interictal epileptiform activity contribute directly to a regression in diverse neurodevelopmental skills affecting cognitive, language, and social skills. Two childhood disorders associated with regression and severe intellectual disability, and both historically associated with ASD, are Rett's syndrome and childhood disintegrative disorder.

The association of developmental regression in ASD to epilepsy and IEDs became a topic of increased interest after Hagberg and colleagues [Hagberg et al., 1983] published a report of 35 girls with regression in higher brain functions, stereotypical hand movements, and ASD, with a significant proportion of the girls having epilepsy. Childhood disintegrative disorder is characterized by late-onset autistic and cognitive regression that can include motor regression and loss of bowel and bladder function, usually occurring after age 3 [Rapin, 1995]. Childhood disintegrative disorder is based on the description, in the early 1900s, of children with normal development until age 3 or 4 years, who regressed in multiple developmental areas. This entity was first described by Heller in 1908 [Mouridsen, 2003], and differentiation from autism, especially from autistic regression, is still in progress [Kurita et al., 2004]. Disintegrative disorder is very rare, with a prevalence of 2 in 100,000 [Fombonne, 2009].

The prevalence of epilepsy in Rett's syndrome and in childhood disintegrative disorder is greater than 70 percent, both disorders have EEGs with marked IEDs, and both featuring regression of cognitive, language, and social skills [Mouridsen et al., 1999; Steffenburg et al., 2001]. Some children with childhood disintegrative disorder overlap with those having epilepsy and CSWS [Roulet Perez et al., 1993]. To what extent the high rate of seizures in these groups is secondary to the severe cognitive impairment present in Rett's syndrome and childhood disintegrative disorder, or what influence other specific variables, such as metabolic or molecular factors (i.e., the role of *MECP2*), have in the development of seizures remains unknown.

The developmental trajectory in approximately 30 percent of children with ASD is characterized by a regression of the few words acquired and a loss of nonverbal communication skills, usually occurring prior to 24 months of age [Goldberg et al., 2003; Lord et al., 2004]. This regression has been termed autistic regression. The relation of autistic regression to epilepsy or to an epileptiform EEG without seizures remains controversial, with some studies reporting higher rates of epilepsy in children with ASD and regression [Kobayashi and Murata, 1998; Hrdlicka et al., 2004], and others showing no relation between ASD, epilepsy, and regression [Tuchman and Rapin, 1997; Baird et al., 2008]. A recent study found that children with autistic regression had more disrupted sleep, as compared to those with autism without regression, and were more likely to have epilepsy [Giannotti et al., 2008]. In addition, Giannotti and colleagues found that epileptiform activity did not differ among those with and without regression, except that those with autistic regression were more likely than those without regression to have more "frequent epileptiform EEGs." There is evidence to suggest that, in a subgroup of children with ASD and without convulsive seizures, an epileptiform EEG is significantly more likely to be associated with a history of regression in language [Tuchman and Rapin, 1997]. However, these data must be put into perspective, as they represent a very specific subgroup of children with autism, and because at the present time there are no data regarding the number of children in the general population without seizures and cognitive and behavioral impairments who have interictal epileptiform abnormalities on an overnight EEG study. Others have found no differences in regression in those with epileptiform EEGs and epilepsy and those without seizures and a normal EEG [Canitano et al., 2005]. Children with autistic regression and an epileptiform EEG (AREE) should be differentiated from those with LKS-CSWS, and these differences are highlighted in Table 55-1.

The mean age of onset of language regression in ASDs is 21 months, and over 90 percent of children with autism who undergo a regression do so before age 3 years [Tuchman and Rapin, 1997]. By contrast, in LKS, only 12–14 percent of children experience regression before age 3 years [Bishop, 1985]. The peak age of onset of symptoms in LKS is between 5 and 7 years [Bureau, 1995]. In only 5 percent of individuals does LKS begin after age 9 years and it appears to occur rarely, if ever, after age 12 years [Bureau, 1995]. In children with the CSWS, the first symptoms occur in up to 20 percent of children between 9 and 12 years of age [Bureau, 1995].

Children with ASD are more likely to regress earlier, usually prior to age 2, as contrasted to those with LKS who have a regression in language usually after age 3 years, and seizures are more likely to occur in children who regress in language after age 3 years [Klein et al., 2000; Shinnar et al., 2001; Wilson et al., 2003]. In addition, children with isolated language regression have a higher frequency of epileptiform

Table 55-1 Landau–Kleffner Syndrome-Continuous Spike Waves During Slow-Wave Sleep Versus Autistic Regression with Epileptiform EEG

	Landau–Kleffner Syndrome-Continuous Spike-Waves During Slow-Wave Sleep (LKS-CSWS)	Autistic Regression with Epileptiform EEG (AREE)
Age of regression/ (symptoms)	Usually after 3 years. Peak age 3–5 years. In CSWS may be as late as 12 years of age	Usually prior to age 2 years with a mean age of regression of 21 months
Seizures	Usually not frequent or intractable. In approximately 25 percent, seizures are not present	Seizures are not part of phenotype. In autistic spectrum disorders, when seizures occur, they are usually not frequent and responded well to antiepileptic medications
EEG	Spikes, sharp waves, or spike-and-wave discharges, usually bilateral and occurring predominantly over the temporal regions. They increase during sleep; EEG pattern of electrical status epilepticus during slow-wave sleep is common	Infrequent spikes, usually centrotemporal. Rarely associated with CSWS. No clear correlation with interictal epileptiform discharges and improvement or worsening of underlying language and social dysfunction
Treatment	See Box 55-1. Case reports, mostly with use of steroids, suggest improvement in language. Surgical outcomes with multiple subpial transections are variable. No controlled clinical trials	No evidence that present medical interventions (antiepileptic medications) or surgical interventions are indicated
Outcome/ Comments	Improvement occurs in late childhood/early adolescence. Approximately one-third recover. Prognosis for seizure control is excellent but recovery of language is variable and not as good as for seizures	Improvement seems related to cognitive skills. No data to determine if interictal discharges combined with regression are marker for worse prognosis

discharges and seizures than children with both language and autistic (social and behavioral) regression [McVicar et al., 2005]. Furthermore, electrical status epilepticus during slow-wave sleep, the EEG pattern associated with LKS and CSWS, is almost exclusively found in those children with isolated language regression [McVicar et al., 2005], and CSWS with autistic regression is a rare occurrence [Tuchman, 2009]. The age of symptom onset seems to be an important indicator of outcome, at least in LKS. In one study, the prognosis for recovery was worse in children with LKS who lost their language at an early age [Bishop, 1985]. In a series of studies, age of language regression differentiates autistic regression from LKS.

In LKS, improvement occurs usually toward late childhood or early adolescence. Approximately one-third of affected children make a good recovery [Mantovani and Landau, 1980]. The prognosis for seizure control and normalization of the EEG is excellent, but prognosis for recovery of language and cognitive function is variable and in general not as good as it is for the seizures [Smith and Hoeppner, 2003]. In the group of children with regression and global cognitive deficits in the context of electrical status epilepticus during slow-wave sleep (ESES), a significant majority is left with some degree of neurological impairment [Rossi et al., 1999; Robinson et al., 2001]. In childhood disintegrative disorder, the prognosis is generally poor [Gillberg, 1991]. In general, children with autistic regression have significant long-term morbidity [Wilson et al., 2003]. What is still not known is whether children with autistic epileptiform regression have a poorer prognosis than those with regression without an epileptiform EEG.

An emerging concept of epileptic encephalopathy suggests a continuum of disorders in which the interictal epileptiform activity activated by sleep may account for regression in varying neurodevelopmental domains (Figure 55-1). This hypothetical model may provide a framework to understand the impact of seizures and interictal epileptiform activity on the developing brain, as well as to unravel the common complex genetic predisposition of these childhood epilepsies [Rudolf et al., 2009]. It also has important implications for the development of pharmaceutical agents that can target and suppress IEDs.

Etiology and Pathophysiology

As a group, the epileptic encephalopathies are associated with regression or slowing of cognitive, language, or behavioral development; the hypothesis is that seizures or the interictal

epileptiform activity are responsible for the deterioration [Nabbout and Dulac, 2003]. There are differences between the epileptic encephalopathies in terms of timing, frequency, and severity of the seizures or IEDs, despite the fact that, as a group, they are associated with poor developmental outcomes. In Dravet's syndrome, the seizures are more predominant than the IEDs, while in infantile spasms the epileptiform activity on the EEG is a more dramatic and likely important determinant of developmental outcome than the seizures. In Lennox–Gastaut syndrome, both the seizures and interictal epileptiform activity seem to play a critical role in terms of neurodevelopmental outcome. To date, studies have failed to dissect the effect of seizures per se from that produced by the underlying disease. A case in point is that individuals with infantile spasms of unknown cause have a better intellectual outcome than those individuals in whom a structural or metabolic etiology is determined.

Numerous etiologies are associated with LKS and CSWS, including neurocysticercosis [Otero et al., 1989], sylvian arachnoid cyst [De Volder et al., 1994], left temporal astrocytoma [Nass et al., 1993; Solomon et al., 1993], and inflammatory demyelinating disease [Perniola et al., 1993], suggesting that this syndrome may result from unilateral brain lesions present during a critical age of development and affecting areas essential for language development, or from multiple and diffuse lesions. In addition, an association between congenital hydrocephalus and CSWS and LKS has been reported [Ben-Zeev et al., 2004], and children with shunted hydrocephalus who develop language or behavioral deterioration may be at high risk for CSWS [Caraballo et al., 2008]. Reports of siblings [Nakano et al., 1989] with LKS have raised the possibility of a genetic basis for this disorder, but other reports of LKS occurring discordantly in monozygotic twins suggest an "environmental trigger" [Feekery et al., 1993]. A variety of different triggers, including an autoimmune process [Nevsimalova et al., 1992], an infectious or inflammatory process [Connolly et al., 1999], and a possible role for an arteritis [Pascual-Castroviejo et al., 1992], have all been proposed as etiologies for LKS. No evidence of encephalitis was found in two patients with LKS who underwent temporal lobectomy [Cole et al., 1988]. LKS, as with other childhood epileptic encephalopathies, has more than one etiology, and what may be important in determining the impact of the epileptic activity on the nervous system and the subsequent neurodevelopmental disorder is the timing of the insult and the extent to which the neural network is affected.

The pathophysiology of epileptic encephalopathies differs and remains poorly understood, but it is likely that the etiology of the epileptic activity, as well as the frequency or location of IEDs alone or in combination, could lead to a specific epileptic encephalopathy. LKS has become the model for understanding the functional mechanisms leading to an epileptic encephalopathy. Findings on functional neuroimaging studies in LKS have been consistent with temporal lobe abnormalities. A study using fluorodeoxyglucose positron emission tomography (PET) during sleep in three males with LKS demonstrated metabolic disturbances that varied among children but predominated over the temporal lobes [Marescaux et al., 1990]. Studies using single photon emission computed tomography imaging (SPECT) have found abnormal perfusion in the left temporal lobe only in LKS [O'Tuama et al., 1992; Guerreiro et al., 1996]. Temporal lobe metabolic abnormalities, as

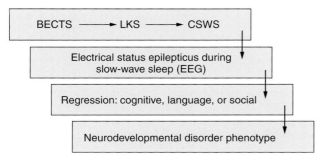

Fig. 55-1 Spectrum of Interictal Epileptiform Discharges and Neurodevelopmental Phenotypes. BECTS, Benign epilepsy with centrotemporal spikes; CSWS: Continuous spikes and waves during slow-wave sleep; LKS: Landau–Kleffner syndrome.

determined with PET scanning in children with LKS, have also been found in association with CSWS [Rintahaka et al., 1995]. A study of four children with LKS demonstrated a reduction in the cortical volume of the superior temporal areas, corresponding to the auditory association cortex with magnetic resonance imaging (MRI) volumetric analysis, with the difference greatest in the two children who had the most frequent temporal lobe epileptiform activity. Although these results do not allow determination of whether the atrophy is the cause of the LKS or the consequence of excitoxicity from the epileptiform discharges, they do support the concept that epileptiform activity may account for language regression in LKS. There is also evidence from magnetoencephalography (MEG) that, in LKS, bilateral discharges are generated in auditory and language areas of the perisylvian cortex, and that 20 percent of children have a unilateral perisylvian pacemaker that triggers bilateral synchrony of the spike discharges [Paetau, 2009].

Two areas of critical importance in understanding the pathophysiology of epileptic encephalopathies are the developmentally related effects of IEDs and seizures, and the common molecular mechanisms that could account for both epilepsy and the neurodevelopmental disorder. Gene defects can affect numerous processes in brain development, such as molecular derangement of ion channels, patterns of cortical neurogenesis leading to malformations of cortical development, and specific protein products, all of which have been implicated in the development of epilepsy and neurodevelopmental disorders [Wisniewski et al., 2001; Crino et al., 2002; Paredes and Baraban, 2002; Noebels, 2003; Muhle et al., 2004]. Genetic abnormalities may be responsible for the EEG pattern and the cognitive dysfunction in children with epilepsy or neurodevelopmental disorders [Roubertie et al., 2003], and the seizures themselves may change neurotransmitter release and gene expression [Kovacs et al., 2003].

Animal model studies have shown that the developmental age at which seizures and IEDs develop is a crucial factor in determining outcome, and that the effects of seizures or IEDs on the developing brain are further modified by age, sex, and underlying pathology [Galanopoulou and Moshe, 2009]. Frequent and prolonged seizures or interictal epileptiform activity are also key factors in determining developmental outcome and likely explain the poor developmental outcomes associated with epileptic encephalopathies [Ben-Ari and Holmes, 2006; Holmes and Lenck-Santini, 2006]. From a treatment perspective, there is animal model evidence that environmental enrichment may ameliorate or reverse the altered gene expression, as well as the cognitive and behavioral aspects caused by the effect of seizures and IEDs on the developing brain [Koh et al., 2005].

Tuberous sclerosis complex (TSC), a neurological disorder commonly associated with both ASD and epilepsy, provides an informative example of common mechanisms that could account for epilepsy and neurodevelopmental disorders [Napolioni et al., 2009]. TSC occurs in about 1 in 6000 live births and is an autosomal-dominant disorder, although up to 60 percent of affected children carry spontaneous mutations of one of two different genes causing the disorder, *TSC2* and *TSC1* [Curatolo, 2003]. Some 40 percent of individuals with TSC have an IQ below 70 and 30 percent have an IQ below 30; the likelihood of cognitive impairment is associated with a history of seizures and particularly infantile spasms [Joinson et al., 2003]. Even in children with TSC and normal cognitive development, careful neuropsychological testing reveals deficits more commonly than in a control sample of children [Harrison et al., 1999].

Epilepsy occurs in approximately 80–90 percent of children with TSC and is often intractable [Holmes and Stafstrom, 2007]. A retrospective study looking at epileptic risk factors for the development of ASD in TSC found that tubers in the temporal lobes predisposed to ASDs and, more specifically, that it was temporal lobe epileptiform discharges, a history of infantile spasms, and onset of seizures in the first 3 years of life that determined whether or not an individual with TSC developed an ASD [Bolton et al., 2002]. Thus, the relation of epilepsy to neurodevelopmental disorders is complex and determined by underlying pathology, as well as by genetic and epigenetic factors combined with the developmental age, location, frequency, and duration of the epileptic activity.

Management

Management of the child with epilepsy and a neurodevelopmental disorder should be individualized. One needs to weigh the advantages of treating the seizures or IEDs with the potential cognitive and behavioral effects of the antiepileptic medications [French et al., 2004]. This consideration should be balanced with an understanding of the psychotropic mechanisms of action of antiepileptic medications and their role in treating children with epilepsy and coexisting mood and behavioral disorders [Di Martino and Tuchman, 2001; Ettinger, 2006].

Treatment of epileptiform discharges in the absence of clinical seizures remains controversial. The classic teaching is not to treat the EEG but to treat the patient. A degree of skepticism is appropriate when attempting to correlate an epileptiform EEG with specific cognitive, language, or behavioral dysfunction. Evidence from clinical case studies and the occurrence of transient cognitive impairment in some patients suggest that, if appropriate testing is done with concurrent EEG monitoring, a reliable correlation can be made between epileptiform discharges and performance on numerous tasks. The controversy is whether treating this group of children in the absence of seizures is justifiable [Binnie, 2003; Pressler et al., 2005]. Despite the higher prevalence of epileptic activity in neurodevelopmental disorders, such as specific language impairment and ASDs, there is no evidence that treatment of the seizures or the IEDs has a positive impact on language, social, cognitive, or behavioral outcomes [Tharp, 2004; Tuchman, 2004].

Most clinicians would agree that, in the epileptic encephalopathies, such as Dravet's syndrome, infantile spasms, Lennox–Gastaut syndrome, and LKS-CSWS, early and aggressive treatment is indicated [Arts and Geerts, 2009]. Interventions commonly used in this group of children include antiepileptic drugs, corticosteroids and adrenocorticotropic hormone (ACTH), immunoglobulins, vagal nerve stimulation, the ketogenic diet, and epilepsy surgery (Box 55-1). In LKS-CSWS, several case reports with poorly defined endpoints suggest that corticosteroid therapy improves language [Hirsch et al., 1990; Lerman et al., 1991; Tsuru et al., 2000; Sinclair and Snyder, 2005; Gallagher et al., 2006]. In addition, a number of case reports using a variety of interventions, including nicardipine

Box 55-1 Treatments for Landau–Kleffner Syndrome-Continuous Spike Waves During Slow-Wave Sleep

- Valproic acid
- Lamotrogine
- Levetiracetam
- Clobazam
- Sulthiame
- Topiramate
- High-dose benzodiazepines
- Adrenocorticotropic hormone (ACTH)/steroids
- Immunoglobulins
- Vagus nerve stimulator
- Ketogenic diet
- Epilepsy surgery

[Pascual-Castroviejo et al., 1992], vigabatrin [Appleton et al., 1993; Wakai et al., 1997], sulthiame, clobazam [Gross-Selbeck 1995], levetiracetam [Kossoff et al., 2003], diazepam [Mikati and Shamseddine, 2005] immunoglobulins [Mikati et al., 2002], and ketogenic diet [Kossoff et al., 2009; Nikanorova et al., 2009], have been associated with improvements in behavioral and language functioning in children with LKS-CSWS. There are no controlled clinical trials of interventions for children with LKS-CSWS, limiting the ability to make rational decisions regarding appropriate intervention [Lagae, 2009].

In children with ESES exclusive of LKS, the most effective treatment is corticosteroids, which, in one study, were reported to abate the EEG discharges successfully in 65 percent of children; other treatments, such as intravenous immunoglobulin infusions and administration of antiepileptic drugs, were successful in less than 50 percent of cases [Kramer et al., 2008]. In infantile spasms, one study suggested that the use of vigabatrin in children with infantile spasms and tuberous sclerosis improved developmental outcome [Jambaque et al.,

2000]; however, there is no substantial evidence that current intervention strategies for infantile spasms improve developmental outcomes [Mackay et al., 2004]. Etiology may be the most reliable predictor of developmental outcome in children with infantile spasms, regardless of intervention [Lux and Osborne, 2006].

Multiple subpial transection (MST) has been the most common neurosurgical treatment for LKS, with multiple reports suggesting postoperative improvement in language function [Sawhney et al., 1995; Grote et al., 1999; Irwin et al., 2001; Guenot, 2004]. What is less clear is whether successful surgical treatment of seizures or epileptiform discharge abatement improves the developmental trajectories of these children [Caplan et al., 1992; Kanner, 2000]. Intellectual capacity influences response to interventions, at least in children with ASD and epilepsy, and current medical and surgical interventions do not appear to alter intellectual ability dramatically [Danielsson et al., 2009], even when surgical elimination of seizures occurs at an early age.

In the management of the epileptic encephalopathies, there is no consensus on which medication to use, when to start one particular treatment compared to another, and what to use as an endpoint for success [Guerrini, 2006; Arts and Geerts, 2009]. There are no comprehensive studies using a multidisciplinary approach that combines medications or surgery to eliminate the seizures or interictal epileptiform activity, with early intensive educative interventions that target communication, behavioral, and educational deficits. If seizures or interictal epileptiform activity interfering with the normal trajectory of development is eliminated, then intensive, frequent, and structured interventions may allow for the plasticity of the brain, now unburdened of the epileptic activity, to overcome the neurodevelopmental deficits.

 The complete list of references for this chapter is available online at **www.expertconsult.com**.
See inside cover for registration details.

Myoclonic Seizures and Infantile Spasms

Kendall Nash and Joseph Sullivan

Introduction

Myoclonus, myoclonic seizures, and infantile spasms share many common features yet are seen in a wide variety of neurologic conditions. Myoclonus is not a diagnosis, but rather a sign that can have many underlying etiologies. The precise definitions of each of these terms has also been somewhat controversial, but for the purpose of this chapter we will use the definition proposed by Victor and Adams [Ropper and Samuels, 2009] and define myoclonus simply as a "shock-like irregular jerk," with myoclonic seizures having a similar clinical appearance but also accompanied by neurophysiologic evidence of being cortically generated. While these definitions each have their own potential flaws, the distinction between a cortically generated movement (myoclonic seizure) and a subcortically generated movement (myoclonus) is extremely important, especially when thinking about some of the progressive myoclonic epilepsies, as many of these patients can manifest both myoclonus and myoclonic seizures. Infantile spasms, however, should not be confused with either, as the spasm itself is often a more complex constellation of movements with a myoclonic component.

Given this overlap, it is fitting to present myoclonic seizures and infantile spasms together as a continuum of events that occur in a developing nervous system disorder. Our approach will be to present each of the specific conditions as they occur across the age spectrum. Progressive myoclonic epilepsies (PME) will be characterized by their individual features with an emphasis on recent genetic discoveries. Infantile spasms will be elaborated on in more detail, given the wide variety of underlying etiologies, treatments, and outcomes seen in this condition.

Epilepsy Syndromes with Prominent Myoclonic Seizures

Myoclonic seizures can occur in a wide variety of pediatric epilepsy syndromes, including Lennox–Gastaut syndrome and childhood absence epilepsy, which are discussed elsewhere in Part VIII. Our focus will be on those syndromes in which myoclonus is a critical feature for the diagnosis. This coverage includes benign myoclonic epilepsy in infants (BME), severe myoclonic epilepsy in infancy (SMEI/Dravet's syndrome), idiopathic epilepsy with myoclonic-astatic seizures (IEMAS), and juvenile myoclonic epilepsy (JME) (Table 56-1).

Benign Myoclonic Epilepsy of Infancy

BMEI was first described by Dravet and Bureau in 1981 [Dravet and Bureau, 1981]. The syndrome is characterized by brief, generalized myoclonic seizures, with the predominant area of muscle involvement being the proximal upper extremities [Hirano et al., 2009], and usually occurs in children between the ages of 4 months and 3 years, although cases have been described with onset up to 4 years 8 months [Rossi et al., 1997]. These attacks often occur multiple times per day. Detailed electroencephalography (EEG) and polygraphic electromyography (EMG) recordings have shown that the myoclonic seizures are often associated with a flexor postural change and approximately 80 percent of attacks involve the upper limbs [Hirano et al., 2009]. A history of febrile seizures (30 percent) and a family history of epilepsy (39 percent) is relatively common [Roger et al., 2002].

EEG Findings

The ictal EEG discharge is often a generalized spike wave (GSW) that may be slower than 3 Hz [Hirano et al., 2009]. Occasionally, the myoclonic seizures can be massive and result in a fall, or they may occur in a cluster. Some infants may exhibit photosensitivity at the onset of the syndrome, and the photic-induced myoclonic seizures are often more prominent than those that occur spontaneously [Capovilla et al., 2007]. Other infants may be sensitive to acoustic or tactile stimuli, leading some to argue for a distinctly separate epilepsy syndrome [Ricci et al., 1995]. We and others [Roger et al., 2002] do not believe this is a clinically distinct syndrome, but rather that the syndrome of BME may include both photosensitive and stimulus-provoked seizures in addition to spontaneous myoclonic seizures. In both groups, the waking EEG in between seizures is often normal but may contain rare generalized spike/wave discharges [Ricci et al., 1995; Capovilla et al., 2007], and the ictal EEG findings are indistinguishable.

Treatment and Outcome

The overall prognosis of myoclonic seizures is excellent, with complete resolution in almost all children usually within 1–2 years of diagnosis. In those who demonstrate photosensitivity, these seizures may be more difficult to control and may persist for a longer period of time [Roger et al., 2002]. The majority of children also have normal neurodevelopmental outcomes [Caraballo et al., 2009], although some studies have reported

Table 56-1 Common Pediatric Epilepsy Syndromes with Prominent Myoclonic Seizures

	Benign Myoclonic Epilepsy of Infancy (BMEI)	Severe Myoclonic Epilepsy of Infancy (SMEI/Dravet's syndrome)	Myoclonic-Astatic Epilepsy (MAE/Doose's syndrome)	Juvenile Myoclonic Epilepsy (JME)
Age at presentation	4 months–3 years	<1 year	1.5–5 years	8–26 years
Psychomotor development	Normal	Slow	Variable	Normal
Family history of epilepsy	50–60%	30%	30–50%	5–10%
Seizure types	Myoclonic seizures only (may be provoked by noise or contact) Febrile seizures (rare)	Febrile seizures Hemiconvulsions Generalized tonic-clonic Partial Myoclonic Atypical absence	Astatic/atonic Myoclonic Atypical absence Tonic (rare)	Myoclonic Generalized tonic-clonic Absence
EEG	Normal background Generalized polyspike/ spike-wave discharges (rare when awake, augmented in sleep) Absence of focal discharges	Normal background at onset, later background slowing Multifocal or generalized spikes/waves	Normal background or excessive slowing at onset (especially biparietal theta) Irregularly generalized 3–6-Hz spike/polyspike wave discharges	Normal background 4–6-Hz polyspike/wave discharges, or 3-Hz spike/wave discharges May have "shifting" focal features
Prognosis	Favorable – likely remits	Unfavorable – medically refractory seizures, mental retardation, ataxia	Variable and somewhat dependent on response to treatment – may remit or evolve into Lennox–Gastaut	Favorable –most require life-long AEDs but some spontaneous remissions

impaired psychomotor development and behavioral disturbances if the child is not treated or if onset of the syndrome is at less than 2 years of age [Mangano et al., 2005]. Those children with a prominent reflex component may have a more favorable neurodevelopmental outcome [Zuberi and O'Regan, 2006].

The medication of choice appears to be valproic acid (VPA), with 80–90 percent responding to VPA monotherapy, although high serum levels (>100 mg/L) may be necessary. When VPA monotherapy does not provide complete control, adjunctive use of a benzodiazepine, such as clonazepam or clobazam, can be helpful [Rossi et al., 1997].

Severe Myoclonic Epilepsy in Infancy

First described in 1978 by Charlotte Dravet, SMEI occurs in normally developing children who experience prolonged febrile (>20 minutes) or afebrile seizures, including hemiconvulsions, during the first year of life. Afebrile, mixed seizures follow, and the emergence of myoclonic seizures is common but not necessary for the diagnosis (borderline variant). For this reason, the syndrome is better referred to as Dravet's syndrome, as the name severe *myoclonic* epilepsy of infancy may mislead clinicians and cause them not to suspect the diagnosis if myoclonic seizures are absent. The syndrome was once thought to be exceedingly rare, with an incidence of 1 in 40,000 children [Hurst, 1990], but with heightened awareness of the clinical spectrum and the availability of genetic testing, this may be an underestimation of the true incidence.

Mutations in the SCN1A Gene

The importance of *SCN1A* gene mutations as an underlying etiology in epilepsy first became apparent when Scheffer and Berkovic reported missense mutations in two families with the syndrome of generalized epilepsy with febrile seizures plus (GEFS+) [Scheffer and Berkovic, 1997]. Due to the common occurrence of febrile seizures in both GEFS+ and Dravet's syndrome, Claes et al. screened seven patients with Dravet's syndrome and found de novo missense mutations in all seven patients [Claes et al., 2001]. Testing for mutations in the *SCN1A* gene is clinically available, and hundreds of patients with Dravet's syndrome with *SCN1A* mutations have been reported [Depienne et al., 2009]. The main difference between individuals with a GEFS+ phenotype and a Dravet phenotype appears to be that the former often have a missense mutation with reduced penetrance, whereas patients with Dravet have mutations that occur in isolated patients (arise de novo) [Claes et al., 2001].

Mutations in the SCN1A gene are seen in approximately 70–85 percent of patients with Dravet's syndrome [Harkin et al., 2007], and therefore it remains a clinical diagnosis based on age of onset and clinical phenotype. One should not exclude the diagnosis on the basis of a negative result on *SCN1A* mutation testing. Approximately 200 different point mutations in the *SCN1A* gene were identified in 271 probands with a strict clinical diagnosis of Dravet's syndrome [Depienne et al., 2009]. Of those probands without a point mutation, the multiplex ligation-dependent probe amplification (MPLA) technique found an additional 14 micro-rearrangements of *SCN1A* [Depienne et al., 2009]. An *SCN1A* variant database was published in 2009, listing each type of mutation and the associated epilepsy syndrome [Claes et al., 2009]. As of 2009, 648 point mutations have been reported, of which 582 (90 percent) are in subjects with Dravet's syndrome. An additional 67 genomic rearrangements were reported, with 46 (7 percent) of these occurring in patients with Dravet's syndrome. The remaining clinical phenotypes with *SCN1A* mutations are wide and varied [Harkin et al., 2007]. In Dravet's syndrome, the end result of each of these mutations appears to be a total loss of function of the mutated allele, most commonly caused by a missense mutation that leads to an abnormality in the pore-forming unit of the sodium channel [Claes et al., 2009]. While specific mutation genotype–phenotype correlations within Dravet's syndrome are not yet available, further research in this area may lead to particular treatment strategies for specific genotypes.

Seizure Semiologies

Patients with Dravet's syndrome have many different seizure semiologies, often occurring in the same patient. The most common presenting seizure type is a prolonged febrile convulsion lasting longer than 25 minutes, but afebrile seizures can be the presenting seizure type in as many as 35 percent [Roger et al., 2002]. Japanese authors have observed that hot water immersion can trigger seizures in these patients [Fujiwara et al., 1990], and this feature is one part of a clinical screening test aimed at predicting the diagnosis of Dravet's syndrome [Hattori et al., 2008]. Other convulsive seizure types include generalized tonic-clonic seizures, hemiclonic seizures, and "falsely generalized," seizures as described by Dravet [Roger et al., 2002]. The latter has a complex semiology, with a high degree of discrepancy between the clinical and EEG findings. Seizures often start in one part of the body, spread to another (on the opposite side), and then potentially return to the original side of origin, only to involve a new body part.

Nonconvulsive seizures are also common and include simple partial, complex partial, atypical absence, and myoclonic types. The specific semiologies of each of these seizure types are similar to that seen in other forms of childhood epilepsy. Tonic seizures are rare. A unique seizure type, termed "obtundation status," is unique to the syndrome. The semiology of this seizure type consists of variable impairment in consciousness, and fragmentary and erratic segmental myoclonias involving the limbs and face. Patients may still be able to engage in simple activities, such as eating or playing with a toy. These episodes may last several hours to days and can either be initiated by, or conclude with, a convulsion [Roger et al., 2002]. The EEG during these episodes is not a pattern of classical atypical absence status, but rather is characterized by a diffuse dysrhythmia with focal or diffuse spikes [Roger et al., 2002]. We have observed one patient, who would begin with this type of clinical phenomenon, including prominent eyelid myoclonia that was dramatically accentuated with eye closure, and would remain in this state for 2–3 days, culminating in a generalized convulsion, after which her mental status cleared. She would remain clear for 2–3 weeks, and then repeat the same cycle over again.

EEG Findings

The EEG is invariably normal early in the course of the disease, and therefore, in contrast with other epilepsy syndromes, the diagnosis must be suspected on clinical grounds. As the disease

Table 56-2 Clinical Screen for Dravet's Syndrome

Clinical Score	Risk Score
Onset <7 months	2
More than 5 seizures prior to 12 months of age	3
Hemiconvulsion	3
Focal seizure	1
Myoclonic seizure	1
Prolonged seizure (>10 minutes)	3
Hot water-induced seizure	2

(Adapted from Hattori J et al. A screening test for the prediction of Dravet syndrome before one year of age. Epilepsia 2008;49(4):626–633.)

progresses, the EEG background becomes slow but often continues to manifest normal sleep architecture [Roger et al., 2002]. Some authors have observed rhythmic 5–6-Hz centro-parietal theta but this is not specific to the syndrome [Doose et al., 1998]. Over time, the interictal EEG can show both generalized and multifocal spikes, or may not show any of these features despite frequent seizures of multiple types, further highlighting the lack of specificity of EEG findings. Given this lack of specificity, a screening test for predicting the diagnosis of Dravet's syndrome under 1 year of age has been developed, with a positive predictive value as high as 94 percent [Hattori et al., 2008]. This screening test uses simple clinical features, as shown in Table 56-2. A sum score of 6 or greater is associated with a high risk of having Dravet's syndrome, and therefore *SCN1A* testing should be done in those cases. Even if the hot water-induced risk factor is excluded, a score of 5 or higher is still indicative of a high-risk patient.

Imaging

Magnetic resonance imaging (MRI) studies are usually normal but may show nonspecific cerebral or cerebellar atrophy or isolated ventricular enlargement. Interestingly, these findings, specifically diffuse brain atrophy, appear to be more common in those children without associated *SCN1A* mutations. Furthermore, despite having frequent prolonged febrile and afebrile convulsions, mesial temporal sclerosis is rare, reported in only 1 of 58 patients [Striano et al., 2007].

Treatment

Until recently, treatment strategies were generally unsuccessful, with poor seizure control despite polytherapy. Many have observed that certain antiepileptic drugs (AEDs) exacerbate seizures, with the most notorious agents being carbamazepine (CBZ) and lamotrigine (LTG) [Wakai et al., 1996; Guerrini et al., 1998]. Some authors have recommended using CBZ as a means of "confirming" the diagnosis when there is a high index of clinical suspicion [Wakai et al., 1996]. Given the availability of genetic testing, we do not endorse this practice.

A study by Chiron et al. and a subsequent meta-analysis pooling these data with unpublished data showed that combination therapy with valproate (VPA) + stiripentol (STP) + clobazam (CLB) resulted in a 70 percent decrease in seizure frequency, with 43 percent of patients becoming seizure-free [Chiron et al., 2000; Kassai et al., 2008]. In this study, the

STP dose began at 50 mg/kg/day divided in 2–3 doses, but could be titrated up to 100 mg/kg/day. The maximum recommended dose is 3500 mg/day [Chiron et al., 2000].

One proposed mechanism for the effect of STP is the potent inhibition of the p450 cytochrome system, resulting in higher levels of VPA and CLB. Plasma levels of CLB were significantly higher but levels of VPA were not [Chiron et al., 2000]. Interestingly, one other result of p450 inhibition is lower levels of metabolites, some of which are thought to explain some of the adverse toxic effects of AEDs. This finding perhaps explains why patients are able to tolerate the higher doses of certain AEDs [Chiron, 2005]. These observations, however, raise the possibility that STP has other mechanisms of action independent of its effects on the p450 system, including enhancement of gamma-aminobutyric acid (GABA)ergic transmission [Quilichini et al., 2006].

Of the newer agents, topiramate (TPM) appears to be very effective, especially if added to STP, resulting in 50 percent reduction of seizures in 78 percent of patients at a modest optimal dose of 3.2 mg/kg/day. Seventeen percent of patients remained seizure-free for at least 4 months [Kroll-Seger et al., 2006].

Bromide therapy has also shown promise in several studies [Oguni et al., 1994], specifically in reducing the number of convulsions. The ketogenic diet may be helpful in some patients [Caraballo et al., 1998].

Our strategy has been to start with VPA or TPM, followed by add-on therapy with a benzodiazepine in the form of clonazepam, clorazepate, or clobazam. When seizures prove to be refractory to this combination, STP is then added. If STP were more readily available in the United States and the cost were not prohibitive, we would very likely be able to utilize this medication earlier in the treatment algorithm.

Aggressive treatment of acute seizures and prevention of status epilepticus is critical, as some small studies have shown a trend towards improved neuropsychologic outcomes in those children with less frequent convulsive seizures [Chipaux et al., 2008]. Each patient should have a clearly defined "emergency plan," and the clinician should ask each family if a particular treatment regimen has been particularly effective for their child [Nolan et al., 2006]. Parents should be educated about the inevitability of seizures, especially prolonged seizures in the setting of fever. Early use of high doses of benzodiazepines, either in the form of rectal diazepam (as high as 1 mg/kg per dose) or buccal midazolam, should be the first-line therapy. Some physicians have recommended insertion of a central venous port for those children who have proven to have difficult intravenous access and multiple episodes of status epilepticus [Dooley et al., 1995]. In these specific cases, families are able to cope much better, knowing that multiple intravenous attempts will not be necessary and appropriate treatment can be initiated to terminate the seizure faster.

Outcome

Long-term outcome with regard to seizure control and neuropsychological development is variable but generally poor. By definition, all children with Dravet's syndrome have normal development at onset. Around 50 percent of children walk unsupported by a mean of 16 months of age; however, it is rare for children to utilize two-word sentences at the normal age of around 2 years [Wolff et al., 2006]. At around 2 years of age,

there appears to be a gradual decline, and then there is a relative stabilization between the ages of 4 and 6 years [Wolff et al., 2006]. A trend was noted that fewer convulsive seizures often resulted in higher developmental quotients. Subsequent small cohorts have reported patients with normal or near-normal IQs and this favorable outcome is attributed to early diagnosis and appropriate management [Chipaux et al., 2008]. It remains to be seen in larger prospective studies whether early diagnosis and appropriate management with the medications outlined above will lead to improved seizure control and a subsequent improvement in neurodevelopmental outcome.

Myoclonic-Astatic Epilepsy of Doose

Some children may present in early childhood with myoclonic seizures very similar to those seen in Dravet's syndrome, but with a prominent astatic component leading to falls. This constellation of findings is what is seen in MAE. Unlike those with Dravet's syndrome, children with MAE usually do not have a dramatic history of prolonged febrile convulsions. While this syndrome does not always have a poor neurodevelopmental outcome, it remains an epileptic encephalopathy; if not appropriately treated, it can progress and lead to permanent neurodevelopmental sequelae or evolution into Lennox–Gastaut syndrome.

Etiology

Genetic factors clearly play a role in the pathogenesis of MAE, based on the high incidence of seizures (32 percent) in probands' siblings and parents; the most common seizure type is absence seizures. Despite the initial discovery of the *SCN1A* gene in a family with GEFS+ that included a family member with MAE [Scheffer and Berkovic, 1997], only a small number of patients with mutations in the *SCN1A* gene have been identified in patients with MAE [Ebach et al., 2005; Harkin et al., 2007]. Further genotype–phenotype correlation studies are necessary to determine if there are underlying genetic factors that would be able to predict response to treatment and outcome.

Seizure Semiologies

Onset of MAE is often between the ages of 2 and 6 years, and children are usually developmentally normal [Kaminska et al., 1999]. These children may begin experiencing unexplained "jerks" and "falls," which occur multiple times per day. These myoclonic seizures can take place in isolation, but often are followed by a brief period of atonia that results in a dramatic fall in which the child appears to be propelled to the ground. Polygraphic studies have documented that atonic falls can occur with or without the preceding myoclonus, and occur in about 64 percent of patients [Oguni et al., 2002]. Although atonic falls are not necessarily seen in all patients, more subtle myoclonic/atonic seizures are common. The only manifestation of these may be a brief head nod or "head drop," with or without a myoclonic jerk of the upper extremities. When head drops occur in clusters with an associated alteration in level of consciousness, nonconvulsive status should be suspected. EEG findings during these episodes are always abnormal, with frequent runs of generalized spike/wave and slow spike-and-wave complexes. Absence seizures are quite common and may be similar to those seen in typical childhood absence epilepsy, but often are accompanied by more prominent myoclonus of the proximal upper extremities.

EEG Findings

The interictal EEG findings are varied and can be normal. The most common findings are generalized 3-Hz spike/wave discharges, as well as rhythmic 4–7-Hz biparietal theta activity. Some patients may also show occipital intermittent rhythmic delta activity (OIRDA) that characteristically attenuates with eye opening. Activation of generalized discharges during sleep is common, but generalized fast rhythms, such as generalized periodic fast activity (GPFA), are uncommon.

Treatment

Early recognition of the syndrome allows treatment to be focused on the broad-spectrum agents that have been shown to be particularly effective. The most commonly used and most effective AEDs have been VPA, LTG, levatiracetam, TPM and various benzodiazepines (clonazepam, clobazam, clorazepate). When absence seizures are frequent, ethosuximide (ETX) can be effective and has also been reported to decrease the frequency of myoclonic seizures; however, it is rarely used as monotherapy for this indication [Oguni et al., 2002]. The combination of VPA/ETX may be particularly effective, especially if high doses of VPA are used.

In those children who are refractory to medical management, a trial of the ketogenic diet should be considered early. The ketogenic diet has been shown to be as effective as other first-line agents in children with MAE [Kilaru and Bergqvist, 2007], and given this efficacy, we consider the ketogenic diet early in our treatment algorithm, especially if there is associated neurodevelopmental decline.

Outcome

The outcome with regard to cognitive development is highly variable but appears to be somewhat dependent on degree of seizure control. Some children may have fairly frequent seizures of multiple types and still have spontaneous remission, usually after approximately 3 years [Kaminska et al., 1999; Oguni et al., 2002]. In some children, the multiple seizure types remain intractable and these children have a higher risk of both cognitive and behavioral disturbances [Oguni et al., 2002]. The occurrence of tonic seizures has been described as a negative prognostic sign, although it remains unclear if these children may actually have an atypical form of Lennox–Gastaut syndrome rather than an atypical form of MAE [Kaminska et al., 1999].

Juvenile Myoclonic Epilepsy

JME is an idiopathic generalized epilepsy (IGE) syndrome characterized by myoclonic seizures, generalized tonic-clonic seizures, and absence seizures. It is extremely common, accounting for 26 percent of IGE and 10 percent of all epilepsies [Janz and Durner, 1998], although this may still be an underestimation; it is very likely underdiagnosed, as many clinicians may not inquire about the presence of myoclonic seizures [Renganathan and Delanty, 2003]. Mean age at onset is highly variable and difficult to determine truly, as some children with childhood absence epilepsy may evolve into the syndrome of JME. Excluding this population, the average age of onset is 15.1 years (7–28 years), with a slight female predominance [Martinez-Juarez et al., 2006].

Seizure Semiologies

In the classic syndrome of JME, myoclonic seizures may precede the first generalized tonic-clonic (GTC) seizure by 6–12 months, although GTCs occur as the first seizure type in approximately one-third of patients [Martinez-Juarez et al., 2006]. Some have proposed specific subgroups of JME, separating those patients who present with typical childhood absence or juvenile absence seizures, although this is much less common than the classical presentation of JME, accounting for only 10 percent of cases. The impact this distinction has on outcome will be discussed below. Photosensitivity is relatively common, occurring in approximately 30 percent of patients [Zifkin et al., 2005].

Myoclonic seizures often occur in the early morning hours shortly after awaking. Transcranial magnetic stimulation studies in patients with JME have demonstrated increased cortical excitability that is not present in other patients with focal epilepsy [Badawy et al., 2006]. Provocation of myoclonic seizures has been linked to higher cognitive tasks requiring higher-order thinking, such as writing or written calculation [Matsuoka et al., 2000].

Specific lifestyle features have been commonly associated with breakthrough seizures, including sleep deprivation, stress, alcohol, and menses [Martinez-Juarez et al., 2006].

EEG Findings

Patients with JME often have abnormal interictal EEGs, with the most common finding being generalized 4–6-Hz polyspike-and-wave (61 percent) or 3-Hz spike-and-wave discharges (14 percent) [Martinez-Juarez et al., 2006]. More prolonged (1–6 days; average 1–2 days) video EEG studies have shown EEG abnormalities of JME in 88 percent of patients [Park et al., 2009]. Other series have reported on the increased yield of an early morning EEG compared to an afternoon EEG (generalized epileptiform activity in 69 percent and 25 percent, respectively) [Labate et al., 2007]. A photoparoxysmal response in treatment-naive patients is also common and has been seen in as many as 35 percent of patients [Specchio et al., 2008].

Pathophysiology

It has long been accepted that the IGEs have a strong genetic component [Berkovic et al., 1998], and given the incidence of JME as a subtype of IGE, much research has been done to understand the underlying genetic basis of JME better. While JME appears to be a relatively homogeneous epilepsy syndrome, there are a number of studies implicating various genetic abnormalities. These include mutations in many different ion channels, including calcium, potassium, and chloride channels linked to at least seven different loci. There are also nonionic mechanisms that relate to neural migration during cortical development, and may explain some of the imaging and postmortem pathologic findings seen in these patients [de Nijs et al., 2009]. For further details about the specific genetic mutations and channels involved, please refer to Chapter 52.

Imaging

Imaging studies in patients with JME have indicated subtle structural changes in mesiofrontal cortex, with an increase in cortical gray matter [Woermann et al., 1999], although this has not been replicated in subsequent studies [Roebling et al., 2009]. These findings are interesting, given that the generalized discharges seen on routine EEGs often have a frontal predominance. This has been further investigated with dense array EEG, which further localized typical 4–6-Hz epileptiform activity to the orbitofrontal/medial frontopolar cortex, whereas some patients also demonstrated basal-medial-temporal sources [Holmes et al., 2010]. These electrophysiologic and anatomic abnormalities appear to be concordant with some of the neuropsychological deficits that are seen in patients with JME. Specific attention has been paid to executive dysfunction that has been demonstrated to correlate with smaller thalamic volumes and more frontal cerebrospinal fluid volumes in children with recent-onset JME when compared to children with benign rolandic epilepsy [Pulsipher et al., 2009].

Treatment

Valproate has long been considered the first-line agent, with reports of up to 86 percent of patients becoming seizure-free for at least 1 year [Penry et al., 1989]. Valproate has also been shown to be particularly effective in those patients with photosensitivity [Covanis et al., 2004]. Despite this efficacy, valproate has many side effects that may lead to significant comorbidities, including weight gain, hyperactivity, transaminitis, thrombocytopenia, pancreatitis. Women of child-bearing age must also consider the possible long-term cognitive effects on a fetus [Meador et al., 2009]. Due to these concerns, many newer AEDs are also commonly used, including lamotrigine, topiramate, zonisamide, and levetiracetam.

Lamotrigine is now accepted to be a broad-spectrum AED that is effective against both partial and generalized seizures [Biton et al., 2005]. Small studies have also shown it to be effective specifically in the management of patients with JME, both as monotherapy and polytherapy, resulting in seizure-free rates between 40 and 83 percent [Buchanan, 1996; Prasad et al., 2003]. LTG is also very well tolerated; however, it does have the potential for exacerbating myoclonic seizures [Prasad et al., 2003; Crespel et al., 2005]. The combination of LTG and VPA has been reported to be particularly effective in both partial and generalized epilepsy, including JME, and suggests the possibility of a synergistic effect [Brodie and Yuen, 1997].

Topiramate is also a broad-spectrum AED that has been shown to be effective in patients with JME, although there are no published studies on its use as monotherapy [Biton and Bourgeois, 2005]. It appears to be equally effective as LTG and VPA when used as polytherapy, although there is a suggestion that tolerability may be inferior [Prasad et al., 2003].

Zonisamide (ZNS) is another broad-spectrum AED with multiple proposed mechanisms of action. Small studies have shown ZNS to be broadly effective against all of the seizure types in JME, with 69, 62, and 38 percent of patients being free of GTC, myoclonic, and absence seizures, respectively [Kothare et al., 2004].

Levetiracetam is gaining a reputation as a broad-spectrum agent, as it has shown to be effective in patients with various forms of idiopathic generalized epilepsies including epilepsy with eyelid myoclonias and absence [Striano et al., 2009], as well as JME [Specchio et al., 2006; Noachtar et al., 2008]. In a study of 120 patients (93 percent of whom had JME) randomized to add-on levetiracetam or placebo, 25 percent were free of myoclonic seizures and 21.7 percent were free of all seizures, including GTCs, during the 12-week treatment phase [Noachtar et al., 2008]. In another open-label study of 48 patients with JME (10 newly diagnosed and 38 resistant to prior treatment), 73 percent were free of GTCs and 37.5 percent were free of myoclonic seizures over the study period, with a mean follow-up of 19 months [Specchio et al., 2006].

Benzodiazepines are widely accepted as having excellent antimyoclonic effects. This is also true of the myoclonic seizures seen in JME, with up to 88 percent of patients on clonazepam having complete control of myoclonic seizures but only 43 percent becoming free of GTCs [Obeid and Panayiotopoulos, 1989]. For this reason, benzodiazepines are not recommended as monotherapy for patients with JME, but can be extremely successful as add-on therapy when myoclonic seizures persist.

Outcomes

It has been widely accepted that JME is a lifelong condition with a high rate of relapse if weaned off AED therapy; however, some recent long-term follow-up studies have shown conflicting results [Martinez-Juarez et al., 2006; Baykan et al., 2008; Camfield and Camfield, 2009]. Furthermore, one must look at specific seizure types, as it appears the natural history of myoclonic seizures decreases after the fourth decade of life, independent of the on-going occurrence of the other seizure types [Baykan et al., 2008].

In the study by Martinez-Juarez et al., 257 patients were followed for a mean of 11 ± 6 years, and all patients were given a specific subtype of JME, including classic JME (72 percent), childhood absence epilepsy (CAE) evolving into JME (18 percent), JME with adolescent absence (7 percent), and JME with astatic seizures (3 percent). During a mean follow-up of 12.4 years in the classic JME group, 58 percent were free from all seizure types, with 91 percent of these patients remaining on AED treatment and only 9 percent seizure-free off medications. Treatment with VPA monotherapy (65 percent) was most common. The remaining 42 percent continued to have seizures despite AED treatment.

In contrast, patients in the CAE evolving into JME group fared much worse, with only 3 of 35 individuals achieving complete seizure freedom [Martinez-Juarez et al., 2006]. Although GTCs were controlled with medications in about 66 percent of patients, absence seizures persisted in 63 percent. These data support the conclusion that JME does appear to be a lifelong disease, specifically in the subgroup of patients with CAE evolving into JME. However, there is still a small subgroup (9 percent) of patients in whom the disease may not be lifelong, and based on these data, it is uncertain whether some of the patients who have been seizure-free on monotherapy for many years would be able to come off AED treatment successfully.

The study by Camfied and Camfield seems to suggest that this indeed may be a possibility. In 24 JME patients with a follow-up period of 25.8 years, 4 individuals (17 percent) were free of all seizures and off AEDs. The mean duration of therapy was 6.5 years before discontinuation. Two additional patients attempted to come off AEDs; they relapsed but later were able to be successfully weaned off medication and remain seizure-free. Another three patients (12.5 percent) had myoclonus only [Camfield and Camfield, 2009]. These results suggest that some patients with JME can successfully discontinue medications. Unfortunately, there do not appear to be clinical or EEG variables that can predict which patients will achieve this result. The decision to discontinue AEDs should be individualized for every patient, and a detailed discussion, with specific attention to the frequency of lifestyle provoking factors, is necessary in order to arrive at a safe and well-informed decision.

Progressive Myoclonic Epilepsies

The PME's are a group of genetically inherited disorders characterized by both epileptic and nonepileptic myoclonus, generalized tonic-clonic seizures, and progressive neurological deterioration, resulting in dementia, ataxia, and various forms of tremor. Recent advances in the genetic basis of these disorders are leading to a better understanding of how each of the disease processes differs. The four most common PMEs will be discussed (Table 56-3).

Unverricht–Lundborg Disease (ULD)

Unverricht–Lundborg disease (ULD) is the most common PME. It usually presents between the ages of 6 and 15 years, with the hallmark presenting symptom being stimulus-sensitive or action myoclonic jerks, which occur in up to half of patients [Lehesjoki, 2002]. Generalized tonic-clonic seizures are also a common feature early in the disease. At initial presentation, neurological examination and EEG studies may be normal, or the EEG may show generalized spike/wave discharges similar to those seen in IGE. It is not until the patient shows signs of progressive ataxia, intention tremor, and dysarthria that one begins to suspect PME clinically. As the disease progresses, the EEG becomes slow, with more frontally predominant polyspike/wave or spike-wave discharges, ranging in frequency between 2 and 6 Hz [Kyllerman et al., 1991]. MRI findings may be normal or may show nonspecific findings, such as cerebellar atrophy and reduced bulk of the basis pontis and medulla [Mascalchi et al., 2002].

The underlying cause of ULD is linked to an abnormality in the cystatin B gene on chromosome 21q22.3 [Lehesjoki et al., 1991]. Although the exact pathophysiology is unknown, mutations in cystatin B appear to lead to accelerated apoptosis, which may explain the progressive neurologic decline [Delgado-Escueta et al., 2001].

The diagnosis of ULD can be made by mutation testing of the cystatin B gene. There is no specific treatment for ULD, but improvements in seizure management with newer-generation AEDs has improved overall prognosis. VPA has been the mainstay of initial treatment; however, recent studies have shown a beneficial effect of levetiracetam, especially if started early [Magaudda et al., 2004].

Lafora's Disease

Lafora's disease (LD) has slightly later onset than ULD but has a more rapid decline, with many patients dying within 10 years of onset. Patients share similar clinical characteristics with other PMEs featuring seizures and myoclonus, but have a more prominent dementing component. Seizure types can be varied, but one peculiar type is that of occipital seizures with hallucinations and transient blindness [Minassian, 2001]. All patients are initially normal neurologically, but may have seizures indistinguishable from IGE until progressive neurological decline is noted. EEG findings early in the course may also resemble IGE, including photosensitivity, but the photosensitivity appears to be maximal at low frequencies between 1 and 6 Hz [Kobayashi et al., 1990]. As the disease progresses, the EEG background becomes slow and disorganized, and there is an evolution of the spike/wave discharges, the 3 Hz discharges becoming faster 6–12 Hz ones [Yen et al., 1991].

The underlying cause of LD is linked to two different sites on chromosome 6 – 6q24 and 6p22 – coding for two different genes: *EPM2A* (larforin) and *NHLRC1* respectively [Minassian et al., 1998; Chan et al., 2003]. The former appears to be involved in regulation of protein folding and the latter may play a role in dendritic transport in neurons. How dysfunction in each of these functions leads to the disease remains unclear.

The diagnosis of LD can be made by testing for mutations in the *EPM2A* gene that accounts for 80 percent of cases [Minassian et al., 1998]. In those cases where mutation testing is negative but the clinical phenotype is giving cause for concern, Lafora bodies can be detected in skin biopsy specimens. Treatment remains palliative.

Myoclonic Epilepsy with Ragged-Red Fibers (MERRF)

Myoclonic epilepsy with ragged-red fibers (MERRF) is a mitochondrial disease characterized by myoclonic epilepsy, ataxia, and ragged-red fibers on muscle biopsy. Multiple other clinical signs commonly seen in mitochondrial disorders may also be

Table 56-3 Differentiating Features of Progressive Myoclonic Epilepsies

Disease	Age at Onset (Years)	Cerebellar Signs	Dementia	Fundi
Unverricht–Lundborg disease (ULD)	6–15	Late	Late or absent (mild)	Normal
Lafora's disease	12–17	Early	Early (severe)	Normal
Myoclonic epilepsy with ragged-red fibers (MERRF)	Variable	Variable	Variable	With or without optic atrophy or retinopathy
Late-infantile neuronal ceroid-lipofuscinosis (LINCL)	2–5	Variable	Rapidly progressive	Subtle visual loss at onset, later blindness with retinal atrophy

(Adapted from Shahwan A, et al. Progressive myoclonic epilepsies: a review of genetic and therapeutic aspects. Lancet Neurol 2005;4(4):239–248.)

seen, such as myopathy, hearing loss, short stature, neuropathy, and optic atrophy [Chinnery et al., 1997]. EEG findings early in the disease are similar to the other PMEs, with 2–5-Hz generalized spike-wave discharges, and gradual background slowing as the disease progresses [So et al., 1989]. Imaging findings include basal ganglia calcifications and brain atrophy [DiMauro et al., 2002]. The key to differentiating MERFF from other PMEs is the constellation of other peripheral nervous system findings.

Diagnosis is made by genetic testing for the most common mutation in the tRNA (*MTTK*) gene of the mitochondrial DNA, which is seen in 90 percent of typical patients [Shoffner et al., 1990]. There is no specific treatment for MERRF although various antioxidants are commonly prescribed, as is customary in other mitochondrial disorders. VPA can be used, although L-carnitine supplementation is recommended [Tein et al., 1993].

Neuronal Ceroid-Lipofuscinoses

There are multiple types of neuronal ceroid-lipofuscinoses (NCLs) that vary in their age and mode of presentation. The most common type that presents with myoclonic seizures is the classical late-infantile type (LINCL; Jansky–Bielschowsky disease). Typical age at presentation is between 2 and 5 years. Multiple types of generalized seizures may occur, including myoclonic, atypical absence, atonic, and generalized tonic-clonic. Most children are previously normal, although nonspecific speech delay commonly precedes the onset of seizures. Shortly after or coincident with onset of seizures, patients become ataxic and psychomotor regression begins. Blindness eventually develops, due to retinal atrophy, but visual impairment is often subtle or incomplete early in the course of the disease [Williams et al., 2006]. Disease progression is variable but children are often bedridden and die within 5 years of the diagnosis.

Early in the course of the disease, the EEG often shows background slowing with generalized epileptiform discharges. The EEG response to photic stimulation is very characteristic, revealing posterior predominant spikes during low-frequency photic stimulation; a photoconvulsive response may be elicited. Imaging findings include cerebellar and cerebral atrophy with nonspecific T2 hyperintensity of the white matter [D'Incerti, 2000].

The gene responsible for LINCL has been mapped to chromosome 11p15, which codes for a protein called tripeptidyl peptidase 1 (TTP1) [Gardiner, 2002]. The protein is involved in lysosomal protein degradation, but it remains unclear how dysfunction in this protein specifically leads to the phenotype of LINCL. Diagnosis is made possible by testing for TTP1 enzyme activity; if this is absent or severely reduced, it is diagnostic of the disease.

Treatment at this time remains supportive. Trials of valproate (particularly at low doses), together with a benzodiazepine (usually clonazepam), can be helpful. Avoidance of carbamazepine and phenytoin is recommended. Trials are under way utilizing both stem cells and gene transfer vectors, with the aim of restoring some TTP1 activity (http://www.clinicaltrials.gov). These studies involve direct intracranial administration of stem cells or a viral vector. The preliminary studies have shown each of these techniques to be safe; however, disease progression appears to continue at the same rate.

Infantile Spasms

Infantile spasms constitute an age-dependent epilepsy syndrome that presents during infancy and is typically identified by clusters of spasms and an interictal EEG pattern known as hypsarrhythmia. As William West first described in his own son, in a letter to the *Lancet* in 1841 [Lux, 2001], the onset of spasms is often accompanied by psychomotor deterioration, thus meeting criteria of an epileptic encephalopathy. West's syndrome refers to the classic triad of spasms, hypsarrhythmia, and psychomotor arrest or regression. With a worldwide incidence of approximately 1 per 3000 live births, infantile spasms is the most prevalent epilepsy syndrome of infancy, and its emotional and financial costs to society are enormous [Pellock et al., 2008].

Despite over 150 years of interest in this disorder, various aspects, from terminology to treatment, remain controversial, in large part because the pathogenesis is unknown. This section focuses on the clinical presentation and prognosis, diagnostic evaluation, associated etiological factors, proposed pathophysiological mechanisms, and current treatment options.

Electroclinical Features

Regardless of etiology, the syndrome manifests during a specific period of brain maturation, most often between 4 and 8 months of life and nearly always before 2 years [Pellock et al., 2008; Riikonen, 1982]. The unique clinical spasms in the setting of hypsarrhythmia or its variants, lack of response to conventional antiepileptic agents, and generally poor outcome distinguish infantile spasms from similar epilepsies of infancy [Aicardi, 1986; Lombroso, 1990].

SPASMS

The classic seizure type, referred to as an epileptic spasm, is characterized by symmetric, bilateral, brief contraction of the axial muscle groups. The EMG tracing during a spasm reveals an abrupt phasic contraction lasting less than 2 seconds, which may be followed by a less intense tonic contraction lasting from 2 to 10 seconds [Kellaway et al., 1979]. Therefore, this unique seizure type is longer than a myoclonic jerk and yet shorter than a tonic seizure.

Depending on which muscle groups are predominantly involved, a spasm is classified as mixed flexor-extensor, flexor, or extensor, in order of their relative frequency [Kellaway et al., 1979]. Most affected infants have more than one type. The flexor spasm consists of sudden flexion of the neck, trunk, and/or extremities. When involved, the legs are commonly held in adduction, whereas the arms may be adducted or abducted. The specific flexor muscles involved and force of contraction vary between spasms, leading to a range of clinical manifestations from massive "jackknife" spasms to more subtle spasms consisting of head-bobbing or shoulder-shrugging. Extensor spasms are marked by abrupt extensor muscle contractions of the same muscle groups. Mixed flexor-extensor spasms reveal a combination of flexor and extensor contractions, most commonly flexion of the neck, trunk, and arms, with extension of the legs. Whether a spasm is flexor, extensor, or mixed does not suggest etiology or influence prognosis. In contrast, asymmetric spasms, which occur in approximately 5–25 percent of all patients, are more likely to be associated with a structural brain abnormality [Kellaway et al., 1979; Gaily et al., 1995, 2001; Fusco and Vigevano, 1993].

Spasms typically occur in clusters, with a 5- to 30-second interval between successive spells [Kellaway et al., 1979]. Often, the intensity of the spasms within a cluster builds to a peak and then declines. The frequency of spasms may vary, from only a few to several hundred per day [Guzzetta et al., 2007]. One common feature to note when taking a history is the common occurrence of spasms upon awakening and their rare occurrence during sleep [Kellaway et al., 1979; King et al., 1985], although the frequency of spasms during day and night is similar, owing to frequent awakenings in affected infants. No obvious precipitating stimuli or circumstances are observed in most patients.

Various clinical phenomena are seen in association with spasms. A behavioral arrest may follow a spasm for up to 90 seconds, but rarely occurs as an independent ictal event without an associated spasm [Kellaway et al., 1979; King et al., 1985]. Crying frequently follows a spasm, which, together with the preceding movements, often leads parents and general practitioners mistakenly to suspect abdominal colic or an exaggerated startle response. Eye movements, consisting of deviation alone or followed by rhythmic nystagmoid movements, are also commonly seen during spasms. Changes in respiratory rhythm occur in the majority of patients, while alterations in heart rate are rare [Kellaway et al., 1979].

HYPSARRHYTHMIA AND THE ICTAL EEG

The EEG hallmark of infantile spasms is hypsarrhythmia, a disorganized interictal pattern consisting of "random high-voltage slow waves and spikes" [Gibbs et al., 1954] (Figure 56-1). The spike discharges are usually multifocal, but when generalized, they are never rhythmically repetitive. A state-dependent EEG pattern, hypsarrhythmia is often present during wakefulness and quiet (non-rapid eye movement [REM]) sleep, and may be reduced or even absent during active (REM) sleep

[Hrachovy et al., 1981]. The classic pattern is usually seen in the early stages of infantile spasms, and in patients younger than 1 year of age. In addition to the classic pattern, there are several hypsarrhythmia variants, which have been grouped together and given the term "modified hypsarrhythmia," all of which have some elements of the classic pattern seen with typical epileptic spasms [Hrachovy et al., 1984]. These modified patterns include increased interhemispheric synchronization, asymmetrical or unilateral hypsarrhythmia, focal features, slow waves without spikes, and generalized background burst suppression. Modified hypsarrhythmia may occur more frequently than classic hypsarrhythmia [Kramer et al., 1997]. Hypsarrhythmia or modified hypsarrhythmia is seen in about two-thirds of cases, while other patterns, such as multifocal independent spike discharges, are present in the remainder [Shields, 2006]. Children with severe brain abnormalities, such as tuberous sclerosis, Aicardi's syndrome, and lissencephaly, do not usually generate the typical hypsarrhythmic pattern. Asymmetric hypsarrhythmia may indicate the presence of a focal central nervous system lesion [Drury et al., 1995]. Regardless of the specific pattern, however, any significant EEG background abnormality in a patient with clinical spasms may contribute to the epileptic encephalopathy, and all patterns should be viewed equally when considering approach to treatment. The chaotic pattern becomes more organized with time and, by the first several years of life, may evolve into the pattern of Lennox–Gastaut syndrome.

The ictal EEG pattern varies, although typically depicts a generalized, high-voltage, slow-wave transient followed by an abrupt voltage attenuation (see Figure 56-1) [Fusco and Vigevano, 1993]. There is no correlation between the ictal pattern and type of spasm, although longer ictal episodes are usually associated with behavioral arrest. Some children have partial seizures that are temporally related to clusters of spasms, a phenomenon that should raise suspicion for a structural brain abnormality [Pachatz et al., 2003], and possibly a focal abnormality with EEG concordance [Ohtsuka et al., 1996]. Among 92 patients with infantile spasms, 36 had partial

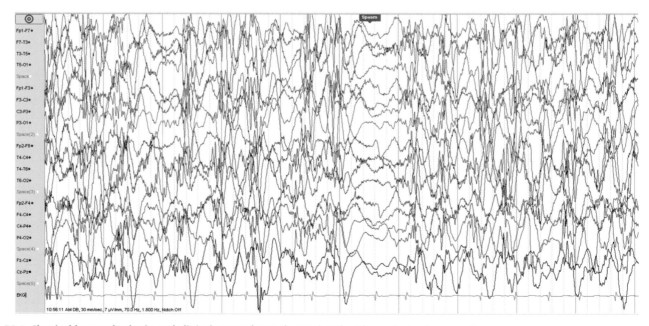

Fig. 56-1 Classical hypsarrhythmia and clinical spasm (center) associated with an electrodecrement.

seizures at some point (before spasm onset, concurrent with spasms, or after spasm cessation). The presence of partial seizures was associated with asymmetrical spasms, hemiparesis, asymmetric hypsarrhythmia, and persistence of seizures, and there was a trend toward increased focal structural imaging findings among these patients.

Classification

The classification of infantile spasms has been debated for years and is currently under revision. Both in studies and in clinical practice, infantile spasms have traditionally been classified as symptomatic, cryptogenic, or idiopathic. This classification is determined on the basis of the developmental history prior to onset of clinical spasms, clinical signs, and diagnostic studies.

SYMPTOMATIC GROUP

The symptomatic group consists of children who have evidence of neurologic injury at the time of onset or a known associated disorder. This group accounts for approximately 80 percent of patients with infantile spasms [Matsumoto et al., 1981; Riikonen, 2009; Partikian and Mitchell, 2009], although a study of 140 affected patients who were evaluated by computed tomography (CT), MRI, and/or positron emission tomography (PET) reported that 96 percent were symptomatic [Chugani and Conti, 1996], highlighting the importance of multimodal neuroimaging in the evaluation of these infants, especially if they do not respond to therapy.

CRYPTOGENIC AND IDIOPATHIC GROUPS

Cryptogenic and idiopathic are often used interchangeably to represent children without an apparent cause on history, examination, or diagnostic studies. Without other neurologic disorders that alone predict poor prognosis, children with cryptogenic or idiopathic infantile spasms have the best outlook for normal future development. At this point, most investigators favor the term cryptogenic, with the idea that all cases must have an underlying cause, even when the cause is unknown [Lux and Osborne, 2006]. However, Vigevano et al. found that 55 percent of 31 patients with cryptogenic infantile spasms had normal neurodevelopmental outcomes and either a family history of idiopathic epilepsy or febrile convulsions or an EEG genetic trait, thus arguing for a truly idiopathic group [Vigevano et al., 1993]. Other investigators have proposed that an idiopathic group can be defined by specific EEG findings, including reappearance of hypsarrhythmia between consecutive spasms of a cluster, and normal neurodevelopmental outcomes [Dulac et al., 1993]. Even if an idiopathic group does exist, however, an idiopathic classification can only be assigned retrospectively, which limits its use at the time of diagnosis.

Etiology

Although the unifying epileptogenic mechanism is unknown, various underlying disorders give rise to infantile spasms. These disorders are often categorized into prenatal, perinatal, and postnatal groups. Accounting for over 40 percent of total cases [Ohtahara et al., 1993], prenatal etiologies include central nervous system malformations (focal cortical dysplasia, lissencephaly, holoprosencephaly, hemimegalencephaly, callosal agenesis/Aicardi's syndrome), chromosomal abnormalities (trisomy 21, Miller–Dieker syndrome), single-gene errors (*ARX*, *CDKL5/STK9*), neurocutaneous syndromes (tuberous sclerosis, neurofibromatosis type 1, incontinentia pigmenti), congenital central nervous system infections (TORCH, toxoplasmosis, rubella, cytomegalovirus, herpes simplex), and rarely, inborn errors of metabolism (phenylketonuria*, mitochondrial disorders, nonketotic hyperglycinemia, pyridoxine dependency*, sulfite oxidase deficiency, Menkes' disease*, biotinidase deficiency*) (the asterisked conditions represent treatable metabolic disorders). Perinatal precipitants include hypoxic ischemic encephalopathy (including periventricular leukomalacia in infants who were born prematurely) and hypoglycemia. Finally, postnatal factors include intracranial hemorrhage from trauma, acquired central nervous system infections, hypoxic-ischemic insults (near-drowning, cardiac arrest, stroke), and brain tumors [Frost et al., 2003; Watanabe, 1998]. Overall, cortical malformations, tuberous sclerosis, and hypoxia-ischemia are the most common known associated disorders.

Diagnostic Evaluation

Our approach to the evaluation of infantile spasms is outlined in Figure 56-2. First, in a child with suspected infantile spasms, an EEG is needed to confirm the presence of hypsarrhythmia. Given the state-dependence of hypsarrhythmia, an extended EEG recording that captures at least one full sleep–wake cycle should be performed in all cases. If the EEG remains normal with no features of hypsarrhythmia or its variants, the EEG should be repeated in 1–2 weeks, again capturing at least one full sleep–wake cycle. Once the diagnosis of infantile spasms is established, the evaluation shifts to classification and determination of underlying etiology. When the history is being taken, special attention should be paid to perinatal issues and prior development. Examination may reveal dysmorphic features, neurologic signs, or neurocutaneous stigmata. Neuroimaging is the most important diagnostic test, leading to confirmation of etiology in approximately 70 percent of cases [Wyllie et al., 2005]. MRI is the initial neuroimaging modality of choice, with higher sensitivity in detecting subtle structural abnormalities than CT [van Bogaert et al., 1993]. In addition, an MRI itself may inform prognosis, as patients with a normal MRI have been shown to have better motor outcomes compared to those with abnormalities [Saltik et al., 2002]. While not indicated in the initial evaluation of infantile spasms, PET imaging is helpful in identifying abnormalities that are not appreciated by MRI or CT [Chugani et al., 1993; Chugani and Conti, 1996]. This technique should be considered in medically intractable cases when focal EEG or clinical exam findings raise suspicion for a focal central nervous system process that may be amenable to surgical resection. If neuroimaging or clinical examination raises suspicion for a genetic disorder, then targeted genetic testing may be indicated (for instance, in the case of Down syndrome or lissencephaly). Results of metabolic (serum and cerebrospinal fluid) and genetic testing combined may determine the etiology in an additional 10 percent of cases [Wyllie et al., 2005]. Of these, genetic testing has been found to be most helpful, while metabolic testing is often low-yield [Trasmonte and Barron, 1998; Jacobson and Conry, 2009]. However, if the examination and neuroimaging are unrevealing, we recommend a basic metabolic screen, including electrolytes, glucose, lactate, pyruvate,

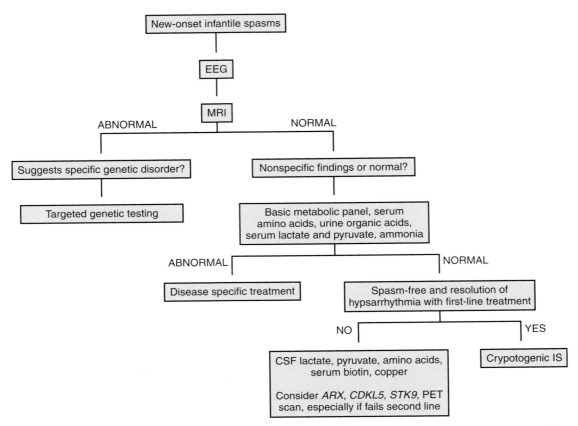

Fig. 56-2 Suggested clinical evaluation and work-up of infantile spasms. IS, infantile spasms; PET, positron emission tomography.

ammonia, plasma amino acids, and urine organic acids. If a patient without a known cause fails initial medical therapy, a lumbar puncture (cell count, glucose, protein, lactate, pyruvate, and amino acids – specifically glycine) should be performed, and serum testing for rare but treatable metabolic disorders that are not diagnosed on first-pass screening (copper for Menkes' disease, biotin for biotinidase deficiency) should be considered. Finally, genetic testing may be revealing in refractory cases without a known cause. Specifically, *ARX* (in male infants) and *CDKL5/STK9* (in female infants, particularly those with Rett's syndrome-like features) should be considered. While the frequency of these gene mutations in infantile spasms is unknown, their contribution to this syndrome is likely appreciable. A recent study screened 177 patients with early-onset seizures of unknown etiology for *CDKL5* mutations, including 30 men and 10 girls with Aicardi's syndrome, for which screening was negative. Of 32 female patients with a history of infantile spasms, 9 (28 percent) had a *CDKL5* mutation [Nemos et al., 2009].

Course and Prognosis

Spontaneous remission of spasms and disappearance of hypsarrhythmia in untreated patients have been reported in 25 percent of children by 1 year of age [Hrachovy et al., 1991]. Natural history is incompletely understood, as most studies involve patients who have been treated with medications that alter the course of infantile spasms. Regardless of treatment, however, it appears that clinical spasms and hypsarrhythmia disappear in one-half of children by 2 years of age and in nearly all

children by 5 years of age [Jeavons et al., 1973]. Approximately 50 percent of children will develop other seizure types, although rates are lower for children with cryptogenic infantile spasms [Koo et al., 1993]. In many patients who exhibit diffuse or multifocal cerebral dysfunction, the disorder evolves into Lennox–Gastaut syndrome. Among infants with focal lesions, such as those seen in tuberous sclerosis, the spasms often evolve into a symptomatic partial epilepsy [Curatolo et al., 2008].

Overall, the developmental outcome in infantile spasms is poor. In a cohort study of 214 patients treated with adrenocorticotropic hormone (ACTH) who were followed for 20–35 years or until death, cognitive outcome was normal or mildly abnormal in 24 percent of survivors [Riikonen, 1996]. Approximately 50 percent have long-term motor impairment [Jeavons et al., 1973; Matsumoto et al., 1981]. Several predictive factors of outcome have been proposed. Most certainly, the pathological process underlying the syndrome heavily influences the prognosis of infantile spasms. Of children classified as symptomatic, only 5–20 percent have normal or mildly impaired development, compared to 50–80 percent who are classified as cryptogenic [Riikonen, 2009; Cowan and Hudson, 1991]. Among the symptomatic group, children with severe brain malformations tend to have worse prognosis. Better initial control of spasms has been associated with improved neurodevelopmental outcome [Riikonen, 1996; Partikian and Mitchell, 2009], even when only evaluating cryptogenic infantile spasms without confounding underlying diagnoses [Lux et al., 2005]. Observational studies have suggested that neurodevelopmental outcomes are improved in infants who have had shorter duration of spasms at time of initial treatment, specifically in infants with cryptogenic infantile spasms treated within 1 month of spasm onset [Kivity et al., 2004; Riikonen, 2009; Cohen-Sadan et al., 2009], and children with infantile spasms and Down syndrome treated within 2 months [Eisermann et al., 2003]. Finally, it has been proposed that a classic hypsarrhythmic pattern in infants with cryptogenic infantile spasms may be associated with improved outcomes, although this remains uncertain [Pellock et al., 2008].

Pathophysiology

Despite it being over 150 years since the clinical recognition of infantile spasms, our understanding of its biological basis is still limited. That this specific epilepsy phenotype is associated with many diverse etiologies points toward a "final common pathway," although historically no suitable animal model existed.

Several hypotheses have been proposed, including brainstem dysfunction due to either disruption of serotonergic neurons [Langlais et al., 1991], or abnormal interaction between the brainstem and a focal or diffuse cortical abnormality [Chugani et al., 1990, 1992], abnormalities in cortical-subcortical interactions [Lado and Moshe, 2002], and immunologic dysfunction.

Alteration in the hypothalamic-adrenal-pituitary (HPA) axis has also been explored. One hypothesis proposes that stress from variable causes during early development results in the release of corticotropin-releasing hormone (CRH), which then leads to increased neuronal excitability and seizures [Brunson et al., 2001]. Supporting evidence for this CRH excess hypothesis includes decreased levels of ACTH found in the cerebrospinal fluid of patients with infantile spasms [Baram et al., 1992b, 1995], and the known effectiveness of ACTH and glucocorticoids in the treatment of infantile spasms. In addition, it has been shown that the CRH receptors are most abundant during infancy, which argues for increased susceptibility to stress during this developmental period [Avishai-Eliner et al., 1996]. However, while it has been shown that injecting CRH into the brains of infant rats produces acute seizures, the ictal semiology and EEG features are not typical of the human infantile spasms phenotype [Baram et al., 1992a]. In addition, CRH levels are not elevated in the cerebrospinal fluid of patients with infantile spasms. While this model accounts for the phenotypic convergence of various etiologies and is supported by the efficacy of hormonal therapy, its usefulness as an animal model is limited. Another hypothesis involving the HPA axis proposes that the protective action of ACTH in infantile spasms could be related, at least in part, to neurosteroids [Rho et al., 2004]. ACTH stimulates adrenal synthesis of both cortisol and deoxycorticosterone (DOC), the latter resulting in increased levels of circulating DOC-derived neurosteroids. In a nonrandomized study, ganaxolone (a neuroactive steroid that modulates GABA receptors via a unique recognition site) as add-on therapy was associated with a 50 percent reduction of spasms in 33 percent of patients with intractable infantile spasms [Kerrigan et al., 2000]. However, corticosteroids are not converted into neurosteroids and yet are also effective in stopping spasms, arguing for a broader underlying mechanism.

In recent years, several new animal models have emerged, spanning the etiological spectrum from acquired to genetic factors. The *N*-methyl-D-aspartate (NMDA) model (injection of NMDA after prenatal exposure to betamethasone) [Velisek et al., 2007] and the Ts65Dn Down syndrome model (injection of GABA agonists) [Cortez et al., 2009] both produced acute spasms with associated electrodecremental EEG changes. However, spasms did not occur spontaneously in either of these models, and therefore they do not address the underlying question of how spasms are generated. Three other animal models do have spontaneous spasmlike seizures. First, the tetrodoxin (TTX) model [Lee et al., 2008] tests the developmental desynchronization hypothesis, which states that infantile spasms result from a particular temporal desynchronization of two or more developmental processes, resulting in brain dysfunction [Frost and Hrachovy, 2005]. TTX is a sodium channel blocker that blocks normal neuronal activity. While the seizures do not develop until the animals are in late adolescence, this model does support the concept of a final common pathway, as multiple genetic and environmental factors could disrupt the developmental process. Another interesting animal model utilizes three toxic compounds (doxorubicin, lipopolysaccharide, and p-chloro-phenylalanine), which, given in short succession, result in cortical and subcortical brain injury and serotonin depletion [Scantlebury et al., 2009]. These pups manifest early spontaneous spasms with associated EEG changes, as well as behavioral changes after spasm onset. Although this model mimics common etiologies, such as neonatal hypoxic-*ischemic* encephalopathy, the induced brain injury is a confounding factor.

Finally, two new ARX mouse models have recently been published [Marsh and Golden, 2009; Price et al., 2009]. The Aristaless-related homeobox (*ARX*) gene encodes a transcription factor involved in cortical development, including GABAergic interneuron migration in the brain [Kitamura et al., 2002; Friocourt et al., 2008]. *ARX* mutations have been found to be associated with a spectrum of neurologic disorders involving mental retardation and epilepsy, including X-linked lissencephaly with ambiguous genitalia, nonsyndromic X-linked mental retardation, and X-linked infantile spasms [Sherr, 2003]. An apparent phenotype–genotype correlation exists, with loss-of-function mutations typically resulting in cortical malformations, and with insertion/duplication mutations resulting in the other *ARX*-related diseases, including infantile spasms. The prevalence of *ARX* mutations in infantile spasms is unknown. Previously, it had been shown that *ARX* knockout mice exhibit a profound GABAergic interneuron migration defect [Kitamura et al., 2002], resulting in a significant deficit of GABAergic interneurons in the neocortex, hippocampus, and striatum. This finding gave rise to the "interneuronopathy" hypothesis, which proposes that the severe epilepsy phenotype in children with *ARX* mutations results largely from cortical interneuron dysfunction [Kato and Dobyns, 2005]. Since the previous *ARX* knockout mice die at birth, limiting postnatal evaluation, investigators have created two new viable mouse models. One is a conditional knockout mouse model (selective deletion of *ARX* from interneurons) [Marsh and Golden, 2009], which produces spasms with associated electrodecrement on EEG, although spasms occur at a later age than in human equivalents and no cognitive changes have been shown. The second is a polyalanine knockin mouse model (targeted expansion of the first polyalanine tract from 16 to 23 alanine codons, the human mutation most commonly associated with X-linked infantile spasms), which produces typical spasms and EEG changes, as well as cognitive sequelae [Price et al., 2009]. Further studies are required to elucidate the role of interneurons in brain development and developmental epilepsies better.

Treatment

The goal of treatment is to prevent or ameliorate the encephalopathy by stopping the spasms and improving the EEG background. Despite numerous published reports on the treatment of infantile spasms over the past half-century, interpretation has been limited due to methodological shortcomings [Lux and Osborne, 2006]. Therefore, at present, there is no consensus regarding optimal treatment, and there is no conclusive evidence that current medical therapies alter neurocognitive or epilepsy outcomes [Hancock et al., 2008]. The most commonly used medical therapies for treatment of infantile spasms are ACTH or oral corticosteroids in the United States, vigabatrin in the UK, and pyridoxine in Japan. With the recent Food and Drug Administration (FDA) approval of vigabatrin in 2009, its use may increase, particularly for infants with tuberous sclerosis or pre-existing cortical blindness. Conventional antiepileptic agents, as well as the ketogenic diet, have been used with incomplete success when first-line agents fail. Finally, fueled by advances in neuroimaging, surgical resection of focal lesions has emerged as a promising option for patients with medically intractable infantile spasms.

We propose a treatment algorithm for infantile spasms based on available evidence and potential known side effects (Figure 56-3).

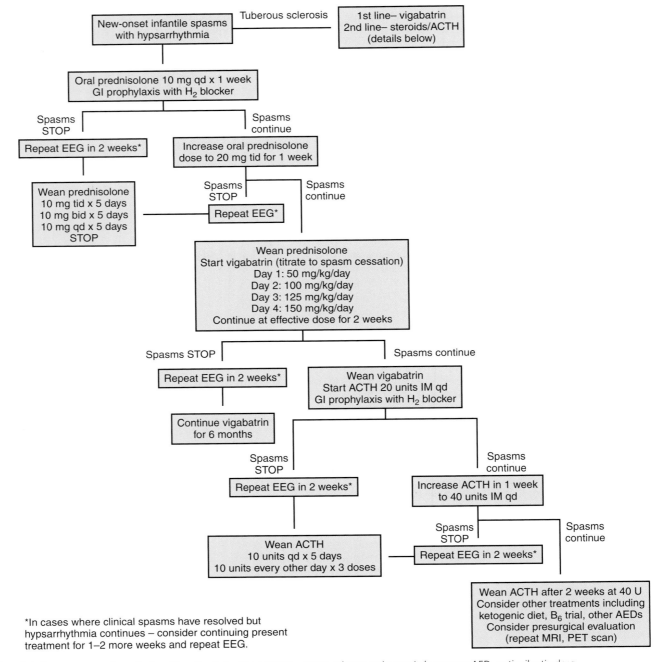

Fig. 56-3 Proposed treatment algorithm for infantile spasms. ACTH, adrenocorticotropic hormone; AED, antiepileptic drug.

Considering some evidence that suggests improved cognitive outcomes in children with cryptogenic infantile spasms or Down syndrome who are treated promptly, we recommend prompt evaluation and treatment of all patients with infantile spasms. In addition, it has been reported that infantile spasms in tuberous sclerosis are independently associated with a reduced IQ, and that the risk of mental retardation increases with prolonged duration of spasms, highlighting the importance of prompt and effective therapy, even in symptomatic cases [O'Callaghan et al., 2004; Goh et al., 2005]. Following the UKISS trial looking at medication schedules for hormonal therapy and vigabatrin, our proposed algorithm supports rapid crossover to an alternate therapy if a complete response has not been achieved with initial therapy. This strategy is supported by the UKISS trial, which showed a high response rate for those who initially did not respond to the allocated treatment but who subsequently received the alternate therapy (74 percent and 75 percent for crossover to hormonal therapy and vigabatrin, respectively) [Lux et al., 2004].

HORMONAL THERAPY

Since initial reports in 1958 describing the effectiveness of ACTH and corticosteroids in stopping the spasms and improving the EEG, hormonal therapy has been the mainstay of treatment for infantile spasms in the United States [Sorel and Dusaucy-Bauloye, 1958]. The recent UKISS trial reported that hormonal therapy (either synthetic ACTH or corticosteroids) stopped the spasms in 73 percent of infants (without tuberous sclerosis) after 2 weeks, compared with vigabatrin in 54 percent [Lux et al., 2004]. While absence of spasms did not differ by treatment group in the follow-up study at 14 months (75 percent versus 76 percent, respectively), there was a clinically significant trend toward better developmental outcomes at 14 months in cryptogenic patients initially treated with hormonal therapy compared to vigabatrin [Lux et al., 2005], highlighting the importance of early spasm cessation and EEG improvement to mitigate the associated encephalopathy. In 2004, a Practice Parameter by the American Academy of Neurology and Child Neurology Society deemed ACTH "probably effective," reaffirming the prevailing consensus that ACTH was the gold standard [Mackay et al., 2004]. In recent years, however, considering the subanalysis results from UKISS (see below), the escalating cost of ACTH, and the severe known potential side effects of ACTH therapy, a national discussion about oral corticosteroids as first-line therapy has emerged.

ACTH

Two forms of adrenocorticotropic hormone (ACTH), natural H.P. Acthar Gel Repository Injection and synthetic cosyntropin (Synacthen Depot), have been used in the United States for the treatment of infantile spasms, but neither is FDA-approved. Unlike H.P. Acthar Gel, Synacthen is not FDA-approved for any purpose and therefore it is only available through a compassionate-use program.

Several prospective, randomized trials of ACTH or cosyntropin of varying doses have shown that 42–87 percent of patients experienced cessation of spasms within 2 weeks of initiating therapy [Baram et al., 1996; Hrachovy et al., 1983, 1994; Vigevano and Cilio 1997; Yanagaki et al., 1999]. Hypsarrhythmia resolved in 20–90 percent of patients, and relapse rates were 15–33 percent. While there is no agreement about dose or duration of treatment, two randomized controlled trials

comparing high-dose ACTH with low-dose ACTH did not show a significant difference in terms of spasm cessation. In a long-term follow-up study, there was no clear benefit of 150 IU/day compared with 40 IU/day [Riikonen, 1982]. Given the lack of evidence to support high-dose ACTH, and considering the dose-dependent potential severe side effects, we recommend lower doses and a short treatment course. A prospective study comparing ACTH and vigabatrin for all patients with infantile spasms showed superior short-term spasm cessation in the ACTH group (74 percent versus 48 percent, respectively) [Vigevano and Cilio, 1997], and the UKISS study showed similar short-term results comparing hormonal therapy with vigabatrin in non-tuberous sclerosis patients [Lux et al., 2004]. Based on these and other studies, a recent Cochrane review concluded that hormonal treatment is more effective than vigabatrin in the short-term treatment of non-tuberous sclerosis-related infantile spasms [Hancock et al., 2008]. ACTH side effects are significant and should be carefully considered when determining the most appropriate form of hormonal therapy for the patient. Cushingoid obesity and irritability develop in most patients. More serious side effects appear to be dose-dependent and include arterial hypertension, cardiomyopathy, electrolyte imbalance, gastric ulcer, immunosuppression, and growth retardation [Shields 2006].

CORTICOSTEROIDS

Corticosteroids result in short-term spasm cessation in 29–70 percent of patients with infantile spasms [Mackay et al., 2004] [Lux et al., 2004]. Except for UKISS, these studies evaluated low-dose corticosteroids. One randomized controlled trial reported that low-dose oral corticosteroids was less effective than ACTH in stopping spasms (29 percent vs 87 percent, respectively) [Baram et al., 1996], while another similar study did not show a significant difference between the two groups (33 percent vs 42 percent, respectively) [Hrachovy et al., 1983]. Based on varying study results, the 2004 Practice Parameter concluded that there was insufficient evidence to recommend oral corticosteroids. Since that time, the UKISS trial subanalysis showed that oral prednisolone was equivalent to synthetic ACTH (70 percent vs 76 percent spasm-free after 14 days, respectively). While this study was not powered to determine a significant difference between the two groups, it had more subjects than prior studies and represents the only randomized controlled trial evaluating the effectiveness of high-dose oral corticosteroid. Incorporating UKISS results, a 2008 Cochrane review concluded that, should oral prednisolone be used, "high dose" is recommended [Hancock et al., 2008]. The difference in dose may explain the significantly lower spasm-free rate of oral prednisone reported in the 1983 and 1996 studies mentioned above. In those studies, prednisone was used at a dose of 2 mg/kg/day, which is roughly half of the UKISS starting dose of 10 mg four times daily.

Of note is the fact that, in August 2007, the price of H.P. Acthar Gel increased 15-fold and a full course of treatment now costs roughly $100,000 [Gettig et al., 2009]; this does not include the specialized nursing training and sometimes brief inpatient admission necessary to train caregivers on how to administer an injectable medication. In comparison, a course of oral prednisolone costs a few hundred dollars and is much easier to administer. Given these circumstances, we and many centers have moved towards using oral prednisolone as first-line therapy [Kossoff et al., 2009], but an adequately powered study comparing prednisolone and ACTH is still warranted.

VIGABATRIN

The first AED to be developed on the basis of a targeted mechanism of action, vigabatrin is an irreversible inhibitor of the enzyme gamma-aminobutyric acid transaminase. Inhibition of this enzyme results in increased levels of GABA in the brain. Vigabatrin has been shown to be effective in the short-term treatment of infantile spasms, particularly in patients with tuberous sclerosis as the underlying cause. In a multicenter retrospective study, suppression of spasms was achieved within a mean of 6 days in 69 percent of all infants and in 96 percent of those with tuberous sclerosis [Aicardi et al., 1996]. In a small study, Chiron et al. reported a 100 percent response rate in patients with tuberous sclerosis treated with vigabatrin (150 mg/kg/day), compared to 45 percent treated with hydrocortisone at 1-month follow-up [Chiron et al., 1997]. Later studies have confirmed the particular efficacy of vigabatrin in patients with infantile spasms due to tuberous sclerosis. In contrast, short-term efficacy rates for all or non-TS infantile spasms range from 35 to 54 percent [Lux et al., 2004; Vigevano and Cilio, 1997; Appleton et al., 1999]. We recommend vigabatrin as first-line therapy for patients with infantile spasms due to tuberous sclerosis. Considering that 75 percent of patients in the UKISS trial, who initially failed hormonal therapy but then were treated with vigabatrin, were spasm-free at 14 months [Lux et al., 2005], we support the use of vigabatrin as second-line therapy in patients without tuberous sclerosis.

In August 2009, vigabatrin was approved by the FDA to treat infantile spasms in children aged 1 month to 2 years. It had been available in many countries for nearly two decades, but was previously unavailable in the U.S. due to concern about an irreversible, cumulative dose-dependent peripheral visual field defect (VFD). In various studies, the prevalence of the vigabatrin-induced peripheral VFD ranged from 25 to 50 percent in adults, 15 percent in children, and 15 to 31 percent in infants [Willmore et al., 2009]. The earliest onset of VFD in infants was found to be 3.1 months. The VFD is a bilateral, concentric, predominantly nasal constriction of the visual field. Visual acuity is not affected, and patients are often asymptomatic until the defect has encroached into the central vision. Perimetry, visual-evoked potentials, and electroretinography testing has been used in adults and children to detect peripheral VFD. In infants, however, electroretinography is the only sensitive technique, and the required sedation limits its use. A recent report recommends using "age-appropriate" visual field testing in infants at baseline and then every 3 months until 18 months of treatment, and then every 6 months thereafter [Willmore et al., 2009]. Unfortunately, there is no viable age-appropriate option for visual field testing in this population, and emphasis is instead placed on informed consent and weighing the risks of anesthesia required for electroretinography against unidentified VFD with drug continuation. To avoid unnecessary exposure, we recommend discontinuation of vigabatrin if a response is not obtained within 2 weeks. If a response is achieved, the infant should have a formal ophthalmologic examination at 3 months and electroretinography should be discussed with the family and ophthalmologist. Some centers that follow electroretinography every 3–4 months also recommend an electroretinogram 6 months after the vigabatrin has been stopped [AES, 2009]. Given the natural history of the disorder, we generally recommend discontinuation of vigabatrin at 6 months, although the benefits of continuation may outweigh the risks in some cases such as pre-existing cortical blindness.

SURGICAL THERAPY

Facilitated by advances in structural and functional neuroimaging techniques, surgical resection of focal or unilateral central nervous system lesions has emerged as an effective epilepsy treatment option in selected patients with intractable infantile spasms. Epilepsy surgery for infantile spasms was fueled by the observation that PET of glucose metabolism could identify focal cortical lesions localized to epileptogenic regions in infants with cryptogenic infantile spasms whose functional imaging was unrevealing, and that surgical resection was associated with a favorable outcome [Chugani et al., 1990]. Following this report, Chugani et al. reported on 23 patients with infantile spasms who underwent cortical resection or hemispherectomy. In 14 of the 23 patients, PET was the only imaging modality that showed the regional abnormality [Chugani et al., 1993]. These and later series have shown that surgical resection of a focal cortical lesion for intractable infantile spasms results in complete seizure control in 50–60 percent of patients [Chugani et al., 1993; Wyllie et al., 1998]. When focal resections are performed on cortical areas showing abnormal metabolism or perfusion on PET or single photon emission computed tomography (SPECT), neuropathological examination of the resected tissue usually reveals cortical dysplasia [Chugani et al., 1990; Vinters, 2002]. The impact of surgery on long-term development is uncertain, although limited evidence points toward improved outcomes, particularly in cases of early surgical intervention [Asano et al., 2001]. While further studies are required to determine the impact of surgery on developmental outcomes, surgical resection of focal cortical regions is an important therapeutic option, and specialized presurgical evaluation should be considered in patients with localizing clinical or EEG signs, specifically asymmetrical spasms, hemihypsarrhythmia, and partial seizures, even in the absence of a well-defined MRI lesion.

OTHER TREATMENTS

There are no randomized controlled trials of other antiepileptic medications or alternative therapies for the treatment of infantile spasms, although limited evidence suggests that valproate, topiramate, zonisamide, pyridoxine, and the ketogenic diet may provide additional benefit in reducing spasms and, therefore, are often used after hormonal therapy and vigabatrin. The impact of these therapies on neurodevelopmental outcome is unknown. Without strong evidence to support a particular agent, the potential risks of each therapy should influence individual treatment decisions.

As an effective broad-spectrum agent for generalized seizure types that may follow infantile spasms, valproate is a reasonable choice after first-line treatments fail, although the increased risk of hepatotoxicity in children under 2 years of age should be considered. Valproate may benefit 40 percent of patients who do not respond to ACTH [Bachman, 1982]. In a recent abstract, 5 out of 5 patients with Down syndrome treated with valproate (doses 30–45 mg/kg/day) after failing at least one other medication were spasm-free at 2 years, and 4 of 5 had resolution of hypsarrhythmia within 2–4 weeks [Patterson et al., 2009]. Further studies are required to determine if valproate is particularly effective in this group of patients. In terms of valproate monotherapy for infantile spasms, one uncontrolled prospective open-label study reported cessation of spasms in 73 percent and resolution of hypsarrhythmia in 91 percent of 22 children at 6 months follow-up, with cessation of spasms in 50 percent within 4 weeks [Siemes et al., 1988]. The 6-month cessation rate is difficult to interpret, however, because dexamethasone therapy was added at 4 weeks if valproate monotherapy was ineffective.

Several open-label studies evaluating topiramate as monotherapy or adjunctive therapy in the treatment of infantile spasms [Peltzer et al., 2009; Glauser et al., 1998] have reported seizure cessation rates of 20–50 percent within variable follow-up periods, with mean maintenance doses of approximately 15 mg/kg/day. A survey of 41 U.S. pediatric epileptologists reported that topiramate is the most commonly used agent after hormonal therapy in patients with symptomatic infantile spasms not associated with tuberous sclerosis [Wheless et al., 2005].

Zonisamide has also been used for infantile spasms. In the largest series, 33 percent of the 27 patients treated with zonisamide (mean dose 8 mg/kg/day) monotherapy or add-on therapy had spasm cessation and 75 percent had resolution of hypsarrhythmia at a mean of 5 days after initiation of treatment, although the relapse rate was 44 percent [Yanai et al., 1999]. Another similar study reported spasm cessation in 26 percent of 23 patients treated with zonisamide monotherapy or add-on therapy, without any relapses at 6 months

[Lotze and Wilfong, 2004]. Suzuki et al. reported that 20 percent of 54 infants given zonisamide after failing vitamin B_6 had cessation of spasms within 3 weeks, although 27 percent relapsed shortly after initial cessation [Suzuki, 2001]. High-dose vitamin B_6 has been the treatment of choice for symptomatic and cryptogenic infantile spasms in Japan, although there are no randomized controlled trials. In two uncontrolled, prospective open-label studies, spasm cessation was achieved in 13–29 percent of patients treated with variable doses of pyridoxine within several weeks [Pietz et al., 1993]. With a mild side effect profile and the possibility of pyridoxine-dependent seizures, a brief trial of pyridoxine should be considered when first-line therapy fails. While an intravenous bolus of pyridoxine during the initial EEG recoding is optimal, this is often not technically feasible. Given the recent evidence that pyridoxine-dependent seizures and folinic-responsive seizures are allelic [Gallagher et al., 2009], folinic acid should be co-administered with pyridoxine. Response to this treatment should be re-evaluated at 1–2 weeks. Finally, there is limited evidence that the ketogenic diet may help control spasms in refractory cases, and possibly even as first-line therapy, although additional studies are required [Kossoff et al., 2002, 2008]. We recommend consideration of the ketogenic diet after hormonal therapy and vigabatrin have failed; whether it is attempted prior to initiation of another medication is based on family preferences and an informed discussion about known side effects of each therapy.

 The complete list of references for this chapter is available online at **www.expertconsult.com**.
See inside cover for registration details.

Febrile Seizures

Shlomo Shinnar

Febrile seizures are a form of acute symptomatic seizures. They occur in 2–5 percent of children and are the most common form of childhood seizures. In the past, it was believed that most febrile seizures represented a form of epilepsy and that the prognosis was not favorable [Lennox, 1949, 1953; Livingston et al., 1947; Taylor and Ounsted, 1971]. Febrile seizures were believed to cause brain damage and subsequent epilepsy [Fowler, 1957; Taylor and Ounsted, 1971; Wallace, 1980]. One author summarized this view of prognosis in an article titled "They Don't Do Very Well" [Wallace, 1980]. This pessimistic view was based on a selected population of children seen in tertiary care centers and on patients with refractory epilepsy seen at these centers who had a history of febrile seizures [Bruton, 1988; Falconer, 1971; Falconer and Serafetinides, 1964; Livingston et al., 1947]. These patients, however, were not representative of a majority of children with febrile seizures [Ellenberg and Nelson, 1980].

Over the past 25 years, much more information on febrile seizures has accumulated from both human and animal studies [Baram and Shinnar, 2002]. The prognosis for febrile seizures usually has been found to be good. Such seizures are not associated with any detectable brain damage [Ellenberg and Nelson, 1978; Knudsen et al., 1996; Maytal and Shinnar, 1990; National Institutes of Health (NIH), 1980; Nelson and Ellenberg, 1978; Verity and Golding, 1991; Verity et al., 1985b, 1993; Wolf and Forsythe, 1989], and epilepsy will eventually develop in only a small minority of children who have had febrile seizures [Annegers et al., 1979, 1987; Berg, 1992; Berg and Shinnar, 1996b; Knudsen et al., 1996; Nelson and Ellenberg, 1976, 1978; van den Berg and Yerushalmi, 1969; Verity and Golding, 1991; Verity et al., 1985b, 1993; Wolf and Forsythe, 1989]. This understanding is based on large epidemiologic studies [Annegers et al., 1979, 1987; Berg, 1992; Nelson and Ellenberg, 1976, 1978; van den Berg and Yerushalmi, 1969; Verity and Golding, 1991; Verity et al., 1985b, 1993], as well as on prospective studies from emergency departments not selected for tertiary referral bias [Berg et al., 1992; Knudsen, 1985a, 1985b; Wolf and Forsythe, 1989]. It also has been learned that, although antiepileptic drugs can prevent recurrent febrile seizures, they do not alter the risk of subsequent epilepsy [American Academy of Pediatrics (AAP), 1999; Berg and Shinnar, 1997; Knudsen et al., 1996; Rosman et al., 1993b; Shinnar and Berg, 1996; Wolf and Forsythe, 1989]. This finding has led to a changing view of the treatment of these common and largely benign seizures [AAP, 1999; Knudsen, 2002].

This chapter reviews the current understanding of the prognosis and management of febrile seizures.

Definitions

A febrile seizure is defined by the International League against Epilepsy as a seizure occurring in association with a febrile illness in the absence of a central nervous system (CNS) infection or acute electrolyte imbalance in children older than 1 month of age without prior afebrile seizures [Commission on Epidemiology and Prognosis, 1993]. This definition is similar to the one adopted earlier by the National Institutes of Health (NIH) Consensus Conference [1980]. The febrile illness must include a body temperature of more than 38.4°C, although the increased temperature may not occur until after the seizure. The child may be neurologically normal or abnormal. In the International League against Epilepsy guidelines for epidemiologic research [Commission on Epidemiology and Prognosis, 1993], febrile seizures and, by extension, febrile status epilepticus are further divided into those occurring in children without prior neonatal seizures and those in children with prior neonatal seizures. In earlier epidemiologic studies, the lower age range used was either 1 month [Annegers et al., 1979, 1987, 1990; Berg et al., 1990, 1992, 1997; Verity et al., 1985a] or 3 months [Nelson and Ellenberg, 1976, 1978]. No specific upper age limit is used. Febrile seizures are most common, however, between the ages of 6 months and 3 years, with peak incidence at approximately 18 months of age. Onset after the age of 7 years is uncommon.

Febrile seizures are further classified as simple or complex. A febrile seizure is complex if it is focal, prolonged (lasting for more than either 10 minutes [Annegers et al., 1979, 1987, 1990; Berg and Shinnar, 1996a; Berg et al., 1992, 1997] or 15 minutes [Berg and Shinnar, 1996a; Nelson and Ellenberg, 1976, 1978]), or multiple (occurrence of more than one seizure during the febrile illness). Conversely, it is simple if it is an isolated, brief, generalized seizure. Although neurologically abnormal children are more likely to experience complex febrile seizures and have a higher risk for subsequent afebrile seizures, the child's prior neurologic condition is not used to classify the seizure as simple or complex [Commission on Epidemiology and Prognosis, 1993; NIH, 1980]. When a careful history is obtained, approximately 30 percent of patients with febrile seizures presenting to the emergency department are found to have complex features [Berg and Shinnar, 1996a].

Epidemiology

Febrile seizures are the most common form of childhood seizures. The peak incidence is at the age of approximately 18 months. In the United States and Western Europe, they occur in 2–4 percent of all children [AAP, 1996; Annegers et al., 1990; Berg, 1995; Nelson and Ellenberg, 1978; van den Berg and Yerushalmi, 1969; Verity et al., 1985a]. In Japan, however, 9–10 percent of all children experience at least one febrile seizure [Tsuboi, 1984], and rates as high as 14 percent have been reported from the Mariana Islands in Guam [Stanhope et al., 1972].

Traditionally, it was thought that febrile seizures most commonly occur as the first sign of a febrile illness. More recent studies, however, found that only 21 percent of the children experienced their seizure either before or within 1 hour of the onset of the fever, 57 percent had a seizure after 1–24 hours of fever, and 22 percent experienced their febrile seizure more than 24 hours after the onset of the fever [Berg et al., 1992, 1997].

Some children are at increased risk of experiencing a febrile seizure. In a case-control population-based study, Bethune et al. [1993] examined risk factors for a first febrile seizure and found that the following four factors were associated with an increased risk of febrile seizures:

1. a history of febrile seizures in a first- or second-degree relative
2. a neonatal nursery stay of more than 30 days
3. developmental delay
4. attendance at day care.

Children with two of these factors had a 28 percent chance of experiencing at least one febrile seizure.

In another case-control study using febrile controls matched for age, site of routine pediatric care, and date of visit, Berg et al. [1995] examined the issue of which children with a febrile illness were most likely to experience a febrile seizure. On multivariate analysis, significant independent risk factors were the height of the peak temperature and a history of febrile seizures in an immediate relative. Gastroenteritis as the underlying illness had a significant inverse (i.e., protective) association with febrile seizures. Similar results on the importance of the peak temperature were reported from a hospital-based study [Rantala et al., 1995].

The majority of febrile seizures are simple seizures. In a recent study of 428 children with a first febrile seizure, Berg and Shinnar [1996a] found that 35 percent had at least one complex feature, including focality in 16 percent, multiple seizures in 14 percent, and prolonged duration (longer than 10 minutes) in 13 percent. Approximately 6 percent of children had at least two complex features, and 1 percent had all three complex features. Of most concern have been prolonged febrile seizures. In that study, 14 percent of the children had seizures lasting longer than 10 minutes; 9 percent, longer than 15 minutes; and 5 percent, longer than 30 minutes, or febrile status epilepticus. Although febrile status epilepticus accounts for only 5 percent of febrile seizures, it accounts for approximately 25 percent of all cases of childhood status epilepticus [Aicardi and Chevrie, 1970; DeLorenzo et al., 1996; Dodson et al., 1993; Dunn, 1988; Maytal et al., 1989; Shinnar et al., 1997], and for more than two-thirds of cases of status epilepticus in the second year of life [Shinnar et al., 1997].

Initial Evaluation

As implied by the definition, to make the diagnosis of a febrile seizure, one must exclude meningitis, encephalitis, serious electrolyte imbalance, and other acute neurologic illnesses. These exclusions usually are feasible and are based on a detailed history and physical and neurologic examination. The most common issue in the emergency department is whether a lumbar puncture is necessary to exclude CNS infection, particularly meningitis or encephalitis. As reported in several studies, the incidence of meningitis in children with an apparent febrile seizure is between 2 and 5 percent [AAP, 1996; Heijbel et al., 1980; Jaffe et al., 1981; Joffe et al., 1983; Lorber and Sunderland, 1980; McIntyre et al., 1990; Rutter and Metcalf, 1978; Rutter and Smales, 1977; Wears et al., 1986]. In all of the reported series, however, a majority of the children with meningitis had identifiable risk factors. In one series, Joffe et al. [1983] reported that the children with meningitis had one of the following four features: a visit for medical care within the previous 48 hours, seizures on arrival to the emergency room, focal seizures, or suspicious findings on physical or neurologic examination. Other authors also have found a low yield on routine lumbar puncture in the absence of risk factors [AAP, 1996; Lorber and Sunderland, 1980; McIntyre et al., 1990; Rossi et al., 1986; Wears et al., 1986].

The AAP [1996] issued guidelines for the neurodiagnostic evaluation of the child with a simple febrile seizure between the ages of 6 months and 5 years. It recommended that a lumbar puncture be strongly considered in the infant younger than 12 months of age. The child between 12 and 18 months of age needs careful assessment, because the signs of meningitis may be subtle. In the absence of suspicious findings on history or examination, a lumbar puncture is not necessary in a child older than 18 months. A lumbar puncture is still recommended in children with a first complex febrile seizure, as well as in any child with persistent lethargy. It also should be strongly considered in a child who has already received prior antibiotic therapy. A lumbar puncture also should be considered in the child older than 5 years of age who presents with an apparent first febrile seizure, to exclude the possibility of encephalitis, as well as meningitis.

In the absence of suspicious findings in the history (e.g., vomiting, diarrhea) or on physical examination, routine blood cell counts and determination of serum electrolyte, calcium, phosphorus, magnesium, or blood glucose levels are of limited value in the evaluation of a child older than 6 months of age with a febrile seizure [AAP, 1996; Gerber and Berliner, 1981; Heijbel et al., 1980; Jaffe et al., 1981; Rutter and Smales, 1977].

Skull radiographs are of no value. Computed tomography (CT) scans also are of limited benefit in this clinical setting. Magnetic resonance imaging (MRI) scans are not indicated in children with a simple febrile seizure [AAP, 1996]. Whether an MRI study is indicated in the evaluation of a child with a prolonged or focal febrile seizure remains unclear [Lewis et al., 2002; Mitchell and Lewis, 2002; Rosman, 2002; VanLandingham et al., 1998]. MRIs often are clinically indicated in the diagnostic evaluation of the child who presents with status epilepticus, whether febrile or not [Dodson et al., 1993].

Electroencephalograms (EEGs) are of limited value in the evaluation of the child with febrile seizures [AAP, 1996; Koyama et al., 1991; Maytal et al., 2000; Millichap, 1991; Sofianov et al., 1983, 1992; Stores, 1991]. They are more likely to be abnormal in the older child with febrile seizures and in children with a family history of febrile seizures, with a complex febrile seizure, or with pre-existing neurodevelopmental abnormalities [Doose et al., 1983; Frantzen et al., 1968;

Koyama et al., 1991; Millichap et al., 1960; Sofianov et al., 1983, 1992; Tsuboi, 1978]. Although EEG abnormalities may be present in these children, their clinical significance is unclear. There is no evidence that they help predict either recurrence of febrile seizures or the development of subsequent epilepsy [AAP, 1996; Doose et al., 1983; Frantzen et al., 1968; Koyama et al., 1991; Kuturec et al., 1997; Maytal et al., 2000; Millichap et al., 1960; Sofianov et al., 1983, 1992; Tsuboi, 1978]. In most cases, they are of limited clinical value in the evaluation of the child with a febrile seizure. EEGs are indicated in the diagnostic evaluation of status epilepticus of all types, including febrile [Riviello et al., 2006], and may be of particular interest in the child with febrile status epilepticus, as they may have predictive value for the development of subsequent epilepsy [Frantzen et al., 1968; Nordli et al., 2009].

Pathophysiology

The pathophysiology of febrile seizures remains unclear. An age-specific increased susceptibility to seizures induced by fever is likely. Although it was thought that the rate of rise of the temperature was the key factor [Livingston et al., 1947], more recent data suggest that it is the actual peak temperature [Berg, 1993; Berg et al., 1995; Rantala et al., 1995]. Although, by definition, CNS infections are excluded, the nature of the illness does appear to play a role. Gastroenteritis is associated with a lower incidence of febrile seizures [Berg et al., 1995], and herpesvirus-6 and herpesvirus-7 infections have had a high reported rate of association with febrile seizures [Barone et al., 1995; Caserta et al., 1998; Hall et al., 1994; Kondo et al., 1993; Theodore et al., 2008]. There is increased interest in the role of herpesvirus-6 in the pathogenesis of prolonged febrile seizures and subsequent temporal lobe epilepsy [Theodore et al., 2008]. Animal models of febrile seizures also reveal an age-dependent effect [Baram et al., 1997; Germano et al., 1996; Holtzman et al., 1981; Olson et al., 1984]. In addition, in vitro preparations demonstrate induction of epileptiform activity by temperature elevation in hippocampal slices in young rats [Tancredi et al., 1992]. Animal data suggest that young rats with neuronal migration disorders are more susceptible to hyperthermia-induced seizures and also are more susceptible to hippocampal damage [Germano et al., 1996]. Of interest, in this model, hippocampal damage occurs with hyperthermia, even in the absence of seizures.

An animal model developed by Baram et al. [1997] mimics the age-specific human condition and has been providing many insights into the pathophysiology and physiologic consequences of febrile seizures. In this model, febrile seizures appear to be of limbic origin [Baram et al., 1997; Chen et al., 1999; Dube et al., 2000; Toth et al., 1998]. As in humans, brief febrile seizures have no detectable anatomic or physiologic sequelae [Chen et al., 1999; Dube et al., 2000; Toth et al., 1998]. Febrile seizures lasting longer than 20 minutes, however, although not causing cell death [Toth et al., 1998], are associated with long-lasting changes in h-channels, The h-channel is the hyperpolarization-activated cation channel, also known as the pacemaker channel, which can be either "excitatory" or "inhibitory" [Poolos, 2004]. These changes are associated with increased susceptibility to seizures, although not with spontaneous seizures [Chen et al., 1999; Dube et al., 2000]. A full review of the findings from this model is outside the scope

of this chapter, and the interested reader is referred to a recent monograph on this rapidly evolving field [Baram and Shinnar, 2002].

Related Morbidity and Mortality

The mortality associated with febrile seizures is extremely low. No deaths were reported from the National Collaborative Perinatal Project [Nelson and Ellenberg, 1978, 1976] or the British Cohort Study [Verity et al., 1985a, 1985b, 1993]. Even in cases of febrile status epilepticus, which represents the extreme end of complex febrile seizures, the mortality rates in recent series are extremely low [DeLorenzo et al., 1996; Dodson et al., 1993; Dunn, 1988; Maytal and Shinnar, 1990; Maytal et al., 1989; Shinnar et al., 2001; Towne et al., 1994; Verity et al., 1993]. In one recent report of 172 cases of febrile status epilepticus, only one death occurred, which in retrospect likely was related to *Shigella* encephalopathy, rather than to the febrile seizure [Shinnar et al., 2001]. Neither the National Perinatal Project nor the British studies found any evidence of permanent motor deficits after febrile seizures. This finding coincides with a recent series of febrile status epilepticus studies [DeLorenzo et al., 1996; Dunn, 1988; Maytal et al., 1989; Shinnar et al., 2001; Towne et al., 1994; Verity et al., 1993].

The cognitive abilities of children with febrile seizures have been extensively studied. No reports describe acute deterioration of cognitive abilities after febrile seizures, even when studies limited to status epilepticus are included [Dunn, 1988; Ellenberg and Nelson, 1978; Hirtz, 2002; Maytal and Shinnar, 1990; Maytal et al., 1989; Shinnar et al., 2001; Verity et al., 1993]. Cognitive abilities and school performance of children with febrile seizures were found to be similar to those of controls in three large studies [Ellenberg and Nelson, 1978; Ross et al., 1980; Verity et al., 1985b, 1993]. The Collaborative Perinatal Project found no difference in IQ scores or performance on the Wide Range Achievement Test at the age of 7 years between children with febrile seizures and their siblings [Ellenberg and Nelson, 1978]. The British National Child Development Study reported that children with febrile seizures performed as well in school at 7 and 11 years of age as their peers without a history of febrile seizures [Ross et al., 1980]. The more recent British Cohort Study also found no difference between 5-year-olds with febrile seizures and 5-year-olds without a history of febrile seizures on a variety of performance tasks [Verity et al., 1985b, 1993]. A recent study from Taiwan, in addition to comparing intelligence and behavior, also found no difference in memory between children with febrile seizures, including complex ones, and population-based controls [Chang et al., 2000, 2001]. This finding is of particular interest because febrile seizures appear to be of limbic origin [Baram et al., 1997; Dube et al., 2000], and memory is subserved by the hippocampus.

Even prolonged febrile seizures do not appear to be associated with adverse cognitive outcomes [Ellenberg and Nelson, 1978; Shinnar and Babb, 1997; Shinnar et al., 2001; Verity et al., 1993]. In the British Cohort Study, no differences were found between 5-year-olds with and those without febrile seizures, even when the analysis was limited to complex febrile seizures [Verity et al., 1985b, 1993]. Ellenberg and Nelson [1978] examined 27 children with febrile convulsions lasting more than 30 minutes and found no differences in cognitive function at 7 years of age between them and their siblings. Insufficient data are available on memory function in children who experienced prolonged febrile seizures, although memory is known to be impaired in those with chronic temporal lobe epilepsy [Bell and Davies, 1998].

Recurrent Febrile Seizures

Approximately one-third of children with a first febrile seizure will experience a recurrence, and 10 percent will have three or more febrile seizures [AAP, 1996; Annegers et al., 1990; Berg, 2002; Berg et al., 1990, 1992, 1997; Knudsen, 1985b; Nelson and Ellenberg, 1976, 1978; Offringa et al., 1992, 1994; van den Berg, 1974; Verity et al., 1985a]. Factors associated with a differential risk of recurrent febrile seizures are summarized in Table 57-1. The most consistent risk factors reported are a family history of febrile seizures and age at first febrile seizure (before age 18 months) [AAP, 1996; Annegers et al., 1990; Berg, 2002; Berg et al., 1990, 1992, 1997; Knudsen, 1985b; Nelson and Ellenberg, 1978; 1976; Offringa et al., 1992, 1994; van den Berg, 1974]. This relation appears to be due to the longer period during which a child with a younger age at onset will be in the age group at risk for febrile seizures, rather than to a greater tendency to have seizures with each specific illness [Offringa et al., 1992, 1994; Shirts et al., 1987].

In studies that examined features of the acute illness, the peak temperature [Berg et al., 1990, 1992, 1997; El-Rahdi and Banajeh, 1989; Offringa et al., 1992, 1994] and also the duration of the fever before the seizure [Berg et al., 1992, 1997] were associated with a differential risk of recurrent febrile seizures. The higher the peak temperature, the lower the chance of recurrence. In the studies by Berg et al. [1992, 1997], patients with a peak temperature of 101°F had a 42 percent recurrence risk at 1 year, compared with 29 percent for those with a peak temperature of 103°F and only 12 percent for those with a peak temperature of 105°F or greater. The shorter the duration of recognized fever, the higher the chance of recurrence. For those with a febrile seizure within an hour of recognized onset of fever, the recurrence risk at 1 year was 46 percent, compared with 25 percent for those with prior fever lasting 1–24 hours and 15 percent for those with more than 24 hours of recognized fever before the febrile seizure. The fact that those infants in whom the febrile seizure occurs at the onset of fever have the highest risk of recurrence has implications for prophylactic strategies that rely on giving medications at the onset of the febrile illness.

The data regarding a family history of unprovoked seizures or epilepsy are conflicting. A large study in Rochester, Minnesota, found no difference in recurrence risk between children with a family history of epilepsy (25 percent) and those with no such family history (23 percent) [Annegers et al., 1990]. Other studies have found more equivocal results [Berg et al., 1992, 1997; Offringa et al., 1992, 1994]. However, even those studies that report an increased risk of recurrence in children with a family history of unprovoked seizures found only a modest increase in risk. A complex febrile seizure is not associated with an increased risk of recurrence in most studies [Annegers et al., 1990; Berg et al., 1990, 1992, 1997; Berg and Shinnar, 1996a; Nelson and Ellenberg, 1978; Offringa, 1992, 1994]. If the initial febrile seizure is prolonged, however, a recurrent febrile seizure also is more likely to be prolonged [Berg and Shinnar, 1996a; Offringa et al., 1994]. The presence of a neurodevelopmental abnormality in the child also has not been demonstrated to be significantly associated with an increased risk of subsequent febrile seizures [Annegers et al., 1990; Berg et al., 1990, 1992, 1997; Offringa et al., 1992, 1994]. Ethnicity and gender also have not been associated with a clear differential risk of recurrent febrile seizures.

Children with multiple risk factors are at highest risk for recurrence [Berg, 2002; Berg et al., 1997; Offringa et al., 1994]. A child with two or more risk factors has a greater than 30 percent recurrence risk at 2 years, and the child with three or more risk factors has a greater than 60 percent recurrence risk [Berg et al., 1997]. By contrast, the child older than 18 months with no family history of febrile seizures who experiences a first febrile seizure associated with a peak temperature higher than 40°C after a recognized fever longer than 1 hour in duration (i.e., no risk factors) has a 2-year recurrence risk of greater than 15 percent [Berg et al., 1997; Offringa et al., 1994].

Table 57-1 Risk Factors for Recurrent Febrile Seizures and for Epilepsy after a Febrile Seizure

Recurrent Febrile Seizures	Epilepsy
DEFINITE RISK FACTOR	
Family history of febrile seizures	Neurodevelopmental abnormality
Age younger than 18 months	Complex febrile seizure
Height of peak temperature	Family history of epilepsy
Duration of fever	Duration of fever
POSSIBLE RISK FACTOR	
Family history of epilepsy	More than one complex feature
NOT A RISK FACTOR	
Neurodevelopmental abnormality	Family history of febrile seizures
Complex febrile seizure	Age at first febrile seizure
More than one complex feature	Height of peak temperature
Gender	Gender
Ethnicity	Ethnicity

(Data from Annegers et al., 1979, 1987, 1990; Berg and Shinnar, 1996b; Berg et al., 1990, 1992, 1997; El-Rahdi and Banajeh, 1989; Knudsen, 1985b; Nelson and Ellenberg, 1976, 1978; Offringa et al., 1992, 1994; van den Berg, 1974; Verity and Golding, 1991.)

Febrile Seizures and Subsequent Epilepsy

Data from five large cohorts of children with febrile seizures indicate that epilepsy subsequently develops in 2–10 percent of children who experience febrile seizures [Annegers et al., 1979, 1987; Berg and Shinnar, 1996b; Nelson and Ellenberg, 1978; van den Berg and Yerushalmi, 1969; Verity and Golding, 1991]. The higher number comes from the study by Annegers et al. [1987], which had the longest follow-up period. In addition, in population- and community-based studies, 15–20 percent of children and adults with epilepsy have a history of prior febrile seizures [Berg et al., 1999; Camfield et al., 1994; Hamati-Haddad and Abou-Khalil, 1998; Rocca et al., 1987a, 1987b, 1987c; Sofianov et al., 1983]. In most studies, the risk of developing epilepsy after a single simple febrile seizure is not substantially different from the risk for this disorder in the general population [Annegers et al., 1979, 1987; Berg and Shinnar, 1996b; Nelson and Ellenberg, 1978; van den Berg and Yerushalmi, 1969; Verity and Golding, 1991].

The risk factors for the development of epilepsy after febrile seizures are summarized in Table 57-1. In all five studies that have examined the issue, presence of a neurodevelopmental abnormality, the occurrence of a family history of epilepsy, and the occurrence of complex febrile seizures are associated with an increased risk of subsequent epilepsy [Annegers et al., 1979, 1987; Berg and Shinnar, 1996b; Nelson and Ellenberg, 1978; van den Berg and Yerushalmi, 1969; Verity and Golding, 1991]. Two studies also have found that the occurrence of multiple febrile seizures was associated with a slightly but statistically significant increased risk of subsequent epilepsy [Annegers et al., 1987; Berg and Shinnar, 1996b]. In addition, in the one study that examined this issue, febrile seizures that occurred within 1 hour of a recognized fever (i.e., at onset) were associated with a higher risk of subsequent epilepsy [Berg and Shinnar, 1996b].

Some controversy exists regarding whether the number of complex features affects the risk of recurrence. Two studies have examined this issue in detail. Both found that prolonged febrile seizures (i.e., febrile status epilepticus) were associated with an increased risk of subsequent epilepsy above that for a complex febrile seizure that was less prolonged [Annegers et al., 1987; Berg and Shinnar, 1996b]. The study by Annegers et al. [1987], however, found that the presence of two complex features (e.g., prolonged and focal) further increased the risk of subsequent epilepsy, whereas this association was not found in the study by Berg and Shinnar [1996b]. Note that these two factors are not independent because prolonged febrile seizures are more likely to be focal [Annegers et al., 1987; Berg and Shinnar, 1996a; Chevrie and Aicardi, 1975; Shinnar et al., 2001].

Age at first febrile seizure, the height of peak temperature at first seizure, and a family history of febrile seizures, all of which are associated with a differential risk of recurrence for febrile seizures, are not associated with a differential risk of developing epilepsy (see Table 57-1) [Annegers et al., 1979, 1987; Berg and Shinnar, 1996b; Nelson and Ellenberg, 1978; Verity and Golding, 1991]. Duration of fever before the febrile seizure appears to be the only common risk factor for both recurrent febrile seizures and subsequent epilepsy [Berg et al., 1992, 1997; Berg and Shinnar, 1996b]. It may well be a marker for overall seizure susceptibility.

The type of epilepsy that develops after febrile seizures is variable [Annegers et al., 1987; Berg et al., 1999; Camfield et al., 1994]. Annegers et al. [1987] report that, in persons with generalized febrile seizures, generalized epilepsies usually develop, whereas focal epilepsies develop in those with focal seizures. This finding suggests that the febrile seizures may be an age-specific expression of seizure susceptibility in patients with an underlying seizure diathesis [Annegers et al., 1987; Shinnar and Moshe, 1991]. Febrile seizures also can be the initial manifestation of specific epilepsy syndromes, such as severe myoclonic epilepsy of infancy [Dravet et al., 2002].

In general, the types of epilepsy that occur in children with prior febrile seizures are varied and not very different from those that occur in children without such a history [Berg et al., 1999; Camfield et al., 1994; Sofianov et al., 1983]. Whether febrile seizures are simply an age-specific marker of future seizure susceptibility or have a causal relationship with the subsequent epilepsy remains a matter of controversy [Berg and Shinnar, 1997; Shinnar, 2003, 2002]. The weight of the epidemiologic data is against a causal association in a majority of cases. Populations with a cumulative incidence of febrile seizures of 10 percent, such as in Tokyo, Japan, do not have an increased incidence of epilepsy [Tsuboi, 1984]. Moreover, evidence that treatment of febrile seizures alters the risk of subsequent epilepsy is lacking [AAP, 1999; Berg and Shinnar, 1997; Knudsen et al., 1996; Rosman et al., 1993b; Shinnar and Berg, 1996; Wolf and Forsythe, 1989]. The data regarding the association between prolonged febrile seizures and subsequent epilepsy are discussed later on.

Febrile Seizures, Mesial Temporal Sclerosis, and Temporal Lobe Epilepsy

One of the most controversial issues in epilepsy is whether prolonged febrile seizures cause mesial temporal sclerosis and mesial temporal lobe epilepsy [Shinnar, 2002, 2003]. Falconer et al., [1964, 1971] described a series of 100 patients with intractable temporal lobe epilepsy, 47 percent of whom had mesial temporal sclerosis on pathologic review. Of the patients with mesial temporal sclerosis, 40 percent had a history of prolonged convulsions in infancy. Since then, a number of retrospective studies from tertiary epilepsy centers report that many adults with intractable mesial temporal lobe epilepsy had a history of prolonged or atypical febrile seizures in childhood [Abou-Khalil et al., 1993; Bruton, 1988; Cendes et al., 1993a, 1993b; French et al., 1993; Sagar and Oxbury, 1987; Taylor and Ounsted, 1971]. Population-based studies, however, have failed to find this association, as have prospective studies of febrile seizures [Annegers et al., 1987; Berg and Shinnar, 1996b, 1997; Nelson and Ellenberg, 1978; van den Berg and Yerushalmi, 1969; Verity et al., 1985a, 1993]. This lack of association may be in part due to the low incidence of febrile seizures sufficiently prolonged to cause damage.

Maher and McLachlan [1995] described a large family with a high rate of both febrile convulsions and temporal lobe epilepsy. The mean duration of the febrile seizures in family members in whom temporal lobe epilepsy subsequently developed was 100 minutes. VanLandingham et al. [1998] reported that, in rare cases, prolonged focal febrile seizures can be associated with mesial temporal sclerosis. A few children with prolonged (mean duration of 100 minutes) focal febrile seizures had acute changes on MRI, which in some cases were followed by later chronic changes. These MRI changes occurred in only a small minority of their patients, however. Furthermore, all cases of mesial temporal sclerosis in this study occurred in patients who had focal seizures, some of whom also had focal lesions, which raises the question of pre-existing focal pathology. The frequent finding of associated heterotopias and subtle migration defects in patients with mesial temporal sclerosis and intractable complex partial seizures whose temporal lobes are resected supports this concept [Mathern et al., 1995a, 1995b; Shinnar, 1998, 2003].

Although prolonged febrile seizures may in some cases produce mesial temporal sclerosis, the epidemiologic data suggest that febrile seizures are not likely to account for a majority of cases of mesial temporal sclerosis. Febrile seizures lasting more than 90 minutes are rare, and are uncommon even in series of patients with febrile status epilepticus [Annegers et al., 1987; Berg and Shinnar, 1996a, 1996b; Chevrie and Aicardi, 1975; Dunn, 1988; Ellenberg and Nelson, 1978; Maytal and Shinnar, 1990; Maytal et al., 1989; Nelson and Ellenberg, 1978; Shinnar et al., 2001; VanLandingham et al., 1998; Verity et al., 1993]. Prolonged febrile seizures also are usually focal [Berg and Shinnar, 1996a; Chevrie and Aicardi, 1975; Shinnar et al., 2001; VanLandingham et al., 1998]. Note that, even in cases of febrile status epilepticus, imaging abnormalities are relatively uncommon [VanLandingham et al., 1998]. Mesial temporal sclerosis also can be found in many patients who have no prior history of febrile seizures [Falconer, 1971; Falconer et al., 1964; Mathern et al., 1995a, 1995b, 1995c, 1996]. Clinicopathologic studies have provided evidence for multiple potential causes of mesial temporal sclerosis and for the frequent presence of dual pathology, such as coexistent subtle migration defects [Mathern et al., 1995a, 1995b, 1995c, 1996]. As previously discussed, in many cases febrile seizures may be an age-specific marker for future seizure susceptibility [Shinnar and Moshe, 1991].

With all of these caveats, it is increasingly clear, from both animal and human data, that prolonged febrile seizures are associated with physiologic and anatomic changes that may lead to subsequent epilepsy in some cases. More recent imaging findings suggest that as many as 30–40 percent of children with prolonged febrile seizures have acute changes on MRI [Lewis et al., 2002; Mitchell and Lewis, 2002; Shinnar, 2003]. Moreover, the presence and severity of these acute changes are predictive of subsequent anatomic mesial temporal sclerosis that may occur before the development of clinical seizures [Lewis et al., 2002; Mitchell and Lewis, 2002; Shinnar, 2003]. These findings offer an opportunity to resolve this controversy. A multicenter study is under way to address prospectively whether or not and under what circumstances prolonged febrile seizures cause mesial temporal sclerosis. Preliminary findings from this study indicate that prolonged febrile seizures are likely to be focal, are much longer than previously thought, with a median duration of an hour, and usually do not stop on their own but require the administration of a benzodiazepine [Shinnar et al., 2008]. Early results from this study confirm in a more systematic fashion the results of VanLandingham and colleagues [VanLandingham et al., 1998].

Genetics

Genetic influences clearly play a major role in febrile seizures. Children with a positive family history of febrile seizures are more likely both to experience a febrile seizure [Berg et al., 1995; Bethune et al., 1993] and to experience recurrent febrile seizures [Annegers et al., 1990; Berg et al., 1990, 1992, 1997; Nelson and Ellenberg, 1978; Offringa et al., 1992, 1994] than children without such a family history. In a study of 32 twin pairs and 673 sibling relationship cases, Tsuboi [1987] reported a concordance rate of 56 percent in monozygotic twins and 14 percent in dizygotic twins. Concordance for clinical symptoms, including age at onset and degree of fever, was higher in

the twin pairs than in the sibling relationship patients. The results were consistent, with a multifactorial mode of inheritance for febrile convulsions in an analysis of the Rochester, Minnesota, data set [Rich et al., 1987]. In population-based studies, a majority of children with febrile seizures do not have a first- or second-degree relative with a history of febrile seizures [Bethune et al., 1993].

At this time, no definitive identification of a gene or locus for febrile seizures has been established. Although gene-mapping studies have demonstrated significant linkages between risk for febrile seizures and five regions of the genome [Johnson et al., 1998; Nabbout et al., 2002; Nakayama et al., 2000; Peiffer et al., 1999; Wallace et al., 1996], the specific loci involved in determining the risk for febrile seizures have yet to be identified. It is also clear that these loci account for only a small fraction of cases of febrile seizures [Greenberg and Holmes, 2002; Racacho et al., 2000]. An autosomal-dominant mode of inheritance has been postulated for a subset of children with febrile seizures [Greenberg and Holmes, 2002; Johnson et al., 1998; Rich et al., 1987], but such cases are relatively rare. Candidate genes in these autosomal-dominant families include both sodium [Baulac et al., 1999] and gamma-aminobutyric acid (GABA) [Wallace et al., 1996] channel mutations. A related syndrome of generalized epilepsy with febrile seizures plus also has been mapped to several different loci in different families and has been associated with mutations in sodium, potassium, and GABA channels [Baulac et al., 1999; Chou et al., 2002; Greenberg and Holmes, 2002; Heuser et al., 2010; Lopez-Cendes et al., 2000; Moulard et al., 1999; Peiffer et al., 1999; Racacho et al., 2000].

Rapid advances in this area in the next 5 years are anticipated. Febrile seizures represent a good example of the interplay between genetic susceptibility and environmental factors. Most likely, all children have some increased susceptibility to seizures from fever at the specific age window. The degree of this susceptibility is influenced by a number of factors, including genetic ones. A febrile illness during the susceptibility period, however, is required for a febrile seizure to occur. Given the appropriate illness with a high enough fever, many 18-month-old infants will have a febrile seizure. Genetic influences are therefore likely to account for some but not all of the cases.

Treatment

Treatment of febrile seizures is a controversial subject. Two major rationales for treatment have evolved, each of which leads to different approaches. The first approach is based on the old idea that febrile seizures are harmful and may lead to the development of epilepsy; treatment is aimed at preventing febrile seizures, using either intermittent or chronic treatment with medications [Hirtz et al., 1986; Millichap, 1991; Millichap and Colliver, 1991]. The second approach is based on the epidemiologic data that febrile seizures are, by and large, benign. Therefore, the only concern is about prolonged febrile seizures. This singular concern leads to a therapeutic approach that does not treat brief febrile seizures [AAP, 1999, 2008; Knudsen, 2002]. Preventing or aborting prolonged febrile seizures to prevent status epilepticus with its attendant complications, however, remains a rational goal [Knudsen, 2002]. The following section reviews the current data regarding available treatments of febrile seizures and their efficacy.

Terminating a Febrile Seizure

In-Hospital Management

If seizure activity is on-going when the child arrives at the emergency department, treatment to terminate the seizure is mandatory. Intravenous diazepam or lorazepam is effective in most cases [Dodson et al., 1993; Maytal and Shinnar, 1995]. Rectal diazepam or diazepam gel also is appropriate for use in a prehospital setting, such as an ambulance, and in cases in which intravenous access is difficult [Camfield et al., 1989; Dodson et al., 1993; Knudsen, 1979, 2002; Morton et al., 1997]. Other benzodiazepines, such as lorazepam, also may be effective but have not been adequately studied, and their absorption properties are such that they are less suitable for rectal administration [Dodson et al., 1993; Graves et al., 1987; Knudsen, 2002]. If the seizure activity continues after an adequate dose of a benzodiazepine, then a full status epilepticus treatment protocol should be used [Dodson et al., 1993; Maytal and Shinnar, 1995].

Home Management

A majority of febrile seizures are brief, lasting less than 10 minutes, and no intervention is necessary. Rectal diazepam has been demonstrated to be effective in terminating febrile seizures [Camfield et al., 1989; Knudsen, 1979, 2002; Morton et al., 1997]. It is widely used in Europe, Canada, and Japan, and now has been widely accepted in the United States. Now that rectal diazepam gel is available in the United States [Morton et al., 1997], use of this agent would seem a rational therapy in those situations in which acute treatment of a febrile seizure at home is appropriate [O'Dell, 2002; O'Dell et al., 2000, 2003]. This approach has the obvious advantage of minimizing drug exposure. It should be used with caution, however, and only with reliable caregivers who have been trained in its use. Candidates for this treatment include children at high risk for prolonged or multiple febrile seizures [Berg and Shinnar, 1996a; Knudsen, 2002; O'Dell, 2002] and those who live far from medical care.

Preventing a Febrile Seizure

Intermittent Medications at Time of Fever

ANTIPYRETICS

Because febrile seizures, by definition, occur in the context of a febrile illness, aggressive treatment with antipyretic medication could be expected to reduce the risk of having a febrile seizure. In support of use of these agents, studies [Berg et al., 1995; Rantala et al., 1995] find that the risk of a febrile seizure is directly related to the height of the fever. Little evidence, however, is available to suggest that antipyretic agents reduce the risk of a recurrent febrile seizure [Knudsen, 2002]. In one study, a group of patients who received aggressive antipyretic therapy had a 25 percent risk of recurrence [Camfield et al., 1980]. Another study found that 50 percent of children who experienced a febrile seizure had received antipyretic medication before the seizure [Rutter and Metcalf, 1978]. The children in whom the febrile seizure occurs at the onset of the fever have the highest risk of recurrent febrile seizures [Berg et al., 1992, 1997]. Recommendations for antipyretic therapy should recognize its limitations and avoid creating undue anxiety and feelings of guilt in the parents [Knudsen, 2002; O'Dell, 2002].

BENZODIAZEPINES

Diazepam given orally or rectally at the time of onset of a febrile illness will reduce the probability of a febrile seizure [Autret et al., 1990; Knudsen, 1985a, 1985b; Knudsen and Vestermark, 1978; McKinlay and Newton, 1989; Rosman et al., 1993a]. Although the effect is statistically significant, it is clinically modest. In one large randomized trial comparing placebo with oral diazepam in a dose of 0.33 mg/kg every 8 hours with fever), recurrence by 36 months was noted in 22 percent of the diazepam treatment group, compared with 31 percent of the placebo treatment group [Rosman et al., 1993a]. This modest reduction in seizure recurrence must be weighed against the side effects of sedating children every time they have a febrile illness [Knudsen, 2002].

BARBITURATES

Intermittent therapy with phenobarbital at the onset of fever is ineffective in reducing the risk of recurrent febrile seizures [Knudsen, 2002; Pearce et al., 1977; Wolf et al., 1977]. Nevertheless, it is still fairly widely used for this purpose [Hirtz et al., 1986; Millichap, 1991; Millichap and Colliver, 1991].

Daily Medications

BARBITURATES

Phenobarbital, given daily at doses that achieve a blood level of 15 µg/mL or higher, was effective in reducing the risk of recurrent febrile seizures in several well-controlled trials [Anthony and Hawke, 1983; Bacon et al., 1981; Camfield et al., 1980; Herranz et al., 1984; Knudsen and Vestermark, 1978; McKinlay and Newton, 1989; Newton, 1988]. In those studies, however, a substantial proportion of the children demonstrated adverse effects, primarily hyperactivity, that required discontinuation of therapy [AAP, 1995; Camfield et al., 1979; Wolf and Forsythe, 1978]. More recent studies have cast some doubt on the efficacy of the drug in this setting and, of greater importance, have raised concerns about potential long-term adverse effects on cognition and behavior [AAP, 1995; Farwell et al., 1990]. Prolonged phenobarbital therapy is rarely indicated because the risks seem to outweigh the benefits in most cases [AAP, 1999; Knudsen, 2002].

VALPROATE

Daily treatment with valproic acid also has been found to be effective in reducing the risk of recurrent febrile seizures in both human and animal studies [Herranz et al., 1984; McKinlay and Newton, 1989; Newton, 1988; Olson et al., 1984]. It is rarely used, however, because the children who would be considered most often for prophylaxis (young and/or neurologically abnormal) also are the ones at highest risk for fatal idiosyncratic hepatotoxicity [AAP, 1999; Dreifuss et al., 1987, 1989; Knudsen, 2002].

OTHER ANTIEPILEPTIC DRUGS

Although benzodiazepines have been used in intermittent therapy, experience with chronic use for treatment of febrile seizures is lacking. These agents may well be effective, but their toxicity and adverse effect profile preclude widespread use in this setting. Phenytoin and carbamazepine are ineffective in preventing recurrent febrile seizures in humans and in animal models of hyperthermia-induced seizures [Anthony and Hawke, 1983; Bacon et al., 1981; Camfield et al., 1982; Olson et al., 1984]. Published data are lacking on the efficacy of the newer antiepileptic drugs, such as gabapentin, lamotrigine, levetiracetam, topiramate, tiagabine, vigabatrin, or zonisamide, in the treatment of febrile seizures. Although, on a theoretical basis, some of these drugs would be expected to have efficacy in preventing recurrent febrile seizures, available data are insufficient to justify their use in this setting. Moreover, long-term antiepileptic drug therapy is rarely indicated in the treatment of febrile seizures [AAP, 1999; Knudsen, 2002].

Preventing Epilepsy

One reason often given for treating febrile seizures is to prevent future epilepsy [Hirtz et al., 1986; Millichap, 1991; Millichap and Colliver, 1991]. Unfortunately, prevention of febrile seizures has not been found to reduce the risk of subsequent epilepsy. Three studies comparing placebo with treatment, either with daily phenobarbital or with diazepam administered at the onset of fever, demonstrated that treatment significantly and substantially reduced the risk of febrile seizure recurrence [Knudsen, 1985b; Rosman et al., 1993a; Wolf et al., 1977]. In all three studies, the risk of later development of epilepsy was no lower in the treatment groups than in the control groups [Knudsen et al., 1996; Rosman et al., 1993b; Shinnar and Berg, 1996; Wolf and Forsythe, 1989]. Two of these studies include more than 10 years of follow-up and found no difference between the treatment group and the control group in the occurrence of epilepsy or in school performance and other cognitive outcomes [Knudsen et al., 1996; Wolf and Forsythe, 1989]. In general, antiepileptic drugs are effective in lowering the risk of a recurrent seizure, whether febrile or afebrile, but are ineffective in preventing the development of subsequent epilepsy, whether in the setting of febrile seizures [AAP, 1999, 2008; Shinnar and Berg, 1996] or acute post-traumatic seizures [Temkin et al., 1990], or after a first unprovoked seizure in childhood [Hirtz et al., 2003; Musicco et al., 1997]. Their lack of efficacy in altering long-term prognosis has considerably diminished the enthusiasm for use of these agents for febrile seizures.

Guidelines for Therapy

Febrile seizures, although a frightening event, usually are benign. Treatment is only rarely indicated for a simple febrile seizure [AAP, 1999]. Even in most children with complex febrile seizures or recurrent febrile seizures, no treatment is needed [Knudsen, 2002]. In view of the available data, a rational goal of therapy would be to prevent prolonged febrile seizures. Therefore, when treatment is indicated, particularly in children at risk for prolonged or multiple febrile seizures [Berg and Shinnar, 1996a] or those who live far from medical care, use of rectal diazepam or diazepam gel at the time of seizure as an abortive agent would seem the most logical choice

[Camfield et al., 1989; Dodson et al., 1993; Knudsen, 1979, 2002; Maytal and Shinnar, 1995; Morton et al., 1997; O'Dell, 2002; O'Dell et al., 2000, 2003].

Counseling and Education

In a majority of cases, counseling and education will be the sole treatment. Education is key to empowering the parents, who have just experienced a frightening and traumatic event [O'Dell, 2002]. Many parents are afraid that their child could have died [Baumer et al., 1981]. Parents need to be reassured that the child will not die during a seizure and that keeping the child safe during the seizure generally is the only action that needs to be taken.

The basic facts about febrile seizures should be presented to the family [O'Dell, 2002]. The recommended amount of information and level of content depend in large part on the medical sophistication of the parents and on their ability to attend to the information given them at that particular time. The parents' perception of their child's disorder will be an important factor in their later coping and will ultimately affect their perception of quality of life.

Parents usually will be interested in information that will help them manage the illness or specific problems; lengthy explanations usually are not helpful. It also is important for the physician to provide information about how to manage further seizures, should they occur. This includes what should be done during a seizure, when it may be necessary to call the physician, and when the child should be taken to the emergency department. In those cases in which rectal diazepam or rectal diazepam gel is being recommended for a subsequent seizure, explicit instructions regarding its use should be given. Because it is difficult to absorb all of this information in an emergency department setting, it usually is advisable for the physician to see the family again a few weeks later, to review the information and answer any additional questions.

Febrile seizures are a common and mostly benign form of childhood seizures. An understanding of the natural history and prognosis will enable the physician to reassure the families of affected children and to provide appropriate counseling and management while avoiding unnecessary diagnostic and therapeutic interventions. More studies are needed on the outcome of prolonged febrile seizures and their optimal treatment. Advances in basic science, genetics, and imaging are providing new insights into this common pediatric disorder that continues to be the subject of active research.

Acknowledgments

Supported in part by grant IR01 NS43209 (S. Shinnar) from the National Institute of Neurological Disorders and Stroke, Bethesda, MD.

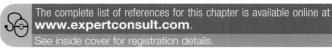

The complete list of references for this chapter is available online at **www.expertconsult.com**.
See inside cover for registration details.

Status Epilepticus

Lawrence D. Morton and John M. Pellock

The spectrum of seizure events extends from isolated, brief seizures to status epilepticus (SE), incorporating a full range of recurrent unprovoked seizures and prolonged or acute repetitive seizures. Typically, seizures are brief and self-limited. There has been considerable research directed at efforts to explain the mechanisms underlying seizure termination, as well as perpetuation, in SE. SE is a pediatric and neurologic emergency associated with significant morbidity and mortality [Dodson et al., 1993; Mitchell, 1996; Pellock, 1993a, 1994; Towne et al., 1994; Weise and Bleck, 1997; Wilson and Reynolds, 1990]. Its prompt recognition and management lead to the best chance of successful outcome. SE may represent the brain's reaction to an acute insult, or it may be a manifestation of already existing epilepsy, either as the initial symptom or as a prolonged exacerbation of seizures [DeLorenzo et al., 1992, 1995, 1996].

Although the definition and classification of SE have been changed numerous times, the term refers to seizures that continue for a prolonged period. Studies suggest that SE frequently goes unrecognized, and that its occurrence has been underestimated in the general population [Treiman, 1993]. One study [O'Dell et al., 2005a] documented that 34 percent of cases of febrile SE presenting in emergency departments across five centers were not recognized as such by the hospital personnel assigned to treat them. Based on this finding, febrile SE has only a 2 out of 3 chance of being recognized in an emergency treatment setting.

This chapter reviews the pathophysiology, definition, classification, epidemiology, etiology, treatment, and prognosis of SE as it occurs in children. The mortality associated with SE is greater in adults than in children, but morbidity and mortality in children are considerable without treatment. Accordingly, current thinking about optimal management uses a more aggressive clinical approach to this neurological emergency, including prompt recognition and initiation of therapy and accelerating the progression of treatment for more rapid termination of the episode [Millikan et al., 2009].

Pathophysiology

A distinguishing feature of SE is the self-sustaining seizure condition. The pathophysiology and biochemical changes underlying the evolution from discrete seizure to SE remain unclear [Lowenstein and Alldredge, 1998; Pellock, 1994; Wasterlain et al., 1993]. Pathophysiological changes that accompany SE can be divided into neuronal (cerebral) and systemic effects. The mechanisms involved in the initiation and maintenance of SE may be different. Ultimately, SE results from a failure of inhibitory mechanisms.

Gamma-aminobutyric acid (GABA) is the most prevalent inhibitory neurotransmitter in the brain. $GABA_A$ receptors are postsynaptic ionotropic receptors that bind directly to chloride channels, producing a fast inhibitory postsynaptic potential (IPSP). $GABA_A$ receptors are the binding sites for the benzodiazepines and it is the activation of this receptor that accounts for its antiseizure effect. A unique feature of SE compared to brief seizures is the time-dependent development of pharmacoresistance to benzodiazepines [Mazarati et al., 1998]. In animal models, investigators studied $GABA_A$ receptor currents by whole-cell patch-clamp techniques in CA1 pyramidal neurons acutely dissociated from rats undergoing lithium/pilocarpine-induced limbic SE and from naive rats [Kapur and Coulter, 1995]. The $GABA_A$ receptor current was absent in 47 percent of SE neurons and reduced in 55 percent of the remainder, compared with naive neurons, thus aiding in seizure perpetuation. Kapur et al., using a paired-pulse technique in an electrogenic model of experimental SE, showed that a marked deterioration of GABA-mediated inhibition occurs during continuous hippocampal stimulation [Kapur et al., 1989].

Additionally, more recent work has demonstrated the development of benzodiazepine pharmacoresistance shortly after the onset of ictal spike wave activity [Jones et al., 2002] and in young naive rats [Goodkin et al., 2003]. Treiman et al. reported similar loss of inhibition in hippocampal slices obtained during various electroencephalography (EEG) stages in lithium-/pilocarpine-induced SE [Treiman et al., 2006]. Altered receptor function and changes in representation affect both seizure representation and consequences in the neonatal brain. $GABA_A$ receptors are heteromeric protein complexes that mediate most fast synaptic inhibition in the forebrain and have many distinct subtypes. Adult rats that develop epilepsy following pilocarpine-induced SE and adult patients with refractory temporal lobe epilepsy demonstrate significant alterations in $GABA_A$ receptor properties in hippocampal dentate granule neurons [Gibbs et al., 1997; Brooks-Kayal et al., 1998, 1999]. In rat pups exposed to pilocarpine-induced SE, different changes are seen in α-1 subunit expression and augmentation compared with those in adult rats. This produced the opposite effect and may serve to enhance inhibition; the rat pups did become epileptic, unlike the adult rats who developed recurrent spontaneous seizures [Zhang et al., 2004a]. Nevertheless, changes in the function of the immature $GABA_A$ receptor, from the dual role of excitatory-inhibitory to inhibitory as the rat matures in infancy, may contribute to increased excitability and hence more seizure susceptibility in the neonate

[(Khazipov et al., 2004]. Additionally, alteration in glutamate receptor representation may alter seizure susceptibility. Alpha-amino-3-hydroxy-5-methyl-4-isoxazolepropionic acid (AMPA) receptors are over-represented in the premature brain, initially in the oligodendrocytes; later they shift their main representation to neurons in the cortex and hippocampus. This condition may partly explain increased risk of periventricular leukomalacia in the preterm infant and increased seizure susceptibility in the term infant [Jensen, 2002]. In one study the effect of SE induced by lithium/pilocarpine in 10-day-old rats demonstrated that pilocarpine-induced prolonged SE caused long-term changes in both glutamate receptors and transporters in hippocampal dentate gyrus. These include a decrease in glutamate receptor 2 mRNA expression and protein levels, as well as an increase in protein levels of the excitatory amino acid carrier 1[Zhang et al., 2004b].

Different studies provide evidence suggesting that endocytosis of GABA$_A$ receptors takes place as a seizure transitions to SE. This leads to a decrease in the number of GABA$_A$ receptors on the synaptic membrane and therefore a decreased response to benzodiazepines [Naylor et al., 2005; Goodkin et al., 2008]. Resistance to other antiseizure medications, such as phenytoin, has also been demonstrated. In addition to GABA$_A$ receptor trafficking, changes in receptor expression and phosphorylation have been shown [Brooks-Kayal et al., 1998, 1999; Terunuma et al., 2008]. Functional changes in voltage-dependent sodium channels have also been described after pilocarpine-induced SE in rats [Remy and Beck, 2006].

Glutamate is the primary excitatory amino acid neurotransmitter and binds to several neuronal receptors, including the *N*-methyl-D-aspartate (NMDA) receptor, which is activated by depolarization, as well as the AMPA receptor, which mediates fast synaptic transmission in the central nervous system. Using a paired-pulse method in a continuous hippocampal stimulation-induced SE model, NMDA receptors become activated during continuous hippocampal stimulation, and NMDA antagonists block the deterioration of GABA-mediated inhibition [Kapur and Lothman, 1990]. During SE, both NMDA and AMPA receptor subunits increase at the synaptic surface [Mazarati et al., 1998; Wasterlain et al., 2002a]. This increase in glutamate receptors further enhances excitability and is proconvulsant in the midst of uninhibited seizures. In a model of self-sustaining SE, seizures are abolished by NMDA receptor antagonists [Wasterlain et al., 2000].

Neuropeptides have emerged as having a role in SE. Substance P agonists facilitate the initiation of SE in animal models. During the course of SE, the de novo expression of substance P occurs in the cells, such as dentate granule cells, that do not usually express it, possibly playing a role in maintenance of SE [Wasterlain et al., 2002b]. In addition, galanin, a 29–30 amino acid peptide, suppresses hippocampal excitability by post- and presynaptic actions [Mazarati et al., 2000]. However, galanin appears to be depleted by SE.

Laminar necrosis and neuronal damage after prolonged seizures are similar to those after cerebral hypoxia. Neuronal injury and cell death from SE are most prominent in areas rich in NMDA glutamate receptors, including the limbic region. The increase in intracellular calcium is critical to cell death, and calcium activates proteases and lipases that degrade intracellular elements, leading to mitochondrial dysfunction and fatal cellular necrosis. Although young animals may be less likely to develop brain damage from SE [Holmes, 1997; Moshè,

1987], studies using alternative models demonstrate hippocampal cellular injury, even in immature rodents [Sankar et al., 1997; Thompson and Wasterlain, 1994]. It is believed that the glutamate-initiated calcium-dependent cascade is mechanistically similar to the NMDA receptor-mediated cell death occurring during cerebral ischemia. In SE, the degree of neuronal injury is related to seizure duration. In a study of limbic SE induced in adult rats using perforant path stimulation, when animals were allowed to recover, there was evidence of mitochondrial injury and dysfunction demonstrated possibly through a free radical mechanism of injury [Cock et al., 2002]. Further evidence suggests that acute and long-term changes in gene expression may occur after prolonged seizures. These changes in the expression of messenger RNA (mRNA) may lead directly to some of the observed hyperexcitability [Rice and DeLorenzo, 1998].

In animal studies using adolescent baboons, induced SE lasting 1.5–5 hours produced neuronal loss in the hippocampus, cerebellum, and neocortex. Significant cell loss continued to occur, although to a lesser extent if the animals were paralyzed and ventilated with maintenance of oxygen, carbon dioxide, serum glucose, body temperature, and blood pressure [Meldrum, 1974, 1983]. Similar changes have been produced in rat models, as well [Cavalheiro et al., 1987; Sperber et al., 1989].

There are limited data in humans. However, evidence from neuropathology, as well as imaging, has been presented in a pediatric case with direct excitotoxic injury in the absence of hypoxia-ischemia [Tsuchida et al., 2007].

Generalized convulsive SE is associated with serious systemic effects resulting from the metabolic demands of prolonged seizures and the autonomic changes that accompany them: alterations in blood pressure and heart rate, incontinence, emesis, acidosis, hypoxia, changes in respiratory function and body temperature, leukocytosis, rhabdomyolysis, and extreme demands on cerebral oxygen and glucose use [Simon et al., 1997]. Circulating catecholamines increase during the initial 30 minutes of SE, resulting in a hypersympathetic state. Tachycardia, sometimes associated with more severe cardiac dysrhythmias, occurs and may be fatal, but this seems more common in adults [Boggs et al., 1993]. Cardiac output also diminishes, and total peripheral resistance increases, along with mean arterial blood pressure, perhaps because of the sympathetic overload. Hyperpyrexia may become significant during the course of SE, even without prior febrile illness in both children and adults, and may persist for some time. Fever may influence the process of neuronal injury [Liu et al., 1993].

In addition, serum pH and glucose levels frequently are abnormal because lactic acidosis increases from increased anaerobic metabolism. Associated respiratory acidosis also may occur as a result of hypoventilation, hypoxia, and pulmonary edema. An increase in the peripheral white blood cell count frequently occurs in the absence of infection. Rhabdomyolysis may compromise renal function. Thus, the cerebral physiologic changes linked to SE are accompanied by increased metabolic demand for oxygen and glucose, and are further complicated by a variety of systemic changes, along with the pathology responsible for SE. As the cascade of neurophysiologic changes occurs, increased lactate from anaerobic metabolism continues, and excitatory neurotransmitters bombard cells, which accelerates metabolic activity and leads to overall neuronal failure. Recovery from this complicated derangement of metabolism is time-dependent; more prolonged seizures produce further neuronal injury and death.

Unlike in adults, in whom biology is more static, the effect of growth and development influences the impact of seizures, both in clinical presentation and in the biologic consequences for the developing brain. Most of our knowledge derives from animal models, so its applicability to the human situation is unclear. Experimental models of seizures in immature animals suggest comparatively less vulnerability to seizure-induced brain injury than in mature animals [Wong and Yamada, 2001]. Repetitive or prolonged neonatal seizures may increase the susceptibility of the developing brain to experience subsequent seizure-induced brain injury later in life. This susceptibility appears to be more closely related to alterations in neuronal connectivity and network properties, rather than to increased cell death during the neonatal period [Holmes et al., 1998; Koh et al., 1999; Schmid et al., 1999].

Rats exposed to early-life seizures demonstrate persistent changes in CA1 hippocampal pyramidal cells, possibly leading to long-term changes in behavior and learning and in epileptogenicity [Villeneuve et al., 2000].

Definition

SE is best considered as a state produced by continuous or repetitive seizures, which has the potential to produce significant systemic or neuronal injury if not aborted. This definition, however, does not provide a clinically useful treatment guideline.

SE is internationally classified as a seizure lasting more than 30 minutes or recurrent seizures producing more than 30 minutes during which the patient does not regain consciousness [ILAE, 1981]. The World Health Organization previously defined SE as "a condition characterized by epileptic seizures that are so frequently repeated or so prolonged as to create a fixed and lasting condition" [Gastaut, 1982]. Lack of recovery for a fixed period, possible frequent repetition, prolongation, and possible propagation of further seizures are inherent in this definition. In the past, the definition of SE required 1 hour of continuous seizures, but more recent studies have used a 30-minute duration of continuous or recurrent seizures without full recovery as the standard clinical and electrographic definition of SE. The recognition that longer duration of seizures increases risk for long-term injury and the risk for fracture during seizures and their treatment has required a definition implying need for expediency in stopping prolonged seizures. Lowenstein and associates proposed an "operational" definition of 5 minutes or more of continuous seizures or "two discrete seizures between which there is incomplete recovery of consciousness" in adults and children older than 5 years of age [Lowenstein et al., 1999]. This definition applies primarily to generalized convulsive SE and may be used to direct treatment to avoid refractory SE, as well as its sequelae. Aggressive early treatment is justified by recent work demonstrating a 10-fold lower rate of mortality for seizures of 10–29 minutes' duration versus those lasting longer than 30 minutes [DeLorenzo et al., 1999].

Because of the difficulty in diagnosing and quantifying seizures in the neonate, no broadly accepted definition of SE in the neonate exists. A proposed definition is either 30 minutes of continuous electroencephalographic seizures or presence of seizure activity for 50 percent of the EEG recording time, with or without the expression of coincident clinical signs (Scher et al., 1993b). Debate continues regarding what constitutes a neonatal seizure. Neonatal seizures can be broken down into three categories: electroclinical, electrographic, and clinical only. Controversy still exists about whether episodic abnormal movements seen in some infants, not accompanied by simultaneous ictal discharges on the EEG, are true seizures. Many neonatal paroxysmal events classified as "subtle seizures" have no EEG correlate [Mizrahi and Kellaway, 1998]. Typical subtle seizures include movements of progression, such as bicycling, oral-buccal-lingual movements, such as chewing and tongue thrusting, and other movements, such as random eye movements. Other movements that typically have no EEG correlate include generalized tonic posturing. Movements typically demonstrating simultaneous ictal discharges on EEG include focal clonic, multifocal clonic, and focal tonic; myoclonic movements may or may not have an EEG correlate [Mizrahi and Kellaway, 1998].

Classification

Any type of seizure may become prolonged and thus develop into SE (Box 58-1). Classification of SE should be performed by observing the clinical events and combining electrographic information when possible. The fundamental distinction between seizures is that some are generalized from onset, whereas others are partial in onset. The latter type may or may not then secondarily generalize. From a management standpoint, however, it may be more useful to consider whether the event is convulsive or nonconvulsive, as this may impact more directly on ready recognition and intervention.

Generalized tonic-clonic SE is the most dramatic and life-threatening form of SE. Myoclonic, generalized clonic, and

---

Box 58-1 Proposed Classification of Status Epilepticus

Partial

Convulsive
- Tonic: hemiclonic SE, hemiconvulsion-hemiplegia-epilepsy
- Clonic hemi–convulsive, generalized convulsive, status epilepticus

Nonconvulsive
- Simple: focal motor status, focal sensory, epilepsia partialis continuans, adversive SE
- Complex partial: epileptic fugue state, prolonged epileptic stupor, prolonged epileptic confusional state, temporal lobe SE, psychomotor SE, continuous epileptic twilight state

Generalized

Convulsive
- Tonic-clonic: generalized convulsive, epilepticus convulsivus
- Tonic
- Clonic
- Myoclonic: myoclonic SE

Nonconvulsive
- Absence: spike-and-wave stupor, spike-and-slow-wave or 3/second spike-and-wave SE, petit mal, epileptic fugue, epilepsia minora continua, epileptic twilight state, minor SE
- Undetermined
  - Subtle: epileptic coma
  - Neonatal: erratic SE

generalized tonic SE occur primarily in children. These children usually have encephalopathic epilepsies [Lockman, 1990; Pellock, 1994; Treiman, 1993], and their consciousness may be preserved throughout the attacks. About one-half of the cases of generalized clonic SE occur in normal children, in whom it is associated with prolonged febrile seizures; the remaining half are distributed among those children with acute and chronic encephalopathies [DeLorenzo et al., 1992]. Generalized tonic SE appears most frequently in children, particularly those with the Lennox–Gastaut syndrome. Prolonged generalized tonic convulsions have been precipitated by benzodiazepine administration.

Nonconvulsive SE also may include complex partial, simple partial, and absence seizures that continue for more than 30 minutes [Kaplan, 1996; Scholtes et al., 1996; Stores et al., 1995]. Complex partial SE may be manifested as an epileptic twilight state marked by a cyclic variation between periods of partial responsiveness and episodes of seemingly motionless staring and complete unresponsiveness accompanied, at times, by automatic behavior [Delgado-Escueta and Treiman, 1987; Privitera, 1997; Scher et al., 1993a; Treiman, 1993]. Simple partial SE is characterized by focal seizures that may persist or be repetitive for at least 30 minutes without impairment of consciousness. When this condition lasts for hours or days, it is termed epilepsia partialis continua [Cockerell et al., 1996; Takahashi et al., 1997]. Absence, or petit mal, status also has been referred to as spike-wave stupor. This type of nonconvulsive SE may be extremely difficult to differentiate from complex partial SE without the aid of an EEG. Classically, features of absence status include a continuous alteration of consciousness without the cyclic variations seen with complex partial SE [Grin and DiMario, 1998]. The EEG recording exhibits prolonged, sometimes continuous, generalized synchronous 3-Hz spike-and-wave complexes, rather than focal ictal discharges, which characterize partial SE [Porter and Penry, 1983; Treiman, 1993]. Absence status does not appear to cause permanent neurological damage [Drislane, 1999]. The child presenting with a prolonged confused state, with a fluctuating level of consciousness or with prolonged unconsciousness, may require both clinical and EEG evaluations in addition to other studies.

Nonconvulsive SE is most likely not rare but simply underdiagnosed. A special category of nonconvulsive SE is subtle SE [Treiman, 1990, 1993]. These patients have severe encephalopathies stemming from a variety of intracranial processes or prolonged uncontrolled convulsive seizures. This type of SE is manifested clinically by the occurrence of mild motor movements, such as nystagmus, or by clonic twitches, which may be unilateral and are intermittent, brief, and without a true sequential pattern. These subtle movements are associated with marked impairment of consciousness, usually with continuous bilateral EEG ictal patterns. These continuing electrographic seizures that are not accompanied by clinical manifestations demonstrate a true "electroclinical dissociation," and may be seen not only in neonates but also in severely ill children and adults [Mizrahi and Kellaway, 1987; Scher et al., 1993a]. The EEG progressively becomes uniform to produce a pattern of continuous ictal discharges, which then becomes interrupted by periods of relative flatness and then severe cortical depression. In a study of children, nonconvulsive SE most commonly followed a bout of convulsive SE or briefer convulsive seizure but with prolonged alteration in mental status [Tay et al., 2006], and is more likely to occur in children with a prior

history of epilepsy [Abend et al., 2007] and remote risk factors for seizures [Classen et al., 2004]. In general, these patients respond poorly to traditional treatment with antiepileptics.

Febrile SE, which is unique to children, represents the extreme end of the complex febrile seizure spectrum. Febrile SE has long been suspected of having a relationship to the development of mesial temporal sclerosis. Patients with intractable temporal lobe epilepsy and mesial temporal sclerosis often have histories of severe febrile convulsions as infants. Diagnostic advances made possible by magnetic resonance imaging (MRI) have shown that very prolonged febrile convulsions may produce hippocampal injury [Lewis, 1999]. More recent studies support the link to the development of mesial temporal sclerosis [Provenzale et al., 2008]. Neuroimaging studies generally show hippocampal swelling during the acute stage [Scott et al., 2002, 2006]. A prospective study investigating long-term outcome in febrile SE found that most were partial (67 percent), and SE was unrecognized in the emergency department about a third of the time [Shinnar et al., 2008]. Human herpesvirus-6B appears to be the most common cause of febrile SE and may play an important pathogenic role in the etiology of mesial temporal lobe epilepsy [Theodore et al., 2008].

Epidemiology

It is projected that between 102,000 and 152,000 events occur in the United States annually, an incidence 2–2.5 times greater than that previously proposed by Hauser [1990], who reported that SE occurs annually in 50,000–60,000 persons in the United States [DeLorenzo et al., 1996; Hauser et al., 1990]. More recent work continues to demonstrate a high incidence of SE varying between 20 and 41 patients per year per 100,000 population [Govoni et al., 2008; Chin et al., 2006; Coeytaux et al., 2000].

Approximately one-third of cases manifest as the initial seizure of a developing epilepsy, one-third occur in patients with previously established epilepsy, and one-third occur as the result of an acute isolated brain insult. Among those previously diagnosed as having epilepsy, estimates of SE occurrence range from 0.5 to 6.6 percent [DeLorenzo et al., 1996].

Hauser reported that up to 70 percent of children who have epilepsy that begins before the age of 1 year will experience an episode of SE [Hauser, 1990]. Also, within 5 years of the initial diagnosis of epilepsy, 20 percent of all patients will experience an episode of SE. Although the subsequent development of epilepsy is likely in adults with SE as their first unprovoked seizure [Hauser et al., 1990], a prospective study of children with SE found only a 0.3 probability plotted on a Kaplan–Meier curve that epilepsy will develop after ≥9 months in those who initially presented with SE [Maytal et al., 1989].

Among children, SE is most common in infants and young toddlers, with more than 50 percent of cases of SE occurring in children younger than 3 years of age [Shinnar et al., 1995]. In a study in Richmond, Virginia, total SE events and incidence per 100,000 population per year demonstrated a bimodal distribution, with the highest values during the first year of life and during the decades beyond 60 years of age [DeLorenzo et al., 1992, 1995, 1996]. Infants younger than 1 year of age represent a subgroup of children with the highest incidence of SE, whether events, total incidents, or recurrences are counted. The recurrence rate for SE in the Richmond study was 10.8 percent [DeLorenzo et al., 1996], but 38 percent of patients younger than 4 years of age had repeat episodes. Children have a much lower mortality rate than adults after adequate treatment [Dunn, 1988; Maytal et al., 1989; Pellock, 1993b; Phillips and Shanahan, 1989; Shinnar et al., 1995]. Age, etiology, and duration directly correlate with mortality [DeLorenzo et al., 1996; Towne et al., 1994].

Etiology

SE usually is a manifestation of an acute precipitating event that affects the central nervous system (CNS) or is an exacerbation of symptomatic epilepsy. Less than 10 percent of cases of SE in adults and children are truly idiopathic in that no precipitating or associated cause can be identified [DeLorenzo et al., 1995, 1996]. Acute symptomatic causes are those most commonly associated with prolonged SE lasting for longer than 1 hour [DeLorenzo et al., 1996]. Thus, a full evaluation for etiology must be undertaken in every case of SE [Dodson et al., 1993; Pellock, 1994]. In patients with pre-existing epilepsy, a precipitating or associated factor may be clearly identified. Identification of this factor may help in treating the episode of SE, preventing further consequences of SE, and perhaps preventing future recurrences.

Although, typically, a precipitant to SE can be identified, a genetic susceptibility may predispose certain persons to develop prolonged seizures in response to an acute insult. Recent work in twins demonstrated a higher incidence in monozygotic twins than in dizygotic twins, providing evidence for a genetic contribution to the risk for SE [Corey et al., 2004]. Seizure type and specific epilepsy syndrome may differ between monozygotic twins, however, and SE may not be a function of the seizure type or syndrome experienced by each person.

A clear difference between causative disorders of SE in adults (Table 58-1) and those in children (Table 58-2) has been

Table 58-2 Etiologies of Status Epilepticus in Children

Etiology	Percentage
Remote symptomatic epilepsy	33%
Acute symptomatic seizures	26%
Febrile	22%
Cryptogenic	15%
Central nervous system infection	13%
Acute metabolic disorders	6%

(From Riviello JJ et al. Practice Parameter: Diagnostic assessment of the child with status epielpticus [an evidence based review]. Neurology 2006;67:1542.)

identified [Pellock and DeLorenzo, 1997; Riviello et al., 2006]. A major cause of SE in children is that associated with fever secondary to non-CNS infections, an etiology that essentially does not exist in adults. Inadequate antiepileptic drug levels and remote causes, including congenital malformations, also account for a significant number of episodes of SE in children, although some studies have found that patients may have had reasonable drug levels when SE occurred [Maytal et al., 1996]. Of note, many patients with subtherapeutic levels of antiepileptic drugs closely followed the instructions of their physicians and recently had drug-dosage alterations.

The distribution of causes associated with SE in children is highly age-dependent [Shinnar et al., 1995]. More than 80 percent of children younger than 2 years of age have SE from a febrile or acute symptomatic cause, whereas cryptogenic or remote symptomatic causes were more common in older children. By contrast, in adults, subtherapeutic levels of antiepileptic drugs, remote causes, and cerebrovascular accidents represent the three most common causes of SE [Pellock and DeLorenzo, 1997]. In adults, SE resulting from remote causes occurred primarily in relation to stroke, so that both acute and previously occurring strokes account for a significant proportion of adult episodes of SE. Stroke is the etiologic disorder in approximately 10 percent of childhood SE episodes, either as the primary acute cause or as a remote event.

Recurrence rates for SE are age-specific, as illustrated in Figure 58-1. Repeat occurrences are much more common in children younger than 1 year of age. In the prospective Richmond study of SE, pediatric, adult, and elderly recurrence rates were 35 percent, 7 percent, and 10 percent, respectively [DeLorenzo et al., 1996]. Recurring SE is more frequent in children with remote symptomatic encephalopathy or progressive degenerative disease [DeLorenzo et al., 1995, 1996]. The extent of clinical and laboratory evaluation that should be performed in each child with recurrent SE will depend on the presentation, signs and symptoms, and underlying medical condition of the patient. For example, a child with recurring SE who has an indwelling shunt for hydrocephalus will almost always need to be evaluated for the possibility of shunt malfunction or infection.

Recently, CNS or systemic autoimmune disorders have been recognized as causes of SE [Shorvon and Tan, 2009]. In some cases, the diseases may be paraneoplastic, but for many, no cause has been determined. Since patients with these etiologies usually are described in case reports or small series, the contribution of the disorders to the epidemiology of SE is difficult to assess, but they appear to represent a fraction of the cases

Table 58-1 Cause and Mortality Data for Status Epilepticus in Adults

Etiologic Disorder/Condition	% of Cases	Mortality Rate (%)
Anoxia	5	71
Hypoxia	13	53
Cerebrovascular accident	22	33
Hemorrhage	1	0
Tumor	7	30
Infection	7	10
Central nervous system infection	3	0
Metabolic	15	30
Low antiepileptic drug level	34	4
Drug overdose	3	25
Alcohol withdrawal	13	20
Trauma	3	25
Remote	25	14
Idiopathic	3	25

(From Pellock JM, DeLorenzo RJ. SE. In: Porter RJ, Chadwick D, eds. The epilepsies 2. Boston: Butterworth–Heinemann, 1997;267.)

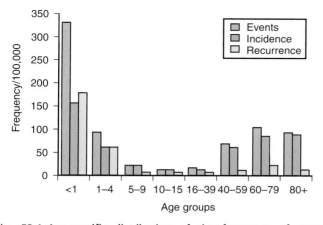

Fig. 58-1 Age-specific distribution of the frequency of status epilepticus (SE) events, the incidence of SE, and the frequency of SE recurrence per year per 100,000 population in Richmond, Virginia. The population in each group was determined from the National Census Bureau data on the demographics of Richmond, 1990. SE events included all episodes of SE per 100,000 population per year. The incidence of SE represents the number of patients per 100,000 in whom SE developed in Richmond, and did not include recurrent episodes of SE. *(Reprinted from DeLorenzo RJ et al. A prospective, population-based study of SE in Richmond, Virginia. Neurology 1996;46:1029.)*

Box 58-2 Goals of Emergency Management for Status Epilepticus

- Ensure adequate brain oxygenation and cardiorespiratory function
- Terminate clinical and electrical seizure activity as rapidly as possible
- Prevent seizure recurrence
- Identify precipitating factors, such as hypoglycemia, electrolyte imbalance, lowered drug levels, infection, and fever
- Correct metabolic imbalance
- Prevent systemic complications
- Further evaluate and treat cause of SE

(From Pellock JM, DeLorenzo RJ. SE. In: Porter RJ, Chadwick D, eds. The epilepsies 2. Boston: Butterworth–Heinemann, 1997:267.)

---

previously diagnosed as infectious, since the patients often have a syndrome qualifying as an encephalitis.

A recently described entity with seizures and persistently altered mentation, including a fluctuating level of consciousness or with prolonged unconsciousness, is anti-NMDA-receptor encephalitis [Dalmau et al., 2008]. Anti-NMDA-receptor encephalitis is a disorder with antibodies against the NR1 subunit of the receptor. This disorder largely affects young people, and its diagnosis is facilitated by the characteristic clinical picture that develops in association with cerebrospinal fluid pleocytosis. Only about half the patients had MRI abnormalities. Recovery from this disorder is typically slow, and symptoms may relapse. The mainstay of treatment is immunotherapy with steroids, plasma exchange, or intravenous immunoglobulin. These immunotherapies may be given individually or in combination [Dalmau et al., 2008]. Other possible autoimmune illnesses include systemic lupus erythematosus, antineuronal antibody syndromes with limbic encephalitis, limbic encephalitis following various systemic viral infections, and Hashimoto's encephalopathy (autoimmune thyroid encephalopathy).

Management and Therapy

Overview

SE is a neurologic and medical emergency. Therapy includes maintenance of respiration, general medical support, and specific treatment aimed at stopping both electrographic and clinical seizures while the cause of the event is investigated [Epilepsy Foundation of America, 1993]. Prompt diagnosis and management provide the best outcome [DeLorenzo, 1990; Pellock, 1993a, 1993b, 1994; Pellock and DeLorenzo, 1997; Rider and Thapa, 1995; Treiman, 1993].

A single generalized convulsion in a child with a prolonged period of impaired consciousness is much more difficult to diagnose, and an EEG should be obtained urgently. If on-going ictal discharges or electrographic seizures are noted, the patient should be considered to be in electrographic SE, and prompt treatment is indicated. The goals of SE emergency management are listed in Box 58-2. Clinical and electrographic seizure activity must be rapidly terminated while ensuring optimal oxygenation and metabolic balance. Both clinical and electrical seizure activity should be terminated as soon as possible [Treiman, 1990]. The longer an episode of SE continues, the more likely it is to result in permanent neurologic damage and to become refractory to treatment [DeLorenzo, 1990; DeLorenzo et al., 1996; Hauser, 1990; Pellock and DeLorenzo, 1997; Towne et al., 1994; Treiman, 1990; Treiman et al., 1992, 1994].

Rapid initiation of care is essential to ensure the best possible outcome. Increased seizure duration commonly is regarded as an important factor contributing to increased morbidity and mortality. Prolonged seizures of any type are associated with an increased risk of complications [Lowenstein et al., 1999]. In a study in adults and children, the mortality rate in SE was 34.8 percent when seizures lasted longer than 1 hour, compared with 3.7 percent when seizure duration was less than 1 hour [DeLorenzo et al., 1992]. Therefore, limiting the time from seizure onset to initial treatment and attainment of control is essential to minimize the complications of prolonged seizures. In a retrospective study, patients with SE may not arrive at the emergency department for 30 minutes or longer, and treatment initiation may not occur for 40–263 minutes, thereby increasing risk for prolonged seizures [Jordan, 1994]. The Veterans Affairs Cooperative Study reported that the mean delay before treatment of SE was 2.8 hours in generalized convulsive SE and 5.8 hours in subtle SE; this study involved exclusively adult patients [Treiman et al., 1998]. In a prospective study of 889 patients (625 adults, 264 children), 41.5 percent received treatment within 30 minutes and 70.9 percent within 60 minutes of seizure onset; 18.1 percent did not have treatment initiated until after 90 minutes of seizures. This latter group of patients, however, included patients in coma diagnosed with subtle or nonconvulsive SE [Pellock et al., 2004].

Supportive Care

In children in SE, cardiorespiratory function must be assessed immediately by vital sign determination, auscultation, airway inspection, and determination of arterial blood-gas concentrations, with suctioning when necessary. Although these children may appear to be breathing spontaneously on arrival at the emergency department, they may already be hypoxic, with respiratory and metabolic acidosis, apnea, aspiration, or central respiratory depression. The need for ventilatory support depends not only on the respiratory status at the time of presentation but also on the conditions before arrival and the ability to maintain adequate oxygenation throughout on-going seizures and during the intravenous administration of large doses of antiepileptic drugs, all of which may cause respiratory depression. In the neurologically depressed patient, elective intubation and respiratory support are recommended. Placement of an oral airway or nasal oxygen cannula will prove to be insufficient in most patients, because respiratory drive is depressed [Pellock, 1994]. Respiratory arrest and depression are principal factors contributing to morbidity and mortality [DeLorenzo et al., 1996]. Rapidly assessing vital signs and performing a general neurologic examination may provide clues to the etiology of SE.

Laboratory Testing

Blood should be drawn for the determination of blood gases, glucose, calcium, electrolytes, complete blood count, and antiepileptic drug levels, as well as for cultures (bacterial and viral) if indicated. Urine drug and metabolic screening should be performed whenever the etiology cannot be determined. As previously noted, a common etiologic or associated factor found in children with SE is intercurrent infection. In a small number of these children, the clinical presentation will include manifestations similar to the initial symptoms of CNS infection. Lumbar puncture should be done early in the course of management, although not necessarily during the initial phase of stabilization [Rider et al., 1995]. In most children, only rarely should the clinician wait to obtain neuroimaging studies before performing a lumbar puncture. Hyperpyrexia may become significant during the course of SE, even in the absence of a febrile illness. Rectal temperatures should be monitored and fever aggressively treated; significant elevations of temperature may contribute to brain damage [Dodson et al., 1993].

Bradyarrhythmias are commonly noted in children when large doses of antiepileptic drugs are administered. In adults, changes range from evidence of myocardial ischemia to tachyarrhythmia [Boggs et al., 1993, 1994; Tigaran et al., 1997]. These are less frequently noted in children. In children with known congenital heart disease or dysrhythmias, electrocardiographic monitoring must be implemented and continued.

Use of Neuroimaging

The decision to perform neuroimaging studies in the child presenting with SE needs to be individualized according to the available history, general physical and neurologic examination findings, and the possibility of significant structural intracranial pathology or increased intracranial pressure, or the presence of lateralizing findings. A Practice Parameter for imaging the child with SE recommends that, if etiology is unknown or it is clinically indicated, imaging should be performed after SE has been controlled and the patient stabilized [Riviello et al., 2006]. Clinical indications would be similar to the indications for neuroimaging in the emergency patient presenting with a seizure [Practice Parameter, 1996].

The incidence of imaging abnormalities, presumably in patients with clinical indication rather than in all patients, ranges from 29 to 70 percent in class III studies. Common findings were cerebral edema (14 percent), atrophy (12.1 percent), infection (4.6 percent), dysplasia, infarction (2.9 percent), tumor and hematoma (2.3 percent each), and trauma and arteriovenous malformation (1.2 percent each) [Riviello et al., 2006]. MRI is more sensitive and specific than CT. Transient focal findings may be seen [Kramer et al., 1987] and diffusion weighted imaging may reveal vasogenic and cytotoxic edema [Scott et al., 2002]. A recent review of neuroimaging in the emergency department demonstrates that CT of the brain in children with a first seizure changes acute management 3–8 percent of the time [Harden et al., 2007].

A growing literature recognizes peri-ictal changes on neuroimaging and discusses their significance. Local and immediate findings have been described in children. Local swelling of the hippocampus has been described in children with prolonged febrile convulsions [Scott et al., 2002, 2006; VanLandingham et al., 1998]. At follow-up evaluation in some patients, edematous areas later appeared atrophic [Scott et al., 2002]. However, there is some evidence that an underlying, predisposing hippocampal abnormality may be present [Scott et al., 2006]. Prolonged seizure as a potential causative pathophysiological sequence to the development of temporal lobe epilepsy has been extensively investigated in animal models in which SE is induced by chemical [Meldrum, 1997; Ben Ari, 1985; Cavalheiro, 1995] or electrical [Lothman et al., 1989] means. Most recently, a study of 11 children with a history of febrile SE with MRI within 72 hours of SE and follow-up 2 years later found that seven demonstrated MRI signal hyperintensity in the hippocampus. On follow-up imaging, five children had hippocampal volume loss and increased signal intensity, meeting the criteria for mesial temporal sclerosis. Four children had developed focal-onset epilepsy [Provenzale et al., 2008].

Focal edema with effacement of gyri [Silverstein and Alexander, 1998] can develop, with subsequent atrophy [Meierkord et al., 1997]. This finding appears to represent cytotoxic edema; in animal models, increased lactate has been found, and this increase correlates with the degree of histologic damage [Najm et al., 1998].

More confounding is the finding of lesions remote from the ictal focus. The lesions may be remote in time, such as in cases in which transient lesions develop days after SE [Hisano et al., 2000], or remote anatomically. These remote lesions typically are associated with transient focal findings on examination, such as weakness [Hisano et al., 2000] or personality changes. Lesions in the splenium have been associated with psychiatric disease [Cole, 2004].

Use of Electroencephalographic Monitoring

EEG monitoring allows optimal management of SE and should be used whenever available. EEG monitoring is extremely useful, but under-utilized, in initial and subsequent management of SE [Jaitly et al., 1994; Pellock, 1993a, 1993b; Pellock and DeLorenzo, 1997; Treiman, 1993]. A recent prospective study looked at the utility of emergency EEG. The most common indication was diagnosis of convulsive SE or follow-up of SE. In 77.5 percent of the cases, the clinician considered the EEG had contributed to the diagnosis. Overall, the EEG resulted in a modification in treatment in 37.8 percent of the cases

[Praline et al., 2007]. Classification of seizure type and evidence regarding etiology and prognosis may be determined from the EEG. Especially useful are the findings in patients with pseudo-seizures and those associated with medication overdoses or focal pathologic entities [Dodson et al., 1993; Riviello et al., 2006; Sonnen, 1997].

In children with prolonged coma or confusional states, nonconvulsive SE can sometimes be diagnosed only with the use of EEG recordings. The EEG is essential; motor findings may be subtle facial or limb movement, or isolated eye movements, or the movements may be absent altogether [Drislane et al., 2008]. Researchers in one study used EEG to diagnose SE in 37 percent of patients with altered consciousness whose diagnosis was unclear clinically [Privitera et al., 1994]. In another study, 8 percent of coma patients met the criteria for nonconvulsive SE [Towne et al., 2000]. In a study in children with unexplained decrease in level of consciousness or suspected subclinical seizures, 19 percent were found to be experiencing seizures by continuous EEG monitoring [Classen et al., 2004].

EEG can help to confirm that an episode of SE has ended. When use of neuromuscular blocking agents is contemplated or when recurrence of seizures cannot be documented by clinical observation (i.e., because of coma or large doses of medication), EEG monitoring is mandatory. Electroclinical dissociation may result from the administration of large doses of antiepileptic drugs in newborns and older children. In one study, 50 percent of patients continued to experience electrographic seizures with no clinical correlate in the 24 hours following cessation of SE [DeLorenzo et al., 1998]. Patients with SE who fail to recover rapidly and completely should be monitored with EEG for at least 24 hours after an episode to ensure that recurrent seizures are not missed. The presence of periodic discharges in these patients suggests the possibility of preceding SE, and careful monitoring may clarify the etiology of these discharges and allow detection of recurrent SE. Conversely, patients whose clinical condition has not returned to baseline may have abnormal movements or postures that, without EEG monitoring, may lead to overtreatment [Ross et al., 1999].

The EEG may provide prognostic information as well. The presence of periodic epileptiform discharges during or after SE is associated with a higher risk of poor outcome [Nei et al., 1999]. Additionally, in refractory SE in children, outcome is poorer with multifocal or generalized abnormalities than with a focal abnormality on the initial EEG [Sahin et al., 2001].

There is increasing use of continuous EEG, primarily for the diagnosis and management of nonconvulsive SE. Seizures, predominantly nonconvulsive seizures, are common in the critically ill child, with one study showing in incidence of 44 percent [Jette et al., 2006]. In this study a 1-hour recording only captured seizures in half the patients ultimately diagnosed with on-going seizures, but this rose to 80 percent with a 24-hour recording, demonstrating the importance of continuous EEG in the critically ill child. The incidence of nonconvulsive SE in children has been estimated to be 23–35 percent of patients monitored [Hosain et al., 2005; Tay et al., 2006; Abend et al., 2007], with prior epilepsy, hypoxic-ischemic injury, and stroke identified as the most common etiologies. While we often become concerned about nonconvulsive SE following convulsive SE, this may not occur with any regularity. Undiagnosed nonconvulsive SE often was found only in the case of brief convulsive seizures followed by persistently altered level of consciousness [Tay et al., 2006]. In a study of

hypothermia for neurological protection following cardiac arrest in 19 children, continuous EEG was used and found seizures in 47 percent of patients, and nonconvulsive SE in 32 percent [Abend et al., 2009a].

Medical Therapy

Prehospital

The majority of SE begins outside of the hospital. Traditionally, rapid treatment focused on recognition and rapidity of transport to an appropriate emergency department. Over the last few decades, however, the focus has shifted to initiating treatment in the prehospital setting. Early intervention with first-line drug therapy has been associated with an 80 percent response rate; response rates decline progressively the longer treatment is delayed [Lowenstein et al., 1993]. Seizures of longer duration are associated with significantly increased morbidity, which include more intensive treatment in the emergency department, and admission to an intensive care unit. There is evidence that prehospital treatment with diazepam, whether intravenous or rectal, is effective for decreasing the complications of prolonged seizures [Lowenstein et al., 1993]. Treatment outside of the hospital has been associated with decreased emergency department visits [Kriel et al., 1991; O'Dell et al., 2005b]. A review of 45 children indicated that prehospital treatment was associated with a shorter duration of SE (32 minutes versus 60 minutes) and a lower incidence of recurrence of seizures in the emergency department [Allredge et al., 1995].

Rectal administration is effective and has been studied more comprehensively than any other alternative route. Alternatives such as intranasal midazolam or buccal midazolam may be as or more effective than rectal diazepam in the out-of-hospital setting. This is reviewed below.

Initial Therapy in the Emergency Department

Treatment should begin with placement of an intravenous line. Fluid restriction is rarely necessary. In children, immediately after placement of the intravenous line, 25 percent glucose (2–4 mL/kg) should be given by bolus if hypoglycemia is suspected. In adolescents and adults, the intravenous line typically is kept open with normal saline, and the patient is given 100 mg of thiamine, followed by 50 mL of 50 percent glucose by slow intravenous push if hypoglycemia is documented [Pellock and DeLorenzo, 1997; Treiman, 1993]. Whenever the intravenous route cannot be established, the intraosseous route can be used efficiently for fluid and medication administration [Orlowski et al., 1990].

The most frequent error committed in the treatment of SE is the initial administration of inadequate doses of an antiepileptic drug. This suboptimal regimen is then followed by a waiting period until more seizures occur before administration of the necessary total dose [Dodson et al., 1993; Pellock and DeLorenzo, 1997]. Management of SE is best accomplished by use of a predetermined protocol in most settings [Pellock, 1994; Pellock and DeLorenzo, 1997; Treiman, 1990]. In almost all situations in which it is medically possible, drugs should be administered intravenously to ensure the most rapid delivery of maximal doses to the brain. The ideal antiepileptic drug for the treatment of SE should optimally have the following properties:
1. rapid onset of action
2. wide spectrum of activity

3. intravenous preparation
4. ease of administration
5. minimal redistribution from the CNS
6. short elimination half-life
7. wide therapeutic safety margin [Pellock, 1993a].

Rapid onset of action and bioavailability of parenteral forms have made benzodiazepines the preferred initial agent for treatment of SE. Lorazepam has become popular in many centers as the initial agent because of its overall advantages over diazepam of rapid onset of action and longer pharmacologic effect [Appleton et al., 1995; Pellock, 1994; Pellock and DeLorenzo, 1997; Treiman, 1990]. When SE continues after the initial dose of benzodiazepines is administered and persists after a primary antiepileptic drug, such as phenytoin, fosphenytoin, or phenobarbital is given, a second benzodiazepine dose should be administered before changing to an alternative antiepileptic drug. A protocol currently used for the management of SE in children by investigators at the Medical College of Virginia at the Virginia Commonwealth University is outlined in Table 58-3 (modified from Pellock and DeLorenzo [1997]). Similar protocols are becoming universally accepted. Recently, in the United Kingdom a committee investigating ideal therapy for SE in children recommended a protocol using a rapid-onset medication, such as a benzodiazepine after initial stabilization, followed by phenytoin or phenobarbital, and then, if necessary, an anesthetic [Appleton et al., 2000].

The choice of the optimal pharmacologic agent may not be identical for every patient with SE. Benzodiazepines and phenytoin (or fosphenytoin) as initial therapy are preferred by some clinicians, but others may wish to use alternative agents if the patient is known to be on maintenance therapy or already has received smaller doses of phenytoin or phenobarbital [Holmes, 1990; Pellock and DeLorenzo, 1997]. Lorazepam, diazepam, phenytoin or fosphenytoin, and phenobarbital are accepted agents for initial and continued therapy of SE. The large SE treatment study done in adults and sponsored by the U.S. Veterans Administration compared four intravenous drug regimens:

1. diazepam, 0.15 mg/kg plus phenytoin, 18 mg/kg
2. lorazepam, 0.1 mg/kg
3. phenobarbital, 15 mg/kg
4. phenytoin, 18 mg/kg.

The first three regimens were found to be superior to phenytoin alone for initial management of generalized convulsive SE in adults [Treiman et al., 1994]. The choice of an initial agent may depend on individual patient characteristics, prior antiepileptic drug therapy, and physician preference. Typically, however, lorazepam has become the first-line treatment of choice. Less uniformity exists in the choice of the second-line agent. Currently, there is no evidence to guide the treating physician in choosing among phenytoin plus phenobarbital, valproate, or levetiracetam [Shorvon et al., 2008].

Table 58-3 Medical College of Virginia Status Epilepticus Treatment Protocol for Children*

Step	Elapsed Time[†]	Procedure
1	0–5 min	Determination of SE. As soon as the diagnosis is made, institute monitoring of temperature, blood pressure, pulse, respirations, ECG, and EEG. Insert oral airway and administer oxygen if necessary. Insert an intravenous catheter and draw venous blood for levels of antiepileptics, glucose (check Dextrostix), electrolytes, calcium, BUN, CBC. Draw arterial antipyretics (acetaminophen). Perform frequent suction
2	6–9 min	Place an intravenous line with normal saline. Administer a bolus of 2 mL/kg 50% glucose
3	10–30 min	Initial treatment consists of an infusion of intravenous lorazepam given at a rate of 1–2 mg/min (0.1 mg/kg) to a maximum dose of 8 mg. This is followed by intravenous phenytoin (fosphenytoin; PHT [FPHT]), 18–20 mg/kg, infused at a rate not to exceed 1 mg/kg/min or 50 mg/min. Monitor ECG and blood pressure. May repeat phenytoin (FHPT), 10 mg/kg before proceeding to next step. Alternatives to phenytoin includes intravenous valproate, 20–40 mg/kg at rates of 3–6 mg/kg/min or levetiracetam 30–60 mg/kg intravenous over 15 minutes
4	31–59 min	If seizures persist, administer a bolus infusion of phenobarbital at a rate not to exceed 50 mg/min until seizures stop or to a loading dose of 20 mg/kg
5	60 min	If control is still not achieved, other options include the following: (1) Midazolam with an initial intravenous loading dose of 0.15 mg/kg, followed by a continuous infusion of 1–2 µg/kg/min titrating every 15 minutes to produce seizure control on EEG. Treatment is typically 12–48 hours (2) Pentobarbital with an initial intravenous loading dose of 5 mg/kg with additional amounts given to produce a burst-suppression pattern on EEG. Maintenance of pentobarbital anesthesia is continued for approximately 4 hours by an infusion of 1–5 mg/kg/hr. The patient is then checked for the reappearance of seizure activity by decreasing the infusion rate. If clinical seizures and/or generalized discharges persist on EEG, the procedure is repeated; if not, the pentobarbital is tapered over 12–24 hours
6	61–80 min	If seizures are still not controlled, call the anesthesia department to begin general anesthesia with halothane and neuromuscular blockade

* Note: Continuous monitoring of EEG is recommended in an obtunded patient to ensure that SE has not recurred. For management of intractable cases, a neurologist who has expertise in SE should be consulted, and advice from a regional epilepsy center should be sought.
† Time from beginning of intervention.
Lumbar puncture should be performed as soon as possible, especially in a febrile child or infant younger than 1 year of age. For infants with a history of neonatal seizures, infantile spasms, or early-onset seizures, pyridoxine 100 mg should be administered intravenously while EEG monitoring is being performed, for both diagnosis and treatment of seizures due to a vitamin B_6 deficiency (a rare cause).
BUN, blood urea nitrogen; CBC, complete blood count; D5W, 5% dextrose in water; ECG, electrocardiogram; EEG, electroencephalogram.
(Adapted from Pellock JM, DeLorenzo RJ. SE. In: Porter RJ, Chadwick D, eds. The epilepsies 2. Boston: Butterworth–Heinemann, 1997;267.)

Benzodiazepines

Intravenous lorazepam and intravenous diazepam have been found to be of equal efficacy in children [Qureshi et al., 2002], but intravenous lorazepam has a longer half-life and less respiratory depression [Appleton et al., 1995; Treiman et al., 1998]. The availability of a rectal preparation provides an alternative when intravenous access cannot be obtained. Intubation is less often required with rectal diazepam than with intravenous diazepam, and seizure recurrence is reduced [Diekmann, 1994]. Diazepam rectally may be used in many out-of-hospital settings for patients with recurrent SE, prolonged seizures, or acute repetitive seizures [Camfield et al., 1989; Dooley, 1998; Pellock, 1998]. Based on the long history of use of rectal diazepam in Europe, as well as experience in the United States and Canada, the following dosages are recommended: age 2–5 years, 0.5 mg/kg/dose; age 6–11 years, 0.3 mg/kg/dose; and age 12 years and older, 0.2 mg/kg/dose. These dosages yield an effective minimum plasma concentration of approximately 150–500 ng/mL [Morton et al., 1997b]. Although midazolam is rarely used in the U.S. for initial treatment of SE, it is efficacious and offers alternative administration routes. Unlike other benzodiazepines, midazolam is water-soluble, allowing for intramuscular injection. The intramuscular administration of midazolam may be particularly useful when intravenous access is unavailable or for prehospital treatment. A prospective, randomized study compared intramuscular midazolam with intravenous diazepam in the emergency department. In evaluating time to seizure control after administration, a 4-minute difference favoring midazolam was found [Chamberlain et al., 1997]. Nasal administration is possible, but absorption may be affected by nasal secretions [Wallace, 1997]. Liquid midazolam is rapidly absorbed through the buccal mucosa and is as effective as rectal diazepam [Scott et al., 1999].

Phenytoin/Fosphenytoin

Fosphenytoin is a water-soluble prodrug of phenytoin delivered in a neutral pH solution [Browne, 1997; Leppik et al., 1987; Ramsay and DeToledo, 1996]. This prodrug is replacing the present injectable phenytoin preparation [Pellock, 1996]. Dosing is safe at 150 mg/min (3 mg/kg/min), a rate three times more rapid than that for phenytoin. Fosphenytoin is quickly converted to phenytoin by systemic phosphatases, and higher unbound phenytoin peak levels are more rapidly attained after the intravenous infusion of fosphenytoin than with the older phenytoin preparation. Studies of infants and children furthermore demonstrate no significant difference among conversion rates for infants, children, and adults [Morton et al., 1997a].

Fosphenytoin is administered in "phenytoin equivalents" to obtain similar phenytoin levels, so that 20 mg/kg of fosphenytoin administered is the amount of fosphenytoin that has to be given so as to yield the amount of phenytoin equal to an administered dose of 20 mg/kg of phenytoin. This compound does not cause local irritation or tissue destruction and therefore may be given intramuscularly or intravenously. Intramuscular administration of fosphenytoin may be of particular advantage because it allows expeditious initiation of therapy when intravenous access is not available and prehospital treatment in other settings.

Recommended doses for intravenous administration of medications for the treatment of SE are given in Table 58-4 [Pellock, 1993a]. Recommended doses for fosphenytoin are identical to those for phenytoin in mg/kg phenytoin equivalent units. Rectal diazepam is administered according to age and weight.

Table 58-4 Recommended Initial Intravenous Doses of Antiepileptic Drugs for Status Epilepticus

Drug	Dose	Rate
Lorazepam	0.1 mg/kg	IV push
Diazepam	0.3 mg/kg	IV push
Phenobarbital	20 mg/kg	2 mg/kg/min
Phenytoin	20 mg/kg)	1 mg/kg/min
Fosphenytoin	20 PE*/kg/min	3 PE/mg/kg/min
Valproate[†]	20–40 mg/kg	3–6 mg/kg/min
Levetiracetam	30–60 mg/kg	Over 5 min

* PE = phenytoin equivalents, which equals 1 mg.
[†] Use with caution in children under the age of 2 years as there is a dramatically higher association with hepatic dysfunction.

Valproic Acid/Valproate

Valproate (valproic acid; VPA) is useful in the management of both generalized and partial epilepsy, and particularly useful in absence SE [Holle et al., 1995; Pellock, 1993a]. In the past, administration of valproate by the oral, nasogastric, or rectal route followed benzodiazepine administration. The U.S. Food and Drug Administration approved intravenous valproate for use in 1997. Although the drug is not approved for treatment of SE, reports of effective and rapid seizure control with good tolerability have been published. In one study of 20 patients with generalized and partial motor seizures, 15 mg/kg of valproate achieved control within 30 minutes [Czapinski and Terczynski, 1998]. Several studies have been carried out in children, demonstrating efficacy in a wide variety of seizures using loading doses of 20–40 mg/kg [Campistol et al., 1999; Kian-Ti et al., 2003; Uberall et al., 2000]. The manufacturer recommends administering VPA over 60 minutes at less than 20 mg/min. However, recent work has confirmed that intravenous valproate may be infused rapidly at higher rates. A study of 18 children reported that, when VPA was administered intravenously at 1.5–11 mg/kg/min, there were no severe infusion-site complications and no changes in vital nor other systemic side effects: specifically no arrhythmias, nor hypotension, nor respiratory suppression [Morton et al., 2007]. Its role in the treatment of SE is being defined [Devinsky et al., 1995]. Intravenous valproate conveys some advantages over intravenous phenobarbital due to its lack of sedation, lack of respiratory suppression, and low risk of hypotension. In addition, valproate may be the drug of choice in certain seizures, or second-line following a benzodiazepine.

In a study of adult and children, one study compared intravenous valproate with intravenous phenytoin as first-line treatment. Seizures were controlled in 66 percent of the valproate group, compared to 42 percent in the phenytoin group [Misra et al., 2006]. The valproate group received sodium valproate 30 mg/kg, compared to the phenytoin group, which received phenytoin at 18 mg/kg. A retrospective study of children with acute repetitive seizures and SE found intravenous valproate to be successful in 39 out of 40 patients, with loading doses typically of 25 mg/kg at an infusion rate of approximately 3 mg/kg/min. No adverse effects were appreciated [Yu et al., 2003]. One randomized, open-label study compared intravenous VPA with diazepam in 40 children with refractory SE, failing initial dosing of diazepam followed by phenytoin, and demonstrated that seizures were terminated equally with both medications (80 percent for VPA and 85 percent for diazepam), but the result was more rapid with VPA [Mehta et al., 2007]. In this study, loading doses of 30–40 mg/kg were employed. Most commonly reported doses were 15–45 mg/kg loading dose, followed by a 1 mg/kg/hour continuous infusion. A recent European consensus statement listed intravenous valproate as an option for the treatment of convulsive SE when benzodiazepines have failed [Shorvon et al., 2008].

In one study of patients with recurrent episodes of absence SE as a manifestation of their primary generalized epilepsy, chronic therapy with valproate markedly reduced seizure recurrence [Berkovic et al., 1989]. The intravenous formulation has been used for the treatment of absence SE [Chez et al., 1999; Alehan et al., 1999; Uberall et al., 2000]. Also reported is a case series indicating its utility in myoclonic SE [Sheth et al., 2000; Wheless, 2003].

Levetiracetam

Levetiracetam is a unique antiepileptic drug that is effective in focal and generalized epilepsies. In 2006, the intravenous formulation was approved. It is not licensed for the treatment of SE, however. Levetiracetam has several properties that make its exploration for the treatment of SE tempting. Studies suggest that levetiracetam is safe to administer in critically ill children with absence of destabilization [Abend et al., 2009b]. There is minimal metabolism of the medication and no appreciable pharmacokinetic drug interaction. Clearance of the drug is renal, and therefore dosing adjustments need to be made in patients with evidence of renal impairment. Dialysis will markedly reduce serum levels.

The available studies in pediatric patients focus on patients with refractory SE and/or uncontrolled retrospective studies. One study looked at patients ranging from three weeks to 19 years of age. Initial loading doses up to 40 mg/kg were used, with a mean total loading dose of 50 mg/kg, though doses as high as 118 mg/kg were recorded. Administration was safe and in no case was the drug discontinued because of side effects [Goraya et al., 2008]. An additional study evaluating levetiracetam for refractory SE in children found the drug to be effective 45 percent of the time [Gallentine et al., 2009]. No patients responded at loading doses less than 30 mg/kg and doses up to 70 mg/kg were utilized. A review of all available series of case studies demonstrated a response rate of 64 percent in refractory SE treated with levetiracetam [Trinka et al., 2009].

Ideally, a drug used to treat SE must be effective, safe, and able to be administered with few side effects. Recent work has focused on rapid infusion, giving large doses of up to 2500 mg in adults in as little as 5 minutes [Uges et al., 2009].

Topiramate

There have also been reports of topiramate being efficacious in refractory SE in adults and children. Topiramate is safe and well tolerated, with sedation being the primary adverse effect [Kahriman et al., 2003; Towne et al., 2003]. High doses (e.g., 10 mg/kg/day) have demonstrated efficacy within 1 day, but experience is limited [Perry, 2006]. The role of topiramate in the treatment of SE is unclear, and limited by the lack of a commercially available parenteral formulation. Most likely it will have a role in refractory SE but not as a first- or second-line agent.

Lacosamide

Data regarding the efficacy of lacosamide in seizure emergencies and SE is restricted to single case reports without pediatric experience. Therefore, at this juncture its future role in the management of SE is unclear. However, lacosamide is effective in the pilocarpine, cobalt-homocysteine, and electrical stimulation models of SE [Stöhr et al., 2007; Bialer et al., 2009]. A single case report described an adult in SE who had failed benzodiazepines, levetiracetam, and etomidate, but responded to 300 mg of lacosamide [Tilz et al., 2009].

SE resistant to therapy with first-line agents requires urgent treatment with agents that depress cerebral activity. Current recommendations for the management of refractory SE include the use of intravenous midazolam, pentobarbital, propofol, thiopental, and valproic acid. These medications are not without significant risk, including the need for prolonged mechanical ventilation, hemodynamic instability, and metabolic syndrome. No randomized controlled trials for any of these medications have been performed in either adults or children with refractory SE. In each case, the dose is regulated such as to control all clear-cut clinical or electrographic seizures and to maintain a suppression-burst pattern in the EEG. Therefore, continuous bedside EEG is monitored. There is no consensus as to the duration of "burst" and "flat" periods that signify optimal dosing [Krishnamurthy et al., 1999]. Most consider that establishing and maintaining any degree of burst-suppression is adequate.

Anesthetic Agents

Continuous infusion with high-dose pentobarbital is most commonly used [Pellock and DeLorenzo, 1997; Eriksson and Koivikko, 1997; Kinoshita et al., 1995] (see Table 53-3). Continuous benzodiazepine infusion with diazepam, midazolam [Nordt and Clark, 1997; Lal Koul et al., 1997; Chamberlain et al., 1997], or lorazepam may also be used. Continuous infusion with midazolam has been demonstrated to be as efficacious as pentobarbital infusion but with fewer cardiovascular adverse effects overall [Gilbert et al., 1999; Holmes et al., 1999; Igartua et al., 1999]. The choice depends on the practitioner's level of comfort with the various agents, as well as their specific treatment-related complications. Propofol anesthesia [Singhi et al., 1998; Stecker et al., 1998; Harrison et al., 1997] has also been effective. However, there have been some concerns that it may be proconvulsant in some patients [Makela et al., 1993], and can lead to metabolic acidosis [Niermeijer et al., 2003]. A recent retrospective study using propofol was noted to have a high mortality rate in refractory SE [Prasad et al., 2001]. However, a study in which 22 children received propofol found that it was successful in 64 percent and there were no safety concerns raised unless the dose exceeded 5 mg/kg/hour. Dosing was typically started with 1–2 mg/kg/hour [van Gestel et al., 2005]. Ketamine, an NMDA antagonist, has not been studied beyond small series [Sheth and Gidal, 1998; Prüss and Holtkamp, 2008]. Ketamine has not been useful early in the treatment of SE, but may become effective later when GABAergic agents generally are no longer effective [Prüss and Holtkamp, 2008].

Nonpharmacological Approaches

In a few extraordinary circumstances, nonpharmacologic treatment options may be available. If a definite seizure focus can be determined, resective surgery may be an option in selected cases (see Chapter 61). In one series of 10 children with pre-existing epilepsy, refractory SE was terminated in all and 7 remained seizure-free at 4 months to 6.5 years of follow-up [Alexopoulos et al., 2005]. Additionally, acute implantation of a vagus nerve stimulator has been reported in refractory SE [De Herdt et al., 2009].

There have been a limited number of cases utilizing the ketogenic diet for the treatment of refractory SE [Francois et al., 2003].

Therapeutic hypothermia is increasingly used in postanoxic patients. Hypothermia may also be useful in the treatment of refractory SE. Hypothermia to 31–35°C for 20–61 hours was reported to terminate SE refractory to multiple agents in 2 adult patients of 4 studied [Corry et al., 2008]. One study demonstrated control of refractory SE in three children with a combination of hypothermia to 30–31°C combined with thiopental [Orlowski et al., 1984].

Medical Complications of Status Epilepticus

The treatment of SE requires close monitoring of physiologic variables and excellent nursing to prevent secondary complications [Pellock, 1993b, 1994; Treiman, 1993]. Besides underlying or precipitating disease states associated with SE, other medical complications are quite common. Pulmonary care, proper positioning, and careful observation of seizures to note possible changes in seizure pattern are mandatory. Constant maintenance of intravenous fluids with adequate glucose and electrolyte administration and appropriate corrections, particularly in neonates and small infants, is essential. Optimal oxygenation, expectant observation, and treatment for hyperthermia and other medical complications lead directly to a lessening of morbidity and mortality. Cardiovascular, respiratory, and renal effects may be severe. Medical complications of SE that may occur in both infants and older children are listed in Box 58-3.

When hyperthermia is resistant to rectally administered antipyretics and cooling blankets, use of neuromuscular blocking agents may be necessary. EEG monitoring is necessary when these agents are used. A physiologic rise in blood pressure may accompany seizures but rarely requires antihypertensive medications unless the child is at risk for malignant hypertension. Treatment, unfortunately, may result in hypotension and reduced cerebral perfusion pressure. Very infrequently does cerebral edema or increased intracranial pressure become problematic in most children with SE that is not associated with an intracranial mass. Use of osmotic diuretics and corticosteroids is rarely indicated in the treatment of SE.

Prognosis

SE is recognized as a medical and neurologic emergency because of associated significant morbidity and mortality. Common sequelae of SE include intellectual dysfunction, permanent neurologic deficits, and continuing recurrent seizures. Neuropathologic studies in animals have demonstrated that

Box 58-3 Medical Complications of Status Epilepticus

- Tachycardia
- Bradycardia
- Cardiac dysrhythmia
- Cardiac arrest
- Conduction disturbance
- Congestive heart failure
- Hypertension
- Hypotension
- Altered respiratory pattern
- Pulmonary edema
- Renal tubular necrosis
- Lower nephron nephrosis
- Rhabdomyolysis
- Increased creatine kinase
- Myoglobinuria
- Carbon dioxide narcosis
- Intravascular coagulation
- Metabolic and respiratory acidosis
- Cerebral edema
- Excessive perspiration
- Dehydration
- Endocrine failure
- Altered pituitary function
- Elevated prolactin
- Elevated vasopressin
- Hyperglycemia
- Hypoglycemia
- Increased plasma cortisol
- Autonomic dysfunction
- Fever

(Modified from Pellock JM. SE. In: Pellock JM, Meyer EC, eds. Neurologic emergencies in infancy and childhood, 2nd edn. Boston: Butterworth–Heinemann, 1993.)

prolonged electrical activity results in irreversible neuronal damage to the CNS [Meldrum, 1983a]. Experimental studies suggest that seizures lasting for less than 30–60 minutes may produce neuronal injuries that are reversible. Seizures lasting longer than 1 hour produce neuronal death [Meldrum, 1983b; Simon, 1985]. As noted previously, prolonged seizures are associated with inadequate blood flow, decreased glucose use and oxygen consumption, and increased excitatory amino acid release, all of which lead to impaired mitochondrial function and neuronal destruction [Dwyer et al., 1986; Lothman, 1990; Wasterlain et al., 1983]. The duration of the SE episode, the patient's age, and the causative disorder all influence the resultant insult to involved neuronal populations.

In the aforementioned prospective population-based epidemiologic study [DeLorenzo et al., 1996, the annual incidence of SE was 41 cases per 100,000 population, and the annual incidence of total SE episodes was 50 per 100,000. The mortality rate was 22 percent, suggesting that, for the approximately 126,000–195,000 SE events, 22,000–42,000 deaths per year will occur in the United States. A majority of patients with SE have no previous history of epilepsy. The highest mortality rate is among the elderly, and the lowest is seen in healthy children or those with febrile SE [van Esch et al., 1996]. Although the overall mortality is extremely low in pediatric patients, younger children are at highest risk, with a mortality rate of 17.8 percent for those younger than 1 year in one study [Morton et al., 2001]. Mortality in these children typically is associated with specific underlying disorders, such as severe brain damage secondary to hypoxia.

Recurrences of SE are common in young children. These patients usually have chronic neurologic disabilities. In those patients who die, death rarely occurs during the acute episode of SE. Rather, most deaths occur 13–30 days after onset of the SE episode. Children with epilepsy and low antiepileptic drug levels have the lowest mortality rate. One reason for the low mortality rate in children is that they are less likely than adults to have systemic diseases. However, in one study, two independent risk factors for increased mortality in children, after excluding progressive or acute neurological insult, were duration of seizures in excess of 2 hours and a history of asthma [Maegaki et al., 2005]. In the elderly, cardiovascular decompensation occurring during the stress of SE may play an important role in the higher mortality rate [Boggs et al., 1993, 1994].

The morbidity associated with SE in children was examined in a database from Virginia [Fortner et al., 1993]. Before their SE event, 81 percent of children with no prior seizures were neurologically normal, in contrast with only 31 percent of children with seizure histories. Of the neurologically normal children with no prior seizures, more than 25 percent deteriorated after their first SE event, in comparison with less than 15 percent of neurologically normal children with a seizure history. Children who were neurologically abnormal without prior seizures deteriorated less frequently (6.7 percent), compared with 11.3 percent of the children who were neurologically abnormal who had a seizure history. In some children, neurologic deficits, such as mild ataxia, incoordination, or mild motor deficits, are transient. Symptoms usually can be attributed to the acute therapies or clinical changes after prolonged seizures.

Determining whether language deficits or school performance difficulties will be transient or more permanent is much more difficult. A previous retrospective study yielded a high rate of morbidity of nearly 30 percent, suggesting a sampling bias [Fortner et al., 1993]. In a prospective study, only 11–15 percent of affected patients had significant morbidity after an episode of SE [Morton et al., 1998]. These more recent findings suggest that the neurologic morbidity is substantially lower than the "greater than 50 percent" rate previously reported in children with SE [Aicardi and Chevrie, 1987]. The morbidity and mortality rates in sick infants, however, are higher than those in older children [Morton et al., 1998].

Patients with refractory SE represent a special population at particularly high risk for mortality and morbidity. Refractory SE typically is diagnosed when seizures have persisted for longer than 60 minutes and have not responded to use of three or more medications. Several series have demonstrated mortality rates ranging from 16 to 32 percent [Gilbert et al., 1999; Kernitsky et al., 2002; Sahin et al., 2001; Singhi et al., 1998] – much higher than the rate typical for childhood SE of approximately 3 percent [DeLorenzo et al., 1996; Maytal et al., 1989; Towne et al., 1994]. In addition, the morbidity rate was quite

high in this population, with 34 percent experiencing developmental deterioration after refractory SE [Sahin et al., 2001].

The consequences of SE for the developing brain are not clearly known. This issue, however, has been difficult to approach in clinical research studies, as multiple factors are all potential contributors to cognitive dysfunction in children with epilepsy. In addition to the seizures themselves, medications, underlying brain malformations, and pre-existing learning problems are all potential contributors to cognitive dysfunction. Studies of laboratory animals experiencing convulsive SE also have revealed an age dependence in vulnerability to neurocognitive impairment [Lui et al., 1994]. While evidence in humans at times is unclear or contradictory, recent work suggests some age-dependent effect. Neonatal SE seems to be an independent risk factor for adverse outcome in full-term newborns compared to similar newborns with seizures [Pisani et al., 2007]. There is some evidence that both recurrent seizures and SE may affect the developing brain in myriad ways, ranging from injury and altered neurogenesis to plasticity leading to epileptogenicity and the development of behavioral and cognitive consequences, even in the absence of readily discernible injury. Using animal models, it is reasonable to estimate that P14–P21 rat pups represent toddlers and young children, and P28 rats represent older children prior to puberty. A 3 mg/kg dose of kainic acid produces very severe seizures in the 15-day-old rats. When subjected to kainic acid again at postnatal day 15, test subjects experienced more severe brain damage and performed worse in spatial learning tasks than their control counterparts [Koh et al., 1999]. Emerging evidence suggests that early-life seizures can alter the function of neurotransmitter systems and intrinsic neuronal properties in the brain, possibly contributing to cognitive and learning impairments. Enhancement of $GABA_A$ receptor function with benzodiazepines disrupts long-term potentiation and memory formation [Seabrook et al., 1997] and hippocampal-dependent spatial learning [Rudolph and Mohler, 2004].

SE constitutes a neurologic emergency that must be treated aggressively. Children may suffer significant morbidity and mortality associated with SE. In addition to treating the seizures, the clinician must investigate the cause of SE and design specific treatments depending on the etiology. An emergency SE treatment and evaluation plan should be established and followed to ensure expedited care. Antiepileptic agents, although successful in treating a majority of SE cases, are not completely successful, and new agents must be developed. In addition, since SE has detrimental effects systemically (e.g., ventilation, blood pressure, cardiac function), future therapies may well include agents that provide systemic as well as nervous system protection to decrease the morbidity and mortality associated with SE. Rapid recognition and treatment of SE offer the best opportunities to improve the outcome in those afflicted with this neurologic emergency worldwide.

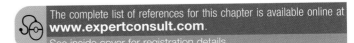

Antiepileptic Drug Therapy in Children

Jeannine M. Conway, Ilo E. Leppik, and Angela K. Birnbaum

Rational management of antiepileptic drug therapy in children requires an understanding of pharmacokinetics, pharmacodynamics, and toxicology of these agents. Pharmacokinetics is the study of drug absorption, distribution, metabolism, and elimination: that is, what the body does to a drug. Pharmacodynamics is the study of a drug's biochemical and physiologic effects: that is, what the drug does to the body. Children, much more than adults, have widely varying abilities to absorb, distribute, metabolize, and eliminate drugs [Rane and Wilson, 1976]. Evidence also exists that antiepileptic drug pharmacodynamics in children differ from those in adults [Henriksen, 1988]. Application of basic pharmacokinetic and pharmacodynamic principles to antiepileptic drug therapy facilitates the attainment and maintenance of targeted serum concentrations, clinical response, control of drug interactions, and optimization of clinical response.

Adverse reactions often dictate the choice of an antiepileptic drug and subsequent adjustment of therapy. An understanding of these reactions, including their differences and similarities among various antiepileptic drugs, and the application of appropriate clinical and laboratory monitoring provide the tools needed for the clinician to prescribe antiepileptic drug therapy rationally.

Pharmacokinetic Principles

Antiepileptic drug pharmacokinetics differ qualitatively and quantitatively between children and adults. Compared with adults, children, particularly neonates, have greater variability in their ability to absorb and eliminate antiepileptic drugs. Potential sources of variability are numerous, and include drug formulation, behavior (compliance, diet, substance abuse), environment, and physiology. Physiologic variability may be correlated with the general health of the patient, but also with specific factors such as gender, age, maturation, and, in a few cases, pregnancy. In the management of pediatric patients with seizures, there is a concern with the effects of age and maturation on the pharmacokinetic profile of the antiepileptic drugs. A drug's effect on a child's learning and behavior should also be a major determinant influencing the choice of an antiepileptic drug. Age has the most influence on antiepileptic drug elimination, metabolic pathways, and absorption. Factors such as protein binding and enzyme induction and/or inhibition are similar for children and for adults.

This chapter will review general pharmacokinetic principles and discuss the clinically relevant features of specific antiepileptic drugs. For quick reference, pharmacokinetic information for the antiepileptic drugs is summarized in tables, with absorption characteristics provided in Table 59-1, and volume of distribution, protein binding, half-life, and metabolites presented in Table 59-2 and Table 59-3.

Absorption

Absorption is a complex phenomenon controlled by the physicochemical properties of the drug, the formulation, and the physiologic conditions at the sites of absorption: stomach, small intestine, colon, rectum, buccal and nasal mucosa, and muscle. Most drugs are given orally as solid formulations, which must first disintegrate into small particles that are then dissolved in the gastrointestinal fluid. Only after a drug is dissolved is it available for absorption. Most drugs are absorbed by passive diffusion of the unionized form but some drugs use active transport mechanisms. Gastrointestinal absorption is influenced by age-dependent changes in physiologic variables, such as gastric emptying time, stomach and intestinal pH, absorptive area, and gastrointestinal transit time. Food intake may affect antiepileptic drug pharmacokinetics, especially absorption. Although there is concern that the ketogenic diet may alter dosing requirements, a recent study indicated that there are no significant changes in the concentrations of several antiepileptic drugs (valproate – free or total, topiramate, phenobarbital, lamotrigine, clonazepam) during the ketogenic diet [Dahlin et al., 2006].

Absorption is described in terms of rate and extent. The term absorption half-life describes the rate at which drug reaches the systemic circulation. An indirect measure of absorption rate is the T_{max}. This measure is useful in comparing the rates of absorption of different brands or formulations of the same drug. A lower (i.e., earlier) T_{max} usually is an indication of a faster rate of absorption. When all other pharmacokinetic parameters are constant, a faster rate of absorption will result in a lower T_{max} and higher maximum concentration (C_{max}).

The extent of absorption describes the amount of a drug that reaches the blood relative to the dose. It is termed oral bioavailability (F) and is the fraction of the dose that reaches the systemic circulation. Absolute bioavailability of a drug is

Table 59-1 Formulations, Routes of Administration, and Bioavailability of Antiepileptic Drugs

Medication	Available Formulation(s)	Possible Route(s)*	T_{max} (Hr)	Fraction Absorbed (F)	Special Problems
Acetazolamide	Tablet	PO	1–4	N/a	
	ER capsule	PO	3–6	N/a	
	Injectable	IV, IM	0.25	N/a	
Carbamazepine	Tablet	PO	3–8	0.79	Prolonged absorptive phase with variable T_{max}; induction results in earlier T_{max}
	Chewable tablet	PO	2	0.79	
	Suspension	PO, PR	0.5–3	0.7–0.9 estimate	Earlier T_{max} results in higher C_{max}, which can produce transient side effects
	ER tablet	PO	3–12	0.89 relative to susp.	Tablet must be swallowed whole; do not crush or chew
	ER capsule	PO	4–8	0.79	Capsules may be opened and the beads sprinkled over food, such as a teaspoon of applesauce or other similar food products. Capsules or their contents should not be crushed or chewed
Clonazepam	Tablet	PO	1–8	0.85	
Clorazepate	Tablet	PO	0.7–1.5	0.91	
Diazepam	Tablet	PO	0.5–2	0.8–1	
		PO	0.1–0.5	0.8–1	
	Gel	PR	0.75	0.9	
	Injectable	IM, IV	1–1.5	0.8–1	IM absorption is slow and variable
Ethotoin	Tablet	PO	2	N/a	
Ethosuximide	Capsule	PO	1.5–4	N/a	
		PO	3–7	N/a	
Felbamate	Tablet	PO	1–4	N/a	
		PO	3.7	N/a	
Fosphenytoin	Injectable	IV, IM	0.5 (IM)	1	Fosphenytoin concentrations after IM administration are lower but more sustained than those after IV administration owing to time required for absorption of fosphenytoin from injection site
Gabapentin	Capsule	PO	2–4	0.6–0.27	Gabapentin bioavailability decreases as dose increases
	Tablet	PO	2–4	0.6–0.27	
		PO	2–4	0.6–0.27	
Lacosamide	Tablet	PO	1–4	1	
	Solution	PO	1–4	1	
	Injectable	IV	End of infusion	1	
Lamotrigine	Compressed tablet	PO	0.5–4	0.98	
	Dispersible tablet	PO, PR	0.5–4	0.98	
Levetiracetam	Tablet	PO	0.3–2	0.95–1	
	Solution	PO	0.3–2	0.95–1	
Lorazepam	Tablet	PO	1–2.5	0.85–1	
	Injectable	IM, IV, PR	0.75–2	0.85–1	
	Concentrated oral solution	PO	1	0.90	
	Buccal	PO	N/a	N/a	
Methsuximide	Tablet	PO	N/a	N/a	
Oxcarbazepine	Tablet	PO	4.5	1	
		PO	6	1	
Paraldehyde	Solution	PR, PO	1.5–2 (PR)	N/a	Do not use discolored solution; avoid plastic equipment Withdrawn from U.S. market
Phenobarbital	Syrup	PO (PR)	1	0.8–1	Unpleasant taste, rejected by many
	Tablet	PO	0.5–8.6	0.8–1	
	Injectable	IM, IV	0.25–1	1	

Table 59-1 Formulations, Routes of Administration, and Bioavailability of Antiepileptic Drugs—cont'd

Medication	Available Formulation(s)	Possible Route(s)*	T_{max} (Hr)	Fraction Absorbed (F)	Special Problems
Phenytoin	Suspension (phenytoin acid)	PO	6–12	0.9–1	Patients should use accurate measuring device; dosing errors possible if suspension not adequately resuspended; strength of suspension must be clearly emphasized when prescribing
	Chewable tablet (phenytoin acid)	PO	4–8	0.9–1	T_{max} dependent on C_{max}
	Prompt-release capsule (phenytoin sodium)	PO	2–6	0.9–1	
	ER capsule (phenytoin sodium)	PO	2–10	0.9–1	T_{max} dependent on C_{max}
	Injectable (phenytoin sodium)	IV, IM	0.25–0.5	0.9–1	IM injection not recommended; absorption is slow and erratic; injection is painful and must be diluted with normal saline without glucose and slowly administered
Pregabalin	Capsule	PO	1.3	0.89–1	
	Solution	PO	1.3	0.89–1	
Primidone	Suspension	PO	4–6	N/a	
	Tablet	PO	4–6	N/a	
Rufinamide	Tablet	PO	4–6	<0.85	Rufinamide bioavailability decreases as dose increases
	Suspension	PO	4–6	<0.85	
Tiagabine	Tablet	PO	0.75–3	0.9	
Topiramate	Tablet	PO, PR	1.4–4.3	0.8	
	Sprinkle capsule	PO	1.4–4.3	0.8	Capsules may be opened and the beads sprinkled over food, such as a teaspoon of applesauce or other similar food products. Capsules or their contents should not be crushed or chewed
Valproate	Capsule	PO	1–3	0.9–1	Capsule filled with liquid valproic acid; avoid opening
	Enteric-coated tablet	PO	2–6	0.9–1	Food delays T_{max}
	Sprinkle capsules	PO	4–6	0.9–1	Capsules may be opened and the beads sprinkled over food, such as a teaspoon of applesauce or other similar food products. Capsules or their contents should not be crushed or chewed
	ER tablet	PO	4–17	0.9	
	Syrup	PO, PR	0.5–1	0.9–1	Valproate has objectionable aftertaste
	Injectable	IV	1	1	May not give IM
Vigabatrin	Tablet	PO	1	1	
	Solution	PO	1–2.5	1	
Zonisamide	Capsule	PO	2–6	1	

* Primary and alternates.
C_{max}, maximum plasma concentration; ER, extended-release; N/a, not available; T_{max}, time to maximum plasma concentration.

determined by comparing the area under the concentration vs. time curve after an oral (or rectal, intramuscular, and so on) dose with the area under the concentration vs. time curve after intravenous (IV) administration of the same drug. However, because many antiepileptic drugs do not have IV formulations, an absolute biovailability cannot be determined. Rather it can be estimated by comparing available oral formulations, termed relative bioavailability. Relative bioavailability is determined by comparing the area under the concentration vs. time curve for a specific formulation to that of a reference product. For

Table 59-2 Pharmacokinetics of Phenytoin

Age Group	V_d (L/kg)	Protein Binding (%)	V_{max} (mg/kg/day)	K_m (mg/L)	$t_{1/2}$(hr)	Initial Maintenance Dose (mg/kg/day)	Comments	Routes of Elimination
Neonates	0.7–1.2	74–90			3–140	4–6	Half-life varies with concentrations	
0.25–3 years		85–91	13.9	4–6.6	1.2–31.5	6–10		Hepatic 95%
4–6 years			11	4–6.8		5–7		
7–9 years			9.75	3.6–6.5		4–7		Renal 5%
>10 years	0.7–0.8	87–93	8.1	3–5.7	6–60	4–6		

K_m, concentration at which metabolism occurs at half the maximum rate; $t_{1/2}$, half-life; T_{max}, time to maximum plasma concentration; V_d, volume of distribution; V_{max}, maximum velocity for metabolism of drug.

example, the relative bioavailability of a generic brand of phenytoin sodium 100-mg capsule is measured by comparing its area under the concentration vs. time curve with that for brand phenytoin (Dilantin 100-mg capsule).

Because the hepatic portal system drains the entire gastrointestinal system (except for the distal rectum and buccal and nasal mucosa) all drugs swallowed are first delivered to the liver after crossing the gastrointestinal mucosa. Thus, a fraction of these drugs may be metabolized before entering the systemic circulation. The average plasma concentration is determined by the bioavailability and the rate of elimination (clearance) by the following relationship:

$$\text{Average drug concentration at steady state} = (\text{Bioavailability} \times \text{Daily Dose})/\text{Clearance}$$

Therefore, changes in bioavailability of a drug from alterations in drug formulation, alterations in gastrointestinal physiology, or interactions with inhibitors or inducers can result in clinically significant increases or decreases in drug concentrations in plasma or at the receptor site.

Descriptors of absorption, such as C_{max} and T_{max}, and the bioavailability, may vary considerably among different formulations of the same drug. The relative rates of absorption, and thus T_{max} and C_{max}, adhere to the following order of most rapid to slowest, and highest peak concentration to lowest: solutions > suspensions > capsules > tablets > extended-release formulations [Garnett and Cloyd, 1993]. Formulation-related differences in absorption characteristics are greatly influenced by the composition of the inactive ingredients (e.g., filler, particle size of drug) and nature of the capsule or tablet coating).

Volume of Distribution

Volume of distribution (V_d) is a measurement of how the drug is distributed throughout the body (tissues and blood), and is expressed in terms of liters or liters per kilogram. Mathematically, it is expressed as the following:

$$V_d(\text{L/kg}) = \text{Dose (mg/kg)}/C_{max}(\text{mg/L})$$

where V_d is the volume of distribution and C_{max} corresponds to the concentation immediately after IV administration, if this was the route of administration. Because many antiepileptic drugs do not have an IV formulation, the V_d of these is estimated from the concentration at T_{max}. V_d values may differ markedly among antiepileptic drugs because drugs distribute

to tissues with different binding characteristics. For example, drugs that concentrate in fat tissue have relatively low plasma concentrations, but may have a V_d value measured in the hundreds of liters because the C_{max} is low. Changes in body composition, such as increases or decreases in fat, muscle, or water, may thus alter V_d values.

V_d is very useful for calculating loading doses. The purpose of a loading dose is to fill body compartments rapidly to reach a targeted plasma concentration and thus a targeted concentration at the site of action. The equation for calculating a loading dose is the following:

$$\text{Loading dose (mg/kg)} = \text{Desired change in plasma concentration (mg/L)} \times \text{Volume (L/kg)}$$

The change in plasma concentration term denotes the desired increase after administration of the loading dose. For example, if a patient has a plasma concentration of 5 mg/L and the target concentration is 20 mg/L, the desired change in concentration is 15 mg/L. For phenytoin, the V_d is approximately 0.75 L/kg, so an IV dose of 11.25 mg/kg is required. When loading doses are administered intramuscularly, orally, or rectally, resultant maximum plasma concentrations are usually less than after IV loading, owing to slower and incomplete absorption and the elimination of some drug during the absorption phase. Table 59-4 presents loading dose information for six major antiepileptic drugs.

Protein Binding

Several antiepileptic drugs are highly bound to one or more plasma proteins, most commonly albumin or α_1-acid glycoprotein. Drug assays usually measure the total concentration of drug, which is the sum of the bound and unbound concentrations. The free fraction is the ratio of unbound to total plasma drug concentration:

$$\text{Free fraction (\%)} = (\text{Unbound concentration}/\text{Total concentration}) \times 100$$

In general, only the unbound drug is able to cross the blood–brain barrier and is in equilibrium with brain and spinal fluid (Figure 59-1; see also Table 59-3). Consequently, clinical response and toxicity correlate better with the unbound drug concentration than with the total drug concentration. For drugs

Table 59-3 Pharmacokinetics of Other Antiepileptic Drugs

Drug	Age Group*	V_d (L/kg)	Protein Binding (%)	t½ (hr)	Route(s) of Elimination	Active Metabolites	Initial Maintenance Dose (mg/kg/day)	Comments
Carbamazepine	N	1.1–2.6	65–70	7.2–27	Hepatic	Carbamazepine-10,11-epoxide	5–20	Therapy should be initiated at 30–50% of initial dose and increased as autoinduction occurs
	C	0.8–2.0	75–85	5–26			15–20	
Clonazepam	C	1.5–4.4	80–90	22–33	Hepatic	None	0.05–0.2	Tolerance to antiepileptic effect frequently occurs
Eslicarbazepine acetate (ESL)	C	0.8–1	40 (A)	6–8	Hepatic	Acetate (ESL) eslicarbazepine	5–30†	
Ethosuximide	N	0.69	<10	32–41	Hepatic	None	15–40	
	C	0.7		15–68				
Felbamate	C	0.73–0.82 (A)	30	14–21 (A)	Hepatic 50–55%; renal 45–50%	None	15–45	
Gabapentin	C	0.6–0.8 (A)	0	5–7	Renal	None	10–15	
Lacosamide	A	0.6	<15	13	Renal 40%; hepatic 60%	None	8–12†	
Lamotrigine	1–4 years	0.9–1.4	55	+ ind: 8 + VPA: 45	Hepatic	None	With VPA 1–5 With enzyme inducer 5–15	Slow-dose titration is necessary to lessen incidence of rash; see product information packet for details about titrating
	5–10 years			+ ind: 7 + VPA: 66 24–31 (A)				
Levetiracetam	C	0.5–0.7	<10	5	Renal	None	10–60	
Oxcarbazepine	C	0.7–0.8	40 (MHD) 4.8–9.3 (MHD)	37–73	Hepatic	10-hydroxy-metabolite (MHD)	8–10	
Phenobarbital	N	0.8–1	32	82–199	Hepatic 50–80%; renal 20–50%	None	3–4	
	I	0.6–0.9	40–55	37–73			4–5	
	C	0.7		21–75			2–3	

Continued

Table 59-3 Pharmacokinetics of Other Antiepileptic Drugs—cont'd

Drug	Age Group*	V_d (L/kg)	Protein Binding (%)	$t_{1/2}$ (hr)	Route(s) of Elimination	Active Metabolites	Initial Maintenance Dose (mg/kg/day)	Comments
Pregabalin	A	N/a	0	4.6–6.8	Renal > 90%; hepatic <10%	None	No pediatric data Adult dose 150–600/day	
Primidone	C	0.43–1.1 (A)	20	4.4–11	Hepatic 60–70%; renal 30–40%	Phenobarbital PEMA	10–15	Therapy should be initiated at 30–50% of initial maintenance dose
Rufinamide	C	0.8–1.2	34	6–10	Hepatic	None	10	
Tiagabine	A	0.74–0.85	96	5–13 Healthy (A)	Hepatic	None	0.375–1.3	
Topiramate	C	0.6–0.8	15	20–30 (A)	Renal >80%; hepatic <20%	None	1–3	
Valproate (valproic acid [VPA])	N	0.28–0.43	68–89	17–40	Hepatic 95%; renal 5%	2-en-VPA, 4-en-VPA, 2, 4-dien-VPA	5–10	
	I	0.2–0.34		6–8			10–20 (monotherapy), 20–30 (induced)	
	C	0.1–0.3	80–95	4–15			10–20 (monotherapy), 20–30 (induced)	
Vigabatrin	I	1.1	0	5.7	Renal	None identified	50–100	Vigabatrin is available as a racemic mixture; the S(+) enantiomer is the active enantiomer
Zonisamide	A	0.8–1.6 h	40–60 h	63–69	Renal 40–50%; hepatic 50–60%	None	2–12 (C)	

* A, adults; C, children; I, infants; N, neonates.
† Being studied, not approved.
MHD, monohydroxy derivative of oxcarbazepine; PEMA, phenylethyl malonamide; $t_{1/2}$, half-life; V_d, volume of distribution.

Table 59-4 Loading Doses of Antiepileptic Drugs

Drug	V_d (L/kg)	Loading Dose (mg/kg)	Route, Formulation	C_{max} (mg/L)	T_{max} (hr)
Carbamazepine	0.8	10	PO, suspension	6–9	2–6
Fosphenytoin	0.75 PE	10–20 PE	IV, IM	15–25 (PHT)	<0.25
Levetiracetam	0.7	50	IV, PO	47–128	Immediate
Phenobarbital	0.8	20	IV	15–25	Immediate
Phenytoin (PHT)	0.75	20	IV	20–30	Immediate
	0.75	20	PO, prompt-release capsule	15–25	8–12
	0.75	20	PO, ER capsule	10–20	10–36
Valproate	0.15–0.25	20	PO, syrup	60–100	0.5–2
	0.15–0.25	15–25	IV	90–100	Immediate

C_{max}, maximum plasma concentration; ER, extended-release; PE, phenytoin equivalents; T_{max}, time to maximum plasma concentration; V_d, volume of distribution.

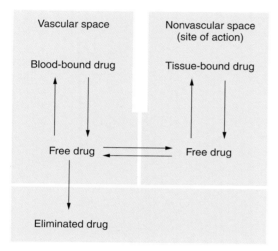

Fig. 59-1 Relationship of unbound drug in vascular and nonvascular compartments.

that have limited protein binding (less than 50 percent) or a constant ratio of unbound to total concentration, measurement of total plasma concentrations is a reliable indicator of response. However, if a drug is highly protein-bound (greater than 85 percent), measurements of total concentrations may be an unreliable guide to clinical outcomes. The fraction bound may change because of illness, age, or other drugs that compete for binding sites. In these circumstances, it may be necessary to measure the free concentration to understand the clinical effect better. Low-extraction drugs are those that have only a small portion of the drug metabolized by each pass through the liver. Most of the antiepileptic drugs are low-extraction drugs and alterations in protein binding do not affect the steady-state concentration of the *unbound* drug. Thus, adjustments in dose generally are not necessary when protein binding is altered because the unbound concentrations remain unchanged. Erroneously increasing the dose when total levels are low, but unbound levels have not changed, will likely result in toxicity.

Metabolism and Elimination

Antiepileptic drugs are eliminated from the body through metabolism and renal excretion. Clearance (Cl) and elimination half-life ($t_{1/2}$) are the pharmacokinetic terms that quantitatively

describe drug elimination. Clearance describes the rate of elimination and defines dosage requirements, whereas $t_{1/2}$ is useful in determining time to steady state and dosing intervals.

Clearance is the volume of blood from which drug is removed (cleared) per unit of time. It is identical conceptually and mathematically to the more familiar physiologic parameter of creatinine clearance. For antiepileptic drugs that are eliminated by the liver, clearance is determined by the free concentration of the drug and the intrinsic ability of hepatic enzymes to metabolize the unbound drug. Although, for most drugs, clearance is proportional to dose, some drugs exhibit nonlinear pharmacokinetics in which clearance changes with concentration (Figure 59-2).

The following points are important to remember:

- Clearance and absorption determine the amount of drug a patient requires to maintain a targeted steady-state plasma concentration.
- Changes in clearance lead to changes in concentration and in the resultant pharmacologic response.
- Changes in protein binding can affect total drug concentration without affecting unbound drug concentration.
- Changes in total drug concentration without a corresponding change in unbound concentration do not require a dosage adjustment.
- Addition or removal of other drugs can induce or inhibit metabolism and alter hepatic clearance.

The $t_{1/2}$ is the time required for the plasma concentration to decline by 50 percent. Half-life is determined by both distribution volume and clearance:

$$t_{1/2} = (0.693 \times V_d)/Cl$$

Thus, $t_{1/2}$ is not a direct measure of Cl, but is useful in calculating the time to reach steady state or the time required for drug elimination. After initiation or modification of therapy or after any change in clearance, 5 half-lives must elapse for a new steady-state plasma concentration to be reached (see Figure 59-2). The time required to attain steady state can be explained by using the definition of $t_{1/2}$. The plasma concentration in the body declines 50 percent in 1 $t_{1/2}$; therefore, the percentage of drug remaining in the body, as indicated by the plasma concentration after 2, 3, 4, and 5 half-lives, is 75 percent, 87.5 percent, 93.75 percent, and 96.875 percent, respectively. The actual amount of drug remaining in the body and the additional amount of drug removed in subsequent half-lives are so small (after 5

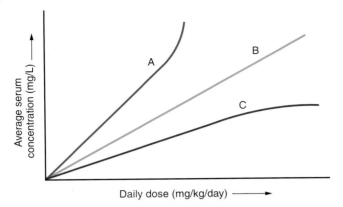

Fig. 59-2 Effect of dose on elimination kinetics. Curve A plots nonlinear pharmacokinetics (of the Michaelis–Menten type) in which clearance decreases with increasing dose, as with phenytoin. Curve B plots linear pharmacokinetics, in which clearance remains the same with increasing dose, as with phenobarbital, felbamate, vigabatrin, tiagabine, topiramate, and valproic acid (unbound drug). Curve C plots nonlinear pharmacokinetics in which clearance increases with dose, as with valproic acid (total), carbamazepine, and lamotrigine.

half-lives) that, for practical purposes, it can be ignored. However, the rate of decline is most rapid in the first two half-lives, and the risk of seizures is greatest during this period.

Biotransformation (metabolism) of medications is accomplished through biochemical reactions. These reactions create compounds that are more polar (more water-soluble) and are eliminated from the body, usually through the kidneys. Phase I reactions (e.g., using the cytochrome P-450 system) involve oxidation and reduction. Phase II reactions (noncytochrome P-450-mediated) couple the drug or its metabolite with endogenous substrates by conjugation or synthesis. The endogenous substrate may be glucuronic acid, glutathione, glucose, sulfate, or acetate, making the drug more polar and hence water-soluble [Capparelli, 1994]. Antiepileptic drugs may undergo metabolism by phase I or II reactions, or a combination of both. As persons mature, the pathways may change and the metabolite profile will be altered.

In the neonate, phase I reactions, such as hydroxylation and, to a lesser extent, dealkylation, are significantly depressed [Anderson and Lynn, 2009]. In older children, however, phase I activity generally exceeds that in adolescents or adults. As a general rule, the rate of drug metabolism reaches a peak at 0.5–2 years of age and then declines in an exponential manner, reaching adult values in early adolescence. As an example, the clearance of valproic acid, in which metabolism includes both phase I and phase II reactions, is fastest in young children and then declines to reach adult values at the age of approximately 12–15 years. Also, its metabolism shifts from phase II to phase I reactions.

For most drugs, the evaluation of maturation-related (as contrasted with chronologic age-related) enzymatic clearance has not been studied systematically. It is likely that some of the variance in drug clearance noted in children of the same age is due to differences in maturational development. As children grow, the dose may need to be increased to compensate for the increased body (and liver) mass, but later re-adjusted for the decline in phase I and II reactions.

Active metabolites formed after biotransformation of the parent compound can contribute significantly to desired and toxic effects of the parent drug. Metabolites exist in both bound and unbound states. Only the unbound metabolite is available for elimination or biotransformation to an inactive metabolite. As with unbound parent drug, the unbound metabolite concentration in the plasma most closely correlates with the concentration of metabolite at the site of action. The presence of active metabolites complicates interpretation of plasma drug concentrations and clinical response. As with the parent drug, the relationship between unbound and total metabolite concentrations can be disrupted by displacement from serum proteins or changes in metabolism. In fact, parent or metabolite concentrations may be altered independently by drug interaction or physiologic change in metabolism. Table 59-5 displays the cytochrome P-450 isoform families involved in antiepileptic drug metabolism, along with known inducers and inhibitors.

Table 59-5 Antiepileptic Drug Involvement with Cytochrome P-450 System

Metabolic Pathway	CYP1A2	CYP2C	CYP3A	Glucuronidation	Not Determined	Renal
Antiepileptic drug substrates	Carbamazepine	Phenytoin Diazepam Barbiturates Lacosamide	Carbamazepine Diazepam Tiagabine Zonisamide	Eslicarbazepine Lamotrigine Valproic acid	Topiramate	Gabapentin Lacosamide Levetiracetam Pregabalin Vigabatrin
Inducers	Carbamazepine Cigarette smoke Omeprazole	Carbamazepine Rifampin Phenobarbital Phenytoin	Carbamazepine Oxcarbazepine Phenobarbital Phenytoin Rifampin Rufinamide	Barbiturates Cigarette smoke Phenytoin		
Inhibitors	Cimetidine Fluoroquinolones Fluvoxamine	Cimetidine Felbamate Fluoxetine Proton pump inhibitors Oxcarbazepine Topiramate	Antifungals Cimetidine Diltiazem Erythromycin Fluoxetine Nefazodone Verapamil	Valproate		

Renal elimination is accomplished by glomerular filtration and/or renal tubular secretion. Glomerular filtration rate and renal tubular function in newborns are less efficient than in adults [Linday, 1994]. After 1 year of age, glomerular filtration rate, corrected for body surface area, is the same as for older children and young adults. Renal tubular function reaches adult values, normalized to body surface areas, within several months. Decreases in clearance can be better correlated with sexual maturity than with chronologic age. Making correlations with physiologic or sexual maturation and developmental age, rather than chronologic age, may be helpful in accounting for the variability observed in clearance of drugs that are renally eliminated [Finkelstein, 1994].

Specific Antiepileptic Drugs

Barbiturates

Phenobarbital, primidone, and methobarbital were the mainstay of the treatment of epilepsy for many years. Primidone itself is active and is metabolized to the active metabolites PEMA and phenobarbital. Because phenobarbital has a half-life measured in days and the other metbolites have relatively short half-lives, phenobarbital is considered to be the primary active agent during primidone use. Methobarbital is also metabolized to phenobarbital. Side effects of this group, including paradoxical hyperactivity in children, have markedly reduced the use of these medications.

Benzodiazepines

As a group, the benzodiazepines are rapidly (T_{max} of 30–180 minutes) and completely absorbed when given orally. The exception to this is midazolam, which is subject to a high first-pass effect when administered orally. Intramuscular administration of diazepam or lorazepam is not recommended because of slow or erratic absorption, but midazolam is more consistently and rapidly absorbed by this route. Diazepam is also absorbed rectally.

The benzodiazepines rapidly cross the blood–brain barrier. Brain concentrations reach equilibrium with plasma concentrations within seconds after IV administration. But the highly lipid-soluble nature of diazepam and lorazepam causes them to redistribute to other body tissues, resulting in a rapid decrease in brain concentrations and a very high V_d. This redistribution is responsible for the short duration of action after a single dose [Greenblatt et al., 1989; Leppik et al., 1983]. The benzodiazepines are metabolized by the liver and have linear elimination kinetics. Some of the metabolites exhibit antiepileptic activity and also may contribute to toxicity. Because the active metabolites have very long half-lives, repeated administration of these drugs, culminating in large total doses, may lead to long periods of sedation, usually most problematic for diazepam and chlorazepate.

Carbamates

The carbamates are organic compounds derived from carbamic acid, NH_2COOH. Some have been found effective for the treatment of epilepsy. Carbamazepine is the oldest of this class; oxcarbazepine and, more recently, eslicarbazepine acetate, have been added to this category.

Carbamazepine

Carbamazepine is a very water-insoluble, neutral compound with a slow dissolution rate in gastrointestinal fluid. The relative bioavailability is similar for all four formulations (i.e., suspension, chewable tablet, extended-release, and regular tablet), ranging from 75 to 90 percent, although marked intrapatient and interpatient variability has been observed [Faigle and Feldmann, 1975; Maas et al., 1987]. In children on maintenance therapy, the rate of absorption is much faster for the suspension than for tablet formulations, resulting in a significantly earlier T_{max} and higher C_{max} (Figure 59-3). This property occasionally produces transient concentration-dependent central nervous system side effects. Administering the same daily dose in smaller amounts and giving it more frequently may correct this problem. Sustained-release preparations may permit twice-a-day dosing, eliminating the need for administration of medications during school hours. This improves medication compliance and decreases central nervous system side effects because peak concentrations will be lower. Studies conducted by the U.S. Food and Drug Administration have demonstrated that carbamazepine tablets are significantly less well absorbed after being exposed to high humidity [Meyer et al., 1992; Wang et al., 1993]. These findings emphasize the importance of storing all antiepileptic drugs at room temperature in a dry location.

The V_d in children for carbamazepine based on oral preparations ranges from 0.8 to 2.0 L/kg. Both carbamazepine and its active metabolite, carbamazepine-10,11-epoxide, are bound to several plasma proteins [Eichelbaum et al., 1975; Rawlins et al., 1975]. Approximately 65–85 percent of carbamazepine and 30–60 percent of carbamazepine-10,11-epoxide are bound to albumin. Both also bind to the reactant protein α_1-acid glycoprotein. Binding to α_1-acid glycoprotein increases after physiologic stress, such as from burn injuries or inflammatory diseases (e.g., juvenile rheumatoid arthritis). Increased binding to α_1-acid glycoprotein can increase total carbamazepine and carbamazepine-10,11-epoxide concentrations without necessarily increasing the unbound drug concentrations. In such situations, patients may have total concentrations above the desired range but have no side effects. Adjusting dosage is not necessary; plasma concentrations return to baseline as α_1-acid glycoprotein declines.

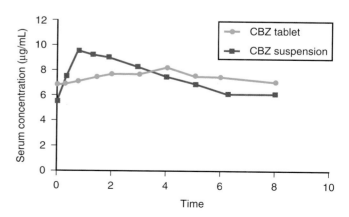

Fig. 59-3 Comparison of serum concentration–time curves after administration of carbamazepine (CBZ) tablets and suspension. Data are from a crossover study in a child with epilepsy on steady-state, maintenance therapy.

Carbamazepine is eliminated primarily by phase I cytochrome P-450-mediated metabolism (see Table 59-5), forming an active metabolite (10,11-epoxide). Carbamazepine displays dose-dependent elimination pharmacokinetics, in which dosage increases produce a less than proportionate increase in steady-state total concentration (see Figure 59-2). Carbamazepine metabolism undergoes autoinduction, in which clearance increases over time after exposure to the drug. Within 30 days after beginning therapy, carbamazepine clearance may increase by as much as 300 percent. Further increases in maintenance doses may result in further induction [Kudriakova et al., 1992]. In some children, induction causes plasma carbamazepine concentrations to remain unchanged or even decline, despite increasing doses up to 40–50 mg/kg per day [Curatolo et al., 1988]. Carbamazepine and carbamazepine-10,11-epoxide metabolism also can be induced by phenytoin or phenobarbital, resulting in as much as a 100 percent increase in clearance [Kerr and Levy, 1989]. Initial carbamazepine $t_{1/2}$ ranges from 10 to 20 hours, but the $t_{1/2}$ decreases because of autoinduction to 4–12 hours. Consequently, many children require three or four doses a day to maintain targeted plasma concentrations. Sustained-release preparations help overcome this problem.

Oxcarbazepine

Oxcarbazepine is rapidly absorbed, with a T_{max} of less than 1 hour after a single oral dose. Absorption is nearly 100 percent. It is a prodrug that is converted extensively to 10,11-dihydro-10-hydroxy-carbamazepine (the monohydroxy derivative), which is the active compound. Less than 2 percent of the area under the concentration–time curve is attributed to the parent compound, and approximately 70 percent to the monohydroxy derivative. Only the monohydroxy derivative is measured for therapeutic monitoring [Theisohn and Heimann, 1982]. Co-administration of oxcarbazepine and food leads to an increase in the bioavailability and maximum plasma concentration; however, T_{max} remains unchanged. The slight changes in the absorption parameters with food administration do not appear to be clinically significant [Degen et al., 1994].

The major advantage of oxcarbazepine is that it is not metabolized to the active epoxide metabolite, which is believed to contribute to the side-effect profile of carbamazepine. Both the parent drug and its metabolite are lipophilic, which facilitates their movement across the blood–brain barrier. The monohydroxy derivative has a volume of distribution of 0.7–0.8 L/kg [Feldmann et al., 1977; Theisohn and Heimann, 1982], and both oxcarbazepine and the monohydoxy derivative bind to plasma proteins at approximately 60 percent and 40 percent, respectively [Klitgaard and Kristensen, 1986; Patsalos et al., 1990].

Approximately 96 percent of an oral dose is eliminated in the urine, with less than 1 percent of oxcarbazepine being excreted unchanged. The greater part of the dose is conjugated and excreted as the glucuronide (9 percent oxcarbazepine glucuronide and 49 percent monohydroxylated glucuronide) [Lloyd et al., 1994; Schutz et al., 1986]. Unlike carbamazepine, oxcarbazepine does not appear to induce its own metabolism [Larkin et al., 1991].

Eslicarbazepine

Eslicarbazepine acetate is a voltage-gated channel blocker that was approved in Europe in 2009. Approval in the US is still pending. Its chemical structure is similar to both carbamazepine and oxcarbazepine [Benes et al., 1999]. It differs from carbamazepine in that it does not produce an epoxide metabolite or exhibit autoinduction. Eslicarbazepine acetate is a prodrug that undergoes first-pass hydrolytic metabolism to cleave the acetate group to form the active entity – eslicarbazepine, which is the S(+) enantiomer of licarbazepine (also known as the S(+)10-monohydroxy metabolite of oxcarbazepine) [Almeida et al., 2008b]. It appears to exhibit linear pharmacokinetics and is metabolized to a glucuronidated metabolite via several uridine diphosphate glucuronosyltransferases [Loureiro and Fernandes-Lopes, 2008]. One study in 29 children and adolescents (ages 2–17 years) shows dose-proportional pharmacokinetics [Almeida et al., 2008a]. Both a suspension and scored tablets of strengths 200 mg, 400 mg, 600 mg, and 800 mg were available in the study. The daily doses used in the study ranged from 5 to 30 mg/kg/day. The T_{max} was between 0.5 and 3 hours. Eslicarbazepine acetate was cleared faster in younger children as compared to adolescents, although C_{max} was similar among all age groups.

Felbamate

Approximately 95 percent of a dose of felbamate is absorbed in adults after oral administration. Absorption of the drug is fairly rapid, with T_{max} values ranging from 1 to 4 hours [Wilensky et al., 1985]. The V_d of felbamate is approximately 0.8 L/kg [Devinsky et al., 1994; Wilensky et al., 1985]. Distribution of felbamate is fairly uniform throughout the entire body. It binds mainly to albumin (22–25 percent), and the amount of binding is dependent on albumin concentration [Perhach and Shumaker, 1995].

About 90 percent of felbamate is eliminated in the urine. Approximately 40–50 percent of the absorbed dose is eliminated as the unconjugated parent compound, and up to 58 percent is found as metabolites and conjugates [Shumaker et al., 1990]. Felbamate is cleared at a faster rate in children. Population pharmacokinetic analysis of data from 139 pediatric patients gives clearance values approximately 40 percent higher in younger children (2–12 years of age) than those in older children and adults (13–65 years).

Gamma-Aminobutyric Acid Analogues

Gabapentin and pregabalin were initally conceived as drugs that may modulate gamma-aminobutyric acid (GABA) receptors. However, this is not their main mechanism of action.

Gabapentin

The absolute bioavailability after oral administration of gabapentin is 60 percent [Vollmer et al., 1986]. Absorption is linear up to daily doses of 1800 mg, after which bioavailability begins to decline, decreasing to 35 percent at daily doses of 4800 mg [Richens, 1993]. Gabapentin uses the L-amino acid transporter system in the gut to enter the body. This system is saturable and the dependence of gabepentin on it may explain the decrease in bioavailability with increasing doses above 1800 mg [Stewart et al., 1993].

Gabapentin has a V_d of approximately 0.6–0.8 L/kg [Richens, 1993] and does not bind to plasma proteins [Vollmer et al., 1986]. To enter the brain, gabapentin uses the L-amino acid transporter system, which is also saturable [Luer et al., 1999].

Gabapentin is eliminated renally. Clearance in children aged 1 month to 12 years was well correlated with creatinine clearance. Clearance was higher in children younger than 5 years of age, necessitating a 30 percent higher dose to attain equivalent concentrations as observed in children age 5 and older and in adults [Haig et al., 2001; Ouellet et al., 2001]. It does not have any significant pharmacokinetic interactions.

Pregabalin

Pregabalin is rapidly absorbed. Its bioavailability is greater than 90 percent. Unlike gabapentin, pregabalin demonstrates no changes in absorption as dose increases. Pregabalin does not bind to plasma proteins and is not metabolized in humans, with 98 percent of the dose recovered unchanged in urine [Brockbrader et al., 2000]. Like gabapentin, it does not appear to interact with other antiepileptic drugs. There were no changes in trough steady-state concentrations of concomitant antiepileptic drugs (phenytoin, lamotrigine, or valproic acid) when pregabalin was co-administered. Likewise, there were no changes in pregabalin concentrations after administration of carbamazepine, phenytoin, lamotrigine, or valproic acid [Brodie et al., 2005]. It should be noted that there did appear to be a decrease in pregabalin exposure when it was given with phenytoin; however, this was thought to be due to a possible food effect with pregabalin. Because pregabalin is eliminated mostly via the kidneys, doses may need to be adjusted in children with decreased renal function.

Hydantoins

The hydantoins include ethytoin, mephenytoin, and phenytoin and its prodrug fosphenytoin. Although used in the past, ethytoin and mephenytoin are not widely used now.

Phenytoin

Phenytoin is a poorly water-soluble compound and is often formulated as a sodium salt. It is available as a suspension, chewable tablet, capsule, and a parenteral formulation. The nonlinear, saturation pharmacokinetics of phenytoin can make even small differences in dose clinically significant. The chewable tablet and the suspension contain phenytoin acid, whereas the capsules and the IV formulation contain phenytoin sodium, which is equivalent to only 92 percent of the acid (see Table 59-1). Thus, two 50-mg chewable tablets deliver 8 percent more phenytoin than a 100-mg phenytoin sodium capsule. The suspension is available in a 125-mg/5-mL strength. In the past, the reliability of the suspension has been questioned owing to its tendency to settle. It has been demonstrated that some agitation is sufficient to permit delivery of the specified amount of drug [Sarkar et al., 1989]. Unexpected fluctuations in plasma phenytoin concentrations associated with the use of suspensions likely have been the result of pharmacokinetics rather than formulation problems. Intramuscular injection of the parenteral solution (with a pH of 11) is contraindicated because it results in precipitation of drug that is then slowly and erratically absorbed [Kostenbauder et al., 1975]. It is also painful and causes tissue necrosis [Serrano and Wilder, 1974]. Phenytoin capsules are available in both prompt-release and extended-release formulations. Patient and family education about the differences in phenytoin dosage forms is important to maintain optimal therapy.

Bioavailability, T_{max}, and C_{max} are altered when large amounts of phenytoin are given as a single oral loading dose, presumably because of the formation of a multicapsule concretion. In a study involving six healthy adults, absorption was reduced by 10–15 percent and T_{max} increased from 18 to 32 hours, when phenytoin sodium capsules were given in single dose of 10 mg/kg or more [Jung et al., 1980]. Dividing the total loading dose into 5-mg/kg doses given every 2–3 hours overcomes this problem. The most rapid way to attain therapeutic plasma concentrations after oral loading is to use prompt-release phenytoin sodium capsules or suspension [Goff et al., 1984].

Some reports have suggested that phenytoin is poorly absorbed in newborns because of irregular gastric emptying time, relatively high gastric pH (greater than 4), or decreased absorptive surface [Morrow and Richens, 1989; Morselli, 1983; Painter et al., 1978]. Other evidence indicates that formulation-related differences in absorption, nonlinear pharmacokinetics, and age-dependent changes in elimination account for much of the variability in plasma concentrations [Dodson, 1984].

Phenytoin V_d in children and adolescents is approximately 0.7 ± 0.1 L/kg [Koren et al., 1984]. The relatively small variability in phenytoin V_d permits precise calculation of loading doses. For example, a 15-mg/kg loading dose given intravenously will result in a postinfusion mean concentration of 20 mg/L, with a range of 15–25 mg/L. Phenytoin is also highly protein-bound to albumin.

Phenytoin undergoes extensive hepatic metabolism. A small fraction, 5 percent or less, is excreted unchanged [Battino et al., 1995]. It is metabolized by a saturable cytochrome P-450 enzymatic pathway. Phenytoin follows Michaelis–Menten or saturable elimination kinetics (see Figure 59-2). As the plasma concentration rises, phenytoin clearance decreases, owing to saturation of enzymatic metabolism. Therefore, increases in dose result in disproportionately greater increases in steady-state plasma concentration.

Phenytoin half-life also varies with plasma concentration. As plasma concentration rises, the half-life increases. Half-life ranges from 8 to 12 hours at low concentrations to more than 60 hours at concentrations above 20 mg/L. At concentrations within or above the therapeutic range, 1–4 weeks may be required to reach steady state.

Phenytoin metabolism in neonates is reduced compared with that in older children. Within days to weeks after birth, the rate of metabolism accelerates, reaching a maximum in the 0.5- to 3-year age range. Children in this age group require the highest mg/kg daily doses (Figure 59-4). Thereafter, metabolism and dosage requirements decline gradually, reaching adult values during adolescence. Figure 59-5 illustrates that even minor alterations in dosage produce disproportionately large changes in plasma concentration. Therefore, small adjustments in daily dose are indicated as the plasma concentration approaches or exceeds K_m, which usually falls in the range of 5–10 mg/L. Use of the scored 50-mg chewable tablet, the 30-mg phenytoin sodium capsule, or the suspension facilitates making such adjustments in dose.

Fosphenytoin

Fosphenytoin is a prodrug of phenytoin that is rapidly hydrolyzed by tissue and red blood cell alkaline phosphatases to phenytoin. Due to the rapid conversion to phenytoin, the

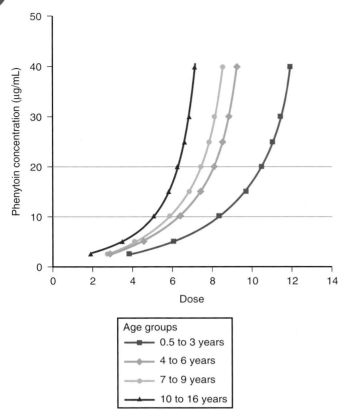

Fig. 59-4 Phenytoin dosing requirements in children. Curves were derived from data of maximum capacity of the enzyme system to metabolize phenytoin (V_{max}) and the plasma concentration at which the rate of metabolism is 50 percent of maximum capacity for children (K_m) (see Table 59-2).

pharmacokinetic information for phenytoin and not fosphenytoin is what is clinically relevent. Fosphenytoin is water-soluble and is formulated as a nontoxic, parenteral solution. The pharmacokinetics of phenytoin derived from fosphenytoin are identical to phenytoin given directly [Leppik et al., 1989]. Fosphenytoin is packaged as milligram phenytoin equivalents and is well tolerated when given intramuscularly.

Fosphenytoin absorption, not its conversion to phenytoin, appears to be the rate-limiting step in achieving therapeutic phenytoin levels. The mean half-life of fosphenytoin is 8 minutes after IV administration [Donn et al., 1987; Gerber et al., 1988; Leppik et al., 1989] and 33 minutes after intramuscular injection [Leppik et al., 1990]. Age does not affect the phosphatase enzyme responsible for the conversion of fosphenytoin to phenytoin. Fosphenytoin is more avidly bound to albumin, compared with phenytoin, resulting in brief increases of free phenytoin concentrations after infusion [Hussey et al., 1990; Jamerson et al., 1990]. The observed decrease in total phenytoin concentrations returns to those expected when the conversion from fosphenytoin to phenytoin is completed; therefore, monitoring of plasma concentrations should be done about 1 hour after IV administration of fosphenytoin. Unlike phenytoin, fosphenytoin can be given intramuscularly and avoids serious tissue necrosis from extravasation of IV phenytoin. Its major uses are treatment of status epilepticus and maintenance therapy when oral administration is not possible.

Lacosamide

Lacosamide (known as harkoside in earlier studies) was approved for use in the United States during 2009. It is completely and rapidly absorbed with a bioavailability of 100 percent [Hovinga, 2003]. Lacosamide appears to follow linear pharmacokinetics and its C_{max} is between 1 and 4 hours after an oral dose [Hovinga, 2003]. There does not seem to be a food effect on lacosamide pharmacokinetics [Kellinghaus, 2009]. Protein binding has been shown to be less than 15 percent. Lacosamide is metabolized to an inactive desmethyl metabolite, which is then cleared along with the parent drug via the kidney. Lacosamide is not approved for use in young children at this time; however, there is at least one clinical trial that is investigating the safety and pharmacokinetics in children with partial seizures between the ages of 2 and 17 years. Doses being studied are 8–12 mg/kg/day.

Lamotrigine

Lamotrigine has a bioavailability approaching 100 percent. Its T_{max} occurs 2–3 hours after administration of a single oral dose. With doses in the range of 15–240 mg, T_{max} and area under the

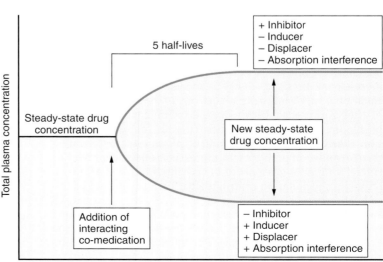

Fig. 59-5 Schematic of steady-state plasma concentrations of antiepileptic drugs when a particular antiepileptic drug is given alone or in combination with other medications. *(We wish to thank Nina Graves, Pharm.D., for her contribution to this figure.)*

concentration–time curve are directly proportional to dose [Yuen and Peck, 1987]. The V_d of lamotrigine is approximately 1.5 L/kg in children [Chen et al., 1999]. It is distributed uniformly throughout the body, and approximately 55 percent of lamotrigine is bound to plasma proteins [Garnett, 1997].

Lamotrigine is extensively metabolized to an inactive glucuronide by an inducible uridine diphosphate (UDP) glucuronyl-transferase reaction [Lamictal, 2004]. Clearance is greater in younger children [Battino et al., 2001]. Infants (younger than 2 months of age) metabolize lamotrigine more slowly, and metabolic rates increase during the first year of life [Mikati et al., 2002]. Estrogen-containing oral contraceptives may cause dramatic cyclical fluctuations of blood levels (decreasing during the estrogen phase and rebounding in the placebo week), and levels decrease dramatically during pregnancy [Pennell et al., 2008]. There may be an impact of age on lamotrigine concentrations [Reimers et al., 2007]. However, data for weight were not available in a majority of the patients and the effect of age could be due to the fact that older children weigh more than younger children [Reimers et al., 2007].

Levetiracetam

Levetiracetam is extremely water-soluble and has an oral bioavailability of close to 100 percent. Its C_{max} is within 2 hours of dose administration. When the drug is administered with food, the rate of absorption is decreased, but the extent of absorption is unchanged. Therefore, levetiracetam can be administered without regard to timing of meals. Levetiracetam also exhibits linear pharmacokinetics after single doses ranging from 250 up to 5000 mg [Patsalos, 2000]. The V_d for levetiracetam is 0.5–0.7 L/kg, and protein binding is less than 10 percent. Two-thirds of a dose is eliminated unchanged and the rest is eliminated as an inactive metabolite in the urine [Keppra package insert, 2004]. The clearance is 30–40 percent higher in children than in adults [Chhun et al., 2009; Glauser et al., 2007; May et al., 2003; Pellock et al., 2001]. Results are now available from studies in children as young as 2 months old and they confirm that the half-life of levetiracetam in younger children is approximately 5–6 hours, shorter than that seen in adults [Glauser et al., 2007]. An IV formulation and a sustained-release formulation are now on the market. It may be possible to give levetiracetam rapidly. Patients (4–32 years of age) who temporarily lost the ability to take medications by mouth were given an IV loading dose of levetiracetam via rapid infusion (given within 6 minutes). Levetiracetam concentrations ranged from 14 to 189 µg/mL and no significant changes in blood pressure or significant abnormalities in the electrocardiogram were experienced [Wheless et al., 2009]. There were also no local infusion site reactions noted; however, the formulation was diluted 1:1 with normal saline or dextrose 5 percent in water (D5W).

Drug–drug interaction information in children indicates that the concentrations of carbamazepine, valproic acid, topiramate, or lamotrigine are similar between study groups who receive levetiracetam or placebo [Otoul et al., 2007].

Rufinamide

Rufinamide is slowly absorbed due to the fact that it is lipophilic and dissolves slowly in aqueous solutions. The bioavailability is nonlinear and decreases at higher doses, with doses of 1600 mg producing less than proportional concentrations. Steady-state doses of 200, 400, and 800 mg produced morning trough concentrations of 2.81, 5.23, and 11.0 µmol/L, whereas 1600-mg doses resulted in a mean trough concentration of 19.6 µmol/L (4.7 mg/L) [Elger et al., 2010; Limite, 2005; NoAuthors, 2005]. Dissolution is the rate-limiting step in absorption; therefore, changes in gastrointestinal environment, such as with the presence of food, could have an effect on the absorption of rufinamide. It is suggested that rufinamide be administered with food. Rufinamide exposure is increased by 31–34 percent and the C_{max} by 36–56 percent when the drug is given after high-fat meals [Perucca et al., 2008]. Rufinamide is metabolized to inactive metabolites via the carboxylesterase pathway. Although rufinamide does not appear to be metabolized via the cytochrome P-450, the carboxylesterase enzymes can be induced by inducers of the CYP450 enzymes. Rufinamide also appears to be a weak inhibitor of CYP2E1 and a weak inducer of CYP3A4.

Pharmacokinetic data in children are beginning to appear in the literature. The majority of the data concerning rufinamide is on file with the manufacturer; however, data on these trials have been summarized in Perucca et al. [2008]. A dosing regimen for children has been simulated from several phase II and III clinical studies involving patients with partial or generalized seizures and one study with Lennox–Gastaut syndrome patients. The simulation included 119 children (aged less than 12 years) and 99 adolescents (12–17 years) [Marchand et al., 2010], and was used in supporting material presented to the European Agency for the Evaluation of Medicinal Products. These studies involved patient populations and the presence of inducing and inhibiting polytherapy. Children who weigh less than 30 kg had greater variability in simulated rufinamide exposure measures than those children who were heavier than 30 kg. In addition, the co-administration of valproate resulted in higher rufinamide plasma concentrations. This study proposed a maximum daily dose of 600 mg for children who also receive valproic acid, and a maximum daily dose of 1000 mg for those children who do not also receive valproic acid. Indeed, valproic acid increased rufinamide steady-state plasma concentrations from 54.9 percent in male children and 70.1 percent in female children in a population pharmacokinetic study that is on file at Eisai [Perucca et al., 2008]. The increase in concentrations when valproic acid was a co-medication was approximately 3 times higher in children than in adults. (Adult concentrations were 15 percent higher.) Population studies involving children have also identified increases in rufinamide's apparent clearance values due to the presence of inducing co-medications. Known antiepileptic drug inducers, such as carbamazepine, phenobarbital, phenytoin, or primidone, as well as vigabatrin, decreased rufinamide steady-state plasma concentrations in children from 23 to 46 percent [Perucca et al., 2008].

Tiagabine

Oral bioavailability of tiagabine is greater than 90 percent, and the bioavailability of tablets and that of the oral solution appear to be similar [Mengel et al., 1991a]. The absorption rate for tiagabine is reduced up to 65 percent when the drug is administered with food, although the extent of absorption is not affected [Mengel et al., 1991b]. Tiagabine has a V_d of 0.74–0.85 L/kg [Gustavson et al., 1997], and protein binding is approximately 96 percent [Gustavson et al., 1997; Ostergaard et al., 1995]. Tiagabine has a half-life of 5–9 hours [Gustavson and Mengel, 1995]. Tiagabine undergoes extensive metabolism by means of the cytochrome P-450 3A isoform, but no active metabolites have been identified. As observed with other drugs, clearances in children are faster than in adults; adjusting both V_d and clearance values according to body size gives values similar to those seen in adults [Gustavson et al., 1997].

Topiramate

Oral tablets of topiramate have a relative bioavailability of approximately 80 percent that of an oral solution. It is rapidly absorbed, with a T_{max} of approximately 2 hours [Easterling et al., 1988]. Overall absorption is not affected by co-administration with food [Doose et al., 1992]. The protein binding of topiramate is less than 15 percent [Ben-Menachem, 1995a], and its V_d is 0.6–0.8 L/kg [Johannessen, 1997]. Elimination is mainly through the kidney, although a portion of the dose is removed by the liver [Ben-Menachem, 1995a]. Preliminary observations in pediatric patients indicate that the mean oral topiramate clearance is 44–55 percent higher in children, and they may need a higher dose than adults to achieve a similar plasma concentration [Adin et al., 2004; Glauser, 1997].

Valproic Acid

Valproic acid appears to be completely absorbed from all the available products (except for the extended-release formulation), but the rate of absorption varies significantly with dosage form (see Table 59-1). Its T_{max} is 0.5–1 hour after ingestion for the syrup, 0.5–2 hours after the capsule, 1–6 hours for the enteric-coated tablet, and 3–6 hours for the sprinkle capsule [Cloyd et al., 1983, 1985, 1992]. Absorption after ingestion of the enteric-coated tablet is delayed for several hours; during this lag phase, plasma concentrations may continue to decline. Food further delays, but does not decrease, valproic acid absorption from the enteric-coated tablet [Fischer et al., 1988]. The extended-release tablet has an absolute bioavailability of 90 percent [Dutta et al., 2004]. The extended-release tablets and the enteric-coated tablets are not interchangeable. The extended-release tablets need to be prescribed at a dose that is 8–20 percent higher than the enteric-coated dose to attain similar plasma concentrations [Dutta and Zhang, 2004]. An IV formulation is also available and has been studied in children. The IV formulation should not be given intramuscularly due to toxic muscle necrosis [Gallo et al., 1997].

Valproic acid distribution volumes vary more than those of carbamazepine, phenobarbital, or phenytoin, and range from 0.12 to 0.49 L/kg. When loading doses are calculated, a volume of 0.2 L/kg is recommended. Valproic acid protein binding to albumin is saturable. At concentrations below 40–50 mg/L, the bound fraction averages 90–95 percent. As total concentration rises to the upper boundary of the therapeutic range, the percentage bound falls to 80–85 percent. Saturable protein binding results in a nonlinear relationship between total valproic acid concentration and dose. Unbound valproic acid concentrations, however, remain linear with dose [Cloyd et al., 1993; Riva et al., 1983]. The percentage of unbound valproic acid can be unpredictable and unusually high after rapid infusion in children who are critically ill [Birnbaum et al., 2003].

Valproic acid is extensively metabolized to both active and inactive metabolites. Principal pathways include glucuronidation, β-oxidation in the mitochondria, and oxidation through cytochrome P-450. The monounsaturated metabolites 2-ene-valproic acid and 4-ene-valproic acid possess anticonvulsant activity; the 2-ene-valproic acid achieves pharmacologically relevant concentrations in the brain. 2-Ene-valproic acid accumulates in the brain more slowly than does valproic acid, which may account for the slow onset and cessation of valproic acid anticonvulsant activity. Although the diunsaturated metabolite 2,4-diene-valproic acid, is a potent hepatotoxin, its role in valproic acid hepatotoxicity remains unclear.

The elimination half-life of valproic acid is short. In the first few weeks after birth, half-life ranges from 17 to 40 hours, but rapidly declines from 3 to 20 hours in infants and young children. The full antiepileptic effect of valproic acid is obtained days to weeks after steady state is reached, and this effect continues for some time after the drug is discontinued. The lingering effect may be partly the result of its inhibitory effect on the enzymes responsible for the degradation of GABA, or may be due to the accumulation of 2-ene- valproic acid. This prolonged duration has prompted some investigators to propose single daily dosing [Stefan et al., 1984]; however, with other proposed mechanisms of action, seizure control is related to plasma valproic acid concentrations. Under these circumstances, dosing at least every half-life is indicated to minimize fluctuations in plasma concentrations. When valproic acid is given as monotherapy, the half-life may be long enough to maintain therapeutic concentrations for up to 24 hours in some children. Such children may be able to take valproic acid once a day [Cloyd et al., 1985].

Vigabatrin

Vigabatrin is a 50:50 racemic mixture of R(−) and S(+) enantiomers, with the S(+) enantiomer responsible for the drug's pharmacologic activities and toxic effects [Haegele et al., 1983; Rey et al., 1990]. Bioavailability is approximately 75 percent in adults when the drug is given orally and is similar for both the tablet and the solution [Hoke et al., 1991]. Administration of vigabatrin with food does not significantly affect vigabatrin pharmacokinetics [Frisk-Holmberg et al., 1989]. Vigabatrin has been studied in children [Rey et al., 1989, 1990], and bioavailability appears to be somewhat lower in children than in adults [Rey et al., 1992]. Vigabatrin does not bind to plasma proteins, and it has an apparent V_d of 0.8 L/kg [Ben-Menachem, 1995b]. Clearance or the dose to concentration ratio of vigabatrin appears to be greater in children than in adults, indicating that a higher dose is needed in children to achieve a particular concentration when compared to adults [Armijo et al., 1997].

Most of a vigabatrin dose appears unchanged in the urine. Studies in infants and children show that the half-life of the inactive R(−) enantiomer, but not the half-life of the active S(+) enantiomer, increases with linear age. Vigabatrin exerts its pharmacologic effect by irreversible inhibition of GABA transaminase, causing increases in synaptic GABA concentrations by inhibiting its breakdown. Because the half-life of GABA transaminase is much longer than that of vigabatrin itself, the pharmacologic effect is determined by the half-life of the enzyme [Ben-Menachem, 1995b; Jung et al., 1977].

Zonisamide

Absolute bioavailability of zonisamide has not been assessed owing to the lack of an IV formulation. The drug reportedly is nearly completely absorbed, as indicated by early studies in which radioactive drug was measured in the urine and bile of rats [Matsumoto et al., 1983]. Human data indicate that, after multiple doses, 65 percent of zonisamide is recovered in urine (62 percent) or feces (3 percent). Food does not affect bioavailability [Zonegran Product Information, 2004]. Zonisamide is only 40 percent bound to plasma proteins, and its apparent V_d is approximately 1.45 L/kg [Zonegran Product Information, 2004]. Zonisamide is highly bound to erythrocytes, resulting in whole-blood concentrations that are higher than plasma concentrations. Binding to erythrocytes causes nonlinearity in plasma concentrations after a dose of greater than 400 mg [Matsumoto et al., 1989]. Zonisamide is eliminated by renal and hepatic routes. The metabolism of zonisamide is mediated in part by cytochrome P-450 3A4 [Zonegran Product Information, 2004]. Zonisamide–carbamazepine interaction was identified in a study including 12 children (5–16 years of age); trough concentrations decreased by 37 percent and carbamazepine-10,11-epoxide by 13 percent when carbamazepine was added to zonisamide monotherapy. The mean trough concentrations observed in 72 children undergoing zonisamide monotherapy were 27.0 ± 9.4 mg/L for a dose of 11.1 ± 2.5 mg/kg/day [Miura, 2004].

Generic Formulations

Absorption may differ among similar formulations (such as tablets) from various manufacturers (e.g., carbamazepine) [Kauko and Tammisto, 1974; Pynnonen et al., 1978; Sillanpaa, 1981]. Significant changes in serum phenytoin concentrations have been observed when the same maintenance doses of medication are taken from different manufacturers [Burkhardt et al., 2004]. Eight adult patients (ages 34 ± 49) had mean total phenytoin concentration of 17.7 ± 5.3 mg/L while on branded drug, which decreased to 12.5 ± 2.7 mg/L with generic and then increased to 17.8 ± 3.9 mg/L after the branded drug was re-introduced. Brand and generic phenytoin do not yield equivalent concentrations in some patients and substitution should not be permitted without prescriber and patient notification. For drugs with nonlinear pharmacokinetics such as phenytoin, such increases can lead to clinical toxicity or seizures [Mikati et al., 1992]. Generic medications can create significant cost savings for patients; however, the risks associated with possible changing drug concentrations need to be considered against the monetary advantages. Substitution of drugs made by differing manufacturers (brand to generic, generic to brand, or generic to generic) may lead to problems, especially when drugs with narrow therapeutic ranges or nonlinear pharmacokinetics are used. Therefore, counseling patients to keep taking medication prepared by the same manufacturer, whenever possible, usually is advisable [Nuwer et al., 1990]. Problems usually arise within 2 weeks of formulation change, so patients and parents should be particularly vigilant during this period. Most of the data available concerning generic substitution of antiepileptic drugs consists of surveys, retrospective database collection, or case studies, and are not prospectively designed to compare brand against generic medications directly.

Pharmacodynamics

Dose-Response or Concentration-Response Concept

Substantial evidence exists that both the number of patients experiencing seizure control increases and the degree of seizure control for a given patient improves with higher antiepileptic drug concentrations [Porter, 1989; Schmidt and Haenel, 1984]. The minimum effective concentration defines the concentration at which the desired pharmacologic response is first observed in *some* patients. The intensity of response increases in direct proportion to drug concentration, until a response is maximized. This result is the maximum pharmacologic effect for that drug. With some drugs, such as phenytoin, further increases in concentration may reduce response (e.g., phenytoin-induced exacerbation of seizures) [Troupin and Ojemann, 1975]. It is not known whether other antiepileptic drugs share this property but there are anecdotal reports of seizures increasing as antiepilpetic drugs are stepped up.

The incidence and severity of side effects also increase with drug concentration. The concentration at which side effects appear is usually, but not always, greater than the concentrations needed to achieve seizure control. The difference between concentrations that produce desired responses and those that produce toxic responses defines the therapeutic range. Optimal ranges, representing population averages, for commonly used antiepileptic drugs are listed in Table 59-6.

Tolerance

Tolerance is a phenomenon in which pharmacologic or toxicologic effect diminishes with chronic use, even at the same or increasing plasma concentrations. Different mechanisms for the development of tolerance have been recognized [Froscher and Engels, 1986; Koella, 1986]. One mechanism is the result of biochemical adaptation (e.g., upregulation or downregulation of receptor sites). For example, the effectiveness of benzodiazepine therapy diminishes over time, necessitating even larger doses. Animal studies have demonstrated that chronic exposure to benzodiazepines causes a downregulation of benzodiazepine receptors, which reduces their anticonvulsant effect.

Another mechanism of tolerance is behavioral. The patient becomes progressively insensitive to drug effect without any apparent biochemical change [Siegel, 1986]. For example, many patients initiated on phenobarbital or primidone exhibit mild neurotoxicity even at low plasma concentrations but later, at the same concentration, have no symptoms [Leppik et al., 1984].

Tolerance can produce changes in clinical response that mimic certain drug interactions. For example, loss of seizure control may result from either tolerance, as in the case of clonazepam, or enzyme induction, which decreases concentrations of many antiepileptic drugs. Differentiating between these phenomena is important in considering adjustments in drug therapy.

Physiologic Factors Affecting Drug Disposition in Children

General Considerations

Antiepileptic drug pharmacokinetics and dosage requirements are influenced by the changing physiology of children as they age. Table 59-7 summarizes the effect of various developmental

Table 59-6 Optimal Target Ranges for Commonly Prescribed Antiepileptic Drugs

Drug	Target Drug Level Total (mg/L)	Free (mg/L)
Carbamazepine	4–12	0.5–3.6
Eslicarbazepine	N/A	N/A
Ethosuximide	40–100	
Felbamate	40–100	
Gabapentin	4–16	
Lacosamide	0–15*	
Lamotrigine	2–20*	1–9*
Levetiracetam	5–45*	
MHD (oxcarbazepine active metabolite)	10–35	
Phenobarbital	15–40	6–20
Phenytoin	10–20	1–2
Primidone	5–12 (15–40 PB)	
Pregabalin	0–10*	
Rufinamide	0–60*	
Tiagabine	0–0.235*	
Topiramate	2–25*	
Valproic acid	50–150	6–20
Vigabatrin	20–160*	
Zonisamide	7–40*	

* Range is not defined, and values are concentrations found in clinical trials. PB, phenobarbital.

Table 59-7 Drug Disposition at Different Ages

	Neonates	Infants, Children	Adolescents
Absorption	↓	↑	A
Plasma protein binding	↓	↓	↓→A
Metabolism	↓	↑	↓→A
Excretion	↓	A	A

↑, Increased from adult levels; ↓, decreased from adult levels; A, equivalent to adult levels.
(From Morrow JI, Richens A. Disposition of anticonvulsants in childhood. Clin Pharmacokin 1989;17 [Suppl 1]:89.)

stages on absorption, protein binding, metabolism, and excretion. The physiologic changes associated with maturation produce marked alterations in antiepileptic drug pharmacokinetics. The variability with which children reach developmental milestones, along with genetic and environmental factors, causes antiepileptic drug pharmacokinetics to vary substantially, even in children of the same age. As a result of the differences between children and adults, children require more frequent and larger doses relative to body size to attain targeted plasma concentrations. Although important

age-related, quantitative differences in antiepileptic drug pharmacokinetics are recognized, the pattern of drug-specific pharmacokinetics, such as saturation of absorption, protein binding, metabolism, and enzyme induction, is similar for children and for adults.

A number of physiologic and pathophysiologic processes can alter antiepileptic drug pharmacokinetics. Gastrointestinal disorders, particularly those that increase transit time, can alter the endothelial lining and decrease absorption. Antiepileptic drugs that are slowly absorbed, such as carbamazepine and phenytoin, are most likely to be affected. Physiologic stress, such as that associated with myocardial infarction, burns, traumatic injury, chronic inflammation, and surgery, increases α_1-acid glycoprotein, resulting in greater binding with carbamazepine and carbamazepine-10,11-epoxide [MacKichan, 1992]. Febrile illnesses may produce increases in phenytoin clearance that persist for several weeks, resulting in lowering of plasma concentrations by as much as 50 percent [Leppik et al., 1986].

Renal failure can affect the excretion of antiepileptic drugs for which the kidney is the primary route of elimination. Both clinical response and plasma antiepileptic drug concentrations should be carefully assessed in patients with renal disease. Severe liver disease can alter the metabolism of antiepileptic drugs, resulting in accumulation of the parent drug [Kutt, 1983]. Antiepileptic drug metabolism appears to be well preserved in mild to moderate liver disease. Clinical response may vary, depending on the particular antiepileptic drug.

Plasma antiepileptic drug concentrations can fluctuate over a 24-hour cycle. A day–night cycle, in which both valproic acid and carbamazepine concentrations decrease at night, exists [Lockard and Levy, 1990; Pisani et al., 1990]. The mechanism for this alteration is presumed to be a circadian rhythm in clearance. Absorption of enteric-coated valproic acid tablets may be reduced at night [Cloyd, 1991]. In either case, considering the effect of night-time plasma antiepileptic drug concentrations when designing dosing strategies for patients with poorly controlled nocturnal seizures may be helpful.

Neonates

Gastric emptying time is irregular, absorption area is reduced, and biliary function is underdeveloped for several months or more after birth. These factors can contribute to erratic drug absorption [Morselli, 1983]. In addition, gastric pH is elevated, which may reduce the absorption of certain drugs, such as clonazepam [Meyer and Straughn, 1993]. In contrast with the oral route, rectal absorption is reliable and efficient. Protein binding is reduced because of lower plasma albumin concentrations, whereas greater extracellular water and less adipose tissue can either increase or decrease V_d. Neonatal drug metabolism and renal excretion are reduced. Reactions mediated by hepatic cytochrome P-450 enzymes reach and then exceed adult values within a few weeks after birth. By contrast, renal elimination of drugs and active metabolites may be lower than in adults until the age of 6 months.

Infants and Children

Gastric emptying time and intestinal motility are increased as children grow. Absorptive area, microbial flora, and biliary function begin to approach those in the adult. Also, gastrointestinal blood flow is greater than in adults. These physiologic characteristics contribute to faster absorption of most drugs, resulting in earlier T_{max}. Plasma albumin levels are lower than adult values, particularly in infancy, resulting in an increased free fraction. Infants and children are capable of synthesizing α_1-acid glycoprotein, which will alter the free fraction of drugs bound to this protein. Metabolism remains elevated for the first 2 years of life; in some cases, drug clearances may be 2–3 times the values seen in adults. Thereafter, metabolism slowly declines, reaching adult values at puberty. After the first 6 months of life, renal excretion is comparable with that in adults.

Antiepileptic Drug Interactions

Interactions involving antiepileptic drugs may alter pharmacokinetics (see Figure 59-5). The clinical significance of pharmacokinetic interactions is determined by several factors, including concentration of the interacting drugs, the patient's seizure control, and presence of toxicity.

Absorption

Concomitant therapy may influence absorption of antiepileptic drugs. For example, continuous tube feedings interfere with phenytoin absorption [Maynard et al., 1987]. Calcium- and magnesium-containing antacids appear to complex with phenytoin, decreasing its rate and extent of absorption. They should not be administered concurrently [Cacek, 1986; Fischer et al., 1988]. Gastric pH affects the rate and extent of benzodiazepine absorption; thus, use of antacids and histamine H_2 blockers may decrease the plasma concentration of these drugs [Meyer and Straughn, 1993].

Protein Binding

Valproic acid and phenytoin compete for the same binding sites. Concurrent administration may decrease valproic acid and phenytoin binding. When this occurs, unbound concentrations briefly rise, potentially leading to clinical toxicity. Total phenytoin and valproic acid concentrations decrease; however, unbound concentrations rapidly re-equilibrate to the original concentration. In general, phenytoin and valproic acid dosing does not have to be adjusted in these circumstances. [Scheyer and Cramer, 1990]. Aspirin and other highly protein-bound drugs can have a similar effect, and measuring unbound concentrations in these circumstances can be very helpful in guiding treatement.

Metabolism

Drugs interact in many ways, such as induction and inhibition of liver enzymes. Information on how drugs are metabolized may provide insight into the potential for a drug interaction. For example, if a drug is known to be an inducer or an inhibitor of a particular P-450 isoenzyme, it may be possible to predict if a medication will affect the plasma concentrations of a second drug that is metabolized by that P-450 particular isoenzyme when the drugs are given concomitantly. This approach may be particularly useful in predicting the interaction between the many new antiepileptic drugs being developed and other possible concomitant medications (see Table 59-5).

Mechanism of Action of Antiepileptic Drugs

Epilepsy can be thought of as an imbalance of excitatory and inhibitory activity in the nervous system that can involve alterations in synaptic function or intrinsic membrane properties. Antiepileptic drugs can be used to compensate or correct for this imbalance in opposing activities. Although the mechanism of action of most antiepileptic drugs was discovered after their potential for use as an anticonvulsant was determined, their type of action at the neuronal level can still be placed into these two types of actions: those that increase inhibitory actions and those that decrease excitatory actions.

Decrease of excitatory responses may be effected by mimicking antagonists to excitatory amino acid receptors, inhibiting excitatory neurotransmitter release into the synapse, or inhibiting an enzyme needed in the synthesis of the excitatory neurotransmitter. By contrast, drugs can be used to increase inhibitory activity at the synaptic level, such as increasing GABA release into the synapse, increasing synthesis of GABA, or using an antiepileptic drug that has a GABA agonist effect. Activity at sodium or calcium channels can result in bursts of action potentials (e.g., an excitatory response) or in a release of neurotransmitter. The latter activity can be inhibitory or excitatory, depending on the neurotransmitter involved (e.g., glutamate, an excitatory neurotransmitter, versus GABA, an inhibitory neurotransmitter). The newer antiepileptic drugs appear to have multiple and/or more unique mechanisms for seizure control. Use of drugs with different mechanisms of action may lead to control of additional types of seizures. Moreover, drugs that have multiple mechanisms of action also can be advantageous because they increase the possibility of controlling seizures in patients with multiple seizure types with one or at least fewer drugs. This practice can result in fewer side effects and lower drug costs. Table 59-8 presents the mechanisms of action proposed for both the older and the newer antiepileptic drugs.

Dosage Formulations and Routes of Administration

Antiepileptic drugs are most commonly and conveniently given orally. In many circumstances, however, use of an alternative route of administration is necessary. Oral administration is not possible, for example, before and during surgery, with acute severe trauma, an inability to swallow when consciousness is impaired, or gastrointestinal illnesses. Interruption of oral administration occurs in children during frequent bouts of vomiting and diarrhea. In acute emergencies, especially within medical facilities, some antiepileptic drugs can be given by intravenous or intramuscular administration. Unfortunately, parenteral formulations are not available for most antiepileptic drugs because of their poor solubility in water. This creates a significant dilemma for those persons on maintenance antiepileptic therapy when oral administration cannot be continued. The rectal route of administration has been extremely useful for those situations, but water-insoluble antiepileptic

Table 59-8 Antiepileptic Drug Mechanisms of Action

	BZD	CBZ	ESL	ESM	FBM	GBP	LCM*	LEV	LTG	PB/PRM	PGB	PHT	RUF	TGB	TPM	VGB	VPA	ZNS
Sodium	+	++	++	–	++	?	+	–	++	+	–	++	++	–	++	?	++	++
Calcium	–	–	–	++	?	++	–	+	+	–	++	–	–	–	?	?	+	++
GABA	++	–	–	–	+	+/?	–	?	+	+	–	–	–	++	+	++	+/?	–
EAA	–	–	–	–	+	–	–	–	?	–	–	–	–	–	+	?	–	–

BZD, benzodiazepines; CBZ, carbamazepine; EAA, excitatory amino acid system; ESL, eslicarbazepine; ESM, ethosuximide; FBM, felbamate; GABA, gamma-aminobutyric acid; GBP, gabapentin; LCM, lacosamide (*also binds to collapsin response mediator protein-2); LEV, levetiracetam; LTG, lamotrigine; PB/PRM, phenobarbital/primidone; PBG, pregabalin; PHT, phenytoin; RUF, rufinamide; TGB, tiagabine; TPM, topiramate; VGB, vigabatrin; VPA, valproic acid; ZNS, zonisamide, +, minor mechanism of action; ++, main mechanism of action;?, inconclusive evidence; –, not a mechanism of action.

drugs are generally not well absorbed rectally [Graves and Kriel, 1987].

Intravenous and Intramuscular Administration

Intravenous administration is a good alternative to oral therapy when patients are hospitalized. Phenytoin is very insoluble in water and thus is formulated with ethanol and propylene glycol, and adjusted to a pH of around 11. This formulation should not be given intramuscularly. Fosphenytoin, a phenytoin prodrug, is not formulated in propylene glycol and is maintained at close to physiological pH. It can be given intramuscularly, and the drug can be infused more rapidly than is possible with phenytoin, with fewer adverse effects [Leppik et al., 1989]. Other antiepileptic drugs that are available for intravenous administration include valproic acid, diazepam, lorazepam, lacosamide, levetiracetam, and phenobarbital. Rapid infusion (less than 15 minutes) of some antiepileptic drugs has been shown to be safe, making them more suitable for loading doses, as well as for bridging therapy.

Rectal Administration

When administered as a solution, diazepam is rapidly absorbed rectally, reaching the T_{max} within 5–20 minutes in children [Lombroso, 1989]. By contrast, rectal administration of lorazepam is relatively slow, with a T_{max} of 1–2 hours [Graves et al., 1987]. Table 59-9 provides a comprehensive list of antiepileptic drugs available for rectal administration and recommendations for use. Only one rectal formulation is available commercially (Diastat). The bioavailability of carbamazepine oral suspension diluted with an equal amount of water given rectally is similar to that of the oral tablet [Graves and Kriel, 1987]. The bioavailability of topiramate tablets crushed in water and given rectally is similar to that of oral tablets [Conway et al., 2003]. The availability of lamotrigine tablets crushed in water and given rectally is about half that of oral tablets [Birnbaum et al., 2000, 2001].

Some drugs cannot be administered rectally owing to factors such as poor absorption or poor solubility in aqueous solutions. The relative rectal bioavailability of gabapentin, oxcarbazepine, and phenytoin is so low that the current formulations are not considered to be suitable for administration by this route [Clemens et al., 2007; Fuerst et al., 1988; Kriel et al., 1997; Kvan and Johannessen, 1975; Moolenaar et al., 1981]. The dependence of gabapentin on an active transport system,

and the much-reduced surface area of the rectum compared with the small intestine, may be responsible for its lack of absorption from the rectum.

Intranasal Administration

Intranasal administration is a potentially attractive alternative route when intravenous administration is impossible or impractical. Nasal access is readily available, even when a patient is having a seizure; requires little, if any, caregiver training; and, under the right circumstances, allows rapid drug absorption. Although the absorptive area of the nasal cavity is approximately the same as that of the rectum, the volume of solution that can be instilled is 0.5 mL or less [Romeo et al., 1998]. Several studies comparing intranasal midazolam with intravenous diazepam have been carried out in children. In summary, both drugs had similar onset of effect and seizure control, although intranasal midazolam has been used for preoperative sedation. Several disadvantages are associated with intranasal midazolam administration:

1. Many patients complain of significant nasal discomfort, presumably owing to the acidic pH of the solution.
2. The volume of a clinically relevant dose is too large for many patients.
3. Bioavailability after intranasal administration is intermediate and variable.
4. Its elimination half-life in children is short [Burstein et al., 1997].

The rapid elimination half-life may explain the reports of seizure breakthrough within a few hours after intranasal delivery of midazolam [Scheepers et al., 2000]. Absorption of diazepam has been demonstrated after intranasal delivery [Lindhardt et al., 2001]. There are currently no commercial intranasal formulations available.

Other Routes of Administration

Lorazepam is absorbed after sublingual administration and can be useful in treatment of serial and prolonged seizures [Yager and Seshia, 1988]. Delivery of antiepileptic agents directly into the cerebral subarachnoid or intraventricular space is being investigated. Spinal intrathecal administration of baclofen for control of spasticity is currently used for persons with spinal cord disease and cerebral palsy, and can be administered by a programmable continuous pump surgically placed in the abdomen [Albright et al., 1993; Penn et al., 1989].

Table 59-9 Antiepileptic Drugs Available for Rectal Administration

Drug	Treatment Usefulness	Dose (mg/kg/dose)	Preparation	Pharmacokinetics	Comments
Carbamazepine (CBZ)	Maintenance	Same as oral	Oral suspension (dilute with equal volume of water) *Suppository gel (CBZ powder dissolved in 20% alcohol and methylhydroxy cellulose)	Peak concentration 4–8 hr; 80% absorbed	Definite cathartic effect
Clonazepam	?Acute	0.02–0.1 mg	Suspension	Peak concentration 0.1–2 hr	Onset may be too slow for acute use
Diazepam	Acute	0.2–0.5 mg	Gel	Peak concentration in ~45 min; concentration >200 ng/mL reached in 15 min	Well tolerated; nordiazepam accumulates with repeated doses
Lamotrigine	?Maintenance	1.5–2 × oral dose	100-mg tablet crushed and suspended in 10 mL of water		Well tolerated
Lorazepam	Acute	0.05–0.1 mg	Parenteral solution	Peak concentration 0.5–2 hr	Well tolerated
Paraldehyde	Acute	0.3 mL	Oral solution (dilute with equal volume of mineral oil)	Effect in 20 min; peak concentration 2.5 hr	Moderate cathartic effect; use glass syringe
Phenobarbital	?Acute	10–20 mg	Parenteral solution	Peak concentration 4–5 hr; 90% absorbed	Onset may be too slow for acute use
	Maintenance	Same as oral	Same as acute	Same as for acute	
Secobarbital	Acute	5 mg	Parenteral solution	Peak concentration 0.5–1.5 hr	
Topiramate	?Maintenance	Same as oral	200 mg tablet crushed and suspended with 20 mL of water	Peak concentration 2–3 hr; 95% absorbed	Well tolerated
Valproic acid (VPA)	Acute	5–25 mg	Oral solution (dilute with equal volume of water)	Peak concentration 1–3 hr	Definite cathartic effect
	Maintenance	Same as oral	*VPA liquid from capsules mixed into Supocire C lipid base	Peak concentration 2–4 hr; 80% absorbed	Well tolerated

* Extemporaneously prepared using commercial product; all other preparations are commercial products given rectally.
(Adapted from Graves NM, Kriel RL. Rectal administration of AEDs in children. Pediatric Neurol 1987;3:321; and Garnett, WR, Cloyd JC. Dosage from considerations in the treatment of epilepsy. In: Dodson WE, Pellock JM, eds. Pediatric epilepsy: Diagnosis and therapy. New York: Demos, 1993;373–385. Additional data from Birnbaum AK et al. Rectal absorption of lamotrigine compressed tablets. Epilepsia 2000;41[7]:850–853; Birnbaum AK et al. Relative bioavailability of lamotrigine chewable dispersible tablets administered rectally. Pharmacotherapy 2001;21[2]:158–162; Conway JM et al. Relative bioavailability of topiramate administered rectally. Epilepsy Res 2003;54[2–3]:91–96.)

Monitoring of Patients on Antiepileptic Drug Therapy

Clinical Monitoring of Efficacy

Clinical assessment of patients is of paramount importance in the assessment of the effectiveness of therapy. The ideal response would be the total elimination of seizures without any adverse effects of therapy. A satisfactory clinical response for many patients, however, might be substantial reduction of seizures with elimination of or decrease in adverse effects.

One of the most common clinical errors is the premature interpretation of the clinical response. Assessment of seizure control requires an accurate record of seizure frequency and severity before and during therapy. Seizures may be eliminated, reduced, or increased in frequency, and more or less severe during therapy. Patients with epilepsy have varying seizure frequency rates before therapy. The length of time required

to assess clinical response varies with the frequency of seizures observed before beginning therapy. Patients with infrequent seizures need a longer period of observation on therapy to permit assessment of clinical response.

Statistical interpretation of the change in seizure frequency based on modified sequential analysis has been proposed [Leppik et al., 1989]. In addition, achievement of steady state with the new drug regimen is necessary to determine if a medication has been given an adequate trial at any specific dose. The time to achieve a steady state varies considerably from drug to drug, depending on the drug's half-life. In every case, 5 half-lives must elapse before a steady state is reached.

Interpretation of clinical response in patients in whom polypharmacy is necessary is especially difficult. Clinical improvement or deterioration after the addition of a second antiepileptic drug could be due to numerous factors. Such factors include the additive or synergistic effect of the two medications, the effect of the second drug alone, and the effect of the second drug on the metabolism and/or displacement of the initial drug. It is important to make clinical conclusions only after a steady state is reached with the new drug regimen. If improvement is obtained after the addition of the second medication, the clinician should attempt to taper and discontinue the first medication, to determine whether the clinical improvement is an effect of synergistic therapy or that of the second medication itself. Finally, it is necessary to remember that withdrawal of co-medication might have an effect on the disposition of the remaining drug(s), which could influence clinical response (see Figure 59-5).

Clinical Monitoring of Adverse Effects

The clinical state of the patient is more important than laboratory testing for the assessment of adverse effects. It is possible to monitor clinical states continuously, whereas laboratory tests generally are obtained at arbitrary times; therefore, impending organ dysfunction often may be detected earlier by clinical changes, rather than by laboratory tests. The most frequent adverse effects are dose-related and often involve the nervous system. Common manifestations of adverse effects are cognitive changes and drowsiness, impaired attention, incoordination, ataxia, and diplopia. In addition to central nervous system adverse reactions, the liver also may produce signs of toxicity. Early signs of liver failure include anorexia, nausea, vomiting, lethargy, and abdominal pain.

Monitoring of Drug Concentrations

The ability to measure blood levels of antiepileptic drugs has been a major advance in the understanding of drug metabolism and disposition, and has led to more rational drug therapy. The influence of periodic monitoring of blood levels may reduce the number of therapeutic failures by 50 percent [Kutt and Penry, 1974]. As expected, drug concentrations generally are related to the dose administered; however, unexpected results may occur, especially in cases of patient noncompliance or with drugs that follow nonlinear kinetics.

Interpretation of "Optimal Therapeutic Ranges"

Numerous factors should be considered in the interpretation of drug concentrations. Medications that have rapid absorption and clearance have wide fluctuation between dosing intervals. For example, the liquid formulation of valproic acid, especially when given to a child also receiving enzyme-inducing co-medications, is rapidly absorbed and eliminated; therefore, a twofold fluctuation during dosing intervals is possible. Recording the time of the blood sample in relation to the last dose is needed to interpret laboratory results properly. Unexpectedly low concentrations are most frequently the result of poor compliance; however, they might be seen after the addition of an enzyme-inducing co-medication. Very high drug concentrations are seen with administration of high doses, in persons with genetically low clearance or some disease states, or with use of enzyme-inhibiting co-medications such as valproic acid [Perucca et al., 2001].

The terms optimal drug concentration and target range are preferred over therapeutic range, for several reasons. First, these newer terms express the concept that the optimal dose

and drug concentration need to be determined for each individual patient. The ideal or optimal dose and drug concentration would be those associated with complete control of seizures with no adverse effects. Clinical effects and toxicity of antiepileptic drugs correlate better with drug concentrations than with total daily dosage [Glauser and Pippenger, 2000]. Published "optimal drug concentrations" are attempts to report ranges of concentrations at which many patients have improved seizure control without significant adverse effects. These ranges generally have not been determined by controlled studies in large populations. Obviously, more clinical experience correlating clinical response with drug concentrations is available for the older antiepileptic drugs. Although measurement of drug concentrations has contributed greatly to the development of rational drug management, routine monitoring may not be beneficial. In a randomized controlled trial of the impact of drug monitoring, no benefit with regard to improved seizure control or reduced adverse effects was observed in the study group in which levels were routinely sampled [Jannuzzi et al., 2000]. A retrospective study of antiepileptic drug monitoring in a pediatric emergency room setting failed to find a correlation between drug concentrations and clinical decisions [Kozer et al., 2003].

When to Obtain Drug Concentrations

Although enthusiasm for routine monitoring of drug concentrations has moderated, this assistance from the laboratory is helpful in clinical management when used appropriately. Laboratory specimens collected for measurement of drug concentrations should be obtained after the drug is at steady state. The time after dose of when the sample was drawn should be recorded in order to interpret where the concentration would be on a pharmacokinetic profile. Recommendations with regard to specific clinical situations in which determination of drug concentration is useful are listed in Box 59-1 [Glauser and Pippenger, 2000]. It is useful to measure the antiepileptic drug concentration after the patient has reached steady state dosing and optimal clinical outcome has been obtained. This level could be considered the "optimal drug concentration" or the "target level" for the individual patient. Then a level should be obtained when a breakthrough of the seizure pattern occurs (i.e. a single seizure in a person usually well controlled, or a doubling of the usual seizure rate). If the level is lower than the "target value," one needs to consider noncompliance or alteration in pharmacokinetics.

Box 59-1 Clinical Indications for Obtaining Antiepileptic Drug Concentrations

- Establishing baseline effective concentration
- Change in dosage
- Addition or elimination of another antiepileptic drug
- Evaluation of lack of efficacy (noncompliance or fast metabolizer)
- Evaluation of toxicity (excessive dose, drug interaction, slow metabolizer, renal or liver failure)
- Evaluation of loss of efficacy (compliance, drug interaction, change in formulation, pregnancy)
- Estimation of the "room to move"

Noncompliance is by far the most common cause of deviation from the "target value." In these cases, the dose should not be changed, but steps should be taken to increase compliance (pill box, education, and so on). Illnesses affecting absorption or clearance can also be detected by comparing the current value with the "target level." Also, levels should be measured after changes in co-medication once a new steady state has been reached to determine if any changes in the levels have occurred. If a patient experiences an increase in seizures but the current concentration is at the "target," it is possible that the seizure threshold has changed or was underestimated, and changes in dose may be needed and a new "target level" should be established.

What to Measure

Total drug concentrations generally are measured; however, it also is possible to determine levels of free or unbound drug, as well as of metabolites of the administered drug. Free drug concentrations correlate best with clinical effect and toxicity; however, they are more expensive and difficult to obtain. In most cases, the ratio of free to bound drug is relatively constant for a particular patient; therefore, total drug concentrations usually are adequate. In certain instances, however, particularly with critically ill patients under intensive care, determination of free drug levels, especially for phenytoin and valproic acid, is essential. In such patients, many drugs are typically administered, increasing the likelihood that antiepileptic drugs will be displaced from protein-binding sites. The percentage of unbound valproic acid increases with higher drug concentrations and with co-medication [Cloyd et al., 1992], or when valproic acid is rapidly administered [Birnbaum et al., 2003]. When the bound fraction is doubled, the valproic acid free fraction may be eight times higher [Fenichel, 1986].

Occasionally, measurement of antiepileptic drug metabolites is useful. With several antiepileptic drugs, metabolites are clinically active and contribute to both response and toxicity. Phenobarbital is an active metabolite present during primidone therapy. Carbamazepine-10,11-epoxide is a derivative of carbamazepine and contributes to toxicity [Schoeman et al., 1984]. Clinical monitoring of oxcarbazepine and eslicarbazepine acetate treatment is evaluated by measuring their primary metabolites.

Laboratory Tests for Idiosyncratic Reactions

In an effort to identify patients in whom serious or potentially life-threatening adverse effects may develop, obtaining complete blood counts and chemistry profiles at routine intervals has become common practice. The cost for this routine monitoring can exceed the costs of medication [Hart and Easton, 1982]. Moreover, it is very debatable whether routine laboratory monitoring can actually identify patients at risk for serious reactions or can identify significant adverse events better than clinical monitoring. Identification of life-threatening reactions is rarely made by routine laboratory screening of asymptomatic children [Camfield et al., 1986]. Fulminant or irreversible hepatic failure during valproic acid therapy is not reliably predicted by laboratory monitoring [Willmore et al., 1991]. Many reports, therefore, indicate that routine laboratory screening of asymptomatic patients is of little value [Camfield et al., 1989; Pellock and Willmore, 1991]. However, complete blood counts and chemistry profiles before, and then

after, initiation of antiepileptic drug therapy are reasonable [Harden, 2000]. It is much more effective to caution patients and parents to obtain these tests immediately whenever there are signs of any possible reaction, such as unusual bleeding or bruising, significant loss of appetite, jaundice, and so on. Testing for inborn errors of metabolism may be useful for identifying young children at risk for hepatic dysfunction from valproic acid.

Adverse Drug Reactions to Antiepileptic Drugs

Adverse drug reactions are defined by the World Health Organization as "any response to a drug that is noxious or unintended, and which occurs at doses used in man for prophylaxis, diagnosis, or therapy" [Venulet and ten Ham, 1996]. The most frequent adverse drug reactions to antiepileptic drugs are dose-related, mild, and reversible. Less frequently observed but potentially more serious are the idiosyncratic adverse reactions, which generally are not related to dosage but may be due to individual peculiarities of drug metabolism, i.e., lack of pathways to process toxic metabolites. Idiosyncratic reactions are almost never seen with antiepileptic drugs that are not metabolized.

Central Nervous System Adverse Reactions

The central nervous system adverse reaction profile for children is similar to that for adults. Most of the older antiepileptic drugs – phenytoin, phenobarbital, primidone, carbamazepine, and valproic acid – and their active metabolites have similar side-effect profiles, comprising of cognitive impairment, sedation, dizziness, diplopia, ataxia, headaches, and effects on somnolence. The effects of antiepileptic drugs on cognitive function generally are concentration- (and dose-) dependent. Drug therapy is known to contribute to cognitive deficits, especially treatment with multiple drugs [Thompson and Trimble, 1982]. Removal of antiepileptic drugs frequently results in improved cognitive function and motor skills [Duncan et al., 1990]. It is important to recognize that reaction times, disordered attention, and impulsivity, even in untreated children with epilepsy, differ from those in control subjects. The differences in attention and reaction time, however, are small between children with mild as opposed to severe seizure disorders [Mitchell et al., 1992].

Side effects frequently occur in children who are given phenobarbital. Phenobarbital has been associated with a significant depression of cognitive function when it is used for treatment of febrile seizures in children. In a randomized, placebo-controlled, prospective study, children had lower mean intelligence quotient (IQ) scores both during and 6 months after stopping therapy with phenobarbital [Farwell et al., 1990]. Clinical tolerance does develop to some degree; however, an unacceptably high frequency of adverse effects from phenobarbital commonly is observed in children [Farwell et al., 1990; Wolf and Forsythe, 1978]. The adverse effects are reminiscent of complaints present in attention deficit disorders and include overactivity, aggressiveness, inattention, and irritability. The behavioral disorders are observed in 20–50 percent of children receiving phenobarbital for febrile seizures, and result in discontinuation of therapy in 20–30 percent of children [Herranz et al., 1984].

The presence of pre-existing behavior problems, especially hyperactivity, is strongly predictive of adverse reactions during phenobarbital therapy. In a study of children receiving phenobarbital for febrile seizures, 80 percent of those with abnormal behavior before drug therapy reported aggravation of pre-existing hyperactive behavior with phenobarbital, versus only 20 percent for children with normal preseizure behavior [Wolf and Forsythe, 1978]. In some cases, these adverse effects may resolve with continuation or with a lower dose of phenobarbital; however, discontinuation of therapy or alternative medication should be considered.

The newer antiepileptic drugs – gabapentin, felbamate, topiramate, lamotrigine, tiagabine, oxcarbazepine, levetiracetam, vigabatrin, and zonisamide – are thought to have fewer and less severe adverse effects; however, their adverse central nervous system effects are similar to those of the older antiepileptic drugs. Although gabapentin has a good safety profile and seems well tolerated in adults, significant behavioral side effects are observed in some children. In a nonblinded, uncontrolled series, adverse behavioral effects were reported in 47 percent of children given gabapentin for add-on therapy; however, only 12 percent of children were withdrawn from gabapentin because of these problems [Khurana et al., 1996]. In other reports, aggression, hyperactivity, temper tantrums, and increased oppositional behavior developed in 12 children taking the drug [Lee et al., 1996; Tallian et al., 1996; Wolf and Forsythe, 1978]. Most, but not all, of these children had pre-existing cognitive dysfunction, such as mental retardation, autistic features, or behavioral difficulties. The adverse cognitive changes resolved with discontinuation of gabapentin; if administration of the drug was resumed, the adverse cognitive changes tended to recur. In one 6-year-old female, the drug was clinically effective in controlling seizures as monotherapy and was well tolerated for 6 months before the aggressiveness developed [Tallian et al., 1996].

In limited pediatric trials, 36 percent of children taking tiagabine have experienced treatment-emergent adverse effects, most commonly somnolence [Gustavson et al., 1997]. In approximately 15 percent of children, decreased functioning in school, aggression, and other cognitive changes occurred within the first 4 months of initiation of topiramate therapy [Gerber et al., 2000]. A previous history of behavioral changes and concurrent lamotrigine therapy were associated factors. Central nervous system-related adverse effects from topiramate tend to decrease over time [Ritter et al., 2000]. Of greater concern are reports of the development of major depression, schizophrenic-like reactions, and organic psychoses in adults taking vigabatrin [Ferrie et al., 1996; Ring et al., 1993]. A reversible acute psychosis has been reported in a child taking vigabatrin [Canovas Martinez et al., 1995]. Development of hyperkinesia, somnolence, and insomnia in children taking vigabatrin has been reported by a number of investigators [Aicardi et al., 1996; Dalla Bernardina et al., 1995; Dulac et al., 1991]. Generally, these effects have not led to discontinuation of the drug. Meador et al. recently reported that, when compared with other antiepileptic drugs, valproic acid can significantly lower, in a dose-related fashion, the IQ of children of 3 years of age who have been exposed to valproic acid in utero [Meador et al., 2009].

Gastrointestinal Effects

Weight Gain

A survey in children and adolescents taking valproic acid found the most common side effect to be weight gain; however, for many patients, the weight gain was "beneficial." The incidence of unwanted weight gain was 26 percent in adults and 15 percent in children and adolescents. An increase in weight was observed more than twice as frequently in females [Clark et al., 1980; Wirrell, 2003]. Weight increase was independent of dose [Covanis et al., 1982]. Weight gain also was reported in children during therapy with carbamazepine [Herranz et al., 1988; Hogan et al., 2000] and vigabatrin [Dalla Bernardina et al., 1995; Dulac et al., 1991]. Weight gain has been reported in adults taking gabapentin [DeToledo et al., 1997].

Weight Loss

Sustained weight loss was reported in children on maintenance topiramate therapy [Reiter et al., 2004]. Seventy-five percent of children and adults during clinical research trials reported a loss of appetite and decrease in body weight while taking felbamate [Bergen et al., 1995]. Zonisamide also is associated with weight loss in children [Kothare et al., 2006].

Gastric Irritation

Signs of gastric irritation, with heartburn and indigestion, are seen with use of some antiepileptic drugs. Gastric irritation during valproic acid therapy can be reduced with administration of lower doses or by taking medication with food. Use of enteric-coated preparations of valproic acid will enable most patients who did not tolerate valproic acid because of gastrointestinal symptoms (nausea/vomiting, eructation, heartburn) to resume valproic acid therapy [Clark et al., 1980; Wilder et al., 1983]. Aggressive medical intervention with antacids and H_2 receptor antagonists (other than cimetidine) has been helpful for some children with clinical signs of gastritis, allowing valproic acid therapy to continue [Marks et al., 1988].

Approximately 20 percent of patients receiving ethosuximide will demonstrate dose-related adverse effects, primarily gastric distress, vomiting, hiccups, and anorexia [Sherwin, 1983]. Gastrointestinal disturbances also are encountered in 14 percent of patients taking carbamazepine, with symptoms of nausea, vomiting, anorexia, and constipation [Herranz et al., 1988]. Nausea and vomiting commonly are observed with felbamate [Dodson, 1984; Theodore et al., 1991].

Gingival Hyperplasia

Gingival hyperplasia occurs in 10–20 percent of persons treated with phenytoin and is more frequent in young persons. It is observed more frequently in persons taking higher dosages, often appears 2–3 months after beginning therapy, and reaches its maximum severity in 12–18 months [Babcock, 1965; Little et al., 1975]. Gingival hyperplasia generally resolves within 2–5 months after discontinuation or a reduction in medication [Little et al., 1975]. A vigorous program of good oral hygiene started before and continued during phenytoin therapy can be effective in minimizing gingival enlargement [Modeer and Dahllof, 1987; Pihlstrom et al., 1980]. Drugs other than antiepileptic drugs, including nifedipine and cyclosporine, have been associated with the development of gingival hyperplasia [Butler et al., 1987].

Increased Seizures

Some patients, especially those with generalized or absence seizures, may experience an increase in seizure activity when carbamazepine or phenytoin is added [Horn et al., 1986; Perucca et al., 1998; Snead and Hosey, 1985]. Vigabatrin also has been reported to increase seizure activity and even lead to status epilepticus [de Krom et al., 1995]. Aggravation of seizures occurred in 3 percent of children with generalized seizures, most often in those with nonprogressive myoclonic epilepsy, and was extremely unusual in children with partial epilepsies and infantile spasms [Lortie et al., 1997]. Oxcarbazepine has been reported to increase myoclonic jerks and absence seizures [Gelisse et al., 2004]. Phenytoin and carbamazepine may increase seizures associated with the Lennox–Gastaut syndrome, and gabapentin and pregabalin can increase or induce myoclonic seizures.

Osteomalacia

Osteomalacia (rickets) may occur in patients taking antiepileptic drugs. In a survey of institutionalized patients, 52 of 144 patients with a developmental cognitive disability ranging in age from 3 to 26 years, who were on antiepileptic drug therapy for at least 2 years, had elevations of serum alkaline phosphatase levels greater than 2 standard deviations above normal. Most patients were taking phenytoin or phenobarbital [Hunt et al., 1986]. The cause of osteomalacia during antiepileptic drug therapy appears to be multifactorial [Farhat et al., 2002]. Many antiepileptic drugs presumably enhance hepatic conversion of 25-hydroxyvitamin D to biologically inactive metabolites. Clinically significant rickets seldom develops in ambulatory children on antiepileptic drug therapy, or in institutionalized children who are not taking medication. On the other hand, clinically overt rickets was observed in 10 percent of institutionalized children on phenobarbital and/or phenytoin. In these patients, sunlight was more important for the maintenance of serum 25-hydroxyvitamin D than were supplements of vitamin D [Morijiri and Sato, 1981].

Current evidence indicates that antiepileptic drugs may decrease bone mineral density in adults. In adults, correlation with 25-hydroxyvitamin D levels was poor [Farhat et al., 2002]. In children, no correlation was observed between duration of antiepileptic drug therapy and 25-hydroxyvitamin D levels. Bone mineral density measurements tended to be lower in patients on older antiepileptic drugs than in patients on newer antiepileptic drugs, but were lower in all patients on any antiepileptic drug than in the control population. It was previously thought that older antiepileptic drugs resulted in induction of vitamin D metabolism, resulting in decreased bone mineral density; however, the lack of correlation between vitamin D levels and bone mineral density suggests that other mechanisms are operative.

Some authors recommend routine bone mineral density monitoring for patients on chronic antiepileptic drug therapy [Farhat et al., 2002]. Consensus is lacking on treatment of patients who have low bone mineral density secondary to antiepileptic drug therapy. Other factors may contribute to decreased bone mineral density, such as lack of exercise and sunlight.

Tremor and Movement Disorders

A benign essential type of tremor has been observed with use of valproic acid, beginning within 1 month of initiating therapy. It is dose-dependent, occurring in some patients with blood valproic acid levels greater than 40 mg/mL. Reduction of tremor may occur with reduction of dose [Karas et al., 1982]. Tremor also has been seen with use of lamotrigine and gabapentin [Schmidt and Kramer, 1994]. Oculogyric crises and choreoathetotic movements have developed in several adults while taking gabapentin [Buetefisch et al., 1996; Reeves et al., 1996].

Other Effects

Hair changes have been associated with antiepileptic drug treatment. Hair changes (thinning or wavy hair) are seen in 12 percent of children during valproic acid therapy [Clark et al., 1980]. Additional dose-related adverse effects of phenytoin include hirsutism, coarse facial features, and acne, especially in children and teenagers. Pancreatitis has been associated with valproic acid therapy [Coulter and Allen, 1980; Wyllie et al., 1984]. Visual field changes, which may be irreversible, may occur with vigabatrin treatment [Krauss et al., 1998]. Topiramate has been reported to cause acute myopia and secondary angle closure glaucoma. Patients present with decreased visual acuity and ocular pain. In a majority of cases, immediate discontinuation of topiramate results in a resolution of symptoms [Sankar et al., 2001; Thambi et al., 2002]. Hyponatremia occasionally is encountered in patients taking carbamazepine and oxcarbazepine [Borusiak et al., 1998; Holtmann et al., 2002; Koivikko and Valikangas, 1983]. Hyperthermia and oligohydrosis have been reported in several children taking topiramate and zonisamide. Clinical signs included fever, decreased sweating, and exercise intolerance, which resolved in a majority of cases when topiramate or zonisamide was discontinued [Arcas et al., 2001; Knudsen et al., 2003]. Topiramate and zonisamide may cause nephrolithiasis. The risk is increased with topiramate or zonisamide treatment and the ketogenic diet [Kossoff et al., 2002].

Anticonvulsant Hypersensitivity Syndrome in Children

Clinical Features

The hypersensitivity syndrome is characterized by rash, fever, and malaise, generally occurring within the first several months of therapy. Certain types of rash may be particularly alarming, such as those of Stevens–Johnson syndrome or toxic epidermal necrolysis. Often hepatic involvement is part of the syndrome, and the liver is the most frequently involved internal organ. Affected children may present with hepatomegaly and elevations in serum transaminase levels. The involvement may progress to hepatic necrosis. Other systems may be involved, including kidney, lungs, bone marrow, and the lymphatic system [Handfield-Jones et al., 1993].

Pathogenesis

Although the mechanism of the hypersensitivity syndrome is not completely understood, current evidence implicates toxic metabolites [Glauser, 2000; Verrotti et al., 2002]. The aromatic AEDs (phenobarbital, phenytoin > carbamazepine > oxcarbazepine), lamotrigine, and felbamate have been more frequently implicated in causing this syndrome. Presumably, accumulation of toxic metabolites, such as reactive aromatic epoxide intermediates, precipitates the syndrome [Glauser, 2000].

Prevention

Routine laboratory monitoring (i.e., with complete blood counts or liver function tests) will not prospectively identify which patients are at high risk for the development of an acute hypersensitivity reaction. Nevertheless, certain factors place some patients at high risk. Clinical profiles that identify patients at high risk for hypersensitivity reactions differ for specific antiepileptic drugs (valproic acid, felbamate, and lamotrigine) (Box 59-2). When one of these drugs is being considered for a patient at high risk, one should proceed with caution. Alternative therapy, if possible, should be considered. Additional laboratory tests to screen for inborn errors of metabolism may be indicated when use of valproic acid is under consideration in children younger than 2 years of age. Families need to be advised that the child is in a high-risk category and counseled on the early recognition of the syndrome.

Although the identification of a high-risk clinical profile is the most inexpensive and practical way available to reduce the risk of hypersensitivity syndrome, various biomarkers also have been identified [Glauser, 2000]. These biomarkers may indicate that some patients have genetic susceptibility to the accumulation of toxic metabolites due to deficient detoxification pathways. The biomarkers that have been investigated include deficient epoxide hydrolase activity and deficiencies in free radical-scavenging enzyme activity. Studies in patients of Chinese ancestry indicate a strong association between the risk of developing toxic epidermal necrolysis and Stevens-Johnson Syndrome and the presence of HLA-B* 1502. Clinicians may want to avoid use of carbamazepine in this population.

Managing Adverse Effects

The clinician and the patient are faced with adverse effects approximately 30 percent of the time when antiepileptic drugs are used, especially during initiation of therapy. In many instances, this rate is acceptable, especially when the patient and the physician mutually agree on which problems are most important to avoid. When no urgency exists, many adverse effects can be avoided during initiation of therapy by gradually increasing doses. In general, management of adverse effects depends on the problem. Most adverse effects are concentration-dependent, and are less prominent at lower doses and blood concentrations. Seizure control may or may not be maintained at the lower dose; if not, the clinician and the patient need to consider whether a compromise is acceptable with regard to either increased seizures or increased adverse effects, or if alternative medication should be considered.

At times, toxicity is encountered only with high drug concentrations and is seen only at peak times; for these patients, it may be possible to avoid toxicity by more frequent and lower doses or by the use of extended-release formulations. Gastric irritation generally is dose-dependent and may be managed in several ways. The amount of drug can be reduced; the effective dose to the gastric mucosa can be lowered by use of enteric-coated formulations; or the patient can be protected by use of H_2 receptor antagonists.

Idiosyncratic reactions pose another problem. Mild, asymptomatic elevations of liver enzymes do not mandate discontinuation of therapy if not in excess of 2–3 times normal values. On the other hand, Stevens–Johnson syndrome and toxic epidermal necrolysis, clinically symptomatic hepatotoxicity, pancreatitis, and most rashes are indications for immediate cessation of the responsible medication. If the rash was mild, however, and especially if the patient had an otherwise favorable clinical response to the drug, a cautious rechallenge might be considered. Successful resumption of therapy has been reported in a number of patients, especially with valproic acid after that drug was discontinued, when a more gradual dose escalation was used [Schlumberger et al., 1994; Tavernor et al., 1995].

Selection of Drugs for Initiation of Antiepileptic Drug Therapy

The selection of a specific drug for the treatment of epilepsy is based primarily on the criteria of therapeutic efficacy expected for the patient and seizure type. Certain epileptic syndromes

---

Box 59-2 Clinical Profiles for Patients at High Risk for Idiosyncratic Reactions to Valproic Acid, Lamotrigine, and Felbamate

Valproic Acid: Hepatotoxicity

- Children younger than 2 years of age
- Multiple concomitant antiepileptic drugs
- Underlying metabolic disease
- Developmental delay

Felbamate: Aplastic Anemia

- Caucasians
- Adults more than children
- Females more than males
- Previous cytopenia

- History of antiepileptic drug allergy or toxicity
- History of immune disorder
- On felbamate less than 1 year

Lamotrigine: Stevens–Johnson Syndrome and Toxic Epidermal Necrolysis

- Children more than adults
- Concurrent valproic acid use
- High starting dose
- Rapid titration
- On lamotrigine less than 1 year

(From Glauser TA. Idiosyncratic reactions: New methods of identifying high-risk patients. Epilepsia 2000;41 [Suppl 8]:S16.)

require specific therapy. For most patients and seizure types, however, efficacy differences are minimal, and the selection of the initial drug for antiepileptic therapy is guided equally by a consideration of potential adverse effects. Although highly effective, phenytoin is rarely a drug of first choice in children because of a higher incidence of dysmorphic effects. In children, especially those with pre-existing tendencies for attention-deficit disorders, an unacceptable incidence of behavioral problems, as well as of cognitive dysfunction, has been noted with barbiturate therapy. The principles to be used during initiation and selection of antiepileptic drug therapy in children have been summarized [Crumrine, 2002; Fenichel, 1986].

Discontinuation of Antiepileptic Drug Therapy

The decision to discontinue antiepileptic drug therapy often is as challenging as the decision to initiate and continue long-term drug therapy. Most commonly, the question arises after a patient has done well and has become seizure-free for some substantial period. At other times, the question arises because of chronic noncompliance, or because no therapy has had a measurable effect on seizure control. Many factors are considered in making these decisions, including the length of the seizure-free interval, drug history, presence of adverse effects, and the neurologic and epilepsy syndrome diagnosis of the patient. Numerous retrospective and prospective investigations are available. Ultimately, the decision to withdraw or to continue antiepileptic drug therapy is that of the patient and family, and their perception of acceptable risk of recurrence often differs from that of the treating physician [Gordon et al., 1996].

Benefits of Drug Discontinuation

The potential benefits of drug discontinuation are numerous. Most obvious is the immediate reduction in cost to the family and third-party payer with elimination of drug therapy and usually the reduction in associated expenses incurred by laboratory tests and physician and clinic charges. In addition, in many patients, the adverse, sometimes previously unrecognized effects of antiepileptic drug therapy are reversed. Patients who had been on phenobarbital, phenytoin, valproic acid, and topiramate had subtle improvement in various psychometric tasks, such as memory, vigilance attention, and visual motor performance [Gallassi et al., 1992; Lee et al., 2003], and in psychomotor speed [Aldenkamp et al., 1993], when therapy was discontinued.

Risks of Drug Discontinuation

The obvious risk of stopping antiepileptic drug therapy is the recurrence of seizures. In most cases, seizure control can be regained with resumption of the previous drug therapy. Response to therapy after a relapse may be rapid and satisfactory [Arts et al., 1988]. Chadwick and colleagues observed that approximately 90 percent of patients who experience seizures after antiepileptic drug discontinuation have a 2-year remission after therapy is resumed [Chadwick et al., 1996]. Thus, control was usually but not always regained despite increasing doses of a previously successful drug regimen.

A guideline has been published to assist the physician and the family considering discontinuation of antiepileptic drug therapy. The conclusions were based on a MEDLINE search [Camfield and Camfield, 2008].

Children who were seizure-free for 2 or more years while on antiepileptic drugs, who had a single type of partial or generalized seizure, who had a normal IQ and normal findings on neurologic examination, and a normalized electroencephalogram (EEG) on therapy had a 69 percent chance of discontinuing antiepileptic drug therapy without seizure recurrence. A similar conclusion was reached by another meta-analysis, in which 75 percent of "relatively unselected" patients were seizure-free 1 year after discontinuation, and 71 percent 2 years after discontinuation of antiepileptic drug therapy [Berg and Shinnar, 1994]. Children with remote symptomatic seizures and those with seizure onset in adolescence (rather than earlier) were at greatest risk of recurrence.

Although relapse was observed in every study, in one prospective series, relapse rates were slightly higher in children who had epileptiform activity on the last EEG before antiepileptic drug discontinuation [Andersson et al., 1997]. The authors concluded that the persistence of 3-Hz spike-wave activity during therapy also was an unfavorable prognostic sign. Children more frequently had recurrences of seizures when antiepileptic drugs were stopped after 1 year versus 3 years of therapy. In another randomized, prospective study of 6 versus 12 months of antiepileptic drug therapy in children who became seizure-free on antiepileptic drug therapy, no difference between relapse rates was observed [Peters et al., 1998]. That report again presented the predictive variables for relapse, which were partial epilepsy, a remote symptomatic etiology, an older age at onset (12 years and older), and an epileptiform EEG during therapy.

Families should discuss withdrawing antiepileptic drugs with their neurologist once children have become free of seizures for 1 year or longer while on antiepileptic drug therapy. Children whose EEGs have become normal have a somewhat better chance of successful withdrawal of therapy. However, there are critical life transitions when the risk of discontinuing therapy outweighs continuation. These are when children have been seizure-free and are eligible to begin driving, and when they are leaving home and transitioning to college or independent living. Finally, for some patients, withdrawal of antiepileptic drugs is rarely successful – for example, those with abnormalities on neurologic examination or with certain seizure syndromes such as juvenile myoclonic epilepsy, Lennox–Gastaut syndrome, or infantile spasms [Peters et al., 1998; Shinnar et al., 1994].

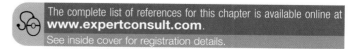

The Ketogenic Diet

James W. Wheless

The incidence of epilepsy in children and adolescents ranges from 50 to 100 per 100,000 [Hauser and Hesdorffer, 1980; Hauser, 1994]. Antiepileptic drugs (AEDs) are the primary treatment modality and provide good seizure control in most children. However, more than 25 percent of children with epilepsy have either intractable seizures or suffer treatment-limiting adverse medication effects [Pellock, 1993, 1995, 1996; Heller et al., 1993; Pellock and Pippenger, 1993; Patsalos and Duncan, 1993]. Only a limited number of these children benefit from surgical therapy.

Uncontrolled seizures pose a variety of risks to children, including higher rates of mortality, accidents, and injuries, a greater incidence of cognitive and psychiatric impairment, poorer self-esteem, higher levels of anxiety and depression, and social stigmatization or isolation [Fisher et al., 1996]. Thus, effective treatment to control seizures is fundamental to improving overall outcome in childhood epilepsy. The ketogenic diet has proven to be an effective treatment for many children with epilepsy [Wheless, 1995a, b; Lefever and Aronson, 2000; Levy and Cooper, 2003]. In this chapter, the history of the development of the diet, current understanding of the biochemistry of ketone body formation and its relation to the anticonvulsant effect of the diet, considerations related to patient selection, and diet efficacy, complications, advantages, and disadvantages are reviewed.

History

For centuries, fasting has been used to treat many diseases, including seizures; it was even used in biblical times [Bible, The King James Version, 1982; Livingston, 1972].

Contemporary accounts of fasting (Table 60-1) include a child who did not respond to the conventional treatment of the day [Hendricks, 1995; Freeman et al., 1994], which was a combination of bromides and phenobarbital [Lennox and Lennox, 1960]. This child's seizures were managed with prayer and fasting, producing dramatic improvement in seizure control during the period of starvation. However, when the period of starvation was terminated, the seizures returned [Conklin, 1922; Freeman et al., 1994; Bridge, 1949]. The child's uncle, a pediatrician, enlisted the aid of John Howland at Johns Hopkins Hospital to understand how starvation and fasting controlled seizures and how one could maintain the beneficial effects of fasting [Lennox and Lennox, 1960]. Concurrently, Wilder at the Mayo Clinic suggested that a diet high in fat and low in carbohydrates could maintain ketosis and its accompanying acidosis longer than fasting [Freeman et al., 1994; Schwartz et al., 1989b]. Wilder was also the first to coin the term ketogenic diet. (See Wheless [2004] for a review of the

ketogenic diet history.) The beneficial effects of this diet were initially recorded by investigators from Johns Hopkins University, the Mayo Clinic, and Harvard University. Use of the ketogenic diet was included in almost every comprehensive textbook on epilepsy in childhood that appeared between 1941 and 1980 [Penfield and Erickson, 1941; Lennox, 1941; Bridge, 1949; Livingston, 1954, 1963, 1972; Lennox and Lennox, 1960; Keith, 1963; Livingston et al., 1977; Withrow, 1980; Bower, 1980].

Until 1938, the ketogenic diet was one of the few available therapies for epilepsy, but it fell into disfavor when researchers turned their attention to the development of new AEDs [Livingston and Pauli, 1975]. After the introduction of sodium valproate, it was believed that this branched-chain fatty acid would treat those children previously placed on the ketogenic diet and that the diet could no longer be justified [Aicardi, 1994]. Use of the ketogenic diet decreased greatly until it received national media attention [NBC Dateline, 1994; Hendricks, 1995; Schneider and Wagner, 1995; Charlie Foundation to Help Cure Pediatric Epilepsy, 1994a; Freeman et al., 1990, 1994, 2000]. After an almost two-decade hiatus, renewed public and scientific interest has led to a better understanding and increased worldwide use of the ketogenic diet [Kleinman, 2004; Stafstrom and Rho, 2004; Kossoff et al., 2009b; Kossoff and McGrogan, 2005a].

Efficacy

As presented in Table 60-2, initial reports began to appear in the 1920s and 1930s that documented the efficacy of the ketogenic diet [Geyelin, 1921; Wilder, 1921; Peterman, 1925; Helmholz, 1927; McQuarrie and Keith, 1927; Lennox and Cobb, 1928; Barborka, 1928a, 1929; Helmholz and Keith, 1930, 1932; Pulford, 1932; Fischer, 1935; Wilder and Pollack, 1935; Helmholz and Goldstein, 1937; Wilkins, 1937]. Over the next 60–70 years, many more clinical reports appeared (Table 60-3) [Keith, 1942; Prasad et al., 1996]. About one-third to one-half of children appeared to have had an excellent response to the diet, defined by cessation or marked reduction in seizure activity. About 10 percent of children become seizure-free after initiation of the ketogenic diet, and typically stop the diet after 2 years. Of those children who become seizure-free, a minority have recurrence after the diet is stopped [Martinez et al., 2007]. Risk factors that increase the likelihood of recurrence are epileptiform abnormalities on electroencephalograms (EEGs) obtained within 12 months of diet discontinuation, a focal abnormality on magnetic resonance imaging (MRI), lower initial seizure frequency, and tuberous sclerosis

Table 60-1 Efficacy of Fasting (1921–1928)

Author	No. of Patients	Age (Yrs) of Patients	Seizure Type	Diet	% Success Rate	Comments
Geyelin [1921]	30	3.5–35	PM, GM	Fasting	87% seizure-free	Results based on 20-day fast, no long-term follow-up
Weeks et al [1923]	64	7–61	PM, GM	Fasting	47% seizure-free during fast	Patients fasted for 3 weeks, all had seizures after return to regular diet
Talbot et al [1926]	23	Children	UN	Fasting	Seizure-free during fast	Seizures returned in all after fast
Lennox [1928]	27	13–42	UN	Fasting	50% had marked reduction in seizures during fast	PB stopped on admit, fast lasted 4–21 days

GM, grand mal; PB, phenobarbital; PM, petit mal; UN, unknown.

Table 60-2 Efficacy of the Ketogenic Diet (1921–1976)

Author	No. of Patients	Age (Yrs) of Patients	Seizure Type	Diet	% Success Rate	Comments
Peterman [1925]	37	2.25–14.5	PM, GM	KD	60% seizure-free 34.5% improved 5.5% not improved	All idiopathic etiology. Follow-up 0.33–2.5 years. Only 2 on PB
Talbot et al [1926]	12	Children	PM, GM	KD	50% seizure-free 33% improved 17% no change	Follow-up period 3–6 months. All idiopathic etiology
Cooder [1933]	38	≤12	GM, SP PM	KD	50% seizure-free 34% improved 16% not improved	>3-month follow-up
Helmholz and Goldstein [1937]	501	Children	UN	KD	Idiopathic etiology: 31% seizure-free 16% definite improvement 53% not improved Symptomatic etiology: 11% seizure-free	92 had symptomatic epilepsy and 142 could not maintain diet. All children had >1-year follow-up. Results from children treated between 1922 and 1936. 1 child developed pellagra
Wilkins [1937]	30	3–14	GM, PM, MM	KD	27% Seizure-free 50% No benefit	Idiopathic etiology. Follow-up >1.5 years. All seizure-free patients resumed a normal diet
Keith [1963]	729	UN	UN	KD	Of 530 idiopathic patients: 31% seizure-free 24% improved 39% no benefit	Patients treated between 1922 and 1944. Follow-up 1–30+ years (some included in Helmholz and Goldstein [1937]). Excluded 84 with symptomatic epilepsy. 115 unable to follow diet. No deaths due to diet
Hopkins and Lynch [1970]	34	1–13	GM, MM	KD	29% successful (seizure-free or much reduced) 32% unsuccessful 26% inadequate trial	1 renal calculus
Livingston [1972]	1001	UN	UN	KD	52% seizures controlled 27% seizures marked improvement 21% no improvement	
Dodson et al [1976]	50	0.5–38	UN	KD	50% seizure-free 20–30% seizures improved considerably	

GM, grand mal; KD, classic ketogenic diet; MM, minor motor; PB, phenobarbital; PM, petit mal; SP, simple partial; UN, unknown.

complex [Martinez et al., 2007]. When the diet has been discontinued, it has usually been due to lack of efficacy. It appears that younger children are more likely to have a more favorable response than older children [Freeman et al., 1998a].

Recent studies attest to the efficacy and safety of the ketogenic diet in infants [Nordli et al., 2001; Kossoff et al., 2002; Klepper et al., 2002; Kang et al., 2005; Eun et al., 2006]. Nordli et al. retrospectively reviewed their experience with 32 infants who had been treated with the ketogenic diet, 17 of whom had infantile spasms [Nordli et al., 2001]. Most infants (71 percent) were able to maintain robust ketosis. The overall effectiveness of the diet in infants was similar to that

Table 60-3 **Efficacy of the Ketogenic Diet (1989–Present)**

Author	No. of Patients	Age (Yrs) of Patients	Seizure Type	Diet*	% Success Rate	Comments
Schwartz [1989b]	59	<5–54	M, A, IS, GTC, AB SP, CP	KD-24 MCT-22 Mod. MCT-13	81% had a >50% reduction of seizures	MCT diet more unpalatable; prospective series
Kinsman et al [1992]	58	1–20	80% multiple seizure type	KD	29% seizure controlled 38% had ≥50% seizure reduction 29% no improvement	All had severe neurology handicaps: MR (84%), cerebral palsy (45%), microcephaly (15%), 3 renal stones
Vining [1998]	51	1–8	230 seizures/mo average (IS SP, GTC, AB, CP, A, M)	KD	At 1 yr: 53% off diet (one-half with poor seizure control, one-half with poor tolerance) 40% of original group had ≥50% decrease in seizure frequency 10% seizure-free	Prospective, multicenter trials; patients failed average of 7 drugs previously
Swink [1997a]	18	0.5–1.75	934 seizures/mo average	KD	At 6 mo: 50% seizure-free 42% had ≥50% seizure reduction Only 1 discontinued diet	Prospective; all children <2 yr old at enrollment
Freeman et al [1998]	150	1–16	410 seizures/mo average (AB, M, A, IS, GTC)	KD	At 1 yr: 55% remained on diet 43% of original group had ≥50% decrease in seizure frequency 7% seizure-free	Prospective; 70% had IQ or DQ <69; prior trials 6.2 AEDs (average)
Hassan et al [1999]	52	5.5 (mean)	81% mixed seizure types	KD-49 MCT-3	Only 13.5% continued diet >12 mo	Retrospective; all had cognitive impairment; mean duration 6.8 mo
Freeman and Vining [1999]	17	Children	LGS – M, A	KD	100% had ≥50% decrease in seizure frequency by fifth day	Inpatient – 5-day duration
Kaytal et al [2000]	48	1–15	Multiple seizure types	KD	46% remained on diet >1 yr Of those on at least 45 days: 38% had >90% seizure reduction 33% had 50–90% reduction	Retrospective; duration >45 days on diet (mean, 350 days)
Hemingway et al [2001]	150	1–16 (mean 5.3)	Multiple seizure types	KD	83 on diet at 1 yr 58 on at >24 mo 30 on >3 yr Of original 150: 13% seizure-free 14% had 90–99% seizure decrease Many off AEDs or on fewer AEDs	Prospective; 3- to 6-yr follow-up of Freeman et al [1998]
Maydell et al [2001]	143	0.34–29 (mean 7.5)	Multiple types: 34 focal onset, 100 generalized Average 23.8 seizures/day	KD	68% on at 1 yr: 16% seizure-free 10% had 90–99% seizure decrease 47% on fewer AEDs	Retrospective; 83 patients had MR
Nordli et al [2001]	32	All <2 (mean 1.15)	Partial, IS, generalized	KD	19% seizure-free 35.5% had improvement	Retrospective; IS responder better than other seizure types
Kossoff et al [2002]	23	0.4–2	IS	KD	At 6 mo: 18 on diet 3 seizure-free 4 >90% improved 6 >50%, <90% improved	Retrospective; age <1 yr and exposure to ≤3 AEDs predicted improvement

Table 60-3 Efficacy of the Ketogenic Diet (1989–Present)—cont'd

Author	No. of Patients	Age (Yrs) of Patients	Seizure Type	Diet*	% Success Rate	Comments
DiMario and Holland [2002]	24	1–15 (mean 6.5)	Not given	KD	At 12 mo: 18 on diet 22% seizure-free 39% had >50% seizure reduction	Retrospective
Coppola [2002]	56	1–23 (mean 10.4)	CP, GTC, LGS, M, GT, SMEI AA	KD	Mean duration 5 mo At 12 mo: 5 patients (8.9%) on diet and all had a >50% to <90% seizure reduction None seizure-free	Prospective, multicenter; 96.4% had MR, 67% had cerebral palsy, and 16% had microcephaly
Kang et al [2005]	199	0.5–17.5	IS, LGS, PE, GE, SMEI, LKS, EIEE	KD	At 1 yr: 54% off diet (~half had intolerance or side effects, half had poor seizure control) 41% of original group had ≥50% decrease in seizure frequency 25% seizure-free	Retrospective, Korea; partial onset and etiology had frequent relapse after discontinuation
Rizzutti et al [2007]	46	1.75–17	PE, LGS, UE	KD	At 1 yr: 72% remained on diet 17.4% seizure-free 67% had ≥50% reduction in seizure frequency	Prospective, Brazil; half started as outpatients
Freitas et al [2007]	54	1–12	PE, GE	KD	At 1 yr: 72% remained on diet 72% had >75% seizure reduction 97% had ≥50% reduction in seizure frequency All had improved cognition	Brazil, prospective
Freeman [2009]	20	1–7	LGS – AT	KD	At 1 year: 60% remained on diet 65% of those had ≥50% seizure reduction 30% were seizure-free	Prospective
Neal et al [2009]	73	2–16	LGS, IS, PE, AT, ME, GE	KD, MCT	3-mo trial; at that time 54 of 73 on KD: 38% of total had >50% seizure reduction 7% had >90% improvement 1 child seizure-free	UK, prospective, randomized trial of KD vs. current treatment. Mean, 11.6 seizures/day at baseline
Nathan et al [2009]	105	0.33–18	PE, GE, ME, AT	KD	Median 17 mo follow-up: 37% seizure-free 22% had 90–99% seizure reduction	India, prospective
Hong et al [2010]	104	1.2 (mean)	IS	KD	37% spasm-free for 6 mo within 2.4 mo (median) of starting diet 18% had EEG normalize and 17% had resolution of hypsarrhythmia	Prospective

* Hyphenated numbers indicate the number of patients on the diet.

A, atonic; AA, atypical absence; AB, absence; AEDs, antiepileptic drugs; AT, atonic; CP, complex partial; DQ, development quotient; EIEE, early infantile epileptic encephalopathy; GE, genaralized epilepsy; GT, generalized tonic; GTC, generalized tonic clonic; IQ, intelligence quotient; IS, infantile spasms; KD, classic ketogenic diet; LGS, Lennox–Gastaut syndrome; LKS, Landau–Kleffner syndrome; M, Myoclonic; MCT, medium-chain triglyceride ketogenic diet; ME, myoclonic epilepsy; Mod. MCT, modified MCT diet; MR, mental retardation; PE, partial epilepsy; SMEI, severe myoclonic epilepsy of infancy (Dravet's syndrome); SP, simple partial; UE, undetermined epilepsy type.

reported for older children; 19.4 percent became seizure-free, and an additional 35.5 percent had a greater than 50 percent reduction in seizure frequency. The diet was particularly effective for children with infantile spasms. Kossoff et al. retrospectively reviewed their experience with the ketogenic diet as a treatment for infantile spasms during a 4-year period [Kossoff et al., 2002]. Twenty-three children, aged 5 months to 2 years, 39 percent of whom had symptomatic infantile spasms and 70 percent of whom had hypsarrhythmia, were started on the ketogenic diet. The children had been previously exposed to an average of 3.3 AEDs (range 0–7), and 74 percent had previously failed or relapsed after adrenocorticotropic hormone (ACTH) or steroids. The average time on the diet was 1.6 years, with 56 percent remaining on the diet at 12 months, 46 percent of whom were over 90 percent improved (three were seizure-free), and 100 percent were over 50 percent improved. Factors that predicted greater than 90 percent improvement at 12 months were age less than 1 year (p = 0.02) and exposure to ≤3 AEDs (p = 0.03). Improvement in development was related to seizure control. The same authors retrospectively reviewed their experience with the ketogenic diet as initial monotherapy for infantile spasms [Kossoff et al., 2008e]. At the end of 1 month, 8 of 13 (62 percent) infants were seizure-free (by parental report); however, the EEG normalization did not occur for 2–5 months. Time to spasm freedom was 6.5 days, suggesting that, if the ketogenic diet is used as initial treatment, a 2-week trial period is sufficient to judge efficacy for infantile spasms. In 2010, the same authors reported their 14-year experience with 104 consecutive infants prospectively started on the ketogenic diet [Hong et al., 2010]. Thirty-seven percent became spasm-free for at least a 6-month period, within a median 2.4 months of starting the ketogenic diet. A normal EEG was eventually obtained in 18 percent, and 17 percent demonstrated resolution of hypsarrhythmia. Eun et al. reviewed their experience treating 43 children with intractable infantile spasms (mean duration 13.4 months) with the ketogenic diet. Retrospective

analysis revealed that the diet resulted in 53.5 percent of the patients being seizure-free; 81 percent had a greater than 50 percent reduction in seizure frequency after a mean duration of 9 months [Eun et al., 2006]. Complete seizure control was obtained within 4 weeks in 78.3 percent of the children who obtained seizure-freedom. The improvements in seizure control correlated with improvements in EEG findings. As part of the Korean multicentered experience, Kang et al. retrospectively reviewed efficacy in 49 infants treated with the ketogenic diet [Kang et al., 2005]. Only 1 of 14 children with severe myoclonic epilepsy of infancy was seizure-free at 12 months, but 56 percent had a greater than 50 percent seizure reduction. Carraballo et al. reported similar results, with 10 percent seizure-free, and 55 percent achieving a greater than 50 percent seizure reduction at 12 months [Carraballo et al., 2005]. In a small study (n = 3) of patients with a diagnosis of early infantile epileptic encephalothopy, none achieved seizure control [Kang et al., 2005].

A few early studies evaluated use of the ketogenic diet in adults (Table 60-4). Some revealed improved seizure control [Barborka, 1928b, 1930], but subsequent reports concluded that the diet is not particularly beneficial in adolescents and adults with epilepsy [Notkin, 1934; Lennox, 1941; Bridge, 1949; Livingston, 1954, 1963, 1972; Withrow, 1980; Mosek et al., 2009]. Reasons cited for this were poor dietary compliance, types of seizures seen in these age groups, and the

Table 60-4 Efficacy of the Ketogenic Diet in Adolescents and Adults

Author	No. of Patients	Age (Yrs) of Patients	Seizure Type	Diet	% Success Rate	Comments
Barborka [1928b]	49	17–42	GM, PM	KD	16% seizure-free 22% improved 27% did not benefit 35% did not cooperate and stay on diet	No patients with symptomatic epilepsy; only 5 on an AED (PB); 3–36-mo follow-up
Barborka [1930]	100	16–51	GM, PM	KD	12% seizure-free 44% improved 44% did not benefit	No patients with symptomatic epilepsy; 3–60-mo follow-up
Bastible [1931]	45	19–57	GM, PM	KD	Of those staying on diet: 7% seizure-free 72% improved 21% seizures increased 16 of 45 unable to maintain diet	All institutionalized females, diagnosed with "epileptic insanity," without known etiology; 6-mo follow-up; best response seen in those with least "mental disorder"
Notkin [1934]	20	22–47	GM	KD	No improvement in any 90% had an increase in seizure number	All institutionalized patients, and off AEDs; no known etiology; average time on diet 11 mo
Sirven et al [1999]	11	19–45	PE, GE	KD	9% seizure-free 46% had >50% decrease in seizure number 9% had slight seizure decrease 36% discontinued diet	All symptomatic epilepsy; 8-mo follow-up
Mady et al [2003]	45	12–19	MT, LGS, CP, GTC, A, M, AT, SP	KD	Of 20 who remained on diet at 1 yr: 6 had >90% efficacy 7 had 50–90% efficacy	Average duration 1.2 yr
Mosek et al [2009]	9	23–36	PE	KD	None seizure-free 2 of 8 had >50% seizure reduction at 12 weeks	Only 2 maintained for 12 weeks (dependent on family members for food supply)

A, atonic; AED, antiepileptic drug; AT, atonic; CP, complex partial; GE, generalized epilepsy; GM, grand mal; GTC, generalized tonic clonic; KD, classic ketogenic diet; LGS, Lennox–Gastaut syndrome; M, Myoclonic; MT, multiple seizure types; PB, phenobarbital; PE, partial epilepsy; PM, petit mal; SP, simple partial.

developmental differences in the ability of the brain to use ke-tone bodies. As a result, past studies suggested that the optimum age of response to the diet may be in young children before the onset of adolescence. Recent studies have challenged the belief that older patients could not maintain therapeutic ketosis or comply with the rigors of the diet, and that the ketogenic diet was less efficacious in this age group. Sirven et al. [1999] reviewed the tolerability, efficacy, and adverse events in 11 adult patients prospectively begun on the classic ketogenic diet for refractory symptomatic epilepsy. All were on stable medication, and had not achieved seizure control with two or more medications; four had prior surgery. At eight months of follow-up, 1 patient was seizure-free, 5 patients had a greater than 50 percent decrease in seizure frequency, 1 patient had a less than 50 percent seizure decrease, and 4 patients discontinued the diet. Common adverse events included gastrointestinal complaints (100 percent), menstrual irregularities in all women, and increased serum cholesterol and cholesterol high-density lipoprotein (HDL) ratios. Subjective improvements in thinking and mood, without a decrease in AEDs, were reported in 7 patients, 1 without improved seizure control. Mady et al. reviewed their experience with 45 adolescents who had been on the ketogenic diet for an average duration of 1.2 years [Mady et al., 2003]. They found no evidence to support the belief that the diet was not efficacious and was too restrictive in this age group. Adolescents with multiple seizure types did best, and those with simple and complex partial seizures had the poorest response. The retention rate for motivated adolescents on the diet was not significantly different than reports in younger children.

Recent studies have critically re-examined the benefits of the diet in selected groups of patients (see Table 60-3). Schwartz et al. [1989a, 1989b] reported on the results of metabolic profiles and seizure control in 59 epileptic children receiving a normal diet or one of three forms of the ketogenic diet:

1. a classical diet (four-to-one ratio of fat to protein and carbohydrate)
2. a medium-chain triglyceride (MCT) diet
3. a modified medium-chain triglyceride diet.

Patients fasted for 18 hours and then were placed on one of the diets and monitored for 6 weeks. All three diets produced a significant increase in total ketone body (aceto-acetate, β-hydroxybutyrate) levels that was most marked using the classical ketogenic diet [Freeman et al., 2000]. Ketone body concentrations reached a maximum in the afternoon and were frequently lower in the morning. Urinary ketones were measured and reflected changes noted in the serum. All three diets improved seizure control and none was superior to the others during the 6 weeks of observation. The first randomized trial of the classical and medium-chain triglyceride ketogenic diets was performed about 20 years later, and confirmed comparable efficacy over a longer follow-up period (1 year) [Neal et al., 2009]. Overall, these investigators found that 81 percent of patients had greater than a 45 percent reduction in seizures. Drowsiness, which occurred in 25 percent of patients during initiation of the diet, usually resolved. The medium-chain triglyceride diet was considered less palatable and associated with more side effects, including diarrhea and vomiting.

Kinsman et al reviewed 59 patients with severe intractable epilepsy; 80 percent had multiple seizure types; and 88 percent were on multiple AEDs [Kinsman et al., 1992]. Improved seizure control occurred in 67 percent of patients; 64 percent were able to reduce the amount of AEDs they were taking; 36 percent became more alert; and 23 percent had better behavior. Comorbid neurologic conditions in this group of patients with refractory epilepsy included mental retardation (84 percent), microcephaly (15 percent), and cerebral palsy (45 percent). Seizure type did not predict success with the diet. Additionally, 75 percent of the improved patients continued the diet for at least 18 months, confirming the efficacy and palatability of the diet and willingness to continue administration of the diet on the part of patients and their families. This study confirmed the earlier work by Livingston, demonstrating that 52 percent of patients had complete control and an additional 27 percent had improved control [Livingston, 1972].

The first multicenter prospective study of the efficacy of the ketogenic diet was based on data collected at seven comprehensive epilepsy centers [Vining et al., 1998]. All children in this study had intractable epilepsy, averaging 230 seizures per month. It was found that 10 percent of treated patients were seizure-free at 1 year. A greater than 50 percent decrease in seizure frequency was observed at 3 months in 54 percent of patients. This improvement was maintained at 6 (53 percent controlled) and 12 months (49 percent controlled) after initiation of the diet. Patient age, seizure type, and EEG abnormalities were not related to outcome. Approximately 47 percent remained on the diet for at least 1 year. Reasons for discontinuation included insufficient seizure control, intolerable side effects, concurrent medical illnesses, or inability to tolerate the restrictive nature of the dietary regimen. Although the number of patients was small, the study demonstrated that the diet could be used effectively in different epilepsy centers with different support staff, and that children and their families were able to comply with the diet when it was effective.

The first large prospective evaluation of the ketogenic diet was conducted in 150 consecutive children aged 1–16 years (mean age 5.3 years) [Freeman et al., 1998a]. The children were followed for a minimum of 1 year, had previously been on an average of 6.24 medications, and were on a mean of 1.97 medications at the diet's initiation. Seventy percent of children had an intelligence or developmental quotient of <69. The children averaged 410 seizures per month before the ketogenic diet. At 6 months, 71 percent remained on the diet and 32 percent had a greater than 90 percent decrease in seizures. At 1 year, 55 percent remained on the diet, 7 percent were seizure-free, and 27 percent had a greater than 90 percent decrease in seizure frequency. There was no statistically significant difference in seizure control based on age, sex, or seizure type, although none of the patients had only partial seizures. Most of those discontinuing the diet did so because it was either insufficiently effective or too restrictive.

All of the prior reports of efficacy of the ketogenic diet described open-label trials. Only one randomized, blinded crossover study has been performed. This study evaluated the efficacy of ketogenic diet for atonic-myclonic or drop seizures associated with Lennox–Gastaut syndrome [Freeman and Vining, 1999; Freeman, 2009; Freeman et al., 2009b]. Twenty children, experiencing at least 15 atonic seizures per day, were fasted for 36 hours, and then received the ketogenic diet for 1 week, in conjunction with a solution of glucose or saccharin. They then crossed over to the other study arm for an additional week. Physicians and parents were blinded to the solution composition and level of ketosis. Fasting and the ketogenic diet resulted in a decrease in the numbers of atonic seizures, which was only partially reversed with the addition of the glucose solution. The improvement in seizure control seen even in the glucose arm may explain the effectiveness of the less restrictive diets (Atkins-like and low glycemic).

A single randomized controlled trial of the ketogenic diet has been performed in children aged 2–16 years [Neal et al., 2008a]. Children with various seizure types or epilepsy syndromes experiencing daily seizures were recruited. They were randomly assigned to receive the ketogenic diet immediately (n = 73), or after a 3-month delay, with no other changes in their treatment (n = 72, control group). Children were also randomly assigned to the classic or the MCT ketogenic diet. After 3 months, the percentage of patients with baseline numbers of seizures despite treatment was significantly lower (p <0.0001) in the diet group (62 percent) than in the controls (136.9 percent). The children in the diet group had a mean of 13.3 seizures per day at baseline, and after 3 months of treatment, 1 was seizure-free; 28 (38 percent) had a greater than 50 percent reduction in seizures and 5 (7 percent) had a greater than 90 percent reduction. Efficacy was the same for symptomatic generalized or symptomatic focal epilepsies. The most common adverse events were constipation, vomiting, lack of energy, and hunger.

The same authors reported on the 1-year follow-up of those children randomized to the classic or MCT versions of the ketogenic diet [Neal et al., 2009]. Of the 125 children who started the diets, data from 64 were available at 6 months, and from 47 at 12 months. At 12 months, there was no significant difference between groups in number achieving greater than 50 percent (17.8 vs. 22.2 percent) or 90 percent (9.6 vs. 9.7 percent) seizure reduction. There was no significant difference in tolerability of the diet, except increased reports of lack of energy after 3 months, and vomiting after 12 months, both in the classical group.

In recent years, two alternative diet regimens that are less restrictive and perhaps more palatable have emerged: the modified Atkins diet [Kossoff and Dorward, 2008a] and a low glycemic index treatment [Pfeifer et al., 2008] (Figure 60-1). No prospective, comparative trials have been performed with the three treatments to evaluate relative efficacy and side-effect profiles. The Atkins diet is less restrictive than the ketogenic diet. The modified Atkins diet is similar in fat composition to a 1:1 ketogenic ratio diet, with approximately 65 percent of the calories from fat sources; it can be started as an outpatient, with guidance from a nutritionist. Three out of 6 patients studied on this diet had a greater than 50 percent seizure reduction; 2 were seizure-free [Kossoff et al., 2003]. Subsequent studies in children, adolescents, and adults reveal that 45 percent have a 50–90 percent seizure reduction, and slightly over

25 percent have a greater than 90 percent seizure reduction (Table 60-5) [Kossoff et al., 2003, 2006, 2007, 2008b, 2008d; Kang et al., 2007b; Carrette et al., 2008; Ito et al., 2008; Weber et al., 2009; Porta et al., 2009; Kumada et al., 2010].

The low glycemic index treatment [Pfeifer et al., 2005; Pfeifer et al., 2008] includes approximately 20–30 percent of calories from protein and 60–70 percent from fat. Total carbohydrates are gradually decreased to 40–60 g/day (about 10 percent of calories), using foods with a low glycemic index [Foster-Powell et al., 2002]. A retrospective review of the efficacy of the low glycemic treatment demonstrated 50 percent of patients (n = 20) with refractory epilepsy experiencing a greater than 90 percent in seizure reduction [Pfeifer et al., 2005]. Of these 20 patients, 9 were transitioned from the ketogenic diet and 11 were initiated on the low glycemic treatment. Those with a greater than 90 percent seizure reduction had an average blood glucose level of 72.6 mg/dL. In a second retrospective review, 76 children on the low glycemic index diet – 42, 50, 54, 64, and 66 percent, respectively – achieved a greater than 50 percent seizure reduction from baseline seizure frequency at follow-up intervals •of 1, 3, 6, 9, and 12 months [Muzykewicz et al., 2009]. Efficacy did not differ between partial onset and generalized seizure types. Increased efficacy was correlated with lower serum glucose levels at the 1- and 12-month follow-up visits. Side effects were minimal, with only three patients reporting transient lethargy. Children were placed on the low glycemic treatment for several reasons:

1. Families thought their child could not comply with the ketogenic diet
2. There was a more than 2-week wait for admission to initiate the ketogenic diet
3. The child and family were unable to tolerate the restrictive ketogenic diet

These reports raise important questions about the level of restrictiveness of protein and calorie intake necessary for seizure control.

Mechanism of Action

While clinical reports support the efficacy of the ketogenic diet, several theories have emerged to explain the diet's mechanism of action [Schwartzkroin, 1999]. Four major areas have been investigated: cerebral acidosis; water balance; the direct effect of ketones or lipids; and alteration in brain energy substrates. The importance of ketone body formation was recognized early in the search for the mechanism of action of the ketogenic diet [McQuarrie and Keith, 1927]. Initially, acidosis and partial dehydration were considered likely contributors to its success [Lennox, 1928; Bridge and Lob, 1931]. Even recently, the diet's effects on water and electrolyte metabolism were thought

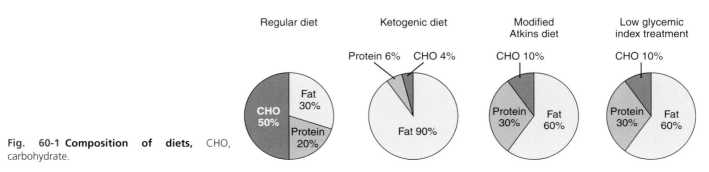

Fig. 60-1 Composition of diets, CHO, carbohydrate.

Table 60-5 Efficacy of the Modified Atkins Diet

Author	No. of Patients	Age (Yrs) of Patients	Seizure Type	% Success Rate	Comments
Kossoff et al [2003]	6	7–52	CP, GA, A, GTC, multiple	3/6 had seizure reduction 2 seizure-free for over 4 mo	Retrospective
Kossoff et al [2006]	20	3–18 (mean 8.1)	Not given	16/20 (80%) completed 6 mo; 11/20 remained on diet at 10 mo At 6 mo: 65% had >50% improvement 35% had >90% improvement 4/7 seizure-free	Prospective
Kang et al [2007b]	14	2–14	CP, LGS, Doose's syndrome	At 6 mo: 7 on diet 5/7 (36%) had >50% seizure reduction 3/7 seizure-free	Prospective
Kossoff et al [2007]	20	4–15 (mean 7.5)	CP, Generalized or multifocal epilepsy	12 completed 6-mo trial: 10 (50%) had >50% improvement 7 (35%) had >90% improvement 2 seizure-free	Prospective, randomized, crossover study (10 vs. 20 g of carbohydrate/day); 10 g/day more likely to have >50% seizure reduction at 3 mo
Carrette et al [2008]	8	31–55 (mean 41.8)	CP, LGS	3 completed 6-mo trial: 1/3 (12.5%) had >50% seizure reduction	Prospective
Kossoff et al [2008d]	30	18–53 (median 31)	CP, A, multiple types	14 completed 6-mo study: 8 (30%) had >50% improvement 1 seizure-free	Prospective, open-label
Kossoff et al [2008b]	1	2	LGS	At 15 mo: Seizures >90% decreased	
Ito et al [2008]	1	7	GTC		Used as replacement for ketogenic diet, to treat glucose transporter type 1 deficiency syndrome
Weber et al [2009]	15	2/17 (median 10)	CP, LGS, A, JME, Doose's syndrome	12 completed 6-mo study: 6 (40%) had >50% improvement 2 (13%) had >90% improvement	Prospective, open label
Porta et al [2009]	10	0.5–15	CP, IS, LGS, GTC	5 completed, median duration 3 mo: 2 (20%) had >50% improvement at 6 mo	Retrospective
Kumada et al [2009]	2	4–5	Nonconvulsive status epilepticus	Free of status epilepticus for 4 and 19 mo respectively	Retrospective

A, absence; CP, complex partial or partial onset ± secondary generalization; GA, generalized atonic; GTC, generalized tonic clonic; IS, infantile spasms; JME, juvenile myoclonic epilepsy; LGS, Lennox–Gastaut syndrome.

responsible for its efficacy [Millichap et al., 1964]. Animal studies show no change in intracellular pH of the cerebral cortex on the ketogenic diet [Al-Mudallal et al., 1996; Harik et al., 1997]. Preliminary studies using MR spectroscopy have demonstrated that children on the diet do not develop alteration of brain water and electrolyte distribution [Seymour et al., 1999] or cerebral acidosis [Marks et al., 1997; Seymour et al., 1999]. This suggests that, although ketoacidosis occurs in these children, changes in brain pH may not be a critical factor. Animal models and human evidence suggest a prominent role of ketonemia [Uhlemann and Neims, 1972; Appleton and DeVivo, 1973, 1974; DeVivo et al., 1975; Al-Mudallal et al., 1995; Stafstrom, 1999a]. One study considered elevated plasma lipids a predictor of seizure control in children [Dekaban, 1966]. A subsequent analysis of blood metabolites in nine children on the ketogenic diet revealed that a rise in total serum arachidonate correlated with improved seizure control [Fraser et al., 2003]. Despite its long history of use and proven value, the exact mechanism of action of the diet remains unknown [Nordli and DeVivo, 1997].

Oxidation of Fatty Acids: Ketogenesis

Ketonemia is essential for the ketogenic diet to work. Ketonemia occurs as a result of fatty-acid oxidation during fasting or while on the ketogenic diet [Hawkins and Biebuyck, 1980; DeVivo, 1980; Cahill, 1982; Mayes, 1996a, 1996b]. Fatty-acid biosynthesis (lipogenesis) takes place in the cytosol, whereas fatty-acid oxidation occurs in mitochondria and generates adenosine triphosphate (ATP) [Roe and Coates, 1995]. The oxidizable substrate may come from dietary sources (ketogenic

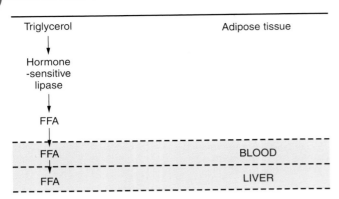

Triglycerol   Adipose tissue

Hormone
-sensitive
lipase

FFA

FFA   BLOOD

FFA   LIVER

Fig. 60-2 **Initial steps in ketogenesis: lipolysis.** FFA, frce fatty acids.

diet) or from mobilization of peripheral adipose stores (starvation) (Figure 60-2). The brain does not directly use fatty acids but readily oxidizes ketone bodies [Hawkins and Biebuyck, 1979, 1980]. Increased fatty-acid oxidation leading to ketone body formation by the liver is characteristic of starvation or the ketogenic diet (Figure 60-3) [Mayes, 1996a]. Glucose, present in small concentrations, is necessary to facilitate ketone body metabolism. This is referred to as the permissive effect of glucose. Acetoacetate, a ketone body constituent, continually undergoes spontaneous decarboxylation to yield acetone that is volatilized in the lungs and gives the breath its characteristic odor.

The liver is the only organ capable of synthesizing significant quantities of ketone bodies that are released into the blood (see

Figure 60-3). The liver is equipped with an active enzymatic mechanism for the production of acetoacetate. Once formed, acetoacetate cannot be significantly metabolized back to fatty acids in the liver because it lacks the enzyme 3-oxoacid-CoA transferase. This accounts for the net production of ketone bodies by the liver. Ketone bodies are then transported to and oxidized in extrahepatic tissues proportionately to their concentration in the blood. Oxidation and brain influx rates of ketone bodies are proportional to their blood concentration of approximately 12 mmol/L. At this level, the oxidative machinery and uptake mechanisms of the cell are saturated [Mayes, 1996a].

Glucose is the principal substrate for brain metabolism. Under certain conditions (e.g., fasting, ketogenic diet), the human brain uses ketone bodies for fuel [Owen et al., 1967]; the movement of ketone bodies into the brain is dependent on a monocarboxylic transport system [DeVivo, 1980]. Acetoacetate and β-hydroxybutyrate (BHB), the two constituents of ketone bodies, are metabolized primarily in the mitochondrial compartment. In the brain, the main pathway for the conversion of acetoacetate to acetoacetyl-CoA involves succinyl-CoA (Figure 60-4). Acetoacetyl-CoA is split to acetyl-CoA and oxidized in the tricarboxylic acid cycle. The enzymes that break down BHB and acetoacetate into acetyl CoA are regulated developmentally, with maximal expression early in life [Hawkins et al., 1971; Dahlquist et al., 1972; Nehlig, 1999]. This is consistent with the higher utilization of ketones by the brain in children compared to adults [Kraus et al., 1974]. Ketone bodies not only serve as a source of energy, but also contribute to the synthesis of the neurotransmitters, glutamate and

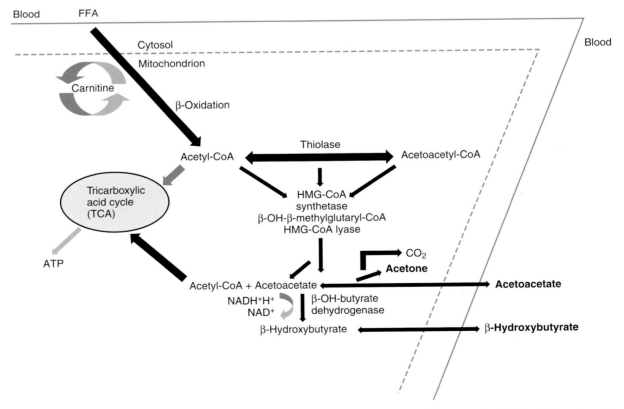

Fig. 60-3 **Ketogenesis in the liver.** Free fatty acids (FFA) from the circulation enter the hepatocyte and then cross the mitochondrial membrane by carnitine transport (long-chain fatty acids) or diffusion (short- and medium-chain fatty acids). ATP, adenosine triphosphate.

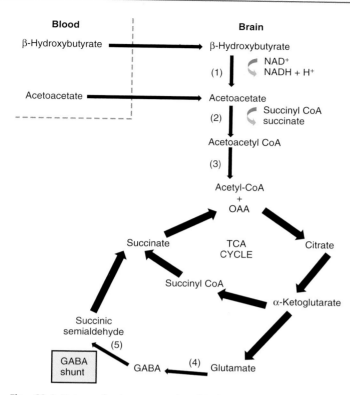

Fig. 60-4 Ketone body use and oxidation in the brain. 1, β-hydroxybutyrate dehydrogenase; 2, 3-oxoacid coenzyme A (CoA) transferase; 3, acetoacetyl-CoA thiolase; 4, glutamic acid decarboxylase (GAD); 5, γ-aminobutyric acid (GABA). OOA, oxaloacetate; TCA, tricarboxylic acid cycle.

gamma-aminobutyric acid (GABA), cerebral metabolic pathways normally dependent on glucose metabolism [Cremer, 1971; Sokoloff, 1973; DeLorey and Olsen, 1994; Rodwell, 1996; Cooper et al., 1996; Yudkoff et al., 2007; Lund et al., 2009]. Furthermore, fatty-acid oxidation increases brain ATP concentration [Mayes, 1996a, 1996b]. Elevation of brain ATP concentration has been verified in an animal model of the ketogenic diet [DeVivo et al., 1978; Nakazawa et al., 1983], suggesting that the ketogenic diet improves cerebral energetics. Increased alpha-ketoglutarate on the diet may also increase activity of the GABA$_A$ shunt [DeVivo, 1980; McGeer and McGeer, 1989; Peng et al., 1993]. Although whole-brain GABA levels are not changed in an animal model of chronic ketosis [Al-Mudallal et al., 1996; Harik et al., 1997], local changes in GABA concentration may occur [Rho et al., 1999b; Yudkoff et al., 2001a]. Two children studied with a new technology, two-dimensional double-quantum MR spectroscopy, showed low initial GABA levels that increased over time on the ketogenic diet [Wang et al., 2003]. The addition of acetoacetate or BHB to rat synaptosomes increased the rate of GABA formation by 35 and 43 percent, respectively [Erecinska et al., 1996]. The addition of β-hydroxybutyrate to cultured rat astrocytes suppresses GABA-transaminase in time- and dose-dependent manners [Suzuki et al., 2009]. This suppression of astrocytic GABA degradation may be another mechanism for increased GABA concentration. At the same time, the conversion of glutamate to aspartate, which has excitatory properties in the brain, is reduced [Erecinska et al., 1996; Yudkoff et al., 1997; Yudkoff et al., 2001b]. Thus, improved cerebral energetics,

along with decreased excitatory (glutamatergic) and increased inhibitory (GABAergic) neurotransmission, may contribute to the efficacy of the ketogenic diet [Peyron et al., 1994; Greene et al., 2003].

Clinical Studies

Ketonemia is necessary but not sufficient for ketogenic diet-induced seizure control [Vining, 1999b; Stafstrom and Spencer, 2000]. Urine ketones are the only readily available inexpensive approach to ketone assessment, and typically the desired range is 80–160 mmol/L. Seizure control correlates significantly (p = 0.03) with serum BHB levels greater than 4 mmol/L, although urine ketones of 160 mmol/L can be found when blood BHB levels exceed 2 mmol/L [Gilbert et al., 2000]. Although serum ketones, particularly BHB, are believed to reflect the immediate state of ketosis more accurately, it is not certain if it is the presence of these ketone bodies that produces the antiseizure effect. Brown et al. [1998] measured serum BHB levels during routine clinic visits and during illness in 12 children. Eight experienced an increase in seizures and decrease in BHB during illness, and 4 had no seizure increase and no lowering of BHB levels. This suggests that BHB levels are important for the anti-seizure effect. Subsequently, Freeman et al. [1998] evaluated serum BHB levels of 35 children 3 months after diet initiation. There was a significant correlation between higher levels of BHB and seizure control. The mean serum BHB level in patients with greater than 90 percent seizure control was over 6 mM.

It is also accepted that the classic ketogenic diet produces the most ketone bodies [Schwartz et al., 1989a]. Despite the fact that ketone bodies partially replace glucose for cerebral metabolism [DeVivo, 1980; Haymond et al., 1983], cerebral glucose levels are unaltered [DeVivo et al., 1978; Al-Mudallal et al., 1995]. Ketones from the circulation are transported across the blood–brain barrier by facilitated diffusion, using a monocarboxylate transport system [Moore et al., 1976; Pellerin et al., 1998]. The efficacy of the diet in childhood and the apparent slightly lower efficacy in older children and adults may be due to maturational changes in this transport system [Persson et al., 1972; Kraus et al., 1974; Dodson et al., 1976; Dahlquist and Persson, 1976; DeVivo, 1980; Williamson, 1985]. A child's ability to extract ketones from the blood into the brain is 4–5 times greater than that seen in adults [DeVivo, 1983]. However, even adult animals placed on the ketogenic diet can upregulate brain monocarboxylate transporter levels [Leino et al., 2001]. MR spectroscopy has documented the fact that both fasting and intravenous BHB infusion in humans increase brain BHB levels [Pan et al., 2000, 2001]. However, proton MR spectroscopy (^{1}H-MRS) performed in occipital gray matter in five children on the ketogenic diet demonstrated a single resonance identified as acetone, and no detectable BHB or acetoacetate [Seymour et al., 1999]. Subsequent experiments in rats and mice showed that acetone is an anticonvulsant and that chronic administration may enhance its action [Likhodii et al., 2002, 2003; Rho et al., 2002]. MR spectroscopy has also been used to study changes in cerebral energetics induced by the ketogenic diet. Alteration of tricarboxylic acid cycle activity by ketosis, resulting in an increased adenosine triphosphate to adenosine diphosphate (ATP:ADP) ratio or greater cerebral energy, has been hypothesized to have an anticonvulsant effect [Masino and Geiger, 2008]. This hypothesis is supported by recent experiments in patients with

Lennox–Gastaut syndrome that used MR spectroscopy (^{31}P) to document improvement in cerebral energy metabolism on the ketogenic diet [Pan et al., 1999].

Additionally, during chronic ketosis, adaptive mechanisms are active that increase the cerebral extraction of ketone bodies [Gjedde and Crone, 1975]. These mechanisms may be why ketosis develops promptly within several days after initiation of the diet, but the anticonvulsant effect may be delayed for 1–2 weeks [Appleton and Devivo, 1973, 1974]. This observation suggests that ketosis per se is insufficient to explain the anticonvulsant effect. Once ketone bodies are extracted, it is postulated that there is a secondary biochemical change or a cascade of biochemical effects that has some form of anticonvulsant effect [Prasad et al., 1996].

The importance of ketosis was demonstrated by Huttenlocher in 1976. He studied two children with a prior history of myoclonic seizures, who were seizure-free on the ketogenic diet. After a 50-minute infusion of glucose, the first patient's serum ketones decreased 67 percent, with no change in serum pH, and a seizure occurred. The second child's EEG changed from normal to diffuse polyspike and slow-wave complexes accompanied by myoclonic jerks after 90 minutes of intravenous glucose. Another study, involving nine children with intractable atypical absence seizures treated with the MCT diet, noted a significant decrease in the mean number of epileptiform discharges in treated patients [Ross et al., 1985]. A rise in serum ketones was the only prominent early biochemical change. DeVivo et al. also reported two children suffering from seizures resulting from a glucose transporter type I defect who were treated with the ketogenic diet and achieved complete control of seizures and improvement in neurologic development [DeVivo et al., 1991]. These observations and others suggest a pivotal role for ketone bodies in providing an alternative energy source and in achieving a still unknown role in seizure control [DeVivo, 1983; Schwartz et al., 1989b; Huttenlocher, 1976; Livingston, 1954; Aicardi, 1992; DeVivo et al., 1978; Withrow, 1980; Millichap et al., 1964; Lamers et al., 1995].

Experimental studies

At the present time, there are several animal models used to study the effects of the ketogenic diet. (For review, see Stafstrom [1999a]; Bough et al. [2002]; Stafstrom and Bough [2003]; Bough and Stafstrom [2004]; Hartman et al. [2007]; Hartman et al. [2008]; Raffo et al. [2008].) In general, these animal models demonstrate that the ketogenic diet provides protection for partial-onset seizures with secondary generalization and generalized myoclonic, tonic, and tonic-clonic seizures. The mechanism appears to be a lowering of neuronal excitability and raising of seizure threshold [Thavendiranathan et al., 2003]. However, some studies have failed to show a protective effect of the ketogenic diet in models where animals were acutely challenged with a convulsant stimulus [Bough et al., 2000a, 2002; Thavendiranathan et al., 2000; Samala et al., 2008]. Differential efficacy in animal models undoubtedly relates to regional differences in protein phosphorylation and the concentration of GABA and other neurotransmitters, and differences between provoked and spontaneous seizures [Szot et al., 2001; Ziegler et al., 2002; Martillotti et al., 2006].

A limited number of animal studies have investigated the effect of age at diet onset versus efficacy. The diet provides a greater level of seizure protection to younger animals [Bough et al., 1999c; Rho et al., 1999a], but older animals also demonstrate an elevated seizure threshold [Appleton and DeVivo, 1974; Hori et al., 1997; Bough and Eagles, 1999b]. While it would seem intuitive that increasing ketonemia would correlate with efficacy of the ketogenic diet, experimental studies have not revealed a positive correlation between them [Bough et al., 1999a, 2000b; Likhodii et al., 2000]. However, rats that developed higher levels of ketosis also showed higher thresholds for seizure induction [Bough and Eagles, 1999b]. Caloric restriction can significantly influence seizure threshold and augment the effects of the ketogenic diet on seizure control [Bough et al., 2000a, 2002, 2003; Greene et al., 2001; Eagles et al., 2003; Mantis et al., 2004; Cheng et al., 2004]. A role for enhanced cerebral energetics in efficacy of the ketogenic diet was first proposed by DeVivo et al. [1978]. Bough et al. [2006] used gene expression profiling to confirm a coordinated upregulation of transcripts for genes encoding proteins involved in energy metabolism in adolescent rat hippocampus, including those specific to mitochondria, after maintenance on a ketogenic diet [Bough et al., 2006]. These data support the hypothesis that a ketogenic diet enhances brain metabolism. Several animal models provide evidence that the ketogenic diet can prevent epileptogenesis [Muller-Schwarze et al., 1999; Stafstrom et al., 1999b; Rho et al., 1999c, 2000; Su et al., 2000; Todorova et al., 2000; Bough et al., 2003; Kossoff and Rho, 2009a; Kossoff et al., 2009c] and mediate neuroprotection [Zieglar et al., 2003; Sullivan et al., 2004; Noh et al., 2005; Gasior et al., 2006; Maalouf et al., 2007; Kim and Rho, 2008; Maalouf et al., 2009]. These studies also support the clinical observation that children can be gradually weaned off the ketogenic diet, resume a normal diet, and not experience loss of seizure control.

Selection of Candidates for the Diet

Despite the fact that several thousand patients have been treated, there currently are no consensus criteria as to which patients are candidates for the diet [Maria et al., 1997] (see Tables 60-1 to 60-4). Many seizure types appear to respond to the ketogenic diet. In general, several groups of children are potential candidates for treatment. These include the following children:
1. those with medically intractable seizures
2. those with poor tolerance of or significant side effects from AEDs
3. those with intractable seizures who are being considered for epilepsy surgery (i.e., callosotomy; nonlesional, extratemporal resections)
4. those with specific neurometabolic disorders or neurologic syndromes (Box 60-1).

One must also consider the age of the patient. As previously discussed, successful outcomes have been experienced in children aged 1–12 years. In older children, it is often more difficult to maintain ketosis. The ketogenic diet is a strictly regulated medical diet. Its success depends on the accuracy and consistency with which the regimen is carried out within the home. Continued support, monitoring, and education by an interdisciplinary team of professionals are necessary.

Little is known about whether the ketogenic diet should be considered in patients who are being evaluated for epilepsy

Box 60-1 Specific Conditions Treated with the Ketogenic Diet

- Glucose transporter deficiency syndrome (GLUT1-DS, *SLC2A1* gene, McKusick 138140)*
- Pyruvate dehydrogenase complex deficiency (McKusick 312170)*
- Associated with Leigh's syndrome
- Associated with lactic acidosis and cerebral dysgenesis
- Succinic semialdehyde dehydrogenase (SSADH) deficiency†
- Phosphofructokinase deficiency
- Mitochondrial respiratory chain complex defects
- Ketotic hypoglycemia
- Glycogenosis type V (McArdle's disease)
- Acquired epileptiform opercular syndrome
- Acquired epileptic aphasia (Landau–Kleffner syndrome)
- Rett's syndrome
- Tuberous sclerosis complex

---

* The ketogenic diet is specifically indicated for these two metabolic disorders.
† Documented improvement in mouse model [Nylen et al., 2009].

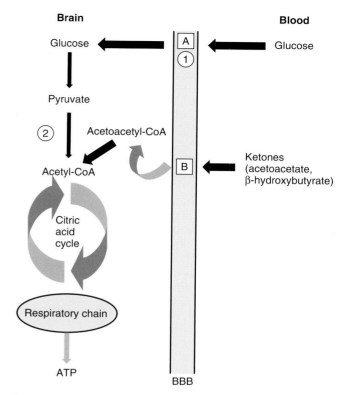

Fig. 60-5 Metabolic defects and the ketogenic diet. Glucose enters the brain by the glucose transporter, GLUT1 (A); ketones penetrate the blood-brain barrier (BBB) by the medium-chain triglyceride transporter (MCT1) (B). GLUT1 deficiency syndrome is caused by a defect in glucose transport into the brain (1). Pyruvate dehydrogenase deficiency impairs acetyl-CoA production (2). The ketogenic diet bypasses these two defects and provides acetyl-CoA for brain energy production. ATP, adenosine triphosphate.

surgery. Forty-seven children with intractable epilepsy and surgically remediable focal malformations of cortical development were treated with the ketogenic diet [Jung et al., 2008b]. Those seizure-free at 3 months continued on the diet, while the rest underwent surgery. The seizure-free rate at 2 years was similar between the two groups, leading the authors to suggest that, in potentially surgically remediable epilepsy, a 3-month trial of the ketogenic diet may be an option. However, in those patients in whom a malignancy or vascular malformation is detected, surgery is preferable. The ketogenic diet may be the preferred initial therapy in children with seizures and specific metabolic defects or seizures associated with specific neurologic syndromes (see Box 60-1 and Figure 60-5) [DeVivo et al., 1973, 1991; Haas et al., 1986; Wijburg et al., 1992; Shafrir and Prensky, 1995; Melvin et al., 1996; Wexler et al., 1997; Bergqvist et al., 1999b; Weber et al., 2001; Klepper et al., 2002, 2004; Liebhaber et al., 2003; Busch et al., 2005; Kang et al., 2005, 2007a; Kossoff et al., 2005b; Lee et al, 2008; Brockmann, 2009, Joshi et al., 2009; Mantis et al., 2009 – mouse model Rett's syndrome; Nylen et al., 2009 – mouse model SSADH; Seo et al., 2010]. These specific metabolic disorders are reviewed in other sections of this book.

For some patients, the ketogenic diet is contraindicated (Box 60-2). Children with acute intermittent porphyria should not be treated with the ketogenic diet because carbohydrate restriction can be harmful in this condition. The ketogenic diet may also worsen some mitochondrial diseases, pyruvate carboxylase deficiency, or organic acidurias [Demeritte et al., 1996b; Nordli, 2000; Kleinman, 2004; Kossoff et al., 2009b]. When indicated, metabolic screen, including urine amino and organic acids, serum amino acids, lactate, pyruvate, and carnitine profile, should be performed before starting the ketogenic diet [Wheless, 2001]. In addition, the combination of the use of the ketogenic diet with topiramate or zonisamide appears to be associated with an increased risk of acidosis.

Box 60-2 Specific Contraindications to the Ketogenic Diet

- Pyruvate carboxylase deficiency
- Organic acidurias
- Selected mitochondrial disease
- Porphyria
- Defects in fatty acid oxidation
  - Short-chain acyl dehydrogenase deficiency (SCAD)
  - Medium-chain acyl dehydrogenase deficiency (MCAD)
  - Long-chain acyl dehydrogenase deficiency (LCAD)
  - Medium-chain 3-hydroxyacyl CoA deficiency
  - Long-chain 3-hydroxyacyl CoA deficiency
- Carnitine deficiency (primary)
- Carnitine palmitoyltransferase (CPI) I or II deficiency
- Carnitine translocase deficiency
- Glutaric aciduria, type II
- Pyruvate dehydrogenase phosphate deficiency

Candidate Selection and the EEG

The predictive value of an EEG obtained before, during, or after initiation of the ketogenic diet is unknown. In a cohort of 29 children, 90 percent of children with normal pretreatment EEGs responded favorably to the diet, compared with only

12 percent with abnormal pretreatment EEGs [Eley, 1933]. Penfield and Erickson [1941] determined that those patients with abnormal hyperventilation studies were more likely to respond to the diet. Livingston [1954] reported on the EEG findings in 102 patients and found that those patients who did best on the diet had petit mal variants. Compared to other children with epilepsy, children with multifocal spikes did less well at 3 months, but showed no difference at 6 or 12 months [Vining et al., 1998].

Many studies, including the original works of Bridge [1949], Livingston [1954], and Keith [1963], have suggested improvement or normalization of the EEG after the diet has been implemented. Nellhaus [1971] correlated normalization of the EEG with the onset of ketosis, clinical improvement, and prognosis. Others have noted that EEG improvement may be seen with clinical improvement in patients with minor motor and petit mal seizures, but not in those with focal or grand mal seizures [Janaki et al., 1976]. Children with atypical absence seizures demonstrated a significant decrease in the number of epileptiform discharges at initiation of MCT therapy. However, their EEGs were unchanged from baseline at the end of a 10-week treatment period, despite two-thirds having a greater than 50 percent decrease in seizure frequency [Ross et al., 1985]. In one study, background EEG improvements correlated with a significant reduction in seizures [Demeritte et al., 1996a]. Kang et al. showed improvement in generalized epileptiform abnormalities more often than focal epileptiform discharges, and a correlation between seizure control and EEG improvement [Kang et al., 2005]. Carraballo also reported improvement in the EEG epileptiform abnormalities in children responding to the diet [Carraballo et al., 2005]. Correlation between EEG improvement and reduction in clinical seizures, and between improvement in interictal discharges and improvement in background, was variable in studies of ambulatory 24-hour EEGs [Freeman and Vining, 1999; Hallbook et al., 2007a; Remahl et al., 2008], perhaps because of differences in seizure type and patient population among these studies.

Initiation and Maintenance

A comprehensive monograph on the evaluation and management of patients being considered for placement on the ketogenic diet was published [Freeman et al., 1994] and subsequently revised [Freeman et al., 2000]. In addition, a videotape, "The Ketogenic Diet for Families, Dietitians, Nurses and Physicians," and other resource material are available from The Charlie Foundation (www.charliefoundation.org). The following is a brief overview of how the diet can be implemented.

Prehospital evaluation

Once a child is considered a candidate for the diet, a screening evaluation by selected members of the team responsible for implementing the diet is initiated. This screening usually includes a comprehensive evaluation by the dietitians and nursing staff. The purpose of this evaluation is to educate the family and to assess their ability, on many levels, to carry out the rigorous and exacting program necessary to maximize the diet's success. At the same time, the different types of meal plans and foods that the child can eat are discussed, along with their preparation. Issues involved in this evaluation are carefully considered and reviewed by Casey et al. [1999] and Freeman et al. [2000].

Hospitalization

The child is typically scheduled for elective admission to the hospital for initiation of the ketogenic diet (Box 60-3). However, in recent years, both retrospective [Vaisleib et al., 2004] and prospective studies [Rizzutti et al., 2007] have documented the feasibility of initiating the diet as an outpatient. The intense educational process afforded by inpatient initiation may be preferable for some families and ketogenic diet centers. Additionally, inpatient initiation allows observation of the child to gauge the initial response to and adverse effects of the diet. Parents are told to view this treatment as a 6–8-week trial. When effective, the ketogenic diet works quickly, typically within the first 1–2 weeks [Kossoff et al., 2008c]. The time to improvement is significantly quicker (mean 5 vs. 14 days, $p < 0.01$) in those children who are fasted at onset, but there is no effect of initial fasting on long-term outcome. If there is no seizure reduction after 6–8 weeks, the ketogenic diet can be discontinued. During this time, patients must adhere strictly to the diet, with proof of persistent ketosis. The frequency of seizures usually decreases gradually, but reversal of the effect can occur rapidly. Weeks of hard work can be undone if a child eats a cookie or a piece of candy. If the seizures are improved, this usually is sufficient motivation for the parents to have the child adhere to the diet. If the child might have an underlying metabolic disease that could be exacerbated by the initial fast, an appropriate evaluation should be performed before initiating the diet. Valproate has been demonstrated experimentally to reduce fasting ketonemia [Turnbull et al., 1986; Thurston et al., 1983]. Clinically, valproate has not impaired the ability to initiate the ketogenic diet or achieve adequate ketosis, nor has it altered the diet's side-effect profile or efficacy [Lyczkowski et al., 2005].

Box 60-3 Initiation of the Ketogenic Diet

Hospitalization for 3 Days

Day 1
- Maintenance fluids
- Check urine ketones each void
- Check fingerstick blood glucose every 6 hr
- Initial EEG, laboratory tests
- Simplify antiepileptic drug (AED) regimen; change to low carbohydrate or carbohydrate-free formulation
- Dietitian consultation
- Education

Day 2
- 4:1 ratio (3:1 in infants), with one-third of total calories using eggnog for 2–3 meals
- Then two-thirds of total calories for 2–3 meals
- Stop fingerstick blood glucose checks

Day 3
- First regular meal on 4:1 ratio
- Discharge – AED regimen
- B vitamins, sugar-free multivitamin
- Calcium supplements

The day before hospital admission, the parents are asked to eliminate carbohydrates from the child's diet. The child eats foods that contain only protein or fat. After dinner, the child begins fasting, with only noncaloric, noncaffeinated beverages given. On the first hospital day, an awake-and-sleeping EEG may be performed. Laboratory studies (complete blood count, platelet count, chemistry panel, and AED levels) are obtained, either before or at the time of admission. During this time, the child receives maintenance fluids and may have one caffeine-free diet drink per day. Blood glucose levels are checked every 6 hours. The dietitian uses this time for further review of meal plans and the child's food preferences and eating habits with the parents [Lasser and Brush, 1973]. Recent studies [Vaisleib et al., 2004; Kim et al., 2004; Bergqvist et al., 2005; Kang et al., 2005; Kossoff et al., 2008c] have suggested no improvement in seizure control with initial fasting or fluid restriction, and fewer adverse events with a nonfasting, gradual initiation. On day one, the child is started on the ketogenic diet, using a 3:1 or 4:1 ratio (fat to protein plus carbohydrate), depending on the child's age. A ketogenic eggnog is used for the initial feedings. The child receives three meals at one-third of the total calories, is advanced as tolerated to two-thirds of the total calories for three meals (day 2), and then eats his or her first full meal. Before discharge, the parents prepare their first ketogenic meal for their child under the supervision of the dietitian. At discharge, the parents have several meal plans for their child and are instructed to monitor the urine ketones on a daily basis and record all occurrences of seizures. Individual decisions are made during the hospital stay as to whether the AED regimen will be simplified. The child is given a prescription for sugar-free multivitamin, mineral, and calcium supplementation and instructed to begin this at home. Vitamin B supplements are given to prevent optic nerve dysfunction [Hoyt and Billson, 1979]. Vitamin D supplementation and calcium prevent osteomalacia while on the ketogenic diet [Hahn et al., 1979]. Inadvertent administration of carbohydrates may occur when intercurrent illnesses are treated. Parents and pediatricians must appreciate that decongestants, antipyretics, and antibiotics are often contained in carbohydrate-containing vehicles [Feldstein, 1996; Freeman et al., 2000; Lebel et al., 2001; McGhee and Katyal, 2001]. The child is then seen regularly for follow-up (Box 60-4). Special attention should be paid to the serum albumin and total protein concentration to make sure that the diet is providing enough protein. Cholesterol and triglyceride levels typically rise when the diet is started, but the diet may be continued unless the cholesterol level rises above 1000 mg/dL and consistently stays there. It is not known whether cholesterol-reducing drugs could be safely given while the child is maintained on the diet. It is not unusual to see minor elevations in the direct bilirubin. Decisions regarding withdrawal of AEDs depend on the child's response to the diet and the family's wishes. Early reduction (during diet initiation or the first month afterward) of AEDs appears to be safe and well tolerated; however, it offers no definite advantage compared with a late taper [Kossoff et al., 2004]. At follow-up, the dietitian also reviews the parental concerns about implementing the diet, and makes adjustments in the meal plan, as necessary, to maintain the child in maximum ketosis. If the child is in apparent maximum ketosis (i.e., urine ketones are more than 160 mg/dL) and seizures recur, this might be the result of caloric excess, which may be manifested by excessive weight gain. Lowering the total caloric and carbohydrate intake may help reduce the number of seizure

Box 60-4 Ketogenic Diet Maintenance

1. Month
- Neurologist, dietitian, nurse, social worker
- Adjust diet as needed
- Laboratory tests – complete blood count (CBC), platelets; SMA20; antiepileptic drug (AED) level(s); serum lipid and carnitine profiles
- Urine calcium, creatinine

3, 6, and 12 Months
- Neurologist, dietitian, nurse
- Laboratory tests – CBC, platelets, SMA20; serum lipid and carnitine profiles
- AED level(s), if needed, and urine calcium, creatinine
- New meals

Maintain for 2 Years (Seizure-Free)
- (Shorter time interval for infantile spasms)

Wean over 1 Year
- 3-5:1–3 months → 3:1–3 months →
- 2.5:1–3 months → 2:1–3 mohths →
- Off

recurrences. If the child is not in maximum ketosis, this may be due to a break in the diet (e.g., "cheating" or taking medicine with sugar) or a lower than 4:1 ratio of fat to protein and carbohydrate. In children who can be successfully withdrawn from AED therapy and are seizure-free for 2 years on the ketogenic diet (about 10 percent of treated children), an EEG is repeated and the ketogenic diet is slowly withdrawn over 1 year. Many of these families elect to continue a low-carbohydrate diet, concerned that seizures may recur.

Complications

It needs to be stressed to parents that the diet is a form of medical therapy, and as such, although it is relatively safe, it is not without side effects (Box 60-5 and Box 60-6) [Ballaban-Gil et al., 1996; Wheless, 2001; Kang et al., 2004]. However, only

Box 60-5 Possible Adverse Events During Initiation of the Ketogenic Diet

Adverse Event	Monitoring/Treatment Strategy
Dehydration	Encourage fluids (do not limit fluids to less than 75% of maintenance); intravenous fluids if necessary (without dextrose)
Hypoglycemia	Check blood sugars every 6 hr until diet is initiated; if symptomatic or blood sugar <30 mg/dL, give orange juice. Screen for metabolic errors in advance
Vomiting	Intravenous fluids; give orange juice

Box 60-6 Possible Adverse Events During Maintenance of the Ketogenic Diet

Adverse Event	Monitoring/Treatment Strategy
■ Constipation	■ Polyethylene glycol, mineral oil, suppositories
■ Exacerbation of gastroesophageal reflux disease	■ Medical management
■ Poor growth	■ Check albumin, total protein ■ Adequate protein ■ Monitor height, weight
■ Kidney stones	■ Urine dipstick for blood, renal ultrasonography ■ Analyze stone (specific treatment) ■ Increase fluids, alkalinize urine
■ Dyslipidemia, hyperlipidemia	■ Check liver function tests, lipid profile; if sustained elevations of cholesterol/ triglycerides, adjust diet and/or treat
■ Prolonged QT interval, cardiomyopathy	■ Electrocardiography, echocardiography, check selenium
■ Excessive bruising	■ Complete blood count, platelet count
■ Optic neuropathy	■ B vitamins
■ Elevated very-long-chain fatty acids	■ Check prior to ketogenic diet if clinically suspected
■ Vitamin D deficiency, osteomalacia	■ Vitamin D, calcium, bone mineral density/densitometry
■ Trace mineral deficiencies	■ Copper, selenium, zinc

6–17 percent of patients discontinue the diet for medical reasons [Thompson et al., 1998; Vining et al., 1998; Kang et al., 2004; Henderson et al., 2006]. If the child has an unrecognized metabolic defect, a catastrophic event could occur during the fasting phase (see Box 60-2). Other adverse events can occur during the initial hospital stay, and, if recognized, are usually easily treated (see Box 60-6). A number of adverse events can occur during the maintenance phase. Many can be prevented with close monitoring, vitamin supplementation, and anticipatory treatment. The most common side effect encountered is constipation, which can be reduced if a calcium supplement with magnesium is given. Many of the children who begin the diet are already prone to this problem because of limited mobility, hypotonia, or spasticity. Constipation can be treated with regular doses of polyethylene glycol, mineral oil, intermittent pediatric-dose enemas, or magnesium hydroxide. Renal stones have occurred in less than 5–10 percent of patients, and can usually be easily managed [Herzberg et al., 1990; Freeman et al., 1994, 2000; Casey et al., 1999; Chesney et al., 1999; Furth et al., 2000; Kaytal et al., 2000; Kielb et al., 2000; Maydell et al., 2001; Nordli et al., 2001; Kossoff et al., 2002; Sampath et al., 2007]. The risk of stone formation may be increased in younger patients (<3 years of age), and those with hypercalciuria and low urine volume [Furth et al., 2000;

Sampath et al., 2007]. Children can be screened for hypercalciuria (urine creatinine: calcium), and fluid intake can be maximized to minimize risk of nephrolithiasis. Even children who develop renal calculi, however, may be able to remain on the ketogenic diet. Evaluation to determine the type of renal stone and the patient's urinary calcium–creatinine ratio is necessary [Gillespie and Stapleton, 2004]. If renal stones appear to be due to hypercalciuria, then the patient can be treated with hydrochlorothiazide (2 mg/kg/day), given polycitra to alkalinize the urine, and monitored with repeated urinary studies and renal ultrasound. If the calcium–creatinine ratios normalize or dramatically improve and no additional renal stones occur, then the diet can be maintained. Oral potassium citrate as a preventative supplement results in urine alkalinization, decreasing the prevalence of kidney stones [Sampath et al., 2007]. Universal supplementation appears to be warranted.

Acetazolamide, which is sometimes used to treat certain forms of seizures, should not be used during initiation of the diet for fear of producing symptomatic metabolic acidosis [Dodson et al., 1976]. Topiramate and zonisamide are weak carbonic anhydrase inhibitors, which, when combined with the ketogenic diet, predispose to metabolic acidosis. The ketogenic diet can be cautiously initiated in children on these drugs. However, the physician should be aware that, in some children, this may cause worsening of their metabolic acidosis, especially during ketogenic diet initiation, and may require adjustments in the drug dose, adjustments in the diet, or addition of polycitra [Takeoka et al., 2002]. To date, no increased risk of nephrolithiasis has been reported in patients on topiramate or zonisamide and the ketogenic diet [Kossoff et al., 2002; Takeoka et al., 2002]. All children on one of these medicines should be treated with increased hydration and monitoring of their urine calcium–creatinine ratio; if the latter is elevated, urine alkalinization should be carried out.

Fatigue occurs in many children during initiation of the diet but is prolonged in only a small number. Children with gastroesophageal reflux, especially if they have cerebral palsy, may have increased gastroesophageal reflux while on the diet. The high fat content decreases gastric emptying, which promotes gastroesophageal reflux. This problem usually can be managed medically [Jung et al., 2008a]. Use of the ketogenic diet in infants to treat their seizure disorders or selected metabolic disorders has rarely been associated with fat malabsorption and secondary failure to thrive due to physiologic pancreatic insufficiency [Goyens et al., 2002]. This has been corrected by alteration of the diet via use of MCT and pancreatic extract. Close attention to growth measurements, laboratory data, and medical supervision is indicated in infants on the ketogenic diet. Only short-term information on growth in a limited number of patients had previously been available [Couch et al., 1999; Kossoff et al., 2002; Williams et al., 2002; Liu et al., 2003]. A prospective cohort study of 237 children, with an average length of follow-up of 308 days, analyzed height and weight measurements over time on the ketogenic diet [Vining et al., 2002]. A small decrease in height scores was observed in the first 6 months, with bigger changes by 2 years. There was a drop in weight in the first 3 months, and after this, the weight remained constant in children who started the diet below the 50th percentile for their weight, while it continued to decrease in children starting above the 50th percentile. Very young children (0–2 years) grew poorly on the diet, while older children (7–10 years) grew almost normally. A subsequent prospective study of 75 children, followed for 12 months, examined growth in children on classical and MCT ketogenic diets [Neal et al., 2009]. Both weight and height percentiles decreased, and by 12 months, there was no difference in outcome between classical and MCT protocols, despite the increased protein in the latter diet.

Twenty-two children had growth parameters monitored for 1 year prior to initiation of the ketogenic diet, and then for 1 year on the diet [Spulber et al., 2009]. Additionally, serial measurements of serum ketones and insulin-like growth factor I (IGF-I) were performed. Weight and height percentiles, body mass index, and height velocity all decreased significantly (p <0.05). Height velocity correlated negatively with serum β-hydroxybutyric acid levels, and was most affected in those with pronounced ketosis. Serum IGF-I decreased immediately at diet initiation, but then reached stable levels at around 3 months after diet initiation.

Several laboratory abnormalities have been reported in children on the ketogenic diet, although none has been found to have clinical significance. Patients on the ketogenic diet are in a chronic acidotic state, putting them at risk for osteopenia. A single longitudinal study has evaluated the effect of the ketogenic diet on bone density, serum hydroxyvitamin D, and parathyroid hormone [Bergqvist et al., 2007, 2008]. At baseline, the children with intractable epilepsy had suboptimal growth status and poor bone health. A progressive loss of bone mineral content, resulting in osteopenia and osteoporosis, occurred with ketogenic diet treatment, despite improved serum vitamin D concentrations. Supplementation of vitamin D and calcium was not sufficient to prevent bone mineral content loss. Increased supplementation and periodic surveillance with dual energy x-ray absorptiometry may be needed to prevent or treat the loss of bone mineral content in children treated with the ketogenic diet [Bergqvist et al., 2008]. This compensated metabolic acidosis puts the young child, who becomes ill, at risk of becoming markedly acidotic, ketotic, or dehydrated. This can be addressed by forewarning parents to increase fluid intake during illness. Serum cholesterol and triglycerides may increase, especially during the first 6 months; they tend to plateau by 6 months, then decline and require routine monitoring [Dekaban et al., 1966; Bergqvist et al., 1998; Chesney et al., 1999; Vining, 1999a; Kang et al., 2004]. Adjustments to the diet (e.g., increased protein and polyunsaturated fat) can be made in children with significantly high cholesterol and triglyceride concentrations. Impaired neutrophil function was described in ketotic children, but only one child had severe, recurrent infections [Woody et al., 1989]. This finding has not been replicated. Slight to significant prolongation of the bleeding time and abnormal platelet aggregation, despite normal platelet count and partial thromboplastin time (PTT), was reported in six children [Berry-Kravis et al., 2001b]. Patients on the diet and undergoing surgery should be evaluated for symptoms of bleeding tendency. Elevated very-long-chain fatty acids were found in one center in 59 percent of patients on the diet, and subsequently raised concerns about confusing this side effect with peroxisomal disorders [Theda et al., 1993]. Changes in the serum carnitine concentrations have also been described. Some believe a carnitine supplement should be given routinely [Demeritte et al., 1996b]. However, a prospective study of 11 children showed no substantial change over 1 year after initiation of the ketogenic diet [Coppola et al., 2006]. Carnitine status

should be monitored, although most children do not need supplementation [Berry-Kravis et al., 1998, 2001a; Lin et al., 1998]. Carnitine supplementation may have conflicting effects; carnitine deficiency may restrict fatty-acid beta-oxidation, and carnitine may also improve glucose transport into cells. Supplementation with magnesium, zinc, calcium, vitamin D, and B vitamins is recommended to avoid deficiency-related disease states [Hahn et al., 1979; Hoyt et al., 1979]. The ketogenic diet is deficient in several trace minerals, and if children are maintained on the diet for more than 2 years, these need to be supplemented [Goodwell et al., 1998; Chee et al., 1998; Bergqvist et al., 1999, 2003].

Serious complications of the ketogenic diet are rare and typically have only been described in single reports, including those of Fanconi's renal tubular acidosis (in co-treatment with valproate) [Ballaban-Gil et al., 1996], severe hypoproteinemia [Ballaban-Gil et al., 1998], marked increase in liver function tests (in co-treatment with valproate) [Ballaban-Gil et al., 1998], cardiomyopathy [Ballaban-Gil, 1999; Best et al., 2000; Bergqvist et al., 2003; Kang et al., 2004; Bank et al., 2008], prolonged QTc [Best et al., 2000], acute hemorrhagic pancreatitis [Stewart et al., 2001], basal ganglia injury [Erickson et al., 2002], scurvy [Willmott and Bryan, 2008], lipoid pneumonia [Kang et al., 2005], and fatal propofol infusion syndrome [Baumeister et al., 2004].

A single retrospective chart review reports maintenance of efficacy and tolerability with long-term use of the ketogenic diet (duration of 6–12 years, n = 28) [Groesbeck et al., 2006]. However, side effects of decreased growth (23 out of 28), kidney stones (7 out of 28), and fractures (6 out of 28) occurred, and careful monitoring with strategies to minimize these complications is suggested.

Advantages and Disadvantages

Advantages

The ketogenic diet has several advantages when compared with other medical therapies. Anecdotal reports have indicated that many of the children who are maintained on the diet are able to have their AEDs decreased or withdrawn. This typically results in the child being more alert and exhibiting better behavior [Maydell et al., 2001; Nordli et al., 2001]. However, even children whose AEDs cannot be substantially lowered or withdrawn may have marked behavioral or cognitive improvements [Katyal et al., 2000]. This has occurred in children who have become seizure-free on the diet and had AEDs withdrawn, as well as in those whose seizures are only minimally improved and who have not had dramatic changes in their AED regimen.

Parents are concerned about cognitive side effects, and, although the newer AEDs tend to have fewer such side effects, there are none with the diet. A prospective pilot study assessed the effects of the ketogenic diet on development and behavior in 65 children with intractable epilepsy [Pulsifer et al., 2001]. Formal evaluation of development, behavior, and paternal stress using parental report measures was performed before diet initiation and 1 year later. At follow-up, mean developmental quotient showed statistically significant improvement (p <0.05), with significant (p <0.05) behavioral improvements in attention and social functioning. The observed developmental and behavioral improvements were not statistically related to reductions in seizure frequency or AEDs. Parental stress was essentially unchanged. This preliminary report supports the prior anecdotal observations of the beneficial effects of the diet on cognition and behavior. Hallbook et al. [2007b] evaluated 18 children with polysomnographic recordings, and quality of life, attention, and behavior scales at baseline, then after 3 and 12 months on the ketogenic diet in a prospective manner on stable AEDs. Eleven children continued with the ketogenic diet for 12 months. They showed improved sleep quality, a decrease in daytime sleep, and significant improvement in attention and quality of life. Experiments in rats have shown no adverse effect of the ketogenic diet on spatial learning and memory, the animal's response to a novel environment, or a battery of behavioral tests [Hori et al., 1997; Bough et al., 2000b]. These reports of a positive cognitive effect of the diet in children and experimental models are in contrast to the single study of cognition in rats [Zhao et al., 2004] and one weight loss study in adults [Wing et al., 1995]. Adults on the ketogenic diet for weight loss performed more poorly on some neurocognitive tasks than did nontreated controls [Wing et al., 1995]. These concerns have not been raised by any study of human beings but should be pursued in experimental and clinical research arenas [Snead, 2004]. In addition, with the ketogenic diet, there appear to be no concerns about organ failure or toxicity.

For many families, the ketogenic diet provides a dramatic change in their role in the treatment of their children's epilepsy. The requirement for preparation and monitoring gives the parents an active role in the treatment of their children and a sense that what they are doing is impacting their children's epilepsy and psychosocial well-being. Only if the diet is ineffective can this become a disadvantage. Finally, rarely, parents may not want to stop the ketogenic diet, even if it is not working. This is the first therapy for their children's seizures of which they are in charge, and the parents may not want to lose this empowerment.

Disadvantages

The most common reasons cited for discontinuation of the ketogenic diet are lack of efficacy, complications, noncompliance (especially in older children), and caregiver concerns [Lightstone et al., 2001]. The ketogenic diet is a strictly regulated medical diet that requires an epilepsy team for success. It requires active participation by the parents and children. The work required on the part of the parents to initiate and maintain this rigorous diet may be considered a disadvantage.

In the 1930s and 1940s, the cost of the diet was considered a major disadvantage. However, at that time the diet was compared with the cost of bromides or phenobarbital. Currently, the child with intractable epilepsy can incur costs of around $5000 per year or more for new AEDs. A retrospective study of medical costs in 15 children with intractable epilepsy who were placed on the ketogenic diet showed a saving of over $10,000 per child for the 1–2-year period after initiation of the diet, compared to the same time period prior to the diet [Mandel et al., 2002]. Successful maintenance on the ketogenic diet can provide a substantial financial benefit.

Many physicians perceive the diet as unpalatable and difficult to initiate and maintain. However, modern nutritional labeling requirements and the use of computers allow the

dietitian to construct a palatable diet, keeping the patient's food preferences in mind, and this permits a much more varied meal plan [Brake and Brake, 1997].

The Ketogenic Diet in the Twenty-First Century

More than 80 years have passed since the ketogenic diet was initially used, and many more therapies are now available for children with epilepsy. The ketogenic diet compares favorably with other new treatments that have been introduced to treat children with epilepsy [The Felbamate Study Group, 1993; George et al., 1994; The Vagus Nerve Stimulation Study Group, 1995; LeFever et al., 2000]. Studies on the newer AEDs, such as zonisamide, lamotrigine, tiagabine, gabapentin, topiramate, oxcarbazepine, lacosamide, pregabalin, and levetiracetam, typically indicate that only 3–10 percent of all intractable patients achieve complete relief of seizures. The question that remains unanswered is, "When, in the course of therapy for a child with intractable epilepsy, should the ketogenic diet be used?" Currently, it is not used until children have failed multiple medications and if they are not considered surgical candidates. However, in some epilepsy syndromes, the diet should be offered as a treatment strategy after failure of one or two drugs. If the child has an epilepsy syndrome that is often resistant to current therapy and if the seizures are not controlled on medication, the ketogenic diet should be mentioned as an alternative therapy at the time of the initial therapeutic discussions. This is especially true in children who are not good candidates for epilepsy surgery or whose parents do not wish their children to have epilepsy surgery. The renewed interest in the ketogenic diet has, once again, raised several research questions that, if answered, have the potential to improve our understanding of the neurochemistry of epilepsy and allow better treatment of all patients with epilepsy [Nordli and DeVivo, 1997; Prasad et al., 1996].

In addition to the need to gain a better understanding of the underlying neurochemical changes induced with the ketogenic diet, several other clinical questions remain. Specifically, for what seizure types or epilepsy syndromes does this diet have a higher chance of being a successful short- or long-term treatment? It would be helpful to have more long-term (i.e., 10–20 years) follow-up data on those patients who appear not to have a return of seizures after the diet is stopped [Keith, 1963].

Issues that require investigation include the risk of late seizure recurrence once the diet is terminated, presence of any long-term effects of the diet on growth and development, and whether the response to treatment is because the patient has a specific subset of known seizure type or epilepsy syndrome. Feasibility of prolonged treatment also needs to be determined. Many children who are not seizure-free or who are not able to come off all AEDs are improved on the ketogenic diet. The improvement in seizure control or behavior and cognitive abilities is such that parents wish to continue the ketogenic diet. How long can we safely maintain these children on the ketogenic diet without encountering new side effects because of micronutrient deficiency? What is the feasibility of prolonged therapy? If no other therapy works better, how do we counsel parents about patients remaining on the diet, when there is no apparent chance of withdrawing it? This same set of questions could be raised in a child who is seizure-free on the diet for 2 years but then does not tolerate withdrawal without recurrence of seizures. The effects of the ketogenic diet on family dynamics also are not known. Are there different psychosocial effects on the siblings of the child with epilepsy who is dependent on this form of therapy?

Additional questions relate to the role of the ketogenic diet in treating less affected or normal children with epilepsy. How does the risk–benefit ratio of the ketogenic diet compare with other therapies? Finally, many adults with intractable epilepsy wish to know if there is any group of adults that could benefit from the ketogenic diet. The ketogenic diet might be useful in other childhood neurologic disorders, such as alternating hemiplegia of childhood or tumors of the nervous system [Nebeling et al., 1995]. There is an expanding experimental literature suggesting that the ketogenic diet may treat several neurologic conditions [Kossoff et al., 2009c; Santra et al., 2004; Murphy et al., 2004].

The ketogenic diet is a therapy that was first used at the beginning of the 20th century and appears still to have a definitive role in the treatment of childhood epilepsy into the 21st century. The preferred sequence of treatments for children with epilepsy will continue to need reassessment and redefinition. It will likely be several years before the exact roles for all current therapies are defined. Until then, it is critical that those taking care of children with seizures be aware of all the treatment options and refer children whose seizures are not controlled to centers specializing in the care of such children [The National Association of Epilepsy Centers, 1990]. For many such children, the ketogenic diet continues to represent a therapeutic alternative.

 The complete list of references for this chapter is available online at **www.expertconsult.com**.
See inside cover for registration details.

Epilepsy Surgery in the Pediatric Population

Mary L. Zupanc and Charles J. Marcuccilli

Epilepsy is one of the most common chronic disorders facing children and adolescents. The overall prevalence of epilepsy has been estimated to be 5–8 per 1000 [Hauser et al., 1975, Hauser, 1994, 1996, 1998; Olafsson et al., 1996; Osuntokun et al., 1987]. Extrapolating the Hauser data from Rochester, Minnesota, of 6.66 per 1000 to the total population in 2004, approximately 2.3 million persons in the United States have epilepsy [Hauser et al., 1991]. In children, there are approximately 10.5 million worldwide with epilepsy. The annual incidence of epilepsy in children is reported to be 61–124 per 100,000 in developing countries and 41–50 per 100,000 in developed countries [Guerrini, 2006]. The cumulative risk of developing epilepsy from birth through adolescence is 1 percent [Hauser et al., 1991, 1994]. Unfortunately, only 60–70 percent of patients will achieve seizure freedom with antiepileptic medications [Kwan and Brodie, 2000; Mohanraj and Brodie, 2006]. The introduction of several new antiepileptic drugs over the past 15 years has not changed the fact that approximately 30–40 percent of patients with epilepsy will be medically refractory [Perucca et al., 2007; Mohanraj and Brodie, 2006].

The identification of a specific epilepsy syndrome is one of the best determinants of prognosis. Some epilepsy syndromes are genetically determined, known channelopathies and may have an excellent prognosis for remission. Other epilepsy syndromes, particularly the lesional epilepsies, are life-long chronic disorders. As an example, benign rolandic epilepsy is characterized by nocturnal focal motor seizures with age of onset between 3 and 8 years, normal findings on neurologic examination, and sleep-activated central-temporal epileptiform discharges on the electroencephalogram (EEG). In this case, the parents can be reassured that their child's epilepsy will often remit by puberty. On the other hand, predictors for the low probability of epilepsy remission include:

1. the presence of a symptomatic localization-related epilepsy secondary to a remote central nervous system injury
2. abnormalities on neurologic examination or cognitive/motor delays
3. persistent epileptiform abnormalities on EEG
4. older age at onset [Arts et al., 1988; Berg et al., 2001; Camfield and Camfield, 2003; Emerson et al., 1981; Hauser et al., 1996, 1998; Juul-Jensen and Foldsprang, 1983; Schmidt et al., 1983; Shafer et al., 1988; Sillanpaa et al., 1998; Sofijanov, 1982; Todt, 1984].

In addition, the longer epilepsy persists without control, the less likely is the chance of remission. Specifically, if seizures remain inadequately controlled for longer than 4 years, the chance of remission decreases to approximately 10 percent [Annegers et al., 1979]. Seizure duration of over 10 years also decreases the likelihood of achieving control in patients who undergo surgery. The presence of multiple seizure types and frequent generalized tonic-clonic seizures also lessens the chance for complete remission. As stated above, 30–40 percent [Mohanraj and Brodie, 2006] of all persons with epilepsy will be intractable. There are approximately 20,000 cases of new-onset epilepsy annually. Therefore, 6000–8000 cases of new-onset epilepsy are intractable each year. In the United States, the number of patients with drug-resistant epilepsy – adult and pediatric – is estimated to be 700,000, a higher number than the number of individuals affected with Parkinson's disease and multiple sclerosis combined [Hiritiz et al., 2007]. Approximately 60 percent of these patients will have partial seizures. Estimates by several investigators suggest that many of these patients are epilepsy surgery candidates [Hauser, 1993; Unnwongse et al., 2010]. This figure may increase as new technologies enable more precise identification of an underlying epileptogenic focus. Additionally, as medical intractability for children with epilepsy is further defined, the number of pediatric epilepsy surgical procedures will probably increase. However, currently, epilepsy surgery is underutilized in the treatment of intractable epilepsy. In fact, over the past 15 years, the mean duration of epilepsy before referral to a tertiary care epilepsy center for evaluation for epilepsy surgery has been over 20 years [Engel et al., 2003; Unnwongse et al., 2010; Choi et al., 2009].

An increasing number of pediatric comprehensive epilepsy centers are equipped to handle the complexities of the preoperative evaluation in children and infants. Many issues must be addressed before a child becomes a candidate for epilepsy surgery. The number of children undergoing epilepsy surgery in the United States is rising, with more than 300 pediatric epilepsy surgical procedures performed annually.

The developing brain is highly susceptible to recurrent seizures. Until recently, the brain was believed to be relatively resistant to injury. A growing body of evidence in animal models, however, suggests that early seizures, even if brief and recurrent, can result in demonstrable structural and physiologic changes in the developing brain's circuitry, resulting in aberrant excitation and inhibition. Clinically, these defects produces spontaneous seizures (epilepsy) and cognitive impairments [Holmes and Ben-Ari, 1998; Holmes et al., 1998;

Stafstrom et al., 2000; Galanopoulou and Moshé, 2009], with the possibility of missed windows of developmental opportunity. Thus, plasticity of the brain in a young infant and child is a "double-edged sword". It protects the brain from the neurologic consequences of destructive lesions and status epilepticus; however, recurrent seizures, or even frequent interictal epileptiform discharges, in this age group can produce permanent abnormal neuronal circuitry, resulting in long-term developmental delays and continued, intractable seizures [Holmes and Lenck-Santini, 2006]. In addition, chronic uncontrolled epilepsy in infants and children poses a significant risk for emotional, behavioral, social, cognitive, and family dysfunction. Population studies have demonstrated that epilepsy reduces life expectancy, and poorly controlled seizures further increase the risk of death in children and adults [Nashef et al., 1995; Hitiris et al., 2007]. In population-based studies, the estimated risk of sudden unexpected death in epilepsy (SUDEP) is estimated to be between 1:500 and 1:1000 per year. For those with uncontrolled epilepsy, the rate of SUDEP is approximately 1:200 per year. [Harvey et al., 1993c; Hauser et al., 1980; Meyer et al., 2010; So et al., 2009]. It should be noted that patients being evaluated for epilepsy surgery have the highest risk of SUDEP, estimated at between 2.2 and 9.3 per 1000 patient-years [Hiritiz et al., 2007].

Several studies have examined outcomes after epilepsy surgery. A majority of these studies has been performed in older adolescents and adults. The focus of these studies has been primarily on the improvement of seizure control, with 64–69 percent of patients having seizure-free outcomes [Engel, 1996; Wyllie, 1998; Wyllie et al., 1998]. These studies have placed less emphasis on improvement in quality of life – for example, enhancement of self-image, improvement in academic performance and psychosocial functioning, and increased independence in activities of daily living [Spencer, 1996; Taylor et al., 1997]. An increasing number of long-term follow-up studies have concentrated on infants and young children. Malformations of cortical development are the most frequently cited pathologic abnormalities in pediatric surgical patients [Duchowny et al., 1996; Wyllie et al., 1998; Harvey et al., 2008; Zupanc et al., 2010]. The overall outcome of pediatric epilepsy surgery in young infants and children is roughly comparable to that in the older adolescent and adult population. In infants, 61–65 percent have seizure-free outcomes [Chugani et al., 1993; Duchowny et al., 1998; Sinclair et al., 2003; Wyllie et al., 1996, 1998; Zupanc et al., 2010]. In young children, the rate of seizure-free outcomes varies, ranging from 58 to 74 percent [Paolicchi et al., 2000; Sinclair et al., 2003; Wyllie et al., 1998; Cossu et al., 2008; Kan et al., 2008; Kim et al., 2008; Zupanc et al., 2010]. The etiology of the epilepsy appears to play the major role in determining prognosis, regardless of location (temporal versus extratemporal). In one study, children with malformations of cortical development had a seizure-free outcome of 58 percent, whereas patients with other pathologies had a 77 percent seizure-free outcome. Temporal lobectomies were more commonly performed in our older adolescent patients, consistent with other studies, and demonstrated a seizure-free outcome of 84 percent. Patients who had modified lateral hemispherectomies also demonstrated a high seizure-free outcome (i.e., approximately 100 percent), even those with cortical dysplasias [Zupanc et al., 2010].

Several studies have reported on cognitive function after surgery in children who have undergone temporal lobectomy (predominantly older children and adolescents) [Gillam et al., 1997; Gleissner et al., 2002; Mabbott and Smith, 2004; Meyer et al., 1986; Szabo et al., 1998; Westerveld et al., 2000; Lah, 2004]. These studies have generally found that memory and intelligence are unchanged. Some reports note a decline in verbal memory and improvements in language, attention, and memory, while other studies have reported that good seizure outcomes have been associated with an increase in IQ [Lah, 2004]. Reports on the cognitive effects of extratemporal resections have been relatively few, in part because of the young age of those having surgery. In a follow-up study of 24 children operated on before 3 years of age, younger age at surgery was correlated with an improvement in developmental quotients [Loddenkemper et al., 2007]. In patients who have undergone successful frontal lobe resection, outcomes include improvements in attention and concentration but no change in executive functions, manual coordination, and language [Blanchette and Smith, 2002; Lendt et al., 2002]. Studies on postoperative psychosocial functioning in children have been relatively rare, almost exclusively retrospective, and based on subjective measures. In children who have undergone temporal lobectomies, studies indicate improvement in behavior, mood, and self-esteem, with the changes linked to improvement in seizure control [Danielsson et al., 2002; Davidson and Falconer, 1975; Duchowny et al., 1992; Meyer et al., 1986; Zupanc et al., 2010]. Of children who have undergone extratemporal resections, improved social behavior was found in about 50 percent [Adler et al., 1991]. Other retrospective studies that combine temporal and extratemporal cases suggest that reduction of seizure frequency, although not necessarily complete elimination of seizures, resulted in improved family life, socialization and behavior, and quality of life [Adler et al., 1991; Keene et al., 1998; Lendt et al., 2002; Mihara et al., 1994; Smith et al., 2004; Whittle et al., 1981; Zupanc et al., 1996, 2010]. Other reports indicate that a reduction in seizures may result in a favorable and significant improvement in the quality of life, with behavioral and developmental "catch-up" progress [Asarnow et al., 1997; Bourgeois et al., 1999; Chugani et al., 1990b; Duchowny et al., 1990, 1992; Wyllie et al., 1996; Jonas et al., 2004; Zupanc et al., 2010]. More recent studies indicate that shorter seizure durations and earlier surgical intervention result in better seizure outcome and quality of life [Jonas et al., 2004; Loddenkemper et al., 2007; Zupanc et al., 2010].

Historical Background

Epilepsy has always been a part of human existence. A generalized tonic-clonic seizure was first described in Akkadian, the oldest written language, more than 3000 years ago [Goldensohn et al., 1997]. Since that time, many descriptions of epilepsy appear in literature, including the Bible. In "On the Sacred Disease", written in the 5th century, Hippocrates stated that epilepsy was a brain disease caused by an excess of phlegm that resulted in an abnormal brain consistency. He proposed diet and drugs as therapy [Scott, 1993]. Until the late 19th century, the treatment of epilepsy was surrounded by superstition, exorcism, magic, and alchemy. Caton's (1842–1926) discovery in 1875 of spontaneous electrical activity of the brain and evoked potentials suggested that seizures might be the result of aberrant electrical activity in the brain [Caton, 1875].

The first effective treatment for epilepsy was potassium bromide, introduced in 1857 [Locock, 1857]. In 1886, Horsley performed the first epilepsy surgery on a patient with intractable post-traumatic epilepsy. Several decades later, the antiepileptic drug phenobarbital was introduced in 1912, followed by phenytoin in 1937. Epilepsy surgery did not advance until 1950, when Penfield published his article on 70 cases of temporal lobectomy [Flanigin et al., 1991; Penfield and Flanigin, 1950]. His neurosurgical career was devoted to the study of seizure semiology (i.e., clinical description) and its correlation with the brain cortex. He used cortical mapping and stimulation in much the same way in which it is used today. He also recognized the substrates of epilepsy, particularly trauma and infection. His seminal clinical research has been instrumental in guiding the hands of contemporary epileptologists and neurosurgeons interested in the surgical approach to epilepsy.

Epilepsy surgery was not regarded as a conventional treatment for intractable epilepsy until recently. In the past 30 years, dramatic improvements in brain imaging that identify specific anatomic substrates of epilepsy have sparked renewed interest in epilepsy surgery. Temporal lobectomy with amygdalo-hippocampectomy has become the standard of care in adult patients with intractable epilepsy emanating from the temporal lobe. The surgical success rate for a seizure-free outcome in these carefully selected patients approaches 80–90 percent [Duchowny et al., 1992; King et al., 1986; Penfield and Flanigin, 1950]. In a randomized, controlled trial of surgery for temporal lobe epilepsy compared to treatment with antiepileptic drugs, 58 percent of patients demonstrated seizure freedom after 1 year compared to only 8 percent of patients treated with medications [Wiebe et al., 2001]. Unfortunately, surgical success does not necessarily translate to an improved quality of life. The accumulation of years of low self-esteem, loss of independence, poor peer relations, and academic failure, coupled with high financial costs, often without benefit of full insurance coverage, translates to continued lack of employment and depression [Reeves et al., 1997]. The lifetime cost of epilepsy for an estimated 181,000 people with onset in 1995 is projected at $11.1 billion, and the annual cost for the estimated 2.3 million people with epilepsy is estimated at $12.5 billion [Bazil, 2004; Begley et al., 1994, 2000; Hathaway et al., 1995]. In one recent study, the calculated total aggregated annual economic impact of epilepsy on the U.S. economy was $9.6 billion in direct medical costs. This analysis did not consider the indirect costs of loss of productivity, quality of life, and comorbidities [Yoon et al., 2009]. With respect to children, it is estimated that the annual cost of medical care for a child with epilepsy is $6379, compared to $1032 for peers without epilepsy [Yoon et al., 2009]. Indirect costs probably account for 80–85 percent of the total costs, and include delayed or missed educational opportunities, psychiatric and social service needs, and lost employment. The direct costs of epilepsy are concentrated in the patients with intractable epilepsy. The growing recognition of the real costs of epilepsy – medical, psychological, educational – has led to increased interest in the early identification of children who might benefit from epilepsy surgery [Jalava et al., 1997]. In older children and adolescents, temporal lobectomies are common epilepsy surgical procedures [Harvey et al., 2008]. In younger children and infants, however, extratemporal resections, including multilobar resections and hemispherectomies, are the more typical procedures [Harvey et al., 2008].

In recent studies, it has been shown that the costs of epilepsy surgery are offset by a decline in health-care costs after successful surgery. One study documented that the total costs for adult patients who were seizure-free following epilepsy surgery declined by 32 percent by 2 years following surgery. In the 24 months after surgery, epilepsy-related costs were $2068–2094 in patients with persisting seizures, as opposed to $582 in patients who were seizure-free following surgery [Langfitt et al., 2007]. In addition, in adult patients, it appears that epilepsy surgery increases quality-adjusted life expectancy by 7.5 years [Choi et al., 2008]. In the pediatric population, additional benefits of epilepsy surgery appear to be improved long-term developmental outcomes and quality of life [Loddenkemper et al., 2007; Zupanc et al., 2010].

Indications for Epilepsy Surgery

Criteria have been proposed for referral and evaluation of children for epilepsy surgery, although there is currently insufficient class I evidence to produce a practice guideline [Cross et al., 2006]. Practice guidelines for temporal lobe and localized neocortical resections for epilepsy have been proposed for adults [Engel et al., 2003]. In determining whether a child is a candidate for epilepsy surgery, several key issues must be considered. The decision-making task must take into account the following:

- Failure of two or three antiepileptic medications in achieving complete seizure control in a child or adolescent.
- Natural history of the epilepsy syndrome. (Likelihood of continued intractability usually can be determined on the basis of the identification of a specific epilepsy syndrome. For example, symptomatic localization-related epilepsy on the basis of an underlying central nervous system lesion is unlikely to go into remission.)
- Identification of a known epileptogenic substrate. Lesional epilepsy in a young infant should prompt an evaluation for epilepsy surgery earlier, as the first antiepileptic medication is started. These young infants are particularly vulnerable to the catastrophic effects of epilepsy in the developing brain.
- Impact of epilepsy on the quality of life, as defined by cognitive and developmental parameters – now and in the future.

The proper classification of seizure type and epilepsy syndrome is crucial in the determination of whether or not a patient is an appropriate epilepsy surgery candidate [Aicardi, 1994; Holmes, 1993]. The benign seizure disorders, such as benign rolandic epilepsy or benign epilepsy with centrotemporal spikes, must be recognized. With rare exceptions, these syndromes usually are easily treated, and affected patients do not present to tertiary epilepsy centers.

The catastrophic epilepsies of infancy and childhood are recognizable early, and affected patients should be referred to a tertiary epilepsy center for consideration for epilepsy surgery. These epilepsy syndromes are characterized by the tetrad of:

1. multiple daily seizures
2. medical intractability to the standard antiepileptic drug therapies
3. cognitive/developmental stagnation or decline

4. presumed or known epileptogenic pathology.

The patients should be surgically treated at an early age, as soon as these catastrophic epilepsies are recognized and the preoperative evaluation can be completed with confidence. The catastrophic epilepsies of infancy and childhood include:

1. Sturge–Weber syndrome
2. large unilateral or focal malformations of cortical development, such as hemimegalencephaly or unilateral schizencephaly
3. symptomatic infantile spasms with focal malformations of cortical development, typically temporal-parietal-occipital dysplasias
4. Rasmussen's syndrome.

Children with Sturge–Weber syndrome who have frequent, medically refractory seizures accompanied by progressive hemiparesis and cognitive impairment should be evaluated promptly for hemispherectomy [Thomas-Sohl et al., 2004; Vining et al., 1997]. Clinical outcome studies indicate that early surgical resection can result in the elimination of seizures, improvement in cognitive abilities, and overall improvement in quality of life, despite hemiparesis and visual field defect as residual neurologic deficits [Erba and Cavazzuti, 1990; Hoffman et al., 1979; Ogunmekan et al., 1991; van Empelen et al., 2004].

Children with hemimegalencephaly, a unilateral or focal malformation of cortical development, can present in infancy with multiple daily seizures, developmental stagnation or decline, and hemiparesis. Hemispherectomy provides relief from seizures (especially in those patients with unilateral epileptiform abnormalities) and improved developmental outcome [Andermann et al., 1993; Vigevano and DiRocco, 1990; Vigevano et al., 1989; Jonas et al., 2004]. The patients with symptomatic infantile spasms who have underlying focal cortical dysplasias, usually temporal-parietal-occipital, should be considered for early focal cortical resection. University of California at Los Angeles investigators have provided the

seminal clinical research in this area and have documented a significant improvement in seizure control and enhanced developmental gains following epilepsy surgery, greater than would have been predicted using the natural history of infantile spasms as a comparison [Asarnow et al., 1997; Chugani et al., 1990a, 1993; Duchowny et al., 1990].

Rasmussen's encephalitis is characterized by intractable focal motor seizures, often evolving into epilepsia partialis continua, cognitive decline, and progressive hemiparesis. Recent findings of glutamate receptor antibodies in some patients with Rasmussen's encephalitis implicate a possible autoimmune pathophysiology [Antel and Rasmussen, 1996; Pardo et al., 2004; Rogers et al., 1994]. Although initial trials of intravenous immunoglobulin and plasmapheresis have been encouraging, long-term studies have not confirmed efficacy [Andrews et al., 1996; Hart et al., 1994; Krauss et al., 1996]. Therefore, the only definitive treatment for Rasmussen's encephalitis remains hemispherectomy [van Empelen et al., 2004; Jonas et al., 2004].

In addition to those with the catastrophic epilepsies of infancy and childhood, all children with tumors and concomitant localization-related epilepsy should be considered for early surgical intervention. Compelling reasons for such intervention exist. Most tumors need to be biopsied or excised. Additionally, although the tumors associated with epilepsy usually are slow-growing, cortical, and well circumscribed, some tumors, especially astrocytomas, are not necessarily benign and can undergo malignant change [Jack, 1995]. Without resection, the natural history of these tumor-associated epilepsy syndromes is one of continued seizures with little hope of remission. Antiepileptic drugs produce side effects that can affect cognitive function and behaviors, with concomitant impact on psychosocial development [Meador, 2002] Examples of tumors that usually are easily resectable are the gangliogliomas and dysembryonic neuroectodermal tumors, which have a predilection for the temporal lobe (Figure 61-1) [Duchowny et al., 1992; Tice et al., 1993; Vali et al., 1993].

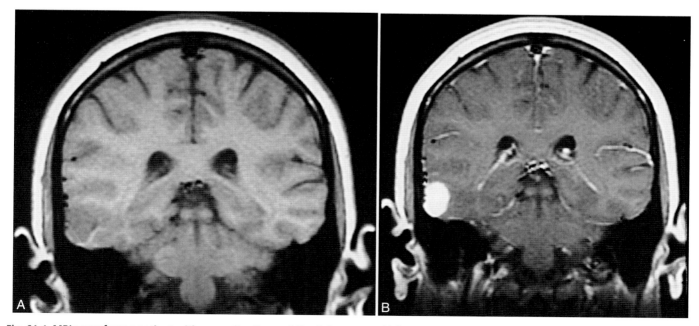

Fig. 61-1 MRI scans from a patient with a ganglioglioma of the right temporal lobe. A, T1-weighted imaging without gadolinium (TR = 500 msec/TE = 16 msec). **B,** T1-weighted imaging with gadolinium (TR = 500 msec/TE = 16 msec). TE, echo time; TR, recovery time.

Children with other types of lesional symptomatic localization-related epilepsy also should be considered as epilepsy surgery candidates. Common substrates of epilepsy include encephalomalacias, vascular malformations, tubers, and malformations of cortical development [Harvey et al., 2008; Zupanc et al., 2010].

Patients who have generalized epilepsy syndromes may also be candidates for epilepsy surgery. The presence of generalized or multifocal epileptiform discharges on surface EEG monitoring should not necessarily exclude someone from epilepsy surgery. Children with generalized or multifocal epilepsy should be considered for epilepsy surgery, if data suggest an underlying focal generator for the epileptic condition [Wyllie, 1995; Wyllie et al., 2007; Zupanc et al., 2010]. Specifically, in the presence of a lesion on magnetic resonance imaging (MRI), the epilepsy syndrome is most likely to be due to a symptomatic localization-related epilepsy with rapid secondary bisynchrony. The mechanisms of underlying generalized epileptiform discharges in focal cerebral lesions can be seen as a form of "maladaptive plasticity" of the immature brain, whereby the lesions in the immature neural network of the young brain permanently alter the neural circuitry, producing spontaneous hypersynchrony and generalized discharges [Sutula, 2004]. These generalized discharges may also involve the thalamocortical network, resulting in generalized rhythmic discharges [Van Hirtum-Das et al., 2006]. Approximately 10–15 percent of children with Lennox–Gastaut syndrome, one of the most common symptomatic "generalized" epilepsy syndromes, have underlying focal malformations of cortical development and should be evaluated carefully for epilepsy surgery. In one study, children who had generalized discharges and focal lesions had identical seizure-free outcomes (72 percent seizure-free) to children with similar lesions and ipsilateral focal epileptiform discharges [Wyllie et al., 2007]. In addition, children with intractable epilepsy who have tonic-atonic seizures associated with generalized spikes/polyspikes (usually Lennox–Gastaut syndrome) and no identifiable lesion on neuroimaging may respond to a complete corpus callosotomy, a palliative treatment that can have a significant impact on quality of life [Wyllie et al., 1993; Zupanc et al., 2010]. An alternative approach is that of a multistaged epilepsy surgery, initially performing a complete corpus callosotomy, then placing lateralizing strip electrodes with the hope of identifying epileptogenic cortex that can be resected. In one study of 14 patients undergoing this approach, 9 went on to have a focal cortical resection and 5 out of 9 (56 percent) were seizure-free [Zupanc et al., 2011].

Patients with tuberous sclerosis and medically refractory, symptomatic, localization-related epilepsy should also be considered for epilepsy surgery. In patients with multiple tubers, emerging neuroimaging techniques, particularly interictal α-[^{11}C]methyl-L-tryptophan (AMT) positron emission tomography (PET) scans, offer promise in identifying the most highly epileptogenic tuber [Asano et al., 2000; Chugani et al., 1998; Juhasz et al., 2003]. If the presurgical evaluation points to a specific tuber, studies have shown that it can be successfully removed, with a significant improvement in seizure control [Bebin et al., 1993; Koh et al., 2000; Romanelli et al., 2004]. There is also precedent for removing multiple tubers in the brain, as several tubers may be producing medically refractory seizures [Weiner et al., 2006].

In summary, factors that favor early intervention with epilepsy surgery include the following:

1. seizure recurrence despite an adequate trial of two or three antiepileptic drugs

2. seizures severe enough to interfere with development or overall quality of life

3. central nervous system lesion identified on MRI, such as tumors, infarctions, and identifiable malformations of cortical development.

Even if the lesion is outside the temporal lobe, in carefully selected patients, epilepsy surgery can generally be performed with little risk of neurologic sequelae and a high rate of surgical success [Britton et al., 1994; Cascino et al., 1990, 1992, 1993, 1994; Montes et al., 1995; Paolicchi et al., 2000; Zupanc et al., 2010].

The suspected central nervous system pathology, based on MRI, may also have an impact on whether or not a patient is an epilepsy surgery candidate. For example, patients with low-grade tumors, infarctions, and mesial temporal sclerosis are likely to undergo remission of their epilepsy and typically have an excellent seizure-free outcome. If the epilepsy is temporal in onset and pathologic features include associated hippocampal formation atrophy or mesial temporal sclerosis, the surgical success rate approaches 80–90 percent [Cascino et al., 1993; Sinclair et al., 2001] (Figure 61-2). Data from our own retrospective study and from the work of Palmini and co-workers suggest that malformations of cortical development, no matter where the cortical location, carry a significant risk for status epilepticus and intractability [Laoprasert et al., 1997; Palmini et al., 1997]. Epilepsy surgery in patients with underlying malformations of cortical development have a lower seizure-free outcome, but it is still close to 60 percent, which is significantly better than additional trials of antiepileptic

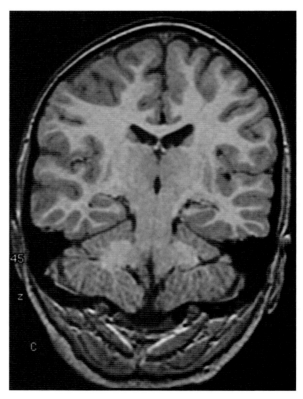

Fig. 61-2 MRI scan from a patient with left temporal hippocampal atrophy. The scan shows a coronal cut obtained with T1-weighted imaging (TR = 24 msec/TE = 9 msec).

medication. Patients with mild malformations of cortical development, such as focal cortical dysplasia (FCD) type 1a, fared better than patients with more severe malformations of cortical development, such as FCD type 2a [Fauser et al., 2004]. In addition, the patients with known central nervous system lesions can be identified early, with detailed MR imaging.

Those children with intractable nonlesional extratemporal localization-related epilepsy represent the biggest challenge to the epileptologist but should still be considered for epilepsy surgery if their seizures remain intractable. The benefits of surgery must be weighed against the risks, especially the risk of neurologic deficits. As an example, localization-related epilepsy emanating from the sensorimotor cortex demands a more conservative approach. Several antiepileptic drugs and suitable investigational antiepileptic drugs should be tried before embarking on a surgical approach with its attendant risks of hemiparesis. On the other hand, if a child has severe, frequent seizures with developmental stagnation and the preoperative evaluation demonstrates congruence of data from seizure semiology, EEG, MRI, single-proton emission computed tomography (SPECT), PET, magnetoencephalography (MEG), and/or MR spectroscopy, epilepsy surgery can be performed.

Preoperative Evaluation

Once a child has been selected as a possible epilepsy surgery candidate, further questions need to be addressed before epilepsy surgery can take place:

1. Can the epileptogenic zone be identified using video EEG, neuroimaging, and other modalities? Is there congruence of the data?
2. Will removal of the epileptogenic zone result in seizure freedom?
3. Can the epileptogenic focus be removed without causing unacceptable neurologic deficits? This requires accurate anatomic localization of eloquent cortex.
4. Will a delay in epilepsy surgery cause loss of developmental plasticity? The evidence would indicate yes, as discussed above.

A multidisciplinary team is required to address the many issues surrounding the prospect of surgery in a child with chronic epilepsy. Epilepsy surgery itself may cure the seizures but will not necessarily address the family's other needs. A child with medically intractable epilepsy and the child's family have complex and diverse problems – not just medical but also developmental, educational, psychosocial, economic, and relational. The coordinated services of a pediatric neurologist or epileptologist, child psychiatrist, pediatric neurosurgeon, pediatric neuropsychologist, speech and language pathologist, and pediatric neuroradiologist, along with diagnostic studies including EEG, neuroimaging, and nuclear isotopic scanning, are required to evaluate the medical aspects before surgery is considered. Clinical nurse specialists are integral, often acting as the case managers and coordinators of the care designed to meet patient and family needs. The social worker is a critical part of the team, providing families with avenues for financial assistance, counseling families, and assisting with transitional services from hospital and clinic to the home environment. In addition, networking with other families who have undergone similar evaluations and treatment also is a critical aspect of the multidisciplinary evaluation, which cannot be effectively carried out without the integration of these services.

Techniques and Technologies
Seizure Semiology

Seizure semiology can provide insightful clues to the lateralization and localization of the underlying epileptogenic focus. The presence of versive head movements, unilateral motor clonic activity, and eye deviation may constitute critical lateralizing information. Specifically, versive head movements indicate that the epileptogenic zone resides in the contralateral hemisphere. In similar fashion, seizures consisting of olfactory or gustatory hallucinations, followed by complex motor automatisms and staring unresponsively, are virtually diagnostic of involvement of the temporal lobe. These seizures generally are seen in older children or adolescents, but also may occur in younger children. It should be noted, however, that seizures emanating from the temporal lobe in infants and young children commonly are associated with behavioral arrest, motor dystonic posturing, and fewer automatisms [Brockhaus and Elger, 1995; Jayakar and Duchowny, 1990; Wyllie et al., 1993]. Additionally, young children are typically incapable of describing the premonitory symptoms before the onset of the more overt clinical seizure. Video EEG monitoring has been helpful in fully elucidating the seizure semiology in these patients. Children with infantile spasms may have partial seizures before, during, or after the onset of the infantile spasms [Kobayashi et al., 2001; Watanabe et al., 2001]. Partial seizures can be a helpful clue that prompts the epileptologist to screen carefully for an underlying focal abnormality, such as a tuber or focal cortical dysplasia.

Physical Examination

The physical examination can also provide very valuable lateralizing information. As with seizure onset or its evolution, a focal abnormality on physical examination may point to an underlying focal structural lesion. For example, a child with schizencephaly and partial seizures may have a subtle hemiparesis, effectively demonstrating the affected hemisphere.

Electroencephalography

The surface EEG is a critical element in the evaluation of children with epilepsy. The advent of computerized prolonged video EEG monitoring has ushered in a new era in the evaluation and management of epilepsy. The digital format allows for easier use of multiple montages to assist in localization of the epileptogenic zone. This technique is used for many purposes, including:

1. differentiation of epileptic and nonepileptic events
2. seizure classification
3. recognition of specific epilepsy syndromes
4. preoperative evaluation with identification of the epileptogenic zone
5. determination of seizure frequency
6. management of status epilepticus.

In the adult preoperative evaluation, prolonged video EEG monitoring provides the baseline data with which all of the other data are compared. In children, however, it is becoming increasingly clear that the surface EEG data may be poorly localized and at times misleading in the preoperative evaluation [Wyllie, 1995]. Therefore, this modality may be less important in localizing the epileptogenic focus. In these children, other modalities, particularly neuroimaging studies (MRI, MR spectroscopy, PET, and SPECT), may provide the pivotal information that determines the location of the epileptogenic zone and may reduce the need for invasive subdural EEG monitoring. Indeed, in the near future, the improvement of noninvasive functional brain imaging techniques may obviate the need for invasive EEG monitoring. Even now, invasive EEG monitoring may be deferred if surface EEG monitoring and MRI data are congruent [Wyllie et al., 1998; Zupanc et al., 2010].

Magnetic Resonance Imaging

MRI scans have greatly enhanced the ability to visualize intraparenchymal brain structures. The linkage between intracranial abnormalities and epilepsy is well accepted [Zupanc, 1997a]. The mechanism(s) involved in the production of epilepsy is an area of intense research and involves structural changes, synaptic reorganization, stimulation of mossy fibers, astroglial proliferation with neuronal cell loss, and neurotransmitter or corresponding receptor changes. With the recent advances in MRI technology, the ability to identify the substrates of epilepsy has been greatly enhanced. This modality provides some of the most sensitive and specific neuroimaging data for localization of the epileptogenic zone [Brooks et al., 1990; Cascino, 1994; Cascino et al., 1989, 1991; Kuzniecky et al., 1993a, 1993c; Madan and Grant, 2009]. The following new technologies are exciting and innovative [Jack, 1995; Madan and Grant, 2009]:

- Use of thin contiguous cuts of 1.5–1.6 mm in multiple sections of the cortex, in combination with a three-dimensional volumetric pulse sequence, provides the necessary resolution to detect small lesions that would be missed with conventional MRI scans. Specific areas can be targeted, and images can be reformatted to correct for head rotation and other perturbations in data collection. This technique has allowed detection of even small amounts of unilateral hippocampal atrophy (see Figure 61-2), as well as identification of small areas of focal cortical dysplasia.

- The ability to conduct quantitative volumetric analysis of the hippocampus has resulted in the determination of unilateral or bilateral hippocampal atrophy. In patients with epilepsy emanating from the temporal lobe, the identification of unilateral hippocampal atrophy combined with concordant surface ictal EEG data is sufficient to allow a temporal lobectomy with amygdalohippocampectomy to proceed without invasive EEG monitoring.

- The fluid-attenuated inversion recovery imaging (FLAIR) technique highlights lesions such as mesial temporal sclerosis and malformations of cortical development and allows detection of previously unidentifiable small lesions. This sequence produces a T2-weighted image that subtracts the cerebrospinal fluid signal (white and bright on T2), but keeps the T2 signal from intraparenchymal structures (Figure 61-3 and Figure 61-4).

- Diffusion tensor imaging is an MRI imaging technique that can identify white-matter tracts [Rugg-Gunn et al., 2001] that may be disrupted in areas of cortical dysplasia.

- Multichannel coils (32 phased array and beyond and higher field strengths (3 Tesla, 7 Tesla, and greater), coupled with newer imaging sequences, including arterial spin labeling (ASL) and susceptibility weighted imaging (SWI), as well as diffusion tensor imaging (DTI/DSI), are likely to increase our detection of focal cortical dysplasias [Madan and Grant, 2009].

With use of these techniques, MRI scans can identify many substrates of epilepsy, including malformations of cortical development, tumors, vascular malformations, and encephalomalacias secondary to trauma, infection, and infarction. Malformations of cortical development are increasingly recognized as being highly epileptogenic [Kuzniecky and Ruben, 1995; Kuzniecky and Barkovich, 2001; Palmini et al., 1995; Raymond et al., 1995]. Advances in MRI technology have greatly improved the ability to identify these abnormalities. They may account for more than 60 percent of the intractable localization-related epilepsies of childhood [Kuzniecky et al., 1993c]. These malformations can be small and difficult to detect, even with sophisticated MRI scans of the brain, or can be widespread and diffuse, as with lissencephaly [Dobyns

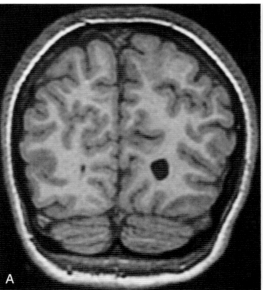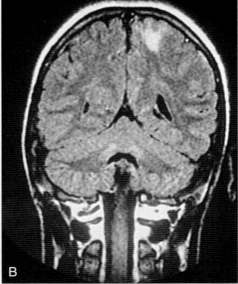

Fig. 61-3 MRI scans from a patient with focal cortical dysplasia of the posterior left parasagittal region. A, With T1-weighted imaging (TR = 24 msec/TE = 9 msec), thickening of the cortex and blurring of the white/gray matter are evident. **B,** The dysplasia is seen more clearly with fluid-attenuated inversion recovery imaging (FLAIR) sequencing (TR = 1100 msec/TE = 142 msec/TI = 2600 msec) (see text). TE, echo time; TI, inversion time; TR, recovery time.

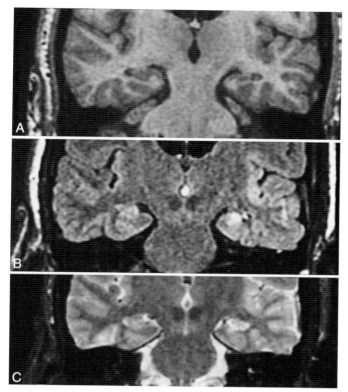

Fig. 61-4 MRI scans showing coronal cuts through the temporal lobes, from a patient with left temporal hippocampal atrophy. A, The atrophy is seen best with T1-weighted imaging (TR = 24 msec/TE = 9 msec). **B,** Concomitant left temporal mesial temporal sclerosis is seen best with fluid-attenuated inversion recovery imaging (FLAIR) sequencing (TR = 1100 msec/TE = 142 msec/TI = 2600 msec). **C,** Middle panel represents the picture created on T2-weighted imaging (TR = 2000 msec/TE = 80 msec).

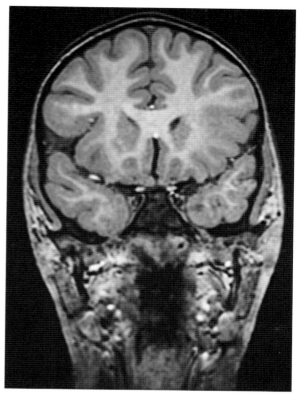

Fig. 61-5 MRI scan from a patient with focal cortical dysplasia of the left frontal region. With T1-weighted imaging (TR = 24 msec/TE = 9 msec), thickening of the cortex and blurring of the white/gray matter are seen.

and Truwit, 1995; Dobyns et al., 1996] (Figure 61-5 and Figure 61-6). The unilateral and focal malformations of cortical development are most often targeted for surgical excision. Clinically, information on the natural history of the malformations of cortical development is emerging. Status epilepticus is a common initial presentation, usually in the latter half of the first decade of life [Laoprasert and Zupanc, 1997]. Many of the malformations of cortical development produce an epilepsy syndrome that is intractable to medical management [Palmini et al., 1997].

Finally, although mesial temporal sclerosis and hippocampal atrophy are not commonly found in children with intractable epilepsy who are younger than 10 years of age, identification of these abnormalities is a powerful indicator of the zone of epileptogenesis [Cascino, 1994; Cascino et al., 1991; Jack, 1995; Swartz et al., 1992]. The pathophysiology of mesial temporal sclerosis and hippocampal formation atrophy is poorly understood. Do the seizures themselves cause mesial temporal sclerosis and hippocampal formation atrophy? Does an underlying malformation of cortical development cause the initial seizures, ultimately resulting in mesial temporal sclerosis and hippocampal formation atrophy [Cendes et al., 1993; Kuks et al., 1993; Trenerry et al., 1993]? Prolonged febrile seizures, head injury, nonfebrile status epilepticus, encephalitis, hypertensive encephalopathy, and viruses, including human

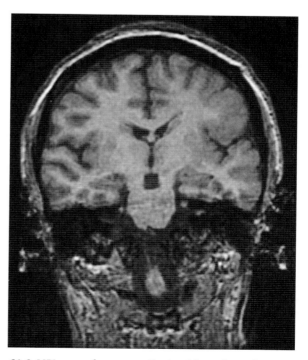

Fig. 61-6 MRI scan from a patient with unilateral perisylvian dysplasia with polymicrogyria (left hemisphere). T1-weighted imaging (TR = 24 msec/TE = 9 msec) was used.

herpesvirus 6 (HHV6), have also been implicated as potential causes of mesial temporal sclerosis [Scott et al., 2001; Solinas et al., 2003; Donati et al., 2003; Theodore et al., 2008]. These questions have not yet been clearly answered. It is known, however, that the degree of volume loss correlates with the amount of cellular loss, as measured in pathologic specimens [Cascino et al., 1991]. The neuronal cell loss, coupled with the presence of aberrant mossy fibers, and synaptic reorganization and excessive glutamatergic activity, probably accounts for the recurrent, recalcitrant seizures [Fuerst et al., 2003; Holmes and Ben-Ari, 1998; Jokeit et al., 1999; Kalviainen et al., 1998; Kotloski et al., 2002; Sutula et al., 1988, 1989; Tasch et al., 1999; Eid et al., 2008].

Co-registration of scalp EEG and MRI data has become an important tool in the determination of source localization relative to the patient's brain anatomy [Lamm et al., 2001]. This technique provides a three-dimensional rendition of the topographic EEG activity on to the patient's head, taking into consideration anatomical differences specific to the patient. More recently, co-registration of the intracranial EEG and MRI data has provided the epileptologist and neurosurgeon with a three-dimensional map of electrode placement used to define the epileptogenic zone, and hence, the boundaries of surgical resection [LaViolette et al., 2011] (Figure 61-7).

Single-Photon Emission Computed Tomography

SPECT also has enhanced the ability to identify the epileptogenic zone. Penfield and colleagues observed relative hyperperfusion in the epileptogenic zone during a seizure [Penfield, 1958]. Interictally, blood flow and metabolism decrease. SPECT scan technology enables quantification of cerebral blood flow and identification of areas of relative blood flow change. SPECT images are reconstructed from data obtained by recording photon emissions from radiotracers injected intravenously. These radiotracers rapidly cross the blood–brain barrier because of their lipophilic nature and bind within minutes to the brain, producing an instantaneous picture of cerebral blood flow [English and Brown, 1990]. Clinical research has focused on both interictal and ictal SPECT scans, with a substantial portion of the clinical research using the radioisotope ^{99m}technetium-hexamethylpropyleneamine oxime (^{99m}Tc-HMPAO) [Cross et al., 1995, 1997; Harvey et al., 1993a, b]. More recently, ^{99m}Tc ethyl cysteinate dimer (ECD) (i.e., ^{99m}Tc-N,N'(1,2-ethylenediyl)bis-L-cysteine diethyl ester), prepared as technetium ^{99m}Tc bicisate (Neurolite), has been introduced [Lanceman et al., 1997]. Logistically, Neurolite provides distinct advantages for ictal SPECT scans because it is a stable isotope tracer that can be mixed well ahead of the time of injection, as opposed to ^{99m}Tc-HMPAO, which decomposes quickly in vitro and must be used less than 30 minutes after it is reconstituted. For ictal SPECT scans, a technologist or nurse trained in the delivery of these radioisotopes can sit at the bedside and deliver the Neurolite within seconds after the onset of a seizure. Spatial resolution with SPECT scans also has improved because of the development of gamma cameras with multiple detectors that provide more data points, with subsequent enhanced sensitivity.

Interictal SPECT scans have been used for longer than 10 years as a method of identifying the epileptogenic focus in patients with medically intractable localization-related epilepsy who are candidates for epilepsy surgery. With interictal SPECT scans, the epileptogenic zone can be identified by a regional area of reduced cerebral blood flow [Adams et al., 1992; Berkovic et al., 1992, 1993; Cordes et al., 1990; Coubes et al., 1993; Denays et al., 1988; Dietrich et al., 1991; Grunwald et al., 1991; Hajek et al., 1991; Kuzniecky et al., 1993b; Lamanna et al., 1989; Launes et al., 1992; Lee et al., 1988; Rowe et al., 1989, 1991; Ryding et al., 1988; Ryvlin et al., 1992; Shen et al., 1990; Verhoeff et al., 1992]. Clinical research clearly indicates that interictal studies alone have a relatively low sensitivity for identification of the epileptogenic focus in adults with temporal lobe epilepsy and even lower sensitivity with extratemporal epilepsy. Data pooled from several studies yield estimates of interictal SPECT sensitivity of 66 percent for temporal lobe epilepsy and 60 percent for extratemporal epilepsy localized by EEG [Spencer, 1994; Knowlton, 2006].

Ictal SPECT scan data, however, have proved valuable with respect to localization of the epileptogenic focus. Ictal SPECT

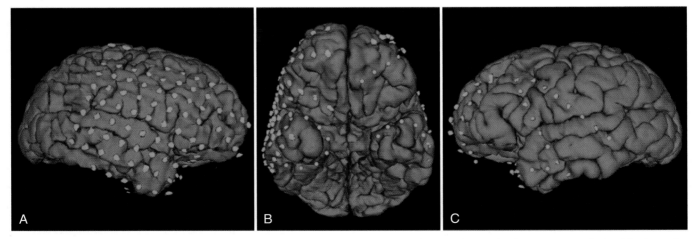

Fig. 61-7 **Three-dimensional CT-derived electrode model overlaid on patient-specific post-electrode placement MRI-derived brain surface used in planning of subsequent resective surgery. A,** Right hemisphere showing 8 × 8 electrode grid complemented by frontal and temporal strip electrodes. **B,** Anterior view showing medial temporal ventral frontal strips. **C,** Lateral left hemisphere view depicting frontal/temporal electrodes. *(Courtesy of Peter LaViolette, Medical College of Wisconsin, Milwaukee, Wisconsin.)*

scans typically reveal an area of regional hyperperfusion that corresponds to the underlying epileptogenic focus, as verified by surgical pathology and surface EEG localization [Bauer et al., 1989; Grunwald et al., 1991; Ho et al., 1994; Hwang et al., 1990; Katz et al., 1990; Lee et al., 1988; Marks et al., 1992; Newton et al., 1992b; Rowe et al., 1989, 1991; Shen et al., 1990; Stefan et al., 1990]. Using data pooled from several centers, the sensitivity of ictal SPECT (as judged by EEG correlation) has been estimated at 90 percent for temporal and 81 percent for extratemporal epilepsy, with specificity at 77 percent and 93 percent, respectively [Spencer, 1994; Knowlton, 2006]. Critical to the efficacy of the ictal SPECT scan is the timing of the injection. If the injection can be given within 30 seconds of the seizure onset, the isotope remains localized and can "capture" the epileptogenic focus or generator before the epileptogenic discharge spreads [Newton et al., 1995]. If the seizure propagation is rapid, ictal injections are less sensitive and unreliable.

Comparison of ictal and interictal scans also is important in determining whether any abnormality in blood flow is significant. With the assistance of computerized technology and surface matching techniques, co-registration of the ictal SPECT scan to the volumetric MRI scan has demonstrated a close relationship between the region of ictal hyperperfusion and MRI structural lesions [Hogan et al., 1996; Mountz et al., 1994]. A technique has been developed whereby the ictal and interictal SPECT scan data are co-registered with one another and the interictal image is subtracted from the ictal image, producing the area of true ictal hyperperfusion [Zubal et al., 1995]. This difference image, called a subtraction SPECT scan, is then co-registered with a three-dimensional representation of the MRI scan. In nonlesional extratemporal epilepsy, this information has been proven to be especially helpful in either

guiding placement for subdural invasive EEG monitoring or obviating the need for invasive monitoring altogether. Several studies have demonstrated that peri-ictal subtraction SPECT provides useful information for seizure localization in patients with focal malformations of cortical development, even when the MRI study is nonlocalizing (i.e., "nonlesional") [O'Brien et al., 1998, 2000, 2004; Tan et al., 2008]. In a large series involving pediatric and adult epilepsy patients, if the site of the surgical resection was concordant with the subtraction SPECT localization (using SISCOM technology, a Mayo Clinic-patented computer program that performs subtraction SPECT and then co-registers the results to a volumetric MRI scan of the brain), postoperative seizure frequency scores were significantly lower and postoperative improvement was greater [O'Brien et al., 1998] (Figure 61-8). A recent multicenter study further confirmed the incremental benefit of the SISCOM technology over traditional side-by-side comparison in the presurgical evaluation, particularly in patients with extratemporal lobe epilepsy [Matsuda et al., 2009].

In summary, SPECT scan technology, particularly subtraction SPECT, holds great merit for localization of the epileptogenic zone, is widely available, and is reasonable in cost. Additionally, the new stable tracers have simplified the procedure and improved the ability to obtain accurate ictal scans. These advances, coupled with increasing resolution of the image scanners, ensure that SPECT scan technology will gain increasing prominence.

Positron Emission Tomography

PET is another imaging modality used for localization of the epileptogenic focus [Mohan et al., 1999]. It uses radiotracers labeled with specific positron-emitting isotopes (^{11}C, ^{15}O,

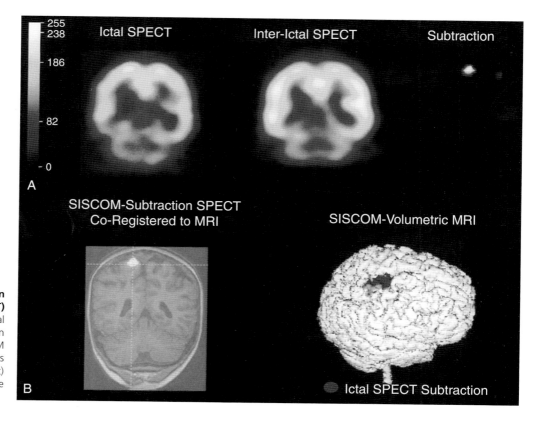

Fig. 61-8 Single-photon emission computed tomography (SPECT) scans. A, Ictal (left) and interictal (middle) scans, along with subtraction SPECT scan (right). **B,** Using SISCOM software (see text), subtraction scans co-registered to the MRI study (left) and with volumetric MRI (right) were obtained.

and ^{18}F) to measure a variety of biochemical brain functions. With the aid of computerized technology and mathematical modeling, the source and concentration of the emission are either qualitatively or quantitatively plotted on a three-dimensional representation of the brain. Cerebral glucose metabolism is the most commonly measured parameter, using ^{18}F-fluorodeoxyglucose (FDG) (Figure 61-9). Other tracers also can be used to measure cerebral blood flow, benzodiazepine and opiate receptors, pH, serotonin metabolism, and amino acid transport [Henry et al., 1993; Mohan et al., 1999; Shah et al., 1995].

FDG PET images are averaged over a 40-minute time interval, suggesting the limited value of this technique for ictal studies. The interictal images, on the other hand, are highly sensitive in complex partial seizures emanating from the temporal lobe. In several studies in adult patients with medically refractory epilepsy of temporal lobe origin, glucose hypometabolism in the temporal lobe correlated highly with localized ictal EEGs and MRI abnormalities in this region [Abou-Khali et al., 1987; Chugani et al., 1990b; Coubes et al., 1993; Debets et al., 1990; Engel et al., 1982; Hajek et al., 1993; Henry et al., 1993; Leiderman et al., 1992; Radtke et al., 1993; Sackellares et al., 1990; Stefan et al., 1987, 1990; Swartz et al., 1992; Theodore et al., 1986, 1990; Valk et al., 1993]. Glucose hypometabolism in the temporal lobe, as obtained on interictal FDG PET scan, has been found to have an overall sensitivity of 84 percent and a specificity of 86 percent [Spencer, 1994; Knowlton, 2006].

In a study by Theodore et al. [1997], the presence of temporal lobe glucose hypometabolism in the presence of a nonlocalizing surface ictal EEG predicted successful outcome with temporal lobectomy. Localization to the temporal lobe was confirmed with invasive EEG monitoring but the authors make the point that invasive EEG monitoring may be unnecessary and may even provide false localizing information in some

patients being evaluated for epilepsy surgery. As technology improves, concordance of noninvasive neuroimaging techniques may be all that is necessary before proceeding with the surgery.

Analysis of nonlesional extratemporal epilepsy in adult patients undergoing PET scans has provided data that have been less definitive [Chugani et al., 1990a; Sackellares et al., 1990; Stefan et al., 1990]. In one recent analysis, the sensitivity and specificity of FDG PET scans decreased to 40 percent in MRI-negative extratemporal cases [Yun et al., 2006]. In children with refractory epilepsy, however, with poor localization on surface EEG and negative findings on MRI scans of the brain, FDG PET scans may still provide useful information in identifying an underlying epileptogenic focus. Specifically, University of California at Los Angeles investigators were the first to recognize a small subset of children with intractable infantile spasms and underlying deficits of focal glucose metabolism [Chugani et al., 1988, 1990a; Olson et al., 1990]. These deficits usually were temporal-parietal-occipital in origin. Many of these patients had partial seizures before, during, or after the onset of their infantile spasms, often providing a clue to localization. Additionally, interictal surface EEG examined retrospectively often disclosed focal delta slowing or an asymmetry in beta activity. Large cortical resections of the underlying epileptogenic zone were performed, guided by PET scan data and electrocorticography. After surgery, the seizures (infantile spasms and/or partial seizures) disappeared. Results indicate, not only that seizure control improved, but also that these patients' development improved at a faster rate and to a greater degree than would have been predicted without surgery [Asarnow et al., 1997; Chugani et al., 1988].

Newer ligands also have been developed. In flumazenil PET scans, the flumazenil binds to benzodiazepine receptors [Juhasz et al., 1999; Mohan et al., 1999]. In the area of the epileptogenic zone, benzodiazepine binding appears to

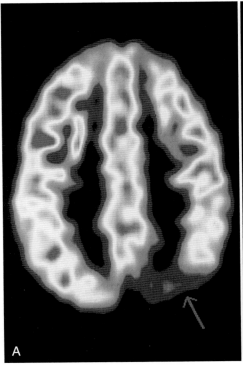
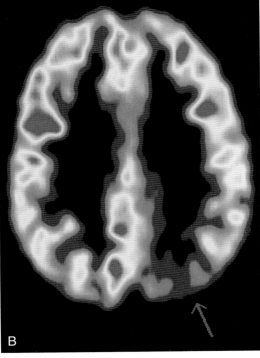

Fig. 61-9 Fluorodeoxyglucose positron emission tomography (FDG PET) scan from a 12-year-old girl with complex partial seizures, showing a focal decrease in glucose metabolism in the left parietal and, to a lesser extent, the left occipital cortex. **A** and **B,** The images were obtained at two different horizontal levels of the brain. EEG performed during the scan demonstrated occasional sharp-wave discharges over the left parietal and central regions. *(Courtesy of Dr. HG Chugani and Children's Hospital of Michigan PET Center, Wayne State University, Detroit, Michigan.)*

be decreased. In one clinical study, the flumazenil PET scan demonstrated a more restricted area of decreased binding than was apparent on the FDG PET scan; the resection of this cortical region was associated with good surgical outcome [Juhasz et al., 2000]. In addition, diffuse cortical abnormalities on flumazenil PET scans predict poor seizure control following epilepsy surgery [Juhasz et al., 2001].

C-alphamethyl-L-tryptophan (AMT) PET scans also have been studied. AMT is an analog of trytophan and a precursor for serotonin synthesis [Chugani et al., 1998; Juhasz et al., 2003]. Data suggest that the AMT PET scans may be useful in identifying the most epileptogenic tuber in patients with tuberous sclerosis, multiple tubers, and medically intractable epilepsy. Concordance of the epileptogenic tuber with increased AMT uptake has been observed in PET scans [Asano et al., 2000; Chugani et al., 1998, Chugani and Muzik, 2000]. In addition, AMT PET scans may also be helpful in reevaluating patients in whom epilepsy surgery has failed to improve seizure control. In the patients studied with AMT PET, the area of increased AMT binding correlated closely with the epileptogenic zone [Juhasz et al., 2004].

Magnetic Resonance Spectroscopy

MR spectroscopy has been used in the study of patients with intractable epilepsy [Kuzniecky et al., 1992; Laxer et al., 1992; Matthews et al., 1990; Novotny, 1995; Connelly et al., 1994]. Specifically, phosphorus MR spectroscopy measures phospholipid metabolism. In the region of the epileptogenic focus, investigators have found abnormal phosphocreatine to inorganic phosphate ratios. Phosphocreatine (Pcr), intracellular pH, and inorganic phosphorus (Pi) increase during a seizure. The adenosine triphosphate concentration, however, only decreases slightly [Duncan, 1997; Prichard, 1994]. Proton MR spectroscopy can also measure regional abnormalities in lactate, N-acetyl-aspartate (NAA), creatine (Cr), and choline (Cho). Lactate levels increase during a seizure and remain elevated for several hours. Data also indicate reductions in the NAA/Cho and NAA/Cr ratios in the region of the epileptogenic zone, presumed to reflect neuronal loss and reactive astrocytosis [Petroff et al., 1984, 1986; Prichard, 1994]. Therefore, abnormal NAA/Cr and NAA/Cho ratios may serve as indices of regional cellular pathology. MR spectroscopy holds promise as an important adjunctive noninvasive technique for assisting with the identification of the underlying epileptogenic zone.

Magnetoencephalography

MEG is another technology that has been developed to improve the ability to identify epileptogenic foci. It measures tiny magnetic fields in the brain that are created by the electrical activity of the brain. Most institutions are using 128-channel MEG technology to enhance resolution. MEG offers several advantages over EEG. First, the magnetic fields are not attenuated by the skull, scalp, and skin, as are electrical potentials. Therefore, the MEG signal contains fewer distortions or changes [Barth, 1993]. Second, MEG is a monopolar measure and does not require a dipolar montage, eliminating the possibility of artifact associated with an "active reference." Third, MEG provides high temporal resolution, which can be useful in determining the functional activity of different brain areas (i.e., motor cortex) or propagation of seizure activity.

Finally, and of greatest importance, MEG measures postsynaptic intracellular currents in the dendrites of neurons situated tangentially to the skull, whereas the EEG measures the extracellular postsynaptic ionic currents [Tovar-Spinoza et al., 2008; Barth, 1993; Barth et al., 1984].

Clinical research suggests that, although surface interictal EEG spike recordings may indicate multifocal activity, MEG can more precisely localize the underlying epileptogenic focus [Barth, 1993; Stefan et al., 2003; Sutherling et al., 1988; Wheless et al., 1999]. In this regard, MEG provides complementary data to EEG and there is a growing belief that combined MEG/EEG data should be used routinely in the presurgical evaluation of patients with intractable epilepsy [Funke et al., 2009]. MEG has provided pivotal information and may become the most precise way of identifying the size, location, and dipole orientation of the epileptogenic zone [Minassian et al., 1999; Stefan et al., 2003; Wheless et al., 1999, 2004]. In particular, there is widespread agreement that MEG provides the best tool to distinguish a temporal from an extratemporal epileptogenic zone [Funke et al., 2009]. In fact, MEG has been employed in children with intractable epilepsy to provide spatial information to be used in planning the excision area [Iida et al., 2005]. MEG spike source clusters have been used to indicate the epileptogenic zone [Iida et al., 2005]. Figure 61-10 demonstrates simultaneously recorded MEG and EEG data obtained at our center and used to map the epileptogenic focus of a child with frontal lobe epilepsy. As shown in Figure 61-10A and B, a left frontal MEG spike is observed while the EEG demonstrates theta range activity without clear epileptiform activity. Figure 61-10C demonstrates the distributed source estimates for the MEG data displayed on a representation of the cortical surface reconstructed from MRI data from the same patient. Note the basomesial frontal location of the epileptogenic zone, which would have been difficult to observe on scalp EEG. In addition, MEG may be a very useful tool in children with respect to functional imaging, particularly imaging language cortex [Stufflebeam et al., 2009; Tovar-Spinoza et al., 2008; Papanicolaou et al., 2004; Simos et al., 1999]. Figure 61-11A demonstrates locations of the equivalent current dipoles (ECD) for the MEG data for a visual reading task displayed in sagittal slices of an anatomical representation of the same patient's brain as in Figure 61-10. The high temporal resolution of MEG allows for the dissociation of functional brain activity in different areas. The patient's language was localized to the left hemisphere, based on the Wada procedure (see below). The extraordinary temporal resolution of MEG also enables us to understand the propagation patterns of interictal activity occurring over a period of 50 msec or less (Figure 61-11B)!

Functional Mapping

If an underlying epileptogenic focus is identified, the next question to consider is whether the epileptogenic zone can be removed without causing unacceptable neurologic deficits. In infants and young children, this proves to be less problematic because of brain plasticity.

Classically, in the older child and adolescent, the sodium amytal test (Wada test) is used in the preoperative evaluation for the localization of speech and language and to determine whether memory can be supported in the contralateral hemisphere [Loring, 1997; Wyllie et al., 1990]. This test involves injecting sodium amytal into either the left or the right

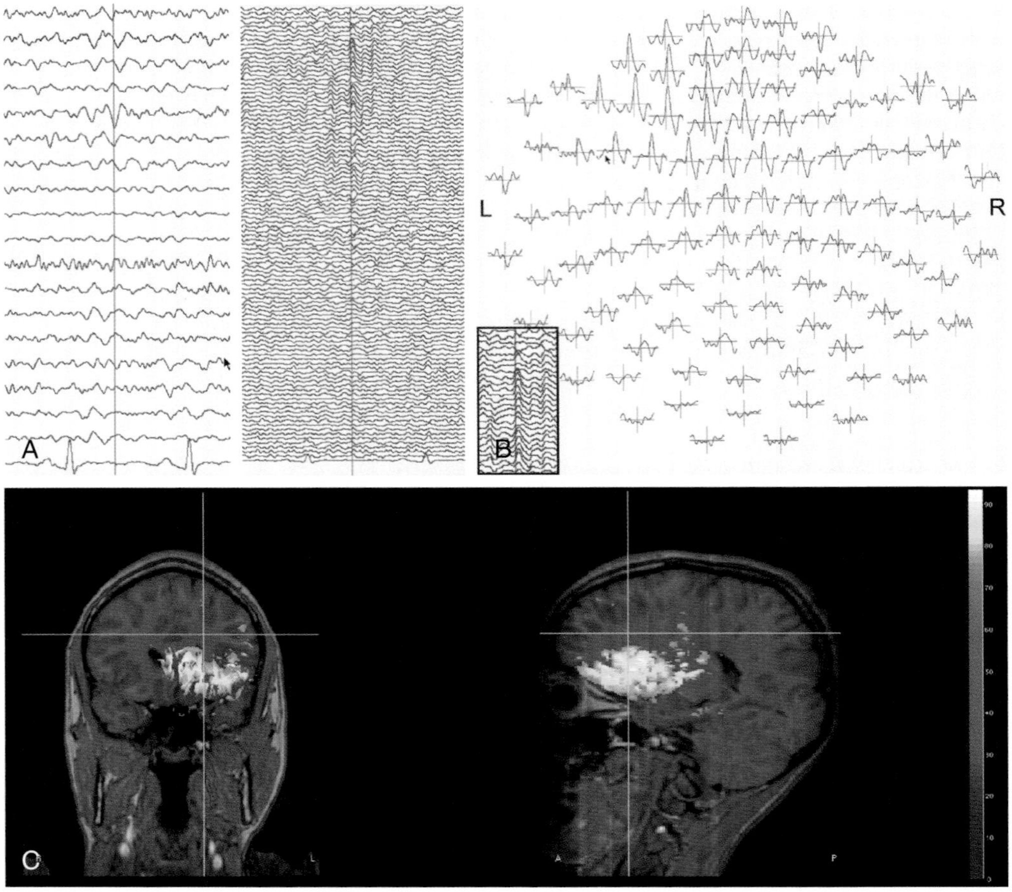

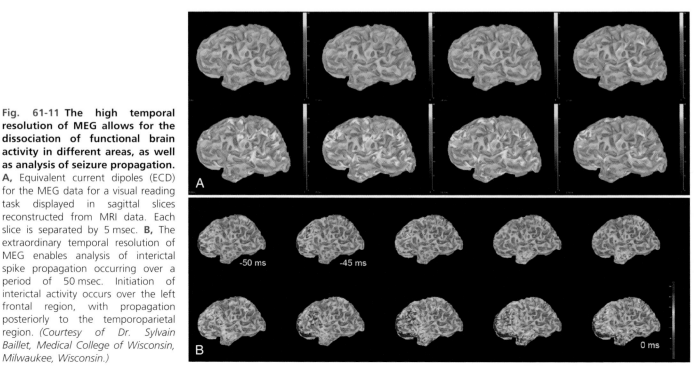

Fig. 61-10 Magnetoencephalography (MEG) complements EEG data in the presurgical evaluation. A, Simultaneously recorded EEG (left tracings) and MEG recordings (right tracings) from a patient with frontal lobe epilepsy. **B,** Distribution of MEG sensors demonstrating left frontal MEG spikes at t = 0 (green line in panel A). Inset demonstrates source MEG data. **C,** Distributed source estimates for MEG data displayed on a representation of the cortical surface reconstructed from MRI data. *(Courtesy of Dr. Sylvain Baillet, Medical College of Wisconsin, Milwaukee, Wisconsin.)*

Fig. 61-11 The high temporal resolution of MEG allows for the dissociation of functional brain activity in different areas, as well as analysis of seizure propagation. A, Equivalent current dipoles (ECD) for the MEG data for a visual reading task displayed in sagittal slices reconstructed from MRI data. Each slice is separated by 5 msec. **B,** The extraordinary temporal resolution of MEG enables analysis of interictal spike propagation occurring over a period of 50 msec. Initiation of interictal activity occurs over the left frontal region, with propagation posteriorly to the temporoparietal region. *(Courtesy of Dr. Sylvain Baillet, Medical College of Wisconsin, Milwaukee, Wisconsin.)*

internal carotid artery, in an attempt to ameliorate ipsilateral hemispheric function chemically and to determine which hemisphere is "dominant" (i.e., responsible for speech and language function and, to a lesser extent, memory). It is a time-consuming test that is invasive and provides a broad but nonspecific overview of hemispheric function. Additionally, controversy continues over its interpretation and its ability to predict postoperative function, particularly with respect to memory [Loring et al., 1992; Perrine, 1994]. As an example, language is a complex function. Although speech arrest after sodium amytal injection usually is in the dominant hemisphere, this is not always the case [Loring et al., 1992]. Language involves spontaneous speech, repetition, comprehension, reading, and counting. These aspects of language are all interactive, but their corresponding cortical areas may be located in different areas of the brain, making it difficult to relegate language to one specific hemisphere or region. In younger children, the Wada test can be even more challenging and technically difficult. Obtaining full cooperation from a child requires preparation, time, and patience. If the child becomes frightened during the test, test validity becomes questionable. Two other techniques also used frequently to identify eloquent cortex (i.e., cortex controlling vital motor, language, or memory functions) are somatosensory-evoked potentials and stimulation mapping. The measurement of somatosensory-evoked potentials has the advantage of being able to be applied successfully, regardless of the state of the patient. This modality can be used in the operating room in the anesthetized patient, or in an awake and cooperative patient. Somatosensory-evoked potentials are used primarily to identify the sensorimotor cortex. Stimulation mapping involves the application of subdural electrodes followed by sequential electrical stimuli at various intensities and durations. Penfield pioneered this technique during the 1930s through the 1950s to localize language and motor functions intraoperatively, in order to avoid postoperative neurologic deficits. Subsequent investigators have used cortical stimulation preoperatively (using implanted grid electrodes) and intraoperatively to map out functional cortex, such as the sensorimotor cortex or expressive language cortex [Ojemann, 1978, 1979, 1993; Ojemann and Dodrill, 1987]. Although cortical stimulation mapping has yielded a tremendous amount of information about the localization of functions,

several other emerging techniques are providing valid, noninvasive methods for mapping out functional areas of the brain. These techniques include functional MRI (fMRI) scans, MEG and magnetic source imaging, and transcranial magnetic stimulation [Binder, 1997; Detre, 2004; Knowlton and Shih, 2004; Peresson et al., 1998; Perrine, 1994; Powell et al., 2004; Sabsevitz et al., 2003; Wheless et al., 2004]. In view of the limitations of the previously described techniques for functional mapping, these noninvasive techniques, which might provide more specific and salient information, are being developed. fMRI scans are being used in a number of epilepsy centers as adjunctive techniques to define eloquent cortex [Kwong et al., 1992; Lee et al., 1996; Ogawa et al., 1992].

fMRI is based on the fact that performance of a specific act will activate the anatomically appropriate cortex in the brain. With activation, a concomitant increase in blood flow occurs, resulting in a change in the paramagnetic properties of the affected cortex. This produces a signal that can then be detected by the MRI scanner. fMRI is a technique that will be increasingly used to map out eloquent functions, such as sensorimotor cortex and speech and language centers [Logan et al., 1995, 1997, 1998; Sachs et al., 2003; O'Shaughnessy et al., 2008]. It is still not suitable for the young, uncooperative infant or child, except for fMRI of the sensorimotor cortex, which can be performed under sedation. Language and memory testing using fMRI can be utilized in cooperative older children and adolescents. In fact, clinical research has yielded increasing proof that fMRI can provide important localization data. With respect to language lateralization, fMRI language examinations, in combination with comprehensive neuropsychometric testing, can play a very important role in estimating the risk for postoperative cognitive changes and in selecting patients for invasive functional mapping procedures [Sachs et al., 2003; O'Shaughnessy et al., 2008; Liegeois et al., 2002; Hertz-Pannier et al., 1997; Stapleton et al., 1997; Anderson et al., 2006]. In the young infant and child, functional studies are less likely to alter the surgical plan because brain plasticity in these age groups makes localization less critical [Shields, 2000; Stafstrom et al., 2000; Wyllie, 1998, Liegeois et al., 2004; Kadis et al., 2007].

An example of a functional MRI scan is illustrated in Figure 61-12.

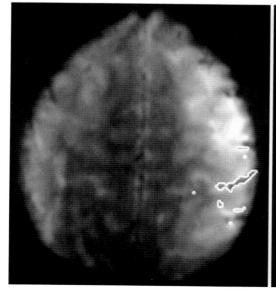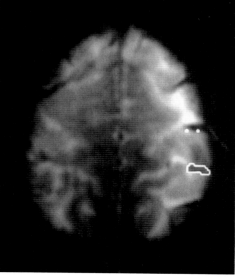

Fig. 61-12 Functional magnetic resonance imaging scan. Identification of left hemisphere motor cortex was achieved by asking the patient to open and close his right hand repetitively. Functional activity (in white) is superimposed on gray scan multishot echo planar images.

Concept of Congruence

Under ideal conditions, identification of the epileptogenic focus is made by the congruence of data obtained during the preoperative evaluation, with the precise localization based on seizure semiology, physical examination, surface ictal and interictal EEG monitoring (and, if necessary, invasive-depth electrodes or subdural electrode strips or grid), MRI scan of the brain, ictal and interictal SPECT scans, interictal PET scan, MEG, fMRI scan, and/or MR spectroscopy. Each case must be individualized, with some cases requiring the acquisition of data from all of these studies. Other cases may be resolved with a less complicated approach. At a minimum, seizure semiology, surface ictal EEG monitoring, and MRI scan of the brain should be congruent. With lesional localization-related epilepsy, the use of invasive EEG monitoring may not be necessary. Electrocorticography at the time of surgery usually can assist with identifying the dimensions of the epileptogenic zone. The sensorimotor cortex can be identified intraoperatively using motor-evoked potentials, somatosensory-evoked potentials, or direct electrical cortical stimulation mapping. In a cooperative patient, fMRI brain imaging or MEG may be able to identify the sensorimotor cortex accurately and display it on a three-dimensional volumetric MRI scan of the brain. If the surgical excision is near functional speech and language cortex, older children and adolescents usually can be cooperative enough to tolerate an awake surgical procedure. In addition, in older cooperative children and adolescents, fMRI has also been very helpful in identifying cortex involved with receptive and expressive language. In younger children (before the age of 5–6 years), brain plasticity is still adequate, so that removal of primary speech and language cortex will result in transition of these functions to the contralateral hemisphere [Peacock, 1995; Shields, 2000].

The most complex cases are those of nonlesional extratemporal epilepsy. The patients usually require an interictal PET scan, subtraction SPECT scan, MR spectroscopy, or MEG, to look for evidence of a localized abnormality. In these patients, placement of invasive subdural strips or grids is generally necessary for precise localization of the epileptogenic focus. However, the advanced neuroimaging techniques allow one to place the invasive subdural strips and grids more accurately, maximizing the opportunity to identify the epileptogenic zone.

Types of Surgery

Several types of epilepsy surgery are performed in children and adults, depending on the identification of the epileptogenic focus and its location and extent [Zupanc, 1997b]. The most common surgical procedures are:
1. temporal lobectomy
2. cortical resection – lobar and multilobar
3. stereotactic lesionectomy
4. hemispherectomy – either functional, modified hemispherectomy or anatomic hemispherectomy
5. multiple subpial transection
6. corpus callosotomy
7. implantation of a vagus nerve stimulator.
Implantation of a vagus nerve stimulator accounts for approximately 16 percent of the total number of operations, while multiple subpial transections are relatively uncommon procedures, accounting for only 0.6 percent [Harvey et al., 2008].

Temporal lobectomy is the most common epilepsy surgery performed in adolescents and adults. This procedure is almost exclusively a temporal lobectomy with amygdalohippocampectomy, because removal of the mesial temporal structures is correlated with a better surgical outcome. Often an associated abnormality or lesion, such as a tumor (dysembryoplastic neuroepithelial tumor [DNET] or ganglioglioma), mesial temporal sclerosis, hippocampal formation atrophy, or malformation of cortical development, is found to be present. The new MRI technologies have been helpful in identification of these substrates of epilepsy. Those patients with mesial temporal sclerosis or hippocampal atrophy concordant with ictal surface EEG abnormalities have an excellent prognosis for successful epilepsy surgery, with a 90 percent chance of becoming seizure-free [Duchowny et al., 1992; Falconer, 1970; Mizrahi et al., 1990]. Younger children do not commonly have mesial temporal sclerosis or hippocampal atrophy [Ng et al., 2004]. Many of the intractable epilepsies in childhood are extratemporal and nonlesional.

Extratemporal cortical resection is more commonly performed in children, often involving extensive lobar or multilobar resections. The extent of the resection is dictated primarily by the extent of the lesion: e.g., a tuberectomy in a patient with tuberous sclerosis versus a multilobar resection in a child with infantile spasms and an underlying focal cortical dysplasia involving the temporal-parietal-occipital lobes. As the ability to identify focal cortical dysplasias and the concomitant epileptogenic zone improves, epilepsy surgical outcomes also will improve. Focal cortical dysplasias are a common cause of intractable partial epilepsy in children, accounting for 60 percent of the cases [Kuzniecky and Barkovich, 2001; Kuzniecky et al., 1993c]. The best predictive factors in successful surgical outcome in focal cortical dysplasia are completeness of the resection and the presence of an identifiable lesion on MRI brain imaging [ILAE Pediatric Epilepsy Surgery Consortium data, submitted for publication].

Stereotactic lesionectomy is performed in highly selected cases in children and adults, with a reported 50–60 percent chance of rendering the patient seizure-free [Britton et al., 1994; Cascino et al., 1990, 1992, 1993, 1994]. Outcome is improved if intraoperative electrocorticography is used to remove not only the lesion, but also the surrounding "epileptogenic zone" [Jooma et al., 1995; Montes et al., 1995; Palmini et al., 1995; Pilcher et al., 1993]. To date, no prospective, controlled studies of statistically significant numbers of patients have critically compared the different operative strategies with respect to outcome [Shields, 2000; Tonini et al., 2004; Wyllie, 1998]. The surgical outcome in these patients may vary, depending on the age of the patient, the location of the lesion, and most important, the type of lesion. In a review of 47 published articles about epilepsy surgery outcome, the best predictors for seizure-free outcome included a history of febrile seizures as a child, mesial temporal sclerosis, tumors, EEG and MRI data concordance, and an extensive surgical resection [Tonini et al., 2004].

Hemispherectomy also is performed in young children [Vining et al., 1997]. The indications for this type of surgery are catastrophic epilepsies in which the substrate of epilepsy is limited to one hemisphere. Epilepsy syndromes that frequently meet these criteria include the following:
1. Sturge–Weber syndrome
2. hemimegalencephaly or other extensive hemispheric malformation of cortical development
3. Rasmussen's encephalitis.

In Sturge–Weber syndrome, the pathologic features consist of unilateral leptomeningeal angiomatosis, frequently resulting in changes in the involved hemisphere with concomitant focal seizures, progressive hemiparesis, and cognitive decline [Roach et al., 1994]. Hemimegalencephaly, by definition, is a malformation of cortical development involving one hemisphere, and is characterized by general disorganization and overgrowth of the neuronal tissue. Early hemispherectomy, particularly if the EEG reveals unilateral discharges, can significantly alter the prognosis in affected children [Andermann et al., 1993; Vigevano et al., 1989; Vigevano and DiRocco, 1990]. With Rasmussen's encephalitis, children have intractable focal seizures, often progressing to epilepsia partialis continua, accompanied by progressive hemiparesis and cognitive decline. Although debate is on-going about the pathophysiology (autoimmune versus infectious), the only long-term successful treatment has been hemispherectomy [Antel and Rasmussen, 1996].

Multiple subpial transection is a newer surgical technique that is used when the epileptogenic zone overlies an area of functional cortex. Multiple subpial transection involves the disruption of connecting horizontal fibers, rather than resection of actual tissue [Blount et al., 2004; Devinsky et al., 2003; Schramm et al., 2002; Spencer et al., 2002]. This technique has been used in the treatment of Landau–Kleffner syndrome [Morrell et al., 1995]. Children with this syndrome have an acquired epileptic aphasia, often intractable to medication. The multiple subpial transection technique has been used over the area deemed to be the epileptogenic zone on electrocorticography. Although good surgical results have been reported, the technique remains controversial. Multiple subpial transection also is being used in areas involving functional cortex. Data indicate that, although multiple subpial transection may be an appropriate adjunctive surgical technique, it will not eliminate seizures if the primary epileptogenic focus is not completely removed [Hufnagel et al., 1997; Spencer et al., 2002].

A complete corpus callosotomy is a palliative surgery that can reduce the seizure burden in carefully selected patients. It most commonly is used in children with Lennox–Gastaut syndrome, with the goal being reduction of tonic and atonic seizures. It can be highly effective [Carson, 2000; Maehara and Shimizu, 2001; McInerney et al., 1999; Sassower et al., 2001; Sorenson et al., 1997; Wyler, 1993]. It is now known that sectioning of the anterior two-thirds corpus callosotomy is rarely effective in controlling seizures long-term. The use of a complete corpus callosotomy, coupled with lateralizing strips, has been demonstrated to be very effective in identifying an epileptogenic zone as part of a multistage surgery [Zupanc et al., 2011].

Goals of Surgery

With use of innovative, noninvasive technologies, the ability of the clinician to identify the underlying epileptogenic zone has improved. In patients with medically intractable epilepsy, this ability allows one of the principal goals of epilepsy surgery to be achieved – that is, the elimination of seizures. The goals of epilepsy surgery, however, may vary, depending on the epilepsy syndrome, the underlying pathophysiology, the cognitive and developmental status of the child or adolescent, and the

identification and location of an epileptogenic zone [Taylor et al., 1997]. Specifically, if a cognitively normal patient has temporal lobe epilepsy, as documented by congruence of seizure semiology and EEG and MRI data, the goals of epilepsy surgery are clear: elimination of seizures and improvement in psychosocial, behavioral, emotional, and family functioning without significant loss of cognitive abilities. On the other hand, a cognitively impaired patient with an extensive bilateral malformation of cortical development might be considered for a corpus callosotomy. In this case, the primary goals of epilepsy surgery would be palliative, with the reduction of seizures and possible improvement in cognitive and behavioral functions. Although improvement in cognition, development, and behavior usually is achieved by virtue of decreased seizure frequency and reduction of antiepileptic drug doses, such results are not always obtained, and outcomes will vary with each patient, depending on the epilepsy syndrome and the identified etiology for the epilepsy. The goals of epilepsy surgery and potential limitations of the results of surgery need to be discussed openly with the family before any decision is made.

In patients with malformations of cortical development (in children, typically extratemporal), epilepsy surgery usually has involved lobar or multilobar resections, as well as hemispherectomies. Approximately 60–65 percent of these patients are seizure-free after surgery, and a majority achieves a significant reduction in seizure burden [Shields, 2000; Wyllie, 1998; Zupanc et al., 2010]. At critical stages of development, this reduction in seizure burden is associated with an improvement in development that appears to be sustained. In patients with malformations of cortical development and medically refractory epilepsy who undergo surgical resection, withdrawal of antiepileptic medication is rarely successful. The cortical dysplasia often is very extensive, involving multiple lobes. On the other hand, children with lesions such as mesial temporal sclerosis, low-grade tumors, or middle cerebral artery infarctions can achieve seizure-free status, with eventual discontinuation of antiepileptic medication.

Deep Brain Stimulation

Deep brain stimulation has been known to be effective in the treatment of movement disorders for years. However, there is increasing interest in deep brain stimulation in the treatment of epilepsy [Kahane and Depaulis, 2010]. Several neurology and neurosurgical groups have applied this technique in the treatment of pharmacoresistant epilepsy. Recently, the SANTE study group has published their results. This was a multicenter, double-blind, randomized trial of bilateral stimulation of the anterior nuclei of the thalamus for localization-related epilepsy. The stimulation of the anterior nucleus of the thalamus was chosen because it projects to both the superior frontal and the temporal lobe structures commonly involved in epileptic seizures, produces discrete EEG changes, and inhibits chemically induced seizures in animal models. In this study, which involved adult patients only, with localization-related epilepsy, bilateral stimulation of the anterior nuclei of the thalamus significantly reduced seizure frequency. Specifically, by 2 years, there was a 56 percent median reduction in seizure frequency; 54 percent of patients had a seizure reduction of at least 50 percent. Fourteen patients were seizure-free for over 6 months [Fischer et al., 2010].

In addition to the anterior nucleus, the centromedian nucleus has also been the subject of both clinical and experimental interest. This nucleus is part of the reticulothalamocortical system, which modulates cortical excitability. There have been several studies that have documented significant improvement in seizure control, particularly in patients with generalized tonic-clonic seizures and atypical absence seizures found in Lennox–Gastaut syndrome [Velasco et al., 1997, 2006; Cukiert et al., 2009].

In the future, deep brain stimulation may be very useful in the treatment of medically refractory epilepsy in children. Further clinical trials are required before it will be utilized in the pediatric population.

Research Issues: Trends for the Future

There are many unanswered questions that still need to be addressed in the pursuit of helping children with intractable epilepsy:

- What are the age-specific developmental mechanisms in childhood epilepsy? Can they be targeted for the development of new and more effective antiepileptic drugs or surgical therapy?
- In children with similar electrographic findings and seizure semiology, why do some respond to antiepileptic drugs, whereas others do not? What clues might this information provide about the mechanisms of epilepsy and possible treatments?
- What is the definition of seizure intractability in children? This concept is in evolution and likely depends on multiple factors, including the natural history of the epilepsy syndrome, etiology of the seizures, seizure frequency, and the degree to which the seizures and antiepileptic drug therapy impact the quality of life.

- Does a time frame exist during which specific epilepsy syndromes mandate intervention, because of either (1) windows of developmental opportunity or (2) diminishing capabilities of neural plasticity? What can we learn about the dimensions of neural plasticity?
- Do seizures contribute to the development of cognitive impairments and to what degree? Can prompt surgery in patients with catastrophic epilepsy ameliorate cognitive impairments? There is increasing evidence that the answer to this questions is "yes." However, formal neuropsychometric testing has produced mixed results.
- Can early successful intervention, with either antiepileptic drugs or epilepsy surgery, result in an improvement in the quality of life for patients with epilepsy?

Future trends for exploration will involve several avenues of research: source localization and predictive EEG patterns for identification of the epileptogenic zone [Smart et al., 2004; Worrell et al., 2004]; implantable devices that can detect predictive EEG patterns before a clinical seizure and deliver either an abortive dose of antiepileptic medication or an abortive electrical stimulus; deep brain cortical-thalamic stimulation to diminish seizure frequency in those patients with subcortical-cortical epileptogenic networks (intractable nonlesional, generalized epilepsy syndromes); and, finally, "designer" antiepileptic drugs targeting specific mechanisms of epilepsy – most likely sodium, potassium, calcium, and Gamma-aminobutyric acid (GABA) channels – to be delivered locally or systemically.

The complete list of references for this chapter is available online at **www.expertconsult.com**. See inside cover for registration details.

Behavioral, Cognitive, and Social Aspects of Childhood Epilepsy

Wendy G. Mitchell, Michèle Van Hirtum-Das, Jay Desai, and Quyen N. Luc

Children and adolescents with epilepsy and adults with childhood-onset epilepsy often are reported to have social maladjustment, including poor educational attainment, lower than expected occupational status, poorer perceived health and fitness, more frequently reported behavior problems, lower rates of marriage as adults, and higher rates of social isolation at all ages [Camfield et al., 1993; Clement and Wallace, 1990; Hoare, 1984; Jalava and Sillanpaa, 1997; Rutter et al., 1970; Sillanpaa, 1990]. These poor outcomes have multiple causes. In any particular patient, one or more causes of poor functioning may be identified and, at times, remedied. In general, neither epilepsy nor the seizures themselves are the most important cause of cognitive or behavioral disability. The underlying causes of cognitive and behavioral dysfunction may be subtle or obvious, but generally are complex and multifactorial. In some instances, underlying neurologic structural lesions cause both epilepsy and other disabilities, including cognitive dysfunction. In others, such as benign focal epilepsy of childhood, learning and behavioral disorders are more difficult to explain, and the relationship with epilepsy is almost certainly not causal.

Cognitive and Behavioral Disorders

Cognitive Disabilities in Children with Epilepsy

Although not all children with epilepsy have cognitive impairment, epilepsy is more frequent in cognitively handicapped children than in the general population [Britten et al., 1986; Forsgren et al., 1990; Sillanpaa, 1992]. Various population-based prospective and cohort studies of mentally retarded children have documented the prevalence of epilepsy to be 15–35 percent. Children with severe mental retardation and cerebral palsy have the highest rates of epilepsy. Table 62-1 contains information from selected population-based or cohort studies that estimate the prevalence of epilepsy in mentally retarded populations. Caution must be used in interpreting this information, since definition of both epilepsy and mental retardation varies. Several studies divide mentally retarded groups into mild (intelligence quotient [IQ] of 50–70) and moderate to severe mental retardation (IQ under 50). Epilepsy is

substantially more prevalent in severely retarded cohorts. Prevalence of epilepsy is highest in cohorts of mentally retarded children with associated cerebral palsy [Curatolo et al., 1995; Sussova et al., 1990]. Even excluding children with major structural brain disease causing epilepsy and associated disabilities, mental retardation is more common in children with epilepsy than in children without epilepsy, with or without other chronic illnesses. Table 62-2 lists selected studies of the prevalence of mental retardation in cohorts of children with epilepsy or in populations surveyed for both mental retardation and epilepsy. Again, definition of both epilepsy and mental retardation is not uniform.

Cognitive Function in Benign Childhood Epilepsy Syndromes

Many studies have noted subtle cognitive dysfunction in children with epilepsy syndromes known to have a good prognosis, easily attainable seizure control, and no structural brain disease, such as childhood absence epilepsy and benign focal epilepsy of childhood [D'Allessandro et al., 1990; Dieterich et al., 1985; Olsson and Campenhausen, 1993; Piccirilli et al., 1994; Singhi et al., 1992]. The cognitive dysfunction detected in children with childhood absence epilepsies includes deficits in visual sustained attention and execution of visual-motor tasks [Levav et al., 2002], verbal memory and word fluency [Henkin et al., 2005], and nonverbal memory and delayed recall [Pavone et al., 2001]. Children with benign childhood epilepsy with centrotemporal spikes have been documented as having difficulties in memory and phonologic processing skills [Northcott et al., 2005]. Furthermore, this condition has been shown to be strongly comorbid with reading disability and speech sound disorder (development of motor control of speech). These deficits are thought to be independently inherited traits rather than a consequence of the epilepsy itself, with increased odds amongst relatives of the proband [Clarke et al., 2007]. Benign childhood epilepsy with occipital paroxysms has been found to be associated with selective dysfunction in perceptive-visual attentional ability, verbal and visual-spatial memory abilities, visual perception, visual-motor integration, some language tasks, reading, writing abilities, and arithmetic abilities [Germano et al., 2005].

Table 62-1 Rates of Epilepsy in Cognitively Impaired Children and Adolescents: Population and Cohort Studies

Study Locale [Author(S), Year]	Age (Years)	% with Epilepsy	Severity of Retardation
Sweden [Gustavson et al., 1977]	5–16	30	Severe
Sweden [Blomquist et al., 1981]	8–19	16	Mild
Sweden [Hagberg et al., 1981]	8–12	12	Mild
United States [Jacobson and Janicki, 1983]	0–21	23	Undefined
Scotland [Goulden et al., 1991]	0–22	15	Undefined
Australia [Wellesley et al., 1992]	6–16	11	Mild
Same as above		15	Moderate
Sweden [Steffenburg et al., 1996]	6–13	15	Mild
Same as above		44	Severe

(Adapted from Steffenburg S et al. Psychiatric disorders in children and adolescents with mental retardation and active epilepsy. Arch Neurol 1996;53:904; Hauser WA, Hesdorffer DC. Seizures and the developmental disabilities. In: Hauser WA, Hesdoffer DC, eds. Epilepsy: Frequency, causes and consequences. New York: Demos Publications, 1990.)

Table 62-2 Frequency of Cognitively Impaired in Children with Epilepsy: Population and Cohort Studies

Study Locale [Author(s), Year]	Age (Years)	% Mentally Retarded	Epilepsy Definition
USA [van den Berg et al., 1969]	0–7	29	Two or more unprovoked seizures
Sweden [Brorson, 1970]	6–13	35	Active epilepsy with one or more seizures in prior 3 years
England [Ross et al., 1980]	11	33	Two or more unprovoked seizures
Finland [Sillanpaa, 1992]	4–15	31	Two or more unprovoked seizures
USA [Murphy et al., 1995]	10	30	Two or more unprovoked seizures on separate days
Sweden [Sidenvall et al., 1996]	0–16	40	Active epilepsy with one or more seizures in prior 5 years
Sweden [Steffenburg et al., 1996]	6–13	38	Active epilepsy with one or more seizures in prior 5 years
Croatia [Bielen et al., 2007]	0–18	28	Active epilepsy with at least one seizure in previous 5 years
USA [Berg et al., 2008	0–16	26	Undefined

(Adapted from Steffenburg S et al. Psychiatric disorders in children and adolescents with mental retardation and active epilepsy. Arch Neurol 1996;53:904.)

Cognitive Dysfunction Due to Interictal Epileptiform Discharges

Conflicting evidence exists regarding the role of interictal epileptiform discharges in cognitive function, as distinct from ictal effects and from the long-term stable interictal effects caused by the clinical syndrome or the underlying etiology [Aldenkamp et al., 2004]. Studies using sophisticated computerized cognitive test batteries time-locked to electroencephalography (EEG) discharges have noted transient cognitive impairment with slowing of reaction times and decreased perceptual accuracy during epileptiform discharges [Aldenkamp et al., 1996; Binnie, 2003, 1993; Shewmon and Erwin, 1989]. At least one study has shown low incidence of such impairment and questioned its clinical significance [Fonseca et al., 2007]. Refinement of methodology has suggested that a larger proportion of presumed transient cognitive impairment can be attributed to subtle seizures, while interictal epileptic activity has a smaller effect upon cognitive functioning [Aldenkamp et al., 2004]. Finally, the effects of such transient cognitive impairment on more stable tasks, such as reading or intelligence, have not been studied and are unknown.

Learning Disabilities and Academic Underachievement

Learning disability is diagnosed when one or more areas of learning are significantly below expectations, and not explained by overall cognitive level, sensory abnormalities, or lack of opportunity or teaching (see Chapters 43 and 45). Learning disabilities are reported to be more frequent in children with epilepsy. Studies have shown that children with epilepsy are at higher risk for repeating a year in school and over half require special education services. Although the frequency of special education placement was significantly higher in the children with remote symptomatic epilepsy and epileptic encephalopathies, in one study 48.9 percent of those considered neurologically normal received some form of special educational services [Berg et al., 2005].

Educational underachievement in reading, writing, and math has been reported in a variety of settings, comparing children with epilepsy both with their normal peers and with children with other chronic illnesses, such as asthma [Bagley, 1970; Fastenau et al., 2004; Holdsworth and Whitmore, 1974; Mitchell et al., 1991; Seidenberg et al., 1986; Selassie et al., 2008; Stores, 1981;

Stores and Hart, 1976; Sturniolo and Galletti, 1994; McNelis et al., 2007]. It is unclear whether the relationship is a direct one, in which the epilepsy, seizures, or medications themselves cause learning disability, or an indirect one, in which an underlying neurologic condition causes both seizures and abnormalities in perception, memory, and visual-motor skills. Educational underachievement may be excessive in subjects drawn from inner-city teaching hospitals because of social factors entirely unrelated to medical conditions [Mitchell et al., 1991]. Parental expectations for a child with epilepsy are often lowered, at times inappropriately [Chavez, 1985; Hartlage and Green, 1972; Hoare and Kerley, 1991; Long and Moore, 1979]. Even after the effects of sociocultural variability have been accounted for, at least some children with epilepsy manifest learning disabilities. In one study comparing children with newly diagnosed epilepsy to children with recently diagnosed moderate asthma, academic underachievement was significantly more common in children with epilepsy, particularly boys with severe epilepsy [Austin et al., 1998]. Earlier seizure onset, generalized nonabsence seizures, and comorbid attention-deficit hyperactivity disorder (ADHD) appear to be risk factors for learning disability amongst children with epilepsy. However, a diagnosis of epilepsy, even when seizures are less severe and controlled, should provide sufficient cause to screen children for learning disability and to monitor academic performance continuously [Fastenau et al., 2008].

Detailed neurocognitive batteries in children with epilepsy demonstrate higher than expected rates of dyslexia, visuospatial difficulties, nonverbal learning difficulties, attention/executive/construction difficulties, verbal memory and learning problems, language difficulties, and slowed processing speeds [Mitchell et al., 1992; Fastenau et al., 2009]. With psychometric testing, almost half of the children with epilepsy met criteria for a learning disability [Seidenberg et al., 1986; Fastenau et al., 2008]. Some of these findings may be related to subtle or overt underlying structural lesions causing both the epilepsy and the learning disability, but not all can be readily explained. Numerous studies attempting to identify demographic, neurological, and seizure-related risk factors for academic underachievment have shown inconsistent results. Inadequate seizure control, early age of onset, longer duration of disorder, and polytherapy have not universally been shown to be associated with academic underachievement. Additionally, in children with normal IQ, no significant relationship between epilepsy type/syndrome and educational problems has been found [Mitchell et al., 1991; Oostrom et al., 2005; McNelis et al., 2007].

Attention Deficit, Impulsivity, and Overactivity

Attention, impulsivity, and activity level can be measured in various ways, ranging from parent and teacher questionnaires to psychometric testing to computerized continuous performance tasks. Regardless of methods used, most studies of children and adults with epilepsy demonstrate an excess incidence of inattention, impulsivity, and slowed reaction time [Kinney et al., 1990; Mitchell et al., 1992; Stores, 1978]. These findings should not imply that clinical ADHD is extremely common in children with epilepsy, although the prevalence is probably somewhat higher than in the general population. As with overall cognitive function in children with epilepsy, simple cause

and effect relationships are uncommon. Underlying neurologic conditions may cause both ADHD and epilepsy [Kinney et al., 1990]. Antiepileptic medications may affect attention and impulsivity, both positively and negatively, at least in some persons [Mitchell et al., 1993; Riva and Devoti, 1996]. Measured effects on attention are small, and may not be clinically significant. In rare instances, frequent seizures may affect attention, and seizure control may eliminate an apparent attention deficit. There is some evidence that frequent epileptiform discharges may disrupt attention, which may improve with antiepileptic treatment [Gordon et al., 1996].

Autism and Autistic Spectrum Disorders

Autistic spectrum disorders are associated with an increased incidence of epilepsy, but evidence that one causes the other is lacking [Carlton Ford et al., 1995; Cavazzuti and Nalin, 1990; Olsson et al., 1988; Steffenburg et al., 1996; Wong, 1993]. A number of syndromes are associated with a high incidence of both autistic behavior and seizures (e.g., Angelman's syndrome, tuberous sclerosis), but the coincidence of seizures and behavioral disorder is due to the underlying condition. A possible rare exception is the child in whom autistic behavior develops along with language regression, accompanied by an epileptiform EEG (continuous spike-and-wave pattern during sleep) [Hirsch et al., 1990; Kyllerman et al., 1996; Perez et al., 1993; Roulet et al., 1991]. This condition has been considered to be a variant of Landau–Kleffner syndrome. Behavior and language may improve with treatment with antiepileptics (rarely), corticosteroids, or corticotropin, or after subpial transection of epileptogenic cortex [Hirsch et al., 1990].

Psychiatric Disorders in Childhood Epilepsy

Little evidence exists to support the notion that severe psychiatric disorders are more common in children with epilepsy. Although major psychiatric illnesses, such as schizophrenia, obsessive-compulsive disorder, or affective disorders, may coexist with childhood epilepsy, the prevalence is not higher than in the general population. Treatment of coexisting severe psychiatric disorder and epilepsy may be complex. Some antiepileptics (carbamazepine, valproic acid) are reported to be beneficial in treatment of certain psychiatric disorders, most notably bipolar affective disorder [Fenn et al., 1996]. In general, however, treatment of epilepsy does not relieve symptoms of major psychiatric illness. Occasionally, "paradoxical normalization," or "forced normalization," is reported in children who experience a decrease in psychiatric symptoms when seizures are uncontrolled, with worsening of symptoms when seizures are in good control [Amir and Gross-Tsur, 1994].

Depressive disorders and mood disturbances have been reported more frequently in adolescents and adults with epilepsy than in healthy peers. Prevalence of depression in children and adolescents with epilepsy is significantly higher than in the general pediatric population [Dunn et al., 1999; Ettinger et al., 1998]. Moreover, depressive disorders are often underdiagnosed and undertreated in patients with pediatric epilepsy [Plioplys, 2003]. A number of studies have clearly highlighted that suicidal ideation and attempts are more likely to be seen in children and adolescents with epilepsy than in the general pediatric population [Baker, 2006; Oguz et al., 2002; Thome-Souza et al., 2007]. In addition to depression, anxiety disorders are frequent comorbidities in childhood epilepsies [Ekinci et al., 2009]. The etiology of depressive symptoms may be complex; social stigma, lack of employment opportunities, and lack of social contacts may contribute to depression. Self-reported quality of life is lower in adolescents with epilepsy than in adolescents with asthma. Although this difference was more striking for young persons with active epilepsy, quality of life measures were low, even when seizures were fully controlled or inactive [Austin et al., 1996].

Behavioral Problems, Conduct Disorders, and Delinquency

Behavioral disturbances in children and adolescents with epilepsy may be due to family factors and parental anxiety about epilepsy, rather than a primary result of epilepsy or of the underlying neurologic disorder [Austin et al., 1992; Carlton Ford et al., 1995; Gortmaker et al., 1990; Hoare and Kerley, 1991; Lothman and Pianta, 1993; Mitchell et al., 1994; Pianta and Lothman, 1994]. Self-esteem is reported to be lower and behavioral problems are more frequent in children and adolescents with epilepsy than in peers with or without chronic illnesses such as asthma or diabetes [Apter et al., 1991; Austin, 1989; Hoare and Mann, 1994; Matthews et al., 1982; Westbrook et al., 1991]. When children with epilepsy are assessed at the time of first seizure diagnosis, behavior problems are frequently reported by parents and teachers, particularly in children who had previously unrecognized seizures [Austin et al., 2001, 2002]. Children with epilepsy have higher rates of oppositional-defiant disorder [Dunn et al., 2009; Jones et al., 2007] and conduct disorder [Davies et al., 2003; Dunn et al., 2009] compared to the general population.

Adolescents and young adults with childhood-onset epilepsy have slightly higher than expected rates of delinquency in some studies [Camfield et al., 1993]. It is uncertain whether this propensity is due to underlying brain disease with poor impulse control, stigma, lack of opportunity, or other sociocultural factors. A population-based study in Finland, however, failed to find a relationship between delinquency and epilepsy in males up to age 22 years, although delinquency was associated with a history of central nervous system trauma [Rantakallio et al., 1992].

Cognitive and Behavioral Outcome of Specific Epilepsy Syndromes

Infantile Spasms

Certain pediatric epilepsy syndromes have been associated with significant, sometimes devastating, cognitive or behavioral declines. Perhaps the best studied of the catastrophic childhood epilepsies is infantile spasms. Mental retardation has been reported in up to 80 percent of children with infantile spasms and is described as severe in more than half of the cases [Jambaqué, 1994]. Although many patients exhibit global arrest of development, specific cognitive deficits, such as speech difficulties and impaired visuospatial abilities, have been noted in others [Besag, 2004]. Thirteen percent of those with cryptogenic infantile spasms were reported to exhibit persistent autistic features. In children with infantile spasms due to tuberous sclerosis, rate of autism is higher (58 percent) [Bolton et al., 2002; Hunt and Dennis, 1987; Riikonen and Amnell, 1981].

Effective early treatment of both cryptogenic and symptomatic spasms may improve cognition and behavior [Caplan et al., 2002; Jambaqué et al., 2000; Kivity et al., 2004]. Other prognostic factors for a better cognitive outcome include sustained seizure control with the first medication [Partikian and Mitchell, 2009], age at onset equal to or greater than 4 months, and absence of atypical spasms and partial seizures [Riikonen, 2009].

Epileptic Encephalopathies of Infancy

Many of the epileptic encephalopathies with neonatal or infantile onset are associated with frequent seizures that are notoriously refractory to treatment with both conventional and newer antiepileptic medication. Included in this group are severe myoclonic epilepsy of infancy (Dravet's syndrome), early infantile epileptic encephalopathy (Ohtahara's syndrome), neonatal myoclonic encephalopathy (or early infantile myoclonic encephalopathy), and migrating partial seizures of infancy. Delayed development usually is seen by the second year, and interpersonal relationships rarely progress past a level expected for that of a 2-year-old [Besag, 2004]. Behavior in the affected child typically is hyperactive with autistic features. It is difficult to attribute the abnormalities in cognition and behavior fully to the frequent seizures and paroxysmal findings on EEG, when an undiagnosed metabolic or genetic etiology may play a causative or contributory role. In children with tuberous sclerosis or Sturge–Weber syndrome, early control of seizures is associated with a more favorable neurodevelopmental and behavioral outcome [Jambaqué et al., 2000; Kramer et al., 2000].

Lennox–Gastaut Syndrome

Lennox–Gastaut syndrome frequently has been associated with autistic features and cognitive deficits, although published literature specific to this topic is sparse [Besag, 2004]. Long-term follow-up evaluation of these patients commonly reveals slowness of intellectual ability and motor speed, apathy (possibly better described as an inability to engage with the environment secondary to frequent epileptiform discharges), and perseverative behavior [Kieffer-Renaux et al., 2001].

Electrical Status Epilepticus in Sleep and Landau–Kleffner Syndrome

Electrical status epilepticus in sleep is an EEG pattern detected in some cases of pediatric epilepsy that often is associated with specific cognitive and language dysfunction. It frequently is encountered in those syndromes described as continuous spikes and waves (during slow-wave sleep and Landau–Kleffner syndrome). With continuous spike-and-wave activity in sleep, a typical decrease in the IQ or developmental quotient is noted by most investigators [Boel and Casaer, 1989; Roulet-Perez et al., 1993]. Of interest, some 40–60 percent of children with continuous spike-wave sleep exhibit an expressive aphasia, which is in contrast with children with Landau–Kleffner syndrome, who tend to present with a verbal or auditory agnosia [Galanopoulou et al., 2000]. In patients with Landau–Kleffner syndrome, language may recover spontaneously, partially improve with therapy, or unfortunately remain permanently affected despite improvement of the EEG abnormality [Besag, 2004].

Benign Focal Epilepsies of Childhood

Of specific note is the syndrome termed benign childhood epilepsy with centrotemporal spikes (benign rolandic epilepsy). Although this disorder was once thought of as a universally benign syndrome, increasing evidence suggests that a subpopulation of children may present with recent impairment of overall cognitive functioning, or difficulties with visual perception, concentration, and short-term memory [Weglage et al., 1997].

Family, Community, and Cultural Perceptions of Epilepsy

Social acceptance and inclusion of children and adolescents with epilepsy are far from complete, even when seizures are infrequent or fully controlled. In some cultural settings, it is not generally disclosed to friends or extended family that a child has epilepsy [Ju et al., 1990]. Some children are not sent to school if seizures are uncontrolled. Despite laws guaranteeing disabled and medically impaired children full access to education, some schools discourage attendance by children with active seizure disorders. All of these prejudices may further impair social and academic function in children with epilepsy. Fear of stigmatization may contribute to the high frequency of nondisclosure of epilepsy among adolescents [MacLeod and Austin, 2003]. It has been suggested that society's understanding of epilepsy, as reflected through literature, has changed over time, and the ancient belief that seizures were a supernatural force has given way to the present understanding that epilepsy represents a medical condition [Jones, 2000]. However, a survey of a newer medium, movies released between 1937 and 2003 from four continents, found portrayal of all of the ancient beliefs about epilepsy, including demonic or divine possession, genius, lunacy, delinquency, and general "otherness" [Baxendale, 2003].

Social Adjustment of Adults with Childhood-Onset Epilepsy

Population-based studies from several countries document that social functioning is impaired in adults who had childhood-onset epilepsy, compared with their healthy peers [Farmer et al., 1992; Sillanpaa, 1990]. Marriage is less frequent, employment is less frequent and at less skilled occupations, and social isolation is more frequent. Differences are more striking when adults have on-going seizures, but are present even when complete remission or control has been obtained. Even when studies were restricted to adults with childhood-onset absence epilepsy, a disorder thought to be benign and likely to remit, social functioning continued to be impaired in comparison with that in nonepileptic peers [Dieterich et al., 1985]. Other studies of outcome in adults with childhood-onset epilepsy find substantial maladaptation as well, particularly in social and vocational function. Social functioning is generally much more impaired in the subgroup of adults with on-going seizures than in those who attain complete remission. A population-based study of adults in Nova Scotia, evaluated 25 years after a diagnosis of juvenile myoclonic epilepsy, documented a high frequency of social isolation, unemployment and social impulsiveness, with 74 percent having at least one major unfavorable social outcome [Camfield and Camfield, 2009].

In long-term follow-up (30 years) of a population-based cohort of children with epilepsy in Finland, about 60 percent of subjects were independent in activities of daily living, and 57 percent were employed, most in manual labor or semiskilled positions [Sillanpaa and Helenius, 1993]. Several studies are notable for including only adults with childhood-onset absence [Olsson and Campenhausen, 1993] or mixed generalized seizures (absence plus generalized tonic-clonic) [Dieterich et al., 1985]. Young adults with persisting absence seizures since childhood or adolescence, originally identified during a population-based study of absence epilepsy, were compared with a Swedish reference sample of young adults, assessing the impact of epilepsy on schooling, occupation, leisure-time activities, friends, daily routines, and housing. Although the overall employment rate did not differ from that in the reference subjects, persons with epilepsy were more likely to be employed in an unskilled job or in an occupation below that expected for educational level. Social isolation was reported in 34.5 percent, compared with 7.9 percent of the reference group. A high percentage of subjects (74 percent) reported that epilepsy had affected at least one area of their social functioning [Olsson and Campenhausen, 1993]. In a Finnish study of adults who had uncomplicated childhood-onset epilepsy, quality of life of adults with epilepsy in remission on medication was lower, and rates of unemployment were higher, than in comparison subjects or in adults whose epilepsy was in remission after withdrawal of medication [Sillanpaa et al., 2004].

Effects Of Antiepileptic Drugs on Behavior, Attention, and Mood

General Effects of Antiepileptic Drugs

Cognitive, psychiatric, and behavioral abnormalities in children with epilepsy often are attributed to antiepileptic medications. Most of these effects are unsupported by data from well-controlled, randomized, prospective clinical research. It is clear, however, that idiosyncratic adverse behavioral and cognitive responses can occur with any antiepileptic drug (see Chapter 59). In addressing issues of abnormal cognition and behavior in the management of pediatric epilepsy, several factors need to be recognized. Epilepsy occurring in the developing brain is likely to be substantially different from that in an adult in both its qualities and response to treatment. In addition, the most refractory epilepsies are likely to begin in childhood. The management of severe childhood epilepsy may prove challenging in that the choice of antiepileptic medication depends on the type of syndrome in which the seizures occur, as well as the cognitive and behavioral abnormalities that may occur with these syndromes. Finally, treating a combination of several seizure types in one patient may be difficult, because some anticonvulsants that are effective in treating one type of seizure may be ineffective or even exacerbate another seizure type.

In well-designed, controlled studies, evidence of long-term adverse cognitive effects of antiepileptic medications is generally slight or difficult to document objectively. A few studies have randomized subjects at the onset of seizures to receive one of several antiepileptic drugs [Aikia et al., 2006; Fritz et al., 2005; Forsythe et al., 1991; Mitchell and Chavez, 1987]. Most studies, however, examine patients assigned nonrandomly to receive various antiepileptic drugs when medication is started, changed, or withdrawn [Aldenkamp et al., 1993; Aman et al., 1994; Chen et al., 1996; Mitchell et al., 1993; Sabers et al., 1995; Stores et al., 1992]. The only double-blind, placebo-controlled, long-term studies of the behavioral effects of monotherapy with antiepileptic drugs are limited to studies of phenobarbital for febrile seizures in infants and toddlers [Farwell et al., 1990; Camfield et al., 1979]. There are many observational studies addressing cognitive and behavioral side effects, often comparing newer antiepileptic agents with older ones. These are typically limited to small patient cohorts and short-term follow-up. Comparative, blinded trials of anticonvulsant monotherapy in pediatrics are extremely limited. One exception is a recently completed comparative trial of monotherapy for childhood absence epilepsy compared ethosuximide, lamotrigine and valproic acid [Glauser et al., 2010]. While efficacy was similar for ethosuximide and valproic acid, negative behavioral effects were more frequent with valproate, particularly affecting attention.

Antiepileptic Drugs and Motor Speed

In older children and adults, the major effect of most antiepileptic medications on cognitive function appears to be a slowing of motor and cognitive processing speed. Early reports that phenytoin caused generalized decline in cognitive function were later disputed when further data analysis and research found that the major effect of phenytoin was on motor speed [Aldenkamp et al., 1994; Dodrill and Tempkin, 1989; Duncan et al., 1990]. Other cognitive functions are relatively spared, if analyzed independent of response speed. Many standardized cognitive tests are at least partly dependent on timed performance. Thus, IQ may appear to be lowered by medications, whereas the primary effect is on motor speed. Nevertheless, some patients perceive that their responses are slower and are bothered by this, despite otherwise normal functioning by most other measures.

Conversely, improvements in cognitive function, impulsivity, and behavior have been reported with several antiepileptic drugs. This improvement may occasionally be dramatic, resulting from control of frequent seizures, such as when a child with frequent absence seizures is started on anticonvulsants. Improved behavior and cognitive function as a direct result of antiepileptic medication also has been documented for some antiepileptic drugs, most consistently carbamazepine, lamotrigine, and levetiracetam [Aldenkamp et al., 2002; Aman et al., 1994; Gillham et al., 2000; Mitchell et al., 1993]. Effects are slight, however, and probably not clinically significant in most instances; they may even be disputed [Seidel and Mitchell, 1999].

Excitement or Agitation Due to Sedative Antiepileptic Drugs

Most sedative drugs have the potential for causing excitement and agitation when they are first initiated, but this effect dissipates in most children over a few weeks. Phenobarbital causes sustained behavioral difficulties, primarily overactivity, in some children, and can cause irritability and disturbed sleep, particularly in infants and toddlers [Camfield et al., 1979; Wolf et al., 1977]. Estimates of the number of children who do not tolerate phenobarbital because of resulting overactivity range from 5 to 25 percent. This effect is more frequent in toddlers and preschool-aged children but may occur at any age.

Published case reports document a variety of idiosyncratic behavioral adverse reactions to virtually all antiepileptic drugs. Valproic acid occasionally causes a confused state or psychosis [Papazian et al., 1995]. Felbamate also has been reported to cause agitation and significant behavioral effects early in treatment, although overall this drug tends to improve behavior with prolonged treatment [Gay et al., 1995].

Behavioral and Cognitive Effects of the Newer Antiepileptic Agents

Newer medications formulated in the last 20 years for use as antiepileptic drugs generally have undergone at least add-on trials in children, with some studies including behavioral and cognitive assessment. These newer antiepileptic drugs have been reported to cause behavior change, both positive and negative. Very few have included behavioral or cognitive measures in properly designed, blinded monotherapy studies, either in comparison with placebo or in comparison with another antiepileptic. Comparison across studies of antiepileptic drugs is further hampered by varying criteria for selection of participants for studies, and use of differing neuropsychologic tests and study designs [Brunbech and Sabers, 2002]. A recent review of the literature regarding anticonvulsant effects in children summarizes published studies, nearly all of which examined phenobarbital, carbamazepine, or valproic acid [Loring and Meador, 2004]. Several other reviews addressing the effects of the newer antiepileptic agents are limited to the adult patient population [Aldenkamp et al., 2006; Kennedy and Lhatoo, 2008].

Specific Medications

Topiramate

Topiramate has been reported in adult epileptic and nonepileptic persons to cause significant cognitive difficulties, primarily involving word-finding and verbal memory, particularly during initial treatment and titration [Fisher and Blum, 1995; Gomer et al., 2007; Huppertz et al., 2001; Lee et al., 2003; Martin et al., 1999; Thompson et al., 2000]. These adverse effects appeared to dissipate over time, particularly if the dosage is increased slowly, although they may persist [Aldenkamp et al., 2003; Tatum et al., 2001]. However, subsequent studies have shown that a gradual introduction of topiramate does not necessarily prevent effects on cognition, that there is no clear relation between daily dosage and cognitive side effects, and that adverse effects on verbal fluency, verbal memory and cognitive speed may persist until withdrawal of the medication [Gerber et al., 2000; Gomer et al., 2007; Huppertz et al., 2001; Kockelmann et al., 2003]. No clear at-risk group or predicting factor has been identified. In one double-blind, randomized, placebo-controlled trial of topiramate for add-on therapy in 86 children with partial epilepsy, children receiving topiramate had an increased frequency of emotional lability, difficulties with concentration, and fatigue, but the changes were not severe enough to cause any subject to discontinue treatment [Elterman et al., 1999].

Lamotrigine

Since its introduction in the United States in 1994, lamotrigine has received much attention with respect to its potential positive psychotropic effects [Brunbech and Sabers, 2002]. Significant improvements in behavior, cognition, and motor skills (unrelated to seizure control) are noted in pediatric patients, although these effects have not yet been formally studied [Culy and Goa, 2000; Meador and Baker, 1997]. Lamotrigine has been reported to have fewer cognitive effects in adults with newly diagnosed epilepsy than those described for carbamazepine, phenytoin, and topiramate [Blum et al., 2006; Brodie et al., 1995; Meador et al., 2001; Steiner et al., 1999]. A short-term treatment study performed on healthy volunteers using low-dose lamotrigine revealed improvement in cognitive activation and mood, and reported subjective positive effects on quality of life relative to that achieved with use of valproate [Aldenkamp et al., 2002]. In a trial of lamotrigine for add-on therapy in children with Lennox–Gastaut syndrome, responders with improved seizure control were noted to be more alert and attentive, whereas nonresponders were more likely to experience agitation. Lamotrigine exhibited no clinically significant adverse cognitive effects as adjunctive treatment for children with well-controlled or mild epilepsy, when compared to placebo [Pressler et al., 2006].

Clobazam

Clobazam is a 1,5 benzodiazepine, initially formulated as an anxiolytic, but later recognized for its antiseizure potential via open-label, adjunctive trials and double-blind, placebo-controlled, add-on trials [Hentschel and Froscher, 1992]. Clobazam is effective as monotherapy in treating partial seizures with secondary generalization and in some primary generalized tonic-clonic seizures. A randomized, double-blind, prospective multicenter Canadian study addressed the cognitive tolerability of clobazam compared to carbamazepine and phenytoin in children with newly diagnosed epilepsy. There appeared to be no deterioration of intelligence, memory, attention, psychomotor speed, or impulsivity in children on clobazam relative to the other standard monotherapies. Behavioral side effects were similar, as well [Bawden et al., 1999]. There are currently no studies published comparing cognitive or behavioral effects of clobazam to the newer antiepileptic drugs or to placebo in adults or children.

Gabapentin

Gabapentin is similar in structure to gamma-aminobutyric acid (GABA) but does not seem to have effects at the GABA receptors. In both adult volunteer studies and studies with double-blind, randomized, crossover designs, gabapentin produced no significant alteration of psychomotor or memory abilities when used for either monotherapy or add-on treatment [Dodrill et al., 1999; Leach et al., 1997; Martin et al., 1999; Meador et al., 1999]. Gabapentin occasionally has been reported to cause aggressive or agitated behavior [Lee et al., 1996; Tallian et al., 1996]. Children in whom significant adverse behavioral changes occur with use of gabapentin tend to have some degree of documented mental retardation [Khurana et al., 1996]. No published controlled studies have evaluated the cognitive and behavioral effects of gabapentin in children who have epilepsy.

Levetiracetam

Levetiracetam, a structurally and mechanistically novel antiepileptic drug, has a favorable pharmacokinetic profile and is effective in treating partial seizures in both adult and pediatric patients [Callenbach et al., 2008; Dooley and Plosker, 2000; Lagae et al., 2003; Li et al., 2009; Verrotti et al., 2009]. Several observational studies have noted significant improvements in verbal fluency, prospective and working memory, and attention in patients treated with levetiracetam [Gomer et al., 2007; Lopez-Gongora et al., 2008; Piazzini et al., 2006]. However, among adult patients with epilepsy who received levetiracetam, behavioral abnormalities were reported in a significant proportion relative to those patients with anxiety or cognitive disorders but without epilepsy. The behavioral events cited were less common than those reported with other antiepileptic agents [Cramer et al., 2003]. Another recent study reported a dose-independent behavioral change in 59 percent of adult patients, 37 percent of which were negative (loss of self-control, restlessness, sleep disturbance, and aggression) and 22 percent positive (increased energy and activation). The positive effects did not appear to be related to type of epilepsy, co-treatment, dose, or psychiatric history, whereas the negative effects were associated with poorer seizure control, intellectual disability, and underlying impulsiveness [Helmstaedter et al., 2008]. A prospective open-label, add-on trial using levetiracetam to treat refractory partial and generalized seizures in children younger than 16 years of age revealed adverse events in 51 percent of subjects. Most of these events were behavioral in nature, although the majority of children did not require discontinuation of the medication. As with the gabapentin study, many of the children were developmentally delayed or cognitively impaired. In this same study, however, improvement in behavior and/or cognition after the addition of levetiracetam was reported in 25.6 percent [Wheless and Ng, 2002]. A few anecdotal reports have described improved behavior in children with autism treated with levetiracetam, but in the same population, some children experienced an increase in aggressive behavior [Rugino and Samsock, 2002].

Oxcarbazepine

Oxcarbazepine is a keto homolog of carbamazepine, although it has a very distinct metabolic profile. It is labeled for use as monotherapy or adjunctive therapy for partial seizures with or without secondarily generalized seizures in children 6 years of age and older. Although no deterioration in cognitive function test results was reported in one crossover and several comparative monotherapy studies in adult epilepsy patients [Aikia et al., 1992; McKee et al., 1994; Sabers et al., 1995], cognitive function has not been systematically studied in children and adolescents. One open-label comparison study investigating the effect of oxcarbazepine on cognition in children and adolescents aged 6–17 years revealed no differences on cognitive testing relative to carbamazepine and valproate. Results, however, were limited to a 6-month follow-up period [Donati et al., 2006]. A nonrandomized, open-label, observational study using oxcarbazepine as monotherapy in children with benign childhood epilepsy with centrotemporal spikes (BECTS) showed apparent conservation of cognitive functions and behavioral abilities [Tzitiridou et al., 2005].

Tiagabine

Tiagabine acts as a GABA uptake inhibitor in neurons and glial cells, and is effective for add-on therapy in the treatment of refractory partial epilepsy. Data from several randomized, double-blind, placebo-controlled, parallel-group or crossover studies of tiagabine as monotherapy or add-on therapy have been published [Aikia et al., 2006; Dodrill et al., 1997; Kalviainen et al., 1996; Sveinbjornsdottir et al., 1994]. Generally, no significant decline in IQ, reaction speed, attention, or memory has been noted at either low or high doses. One randomized, open, comparative study investigating the cognitive side effects of tiagabine versus topiramate revealed deterioration in verbal memory (delayed free recall) in patients being treated with tiagabine [Fritz et al., 2005]. However, this finding of a decline in only one of three measures of verbal learning and memory was not conclusive evidence that the drug only affects the episodic memory ability, thus suggesting that further study is necessary. No information is available regarding the cognitive effects of tiagabine in the pediatric population.

Zonisamide

No published trials have used formal neuropsychological tests to evaluate cognitive or behavioral function in pediatric patients with either partial or generalized seizures treated with zonisamide. In several observational studies, 26–61 percent of patients reported mild to moderate adverse events, with only a mild development of tolerance over time [Berent et al., 1987; Kothare et al., 2006; Tosches and Tisdell, 2006; Wilfong, 2005]. Cognitive dysfunction, specifically attention, memory, and language changes, was reported in 2–11 percent, often occurring at therapeutic serum levels. One prospective, randomized, open-label investigation of zonisamide as monotherapy in adult patients used several standardized neuropsychological tests for evaluation of cognitive changes. Significantly decreased performance with delayed word recall and verbal fluency were noted, despite the absence of confounding factors, such as intractable epilepsy and polypharmacy [Park et al., 2008]. Reports from Japan, where the medication has been in use for 20 years, suggest that psychotic episodes and behavior changes may occur in children given zonisamide, despite improved seizure control [Hirai et al., 2002; Kimura, 1994].

Vigabatrin

Vigabatrin was recently approved in the United States, after long delays due to reports of vigabatrin-induced retinal toxicity. Approval in the United States is for the treatment of infantile spasms and refractory complex partial seizures in adults. Mild and transient drowsiness, dizziness, and irritability are frequently reported with vigabatrin initiation, but do not appear to affect cognition in a strong, adverse way [Dodrill et al., 1993; McGuire et al., 1992; Monaco et al., 1997]. Both a single review of the cognitive effects of vigabatrin, and a monotherapy study comparing the drug to carbamazepine in adult patients with partial epilepsy, not only revealed an absence of cognitive deterioration, but also reported an improvement in tests of memory, psychomotor speed, and flexibility of mental processing [Monaco, 1996; Kälviäinen et al., 1995].

Rufinamide

Rufinamide is a structurally novel compound that appears to exert its action by limiting the frequency of sodium-dependent neuronal action potentials. Reports during the experimental phase of the drug revealed potential improvement of reaction-timed tests, but a possible impairment of short-term memory at higher doses. One multicenter, double-blind, randomized, placebo-controlled, parallel study of rufinamide in patients aged 15–64 years with partial epilepsy has been performed and revealed no significant deterioration in psychomotor speed, alertness, attention, or working memory [Aldenkamp and Alpherts, 2006]. There have been no published investigations of the cognitive and behavioral effects of this medication in the pediatric population.

Fear of Side Effects and Effective Antiepileptic Drug Use

Despite the relative paucity of documentation of sustained adverse cognitive effects of antiepileptics, sophisticated parents and teachers often are well versed in the possible adverse effects of medications, exaggerated, to some degree, by frightening stories in the lay media and, increasingly, on the Internet. Parents may be under the erroneous impression that a particular antiepileptic drug will "make the child retarded," and may blame developmental problems that subsequently emerge on previous administration of antiepileptic drugs, or may avoid administration of these medications because of fear of disturbing the child's behavior or development.

Treatment of Cognitive, Social, Academic and Behavioral Problems Associated with Epilepsy

As with all medical treatment, care of the child with epilepsy must be individualized. Nevertheless, several general principles apply. The developmental, cognitive, academic, and behavioral status of the child and the social functioning of the family must be integral and on-going concerns in the management of a child with epilepsy. Brief developmental, cognitive, or academic assessment is appropriate at the time of initial evaluation and at follow-up visits. Although treatment generally will not alter the underlying cognitive capacity of the child, early intervention and referral to appropriate community and school resources will maximize function. Appropriate counseling of the family may minimize later behavioral and adjustment difficulties. Group programs to help families with their children with epilepsy may be effective in altering parental attitudes, reducing fears, and improving the children's participation in family and community activities [Lewis et al., 1990]. They may also improve self-management and communication skills and health-related quality of life in the social exclusion dimension [Jantzen et al., 2009].

School Inclusion and Academic Planning

At times, parents report that a child with epilepsy is being excluded from school programs, sent home repeatedly, or placed in a more restrictive class setting than is appropriate for his or her abilities. The treating neurologist or pediatrician may need to intervene with the appropriate authorities if a child is being denied appropriate educational experiences because school personnel are concerned about the possibility of seizures. Having a treatment plan for seizures may be useful in reducing the anxiety of school personnel. Any child with special needs or suspicion of learning disabilities should be thoroughly evaluated by the school, and have an individualized educational plan prepared for him/her.

Local branches of voluntary organizations, such as the Epilepsy Foundation of America, may be helpful in providing informational programs to schools. At least in the United States, federal law mandates inclusion of children with disabilities and medical conditions in educational programs in the least restrictive environment appropriate for the child's needs.

Behavior Problems and Discipline

Behavioral problems and parent–child interaction should be addressed regularly in the management of children with epilepsy. Parents may avoid disciplining a child with epilepsy in an age-appropriate manner out of fear that causing the child to become angry or upset may trigger seizures. Parents must be reassured that this is not the case. Significant abnormalities in behavior, activity, or attention warrant a more detailed evaluation. This may include psychiatric evaluation and/or psychometric testing. Psychometric testing, along with a clinical history gathered from parents, teachers, and patients, may be necessary to differentiate behavioral difficulties associated with coexisting ADHD from those due to family dysfunction, oppositional disorders, inappropriate parental expectations, and other factors.

Treatment of Attention-Deficit Disorders (ADD and ADHD) in Children with Epilepsy

Alteration in antiepileptic treatment may improve behavior and attention if the original treatment has substantially affected behavior. However, ADHD may coexist with epilepsy, independent of antiepileptic treatment. Treatment with stimulants (e.g., methylphenidate, pemoline, dextroamphetamine) or with tricyclic antidepressants (e.g., imipramine, desipramine) generally does not compromise seizure control [Gross-Tsur et al., 1997]. Atomoxetine (a nonamphetamine selective norepinephrine reuptake inhibitor with stimulant properties) does not significantly affect seizure control; nor does it have significant pharmacokinetic interactions with antiepileptic medications. Bupropion, an antidepressant drug occasionally useful for ADHD, particularly when associated with mood disorder,

may increase tendency toward seizures, particularly at high doses. Most pediatric neurologists avoid its use at doses greater than 100 mg per day in children with epilepsy.

Peer Relationships, Teasing, and Social Isolation

Social isolation and poor peer relationships are a particular problem in school-aged and adolescent children with epilepsy and are difficult to address therapeutically. Nonverbal learning disabilities may make the child socially maladroit and target them for teasing by peers. Children may be particularly at risk for teasing and exclusion by peers if they have had seizures at school or are singled out by the need to leave the classroom to take medication during the school day. Therapeutic or educational programs that emphasize social skills and assertiveness training may be helpful in some children and adolescents [Henriksen, 1990; Lewis et al., 1990; Strang, 1990].

Occupational Planning and Adjustment

Occupational adjustment may be poor in adults with childhood-onset epilepsy. Vocational plans and postsecondary education should be discussed with adolescents who have epilepsy, with appropriate goal-setting. Adolescents with well-controlled epilepsy may be assured that their epilepsy will not interfere with career goals, with a few notable exceptions; military service, airlines, and public safety professions (police and fire) generally will exclude applicants with epilepsy, regardless of control. Some states will restrict commercial drivers' licenses, even with good seizure control. Appropriate resources for assessment, training, and placement should be identified in the community. In addition to school-based programs, local Epilepsy Foundation affiliates may be a good resource, as may the state department of vocational rehabilitation.

Headaches in Infants and Children

Donald W. Lewis

Introduction

Headache is a universal affliction of humans from which children are not spared. Headache is the most common reason that children are referred to child neurology practices. It is therefore essential for clinicians to have a thorough, systematic approach to the evaluation and management of the child or adolescent with the complaint of headache.

Headache may be due to primary entities, such as migraine or tension-type, or the pain may result from secondary causes such as brain tumors, increased intracranial pressure, drug intoxications, paranasal sinus disease, or acute febrile illnesses such as influenza. The evaluation of a child presenting with headache follows the traditional medical model, with extraction of the necessary history and performance of a thorough physical and neurologic examination. In most instances, this initial process will yield a diagnosis or determine the need for further ancillary testing. Once the diagnosis is established, a comprehensive treatment program can be put into place, blending pharmacologic and biobehavioral measures, and keeping both physical and emotional factors in mind.

The purpose of this chapter is to explore the symptom of headache, reviewing the epidemiology, current classification system, appropriate evaluation, and differential diagnosis.

Epidemiology

Headaches are common during childhood and become increasing more frequent during adolescence. The prevalence of headache ranges from 37 to 51 percent in 7-year-olds, gradually rising to 57–82 percent by age 15. Recurring or frequent headaches occurred in 2.5 percent of 7-year-olds and 15 percent of 15-year-olds [Bille, 1962]. Before puberty, boys are affected more frequently than girls, but after puberty, headaches occur more frequently in girls [Deubner, 1977; Sillanpaa, 1983; Dalsgaard-Nielsen, 1970; Laurell et al., 2004].

The prevalence of migraine headache steadily increases through childhood and the male:female ratio shifts during adolescence. The prevalence rises from 3 percent at age 3–7 years to 4–11 percent by age 7–11, and up to 8–23 percent during adolescence (Table 63-1). The mean age of onset of migraine is 7.2 years for boys and 10.9 years for girls [Dalsgaard-Nielsen, 1970; Lipton et al., 1994; Mortimer et al., 1992; Valquist, 1955; Small and Waters, 1974; Sillanpaa, 1976; Stewart et al., 1991; Stewart et al., 1992].

Data regarding tension-type headache is limited. Two studies including school-aged children of 7–19 years, and using the International Classification of Headache Disorders (ICHD-2) criteria, found the 1-year prevalence of tension-type headache to be 10–23 percent. The prevalence of tension-type headache increased with age in both boys and girls, up to age 11 years, and thereafter only increased in girls [Laurell et al., 2004; Zwart et al., 2004].

Chronic daily headache, defined as more than 15 headache days/month for more than 4 months, occurs in 1–2 percent of adolescents [Wang et al., 2006, 2009].

Classification

The International Headache Society's comprehensive classification system for the spectrum of primary and secondary headache disorders is available on their website (http://ihs-classification.org/en) (Box 63-1). There are three major categories: the primary headaches, the secondary headaches, and the cranial neuralgias. Each headache category is carefully defined, subclassified, and annotated.

For example, the classification for the primary headache disorder, migraine, is subclassified into migraine without aura, migraine with aura, and the childhood periodic syndromes that are commonly precursors of migraine. Migraine with aura is further divided into subgroups based upon current views of the pathophysiology of migraine. The visual, sensory, motor, or psychic phenomena that herald the onset of a migraine attack are all included under migraine with aura (Box 63-2). A migraine attack accompanied by hemiparesis (e.g., familial hemiplegic migraine [FHM]) falls in the category of migraine with aura, although alternative explanations for hemiparesis with headache must be carefully sought before the diagnosis of FHM can be accepted.

There are several "orphan" pediatric headache disorders, traditionally included within the migraine spectrum, that are omitted from ICHD-2. Alice in Wonderland syndrome is characterized by bizarre visual (e.g., macropsia or micropsia) or perceptual (e.g., prosopagnosia) experiences before the onset of a typical migraine headache. This entity is now viewed as a form of migraine with aura, in which the aura occurs in the parietal or posterior temporal cortical regions, yielding the unusual visuoperceptual phenomena.

Alternating hemiparesis of childhood (AHC) is a rare and bizarre entity, once thought to be a migrainous phenomenon.

Table 63-1 Prevalence of Migraine Headache through Childhood

	Age 3–7 Years	Age 7–11 Years	Age 15 Years
Prevalence	1.2–3.2%	4–11%	8–23%
Gender ratio	Boys > girls	Boys = girls	Girls > boys

Box 63-1 International Classification of Headache Disorders (ICHD-2)

Primary Headache Disorders

1. Migraine
2. Tension-type
3. Cluster headache
4. Other primary headache disorders

Secondary Headaches

5. Headache attributed to head or neck trauma
6. Headache attributed to cranial or cervical vascular disorder
7. Headache attributed to nonvascular intracranial disorder
8. Headache attributed to substance or withdrawal from substances
9. Headache attributed to infection
10. Headache attributed to disorders of homeostasis
11. Headache attributed to disorders of the cranium, neck, eyes, ears, nose, sinuses, teeth, or other facial or cranial structures
12. Headache attributed to psychiatric disorders

Cranial Neuralgias, Central and Primary Facial Pain

13. Cranial neuralgia and central causes of facial pain
14. Other headache, cranial neuralgia, central or primary facial pain

Box 63-2 2003 International Classification of Headache Disorders (ICHD-2): Migraine

- Migraine without aura
- Migraine with aura
  - Typical aura with migraine headache
  - Typical aura with nonmigraine headache
  - Typical aura without headache
  - Familial hemiplegic migraine
  - Sporadic hemiplegic migraine
  - Basilar-type migraine
- Childhood periodic syndromes that are commonly precursors of migraine
  - Cyclical vomiting
  - Abdominal migraine
  - Benign paroxysmal vertigo of childhood
- Retinal migraine
- Complications of migraine
  - Chronic migraine
  - Status migraine
  - Persistent aura without infarction
  - Migrainous infarction
- Probable migraine

AHC is now viewed as a metabolic disorder, probably due to a mitochondrial disorder or a channelopathy. Recently, however, a novel *ATP1A2* mutation within one kindred, with features that bridged the phenotypic spectrum between AHC and FHM, has been reported and may draw AHC back into the migraine spectrum [Swoboda et al., 2004; Bassi et al., 2004].

Ophthalmoplegic migraine no longer falls in the migraine category, but in the group of cranial neuralgias. While paradoxically still labeled as "migraine," this clinical entity is characterized by transient disturbances of cranial nerves III, IV, or VI, coupled with intense peri- or retro-orbital pain, and is viewed as a transient demyelinative process.

Clinical Classification

A useful clinical classification system was proposed by Rothner; it divides headache into five temporal patterns (Figure 63-1): acute, acute recurrent, chronic progressive, chronic nonprogressive, and mixed. Each of these temporal patterns suggests differing pathophysiologic processes and has distinctive differential diagnoses (Box 63-3).

Acute Headache

The acute, sudden onset of headache in an otherwise healthy child is usually due to intercurrent viral infection (e.g., influenza, upper respiratory infection, or pharyngitis). The acute headache with focal neurologic signs must raise concerns for intracranial hemorrhage from aneurysm, vascular malformation, or coagulopathy. Sudden headache with fever warrants consideration of cerebrospinal fluid (CSF) analysis for the possibility of meningitis.

Acute Recurrent Headache

An acute-recurrent pattern implies episodes or attacks of headache, separated by symptom-free intervals. The primary headache disorders, migraine and tension-type, are the most common causes of this pattern, although complex partial seizures, substance abuse, cluster headache, and recurrent trauma can, infrequently, produce recurring headache syndromes.

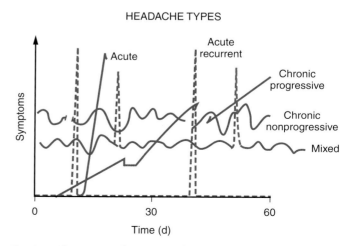

HEADACHE TYPES

Fig. 63-1 Five temporal patterns of pediatric headache.

Box 63-3 Differential Diagnosis of the Five Temporal Patterns

Acute

Generalized
- Fever
- Systemic infection
- Central nervous system infection
- Toxins: lead, CO
- After seizure
- Electrolyte imbalance
- Hypertension
- Hypoglycemia
- Post lumbar puncture
- Trauma
- Embolic
- Vascular thrombosis
- Hemorrhage
- Autoimmune/Collagen vascular disease
- Exertional

Localized
- Sinusitis
- Otitis
- Ocular abnormality (glaucoma)
- Dental disease
- Trauma
- Cranial neuralgia (occipital)
- Temporomandibular joint dysfunction

Acute-Recurrent
- Migraine
- Complex migraine

- Migraine variants
- Cluster
- Paroxysmal hemicrania
- After seizure
- Tic douleureux
- Exertional

Chronic Progressive
- Brain Tumor
- Idiopathic intracranial hypertension
- Brain abscess
- Subdural hematoma
- Hydrocephalus
- Hemorrhage
- Hypertension
- Vasculitis

Chronic Nonprogressive and Mixed*
- Chronic daily headache (chronic migraine)
- Chronic tension-type
- Chronic Hemicrania continuum
- Conversion disorder
- Malingering
- After concussion
- Depression
- Anxiety
- Adjustment reaction

---

* with superimposed migraine.

Chronic Progressive Headache

Chronic progressive headache implies a gradually increasing frequency and severity of headache, and is the most ominous of the five temporal patterns. The pathological correlate is increasing intracranial pressure. Causes of this pattern include brain tumor, hydrocephalus, idiopathic intracranial hypertension (pseudotumor cerebri), chronic meningitis, brain abscess, or subdural hematoma.

Chronic Nonprogressive Headache

Chronic non-progressive or chronic daily headache (CDH) represents a pattern of frequent or near-constant headache. The definition of CDH is: ≥ 4 months with ≥ 15 headaches per month and the headaches lasting ≥ 4 hours. Many adolescents will have continuous, unremitting, disabling daily headache. The most common form of CDH is chronic migraine. Affected patients generally have normal neurologic examinations and there are usually interwoven psychological factors and heightened anxiety about unrecognized, underlying organic causes. Management of

these patients requires a carefully crafted blend of pharmacologic and biobehavioral strategies.

Mixed Headache

A "mixed" headache pattern represents the superimposition of acute recurrent headache (usually migraine) upon a chronic daily background pattern; it is therefore a variant of CDH (see following sections).

Diagnostic Criteria

The ICHD-2 established the diagnostic criteria for the primary headache disorders, incorporating many developmentally sensitive changes compared to previous criteria, and thus improving applicability to children and adolescents while maintaining specificity and improving sensitivity (Box 63-4) [Oleson, 2004]. For example, the criteria accept that pediatric migraine may be brief (approximately 1 hour), as opposed to a 4-hour duration for adults; may be bifrontal in location (under age 15 years); and may have associated symptoms of photophobia and phonophobia, which may be *inferred* by the child's behavior, such as withdrawing to a dark, quiet room to rest during the headache attack.

Box 63-4 ICHD-2 Diagnostic Criteria for the Primary Headache Disorders: Migraine and Tension-Type

Pediatric Migraine without Aura

A. At least five attacks fulfilling criteria B–D
B. Headache attacks lasting 1–72 hours
C. Headache has at least two of the following characteristics:
  1. Unilateral location, may be bilateral or frontotemporal (not occipital)
  2. Pulsing quality
  3. Moderate or severe pain intensity
  4. Aggravation by, or causing avoidance of, routine physical activity (e.g., walking or climbing stairs)
D. During the headache, at least one of the following:
  1. Nausea and/or vomiting
  2. Photophobia and phonophobia, which may be *inferred* from the patient's behavior
E. Not attributed to another disorder

Episodic Tension-Type Headache

A. At least 10 episodes occurring on ≥1, but ≤15 days per month for at least 3 months and fulfilling criteria B–D
B. Headache lasting 30 minutes to 7 days
C. Headache has at least two of the following characteristics:
  1. Bilateral location
  2. Pressing/tightening (non-pulsing) quality
  3. Mild or moderate intensity
  4. Not aggravated by routine physical activity, such as walking or climbing stairs
D. Both of the following:
  5. No nausea or vomiting (anorexia may occur)
  6. Photophobia or phonophobia (but not both)
E. Not attributed to another structural or metabolic disorder

Box 63-5 ICHD-2 Criteria for Cyclical Vomiting Syndrome

Description

- Recurrent episodic attacks, usually stereotypical in the individual patient, of vomiting and intense nausea
- Attacks are associated with pallor and lethargy
- There is complete resolution of symptoms between attacks

Diagnostic Criteria

A. At least five attacks fulfilling criteria B and C
B. Episodic attacks, stereotypical in the individual patient, of intense nausea and vomiting lasting 1–5 days
C. Vomiting during attacks occurs at least five times/hour for at least 1 hour
D. Symptom-free between attacks
E. Not attributed to another disorder. History and physical examination do not show signs of gastrointestinal disease

Box 63-6 ICHD-2 Criteria for Abdominal Migraine

Description

- An idiopathic recurrent disorder seen mainly in children and characterized by episodic midline abdominal pain manifesting in attacks lasting 1–72 hours with normality between episodes
- The pain is of moderate to severe intensity and associated with vasomotor symptoms, nausea and vomiting

Diagnostic Criteria

A. At least five attacks fulfilling criteria B–D
B. Attacks of abdominal pain lasting 1–72 hours
C. Abdominal pain has all of the following characteristics:
  1. Midline location, periumbilical, or poorly localized
  2. Dull or "just sore" quality
  3. Moderate or severe intensity
D. During abdominal pain, at least two of the following:
  1. Anorexia
  2. Nausea
  3. Vomiting
  4. Pallor
E. Not attributed to another disorder. History and physical examination do not show signs of gastrointestinal or renal disease, or such disease has been ruled out by appropriate investigations

ICHD-2 also includes criteria for cyclical vomiting and abdominal migraine (Box 63-5 and Box 63-6).

Evaluation of the Child with Headache

The evaluation of a child with headaches follows the traditional medical model and begins with a thorough medical history and complete physical and neurologic examination. The brief series of questions shown in Figure 63-2 provides a logical framework for evaluating headaches and generally yields sufficient information to diagnose most primary headaches and reveal clues to presence of secondary headache disorders.

The role of ancillary diagnostic studies, such as laboratory testing, electroencephalography (EEG), and neuroimaging,

has been extensively reviewed [Lewis et al., 2002]. This American Academy of Neurology (AAN) Practice Parameter determined that there is inadequate documentation in the literature to support any recommendation as to the appropriateness of routine laboratory studies (e.g., hematology or chemistry panels) or performance of lumbar puncture. Routine EEG is not recommended as part of the headache evaluation. Data compiled from eight studies showed that the EEG was not necessary for differentiation of primary headache disorders (e.g., migraine, tension-type) from secondary headache due to structural disease involving the head and neck, or from headaches due to a psychogenic etiology. In addition, EEG is unlikely to define or determine an etiology of the headache or to distinguish migraine from other types of headaches. Furthermore, in those children undergoing evaluation for recurrent headache who were found to have paroxysmal EEGs, the risk of future seizures is negligible.

The role of neuroimaging is better defined. Data compiled from six pediatric studies permitted the following recommendations:

1. Obtaining a neuroimaging study on a routine basis is *not* indicated in children with recurrent headaches and a normal neurologic examination.
2. Neuroimaging should be considered in children in whom there are historic features to suggest:
  a. recent onset of severe headache
  b. change in the type of headache
  c. neurologic dysfunction.
3. Neuroimaging should be considered in children with an abnormal neurologic examination (e.g., focal findings, signs of increased intracranial pressure, significant alteration of consciousness), and/or the coexistence of seizures.

Care must be taken not to over- or under-interpret these recommendations. Neuroimaging may be considered in children with recurrent headache based upon clues extracted from the medical history or based upon the findings on neurologic examination. The "managed care industry" has focused only upon recommendation number 1 and failed to recognize recommendations 2 and 3, which clearly place the responsibility in the hands of the clinician to make decisions regarding ancillary testing, including neuroimaging, based upon good clinical judgment. The findings of the AAN Practice Parameter support the medical decision to perform scans, or to withhold scans, based upon clinical determinants for the individual patient.

Primary Headache Syndromes

Migraine

Migraine is the most common acute recurrent headache syndrome. The classification of migraine is shown in Box 63-2 and the cardinal diagnostic features are shown in Box 63-4.

Pathophysiology

Incompletely understood, migraine is thought to be a complex, primary, neuroglial process (Figure 63-3) [Pietrobon and Striessnig, 2003; Silberstein, 2004; Goadsby et al., 2009]. The principal underlying phenomenon of migraine is hyperexcitable neurons. Polygenic influences produce disturbances of neuronal ion channels (e.g., sodium, calcium), leading to episodes of cortical spreading depression (CSD) and activation of the "trigeminovascular system."

Key questions to ask in the evaluation of children with headaches Headache Database	
1. How and when did your headache(s) begin?	
2. What is the time pattern of your headache: sudden first headache, episodes of headache, an everyday headache, gradually worsening, or a mixture?	
3. Do you have one type of headache or more than one type?	
4. How often does the headache occur and how long does it last?	
5. Can you tell that a headache is coming?	
6. Where is the pain located and what is the quality of the pain: pounding, squeezing, stabbing, or other?	
7. Are there any other symptoms that accompany your headache: nausea, vomiting, dizziness, numbness, weakness, or other?	
8. What makes the headache better or worse? Do any activities, medications, or foods tend to cause or aggravate your headaches?	
9. Do you have to stop your activities when you get a headache?	
10. Do the headaches occur under any special circumstances or at any particular time?	
11. Do you have any other symptoms between headaches?	
12. Are you taking or are you being treated with any medications (for the headache or other purposes)?	
13. Do you have any other medical problems?	
14. Does anyone in your family suffer from headaches?	
15. What do you think might be causing your headache?	

Adapted from Rothner, 1995

Fig. 63-2 Key questions to ask in the evaluation of children with headaches. *(Adapted from Rothner AD. The evaluation of headaches in children and adolescents. Seminars in Pediatric Neurology 1995; 2:109–118.) [Rothner, 1995]*

CSD represents a slowly propagating wave (approximately 2–6 mm/min) of neuronal excitation, followed by depolarization, and is now viewed as cause of the migraine aura. Clinically, migraine aura represents transient, focal, somatosensory phenomena, such as visual scotomata or distortions, dysesthesias, hemiparesis, or aphasia, and is caused by regional neuronal depolarization, possibly accompanied by some degree of regional oligemia.

While CSD nicely explains the somatosensory aura, only about 30 percent of children and adolescents experience aura, so explanation of the pain requires involvement of other cerebral circuits. Clearly, the processes leading to migraine pain must occur in the absence of a perceived aura. Two mechanisms are thought to be responsible for the generation of the pain of migraine:
1. neurogenic inflammation of the meningeal vessels
2. "sensitization" of peripheral and central trigeminal afferents. Activation of the "trigeminovascular" system by descending cortical, thalamic, hypothalamic, and brainstem nuclei, and, possibly, by ascending cervical neurons, initiates vascular dilatation with extravasation of plasma proteins from dural vessels; this, in turn, activates trigeminal meningeal afferents. These processes set the stage for "neurogenic" inflammation of the

dural and pial vessels, mediated principally by neuropeptides and calcitonin gene-related peptide (CGRP). The inflammatory cascade stimulates nociceptive afferents, leading to pain.

Neurogenic inflammation alone may be an insufficient explanation for the severity and quality of pain in migraine. One of the striking symptoms experienced during an attack of migraine is that seemingly innocuous activities, such as coughing, walking up stairs, or bending over, greatly intensify the pain. This observation, coupled with elegant research, has led to the concepts of "sensitization" of trigeminal vascular afferents, whereby both peripheral and central afferent circuits become exceptionally sensitive to mechanical, thermal, and chemical stimuli. These circuits become so sensitive that virtually any stimulation is perceived as painful: the concept of "allodynia" [Burstein et al., 2000, 2004; Burstein and Jakubowski, 2004].

Therefore, the current view of the pathophysiology of migraine begins with an inherited vulnerability with hyperexcitable neuron–glial networks. A variety of stimuli may trigger episodes of CSD and, separately, activation of the trigeminovascular system, which, in turn, initiates the processes of localized, neurogenic inflammation and sensitization of both peripheral and central afferent circuitry. Controversy exists

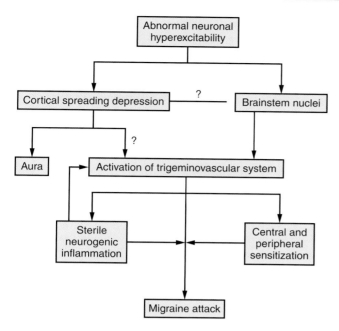

Adapted from Peitrobon and Striessnig 2003

Fig. 63-3 Migraine pathophysiology. *(Adapted from Pietrobon D, Striessnig J. Neurobiology of migraine. Nat Rev 2003;4:386.)*

as to whether CSD is the primary initiating event producing the cascade of downstream effects through the trigeminal vascular networks. The absence of aura in two-thirds of patients calls this into question. Exciting translational research exploring the pathophysiology of migraine continues.

Clinical Manifestations

MIGRAINE WITHOUT AURA

The diagnostic criteria for migraine without aura are shown in Box 63-4.

Migraine without aura is the most frequent form, accounting for 60–85 percent of all migraine in children and adolescents. Patients will often recognize prodromal features: mood changes (euphoria to depression), irritability, lethargy, yawning, food cravings, or increased thirst. Perhaps the most frequent heralding feature is a change in behavioral patterns or withdrawal from activities.

A migraine headache begins gradually and is usually localized to the frontal or temporal region. The pain may be unilateral. The quality is generally described as pounding, pulsing, and throbbing, but the key feature is its intensity. Routine activities will be interrupted. Photophobia and/or phonophobia are common, and may be inferred by the child's desire to seek a quiet, dark place to rest or even to sleep, since sleep often produces significant relief.

Nausea, vomiting, and abdominal pain may be the most disabling features; a student with headache may be able to stay in the classroom with pain, but the onset of nausea or vomiting necessitates a visit to the school nurse.

Migraine headaches typically last for hours, even days (1–72 hours), but do not, generally, occur more frequently than 6–8 times per month. More than 8–10 attacks per month must warrant consideration of alternative diagnoses, such as organic

conditions (i.e., idiopathic intracranial hypertension) or the spectrum of chronic daily headache [Gladstein et al., 1997; American College of Emergency Physicians, 1996].

The time of day when the headache occurs tends to shift through childhood. Younger children will complain in the afternoon, after school. The early teenagers will frequently begin to report their headaches about lunchtime, often precipitated by the chaos of the school cafeteria with its combination of bright lights, loud noise, and peer pressures. Older teens will acquire the more adult patterns of morning headache, which is often a cause for concern since morning occurrence frequently raises suspicion of space-occupying lesions.

While most verbal children can readily relate these symptoms, the developmentally challenged may be unable to express themselves. Caregivers will report repeated, cycling, events of quiet, withdrawn behavior with pallor, regurgitation, vomiting, and desire to rest. These stereotyped episodes may prompt investigation for epilepsy, gastroesophageal reflux, or hydrocephalus, when, in fact, they may represent migraine.

MIGRAINE WITH AURA

Approximately 14–30 percent of children will report visual disturbances, distortions, or obscuration before or as the headache begins (Box 63-7) [Lewis, 1995]. The aura ("cool breeze") is, however, an inconsistent feature in childhood and adolescents. The presence of an aura must be elicited with very specific questions: "Do you have spots, colors, lights, dots in your eyes before or as you are getting a headache?"

Box 63-7 Forms of Migraine Aura

Visual

- Negative scotoma
- "Fortification" scotoma
- Field deficits
  - Hemianopsia
  - Quadrantanopsia
- Photopsia
- Visual distortions
  - Teichopsia
  - Metamorphopsia
  - Prosopagnosia
  - "Alice in Wonderland"

Sensory

- Paresthesias
- Dyesthesias
- Perioral and/or hand numbness (chiro-oral)

Motor

- Hemiparesis
- Monoparesis

Aphasia

Psychic

- Confusion
- Dysphasia
- Amnesia
- Dysequilibrium

Typically, the aura is a visual phenomenon, but, as discussed in the pathophysiology section above, the cortical spreading depression responsible for the aura may disturb virtually any cortical region, including language, motor, or sensory areas. The classic visual symptomatology during migraine includes three dominant visual phenomena:

1. binocular visual impairment with scotoma (77 percent)
2. distortion or hallucinations (16 percent)
3. monocular visual impairment or scotoma (7 percent) [Hachinski et al., 1973].

The onset of the visual aura is gradual and lasts up to 30 minutes. Sudden images and complicated visual perceptions should prompt consideration of complex partial seizures, even if followed by headache. Young adolescents may experience bizarre visual phenomena (distortions, illusions, micropsia, and macropsia) within the spectrum of the "Alice-in-Wonderland" syndrome. Transient visual obscurations – brief episodes of near-complete blindness – are also features of idiopathic intracranial hypertension.

ALICE IN WONDERLAND SYNDROME

Bizarre visual illusions and spatial distortions occasionally precede migraine headaches. Similar to Alice, who experienced visual distortions after eating mushroom in *Through the Looking Glass*, affected children will describe visual distortions before or as the headache is beginning. The children may describe bizarre or vivid visual illusions, such as:

- micropsia: objects appear smaller
- macropsia: objects appear larger
- metamorphopsia: objects (such as faces) appear distorted
- teleopsia: objects appear far away.

These patients are seldom confused or frightened by these illusions and are able to relate the experience in exquisite and enthusiastic detail. This unusual visual symptomatology is best considered as migraine with aura, though, historically, Alice in Wonderland syndrome is included as a distinct variant. This type of visual-perceptual abnormality has been reported with infectious mononucleosis, complex partial seizures, and hallucinogenic drug ingestion.

Retinal Migraine

Also referred to as ocular, ophthalmic, or anterior visual pathway migraine, this variant is uncommon in young children but can occur during adolescence. Affected patients will report brief (seconds to <60 minutes), sudden, monocular, black or gray "outs," or bright, blinding episodes (e.g., photopsia) of visual disturbance before, after, or during the headache. A 60-minute interval between visual symptom and headache may occur. As in ophthalmoplegic migraine, the pain of retinal migraine is often described as retro-orbital and ipsilateral to the visual disturbance.

Examination of the optic fundus during an attack may disclose constriction of retinal vasculature with marked retinal pallor. An occasional patient may suffer significant visual sequelae (e.g. scotoma, altitudinal defects, or monocular blindness) in retinal migraine thought to be due to retinal infarction. Although the patient population with retinal migraine is generally much younger than those who experience amaurosis fugax from atheromatous carotid disease, evaluation for hypercoagulable states, embolic sources, and carotid dissection must be considered.

Basilar-Type Migraine

Also known as basilar artery or vertebrobasilar migraine, this clinical entity is the most common of migraine variants and is estimated to represent 3–19 percent of all migraine [Bickerstaff, 1961; Lapkin and Golden, 1978; Golden and French, 1975]. This wide range of frequency relates to the rigorousness of the definition. Some authors consider any headache with dizziness to be within the spectrum of basilar-type migraine (BTM), whereas others require the presence of clear signs and symptoms of posterior fossa involvement before establishing this diagnosis. The ICHD-2 criteria require two or more symptoms and emphasize bulbar and bilateral sensorimotor features (Box 63-8).

The onset of BTM tends to be in younger children, with the mean age being 7 years; however, the clinical entity probably may appear as early as 12–18 months of age, as episodic pallor, clumsiness, and vomiting, and evolving from one of the periodic syndromes, benign paroxysmal vertigo.

Children with BTM have recurrent attacks of intense dizziness, vertigo, visual disturbances, ataxia, and diplopia. These early, transient features last minutes up to an hour and are then followed by the headache phase. The headache may be occipital in location. The quality of the pain may be ill defined and terms such as pulsing or throbbing may not be used. A small subset of patients with BTM will have their posterior fossa symptoms *after* the headache phase is well established.

The pathogenesis of BTM is not well understood. While focal cortical processes, oligemia, or depolarization can explain the deficits in hemiplegic migraine, the posterior fossa signs of BTM are more problematic. A single case report of a 25-year-old woman with BTM exists, wherein transcranial Doppler and single-photon emission computed tomography (SPECT) were performed through the course of a BTM attack. These data suggest decreased posterior cerebral artery perfusion through the aura phase at a time when the patient described was experiencing transient bilateral blindness and ataxia [La Spina et al., 1997].

The sudden appearance of diplopia, vertigo, and vomiting must prompt consideration of disorders within the posterior fossa, such as arteriovenous malformations, cavernous angiomas,

---

Box 63-8 Signs and Symptoms of Basilar-Type Migraine

Vertigo	73%
Nausea or vomiting	30–50%
Ataxia	43–50%
Visual field deficits	43%
Diplopia	30%
Tinnitus	13%
Vertigo	73%
Hearing loss	*
Confusion	20%
Dysarthria	*
Weakness (hemiplegia, quadriplegia, diplegia)	20%
Syncope	*

* No figures available

tumors (medulloblastoma, ependymoma, brainstem glioma), congenital malformations (e.g., Chiari, Dandy–Walker), or vertebrobasilar insufficiency (e.g., vertebral dissection or thrombosis). Acute labyrinthitis or positional vertigo can mimic BTM. Complex partial seizures and drug ingestions must be considered at any age. Rarely, metabolic diseases such as Hartnup's disease, hyperammonemias (urea cycle or organic acidemias), or disorders of pyruvate/lactate metabolism may present with episodic vertigo, but these inborn errors of metabolism usually have some degree of altered consciousness, even coma.

Hemiplegic Migraine

Familial Hemiplegic Migraine

FHM is an uncommon autosomal-dominant form of migraine headache, in which the aura has a "stroke-like" quality, producing some degree of hemiparesis. The nosology is somewhat misleading since there is actually a wide diversity of focal symptoms and signs that can accompany this migraine variant, beyond motor deficits. Barlow proposed the more appropriate term "hemi-syndrome migraine" to emphasize the diversity of associated symptoms, but this was not adopted [Barlow, 1984]. ICHD-2 clearly requires that "some degree of hemiparesis" must be present.

A series of exciting discoveries into the molecular genetics of FHM have broadened our understanding of the fundamental mechanisms of migraine and demonstrated the overlap with other paroxysmal disorders, such as acetazolamide-responsive episodic ataxia [Joutel et al., 1993]. Genetic linkage to chromosome 19p13 has been identified in half of the known FHM pedigrees. FHM types 2 and 3 are clinically quite similar but have distinctly different molecular mechanisms. FMF type 2 is due to point mutation of the alpha-2 subunit of the sodium-potassium pump (ATP1A2) gene on chromosome 1q21–23, and type 3 is due to a sodium channel gene mutation (SCN1A) [Ophoff et al., 1997; Gardner et al., 1997; Dichgans et al., 2005]. More genotypes will likely be identified with broadening of the phenotype. The chromosome 19 defect (FHM type 1) produces a missense mutation in a neuronal calcium channel gene (CACNA1A), providing compelling evidence that FHM represents a channelopathy. These discoveries have revolutionized our understanding of migraine and may open new territory for pharmacologic interventions.

From the clinical perspective, hemiplegic migraine is characterized by transient episodes of focal neurologic deficits, hemiparesis, hemisensory changes, aphasia, and visual field defects, which precede the headache phase by 30–60 minutes; occasionally, they extend well beyond the headache itself. The headache is often, but not invariably, contralateral to the focal deficit.

The appearance of acute, focal neurologic deficits in the setting of headache in an adolescent necessitates vigorous investigation for disorders such as intracranial hemorrhage, stroke, tumor, vascular malformations, acute disseminated encephalomyelitis, or focal infection. Complex partial seizure or drug intoxication with a sympathomimetic must also be considered. Neuroimaging (magnetic resonance imaging [MRI] and magnetic resonance angiography [MRA]) and EEG may be indicated. Investigations for embolic sources or hypercoagulable states are likewise appropriate. Molecular genetic testing is now available for the three genes known to be associated with FHM: CACNA1A (FHM 1), ATP1A2

(FHM 2), and SCN1A (FHM 3) [http://www.ncbi.nlm.nih.gov/bookshelf/br.fcgi?book=gene&part=fhm].

Sporadic hemiplegic migraine represents a clinically indistinguishable phenomenon, but lacks the identifiable family history.

Alternating Hemiplegia of Childhood

Traditionally, this rare entity has been considered a variant of hemiplegic migraine, but more recent perspectives suggest other mechanisms and the ICHD-2 has omitted it from the migraine spectrum. Affected patients have their initial symptoms before 18 months of life, and have repeated attacks of hemiplegia involving either side of the body, paroxysmal movement disorders (dystonia, oculomotor disorders, autonomic), and a background pattern of developmental delay. Curiously, the symptoms abate upon sleeping.

Children with AHC have attacks of paralysis: hemiparesis, monoparesis, diparesis, ophthalmoparesis, or bulbar paralysis, which may be accompanied by variable tone changes (flaccid, spastic, or rigid). A variety of paroxysmal involuntary movements, including chorea, athetosis, dystonia, nystagmus, and respiratory irregularities (hyperpnea), can be seen. The attacks of paralysis can be brief (minutes) or prolonged (days), and are potentially life-threatening during periods of bulbar paralysis. Curiously, the attacks generally subside following sleep. Affected children are frequently developmentally challenged [Verret and Steele, 1971; Aicardi et al., 1995].

A recent comprehensive report of 103 children who met existing criteria for AHC focused on the earliest manifestations of symptoms and evolution of features over time. Paroxysmal eye movements were the most frequent early symptom, manifesting in the first 3 months of life in 83 percent of patients. Hemiplegic episodes appeared by 6 months of age in 56 percent of infants. Distinct convulsive episodes with altered consciousness, believed to be epileptic in nature, were reported in 41 percent of patients. Static features of AHC included ataxia (96 percent) and cognitive impairment (100 percent). MRI studies were generally normal (78 percent). Treatments included flunarizine, benzodiazepines, carbamazepine, barbiturates, and valproic acid. Flunarizine was the most effective agent, but perceived improvement occurred in only 60 percent of patients [Sweney et al., 2009].

The link to migraine was tenuous, but was based upon the presence of a high prevalence of migraine in the families of affected children and upon cerebral blood flow data that suggest a "migrainous" mechanism. In 1997, an international workshop was conducted to address the various hypotheses surrounding AHC and proposed mechanisms, including channelopathy, mitochondrial cytopathy, and cerebrovascular dysfunction. Channelopathy was suggested as the most likely explanation [Rho and Chugani, 1998]. A novel ATP1A2 mutation in a kindred with features that bridged the phenotypic spectrum between AHC and FHM has been reported. This observation may draw AHC back into the migraine spectrum; however, at this point the underlying molecular mechanisms of AHC are unknown [Wang et al., 2006].

Investigations into the etiology of this entity should include aggressive evaluation for vascular disorders, inborn errors of metabolism, mitochondrial encephalomyopathies, migraine (FHM 1) or epileptic variants.

Management is difficult; it may target the attacks of hemiparesis, or address the associated seizures or movement disorder. For the episodes of hemiparesis, flunarizine (5–10 mg/day), not available through U.S. pharmacies, can be effective in reducing attack frequency and severity.

Confusional Migraine

Omitted from the ICHD-2 classification system is the entity "confusional migraine," which most likely represents a hybrid or overlap between hemiplegic and basilar-type migraine. Perhaps the term "confusional migraine" may disappear in the near future; those patients who have attacks associated with language disturbances, hemiparesis, and confusion are likely to be considered to have hemiplegic migraine, and those with bilateral blindness, vertigo, and confusion will be classified as having basilar-type migraine, dependent upon which symptoms predominate in individual patients.

The clinical entity was first described in 1970 by Gascon and Barlow, who reported a series of children, aged 8–16 years, with acute confusional states lasting 4–24 hours, and associated with agitation and aphasia. The authors suggested that the confusional state was a manifestation of juvenile migraine [Garcon and Barlow, 1970]. Ehyai and Fenichel later introduced the term acute confusional migraine [Ehyai and Fenichel, 1978]. Subsequent reports have broadened the clinical phenomenology to include blindness, paresthesias, hemiparesis, and amnesia. Amnesia can be such a prominent feature that Jenson proposed the term transient global amnesia of childhood, but amnesia is only part of the clinical spectrum [Jensen, 1980].

Affected children, more commonly males, become agitated, restless, disoriented, and, occasionally, combative for minutes to hours. Once consciousness has returned to baseline, the patients may describe an inability to communicate, frustration, confusion, and loss of orientation to time, and may not recall a headache phase at all. A strong family history of migraine is elicited in 75 percent of patients.

There is clear link to head trauma in many cases [Ferrera and Reicho, 1996]. The term "footballer's migraine" is applied in Europe when a soccer player, after "heading" the ball, develops acute confusional state with headache. Similar phenomena may follow other causes of minor head injury. This variant should be viewed within the spectrum of trauma-triggered migraine.

Acute confusional states in children and adolescents warrant aggressive investigation for encephalitis, brain abscess, drug intoxication, cerebrovascular disease, vasculitis, or metabolic encephalopathies [Amit, 1988]. Particular attention must be focused on the possibility of complex partial seizures or postictal states.

Childhood "Periodic Syndromes"

The three curious and pediatric-specific clinical entities described below represent episodic conditions with stereotyped features that are considered precursors of migraine. Benign paroxysmal torticollis, omitted from ICHD-2, is also best discussed in this section and may be introduced to the group of periodic syndromes in future classification systems.

Cyclical Vomiting Syndrome

Cyclical vomiting syndrome (CVS) is a disorder characterized by recurrent, self-limiting-episodes of intense vomiting (more than four emeses/hour), recognizable by their stereotypical time of onset, duration, and symptomatology within the individual (see Box 63-5). The vomiting is uniquely intense and the subjective nausea disabling; the resultant dehydration often necessitates hospital-based treatment. The attacks are accompanied by pallor, listlessness, anorexia, abdominal pain, retching, headache, and photophobia. The interval between attacks is 2–4 weeks and a typical attack lasts 24–48 hours. The children are, by definition, healthy between attacks.

Boys and girls are equally affected by CVS. The usual age of onset is 5 years, but the diagnosis is often delayed until age 8 and many, if not most, children will "outgrow" these attacks by age 10.

A recent practice guideline provides expert opinion regarding the evaluation and treatment of children with CVS [Li et al., 2008]. A thorough diagnostic evaluation must be performed to rule out intermittent bowel obstruction, elevated intracranial pressure, epilepsy, and metabolic disorders, such as urea cycle defects and organic acidurias. There is clearly a subset of children with a cyclic vomiting pattern who have underlying metabolic disorders.

The link to migraine is based upon natural history data that suggest the evolution toward more typical migraine, parallels drawn based upon autonomic data (i.e., "neurocardiac"), and presence of family history of migraine in children with CVS.

The management of CVS involves both acute strategies and preventative measures. For acute treatment of attacks, patients must be volume-replenished with solutions containing glucose (approximately 10 percent). Pharmacologic measures have not been systematically investigated, but anecdotal information suggests a role for antiemetics (e.g., ondansetron, promethazine, or prochlorperazine) and sedation (e.g., diphenhydramine, benzodiazepine). Subcutaneous sumatriptan (2–4 mg) has been used, but no controlled trials have been conducted. Preventive strategies include lifestyle changes plus agents such as cyproheptadine, amitriptyline or nortriptyline, valproate, topiramate, propranolol, or verapamil; these have all been utilized, but again, no clinical trials have been reported.

Abdominal Migraine

Abdominal migraine is an addition to the ICHD-2. The diagnostic criteria for abdominal migraine are listed in Box 63-6. This clinical entity is characterized by recurrent episodes of midline, epigastric abdominal pain lasting 1–72 hours. The pain is of moderate to severe intensity and is associated with vasomotor symptoms (e.g., flushing, pallor), as well as nausea and vomiting. The patients are well between attacks. Thorough gastrointestinal and renal investigations must be conducted before this diagnosis can be entertained. In a recent series of patients with idiopathic chronic abdominal pain collected from an academic pediatric gastrointestinal clinic, 4–15 percent were found to meet diagnostic criteria for abdominal migraine, suggesting that abdominal migraine is an underdiagnosed cause of recurrent abdominal pain in children in the United States.

Benign Paroxysmal Vertigo of Childhood

Benign paroxysmal vertigo of childhood is common and occurs in young children as abrupt, brief episodes of unexplained unsteadiness, with the child appearing to be "off balance" or falling. Careful observation may disclose nystagmus. Older children may be able to report symptoms of dizziness, clumsiness, headache, and nausea. The attacks may occur in clusters and typically resolve with sleep. In a small series of patients with long-term follow-up, most of the children had resolution of the episodes of vertigo, but later developed migraine.

The diagnosis of benign paroxysmal vertigo is one of exclusion. Epilepsy, otologic pathology, and central nervous system pathology should be considered.

Management of benign paroxysmal vertigo can include symptomatic treatment, such as antiemetics, although sleep will abort the attack in most patients. For a child in whom frequent events are occurring, a trial of cyproheptadine prophylaxis may be helpful in aborting attacks. A dosage of 2–4 mg nightly may be all that is required and medication should be discontinued after the attacks have stopped. The majority of patients will not require any treatment. Reassurance regarding the benign nature of the condition may be all that is required.

Benign Paroxysmal Torticollis

Benign paroxysmal torticollis (BPT) is a rare paroxysmal dyskinesia characterized by attacks of head tilt alone or tilt accompanied by vomiting and ataxia, which may last hours to days [Chaves-Carballo, 1996]. Other torsional or dystonic features, including truncal or pelvic posturing, were described by Chutorian [Chutorian, 1974]. Attacks first manifest during infancy, between 2 and 8 months of age.

The original descriptions of BPT by Snyder suggested a form of labyrinthitis and demonstrated abnormal vestibular reflexes [Snyder, 1969]. A recent case series of 10 patients followed longitudinally, plus a literature review of another 93 cases, has expanded our understanding of BPT. The authors found that attacks usually lasted for less than 1 week, but often recurred every few days or every few months. The episodes improved by age 2 years and typically ended by age 3. There was a very frequent family history of migraine. Developmental assessments, available only in the authors' 10 cases, showed accompanying gross motor delays in 50 percent of children, with additional fine motor delays in 30 percent. Curiously, as BPT improved, so did the gross motor delays and the fine motor delays in about one-half to one-third of the children. The authors concluded that BPT is likely an "age-sensitive, migraine-related disorder, commonly accompanied by delayed motor development" [Rosman et al., 2009].

The link to migraine is strengthening. In addition to a frequent family history of migraine, intriguing molecular genetic information has been reported, in which four children with benign paroxysmal torticollis were shown to be linked to familial *CACNA1A* mutations [Giffin et al., 2002]. BPT is likely a migraine precursor within the spectrum of basilar-type migraine and benign paroxysmal vertigo.

The differential diagnosis must include gastroesophageal reflux (e.g., Sandifer's syndrome), idiopathic torsional dystonia, and complex partial seizure, but particular attention must be paid to the posterior fossa and craniocervical junction, where congenital or acquired lesions may produce torticollis. Rarely, trochlear nerve dysfunction produces compensatory head tilt.

The management is unclear; there are no clinical trials reported. There may be no need for treatment in most patients, beyond reassurance. If the episodes are judged to be very frequent or painful, a trial of cyproheptadine may be a safe measure.

Management of Pediatric Migraine

Once the diagnosis of migraine is established and appropriate reassurances have been provided, a balanced and individually tailored treatment plan can be instituted. The first step is to appreciate the degree of disability imposed by the patient's headache. Understanding of the impact of the headache on the quality of life will guide in the decisions regarding the most appropriate therapeutic course [Powers et al., 2003, 2004].

An AAN Practice Parameter has established the general principles for the management of migraine headache. The fundamental goals of long-term migraine treatment include:

1. reduction of headache frequency, severity, duration, and disability
2. reduction of reliance on poorly tolerated, ineffective, or unwanted acute pharmacotherapies
3. improvement in the quality of life
4. avoidance of acute headache medication escalation
5. education and enablement of patients to manage their disease to enhance personal control of their migraine
6. reduction of headache-related distress and psychological symptoms [Silberstein, 2000].

To achieve these goals, it is becoming increasingly clear that a balanced treatment must include biobehavioral strategies and nonpharmacologic methods, as well as pharmacologic measures. Biobehavioral treatments include biofeedback, stress management, sleep hygiene, exercise, and dietary modifications (Box 63-9) [Holroyd and Mauskop, 2003].

Biofeedback has demonstrated effectiveness in the treatment of both adults and children with migraine in controlled trials.

Box 63-9 Complementary and Alternative Treatments

- Identification of migraine triggers
- Biobehavioral
- Biofeedback
  - Electromyographic biofeedback
  - Electroencephalography
  - Thermal hand warming
  - Galvanic skin resistance feedback
- Relaxation therapy
  - Progressive muscle relaxation
  - Autogenic training
  - Meditation
  - Passive relaxation
  - Self-hypnosis
- Cognitive therapy/Stress management
  - Cognitive control
  - Guided imagery
- Dietary measures
  - "Avoidance diets"
  - Caffeine moderation
  - Herbs: feverfew (*Tanacetum parthenium*), ginkgo, valerian root
  - Minerals: magnesium
  - Vitamins: riboflavin (B_2)
- Acupuncture
- Massage therapy
- Aroma therapy

While the physiological basis for its effectiveness is unclear, data suggest that levels of plasma beta-endorphin can be altered by biofeedback therapies [Baumann, 2002]. Biofeedback therapies commonly use electrical devices that provide audio or visual displays to demonstrate a physiological effect. Thermal biofeedback is the most commonly used technique in pediatrics, wherein children are taught to raise the temperature of one of their fingers. These techniques can easily be taught to children and their use is associated with fewer and briefer migraine headaches. Once taught these methods, the children can manage future headaches, allowing them to feel greater control of their health.

Stress management and relaxation therapies use techniques such as progressive relaxation, self-hypnosis, and guided imagery. Controlled trials have reported relaxation therapies to be as effective in reducing the frequency of migraine attacks as the beta-blocker propranolol [Olness et al., 1987].

Sleep disturbances occur in 25–40 percent of children with migraine. One recent study found too little sleep (42 percent), bruxism (29 percent), co-sleeping (25 percent), and snoring (23 percent) in a population of 118 children. When children with migraine were compared to matched controls, statistically significant differences where found in sleep duration, daytime sleepiness, night awakenings, sleep anxiety, parasomnias, sleep onset delay, bedtime resistance, and sleep-disordered breathing [Miller et al., 2003]. It remains unclear, however, whether sleep disturbances increase the occurrence of migraine, whether frequent and intense migraine leads to sleep disturbances, or whether the two are unrelated. Current practice is to recommend good sleep hygiene.

Exercise is recommended for patients with frequent migraines, and a review of Internet websites serving headache sufferers reveals the common endorsement of regular physical activity. A recent study to evaluate the effects of exercise on plasma beta-endorphin levels in 40 migraine patients found beneficial effects on all migraine parameters [Koseoglu et al., 2003].

The role of dietary measures has recently been reviewed, yet the subject remains controversial [Millichap and Yee, 2003]. Between 7 and 44 percent of children and adults with migraine report that a particular food or drink can precipitate a migraine attack [Stang et al., 1992; Van den Bergh et al., 1987]. In children, the principal dietary triggers were cheese, chocolate, and citrus fruits. Other purported dietary precipitants included processed meats, yogurt, fried foods, monosodium glutamate, aspartamine, and alcoholic beverages. For chocolate, the median time interval to the onset of headache following ingestion was 22 hours (3.5–27 hours) [Gibb et al., 1991].

None the less, wholesale dietary elimination of a laundry list of foods is not recommended. Once popular, elimination diets are now judged to be excessive, and generally set the stage for a battleground at home when parents attempt to force a restrictive diet upon an unwilling adolescent, ultimately producing heightened tensions. A more reasonable approach is to review the list of foods thought to be linked to migraine and invite the patient to keep a headache diary and see if a temporal relationship exists between ingestion of one or more of those foods and the development of headache. If a link is found, prudence dictates avoidance of the offending food substance.

In addition to looking at what patients eat, it is important to encourage them to take regular meals and to drink plenty of fluids. Many teenagers routinely skip breakfast. Missing meals

is a common precipitant of migraine and is identified by adolescents as one of the leading triggers [Lewis et al., 1996]. A simple lifestyle modification for adolescents with frequent migraine includes eating three meals a day, including breakfast, and to consume plenty of water.

Overuse of "over-the-counter" analgesics has been a particular focus recently. Recognized in adults some years ago, overuse (more than 5 times per week) of acetaminophen, ibuprofen, and, to a lesser extent, aspirin-containing compounds can be a contributing factor to frequent, even daily, headache patterns. When recognized, patients who are overusing analgesics must be educated to discontinue the practice. Retrospective studies have suggested that this recommendation alone can decrease headache frequency [Reimschisel, 2003; Rothner and Guo, 2004].

Caffeine in coffee and sodas warrants special mention. A link between caffeine and migraine has been established [James, 1998; Mannix et al., 1997]. Not only does caffeine itself seem to have an influence on headache; caffeine may disrupt sleep or aggravate mood, both of which may exacerbate headache. Furthermore, caffeine withdrawal headache, which begins 1–2 days following cessation of regular caffeine use, can last up to a week [Dusseldorp and Katan, 1990]. Every effort must be made to moderate caffeine use.

The pharmacologic management of pediatric migraine has been subjected to thorough review but controlled data are, unfortunately, limited (Table 63-2 and Table 63-3) [Lewis et al., 2004; Victor and Ryan, 2003].

Table 63-2 Acute Treatments for Migraine in Children and Adolescents

Agent	Dose
ANALGESICS	
Ibuprofen	7–10 mg/kg/ every 4–6 hours
Acetaminophen	15 mg/kg/ every 4–6 hours
Naproxen sodium	10–15 mg/kg every 8–12 hours
Ketorolac	10–30 mg IV, PO
TRIPTANS	
Nasal Sprays	
Sumatriptan	5–20 mg
Zolmitriptan	5–10 mg
Oral Forms	
Almotriptan*	6.25, 12.5 mg
Eletriptan	20, 40 mg
Frovatriptan	2.5 mg
Naratriptan	1, 2.5 mg
Sumatriptan	25, 50, 100 mg
Rizatriptan	5, 10 mg (tablet and ODT)
Zolmitriptan	5, 10 mg (tablet and ODT)
Injectable (Subcutaneous)	
Sumatriptan	6 mg

* Approved by the Food and Drug Administration for use in adolescents 12–17 years with migraine ≥ 4 hours.
IV, intravenous; ODT, oral disintegrating tablet; PO, by mouth.

Table 63-3 Evidence Summary for Treatment of Acute Attacks of Migraine in Children and Adolescents

Drug	Evidence Classification*	Study Design	n	Ages (Yrs)	Primary Endpoint	Efficacy	Placebo Response	Clinical Impression of Effect
NSAIDS AND NONOPIATE ANALGESICS								
Ibuprofen	II	DBPC	88	4–16	HA response	68%	37%	+++
	II	DBPC	84	6–12	HA response	76%	53%	+++
	II	DBPCCO	32	10–17	HA relief	69%	28%	+++
Acetaminophen	II	DBPC	88	4–16	HA response	54%	37%	++
TRIPTANS (SEROTONIN$_{1B/1D}$ RECEPTOR AGONISTS)								
Nasal Spray								
Sumatriptan	II	OL	58	4–11	HA relief	78%	–	++
	III	DBPC	14	6–10	HA response	86%	43%	+++
	I	DBPC	510	12–17	2-hr HA response	63–66%	53%	+++
Zolmitriptan	I	SB-DBPC	171	12–17	1-hr HA response	58%	43%	+++
Oral Triptans								
Naratriptan	I	DBPC	300	12–17	4-hr HA relief	64–72%	65%	0
Rizatriptan	I	DBPC	296	12–17	2-hr pain relief	66%	56%	++
	I	DBPC	96	6–17	2-hr HA relief	74%	36%	
Sumatriptan	I	DBPC	302	12–17	2-hr pain relief	N/a	N/a	0
	II	DBPCCO	23	8–16	2 hr >50% decrease	34%	21%	0
Zolmitriptan	IV	OL	38	12–17	HA improvement	88%	–	+
	II	DBPCCO	32	11–17	2-hr pain relief	62%	28%	++
	I	DBPC	850	12–17	2 hr-HA response	53–57%	58%	0
Eletriptan	II	DBPC	267	12–17	2-hr HA response	57%	57%	0
Almotriptan	IV	OL	15	11–17	HA reduction	85%	–	+
	I	DBPC	866	12–17	2-hr pain relief	67%	55%	+++
Subcutaneous								
Sumatriptan	IV	OL	17	6–16	HA response	64%	–	+
Subcutaneous	IV	OL	50	6–18	HA response	78%	–	+

DBPC, double-blind placebo-controlled; DBPCCO, double blind, placebo controlled, cross over; HA, headache; NS, not significant; OL, open label; SB, single blind
Clinical impression of effect:
  0, Ineffective: Most patients get no improvement.
  +, Somewhat effective: Few patients get clinically significant improvement.
  ++, Effective: Some patients get clinically significant improvement.
  +++, Very effective: Most patients get clinically significant improvement.
(Adapted from Lewis D. Pediatric migraine. Neurol Clin 2009 May;27[2]:481–501.)

For the acute treatment of migraine, the most rigorously studied agents are ibuprofen, acetaminophen, and the "triptans" (almotriptan and rizatriptan tablets, sumatriptan and zolmitriptan nasal sprays), all of which have shown safety and efficacy in controlled trials. Almotriptan is the only triptan approved by the Food and Drug Administration (FDA) for use in adolescents. No triptan is approved for children under age 12. For children less than 12 years of age, ibuprofen (7.5–10 mg/kg) and acetaminophen (15 mg/kg) have demonstrated efficacy and safety in the acute treatment of migraine [Hamalainen et al., 1997; Lewis et al., 2002]. Almotriptan demonstrated statistically significant efficacy over placebo in adolescents aged 12–17 (n = 866), with 2-hour headache relief of 73 percent in the 12.5 mg almotriptan tablet group and 52 percent in the placebo group (p <0.01) [Linder et al., 2008]. Zolmitriptan (5 mg) and sumatriptan (5 and 20 mg) in the nasal spray form and rizatriptan (5 and 10 mg) have demonstrated both safety and efficacy in controlled trials in adolescents, but have not yet received FDA approval [Lewis et al.,

2007; Winner et al., 2000; Ahonen et al., 2004, 2006; Ueberall, 2001]. Butalbital preparations are no longer recommended.

For preventative treatment in the population of children and adolescents with frequent, disabling migraine, topiramate and flunarizine (not available in the U.S.) have demonstrated efficacy in controlled trials (Table 63-4 and Table 63-5). In a recent controlled, blinded trial, topiramate (100 mg/day) resulted in a statistically significant reduction in the monthly migraine attack rate from baseline versus placebo (72.2 versus 44.4 percent). Furthermore, a 50 percent reduction in monthly migraine day rate from baseline versus placebo favored topiramate at 100 mg/day (83 versus 45 percent) [Lewis et al., 2009].

Typically, for teenagers, a dose of 15–25 mg of topiramate is initiated as a single bedtime dose (15–25 mg), and then gradually titrated toward 50 mg twice a day incrementally on a weekly or every other week basis. Clinical experience has demonstrated that many patients will respond to doses as low as 25 mg at bedtime, so it is valuable to "titrate to effect."

Table 63-4 Preventative Agents for Treatment of Migraine in Children and Adolescents

Agent	Dose
ANTIDEPRESSANT AGENTS	
Amitriptyline	5–25 mg at bedtime
ANTIEPILEPTIC AGENTS	
Topiramate	15–25 mg hs titrate, up to 50 mg twice daily
Valproic acid	250–500 mg orally twice daily 500–1000 mg ER preparation at bedtime
NONSTEROIDAL ANTI-INFLAMMATORY AGENTS	
Naproxen	250–500 mg orally twice daily (maximum 6 weeks)
ANTIHYPERTENSIVE AGENTS	
Propranolol	60–120 mg orally once a day
ANTIHISTAMINES	
Cyproheptadine	2–8 mg orally divided tid, bid, or twice or three times daily

ER, extended-release; hs, at bedtime.

Cognitive effects must be monitored quite carefully and more evidence is needed to assess the educational impact of topiramate for prevention of adolescent migraine. It is counterproductive to reduce the headache burden at the expense of academic performance.

Uncontrolled data are emerging regarding antiepileptic agents, such as disodium valproate and levetiracetam, as well as the antihistamine cyproheptadine and the antidepressant amitriptyline [Serdaroglu et al., 2002; Miller, 2004; Lewis et al., 2004].

Other Primary Headache Syndromes

Chronic Daily Headache

CDH is formally defined as spanning a period of more than 4 months, during which the patient has more than 15 headaches per month, with the headaches lasting more than 4 hours per day. Many adolescents will report having headaches virtually every single day, sometimes during every waking hour. This chronic, nonprogressive, unremitting, daily or near-daily pattern of headache represents one of the most difficult subsets of headache. The estimated prevalence of CDH in adolescents is about 1–2 percent, and may be as high as 4 percent in the adult population [Abu-Arefeh and Russell, 1994; Lipton and Stewart, 1997; Castillo et al., 1999]. CDH is very common in referral headache centers, where up to 15–20 percent of patients will present with daily or near-daily head pain [Viswanathan et al., 1998].

Understandably, the quality of life of patients with CDH is significantly impaired. The negative impact extends beyond the affected patient to their family, friends, and society as a whole. The extensive disability that results from CDH can be measured in school absences, abstinence from after-school activities, and the family discord that invariably results. Therefore, early diagnosis and management of frequent or chronic daily headaches are essential.

Four primary chronic headache categories have been identified:
1. chronic migraine
2. chronic tension-type
3. new daily persistent headache
4. hemicranium continuum.

Chronic migraine is the most common form of CDH in adolescents, and evolves slowly from an episodic migraine pattern to daily migraine. Similarly, chronic tension-type headaches evolve from episodic tension-type headaches. Quite frequently, there is a mixed pattern, with daily background tension-type headache and interspersed episodes of more typical migraine, but rarely a moment of headache freedom.

The new daily persistent headaches appear to represent a unique entity, in which the daily headache pattern starts quite abruptly, de novo, without any history of previous headache syndrome. Uncommon in children, hemicrania continua represents a cluster variant with daily or continuous unilateral pain and conjunctival injection, lacrimation, rhinorrhea, and, occasionally, ptosis. One of the key features of hemicrania continua is remarkable and prompt responsiveness to indomethacin (25–50 mg orally twice a day).

Each of these four types of CDH is further separated into those with or without superimposed analgesic overuse (>5 doses/week of over-the-counter analgesics). The medications implicated in this analgesic overuse syndrome include most over-the-counter analgesics (e.g., acetaminophen, aspirin, ibuprofen), opioids, butalbital, isometheptene, benzodiazepines, ergotamine, and triptans [Mathew et al., 1990].

Secondary causes of the CDH pattern in children and adolescents include neoplasm, idiopathic intracranial hypertension (pseudotumor cerebri), hydrocephalus, chronic subdural hematomas, chronic sinusitis, glaucoma, malocclusion, and temporomandibular dysfunction, as well as psychological conditions. The "medicolegal headache" will fall into this category, as pending litigation tends to exacerbate stress levels and contribute to prolongation of the headache syndrome. Since the patient and family who present with the complaint of CDH are understandably concerned about the possibility of organic causes, it is critical to consider and exclude possible secondary causes for their headache. No treatment regimen will be successful until clear and confident reassurances as to the absence of serious underlying disease are provided. Parental skepticism can compound the clinical problem immeasurably.

Breaking the cycle of CDH is the principle goal of management. Pharmacologic efforts used in isolation, however, will be uniformly unsuccessful. Therefore, initiation of a multidisciplined approach, with emphasis upon preventive strategies, takes precedence over the use of intermittent analgesics. This population of patients has already likely been overusing over-the-counter analgesic agents, so a fundamental change in treatment philosophy must be taught to the patient and family.

An integral part of the educational process will be the incorporation of wholesale lifestyle changes, such as regulation of sleep and eating habits, regular exercise, identification of triggering factors, stress management biofeedback-assisted

Table 63-5 Summary of Evidence for Preventative Therapies for Migraine in Children and Adolescents

Drug	Class*	Study Design	n	Ages (Yrs)	Primary Endpoint	Efficacy	Placebo Response	Clinical Impression of Effect
ANTIEPILEPTICS								
Divalproex sodium/ sodium valproate	IV	OL	42	7–16	HA/m	81%	–	+
	IV	OL	10	9–17	HA/m	83%	–	+
	IV	OL	23	7–17	HA/m	65% >50% reduction	–	+
Gabapentin	IV	Retrospective OL	18	6–17	HA freq/m	83% >50% reduction	–	++
Topiramate	II	DBPC	44	9–17	HA/m	75%	38%	++
	I	DBPC	51	12–17	HA/m	54–67%	42%	+++
	I	DBPC	85	12–17	HA/m	76%	45%	+++
Levetiracetam	IV	OL	20	6–17	HA/m	90%	–	+
	IV	OL	19	Mean 12	HA/m	67%	–	+
Zonisamide	IV	OL	12	Mean 13	HA/m	75%	–	+
ANTIDEPRESSANTS								
Trazodone	II	DBPC	35	7–18	HA freq	45%	40%	O
Pizotifen	II	DBPCCO	47	7–14	HA/m	15%	16%	O
TRICYCLIC ANTIDEPRESSANTS								
Amitriptyline	IV	OL	192	9–15	HA freq/m	84%	–	++
	IV	OL	73	3–18	HA freq/m	89%	–	++
ANTIHISTAMINES								
Cyproheptadine	II	DBPC	68†	17–53	% improve	75%	–	++
	IV	Retrospective	30	3–18	HA/m	62%	–	++
CALCIUM CHANNEL BLOCKERS								
Flunarizine	II	DBPC	42	7–14	>50% improve	76%	19%	+++
	II	DBPCCO	63	5–11	HA/m	67%	33%	+++
Nimodipine	II	DBPCCO	37	7–18	HA/m	15%	16%	O
ANTIHYPERTENSIVE AGENTS								
Propranolol	II	DBPC	39	3–12	HA freq	58%	55%	O
	II	DBCO	28	7–16	HA freq	71%	10%	++
	II	DBPC	28	6–12	HA freq	NS	NS	O
Timolol	II	DBPCCO	19	6–13	HA/m	38%	40%	O
Clonidine	II	DBPC	43	7–14	HA/6 wks	NS	NS	O
	II	DBPC	54	<15	HA/m	40%	65%	O
NONSTEROIDAL ANTI-INFLAMMATORY DRUGS								
Naproxen sodium	III	DBPC	10	6–17	HA freq	60%	40%	+

† Includes patients >18 years of age.
DBPC, double-blind placebo-controlled; DBPCCO, double blind, placebo controlled, cross over; HA, headache; NS, not significant; OL, open label
(Adapted from Lewis D. Pediatric migraine. Neurol Clin. 2009 May;27[2]:481–501.)

relaxation therapy and biobehavioral programs, and psychological or psychiatric intervention (see Box 63-9) [Rothrock, 1999].

The genesis and persistence of the CDH pattern may have its roots in psychosocial factors. Therefore, a thorough social and educational history must then be obtained. Exploring issues relating to life at school (e.g., bullying, learning disabilities), family conflict (parental discord or impending divorce), grief and loss (grandparent's illness, break-up of personal relationship), drug and alcohol use, and other factors in the teenager's world will help the practitioner, the patient, and the family understand some of the obstacles that may complicate management.

For the CDH population, a group of lifestyle changes must be incorporated into the treatment plan. This essentially constitutes maintenance of a healthy lifestyle, and includes five major components:

1. return to the routine of adolescent "life"; return to school
2. adequate and regular sleep

3. regular exercise (20–30 minutes per day of aerobic exercise)
4. balanced nutrition, including avoidance of skipping meals
5. adequate fluid intake with avoidance of caffeine.

The pharmacologic treatment of CDH requires an individually tailored regimen with the judicious use of appropriate prophylactic and analgesic agents. Recognizing the degree of disability will help guide the aggressiveness of the management. Unfortunately, no controlled studies have explored the pharmacologic management of CDH in children.

For the population of children and adolescents with CDH, preventative therapy takes center-stage and represents the mainstay of drug treatment (see Tables 63-3 and 63-4). Since the majority of children with CDH has chronic migraine or prominent migrainous features, a modification of standard migraine therapy is appropriate, but emphasis must be placed on prevention measures rather than analgesic or abortive strategies. The one exception may be the patients with a recent onset of CDH attributed almost exclusively to analgesic rebound. In this infrequent group, a trial of an analgesic-free period, as noted above, may be the sole successful treatment.

Preventative therapies used for CDH include tricyclic antidepressants, antiepileptic agents, beta-blockers, serotonergic agents, calcium channel blockers, and other miscellaneous treatments; however, none of these medications has been subjected to controlled trials and none is currently approved for the prevention of headaches in children [Redillas and Solomons, 2000].

When making the clinical decision regarding choice of pharmacologic agents, it is important to consider comorbid conditions. For the patient with difficulty falling asleep, amitriptyline at bedtime may provide dual benefits. Similarly, if there are mild to moderate affective issues, amitriptyline, valproic acid, or one of the selective serotonin reuptake inhibitors (SSRIs) may be beneficial. It there is comorbid obesity, topiramate may decrease the appetite. Alternatively, if the patient's appetite is low, valproate often stimulates the appetite.

Antidepressants

The tricyclic antidepressant, amitriptyline, has been widely used for the prevention of migraine headaches. The mechanism of action is unclear, but is thought to be due to a multiple re-uptake inhibitor action. The agents are well tolerated in children and adolescents; side effects are attributable to their anticholinergic effects, and there are additional concerns about cardiac arrhythmias. The most frequently cited side effects include sedation. In order to minimize side effects, a slow taper, starting at 0.25 mg/kg (5–10 mg) and increasing by 5–10 mg every 2–3 weeks until a dose of 1.0 mg/kg (10–25 mg) is reached, results in well-tolerated, effective management [Hershey et al., 2000].

SSRIs have not been studied for CDH, but may have a role in those patients with comorbid depression.

Antiepileptic Drugs

Several antiepileptic drugs have been shown to be effective in preventing adult migraine; however, very limited evidence is available in children. Topiramate has demonstrated efficacy in preventing adult and adolescent migraine [Brandes et al., 2004]. A significant reduction in headache frequency was demonstrated at doses of 50–100 mg b.i.d. Adverse events resulting

in discontinuation in the topiramate groups included cognitive blunting, paresthesias, fatigue, and nausea. One retrospective study assessing the efficacy of topiramate for pediatric headache included 41 evaluable patients. Topiramate at daily doses of 1.4 ($\pm$ 0.74) mg/kg/day was used, and headache frequency was reduced from 16.5 ($\pm$ 10) headaches/month to 11.6 ($\pm$ 10) headaches/month (p < 0.001). Mean headache severity, duration, and accompanying disability were also reduced. Side effects included cognitive changes (12.5 percent), weight loss (5.6 percent), and sensory symptoms (2.8 percent) [Hershey et al., 2002]. This study population consisted predominantly of children with very frequent migraine headaches approaching the spectrum of CDH, as defined by $\geq$15 headaches per month. The most common side effects observed included paresthesias, weight loss, and cognitive problems. The cognitive problems appear to decline with use, and can be minimized by very slow tapering and starting at a very low dose. This starting dose may be as low as 12.5 mg/day, and this may be slowly increased by 12.5–25 mg every 2 weeks to a dose of 50 mg. b.i.d. [Hershey et al., 2002]. The weight loss needs to be monitored, although, for the majority, it does not appear to be significant.

Sodium valproate has been shown to be effective and is approved for the prevention of migraines in adults [Mathew et al., 1995]. It has also been shown to be effective for CDH and is available in an extended-release formulation [Freitag et al., 2001, 2002]. A small study of 42 patients demonstrated that it was effective and well tolerated in 7–16-year-olds [Caruso et al., 2000]. Two of the side effects that may limit its use in adolescents include weight gain and the development of ovarian cysts.

Gabapentin has also been used for prevention of adult headaches. It appears to be well tolerated; however, its effectiveness in children and adolescents is unknown [Mathew et al., 2001].

Antihistamines

The antihistamine cyproheptadine has been widely used for the prevention of migraine headaches in young children, but it has not been studied in CDH [Bille et al., 1977]. It tends to be very well tolerated; its most significant side effects are sedation and weight gain, which specifically limits its tolerability in adolescents.

Beta-Blockers

Both propranolol and atenolol have been approved for the prevention of migraines in adults. There are conflicting data regarding the efficacy of propranolol for migraine in children, and no data regarding its use in CDH. The exact dosing parameters also have not been identified. Two of its more common side effects, of concern for children, are exacerbation of reactive airway disease and depression. This reactive airway disease may be of special concern for the athletic adolescent, who is unaware of it until the combination of exercise and a beta-blocker results in shortness of breath.

Nonsteroidal Anti-Inflammatory Agents

Naproxen sodium was shown to be effective in adolescent migraine in one small (n = 10) trial using a double-blind, placebo-controlled, crossover design [Lewis et al., 1994]. Sixty percent of the patients experienced a greater than 60 percent reduction in headache frequency and severity with naproxen

250 mg twice a day, whereas only 40 percent responded favorably to placebo. No adverse effects were noted in this study. Naproxen should not be used for longer than 8 weeks because of potential gastrointestinal toxicity.

Naproxen is often used in conjunction with amitriptyline or topiramate. Patients are begun on a schedule of 250–500 mg twice a day, and at the same time an evening dose of 5–25 mg of amitriptyline is started. After about 4–6 weeks, the naproxen is discontinued and the amitriptyline continued. Alternatively, naproxen is begun and topiramate titrated upward by 25 mg/week to a target dose of 50–100 mg twice a day. Naproxen is then discontinued after 6–8 weeks and topiramate continued.

Botulinum toxin type A (Botox) by injection has been found to be effective in the treatment of headache disorders in adults. A recent study reported treatment of 12 adolescents (14–18 years) who had Botox injections for migraine and CDH. Six patients (all female) were in long-term treatment and received Botox every 3 months. Effectiveness was evaluated using pain scales and a standardized quality of life survey at baseline and prior to each treatment session. Each patient had 9–63 (average = 42) injections per treatment. All six long-term patients reported improvement in headache symptoms, with decreases on pain scales and an average of 33–75 percent improvement in quality of life. Two long-term patients had complete relief of headaches between injection series. Four patients had only one series of injections with "good results." Two patients had no improvement and refused additional injections. Side effects were mild ptosis (n = 1), blurred vision (n = 1), and a hematoma at injection site with tingling in one arm lasting 24 hours (n = 1). These results warrant a controlled trial evaluation of Botox since it may be an effective option for certain adolescents with intractable migraine and CDH [Chan et al., 2009].

Analgesic Agents in Chronic Daily Headache

The use of analgesic agents for children and adolescents with CDH is controversial, particularly in view of a growing body of literature regarding analgesic overuse in children. Since the children describe continuous or near-continuous pain, it is often difficult to decide when and how to use analgesics in order to avoid the "slippery slope" of analgesic overuse. One approach is to map or make a graph of the pattern of headaches to identify the epochs of intense migraine pain and when it arises from the background daily pain, at which time analgesics, including the "triptan agents," may be most useful. Patients with CDH are often able to report that they may have headache every waking hour, but twice a week they have an intense headache that likely represents the migraine component. Once this is teased out of the history, analgesics can be more rationally employed. Analgesic overuse may be one of the leading precipitants of the phenomenon of CDH, so care must be taken not to kindle the flames further with overuse. The keys for effective use include catching the migraine component of the headache as soon as it starts, using an adequate dose, and avoiding overuse.

Nonpharmacologic Measures for CDH

A variety of vitamins (e.g., riboflavin 400 mg/day), minerals (e.g., magnesium 400 mg/day), and herbal remedies (e.g. butterbur, feverfew) have been attempted for prevention of headaches. Unfortunately, none of these remedies has been thoroughly evaluated in children with CDH, but may play a role, particularly in families where traditional pharmacologic approaches are considered unacceptable (see Box 63-9).

Biofeedback-assisted relaxation training has been shown to be an effective treatment for aborting and preventing recurrent headaches in a large number of studies in children. This technique is typically taught over a multisession analysis. It is also effective in a single session with tape provided for home practicing [Powers et al., 2001]. It does require a degree of motivation in the child, and it is difficult to assess effectiveness in isolation. However, it has low side-effect potential and may provide a benefit, including moderation of stress and sleep-onset difficulties.

Psychological or psychiatric interventions are quite valuable if emotional comorbidity has been demonstrated [Juant et al., 2000]. In addition, if "stress" has been implicated as a possible migraine trigger, psychological or psychiatric intervention, stress management, or self-hypnosis may be beneficial for CDH treatment and management. For many adolescents with CDH, cognitive behavioral therapies take center-stage in management.

Other avenues to consider in management of this difficult subset of patients include acupuncture, chiropractic manipulation, and aromatherapy. It is imperative to be able to discuss complementary and alternative measures comfortably with patients and families dealing with CDH, since oftentimes the patient has already tried multiple therapeutic regimens without success. We must be prepared to consider the spectrum of complementary and alternative measures when attempting to help this refractory group of adolescents.

The outcome of adolescents with CDH is poorly understood. No long-term follow-up data exist. One abstracted report provides short-term follow-up on 24 adolescents (peak age 13 years) with CDH, of whom more than half experienced a greater than 75 percent reduction in headache frequency and one-third a greater than 90 percent improvement in a 6-month follow-up. A wide variety of preventative agents was employed, but amitriptyline and topiramate provided the largest proportion of successful outcomes.

Tension-Type Headache

Tension-type headache (TTH) may be episodic or chronic, the differentiation being a lower frequency (fewer than 15 days/month) in episodic TTH and greater frequency (≥15 days/month) in chronic TTH. Episodic TTH may be the most prevalent type of all primary headaches, but infrequently prompts referral to subspecialty clinics. Pathophysiologically, tension-type and migraine headaches may be similar, and there is a growing appreciation that the two may fall within a spectrum, with milder, less disabling headaches being classed as tension-type, and more severe patterns being classed as migraine. The diagnostic criteria for TTH (Box 63-4) emphasize the distinction from migraine. Generally, nausea and vomiting are not present in TTH; either photophobia or phonophobia may be present, but not both. On occasion, associated symptoms, such as tiredness, sleep disturbances, and lightheadedness, may occur with episodic TTH.

The management of TTH has not been rigorously studied, but simple over-the-counter analgesics are commonly used. Various agents, such as acetaminophen (15 mg/kg), ibuprofen (7–10 mg/kg), or naproxen (7–10 mg/kg), may be very helpful;

however, overuse of these medications (5 doses/week) is a major concern. Chronic TTH is often associated with a significant degree of stress and anxiety for the child and family, given the frequent, unrelenting nature of this type of headache (see CDH above).

Cranial Neuralgias

Ophthalmoplegic Migraine

Once classified as migraine, ophthalmoplegic migraine (OM) is now viewed as a cranial neuralgia, but oddly still called "migraine." This is one of the most dramatic and clinically challenging headache syndromes and, fortunately, one of the least common. Available epidemiological data suggest an annual incidence of 0.7 per million [Hansen et al., 1990]. The two key features are ophthalmoparesis and headache, though the headache may be mild or a nondescript retro-orbital discomfort. Ptosis, adduction defects, and skew deviations are the common objective findings.

The clinical course of OM is quite different from that of the more commonly encountered migraine with aura. Symptoms and signs of oculomotor dysfunction may not appear until well into the headache phase, rather than preceding the headache. The signs may persist for days or even weeks *after* the headache has resolved.

The oculomotor nerve, or its divisions, is most frequently involved, but pupillary involvement is inconsistent, with some authors reporting pupillary involvement in only one-third of patients [Vijayan, 1980]. The oculomotor nerve involvement may be incomplete, with partial deficits in both inferior and superior divisions of the third nerve. Abduction defects, due to abducens nerve involvement, constitute the second most frequently reported variant of OM, while trochlear nerve involvement is the least common.

The mechanism of OM is controversial. The primary theories suggest ischemic, compressive, or inflammatory processes [Stommel et al., 1994]. Lack of pupillary involvement argues for an ischemic mechanism, whereas a higher incidence of pupillary involvement weighs toward a compressive mechanism. Alternatively, recent reports have questioned whether OM may be an inflammatory process within the spectrum of Tolosa–Hunt syndrome, particularly given the steroid-responsiveness of many patients. Furthermore, high-resolution neuroimaging has shown a reversible enhancement of the oculomotor nerve during attacks, which lends further credence to an inflammatory/demyelinating mechanism, validating the ICHD-2 classification as a cranial neuropathy [Mark et al., 1998].

The differential diagnosis for OM includes aneurysm or mass lesion in or around the orbital apex and parasellar region. Imaging study with MRI or MRA is usually indicated.

Repeated attacks of OM can lead to permanent deficits; therefore, acute treatment with steroids and prophylactic treatment must be considered.

Occipital neuralgia is characterized by a stabbing pain in the upper neck or occipital region, often precipitated by neck flexion or head rotation. It may occur post-traumatically. Examination of the craniocervical region may disclose point tenderness, C2 distribution sensory changes, or limitation of motion. MRI of the craniocervical junction is warranted to exclude congenital or pathological processes. Treatments include soft collars, nonsteroidal anti-inflammatory drugs (naproxen), muscle relaxants, local injections, and physical therapy. The prognosis is actually good.

A similar entity is neck-tongue syndrome, wherein head movements trigger occipital pain, accompanied by ipsilateral tongue numbness. Again, craniocervical anomalies must be sought, though the majority of children and adolescents have not demonstrable abnormalities. The syndrome occasionally occurs in families.

Cluster Headache

The trigeminal autonomic cephalalgias (TACs) represent a group of primary headache disorders associated with excruciating head pain, accompanied by autonomic features such as lacrimation, ptosis, rhinorrhea, and vasomotor changes. Cluster headache is an uncommon TAC in children and adolescents. The prevalence of childhood onset of cluster headache is approximately 0.1 percent [Lampl, 2002]. The diagnostic criteria require at least five attacks of severe unilateral orbital pain lasting 15–180 minutes, with a sense of restless agitation accompanied by ipsilateral conjunctival injection, lacrimation, nasal congestion, rhinorrhea, eyelid edema, forehead sweating, miosis, or ptosis. Cluster headaches may be episodic or chronic, and attacks occur in series that last for weeks or even months. A cluster may be precipitated by alcohol, histamine, or nitroglycerine. Males are three times more likely to be affected than females.

The management is difficult. Acute treatments include inhalation of 100 percent oxygen at 8–10 L/min for 10–15 minutes through a non-rebreathing facemask; sumatriptan 6 mg subcutaneous injections or 20 mg intranasally, zolmitriptan nasal spray 5–10 mg; and intravenous, intramuscular, or subcutaneous injections of dihydroergotamine, 0.5–1.0 mg, at headache onset. Prophylactic medications useful in preventing attacks during cluster cycles include verapamil, sodium valproate, topiramate, melatonin, lithium carbonate, methysergide, and ergotamine tartrate [Newman et al., 2001; Rosen, 2009].

Paroxysmal Hemicrania

This TAC is characterized by intense attacks of periorbital pain lasting only 5–30 minutes; these can occur as many as dozens of times per day. In distinction to cluster headaches, the attacks are generally brief and can occur multiple times in succession. Like cluster headaches, there may be accompanying autonomic symptoms (lacrimation, rhinorrhea). The most striking feature is the exquisite responsiveness to indomethacin (25–50 mg/day), which has prompted the alternative nosology, "indomethacin-sensitive" headache. When evaluating a child with brief intense attacks of pain in and around the face or orbit, it is reasonable to consider a trial of oral indomethacin as a diagnostic challenge.

Temporomandibular Joint Dysfunction

Temporomandibular joint dysfunction presents with unilateral pain just anterior or inferior to the ear. The pain is aggravated by chewing, teeth clenching, or yawning. The patients may describe a clicking or locking of their jaw. Family members may describe bruxism and there may be antecedent trauma. Examination reveals tenderness over the temporomandibular joint and limitation of mouth opening. Treatment includes nonsteroidal anti-inflammatory drugs, muscle relaxation, and avoidance of provocative processes like chewing of gum or hard candy. Major oral surgery is rarely necessary.

Specific Secondary Headache Syndromes

Post-Traumatic Headache

Headache following closed head injury or neck trauma in children is one of the most common secondary headache syndromes, but has not been systematically studied. No epidemiological data are available. Post-traumatic headache is divided into acute and chronic, patterns based upon duration of symptoms, less than 3 months being acute and more than 3 months being chronic.

Acute post-traumatic headache must immediately raise concerns for traumatic brain injury, such as cerebral hematoma (subdural or epidural), subarachnoid hemorrhage, cerebral contusion, or skull fracture, and warrants urgent neuroimaging, particularly if associated with alteration of consciousness, seizures, or Glasgow Coma Scale <13. If post-traumatic headache is suspected, emergent noncontrast computed tomography (CT) of the head and cervical spine x-rays are warranted. If focal neurologic symptoms or signs are present, then evaluation for vascular injury (i.e., carotid dissection) may be indicated and detection may require specific MRI sequences (MRA). CSF leaks following meningeal tears can lead to positional, or "low-pressure," headaches.

Post-traumatic headache is defined as headache that begins within 2 weeks of closed head injury. It is, furthermore, divided into acute post-traumatic headache if the symptoms have been present for less than 3 months, and chronic if symptoms have been present for more than 3 months.

Trauma-triggered migraine can be initiated by mild head injury. The key features are aura (e.g., visual, cognitive, motor, or sensory), duration of 1–72 hours, frontal or unilateral location, moderate to severe pain, aggravation by routine activities, nausea and/or vomiting, and photophobia and phonophobia. A particular subset of post-traumatic migraine is termed "confusional" or "footballer's migraine," wherein mild head injury triggers an acute confusional state, often with agitation, and accompanied by a headache with migraine features.

Chronic post-traumatic headache may be part of a global postconcussive syndrome, with behavioral changes (e.g., hyperactivity, hypoactivity), dizziness, tinnitus, vertigo, blurred vision, memory changes, sleep disorder, irritability, and attentional disorders. The duration of symptoms is variable, with some patients having brief, self-limited syndromes, and others suffering from headaches for more than 6–12 months. One retrospective study of 23 children with chronic post-traumatic headache found a mean duration of 13.3 months (range 2–60 months, median 7 months) [Callaghan, 2001]. The headache forms span the spectrum from tension-type, migraine, CDH, neuralgias (e.g., occipital neuralgia), temporomandibular joint dysfunction, and, even, on rare occasions, cluster headache.

A recent prospective study of 117 children (81 males, 36 females; range 3–15 years [mean age 8.5 yrs]) admitted with closed head injury (minor 79 percent, major 21 percent) found that 8 (7 percent) children (5 males, 3 females; mean age 10.5 yrs) reported chronic post-traumatic headache. Five (4 percent) children had episodic tension-type headache and

3 (2.5 percent) had migraine with or without aura. Headache resolved over 3–27 months in all patients [Kirk et al., 2008].

Many athletes competing in contact sports experience post-traumatic headache as part of a postconcussion syndrome. A common question concerns when it is safe to return to full contact. Three organizations – the AAN, the American College of Sports Medicine, and the British Association of Sport and Exercise Medicine – have provided guidelines regarding return to activities, which range from 1 to 4 weeks [Quality Standards Subcommittee, 1997; American College of Sports Medicine, 1991; McCrory et al., 2009]. These guidelines are available online. See http://aappolicy.aapublications.org/cgi/content/full/pediatrics and http://www.acsm.org.

The management of post-traumatic headache requires an appreciation of the degree of disability produced by the headache. Post-traumatic tension-type headaches can generally be managed with nonsteroidal anti-inflammatory agents, such as ibuprofen or naproxen sodium. Post-traumatic migraine is treated as discussed earlier, with a balance of analgesic or "triptan" agents and, if warranted, daily preventative therapies. For patients with frequent or daily headaches, the management strategies discussed in the CDH section apply, with daily preventative programs, both pharmacologic and nonpharmacologic, as well as analgesics for episodes of intense pain.

There are no outcome data on post-traumatic headache in children and adolescents, but typically, 3–6 months is the anticipated course of recovery. Pending litigation may exacerbate stress levels and contribute to prolongation of the headache syndrome.

Idiopathic Intracranial Hypertension

Also known as pseudotumor cerebri, idiopathic intracranial hypertension (IIH) produces a global, daily, pounding headache (approximately 94 percent) and is an important consideration in the differential diagnosis of CDH. The incidence of IIH is 3.5–19 per 100,000, with a majority of patients being female. Neck stiffness (30–59 percent) and transient visual disturbances may be present. The key finding on physical examination is papilledema. Neuroimaging will likely be normal. The pathogenesis of IIH is unclear but somehow involves impairment of CSF reabsorption. IIH can be caused by multiple disorders, including endocrinopathies (e.g., hypothyroidism, Addison's disease, oral steroids), pregnancy, drugs (e.g., tetracycline, oral contraceptive agents), vitamin A intoxication, anemia, systemic lupus erythematosus, chronic sinopulmonary infection, and obesity, or may be idiopathic.

Other secondary headaches that present with CDH include intoxications (lead or other heavy metals), chronic carbon monoxide poisoning, chronic meningitis with such pathogens as tuberculosis, fungi, or spirochetal syphilis, or Lyme disease. A chronic daily pattern can also be seen, with central nervous system leukemia/lymphoma or leptomeningeal metastasis. Rarely, diffuse "butterfly" gliomatosis of the brain can produce this picture, but cognitive decline and pyramidal tract signs would be expected. Uncontrolled hypertension can lead to optic disc changes with headache, but this would be uncommon during adolescents. Chronic sinusitis or venous sinus thrombosis can also produce a pattern of slowly increasing intracranial pressure with normal CT scan.

The diagnostic criteria for IIH in the prepubertal child include normal mental status; symptoms and signs of generalized intracranial hypertension (e.g., papilledema); documented elevated intracranial pressure measured in the lateral decubitus position (<8 years, 180 mm H_2O; ≥ 8 years, 250 mm H_2O); normal CSF composition; absence of evidence of hydrocephalus; mass, structural, or vascular lesion on neuroimaging (narrowing of the transverse sinuses is allowed); and no other identified cause of intracranial hypertension [Rangwala and Liu, 2007]. The diagnostic test of choice for IIH is lumbar puncture, with measurement of opening pressure. Given a normal CT scan, the test can be accomplished safely, even though the examination shows a sixth nerve palsy, since this can be a "false localizing" sign, indicative of diffuse increase in intracranial pressure.

For adolescents, the normal CSF opening pressure is <180 mm H_2O. Patients with IIH may have CSF opening pressure exceeding 200 mm H_2O, and often 400 mm H_2O. CSF must be collected for glucose, protein, cell counts, and cultures (bacterial, fungal, tuberculosis), but special studies, such as cryptococcal antigen, Venereal Diseases Research Laboratory test (VDRL), neuroborreliosis, and CSF cytopathology, may be an option.

The lumbar puncture not only provides critical diagnostic information, but also the relief of pressure usually provides significant decrease in headache symptoms. The volume of CSF to be removed is controversial. Generally, removal of sufficient volume to lower the pressure down to about 200 mm H_2O is valid and safe. Care must be taken to limit the risk of "post-lumbar puncture" headache by keeping the patient recumbent for several hours following the procedure.

Once the diagnosis of IIH is established, the carbonic anhydrase inhibitor, acetazolamide, can be used to lower CSF pressures, probably by a diuretic mechanism. The side effects are few but include paresthesias, polyuria, and sedation. The dose is typically 250 mg twice a day up to 1000 mg per day. There is a once-daily preparation available. The recovery is slow, over weeks or months. If obesity is a contributing factor, a weight loss program is strongly recommended, though difficult to institute. If the visual symptoms are severe or progressive, or if there is visual compromise, ophthalmologic intervention may be necessary, with performance of an optic nerve sheath fenestration.

Intracranial Hypotension

Low-pressure headache may occur following lumbar puncture or other processes that cause a tear in the dura mater, including penetrating trauma or cranial surgery. The cardinal clinical feature is orthostatic or positional headache, in which a severe, pounding, nauseating headache occurs immediately upon standing or sitting up from a reclined position. Importantly, the symptoms resolve when the patient lies back down. Specific ICHD-2 diagnostic criteria include neck stiffness, tinnitus, hyperacusia, and photophobia. The CSF opening pressure will be approximately 60 mm H_2O in the sitting position.

While the majority of post-spinal tap headaches resolve spontaneously, persistence of disabling symptoms may necessitate consideration of a "blood patch" or other technique to repair the source of the CSF leak; this may take 72 hours to be effective.

Brain Tumor Headache

About two-thirds of children with brain tumors will have headache as a presenting symptom. There is, however, no invariable "brain tumor headache" profile. A steady, gradual rise in intracranial pressure typically produces the chronic progressive pattern, but, on occasion, an anaplastic tumor or hemorrhage into tumor may cause an acute pattern (see Figure 63-1). Several historic clues suggest space-occupying lesions, such as brain tumors, but may also be present in other expanding masses, such as brain abscess, hematoma, or vascular anomaly. Morning headache or headaches that awaken the child from sleep are classic symptoms of the dependent edema of intracranial lesions. Likewise, nocturnal or morning emesis, with or without headache, suggests increased intracranial pressure and is a particularly common symptom of tumors arising near the floor of the fourth ventricle. Head pain aggravated by exertion or the Valsalva maneuver suggests a mass lesion. In addition to headache, parents may note behavioral or mood changes, cognitive changes, or declining school performance.

Accompanying symptoms may suggest localized disturbances of neurologic function. Ocular symptoms are common: loss of vision (e.g., craniopharyngioma, optic pathway tumor) or diplopia (e.g., brainstem glioma, medulloblastoma). Disorders of coordination, such as truncal ataxia (e.g., medulloblastoma, ependymoma) or dysmetria (e.g., cerebellar astrocytoma), suggest posterior fossa tumors. The presence of seizures indicates cortical disturbances, often localized to the temporal lobes.

The key physical examination signs that indicate brain tumor include:

- papilledema
- abnormal eye movements
- hemiparesis
- ataxia (truncal or appendicular)
- abnormal tendon reflexes [The Childhood Brain Tumor Consortium, 1991].

As stated in the AAN Practice Parameter, neuroimaging (MRI or CT) is therefore appropriate for children with headache in whom there are historical features to suggest the recent onset of severe headache, a change in the type of headache, or focal neurologic dysfunction. Neuroimaging should also be considered in children with an abnormal neurologic examination (e.g., focal findings, signs of increased intracranial pressure, significant alteration of consciousness) and/or the coexistence of seizures.

Chiari Malformation

Chiari malformations (type I) are, arguably, among the most common incidental findings when performing MRI in children with headache, and are the source of great controversy. Tonsillar ectopia of 5 mm or less is *not* considered pathological. When symptomatic, children with Chiari I malformation may complain of occipital headache, neck pain or stiffness, arm weakness, and gait abnormalities. The headache may be aggravated by neck flexion or extension, or the Valsalva maneuver. Basal skull abnormalities or scoliosis may be identified. In a retrospective MRI analysis of 49 children with Chiari I malformation, 57 percent of children were asymptomatic. Headache and neck pain were the most frequent complaints. Syringomyelia was detected in 14 percent of patients and skull-base abnormalities in 50 percent. The magnitude of tonsillar ectopia (5–23 mm) correlated with severity score (p = 0.04), but not with other clinical measures. Children with greater amounts of tonsillar ectopia on MRI are more likely to be symptomatic [Wu et al., 1999]. Extreme care must be exercised before embarking upon surgical decompression. MRI with CSF flow studies may help to determine whether suboccipital decompression is necessary.

Metabolic Causes of Headache in Children

MELAS

Mitochondrial myopathy, encephalopathy, lactic acidosis, and stroke-like episodes (MELAS) constitute a mitochondrial disorder characterized by migraine-like headaches, episodic hemiparesis, development regression/dementia, short stature, seizures, and cortical blindness. The initial presentation is seizures in 28 percent, recurrent headache in 28 percent, gastrointestinal symptoms (emesis or anorexia) in 25 percent, limb weakness in 18 percent, short stature in 18 percent, and stroke in 17 percent. Onset age is below 2 years in 8 percent, 2–5 years in 20 percent, 6–10 years in 31 percent, 11–20 years in 17 percent, 21–40 years in 23 percent, and over age 40 in only 1 percent [DiMauro and Hirano, 2005].

Diagnosis requires "stroke-like" episodes, encephalopathy with seizures and/or dementia, mitochondrial myopathy (ragged red fibers on muscle biopsy), lactic acidosis, and clinical features including recurrent vomiting. The disorder is caused by a point mutation in the mitochondrial DNA *MT-TL1* encoding tRNA^{Leu}. With expanded genetic testing, the phenotype of MELAS is evolving.

CADASIL

Cerebral autosomal-dominant arteriopathy with subcortical infarcts and leukoencephalopathy (CADASIL) is a mitochondrial disorder that usually affects young adults, but can rarely be seen in adolescents. It should be considered in adolescents with migraine with aura, in whom neuroimaging discloses subcortical infarcts and/or multifocal T2/fluid-attenuated inversion recovery (FLAIR) hyperintensities in the deep white matter. An autosomal-dominant family history of migraine, early stroke, and/or dementia may be present. The clinical spectrum is variable, but migraine headache occurs in more than one-third of patients and may be the only manifestation. A recent case report described a 14-year-old girl with a 3-year history of episodic headaches, three episodes of right hemiparesis, persistent hypertension, negative family history, normal MRI, and a "Notch3" mutation [Golomb et al., 2004]. This case report raises the possibility of screening for CADASIL in children with headaches and hemiplegia episodes (hemiplegic migraine) using skin biopsy and genetic testing for the Notch3 mutation, even when MRI is normal and family history negative.

Conclusion

Headache is a universal affliction from which children are not spared. It is essential for clinicians to have a systematic approach to the evaluation of children or adolescents with the complaint of headache to determine which headaches are primary entities, such as migraine or tension-type, and which result from secondary causes, such as brain tumors, increased intracranial pressure, drug intoxications, paranasal sinus disease, or acute febrile illnesses like influenza.

Migraine, one of the most common primary headache disorders, is chronic, progressive, and debilitating, negatively impacting the lives of millions of human beings. The origins of the disability can be traced into adolescence for the overwhelming majority of adult sufferers. Pediatricians and child neurologists stand in a pivotal position to prevent decades of suffering and diminished quality of life directly attributable to migraine by providing accurate diagnosis, implementing of lifestyle modifications, and aggressive use of pharmacologic measures *during adolescence.*

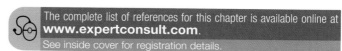

Breath-Holding Spells and Reflex Anoxic Seizures

Sarah M. Roddy

Breath-holding spells and reflex anoxic seizures are non-epileptic paroxysmal events. The events are benign, but can be frightening to parents and others observing an episode. It is important to differentiate these episodes from epileptic seizures so that the child is not inappropriately treated with antiepileptic medication.

Possibly the earliest report of breath-holding spells was published in 1737 by Nicholas Culpepper, who gave the following description: "There is a disease . . . in children from anger or grief, when the spirits are much stirred and run from the heart to the diaphragms forceably, and hinder or stop the breath . . . but when the passion ceaseth, this symptom ceaseth."

The clinical characteristics were well recognized and described in the pediatric literature in the 19th and early 20th centuries. More recent reports have provided a better understanding of the pathophysiology of these events.

Breath-Holding Spells

Clinical Features

The term breath holding is a misnomer and implies that the child is voluntarily holding his or her breath in a prolonged inspiration. Breath-holding episodes actually occur during expiration and are involuntary. Breath-holding spells are not uncommon, with an incidence of 4.6–4.7 percent [Linder, 1968; Lombroso and Lerman, 1967]. The typical age of onset is between 6 and 18 months, although occasionally the onset may occur in the first few weeks of life [Breukels et al., 2002]. Fewer than 10 percent have onset after 2 years of age [DiMario, 1992]. The frequency of episodes ranges from several times daily to once yearly. The spells are often spaced weeks to months apart at onset, and increase in frequency to as many as several per day during the second year of life [Laxdal et al., 1969; DiMario, 2001]. Breath-holding spells are classified by the color change manifested in the child during an event. Cyanotic episodes are more common than pallid episodes. In some instances, there are features of both cyanosis and pallor, and these are termed mixed episodes.

Cyanotic breath-holding spells are often precipitated by emotional stimuli, such as anger or frustration. The child typically cries vigorously but usually for less than 15 seconds, then becomes silent, and holds the breath in expiration. The apnea is associated with the rapid onset of cyanosis. Some episodes may resolve at this point, but there may be loss of consciousness and a brief period of limpness, followed by opisthotonic posturing. Recovery is usually within 1 minute, with the child having a few gasping respirations and then a return to regular breathing and consciousness.

Pallid breath-holding spells are usually provoked by sudden fright or pain. A fall with a minor injury to the head is frequently the precipitating event. An unexpected event or a surprise seems to play a role in triggering the spell. Sometimes the provoking event is not witnessed, and the child is found already in an episode. The child may gasp and cry, although it is usually for only a brief period of time. The child then becomes quiet, loses consciousness, and becomes pale. Limpness and diaphoresis are common. Clonic movements of the extremities and incontinence may occur with more severe episodes. Cyanosis may occur during the episode but is much milder than with cyanotic breath-holding spells. The child typically regains consciousness in less than 1 minute but may sleep for several hours after the episode.

An association between behavior problems, emotional factors, and breath-holding spells has been discussed by many investigators. Breath-holding spells were described by Abt [1918] as occurring in "neuropathic children of neuropathic parents." Bridge et al. [1943] stated that children susceptible to breath holding are usually of the active, energetic type, who react vigorously to situations, and that episodes were precipitated by "spoiled child reactions." Breath-holding spells were felt to be a sign of a disturbed parent–child relationship by Kanner [1935]. Laxdal et al. [1969] reported that 30 percent of the children with breath-holding spells had abnormal behavior, including temper tantrums, hyperactivity, and stubbornness. To investigate the role of behavior and breath holding further, DiMario and Burleson [1993b] studied behavior in children with breath-holding spells compared with controls and found no differences in the behavioral profiles, suggesting that breath-holding spells are nonvolitional and cannot be equated with a temperamentally difficult child.

Breath-holding spells generally decrease in frequency during the second year of life. By 4 years of age, 50 percent of children will no longer have episodes. Almost all will have stopped having episodes by age 7–8 years [DiMario, 1992; Goraya and Virdi, 2001]. Syncopal episodes occur in late childhood or adolescence in as many as 17 percent of patients with breath-holding spells [Lombroso and Lerman, 1967].

Serious complications with breath-holding spells are rare. Taiwo and Hamilton [1993] reported a prolonged cardiac

900

arrest in a patient with breath-holding spells. The few reported deaths may have been precipitated by aspiration or occurred in children who were at the severe end of the spectrum of breath-holders, often with structural abnormalities of the respiratory tract or complicated medical histories [Paulson, 1963; Southall et al., 1987, 1990].

Clinical Laboratory Tests

A detailed history of the event, including the precipitating circumstances, is essential in making the diagnosis of breath-holding spells. If the event was not witnessed from onset, important details may not be available. A video recording by the parents may be helpful in confirming the diagnosis. Usually, no laboratory tests are needed to make the diagnosis. An electroencephalogram (EEG) is usually not indicated, unless the convulsive activity is prolonged or the clinical description is incomplete and epileptic seizures cannot be ruled out. If ocular compression is performed in patients with pallid breath-holding spells, there may be asystole on cardiac monitoring, and slowing or suppression of voltage on EEG [Lombroso and Lerman, 1967; Stephenson, 1978]. Long QT syndrome is rare but should be considered as part of the differential diagnosis in a child with breath-holding spells. Patients with long QT syndrome have episodes of loss of consciousness that may be induced by injury, fright, or excitement. An electrocardiogram should be considered in any patient with breath-holding spells [Breningstall, 1996; Franklin and Hickey, 1995].

Pathophysiology

Cyanotic Spells

The pathophysiology of cyanotic breath-holding spells is complex and not completely understood. Cyanosis occurs early in the episode, which is unusual during voluntary breath holding. In breath-holding spells, the breath is held in full expiration, which also is not typical with voluntary breath holding [Livingston, 1970]. Gauk et al. [1963] studied a child during a cyanotic breath-holding episode with cinefluorography and noted the diaphragm to be high, as would be seen in full expiration, and motionless during the period of apnea. Spasm of the glottis and respiratory muscles, with increased intrathoracic pressure, occurs during expiration. Increased intrathoracic pressure reduces cardiac output, causing a decrease in cerebral perfusion. Lombroso and Lerman [1967] suggested that violent crying could lead to hypocapnia, which would also impair cerebral circulation.

Southall et al. [1985] further evaluated the prolonged expiratory mechanism in nine infants with cyanotic episodes that were usually triggered by noxious stimuli. Arterial oxygen saturation fell below 20 mm Hg within 20 seconds. Loss of consciousness occurred after 30 seconds. Measurements of respiratory movements, airflow, and esophageal pressure, and, in some patients, microlaryngoscopy and chest fluoroscopy were obtained. They documented no inspiratory flow during the period of apnea but continued expiratory muscle activity at low lung volumes with partial or complete glottic closure. No intracardiac shunt could be demonstrated. The rapid fall in arterial oxygen saturation was attributed to lack of ventilation at a maximum expiratory position in the presence of a rapid circulation time. The researchers hypothesized that central and peripheral neural respiratory control was functioning normally but was interfered with by a mechanical defect involving lung-volume maintenance. This defect could occur because of an excessively compliant rib cage, allowing alveolar collapse. This collapse, in turn, could lead to stretching of the airways and their stretch receptors, inappropriately simulating maximum lung volumes and thereby inhibiting inspiration. Southall et al. [1990] did further evaluations of prolonged expiratory apnea with krypton infusion scans and demonstrated krypton outside the lung fields, without evidence of an intracardiac shunt. They felt there was intrapulmonary shunting that contributed to the rapid onset and severity of the hypoxemia.

The relation between breath holding and chemosensitivity has also been investigated. Anas et al. [1985] hypothesized that persons with cyanotic breath-holding episodes have blunted ventilatory chemosensitivity. Because of the difficulty of measuring chemosensitivity in toddlers, they measured ventilatory responses to progressive hypercapnia and to progressive hypoxia in subjects aged 11–50 who had a history of cyanotic breath-holding spells and compared the results with a control group. Contrary to their hypothesis, the majority of persons with a history of cyanotic breath-holding spells had normal ventilatory responses. However, no one with a history of breath-holding spells had high normal responses to hypercapnia or hypoxia, as did some individuals in the control group. They postulated that the difference between the groups might represent the vestige of a disorder of ventilatory chemosensitivity that resolved with maturation.

Kahn et al. [1990] also investigated the relation between breath holding and cardiorespiratory control. The study included 71 infants with a history of breath-holding spells and age- and gender-matched controls. The median age of infants in the study was 14 weeks, which is younger than the typical age for onset of breath-holding episodes. The infants with breath-holding spells were significantly more often covered with sweat during sleep and wakefulness compared with control infants. One-night sleep studies were obtained in each infant. The infants with breath-holding spells had significantly less non-rapid eye movement (REM) stage III sleep, more indeterminate sleep, more arousals, and more sleep-stage changes than the control infants. Airway obstructions during sleep occurred in 41 infants with a history of breath holding, compared with 6 in the control group. The obstructions were generally short and not accompanied by significant bradycardia or oxygen desaturation. The researchers concluded that there was a common underlying mechanism resulting in airway obstruction during breath-holding spells and sleep, which possibly involved the autonomic nervous system because the autonomic nervous system controls the patency of the upper airways. Guilleminault et al. [2007] performed polysomnography in 14 children with cyanotic breath-holding spells and found an abnormal respiratory index in all 14. Examination showed upper airway narrowing, and adenotonsillectomy was performed in 13 with marked improvement in sleep-disordered breathing and resolution of their breath-holding spells.

Kohyama et al. [2000] did polysomnography to evaluate REM sleep in seven children with breath-holding spells and nine normal age-matched controls. The children with breath-holding spells had a significant decrease in ocular activity during REM sleep, especially during the last third of the night, compared with the controls. Relative elevation of cholinergic tone, compared with monoaminergic tone, is considered to be involved in the physiologic increase of REM sleep in the later cycles of the night. The vestibular nucleus and the medioventral caudal pons are believed to be involved in bursts of eye movements during REM sleep. They hypothesized that there was a functional disturbance in the pons of children with breath-holding spells. The study also suggests that the autonomic nervous system is involved because of the more pronounced decrease in eye movement in the later cycles of the night, which are regulated by the autonomic nervous system.

DiMario and Burleson [1993a] used noninvasive methods to evaluate autonomic nervous system function in children with severe cyanotic breath-holding spells. Compared with controls, the breath-holders had a significantly greater increase in pulse rate at 15 seconds of standing after rising from the supine position. Breath-holders also had a greater decrease in diastolic blood pressure without an increase in systolic blood pressure after standing from the supine position. These results suggest that there is autonomic dysregulation in children with cyanotic breath-holding spells. Using the results of this study and prior pieces of work, DiMario and Burleson postulated that, in addition to evidence of parasympathetic excess, children with cyanotic breath holding exhibit subtle sympathetic excess, which mediates vascular resistance, arterial distensibility, and blood flow through the lungs. This sympathetic overactivity could cause the intrapulmonary shunting and subsequent hypoxemia [Southall et al., 1990].

Pallid Spells

Excessive vagal tone leading to cerebral hypoperfusion is the underlying cause of pallid breath-holding spells. Observation of children during a typical episode reveals marked bradycardia or asystole [Bridge et al., 1943]. Ocular compression that triggers the oculocardiac reflex has been used to evaluate vagal tone in children with breath holding [Lombroso and Lerman, 1967; Stephenson, 1978]. This maneuver results in transmission of afferent signals to the brainstem via the ophthalmic division of the trigeminal nerve and efferent parasympathetic signals via the vagus nerve. In 61–78 percent of children with pallid breath-holding spells, ocular compression resulted in asystole of 2 seconds or longer, compared with 23–26 percent of children with cyanotic breath-holding spells [Lombroso and Lerman, 1967; Stephenson, 1978]. Episodes that occurred spontaneously during cardiac monitoring were also associated with asystole [Lombroso and Lerman, 1967; Maulsby and Kellaway, 1964]. The asystole during spontaneous episodes is believed to be vagally mediated. When asystole is prolonged, a reflex anoxic seizure may occur.

The role of underlying autonomic dysfunction in children with pallid breath-holding spells has been investigated in a small number of patients. Measurements of mean arterial pressures, pulse rates, electrocardiograms, and plasma norepinephrine levels were obtained in patients and controls during changes in position. The breath-holders had a statistically significant decrease in mean arterial pressure and an unsustained increase in pulse rate during the prone to standing maneuver. One child with pallid breath-holding spells had a plasma norepinephrine level that was 60 percent below the mean for both groups [DiMario et al., 1990]. Further evaluation of autonomic function was performed in children with either pallid or cyanotic breath-holding spells. Respiratory sinus arrhythmia, which is an established measure of vagal tone, was measured. There were no significant differences between controls and children with cyanotic breath-holding spells. The children with pallid spells, however, had a marked difference in respiratory sinus dysrhythmia, with less variability compared with controls and those with cyanotic episodes [DiMario et al., 1998]. These studies suggest that there may be an underlying parasympathetic dysregulation in children with pallid breath-holding spells.

The role of anemia in the pathophysiology of breath-holding spells was suggested by Holowach and Thurston [1963]. They found that 23.5 percent of 102 children with breath holding had a hemoglobin level less than 8 g/100 mL, compared with 7 percent and 2.6 percent in two control groups. Some studies did not find any significant difference in hemoglobin levels in the breath-holding group, compared with the control group [Laxdal et al., 1969; Maulsby and Kellaway, 1964]. Kolkiran et al. [2005] reported that asystole during breath-holding spells was prolonged in children with iron deficiency. There are reports of children with breath-holding spells and concomitant anemia, who had resolution of their spells with correction of the anemia [Bhatia et al., 1990; Colina and Abelson, 1995; DiMario, 1992; Mocan et al., 1999; Orii et al., 2002]. Tam and Rash [1997] described a child with pallid breath-holding spells associated with transient erythroblastopenia of childhood. The spells resolved after treatment with iron but before the anemia resolved. Daoud et al. [1997] studied 67 children with breath-holding spells to investigate the effect of iron therapy. Treatment and placebo groups were similar with respect to gender, age at onset, and frequency and type of spells, and had similar blood indices, including packed cell volume, mean corpuscular volume, saturation index, total iron binding capacity, and serum iron. At the end of the treatment period, 51.5 percent of the children treated with ferrous sulfate had complete remission of spells, and an additional 36.4 percent experienced a greater than 50 percent reduction. No children in the placebo group had total remission of spells, and only 5.9 percent had a greater than 50 percent reduction. As expected, the treatment group experienced significant improvement in the hemoglobin level and total iron-binding capacity. However, some children who were not iron-deficient had a favorable response to iron therapy, and some who were iron-deficient did not respond. A recent study suggests that checking serum soluble transferrin receptor levels in children with breath-holding spells may be helpful in assessing iron status. An increase in serum soluble transferrin receptor levels is an early change seen in iron deficiency before anemia develops [Handan et al., 2005]. Iron deficiency may play a role in the pathophysiology of breath-holding spells because iron is important for catecholamine metabolism and neurotransmitter function [Daoud et al., 1997].

Genetics

In children with breath-holding spells, there is a positive family history of similar episodes in 23–38 percent, suggesting a genetic influence [Laxdal et al., 1969; Lombroso and Lerman, 1967]. An evaluation of family pedigrees found that 27 percent of 114 proband parents and 21 percent of proband siblings had a history of breath holding. Several families had some members with pallid spells and other members with cyanotic spells. The male to female ratio was 1:1.2 and the risk of transmission from parent to child was 50:50. There were seven instances of father to son transmission, ruling out an X-linked inheritance. Using a regression model for pedigree analysis, the inheritance pattern was consistent with an autosomal-dominant pattern with reduced penetrance [DiMario and Sarfarazi, 1997].

Treatment

The most important aspect of treatment of breath-holding spells is to reassure the family of the benign nature of the spells. It is important to emphasize that the episodes do not lead to mental retardation or epilepsy. Although parents are inclined to pick up a child who is having a breath-holding spell, they should be instructed to place the child in a lateral recumbent position so as not to prolong the period of cerebral anoxia. Initiation of cardiopulmonary resuscitation should be avoided. Although anger and frustration are often precipitants for breath-holding spells, parents should be encouraged not to alter customary discipline for fear of triggering an episode [DiMario, 1992]. Parenting a child with breath-holding spells has been associated with more maternal stress than parenting a child with a convulsive seizure disorder, and parents of children with breath-holding spells are at risk for developing dysfunctional parenting behaviors [Mattie-Luksic et al., 2000]. Referral of parents to professionals to help with stress and parenting skills should be considered.

Treatment with iron therapy should be initiated in any child who has iron deficiency anemia and should be considered in any child with breath-holding spells because children without anemia may have improvement in their breath-holding spells. The convulsive movements seen during breath-holding spells are reflex anoxic seizures, which are not epileptic and do not require antiepileptic treatment. There have been a few patients who have been reported to have prolonged seizures and even status epilepticus from breath-holding spells [Emery, 1990; Kuhle et al., 2000; Moorjani et al., 1995; Nirale and Bharucha, 1991]. It is presumed that these patients have a lowered seizure threshold and that hypoxia-ischemia triggered the seizures [Emery, 1990]. Stephenson [1990] has termed these events anoxic-epileptic seizures. Treatment with antiepileptic medication may stop the seizure activity but not the breath-holding spells. Atropine (0.01 mg/kg two or three times daily) is effective for pallid breath-holding spells, but its use is rarely warranted [McWilliam and Stephenson, 1984; Stephenson, 1980]. Piracetam, which has a chemical structure similar to gamma-aminobutyric acid (GABA), has been used to treat children with breath-holding spells. In a study of 76 children with breath-holding spells, treatment with piracetam for 2 months resulted in 92 percent having no recurrence of episodes for 6 months after treatment, compared with 30 percent who received placebo [Donma, 1998]. Azam et al. [2008] treated 52 children with breath-holding spells using piracetam in doses ranging from 50 to 100 mg/kg/day and iron supplementation in those with hemoglobin less than 10 g/100 mL. In 81 percent of the children the spells completely resolved, and in an additional 9 percent the frequency and intensity were reduced. Piracetam has not received approval from the U.S. Food and Drug Administration and is designated only as an orphan drug for use in myoclonus.

Reflex Anoxic Seizures

Reflex anoxic seizures are nonepileptic events resulting from cardiac asystole of vagal origin [Stephenson, 1990, 2001]. Pain and surprise are common provoking factors for the events [Stephenson, 1980]. Reflex anoxic seizures may occur with pallid breath-holding spells but also have been reported with minor blows to the occiput, expelling hard stools past an anal fissure, venipuncture, intramuscular injections, and seeing an intravenous scalp drip [Braham et al., 1981; Gordon, 1982; Lombroso and Lerman, 1967; Roddy et al., 1983; Stephenson, 1980]. Nonepileptic anoxic seizures may also occur after syncope, cyanotic breath-holding spells, or any event that results in a sudden reduction in cerebral perfusion or hypoxia.

Clinical Features

Reflex anoxic seizures occur a few seconds after the provocation and are characterized by loss of muscle tone initially and later by tonic posturing. There may be opisthotonic posturing in some patients. A few jerks at the onset and end of an anoxic seizure may occur and probably represent myoclonic phenomena. A snoring type of inspiration or snort occurring close to the restoration of the cardiac rhythm is often noted. Urinary incontinence happens in approximately 10 percent of children with anoxic seizures, with bowel incontinence occurring less commonly [Stephenson, 1990]. Other less common features include adversive head movements, limb quivering or twitching, agitation or fear, vomiting, and tongue biting. The color change seen with an anoxic seizure may be cyanosis or pallor, depending on the mechanism producing loss of consciousness. The duration of unconsciousness is almost always less than 1 minute. Most patients experience a rapid recovery of consciousness, but some will be dazed or disoriented for a short period. Some will be drowsy after an episode and may sleep [Stephenson, 1990]. Occasionally, patients will have prolonged seizure activity after syncopal spells. These events, termed anoxic-epileptic seizures, are epileptic seizures triggered by hypoxia in patients with a lowered seizure threshold [Stephenson, 1990]. A positive family history of epilepsy may make some children more prone to anoxic-epileptic seizures [Horrocks et al., 2005].

Pathophysiology

The mechanism of reflex anoxic seizures has been studied by using ocular compression with EEG and cardiac monitoring [Gastaut and Fischer-Williams, 1957; Gastaut and Gastaut, 1958; Lombroso and Lerman, 1967; Stephenson, 1978]. Ocular compression induced asystole in susceptible patients. If asystole lasted 3–6 seconds, there were no clinical symptoms and the EEG demonstrated only desynchronization. When asystole lasted 7–13 seconds, slow waves appeared, usually associated with altered consciousness. If asystole was prolonged for 14 seconds or more, there were often myoclonic jerks or tonic posturing. The EEG during this time reveals no electrocerebral activity. With return of cardiac activity, there was again high-voltage slow-wave activity on the EEG with return of normal activity over 20–30 seconds [Gastaut and Fischer-Williams, 1957]. At no time during EEG monitoring were epileptiform discharges present. Some patients have had spontaneous episodes or episodes triggered by other stimuli, such as venipuncture during EEG and cardiac monitoring, and have demonstrated similar changes to those seen with ocular compression [Braham et al., 1981; Gordon, 1982; Lombroso and Lerman, 1967; Roddy et al., 1983]. Ocular compression increases vagal tone, with the afferent pathway involving fibers from the trigeminal nerve originating from the cornea, iris, and eyelids. In contrast, episodes induced by exteroceptive stimulation, such as pain and emotion, have afferent fibers in various sensory pathways. In both situations, the vagal reflex centers are located in the brainstem in the nucleus ambiguus [Chen and Chai, 1976]. The efferent pathway involves the cardioinhibitory fibers of the vagus nerve.

Clinical Laboratory Tests

Diagnosis of reflex anoxic seizures is usually made by obtaining a history of the episode. Details about the precipitating circumstances and onset are essential. Parents may state that their child had a seizure, and a careful description of the movements and posture, length of the episode, and recovery period will be helpful. Usually, no laboratory tests are needed, although consideration should be given to obtaining an electrocardiogram to evaluate for a cardiac cause if the episodes are not typical. Rarely is it necessary to obtain an EEG. If an EEG is performed, ocular compression may be helpful in confirming the diagnosis.

Treatment

Treatment of reflex anoxic seizures focuses on explaining the nature of the event to the parents and reassuring them that the episodes are not epileptic seizures and do not need treatment with antiepileptic medication. In more severe cases, atropine, theophylline, and transdermal scopolamine have been helpful [Benditt et al., 1983; McWilliam and Stephenson, 1984; Palm and Blennow, 1985; Stephenson, 1979]. Pacemaker implantation has also been useful in the rare patient with severe episodes [Kelly et al., 2001; McLeod et al., 1999; Porter et al., 1994; Sapire et al., 1983]. Children with reflex anoxic seizures are at risk of bradycardia during surgical procedures, and modifications in the anesthesia protocol may be warranted [Onslow and Burden, 2003; Pollard, 1999].

Syncope and Paroxysmal Disorders Other than Epilepsy

Neil R. Friedman, Debabrata Ghosh, and Manikum Moodley

Paroxysmal disorders, including epilepsy and syncope, represent one of the most common neurological problems in the pediatric population. Although the clinical manifestations of paroxysmal disorders are highly heterogeneous, recent advances in molecular genetic analysis have highlighted striking similarities in their molecular pathophysiology [Crompton and Berkovic, 2009]. Paroxysmal disorders other than epilepsy are described in this chapter (Box 65-1). Breath-holding spells, migraine, pseudoseizures, and sleep-related paroxysmal disorders are reviewed elsewhere in this book.

Syncope

Syncope is defined as the temporary loss of consciousness and postural tone resulting from transient and diffuse cerebral hypoperfusion, followed by spontaneous recovery with no neurological sequelae [Feit, 1996]. In the young patient, syncope often results from a fall in systolic pressure below 70 mmHg or a mean arterial pressure of 30–40 mmHg [Kaufmann, 2004]. The event is typically preceded by a prodrome lasting several seconds to 1–2 minutes, which has distinctive premonitory features such as nausea, epigastric discomfort, blurred or tunnel vision, muffled hearing, dizziness, lightheadedness, diaphoresis, hyperventilation, palpitations, pallor, cold and clammy skin, or weakness [Sapin, 2004; Strieper, 2005]. These symptoms may occur in any combination or be variably present in any given patient from one episode to the next. If the prodrome is of sufficient duration, patients may learn to recognize their symptoms and lie down to relieve the symptoms and prevent syncope [McLeod, 2003]. Although syncope is commonly a benign self-limiting event, rarely it may be the first warning sign of a serious underlying cardiac or noncardiac disease.

Epidemiology

Syncope is a common clinical problem affecting an estimated 15–25 percent of children and adolescents prior to adulthood. It is not often brought to medical attention, thus accounting for only about 1 percent of pediatric emergency room visits [Vlahos et al., 2007; Longin et al., 2008]. Its true incidence therefore remains unknown. In the 26-year surveillance of the Framingham study, syncope occurred in 3 percent of men and 3–5 percent of women [Savage et al., 1985]. In the Rochester Epidemiologic Project, Driscoll et al. reported on older children and adolescents studied over two 5-year periods [Driscoll et al., 1997]. In the first 5-year period (1950–1954), the incidence of syncope cases requiring medical attention equaled 71.9 per 100,000 population; the second period of study (1987–1991) reported an incidence of 125.8 cases per 100,000 population, with this incidence peaking among adolescents, in particular females aged 15–19 years [Batra and Balaji, 2005]. According to Sheldon et al., the most common age for a child's first vasovagal syncopal episode is approximately 13 [Sheldon et al., 2006]. The recurrence rate of syncope ranges from 33 to 51 percent when patients are followed for up to 5 years [Kapoor et al., 1983].

Etiology

Syncope may result from cardiovascular or neurological causes (cardiovascular-mediated or neurally mediated syncope). Each of these categories accounts for about 50 percent of adult syncope but, in children, cardiovascular-mediated syncope is less frequent than it is in adults [Kapoor, 2000].

Cardiovascular-Mediated Syncope

Cardiovascular-mediated syncope has a higher mortality and a higher incidence of sudden death than neurally mediated syncope [Kapoor et al., 1983]. It is therefore imperative to distinguish syncope from seizures, and to triage patients with syncope due to malignant cardiac causes for urgent and appropriate investigations and management [Crompton and Berkovic, 2009]. Risk factors that suggest structural or conduction heart defects are given in Box 65-2. If any of these risk factors is present, an urgent referral should be made for pediatric cardiology evaluation. Cardiovascular causes of syncope in children are given in Box 65-3.

Neurocardiogenic Syncope

Neurocardiogenic syncope, previously known as vasodepressor, vasovagal, or neurally mediated syncope, is the most common cause of syncope and also the type most commonly confused with epilepsy [Stephenson, 1990c].

Clinical Features

A diagnosis of syncope rests mainly on clinical grounds [Lerman-Sagie et al., 1994]. The patient's history, physical examination, and electrocardiography (EKG) have a combined

Box 65-1 Syncope and Other Nonepileptic Paroxysmal Disorders

Syncope

- Cardiovascular-mediated syncope
- Neurocardiogenic syncope
- Convulsive syncope
- Reflex syncope
- Psychogenic syncope
- Situational syncope
  - Cough
  - Sneezing
  - Defecation
  - Micturition
  - Deglutition (cold liquids)
  - Carotid sinus hypersensitivity
  - Hair grooming
  - Trumpet playing
  - Suffocation
  - Weight lifting
  - Diving
  - Stretching
- Drug-induced
- Metabolic (hypoglycemia, hypoxia, hyperventilation)

Paroxysmal Dyskinesias

- Paroxysmal kinesigenic choreoathetosis
- Paroxysmal nonkinesigenic choreoathetosis
- Paroxysmal exercise-induced dyskinesia

Childhood Periodic Syndromes

- Benign paroxysmal vertigo
- Benign paroxysmal torticollis
- Cyclic vomiting

Other Nonepileptic Paroxysmal Disorders

- Dopa-responsive dystonia
- Episodic ataxias
- Sandifer's syndrome
- Spasmus nutans
- Paroxysmal tonic upgaze of childhood
- Benign myoclonus of infancy
- Hereditary hyperekplexia
- Shuddering attacks
- Stereotypies, self-stimulation, and masturbation
- Hyperventilation syndrome

Box 65-2 Risk Factors for Cardiac Disease

- History of heart murmur or congenital heart disease
- Acute attacks associated with hyperpnea or cyanosis
- Abrupt loss of consciousness during exercise
- Absence of usual premonitory symptoms or precipitating factors associated with neurally mediated syncope

Box 65-3 Cardiovascular Causes Of Syncope

Arrhythmias

- Compete heart block
- Sick sinus syndrome
- Tachyarrhythmias
  - Supraventricular
  - Ventricular
- Long QT syndrome
  - Wolff–Parkinson–White syndrome
- Channelopathies

Cardiac – Structural

- Aortic stenosis
- Hypertrophic obstructive cardiomyopathy
- Coronary artery anomalies
- Primary pulmonary hypertension
- Eisenmenger's syndrome
- Mitral valve prolapse
- Arrhythmogenic right ventricular dysplasia

diagnostic yield of about 50 percent [Kaufmann, 2004]. A prodromal phase of presyncope consists of lightheadedness, blurred vision, epigastric discomfort, nausea, pallor, or diaphoresis [Manolis et al., 1990; Feit, 1996; McLeod, 2003]. When present, these clinical features help to differentiate syncope from epilepsy. A detailed history usually reveals contributory environmental factors before the loss of consciousness and postural tone. These environmental factors include upright posture, prolonged standing, change in posture (orthostasis), crowding, heat, fatigue, hunger, or a concurrent illness [Sutton, 1996]. Emotional or stress factors, such as venipuncture, public speaking, "fight-or-flight" situations, pain, and fear, are also commonly identified [Driscoll et al., 1997]. The loss of consciousness is usually brief, lasting from a few seconds to 1–2 minutes, followed by rapid spontaneous recovery without neurological deficits. During the ictus the patient may have tonic posturing or a brief clonic seizure, rarely associated with incontinence. Rarely, myoclonic jerks mimicking an epileptic seizure may occur during syncope [Crompton and Berkovic, 2009]. The postictal period may be accompanied by persistent nausea, pallor, diaphoresis, and a generally "washed-out" appearance. Complete recovery usually evolves in less than an hour [McLeod, 2003].

Distinguishing between neurocardiogenic syncope and seizure is the most common clinical dilemma and a frequent source of diagnostic error. Often, interobserver agreement is poor when a retrospective diagnosis is made on information obtained after a single syncopal episode. In distinguishing patients with syncope due to cardiac causes, a history or physical signs of cardiac disease can be 95 percent sensitive for a cardiac etiology [Crompton and Berkovic, 2009]. These features are, however, nonspecific, as neurocardiogenic syncope might occur in patients with heart disease [Crompton and Berkovic, 2009]. Patients with pseudosyncope and pseudoseizures typically use the events consciously or unconsciously to avoid an unpleasant emotional situation [Wieling and Shen, 2008]. Most of these patients are young females. A very high number of events, episodes without injury, and florid symptomatology are typical. Furthermore, in these patients, recovery after a syncopal event is often prolonged (10–30 minutes), despite a supine posture. In true syncope, consciousness returns within 1 minute of lying down, and unconsciousness for more than 5 minutes is rare [Wieling and Shen, 2008].

The evaluation of syncope may therefore result in unnecessary and costly investigations [Landau and Nelson, 1996]. A complete evaluation would include neuroimaging studies, electroencephalography (EEG), EKG, echocardiography, Holter monitoring, selected metabolic testing, and, in certain cases, intracardiac electrophysiologic studies or implantable continuous loop recordings. Despite extensive investigations, more than 40 percent of patients with recurrent syncope do not have a specific diagnosis [Kapoor, 1991; Grubb et al., 1992].

Pathophysiology

Lewis first introduced the term "vasovagal syncope" in 1932 to indicate that the blood vessels (vaso) and the heart (vagal activity) were involved in the syncopal event [Lewis, 1932]. Hence, the classical clinical signs of vasovagal syncope are marked bradycardia and hypotension. There is no consensus concerning the mechanisms underlying the vasovagal reaction, but several theories have been proposed [Abboud, 1993; Kosinski et al., 1995; Grubb and Kosinski, 1996]. The ventricular theory (Figure 65-1) proposes that, among predisposed individuals who experience recurrent syncope, excess peripheral venous pooling on prolonged standing results in diminished venous return. Decreased cardiac ventricular filling activates mechanoreceptors located mainly in the inferoposterior wall of the left ventricle, which send afferent impulses via C-fibers to the dorsal nucleus of the vagus [van Lieshout et al., 1991]. Arterial baroreceptors and carotid sinus afferent activation may also contribute to the complex pathophysiology of syncope [Kinsella and Tuckey, 2001]. These inhibitory cardiac and arterial receptors mediate increased parasympathetic activity, and inhibit sympathetic activity that results in bradycardia, vasodilatation, and hypotension (Bezold–Jarisch reflex) [Kinsella and Tuckey, 2001; Shen and Gersh, 1993]. The normal response during upright posture is an increased heart rate and diastolic pressure, and an unchanged or slightly decreased systolic pressure [Rea and Thames, 1993]. In individuals susceptible to recurrent syncope, a "paradoxical" reflex bradycardia and peripheral vascular dilatation occur [Grubb and Kosinski, 1996]. The previous emphasis on parasympathetic (vagal) output is shifting to sympathetic withdrawal as the main mechanism responsible for the bradycardia or asystole (cardioinhibitory response) and hypotension (vasodepressor response) that accompany neurocardiogenic syncope [Hannon and Knilans, 1993]. Although parasympathetic-mediated bradycardia remains a contributory factor in syncope, the responsible phenomena are vasodilatation and hypotension [Kosinski et al., 1995]. Current hypotheses propose that the primary efferent event is systemic vasodilatation, and that this vasodepressor element is mediated by a profound, centrally mediated sympathetic withdrawal [Kosinski et al., 1995]. The persistence of neurocardiogenic syncope in subjects who had cardiac transplants and, therefore, technically

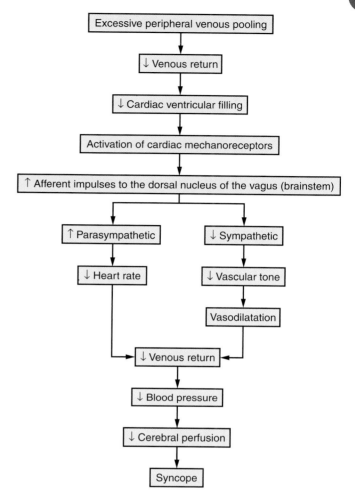

Fig. 65-1 **The pathophysiology of syncope.**

denervated hearts, as well as the findings of increased epinephrine levels during upright position and syncope, are strong evidence supporting a sympathetic withdrawal mechanism in syncope [Fitzpatrick et al., 1993; Njemanze, 1993; Sra et al., 1994]. Altered cerebral autoregulation may also be contributory in neurocardiogenic syncope [Rodriguez-Nunez et al., 1997]. Transcranial Doppler studies have demonstrated cerebral vasoconstriction during tilt-table-induced syncope [Grubb et al., 1991]. These observations may stimulate future research and modify current insight about neurocardiogenic syncope.

Diagnostic Evaluation

The history, clinical examination, and EKG have a combined diagnostic yield of 50 percent [Kaufmann, 2004]. The patient history is the cornerstone on which the diagnosis of syncope is made. Important historical details to take from patients are given in Box 65-4. On clinical examination, blood pressure and heart rate should be taken in the supine and upright positions, noting any orthostatic hypotension with or without an increase in heart rate. Special attention should be paid to detecting cardiac anomalies. An EKG should be obtained on all patients who present with syncope, especially if it is recurrent or occurs with exercise. All patients with recurrent syncope, family history of syncope or sudden unexplained

---

Box 65-4 History in Neurocardiogenic Syncope

Patient

- Hydration status
- Environmental conditions
- Activity immediately before syncopal event
- Frequency and duration of the episode
- Any aura or prodrome before the episode
- Historical data from witnesses
- Complete drug history

Family

- Family history of syncope or cardiac disease
- Sudden unexplained death in children or young adults
- Family history of seizures
- Familial deafness

---

death should be referred to cardiology for further evaluation. This may include echocardiography and a Holter or event monitor. Rarely, cardiac catheterization with right ventricular endomyocardial biopsy may be necessary before a patient can resume activities [Strieper, 2005].

Tilt-Table Testing

Until the mid-1980s, the diagnosis of neurocardiogenic syncope was made primarily by a careful and detailed patient and family history, the physical examination, and EKG. Tilt-table testing as a potential diagnostic tool for neurocardiogenic syncope was introduced only in 1986 after the ground-breaking report by Kenny et al. [Kenny et al., 1986]. A number of reports have since emerged, attesting to the utility of the test in reproducing syncopal episodes in patients who are predisposed to neurocardiogenic hypotension and bradycardia.

Despite criticism that this provocative test suffers from "naïve rationale," lacks patient selection standards, and needs controlled treatment and outcome studies [Landau and Nelson, 1996], the tilt-table test continues to enjoy popularity as a noninvasive and physiologically appropriate neurophysiologic test for the diagnosis of neurocardiogenic syncope [Kapoor, 1999; Dijane et al., 1996].

The test is done by positioning the patient head upright at an angle of 60–80 degrees for 15–60 minutes on a tilt table with a supporting footboard. A tilt-table test result is positive when the symptoms of syncope or presyncope are reproduced [Sra et al., 1991]. If the result is negative, isoproterenol is administered intravenously and the dose increased until the heart rate goes up by at least 20 percent. To standardize the test, the duration of head-up tilting has been increased to 45 minutes or 2 standard deviations (SD) of the mean time required to reproduce syncope [Sneddon and Camm, 1993]. A comprehensive analysis of available tilt-table data suggests that administration of isoproterenol has no added benefit, and 60 degrees for 45–60 minutes is recommended [Kapoor et al., 1994].

Experience with tilt-table test among pediatric populations is limited. Of 35 adolescents who had recurrent presyncope or syncope, 26 had positive tilt-table test results at 60 degrees for 30–60 minutes and isoproterenol infusion from 1 to 5 µg/minute [Thilenius et al., 1991]. Among 54 pediatric patients

who had recurrent syncope, tilt-table testing at 80 degrees for 30 minutes was superior to studies, such as chest radiograph, EKG, echocardiogram, EEG, or neuroimaging, in arriving at a diagnosis of neurocardiogenic syncope [Strieper et al., 1994]. Tilt-table studies in 20 children with unexplained syncope and 10 controls, using 60 degrees for 25 minutes and isoproterenol infusion of 0.02–0.08 µg/kg/minute, were positive in 75 percent of patients and in 10 percent of controls, with a sensitivity of 75 percent and a specificity of 90 percent [Alehan et al., 1996]. The tilt-table test has been used in children as young as 3 years of age [Grubb et al., 1992].

In addition to heart rate and blood pressure monitoring during tilt-table testing, EKG recording may be used to differentiate anoxic from epileptic seizures [Grubb et al., 1992]. More controlled studies and standardization of degree and duration of tilting are necessary to validate the tilt-table test as a safe, practical, and useful diagnostic tool for neurocardiogenic syncope in children [Benditt and Lurie, 1996; Mansourati and Blanc, 1996; Moya et al., 1996a, b; Victor, 1996].

Treatment

The objective of treatment for neurocardiogenic syncope is to prevent recurrent syncope, which leads to impaired quality of life, psychological distress, and substantial morbidity. Once a diagnosis of neurocardiogenic syncope is confirmed, treatment requires counseling of the patient (when appropriate) and his or her parents. The benign nature of these events should be explained to allay concerns about epilepsy or sudden death. Neurocardiogenic syncope almost always resolves within months to 3–5 years after onset [Strieper, 2005]. Most patients presenting after a single uncomplicated syncopal event require simple reassurance, education about the disease, and advice on recognizing prodromal symptoms and how to avoid provocative situations – in particular, prolonged standing, sudden postural changes, dehydration, and irregular meal times. If a prodromal phase is consistently present, the patient may by taught to recline or sit to avoid injury from a fall. Supplemental fluids and electrolytes may be beneficial; up to 1500–2500 mL per day are recommended for adolescents. Patients should be instructed to increase dietary salt, either as salt tablets or liberal use of salt with meals (Box 65-5).

Box 65-5 Nonpharmacologic Treatment of Neurocardiogenic Syncope

- Counseling and reassurance
- Avoid precipitating or triggering factors
- Increase water and salt intake
  - 1.5–2.5 L of water daily (adolescents and adults)
  - At least 5–10 g of salt a day
- Physical countermaneuvers
  - Leg crossing
  - Buttock tensing
  - Squatting
- Head-up sleeping
- Elastic stockings
- Abdominal binders
- Psychological counseling

If, despite these conservative measures, the syncopal episodes become refractory, pharmacologic therapy may be tried. Favorable but not consistent response to treatment has been reported with β-adrenergic receptor antagonists, α-adrenergic receptor agonists, anticholinergic agents, theophylline, serotonin reuptake inhibitors, and mineralocorticosteroids [Milstein et al., 1990; Scott et al., 1995; Raviele et al., 1996; Boehm et al., 1997; Sra et al., 1997] (Box 65-6). Beta blockers, fludrocortisone and midodrine, and an α-adrenergic agonist, are often prescribed in children but none of these agents has shown a consistent therapeutic benefit in clinical trials [Kaufmann and Freeman, 2004; Freeman, 2008]. Low-dose midodrine is promising and is currently recommended as first-line therapy for vasovagal syncope in children by some authorities [Stewart, 2006]. When using fludrocortisone, combine with increased salt intake for an optimal effect. Subjects who require isoproterenol to induce syncope during tilt-table testing or who experience tachycardia before syncope may respond better to beta-blocker therapy [Sra et al., 1992; Leor et al., 1994; Wieling and Shen, 2008].

Prognosis

The prognosis for recovery is excellent in neurocardiogenic syncope. Most patients show spontaneous resolution of their syncope and presyncope within the first year after onset; 5–10 percent will however, continue to show symptoms over an extended period of time, often up to 5 years [Strieper, 2005].

Convulsive Syncope

A brief tonic or, rarely, a clonic seizure may accompany syncope. In a study of blood donors, 0.05 percent suffered a convulsion associated with syncope (convulsive syncope) [Lin et al., 1982]. Among 216 children who had a positive tilt-table test, 25 (11.6 percent) had seizures during the test [Fernandez Sanmartin et al., 2003]. Most convulsions consisted of tonic spasms (65 percent), characterized by eye rolling, nuchal rigidity, arms flexed at the elbow, and fists clenched, followed usually by prompt recovery [Lin et al., 1982]. Other types of convulsions were myoclonic (23 percent), clonic (6 percent), and tonic-clonic (6 percent). No difference was found in the severity of bradycardia or hypotension among those who had syncope associated with convulsion and those who did not [Lin et al., 1982]. In subjects who had cardiac asystole induced by ocular compression, only those who remained asystolic for more than 14 seconds experienced convulsive phenomena [Lin et al., 1982]. Convulsive syncope results from cerebral ischemia and is not indicative of an epileptic predisposition. The EEG reveals diffuse slowing, followed by loss of electrocerebral activity; epileptiform activity is absent [Fernandez Sanmartin et al., 2003; Stephenson, 1990d]. Rarely, an epileptic seizure is triggered by syncope. In such cases, the EEG, in contrast to what is seen in convulsive syncope, reveals epileptiform activity [Stephenson, 1990g].

Reflex Syncope

Syncope that is triggered by specific factors or events is known as reflex or situational syncope. The most common of these among infants and children is breath-holding spells. These are discussed in greater detail in Chapter 64. A related but distinctive type of syncope (known by various names in the past, including pallid breath-holding spells or pallid infantile syncope) is frequently confused with breath-holding spells. A simple and more appropriate designation for this type of paroxysm is reflex syncope.

In reflex syncope, the antecedent event is minor trauma (usually to the head) before loss of postural tone and consciousness, without any audible inspiratory stridor or expiratory cry. Reflex syncopal episodes are easily confused with typical breath-holding spells, but evidence is lacking that these result from transient cerebral hypoxia because of breath holding. The rapid or immediate onset of syncope after minor trauma or other unexpected painful stimuli differentiates reflex syncope from breath-holding spells. In breath-holding spells, several seconds may elapse before loss of consciousness. There is general agreement that reflex syncopal attacks do not represent epileptic seizures, but the mechanism responsible is less clear. Some refer to these events as reflex anoxic seizures [Stephenson, 1978]. According to Stephenson, cardiac arrest is inducible in individuals susceptible to reflex syncope by the ocular compression test. This test is performed by applying pressure over the closed eyelids for 10 seconds during cardiac and EEG monitoring [Stephenson, 1980]. After 7–15 seconds of asystole, a typical paroxysm is reproduced, thus confirming

---

Box 65-6 **Medications for Treatment of Neurocardiogenic Syncope***

Beta-Adrenergic Blockers

- Atenolol 1–2 mg/kg/day
- Esmolol
- Metoprolol 1–2 mg/kg/day
- Nadolol
- Propranolol 0.5–4 mg/kg/day

Anticholinergics

- Disopyramide 10–15 mg/kg/day
- Hyoscine
- Propantheline
- Scopolamine

Alpha-Adrenergic Agonists

- Ephedrine
- Methylphenidate 5–10 mg use three times a day
- Midodrine
- Pseudoephedrine 60 mg use two times a day

Serotonin Receptor Uptake Inhibitors

- Fluoxetine 10–20 mg/day
- Sertraline 25–50 mg/day

Mineralocorticoids

- Fludrocortisone 0.1–0.3 mg/day

* Pediatric doses are given for those medications used in children for which dosages have been recommended.
(Data from Grubb and Kosinski, 1996; Lazarus and Mauro, 1996; Raviele et al., 1996; Sra et al., 1997.)

the diagnosis of reflex syncope. Reproduction of reflex syncope by ocular compression suggests that these children have an exaggerated oculocardiac reflex [Stephenson, 1990f]. Despite assurances about the safety and diagnostic usefulness of the ocular compression test to reproduce this type of syncope [Gastaut, 1974; Stephenson, 1980, 1990f], its acceptance as a provocative test has been limited.

Situational Syncope

Other triggering factors associated with syncope include cough, deglutition (cold liquids), defecation, diving, micturition, sneezing, trumpet playing, weight lifting, and Valsalva maneuver [Hannon and Knilans, 1993]. These events are more common in adults than in children and are referred to as situational syncope. A common denominator in situational syncope is the fact that most of the triggering factors are accompanied by a Valsalva-like maneuver. Hair-grooming syncope is an uncommon type of situational syncope among adolescent females; it is often followed by brief seizure activity [Lewis and Howell, 1986; Igarashi et al., 1988; Lewis and Frank, 1993]. The convulsive syncope is almost invariably preceded by a prodrome of presyncope symptoms of nausea, lightheadedness, diaphoresis, and visual blurring. The reaction is thought to be a variant of neurocardiogenic syncope that is triggered by hair pulling or scalp stimulation, which activates the trigeminal nerve [Kosinski and Grubb, 2005].

Hyperventilation Syncope

If the syncope is preceded by paresthesias, lip tingling, and anxiety or panic, consider hyperventilation as the cause. Loss of postural tone and consciousness during hyperventilation is thought to result from cerebral vasoconstriction induced by hypocapnia. This type of syncope is discussed in more detail later in this chapter (see "Hyperventilation Syndrome").

Suffocation or Strangulation Syncope

Meadow's syndrome (Munchausen's by proxy) is a rarely suspected cause of syncope. A caretaker induces loss of consciousness by obstructing the infant's airway using a pillow or by pressing the infant's face against the caretaker's trunk [Stephenson, 1990e]. In other cases, compression of the neck by strangulation results in cerebral hypoxia and, after repeated attempts, brain damage. A solicitous and omnipresent caretaker should raise suspicion of foul play [Folks, 1995]. The morbid events have been documented in some cases during video/EEG monitoring, but the incriminating evidence may not be admissible in court.

Drug-Induced Syncope

When episodes begin with a slow onset and gradual recovery, consider a toxic or metabolic cause, such as hypoglycemia, alcohol, or drugs (illicit or prescribed) [Olshansky, 2005]. Among the medications that can cause syncope are those that induce ventricular tachycardia or cause hypotension. Cardiovascular medications (vasodilators and antiarrhythmics), psychotropics, diuretics, and glucose-controlling medications are the most common drugs associated with syncope [Lazarus and Mauro, 1996]. Illicit drugs may also cause syncope (particularly alcohol, but also cocaine and marijuana). Alcohol and illicit drugs can cause syncope by several mechanisms, including exacerbation of a supraventricular or ventricular tachyarrhythmia [Strieper, 2005]. Drug-induced syncope is common among the elderly but rare among children. However, illicit drug use is increasing significantly in the younger age group. Toxicology screens often provide clues to this diagnosis.

Psychogenic Syncope

One of the most important causes of syncope in pediatric patients, in particular adolescents, is psychogenic syncope. Several features help distinguish psychogenic syncope from neurocardiogenic syncope [Benbadis and Chichkova, 2006; Thijs et al., 2009]:

1. Episodes are extremely frequent (sometimes several episodes per day).
2. The episodes are usually not associated with injury and lack any of the usual precipitating or triggering factors.
3. Patients experience onset of syncope in the supine position.
4. Patients fail to regain consciousness rapidly after a syncopal event (occasionally taking as long as several hours), during which time there are no cardiovascular or neurologic abnormalities and resumption of the supine posture does not terminate the event.
5. Finally, patients manifest remarkable indifference to their syncope. During tilt-table testing, these patients may suddenly faint without any changes in their heart rate and blood pressure.

A detailed psychosocial history may provide clues about the possible mechanisms involved. Many of these individuals turn out to have conversion reactions, most frequently secondary to sexual abuse. A useful clinical maneuver in the unresponsive patient whose eyes are closed is to touch the eyelashes gently. This touch elicits a blink reflex in the conscious patient and alerts the examiner to the underlying psychopathology. Appropriate referral to a behavioral specialist or pediatric psychiatrist should be made for further evaluation and management.

Paroxysmal Dyskinesias

Paroxysmal dyskinesias are episodic attacks of involuntary hyperkinetic (dystonic, choreoathetoid, or ballistic) movements with preserved consciousness. In 1940, Mount and Reback first described a familial paroxysmal movement disorder manifested by involuntary writhing and posturing of the trunk and extremities, later labeled as paroxysmal dystonic choreoathetosis [Mount and Reback, 1940]. Kertesz introduced the term paroxysmal kinesigenic choreoathetosis to differentiate cases in which the episodes were brief and precipitated by movement, instead of by prolonged immobility or intake of specific beverages (coffee, tea, cola drinks, alcohol), as in the cases of Mount and Reback [Kertesz, 1967]. These hyperkinetic movements or dyskinesias may manifest as dystonia (abnormal distorted posturing), chorea (arrhythmic, bizarre, jerky, dancing movement), athetosis (distal slow, sinuous limb movement), or ballism (violent flailing limb movement). They may occur individually or in various combinations. The most widely used classification system for the paroxysmal dyskinesias is the one proposed by Demirkiran and Jankovic in1995 [Demirkiran and Jankovic, 1995]. The paroxysmal dyskinesias are classified into four types: paroxysmal kinesigenic dyskinesia

(PKD), paroxysmal nonkinesigenic dyskinesia (PNKD), paroxysmal exercise-induced dyskinesia (PED), and paroxysmal hypnogenic dyskinesia (PHD). Each category is further subdivided into idiopathic (familial and sporadic) and, rarely, symptomatic [Blakeley and Jankovic, 2002] secondary to stroke, trauma, multiple sclerosis, central nervous system infections, and other known causes, with resultant abnormality on brain magnetic resonance imaging. The majority of cases are primary or idiopathic, and of the PKD or PNKD type. PHD, though included in this classification scheme due to semiologic similarity, has been proven to consist of nocturnal seizures secondary to autosomal-dominant nocturnal frontal lobe epilepsy (ADNFLE) [Luders, 1996; Phillips et al., 2001].

The etiology, anatomy, physiology, and pathogenesis of the paroxysmal dyskinesias are not yet completely understood. Evidence supports the striatum as the primary area of brain involvement, based on current clinical, radiological, and experimental data. Symptomatic cases have been shown to have structural pathology of the striatum; abnormalities of the striatum have been found on MR spectroscopy, positron emission tomography (PET), and single photon emission computerized tomography (SPECT); and in in vivo experimental studies, using the dt^{sz} mutant hamster animal model of paroxysmal dyskinesia, striatal increase of extracellular dopamine during dystonic episodes has been shown [Ko et al., 2001; Sanger, 2003; Hamann and Richter, 2004]. However, in another animal study using the lethargic mouse model (produced by calcium channel mutation), abnormal cerebellar output was shown to be responsible for the paroxysmal dyskinesia [Devanagondi et al., 2007]. Excess cytochrome oxidase activity in the red nucleus disappeared after surgical removal of the cerebellum. A similar conclusion was reached in the tottering mouse model [Campbell et al., 1999].

The etiology of most of these paroxysmal dyskinesias, as with many periodic syndromes, is thought to be secondary to an underlying channelopathy. They share common clinical characteristics with epilepsy, migraine headaches, periodic paralysis, episodic ataxia with myokymia, including episodic attacks with normal interictal examination, common precipitating mechanisms such as stress, fatigue, diet, alcohol, and caffeine, and treatment response to similar medications. Both hypokalemic and hyperkalemic periodic paralysis and episodic ataxia with myokymia are due to mutations in ion-channel genes. Carbamazepine is effective in certain epilepsies, as in PKD, and acetazolamide is useful in periodic paralysis, myotonia, episodic ataxia, and some paroxysmal dyskinesias [Bhatia et al., 2000; Ptacek and Fu, 2001; Celesia, 2001; Margari et al., 2005; Cannon, 2001]. Genetic mutations in the alpha subunit of calcium-sensitive potassium channel on chromosome 10q22 cause epilepsy and PNKD [Du et al., 2005]. Mutations in voltage-gated neuronal K$^+$ channel K$_v$7 (KCNQ) produces dyskinesia in the dt^{sz} mutant hamster model of paroxysmal nonkinesigenic dyskinesia. Retigabine and flupirtine, which result in opening of the above type of K$^+$ channel, effectively treated the paroxysmal dystonia, proving the role of K$_v$7 channel mutation in the causation of PNKD [Richter et al., 2006]. Interestingly, however, many of the familial PNKDs are caused by the mutation of *MR-1* (myofibrillogenesis regulator 1) gene on chromosome 2. The *MR-1* gene is not involved with an ion channel; rather, it is predicted to be involved in the stress response pathway [Lee et al., 2004; Rainier et al., 2004; Chen et al., 2005a; Hempelmann et al., 2006; Bruno et al., 2007].

Some symptomatic forms of PKDs are caused by the X-linked monocarboxylate transporter 8 (*MCT 8*) gene mutation responsible for transport of T3 (tri-iodothyronin) across the neuronal membrane [Dumitrescu et al., 2004; Brockmann et al., 2005; Fuchs et al., 2009].

The paroxysmal dyskinesias are also described in Chapter 68.

Paroxysmal Kinesigenic Dyskinesia

This is the most common form of all the paroxysmal dyskinesias, although the exact prevalence is unknown. The attacks are brief (usually lasting less than 1 minute) and characterized by dystonic posturing, choreoathetosis, or ballistic movements, either singly or in combination; they affect one or both sides concomitantly [Lance, 1977; Bruno et al., 2004]. The patient remains conscious throughout the episode, without any postictal impairment. In the largest series of 121 cases of paroxysmal kinesigenic dyskinesia, 51 were male and 44 female [Bruno et al., 2004]. Ninety-five cases were familial, and the majority of these were consistent with autosomal-dominant inheritance. Males also outnumbered females in sporadic cases. The mean age at onset was 11.7 ± 3.4 years in the familial cases, and similar for the sporadic ones. The age range, however, varied from 1 to 20 years. The dyskinesias are always triggered by sudden movement; however, an intention to move or startle may also bring them on. Anxiety or stress may also play an important role, causing confusion, at times, with a psychogenic movement disorder with consequent delay in the diagnosis. Spells occur more frequently following physical exertion or during sickness. An aura is present in more than 80 percent of cases. These auras consist of a feeling of tightness, numbness, tingling, or paresthesia in the involved extremities [Lance, 1977; Bruno et al., 2004]. The ictus consists of dystonic posturing in up to two-thirds of all cases. Choreoathetosis or ballistic movements occur in some, and a combination of movements occurs in one-third. In about one-third of cases, the attacks may be focal or unilateral, one-third may have bilateral involvement, and the remainder has either unilateral or alternating bilateral involvement. In focal cases, the movement usually starts with the limb in action. The attacks are typically short, with more than 90 percent lasting less than 30 seconds, and usually never more than a minute. The attacks occur daily in more than 80 percent of cases, and the frequency may reach up to 100 attacks in a day [Lance, 1977; Houser et al., 1999; Bruno et al., 2004].

Associated neurological disorders, like infantile convulsions, are common (11–19 percent) in children with PKD; almost half of their family members had infantile seizure [Margari et al., 2000, 2002; Bhatia, 2001; Bruno, et al., 2004]. This association brought up a homogenous autosomal-dominant syndrome described as infantile convulsions and choreoathetosis (ICCA), with benign seizures in infancy, followed by later-onset paroxysmal kinesigenic dyskinesia [Rochette et al., 2008]. In familial forms of PKD, febrile seizures are seen in 9 percent of the affected individuals and in 30 percent of other family members. Migraine with and without aura occurs in about one-third of all PKD cases and in two-thirds of their family members. Other neurological abnormalities include writer's cramp, essential tremor, and myoclonus [Bruno et al., 2004; Margari et al., 2005].

Differential diagnoses depend on age of onset of the symptoms. These include other forms of paroxysmal dyskinesias, dopa-responsive dystonia, complex motor tics, complex motor stereotypies, seizure, pseudoseizure, psychogenic movement disorder, malingering, shuddering attacks, and Sydenham's chorea. Complex motor stereotypies in younger children are sometimes difficult to distinguish from PKD or PNKD. Excitement precipitating the complex movement pattern and involvement of predominantly the upper limbs or upper part of the body in a child with autistic behaviors or cognitive impairment is suggestive of a complex motor stereotypy rather than PKD. Dopa-responsive dystonia can be distinguished clinically by the predominant involvement of the lower limbs and a diurnal variation, with worsening in the evening. Chorea in Sydenham's chorea may start unilaterally and intermittently on attempted activity, but the preceding history of sore throat, laboratory evidence of streptococcal infection, and self-limiting course of the disorder help in making the diagnosis. The distinguishing features of various types of paroxysmal dyskinesias are shown in Table 65-1. Increased awareness of PKD among clinicians is needed, as the diagnosis is delayed in most cases. The mean time from first seeking medical attention to confirmation of diagnosis is approximately 5 years [Bruno et al., 2004]. Proposed diagnostic criteria for PKD are shown in Box 65-7 [Bruno et al., 2004].

Despite the existence of several PKD gene loci found through linkage studies, no PKD gene has been identified so far. A form of autosomal-dominant PKD with episodic ataxia and spasticity has been mapped at chromosome 1p [Auburger et al., 1996]. ICCA, or ICCA-like syndromes, has been mapped to the pericentromeric region of chromosome 16 (16p12–q12). This involves the *PKC1* or *EKD1* gene locus [Tomita et al., 1999; Swoboda et al., 2000; Bennett et al., 2000; Rochette et al., 2008]. Another locus (*EKD 2*) has been identified on the same

chromosome in an Indian family with PKD [Valente et al., 2000].

Neurophysiology and neuroimaging studies are normal in familial and sporadic idiopathic cases, except for occasional slowing noted on the EEG [Buruma and Roos, 1986]. No epileptiform activity is usually seen, even during an episode. Nevertheless, reports of epilepsy among members of the same family raise the question about the possible association between these disorders [Demirkiran and Jankovic, 1995; Margari et al., 2000, 2002; Rochette et al., 2008]. Lombroso demonstrated ictal discharges emanating from the supplementary sensorimotor cortex and ipsilateral caudate nucleus by invasive long-term monitoring in a female with paroxysmal kinesigenic choreoathetosis [Lombroso, 1995]. Thus, some authors believe that these paroxysmal movement disorders are an expression of subcortical seizures involving cortico-striato-thalamo-cortical circuits [Tan et al., 1998]. The pathology in this circuit underlies the pathophysiology of most

---

Box 65-7 Proposed Diagnostic Criteria for Paroxysmal Kinesigenic Dyskinesia

- Identified kinesigenic trigger for the attacks
- Short duration of the attacks (<1 min)
- No loss of consciousness or pain during attacks
- Exclusion of other organic diseases and normal neurological examination
- Control of attacks with phenytoin or carbamazepine, if tried
- Age of onset between 1 and 20 years, if no family history of paroxysmal kinesigenic dyskinesia

---

Table 65-1 Differential Diagnoses of Various Types of Paroxysmal Dyskinesia

Features	PKD	PNKD MR1+	PNKD MR1−	PED	PHD
Nomenclature	PKC	PDC, FPC	PDC, FPC	PEDt	ADNFLE
Inheritance	AD – 16q	AD – 2q35	AD – 2q13	AD/AR	AD – 20q13, 15q24, 1q21, 8p21
Age of onset (years)	1–20	<1–12	1–23	Usually childhood	Usually childhood
Triggers	Sudden whole-body movement	Coffee, alcohol, stress	Exercise	After 10–15 minutes of exercise	Sleep
Clinical features	Chorea, athetosis, ballismus, dystonia	Chorea, athetosis, dystonia, ballismus	Chorea, athetosis, dystonia, ballismus	Mainly leg dystonia	Wakes up with dystonic posture
Usual duration	<1–5 min	10 min to 1 hr	10 min to 2–3 h	10–15 min	<1 min
Frequency	1–20/day	1/week	1/week	Unclear	Several/night
Associations	Infantile seizures, migraine, writer's cramp, essential tremor	Migraine	Epilepsy	RE-PED-WC	
Medication	Carbamazepine Phenytoin Oxcarbazepine	CLN (clonazepam) Benzodiazepine	CLN (clonazepam) Benzodiazepine	Acetazolamide L-DOPA	Carbamazepine Oxcarbazepine
Prognosis	Excellent	Excellent, worse than PKD	Minimally worse than PNKD MR1+	Poor medication response	Excellent

AD, autosomal-dominant; ADNFLE, autosomal-dominant nocturnal frontal lobe epilepsy; AR, autosomal-recessive; MR1+, myofibrillogenesis regulator 1 positive; MR1−, myofibrillogenesis regulator 1 negative; PDC, paroxysmal dystonic choreoathetosis; PED, paroxysmal exercise-induced dyskinesia; PEDt, paroxysmal exercise-induced dystonia; PHD, paroxysmal hypnogenic dyskinesia; PKC, paroxysmal kinesigenic choreoathetosis; PKD, paroxysmal kinesigenic dyskinesia; PNKD, paroxysmal nonkinesigenic dyskinesia; RE–PED–WC, rolandic epilepsy–paroxysmal exercise-induced dystonia–writer's cramp.

movement disorders in general. In primary (idiopathic or genetic) movement disorders, there is no detectable pathology on MRI of the brain, whereas in secondary or symptomatic cases there is involvement of basal ganglia or thalamus, with or without cortical involvement. Electromyography shows doublet or triplet discharges. Somatosensory-evoked potential (SSEP) shows reduction in amplitude of cortical sensory response. Motor-evoked potential, however, shows an increased motor cortical excitability with diminished stimulation threshold, high amplitude, and motor facilitation. Spinal and brainstem reflexes, like H reflex and blink reflex, suggest lack of inhibition. This phenomenon has led to the alternate hypothesis of spinal or brainstem modulation of central motor activity, producing paroxysmal dyskinesias [Lee et al., 1999].

Once diagnosed, there are only a few neurological disorders with a more satisfying treatment response, with an exquisite sensitivity to antiepileptic medications [Wein et al., 1996]. The attacks can be prevented, even with subtherapeutic levels of phenytoin or carbamazepine. Other medications found to be effective, but to a lesser degree, are barbiturates, benzodiazepines, valproate, lamotrigine, levetiracetam, scopolamine, L-DOPA, belladonna, chlordiazepoxide, and diphenhydramine [Lance, 1977; Kinast et al., 1980; Bruno et al., 2004]. Most children tried with other medication were eventually switched back to either phenytoin or carbamazepine. In a recent report, oxcarbazepine worked very well in four children with PKD [Chillag and Deroos, 2009]. This marked sensitivity to antiepileptic medications has been used to differentiate paroxysmal kinesigenic dyskinesia from the nonkinesigenic type. Whether treated or not, the attack frequency generally decreases with increasing age. More than one-quarter of patients enjoy complete remission by age 20 years, and a further quarter have marked reduction in attack frequency. Females in the idiopathic category have the best prognosis [Bruno et al., 2004].

Paroxysmal Nonkinesigenic Dyskinesia

PNKD is characterized by episodes of dystonia and/or choreoathetosis involving the face, trunk, and extremities, often associated with dysarthria and dysphasia, lasting from minutes to several hours and occurring up to several times a week [Pryles et al., 1952; Lance, 1977; Tibbles and Barnes, 1980; Kinast et al., 1980; Bressman et al., 1988; Demirkiran and Jankovic, 1995]. Historically, in 1940, Mount and Reback reported the first family with PNKD, labeling them as cases of "familial paroxysmal choreoathetosis" [Mount and Reback, 1940]. Various eponyms have been used to describe this condition but, due to overlapping semiologic features, the term paroxysmal nonkinesigenic dyskinesia is preferred. Proposed diagnostic criteria for PNKD are indicated in Box 65-8.

Mutations of the myofibrillogenesis regulator 1 (MR-1) gene (also known as the PNKD1 gene) form a distinct homogenous subset of PNKD [Bruno et al., 2007]. Onset is usually in infancy or early childhood, with a mean of 4 years, but late onset has been reported. This is in contradistinction to the MR-1 gene-negative group, which has a later age of onset with a mean of 12 ± 10.8 years. The attacks begin spontaneously at rest or after intake of caffeine or alcohol. Alcohol and caffeine sensitivity is noted in almost 100 percent of MR-1 gene-positive cases, which is distinctly uncommon in the other group. Stress is another common precipitating factor that occurs in more than 80 percent of the MR-1 gene-positive group. Other

> ### Box 65-8 Proposed Diagnostic Criteria for Paroxysmal Nonkinesigenic Dyskinesia in the *MR*1 Gene Mutation-Positive Group
>
> - Hyperkinetic involuntary movement attacks, with dystonia, chorea, or combination of these, typically lasting 10 minutes to 1 hour, but up to 4 hours
> - Normal neurologic examination results between attacks, and exclusion of secondary causes
> - Onset of attack in infancy or early childhood
> - Precipitation of attacks by caffeine and alcohol consumption
> - Family history of movement disorder meeting above criteria

precipitating factors include fatigue, hunger, chocolate, and excitement. Exercise has been noted to bring on the majority of the attacks in MR-1 gene-negative cases, implicating more heterogeneity in these patients and causing confusion with some cases of paroxysmal exercise-induced dyskinesia. An aura, consisting of focal limb stiffening, twitching, numbness, a generalized "funny feeling," or lightheadedness, has been noted [Williams and Stevens, 1963; Bruno et al., 2007]. About 12 percent present only with dystonia, and the rest with a combination of dystonia and chorea in the MR-1 gene-positive cases, whereas the other group may have dystonia, chorea, a combination of both, and ballism as part of the clinical manifestations. Almost half may have speech involvement. Typical attack duration is 10 minutes to 1 hour, but may last up to 12 hours. Attack frequency is highly variable, but 86 percent have at least one attack every week.

Clonazepam and diazepam are the most effective preventive and abortive agents in 97 percent of cases studied by Bruno et al. [Bruno et al., 2007]. Sleep benefit is also noted in the majority of cases [Byrne et al., 1991; Bruno et al., 2007]. The MR-1-negative group, however, did not have sustained benefit from clonazepam in at least half of the cases treated. Other antiepileptic medications, including valproate, carbamazepine, topiramate, and gabapentin, proved partially beneficial for MR-1-negative patients, but MR-1-positive patients did not respond well. L-DOPA, acetazolamide, and haloperidol did not help either group.

Prognosis is not as good as in PKD; however, almost two-thirds of the mutation-positive group improved with age, with only a minority (18 percent) becoming worse. The prognosis in the mutation-negative group is a little worse than in the mutation-positive group. Migraine is coexistent in 47 percent of cases in the MR-1-positive cases, whereas seizures are reported in 23 percent of the MR-1-negative cases [Kinast et al., 1980; Przuntek and Monninger, 1983; Bruno et al., 2007].

PNKD follows an autosomal-dominant transmission pattern, with almost equal sex distribution. The majority of familial PNKD are caused by the mutation of the MR-1 gene on chromosome 2q35 [Fouad et al., 1996; Fink et al., 1996; Jarman et al., 1997; Raskind et al., 1998]. Recently, linkage studies in a Canadian family with European descent identified a second locus at the 2q31 region [Spacey et al., 2006]. The MR-1 gene is not involved in the ion channel, contrary to previous postulations; rather, it works in the stress response pathway. Although the exact function of MR-1 is unknown, its gene product is homologous to the hydroxyacylglutathione hydrolase (HAGH) of the glyoxalase system. HAGH catalyzes the final step in conversion of methylglyoxal (a byproduct of glycolysis, also found in coffee and alcoholic beverages) to lactic acid and reduced glutathione. This relationship explains the exquisite sensitivity to coffee and alcohol in attack precipitation; emotional stress may also act in a similar manner [Lee et al., 2004; Rainier et al., 2004; Chen et al. 2005a; Hempelmann et al., 2006; Bruno et al., 2007]. Mutations in voltage-gated neuronal K$^+$ channel K$_v$7 (KCNQ) has been shown to produce dyskinesia in dt^{sz} mutant hamster model of PNKD [Richter et al., 2006]. In some patients with coexistent generalized epilepsy and PNKD, a mutation in the alpha subunit of the calcium-sensitive potassium channel (BK channel) located on chromosome 10q22 has been discovered [Du et al., 2005].

Paroxysmal Exercise-Induced Dyskinesia

This interesting autosomal-dominant disorder is not as common or well understood as the others. No specific genetic defect has yet been found. Children or young adults with otherwise normal health develop dystonic posturing, with or without pain, after a prolonged period of exercise, usually more than 10–15 minutes. Fasting and stress can bring on the attacks. The attack may last 10–30 minutes and usually involves the limb/s being used in exercise. Association with absence or complex partial seizures has been described [Plant et al., 1984; Munchau et al., 2000]. In a Sardinian family with rolandic epilepsy, paroxysmal exertional dyskinesia, and writer's cramp, and showing an autosomal-recessive pattern of inheritance, the disorder has been has been mapped to 16p12–11.2, which overlaps the ICCA locus [Guerrini et al., 1999]. Linkage of one family pedigree with typical PED was not established to the PNKD or ICCA loci [Munchau et al., 2000]. PED cases may represent a variant of either PKD or PNKD where there is precipitation by exercise. Cases of dopa-responsive dystonias may pose a great challenge in differential diagnosis when the lower limbs are primarily involved; however, the excellent response to L-DOPA in dopa-responsive dystonias, along with gene testing, should clarify that doubt. The responses to medication in PED are modest at best; drugs used have included acetazolamide, L-DOPA, and trihexyphenidyl.

Dopa-Responsive Dystonia

Only a few disorders in the practice of pediatric neurology provide the opportunity to reverse a disabling condition in the dramatic manner afforded by dopa-responsive dystonia (DRD). The condition was first reported by Segawa in 1971, with an autosomal-dominant mode of inheritance [Segawa et al., 1986]. The estimated prevalence in England and Japan is 0.5 per million [Nygaard, 1993]. The onset is between 1 and 9 years of age (average 5 years). Females outnumber males by 3–4:1. Symptoms usually start with unilateral leg or foot dystonia, precipitated by actions such as walking or running, and improvement with rest. The most characteristic feature is the diurnal variation of the dystonia, which worsens in the evening and improves markedly in the morning. Sleep acts as the most important relieving factor. Classically, the dystonia starts with one foot, spreading to affect the whole of the ipsilateral lower limb. It then spreads to the ipsilateral upper limb, contralateral lower limb, and, finally, the contralateral upper limb, following the pattern of the letter N. The last area involved is the craniocervical region. Involvement spreading

from one lower limb to the other and, finally, involving upper limbs and craniocervical region may occur. It may take 5–6 years from the onset for the dystonia to be generalized [Segawa et al., 1986; Trender-Gerhard et al., 2009]. The periodicity, action induction, fatigability, asymmetry, and diurnal variation may not be very prominent with advancing disease pathology. This is an important point to consider in the history. Dystonic posturing of the big toe (striatal toe) may mimic an upgoing plantar (Babinski) response [Iivanainen and Kaakkola, 1993]. Features of parkinsonism, such as rigidity, bradykinesia, postural instability, action or postural tremor of the arms, and, rarely, a resting tremor, may eventually develop in some cases [Nygaard et al., 1994]. The presence of rigidity and dystonia in the lower limbs may mimic a spastic diplegic form of cerebral palsy, resulting in misdiagnosis. If in doubt, a trial of L-DOPA usually results in dramatic improvement. It is worth noting that the improvement is expected, even if this condition is diagnosed very late. There is a need for a high index of suspicion on the part of the clinician to think about this disease in the clinical context and consider a trial of L-DOPA [Nygaard et al., 1994; Segawa, 2000; Segawa et al., 2003]. Less frequently, DRD may be inherited in an autosomal-recessive fashion with much younger age of onset, but retaining all the other characteristics of the above description. Dystonia as the predominant clinical entity represents the "pure form" of DRD. In a subset of children, often referred to as having DRD plus syndrome, seizures, developmental delay, other dyskinesias, tremor, chorea, and oculogyric phenomena may occur [Schiller et al., 2004; Clot et al., 2009].

Neuroimaging studies are typically normal. PET studies have been normal in most cases [Snow et al., 1993]. Pathologically, there is no cell degeneration in the nigrostriatal dopaminergic system. There is inadequate dopamine synthesis in the striatum secondary to dysfunction of the enzyme tyrosine hydroxylase, either as a primary deficiency or secondary to a lack of the co-factor tetrahydrobiopterin (BH4). There is reduction of the dopamine metabolite homovanillic acid (HVA) in the cerebrospinal fluid. BH4 acts as essential co-factor for tyrosine, phenylalanine, and tryptophan hydroxylases. Defect in the biosynthetic pathway of BH4 causes a reduction of dopamine and serotonin (5-hydroxytryptamine) metabolites, HVA, and 5-hydroxy indole acetic acid (5-HIAA), respectively [Nygaard, 1995]. Neuropathologic data in one case demonstrated marked reduction of dopamine levels in the substantia nigra and in the striatum [Rajput et al., 1994].

Autosomal-dominant DRD is caused by mutations in the GCH1 gene on chromosome 14 (14q22.1–q22.2), which encodes the enzyme guanosine triphosphate cyclohydrolase 1 (GTPCH-1) in the BH4 biosynthetic pathway [Furukawa et al., 1995; Tanaka et al., 1995; Segawa, 2000; Segawa et al., 2003; Clot et al., 2009]. Autosomal-recessive DRD may be secondary to tyrosine hydroxylase (TH) gene mutation. Tyrosine hydroxylase deficiency is associated with a broader phenotype than just a dopa-responsive dystonia and gait disorder, and includes a more severe infantile parkinsonism or progressive infantile encephalopathy phenotype. DRD plus disorders may be due to sepiapterin reductase gene mutation or other defects in the BH4 biosynthesis pathway.

The response to treatment with L-DOPA in typical cases of DRD is dramatic. Fatigability is usually alleviated within a week, and dystonia within 6 weeks of optimum dose. A combination of L-DOPA and dopa decarboxylase inhibitor should be used. Preparations with a higher ratio of dopa decarboxylase inhibitor, e.g., carbidopa-L-DOPA 25–100 mg, are generally preferred to the 10–100 mg preparation. Young adolescents, more particularly females, have much higher dopa decarboxylase activity, thus requiring a higher dose of carbidopa. A dose of 5 mg/kg/day of carbidopa-L-DOPA is effective in most cases. The medication is generally well tolerated and the effect sustained, even after prolonged use of 30 years [Segawa et al., 1986]. The reason for the lack of any significant side effect is the paucity of dopamine synthesis in this condition with preserved structure of the nigrostriatal system with no cell damage or death. The use of L-DOPA is, therefore, the equivalent of supplementing dopamine in the deficient state.

Dopa-responsive dystonia is also described in Chapter 68.

Episodic Ataxias

The episodic ataxias (EA) are a group of autosomal-dominant disorders characterized by recurrent episodes of cerebellar ataxia, vertigo, dysarthria, and nystagmus, starting in childhood and lasting for minutes or hours, with otherwise normal brain functions. Although patients are asymptomatic between attacks, neurologic examination may reveal ocular abnormalities, including downbeating or gaze-evoked nystagmus, abnormal optokinetic nystagmus, hypermetric saccades, saccadic pursuit, or myokymia [Van Dyke et al., 1975; Jen et al., 2004]. Two main forms are recognized: episodic ataxia type 1 (EA1) and type 2 (EA2). The number of identified EA phenotypes and genotypes is, however, expanding, and is now up to seven (EA7). These disorders share some common features: namely, all are channelopathies, with autosomal-dominant inheritance pattern, and are responsive to acetazolamide. Some show spontaneous improvement with advancing age [Rajakulendran et al., 2007; Strupp et al., 2007; Jen et al., 2007]. The differential diagnoses include episodic neurological disorders, such as epilepsy, paroxysmal dyskinesia, and migraine. To make things more complicated, these disorders may frequently coexist in the same patient. Some metabolic disorders, like Hartnup's disease, organic aciduria, and mitochondrial cytopathies, may present with intermittent or episodic ataxia.

Episodic Ataxia Type 1

Historically, EA1 was first described by Van Dyke et al. in 1975 in 11 members spanning three generations of a family that had periodic ataxia and continuous muscle movement [Van Dyke et al., 1975]. Children with EA1 have brief attacks of truncal and limb ataxia, coarse tremor, and titubation lasting seconds to minutes, starting in the first or second decade. The attacks may be associated with nausea, vomiting, dysarthria, or nystagmus. They may have visual symptoms of oscillopsia and visual blurring. The frequency is highly variable, varying from multiple times a day to only a few times a year. Physical exertion, emotional stress, startles, and sudden change in posture may bring on the attacks. Brain MRI scan is normal. Rest and sleep may abort an acute attack. The attack frequency decreases with age. One diagnostic clinical feature is the nearly constant presence of continuous muscle activity, either in a rippling pattern of myokymia, or as neuromyotonia. Myokymia may involve eyelids, facial muscles, or the muscles acting on the fingers. This feature, a manifestation of peripheral nerve hyperexcitability, is present almost all the time, irrespective of the ataxic spell. If it is clinically absent, electromyography invariably shows the changes of myokymia, with or without grouped discharges of doublet, triplet, and multiplets [Hanson et al., 1977]. In some cases, mild ischemia in the muscle tested may bring on the myokymic discharges [Lubbers et al., 1995]. Seizures are seen more commonly in these patients [Brunt and van Weerden, 1990]. Seizures are ten times more common in patients with EA1 compared to the general population [Zuberi et al., 1999].

Early genetic linkage studies mapped the EA1 locus to chromosome 12p13, and studies later confirmed a mutation of the *KCNA1* gene encoding the voltage-gated potassium channel subunit Kvα1.1. This leads to a reduction in potassium permeability that results in prolongation of the action potential and failure to repolarize, thus producing repetitive myokymic discharges [Benatar, 2000]. The pathogenesis of cerebellar ataxia may be related to hyperactivity of the gamma-aminobutyric acid (GABA)ergic basket cell inhibition over cerebellar Purkinje cells [Zhang et al., 1999]. The other pathogenesis is spreading acidification in cerebellar cortex [Chen et al., 2005b]. *KCNA1* gene mutation in the knockout mouse model has been shown to have epilepsy, thus leading to the postulation that *KCNA1* gene mutation may be a susceptibility factor for epilepsy in humans [Smart et al., 1998].

Acetazolamide, a carbonic anhydrase inhibitor, is effective in reducing the frequency of ataxic episodes in some patients. The starting dose is 125–250 mg daily and can be slowly increased to a maximum of 500 mg twice daily. Mechanism of action is postulated to be through increasing pH in the vicinity of the ion channel, causing hyperpolarization of the cell membrane and thus reducing neuronal hyperexcitability. Common side effects include tingling, numbness, altered taste, and some impairment of concentration and memory. One bothersome side effect is renal stones, which can be prevented with proper hydration and drinking citrus juice or potassium chloride [Griggs et al., 1978; Lubbers et al., 1995]. Some patients not responding to acetazolamide may respond to antiepileptic medications, such as carbamazepine, phenytoin, valproic acid, or phenobarbital [Eunson et al., 2000; Klein et al., 2004].

Episodic Ataxia Type 2

EA2 is the most common of all episodic ataxias. The ataxic symptoms start in early childhood. Though ataxic symptoms are the same as in EA1, several features distinguish this condition. The duration of each attack is more prolonged, is measured in hours to days, and is more commonly associated with nausea, vomiting, and vertigo. The attack frequency varies from daily to once a year. These attacks are provoked by exertion, stress, intercurrent illness, or alcohol, and never by sudden movement (common in EA1). More than half have migraine headache during the attack; familial hemiplegic migraine is an allelic disorder coexisting with EA2 at times. Myokymia is not a feature. Interictally, more than 90 percent of patients usually manifest downbeating nystagmus. Weakness during, or preceding, the attack is well described in EA2 secondary to a myasthenic phenomenon due to impaired neuromuscular transmission. Patients with EA2 may develop progressive cerebellar ataxia with time [Baloh et al., 1997; Jankovic and Demirkiran, 2002; Jen et al., 2004], and brain MRI scan often demonstrates anterosuperior vermian cerebellar atrophy [Vighetto et al., 1988]. Decreased phosphate, reduced creatine, increased pH, and high lactate in the cerebellum are the hallmarks on MR spectroscopy [Bain et al., 1992; Harno et al., 2005]. Intermittent rhythmic delta activity, sometimes associated with low-amplitude spikes resulting in irregular spike-and-wave patterns, has been reported in EEG studies [Van Bogaert and Szliwowski, 1996]. Vestibular migraine is the closest differential diagnosis, where vertigo is the predominant symptom and ataxia is typically of a vestibular type (rather than cerebellar type). The associated nystagmus is also of a vestibular type and not downbeating, as is classical for EA2. Peripheral vestibular deficits can be seen in up to 20 percent of cases of vestibular migraine [Jen et al., 2004; Brandt and Strupp, 2006].

The responsible gene has been mapped to the short arm of chromosome 19 [von Brederlow et al., 1995]. Localization of the gene responsible for familial hemiplegic migraine also mapped to chromosome 19p, suggesting that these paroxysmal disorders were allelic [Joutel et al., 1993]. Subsequent studies showed that both EA2 and familial hemiplegic migraine are both associated with loss-of-function mutations in the gene *CACNA1A*, which encodes the alpha$_{1A}$ subunit of voltage-gated neuronal calcium channels located on chromosome 19p13 [Ophoff et al., 1996; Ducros et al., 2001]. This gene encodes the Ca$_v$2.1 subunit of the P/Q-type calcium channel, which acts as the voltage sensor and ion-conducting pore [Shapiro et al., 2001].

Approximately 50–75 percent of all patients with EA2 are responsive to treatment with acetazolamide, regarding both the frequency and the severity of the attacks. Favorable response has been sustained for up to 5 years [Griggs et al., 1978]. The mechanism of action is by alteration of intracellular pH. The attacks are precipitated by high intracellular pH values, precipitated by exercise and stress through hyperventilation and consequent alkalosis [Bain et al., 1992]. Acetazolamide lowers the intracellular pH, which in turn reduces potassium conductance and thereby restores excitability and resting activity of the neurons [Shapiro et al., 2001]. Starting dose is usually 250 mg a day, increasing gradually to a maximum of 1000 mg per day. Sulthiame, another carbonic anhydrase inhibitor, has also been used successfully. It causes fewer side effects, and is most effective in dosages between 50 and 300 mg per day [Brunt and van Weerden, 1990]. Acetazolamide is, however, the choice of treatment. For those who are allergic, intolerant, or unresponsive to acetazolamide, an alternative treatment to consider is 4-aminopyridine (4AP), a potassium channel blocker. At a dose of 5 mg three times a day, 4AP has been shown to be beneficial [Strupp et al., 2004]. Similarly, 3,4 diamino pyridine (DAP) has been shown to improve the downbeating nystagmus often observed with EA2 [Strupp et al., 2003]. The loss-of-function mutations in EA2 lead to the reduction of calcium-dependent neurotransmitter GABA release in Purkinje cells. Aminopyridines increase the release of GABA in the cerebellar Purkinje cells. Increase in excitability of Purkinje cell and the prolongation of the action potential duration by blocking potassium channels have been proven in animal studies [Shapiro et al., 2001; Etzion and Grossman, 2001].

Other Types of Episodic Ataxias

Other types of episodic ataxias are much rarer. EA3 was described in a large Canadian family with episodic vertigo, tinnitus, and ataxia, linked to chromosome 1q42. These patients are normal in between attacks [Steckley et al., 2001; Cader et al., 2005]. EA4 is described in two kindreds from North Carolina with late-onset episodic vertigo and ataxia with persistent interictal nystagmus not responsive to acetazolamide. No gene locus has been detected yet [Farmer and Mustian, 1963; Small et al., 1996]. The EA cases with mutation in the *CACNB4* gene, encoding the beta$_4$ subunit of the P/Q-type voltage-gated calcium channel, have been designated as EA5 [Escayg et al., 2000]. EA6 was first observed in a child with episodic attacks of hemiplegia and migraine in a setting of fever and epilepsy. A mutation in the *SLC1A3* gene encoding glial glutamate transporter, *EAAT1*, has been found [Jen et al., 2005]. A family with EA, triggered by exertion and excitement lasting hours to days, and associated with weakness, vertigo, and slurred speech, mapped to chromosome 19q13, has been designated as EA7 [Kerber et al., 2007].

Childhood Periodic Syndromes

The childhood periodic syndromes include a diverse group of disorders, which have at their core periodic or paroxysmal occurrences with a return to normal baseline functioning and symptom-free interval between attacks. They are believed to be precursors to migraine and are classified as such by the International Classification of Headache Disorders, Second Edition [Headache Classification Committee, 2004]. The term childhood periodic syndromes was first used by Wylie and Schlesinger in 1933 [Wyllie and Schlesinger, 1933] and has gained increasing acceptance in the past decade [Winner, 2005; Cuvellier and Lepine, 2010]. Sometimes referred to as "migraine equivalents," it includes benign paroxysmal vertigo, benign paroxysmal torticollis, and cyclic vomiting syndrome, which are discussed below.

Benign Paroxysmal Vertigo

Benign paroxysmal vertigo (BPV) in childhood is a paroxysmal, nonepileptic event first described by Basser in 1964 [Basser, 1964]. The syndrome is characterized by vertigo of sudden onset lasting seconds to minutes, an inability to maintain posture, stance, or gait without support, and no change in sensorium. The child is usually pale and scared. Nystagmus, vomiting, and diffuse sweating may occur but are uncommon [Fenichel, 1967; Koenigsberger et al., 1968; Dunn and Snyder, 1976; Eeg-Olofsson et al., 1982; Drigo et al., 2001]. The paroxysms tend to be stereotypic and the frequency is variable, ranging from several times a week to once a year. Recovery is rapid and complete. Specific trigger factors are uncommon. BPV is easily overlooked due to its benign, paroxysmal, and transient nature, coupled with the difficulty that a young child has in describing vertiginous sensations. Onset is usually under 4 years of age [Eeg-Olofsson et al., 1982; Drigo et al., 2001], but later age of onset has been described [Abu-Arafeh and Russell, 1995b; Mira et al., 1984b; Mierzwinski et al., 2007]. The episodes gradually abate over months to years. Prevalence data are poor; one population study estimated the prevalence rate at 2.6 percent [Abu-Arafeh, Russell, 1995b], although the population characteristics were not typical for BPV. The neurological examination between spells is normal.

Etiology is unknown but thought to involve the central or peripheral vestibular system. This is supported, in part, by the presence of nystagmus during the acute attack [Eeg-Olofsson et al., 1982]. Normal hearing and caloric test would suggest that central vestibular pathways are more likely to be affected than the peripheral part of the vestibular nerve or inner ear [Mira et al., 1984a; Finkelhor and Harker, 1987]; earlier studies, however, reported abnormal caloric and rotational tests [Basser, 1964; Koenigsberger et al., 1968; Dunn and Snyder, 1976]. A relationship between BPV and migraine has been suggested [Fenichel, 1967; Koehler, 1980; Mira et al., 1984a; Lanzi et al., 1994; Abu-Arafeh and Russell, 1995b], and BPV is often considered a precursor to migraine headaches later on in life. There is a greater prevalence of migraine in BPV patients (24 versus 10.6 percent), and of BPV in migraine sufferers (8.8 versus 2.6 percent), than controls [Abu-Arafeh and Russell, 1995b]. Basilar artery migraine may present with similar symptoms [Golden and French, 1975; Lempert et al., 2009], suggesting a possible vascular basis for the symptoms [Basser, 1964; Fenichel, 1967; Perez Plasencia et al., 1998].

Benign paroxysmal torticollis (BPT) appears to be related to BPV and sometimes precedes it. First described by Snyder in 1969 [Snyder, 1969], the spells tend to occur at a slightly younger age (2–8 months) and are paroxysmal, but may last minutes to days. Spells begin with a sudden onset of torticollis with tilting of the head to one side and rotation of the chin to the opposite side. This may occasionally be accompanied by torsion or dystonia of the trunk or pelvis [Chutorian, 1974]. The frequency and duration of the episodes decline as the child gets older. A number of children will subsequently go on to develop BPV [Dunn and Snyder, 1976; Eeg-Olofsson et al., 1982; Lindskog et al., 1999]. Linkage to the *CACNA1A* gene has been described in four children [Giffin et al., 2002], but for the most part, BPT is also considered a migraine equivalent. This is discussed in more detail in the next section.

The diagnosis of BPV is based on a characteristic history and normal neurological events, but certain differential diagnoses should be considered. The most common differential diagnosis is epilepsy, especially temporal lobe epilepsy, but the brief nature of the spells, their occurrence only in the awake state, and lack of any change in sensorium should all help to differentiate BPV from seizure. Other differential diagnostic considerations include posterior fossa tumors (these usually have other neurological signs and symptoms) and acute vestibular neuronitis (which tends to occur more commonly in adults, is invariably associated with nystagmus, and lasts days to weeks rather than seconds). Ménière's disease is rare in childhood and is usually associated with tinnitus and hearing loss. BPV is differentiated by the postural nature of this syndrome, which precipitates vertigo and nystagmus. The typical age of onset of BPV would make a functional disorder unlikely, although this should be considered in older children [Mierzwinski et al., 2007].

Treatment is reassurance for the family and child that the disorder is completely benign and resolves with time. Meclizine hydrochloride and dimenhydrate have been used with variable success when spells are unusually frequent or severe.

Benign Paroxysmal Torticollis of Infancy

Involuntary twisting of the neck (wryneck or torticollis), with abnormal head positioning, followed by subsequent spontaneous resolution, is characteristic of BPT of infancy. Usual age of onset is the first 6 months of life. The condition may involve either side of the neck, and the side may alternate between spells. In addition to the torticollis, the affected child may develop a pelvic tilt (tortipelvis) or retrocollis [Chutorian, 1974; Rosman et al., 2009]. The episodes may last from 10 minutes

to 30 days (average about 5 days), and may recur every 7 days to 5 months (mean 37 days). The abnormal neck posturing may persist during sleep, which goes against the dystonic theory as to the possible underlying mechanism of BPT [Snyder, 1969; Drigo et al., 2000; Rosman et al., 2009]. An attack may be anticipated by the onset of irritability, distress, or vomiting [Chaves-Carballo, 1996]. There may be associated vertigo, ataxia, pallor, apathy, and gaze abnormalities during an acute attack. Some children are found to have motor developmental delay. The episodes spontaneously remit in most children by 2–3 years of age without treatment. There are few cases of familial occurrence [Gilbert, 1977; Lipson and Robertson, 1978]. Since the original description of BPT by Snyder more than 40 years ago [Snyder, 1969], there have been a further 23 reports of 113 cases described in the medical literature that conform to the features as outlined above [Sanner and Bergstrom, 1979; Hanukoglu et al., 1984; Bratt and Menelaus, 1992; Cataltepe and Barron, 1993; Cohen et al., 1993; Rosman et al., 2009].

The pathophysiology of BPT is subject to speculation. The observation, in some cases, of eye rolling or deviation suggests labyrinthine involvement. Abnormal oculovestibular function was found in 9 of 12 cases [Snyder, 1969], but not reproduced by future studies. Others believe that BPT is a forerunner of migraine, and it is thus considered as migraine equivalent. Evidence supporting this hypothesis includes:
1. a high percentage of family history of migraine (30–90 percent of cases)
2. associated pallor and vomiting
3. future onset of migraine headache or motion sickness in children after the disappearance of paroxysmal torticollis
4. later occurrence of BPV or cyclic vomiting syndrome in some cases on follow-up [Dunn and Snyder, 1976; Deonna and Martin, 1981; Eviatar, 1994; Giffin et al., 2002].

Another theory involves an ion-channel disorder, since two patients in a kindred with familial hemiplegic migraine linked to the *CACNA1A* gene initially presented with BPT [Giffin et al., 2002].

The differential diagnosis includes seizures, vertigo, gastroesophageal reflux, diaphragmatic hernia (Sandifer's syndrome), dystonia, posterior fossa mass, and craniocervical junction abnormalities (basilar impression, platybasia, atlantoaxial instability, Chiari malformation, and Klippel–Feil syndrome). Vestibular testing may be difficult to perform and interpret in young children. Brainstem auditory-evoked potentials may be of interest because hearing impairment may be an associated finding. Neuroimaging studies are necessary to exclude congenital and acquired lesions involving the craniocervical region.

Treatment with diphenhydramine, meclizine, and chlorpromazine has not been successful [Snyder, 1969; Rosman et al., 2009]. The prognosis, however, is excellent, with complete disappearance of torticollis in almost 100 percent of cases by 3 years of age. Motor developmental delay, found in some cases, also improves with time [Dunn and Snyder, 1976; Drigo et al., 2000; Rosman et al., 2009].

Benign paroxysmal torticollis is also described in Chapter 68.

Cyclic Vomiting Syndrome

Cyclic vomiting syndrome (CVS) is a chronic, disabling disorder characterized by "recurrent, discrete, self-limited episodes of vomiting and is defined by symptom-based criteria and the absence of positive laboratory, radiographic, and endoscopic testing" [Li et al., 2008]. First described in the British literature by Gee in 1882 [Gee, 1882], the prevalence has been estimated at 1.9 percent in community-based studies [Abu-Arafeh and Russell, 1995a]. In an Irish study, the incidence was 3.15 per 100,000 children per year, with a median age of onset of symptoms of 4 years (range 0–14 years) [Fitzpatrick et al., 2008]. Onset is typically in early childhood; however, onset in infancy and adults also occurs [Prakash and Clouse, 1999; Fleisher et al., 2005]. Although the majority of cases abate by adolescence, about one-third of individuals continue to experience vomiting during their teenage years [Fleisher and Matar, 1993; Dignan et al., 2001; Fitzpatrick et al., 2007]. It is not known what percentage of persons continue with vomiting into adult life. A female predominance has been reported in CVS [Prakash et al., 2001; Li and Misiewicz, 2003]; however, in the population-based Irish study by Fitzpatrick et al., females accounted for only 49 percent of the cohort [Fitzpatrick et al., 2008].

In a consensus paper from the North American Society for Pediatric Gastroenterology, Hepatology, and Nutrition [Li et al., 2008], an operational definition of CVS was developed that stipulates inclusion of *all* of the following criteria for diagnosis:

- At least five attacks in any interval, or a minimum of three attacks during a 6-month period
- Episodic attacks of intense nausea and vomiting lasting 1 hour to 10 days, and occurring at least 1 week apart
- Stereotypical pattern and symptoms in the individual patient
- Vomiting during attacks that occurs at least four times an hour and lasts for at least 1 hour
- Return to baseline health between episodes
- Not attributed to another disorder.

The term cyclic vomiting syndrome plus (CVS+) has been used to describe a subset of children with CVS who have an underlying neuromuscular or neurological disorder [Boles et al., 2003]. In this group of children, the median age of onset of cyclic vomiting episodes was 4 years – 3 years younger than the children with CVS and no underlying neurological or neuromuscular disorders, suggesting a more severe phenotype [Boles et al., 2006]. Population studies, however, have suggested a similar median age of onset of cyclic vomiting episodes (see above). Maternal inheritance in many cases, mitochondrial DNA mutations in some, and biochemical markers of disturbed electron transport chain/energy metabolism (lactic acidosis, energy-depleted patterns on urine organic acid testing) initially raised the suggestion that CVS+ syndrome was a mitochondrial cytopathy [Boles and Williams, 1999; Wang et al., 2004]. Further analysis of this cohort, and comparisons to CVS children without associated neuromuscular or neurological features, concluded that mitochondrial DNA sequence-related mitochondrial dysfunction is a risk factor for disease development in CVS in general, and is not specific to the CVS+ group [Boles et al., 2005, 2006].

The etiology and pathophysiology of CVS is unknown. Since CVS shares certain characteristics with migraine headaches, it is sometimes referred to as a migraine variant. These characteristics include similar triggers and prodromal symptoms, recurrent, discrete episodes, vasomotor/autonomic changes, and responsiveness to antimigraine medication in CVS. It is one of the childhood periodic syndromes that is a common precursor to subsequent migraine. Migraine headaches have been reported in 11–38 percent of children with CVS [Fleisher and Matar, 1993; Symon and Russell, 1995]. The prevalence rate of migraine in children with CVS is twice that of the general childhood population (21 vs. 10.6 percent) [Abu-Arafeh and Russell, 1995a]. In approximately 22–27 percent of children with CVS, the condition transforms into more typical migraine headaches [Fleisher and Matar, 1993; Dignan et al., 2001; Stickler, 2005]. Mitochondrial dysfunction is felt to play a role in selected cases (see below). Autonomic dysregulation has been shown in a number of studies in children with CVS [Rashed et al., 1999; Chelimsky and Chelimsky, 2007], and sympathetic hyperresponsiveness has been postulated as a potential mechanism contributing to the CVS. The episodic nature and natural history of CVS have led some to postulate that CVS may represent an ion-channel disorder, despite the fact that it is not inherited in a simple mendelian fashion [Ptacek, 1999]. The corticotrophin-releasing factor (CRF) hypothesis proposes that CVS is precipitated by stimuli or factors associated with CRF release, and that the resultant endocrine, autonomic, and visceral changes are reminiscent of CRF activation in the paraventricular nucleus of the hypothalamus and dorsal vagal complex in the brain [Tache, 1999]. Central CRF has been shown to delay gastric emptying and stasis in animal studies [Tache, 1999].

Clinically, the attacks are explosive in onset, with recurrent severe bouts of emesis, retching, and nausea lasting hours to days. The vomiting is often bilious [Li et al., 2008], with a peak median intensity of six emeses per hour [Li, 2001]. Only half of the children with CVS have a "predictable" periodicity, typically every 2–4 weeks [Li, 2001]. Other symptoms include abdominal pain, diarrhea, anorexia, lethargy, pallor, headache, photophobia, and phonophobia [Li, 2001; Prakash et al., 2001; Li and Misiewicz, 2003; Fitzpatrick et al., 2008]. Low-grade fever may be present [Fleisher, 1995; Li, 2001]. The spells often occur in the early hours of the morning or upon waking, and they are frequently triggered by physical or psychological stress or excitement [Fleisher and Matar, 1993; Li et al., 2008]. Onset may be abrupt but a prodrome is reported in 22–38 percent of cases [Prakash et al., 2001; Fitzpatrick et al., 2008]. The paroxysms often end abruptly, much like the onset. For any particular child, the episodes tend to be stereotypical with respect to time of onset, duration, and symptoms. Intravenous hydration is often required [Prakash et al., 2001; Li and Misiewicz, 2003]. There is frequently a very long delay from disease onset to diagnosis [Prakash et al., 2001; Fitzpatrick et al., 2008]. Between episodes, children are completely well.

A family history of migraine in a first- and second-degree relative is common (35–56 percent) [Fleisher and Matar, 1993; Symon and Russell, 1995; Pfau et al., 1996; Stickler, 2005]; a figure of 20 percent was found in one population-based study [Fitzpatrick et al., 2008], although a family history of CVS is uncommon. There appears to be a high prevalence of anxiety and mood symptoms in children with CVS, as well as their parents [Forbes et al., 1999; Tarbell and Li, 2008].

Diagnosis relies on a careful history and exclusion of other serious underlying causes of vomiting. Vomiting in CVS tends to occur with a much higher intensity but lower frequency than other chronic vomiting disorders. There are no specific laboratory or neurophysiologic markers that lead to a diagnosis of CVS. Testing to exclude all of the possible differential diagnoses would subject many children to unnecessary and costly radiographic and endoscopic procedures [Li et al., 2008]. Expert consensus recommends that electrolytes, glucose, and upper gastrointestinal radiographs should be obtained in order to exclude malrotation in all children; in refractory cases, a renal ultrasound should also be performed to exclude transient hydronephrosis [Li et al., 2008]. These studies should preferably be carried out during an acute crisis, and blood work should be done prior to intravenous hydration. Abnormal neurological findings on examination, a history that suggests a possible underlying metabolic disorder (such as an association of the spells with fasting, illness, or certain food groups), or hypoglycemia on presentation warrant further diagnostic evaluation; this should include neuroimaging and testing for inborn errors of metabolism (fatty acid oxidation disorders, urea cycle defects, mitochondrial cytopathies, or amino/organic acidurias). The North American Society for Pediatric Gastroenterology, Hepatology, and Nutrition task force for CVS also recommends a neurometabolic work-up for children under the age of 2 with suspected CVS [Li et al., 2008]. Significant abdominal pain and tenderness, together with bilious vomiting and progressive worsening of symptoms, require further gastroenterology evaluation.

Differential diagnosis is extensive and includes both gastrointestinal and nongastrointestinal disorders. The most common gastrointestinal differential diagnosis is from viral gastroenteritis. Children with CVS are usually substantially sicker, requiring intravenous fluids for dehydration [Li and Misiewicz, 2003]. Nongastrointestinal disorders include neurological, metabolic, renal, and endocrine etiologies.

Treatment includes prevention, prophylaxis, and acute management of vomiting episodes. Prevention depends on the identification of triggers and avoidance of precipitants, if possible. If anticipatory anxiety or stress is a factor, lifestyle changes, behavioral intervention, biofeedback, and counseling may be effective. Prophylactic medication should be considered in children with frequent cycles of emesis, frequent school absences,

and/or severe, debilitating spells. A wide variety of medications have been used for prophylactic treatment of CVS; however, good evidence-based data to support any therapy are lacking [Li et al., 2008]. Table 65-2 is modified from consensus recommendations from a recent expert task force review on CVS [Li et al., 2008]. A recent study showed the effectiveness of valproic acid in a small group of children with refractory CVS, in whom "organic causes" were excluded [Hikita et al., 2009]. There are no evidence-based guidelines to help direct treatment and there is a very high placebo effect [Li and Misiewicz, 2003]. A sequential trial of medications, over an appropriate length of time and vomiting cycles, should be tried. Acute management involves rapid recognition and identification of a spell. If the child experiences a prodrome, efforts should focus on abortive measures to prevent a full-blown attack. Nonsteroidal analgesia (e.g., Ibuprofen) or off-label use of triptans, if appropriate, together with an antiemetic, especially sublingual or oral disintegrating tablets, should be tried [Li et al., 2008]. In the case of an established attack, intravenous fluids containing glucose and intravenous antiemetic medication ($5HT_3$ antagonists) should be administered [Li et al., 2008]. Ketosis should be avoided. Proton pump inhibitors or H_2 receptor antagonists should be considered for children who have prolonged or frequent episodes of vomiting or epigastric discomfort [Forbes et al., 1999; Forbes and Fairbrother, 2008; Li et al., 2008]. The child should be placed in a quiet, dark environment. Sedation may be of some benefit if there is a lot of anxiety or distress. Pain medication may be necessary for severe abdominal pain or headache.

Sandifer's Syndrome

Named for the British neurologist, Paul Sandifer [Sutcliffe, 1969], the full syndrome comprises tonic neck extension, deviation of the head to one side ("spastic torticollis"), and

Table 65-2 Prophylactic Medications for Cyclic Vomiting Syndrome*

	Class of Drug	Drug	Dosage
Age 5 or younger	Antihistamine (first line)	Cyproheptadine	0.25–0.5 mg/kg/day divided two times a day or three times a day
		Pizotifen (available in UK, Canada)	
	Beta blockers (second line)	Propranolol	0.25–1.0 mg/kg/day, most often 10 mg divided two times a day or three times a day
Age 6 or older	Tricyclic antidepressants (first line)	Amitriptyline	Begin 0.25-0.5 mg/kg qhs, increase weekly by 5-10 mg, to max dose of 1-1.5 mg/kg/day
		Alternative: Nortriptyline	
	Beta blockers (second line)	Propranolol	0.25–1.0 mg/kg/day, most often 10 mg divided two times a day or three times a day
Other agents	Antiepileptic drugs	Phenobarbital *Alternatives:* Topiramate Valproic acid Gabapentin Levetiracetam	2 mg/kg/day at bedtime nightly –
	Supplements	L-carnitine	50–100 mg/kg/day divided two times a day or three times a day (max 1 g three times a day)
		Coenzyme Q_{10}	10 mg/kg/day divided two times a day or three times a day (max 100 mg three times a day)

* See text for further details. All recommendations are made for off-label use.
(Adapted from Li BU, et al. North American Society for Pediatric Gastroenterology, Hepatology, and Nutrition consensus statement on the diagnosis and management of cyclic vomiting syndrome, J Pediatr Gastroenterol Nutr 47:379–393, 2008.)

dystonic posturing of the trunk [Kinsbourne, 1964; Mandel et al., 1989]. Torticollis in the absence of truncal dystonia may occur [Murphy and Gellis, 1977], and must be differentiated from other positional torticollis in which there is typically contracture or tightness of the sternocleidomastoid muscles. Apnea, tonic body stiffening, and writhing movements of the limbs may be seen in the neonatal or early infantile period [Werlin et al., 1980; Mandel et al., 1989]. Initially described in association with hiatus hernia [Kinsbourne, 1964; Sutcliffe, 1969; Gellis and Feingold, 1971; Murphy and Gellis, 1977], Sandifer's syndrome more commonly occurs in association with gastroesophageal reflux disease (GERD) [Bray et al., 1977; Werlin et al., 1980; Shepherd et al., 1987; Gorrotxategi et al., 1995]. The abnormal posturing is felt possibly to represent the body's response to discomfort associated with reflux [Werlin et al., 1980; Deskin, 1995].

The incidence is unknown, although the syndrome is said to occur in anywhere from 1 to 8 percent of cases of GERD [Shepherd et al., 1987; Lehwald et al., 2007]. There appears to be no correlation between the degree of reflux or esophagitis and the severity of symptoms [Mandel et al., 1989]. Although Sandifer's syndrome is commonly seen in clinical practice, there are scant reports in the medical literature. In one series of children aged 2 months to 5 years monitored by video EEG for paroxysmal nonepileptic events, approximately 15 percent were found to be due to GERD. Onset is usually in infancy or early childhood, but older-onset cases have been described [Kinsbourne, 1964; Mandel et al., 1989; Lehwald et al., 2007]. The diagnosis can be difficult in children with underlying neurological or metabolic disorders, as the dystonic movements or neck/head posturing is often attributed to their primary underlying disorder [Mandel et al., 1989; Gorrotxategi et al., 1995; Lehwald et al., 2007].

Sandifer's syndrome is most commonly associated with a normal neurological examination, especially in infants. The history should provide clues to the diagnosis, given the intermittent nature of the torticollis, and the relationship to feeding or the immediate postprandial period. Reflux or vomiting of feeds is not always present. Ways to differentiate Sandifer's syndrome from other causes of torticollis (muscular, cervical, and vertebral abnormalities, or posterior fossa tumors) include the intermittent nature of the torticollis, lack of muscle contracture of the sternocleidomastoid, and typical relationship to feeding. Other differential diagnostic considerations include extensor spasms/seizures [Kabakus and Kurt, 2006; Lehwald et al., 2007] or primary movement disorders [Mandel et al., 1989].

Treatment of Sandifer's syndrome is primarily medical and directed at treating the underlying reflux problem. Occasionally, surgery, such as Nissen fundoplication, is needed, especially in the presence of a hiatus hernia.

Spasmus Nutans

Spasmus nutans is a benign, self-limiting condition manifest by an intermittent triad of asymmetric nystagmus, head nodding, and torticollis in infancy. It was first described in the medical literature by Raudnitz in 1897 [Weissman et al., 1987]. Differentiation of spasmus nutans from other similar but more serious disorders has been hampered by the fact that patients often do not demonstrate all of the typical diagnostic features [Gottlob et al., 1990]. Furthermore, clinical detection of asymmetric nystagmus at such a young age may be challenging. The nystagmus, typically, is of low amplitude (3 degrees), high frequency (up to 15 Hz), and horizontal, but may rarely be vertical, oblique, jerky, or pendular. Monocular or dissociated nystagmus may occur in spasmus nutans [Farmer and Hoyt, 1984]. The head nodding possibly corresponds to a compensatory oculovestibular reflex [Gottlob et al., 1992]. The mechanism of head tilt is unclear, possibly related to asymmetry in the type of nystagmus, with partial compensated correction in a specific head posture. The pathophysiology, mechanisms, and substrate involved in spasmus nutans are undetermined. Initial speculation that "spasmus nutans results from environmental deprivation of sunlight" has not been substantiated. Certain demographic populations (African-American and Hispanic ancestry) and low socioeconomic conditions may, however, represent risk factors for the development of spasmus nutans [Wizov et al., 2002].

Numerous cases of spasmus nutans have been associated with chiasmatic lesions [Kelly, 1970; Antony et al., 1980; Farmer and Hoyt, 1984; Albright et al., 1984], diencephalic syndrome, porencephalic cysts [Gottlob et al., 1990], opsoclonus-myoclonus syndrome [Allarakhia and Trobe, 1995], empty sella syndrome [Gottlob et al., 1990], ependymoma [Gottlob et al., 1990], and retinal disorders [Lambert and Newman, 1993; Gottlob et al., 1995a; Kiblinger et al., 2007]. Spasmus nutans should no longer be regarded as a benign entity when first seen until serious ocular, intracranial, or systemic abnormalities are excluded by brain MRI scan and electroretinography [Norton and Cogan, 1954; Hoefnagel and Biery, 1968; Kiblinger et al., 2007].

To differentiate congenital nystagmus from spasmus nutans, eye and head movements were recorded in 23 patients with spasmus nutans, 10 patients with spasmus nutans-like disease (associated with central nervous system lesions), and 25 patients with congenital nystagmus. The mean onset of nystagmus was 8 months and head nodding 15 months in the spasmus nutans group. The following findings helped differentiate spasmus nutans from infantile nystagmus: ocular oscillations were of later onset; head nodding was more frequent, of larger amplitude, and clinically easier to detect; and nystagmus was asymmetric and intermittent in spasmus nutans compared with infantile nystagmus. Opticokinetic nystagmus was usually present in spasmus nutans and absent in most patients with infantile nystagmus. Head tilt was not found to be helpful in the differentiation. The ocular movement recordings were not useful for differentiating idiopathic spasmus nutans from spasmus nutans associated with neurologic abnormalities; neuroimaging studies are required for this [Gottlob et al., 1990]. A normal electroretinogram may help to rule out retinal pathology, thereby substantiating a diagnosis of spasmus nutans [Smith et al., 2000]. Other differential diagnoses include bobble-head doll syndrome, which mimics head nodding but without head tilt or nystagmus, and is secondary to third ventricular tumors or colloid cysts. Long-term follow-up studies are important to substantiate a diagnosis of spasmus nutans. Most patients eventually attain good visual acuity. Subclinical nystagmus persists until at least 5–12 years of age [Gottlob et al., 1990, 1995b].

Spasmus nutans is also described in Chapter 68.

Paroxysmal Tonic Upgaze of Childhood

First described in 1988 as a benign paroxysmal extraocular movement disorder [Ouvrier and Billson, 1988], paroxysmal tonic upgaze of childhood (PTUC) involves transient episodes of sustained tonic upward deviation of the eyes, with or without ataxia. Although it was initially thought to be a benign condition, neurological and developmental abnormalities occur in approximately half of the cases. These include chronic ataxia, persistent mild ocular movement abnormalities (nystagmus, strabismus, and saccadic abnormalities), learning disabilities, pervasive developmental disorder, and cognitive deficits [Hayman et al., 1998; Ouvrier and Billson, 2005]. Most cases are sporadic; however, familial cases have been reported, suggesting an autosomal-dominant mode of inheritance [Campistol et al., 1993; Guerrini et al., 1998; Roubertie et al., 2008]. Etiology remains uncertain, although neurotransmitter depletion affecting the pathways controlling supranuclear vertical eye movements has been postulated [Ouvrier and Billson, 1988]. Others have suggested that it may be the result of an age-dependent immature corticomesencephalic control of vertical eye movement [Hayman et al., 1998]. Abnormal GABA transmission was suggested in one case with coexisting absence epilepsy in which valproic acid seemed to be associated with the development or "unmasking" of PTUC [Luat et al., 2007]. In some instances, brain MRI scan has demonstrated structural abnormalities in the mesencephalic region, including a pinealoma [Spalice et al., 2000] and a vein of Galen malformation [Hayman et al., 1998]. A single case report showed an association between PTUC and a partial tetrasomy of chromosome 15 in a 3-month-old child [Joseph et al., 2005], and mutations in the *CACNA1A* gene have been shown in at least one family pedigree, in which PTUC was an early clinical manifestation in some family members [Roubertie et al., 2008].

Abnormalities of ocular movement typically occur in the first few years of life, often the first year, but may occur as early as the first few weeks of life [Ahn et al., 1989; Mets, 1990; Hayman et al., 1998]. The eye movement abnormalities include brief, conjugate, upward deviation of the eyes lasting seconds to minutes, compensatory neck flexion, and incomplete downward saccades on attempted downgaze [Ouvrier and Billson, 1988; Campistol et al., 1993]. They tend to exacerbate with fatigue and are relieved by sleep. Horizontal eye movements are normal. The episodes tend to dissipate gradually and resolve over years [Hayman et al., 1998; Verrotti et al., 2001]. There is no consistent precipitating factor with regard to onset; however, a relationship to febrile illness and immunization has been raised in some cases [Hayman et al., 1998; Spalice et al., 2000; Verrotti et al., 2001].

Ataxia is a frequent accompaniment of the paroxysmal events and appears to be predominantly truncal in nature. It persists in a significant number of affected cases as a chronic, permanent disability [Ouvrier and Billson, 2005].

In the majority of children, laboratory, neuroimaging, and neurophysiological studies are normal. Metabolic evaluation, including spinal fluid analysis, has been normal, although the specific nature of the work-up has not been well defined [Ouvrier and Billson, 1988; Campistol et al., 1993; Spalice et al., 2000; Lispi and Vigevano, 2001; Verrotti et al., 2001]. In all cases, video EEG has been normal, with captured spells confirming their nonepileptic nature. Neuroimaging studies are typically normal, but a number of different abnormalities have been described, including a pinealoma [Spalice et al., 2000], vein of Galen malformation [Hayman et al., 1998], periventricular leukomalacia [Sugie et al., 1995], and delayed myelination (Luat et al., 2007], suggesting that neuroimaging studies should be a consideration in the evaluation of these children.

Differential diagnosis includes epilepsy, oculogyric crises, opsoclonus-myoclonus, and brainstem disorders (either destructive or compressive).

The paroxysmal episodes are generally brief and self-limiting, making medication unnecessary. Response to L-DOPA has been reported in some cases [Ouvrier and Billson, 1988; Campistol et al., 1993], but this is not consistent [Hayman et al., 1998; Ouvrier and Billson, 2005]. Adrenocorticotropic hormone (ACTH), acetazolamide, and anticonvulsant medications appear to be ineffective [Ouvrier and Billson, 2005].

Paroxysmal tonic upgaze is also described in Chapter 68.

Benign Myoclonus of Infancy

Benign myoclonus of infancy (BMI) was first described in 1976 by Fejerman [Fejerman, 1976]. Infants aged 1–12 months develop sudden onset of flexor or extensor spasms while awake; these usually occur in clusters. The paroxysmal activity resembles infantile spasms, without EEG correlate of hypsarrhythmia and the associated neurologic abnormalities seen in West's syndrome. Development is normal. The clinical features have been best summarized by Caraballo et al. in 2009; their report includes 102 infants with long-term follow-up [Caraballo et al., 2009]. The paroxysmal motor phenomena may involve brief myoclonus or tonic contractions mimicking infantile spasm, shuddering, atonic or negative myoclonus, or a combination of the above. Involved body parts include neck, trunk, upper limbs, head (cephalic myoclonus), or eyes (blinking) [Lombroso and Fejerman, 1977; Maydell et al., 2001; Caraballo et al., 2009]. The myoclonic activity increases for a few weeks or months after onset, then stabilizes and starts decreasing after about 3 months, before disappearing spontaneously by 2 years of age [Lombroso and Fejerman, 1977]. There is no obvious gender predilection, and familial occurrence has only rarely been reported [Galletti et al., 1989]. The etiology is unknown but prognosis is excellent, with no significant morbidity, even after 40 years of follow-up. No specific treatment is needed; however, it is very important to avoid over-investigation in these cases [Caraballo et al., 2009].

The condition should be differentiated from stimulus-sensitive or action myoclonus as seen in posthypoxic encephalopathies, which are severe and disabling, often resulting in the patient falling to the ground on attempted standing or walking. Periodic myoclonus may result from subacute sclerosing panencephalitis, but the myoclonus is a bit slower, as these are reticular in origin. Other differential diagnoses include epileptic cortical myoclonus, secondary to herpes simplex encephalitis, for example; progressive degenerative disorders of gray or white matter, including gangliosidoses; leukodystrophies; and progressive myoclonic epilepsy of early childhood, such as Unverricht–Lundborg and Lafora body diseases [Dravet et al., 1986] or myoclonic epilepsy and ragged red fibers (MERRF). Other protracted but eventually self-limiting disorders, such as hereditary essential myoclonus, benign essential myoclonus, and shuddering attacks, should be considered and excluded. The condition should also be differentiated from benign neonatal sleep myoclonus, which represents an exaggeration of normal physiologic phenomena during sleep [Noone et al., 1995]. EEG studies fail to reveal any epileptiform activity during the paroxysmal episodes of myoclonus; however, more prolonged video EEG monitoring may be required in certain situations to establish the nonepileptic nature of the myoclonus [Bleasel and Kotagal, 1995; Pachatz et al., 1999].

Benign myoclonus of infancy is also described in Chapter 68.

Hereditary Hyperekplexia

An exaggerated startle response may be a component of epilepsy (startle epilepsy) or of a nonepileptiform paroxysmal disorder: namely, hyperekplexia, or startle disease. The term hyperekplexia is derived from Greek, and means excessive jerking or jumping (startle). Kirstein and Silfverskiold first described this entity in 1958 [Kirstein and Silfverskiold, 1958]. It involves a strikingly excessive response to startle elicited by unexpected sudden visual, auditory, or somatosensory stimuli that fail to produce a startle response in most normal individuals. In the normal individual, the startle response is a basic alerting reaction, with stereotyped features consisting of eye blinking, facial grimacing, flexion of the head, elevation of the shoulders, and flexion of the elbows, trunk, and knees. This involuntary reflex appears during infancy at the same time as the Moro reflex [Andermann and Andermann, 1988]. The abnormal or pathologic response consists of an exaggerated startle response associated with generalized muscle stiffness, attaining a fetal position and loss of postural control, causing the subject to fall "en statue" without loss of consciousness [Aicardi, 1992]. The generalized stiffness may compromise breathing in the neonatal and early infantile period, sometimes with fatality; frequent falls are common at a later age which may result in injuries, including head trauma [Kirstein and Silfverskiold, 1958; Andermann et al., 1980; Andermann and Andermann, 1988; Aicardi, 1992; Praveen et al., 2001].

Hyperekplexia presents in its major form during the neonatal period as stiff-baby syndrome ("stiff-man syndrome in the newborn") [Klein et al., 1972; Lingam et al., 1981]. The onset of stiffness becomes evident a few hours after birth. Shoulder girdle muscles are particularly stiff. There may be difficulty in swallowing and frequent choking. Apnea may result from hyperekplexia and may cause death [Kurczynski, 1983; Nigro and Lim, 1992]. The hypertonia usually disappears during sleep, although repetitive and violent movements of the extremities may be seen during the hypnagogic stage, which may lift the child off the bed [Andermann and Andermann, 1988; Aicardi, 1992]. The neonatal form improves spontaneously during the first year of life, although later on there may be absence of crawling and delay in walking. Hip dislocation, as well as umbilical, inguinal, and diaphragmatic hernias, may result from increased intra-abdominal pressure due to generalized muscle stiffness [Aicardi, 1992; Gordon, 1993]. A clinically useful maneuver is to tap the bridge of the nose or the glabella (glabellar tap). This maneuver will elicit an exaggerated, nonhabituating startle response in affected individuals [Shahar et al., 1991; Nigro and Lim, 1992]. Similar results

may be obtained by blowing air directly on the face of neonates and infants with hyperekplexia [Shahar and Raviv, 2004].

Neurophysiologic studies demonstrate that hyperekplexia is not simply an exaggerated normal startle response [Hallett et al., 1986]. Electromyogram latencies are shorter than normal. EEG studies are mostly normal; however, they may reveal an initial myogenic spike, maximally in the frontocentral region, followed by slow waves and desynchronization of background activity corresponding to the phase of apnea, bradycardia, and cyanosis [Andermann and Andermann, 1988; Tohier et al., 1991; Praveen et al., 2001]. Auditory and somatosensory-evoked potentials may be exaggerated or normal [Hallett et al., 1986; Andermann and Andermann, 1988]. Rostrocaudal recruitment of cranial nerve-innervated muscles supports a brainstem reticular origin for the abnormal startle response in hyperekplexia [Brown, 2002].

The condition is familial and transmitted as an autosomal-dominant trait. Linkage analyses initially demonstrate genetic homogeneity in typical cases to the long arm of chromosome 5 [Ryan et al., 1992; Shiang et al., 1993]. Point mutations or deletions in the alpha subunit of the inhibitory glycine receptor (*GLRA1*) gene, located on chromosome 5q33–35, were subsequently found [Shiang et al., 1995; Tsai et al., 2004]. Some sporadic cases of hyperekplexia may show abnormalities in the beta subunit of the glycine receptor (*GLRβ*), located on chromosome 4q32.1 [Hejazi et al., 2001; Rees et al., 2002]. Rare mutations of the genes coding for receptor clustering proteins gephyrin and collybistin have also been described as causing hyperekplexia [Rees et al., 2003; Harvey et al., 2004]. New research suggests that mutation in the genes encoding presynaptic glycine transporter GlyT2 is also a cause of human hyperekplexia [Eulenburg et al., 2006]. Glycine receptors are found primarily in the brainstem and spinal cord [Rajendra et al., 1997]. The main inhibitory neurotransmitter receptor is the GABA type A receptor. Affected individuals usually reveal a favorable response to treatment with clonazepam, an agonist of GABA type A receptors [Shiang et al., 1995].

The differential diagnoses in the neonatal period are congenital stiff-person syndrome, Schwartz–Jampel syndrome, startle epilepsy, myoclonic seizures, neonatal tetany, and phenothiazine toxicity [Andermann and Andermann, 1988; Praveen et al., 2001]. The relationship of hyperekplexia to other nonepileptic startle disorders, such as jumping (jumping Frenchmen of Maine), latah (ticklishness associated with echopraxia and coprolalia in Malaysia), and myriachit (to act foolishly, as reported from Siberia, Asia, and Africa), as discussed over a century ago by Gilles de la Tourette [1884; 1899] in the context of "tic convulsif," remains conjectural.

Treatment is most effective with clonazepam (0.1–0.2 mg/kg/day) but, in some cases, symptoms may not be totally suppressed [Aicardi, 1992; Tijssen et al., 1997]. Valproic acid is recommended in cases of late onset [Dooley and Andermann, 1989]. Vigabatrin did not reduce startle activity among four patients with hyperekplexia [Tijssen et al., 1997]. Phenobarbital, phenytoin, and diazepam have not proved to be effective [Giacoia and Ryan, 1994]. The prognosis is variable. Neonatal hyperekplexia may result in apnea, neonatal encephalopathy, cerebral palsy, and unexpected death [Chaves-Carballo et al., 1999]. Early identification and treatment improve the outcome in most children. A simple maneuver, like forced flexion of the head and legs towards the trunk, is known to be life-saving when prolonged stiffness impedes breathing [Vigevano et al., 1989]. Hypertonia and motor delay improve with increasing age, and muscle tone becomes normal by the age of 3 years. In some families, the exaggerated startle response ameliorates or disappears spontaneously by 2 years of age, although hyperekplexia may persist or reoccur in adult life, resulting in falls [Shahar et al., 1991].

In the minor form of hyperekplexia, there is only an abnormal startle response without generalized stiffness or tonic spasms. The minor form is not associated with neurologic or catastrophic sequelae, and in this group no mutations have been detected in the genes encoding the glycine receptor [Tijssen et al., 1997, 2002].

Hyperekplexia is also described in Chapter 68.

Shuddering Attacks

Shuddering or shivering attacks are uncommon paroxysmal events rarely reported and poorly understood. A retrospective series of paroxysmal nonepileptic events in 666 children found 7 percent of all events to be due to shuddering attacks [Bye et al., 2000]. These may start as early as 4–6 months of age, and rarely occur after the age of 3. They are precipitated or aggravated by excitement, fear, anger, frustration, or embarrassment [Vanasse et al., 1976; Holmes and Russman, 1986]. The episodes last usually for a few seconds, and are characterized by rapid shivering or stiffening of the body with abnormal posturing, with adduction of the knees and arms, flexion of the head, elbows, trunk, and knees, and flexion or extension of the neck. There is no alteration of consciousness with the abnormal movements. The attacks are very frequent, occurring multiple times a day, and in excess of 100 per day in some cases. The pathophysiology of shuddering attacks is unknown. In one series, in 5 of 6 cases, one of the parents had an essential tremor. These children also had some postural tremor on examination [Vanasse et al., 1976]. Electromyography studies have revealed the frequency of these shuddering attacks to be similar to that of essential tremor [Kanazawa, 2000]. Head tremor may evolve from shuddering attacks [DiMario, 2000]. These characteristics suggested that shuddering attacks may represent the expression of an "essential tremor in the immature brain." Later studies, however, failed to find an increased frequency of family history of essential tremor in children with shuddering attacks [Kanazawa, 2000]. The other theory is that shuddering attacks are a variant of benign myoclonus of early infancy [Fejerman, 1997]. The differential diagnoses include generalized seizures or infantile spasm. Ictal EEG is normal [Holmes and Russman, 1986; Kanazawa, 2000]. No symptomatic cases of shuddering attacks have been reported so far. Treatment with antiepileptic mediations has not been effective. Propranolol has been effective in eliminating shuddering attacks [Barron and Younkin, 1992]. Monosodium glutamate has been implicated in some cases, and its avoidance or elimination from the diet has been effective [Reif-Lehrer and Stemmermann, 1975]. The prognosis is favorable; most children improve spontaneously before 10 years of age [Vanasse et al., 1976; Kanazawa, 2000].

Shuddering attacks are also described in Chapter 68.

Stereotypies, Self-Stimulation, and Masturbation

Repetitive stereotyped movements are very common among children with autism, mental retardation, and sensory deprivation; however, they are also observed in nonautistic children with normal cognition. These movements involve rhythmic motor behaviors, self-stimulating movements, and gratification phenomena, an extreme example of which is masturbatory behavior. Examples of self-stimulating movements or gratification phenomena include body rocking, head banging (jactatio capitis), and head rolling [Sallustro and Atwell, 1978]. Rocking motions of the trunk observed among mentally and visually impaired children may represent a form of vestibular stimulation akin to the maternal rocking that effectively comforts a crying, tired, or sleepy infant. The characteristic, purposeless, writhing, repetitive hand movements seen among autistic children and in Rett's syndrome may also be grouped into the category of self-stimulating behavior. Children who have a photoconvulsive response may learn to induce a seizure by repetitive hand movements in front of their eyes as a form of photic stimulation. Broadly, all the above movements fall in the category of stereotypies. More specifically, stereotypies are abnormal involuntary, repetitive, rhythmic, seemingly purposeless, suppressible, distractible, and predictable in regard to pattern, amplitude, and location of the movement. In the majority of cases, emotional excitement precedes the stereotypies. These may take the form of hand flapping, hand waving or rotation, finger wiggling, wing-beating movements of the arm, head/shoulder/body gyration, and ritualistic complex movement pattern, with or without vocalization. Stereotypies may be motor or vocal (associated with sound production). Each type may be simple or complex, depending on the complexity of the movement pattern or content of the vocalization [Harris et al., 2008; Goldman et al., 2009]. Among the vocal stereotypies, common ones involve grunting sounds, hissing, whistling, acting out a movie character, sound of engine, imaginary video game. Very often, complex motor stereotypies may be combined with vocal stereotypies.

Stereotypy and posturing during masturbation are also described in Chapter 68.

Tics, paroxysmal dyskinesias, and complex partial seizures are the major differential diagnoses to be considered. Tics are differentiated from stereotypies by the brevity of the phenomena, tics being much briefer; the majority of the tics affect craniofacial muscles, whereas upper limbs are predominantly affected in stereotypies. Emotional excitement is the prime precipitant for stereotypies, whereas stress/anxiety or relaxation after stress is a major factor in tic production. Distractibility is also more suggestive of stereotypies. Family history is more common with tics and less common in stereotypies. Association with autism, mental retardation, and sensory deprivation also characterizes stereotypies [Singer, 2009]. The pathophysiology of stereotypies is unclear. As in other involuntary movements, the cortico-striato-pallido-thalamic pathway is thought to be involved. Improvement of stereotyped behavior in primates with stereotypies by high-frequency deep-brain stimulation of anterior subthalamic nucleus gives credence to the above hypothesis [Baup et al., 2008]. Medications have not been successful in treating stereotypies. Applied behavioral therapy may be of some help in autistic children [Miller et al., 2006]. Habit reversal was beneficial in reducing motor stereotypies in nonautistic children [Miller et al., 2006]. Prognosis depends on the primary underlying diagnosis. Even in primary stereotypies without underlying autism, mental retardation, or sensory deprivation, stereotypies may persist in 94 percent of cases [Harris et al., 2008].

More difficult to recognize is masturbatory behavior, particularly when this occurs in young children and infants [Fleisher and Morrison, 1990; Nechay et al., 2004]. The repetitive movements usually involve the lower trunk and may be accompanied by pelvic thrusting or contractions of the gluteal muscles. Thighs may adduct and rub against each other. Use of midline seat belts in a car seat or while on a high chair may stimulate the genitalia and provoke this masturbatory behavior. The physical effort may be prolonged until the inciting stimulus is removed or the child is distracted. Other manifestations may include diaphoresis, hyperpnea, flushing, and grunting [Fleisher and Morrison, 1990]. The paroxysms may terminate in fatigue, exhaustion, or sleep. During a typical episode, parents may give a history of partial responsiveness, as it may require a lot of effort to distract the infant or child from a pleasurable act. Differential diagnosis is from an epileptic seizure, paroxysmal dyskinesia, or a dystonic disorder. The prominent hyperventilation and grunting sounds may unnecessarily lead to investigations for asthma. Detailed observation of an episode or review of a videotaped event can be especially helpful in clarifying the event and making the diagnosis, particularly in infants younger than 1 year of age [Casteels et al., 2004]. Any explanation of the benign nature of the paroxysms should take into account unusually sensitive or unbelieving parents, more so in baby girls [Leung and Robson, 1993]. Reassurance that the episodes are benign and self-limiting should help to avoid unjustified concerns and unnecessary investigations [Mink and Neil, 1995].

Hyperventilation Syndrome in Childhood

The hyperventilation syndrome (HVS) may best be defined as a syndrome characterized by "a variety of somatic symptoms induced by physiologically inappropriate hyperventilation and usually reproduced in whole or in part by voluntary hyperventilation" [Lewis and Howell, 1986]. In addition to somatic symptoms, psychological symptoms are also common. The term was first used in by Kerr et al. in 1937 [Kerr et al., 1938]. Hyperventilation as a paroxysmal event may also be a primary manifestation of certain neurological conditions, metabolic disorders, or genetic syndromes but differs from HVS in which, by definition, there is no underlying organic disease.

The incidence of HVS in the general (adult) population is about 5–11 percent; however, in a selected population of patients being evaluated for dizziness, it accounted for 24 percent of the cases [Evans, 1995]. It is more common in females than males [Enzer and Walker, 1967; Joorabchi, 1977; Perkin and Joseph, 1986]. In two small series, age at onset ranged from 5 to 18 years, with just over half occurring in the 13–16-year-old age group [Enzer and Walker, 1967; Herman et al., 1981]. Symptoms may last from several minutes to hours [Enzer and Walker, 1967].

The clinical presentations of HVS are protean [Joorabchi, 1977; Perkin and Joseph, 1986; Hanna et al., 1986; Evans, 1995] and often do not involve the nervous system. Common non-neurological manifestations include symptoms referable to the heart (palpitations, shortness of breath, chest pain), abdomen (abdominal distention, abdominal pain, flatulence, belching, diarrhea), and lungs (shortness of breath, feeling of suffocation, or inability to draw in an adequate breath). Neurological symptoms may involve the autonomic, peripheral, or central nervous system. Autonomic manifestations include palpitations, tachycardia, sweating, and nausea from excessive sympathetic activity. Peripheral nervous system manifestations include numbness, tingling, generalized weakness or muscle stiffness, carpopedal spasm, or generalized tetany. The paresthesias may be asymmetric or even unilateral [Lewis, 1953; Tavel, 1964; Perkin and Joseph, 1986; Evans, 1995] and may involve the distal extremities, face, or trunk. Dizziness, vertigo, ataxia, tinnitus, headache, syncope, tremulousness, and visual disturbances are common central nervous symptoms. Visual symptoms include blurring of vision, loss of vision, and flashing lights. Syncope may result in secondary seizure. Psychological manifestations include nervousness, disorientation, "out of body" sensation, fear, and anxiety.

The pathophysiology underlying HVS includes reduction in arterial PCO_2 with resultant respiratory alkalosis, causing a left shift in the oxygen dissociation curve and increased binding of oxygen to hemoglobin. This results in decreased oxygen delivery to tissue. Hypocapnea also leads to cerebral vasoconstriction, with resultant diminished cerebral blood flow. Alkalosis also causes a reduction of plasma calcium concentration. Hypophosphatemia has also been implicated. Finally, hyperventilation may be triggered by beta-adrenergic stimulation from anxiety or stress [Herman et al., 1981; Evans, 1995]. In a double-blind, placebo-controlled trial, hypocapnea was not necessary to induce symptoms and appeared to be an epiphenomenon or consequence of the attack, suggesting that other mechanisms may be the cause for the symptoms [Hornsveld et al., 1996].

The diagnosis of HVS is often unrecognized or misdiagnosed, as the patients generally do not complain of hyperventilation, the diagnosis is not considered, or the signs and symptoms from the hyperventilation may be atypical [Joorabchi, 1977]. Psychological factors, including stress, anxiety, and panic attacks, commonly underlie HVS [Enzer and Walker, 1967; Herman et al., 1981]. The diagnosis can often be made at the bedside by having the patient breathe rapidly or draw in exaggerated deep breaths, with reproduction of the symptoms. This should not be performed in persons with cardiac or cerebrovascular disease, or in persons with hypercoagulable states or sickle cell disease. The validity of the hyperventilation provocation test has, however, been brought into question [Hornsveld et al., 1996]. EEG is typically normal, although hyperventilation may induce an absence seizure (3 Hertz spike and wave) in a person with absence epilepsy and whose presentation and symptoms, especially transient alteration in consciousness, may be confused with HVS. Other causes should be excluded by appropriate laboratory tests when indicated. Pain, fever, sepsis, and certain drugs (such as caffeine or salicylate toxicity) can result in HVS. Topiramate, an antiepileptic medication, may also cause central hyperventilation due to its inhibition of carbonic anhydrase [Laskey et al., 2000; Philippi et al., 2002]. Neurological causes include brainstem strokes or tumors, malignant hyperthermia, and encephalitis. A number of genetic syndromes cite primary hyperventilation as a clinical manifestation. These include Joubert's syndrome [Joubert et al., 1969; Boltshauser and Isler, 1977]; Pitt–Hopkins syndrome, caused by mutations of the *TCF4* gene on chromosome 18q21 [Pitt and Hopkins, 1978; Giurgea et al., 2008]; Rett's syndrome, caused by a mutation of the *MECP2* gene [Southall et al., 1988; Murakami et al., 1998; Kerr and Julu, 1999]; and Leigh's syndrome, due to *SURF1* gene mutations [Pronicka et al., 2001]. There is also a single case report of two brothers with novel duplication in the *ARX* gene and intermittent hyperventilation [Demos et al., 2009].

The differential diagnosis of HVS depends, in part, on the particular symptoms on presentation and includes seizures, stroke, migraine, multiple sclerosis, causes of central and peripheral vertigo, brain tumors, episodic ataxias, periodic paralysis, and psychosomatic disorders. Non-neurological causes, such as asthma, should also be considered, as they may cause hyperventilation leading to respiratory alkalosis.

Treatment is predominantly supportive and includes reassurance, education, and respiratory control procedures. Nonmedical interventions include breathing exercises, holding one's breath or breathing more slowly, biofeedback, counseling, and occasionally breathing into a paper bag. Medications may occasionally be necessary if there is a significant component of stress, anxiety, or depression. Beta blockers may also be of use in selective cases; however, there is no good evidence-based medicine to support any of these approaches. Signs and symptoms of hyperventilation continued to occur in adulthood in 40 percent in one series [Herman et al., 1981].

The complete list of references for this chapter is available online at **www.expertconsult.com**.
See inside cover for registration details.

Sleep–Wake Disorders*

Suresh Kotagal

Complaints about insufficient or nonrestorative sleep are quite common in childhood and adolescence. In a questionnaire survey of 332 children of 11 through 15 years of age, Ipsiroglu et al. [2001] observed that 28 percent of the subjects had snoring, insomnia, or a parasomnia. In another survey of 472 4- to 12-year-old urban and rural children receiving routine pediatric care, Stein et al. [2001] noted a 10 percent prevalence of sleep disorders. Less than one-half of the parents had discussed the sleep problems with the pediatrician. Childhood sleep disorders can have a significant effect on the quality of life. Many disorders are also easily treatable, thus underscoring the importance of their prompt recognition and management. This chapter covers salient aspects of childhood sleep–wake function and common pediatric sleep disorders.

Sleep Physiology and Ontogeny

Sleep–wake regulation is mediated via a complex set of interactions. There is a dynamic balance between the circadian drive for sleep (process C), which serves to enhance alertness, and the homeostatic drive (process S), which facilitates sleep. Adenosine, an extracellular factor that is secreted by neurons in the basal forebrain, plays a key role in sleep induction. (Caffeine is an antagonist of adenosine.) Neurons of the ventrolateral preoptic nucleus that contain gamma-aminobutyric acid (GABA) and galanin serve to inhibit wakefulness-promoting regions of the forebrain and the laterodorsal pontine tegmentum, and are thus also involved in sleep induction. Sleep onset is further facilitated by melatonin, a light-sensitive hormone that is released from the pineal gland. The principal components of the ascending arousal system are the cholinergic neurons of laterodorsal pontine tegmentum and the nucleus basalis of Meynert. Cells of the dorsolateral hypothalamus produce hypocretin (orexin), which is also an important wakefulness-promoting peptide. The hypocretin neurons project widely to the forebrain and brainstem. There is a tendency for mutual inhibition between the wakefulness-promoting and the sleep-promoting circuits. This phenomenon has been characterized as a "flip-flop" switch [Fuller et al., 2006; Lu and Zee, 2010].

The ultimate command center for the once-a-day (circadian) rhythm of sleep and wakefulness is the suprachiasmatic nucleus of the hypothalamus [Miller et al., 1996; Steriade et al., 1993], which has cells with receptors for melatonin. The suprachiasmatic nucleus is strongly influenced by light-mediated impulses received through the retinohypothalamic tract. *Clock* and *Period* genes, remarkably preserved across various phyla, were studied initially in *Drosophila melanogaster*; they also influence the timing of activity of the suprachiasmatic nucleus cells [Challet et al., 2003; Franken and Dijk, 2009; Hamada et al., 2001]. The mammalian target of rapamycin (mTOR) signaling is involved in modulation of photic entrainment of the suprachiasmatic circadian clock [Cao et al., 2010]. The body temperature rhythm is also regulated by the hypothalamus [van Someren, 2000]; a rise in body temperature leads to postponement of sleep. Conversely, individuals are most sleepy around the nadir of body temperature: that is, around 0400 hours. An artificial increase in body temperature in the 1–2 hours before bedtime, such as through vigorous exercise, may provoke sleep-onset insomnia.

Wakefulness can be differentiated from sleep by 27–28 weeks' postconceptional age in the preterm infant. At this age, sleep is primarily of the active or rapid eye movement (REM) type, which is associated with irregular breathing, phasic electromyographic activity, and low-voltage electroencephalographic (EEG) activity. Cerebral blood flow and metabolism are higher in REM than in non-rapid eye movement (NREM) sleep, which is also termed quiet sleep in newborns. By 40 weeks' postconceptional age, active (REM) sleep decreases to about 50 percent of the total sleep time, with a corresponding rise in the proportion of quiet (NREM) sleep. By 46–48 weeks' postconceptional age, sleep spindles appear during stages N2 and N3 of NREM sleep. By 4–6 months of age, NREM sleep has fully differentiated into N1, N2, and N3 sleep, corresponding respectively with lighter to deeper stages in terms of arousal threshold. N3 is also termed slow-wave sleep. It is characterized by the generalized slow-wave activity in the 0.5–4 Hz range on the EEG (Figure 66-1). The bulk of N3 occurs during the first third of the night. Growth hormone release is closely linked to N3 sleep [Van Cauter et al., 2008], with suppression of the latter leading to impaired growth hormone release. The release of cortisol is suppressed during N3 sleep [van Cauter et al., 2008]. REM sleep decreases gradually over time. By the age of 3 years, it constitutes only about 20–25 percent of total sleep.

Prior to age of 3 months, the transition from wakefulness is initially into REM sleep. After this age, however, the physiologic transition is from wakefulness into NREM sleep, with REM sleep occurring 90–140 minutes later. The physiologic sleep-onset time in elementary school-age children is usually around 8:00–8:30 pm. Around adolescence, there is a physiologic delay in sleep-onset time, which shifts to around 10:30–11:00 pm [Carskadon et al., 1998]. Teenage girls

---

* Portions of this chapter have appeared in Kotagal S. Sleep disorders in childhood. Neurol Clin 2003;21:961;81.

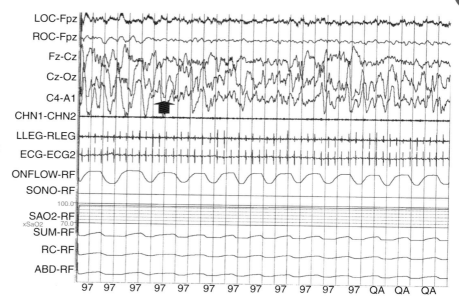

Fig. 66-1 Normal nocturnal polysomnogram during stage III of non-rapid eye movement (NREM) sleep indicating continuous delta (<4 Hz) activity on the EEG (arrow), regular respiration, and tonic chin electromyographic activity. Stage III and stage IV NREM sleep are together also termed "slow wave" sleep, which is most abundant in the first third of the night's sleep. Nocturnal growth hormone release is closely linked to slow-wave sleep. Parasomnias, such as sleepwalking and confusional arousals, generally occur during the transition from slow-wave sleep to the lighter stages of NREM sleep. (Paper speed 10 mm/second.)

generally have their final morning awakening about one half-hour earlier than boys. When juxtaposed with early high-school start times of around 7:30 am, it is easy to understand why most teenagers are chronically sleep-deprived.

The International Classification of Sleep Disorders

The International Classification of Sleep Disorders was introduced in 1990, and has undergone subsequent revisions [American Sleep Disorders Association, 2006]. It was created initially through collaborative efforts of the American Sleep Disorders Association, the European Sleep Research Society, the Japanese Society of Sleep Research, and the Latin American Sleep Society. Primary sleep disorders are separated from those due to medical or psychiatric conditions. Primary sleep disorders are further subdivided into:

1. dyssomnias, or disorders that are accompanied by excessive sleepiness or insomnia
2. parasomnias, or disorders that intrude on to sleep, but are not associated with complaints of insomnia or sleepiness.

Dyssomnias are further subdivided into intrinsic, extrinsic, and circadian rhythm sleep disorders. An abbreviated version of the International Classification of Sleep Disorders-2 is presented in Box 66-1.

Assessment of Sleep–Wake Complaints

Sleep History

The sleep history is provided by the patient, parent, or guardian. It is crucial to the planning of appropriate diagnostic procedures and arriving at a specific diagnosis. Questions relevant to infants and preschool-age children include:

- the sleeping environment (e.g., crib, bassinet, parent's bed)
- the sleeping position (e.g., prone or supine, semi-upright)
- habitual need for sleep aids (e.g., pacifier, rocking, patting)

- the time of going to bed, sleep onset, and the final morning awakening (on school nights and during weekends and holidays)
- sensation of restlessness in the legs before sleep onset, intrusive thoughts or worries that might interfere with sleep onset
- presence of habitual snoring, mouth breathing, observed apnea, restless sleep, sweating, gastroesophageal reflux, and abnormal behavior at night suggestive of seizures or parasomnias
- behavior during the daytime (irritability, inattentiveness, hyperactivity, sleepiness)
- number of daytime naps and their duration
- medications that may affect sleep–wake function (e.g., sedatives, stimulants)
- interventions that the parents have used to improve the child's sleep.

In adolescents, one should also inquire about activities that might interfere with going to bed at a reasonable hour, such as after-school employment, and resorting to vigorous exercise, heavy meals, caffeine, cell phones, computers, television, nicotine, and illicit substances in the late evening or at bedtime. Patients with restless legs syndrome may experience an urge to move their limbs, a feeling of "bugs or spiders crawling on their legs" in the evening hours, exacerbation of this discomfort when the limbs are kept immobile, and relief with movement. Daytime sleepiness assessment should include questions about taking involuntary naps in the classroom, automatic behavior, and the impact of sleepiness on driving, cataplexy, hypnagogic hallucinations, medications used to promote alertness, academic function, behavioral and mood problems, and the number of school days missed because of sleepiness.

The Pediatric Daytime Sleepiness Scale (PDSS) is a simple, validated questionnaire that can be administered to children in the 11–14-year age group [Drake et al., 2003]. It has eight items, each rated on a 0–4 scale. It provides a numerical score for sleepiness; the 50th percentile score on the PDSS is 16, the 75th percentile is 20, and the 90th percentile is 23. Participants who reported low school achievement, high absenteeism, low school enjoyment, low total sleep time and frequent illnesses

Box 66-1 The International Classification of Sleep Disorders

Insomnia (Examples)

- Idiopathic insomnia, paradoxical insomnia, adjustment insomnia, psychophysiologic insomnia, insomnia due to mental disorder, inadequate sleep hygiene, insomnia due to substance abuse, insomnia due to medical condition, behavioral insomnia of childhood – sleep-onset association type, behavioral insomnia of childhood – limit-setting type

Sleep-Related Breathing Disorders (Examples)

- Primary central sleep apnea, Cheyne–Stokes breathing, high-altitude periodic breathing, central sleep apnea due to medical condition, obstructive sleep apnea – adult, obstructive sleep apnea – pediatric, primary apnea – infancy, sleep-related hypo-ventilation, sleep-related hypoventilation/hypoxemia due to neuromuscular and chest wall disorders

Hypersomnia of Central Origin not due to a Circadian Rhythm Sleep Disorder (Examples)

- Narcolepsy with cataplexy, narcolepsy without cataplexy, narco-lepsy due to medical condition without cataplexy, narcolepsy unspecified, recurrent hypersomnia (including Kleine–Levin syn-drome and menstrual-related hypersomnia), idiopathic hyper-somnia with long sleep, idiopathic hypersomnia without long

sleep, hypersomnia due to medical condition, hypersomnia due to drug or substance, sleep-related breathing, behaviorally induced insufficient sleep syndrome disorder, or other cause of disturbed nocturnal sleep

Circadian Rhythm Sleep Disorders (Examples)

- Delayed sleep phase disorder, advanced sleep phase disorder, irregular sleep–wake rhythm, circadian rhythm sleep disorder – non-entrained type, jet lag disorder, shift work disorder, circadian rhythm sleep disorder due to drug or substance

Parasomnias (Examples)

- Confusional arousals, sleepwalking, sleep terrors, REM sleep behavior disorder, recurrent isolated sleep paralysis, nightmare disorder, sleep-related dissociative disorder, sleep-related groan-ing, exploding head syndrome, sleep-related eating disorder

Sleep-Related Movement Disorders (Examples)

- Restless legs syndrome, periodic limb movement disorder, sleep-related leg cramps, sleep-related bruxism, rhythmic movement disorder

Other Sleep Disorders

- Environmental sleep disorder

(From American Sleep Disorders Association, International Classification of Sleep Disorders, 2nd edn, pocket version: Diagnostic and Coding Manual. Westchester, Illinois: American Academy of Sleep Medicine, 2006.)

---

all had higher levels of sleepiness as measured by this scale [Drake et al., 2003]. Another survey tool that is commonly used in clinical practice is the Children's Sleep Habits Questionnaire. It is a 45-item, validated questionnaire that is completed by parents of 4–11-year-olds [Owens et al., 2000]. The questions pertain to sleep–wake function in the preceding 2 weeks, such as "the child sleeps too little" or "the child suddenly falls asleep in the middle of active behavior." The items represent several domains that present as sleep complaints, such as bedtime resistance, sleep-onset delay, sleep duration, sleep anxiety, night awakenings, parasomnias, breathing disturbance, and daytime sleepiness. Responses are rated as rarely (occurring 0–1 time/week; 1 point), sometimes (occurring 2–4 nights/week; 2 points), or usually (occurring 5–7 nights/week; 3 points). Scores of 41 or greater correlate with presence of a sleep disorder. The internal consistency estimate for this ques-tionnaire in a community (nonclinic sample) of 4–10-year-olds is 0.36–0.70. The test-retest reliability over a 2-week period is 0.62–0.79.

Sleep-Related Examination

Height, weight, and body mass index are recorded because obstructive sleep apnea may be associated with poor weight gain during infancy, and with obesity during adolescence [Arens et al., 2010]. The blood pressure should be measured because long-standing and severe obstructive sleep apnea (OSA) can be associated with hypertension. OSA patients may exhibit cranio-facial abnormalities such as micrognathia, dental malocclusion, macroglossia, myopathic face and midface hypoplasia, deviated nasal septum, swollen inferior turbinates, tonsillar hypertrophy and mouth breathing [Brooks, 2002; Hoban and Chervin,

2007]. Consultation with a pediatric otolaryngologist may be required to exclude adenoidal hypertrophy. Inattentiveness, irritability, and mood swings may be clues to daytime sleepiness. Obstructive sleep apnea related to brainstem abnormalities like the Chiari type I or II malformations [Gosalakkal, 2008] can lead to hoarseness of voice, decreased gag reflex, and changes in the amplitude of the jaw jerk relative to that of other tendon reflexes. Neuromuscular disorders, like myotonic dystrophy, may be associated with chronic obstructive hypoventilation from a combination of palatal muscle weakness, high-arched palate, and diminished chest wall–abdominal excursion [Givan, 2002; Misuri et al., 2000]. The parent–child interaction should be observed not only for clues indicating parental anxiety and reluctance to set limits on inappropriate behaviors that perpetu-ate insomnia in toddlers, but also for subtle clues indicating a child maltreatment syndrome. Home videos, if available, may be invaluable in the assessment of restless legs syndrome, parasomnias, and nocturnal seizures.

Nocturnal Polysomnography

This procedure involves the monitoring of multiple physiologic parameters in sleep. It is useful in the evaluation of intrinsic sleep disorders, such as narcolepsy, obstructive sleep apnea, nocturnal spells, and periodic limb movement disorder. It may not be indicated for diagnosing obstructive sleep apnea secondary to *severe* adenotonsillar enlargement, which can be easily recognized on the basis of clinical findings combined with severe oxygen desaturation on simple overnight oximetry in the home environment. The nocturnal polysomnogram usu-ally consists of simultaneous monitoring of 2–4 channels of the EEG, eye movements, chin and leg electromyogram, nasal pressure, thoracic and abdominal respiratory effort, electrocardiogram, and oxygen saturation [Kotagal and Goulding, 1996; Kotagal and Herold, 2002; Sheldon, 2007]. Patients with Down syndrome, neuromuscular disorders, and obesity may exhibit hypoventilation that is characterized by shallow chest and abdominal wall movement, with resultant CO_2 retention. It is therefore important to measure end-tidal CO_2 levels concurrently in these patients. Esophageal pH can be monitored simultaneously when there is a suspicion of gastroesophageal reflux. Criteria for the scoring of sleep and sleep-related events such as apnea, arousals, and periodic limb movements have been recently revised [Iber et al., 2007].

In patients with obvious upper airway obstruction secondary to obesity or neuromuscular disorders like myotonic dystrophy, a therapeutic trial of positive pressure airway breathing can be attempted midway during the course of the sleep recording. A full 16- to 20-channel EEG montage is recommended when parasomnias and seizures are both in the differential diagnosis. Simultaneous video monitoring is standard for all nocturnal polysomnograms. Normative data for common physiologic variables are listed in Table 66-1 [Marcus and Loughlin, 1996]. There is insufficient evidence regarding the utility of ambulatory, in-home polysomnograms, especially in the preschool age group; thus, traditional sleep laboratory monitoring remains the gold standard in pediatric sleep medicine.

Multiple Sleep Latency Test

The Multiple Sleep Latency Test (MSLT) assesses how quickly one is able to fall asleep during the daytime and whether transition from wakefulness is into NREM sleep or into REM sleep. The MSLT can reliably detect sleepiness under clinical and experimental conditions [Littner et al., 2005]. The lower age limit at which one can utilize this test is about 6–7 years. Application of the MSLT to children younger than 6 years is unhelpful because healthy pre-school age children tend to take physiologic daytime naps. In order to be able to derive valid conclusions, the MSLT must be preceded the night before by a polysomnogram in which the total sleep time approximates physiologic sleep. The MSLT consists of the provision of four or five daytime nap opportunities at 2-hour intervals: e.g., at 10:00, 12:00, 14:00, and 16:00 hours. The EEG, chin electromyogram, and eye movements are monitored during each nap opportunity. The patient should be dressed in street clothes. The attending parent or guardian should be available to prevent the child from dozing off involuntarily in between the scheduled nap times. At each planned nap opportunity, the lights are turned off and the patient is asked to try to sleep. The time from "lights out" to sleep onset is measured, and represents the sleep latency. A mean sleep latency is also derived for the four naps. Normative values for the mean sleep latency have been established. The nap opportunity is terminated either 15 minutes after sleep onset, or if the patient does not fall asleep, at 20 minutes after "lights out." The mean sleep latency decreases inversely with an increase in the Tanner stage of sexual development, and ranges between 12 and 18 minutes [Carskadon, 1982]. A mean sleep latency of less than 5 minutes indicates severe daytime sleepiness; a value between 5 and 10 minutes indicates moderate daytime sleepiness. A urine drug screen is obtained in between the naps if illicit drug-seeking behavior is suspected. The occurrence of REM sleep within 15 minutes of sleep onset constitutes a sleep-onset rapid eye movement period (SOREMP). The presence of SOREMPs on two more MSLT nap opportunities in conjunction with a shortened mean sleep latency of less than 5 minutes is highly suggestive of narcolepsy.

In adults, a mean sleep latency of less than 5 minutes in association with two or more SOREMPs is 70 percent sensitive and 97 percent specific for the diagnosis of narcolepsy [Aldrich et al., 1997]. Comparable data on the sensitivity and specificity are not available for children and adolescents. A study by Gozal et al. [2001] suggests that, in prepubertal children, the normal mean sleep latency is 23.7 minutes, plus or minus 3.1 minutes. Palm et al. [1989] also found a mean sleep latency of 26.4 minutes plus or minus 2.8 minutes in 18 prepubertal children. These data suggest that the normal mean sleep latency in children may actually be higher than previously reported,

Table 66-1 Normal Polysomnographic Values in Children

Parameter	Average	Standard deviation
Total sleep time	472 min	42 min
Sleep efficiency	90%	7
Sleep latency	24.1 min	25.6 min
REM latency	87.8 min	41.2 min
REM sleep (% of TST)	21.1%	4.9
Stage N3 sleep (% of TST)	26.3%	4.8
Stage N2 sleep (% of TST)	36%	6.6
Stage N1 sleep (% of TST)	5.2%	2
Apnea hypopnea index (events per hour of sleep)	0.9	0.7
End-tidal CO_2 > 50 mm (% time)	25% or less	
Oxygen saturation (% time < 90%)	0.04%	0.18
Oxygen desaturations > 4% (number/hour of TST)	0.4	0.78

REM, rapid eye movement; TST, total sleep time.
(From Montgomery-Downs HE et al. Polysomnographic characteristics in normal preschool and early school aged children. Pediatrics 2006;117:741.)

and that normative data for the multiple sleep latency test in childhood might perhaps need revision. One of the merits of the multiple sleep latency test is that it provides reliable and quantitative information about the propensity for sleepiness. It has been validated as a measure of daytime sleepiness following episodes of sleep loss [Rosenthal et al., 1993], sleep disruption [Stepanski et al., 1987], and hypnotic drug and alcohol abuse [Billiard et al., 1987; Papineau et al., 1998]. The effects of treatment of daytime sleepiness with stimulants cannot be reliably measured, however. In addition, although one can control ambient noise and light that might affect sleep during the testing process, one cannot control for internal factors, like anxiety and apprehension, that also affect sleep propensity.

Maintenance of Wakefulness Test

The Maintenance of Wakefulness Test (MWT) is the mirror image opposite to the MSLT; one measures the ability to *stay awake* in a darkened, quiet environment during the daytime while the patient is seated in a semireclining position [Littner et al., 2005]. EEG, eye movements, and chin electromyography are monitored in a manner identical to that in the MSLT. The patient is provided four or five nap opportunities. The duration of each session is 40 minutes. The average mean sleep latency for normal adults is 35.2 minutes. Normative values have not been established for children. The test helps assess the effect of stimulant medication treatment on daytime sleepiness [Mitler et al., 2000].

Actigraphy

This technique involves the recording and storing of skeletal muscle activity continuously for 1–2 weeks in the home environment, generally from the nondominant forearm, using a wristwatch-shaped microcomputer device that measures linear acceleration and translates it into a numeric and graphic representation. This numeric representation is sampled frequently – that is, every 0.1 second – and aggregated at a constant interval or epoch length [Acebo and LeBourgeois, 2006]. The device captures signals during periods of muscle activity (generally correlating with wakefulness) and periods of no muscle activity (generally correlating with sleep; Figure 66-2). There is close correlation with polysomnographically determined total sleep time, sleep latency, and sleep efficiency [total sleep time or total time in bed ×100; Kothare and Kaleyias, 2008; van de Water et al., 2010]. Wrist actigraphy should be combined with 1–2 weeks of "sleep logs" that document specific wake-up and sleep-onset times, daytime naps, and so on. Wrist actigraphy is useful in the study of insomnia and circadian rhythm disorders like the delayed sleep phase syndrome [Kothare and Kaleyias, 2008]. In the latter instance, it will depict sleep onset late at night or in the early morning hours and uninterrupted sleep thereafter, with final awakening late in the morning or early afternoon (see Figure 66-1). In patients being evaluated for suspected narcolepsy, 2 weeks of actigraphy before nocturnal polysomnography and the MSLT help exclude the possibility of sleepiness resulting from a circadian rhythm disorder or insufficient sleep at night.

Common Childhood Sleep Disorders

Sleep-Related Breathing Disturbances

In increasing level of severity, the spectrum of sleep-disordered breathing in childhood ranges from snoring without sleep disruption (primary snoring) to the upper airway resistance syndrome (snoring that disrupts sleep continuity but without associated apnea or oxygen desaturation) to classic obstructive sleep apnea and, finally, obstructive hypoventilation (apnea, oxygen desaturation, plus hypercarbia). Between 10 and 12 percent of children snore on a habitual basis [Corbo et al., 2001; O'Brien et al., 2003]. The snoring sound is the result of vibration of the soft palate during inspiration due to narrowing of the oropharynx. Although some guidelines [American Academy of Pediatrics, 2002] suggest that primary snoring may be a "benign condition that does not warrant any specific therapy," a study of 87 children of 5–7 years of age [O'Brien et al., 2004] found that, compared with age-matched nonsnoring children, those with primary snoring performed worse on neuropsychologic measures of attention and had more social

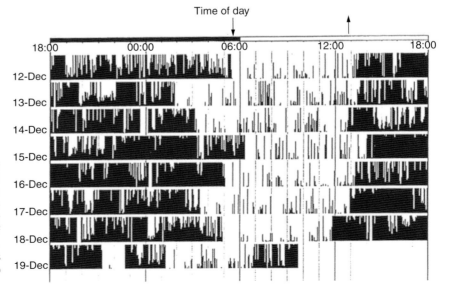

Fig. 66-2 Wrist actigraph demonstrating 2 weeks of sleep–wake recording in a teenager with delayed sleep phase syndrome, who presented with difficulty falling asleep. The dark bars indicate presence of muscle activity, which correlates closely with wakefulness, and the clear areas indicate lack of muscle activity, which generally correlates with sleep. Notice sleep onset late in the early morning hours (down arrow) and awakening in the afternoon (up arrow).

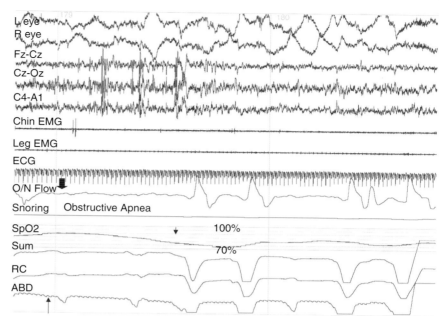

Fig. 66-3 Nocturnal polysomnogram demonstrating obstructive sleep apnea. Notice lack of signal in the nasal pressure channel (bold down arrow), despite persistence of abdominal respiratory effort (upward arrow). The oxygen desaturation resulting from the obstructive apnea event triggers an EEG arousal (small downward arrow). (Paper speed 10 mm/second.)

problems and anxious or depressive symptoms. Community-based studies have determined the prevalence of childhood obstructive sleep apnea at 1.1–2.9 percent [Ali et al., 1993; Brunetti et al., 2001].

OSA is characterized by partial or complete upper airway occlusion, with impaired air exchange despite persistence of thoracic and abdominal respiratory effort. This generally occurs in association with increased resistance to inspiration and transient oxygen desaturation of 3–4 percent (Figure 66-3). In some instances, there is an additional component of hypoventilation due to shallow abdominal and chest wall motion, which leads to hypercarbia. The most common etiologic factors for childhood OSA are adenotonsillar hypertrophy, craniofacial anomalies like micrognathia or maxillary hypoplasia, neuromuscular disorders such as myotonic dystrophy or congenital nonprogressive myopathies, and obesity [Lumeng and Chervin, 2008]. Repetitive occlusion of the upper airway during sleep, with resultant oxygen desaturation, provokes cortical arousals and suppression of REM and N3 sleep. Nocturnal symptoms of childhood obstructive sleep apnea include habitual snoring, restless sleep with snort arousals, bed wetting, excessive sweating, mouth breathing, choking sounds, and parasomnias such as confusional arousals and sleepwalking. Parental reports of snoring that is interrupted by silent pauses, which then terminate with snorting sounds, are characteristic of OSA. A metabolic syndrome, characterized by insulin resistance, hyperglycemia, hypertension, dyslipidemia, abdominal obesity, and proinflammatory and prothrombotic states, may develop as a consequence of OSA [Arens et al., 2010]. Daytime symptoms of OSA include inattentiveness, impaired academic performance, hyperactivity, and sleepiness [Chervin et al., 2002; Gozal, 2008]. The upper airway resistance syndrome is a form of upper airway obstruction in which no frank apneas or oxygen desaturation are observed during sleep, but the airway narrowing leads to recurrent arousals, fragmented sleep, and daytime sleepiness [Guilleminault et al., 1996]. Some patients exhibit subtle posterior displacement of the tongue, narrow nostrils, or a high-arched palate, but others might not have any craniofacial anomalies. The nocturnal polysomnogram may appear superficially normal, with the exception of snoring and increased EEG arousals of 3 or more seconds (normally less than 10–12 per hour of sleep). Simultaneously obtained intraluminal pressures from an esophageal balloon demonstrate a marked increase in the intrathoracic negative pressure during the upper airway resistance syndrome episodes. Nocturnal polysomnography is not needed to confirm the diagnosis in patients who already manifest the classic symptoms of OSA with marked tonsillar hypertrophy; one night of oximetry in the home environment, which documents recurrent oxygen desaturation, is sufficient for establishing the diagnosis in these patients [Brouilette et al., 2000]. Nocturnal polysomnography is, however, indicated when the diagnosis is uncertain or less obvious. It is also indicated when OSA is suspected in the context of multiple neurologic handicaps, such as in Down syndrome or cerebral palsy, and when the patient needs to be considered for a nonsurgical treatment such as a continuous positive airway pressure device. OSA secondary to adenotonsillar hypertrophy may respond in a modestly favorable manner to adenotonsillectomy, but patients younger than 3 years old and those with severe obstructive sleep apnea should be monitored postoperatively in the intensive care unit for respiratory compromise due to postoperative upper airway edema. Patients should generally be re-evaluated clinically and with polysomnography 2–3 months after adenotonsillectomy. Positive airway pressure breathing devices should be considered if there is significant, residual OSA. Weight-reduction measures are indicated in obese patients. Orthodontic consultation and the use of oral appliances during sleep is indicated in those with retrognathia and tongue prolapse [Rondeau, 1998]. Rapid maxillary distraction is a nonsurgical technique that is used in OSA with associated high-arched palate and consequent narrowing of the nasal passages [Abad and Guilleminault, 2009].

Central Hypoventilation Syndromes

Defective automatic control of breathing during sleep as a result of brainstem dysfunction is characteristic of this category of disorders, which presents in infancy or childhood.

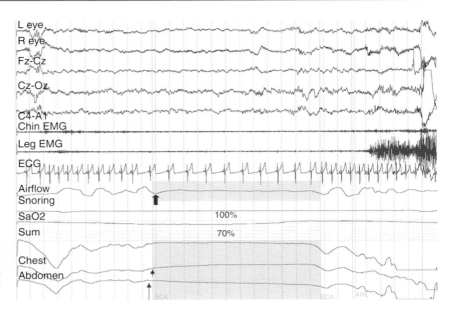

Fig. 66-4 Central sleep apnea in a child with a primary brainstem tumor involving the medulla. Notice the simultaneous cessation of signal in the airflow channel (wide arrow), as well as in the thoracic and abdominal effort channels (thin arrows).

Developmental malformations of the brainstem are common, but may be visible only on microscopic examination. Head injury, bulbar poliomyelitis, syringobulbia, Chiari types I and II malformation [Zolty et al., 2000], and inborn errors of metabolism (e.g., Leigh's syndrome) are some underlying conditions. Polysomnography may reveal central sleep apnea, oxygen desaturation, shallow respiratory effort, and elevated levels of end tidal carbon dioxide (Figure 66-4). Except for surgical decompression in Chiari malformation and syringobulbia-associated hypoventilation, the management is similar to that of primary congenital central alveolar hypoventilation, which is discussed below.

Congenital central alveolar hypoventilation is a disorder in which there is no obvious structural or biochemical etiology for the defective central control of breathing during sleep [Gozal, 2004; Gozal and Harper, 1999]. Onset of symptoms is during infancy or early childhood. The respiratory rate and depth are initially normal during wakefulness, but shallow breathing (hypoventilation), hypercarbia, and oxygen desaturation appear during sleep. The dysfunction is worse in NREM sleep, as compared to REM sleep. Ventilatory challenge with inhalation of a mixture of 5 percent CO_2 and 95 percent O_2 fails to evoke the physiologic, three- to fivefold increase in minute volume. Common sites of neuronal loss and gliosis include the arcuate nucleus in the medulla, the ventrolateral nucleus of the tractus solitarius, nucleus ambiguus, nucleus retroambigualis, the chemosensitive ventral medullary surface, and the nucleus parabrachialis in the dorsolateral pons. Between 15 and 20 percent of congenital central alveolar hypoventilation patients have coexisting Hirschsprung's disease or neural crest tumors, such as neuroblastoma or ganglioneuroma [Roshkow et al., 1988; Swaminathan et al., 1989]. It has been hypothesized that congenital central alveolar hypoventilation is a neural crest disorder because, during fetal development, brainstem neurons that regulate chemosensitivity are derived from the neural crest. The proto-oncogene, receptor tyrosine kinase, is involved in this process [Bolk et al., 1996]. Mutations in the *PHOX2B* gene have been identified in over 90 percent of patients with central hypoventilation syndrome [Traochet et al., 2005]. They generally consist of expansions of the polyalanine tail in this gene, though expansions of non-polyalanine repeats have also been implicated [Weese-Mayer et al., 2010]. Tumors of the neural crest manifest increased prevalence in those with non-polyalanine expansions. Mutations in the *PHOX2B* gene are transmitted in an autosomal-dominant manner. Mosaicism occurs in 5–10 percent of the parents, which emphasizes the importance of molecular testing in parents of the affected child [Weese-Mayer et al., 2010]. A knockout mouse model has been developed, which also have an inability to respond to hypercarbia, depletion of neurons in the retrotrapezoid nucleus and the parafacial respiratory group of neurons [Amiel et al., 2009]. There is no definitive and satisfactory treatment for congenital central alveolar hypoventilation, though acetazolamide and theophylline enhance chemoreceptivity of the brainstem respiratory neurons to a modest degree. Home ventilation via tracheostomy and diaphragmatic pacing are other therapeutic modalities. Patients may die during infancy or childhood. It is recommended that patients with congenital central hypoventilation syndrome undergo an annual hospital admission for a comprehensive, multidisciplinary evaluation that includes 72-hour Holter monitoring, echocardiogram, evaluation of autonomic dysregulation affecting other organ systems, and imaging for neural crest tumors when appropriate [Weese-Mayer et al., 2010].

Narcolepsy

Chronic daytime sleepiness, hypnagogic hallucinations (vivid dreams at sleep onset), sleep-onset paralysis, cataplexy (sudden loss of skeletal muscle tone in response to emotional triggers like laughter, fright, or surprise), and fragmented night sleep are the characteristic clinical features of narcolepsy. The incidence of narcolepsy in the United States is 1.37 per 100,000 persons per year (1.72 for men and 1.05 for women). It is highest in the second decade, followed by a gradual decline. The prevalence is approximately 56 per 100,000 persons [Silber et al., 2002]. A meta-analysis of 235 pediatric cases derived from three studies [Challamel et al., 1994] found that 34 percent of all narcolepsy subjects experienced onset of symptoms before the age of 15 years, 16 percent before the age of 10 years,

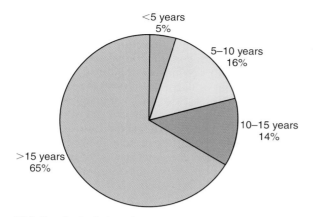

Fig. 66-5 Graph depicting the age of onset of narcolepsy. *(Data derived from Challamel MJ et al. Narcolepsy in children. Sleep 1994;17S:17.)*

and 4.5 percent before age 5 years (Figure 66-5). Although the age of onset is generally in the latter half of the first decade or the second decade, rare cases with onset of extreme sleepiness and cataplexy during infancy have also been reported [Nevsimalova et al., 1986; Sharp and D'Cruz, 2001]. Childhood daytime sleepiness may be overlooked by parents, schoolteachers, and physicians alike. Sleepy children may be mistaken for being "lazy." They may exhibit mood swings and inattentiveness as a consequence of sleepiness-related prefontal cortical dysfunction. Cataplexy is present in about two-thirds of patients. The cataplectic muscle weakness generally lasts for a few seconds to minutes, and is associated with muscle atonia, absence of muscle stretch reflexes, and full preservation of consciousness. Because cataplexy can be subtle, the examiner might need to ask leading questions about sudden muscle weakness in the lower extremities, neck, or trunk in response to laughter, fright, excitement, or anger. Cataplexy is associated with abrupt hyperpolarization of the spinal alpha motor neurons. Fragmentation of night sleep is also common in narcolepsy. Children younger than 7 or 8 years may not be able to provide a reliable history of cataplexy, hypnagogic hallucinations, or sleep paralysis. Patients with narcolepsy exhibit less circadian clock-dependent alertness during the daytime and also less circadian clock-dependent sleepiness at night [Broughton et al., 1998]. Secondary narcolepsy is a rare entity, but may develop as a sequel to closed head injury and in patients with deep midline brain tumors, lymphomas, and encephalitis [Autret et al., 1994]. Obesity and precocious puberty may accompany the onset of narcolepsy-cataplexy in childhood [Perriol et al., 2010; Kotagal et al., 2004; Plazzi et al., 2006].

Stores et al. [2006] assessed the psychosocial difficulties of 42 children with narcolepsy (mean age 12.4, range 7.3–17.9), 18 subjects with excessive daytime sleepiness unrelated to narcolepsy (EDS; mean age 14.2, range 5.1–18.8), and 23 unaffected controls (mean age 11.3, range 6–16.8). They found significantly higher scores on the Strengths and Difficulties Questionnaire in the narcolepsy and EDS groups. The domains of this questionnaire included prosocial, peer problems, hyperactivity, conduct problems, emotional problems, and adverse impact on the family. As compared to healthy controls, both the narcolepsy and the EDS groups scored higher on the Child Depression Inventory. Children with narcolepsy and EDS also had more absences from school (means 6.4 and 5.3 days,

respectively), as compared to controls (mean 1.3), and displayed more problems on a composite educational difficulties score, suggesting that sleepiness in general, rather than narcolepsy per se adversely influences the psychosocial and emotional health of the patients.

The presence of the histocompatibility antigen DQB1*0602 in close to 100 percent of persons with narcolepsy, as compared with a 12–32 percent prevalence in the general population, indicates genetic susceptibility, which by itself is insufficient to precipitate the clinical syndrome. Monozygotic twins have been reported to remain discordant for narcolepsy [Langdon et al., 1986; Mignot et al., 1999, 2001]. In genetically susceptible individuals, acquired life stresses like minor head injury, systemic illnesses such as infectious mononucleosis, and bereavement may play a role in triggering the disorder, and have been reported in close to two-thirds of subjects – "the two-hit hypothesis" [Billiard et al., 1986]. The key pathophysiologic event in human narcolepsy-cataplexy is hypocretin ligand deficiency [Nishino et al., 2000, 2001]. Hypocretin (orexin) is a peptide that is produced by neurons of the dorsolateral hypothalamus. Hypocretins 1 and 2 (synonymous with orexins A and B) are peptides that are synthesized from preprohypocretin. They have corresponding receptors. Whereas the hypocretin type 1 receptor binds only to hypocretin1, the hypocretin type 2 receptor binds to both type 1 and 2 ligands [Hungs et al., 2001]. Hypocretin-producing neurons have widespread projections to the forebrain and brainstem. Hypocretin promotes alertness and increases motor activity and basal metabolic rate [John et al., 2000]. Of significance is the postmortem examination finding in human narcolepsy of an 85–95 percent reduction in the number of hypocretin-containing neurons of the hypothalamus, whereas melanin-concentrating hormone neurons that are intermingled with hypocretin neurons remain unaffected, thus suggesting a targeted neurodegenerative process [Thannickal et al., 2000]. It is hypothesized that an immune-mediated degenerative process affecting the hypocretin-producing cells of the hypothalamus (perhaps linked to HLA DQB1*0602 by mechanisms yet unknown) provokes a decrease in forebrain noradrenergic activation, which in turn decreases alertness. A corresponding decrease of noradrenergic activity in the brainstem leads to disinhibition of brainstem cholinergic systems, thus triggering cataplexy and other phenomena of REM sleep, such as hypnagogic hallucinations and sleep paralysis. The decrease in hypocretin-1 ligand levels that is characteristic of human narcolepsy-cataplexy is also reflected in the cerebrospinal fluid (CSF). Using a radioimmunoassay, Nishino et al. [2000, 2001] found that the mean CSF level of hypocretin-1 in healthy controls was 280.3 ± 33.0 pg/mL; in neurologic controls it was 260.5 ± 37.1 pg/mL; and in those with narcolepsy-cataplexy, hypocretin-1 was either undetectable or less than 100 pg/mL. Low to absent CSF hypocretin-1 levels were found in 32 of 38 narcolepsy-cataplexy patients, who were all also HLA DQB1*0602-positive. Narcolepsy patients who were HLA DQB1*0602 antigen-negative tended to have normal to high CSF hypocretin-1 levels. In another study of narcolepsy with cataplexy, narcolepsy without cataplexy, and idiopathic hypersomnia, Kanbayashi et al. [2002] found nine narcolepsy-cataplexy subjects who were HLA DQB1*0602-positive but CSF hypocretin-1-deficient. In contrast, narcolepsy *without* cataplexy and idiopathic hypersomnia patients exhibited normal CSF hypocretin levels (Figure 66-6). The hypocretin assay

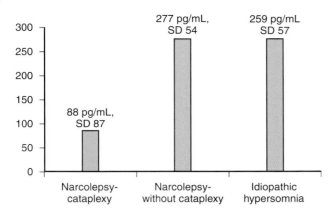

Fig. 66-6 Cerebrospinal fluid levels of hypocretin-1 in patients with narcolepsy-cataplexy, narcolepsy without cataplexy, and idiopathic hypersomnia. *(Data derived from Kanbayashi T et al. CSF hypocretin-1 [orexin-A] concentrations in narcolepsy with and without cataplexy and idiopathic hypersomnia. J Sleep Res 2002;11:91.)*

may be most useful when an HLA DQB1*0602-positive patient with suspected narcolepsy-cataplexy is already receiving central nervous system stimulants at the time of initial presentation, and in whom the discontinuation of these medications for the purpose of obtaining polysomnography and an MSLT is inconvenient or impractical.

A combined battery of nocturnal polysomnogram and MSLT remains the most widely used method to diagnose narcolepsy. The nocturnal polysomnogram demonstrates increased arousals, decreased initial REM latency of less than 70 minutes (time from sleep onset to onset of the first REM sleep epoch; normal value in teenagers is around 140 minutes), and absence of any other significant sleep pathology, such as OSA. Periodic limb movements may be increased. During REM sleep, there may be persistence of tonic electromyographic activity. This phenomenon is called REM sleep without atonia. When persistence of electromyographic activity is combined with physical dream enactment, patients are defined as having a REM sleep behavior disorder. The multiple sleep latency test, which is obtained on the day after the nocturnal polysomnogram, records sleep onset on each of the four nap opportunities within 5 minutes of "lights out," whereas the reference value is approximately 16–18 minutes. Sleep-onset REM periods are also seen during at least 2 out of 4 nap opportunities. Because narcolepsy is a lifelong condition, these diagnostic test results need to be clear and unambiguous for the diagnosis to be confirmed.

Management of narcolepsy requires a combination of lifestyle changes and pharmacotherapy. A planned daytime nap of 20–30 minutes at school and another one in the afternoon upon return home may enhance alertness. The patient should observe regular sleep onset and morning wake-up times, avoid alcohol, and exercise regularly. To minimize the risk of accidents, the patient should avoid sharp, moving objects. Daytime sleepiness is treated pharmacologically with modafinil (100–400 mg/day in two divided doses), or regular or extended-release preparations of methylphenidate (20–60 mg/day in two divided doses) and dextroamphetamine (10–30 mg/day in two divided doses) [Littner et al., 2001]. Cataplexy is treated using clomipramine (25 mg at bedtime), protryptiline (2.5–5 mg/day in two divided doses), or sodium

oxybate (gamma-hydroxybutyrate). Sodium oxybate is administered in two divided doses or at night, and seems to work by stabilizing nocturnal sleep architecture. There are insufficient data on its use in childhood. Emotional and behavioral problems that commonly accompany childhood narcolepsy may require the addition of fluoxetine (10–30 mg every morning) or sertraline (25–50 mg twice daily) and supportive psychotherapy. Teenagers should be counseled against driving if they have uncontrolled sleepiness. They should also avoid work and social situations in which they could endanger themselves or others. There have been anecdotal reports of improvement in narcolepsy-cataplexy following the infusion of intravenous immunoglobulin G [Dauvilliers, 2009], but randomized controlled studies have not been carried out. The Narcolepsy Network (www.narcolepsynetwork.org) is a private, nonprofit resource for patients, families, and health professionals. There is also a National Narcolepsy Registry, more information on which can be found at www.ninds.nih.gov/disorders/narcolepsy. Experimental treatment efforts are focused on hypocretin replacement therapy, gene therapy, and cell transplantation [Ritchie et al., 2010].

Idiopathic Hypersomnia

Idiopathic hypersomnia is associated with a complaint of excessive daytime sleepiness, occurring daily for at least 3 months. Nocturnal polysomnography should have excluded other conditions leading to hypersomnia. In contrast with the mean sleep latency on the MSLT of less than 5 minutes that is typical of narcolepsy, the mean sleep latency in idiopathic hypersomnia is generally in the 5- to 10-minute range. Two or more SOREMPs that are typically seen on the MSLT in patients with narcolepsy are also not present. Patients do not exhibit cataplexy, hypnagogic hallucinations, or sleep paralysis [Frenette and Kushida, 2009]. Two subtypes of idiopathic hypersomnia have been identified. In idiopathic hypersomnia with long sleep, there is prolonged nocturnal sleep lasting 10 or more hours. In idiopathic hypersomnia without long sleep, the major nocturnal sleep period is 6–10 hours in length. In a review of 42 patients evaluated at the University of Michigan over a 10-year period, Basetti and Aldrich [1997] observed that idiopathic hypersomnia began at a mean age of 19 ± 8 years (range 6–43). Almost half of the subjects described restless sleep with frequent arousals. Habitual dreaming was present in about 40 percent of the subjects. They mention that there is substantial clinical overlap between narcolepsy and idiopathic hypersomnia. In a subset of children, idiopathic hypersomnia may represent a transitional phase en route to the development of classic narcolepsy [Kotagal and Swink, 1996].

Restless Legs Syndrome

Restless legs syndrome is an autosomal-dominant, sensorimotor disorder in which the subject complains of a peculiar "creepy or crawling" feeling in the extremities [Picchietti and Picchietti, 2008]. The discomfort appears in the evening and night-time hours, is exacerbated by immobility, and is momentarily relieved by movement of the limb [Allen et al., 2003]. There is also an urge to move the limbs. This discomfort interferes with sleep initiation and maintenance, and may be accompanied by daytime fatigue, inattentiveness, or sleepiness.

A large population-based survey of over 10,000 families in the United Kingdom and the United States found a prevalence of definite restless legs syndrome in 1.9 percent of 8–11-year-olds and in 2 percent of 12–17-year-olds [Picchietti et al., 2007]. Childhood restless legs syndrome may be synonymous with "growing pains" in some children [Walters, 2002]. On nocturnal polysomnography, the patient may or may not demonstrate periodic limb movements, which are defined as a series of four or more rhythmic, electromyographically recorded movements of the legs lasting 0.5–10 seconds that occur 5–90 seconds apart, generally during stages N1 or N2 of sleep. The favorable response to dopamine receptor agonists like pramipexole and carbidopa-levodopa suggests that central nervous system dopamine deficiency is a pathophysiologic feature. There may be an associated systemic iron deficiency in the form of low levels of serum ferritin [Kotagal and Silber, 2004] because iron is a co-factor for tyrosine hydroxylase, which is essential in the synthesis of dopamine. There also appears to be an association between restless legs syndrome and attention-deficit disorder [Chervin et al., 2002; Picchietti et al., 1999]; in a community-based questionnaire survey of 866 children aged 2–13.9 years, Chervin et al. [2002] found an odds ratio for significant hyperactivity and restless legs of 1:9. Besides dopamine agonists, oral iron, clonazepam, gabapentin, gabapentin enacarbil [Bogan et al., 2010], and pregabalin [Allen et al., 2010] have also been used to treat restless legs syndrome, but there has been no randomized controlled trial in childhood to determine efficacy definitely.

Periodic Hypersomnia (Kleine–Levin Syndrome)

Periodic hypersomnia is generally seen in adolescents, with a male predominance. Patients develop 1- to 2-week periods of hypersomnolence, characterized by sleeping 18–20 hours per day, cognitive and mood disturbances in association with compulsive hyperphagia, and hypersexual behavior, with an intervening 2–4 months of normal alertness and behavior [Brown and Billiard, 1995; Frenette and Kushida, 2009]. Incomplete forms of the syndrome have also been recognized. The hyperphagia may be in the form of binge eating, and can actually be associated with a 2–5 kg increase in body weight. Nocturnal polysomnography during the sleepy periods exhibits decreased sleep efficiency, shortened latency to REM sleep, and decreased percentage of time spent in N3 sleep. The MSLT reveals moderately shortened mean sleep latency in the 5–10-minute range, but lacks the two or more SOREMPs that are typically seen in narcolepsy. The episodic hypersomnia gradually diminishes, ultimately resolving completely over 2–5 years or evolving into classic depression, thus bringing up the issue of whether the disorder is a variant of depression. A disturbance of hypothalamic function has been hypothesized but not established. The association of Kleine–Levin syndrome with histocompatibility antigen DQB1*0201, and the occasional precipitation after systemic infections, as well as the relapsing and remitting nature, are suspicious for an autoimmune etiology [Dauvilliers et al., 2002]. There is no satisfactory treatment, although lithium has been reported to be effective in a case report [Poppe et al., 2003]. Modafinil may reduce the duration of the symptomatic episodes [Huang et al., 2010].

Delayed Sleep Phase Disorder

Circadian rhythm disorders are characterized by alteration in the timing of sleep onset and offset relative to the societal norms. Delayed sleep phase disorder [DSPD] is the most common circadian rhythm sleep disorder. The basis for all circadian rhythm disorders is abnormal functioning of a molecular feedback loop between CLOCK and BMAL1 (transcription regulating proteins) and the expression of *Period* genes *Per1*, *Per2*, *Per3*, and *Cryptochrome* genes *Cry1* and *Cry2* [Wulff et al., 2009]. DSPD was described initially in a medical student who was unable to wake up in time to attend his morning classes [Weitzman et al., 1981]. Despite hypnotic use, the patient was unable to fall asleep before the early morning hours and was mistaken initially for having insomnia. Sleep in the laboratory was, however, quantitatively and qualitatively normal. The delay in the timing of occurrence of the sleeping phase of the 24-hour sleep–wake cycle was due to a constitutional inability to prepone sleep, which in turn is secondary to altered function of the circadian timekeeper, i.e., the suprachiasmatic nucleus. The disorder typically has onset in adolescence, with a male predominance. The increased frequency of HLA DR1 and the occasional familial clustering of delayed sleep phase syndrome suggest a genetic predisposition [Garcia et al., 2001]. The condition must, however, be differentiated from school avoidance seen in adolescents with delinquent and antisocial behavior, because these individuals can fall asleep at an earlier hour at night in the controlled sleep laboratory setting. Maintenance of sleep logs and wrist actigraphy for 1–2 weeks is helpful in establishing the diagnosis of delayed sleep phase syndrome (see Figure 66-2). "Bright light" therapy is helpful in advancing the sleep-onset time to an earlier hour [Cole et al., 2002]. It consists of the provision of 2700–10,000 lux of bright light via a "light box" for 20–30 minutes immediately upon awakening in the morning. The light box is kept at a distance of 18–24 inches from the face. The phototherapy leads to a gradual advancement (shifting back) of the sleep-onset time at night. Bright light therapy may be combined with melatonin that is administered about 5–5.5 hours before the required bedtime in a dose of 0.5–1 mg. Another therapeutic option is one of progressively delaying bedtime by 3–4 hours per day until it becomes synchronized with socially acceptable sleep–wake time (chronotherapy), and then adhering to this schedule. Over time, however, all DSPD patients remain at risk for drifting back to progressively later and later bedtimes. Daytime stimulants, such as modafinil (100–400 mg/day in two divided doses), may improve the level of daytime alertness. The physician may also need to write a letter to the school, requesting a mid-morning school start time on medical grounds.

The Relationship between Sleep and Epilepsy

The onset of sleep may be associated with increased interictal spiking, as well as with an increased propensity for clinical seizures. Frontal and temporal lobe seizures are especially prone to occur and to generalize secondarily during sleep [Bourgeois, 1996; Kotagal and Yardi, 2008]. Interictal epileptiform discharges may be observed only during sleep [Shinnar et al., 1994]. Nocturnal seizures are most likely to occur during stage N2, followed by N1, N3, and REM sleep, in that order.

The syndrome of electrical status epilepticus during slow-wave sleep (ESES) is characterized by continuous spike-and-wave discharges during 85 percent or more of nocturnal NREM sleep, along with cognitive and behavioral regression [Nickels and Wirrell, 2008]. There are two different forms of ESES – Landau–Kleffner syndrome and the syndrome of continuous spike-wave stupor. Landau–Kleffner syndrome is characterized by regression in language function, typically in the form of auditory verbal agnosia, in association with continuous epileptiform activity during both REM and NREM sleep [Landau and Kleffner, 1957]. Continuous spike-wave stupor, by contrast, is associated with global regression of cognition. The sleep EEG findings are, however, similar to those of the Landau–Kleffner syndrome. Prolonged daytime and night-time EEG may be needed to establish the diagnosis of either entity. Intravenous lorazepam or diazepam may transiently suppress the epileptiform discharges. Long-term maintenance with valproic acid may be modestly effective. Liukkonen et al. followed 32 children with ESES longitudinally (Liukkonen et al., 2010]. Treatment was with valproic acid alone or valproic acid combined with ethosuximide. Ten of 32 children regained their pre-ESES cognitive levels. Unfavorable cognitive outcome was predicted by younger age at ESES diagnosis, lower IQ at initial diagnosis, and no response to drug treatment.

Sleep deprivation leads to activation of seizures. Ellingson et al. [1984] observed that clinical seizures occurred after sleep deprivation in 19 of 788 (2.4 percent) otherwise healthy subjects. Patterns of epileptiform abnormality are also considerably influenced by sleep [Kotagal and Yardi, 2008]. For example, the three-per-second spike-and-wave complexes of absence seizures are replaced in sleep by single spike-and-waves or by polyspike-and-wave complexes. The hypsarrhythmia of infantile spasms is replaced during sleep by brief periods of generalized voltage attenuation. Patients with Lennox–Gastaut syndrome may manifest long runs of generalized spike-and-wave discharges.

Conversely, seizures also influence sleep by suppressing REM sleep, with a corresponding increase in slow-wave sleep. This effect of slowing of the background EEG frequency may persist for days after a seizure. Frequent nocturnal seizures also tend to disrupt sleep continuity, with an increased number of arousals. Patients with Lennox–Gastaut syndrome frequently exhibit tonic seizures during sleep. Vagus nerve stimulation has been found to result in shortened sleep latency, reduced N1 sleep, and increased N3 sleep [Kotagal and Yardi, 2008]. OSA has also been observed after vagus nerve stimulation [Khurana et al., 2007].

Disorders of sleep can also adversely affect seizure control. Patients with OSA have been documented to manifest poor seizure control, which improves after correction of OSA with positive airway pressure breathing, adenotonsillectomy, or tracheostomy [Britton et al., 1997]. In some instances, the daytime somnolence from sleep apnea may be mistaken as a side effect of antiepileptic therapy. In general, antiepileptic drugs lead to stabilization of sleep with a decreased number of nocturnal arousals. Phenobarbital therapy is associated with suppression in the proportion of time spent in REM sleep and increased stage N3 sleep. Both phenytoin and carbamazepine also increase N3 at the expense of N1 and N2 sleep. Benzodiazepines increase stage N3 sleep at the expense of N1 sleep. Lamotrigine can increase the proportion of time spent in REM sleep, with fewer sleep-stage shifts [Kotagal and Yardi, 2008]. Felbamate has been reported to cause insomnia in about 11 percent of subjects [Cilio et al., 2001].

Sleep in Neurologically Compromised Children

Children with spastic quadriparetic cerebral palsy may exhibit daytime irritability in conjunction with fragmented sleep and frequent night-time awakenings, and oxygen desaturation from OSA due to upper airway collapse or adenotonsillar hypertrophy [Kotagal et al., 1994]. They may also have impaired central arousal mechanisms and be unable to compensate for apnea by changes in body position, making OSA especially problematic for them. Jouvet and Petre-Quadens [1966] have described prolonged initial REM latency and suppression in the proportion of time spent in REM sleep in patients with severe mental retardation. Decreased rapid eye movements and spindle density, as well as the presence of "undifferentiated" sleep, correlate with low levels of intelligence [Zucconi, 2000]. Patients with Leigh's syndrome manifest recurrent central apneas or hypoventilation as a consequence of brainstem involvement [Cummiskey et al., 1987]. Joubert's syndrome is associated with periods of hyperpnea and panting respiration. Rett's syndrome is characterized by deep, sighing respiration during wakefulness and normal breathing patterns during sleep, consistent with impairment of the voluntary, cortical control of breathing, and a normal automatic or brainstem control of respiration [Zucconi, 2000]. Patients with Down syndrome have complicated sleep problems. They may develop OSA from the combination of macroglossia, midface hypoplasia, and hypotonic upper airway musculature [Levanon et al., 1999; Kotagal, 2007]. Superimposed on this may be an element of hypoventilation and consequent retention of carbon dioxide due to shallow movement of intercostal and diaphragm muscles. Sleep architecture is disrupted, with decreased sleep efficiency, increased arousals, suppression of N3, and REM sleep. Patients with achondroplasia may develop OSA in infancy as a result of macroglossia and midface hypoplasia. They may also develop central sleep apnea as a consequence of cervicomedullary compression. There is no correlation between the diameter of the foramen magnum and severity of the sleep apnea, but patients need close follow-up of their neurologic and respiratory function. Zucconi et al. [1996] found sleep-related breathing disorders in close to 75 percent of achondroplasia patients. Certain lysosomal storage disorders, such as the mucopolysaccharidoses like Hurler's syndrome, have been associated with severe OSA that resolves with surgical reduction of macroglossia or bone marrow transplantation. Patients with Niemann–Pick type C disease frequently manifest cataplexy from brainstem involvement, fragmented night sleep, and daytime sleepiness, occasionally in conjuction with reduced CSF levels of hypocretin-1 [Vankova et al., 2003]. Circadian rhythm disorders, like irregular sleep–wake rhythms, are common in patients with severe mental retardation and cerebral palsy; this is especially true if there is associated blindness with impaired light perception that might impair melanopsin activation in the retinal ganglionic cells, and consequent melatonin secretion from the pineal gland and the development of circadian rhythms. Many blind patients with complete lack of light perception fall asleep relatively early in the evening and are wide awake in early morning hours (3 or 4 am), or exhibit multiple periods of daytime sleepiness (irregular sleep–wake rhythms) [Leger et al., 1999]. Melatonin administration and bright light (if light perception is intact) may be used to reset the sleep schedule in these patients.

Parasomnias

Parasomnias are unpleasant or undesirable events that intrude on to sleep, without altering sleep quality or quantity. These events may occur at the transition to sleep, during REM sleep, or at the time of shifting from N3 sleep into the lighter N2/N1 sleep [Kotagal, 2009]. The incidence of parasomnias is variable, though 30 percent of children have at least one episode of sleepwalking, and sleeptalking is noted in about half the population [D'Cruz and Vaughn, 2001]. Frequently, the patient is unaware of the events, but medical attention is sought owing to disruption of the sleep of other family members or after serious injury to the patient. NREM parasomnias, such as confusional arousals, sleepwalking, and sleep terrors, are most commonly seen during N3 sleep and are thus prevalent in the first third of night, when this type of sleep is most abundant. NREM parasomnias occur during attempted transition from N3 into N2 or N1 sleep, with consequent partial arousal and nonepileptic behaviors. Confusional arousals are seen most often in toddlers, whereas sleepwalking and sleep terrors may occur throughout the first decade. Children with confusional arousals may sit up in bed, moan or whimper inconsolably, and utter words like "no" or "go away." Autonomic activation, characterized by flushing, sweating, and piloerection, is minimal to absent. The events generally last 5–30 minutes, after which the patient goes right back to sleep and has no recollection of the events whatsoever upon awakening the following morning. Patients with night terrors and sleepwalking may exhibit flushing of the face, increased sweating, inconsolability, and agitation, but again with complete amnesia for the event in the morning. In all of the three NREM parasomnias, a concurrently obtained EEG will show rhythmic activity in the 2–6-Hz range, consistent with partial arousal from slow-wave sleep. A low dose of clonazepam (0.25–0.5 mg at bedtime) is helpful in preventing most NREM parasomnias. In some NREM parasomnias, the partial arousals may be triggered by underlying sleep apnea, restless legs syndrome, or gastroesophageal reflux. If so, treatment of these underlying disorders will help alleviate parasomnia. Environmental safety measures, such as installing a deadbolt lock on the door, may be necessary in patients with habitual sleepwalking. NREM parasomnias can sometimes be confused with nocturnal seizures, especially those with frontal lobe onset [Zucconi et al., 1998]. In general, however, the seizure events are shorter in duration (often 20–30 seconds), and are accompanied by more prominent head segment automatisms, such as lip smacking, eye deviation, or chewing. Further, the patient may have partial recall of the event and headache upon awakening in the morning. In contrast to the 6-channel EEG montage that is utilized in standard video polysomnography, the study of suspected parasomnias in the sleep laboratory calls for a full 16-channel EEG montage to help distinguish seizures from parasomnias. Most NREM parasomnias subside spontaneously by 10–12 years of age.

Common REM sleep parasomnias include nightmares (scary dreams), terrifying hypnagogic hallucinations, and the REM sleep behavior disorder. Because REM sleep is most abundant during the final third of night sleep, nightmares and REM sleep

behavior disorder tend to occur during the early morning hours. The REM sleep behavior disorder is characterized by actual motoric dream enactment, during which the patient might kick, jump, or struggle against an imaginary assailant as a result of failure of the customary inhibition of skeletal muscle activity in REM sleep by the medullary nucleus reticularis gigantocellularis. The nocturnal polysomnogram reveals increased phasic electromyographic activity during REM sleep. Although REM sleep behavior disorder is relatively infrequent during childhood, sporadic cases do occur. Treatment with clonazepam (0.25–0.5 mg at bedtime) is effective in preventing most REM parasomnias.

Autism and Sleep

Sleep–wake problems occur in 40–80 percent of children with autism. Problems with sleep often develop early around the same time as onset of developmental regression [Miano and Ferri, 2010]. There does not seem to be increased predeliction by gender. Sleep initiation and maintenance difficulty are the most common complaints [Richdale, 1999; Malow et al., 2006]. There seem to be many pathophysiologic mechanisms underlying the insomnia. To begin with, the child with autism has a difficult time with self-regulation of emotions [Johnson et al., 2009]. Children with autism may experience difficulties with comprehension of parental directions and also with verbalizing their apprehensions [Goldman et al., 2011]. The memory of exciting or upsetting experiences from earlier in the day may linger right into bedtime, and at times even through the night. Sometimes, parents inadvertently contribute to sleep initiation and maintenance difficulty by resorting to behaviors such as rocking the child to sleep or holding the child in their arms till sleep has ensued, at which point the child is placed in bed. As a consequence, there is habit-forming to these extraneous stimuli. When the child awakens in the middle of the night, it is hard to fall back to sleep without once again being held or rocked. This entity is termed sleep-onset association disorder [Johnson et al., 2009]. Comorbid seizures can disrupt sleep, as might also agents like benzodiazepines, phenobarbital, and felbamate that are used for their treatment. Further, a genetic susceptibility region for autism has been localized to chromosome 15q. This region also expresses a variety of GABA-related genes, the disruption in function of which might predispose to insomnia [McCauley et al., 2004]. An alteration in the timing of release of melatonin, with low levels at night and higher levels in the daytime, has also been reported [Ritvo et al., 1993]. Systemic disturbances, such as gastroesophageal reflux, could also contribute to sleep initiation and maintenance difficulty.

The clinician should try to determine if the daily schedule of the autistic child is unduly rigorous and thus leading to excessive excitement and anxiety. If so, simplifying the afternoon and evening regimen, and adhering to a consistent and simple evening schedule, with 30–60 minutes of quiet time before bedtime, may be employed. Postponing bed onset time by about an hour, avoiding daytime naps, and use of graduated extinction techniques may be useful in managing the sleep onset association disorder. The help of a child psychologist might be required in this regard. Complete extinction (removing reinforcement to reduce a behavior) and various forms of graduated extinction are commonly utilized by psychologists. Controlled-release formulations of melatonin, provided at bedtime in a dose of 3–6 mg, are used empirically. Clonidine,

0.1–0.2 mg in two divided doses, can be used for its anxiolytic effect. Risperidone, administered in low doses (0.5–1 mg/ day) may have a calming effect on the child as well, but higher doses should be avoided, as the dopamine antagonist effect of risperidone can precipitate restless legs syndrome, with consequent rebound deterioration in sleep. The combination of behavioral techniques and melatonin administration has also been recommended [Miano and Ferri, 2010].

Nocturnal polysomnography is technically challenging in children with autism and generally documents nonspecific abnormalities of sleep fragmentation. Unless there is a strong suspicion of obstructive sleep apnea, it is usually not needed. Two weeks of actigraphy and parental logs of sleep–wake function generally yield useful information about sleep latency, sleep onset time, and total sleep time.

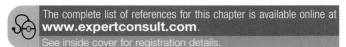

The complete list of references for this chapter is available online at **www.expertconsult.com**.
See inside cover for registration details.

Index

Note: Page numbers followed by *b* indicate boxes, *f* indicate figures and *t* indicate tables. Page numbers preceded by e indicate the material is available online only.